ROBBINS

BASIC PATHOLOGY

ROBBINS
BASIC
PATHOLOGY

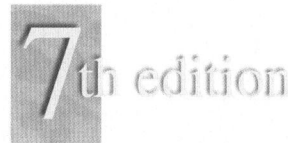

7th edition

VINAY KUMAR, MD, FRCPath
Professor and Chairman
Department of Pathology
The University of Chicago
Pritzker School of Medicine
Chicago, Illinois

RAMZI S. COTRAN, MD*
Formerly, Frank Burr Mallory Professor of Pathology
Harvard Medical School
Chairman, Department of Pathology
Brigham and Women's Hospital
The Children's Hospital
Boston, Massachusetts

STANLEY L. ROBBINS, MD
Consultant in Pathology
Brigham and Women's Hospital
Boston, Massachusetts

With illustrations by
JAMES A. PERKINS, MS, MFA

---

*Deceased

SAUNDERS
An Imprint of Elsevier Science
Philadelphia   London   Toronto   Montreal   Sydney   Tokyo

SAUNDERS

An Imprint of Elsevier Science

The Curtis Center
Independence Square West
Philadelphia, Pennsylvania 19106

ROBBINS BASIC PATHOLOGY

ISBN 0−7216−9274−5
1E ISBN 0−8089−0007−2

Library of Congress Cataloging-in-Publication Data

Robbins basic pathology/[edited by] Vinay Kumar, Ramzi S. Cotran, Stanley L. Robbins; with illustrations by James A. Perkins.—7th ed.
     p.cm.
    Previously published: Basic pathology. 6th ed. 1997.
    ISBN 0−7216−9274−5
    International Edition ISBN 0−8089−0007−2
     1. Pathology. I. Kumar, Vinay. II. Cotran, Ramzi S. III. Robbins, Stanley L. (Stanley Leonard). IV Basic pathology

RB111 .K895 2002
616.07—dc21
2002066971

Acquisitions Editor: William Schmitt
Developmental Editor: Hazel Hacker
Project Manager: Amy Norwitz
Book Designer: Ellen Zanolle

PI/QWK

Printed in China

Last digit is the print number: 9 8 7 6 5 4 3 2

This book is dedicated to

Dr. Ramzi S. Cotran
1932 – 2000

A dear friend,
respected colleague,
irreplaceable coauthor

He left a legacy of excellence
and memories that will long be treasured

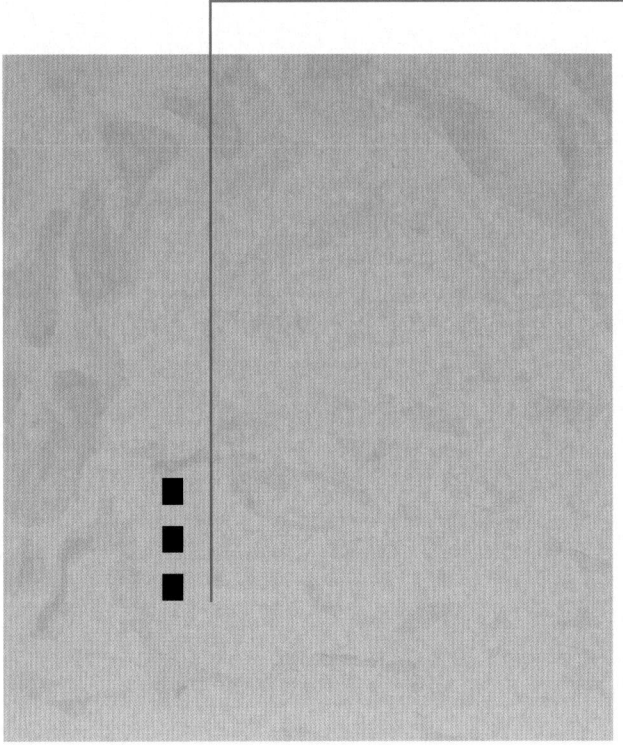

Preface

We launch this seventh edition of *Robbins Basic Pathology* with mixed emotion—excitement over the completion of this long and arduous project tempered by sadness over the loss of our colleague and coauthor, Dr. Ramzi S. Cotran, who passed away before this rewrite was completed. This tragic event spurred us to redouble our efforts to ensure that this edition was worthy of all the earlier ones to which he had contributed.

This edition, like all previous ones, has been extensively revised and in some areas completely rewritten. A few examples of some of the changes are as follows.

■ Almost all of the black-and-white photographs of former editions have been replaced by full-color gross and microscopic illustrations.
■ Many new pieces of four-color art—schematics, flow charts, and diagrammatic representations of disease—have been added to facilitate the understanding of difficult concepts such as the molecular basis of cancer, interactions of HIV with its receptors, and the biochemical basis of apoptotic cell death.
■ More illustrations have been added—62 in all, or an additional 10% of the aggregate.
■ New tables have been devised to better present cumbersome detail.
■ The chapter on disorders of the skin added to the previous edition has been revised. Similarly, in response to apparent need, pediatric disorders have been consolidated further into the chapter on genetic diseases.

■ Although the focus of the text on disease mechanisms remains, the discussion of laboratory diagnosis of selected disorders has been included to highlight the importance of laboratory medicine in the practice of medicine.

Despite the extensive changes and revisions, our goals remain substantially unaltered. As in previous editions, we have strived to provide a balanced, accurate, and up-to-date view of the central body of pathology. The strong emphasis on clinicopathologic correlations is maintained, and wherever understood, the impact of molecular pathology on the practice of medicine is highlighted. Indeed, in the 5 years since the previous edition, spectacular advances, including completion of the human genome project, have occurred. This has impacted all areas of medicine, including pathology. It is now possible, for example, to undertake molecular profiling of tumors, and early studies indicate that this information can provide more precise prognostic information. While many of the "breakthroughs" on the bench have not yet reached the bedside, we have included them in measured "doses" so that the students can begin to experience the excitement that is ahead in their careers.

We continue to firmly believe that clarity of writing and proper usage of language enhance comprehension and facilitate the learning process. Generations of students have told us that they enjoy reading this book. We hope that this edition will be worthy of and possibly enhance the tradition of its forebears.

Acknowledgments

Any large endeavor of this type cannot be completed without the help of many individuals. This is particularly true of this edition because the death of Dr. Ramzi S. Cotran posed new challenges for its timely publication. We are deeply indebted to many who rose to the occasion and provided extra time, at short notice, to help in the completion of this edition. In this regard we are particularly thankful to Drs. Fred Schoen, Helmut Rennke, and Christopher Crum for graciously accepting last-minute assignments to revise chapters in their areas of expertise. They are well known to many readers for their contributions to *Pathologic Basis of Disease*. In addition to revising an extra chapter, Dr. Richard Mitchell helped in editing large portions of the text during the final phases of the publication process, for which he is owed our deep gratitude. The contributors of various chapters are listed in the table of contents as well as in the chapters themselves. To each of them a special thanks.

Beverly Shackelford (UT Southwestern at Dallas), who has assisted one of us (VK) over the past 18 years, continued to be the "mother hen" who made sure that everyone did his or her job and remained on track. Her supervisory and editorial task assumed greater complexity and importance with the translocation of one of us (VK) from Dallas to Chicago. Without her dedication this book could not have been completed. No amount of "thank-yous" can fully capture our indebtedness to her. Vera Davis and Dionne Smith deserve thanks for coordinating the tasks from Chicago.

Many colleagues at University of Chicago have enhanced the text by providing helpful critiques in their areas of interest. Included among them are residents Drs. Lisa Yerian, Robert Anders, and Bretta Warren (neoplasia); and faculty colleagues Drs. John Hart (gastrointestinal tract); Jose Manaligod (kidney); Anthony Montag (male genital system); and Manuel Utset and Sangram S. Sisodia (central nervous system).

We are also extremely grateful to many of our colleagues at the University of Texas Southwestern Medical School at Dallas and the Brigham and Women's Hospital in Boston for providing us with photographic gems from their personal collections. They are individually acknowledged in the credits to their contribution(s). For any unintended omissions we offer our apologies.

Many at W.B. Saunders deserve recognition for their role in the production of this book. This text was fortunate again to be in the hands of Hazel Hacker, the most outstanding developmental editor that we have had the privilege to work with. In her calm and composed voice, she managed to keep the authors "in line" during difficult transitions. Others deserving of our thanks are Amy Norwitz (Project Manager) and Ellen Zanolle (Designer). William Schmitt, Publishing Director of Medical Textbooks, continued to be our cheerleader and friend.

Ventures such as this exact a heavy toll from the families of the authors. We thank them for their tolerance of our absences, physically and emotionally. We are blessed and strengthened by their unconditional support and love, and for their sharing with us the belief that our efforts are worthwhile and useful. We are especially grateful to

Raminder Kumar, who managed the rigors of transition from Dallas to Chicago and provided silent but firm support.

And finally, each of us wishes to salute his coauthors for the shared vision, excitement, and dedication to medical education that keep us united despite differences in opinions and individual styles. With each new edition our mutual respect and friendship grow stronger. Both of us wish to reacknowledge our debt to the late Dr. Ramzi S. Cotran for being a wonderful colleague and friend. Vinay Kumar wishes to salute Dr. Stanley Robbins for having conceived of this text almost 30 years ago and for the privilege of sharing the title page with him. And conversely, Stanley Robbins wishes to tender his deepest gratitude to Vinay Kumar for his dedication to this edition—without him there would be no book.

VK
SLR

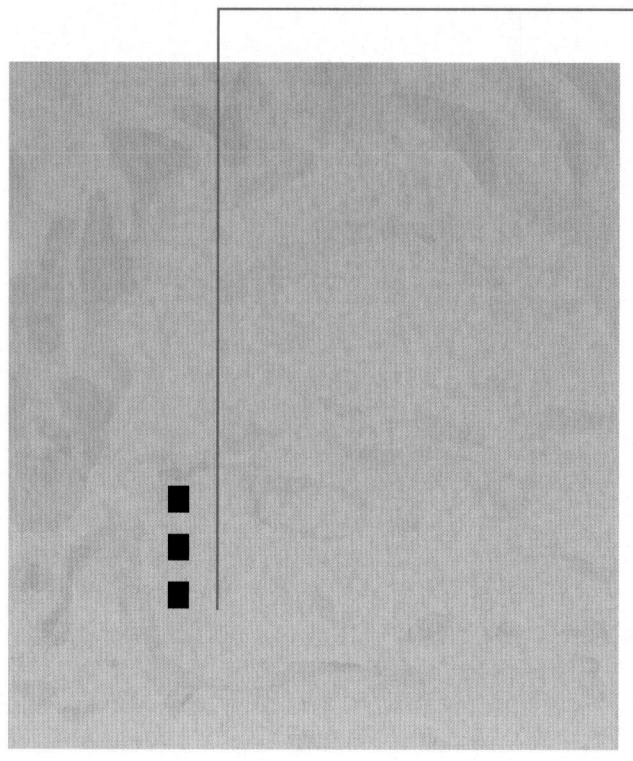

Contents

*Deceased

*Deceased

1

GENERAL
PATHOLOGY

1

Cell Injury, Adaptation, and Death

RICHARD N. MITCHELL, MD, PhD
RAMZI S. COTRAN, MD*

INTRODUCTION TO PATHOLOGY

Literally translated, *pathology* is the study *(logos)* of suffering *(pathos)*. It is a discipline that bridges clinical practice and basic science, and it involves the investigation of the underlying causes *(etiology)* of disease as well as the mechanisms *(pathogenesis)* that result in the presenting signs and symptoms of the patient. To understand the structural and functional changes that occur in cells, tissues, and organs, pathologists use contemporary molecular,

microbiologic, and immunologic techniques. To render diagnoses and guide therapy in the clinical setting, pathologists identify changes in the gross or microscopic appearance *(morphology)* of cells and tissues. Traditionally, the discipline is divided into general pathology and systemic pathology; the former focuses on the fundamental cellular and tissue responses to pathologic stimuli, while the latter examines the particular responses of specialized organs. In this book, we first cover the broad principles of general pathology and then progress to specific disease processes in individual organs.

*Deceased

OVERVIEW OF CELL INJURY

Cells are active participants in their environment, constantly adjusting structure and function to accommodate changing demands and extracellular stresses. Cells tend to preserve their immediate environment and intracellular milieu within a relatively narrow range of physiologic parameters—they maintain normal *homeostasis*. As cells encounter physiologic stresses or pathologic stimuli, they can undergo adaptation, achieving a new steady state and preserving viability. The principal adaptive responses are *atrophy*, *hypertrophy*, *hyperplasia*, and *metaplasia*. If the adaptive capability is exceeded, *cell injury* develops. Within certain limits, injury is *reversible*, and cells return to a stable baseline; however, with severe or persistent stress, *irreversible injury* results, and the affected cells die. Two principal patterns of cell death are recognized; these have distinct mechanisms, but there is also considerable overlap between the two processes:

■ *Necrosis* (typically *coagulative necrosis*) occurs after a loss of blood supply or after an exposure to toxins and is characterized by cellular swelling, protein denaturation, and organellar breakdown. This pathway of cell death may result in considerable tissue dysfunction.

■ *Apoptosis* occurs as a result of an internally controlled "suicide" program, after which the dead cells are removed with minimal disruption of the surrounding tissue. This occurs in physiologic states when unwanted cells are to be eliminated (e.g., embryogenesis), as well as in a variety of pathologic states (e.g., irreparable mutational damage).

The relationships between normal, adapted, and reversibly and irreversibly injured cells are illustrated in Figure 1–1. Myocardium subjected to persistent increased load, as in hypertension or with a stenotic valve, adapts by undergoing *hypertrophy*—an increase in the size of the individual cells and ultimately the entire heart—to generate the required higher pressures. Conversely, in periods of prolonged starvation or in *cachexia* (weight loss, as in the setting of malignant tumors), myocardium undergoes *atrophy*—a decrease in cell size without an appreciable change in number. Myocardium subjected to reduced blood flow (*ischemia*) from an occluded coronary artery may be reversibly injured if the occlusion is incomplete or sufficiently brief, or it may undergo irreversible injury (*infarction*) after complete or prolonged occlusion. Note, too, that stresses and injury affect not only the morphologic appearance but also the *functional* status of cells and tissues. Thus, reversibly injured myocytes are not dead and, in fact, closely resemble normal myocytes; however, they are transiently noncontractile and can therefore have a potentially lethal clinical impact. Whether a specific form of stress induces adaptation or causes reversible or irreversible injury depends not only on the nature and severity of the stress but also on several other variables, including specific cellular vulnerability, differentiation, blood supply, and nutritional status.

The immediately following sections describe the causes of cell injury and the mechanisms by which they exert their effects. Subsequent sections describe cellular and subcellular adaptations to injury, followed by a detailed analysis of the transition from reversible to irreversible injury, and the morphology of injured cells. Finally, there is an expanded discussion of programmed cell death (apoptosis) and the processes contributing to cellular aging (*senescence*).

CAUSES OF CELL INJURY

The stresses that can induce cell injury range from the gross physical trauma of a motor vehicle accident to the single gene defect that results in a defective enzyme underlying a specific metabolic disease. Most causes can be grouped into the following broad categories.

Oxygen Deprivation. *Hypoxia*, or oxygen deficiency, interferes with aerobic oxidative respiration and is an extremely important and common cause of cell injury and death. Hypoxia should be distinguished from *ischemia*, which is a loss of blood supply in a tissue due to impeded arterial flow or reduced venous drainage. While ischemia is the most common cause of hypoxia, oxygen deficiency can also result from inadequate oxygenation of the blood, as in pneumonia, or reduction in the oxygen-carrying capacity of the blood, as in anemia or carbon monoxide (CO) poisoning (CO forms a stable complex with hemoglobin that prevents oxygen binding).

Chemical Agents. Virtually any chemical substance can cause injury; even innocuous substances such as glucose or salt, if sufficiently concentrated, may so derange the osmotic environment that injury or cell death results. Oxygen at sufficiently high partial pressures is also toxic. Agents commonly known as poisons cause severe damage at the cellular level by altering membrane permeability, osmotic homeostasis, or the integrity of an enzyme or cofactor and can culminate in the death of the whole organism. Other potentially toxic agents are encountered daily in our environment; these include air pollutants, insecticides, carbon monoxide, asbestos, and social "stimuli" such as ethanol. Even therapeutic drugs can cause cell or tissue injury in a susceptible patient or in the appropriate setting.

Infectious Agents. These range from submicroscopic viruses to meter-long tapeworms; in between are the rickettsiae, bacteria, fungi, and protozoans. The diverse ways by which biologic agents cause injury are discussed in Chapter 9.

Immunologic Reactions. Although the immune system defends the body against foreign materials, immune reactions intended or incidental can nevertheless result in cell and tissue injury. *Anaphylaxis* to a foreign protein or a drug is a classic example. Moreover, a loss of *tolerance* with responses to self-antigens is the underlying cause of a number of *autoimmune diseases* (Chapter 5).

Genetic Defects. Genetic defects may result in pathologic changes as conspicuous as the congenital malformations associated with Down syndrome or as subtle as the single amino acid substitution in the hemoglobin S of sickle cell anemia. The several inborn errors of metabolism due to congenital

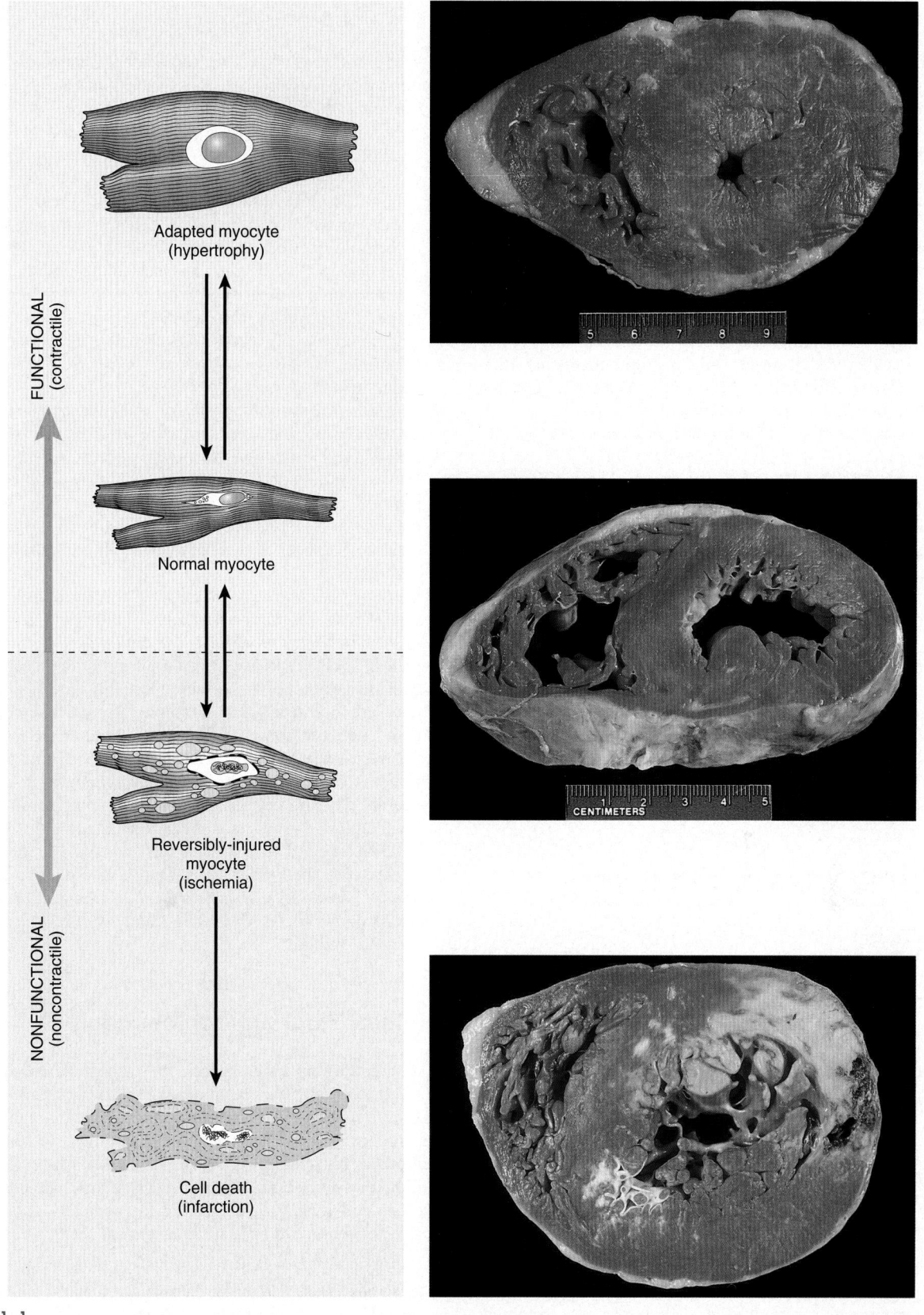

Figure 1-1

The relationship between normal, adapted, reversibly injured, and dead myocardial cells. The cellular adaptation depicted here is hypertrophy, the type of reversible injury is ischemia, and the irreversible injury is ischemic coagulative necrosis. In this example of myocardial hypertrophy *(top cross-section),* the left ventricular wall is over 2 cm in thickness (normal, 1 to 1.5 cm). The cross-section in the middle shows normal myocardium. In reversibly injured myocardium, there are generally only functional effects, without any readily apparent gross or even microscopic changes. In the specimen showing necrosis *(bottom cross-section),* the transmural light area in the posterolateral left ventricle represents an acute myocardial infarction. All three transverse sections of myocardium have been stained with triphenyltetrazolium chloride, an enzyme substrate that colors viable myocardium magenta. Failure to stain is due to enzyme leakage following cell death.

enzymatic deficiencies are excellent examples of cell and tissue damage resulting from frequently "trivial" alterations in deoxyribonucleic acid (DNA). The major genetic abnormalities are discussed in Chapter 7.

Nutritional Imbalances. Even in the current era of burgeoning global affluence, nutritional deficiencies remain a major cause of cell injury. Protein-calorie insufficiency among underprivileged populations is only the most obvious example; specific vitamin deficiencies are not uncommon even in industrialized nations with relatively high standards of living (Chapter 8). Ironically, excesses of nutrition are also important causes of morbidity and mortality; for example, obesity markedly increases the risk for type 2 (formerly called adult-onset, non–insulin-dependent) *diabetes mellitus.* Moreover, diets rich in animal fat are strongly implicated in the development of *atherosclerosis* as well as in increased vulnerability to many disorders, including cancer.

Physical Agents. Trauma, extremes of temperatures, radiation, electric shock, and sudden changes in atmospheric pressure all have wide-ranging effects on cells (Chapter 8).

Aging. As we will see (Chapter 3), healing of injured tissues does not always result in a perfect restoration of structure or function. Repeated trauma can also lead to tissue *degeneration* even in the absence of outright cell death. Moreover, intrinsic *cellular senescence* leads to alterations in replicative and repair abilities of individual cells and tissues. All of these changes result in a diminished ability to respond to exogenous stimuli and injury and, eventually, the death of the organism. The specific mechanisms underlying cellular senescence are covered later in this chapter.

MECHANISMS OF CELL INJURY

Clearly, there are many different ways to induce cell injury. Moreover, the biochemical mechanisms linking any given injury and the resulting cellular and tissue manifestations are complex and tightly interwoven with other intracellular pathways. Thus, dissecting cause and effect may be difficult. Nevertheless, a number of general principles are relevant to most forms of cell injury:

■ *The cellular response to injurious stimuli depends on the type of injury, its duration, and its severity.* Thus, low doses of toxins or a brief duration of ischemia may lead to reversible cell injury, whereas larger toxin doses or longer ischemic intervals may result in irreversible injury and cell death.
■ *The consequences of an injurious stimulus depend on the type, status, adaptability, and genetic makeup of the injured cell.* The same injury has vastly different outcomes depending on the cell type; thus, striated skeletal muscle in the leg accommodates complete ischemia for 2 to 3 hours without irreversible injury, whereas cardiac muscle dies after only 20 to 30 minutes. The nutritional (or hormonal) status can also be important; clearly, a glycogen-replete hepatocyte will tolerate ischemia much better than one that has just

burned its last glucose molecule. Genetically determined diversity in metabolic pathways can also be important; when exposed to the same dose of a toxin, individuals with polymorphisms in enzyme genes may catabolize it with different efficacies, leading to different outcomes. With the completion of the human genome project, much effort is now directed toward understanding the role of genetic polymorphisms on disease susceptibility.
■ Four intracellular systems are particularly vulnerable: (1) cell membrane integrity, critical to cellular ionic and osmotic homeostasis; (2) adenosine triphosphate (ATP) generation, largely via mitochondrial aerobic respiration; (3) protein synthesis; and (4) the integrity of the genetic apparatus.
■ *The structural and biochemical components of a cell are so integrally connected that regardless of the initial locus of injury, multiple secondary effects rapidly occur.* For example, poisoning of aerobic respiration with cyanide results in diminished activity of the sodium-potassium ATPase necessary to maintain intracellular osmotic balance; as a result, the cell can rapidly swell and rupture.
■ *Cellular function is lost far before cell death occurs, and the morphologic changes of cell injury (or death) lag far behind both* (Fig. 1–2). Since the specific activities of a cell typically rely on all systems' being intact, cells lose functional activity relatively quickly even if they are not dead. For example, myocardial cells become noncontractile after 1 to 2 minutes of ischemia, although they do not die until 20 to 30 minutes of ischemia have elapsed. Moreover, changes in the appearance of the cell are evident only after some critical biochemical system has been deranged and sufficient time has passed to manifest the change. The same myocytes that died after 30 minutes of ischemia do not appear dead by *ultrastructural evaluation* (electron microscopy) for 2 to 3 hours, and by *light microscopy* for 6 to 12 hours.

General Biochemical Mechanisms

With certain injurious agents, the pathogenic mechanisms are well defined; thus, cyanide inactivates cytochrome oxidase in mitochondria, resulting in ATP depletion, and certain bacteria can elaborate phospholipases that degrade cell membrane phospholipids. However, with many injurious stimuli, the precise pathogenic mechanisms that ultimately result in cell injury (or death) are incompletely understood. In spite of that, several basic biochemical themes emerge in the causation of injury:

■ *ATP depletion.* The high-energy phosphates of ATP are critical for virtually every process in the cell including the maintenance of cellular osmolarity, transport processes, protein synthesis, and basic metabolic pathways. A loss of ATP synthesis (via either mitochondrial oxidative phosphorylation or anaerobic glycolysis) results in rapid shutdown of most critical homeostatic pathways.

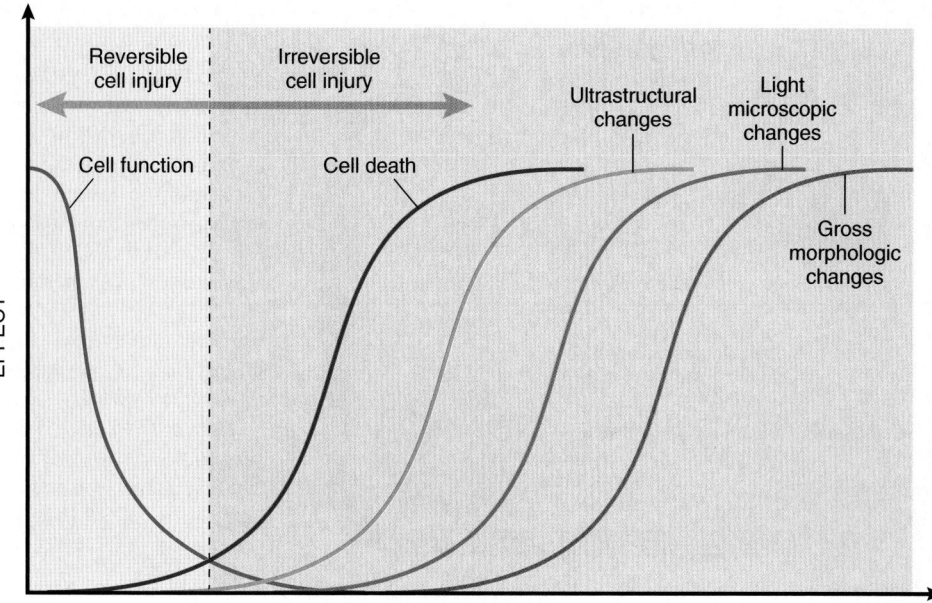

Figure 1–2 ■

Schematic diagram demonstrating the relationship between cellular function, cell death, and the morphologic changes of cell injury. Note that cells may become rapidly nonfunctional after the onset of injury, although they are still viable, with potentially reversible damage; a longer duration of injury may eventually lead to irreversible injury and cell death. Note also that cell death typically precedes ultrastructural, light microscopic, and grossly visible morphologic changes.

■ *Oxygen deprivation or generation of reactive oxygen species.* A lack of oxygen obviously underlies the pathogenesis of cell injury in ischemia, but partially reduced activated oxygen species are also important mediators of cell death (Fig. 1–3). These free radical species cause lipid peroxidation and other deleterious effects on cell structure (see later).

■ *Loss of calcium homeostasis.* Cytosolic free calcium is normally maintained by ATP-dependent calcium transporters at concentrations that are up to 10,000 times lower than the concentration of extracellular calcium or of sequestered intracellular mitochondrial and endoplasmic reticulum calcium. Ischemia or toxins allow a net

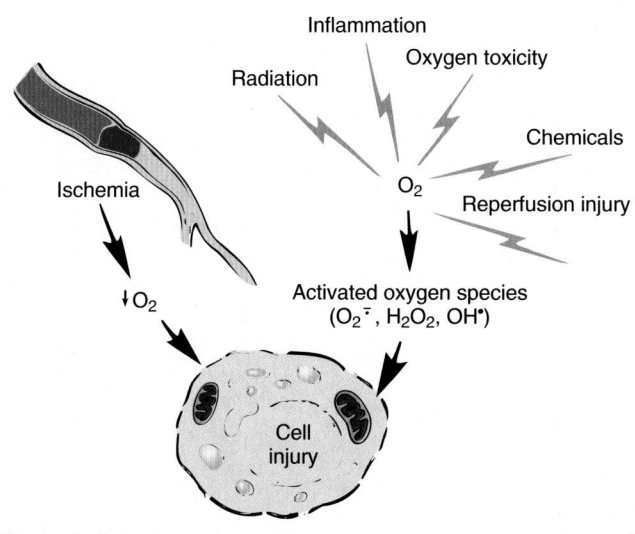

Figure 1–3 ■

The role of oxygen in cell injury. Ischemia causes cell injury by reducing cellular oxygen supplies; other stimuli, such as radiation, induce damage via toxic activated oxygen species.

influx of extracellular calcium across the plasma membrane, followed by the release of calcium from the intracellular stores. Increased cytosolic calcium in turn activates a variety of phospholipases (promoting membrane damage), proteases (catabolizing structural and membrane proteins), ATPases (accelerating ATP depletion), and endonucleases (fragmenting genetic material) (Fig. 1–4). Although cell injury results in increased intracellular calcium, and this in turn mediates a variety of deleterious effects, including cell death, a loss of calcium homeostasis is not always a necessary proximate event in irreversible cell injury.

■ *Defects in plasma membrane permeability.* The plasma membrane may be directly damaged by certain bacterial toxins, viral proteins, complement components, cytolytic lymphocytes, or any of a number of physical or chemical agents. Alterations of membrane permeability may also be secondary, that is, due to a loss of ATP synthesis or resulting from calcium-mediated phospholipase activation. A loss of membrane barriers leads to a breakdown of the concentration gradients of metabolites necessary to maintain normal metabolic activities.

■ *Mitochondrial damage.* Since all mammalian cells are ultimately dependent on oxidative metabolism, mitochondrial integrity is critical for cell survival. It is not too surprising then that mitochondria—either directly or indirectly—end up as targets of most types of injury. Increases in cytosolic calcium, intracellular oxidative stress, and lipid breakdown products all culminate in the formation of high-conductance channels of the inner mitochondrial membrane (also called the *mitochondrial permeability transition*; Fig. 1–5). These nonselective pores allow the proton gradient across the mitochondrial membrane to dissipate, thereby preventing ATP generation. Cytochrome *c* (an important soluble protein in the electron transport chain) also leaks out into the cytosol, where it activates apoptotic death pathways.

Figure 1–4 ■

Sources and consequences of increased cytosolic calcium in cell injury. ATP, adenosine triphosphate.

With these general concepts in mind, we now focus on three common forms of cell injury: ischemic and hypoxic injury, free radical–induced injury, and some forms of toxic injury.

Ischemic and Hypoxic Injury

Ischemia is far and away the most common type of cell injury in clinical medicine, typically occurring because of diminished blood flow in a particular tissue's vascular bed. In contrast to hypoxia, in which glycolytic energy generation can continue (albeit less efficiently than by oxidative pathways), ischemia also compromises the delivery of substrates for glycolysis. Consequently, anaerobic energy generation also ceases in ischemic tissues after potential substrates are exhausted or when glycolysis is inhibited by the accumulation of metabolites that would normally be removed by blood flow. Consequently, *ischemia injures tissues faster than does hypoxia.*

The first effect of hypoxia is on the cell's aerobic respiration, that is, oxidative phosphorylation by mitochondria; as a consequence of reduced oxygen tension, the intracellular generation of ATP is markedly reduced. The resulting depletion of ATP has widespread effects on many systems within the cell (Fig. 1–6).

■ Activity of the plasma membrane ATP-driven "sodium pump" is reduced, with the subsequent accumulation of intracellular sodium and the diffusion of potassium out of the cell. The net gain of sodium solute is accompanied by an isosmotic gain of water, producing *acute cellular swelling*. This is further exacerbated by the increased osmotic load from the accumulation of other

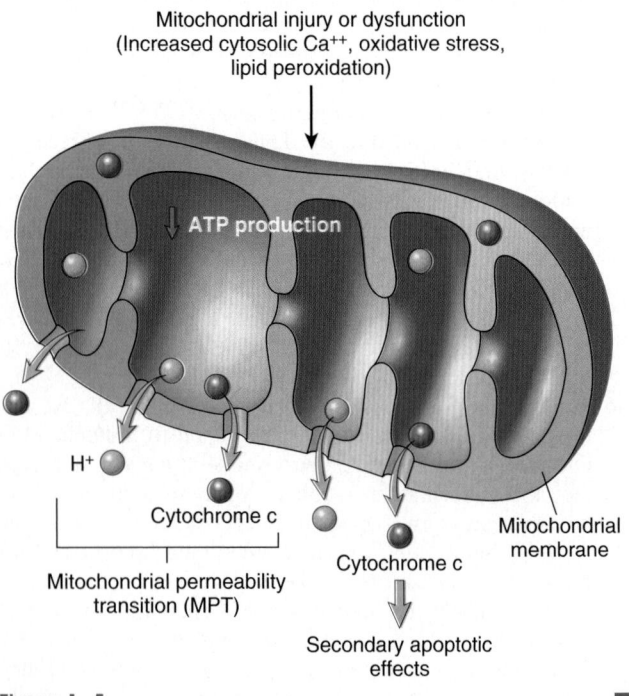

Figure 1–5 ■

Mitochondrial dysfunction, induced by a variety of stimuli, causes a mitochondrial permeability transition, which leads to decay of the proton gradient necessary for ATP generation, as well as releasing cytochrome *c* from the mitochondria into the cytosol.

Figure 1–6 ■

Postulated sequence of events in reversible ischemic injury. Diminished oxidative phosphorylation and reduced ATP levels have a central role in mediating effects on multiple intracellular systems. Note that all these effects are potentially reversible, and the restoration of blood flow eventually allows the cell to recover normal function. ER, endoplasmic reticulum.

metabolites, such as inorganic phosphates, lactic acid, and purine nucleosides.

■ Anaerobic glycolysis increases because of decreased ATP and associated increases in adenosine monophosphate (AMP) that stimulate the enzyme phosphofructokinase. This pathway was evolutionarily designed to maintain the cell's energy by generating ATP from glycogen, and its activation leads to rapid *depletion of glycogen stores*, apparent histologically by reduced staining for carbohydrates (e.g., the periodic acid–Schiff [PAS] stain). Increased glycolysis also results in the accumulation of lactic acid and inorganic phosphates from hydrolysis of phosphate esters, *thus lowering the intracellular pH*.

■ Decreasing pH and ATP levels cause ribosomes to detach from the rough endoplasmic reticulum (RER) and polysomes to dissociate into monosomes, with a resultant *reduction in protein synthesis*.

If hypoxia is not relieved, worsening mitochondrial function and increasing membrane permeability cause further morphologic deterioration. As the cytoskeleton disperses, ultrastructural features such as microvilli are lost, and cell surface "blebs" are formed. Mitochondria, endoplasmic reticulum, and indeed whole cells usually appear swollen owing to a loss of osmotic regulation. *If oxygen is restored, all the above disturbances are reversible*; *however, if ischemia persists, irreversible injury follows* (see later discussion).

Ischemia/Reperfusion Injury

If cells are reversibly injured, the restoration of blood flow can result in cell recovery. However, under certain circumstances, the restoration of blood flow to ischemic but otherwise viable tissues results, paradoxically, in exacerbated and accelerated injury. As a result, tissues sustain the loss of cells *in addition to those that are irreversibly damaged at the end of the ischemic episode*. This so-called *ischemia/reperfusion injury* is a clinically important process that significantly contributes to tissue damage in myocardial and cerebral infarctions, but it is also amenable to therapeutic intervention.

Although the exact mechanisms are unclear, reperfusion into ischemic tissues may cause further damage by the following means:

■ Restoration of blood flow bathes compromised cells in high concentrations of calcium when they are not able to fully regulate their ionic environment; increased intracellular calcium activates the pathways described in Figure 1–4 and causes a loss of cellular integrity.

■ Reperfusion of injured cells results in a locally augmented recruitment of inflammatory cells; these cells release high levels of oxygen-derived reactive species (see later), which promote additional membrane damage as well as the mitochondrial permeability transition (see Figs. 1–5 and 1–20).

■ Damaged mitochondria in compromised but still viable cells yield incomplete oxygen reduction and therefore increased production of free radical species; in addition, ischemically injured cells have compromised antioxidant defense mechanisms.

Free Radical–Induced Cell Injury

As mentioned in the discussion of ischemic reperfusion, free radical–induced injury, particularly that induced by activated oxygen species, is an important mechanism of cell damage. Free radical damage also underlies chemical and radiation injury, toxicity from oxygen and other gases, cellular aging, microbial killing by phagocytic cells (Chapter 9), inflammatory cell damage, tumor destruction by macrophages, and other injurious processes (see Fig. 1–3).

Free radicals are chemical species with a single unpaired electron in an outer orbital. Such chemical states are extremely unstable and readily react with inorganic or organic chemicals; when generated in cells, they avidly attack and degrade nucleic acids as well as a variety of membrane molecules. In addition, free radicals initiate autocatalytic reactions; molecules that react with free radicals are in turn converted into free radicals, further propagating the chain of damage.

Free radicals may be generated within cells by

■ The reduction-oxidation (redox) reactions that occur during normal physiologic processes (Fig. 1–7). During normal respiration, for example, molecular oxygen is sequentially reduced in mitochondria by the addition of four electrons to generate water. In the process, small amounts of toxic intermediate species are generated; these include superoxide radicals (O_2^-), hydrogen peroxide (H_2O_2), and OH·. Further, some intracellular oxidases (such as xanthine oxidase) generate superoxide radicals as a direct consequence of their activity. Transition metals such as copper and iron also accept or donate free electrons during certain intracellular reactions and thereby catalyze free radical formation, as in the Fenton reaction ($Fe^{++} + H_2O_2 \rightarrow Fe^{+++} + OH· + OH^-$). Since most intracellular free iron is in the ferric (Fe^{+++}) state, it must first be reduced to the ferrous (Fe^{++}) form to participate in the Fenton reaction. That reduction step is catalyzed by superoxide ion, and thus iron and superoxide synergize to elicit maximal oxidative cell injury.

■ Nitric oxide (NO), an important chemical mediator normally synthesized by a variety of cell types (Chapter 2) that can act as a free radical or can be converted into highly reactive nitrite species.

■ The absorption of radiant energy (e.g., ultraviolet light, x-rays). Ionizing radiation can hydrolyze water into hydroxyl (OH·) and hydrogen (H·) free radicals.

■ The enzymatic metabolism of exogenous chemicals (e.g., carbon tetrachloride; see later).

Three reactions are particularly relevant to cell injury mediated by free radicals (see Fig. 1–7):

■ *Lipid peroxidation of membranes*. Double bonds in membrane polyunsaturated lipids are vulnerable to attack by oxygen-derived free radicals. The lipid-radical interactions yield peroxides, which are themselves unstable and reactive, and an autocatalytic chain reaction ensues.

■ *DNA fragmentation*. Free radical reactions with thymine in nuclear and mitochondrial DNA produce single-strand breaks. Such DNA damage has been

A. FREE RADICAL GENERATION

Figure 1–7 ■

Generation of free radicals *(A, top),* the cell injury resulting from the action of unopposed free radicals *(B, bottom left),* and their neutralization by cellular antioxidant mechanisms *(C, bottom right). A,* O_2 is converted to superoxide $(O_2^{\cdot-})$ by oxidative enzymes (such as P-450 and b5 oxidases) in the endoplasmic reticulum, mitochondria, plasma membrane, peroxisomes, and cytosol. The $O_2^{\cdot-}$ is converted to H_2O_2 by superoxide dismutase (SOD) and then to $OH^{\cdot}$ by the Cu^{++}/Fe^{++}–catalyzed Fenton reaction *(pink box). H_2O_2* is also derived directly from oxidases in peroxisomes. *B,* The resultant free radicals can damage lipids (peroxidation), proteins, and DNA. Note that superoxide catalyzes the reduction of Fe^{+++} to Fe^{++}, thus enhancing $OH^{\cdot}$ generation by the Fenton reaction. *C,* The major antioxidant enzymes are SOD, catalase, and glutathione peroxidase. Free radicals are also neutralized by scavengers (vitamins E, A, and C, and β-carotene), and the ability of Cu^{++} and Fe^{+++} to form radicals is minimized by binding the ions to carrier proteins (ferritin and ceruloplasmin, respectively). GSH, reduced glutathione; GSSG, oxidized glutathione; NADPH, reduced form of nicotinamide adenine dinucleotide phosphate; NO, nitric oxide.

implicated in both cell killing and the malignant transformation of cells.

■ *Cross-linking of proteins.* Free radicals promote sulfhydryl-mediated protein cross-linking, resulting in enhanced rates of degradation or loss of enzymatic activity. Free radical reactions may also directly cause polypeptide fragmentation.

Besides being a consequence of chemical and radiation injury, free radical generation is also a normal part of respiration and other routine cellular activities, including microbial defense. Fortunately, free radicals are inherently unstable and generally decay spontaneously; superoxide, for example, rapidly breaks down in the presence of water into oxygen and hydrogen peroxide. However, cells have also developed several enzymatic and nonenzymatic systems to inactivate free radicals (see Fig. 1–7).

■ The rate of spontaneous decay is significantly increased by the action of superoxide dismutases (SODs) found in many cell types (catalyzing the reaction $2O_2^{\cdot-}\ 2H \rightarrow H_2O_2 + O_2$).

■ Glutathione (GSH) peroxidase also protects against injury by catalyzing free radical breakdown ($2OH^{\cdot} + 2GSH \rightarrow 2H_2O + GSSG$ [glutathione homodimer]). The intracellular ratio of oxidized (GSSG) to reduced (GSH) glutathione is a reflection of the oxidative state of the cell and an important aspect of the cell's ability to catabolize free radicals.

■ Catalase, present in peroxisomes, directs the degradation of hydrogen peroxide ($2H_2O_2 \rightarrow O_2 + 2H_2O$).

■ Endogenous or exogenous antioxidants (e.g., vitamins E, A, and C, and β-carotene) may either block the formation of free radicals or scavenge them once they have formed.

■ Although free ionized iron and copper can catalyze the formation of reactive oxygen species, these elements are usually sequestered by storage and/or transport proteins (e.g., transferrin, ferritin, and ceruloplasmin).

Chemical Injury

Chemicals induce cell injury by one of two general mechanisms:

■ *Some chemicals act directly by combining with a critical molecular component or cellular organelle.* For example, in mercuric chloride poisoning, mercury binds to the sulfhydryl groups of various cell membrane proteins, causing inhibition of ATPase-dependent transport and increased membrane permeability. Many antineoplastic chemotherapeutic agents and antibiotics also induce cell damage by similar direct cytotoxic effects. In such instances, the *greatest damage is sustained by the cells that use, absorb, excrete, or concentrate the compounds.*

■ *Many other chemicals are not intrinsically biologically active but must be first converted to reactive toxic metabolites, which then act on target cells.* This modification is usually accomplished by the P-450 mixed function oxidases in the smooth endoplasmic reticulum (SER) of the liver and other organs. Although the metabolites might cause membrane damage and cell injury by direct covalent binding to protein and lipids, the most important mechanism of cell injury involves the formation of reactive free radicals. Carbon tetrachloride (CCl_4, used widely in the dry cleaning industry) and acetaminophen belong in this category. CCl_4, for example, is converted to the toxic free radical $CCl_3\cdot$, principally in the liver. The free radicals cause autocatalytic membrane phospholipid peroxidation, with rapid breakdown of the endoplasmic reticulum. In less than 30 minutes, there is a decline in hepatic protein synthesis of both enzymes and plasma proteins; within 2 hours, swelling of the SER and dissociation of ribosomes from the RER have occurred. There is reduced lipid export from the hepatocytes, owing to their inability to synthesize apoprotein to complex with triglycerides and thereby facilitate lipoprotein secretion; the result is the "fatty liver" of CCl_4 poisoning. Mitochondrial injury follows, and subsequently diminished ATP stores result in defective ion transport and progressive cell swelling; the plasma membranes are further damaged by fatty aldehydes resulting from lipid peroxidation in the SER. The end result can be calcium influx and eventually cell death.

As noted previously, injurious stimuli need not be lethal. Obviously, a limited severity or duration of injury allows cells and tissues to eventually return to their normal baselines. As important in the survival equation is the ability of the injured cell to respond and adapt to injury. Before we discuss the pathways and appearances of cellular death, we turn our attention to the adaptive changes that cells and tissues undergo in response to physiologic and pathologic perturbations.

CELLULAR ADAPTATION TO INJURY

As described earlier, even under normal conditions, cells must constantly adapt to changes in their environment. These *physiologic adaptations* usually represent responses of cells to normal stimulation by hormones or endogenous chemical mediators (e.g., the enlargement of the breast and induction of lactation by pregnancy). *Pathologic adaptations* often share the same underlying mechanisms, but they allow the cells to modulate their environment and ideally escape injury. Thus, cellular adaptation is a state that lies between the normal, unstressed cell and the injured, overstressed cell.

Cellular adaptation can proceed by a number of mechanisms. Some adaptive responses involve *up- or down-regulation of specific cellular receptors*; for example, cell surface receptors involved in the uptake of low-density lipoproteins (LDLs) are normally down-regulated when the cells are cholesterol replete (Chapter 7). Other adaptive responses are associated with the *induction of new protein synthesis by the target cell.* These proteins, for example heat shock proteins, may protect cells from certain forms of injury. Still other adaptations involve a switch from producing one type of protein to another, or marked overproduction of a specific protein; such is the case in cells synthesizing various collagens and extracellular matrix proteins in chronic inflammation and fibrosis (Chapter 3). Cellular adaptive responses can thus occur at any of a number of steps, including receptor binding; signal transduction; or protein transcription, translation, or export.

In this section, the adaptive changes in cell growth and differentiation that are particularly important in pathologic conditions are considered. These include *atrophy* (decrease in cell size), *hypertrophy* (increase in cell size), *hyperplasia* (increase in cell number), and *metaplasia* (change in cell type).

Atrophy

Shrinkage in the size of the cell by the loss of cell substance is known as atrophy. When a sufficient number of cells is involved, the entire tissue or organ diminishes in size, becoming atrophic (Fig. 1–8). It should be emphasized that *although atrophic cells may have diminished function, they are not dead.* In contradistinction, apoptotic death may also be induced by the same signals that cause atrophy and thus may contribute to loss of cells in the "atrophy" of an entire organ.

Causes of atrophy include a decreased workload (for example, immobilization of a limb to permit healing of a fracture), a loss of innervation, a diminished blood supply, inadequate nutrition, a loss of endocrine stimulation, and aging. Although some of these stimuli are physiologic (e.g., the loss of hormone stimulation in menopause) and others pathologic (e.g., denervation), the fundamental cellular changes are identical. They represent a retreat by the cell to a smaller size at which survival is still possible; a new equilibrium is achieved between cell size and diminished blood supply, nutrition, or trophic stimulation.

Atrophy represents a reduction in the structural components of the cell; the biochemical mechanisms underlying this process are varied but ultimately affect the balance

Figure 1–8 ■

A, Atrophy of the brain in an 82-year-old man. The meninges have been stripped. *B,* Normal brain of a 25-year-old man, for comparison.

between synthesis and degradation. Decreased synthesis, increased catabolism, or both may cause atrophy. In normal cells, the synthesis and degradation of cellular constituents are influenced by a number of hormones, including insulin, thyroid-stimulating hormone, and glucocorticoids.

The regulation of protein degradation seems to play a key role in atrophy. Mammalian cells contain two proteolytic systems that serve distinct degradative functions:

■ *Lysosomes* contain proteases and other enzymes that degrade *molecules endocytosed* from the extracellular environment, as well as catabolize subcellular components such as *senescent organelles.*

■ The *ubiquitin-proteasome pathway* is responsible for the degradation of many *cytosolic and nuclear proteins.* Proteins to be degraded by this process are typically targeted by conjugation to *ubiquitin,* a 76–amino acid cytosolic peptide. The protein is then degraded within a large cytoplasmic proteolytic complex, the *proteasome.* This pathway is responsible for the accelerated proteolysis in hypercatabolic states (including cancer cachexia) and for the regulation of a variety of intracellular activation molecules.

In many situations, atrophy is accompanied by marked increases in the number of *autophagic vacuoles,* a fusion of lysosomes with intracellular organelles and cytosol that allows the catabolism and turnover of self-components in a given cell. Some of the cell debris within the autophagic vacuole may resist digestion and persist as membrane-bound residual bodies (e.g., *lipofuscin*), described in greater detail later (see p 20).

Hypertrophy

Hypertrophy is an increase in the size of cells and consequently an increase in the size of the organ. In contrast, hyperplasia (discussed next) is characterized by an increase in cell number. Stated another way, in pure hypertrophy, there are no new cells, just bigger cells, enlarged by an increased synthesis of structural proteins and organelles. *Hypertrophy can be physiologic or pathologic and is caused either by increased functional demand or by specific hormonal stimulation.* Hypertrophy and hyperplasia can also occur together, and obviously both result in an enlarged *(hypertrophic)* organ. Thus, the massive physiologic hypertrophy of the uterus during pregnancy occurs as a consequence of estrogen stimulation of both smooth muscle hypertrophy and smooth muscle hyperplasia (Fig. 1–9). In comparison, the avid weight lifter can develop his or her rippled physique only by hypertrophy of individual skeletal muscle cells induced by an increased workload. Examples of pathologic cellular hypertrophy include the cardiac enlargement that occurs with hypertension or aortic valve disease (see Fig. 1–1), and enlargement of residual viable cardiac myocytes after myocardial infarction. In the latter case, hypertrophy compensates for the death of neighboring cells due to ischemia.

The striated muscle cells in both the heart and skeletal muscle can undergo only hypertrophy in response to increased demand because in the adult they cannot divide to generate more cells to share the work. Consequently, the synthesis of more proteins and myofilaments *per cell* putatively achieves a balance between the demand and the cell's functional capacity; it permits an increased workload with a level of metabolic activity per unit volume of cell not different from that borne by the normal cell. However, these adaptive changes may not be completely benign; they can also result in a dramatic change in the cellular phenotype. Thus, in chronic cardiac volume overload, a variety of genes—normally expressed only in the neonatal heart—are reactivated, and contractile proteins switch to fetal isoforms, which contract more slowly. Nuclei in such hypertrophied cells also have a much higher DNA content than that of normal myocardial cells, probably because the cells arrest in the cell cycle without undergoing mitosis.

Figure 1-9

Physiologic hypertrophy of the uterus during pregnancy. *A,* Gross appearance of a normal uterus *(right)* and a gravid uterus *(left)* that was removed for postpartum bleeding. *B,* Small spindle-shaped uterine smooth muscle cells from a normal uterus. Compare this with large, plump hypertrophied smooth muscle cells from a gravid uterus (*C,* same magnification).

The mechanisms driving cardiac hypertrophy involve at least two types of signals: *mechanical triggers,* such as stretch, and *trophic triggers,* such as activation of α-adrenergic receptors. Whatever the exact mechanism or mechanisms of hypertrophy, a limit is reached beyond which the enlargement of muscle mass can no longer compensate for the increased burden; in the case of the heart, cardiac failure ensues. At this stage, a number of "degenerative" changes occur in the myocardial fibers, of which the most important are fragmentation and loss of myofibrillar contractile elements. The factors that limit continued hypertrophy and cause the regressive changes are incompletely understood. There may be finite limits of the vasculature to adequately supply the enlarged fibers, of the mitochondria to supply ATP, or of the biosynthetic machinery to provide the contractile proteins or other cytoskeletal elements.

Hyperplasia

Hyperplasia constitutes an increase in the number of cells in an organ or tissue. Hypertrophy and hyperplasia are closely related and often develop concurrently in tissues, so that both may contribute to an overall increase in organ size (e.g., the gravid uterus). In certain instances, however, even potentially dividing cells, such as renal epithelial cells, undergo hypertrophy but not hyperplasia.

Hyperplasia can be physiologic or pathologic. Physiologic hyperplasia is divided into (1) *hormonal hyperplasia,* exemplified by the proliferation of the glandular epithelium of the female breast at puberty and during pregnancy; and (2) *compensatory hyperplasia,* that is, hyperplasia that occurs when a portion of the tissue is removed or diseased.

For example, when a liver is partially resected, mitotic activity in the remaining cells begins as early as 12 hours later, eventually restoring the liver to its normal weight. The stimuli for hyperplasia in this setting are polypeptide growth factors, produced by remnant hepatocytes as well as nonparenchymal cells found in the liver. After restoration of the liver mass, cell proliferation is "turned off" by various growth inhibitors. Hyperplasia is also a critical response of connective tissue cells in wound healing, by which growth factor–stimulated fibroblasts and blood vessels proliferate to facilitate repair (Chapter 3).

Most forms of pathologic hyperplasia are instances of excessive hormonal or growth factor stimulation. For example, after a normal menstrual period there is a burst of proliferative endometrial activity that is essentially physiologic hyperplasia. This proliferation is normally tightly regulated by stimulation through pituitary hormones and ovarian estrogen and by inhibition through progesterone. However, if the balance between estrogen and progesterone is disturbed, endometrial hyperplasia ensues, a common cause of abnormal menstrual bleeding. Increased sensitivity to normal levels of growth factors may also underlie pathologic hyperplasia. Thus, the common skin wart is caused by an increased expression of various transcription factors by an infecting *papillomavirus;* any minor trophic stimulation of the cell by growth factors results in an overexuberant mitotic activity. It is important to note that in both these situations, the hyperplastic process remains controlled; if hormonal or growth factor stimulation abates, the hyperplasia disappears. This differentiates these processes from cancer, in which cells continue to grow despite the absence of hormonal stimuli. Nevertheless, pathologic hyperplasia constitutes a fertile soil in which cancerous proliferation may eventually arise. Thus, patients with hyperplasia of the endometrium are at increased risk of developing endometrial cancer, and certain papillomavirus infections predispose to cervical cancers (Chapter 19).

Metaplasia

Metaplasia is a reversible change in which one adult cell type (epithelial or mesenchymal) is replaced by another adult cell type. This is cellular adaptation whereby cells sensitive to a particular stress are replaced by other cell types better able to withstand the adverse environment. Metaplasia is thought to arise by genetic "reprogramming" of epithelial stem cells or of undifferentiated mesenchymal cells in connective tissue.

Epithelial metaplasia is exemplified by the squamous change that occurs in the respiratory epithelium in habitual cigarette smokers. The normal ciliated columnar epithelial cells of the trachea and bronchi are focally or widely replaced by stratified squamous epithelial cells. Vitamin A deficiency may also induce squamous metaplasia in the respiratory epithelium. Presumably, the more "rugged" stratified squamous epithelium is able to survive under circumstances that the more fragile specialized epithelium would not tolerate. *Although the adaptive metaplastic epithelium probably has survival advantages, important protective mechanisms are lost,* such as mucus secretion and ciliary clearance of particulate matter. Epithelial metaplasia is therefore a double-edged sword; moreover, *the influences that induce metaplastic transformation, if persistent, may induce cancer transformation in the metaplastic epithelium.* Thus, in a common form of lung cancer, squamous metaplasia of the respiratory epithelium often coexists with cancers composed of malignant squamous cells. Although not proved, it is thought that cigarette smoking initially causes squamous metaplasia, and cancers arise later in some of these altered foci. Metaplasia need not always occur in the direction of columnar to squamous epithelium; in chronic gastric reflux, the normal stratified squamous epithelium of the lower esophagus may undergo metaplastic transformation to gastric or intestine-type columnar epithelium (Fig. 1–10).

Metaplasia may also occur in mesenchymal cells but less clearly as an adaptive response. Thus, bone or cartilage may form in tissues where they are normally not encountered. For example, bone is occasionally formed in soft tissues, particularly (but not always) in foci of injury.

Subcellular Responses to Injury

Thus far, we have largely focused on whole tissue or on the cell as a unit. However, responses to certain conditions are associated with rather distinctive alterations involving only subcellular organelles and cytosolic proteins. Although some of these alterations also occur in acute lethal injury, others represent more chronic forms of cell injury, and still others are adaptive responses. In this section, only some of the more common or interesting of these reactions are discussed.

Figure 1–10 ■

Metaplasia. *A,* Schematic diagram of columnar to squamous metaplasia. *B,* Metaplastic transformation *(arrow)* of the normal adult esophageal stratified squamous epithelium *(left)* to mature columnar epithelium (so-called Barrett metaplasia).

Lysosomal Catabolism. *Primary lysosomes* are membrane-bound intracellular organelles containing a variety of hydrolytic enzymes; these fuse with vacuoles containing material destined for digestion to form *secondary lysosomes,* or *phagolysosomes.* Lysosomes are involved in the breakdown of ingested materials in one of two ways: *heterophagy* or *autophagy* (Fig. 1–11).

Heterophagy. Materials from the external environment are taken up through a process generically called *endocytosis;* uptake of larger particulate matter is called *phagocytosis;* and uptake of soluble smaller macromolecules is denoted *pinocytosis.* Endocytosed vacuoles and their contents eventually fuse with a lysosome, resulting in degradation of the engulfed material. Although it occurs to some extent in all cell types, heterophagy is most conspicuous in the "professional" phagocytes; bacteria are ingested and degraded by neutrophils, and macrophages engulf and catabolize necrotic cells.

Autophagy. In this process, intracellular organelles and portions of cytosol are sequestered from the cytoplasm in an *autophagic vacuole* formed from ribosome-free regions of the RER. This then fuses with preexisting primary lysosomes to form an *autophagolysosome.* Autophagy is a common phenomenon involved in the removal of damaged or senescent organelles and in the cellular remodeling associated with cellular differentiation. It is particularly prominent

HETEROPHAGY   AUTOPHAGY

Figure 1-11 ■

A, Schematic representation of autophagy *(right)* and heterophagy *(left). B,* Electron micrograph of an autophagolysosome containing a degenerating mitochondrion and amorphous material *(arrow).* The asterisk indicates a normal mitochondrion for comparison. (*A,* Redrawn from Fawcett DW: A Textbook of Histology, 11th ed. Philadelphia, WB Saunders, 1986, p 17. *B,* From Cotran RS, Kumar V, Collins T: Robbins Pathologic Basis of Disease, 6th ed. Philadelphia, WB Saunders, 1999.)

in cells undergoing atrophy induced by nutrient or hormonal deprivation, as discussed previously.

The enzymes in the lysosomes can completely catabolize most proteins and carbohydrates, although some lipids remain undigested. Lysosomes with undigested debris may persist within cells as *residual bodies* or may be extruded. *Lipofuscin pigment* granules represent indigestible material resulting from intracellular lipid peroxidation, and certain indigestible pigments, such as carbon particles inhaled from the atmosphere or inoculated pigment in tattoos, can persist in phagolysosomes of macrophages for decades (discussed later).

Lysosomes are also repositories where cells sequester materials that cannot be completely metabolized. Hereditary *lysosomal storage disorders*, caused by deficiencies of enzymes that degrade various macromolecules, result in abnormal collections of intermediate metabolites in the lysosomes of cells all over the body; neurons are particularly susceptible to lethal injury from such accumulations (Chapter 7).

Induction (Hypertrophy) of Smooth Endoplasmic Reticulum. Protracted use of barbiturates leads to increasing tolerance, such that repeated doses lead to progressively shorter durations of sleep. Patients are therefore said to have "adapted" to the medication. This adaptation is due to induction of an increased volume (hypertrophy) of hepatocyte SER, which metabolizes the drug via the P-450 mixed-function oxidase system found there. The purpose of such enzyme modifications is to increase the solubility of various compounds (e.g., steroids, alcohol, aryl hydrocarbons, insecticides) and thereby facilitate their excretion. Although this is frequently described as "detoxification," many compounds are in fact rendered *more* injurious by P-450 modification (recall the effects of CCl_4 breakdown). In any event, the barbiturates and other substances stimulate (induce) the synthesis of more enzymes as well as more SER. In this manner, the cell adapts to be more effective at drug modification. It also follows that cells that have adapted to efficiently metabolize one compound are also more effective at metabolizing others. Thus, patients who increase their alcohol intake while taking phenobarbital for epilepsy may end up with subtherapeutic levels of the antiseizure medication.

Mitochondrial Alterations. As described previously, mitochondrial dysfunction clearly plays an important role in acute cell injury and death. In some nonlethal pathologic conditions, however, various alterations in the number, size, shape, and presumably function of mitochondria may also occur. For example, in cellular hypertrophy there is an increase in the number of mitochondria in cells; conversely, mitochondria decrease in number during cellular atrophy (probably via heterophagy; see Fig. 1-11). Mitochondria may assume extremely large and abnormal shapes *(megamitochondria),* as seen in hepatocytes in various nutritional deficiencies and alcoholic liver disease. In certain inherited metabolic diseases of skeletal muscle, the *mitochondrial myopathies,* defects in mitochondrial metabolism are associated with increased numbers of unusually large mitochondria containing abnormal cristae.

Cytoskeletal Abnormalities. The cytoskeleton consists of actin and myosin filaments, microtubules, and various classes of intermediate filaments; several other nonpolymerized and nonfilamentous forms of contractile proteins also contribute to the cellular scaffolding. The cytoskeleton is important for

■ Intracellular transport of organelles and molecules
■ Maintenance of basic cell architecture (e.g., cell polarity, distinguishing up and down)

■ Conveying cell-cell and cell–extracellular matrix signals to the nucleus
■ Mechanical strength for tissue integrity
■ Cell mobility
■ Phagocytosis

Clearly, cellular hypertrophy and atrophy require a corresponding increase or decrease in cytoskeletal elements. However, it is not sufficient that there be simply more or less of the proteins; these elements must be functionally organized to provide the requisite strength, contractile activity, or other physiologic attributes. Cells and tissues therefore respond to environmental stressors (e.g., shear stress in blood vessels or increased pressures in the heart) by constantly remodeling their intracellular scaffolding.

Abnormalities of the cytoskeleton occur in a variety of pathologic states. Alterations may be reflected by an abnormal cellular appearance and function (hypertrophic cardiomyopathy, Chapter 11), aberrant movements of intracellular organelles, defective cell locomotion, or intracellular accumulations of fibrillar material. Perturbations, as, for example, in the organization of *microtubules*, can cause sterility by inhibiting sperm motility, as well as immobilizing cilia of the respiratory epithelium, resulting in chronic infections due to defective clearance of inhaled bacteria (*Kartagener*, or the *immotile cilia, syndrome*). Microtubules are also essential for leukocyte migration and phagocytosis. Drugs that prevent microtubule polymerization (e.g., colchicine) are therefore useful in treating gout, in which symptoms are due to movement of macrophages toward urate crystals with subsequent frustrated attempts at phagocytosis. Since microtubules form the mitotic spindle, drugs that bind to microtubules (e.g., vinca alkaloids) are also antiproliferative and therefore useful for antitumor therapies.

Heat Shock Proteins. One of the most highly conserved adaptive biologic responses in the phylogenetic hierarchy is the induction of *stress proteins* after potentially injurious stimuli. These were originally called *heat shock proteins (HSPs)* because they were described in fruit fly larvae after slight (4° to 5°C) elevations in temperature; however, the same proteins are elaborated in normal cells and in response to a wide variety of physical and chemical stimuli in all species so far examined. Thus, although somewhat of a misnomer, the term *heat shock proteins* remains sanctified by long usage.

HSPs play important roles in normal intracellular protein "housekeeping," including the process of protein folding, disaggregation of protein-protein complexes, and transport of proteins into various intracellular organelles (*protein kinesis*; Fig. 1–12A). Thus, they are also called *chaperones*. HSPs may be constitutively produced (e.g., *Hsp 60*, and *Hsp 90* family members; the numbers are based on approximate molecular weights), or baseline synthesis may be increased after cellular stress that leads to protein aggregation and denaturation (e.g., *Hsp 70* family members). Those induced after injurious stimuli putatively play a role in refolding denatured polypeptides to restore their function before they can cause serious cell dysfunction or death. Alternatively, when refolding is not successful, *irretrievably denatured* proteins are tagged by binding of the *ubiquitin* HSP molecule; ubiquitin

binding targets these proteins for cytosolic catabolism by *proteasomes*, a particulate cluster of nonlysosomal proteinases (Fig. 1–12B).

HSP chaperones are induced in myocardial infarction and neuronal ischemic injury, and their induction appears to limit tissue necrosis in certain models of ischemia and reperfusion. The fact that they are found so ubiquitously and are strongly induced in the setting of sublethal cellular stresses indicates that they play a role in cell adaptation to injury. Moreover, there is increasing evidence that misfolded or misdirected proteins may play central roles in a variety of diseases including *amyloidosis* (Chapter 5), as well as neurodegenerative disorders such as Creutzfeldt-Jakob disease and Alzheimer disease (Chapter 23).

Intracellular Accumulations

Under some circumstances, cells may accumulate abnormal amounts of various substances. These may be harmless or may cause varied degrees of injury. The location of the substance may be either in the cytoplasm, within organelles (typically lysosomes), or in the nucleus. The substance may be synthesized by the affected cells or may be produced elsewhere.

There are three general pathways by which cells can accrue abnormal intracellular accumulations (Fig. 1–13):

■ A normal substance is produced at a normal or an increased rate, but the metabolic rate is inadequate to remove it. An example of this type of process is fatty change in the liver (see later).
■ A normal or an abnormal endogenous substance accumulates because of genetic or acquired defects in its metabolism, packaging, transport, or secretion. One example is a genetic enzymatic defect in a specific metabolic pathway; the resulting disorders are referred to as storage diseases (Chapter 7). In other cases, mutations cause defective folding and transport and hence accumulation (e.g., α_1-antitrypsin deficiency) of proteins.
■ An abnormal exogenous substance is deposited and accumulates because the cell has neither the enzymatic machinery to degrade the substance nor the ability to transport it to other sites. Accumulations of carbon or silica particles are examples of this type of alteration.

Fatty Change (Steatosis). *Fatty change* refers to any abnormal accumulation of triglycerides within parenchymal cells. Although itself an indicator of reversible injury, fatty change is sometimes encountered in cells adjacent to those that have undergone necrosis. Fatty change is most often seen in the liver, since this is the major organ involved in fat metabolism, but it may also occur in heart, skeletal muscle, kidney, and other organs. Steatosis may be caused by toxins, protein malnutrition, diabetes mellitus, obesity, and anoxia. However, *alcohol abuse is undoubtedly the most common cause of fatty change in the liver (fatty liver) in industrialized nations.*

As shown in Figure 1–14A, free fatty acids from adipose tissue or ingested food are normally transported into

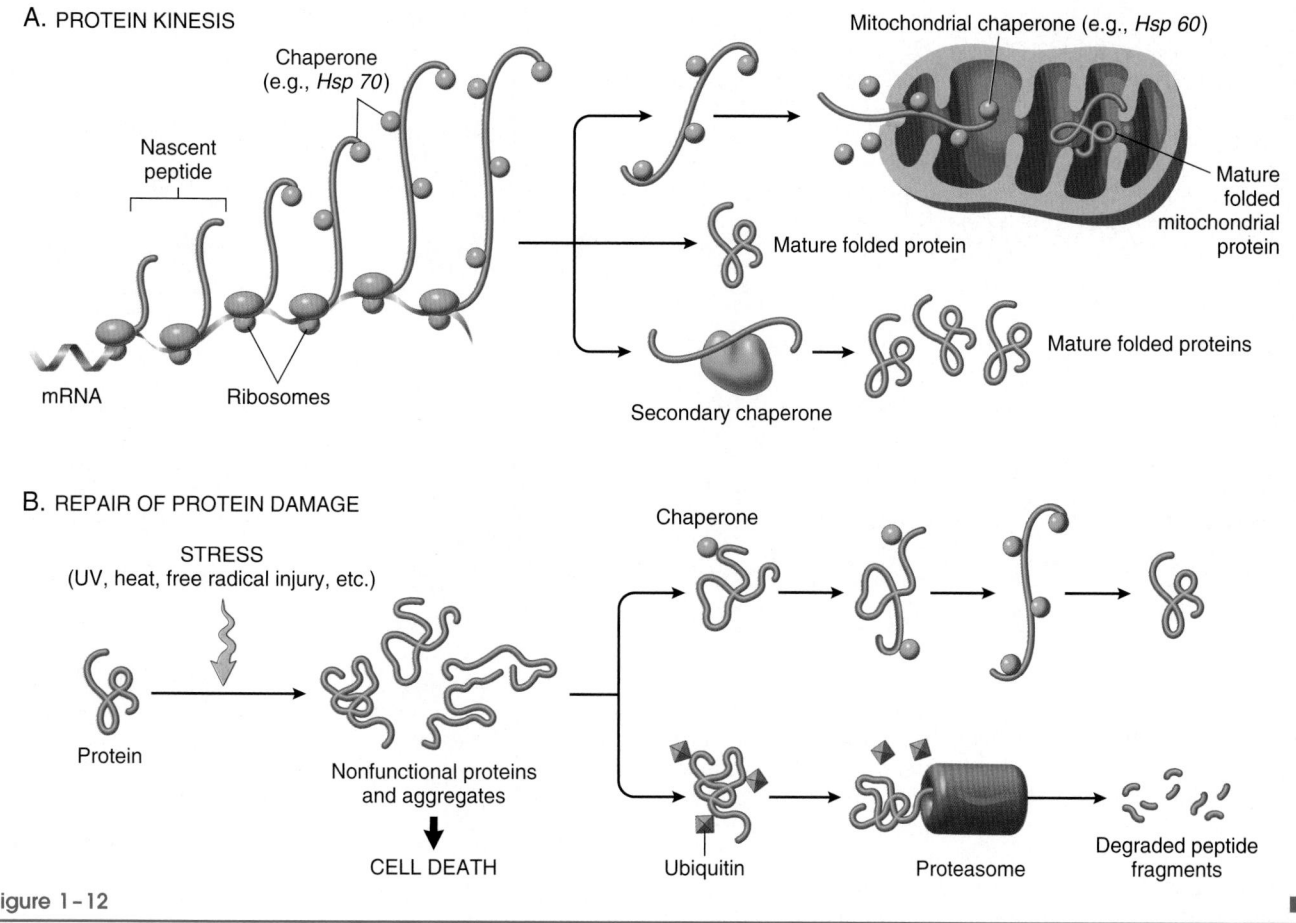

A. PROTEIN KINESIS

B. REPAIR OF PROTEIN DAMAGE

Figure 1-12

Diagram of the roles played by chaperones (heat shock proteins [HSPs]) in normal protein folding and translocation into organelles (protein kinesis) *(A)*, and in repair of damaged proteins, either by refolding or by targeting for degradation via proteasomes *(B)*. mRNA, messenger RNA; UV, ultraviolet radiation.

hepatocytes; there they are esterified to triglycerides, converted into cholesterol or phospholipids, or oxidized to ketone bodies. Some fatty acids are synthesized from acetate within the hepatocytes, as well. Egress of the triglycerides from the hepatocytes requires complexing with apoproteins to form lipoproteins, which may then traverse the circulation (Chapter 7). Excess accumulation of triglycerides may result from defects at any step from fatty acid entry to lipoprotein exit, thus accounting for the occurrence of fatty liver after diverse hepatic insults. Hepatotoxins (e.g., alcohol) alter mitochondrial and SER function; CCl_4 and protein malnutrition decrease the synthesis of apoproteins; anoxia inhibits fatty acid oxidation; and starvation increases fatty acid mobilization from peripheral stores.

The significance of fatty change depends on the cause and the severity of accumulation. When mild, it may have no effect on cellular function. More severe fatty change may transiently impair cellular function, but unless some vital intracellular process is irreversibly impaired (e.g., in CCl_4 poisoning), fatty change is reversible. In a severe form, fatty change may precede cell death, but it should be emphasized that *cells may die without undergoing fatty change.*

MORPHOLOGY

In any site, fatty accumulation appears as clear vacuoles within parenchymal cells. Special staining techniques are required to distinguish fat from intracellular water or glycogen, which can also produce clear vacuoles but have a different significance. To identify fat microscopically, tissues must be processed for sectioning without the organic solvents typically used in sample preparation. Usually, portions of tissue are therefore frozen to enable the cutting of thin sections for histologic examination; the fat is then identified by staining with Sudan IV or oil red O (these stain fat orange-red). Glycogen may be identified by staining for polysaccharides using the periodic acid–Schiff stain (which stains glycogen red-violet). If vacuoles don't stain for either fat or glycogen, they are presumed to be composed mostly of water.

Fatty change is most commonly seen in the liver and the heart. In the **liver,** mild fatty change may not affect the gross appearance. With accumulation, the organ enlarges and becomes progressively yellow until, in extreme cases, it may weigh 3 to 6 kg (1.5–3 times the normal weight) and appear bright yellow, soft, and greasy. Early fatty change is seen by light microscopy as small fat vacuoles in the cytoplasm around the nucleus. In later stages, the vacuoles coalesce to create cleared spaces that displace the nucleus to the cell periphery (Fig. 1–14B). Occasionally, contiguous cells rupture, and the enclosed fat globules unite to produce so-called fatty cysts.

In the **heart,** lipid is found in the form of small droplets, occurring in one of two patterns. Prolonged moderate hypoxia (as in profound anemia) results in focal intracellular fat deposits, creating grossly apparent bands of yellowed myocardium alternating with bands of darker, red-brown, uninvolved heart ("tigered effect"). The other pattern of fatty change is produced by more profound hypoxia or by some forms of myocarditis (e.g., diphtheria) and shows more uniformly affected myocytes.

Cholesterol and Cholesteryl Esters. Cellular cholesterol metabolism is tightly regulated to ensure normal cell membrane synthesis without significant intracellular accumulation. However, phagocytic cells may become overloaded with lipid (triglycerides, cholesterol, and cholesteryl esters) in several different pathologic processes.

Scavenger macrophages in contact with the lipid debris of necrotic cells or abnormal (e.g., oxidized) forms of plasma lipid may become stuffed with lipid because of their phagocytic activities. These macrophages become filled with minute, membrane-bound vacuoles of lipid, imparting a foamy appearance to their cytoplasm (*foam cells*). In *atherosclerosis*, smooth muscle cells and macrophages are filled with lipid vacuoles composed of cholesterol and cholesteryl esters; these give atherosclerotic plaques their characteristic yellow color and contribute to the pathogenesis of the lesion (Chapter 10). In hereditary and acquired hyperlipidemic syndromes, macrophages accumulate intracellular cholesterol; when present in the subepithelial connective tissue of skin or in tendons, clusters of these foamy macrophages form masses called *xanthomas.*

Proteins. Morphologically visible protein accumulations are much less common than lipid accumulations; they may occur because excesses are presented to the cells or because the cells synthesize excessive amounts. In the kidney, for example, trace amounts of albumin filtered through the glomerulus are normally reabsorbed by pinocytosis in the proximal convoluted tubules. However, in disorders with heavy protein leakage across the glomerular filter (e.g., nephrotic syndrome), there is a commensurately increased pinocytic reabsorption of the protein. Fusion of these pinocytic vesicles with lysosomes results in the histologic appearance of pink, hyaline cytoplasmic droplets (Fig. 1–15A). The process is reversible; if the proteinuria abates, the protein droplets are metabolized and disappear. Another example is the marked accumulations of newly synthesized immunoglobulins that may occur in the RER of some plasma cells, resulting in rounded, eosinophilic *Russell bodies.*

Figure 1–13 ■

General mechanisms of intracellular accumulation: (1) abnormal metabolism, as in fatty change in the liver; (2) mutations causing alterations in protein folding and transport, so that defective molecules accumulate intracellularly; (3) a deficiency of critical enzymes responsible for breaking down certain compounds, causing substrates to accumulate in lysosomes, as in lysosomal storage diseases; and (4) an inability to degrade phagocytosed particles, as in carbon pigment accumulation.

Accumulations of intracellular proteins are also seen in certain types of cell injury. For example, the Mallory body, or "alcoholic hyalin," is an eosinophilic intracytoplasmic inclusion in liver cells that is highly characteristic of alcoholic

A

Figure 1-14   ■

A, Possible mechanisms leading to the accumulation of triglycerides in fatty liver. Defects in any of the six numbered steps of uptake, catabolism, or secretion can result in lipid accumulation. *B,* High-power detail of fatty changes of liver. In most cells, the well-preserved nucleus is squeezed into the displaced rim of cytoplasm around the fat vacuole. (*B,* Courtesy of Dr. James Crawford, Department of Pathology, Brigham and Women's Hospital, Boston.)

Figure 1-15   ■

Intracellular protein accumulations. *A,* Protein reabsorption droplets in the renal tubular epithelium; the droplets are contained within pinocytic vacuoles and within lysosomes. *B,* Alcoholic hyalin *(arrow)* (also called Mallory bodies), composed of aggregated intermediate filaments in hepatocytes from an individual with chronic alcohol abuse. Also note the intracellular fat accumulation *(asterisks),* associated with acute alcohol intake. (*A,* Courtesy of Dr. Hemut Rennke, Department of Pathology, Brigham and Women's Hospital, Boston.)

liver disease (Fig. 1–15*B*). Such inclusions are composed predominantly of aggregated prekeratin intermediate filaments that presumably resist degradation. Another example is the neurofibrillary tangle found in the brain in Alzheimer disease; this aggregated protein inclusion contains microtubule-associated proteins and neurofilaments, a reflection of a disrupted neuronal cytoskeleton (Chapter 23).

Glycogen. Excessive intracellular deposits of glycogen are associated with abnormalities in the metabolism of either glucose or glycogen. In poorly controlled diabetes mellitus, the prime example of aberrant glucose metabolism, glycogen accumulates in renal tubular epithelium, cardiac myocytes, and beta cells of the islets of Langerhans. Glycogen also accumulates within cells in a group of closely related genetic disorders collectively referred to as *glycogen storage diseases,* or *glycogenoses* (Chapter 7). In these diseases, enzymatic defects in the synthesis or breakdown of glycogen result in massive stockpiling, with secondary injury and cell death.

Pigments. Pigments are colored substances that are either exogenous, coming from outside the body, or endogenous, synthesized within the body itself.

The most common exogenous pigment is carbon (an example is coal dust), a ubiquitous air pollutant of urban life. When inhaled, it is phagocytosed by alveolar macrophages and transported through lymphatic channels to the regional tracheobronchial lymph nodes. Aggregates of the pigment grossly blacken the draining lymph nodes and pulmonary parenchyma *(anthracosis).* Heavy accumulations may induce emphysema or a fibroblastic reaction that can result in a serious lung disease called coal workers' pneumoconiosis (Chapter 8).

Endogenous pigments include lipofuscin, melanin, and certain derivatives of hemoglobin. *Lipofuscin*, or "wear-and-tear pigment," is an insoluble, brownish-yellow granular intracellular material that accumulates in a variety of tissues (particularly the heart, liver, and brain) as a function of age or atrophy. Lipofuscin represents complexes of lipid and protein that derive from the free radical–catalyzed peroxidation of polyunsaturated lipids of subcellular membranes. It is not injurious to the cell but is important as a marker of past free radical injury. When apparent in tissue grossly, it is called *brown atrophy*. By electron microscopy, the pigment appears as perinuclear electron-dense granules (Fig. 1–16).

Melanin is an endogenous, brown-black pigment formed by melanocytes when the enzyme tyrosinase catalyzes the oxidation of tyrosine to dihydroxyphenylalanine. It is synthesized exclusively by melanocytes, specific cells characteristically found in the epidermis, and acts as an endogenous screen against harmful ultraviolet radiation. Although melanocytes are the only source of melanin, adjacent basal keratinocytes in the skin can accumulate the pigment (e.g., in freckles), or it may be accumulated in dermal macrophages.

Hemosiderin is a hemoglobin-derived granular pigment that is golden-yellow to brown and accumulates in tissues when there is a local or systemic excess of iron. Iron is normally stored within cells in association with the protein *apoferritin*, forming ferritin micelles. Hemosiderin pigment represents large aggregates of these ferritin micelles, readily visualized by light and electron microscopy; the iron can be unambiguously identified by the Prussian blue histochemical reaction. Although usually pathologic, small amounts of hemosiderin are normal in the mononuclear phagocytes of the bone marrow, spleen, and liver, where there is extensive red cell breakdown.

Local excesses of iron, and consequently of hemosiderin, result from hemorrhage. The best example is the common bruise. After lysis of the erythrocytes at the site of hemorrhage, the red cell debris is phagocytosed by macrophages; the hemoglobin content is then catabolized by lysosomes with accumulation of the heme iron in hemosiderin. The array of colors through which the bruise passes reflects these transformations. The original red-blue color of hemoglobin is transformed to varying shades of green-blue by the local formation of biliverdin (green bile) and bilirubin (red bile) from the heme moiety; the iron ions of hemoglobin are accumulated as golden-yellow hemosiderin.

Whenever there is systemic overload of iron, hemosiderin is deposited in many organs and tissues, a condition called *hemosiderosis*. It is found at first in the mononuclear phagocytes of the liver, bone marrow, spleen, and lymph nodes and in scattered macrophages throughout other organs. With progressive accumulation, parenchymal cells throughout the body (but principally the liver, pancreas, heart, and endocrine organs) become "bronzed" with accumulating pigment. Hemosiderosis (Chapter 12) occurs in the setting of (1) increased absorption of dietary iron, (2) impaired utilization of iron, (3) hemolytic anemias, and (4) transfusions (the transfused red cells constitute an exogenous load of iron). In most instances of systemic hemosiderosis, the iron pigment does not damage the parenchymal cells or impair organ function despite an impressive accumulation (Fig 1–17). However, more extensive accumulations of iron result in *hemochromatosis* (Chapter 16), with tissue injury including liver fibrosis, heart failure, and diabetes mellitus.

Figure 1–16   ■

Lipofuscin granules in a cardiac myocyte as shown by electron microscopy. *A,* Low-power magnification. Note the perinuclear, intralysosomal location. *B,* High-power magnification. The electron-dense bodies are composed of lipid-protein complexes.

Figure 1–17

Hemosiderin granules in liver cells. *A,* H & E–stained section showing golden-brown, finely granular pigment. *B,* Prussian blue reaction, specific for oxidized Fe^{+++} iron.

Pathologic Calcification

Pathologic calcification is a common process in a wide variety of disease states; it implies the abnormal deposition of calcium salts, together with smaller amounts of iron, magnesium, and other minerals. When the deposition occurs in dead or dying tissues, it is called *dystrophic calcification; it occurs in the absence of calcium metabolic derangements* (i.e., with normal serum levels of calcium). In contrast, the deposition of calcium salts in normal tissues is known as *metastatic calcification and almost always reflects some derangement in calcium metabolism (hypercalcemia).*

Dystrophic Calcification. Dystrophic calcification is encountered in areas of necrosis of any type. It is virtually inevitable in the *atheromas* of advanced atherosclerosis, areas of intimal injury in the aorta and large arteries characterized by accumulated lipids (Chapter 10). Although dystrophic calcification may only represent evidence of previous cell injury, it is also frequently a cause of organ dysfunction. For example, cuspal calcification can develop in aging or damaged heart valves, resulting in severely compromised valve motion. Dystrophic calcification of the aortic valves is an important cause of aortic stenosis in the elderly (Fig. 1–18).

MORPHOLOGY

Regardless of the site, the calcium salts are grossly seen as fine, white granules or clumps, often felt as gritty deposits. Sometimes, a tuberculous lymph node is essentially converted to stone. Histologically, calcification appears as **intracellular** and/or **extracellular** basophilic deposits. In time, **heterotopic bone** may be formed in the focus of calcification.

The pathogenesis of dystrophic calcification involves *initiation* (or nucleation) and *propagation,* both of which may be either intracellular or extracellular; the ultimate end product is the formation of crystalline *calcium phosphate.* Initiation in extracellular sites occurs in membrane-bound vesicles about 200 nm in diameter; in normal cartilage and bone they are known as *matrix vesicles,* and in pathologic calcification they derive from degenerating cells. It is thought that calcium is initially concentrated in these vesicles by its affinity for membrane phospholipids, while phosphates accumulate as a result of the action of membrane-bound phosphatases. Initiation of intracellular calcification occurs in the mitochondria of dead or dying cells that have lost their ability to regulate intracellular calcium. After initiation in either location, propagation of crystal formation occurs. This is dependent on the concentration of Ca^{++} and PO_4^- in the extracellular spaces, the presence of mineral inhibitors, and the degree of collagenization. Collagen enhances the rate of crystal growth, but other proteins such as *osteopontin* (an acidic, calcium-binding phosphoprotein) are also involved.

Figure 1–18

A view looking down onto the unopened aortic valve in a heart with calcific aortic stenosis. The semilunar cusps are thickened and fibrotic. Behind each cusp are large irregular masses of dystrophic calcification that will prevent normal opening of the cusps.

Metastatic Calcification. Metastatic calcification can occur in normal tissues whenever there is hypercalcemia; clearly, hypercalcemia also exacerbates dystrophic calcification. The four major causes of hypercalcemia are (1) *increased secretion of parathyroid hormone*, due to either primary parathyroid tumors or production by other malignant tumors; (2) *destruction of bone* due to the effects of accelerated turnover (e.g., *Paget disease*), immobilization, or tumors (increased bone catabolism associated with multiple myeloma, leukemia, or diffuse skeletal metastases); (3) *vitamin D–related disorders* including vitamin D intoxication and *sarcoidosis* (in which macrophages activate a vitamin D precursor); and (4) *renal failure*, in which phosphate retention leads to *secondary hyperparathyroidism*.

MORPHOLOGY

Metastatic calcification can occur widely throughout the body but principally affects the interstitial tissues of the vasculature, kidneys, lungs, and gastric mucosa. The calcium deposits morphologically resemble those described in dystrophic calcification. Although they do not generally cause clinical dysfunction, extensive calcifications in the lungs may produce remarkable radiographs and respiratory deficits, and massive deposits in the kidney **(nephrocalcinosis)** can cause renal damage.

REVERSIBLE AND IRREVERSIBLE CELL INJURY

Up to this point, we have focused on the causes and mechanisms of cell injury, as well as the various adaptive responses that cells and tissues can utilize in the face of stress to maintain viability (if not necessarily normal function). In this section, we turn our attention to the pathways underlying the sequence of events whereby *reversible injury becomes irreversible*, and *cell death* occurs.

The molecular mechanisms connecting most forms of cell injury to ultimate cell death have proved elusive. First, there are clearly many ways to injure a cell, not all of them invariably fatal. Second, the numerous macromolecules, enzymes, and organelles within the cell are so closely interdependent that it is difficult to distinguish a primary injury from secondary (and not necessarily relevant) ripple effects. Third, the "point of no return," at which irreversible damage has occurred, is still largely undetermined; thus, we have no precise cutoff point to establish cause and effect. Finally, there is probably no common final pathway by which cells die.

General Pathways

As discussed previously, regardless of the initial cause of injury, four cell systems are particularly vulnerable: (1) cell membrane integrity, critical to cellular ionic and osmotic homeostasis; (2) ATP generation, largely via mitochondrial aerobic respiration; (3) protein synthesis; and (4) the

integrity of the genetic apparatus. Within limits, the cell can compensate for disturbance of any of these and, if the injurious stimulus abates, return to normalcy. Persistent or excessive injury, however, causes cells to pass the threshold into *irreversible injury* (Fig. 1–19). This is associated with extensive damage to all membranes, swelling of lysosomes, and vacuolization of mitochondria, with a resulting reduced capacity to generate ATP. Extracellular calcium enters the cell, and intracellular calcium stores are released, resulting

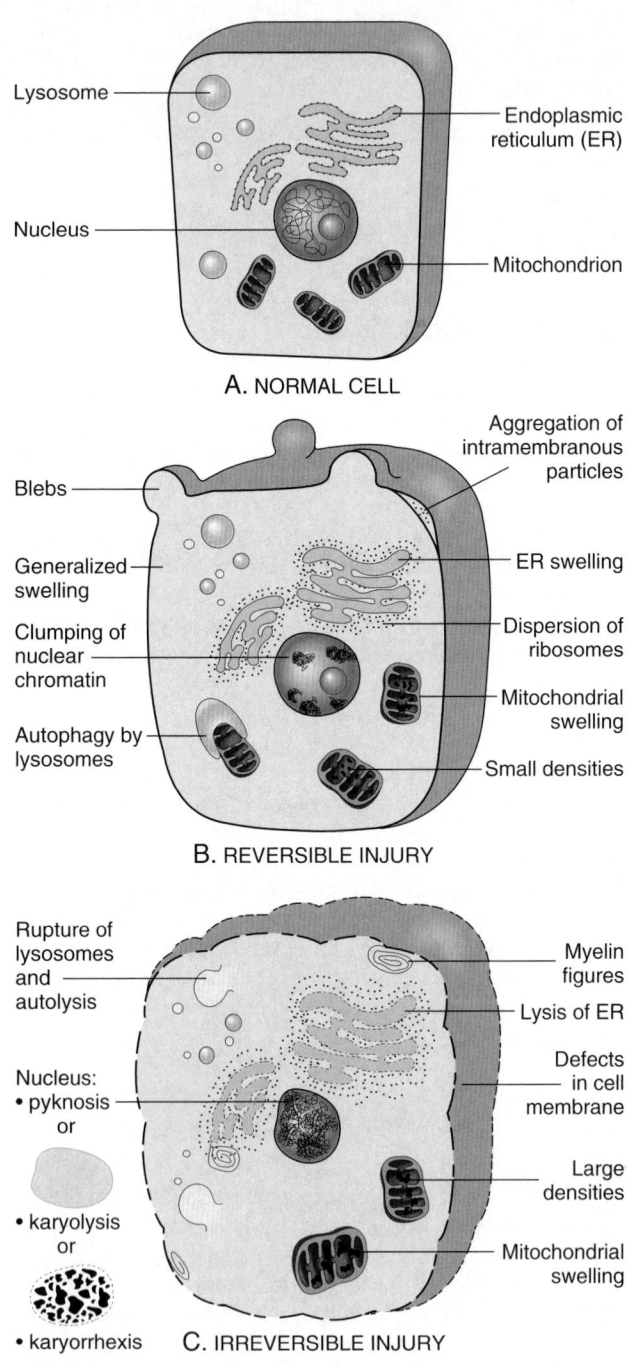

A. NORMAL CELL

B. REVERSIBLE INJURY

C. IRREVERSIBLE INJURY

Figure 1–19 ■

Schematic representations of the ultrastructural features of normal cells *(A)*, and those changes seen in reversible *(B)* and irreversible *(C)* cell injury (see text).

in the activation of enzymes that can catabolize membranes, proteins, ATP, and nucleic acids (see Fig. 1–4). Thus, one of the earliest ultrastructural markers of irreversible injury is the *accumulation of amorphous, calcium-rich densities in the mitochondrial matrix.* After this, there is continued loss of proteins, essential coenzymes, and ribonucleic acids from the hyperpermeable plasma membrane, with cells leaking metabolites vital for the reconstitution of ATP and further depleting intracellular high-energy phosphates. Injury to the lysosomal membranes results in leakage of their enzymes into the cytoplasm; the acid hydrolases are activated in the reduced intracellular pH of the ischemic cell and degrade cytoplasmic and nuclear components.

After cell death, cellular constituents are progressively digested by lysosomal hydrolases; moreover, there is widespread leakage of potentially destructive cellular enzymes into the extracellular space. Dead cells may ultimately be replaced by large, whorled phospholipid masses called *myelin figures.* These phospholipid precipitates are then either phagocytosed by other cells or further degraded into fatty acids; calcification of such fatty acid residues results in the generation of calcium soaps.

It is worth noting that leakage of intracellular proteins across the degraded cell membrane into the peripheral circulation provides a means of detecting tissue-specific cell injury and death using blood serum samples. Cardiac muscle, for example, contains a specific isoform of the enzyme creatine kinase and of the contractile protein troponins; liver (and specifically bile duct epithelium) contains a temperature-resistant isoform of the enzyme alkaline phosphatase. Irreversible injury and cell death in these tissues is consequently reflected in increased levels of such proteins in the general circulation.

To summarize, irreversible cell injury eventually affects oxidative phosphorylation and hence the synthesis of vital ATP supplies; membrane damage is a critical step in the development of lethal cell injury, and calcium is a potential mediator of the final morphologic alterations in cell death.

Mechanisms of Irreversible Injury

The biochemical sequence of events associated with cell injury were described earlier as a continuum from onset to ultimate digestion of the lethally injured cell by lysosomal enzymes. However, where was the "point of no return" beyond which the cell was irretrievably doomed to destruction? And when did the cell actually die? Two phenomena consistently characterize irreversibility. *The first is the inability to reverse mitochondrial dysfunction* (lack of oxidative phosphorylation and ATP generation) even after resolution of the original injury (e.g., restoration of blood flow). *The second is the development of profound disturbances in membrane function.* Although the depletion of ATP in itself might constitute a lethal event, the evidence is conflicting; it has been possible experimentally to dissociate the morphologic changes, as well as ATP depletion, from the inevitability of cell death.

Considerable evidence favors cell membrane damage as a central factor in the pathogenesis of irreversible cell injury. Loss of volume regulation, increased permeability to extracellular molecules, and demonstrable plasma membrane ultrastructural defects occur even in the earliest stages of irreversible injury. There are several potential causes of membrane damage, and all may play a role in certain forms of injury (Fig. 1–20).

Figure 1–20   ■

Mechanisms of membrane damage in ischemia (see text).

■ *Progressive loss of membrane phospholipids.* In ischemic liver, irreversible injury is associated with a marked decrease in membrane phospholipids. One explanation may be increased degradation due to activation of endogenous phospholipases by ischemia-induced increases in cytosolic calcium. Progressive phospholipid loss can also occur secondary to decreased ATP-dependent reacylation or diminished de novo synthesis of phospholipids.

■ *Cytoskeletal abnormalities.* Activation of proteases by increased intracellular calcium may result in damage to the cytoskeleton. In the setting of cell swelling, such injury may cause detachment of the cell membrane from the cytoskeleton, rendering the membrane susceptible to stretching and rupture.

■ *Toxic oxygen radicals.* Partially reduced oxygen species are highly toxic and cause injury to cell membranes and other cellular constituents. Such oxygen radicals are increased in ischemic tissues, particularly after restoration of blood flow by recruitment of leukocytes and other mechanisms discussed in the section "Ischemia/Reperfusion Injury."

■ *Lipid breakdown products.* These catabolic products accumulate in ischemic cells as a result of phospholipid degradation and have a detergent effect on membranes.

Whatever the mechanism or mechanisms of membrane damage, the end result is a massive leak of intracellular materials and a massive influx of calcium, with the consequences described earlier (see Fig. 1–4).

Morphology of Reversible Cell Injury and Cell Death—Necrosis

Recall that *functional changes typically precede any morphologic changes of cell injury.* Moreover, the time lag required to produce the morphologic changes of cell injury and death varies with the sensitivity of the methods used to detect these changes. With histochemical or ultrastructural techniques, changes may be seen in minutes to hours after injury due to various causes; however, it may take considerably longer (hours to days) before changes can be seen by light microscopy or on gross examination (see Fig. 1–2).

MORPHOLOGY

REVERSIBLE INJURY. The ultrastructural changes of reversible cell injury (see Fig. 1–19) include (1) **plasma membrane alterations** such as blebbing; blunting or distortion of microvilli; and loosening of intercellular attachments; (2) **mitochondrial changes** such as swelling and the appearance of phospholipid-rich amorphous densities; (3) **dilation of the endoplasmic reticulum** with detachment of ribosomes and dissociation of polysomes; and (4) **nuclear alterations,** with disaggregation of granular and fibrillar elements.

Two patterns of morphologic change correlating to reversible injury can be recognized under the light microscope: **cellular swelling** and **fatty change.**

Cellular swelling is the first manifestation of almost all forms of injury to cells; it appears whenever cells are incapable of maintaining ionic and fluid homeostasis. It can be a difficult morphologic change to appreciate with the light microscope and may be more apparent at the level of the whole organ. When all cells in an organ are affected, there is pallor, increased turgor, and increased weight. Microscopically, small, clear vacuoles may be seen within the cytoplasm; these represent distended and pinched-off segments of the endoplasmic reticulum. This pattern of nonlethal, reversible injury is sometimes called **hydropic change** or **vacuolar degeneration** (Fig. 1–21); swelling of cells is reversible.

Fatty change, occurring in hypoxic injury and various forms of toxic or metabolic injury, is manifested by the appearance of lipid vacuoles in the cytoplasm (see Fig. 1–15). It is a less universal reaction, principally encountered in cells participating in fat metabolism (e.g., hepatocytes and myocardial cells), and **is also reversible.**

Irreversible Cell Injury—Necrosis. *Necrosis refers to a sequence of morphologic changes that follow cell death in living tissue* (tissue placed in fixative is dead but not necrotic). As commonly used, necrosis is the gross and histologic correlate of cell death occurring in the setting of irreversible exogenous injury. Its most common manifestation is *coagulative necrosis,* characterized by cell swelling,

Figure 1–21 ■

Cellular swelling in hepatocytes in alcoholic liver disease. The nuclei and plasma membranes are largely intact, suggesting viability. The swollen hepatocyte on the left also shows alcoholic hyalin *(arrow).* (Courtesy of Dr. James Crawford, Department of Pathology, Brigham and Women's Hospital, Boston.)

denaturation of cytoplasmic proteins, and breakdown of cell organelles.

The morphologic appearance of necrosis is the result of two essentially concurrent processes: (1) enzymatic digestion of the cell and (2) denaturation of proteins. The hydrolytic enzymes may derive either from the dead cells themselves, in which case the digestion is referred to as *autolysis,* or from the lysosomes of invading inflammatory cells, termed *heterolysis.* These processes require hours to develop, and so there are no detectable changes in cells if, for example, a myocardial infarct causes sudden death. Although subtle ultrastructural changes might be evident 20 to 40 minutes after myocardial cell death, and enzymes leaked from damaged myocardium can be detected in the bloodstream as early as 2 hours after myocardial cell death, the classic histologic features of necrosis are not apparent until 4 to 12 hours after irreversible injury has occurred.

MORPHOLOGY

Dead cells show increased eosinophilia (i.e., pink staining from the eosin dye: the "E" in "H & E"). This is attributable in part to increased binding of eosin to denatured intracytoplasmic proteins, and in part to loss of the basophilia that is normally imparted by the RNA in the cytoplasm (basophilia is the blue staining from the hematoxylin dye: the "H" in "H & E"). The cell may have a more glassy homogeneous appearance than viable cells, due mainly to the loss of glycogen particles. When enzymes have degraded the organelles, the cytoplasm becomes vacuolated and appears moth-eaten. Finally, calcification of the dead cells may occur. Nuclear changes assume one of three patterns (see Fig. 1–19), all due to nonspecific breakdown of DNA. The basophilia of the chromatin may fade (**karyolysis**), presumably secondary to DNAse activity. A second pattern is **pyknosis,** characterized by nuclear shrinkage and increased basophilia; the DNA condenses into a solid shrunken mass. In the third pattern, **karyorrhexis,** the pyknotic nucleus fragments. In 1 to 2 days, the nucleus in a dead cell completely disappears.

Once the dead cells have undergone these early changes, the mass of necrotic tissue may exhibit distinctive morphologic patterns depending on whether enzymatic catabolism or protein denaturation predominates. Although the terms describing patterns of necrosis are somewhat outmoded, they are routinely used, and their meanings are understood by pathologists and clinicians. When denaturation is the primary pattern, so-called **coagulative necrosis** develops. In the instance of dominant enzymatic digestion, the result is **liquefactive necrosis;** in special circumstances, **caseous necrosis** or **fat necrosis** may develop.

Coagulative necrosis implies preservation of the basic structural outline of the coagulated cell or tissue for a span of days. Presumably, the injury or the subsequent increasing acidosis denatures not only the structural proteins but also the enzyme proteins, thus blocking cellular proteolysis. Myocardial infarction is a prime example in which acidophilic, coagulated, anucleate cells may persist for weeks. Ultimately, the necrotic myocardial cells are removed by fragmentation and phagocytosis by scavenger white blood cells. The process of coagulative necrosis, with preservation of the general tissue architecture, is characteristic of hypoxic death of cells in all tissues (Fig. 1–22A) except the brain.

Liquefactive necrosis is characteristic of focal bacterial or sometimes fungal infections, since these provide powerful stimuli for the accumulation of white cells (Fig. 1–22B). For unclear reasons, hypoxic death of cells within the central nervous system also results in liquefactive necrosis. Whatever the pathogenesis, liquefaction completely digests the dead cells. Although **gangrenous necrosis** is not a distinctive pattern of cell death, the term is still commonly used in surgical practice. It refers to ischemic coagulative necrosis (frequently of a limb); when there is superimposed infection with a liquefactive component, the lesion is called "wet gangrene."

Caseous necrosis is a distinctive form of necrosis encountered most often in foci of tuberculous infection (Chapter 13). The term "caseous" is derived from the cheesy, white gross appearance of the central necrotic area (Fig. 1–23A). Microscopically, the necrotic focus is composed of structureless, amorphous granular debris enclosed within a distinctive ring of granulomatous inflammation (Chapter 2, see Fig. 2–23). Unlike coagulative necrosis, the tissue architecture is completely obliterated.

Fat necrosis is another well-accepted term that does not really denote a specific pattern of necrosis. Rather, it describes focal areas of fat destruction, typically occurring after pancreatic injury; these result from pathologic release of activated pancreatic enzymes into adjacent parenchyma or the peritoneal cavity. This occurs in the disastrous abdominal emergency known as **acute pancreatitis** (Chapter 17); activated pancreatic enzymes escape from acinar cells and ducts, liquefying fat cell membranes and hydrolyzing the triglyceride esters contained within them. The released fatty acids combine with calcium to produce grossly visible chalky white aresas (fat saponification), which enable the surgeon or pathologist to identify this disease on simple inspection (Fig. 1–23B). Histologically, only shadowy outlines of necrotic fat cells may be seen, with basophilic calcium deposits and a surrounding inflammatory reaction.

Figure 1–22 ■

A, Kidney infarct exhibiting coagulative necrosis, with loss of nuclei and clumping of the cytoplasm but with preservation of basic outlines of glomerular and tubular architecture. *B,* A focus of liquefactive necrosis in the kidney caused by fungal seeding. The focus is filled with white cells and cellular debris, creating a renal abscess that obliterates the normal architecture.

Figure 1–23 ■

A, A tuberculous lung with a large area of caseous necrosis. The caseous debris is yellow-white and cheesy (hence the name caseous). *B,* Foci of fat necrosis with saponification in the mesentery. The areas of white-yellow chalky deposits represent calcium soap formation at sites of lipid breakdown.

Eventually, in the living patient, most necrotic cells and their debris disappear by a combined process of extracellular enzyme digestion and leukocyte phagocytosis. If necrotic cells and cellular debris are not promptly eliminated, they tend to attract calcium salts and other minerals and undergo *dystrophic calcification,* as discussed earlier.

PROGRAMMED CELL DEATH— APOPTOSIS

Apoptosis is a distinctive and important mode of cell death that should be differentiated from necrosis, although it does share some mechanistic features (Fig. 1–24, Table 1–1). Rather than the cellular "homicide" that occurs in necrotic cell death, apoptosis is a pathway of cellular "suicide." Apoptosis (from root words meaning "a falling away from") is responsible for the programmed cell death in

several important physiologic (as well as pathologic) processes, including

■ The programmed destruction of cells during embryogenesis, as occurs in implantation, organogenesis, and developmental involution

■ Hormone-dependent physiologic involution, such as involution of the endometrium during the menstrual cycle, or the lactating breast after weaning; or pathologic atrophy, as in the prostate after castration

■ Cell deletion in proliferating populations, such as intestinal crypt epithelium, or cell death in tumors

■ Deletion of autoreactive T cells in the thymus (>95% of thymocytes die in the thymus during maturation!), cell death of cytokine-starved lymphocytes, or cell death induced by cytotoxic T cells

■ A variety of mild injurious stimuli (heat, radiation, cytotoxic cancer drugs, etc.) that cause irreparable DNA damage that in turn triggers cell suicide pathways (e.g., via the tumor suppressor protein TP53)

Indeed, failure of cells to undergo physiologic apoptosis may result in aberrant development, unimpeded tumor proliferation, or autoimmune disease.

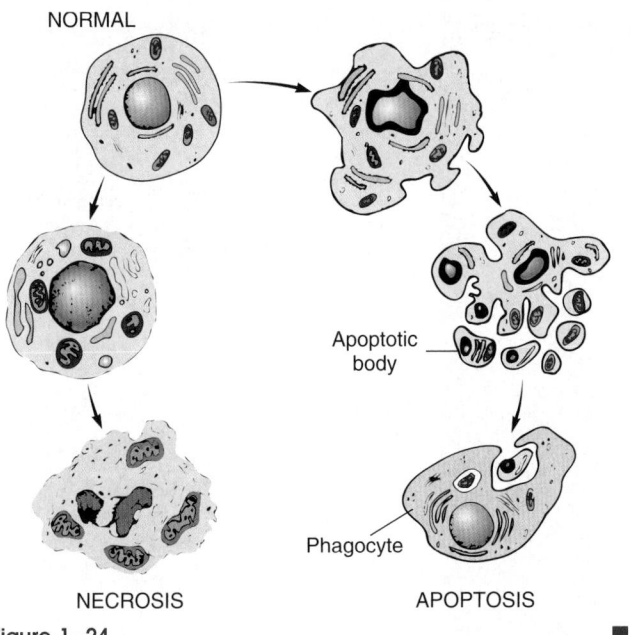

NORMAL

Apoptotic body

Phagocyte

NECROSIS   APOPTOSIS

Figure 1–24 ■

The sequential ultrastructural changes seen in coagulation necrosis *(left)* and apoptosis *(right)*. In apoptosis, the initial changes consist of nuclear chromatin condensation and fragmentation, followed by cytoplasmic budding and phagocytosis of the extruded apoptotic bodies. Signs of coagulation necrosis include chromatin clumping, organellar swelling, and eventual membrane damage. (Adapted from Walker NI, et al: Patterns of cell death. Methods Arch Exp Pathol 13:18, 1988.)

MORPHOLOGY

Apoptosis usually involves single cells or clusters of cells that appear on H & E–stained sections as round or oval masses with intensely eosinophilic cytoplasm (Fig. 1–25A). The nuclear chromatin is condensed, and it aggregates peripherally, under the nuclear membrane, into well-delimited masses of various shapes and sizes. Ultimately, karyorrhexis occurs; at a molecular level, this is reflected in fragmentation of DNA into nucleosome-sized pieces, presumably through the activation of endonucleases (Fig. 1–25B). The cells rapidly shrink, form cytoplasmic buds, and fragment into apoptotic bodies composed of membrane-bound vesicles of cytosol and organelles (see Fig. 1–24). Because these fragments are quickly extruded and phagocytosed or degraded, even substantial apoptosis may be histologically inapparent. Moreover, apoptosis does not elicit an inflammatory response, further hindering microscopic recognition.

Mechanisms of Apoptosis. The mechanisms underlying apoptosis are the subject of extensive and evolving investigation. The basic process can be understood as four separable but overlapping components (Fig. 1–26):

1. *Signaling.* Apoptosis may be triggered by a variety of signals ranging from an intrinsic programmed event (e.g., in development), a lack of growth factor, specific

Table 1–1. SIMPLIFIED FEATURES OF COAGULATION NECROSIS VERSUS APOPTOSIS

	Coagulation Necrosis	Apoptosis
Stimuli	Hypoxia, toxins	Physiologic and pathologic factors
Histologic appearance	Cellular swelling Coagulation necrosis Disruption of organelles	Single cells Chromatin condensation Apoptotic bodies
DNA breakdown	Random, diffuse	Internucleosomal
Mechanisms	ATP depletion Membrane injury Free radical damage	Gene activation Endonucleases Proteases
Tissue reaction	Inflammation	No inflammation Phagocytosis of apoptotic bodies

receptor-ligand interactions, release of granzymes from cytotoxic T cells, or selected injurious agents (e.g., radiation). Transmembrane signals may either suppress preexisting death programs (and are thus survival stimuli) or initiate a death cascade. The most important in this latter group are those that belong to the tumor necrosis factor receptor (TNFR) superfamily of plasma membrane molecules (this includes the FAS surface molecule [Chapter 5]). These plasma membrane receptors share an intracellular "death domain" protein sequence that when oligomerized (typically trimerized) leads to activation of initiator caspases and a cascade of enzyme activation culminating in cell death.

2. *Control and integration.* This is accomplished by specific proteins that connect the original death signals to the final execution program. These proteins are important because their actions may result in either "commitment" or abortion of potentially lethal signals. There are two broad pathways in this stage: (1) direct transmission of death signals by specific *adapter proteins* to the execution mechanism; and (2) regulation of *mitochondrial permeability* by members of the *BCL-2 family of proteins* (Chapter 6). Recall (see Fig. 1–5) that various agonists (Ca^{++}, free radicals, etc.) can affect mitochondria by causing *mitochondrial permeability transitions*. Formation of pores within the inner mitochondrial membrane results in reduction of the membrane potential, with diminished ATP production and mitochondrial swelling; increased permeability of outer mitochondrial membranes releases the apoptotic trigger, cytochrome *c*, into the cytosol. It is speculated that released cytochrome *c* binds certain cytosolic proteins (e.g., *proapoptotic protease-activating factor*, or *Apaf-1*) and activates them, triggering execution caspase activation and setting in motion the proteolytic events that kill the cell. *BCL-2* (found in the mitochondrial membrane) *suppresses apoptosis by preventing increased mitochondrial permeability and by stabilizing proteins like Apaf-1 so*

Figure 1–25 ■

A, Apoptosis of a keratinocyte in the skin, due in this case to an immune reaction *(arrow).* In the H & E–stained section, note the intensely eosinophilic cytoplasm and the condensed, pyknotic nucleus. *B,* Agarose gel electrophoresis of DNA extracted from cultured cells stained with ethidium bromide and photographed under UV illumination. *Lane a,* Viable control culture with DNA all of a large size that migrates minimally into the gel. *Lane b,* Culture with extensive apoptosis showing a laddered pattern of DNA fragmentation. *Lane c,* Culture with massive necrosis showing diffuse smearing of the DNA. Note that these patterns are characteristic of, but not specific for, apoptosis and necrosis, respectively. (*A,* Courtesy of Dr. Scott Granter, Brigham and Women's Hospital, Boston. *B,* From Kerr JFR, Harmon BV: Definition and incidence of apoptosis: A historical perspective. In Tomei LD, Cope FO [eds]: Apoptosis: The Molecular Basis of Cell Death. Cold Spring Harbor, NY, Cold Spring Harbor Laboratory Press, 1991, p 13.)

that caspase activation does not occur. Other members of the BCL-2 family bind to BCL-2 and modulate its antiapoptotic effect; thus, BCL-X$_L$ inhibits apoptosis while BAX and BAD promote programmed cell death (see Fig. 1–26).

3. *Execution.* This final pathway of apoptosis is characterized by a distinctive constellation of biochemical events that result from the synthesis and/or activation of a number of cytosolic catabolic enzymes. It culminates in the morphologic changes described earlier. Although there are subtle variations, the final execution pathways exhibit common themes generally applicable to all forms of apoptosis.

■ *Protein cleavage* by a class of newly recognized proteases named *caspases,* so called because they have an active site *c*ysteine, and cleave after *asp*artic acid residues. In experimental systems, overexpression of *any* of the caspases results in cellular apoptosis, suggesting that under normal circumstances, they must be tightly controlled. Activation of one or more such caspase enzyme putatively leads to a cascade of activation of other proteases, inexorably culminating in cell suicide. For example, down-stream *endonuclease* activation results in the characteristic DNA fragmentation, while cell volume and shape changes may in part result from cleavage of components of the cytoskeleton.

■ *Extensive protein cross-linking* via *transglutaminase activation* converts soluble cytoplasmic proteins and particularly cytoskeletal proteins into a covalently linked condensed shell that readily fragments into apoptotic bodies.

■ *DNA breakdown* into 180– to 200–base pair fragments (the distance between nucleosomes) occurs through the action of Ca^{++}- and Mg^{++}- dependent endonucleases. This may be visualized as a distinctive "laddering" of DNA into discrete-sized pieces on agarose gel electrophoresis; this pattern is often distinguished from the random DNA fragmentation (forming a "smear" on agarose gels) typically seen in necrotic cells (see Fig. 1–25B). It should be noted that laddering may also be seen in early stages of necrosis. Thus, while it is a useful marker for apoptosis, DNA laddering is not diagnostic for programmed cell death.

4. *Removal of dead cells.* Apoptotic cells and their fragments have marker molecules on their surfaces that facilitate uptake and disposal by adjacent cells or phagocytes. This occurs by the flipping of phosphatidylserine from the inner cytoplasmic face of the apoptotic cells to the extracellular face. This and other alterations allow the early recognition and phagocytosis of apoptotic cells without release of proinflammatory mediators. The process is so efficient that dead cells disappear without leaving a trace, and inflammation is virtually absent (see Fig. 1–26).

CELLULAR AGING

Cellular aging is discussed here because it almost certainly represents a progressive accumulation of sublethal injury that compromises cellular function and may lead to cell death, or at least to diminished capacity of cells to respond to injury.

A number of cellular functions decline progressively with age. Mitochondrial oxidative phosphorylation is reduced, as is synthesis of structural, enzymatic, and receptor proteins. Senescent cells have a diminished capacity for nutrient uptake and for repair of chromosomal damage. The morphologic alterations in senescent cells include irregular nuclei, pleomorphic vacuolated mitochondria, diminished endoplasmic

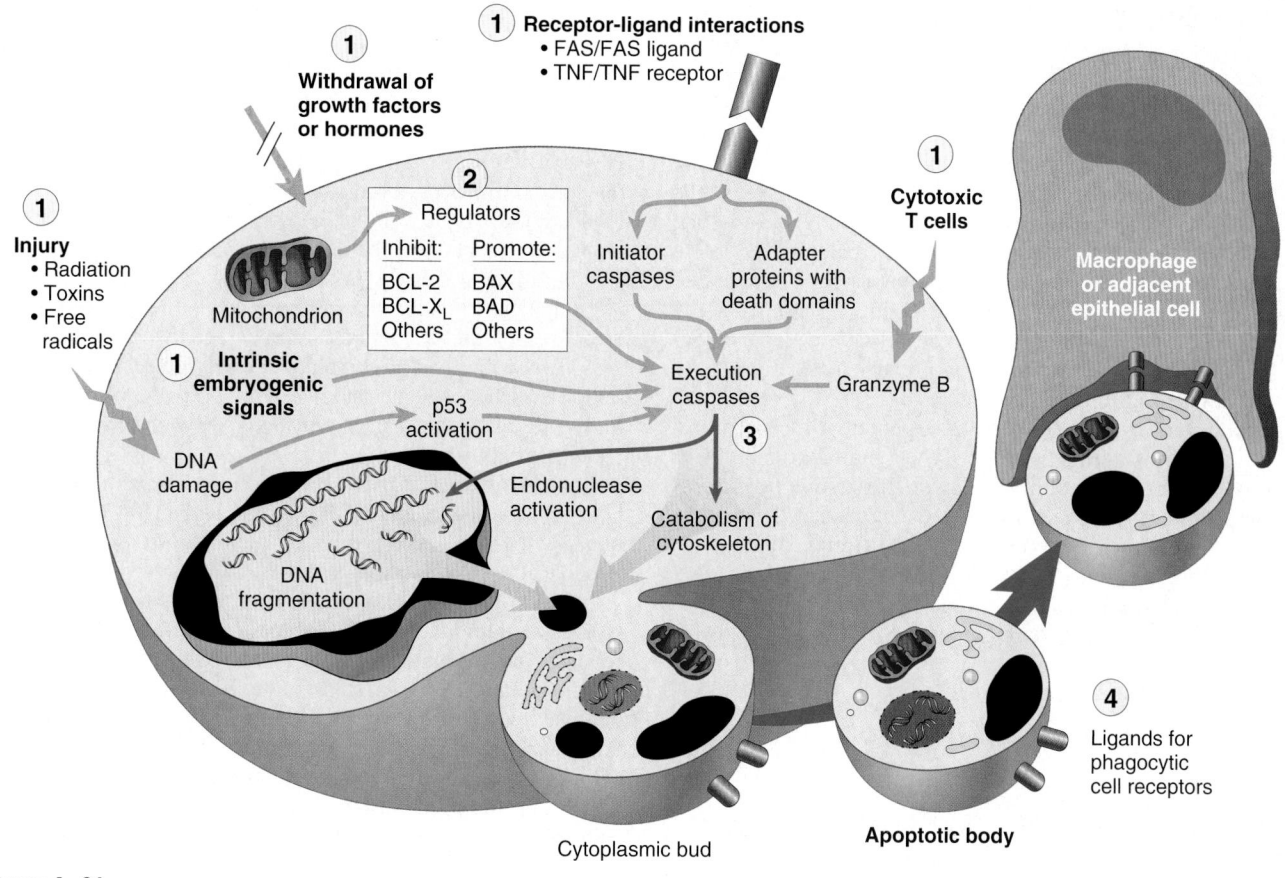

Figure 1–26 ■

Schematic representation of events in apoptosis. A variety of intrinsic or extrinsic triggers (labeled *1*) can induce apoptosis; these triggers include injurious stimuli such as radiation or free radicals (which damage DNA and activate TP53 (p53) pathways), intrinsic activation of programmed cell death pathways (e.g., during embryogenesis), withdrawal of growth factors, receptor ligation (e.g., FAS and tumor necrosis factor [TNF] receptor), or release of granzymes by cytotoxic T cells. Some stimuli (such as cytotoxic T cells) directly activate caspases in the execution pathway. Others act via adapter proteins or through mitochondrial release of cytochrome *c*. Labeled *2* are regulatory proteins of the BCL-2 family that can either inhibit or promote cell death. Labeled *3* are the execution caspases that activate latent cytoplasmic endonuclease and proteases that degrade cytoskeletal and nuclear proteins. This results in a cascade of intracellular degradation, including breakdown of the cytoskeleton and endonuclease-mediated fragmentation of nuclear chromatin. Not shown is the transglutaminase activation that contributes to the catabolism of the cytoskeleton by cross-linking proteins. The end result (*4*) is the formation of apoptotic bodies containing various intracellular organelles and other cytosolic constituents; these bodies express new ligands (e.g., phosphatidylserine) that mediate phagocytic cell binding and uptake.

reticulum, and distorted Golgi apparatuses. Concurrently, there is a steady accumulation of *lipofuscin pigment* (indicating past oxidative damage and membrane injury), *abnormally folded proteins*, and *advanced glycosylation end products* (AGEs; Chapter 17) capable of cross-linking adjacent proteins.

Although there are many theories, it is clear that cellular senescence is multifactorial. It involves the cumulative effects of both an intrinsic molecular clock of cellular aging and the extrinsic stressors of the cellular environment *(wear and tear)*.

The *intrinsic cellular aging* theories hold that cell senescence occurs because of predetermined genetic programming. Such theories are supported by the long-standing observation that normal adult human fibroblasts in culture have a finite life span; they stop dividing and become senescent after about 50 doublings (the so-called Hayflick phenomenon). Fibroblasts from neonates go through about 65 doublings before they cease dividing, while fibroblasts from patients with *progeria*, who age prematurely, exhibit

only 35 or so doublings. While we remain rather ignorant of *why* cells and organisms should have evolved to have a finite number of replications, we have begun to understand *how* cells "know" the number of divisions they've undergone. Two mechanisms are proposed:

■ *Incomplete replication of chromosome ends (telomere shortening).* Because of the mechanisms of DNA replication, every normal cell division results in a slightly truncated copy of each chromosome. Without some mechanism to protect the fidelity of the replication process, genes near the ends of chromosomes would eventually be lost after a number of divisions and cells would presumably cease normal function. The molecular strategy to overcome this problem uses *telomeres*: short, multiply repeated sequences of nontranscribed DNA (TTAGGG) that sit at the ends of chromosomes. Besides providing a buffer of nontranscribed DNA that can be repeatedly shortened without affecting the replication of functional genes, telomere sequences protect chromosome termini from fusion and degradation. When *somatic cells* replicate, a small section of each telomere array is not duplicated, and telomeres become progressively shortened. Eventually, after multiple cell divisions, severely truncated telomeres are thought to signal the process of cellular senescence. However, in *germ cells* and *stem cells* (but not usually in somatic cells), in which indefinite rounds of replication are required, telomere length is restored after each cell division by a specialized enzyme called *telomerase*. Interestingly, telomerase is also activated in immortal cancer cells (Chapter 6), suggesting that preservation of telomere length might be a critical step in tumorigenesis (Fig. 1–27).

■ *Clock genes.* The concept that genetic timers control the tempo of aging is supported by the identification of clock genes, particularly in lower life forms. For example, the *clk-1* gene in the *Caenorhabditis elegans* nematode alters the growth rate and timing of multiple developmental processes. Worms with mutated *clk-1* have a decreased rate of development as well as 50% longer life spans compared with normal worms. Mammalian homologues of these genes are being vigorously pursued.

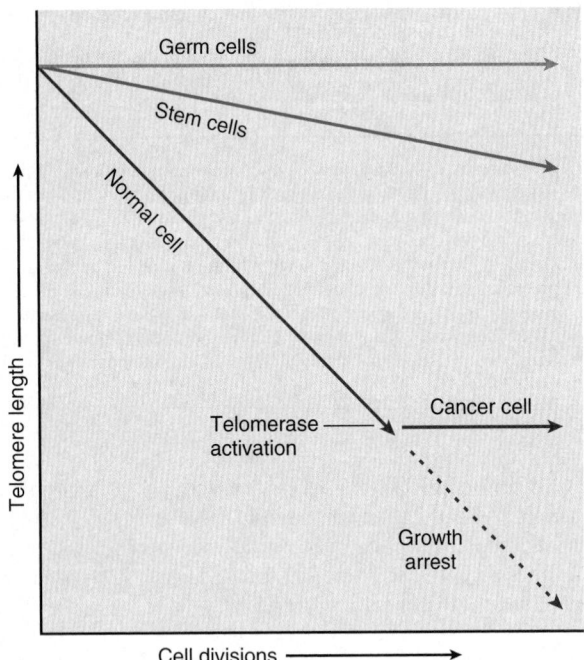

Figure 1–27 ■

Telomere-telomerase hypothesis and proliferative capacity. Telomere length is plotted against the number of cell divisions. In normal somatic cells, there is no telomerase activity, and telomeres progressively shorten with increasing cell divisions until *growth arrest or senescence* occurs. Germ cells and stem cells both contain telomerase activity, but only germ cells have sufficient levels of the enzyme to maintain telomere length indefinitely. Telomerase activation in cancer cells turns off the "telomeric clock" that normally limits the proliferative capacity of somatic cells, resulting in tumor cell immortalization. (Modified and redrawn from Holt SE, et al: Refining the telomere-telomerase hypothesis of aging and cancer. Nature Biotech 14:836, 1996. Copyright 1996, Macmillan Magazines Limited.)

In addition to intrinsic genetic clocks, current theories hold that cellular life span is also regulated by a balance of ongoing injury and the ability of cells to repair damage. These *wear-and-tear theories* suggest that despite robust cellular repair mechanisms (recall, for example, the role of HSPs in refolding damaged proteins), long-term adverse exogenous influences eventually prevail and cells senesce. Preservation of the cellular genetic apparatus is particularly crucial in maintaining cell longevity, and cells expend substantial effort in the recognition and repair of damaged DNA. Although these pathways are extremely efficient, occasional errors persist and accumulate as cells age. Moreover, the rate at which such errors accumulate strongly correlates with cellular senescence. Thus, patients with *Werner syndrome* (one of the diseases that cause *progeria*) show premature aging; these patients have a defective *helicase*, a DNA-unwinding protein involved in DNA replication and repair. Defects in DNA repair also underlie the accelerated aging seen in patients with *Cockayne syndrome* and *ataxia telangiectasia* (Chapter 6).

A favored hypothesis regarding the cause of cellular wear and tear involves *free radical damage*, occurring by repeated environmental exposure to such influences as ionizing radiation, a progressive reduction of antioxidant defense mechanisms (e.g., vitamin E, glutathione peroxidase), or both. The accumulation of lipofuscin in aged cells is a telltale sign of such damage, but there is no evidence that the pigment itself is toxic to cells. Nevertheless, free radicals *can* induce mitochondrial and nuclear DNA damage; free radical injury is estimated to cause some 10,000 base modifications per cell per day. Consistent with this theory of aging are the following observations: (1) longevity among different species is inversely correlated with the rates of mitochondrial generation of superoxide radicals; (2) overexpression of the antioxidative enzymes superoxide dismutase and catalase extends life span in experimental models of aging; and (3) restriction of caloric intake lowers steady-state levels of oxidative damage, slows age-related changes, and extends the maximal life span in mammals.

A second wear-and-tear mechanism involves post-translational modifications of intracellular and extracellular proteins. One such modification is free radical oxidation; another is nonenzymatic glycosylation, leading to the formation of AGEs capable of cross-linking adjacent proteins. Age-related glycosylation of lens proteins underlies senile cataracts, and systemic AGEs are probably responsible for complications of diabetes mellitus (Chapter 17).

In summary, cellular aging mechanisms involve both programmed events and the consequences of progressive environmental injury. Programmed aging assumes a predetermined sequence of events, including the repression and derepression of specific genetic programs, leading ultimately to senescence. However, many changes in gene expression occur during cell aging, and the issue of which of these changes represent a cause for aging rather than an effect of cellular senescence is still unresolved. Moreover, while programmed cell aging is a reasonable explanation of senescence in mitotically active cells, it is not clear how this concept should apply to the aging of postmitotic cells, such as neurons.

BIBLIOGRAPHY

Blackburn EH: Switching and signaling at telomere. Cell 106:661, 2001. (This review describes structure of telomeres and the molecular mechanisms of telomere function.)

Boukamp P: Ageing mechanisms; the role of telomere loss. Clin Exp Dermatol Oct;26(7):562, 2001. (A discussion of the role of telomeres in aging.)

Cristofalo DV, Pignolo RJ: Replicative senescence of human cells in culture. Physiol Rev 73:617, 1993. (A review of the theories of cellular senescence.)

Cummings MC et al: Apoptosis. Am J Surg Pathol 21:88, 1997. (An excellent summary and overview of apoptotic pathways.)

Fuchs E, Cleveland DW: A structural scaffolding of intermediate filaments in health and disease. Science 279:514, 1998. (A succinct overview of the role of cytoskeleton in cell adaptation and disease.)

Granville DJ et al: Apoptosis: Molecular aspects of cell death and disease. Lab Invest 78:893, 1998. (A thorough compendium of apoptosis pathways and associations with disease.)

Gupta S: Molecular steps of death receptor and mitochondrial pathways of apoptosis. Life Sci 69:2957, 2001. (A good summary of the molecular changes in apoptosis.)

Hathway DE: Toxic action/toxicity. Biol Rev Camb Philos Soc 75:95, 2000. (A well-written overview of basic pathways of toxic injury and the intracellular responses to them.)

Holt SE et al: Refining the telomere-telomerase hypothesis of aging and cancer. Nat Biotech 14:836, 1996. (A summary of the role of telomeres in cell death and immortalization.)

Lemasters JJ et al: The mitochondrial permeability transition in toxic, hypoxic, and reperfusion injury. Mol Cell Biochem 174:159, 1997. (A discussion of the mechanisms underlying the role of mitochondria in cell death.)

Macario AJ, Conway de Macario E: Stress and molecular chaperones in disease. Int J Clin Lab Res 30:49, 2000. (An excellent and readable summary of the physiologic and pathologic roles played by chaperone proteins.)

Maclellan WR, Schneider MD: Death by design. Programmed cell death in cardiovascular biology and disease. Circ Res 81:137, 1997. (Apoptosis pathways in cardiovascular injury.)

Majno G, Joris I: Apoptosis, oncosis, and necrosis; an overview of cell death. Am J Pathol 146:3, 1995. (A discussion of the historical and pathologic distinctions in the basic modes of cell death.)

Mergner WJ et al (eds): Cell Death. Mechanisms of Acute and Lethal Cell Injury, Vol 1. New York, Field & Wood Medical, 1990. (A compendium of articles dealing with biochemical mechanisms of cell injury.)

Preisig P: What makes cells grow larger and how do they do it? Renal hypertrophy revisited. Exp Nephrol 7:273, 1999. (A short and readable review of the cellular mechanisms of hypertrophy.)

Reed JC: Double identity for proteins of the Bcl-2 family. Nature 387:773, 1997. (A short review of the regulatory molecules in apoptosis.)

Reed JC: Mechanisms of apoptosis. Am J Pathol 157:1415, 2000. (A good, thorough overview of apoptotic pathways.)

Schoen FJ et al: Calcification: pathology, mechanisms and strategies of prevention. J Biomed Mater Res 22:A1, 1988. (A summary of the mechanisms of calcification.)

Science issue devoted to theories of aging. Science 273:54, 1996. (Reviews on longevity genes, oxidative injury, and replicative senescence.)

Tanaka K, Chiba T: The proteasome: a protein-destroying machine. Genes Cells 3:499, 1998. (An excellent summary of the structure and function of proteasomes.)

Taubes G: Misfolding the way to disease. Science 271:1493, 1996. (A commentary report on developments in protein kinesis, as part of an issue devoted to articles on protein folding and intracellular translocation.)

Toyokuni S: Reactive oxygen species–induced molecular damage and its application in pathology. Pathol Int 49:91, 1999. (A review of mechanisms of free radical injury and associated pathologies.)

Trump BJ, Berezesky I: The reactions of cells to lethal injury: Oncosis and necrosis—the role of calcium. In Lockshin RA et al (eds): When Cells Die—A Comprehensive Evaluation of Apoptosis and Cell Death. New York, Wiley-Liss, 1998, pp 57–96. (A review of theories regarding cell injury and death associated with dysregulation of intracellular calcium.)

2

Acute and Chronic Inflammation

RICHARD N. MITCHELL, MD, PhD
RAMZI S. COTRAN, MD*

OVERVIEW OF INFLAMMATION

The same exogenous and endogenous stimuli that cause cell injury (Chapter 1) also elicit a complex reaction in vascularized connective tissues called *inflammation*. Reduced to its simplest terms, *inflammation is a protective response intended to eliminate the initial cause of cell injury as well as the necrotic cells and tissues resulting from the original insult.* Inflammation accomplishes its protective mission by diluting, destroying, or otherwise neutralizing harmful agents (e.g., microbes or toxins). It then sets into motion the events that eventually heal and reconstitute the sites of injury. Thus, inflammation is also intimately interwoven with *repair processes whereby damaged tissue is replaced by the regeneration of parenchymal cells, and/or by filling of any residual defect with fibrous scar tissue (Chapter 3).*

Although inflammation helps clear infections and, along with repair, makes wound healing possible, both inflammation and repair have considerable potential to cause harm. Thus, inflammatory responses are the basis of life-threatening anaphylactic reactions to insect bites or drugs, as well as of certain chronic diseases such as rheumatoid arthritis and atherosclerosis. Other harmful examples include inflammation in the peritoneum leading to fibrous bands that cause intestinal obstruction, or pericardial inflammation resulting in dense encasing scar that impairs cardiac function.

The inflammatory response has many players. These include circulating cells and plasma proteins, vascular wall

*Deceased

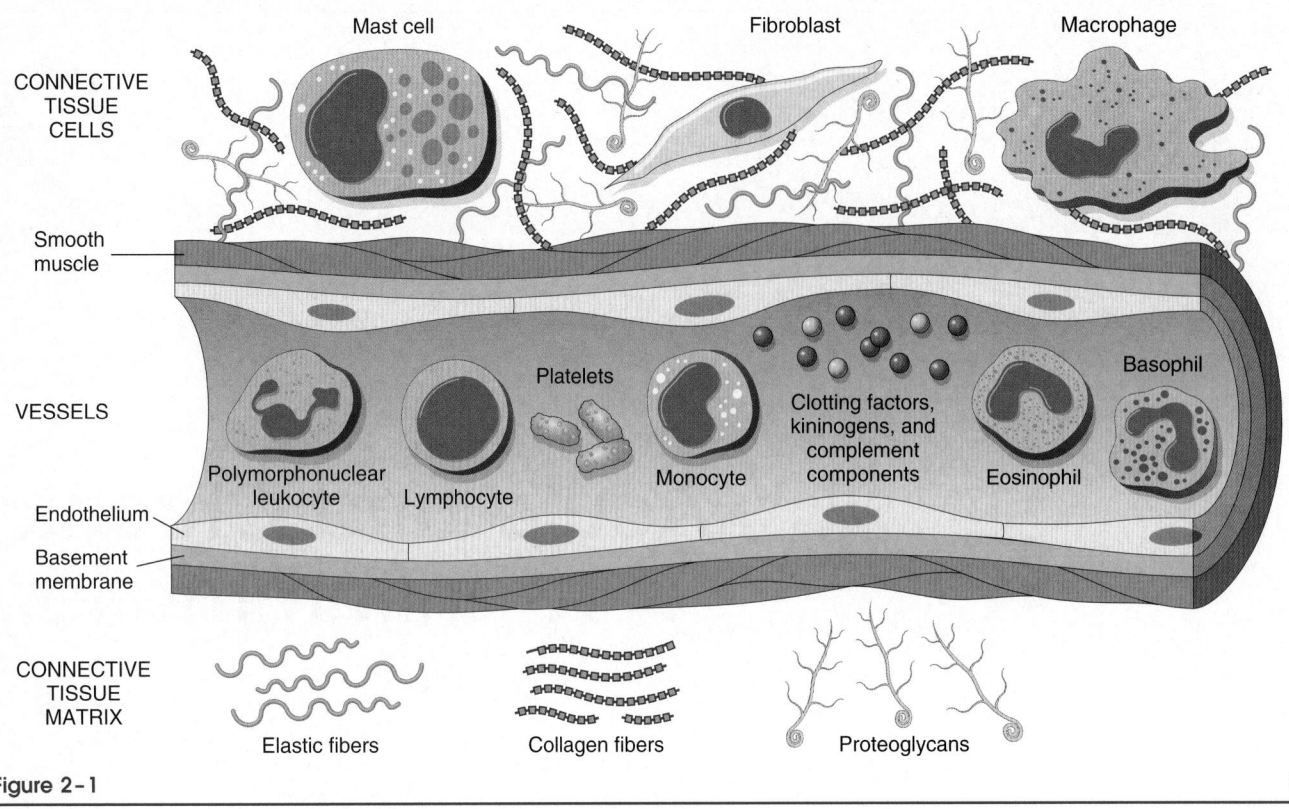

Figure 2-1 ■

The components of acute and chronic inflammatory responses: circulating cells and proteins, vascular wall cells, and the cells and matrix elements of the extravascular connective tissue. Cells and proteins are not drawn to scale.

cells, and cells and extracellular matrix of the surrounding connective tissue (Fig. 2-1). The circulating cells include bone marrow–derived polymorphonuclear leukocytes *(neutrophils), eosinophils, and basophils; lymphocytes and monocytes; and platelets;* the circulating proteins include *clotting factors, kininogens, and complement components,* largely synthesized by the liver. The vascular wall cells include the endothelial cells in direct contact with the blood, as well as the underlying smooth muscle cells that impart tone to the vessels. The connective tissue cells include sentinels to invasion such as *mast cells, macrophages, and lymphocytes,* in addition to the *fibroblasts* that synthesize the extracellular matrix and can proliferate to fill in a wound (Chapter 3). The *extracellular matrix (ECM)* consists of *fibrous structural proteins* (e.g., collagen and elastin), gelforming *proteoglycans,* and adhesive glycoproteins (e.g., *fibronectin*) that are the cell-ECM and ECM-ECM connectors (Chapter 3). As we will see, these all interact to, ideally, resolve a local injury and restore normal tissue function.

While the inflammatory response involves a complex set of highly orchestrated events, the broad outlines of inflammation are as follows. An initial inflammatory stimulus triggers the release of chemical mediators from plasma or connective tissue cells. Such soluble mediators, acting together or in sequence, amplify the initial inflammatory response and influence its evolution by regulating the subsequent vascular and cellular responses. The inflammatory response is terminated when the injurious stimulus is removed and the inflammatory mediators have been dissipated, catabolized, or inhibited.

Inflammation is divided into two basic patterns. *Acute inflammation* is of relatively short duration, lasting from a few minutes up to a few days, and is *characterized by fluid and plasma protein exudation and a predominantly neutrophilic leukocyte accumulation. Chronic inflammation* is of longer duration (days to years) and is *typified by influx of lymphocytes and macrophages with associated vascular proliferation and scarring.* However, as we will see, these basic forms of inflammation can overlap, and many factors modify their course and histologic appearance.

ACUTE INFLAMMATION

Acute inflammation is the immediate and early response to injury designed to deliver leukocytes to sites of injury. Once there, leukocytes clear any invading microbes and begin the process of breaking down necrotic tissues.

This process has two major components (Fig. 2-2):

■ *Vascular changes:* alterations in vessel caliber resulting in increased blood flow *(vasodilation)* and structural changes that permit plasma proteins to leave the circulation *(increased vascular permeability)*
■ *Cellular events:* emigration of the leukocytes from the microcirculation and accumulation in the focus of injury *(cellular recruitment and activation)*

The cascade of events in acute inflammation is integrated by local release of *chemical mediators.* The vascular changes

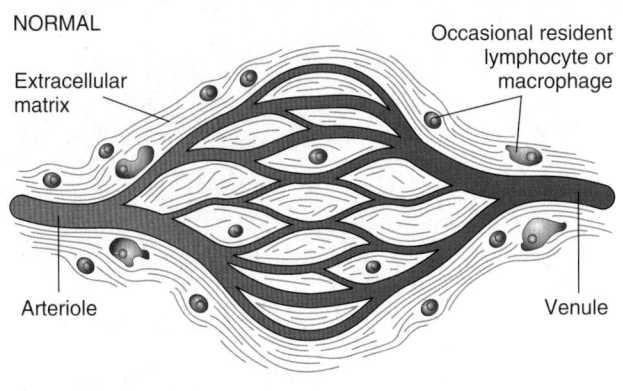

NORMAL

Extracellular matrix

Occasional resident lymphocyte or macrophage

Arteriole

Venule

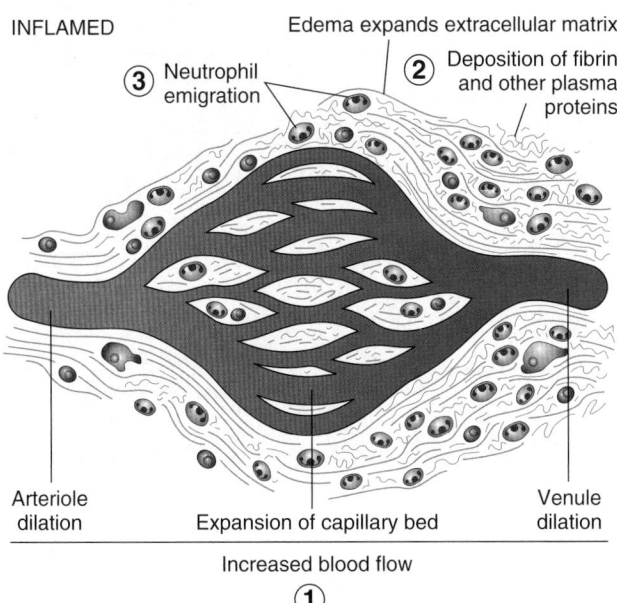

INFLAMED

Edema expands extracellular matrix

③ Neutrophil emigration

② Deposition of fibrin and other plasma proteins

Arteriole dilation

Expansion of capillary bed

Venule dilation

Increased blood flow

①

Figure 2-2   ■

The major local manifestations of acute inflammation: (1) vascular dilation (causing erythema and warmth), (2) extravasation of plasma fluid and proteins (edema), and (3) leukocyte emigration and accumulation in the site of injury.

and cell recruitment account for three of the five classic local signs of acute inflammation: heat *(calor)*, redness *(rubor)*, and swelling *(tumor)*. The two additional cardinal features of acute inflammation, pain *(dolor)* and loss of function *(functio laesa)*, occur as consequences of mediator elaboration and leukocyte-mediated damage (see later).

Vascular Changes

Changes in Vascular Caliber and Flow. These changes begin relatively quickly after injury but may develop at variable rates, depending on the nature and severity of the original injury.

■ After transient (seconds) vasoconstriction, arteriolar *vasodilation* occurs, resulting in locally increased blood flow and engorgement of the down-stream capillary beds. This vascular expansion is the cause of the redness

(erythema) and warmth characteristically seen in acute inflammation (see Fig. 2–2).

■ Subsequently, the microvasculature becomes more permeable, resulting in the movement of protein-rich fluid into the extravascular tissues. This causes the red blood cells to become effectively more concentrated, thereby increasing blood viscosity and slowing the circulation. These changes are reflected microscopically by numerous dilated small vessels packed with erythrocytes, a process called *stasis*.

■ As stasis develops, leukocytes (principally neutrophils) begin to settle out of the flowing blood and accumulate along the vascular endothelial surface, a process called *margination*. After adhering to endothelial cells (see later), the leukocytes squeeze between them and migrate through the vascular wall into the interstitial tissue.

Increased Vascular Permeability. In the earliest phase of inflammation, arteriolar vasodilation and augmented blood flow increase intravascular hydrostatic pressure and the movement of fluid from capillaries. This fluid, called a *transudate*, is essentially an ultrafiltrate of blood plasma and contains little protein. However, transudation is soon eclipsed by increasing vascular permeability that allows the movement of protein-rich fluid and even cells into the interstitium (called an *exudate*). The loss of protein-rich fluid into the perivascular space reduces the intravascular osmotic pressure and increases the osmotic pressure of the interstitial fluid. The net result is outflow of water and ions into the extravascular tissues; this fluid accumulation is called *edema* (Figs. 2–2 and 2–3).

Acute inflammation induces leakiness of endothelial monolayers by a number of pathways. Arterioles, capillaries, and venules are affected differently depending on the mechanisms involved, and the onset, duration, volume, and characteristics *(transudate vs. exudate)* of the resulting fluid (Fig. 2–4).

■ *Endothelial cell contraction leads to intercellular gaps in venules.* The most common form of increased vascular permeability, endothelial cell contraction is a reversible process elicited by histamine, bradykinin, leukotrienes, and many other classes of chemical mediators. Cellular contraction occurs rapidly after binding of mediators to specific receptors and is usually short-lived (15 to 30 minutes); consequently, this is called the *immediate transient response*. Only those endothelial cells lining small postcapillary venules undergo contraction; endothelium in capillaries and arterioles is unaffected—presumably due to fewer receptors for the relevant chemical mediators. Parenthetically, many of the later leukocyte events in inflammation (e.g., adhesion and emigration) also occur predominantly in postcapillary venules.

Endothelial cell retraction is another reversible mechanism resulting in increased vascular permeability. Cytokine mediators (including tumor necrosis factor [TNF] and interleukin 1 [IL-1]) induce a structural reorganization of the endothelial cytoskeleton, so that cells retract from each other and cell junctions are disrupted. In contrast to the immediate transient response, endothelial retraction takes 4 to 6 hours to develop after the initial trigger and persists for 24 hours or more.

A. NORMAL

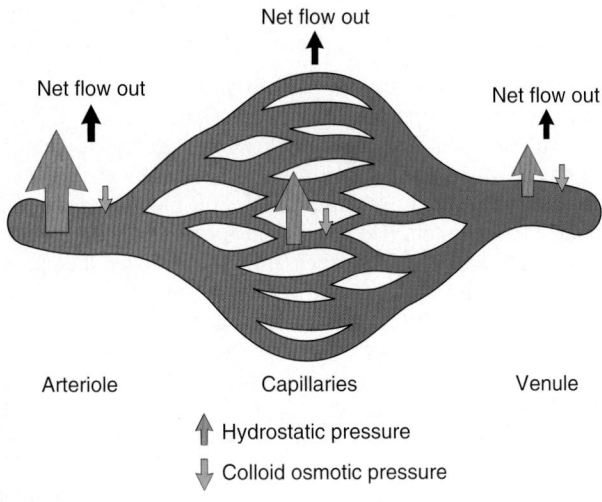

B. ACUTE INFLAMMATION

Figure 2-3 ■

Blood pressure and plasma colloid osmotic forces in normal and inflamed microcirculation. *A,* Normal hydrostatic pressure *(red arrows)* is about 32 mm Hg at the arterial end of a capillary bed and 12 mm Hg at the venous end; the mean colloid osmotic pressure of tissues is approximately 25 mm Hg *(green arrows),* which is equal to the mean capillary pressure. Although fluid tends to leave the precapillary arteriole, it is returned in equal amounts via the postcapillary venule, so that the net flow *(black arrows)* in or out is zero. *B,* Acute inflammation. Arteriole pressure is increased to 50 mm Hg, the mean capillary pressure is increased because of arteriolar dilation, and the venous pressure increases to approximately 30 mm Hg. At the same time, osmotic pressure is reduced (averaging 20 mm Hg) because of protein leakage across the venule. The net result is an excess of extravasated fluid.

■ *Direct endothelial injury* results in vascular leakage by causing endothelial cell necrosis and detachment. This effect is usually seen after severe injuries (e.g., burns or infections), and the endothelial cell detachment is often associated with platelet adhesion and thrombosis. In most cases, leakage begins immediately after the injury and persists for several hours (or days) until the damaged vessels are thrombosed or repaired. Thus, the reaction is known as the *immediate sustained response.* Venules, capillaries, and arterioles can all be affected depending on the site of the injury.

Direct injury to endothelial cells may also induce a *delayed prolonged leakage* that begins after a delay of 2 to 12 hours, lasts for several hours or even days, and involves venules and capillaries. Examples include mild to

Gaps due to endothelial contraction

• Venules
• Vasoactive mediators (histamine, leukotrienes, etc.)
• Most common
• Fast and short-lived (minutes)

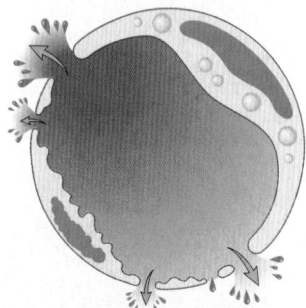

Direct injury

• Arterioles, capillaries, and venules
• Toxins, burns, chemicals
• Fast and may be long-lived (hours to days)

Leukocyte-dependent injury

• Mostly venules
• Pulmonary capillaries
• Late response
• Long-lived (hours)

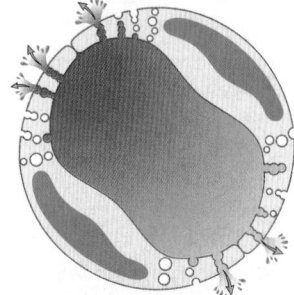

Increased transcytosis

• Venules
• Vascular endothelium–derived growth factor

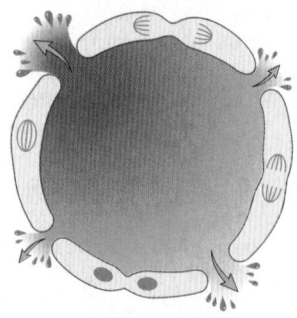

New blood vessel formation

• Sites of angiogenesis
• Persists until intercellular junctions form

Figure 2-4 ■

Diagrammatic representation of various mechanisms underlying increased vascular permeability in inflammation (see text).

moderate thermal injury, certain bacterial toxins, and x- or ultraviolet irradiation (i.e., the sunburn that appears the evening after a day in the sun). Although the mechanism is unclear, both delayed cell damage attributable to apoptosis and the action of cytokines have been suggested.

■ *Leukocyte-dependent endothelial injury* may occur as a consequence of leukocyte accumulation during the inflammatory response. As discussed later, such leukocytes may release toxic oxygen species and proteolytic enzymes, which then cause endothelial injury or detachment. This form of injury is largely restricted to those vascular sites (venules and pulmonary capillaries) where leukocytes can adhere to the endothelium.

■ *Increased transcytosis* via an intracellular vesicular pathway augments venular permeability, especially after exposure to certain mediators (e.g., vascular endothelial growth factor [VEGF]; see later). Transcytosis occurs across channels formed by fusion of uncoated vesicles.

■ *Leakage from new blood vessels.* As described in Chapter 3, tissue repair involves new blood vessel formation *(angiogenesis).* These vessel sprouts remain leaky until proliferating endothelial cells differentiate sufficiently to form intercellular junctions. New endothelial cells also have increased expression of receptors for vasoactive mediators, and certain angiogenic factors (e.g., vascular endothelial growth factor) directly induce increased vascular permeability via transcytosis.

Although these mechanisms are separable, they may all participate in the setting of a particular stimulus. For example, in a thermal burn, leakage results from chemically mediated endothelial contraction as well as from direct injury and leukocyte-mediated damage. Different chemical mediators are also produced in progressive stages of an inflammatory response, resulting in delayed and/or sustained vascular changes. Finally, fluid leaks from new capillaries as the process of healing begins after any injury.

Cellular Events

The sequence of events in the extravasation of leukocytes from the vascular lumen to the extravascular space is divided into (1) margination and rolling, (2) adhesion and transmigration between endothelial cells, and (3) migration in interstitial tissues toward a chemotactic stimulus (Fig. 2–5). Rolling, adhesion, and transmigration are mediated by the binding of complementary adhesion molecules on leukocytes and endothelial surfaces (see later). Chemical mediators—chemoattractants and certain cytokines—affect these processes by modulating the surface expression or avidity of the adhesion molecules.

Margination and Rolling. As blood flows from capillaries into postcapillary venules, circulating cells are swept by laminar flow against the vessel wall. In addition, the smaller, discoid red cells tend to move faster than the larger, spherical white cells. As a result of these effects, leukocytes are pushed out of the central axial column (where they normally flow) and thus have a better opportunity to interact with lining endothelial cells. These interactions are augmented by the increasing vascular permeability that occurs in early inflammation causing fluid to exit the vessel and blood flow to

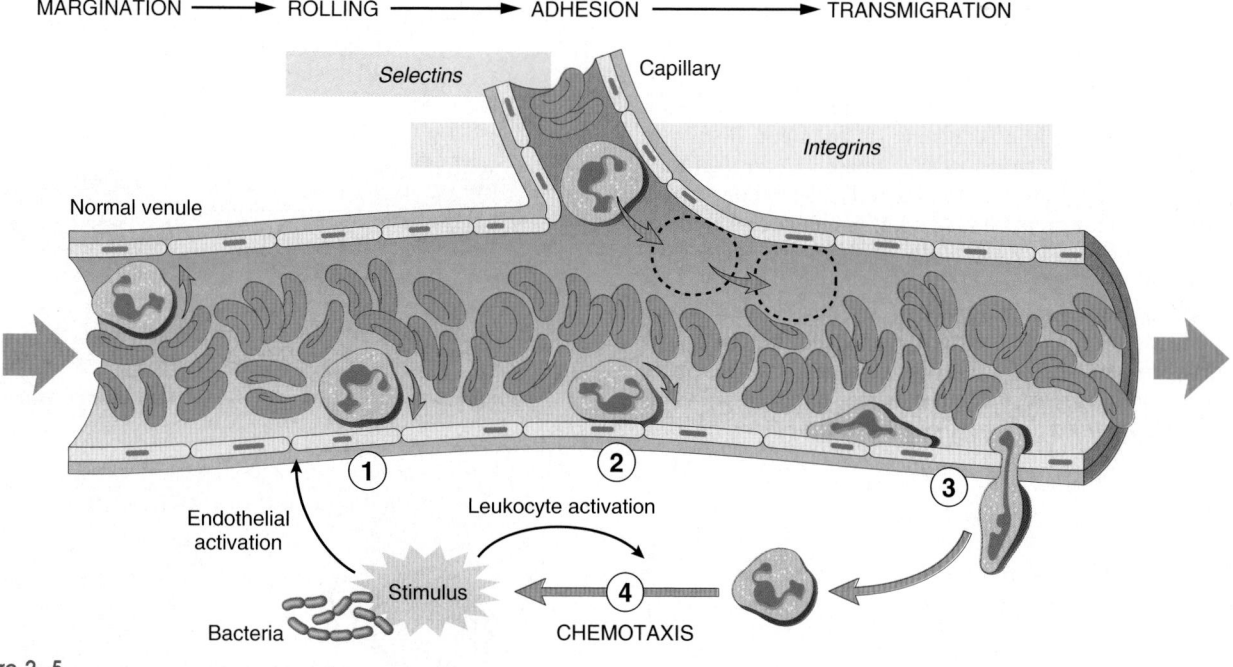

Figure 2-5

Sequence of events in leukocyte emigration in inflammation. Laminar blood flow and the presence of red blood cells tend to push leukocytes against the venular wall, increasing their contact with endothelial cells (see the capillary branch at the top with cells entering the venule flow). The leukocytes (1) roll, (2) arrest and adhere to endothelium, (3) transmigrate through an intercellular junction and pierce the basement membrane, and (4) migrate toward chemoattractants released from a source of injury. The roles of selectins, activating agents, and integrins are also indicated.

■

Table 2-1. ENDOTHELIAL AND LEUKOCYTE ADHESION MOLECULE PAIRS

Endothelial Molecule	Leukocyte Molecule	Major Role
P-selectin	Sialyl–Lewis X–modified proteins	Rolling (neutrophils, monocytes, lymphocytes)
GlyCam-1, CD34	L-selectin	Rolling* (neutrophils, monocytes)
E-selectin	Sialyl–Lewis X–modified proteins	Rolling and adhesion (neutrophils, monocytes, T lymphocytes)
VCAM-1 (immunoglobulin family)	VLA-4 integrin	Adhesion (eosinophils, monocytes, lymphocytes)
ICAM-1 (immunoglobulin family)	CD11/CD18 integrins (LFA-1, Mac-1)	Adhesion, arrest, transmigration (neutrophils, monocytes, lymphocytes)
CD31 (PECAM-1)	CD31 (PECAM-1)	Arrest, transmigration (neutrophils, monocytes, lymphocytes)

ICAM-1, intercellular adhesion molecule 1; PECAM-1, platelet endothelial cell adhesion molecule 1; VCAM-1, vascular cell adhesion molecule 1.

*L-selectin/CD34 interactions are also involved in the "homing" of circulating lymphocytes to the high endothelial venules in lymph nodes.

slow. This process of leukocyte accumulation at the periphery of vessels is called margination. Subsequently, leukocytes tumble on the endothelial surface, transiently sticking along the way, a process called rolling.

The relatively loose and transient adhesions involved in rolling are accounted for by the *selectin* family of molecules. Selectins are receptors expressed on leukocytes and endothelium and characterized by an extracellular domain that binds selected sugars (hence the *lectin* part of the name). These include E-selectin (also called CD62E), confined to endothelium; P-selectin (CD62P), present on endothelium and platelets; and L-selectin (CD62L), on the surface of most leukocytes. Selectins bind sialylated oligosaccharides (e.g., *sialyl–Lewis X on leukocytes*) that decorate mucin-like glycoproteins on target cells (Table 2–1).

The endothelial selectins are typically expressed at low levels or are not present at all on normal cells. They are up-regulated after stimulation by specific mediators. This allows a degree of specificity of binding restricted to sites where there is ongoing injury. For example, in nonactivated endothelial cells, P-selectin is found primarily in intracellular *Weibel-Palade bodies*; however, within minutes of exposure to mediators such as histamine or thrombin, P-selectin is distributed to the cell surface, where it can facilitate leukocyte binding (Fig. 2–6A). Similarly, E-selectin, which is not present on normal endothelium, is induced after stimulation by inflammatory mediators such as IL-1 and TNF (Fig. 2–6B).

Adhesion and Transmigration. Eventually, leukocytes firmly stick to endothelial surfaces (*adhesion*) before crawling between endothelial cells and through the basement membrane into the extravascular space (*diapedesis*). This firm adhesion is mediated by molecules of the *immunoglob-*

ulin superfamily on endothelial cells that interact with *integrins* expressed on leukocyte cell surfaces (see Table 2–1). The endothelial adhesion molecules include ICAM-1 (intercellular adhesion molecule 1) and VCAM-1 (vascular cell adhesion molecule 1); cytokines such as TNF and IL-1

REDISTRIBUTION OF P-SELECTIN

Weibel-Palade bodies

Histamine
Thrombin

A

CYTOKINE INDUCTION OF ENDOTHELIAL
ADHESION MOLECULES
(E-selectin or ICAM-1)

Neutrophil

Cytokines
IL-1
TNF

B

INCREASED AFFINITY OF INTEGRINS

Chemokines
Complement C5a
Platelet-activating factor

C

Figure 2-6   ■

Three general mechanisms mediating increased leukocyte-endothelial adhesion in the setting of inflammatory stimuli. Note that some mechanisms require new protein synthesis (and therefore take longer), compared with others that involve only a redistribution of adhesion molecules or alteration of the configuration of an existing protein complex. *A,* Redistribution of P-selectin. *B,* Cytokine activation of endothelium, resulting in increased de novo synthesis of adhesion molecules. *C,* Increased binding affinity of integrins (see text). ICAM-1, intercellular adhesion molecule 1; IL-1, interleukin 1; TNF, tumor necrosis factor.

induce the expression of both ICAM-1 and VCAM-1. *Integrins* are transmembrane heterodimeric (composed of different α and β chains) glycoproteins that also function as cell receptors for extracellular matrix (Chapter 3). The principal ICAM-1–binding integrins are LFA-1 (CD11a/CD18) and Mac-1 (CD11b/CD18); VCAM-1 binds to the integrin VLA-4 (Table 2–1). Integrins are normally expressed on leukocyte plasma membranes but do not adhere to their appropriate ligands until the leukocytes are activated by chemotactic agents or other stimuli (produced by endothelium or other cells at the site of injury). Only then do the integrins undergo the conformational change necessary to confer high binding affinity for the endothelial adhesion molecules (Fig. 2–6C).

Leukocyte diapedesis occurs predominantly in the venules of the systemic vasculature, although it also occurs in capillaries in the pulmonary circulation. After firm adhesion to the endothelial surface, leukocytes transmigrate primarily by squeezing between cells at intercellular junctions (although *intracellular* movement through endothelial cell cytoplasm has been described). PECAM-1 (platelet endothelial cell adhesion molecule 1, also called CD31), a cell-cell adhesion molecule of the immunoglobulin superfamily, is the dominant protein mediating this process. After traversing the endothelial junctions, leukocytes cross basement membranes by focally degrading them with secreted collagenases.

To summarize (Fig 2–7), the events in leukocyte recruitment at an inflammatory site involve (1) **endothelial activation,** *increasing the expression of selectins and selectin ligands; (2)* **leukocyte rolling,** *facilitated by relatively loose selectin binding to carbohydrate ligands; (3)* **firm adhesion,** *facilitated by chemokine-induced changes in integrin affinity for endothelial ligands; and (4)* **transmigration** *between endothelial cells utilizing PECAM-1 (CD31) interactions.*

Neutrophils, monocytes, eosinophils, and various types of lymphocytes use different (but overlapping) molecules for rolling and adhesion. The type of recruited leukocyte depends on the nature of the inciting stimulus as well as the age of the inflammatory site. Thus, in most forms of acute inflammation, neutrophils predominate for the first 6 to 24 hours and are replaced by monocytes in the subsequent 24 to 48 hours (Fig. 2–8). This pattern is best explained by

---

Figure 2–7   ■

Molecules mediating endothelial-neutrophil interaction. (1) *Initial adhesion* via the selectins and glycosylated proteins. E- and P-selectins on endothelial cells are up-regulated at the inflammatory sites by action of specific mediators. E- and P-selectins bind sialyl–Lewis X oligosaccharide epitopes on certain leukocyte glycoproteins, while L-selectins on leukocytes bind sugar moieties on specific endothelial cell glycoproteins. Note that the various receptors are consistently color-coded (e.g., L-selectin and its ligand are orange, P-selectin is blue, E-selectin is yellow, and sialyl–Lewis X glycoproteins are green). (2) *Activation of leukocytes* by chemokine mediators increases integrin avidity. (3) *Firm adhesion* via integrin–endothelial cell receptor interactions. Leukocyte function–associated antigen 1 (LFA-1) and Mac-1 integrins on leukocytes bind to intercellular adhesion molecule 1 (ICAM-1) on endothelial cells. (4) Homotypic (like-like) interaction of platelet endothelial cell adhesion molecule 1 (PECAM-1) (CD31) on leukocytes and endothelial cells mediates transmigration between cells.

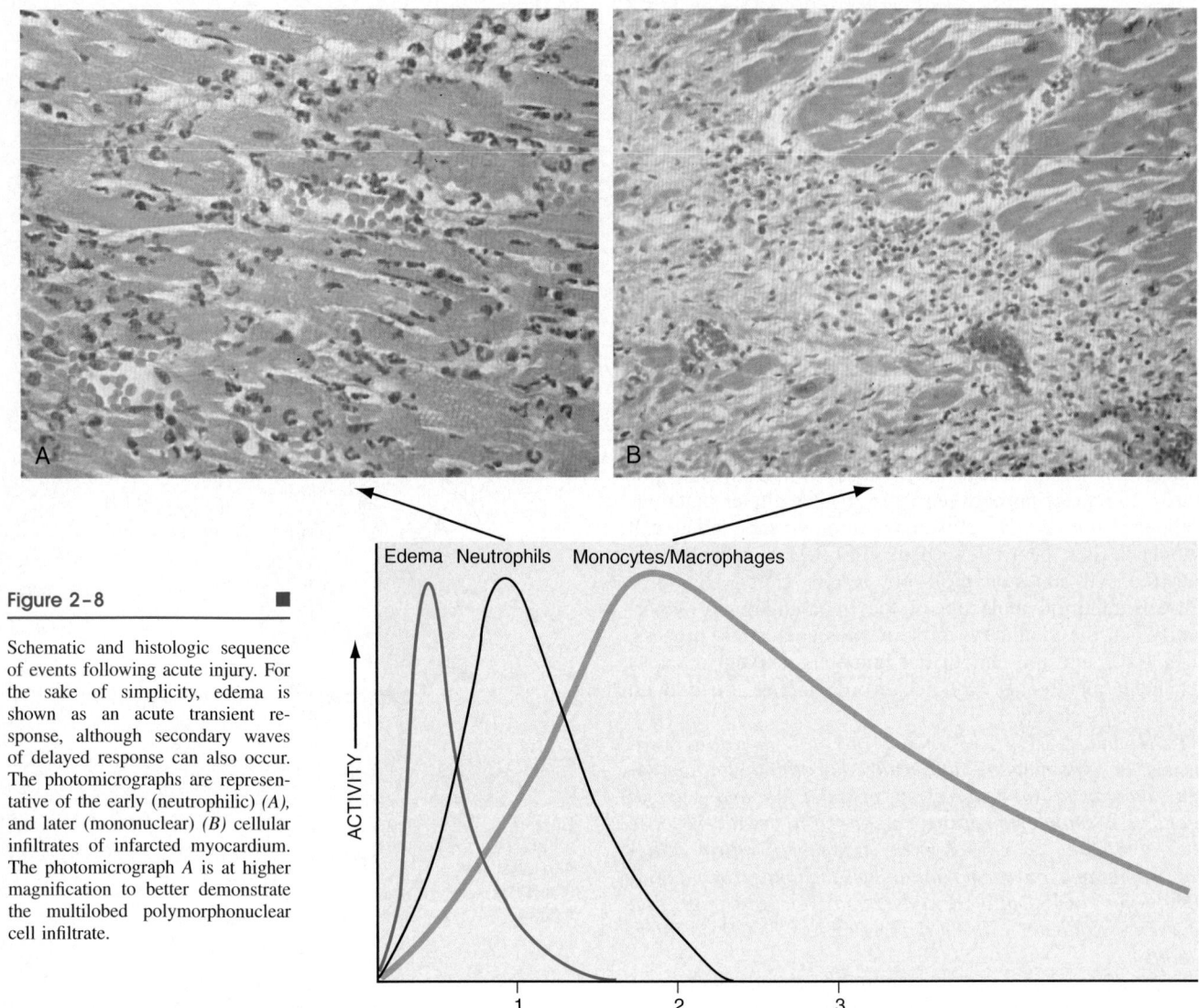

Figure 2-8 ■

Schematic and histologic sequence of events following acute injury. For the sake of simplicity, edema is shown as an acute transient response, although secondary waves of delayed response can also occur. The photomicrographs are representative of the early (neutrophilic) *(A),* and later (mononuclear) *(B)* cellular infiltrates of infarcted myocardium. The photomicrograph *A* is at higher magnification to better demonstrate the multilobed polymorphonuclear cell infiltrate.

the sequential expression of different adhesion molecules and chemotactic factors at different phases of an inflammatory response. In addition, neutrophils are rather short-lived, undergoing apoptosis within 24 to 48 hours after exiting the bloodstream, while monocytes survive substantially longer and may persist for long periods as tissue macrophages.

Chemotaxis and Activation. After extravasating from the blood, leukocytes migrate toward sites of injury along a chemical gradient in a process called *chemotaxis* (see Fig. 2–5). Both exogenous and endogenous substances can be chemotactic for leukocytes, including (1) soluble bacterial products, particularly peptides with *N*-formylmethionine termini; (2) components of the complement system, particularly C5a (p 46); (3) products of the lipoxygenase pathway of arachidonic acid (AA) metabolism, particularly leukotriene B_4 (LTB_4) (p 47); and (4) cytokines, especially those of the *chemokine* family (e.g., IL-8).

Chemotactic molecules bind to specific cell surface receptors, resulting in the G protein–mediated activation of phos-

pholipase C (Fig. 2–9); phospholipase C hydrolyzes plasma membrane phosphatidylinositol bisphosphate (PIP_2) into diacylglycerol (DAG) and inositol triphosphate (IP_3). DAG then causes a number of secondary events (see later), while IP_3 increases intracellular calcium (by release from the endoplasmic reticulum and by extracellular influx). Increased cytosolic calcium triggers the assembly of cytoskeletal contractile elements necessary for movement. Leukocytes move by extending *pseudopods* that anchor to the extracellular matrix and then pull the cell in the direction of the extension. Thus, at the pseudopod's leading edge, actin monomers are polymerized into long filaments; at the same time, actin filaments elsewhere in the cell must be disassembled to allow flow in the direction of the extending pseudopod. The direction of such movement is specified by a higher density of receptor–chemotactic ligand interactions on the leading edge of the cell.

Besides stimulating locomotion, chemotactic factors also induce other leukocyte responses, generically referred to as *leukocyte activation* (see Fig. 2–9):

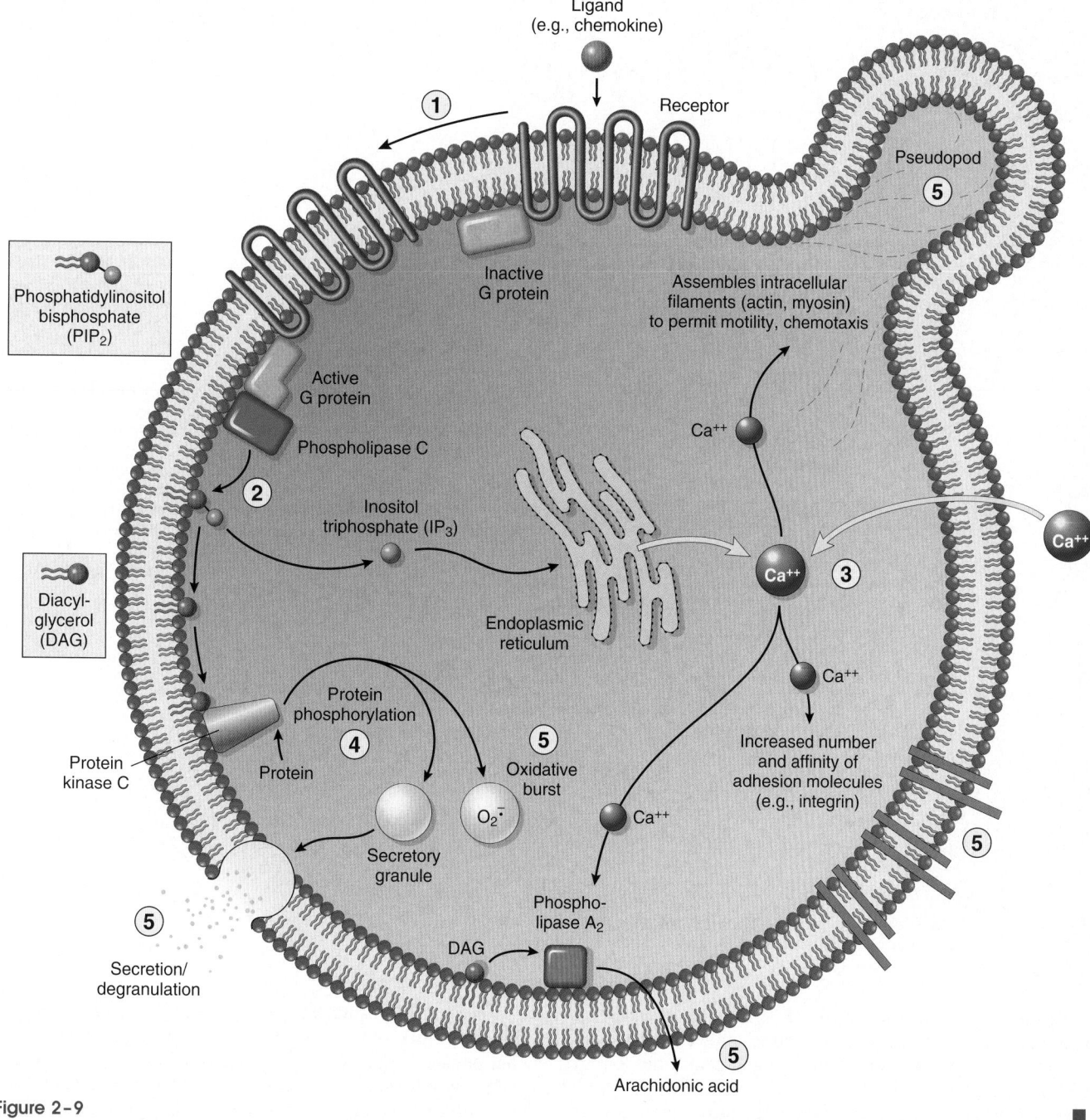

Figure 2-9

Biochemical events in leukocyte activation. The key events are (1) receptor-ligand binding, resulting in activation of the associated G protein; (2) phospholipase C activation, resulting in cleavage of phosphatidylinositol bisphosphate (PIP$_2$) to form inositol triphosphate (IP$_3$) and diacylglycerol (DAG); (3) IP$_3$-induced increases in cytosolic calcium from endoplasmic reticulum and extracellular sites; and (4) DAG-mediated activation of protein kinase C, resulting in the phosphorylation of a variety of intracellular proteins. The biologic activities resulting from leukocyte activation stem from the protein kinase C phosphorylation events, the stimulatory effects of DAG on phospholipase A$_2$, and effects secondary to increased intracellular calcium. These include (5) secretion/degranulation, the oxidative burst, elaboration of arachidonic acid metabolites, modulation of adhesion molecules, and chemotaxis.

■ Degranulation and secretion of lysosomal enzymes, and generation of the oxidative burst via DAG-induced activation of *protein kinase C*

■ Production of AA metabolites via DAG- and calcium-induced activation of *phospholipase A2*

■ Modulation of leukocyte adhesion molecules via increased intracellular calcium, including increased (or decreased) numbers and increased (or decreased) affinities

Phagocytosis and Degranulation. Phagocytosis and the elaboration of degradative enzymes are two major benefits of having recruited leukocytes at the site of inflammation. Phagocytosis consists of three distinct but interrelated steps (Fig. 2–10A): (1) recognition and attachment of the particle to the ingesting leukocyte; (2) engulfment, with subsequent formation of a phagocytic vacuole; and (3) killing and degradation of the ingested material.

A

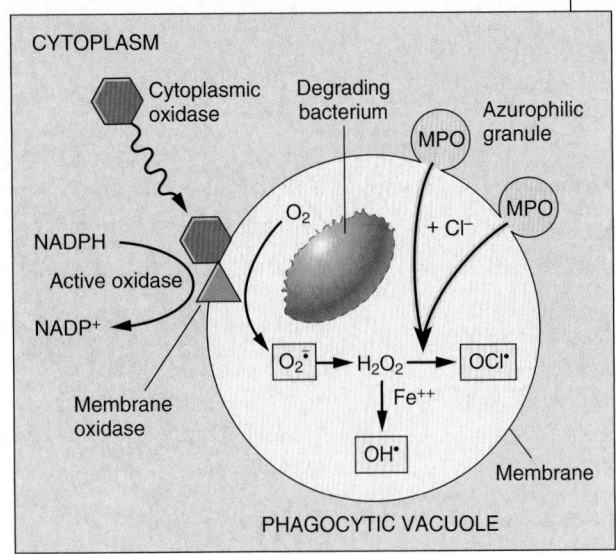

B

Figure 2–10 ■

A, Phagocytosis of a particle (e.g., a bacterium) involves (1) attachment and binding of *opsonins* (e.g., collectins, or C3b and the Fc portion of immunoglobulin) to receptors on the leukocyte surface, followed by (2) engulfment and (3) fusion of the phagocytic vacuole with granules (lysosomes), and degranulation. Note that during phagocytosis, granule contents may be released extracellularly. *B,* Summary of oxygen-dependent bactericidal mechanisms within the phagolysosome. MPO, myeloperoxidase, NADP$^+$ and NADPH, oxidized and reduced forms, respectively, of nicotinamide adenine dinucleotide phosphate.

Recognition and attachment of leukocytes to most microorganisms is facilitated by serum proteins generically called *opsonins*; opsonins bind specific molecules on microbial surfaces and in turn facilitate binding with specific opsonin receptors on leukocytes. The most important opsonins are *immunoglobulin G* (IgG) molecules (specifically the Fc portion of the molecule), the *C3b* fragment of complement (and its stable C3bi form), and plasma carbohydrate-binding lectins called *collectins*, which bind to microbial cell wall sugar groups. In many cases, the binding of IgG is responsible for triggering the activation of the complement cascade that results in deposition of the C3b fragments on the targeted particle; however, a number of stimuli (e.g., microbial surfaces) can directly induce complement activation by an IgG-independent *alternative pathway* (p 46). The corresponding receptors on leukocytes are the Fc receptor (FcR) for IgG, the complement receptors 1, 2, and 3 (CR1, 2, and 3) for complement fragments, and C1q for the collectins.

Binding of opsonized particles triggers *engulfment*; in addition, IgG binding to FcR induces cellular activation that enhances degradation of ingested microbes. In engulfment, pseudopods are extended around the object, eventually forming a phagocytic vacuole. The membrane of the vacuole then fuses with the membrane of a lysosomal granule, resulting in discharge of the granule's contents into the *phagolysosome* and degranulation of the leukocyte (Fig. 2–10A). The biochemical mechanisms of these processes are essentially the same as the IP$_3$- and DAG-mediated pathways described earlier for chemotaxis and activation.

The final step in the phagocytosis of microbes is killing and degradation. Microbial killing is accomplished largely by reactive oxygen species (Fig. 2–10B). Phagocytosis stimulates an *oxidative burst* characterized by a sudden increase in oxygen consumption, glycogen catabolism (glycogenolysis), increased glucose oxidation, and production of reactive oxygen metabolites. The generation of the oxygen metabolites is due to rapid activation of a leukocyte

NADPH oxidase, which oxidizes NADPH (reduced nicotinamide adenine dinucleotide phosphate) and, in the process, converts oxygen to superoxide ion ($O_2^{\cdot-}$).

$$2O_2 + NADPH \xrightarrow[\text{NADPH oxidase}]{} 2O_2^{\cdot-} + NADP^+ + H^+$$

Superoxide is then converted by spontaneous dismutation into hydrogen peroxide ($O_2^{\cdot-} + 2H^+ \rightarrow H_2O_2$). The quantities of hydrogen peroxide produced are generally insufficient to effectively kill most bacteria (although superoxide and hydroxyl radical formation may be sufficient to do so). However, the lysosomes of neutrophils (called *azurophilic granules*) contain the enzyme myeloperoxidase (MPO), and in the presence of a halide such as Cl^-, myeloperoxidase converts H_2O_2 to $HOCl^{\cdot}$ (hypochlorous radical). $HOCl^{\cdot}$ is a powerful oxidant and antimicrobial agent (NaOCl is the active ingredient in chlorine bleach) that kills bacteria by halogenation, or by protein and lipid peroxidation. Fortunately, NADPH oxidase is active only after translocation of its cytosolic subunit to the membrane of the phagolysosome; thus, the reactive end products are generated only within that compartment (Fig. 2–10*B*). After the oxygen burst, H_2O_2 is eventually broken down to water and O_2 by the actions of catalase, and the other reactive oxygen species are also degraded (Chapter 1). *The dead microorganisms are then degraded by the action of the lysosomal acid hydrolases.*

It is important to note that even in the absence of an oxidative burst (see later), other constituents of the leukocyte granules are capable of killing bacteria and other infectious agents. These include *bactericidal permeability-increasing protein* (causing phospholipase activation and membrane phospholipid degradation), *lysozyme* (causing degradation of bacterial coat oligosaccharides), *major basic protein* (an important eosinophil granule constituent with potent cytotoxicity for parasites), and *defensins* (peptides that kill microbes by forming holes in their membranes).

Summary of the Vascular and Cellular Changes in Acute Inflammation. *To review (see Fig. 2–2), the vascular changes in acute inflammation are characterized by increased blood flow secondary to arteriolar and capillary bed dilation (erythema and warmth). Increased vascular permeability, either through widened interendothelial cell junctions of the venules or by direct endothelial cell injury, results in an exudate of protein-rich extravascular fluid (tissue edema). The leukocytes, initially predominated by neutrophils, adhere to the endothelium via adhesion molecules, then leave the microvasculature and migrate to the site of injury under the influence of chemotactic agents. Phagocytosis, killing, and degradation of the offending agent follows.*

Defects in Leukocyte Function

Since leukocytes play a central role in host defense, it is not surprising that defects in leukocyte function, both genetic and acquired, lead to increased vulnerability to infections, often recurrent and life-threatening. Although individually rare, these disorders underscore the importance of the complex series of events that must occur in vivo to protect the human body after invasion by microorganisms (Table 2–2).

■ *Defects in adhesion.* In *leukocyte adhesion deficiency type 1* (LAD-1), defective synthesis of the CD18 β subunit of the leukocyte integrins LFA-1 and Mac-1 leads to impaired adhesion, spreading, phagocytosis, and generation of an oxidative burst. *Leukocyte adhesion deficiency type 2 (LAD-2)* is caused by a general defect in fucose metabolism resulting in the absence of sialyl–Lewis X, the oligosaccharide epitope on leukocytes that binds to selectins on activated endothelium.

■ *Defects in microbicidal activity.* An example is *chronic granulomatous disease (CGD),* a genetic deficiency in one of the several components of the NADPH oxidase responsible for generating superoxide (see earlier). In these patients, engulfment of bacteria does not result in activation of oxygen-dependent killing mechanisms, despite the fact that the myeloperoxidase activity of the cells is normal. Interestingly, this is true even in infections by bacteria that produce hydrogen peroxide, in part because many of them (e.g., *Staphylococcus aureus*) also possess their own catalase, which degrades the H_2O_2 and thus prevents its utilization by the neutrophils.

■ *Defects in phagolysosome formation.* One such disorder, *Chédiak-Higashi syndrome*, is an autosomal recessive disease that results from disordered intracellular trafficking of organelles, ultimately impairing lysosomal degranulation into phagosomes. The secretion of lytic secretory granules by cytotoxic T cells is also affected, explaining the severe immunodeficiency seen in the disorder.

■

Table 2-2. DEFECTS IN LEUKOCYTE FUNCTION

Disease	Defect
Genetic	
Leukocyte adhesion deficiency 1	β chain of CD11/CD18 integrins
Leukocyte adhesion deficiency 2	Sialyl–Lewis X (selectin receptor)
Neutrophil-specific granule deficiency	Absence of neutrophil-specific granules
	Defective chemotaxis
	Decreased oxidative burst
Chronic granulomatous disease	
X-linked	NADPH oxidase (membrane component)
Autosomal recessive	NADPH oxidase (cytoplasmic component)
Myeloperoxidase deficiency	Absent MPO-H_2O_2 system
Chédiak-Higashi syndrome	Membrane protein involved in organelle trafficking
Acquired	
Thermal injury, diabetes, sepsis, etc.	Chemotaxis
Hemodialysis	Adhesion
Leukemia, sepsis, diabetes, malnutrition, etc.	Phagocytosis and microbicidal activity

MPO, myeloperoxidase; NADPH, reduced nicotinamide adenine dinucleotide phosphate.

Chemical Mediators of Inflammation

We will now discuss the chemical mediators that direct the vascular and cellular events in acute inflammation. While the glut of known mediators almost certainly has survival value for organisms (as well as being exceedingly useful for pharmaceutical companies in search of the next new drug), it is neither desirable to review, nor possible to remember, every mediator in detail. Instead, we will emphasize general principles and highlight only some of the more important molecules.

■ *Mediators may be circulating in the plasma* (typically synthesized by the liver), *or they may be produced locally by cells at the site of inflammation* (Fig. 2–11). Plasma-derived mediators (complement, kinins, coagulation factors) circulate as inactive precursors that must undergo proteolytic cleavage to acquire their biologic properties. Cell-derived mediators are normally sequestered in intracellular granules that are secreted upon activation (e.g., histamine in mast cells) or are synthesized de novo in response to a stimulus (e.g., prostaglandins).

■ *Most mediators induce their effects by binding to specific receptors on target cells.* However, some have direct enzymatic and/or toxic activities (e.g., lysosomal proteases or reactive oxygen species).

■ *Mediators may stimulate target cells to release secondary effector molecules.* These secondary mediators may have properties similar to the initial effector molecule, in which case they may amplify a particular response. On the other hand, they may have opposing functions and thereby act to counter-regulate the initial stimulus.

■ *Mediators may act on only one or a very few targets, or they may have widespread activity; there may be widely differing outcomes depending on which cell type they affect.*

■ *Mediator function is generally tightly regulated.* Once activated and released from the cell, most mediators quickly decay (e.g., AA metabolites), are inactivated by enzymes (e.g., kininase inactivates bradykinin), are eliminated (e.g., antioxidants scavenge toxic oxygen metabolites), or are inhibited (complement inhibitory proteins).

■ *A major reason for the checks and balances is that most mediators have the potential to cause harmful effects.*

Vasoactive Amines. *Histamine* is widely distributed in tissues, particularly in mast cells adjacent to vessels, although it is also present in circulating basophils and platelets. Preformed histamine is stored in mast cell granules and is released in response to a variety of stimuli: (1) physical injury such as trauma or heat; (2) immune reactions involving binding of IgE antibodies to Fc receptors on mast cells; (3) C3a and C5a fragments of complement, the so-called *anaphylatoxins* (see later); (4) leukocyte-derived histamine-releasing proteins; (5) neuropeptides (e.g., substance P); and (6) certain cytokines (e.g., IL-1 and IL-8).

In humans, histamine causes arteriolar dilation and is the principal mediator of the immediate phase of increased vascular permeability, inducing venular endothelial contraction and interendothelial gaps. Soon after its release, histamine is inactivated by histaminase.

Serotonin (5-hydroxytryptamine) is also a preformed vasoactive mediator, with effects similar to those of histamine. It is found primarily within platelet dense body granules (along with histamine, adenosine diphosphate, and calcium) and is released during platelet aggregation (Chapter 4).

Figure 2–11

Chemical mediators of inflammation. ECs, endothelial cells.

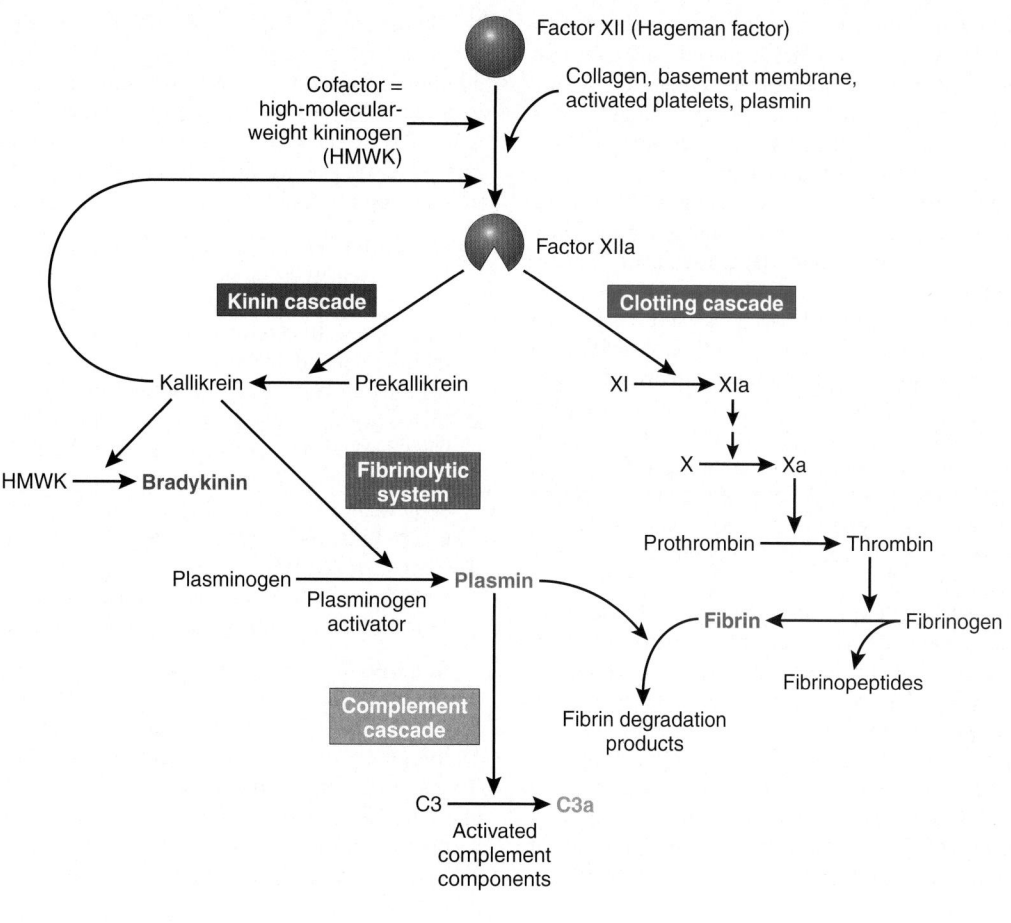

Figure 2–12

Interrelationships between the four plasma mediator systems triggered by activation of factor XII (Hageman factor). See text for details.

Neuropeptides. Like the vasoactive amines, neuropeptides can initiate inflammatory responses; these are small proteins, such as *substance P*, that transmit pain signals, regulate vessel tone, and modulate vascular permeability. Nerve fibers that secrete neuropeptides are especially prominent in the lung and gastrointestinal tract.

Plasma Proteases. Many of the effects of inflammation are mediated by three interrelated plasma-derived factors: the kinins, the clotting system, and complement—all linked by the initial activation of Hageman factor (Fig. 2–12). Hageman factor (also known as *factor XII* of the *intrinsic coagulation cascade*) is a protein synthesized by the liver that circulates in an inactive form until it encounters collagen, basement membrane, or activated platelets (as at a site of endothelial injury). With the assistance of a high-molecular-weight kininogen (HMWK) cofactor, factor XII then undergoes a conformational change (becoming factor XIIa), exposing an active serine center that can cleave a number of protein substrates (see later).

Kinin system activation leads ultimately to the formation of *bradykinin* from its circulating precursor, high-molecular-weight kininogen (see Fig. 2–12). Like histamine, bradykinin causes increased vascular permeability, arteriolar dilation, and bronchial smooth muscle contraction. It also causes pain when injected into the skin. The actions of bradykinin are short-lived because it is rapidly inactivated by degradative kininases present in plasma and tissues. It is important to note that *kallikrein*, an intermediate in the kinin cascade with chemotactic activity, is also a potent activator of Hageman factor and thus allows amplification of the entire pathway.

In the *clotting system* (Chapter 4), the resultant factor XIIa–driven proteolytic cascade causes *thrombin* activation, which in turn cleaves circulating soluble fibrinogen to generate an insoluble *fibrin clot*. Factor Xa, an intermediate in the clotting cascade, causes increased vascular permeability and leukocyte emigration. Thrombin participates in inflammation by enhancing leukocyte adhesion to endothelium (see Fig. 2–6A) and by generating *fibrinopeptides* (during fibrinogen cleavage) that increase vascular permeability and are chemotactic for leukocytes.

While activated Hageman factor is inducing clotting, it is concurrently activating the *fibrinolytic system*. This mechanism exists to counter-regulate clotting by cleaving fibrin, thereby solubilizing the fibrin clot. Without fibrinolysis and other regulatory mechanisms, initiation of the coagulation cascade, even by trivial injury, would culminate in continuous and irrevocable clotting of the entire vasculature (Chapter 4). *Plasminogen activator* (released from endothelium, leukocytes, and other tissues) and *kallikrein* cleave *plasminogen*, a plasma protein bound up in the evolving fibrin clot. The resulting product, *plasmin*, is a multifunctional protease that cleaves fibrin and is therefore important in lysing clots. However, fibrinolysis also participates in multiple steps in the vascular phenomena of inflammation. For example, fibrin degradation products increase vascular permeability, while plasmin also cleaves the complement C3 component to C3a, resulting in vasodilation and increased vascular permeability (see later). Plasmin can also activate Hageman factor, thereby amplifying the entire set of responses.

The complement system consists of a cascade of plasma proteins that play an important role in both immunity and inflammation. They function in immunity primarily by ultimately generating a porelike membrane attack complex (MAC) that effectively punches holes in the membranes of invading microbes. In the process of generating the MAC, a number of complement fragments are produced, including C3b opsonins as well as fragments that contribute to the inflammatory response by increasing vascular permeability and leukocyte chemotaxis.

Complement components (numbered C1 to C9) are present in plasma as inactive forms. Briefly, the most critical step in the elaboration of the biologic functions of complement is the activation of the third component, C3 (Fig. 2–13). C3 cleavage occurs (1) via the *classic pathway,* triggered by fixation of C1 to antigen-antibody complexes; or (2) through the *alternative pathway,* triggered by bacterial polysaccharides (e.g., endotoxin), complex polysaccharides, or aggregated IgA, and involving a distinct set of serum components, including *properdin* and *factors B and*

D. Whichever pathway is involved, *C3 convertase cleaves C3 to C3a and C3b*. C3b then binds to the C3 convertase complex to form C5 convertase; this complex cleaves C5 to generate C5a and initiate the final stages of assembly of the C5 to C9 MAC. The various other complement-derived factors generated along the way affect a variety of phenomena in acute inflammation:

■ *Vascular effects.* C3a and C5a (also called *anaphylatoxins*) increase vascular permeability and cause vasodilation by inducing mast cells to release their histamine. C5a also activates the lipoxygenase pathway of AA metabolism in neutrophils and monocytes (see later), causing further release of inflammatory mediators.
■ *Leukocyte activation, adhesion, and chemotaxis.* C5a activates leukocytes and increases the affinity of their integrins (p 38, see Fig. 2–6C), thereby increasing adhesion to endothelium. It is also a potent chemotactic agent for neutrophils, monocytes, eosinophils, and basophils.
■ *Phagocytosis.* When fixed to a microbial surface, C3b and C3bi act as opsonins, augmenting phagocytosis by cells bearing C3b receptors (neutrophils and macrophages).

The significance of C3 and C5 (and their activation by-products) is further increased by the fact that they can also be activated by proteolytic enzymes present within the inflammatory exudate. These include lysosomal hydrolases released from neutrophils, as well as plasmin. Thus, the chemotactic effect of complement and the complement-activating effects of neutrophils can potentially set up a self-perpetuating cycle of neutrophil emigration.

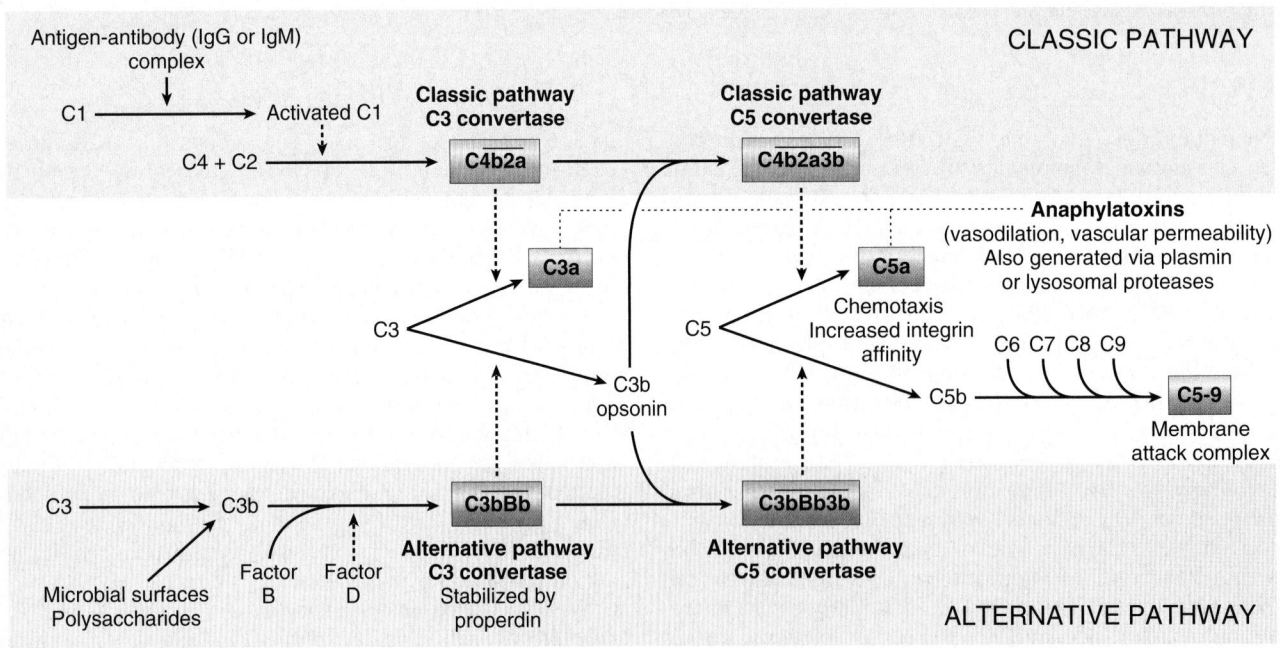

Figure 2–13

Overview of complement activation pathways. The classic pathway is initiated by C1 binding to antigen-antibody complexes; the alternative pathway is initiated by C3b binding to various activating surfaces, such as microbial cell walls. The C3b involved in the initiation of the alternative pathway may be generated in several ways, including spontaneously, by the classic pathway, or by the alternative pathway itself (see text). Both pathways converge and lead to the formation of inflammatory complement mediators (C3a and C5a) and the membrane attack complex. Bars over the letter designations of complement components indicate enzymatically active forms; dashed lines indicate proteolytic activities of various components. IgG, immunoglobulin G; IgM, immunoglobulin M. (Modified from Abbas AK, et al: Cellular and Molecular Immunology, 3rd ed. Philadelphia, WB Saunders, 1995, p 261.)

Overall, a few general conclusions *regarding the plasma proteases* may be drawn:

- *Activated Hageman factor (factor XIIa) initiates four systems involved in the inflammatory response: (1) the kinin system, producing vasoactive kinins; (2) the clotting system, inducing the activation of thrombin, fibrinopeptides, and factor X, all with inflammatory properties; (3) the fibrinolytic system, producing plasmin and degrading thrombin; and (4) the complement system, producing the anaphylatoxins C3a and C5a.*
- *Bradykinin, C3a, and C5a are major mediators of increased vascular permeability.*
- *C5a is a major mediator of chemotaxis.*
- *Thrombin has significant effects on multiple cells and pathways (leukocyte adhesion, vascular permeability, and chemotaxis).*
- *Many of the products of the pathway (e.g., kallikrein and plasmin) can amplify the system by feedback activation of Hageman factor.*

Arachidonic Acid Metabolites: Prostaglandins, Leukotrienes, and Lipoxins. Products derived from the metabolism of AA affect a variety of biologic processes, including inflammation and hemostasis. They can be thought of as short-range hormones that act locally at the site of genera-tion and then rapidly spontaneously decay, or are enzymatically destroyed.

AA is a 20-carbon polyunsaturated fatty acid (four double bonds) derived primarily from dietary linoleic acid and present in the body mainly in its esterified form as a component of cell membrane phospholipids. It is released from these phospholipids via cellular phospholipases that have been activated by mechanical, chemical, or physical stimuli, or by inflammatory mediators such as C5a. AA metabolism proceeds along one of two major pathways: *cyclooxygenase, synthesizing prostaglandins and thromboxanes,* and *lipoxygenase, synthesizing leukotrienes and lipoxins* (Fig. 2–14). AA metabolites (also called *eicosanoids*) can mediate virtually every step of inflammation (Table 2–3); their synthesis is increased at sites of inflammatory response, and agents that inhibit their synthesis also diminish inflammation.

- *Cyclooxygenase pathway.* Products of this pathway include prostaglandin (PG) E_2 (PGE_2), PGD_2, PGF_{2a}, PGI_2 (prostacyclin), and thromboxane A_2 (TXA_2), each derived by the action of a specific enzyme. Some of these enzymes have a restricted tissue distribution. For example, platelets contain the enzyme thromboxane synthase, and hence TXA_2, a potent platelet-aggregating agent and vasoconstrictor, is the major prostaglandin product in

Figure 2–14

Generation of arachidonic acid metabolites and their roles in inflammation. Note the enzymatic activities whose inhibition through pharmacologic intervention blocks major pathways (denoted with a red ×). COX-1, COX-2, cyclooxygenase 1 and 2; HETE, hydroxyeicosatetraenoic acid; HPETE, hydroperoxyeicosatetraenoic acid.

■

Table 2–3. ACTIONS OF EICOSANOIDS IN INFLAMMATION

Action	Metabolite
Vasoconstriction	Thromboxane A_2, leukotrienes C_4, D_4, E_4,
Vasodilation	Prostacyclin (PGI$_2$), PGE$_1$, PGE$_2$, PGD$_2$, lipoxins
Increased vascular permeability	Leukotrienes C_4, D_4, E_4
Chemotaxis and leukocyte adhesion	Leukotriene B_4, lipoxins

PG, prostaglandin.

Figure 2–15   ■

these cells. Endothelium, on the other hand, lacks thromboxane synthase but possesses prostacyclin synthase, which leads to the formation of PGI$_2$, a vasodilator and a potent inhibitor of platelet aggregation. The opposing roles of TXA$_2$ and PGI$_2$ in hemostasis are further discussed in Chapter 4. PGD$_2$ is the major metabolite of the cyclooxygenase pathway in mast cells; along with PGE$_2$ and PGF$_{2\alpha}$ (which are more widely distributed), it causes vasodilation and potentiates edema formation. The prostaglandins are also involved in the pathogenesis of pain and fever in inflammation; PGE$_2$ augments pain sensitivity to a variety of other stimuli and interacts with cytokines to cause fever.

■ *Lipoxygenase pathway.* 5-Lipoxygenase (5-LO) is the predominant AA-metabolizing enzyme in neutrophils, and the products of its actions are the best characterized. The 5-hydroperoxy derivative of AA, 5-HPETE (5-hydroperoxyeicosatetraenoic acid), is quite unstable and is either reduced to 5-HETE (hydroxyeicosatetraenoic acid) (which is chemotactic for neutrophils) or converted into a family of compounds collectively called *leukotrienes* (see Fig. 2–14). The first leukotriene generated from 5-HPETE is called *leukotriene A$_4$* (LTA$_4$), which in turn gives rise to LTB$_4$ by enzymatic hydrolysis or to LTC$_4$ by addition of glutathione. *LTB$_4$ is a potent chemotactic agent and causes aggregation of neutrophils. LTC$_4$ and its subsequent metabolites, LTD$_4$ and LTE$_4$, cause vasoconstriction, bronchospasm, and increased vascular permeability.* Cell-cell interactions are important in leukotriene biosynthesis; AA products can pass from one cell to another, and different cells can cooperate with each other to generate eicosanoids (*transcellular biosynthesis*). In this manner, cells that lack some intermediary enzyme in the synthetic pathway of a particular eicosanoid can nevertheless synthesize it using precursors generated in other cells. One such example of transcellular biosynthesis is the generation of *lipoxins*.

■ *Lipoxins are synthesized using transcellular pathways.* Thus, platelets alone cannot form lipoxins A$_4$ and B$_4$ (LXA$_4$ and LXB$_4$), but they can form the metabolites from the intermediate LTA$_4$ derived from adjacent neutrophils (Fig. 2–15). Lipoxins have both pro- and anti-inflammatory actions. For example, LXA$_4$ causes vasodilation and antagonizes LTC$_4$-stimulated vasoconstriction; other activities inhibit neutrophil chemotaxis and adhesion while stimulating monocyte adhesion. An inverse relation-

Biosynthesis of leukotrienes and lipoxins via cell-cell interaction. Activated neutrophils convert arachidonic acid to leukotriene A$_4$ (LTA$_4$) via 5-lipoxygenase; LTA$_4$ is subsequently converted to LTB$_4$ (a major chemotactic eicosanoid), but neutrophils lack the LTC$_4$ synthase, so that LTC$_4$ (which causes vasoconstriction and increased vascular permeability) cannot be produced. Conversely, platelets lack the 5-lipoxygenase enzyme but can convert neutrophil-derived LTA$_4$ into LTC$_4$ as well as various other lipoxins. (Courtesy of Dr. C. Serhan, Brigham and Women's Hospital, Boston.)

ship between the formation of lipoxins and leukotrienes suggests that *lipoxins may be natural endogenous negative regulators of leukotriene actions.*

The fact that eicosanoids play a central role in inflammatory processes (see Fig. 2–14) is emphasized by the clinical utility of agents that block eicosanoid synthesis. Aspirin and most nonsteroidal anti-inflammatory drugs (NSAIDs), such as ibuprofen, inhibit all up-stream cyclooxygenase activity and thus all prostaglandin synthesis (hence their efficacy in treating pain and fever). Of significant interest, there are two forms of cyclooxygenase (COX), called COX-1 and COX-2. Moreover, COX-1 (but not COX-2) is expressed in the gastric mucosa, and the mucosal prostaglandins generated by COX-1 are protective against acid-induced damage. Thus, inhibition of cyclooxygenases by aspirin and NSAIDs (which inhibit both COX-1 and COX-2) reduces inflammation by blocking prostaglandin synthesis but also predisposes to gastric ulceration. To preserve the anti-inflammatory effects of COX inhibition but prevent the harmful effects on gastric mucosa, highly selective COX-2 inhibitors are now available. Notably, lipoxygenase is not affected by any of the COX inhibitors, and in fact COX blockade may increase substrate access to the lipoxygenase pathways. Glucocorticoids, which are powerful anti-inflammatory agents, act in part by inhibiting the activity of phospholipase A$_2$ (recall that phospholipases are required for the generation of AA from the membrane phospholipids).

Platelet-Activating Factor. Originally named for its ability to aggregate platelets and cause degranulation, platelet-activating factor (PAF) is another phospholipid-derived mediator with a broad spectrum of inflammatory effects. Formally, PAF is *acetyl glycerol ether phosphocholine*; it is generated from the membrane phospholipids of neutrophils, monocytes, basophils, endothelium, and platelets (and other cells) by the action of phospholipase A$_2$. PAF acts directly on target cells via a specific G-protein–coupled receptor. Besides platelet stimulation, PAF causes vasoconstriction and bronchoconstriction and is 100 to 10,000 times more potent than histamine in inducing vasodilation and increased vascular permeability. PAF can elicit most of the features of inflammation, including enhanced leukocyte adhesion (via integrin conformational changes), chemotaxis, leukocyte degranulation, and the oxidative burst; it also stimulates the synthesis of other mediators, particularly eicosanoids.

Cytokines. Cytokines are polypeptide products of many cell types (but principally activated lymphocytes and macrophages) that modulate the function of other cell types. These include *colony-stimulating factors*, which direct the growth of immature marrow precursor cells; many of the classic *growth factors; interleukins*; and *chemokines* that stimulate leukocyte adhesion and directed movement *(chemotaxis)*. They are discussed in detail in Chapter 5, but we review here their general properties and focus on those cytokines specifically involved in inflammation.

Cytokines are produced during immune and inflammatory responses; their *secretion is typically transient and tightly regulated*. Many cell types produce multiple cytokines, and the effects tend to be *pleiotropic* (different cells are affected differently by the same cytokine). Cytokines are also frequently *redundant* in that the same

activity may be induced by many different proteins. They can act on the same cell that produces them (*autocrine* effect), on other cells in the immediate vicinity (*paracrine* effect), or systemically (*endocrine* effect); activities are mediated by binding to specific receptors.

Cytokines may be roughly grouped into five classes based on their actions or target cells.

■ *Cytokines that regulate lymphocyte function* such as activation, growth, and differentiation (e.g., IL-2, which stimulates proliferation, and transforming growth factor β, which inhibits lymphocyte growth).
■ *Cytokines involved in innate immunity*, that is, the primary response to injurious stimuli. These include two major inflammatory cytokines, TNF and IL-1 (see later).
■ *Cytokines that activate inflammatory cells (in particular, macrophages) during cell-mediated immune responses*, such as interferon-γ (IFN-γ) and IL-12.
■ *Chemokines* that have chemotactic activity for various leukocytes.
■ *Cytokines that stimulate hematopoiesis*, including granulocyte-monocyte colony-stimulating factor (GM-CSF) and IL-3.

Interleukin 1 and Tumor Necrosis Factor. Although historically associated with cellular immune responses, various cytokines, in particular IL-1 and TNF, have additional effects that are important in inflammatory responses (Fig. 2–16). Both IL-1 and TNF are produced by activated macrophages (IL-1 can also be synthesized by other cell types), and secretion is stimulated by endotoxin, immune complexes, toxins, physical injury, or a variety of inflammatory mediators. Both IL-1 and TNF

Figure 2–16   ■

Major effects of interleukin 1 (IL-1) and tumor necrosis factor (TNF) in inflammation. PDGF, platelet-derived growth factor; PGE, prostaglandin E; PGI, prostaglandin I.

Bacterial products, immune complexes, toxins, physical injury, other cytokines

MACROPHAGE (and other cell) ACTIVATION

IL-1 / TNF

ACUTE-PHASE REACTIONS

Fever
↑ Sleep
↓ Appetite
↑ Acute-phase proteins
Hemodynamic effects (shock)
Neutrophilia

ENDOTHELIAL EFFECTS

↑ Leukocyte adherence
↑ PGI synthesis
↑ Procoagulant activity
↓ Anticoagulant activity
↑ IL-1, IL-8, IL-6, PDGF

FIBROBLAST EFFECTS

↑ Proliferation
↑ Collagen synthesis
↑ Collagenase
↑ Protease
↑ PGE synthesis

LEUKOCYTE EFFECTS

↑ Cytokine secretion (IL-1, IL-6)

induce *endothelial activation* with increased expression of adhesion molecules, secretion of additional cytokines and growth factors, production of eicosanoids and nitric oxide (NO) (see later), and increased endothelial thrombogenicity. TNF also causes aggregation and activation of neutrophils and the release of proteolytic enzymes from mesenchymal cells, thus contributing to tissue damage. Both cytokines activate tissue fibroblasts, resulting in increased proliferation and production of extracellular matrix.

IL-1 and TNF also induce the *systemic acute-phase responses* typically associated with infection or injury. These include fever, lethargy, hepatic synthesis of various proteins, metabolic wasting *(cachexia),* neutrophil release into the circulation, and release of adrenocorticotropic hormone (inducing corticosteroid synthesis and release). TNF also plays a major role in mediating the hypotensive effects of septic shock, including diminished myocardial contractility and vascular smooth muscle relaxation.

Chemokines. The *chemokines* are a family of small (8 to 10 kD), structurally related proteins that act primarily as activators and chemoattractants for subsets of leukocytes. Unique combinations of chemokines recruit the particular cell populations present in a given inflammatory site (e.g., neutrophils vs. eosinophils vs. lymphocytes). In addition, chemokines can stimulate hematopoietic precursor cells as well as recruit and activate mesenchymal cells such as fibroblasts and smooth muscle cells. Many chemokines bind to extracellular matrix; their presence in the extracellular matrix maintains the chemotactic gradients necessary for the directed migration of recruited cells. Chemokines mediate their activities by binding to specific G-protein–coupled receptors on target cells; two of these chemokine receptors (called CXCR4 and CCR5) are important coreceptors for the binding and entry of the human immunodeficiency virus (HIV) into lymphocytes. There are four general types of chemokines with relatively distinct biologic activities; these are classified according to the arrangement of highly conserved cysteine residues. The two major groups of these are CXC and CC chemokines:

■ CXC chemokines have one amino acid separating the conserved cysteines and act primarily on neutrophils. IL-8 is typical of this group; it is produced by activated macrophages, endothelium, or fibroblasts, mainly in response to IL-1 and TNF.
■ CC chemokines have adjacent cysteine residues and include monocyte chemoattractant protein 1 (MCP-1) and macrophage inflammatory protein 1α (MIP-1α) (both chemotactic predominantly for monocytes), RANTES (*r*egulated on *a*ctivation *n*ormal *T* *e*xpressed and *se*creted) (chemotactic for memory CD4+ T cells and monocytes), and eotaxin (chemotactic for eosinophils).

Nitric Oxide and Oxygen-Derived Free Radicals. *NO* is a short-lived, soluble, free radical gas produced by a variety of cells and capable of mediating a bewildering number of effector functions. In the central nervous system, it regulates neurotransmitter release as well as blood flow. Macrophages use it as a cytotoxic metabolite for killing microbes and tumor cells. When produced by endothelium (where it was originally named *endothelium-*

derived relaxation factor, or *EDRF*), it activates guanylate cyclase in vascular smooth muscle, resulting in increased cyclic guanosine monophosphate (cGMP) and, ultimately, smooth muscle relaxation (vasodilation). Although we are primarily interested here in the effects of NO relevant to the inflammatory response (Fig. 2–17), its ubiquitous generation and diverse effects make it an important mediator in a vast number of physiologic and pathologic states.

Since the half-life of NO is measured in seconds, it can affect only those cells near the source where it is generated. Moreover, the short half-life of NO dictates that its effects are regulated primarily by the rate of synthesis. NO is synthesized de novo from L-arginine, molecular oxygen, and NADPH by the enzyme nitric oxide synthase (NOS). There are three isoforms of NOS, with different tissue distributions, dependence on free Ca^{++}, and constitutive versus inducible modes of expression. Type I (nNOS) is a constitutively expressed neuronal NOS, whose enzyme activity is dependent on elevated intracellular Ca^{++} concentrations. Type II (iNOS) is an inducible enzyme present in many cell types, including hepatocytes, cardiac myocytes, and respiratory epithelium; its activity is independent of intracellular Ca^{++} concentrations. Of significance in inflammation, iNOS is also present in endothelium, smooth muscle cells, and macrophages; it is induced by a number of inflammatory cytokines and mediators, most notably by IL-1, TNF, and interferon-γ, and by lipopolysaccharide (LPS) present in the cell walls of gram-negative bacteria. Type III (eNOS) is a constitutively synthesized NOS found primarily (but not exclusively) within endothelium, with activity that is also dependent on intracellular Ca^{++} concentrations. Calcium-elevating agonists of eNOS activity include bradykinin or thrombin as well as increased shear stress on the endothelial surface.

NO plays multiple roles in inflammation (see Fig. 2–17), including (1) relaxation of vascular smooth muscle (vasodilation), (2) antagonism of all stages of platelet activation (adhesion, aggregation, and degranulation), (3) reduction of leukocyte recruitment at inflammatory sites, and (4) action as a microbicidal agent (with or without superoxide radicals) in activated macrophages.

Oxygen-derived free radicals are synthesized via the NADPH oxidase pathway (see earlier) and are released from neutrophils and macrophages after stimulation by chemotactic agents, immune complexes, or phagocytic activity. Superoxide (O_2^- is subsequently converted to H_2O_2, OH·, and toxic NO derivatives. At low levels, these reactive oxygen species can increase chemokine, cytokine, and adhesion molecule expression, thus amplifying the cascade of inflammatory mediators. At higher levels, these short-lived molecules are implicated in a variety of tissue injury mechanisms, including (1) endothelial damage, with thrombosis and increased permeability; (2) protease activation and antiprotease inactivation, with a net increase in breakdown of the extracellular matrix; and (3) direct injury to other cell types (e.g., tumor cells, erythrocytes, parenchymal cells). Fortunately, a variety of antioxidant protective mechanisms (e.g., catalase, superoxide dismutase, and glutathione) are present in tissues

Vascular smooth muscle relaxation and vasodilation

Figure 2-17   ■

Sources and effects of nitric oxide (NO) in inflammation. Note NO synthesis by endothelial cells (mostly via endothelial cell [type III] NO synthase [eNOS], *left*) and by macrophages (mostly via inducible [type II] NO synthase [iNOS], *right*). NO causes vasodilation and reduces platelet and leukocyte adhesion; NO free radicals are also cytotoxic to microbial and mammalian cells.

and serum to minimize the toxicity of the oxygen metabolites (Chapter 1).

Lysosomal Constituents. The lysosomal granules of neutrophils and monocytes contain multiple molecules that can mediate acute inflammation. These may be released after cell death, by leakage during the formation of the phagocytic vacuole, or by *frustrated phagocytosis* against large, indigestible surfaces, as described later (p 52).

While *acid proteases* have acidic pH optima and are generally active only within phagolysosomes, *neutral proteases*, including enzymes such as elastase, collagenase, and cathepsin, are active in the extracellular matrix and cause destructive, deforming tissue injury by degrading elastin, collagen, basement membrane, and other matrix proteins. Neutral proteases can also cleave C3 and C5 directly to generate the C3a and C5a anaphylatoxins and can promote the generation of bradykinin-like peptides from kininogen.

Thus, if the initial leukocyte infiltration is left unrestrained, substantial vascular permeability and tissue damage may result. These effects are checked, however, by a series of *antiproteases* present in the serum and extracellular matrix. These include α_2-macroglobulin (in the serum) as well as the archetypal antiprotease α_1-antitrypsin, which is the major inhibitor of neutrophil elastase. Deficiencies of these inhibitors may result in sustained activation of leukocyte proteases, potentially resulting in tissue destruction at sites of leukocyte accumulation. In the lung, for example,

inhibitor deficiency can eventually give rise to a severe panacinar emphysema (Chapter 13).

Summary of the Chemical Mediators of Acute Inflammation. Table 2–4 represents an attempt to abstract the most relevant mediators of acute inflammation in vivo. Vasodilation is predominantly regulated by the prostaglandins PGI_2 and TXA_2 and by NO, while increased vascular permeability is probably mediated via histamine, the anaphylatoxins (C3a and C5a), the kinins, PAF, and leukotrienes C, D, and E. Chemotaxis is strongly driven by C5a, LTB_4, and the chemokines. Cytokines and prostaglandins also play a major role in leukocyte and endothelial activation as well as in the systemic manifestations of acute inflammation. Finally, tissue damage is in large part attributable to the effects of NO, oxygen-derived free radicals, and leukocyte lysosomal enzymes (see later).

Inflammation-Induced Tissue Injury

It should be evident from the preceding discussion that the inflammatory response has evolved with many checks and balances. Thus, powerful mediators such as leukotrienes are controlled by equally potent lipoxins. Free radicals are scavenged by antioxidant mechanisms. Nevertheless, limited tissue injury almost always accompanies the inflammatory response. For example, phagocytosis results in the release of lysosomal enzymes not only within the phagolysosome but also potentially into the

■

Table 2-4. EFFECTS OF INFLAMMATION AND THEIR MAJOR MEDIATORS

Vasodilation

Prostaglandins
Nitric oxide

Increased Vascular Permeability

Vasoactive amines (histamine, serotonin)
C3a and C5a (by inducing release of vasoactive amines)
Bradykinin
Leukotrienes C_4, D_4, E_4
Platelet-activating factor

Chemotaxis, Leukocyte Activation

C5a
Leukotriene B_4
Bacterial products
Chemokines (e.g., interleukin 8 [IL-8])

Fever

IL-1, IL-6, tumor necrosis factor
Prostaglandins

Pain

Prostaglandins
Bradykinin

Tissue Damage

Neutrophil and macrophage lysosomal enzymes
Oxygen metabolites
Nitric oxide

---

extracellular space (see Fig. 2–10A), where cell injury and matrix degradation result. This may occur by premature degranulation of lysosomes (before complete closure of the phagocytic vacuole), during attempts by the leukocyte to phagocytose large, flat surfaces (*frustrated phagocytosis),* or because of substances that can lyse lipid membranes (such as urate crystals in gout). In addition, activated leukocytes release reactive oxygen species and products of AA metabolism (see earlier), both of which are potent mediators capable of causing direct endothelial injury and tissue damage. Indeed, leukocyte-dependent tissue injury from persistent and/or excessive leukocyte activation underlies many human diseases, including rheumatoid arthritis and certain forms of chronic lung disease (Chapters 13 and 21).

Outcomes of Acute Inflammation

Although the consequences of acute inflammation are modified by the nature and intensity of the injury, the site and tissue affected, and the ability of the host to mount a response, *acute inflammation* generally has one of three outcomes (Fig. 2–18):

■ *Resolution.* When the injury is limited or short-lived, when there has been no or minimal tissue damage, and when the tissue is capable of replacing any irreversibly injured cells, the usual outcome is restoration to histologic and functional normalcy. This involves neutralization or removal of the various chemical mediators, nor-

malization of vascular permeability, and cessation of leukocyte emigration with subsequent death (by apoptosis) of extravasated neutrophils. Eventually, the combined efforts of lymphatic drainage and macrophage ingestion of necrotic debris lead to the clearance of the edema fluid, inflammatory cells, and detritus from the battlefield (Fig. 2–19).

■ *Scarring* or *fibrosis* (Chapter 3) results after substantial tissue destruction or when inflammation occurs in tissues that do not regenerate. In addition, extensive *fibrinous exudates* (due to increased vascular permeability) may not be completely absorbed and are *organized* by ingrowth of connective tissue with resultant fibrosis. *Abscess formation* may occur in the setting of extensive neutrophilic infiltrates (see later) or in certain bacterial or fungal infections (these organisms are then said to be *pyogenic,* or "pus forming"). Due to the extensive underlying tissue destruction (including the extracellular matrix), the *only outcome of abscess formation is scarring.*

■ *Progression to chronic inflammation* may follow acute inflammation, although signs of chronic inflammation may be present at the onset of injury (e.g., in viral infections or immune responses to self-antigens; see later). Depending on the extent of the initial and ongoing tissue injury, as well as the capacity of the affected tissues to regrow, chronic inflammation may be followed by regeneration of normal structure and function (*regeneration*) or may lead to scarring.

CHRONIC INFLAMMATION

Chronic inflammation can be considered to be inflammation of prolonged duration (weeks to months to years) in which active inflammation, tissue injury, and healing proceed simultaneously. In contrast to acute inflammation, which is distinguished by vascular changes, edema, and a largely neutrophilic infiltrate, chronic inflammation is characterized by the following (Fig. 2–20; see also Fig. 2–18):

■ *Infiltration with mononuclear ("chronic inflammatory") cells,* including macrophages, lymphocytes, and plasma cells

■ *Tissue destruction,* largely directed by the inflammatory cells

■ *Repair,* involving new vessel proliferation (angiogenesis) and fibrosis

As indicated in Figure 2–18, chronic inflammation may progress from acute inflammation. This transition occurs when the acute response cannot be resolved, either because of the persistence of the injurious agent or because of interference in the normal process of healing. For example, a peptic ulcer of the duodenum initially shows acute inflammation followed by the beginning stages of resolution. However, recurrent bouts of duodenal epithelial injury interrupt this process and result in a lesion characterized by both acute and chronic inflammation (Chapter 15). Alternatively, some forms of injury (e.g., viral infections) engender a

Figure 2-18

Causes and outcomes of acute and chronic inflammation (see text).

response that involves chronic inflammation essentially from the beginning. Although the injurious agents mediating chronic inflammation may be less noxious than those that cause acute inflammation, the overall failure to resolve the process may lead to substantially more long-term injury. Fibrosis, in particular—the proliferation of fibroblasts and accumulation of excess extracellular matrix—is a common feature of many chronic inflammatory diseases and is an important cause of organ dysfunction (Chapter 3).

Chronic inflammation arises in the following settings:

■ *Viral infections.* Intracellular infections of any kind typically require lymphocytes (and macrophages) to identify and eradicate infected cells.

■ *Persistent microbial infections*, most characteristically by a selected set of microorganisms including mycobacteria (tubercle bacilli), *Treponema pallidum* (causative organ-

ism of syphilis), and certain fungi. These organisms are of low direct pathogenicity, but typically they evoke an immune response called *delayed hypersensitivity* (Chapter 5), which may culminate in a granulomatous reaction (see later).

■ *Prolonged exposure to potentially toxic agents.* Examples include nondegradable exogenous material such as inhaled particulate silica, which can induce a chronic inflammatory response in the lungs (*silicosis*, Chapter 8), and endogenous agents such as chronically elevated plasma lipid components, which may contribute to *atherosclerosis* (Chapter 10).

■ *Autoimmune diseases*, in which an individual develops an immune response to self-antigens and tissues (Chapter 5). Because the responsible antigens are in most instances constantly renewed, a self-perpetuating immune reaction results (e.g., *rheumatoid arthritis* or *multiple sclerosis*).

Figure 2–19 ■

Events in the complete resolution of inflammation: (1) return to normal vascular permeability; (2) removal of edema fluid and proteins by drainage into lymphatics or (3) by macrophage pinocytosis; (4) phagocytosis of apoptotic neutrophils and (5) necrotic debris by macrophages; and (6) eventual exodus of macrophages. Note the central role of macrophages in resolution. (Modified from Haslett C, Henson PM: In Clark R, Henson PM [eds]: The Molecular and Cellular Biology of Wound Repair. New York, Plenum, 1996.)

Figure 2–20 ■

Chronic inflammation in the lung, showing the three characteristic histologic features: (1) collection of chronic inflammatory cells (*); (2) destruction of parenchyma (normal alveoli are replaced by spaces lined by cuboidal epithelium [arrowheads]); and (3) replacement by connective tissue (fibrosis) (arrows).

Chronic Inflammatory Cells and Mediators

Macrophages. Constituting the critical mainstay and heart of chronic inflammation, *macrophages* are tissue cells that derive from circulating blood *monocytes* after their emigration from the bloodstream. Macrophages, normally diffusely scattered in most connective tissues, may also be found in increased numbers in organs such as the liver (where they are called *Kupffer cells*), spleen and lymph nodes (called *sinus histiocytes*), central nervous system (*microglial cells*), and lungs (*alveolar macrophages*). In these sites, macrophages act as filters for particulate matter, microbes, and senescent cells (the so-called *mononuclear phagocyte system*), as well as acting as sentinels to alert the specific components of the immune system (T and B lymphocytes) to injurious stimuli (Chapter 5).

The half-life of circulating monocytes is about 1 day; under the influence of adhesion molecules and chemotactic factors, they begin to emigrate at a site of injury within the first 24 to 48 hours after onset of acute inflammation, as described previously. When monocytes reach the extravascular tissue, they undergo transformation into the larger macrophages now capable of substantial phagocytosis. Macrophages may also become *activated*, a process resulting in increased cell size, increased content of lysosomal enzymes, more active metabolism, and greater ability to kill ingested organisms. By light microscopy and standard H & E staining, these cells appear large, flat, and pink; this appearance is sometimes similar to that of squamous cells, and these activated cells are therefore called *epithelioid macrophages*. Activation signals include cytokines secreted by sensitized T lymphocytes (in particular IFN-γ), bacterial *endotoxin*, various mediators produced during acute inflammation, and extracellular matrix proteins such as fibronectin. After activation, macrophages secrete a wide variety of biologically active products, that, if unchecked, can result in the tissue injury and fibrosis characteristic of chronic inflammation (Fig. 2–21). These products include

- ■ *Acid and neutral proteases.* Recall that the latter were also implicated as mediators of tissue damage in acute inflammation. Other enzymes, such as *plasminogen activator*, greatly amplify the generation of proinflammatory substances.
- ■ *Complement components and coagulation factors.* Although hepatocytes are the major source of these proteins in plasma, activated macrophages may release significant amounts of these proteins locally into the extracellular matrix. These include complement proteins C1 to C5; properdin; coagulation factors V and VIII; and tissue factor.
- ■ *Reactive oxygen species and NO.*
- ■ *AA metabolites (eicosanoids).*
- ■ *Cytokines,* such as IL-1 and TNF, as well as a variety of *growth factors* that influence the proliferation of smooth muscle cells and fibroblasts and the production of extracellular matrix.

At sites of acute inflammation where the irritant is cleared and the process is resolved, macrophages eventually

Figure 2-21 ■

Maturation of circulating monocytes into activated tissue macrophages. Macrophages may be activated by cytokines (in particular, interferon-γ [IFN-γ] from immune-activated T cells or by nonimmunologic stimuli such as endotoxin. The products made by activated macrophages that mediate tissue injury and fibrosis are indicated. AA, arachidonic acid; FGF, fibroblast growth factor; PDGF, platelet-derived growth factor; TGFβ, transforming growth factor β (see Chapter 3).

die or wander off into lymphatics. In chronic inflammatory sites, however, macrophage accumulation persists, and macrophages can proliferate. Steady release of lymphocyte-derived factors (see later) is an important mechanism by which macrophages are recruited to or immobilized in inflammatory sites. IL-4 or IFN-γ can also induce macrophages to fuse into large, multinucleated cells called *giant cells*.

Lymphocytes, Plasma Cells, Eosinophils, and Mast Cells. Other types of *cells present in chronic inflammation are lymphocytes, plasma cells, eosinophils, and mast cells (see Fig. 2–1).*

Both *T and B lymphocytes* migrate into inflammatory sites using some of the same adhesion molecule pairs and chemokines that recruit monocytes. *Lymphocytes are mobilized in the setting of any specific immune stimulus* (i.e., infections) as well as in non–immune-mediated inflammation (e.g., due to infarction or tissue trauma). T lymphocytes have a reciprocal relationship to macrophages in chronic inflammation (Fig. 2–22); they are initially activated by interaction with macrophages presenting "processed" antigen fragments on their cell surface (Chapter 5). The *activated lymphocytes* then produce a variety of mediators, including IFN-γ, a major stimulating cytokine for activating monocytes and macrophages. Activated macrophages in turn release cytokines, including IL-1 and TNF, that further activate lymphocytes as well as other cell types (as we have seen).

The end result is an inflammatory focus where macrophages and T cells can persistently stimulate one another until the triggering antigen is removed, or some modulating process occurs. *Plasma cells* are the terminally differentiated end

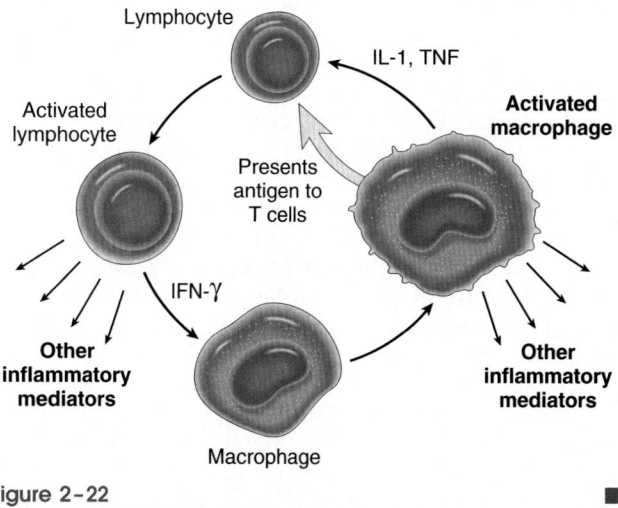

Figure 2-22 ■

Macrophage-lymphocyte interactions in chronic inflammation. Activated lymphocytes and macrophages stimulate each other, and both cell types release inflammatory mediators that affect other cells. IFN-γ, interferon-γ; IL-1, interleukin 1; TNF, tumor necrosis factor.

product of B-cell activation; they can produce antibodies directed against antigens in the inflammatory site or against altered tissue components.

Eosinophils are characteristically found in inflammatory sites around parasitic infections or as part of immune reactions mediated by IgE, typically associated with allergies. Their emigration is driven by adhesion molecules similar to those used by neutrophils, and by specific chemokines (e.g., *eotaxin*) derived from leukocytes or epithelial cells. Eosinophil-specific granules contain major basic protein (MBP), a highly charged cationic protein that is toxic to parasites but also causes epithelial cell lysis.

Mast cells are sentinel cells widely distributed in connective tissues throughout the body and can participate in both acute and chronic inflammatory responses. Mast cells are "armed" with IgE to certain antigens. When these antigens are subsequently encountered, the prearmed mast cells are triggered to release histamines and AA metabolites that elicit the early vascular changes of acute inflammation. IgE-armed mast cells are central players in *anaphylactic shock* (Chapter 5), but they also play a beneficial role in a variety of infections, particularly those involving parasites. Mast cells can also elaborate cytokines such as TNF, thereby participating in more chronic responses.

An important final point: *although neutrophils are the classic hallmarks of acute inflammation, many forms of chronic inflammation may nevertheless continue to show extensive neutrophilic infiltrates, due either to persistent microbes or to mediators elaborated by macrophages or necrotic cells. This is sometimes called acute chronic inflammation.*

Granulomatous Inflammation

Granulomatous inflammation is a distinctive pattern of chronic inflammation characterized by aggregates of activated macrophages that assume a squamous cell–like (epithelioid) appearance. Granulomas are encountered in relatively few pathologic states; consequently, recognition of the granulomatous pattern is important because of the limited number of conditions (some life-threatening) that cause it (Table 2–5). Granulomas can form in the setting of persistent T-cell responses to certain microbes (such as *Mycobacterium tuberculosis*, *Treponema pallidum* causing the syphilitic *gumma*, or fungi), where T-cell–derived cytokines are responsible for persistent macrophage activation; these are discussed further in Chapter 5. *Tuberculosis is the archetypal granulomatous disease due to infection and should always be excluded as a cause when granulomas are identified.* Granulomas may also develop in response to relatively inert foreign bodies (e.g., suture, splinter, breast implant), forming so-called *foreign body granulomas.* Notably, granuloma formation does not always lead to eradication of the causal agent, which is frequently resistant to killing or degradation. Nevertheless, the formation of a granuloma effectively "walls off" the offending agent and is therefore a useful defense mechanism.

Table 2–5. EXAMPLES OF GRANULOMATOUS INFLAMMATION

Bacterial

Tuberculosis (*Mycobacterium tuberculosis*)
Leprosy (*Mycobacterium leprae*)
Syphilitic gumma (*Treponema pallidum*)
Cat-scratch disease (*Bartonella henselae*)

Parasitic

Schistosomiasis (*Schistosoma mansoni, S. haemotobium, S. japonicum*)

Fungal

Histoplasma capsulatum
Blastomycosis
Cryptococcus neoformans
Coccidioides immitis

Inorganic Metals or Dusts

Silicosis
Berylliosis

Foreign Body

Suture, breast prosthesis, vascular graft

Unknown

Sarcoidosis

MORPHOLOGY

In the usual H & E preparations (Fig. 2–23), activated macrophages in granulomas have pink, granular cytoplasm with indistinct cell boundaries. The aggregates of epithelioid macrophages are surrounded by a collar of lymphocytes secreting the cytokines responsible for ongoing macrophage activation. Older granulomas also develop a surrounding rim of fibroblasts and connective tissue, due to cytokines elaborated by the activated macrophages; this rim of scarring is useful in containing the injurious agent that caused formation of the granuloma in the first place, although it may also be a cause of tissue injury and dysfunction. Frequently, but not invariably, multinucleated **giant cells** 40 to 50 μm in diameter are also found in granulomas. They consist of a large mass of cytoplasm and multiple nuclei and derive from the fusion of 20 or more macrophages. In granulomas associated with certain infectious organisms (most classically due to the tubercle bacillus), a combination of hypoxia and free radical injury leads to a central zone of necrosis. Grossly, this has a granular, cheesy appearance and is therefore called **caseous necrosis** (Chapters 1 and 13).

Lymphatics and Lymph Nodes in Inflammation

The system of lymphatics and lymph nodes filters and polices the extravascular fluids. Together with the *mononuclear phagocyte system*, it represents a secondary line of defense that is called into play whenever a local inflammatory reaction fails to contain and neutralize injury.

Figure 2-23   ■

A typical granuloma resulting from infection with *Mycobacterium tuberculosis* showing central *(caseous)* necrosis, activated *epithelioid* macrophages, multiple giant cells, and a peripheral accumulation of lymphocytes.

Lymphatics are extremely delicate channels that are difficult to visualize in ordinary tissue sections because they readily collapse unless they are engorged with edema fluid and/or recirculating leukocytes. They are lined by continuous endothelium with loose overlapping cell junctions, scant basement membrane, and no muscular support except in the larger ducts. Valves are present in the larger collecting lymphatics, allowing lymph content to flow only in the distal-to-proximal direction. Thin fibrils, attached at right angles to the walls of the lymphatic vessel, extend into the adjacent tissues and serve to maintain patency of the channel.

Because the junctions of lymphatics are loose, lymphatic fluid eventually equilibrates with extravascular fluid. Consequently, during inflammation, lymphatic flow is increased and helps drain the edema fluid from the extravascular space (see Fig. 2–19). In addition to fluid, leukocytes and cell debris may also find their way into lymph. Moreover, in the setting of extensive inflammation, the drainage may also transport the offending (microbial or chemical) agent. As a result, the lymphatics themselves may become secondarily inflamed *(lymphangitis)*, as may the draining lymph nodes *(lymphadenitis)*. For example, it is not uncommon in infections of the hand to observe red streaks following the course of the lymphatic channels and extending along the arm to the axilla, accompanied by painful enlargement of the axillary lymph nodes. The nodal enlargement is usually caused by the proliferation of lymphocytes and macrophages in the lymphoid follicles and sinuses, as well as by hypertrophy of the phagocytic cells. This constellation of nodal histologic changes is termed *reactive*, or *inflammatory*, *lymphadenitis*.

The secondary lymph node barriers usually contain the spread of the infection. However, in some instances they are overwhelmed, and infectious organisms drain through progressively larger channels, eventually gaining access to the vascular circulation and resulting in *bacteremia*. The phagocytic cells of the liver, spleen, and bone marrow constitute the next line of defense, but in massive infections, bacteria seed distant tissues of the body. The heart valves, meninges, kidneys, and joints are favored sites of implantation for blood-borne organisms, and in such a fashion endocarditis, meningitis, renal abscesses, and septic arthritis may develop.

MORPHOLOGIC PATTERNS OF ACUTE AND CHRONIC INFLAMMATION

The severity of the inflammatory response, its specific cause, and the particular tissue involved can all modify the basic morphologic patterns of acute and chronic inflammation. Such patterns frequently have clinical significance and are described in greater detail as follows (Fig. 2–24):

MORPHOLOGY

SEROUS INFLAMMATION. This is characterized by the outpouring of a watery, relatively protein-poor fluid **(effusion)** that, depending on the site of injury, derives either from the serum or from the secretions of mesothelial cells lining the peritoneal, pleural, and pericardial cavities. The skin blister resulting from a burn or viral infection is a good example of a serous effusion accumulated either within or immediately beneath the epidermis of the skin (see Fig. 2–24A).

FIBRINOUS INFLAMMATION. This occurs as a consequence of more severe injuries, with a resultant greater vascular permeability allowing larger molecules (specifically, **fibrinogen**) to pass the endothelial barrier. Histologically, the accumulated extravascular fibrin appears as an eosinophilic meshwork of threads or, sometimes, as an amorphous coagulum (see Fig. 2–24B). Fibrinous exudates may be degraded by fibrinolysis, and the accumulated debris may be removed by macrophages, resulting in restoration of the normal tissue structure **(resolution)**. However, failure to completely remove the fibrin results in the ingrowth of fibroblasts and blood vessels, leading ultimately to scarring **(organization)**. For example, organization of a fibrinous pericardial exudate forms dense fibrous scar tissue that bridges or obliterates the pericardial space and restricts myocardial function.

SUPPURATIVE (PURULENT) INFLAMMATION. This is manifested by the presence of large amounts of purulent exudate **(pus)** consisting of neutrophils, necrotic cells, and edema fluid. Certain organisms (e.g., staphylococci) are more likely to induce this localized suppuration and are therefore referred to as **pyogenic**. Abscesses are focal collections of pus that may be caused by deep seeding of pyogenic organisms into a tissue or by secondary infec-

Figure 2-24 ■

Histologic patterns of acute inflammation, *A,* Serous inflammation. A low-power view of a cross-section of a skin blister showing epidermis separated from the dermis by a focal collection of serous effusion. *B,* Fibrinous inflammation. A pink meshwork of fibrin exudate *(right)* overlies the pericardial surface. *C,* Suppurative inflammation. A bacterial abscess in myocardium. *D,* Ulceration. A low-power view of a cross-section of a duodenal ulcer crater with an acute inflammatory exudate in the base.

tions of necrotic foci. Abscesses typically have a central, largely necrotic region rimmed by a layer of preserved neutrophils (see Fig. 2–24C), with a surrounding zone of dilated vessels and fibroblastic proliferation indicative of early repair. In time, the abscess may become completely walled off and eventually replaced by connective tissue.

ULCERATION. This refers to a site of inflammation where an epithelial surface (skin, gastric epithelium, colonic mucosa, bladder epithelium) has become necrotic and eroded, often with associated subepithelial acute and chronic inflammation. This can occur as a consequence of toxic or traumatic injury to the epithelial surface (e.g., peptic ulcers (Chapter 15)) or may be due to vascular compromise (as in foot ulcers associated with the vasculopathy of diabetes (Chapter 17)). The peptic ulcer of the stomach or duodenum (see Fig. 2–24D) illus-

trates the typical findings. There is usually an early intense neutrophilic infiltrate with associated vascular dilation. In chronic lesions where there has been repeated insult, the area surrounding the ulcer develops fibroblastic proliferation, scarring, and the accumulation of chronic inflammatory cells.

SYSTEMIC EFFECTS OF INFLAMMATION

Anyone who has suffered through a severe bout of a viral illness (such as influenza) has experienced the systemic effects of inflammation, collectively called *acute-phase reaction. Fever* is only one of the more obvious of these systemic effects of inflammation; others include increased somnolence, malaise, anorexia, accelerated degradation of skeletal muscle proteins, hypotension, hepatic synthesis of a variety of proteins (e.g., complement and coagulation proteins), and alterations in the circulating white blood cell pool.

The cytokines IL-1, IL-6, and TNF are the most important mediators of the acute-phase reaction. These cytokines are produced by leukocytes (and other cell types) in response to infection, or to immune and toxic injury, and are released systemically, frequently in a sort of cytokine cascade. Thus, TNF induces the production of IL-1, which in turn stimulates the production of IL-6 (Chapter 3). Although there are some differences, TNF and IL-1 cause similar effects (see Fig. 2–16); for example, both act on the thermoregulatory center of the hypothalamus—via local PGE production—to induce fever (hence the efficacy of aspirin and NSAIDs in reducing fever). IL-6 stimulates the hepatic synthesis of several plasma proteins, most notably fibrinogen; elevated fibrinogen levels cause erythrocytes to agglutinate more readily, explaining why inflammation is associated with a higher *erythrocyte sedimentation rate* by objective testing.

Leukocytosis (increased white blood cell count) is a common feature of inflammatory reactions, especially those induced by bacterial infection. The leukocyte count typically increases to 15,000 or 20,000 cells per μL (normal = 4000 to 10,000 cells per μL) but may climb as high as 40,000 to 100,000 cells per μL, a so-called *leukemoid reaction*. Leukocytosis initially results from the release of cells from the bone marrow (caused by IL-1 and TNF) and is associated with an increased number of relatively immature neutrophils in the blood ("left-shift"). Prolonged infection, however, also induces proliferation of precursors in the bone marrow, caused by IL-1– and TNF–driven increases in the production of colony-stimulating factors.

Most bacterial infections induce a relatively selective increase in polymorphonuclear cells *(neutrophilia)*, while parasitic infections (as well as allergic responses) characteristically induce *eosinophilia*. Certain viruses, such as infectious mononucleosis (Chapter 12), mumps, and rubella, engender selective increases in lymphocytes *(lymphocytosis)*. However, most viral infections, as well as rickettsial, protozoal, and certain types of bacterial infections (typhoid fever), are associated with a decreased number of circulating white cells *(leukopenia)*. Leukopenia is also encountered in infections that overwhelm patients debilitated by, for example, disseminated cancer.

Although this concludes our discussion of the cellular and molecular events in acute and chronic inflammation, we still need to consider the changes induced by the body's attempts to heal the damage, the process of *repair*. As described next in Chapter 3, the repair begins almost as soon as the inflammatory changes have started and involves several processes, including cell proliferation, differentiation, and extracellular matrix deposition.

BIBLIOGRAPHY

Baggiolini M: Chemokines in medicine and pathology. J Intern Med 250:91, 2001. (A well-written review.)

Coleman JW: Nitric oxide in immunity and inflammation. Int Immunopharmacol 8:1397, 2001. (Modulation of immunity and inflammation by NO.)

Cotran RS, Briscoe DM: Endothelial cells in inflammation. In Kelley W, et al (eds): Textbook of Rheumatology, 5th ed. Philadelphia, WB Saunders, 1997. (An overview of inflammatory cells and adhesion molecules.)

Cotran RS, Mayadas TN: Endothelial adhesion molecules in health and disease. Pathol Biol 46:164, 1998. (A well-written overview of the molecules mediating leukocyte adhesion and their mechanisms of regulation.)

Dinarello CA: Biologic basis for interleukin-1 in disease. Blood 87:2095, 1996. (Comprehensive summary of the effects and role of IL-1 in pathologic states.)

Dvorak AM, et al: The vesiculo-vacuolar organelle (VVO): A distinct endothelial cell structure that provides a transcellular pathway for macromolecular extravasation. J Leukoc Biol 59:100, 1996. (A description of the transcytosis pathway for increased vascular permeability.)

Everts B, et al: COX-2-specific inhibitors—the emergence of a new class of analgesic and anti-inflammatory drugs. Clin Rheumatol 19: 331, 2000. (Good introduction to the selective cyclooxygenase inhibitors.)

Funk CD: Prostaglandins and leukotrienes: advances in eicosanoid biology. Science 294:1871, 2001. (An update on this family of mediators.)

Goetzl EJ, et al: Specificity of expression and effects of eicosanoid mediators in normal physiology and human diseases. FASEB J 9:1051, 1995. (Reasonably current overview of arachidonic acid mediators.)

Imhof BA, Dunon D: Leukocyte migration and adhesion. Adv Immunol 58:345, 1995. (A comprehensive review of adhesion molecules and mechanisms of leukocyte migration.)

Jaeschke H, Smith CW: Mechanisms of neutrophil-induced parenchymal injury. J Leukoc Biol 61:647, 1997. (Review of the pathways and mediators of neutrophil-mediated injury).

Kaufman DR, Choi Y: Signaling by tumor necrosis factor receptors: pathways, paradigms and targets for therapeutic modulation. Int Rev Immunol 18:405, 1999. (A good review of the pathways of TNF-mediated effects and clinical implications.)

Kaufmann SH: Immunity to intracellular bacteria. Annu Rev Immunol 11:129, 1993. (A comprehensive review of the basic immunology related to intracellular bacterial pathogens and of the role of granulomatous inflammation in normal defense.)

Kelso A: Cytokines: Principles and prospects. Immunol Cell Biol 76:300, 1998. (A reasonably comprehensive and up-to-date overview of a complex and constantly evolving field.)

Laroux FS, et al: Role of nitric oxide in inflammation. Acta Physiol Scand 173:113, 2001. (A review of the multiple actions of NO.)

Luscinskas FW, Gimbrone MA Jr: Endothelial-dependent mechanisms in chronic inflammatory leukocyte recruitment. Annu Rev Med 47:413, 1996. (Review focusing on the specific pathways involved in chronic inflammation.)

Morgan BP: Physiology and pathophysiology of complement: progress and trends. Crit Rev Clin Lab Sci 32:265, 1995. (An excellent review of the various aspects of complement.)

Premack BA, Schall TJ: Chemokine receptors: Gateways to inflammation and infection. Nat Med 2:1174, 1996. (A lucid review of chemokines and their receptors; also includes the current nomenclature of this rapidly expanding field.)

Serhan CN: Lipoxins and novel aspirin-triggered lipoxins: A jungle of cell-cell interactions or a therapeutic opportunity? Prostaglandins 53:107, 1997. (An excellent summary of these newly described mediators and their clinical implications.)

Serhan CN, et al: Lipid mediator networks in cell signaling: update and impact of cytokines. FASEB J 10:1147, 1996. (Comprehensive summary of the pathways of arachidonic acid metabolite signaling and interplay with protein cytokines.)

Tedder TF, et al: The selectins: vascular adhesion molecules. FASEB J 9:866, 1995. (A review of the structure, distribution, and function of selectins.)

Tsokos GC: Lymphocytes, cytokines, inflammation, and immune trafficking. Curr Opin Rheumatol 7:376, 1995. (Cytokine and adhesion molecule interplay in inflammation and pathologic states.)

3

Tissue Repair: Cell Regeneration and Fibrosis

RICHARD N. MITCHELL, MD PhD
RAMZI S. COTRAN, MD*

CELL REGENERATION
    Control of Cell Growth and
      Differentiation
    Soluble Mediators
    Extracellular Matrix and Cell-Matrix
      Interactions
REPAIR BY CONNECTIVE TISSUE (FIBROSIS)
    Angiogenesis
    Fibrosis (Scar Formation)
    Scar Remodeling

**GROWTH FACTORS IN CELL REGENERATION
AND FIBROSIS**
WOUND HEALING
    Healing by First Intention
    Healing by Second Intention
    Wound Strength
PATHOLOGIC ASPECTS OF REPAIR
**OVERVIEW OF THE INFLAMMATORY-
REPARATIVE RESPONSE**

Even as cells and tissues are being injured, events that contain the damage and prepare the surviving cells to replicate are set into motion. Stimuli that induce death in some cells can trigger the activation of replication pathways in others; recruited inflammatory cells not only clean up the necrotic debris but also elaborate mediators that drive the synthesis of new extracellular matrix (ECM). Thus, repair begins very early in the process of inflammation and involves two dichotomous processes:

■ *Regeneration of injured tissue by parenchymal cells of the same type*
■ *Replacement by connective tissue (fibrosis)*, resulting in a scar

Commonly, tissue repair (*healing*) involves a combination of both processes. Interestingly, regeneration and scarring involve essentially similar mechanisms including cell migration, proliferation, and differentiation, as well as matrix synthesis. Although soluble factors control many elements of these processes, interactions with the ECM are also extremely important. In fact, orderly regeneration of epithelium requires an intact basement membrane (BM) matrix; if the ECM has also been destroyed by an injury, tissues can heal only by generating a scar.

*Deceased

CELL REGENERATION

Control of Cell Growth and Differentiation

In general, the number of cells in a given tissue is a cumulative function of the rates at which new cells enter and existing cells exit the population. Entry of new cells into a tissue population is largely determined by their proliferation rates, while cells can leave the population either by cell death or differentiation into another cell type. As shown in Figure 3–1, increased cell number in a particular population may therefore result from either increased proliferation or decreased cell death or differentiation.

Cell proliferation can be stimulated by intrinsic growth factors, injury, cell death, or even mechanical deformation of tissues. Notably, the biochemical mediators and/or mechanical stressors present in the local microenvironment can either stimulate *or inhibit* cell growth. Thus, an excess of stimulators or a deficiency of inhibitors results in net cell growth. Although growth can be accomplished by shortening the length of the cell cycle or decreasing the rate of cell loss, *the most important regulatory control is the induction of resting cells (in G_0) to enter the cell cycle*, as described later. It is also important to remember that the various signals from the local environment may not only change the proliferative rate of cells but can also alter their differentiation and synthetic capacity.

Normal Cell Proliferation: The Cell Cycle. Proliferating cells progress through a series of checkpoints and defined phases called the *cell cycle* (Fig. 3–2A). The cell cycle consists of (in order) the presynthetic *growth phase 1*, or G_1; a DNA-*synthetic phase*, or *S*; the premitotic *growth phase 2*, or G_2; and the *mitotic phase*, or *M*. Quiescent cells are in a physiologic state called G_0. With the exception of tissues composed primarily of terminally differentiated, nondividing cells, which all reside in G_0, most mature tissues consist of cells in some combination of the various states (see later).

Entry and progression of cells through the cell cycle are controlled by changes in the levels and activities of a family of proteins called *cyclins*. The levels of the various cyclins increase at specific stages of the cell cycle, after which they are rapidly degraded as the cell moves on through the cycle. Cyclins accomplish their regulatory functions by complexing with (and thereby activating) constitutively synthesized proteins called *cyclin-dependent kinases (CDKs)*. Different combinations of cyclins and CDKs are associated with each of the important transitions in the cell cycle (schematically represented in Fig. 3–2B), and they exert their effects by phosphorylating a selected group of protein substrates (*kinases phosphorylate* proteins; counter-regulatory proteins called *phosphatases dephosphorylate* proteins). Depending on the protein, phosphorylation can lead to conformational changes that can potentially

■ Activate *or* inactivate an enzymatic activity
■ Induce *or* interfere with protein-protein interactions
■ Induce *or* inhibit binding of a protein to DNA
■ Induce *or* prevent the catabolism of a protein

A specific example involves CDK1, which controls the critical transition from G_2 to M (Fig. 3–2C). As the cell moves into G_2, cyclin B is synthesized, and it binds to CDK1. This cyclin B–CDK1 complex is activated by phosphorylation, and the active kinase then phosphorylates a variety of proteins involved in mitosis, including those involved in DNA replication, depolymerization of nuclear lamina, and mitotic spindle formation. After cell division, cyclin B is degraded by the ubiquitin-proteasomal pathway (see Fig. 1–12B); until there is a new growth stimulus and synthesis of new cyclins, the cells do not undergo further mitosis.

In addition to synthesis and degradation of cyclins, the cyclin-CDK complexes are also regulated by the binding of *CDK inhibitors*. These are particularly important in regulating *cell cycle checkpoints* ($G_1 \rightarrow S$ and $G_2 \rightarrow M$), points at which the cell takes stock of whether its DNA is sufficiently replicated and all mistakes repaired before progressing. Failure to adequately monitor the fidelity of DNA replication leads to the accumulation of mutations and possible malignant transformation. Thus, as an example, when DNA is damaged (e.g., by ultraviolet irradiation), the *tumor suppressor* protein TP53 (formerly p53; a phosphorylated protein of molecular mass 53 kD; Chapter 6) is stabilized and induces the transcription of CDKN1A (formerly p21), a CDK inhibitor. This arrests the cells in G_1 or G_2 until the DNA can be repaired; at that point, the TP53 levels fall, CDKN1A diminishes, and the cells can proceed through the checkpoint. If the DNA damage is too extensive, TP53 will initiate a cascade of events to convince the cell to commit suicide (*apoptosis*; Chapters 1 and 6).

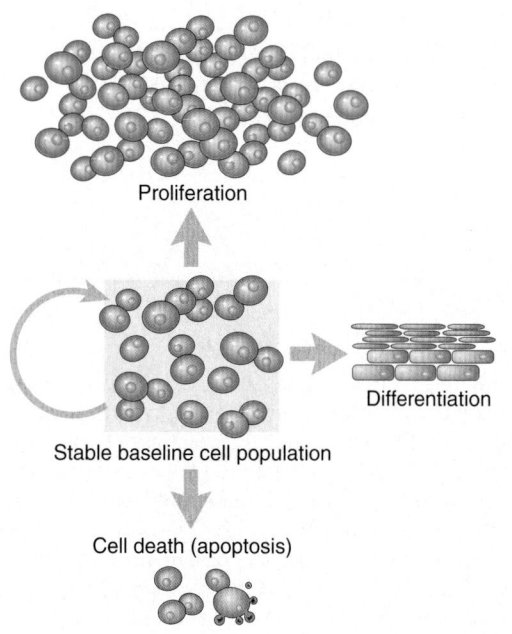

Proliferation

Stable baseline cell population

Differentiation

Cell death (apoptosis)

Figure 3–1 ■

Mechanisms regulating cell populations. Cell numbers can be altered by increased or decreased rates of cell death *(apoptosis)* or by changes in the rates of proliferation or differentiation. (Modified from McCarthy NJ, et al: Apoptosis in the development of the immune system: growth factors, clonal selection and *bcl-2.* Cancer Metastasis Rev 11:157, 1992.)

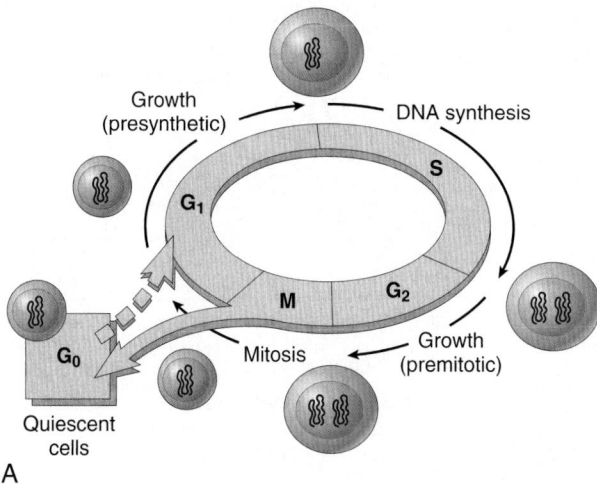

Figure 3–2   ■

The cell cycle. *A,* Stages of the cell cycle. G_1 (presynthetic) and S (synthetic) stages generally constitute the majority of the time of the cell cycle; the M (mitotic) phase is typically brief. Note that while some cell populations continuously cycle and proliferate (e.g., hematopoietic progenitor cells), most cells in the body are quiescent and are in stage G_0. *B,* Control of cell cycle progression. Cyclin-dependent kinases (CDKs) are constitutively synthesized but are activated only when complexed with cyclins. The cyclins (indicated as globular proteins) are synthesized only at certain stages of the cell cycle and then are degraded as the cell progresses into the next phase; as they are degraded the relevant CDK becomes inactive. The names of the cyclins and CDKs here are deliberately simplified and generic; see *C* for a specific example of the actual names for one phase of the cycle. *C,* Regulation of CDK1 kinase activity by cyclin B in the $G_2 \rightarrow$ M transition. Binding of newly synthesized cyclin B to inactive CDK1 kinase at the beginning of G_2 results in a complex that can be activated by phosphorylation. This active kinase complex then phosphorylates a number of proteins important in regulating the $G_2 \rightarrow$ M transition. After mitosis, the cyclin B dissociates from the complex and is degraded, leaving behind the inactive CDK1 kinase, which can re-enter the cycle at the next G_2 stage. (Adapted from Dr. Anindya Dutta, Brigham and Women's Hospital, Boston.)

The Proliferative Potential of Different Cell Types. The cells of the body are divided into three groups on the basis of their regenerative capacity and their relationship to the cell cycle. With the exception of tissues composed primarily of nondividing permanent cells (e.g., cardiac muscle and nerve), most mature tissues contain variable proportions of continuously dividing cells, quiescent cells that occasionally go back to the cell cycle, and nondividing cells

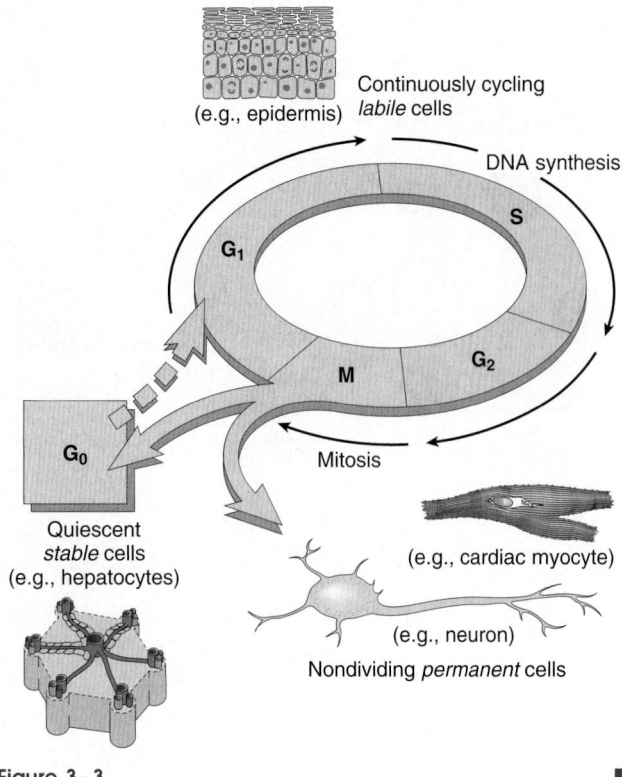

Figure 3-3 ■

Cell populations and cell cycle phases. Constantly dividing labile cells continuously cycle from one mitosis to the next. Nondividing permanent cells have exited the cycle and are destined to die without further division. Quiescent stable cells in G_0 are neither cycling nor dying and can be induced to re-enter the cycle by an appropriate stimulus.

(Fig. 3–3). Note that the ability to proliferate is generally inversely correlated with the degree of differentiation.

■ *Labile cells.* These are continuously dividing (and continuously dying). Regeneration occurs from a population of *stem cells* with relatively unlimited capacity to proliferate. When a stem cell divides, one daughter cell retains the ability to divide (self-renewal), while the other differentiates into nonmitotic cells that carry on the normal function of the tissue. Labile cells include hematopoietic cells in the bone marrow and also represent the majority of surface epithelia including the stratified squamous surfaces of the skin, oral cavity, vagina, and cervix; the cuboidal epithelia of the ducts draining exocrine organs (e.g., salivary glands, pancreas, biliary tract); the columnar epithelium of the gastrointestinal tract, uterus, and fallopian tubes; and the transitional epithelium of the urinary tract.
■ *Stable cells.* These are considered to be quiescent (or have only low-level replicative capacity) in their normal state but are capable of undergoing rapid division in response to injury. Stable cells constitute the *parenchyma* of most solid glandular tissues, including liver, kidney, and pancreas, as well as endothelial cells lining blood vessels, and the fibroblast and smooth muscle connective tissue *(mesenchymal)* cells; the proliferation of fibroblasts and smooth muscle cells is particularly important in response to injury and wound healing.

■ *Permanent cells.* These are considered to be terminally differentiated and nonproliferative in postnatal life. The majority of neurons and cardiac muscle cells belong to this category. Thus, injury to brain or heart is irreversible and results in only scar since the tissues cannot proliferate. Although skeletal muscle is usually categorized as a permanent cell type, satellite cells attached to the endomysial sheath do confer some regenerative capacity. There is also some evidence that heart muscle cells may proliferate after myocardial necrosis.

Soluble Mediators

Overview. *Cell growth and differentiation are dependent on extracellular signals derived from soluble mediators and ECM matrix (see ECM discussion in the following section).* Although many chemical mediators affect cell growth, the most important are *polypeptide growth factors* circulating in the serum or produced locally by cells. Most growth factors have *pleiotropic effects;* that is, in addition to stimulating cellular proliferation, they mediate a wide variety of other activities, including cell migration and differentiation and tissue remodeling, and are therefore involved in various stages of wound healing. The growth factors induce cell proliferation by affecting the expression of genes involved in normal growth control pathways, the so-called protooncogenes. The expression of these genes is tightly regulated during normal regeneration and repair. Alterations in the structure or expression of protooncogenes can convert them into *oncogenes*, which contribute to uncontrolled cell growth characteristic of cancers; thus, normal and abnormal cell proliferation may follow similar pathways (Chapter 6). There is a huge (and ever-increasing) list of known soluble mediators. Rather than attempt an exhaustive cataloguing, later in the chapter we highlight only selected molecules, and these are restricted to those that contribute to the process of *healing.* For now, we discuss general concepts and generic signaling pathways.

Signaling by Soluble Mediators. Signaling may occur directly between adjacent cells, or over greater distances (Fig. 3–4). Adjacent cells communicate via *gap junctions*, narrow, hydrophilic channels that effectively connect the two cells' cytoplasm. The channels permit movement of small ions, various metabolites, and potential second messenger molecules, but not larger macromolecules. *Extracellular signaling* via soluble mediators occurs in four different forms:

■ *Autocrine* signaling, in which a soluble mediator acts predominantly (or even exclusively) on the cell that secretes it. This pathway is important in the immune response *(cytokines)* and in compensatory epithelial hyperplasia (e.g., liver regeneration).
■ *Paracrine* signaling, meaning that mediators affect cells only in the immediate vicinity. To accomplish this, there can be only minimal diffusion, with the signal rapidly degraded, taken up by other cells, or trapped in the ECM. This pathway is important for recruiting inflammatory cells to the site of infection and for the controlled process of wound healing.
■ *Synaptic*, in which activated neural tissue secretes *neurotransmitters* at a specialized cell junction *(synapse)*

GAP JUNCTIONS

AUTOCRINE SIGNALING

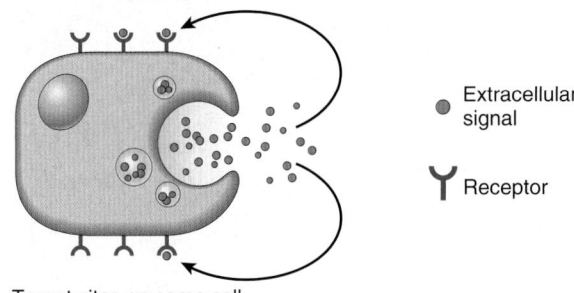

● Extracellular signal

Y Receptor

Target sites on same cell

PARACRINE SIGNALING

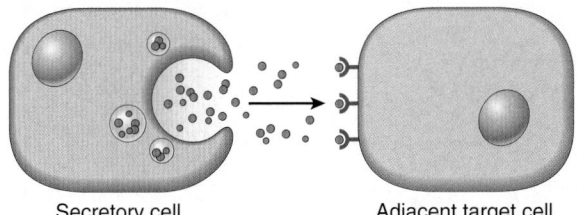

Secretory cell   Adjacent target cell

SYNAPTIC SIGNALING

Muscle cell

Neuron

ENDOCRINE SIGNALING

Blood vessel

Hormone secretion into blood by endocrine gland

Distant target cells

Figure 3–4   ■

General patterns of intercellular signaling (see text). (Modified from Lodish, et al [eds]: Molecular Cell Biology, 3rd ed. New York, WH Freeman, 1995.)

onto target cells such as other nerves or muscle (Chapter 23).

■ *Endocrine,* in which a regulatory substance, such as a hormone, is released into the bloodstream and acts on target cells at a distance.

Since most signaling molecules are present at extremely low concentrations ($\leq 10^{-8}$ M), binding to the appropriate target cell receptor is typically a high-affinity and exquisitely specific interaction. Receptor proteins may be on the cell surface, or they may be intracellular; in the latter case, *ligands* (molecules that bind to receptors) must be sufficiently hydrophobic to enter the cell (e.g., vitamin D, or steroid and thyroid hormones). *For intracellular receptors, ligand binding leads to the formation of receptor-ligand complexes that directly associate with nuclear DNA and subsequently either activate or turn off gene transcription.*

For cell surface receptors, the binding of a ligand leads to a cascade of secondary intracellular events beginning with increased intracellular calcium, cyclic AMP, or inositol triphosphate (IP_3), or the activation of a kinase. The resulting cascade of signals is a way to amplify an initially small number of receptor-mediator interactions. The end result is the translocation of *activated transcription factors* into the nucleus. These transcription factors are proteins that can bind to certain DNA sequences called *promoters* and *enhancers* that lie up-stream of particular genes. Binding of the transcription factors causes DNA conformational changes that modify the down-stream transcription of these genes; depending on the nature of the transcription factor, binding may activate or repress gene transcription.

Cell surface receptors are of four general types (Fig. 3–5):

■ *Ion channel receptors.* Ligand binding alters the conformation of the receptor so that specific ions can flow through it. This results in a change of electric potential across the cell; it may also initiate a cascade of enzymatic activity driven by binding of the particular ion (e.g., calcium). The acetylcholine receptor at the nerve-muscle junction is an example.

■ *Receptors with intrinsic kinase activity.* These are usually dimeric transmembrane molecules with an extracellular ligand-binding domain; ligand binding causes stable dimerization with subsequent mutual phosphorylation of the receptor subunits. Once phosphorylated, the receptors can bind to other intracellular proteins (e.g., RAS, phosphatidylinositol 3-kinase, phospholipase Cγ) and stimulate a cascade of events leading to entrance into S phase or induction of other transcriptional programs. An especially important pathway stimulated by *RAS* activation is the *mitogen-activated protein (MAP) kinase cascade,* which is involved in the intracellular signaling of multiple growth factors, including *epidermal growth factor (EGF)* and *fibroblast growth factor (FGF).*

■ *G-protein–coupled receptors.* These receptors all contain seven transmembrane segments; after binding to their specific ligand, the receptors associate with intracellular GTP-hydrolyzing proteins (hence the name *G-protein–coupled receptors*). Binding of the G proteins to the receptor results in their activation, whereupon they dissociate and can stimulate a variety of other proteins, including adenylate cyclase (to make cyclic AMP) and

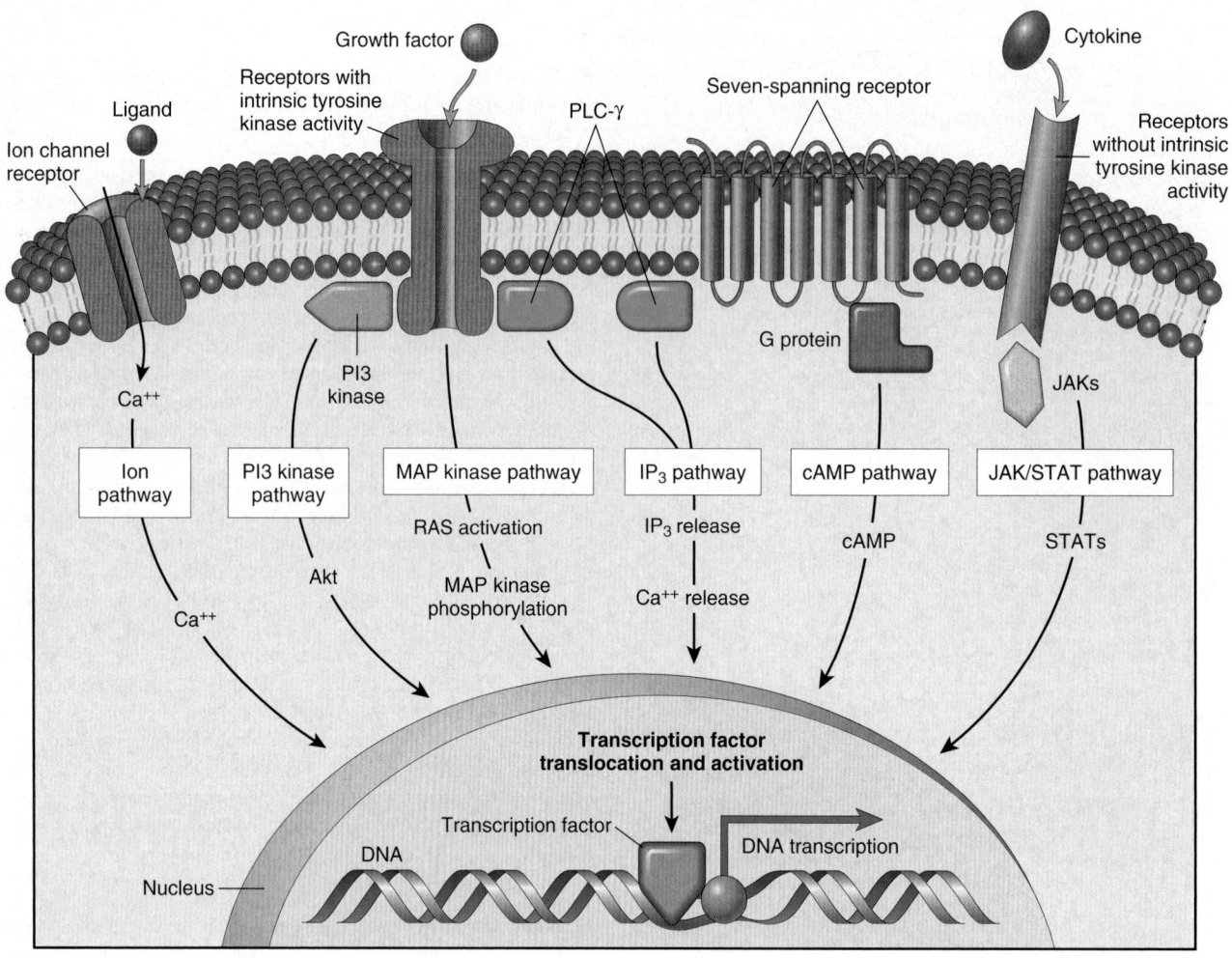

Figure 3-5

Simplified overview of the major types of cell surface receptors and their principal signal transduction pathways leading to transcription factor activation and translocation into the nucleus (see text). cAMP, cyclic adenosine monophosphate; IP_3, inositol triphosphate; JAK, Janus kinase; MAP kinase, mitogen-activated protein kinase; PI3 kinase, phosphatidylinositol 3-kinase; PLC-γ, phospholipase Cγ; STAT, signal transducers and activators of transcription.

phospholipase Cγ. Receptors in this category include those for epinephrine and glucagon, as well as the chemokines (Chapter 2).

■ *Receptors without intrinsic enzymatic activity*. These are usually monomeric transmembrane molecules with an extracellular ligand-binding domain; ligand interaction induces an intracellular conformational change that allows association with, and activation of, intracellular protein kinases. These lead to phosphorylation of the receptor complex and a down-stream activation cascade involving *Janus kinases (JAKs)* and *STATs (signal transducers and activators of transcription)*. These include receptors involved in *cytokine* activation in the immune system, and the erythropoietin receptor.

It is important to note that not all ligands induce stimulatory signals; in fact, growth-inhibitory signals (e.g., inducing *contact inhibition* of growth) are equally important. *Transforming growth factor β (TGF-β)* is a good example; its receptor has intrinsic kinase activity, and when complexed with TGF-β it phosphorylates specific intracellular proteins (*SMADs*), which in turn increase the synthe-

sis of CDK inhibitors and block the activity of transcription factors.

To summarize, polypeptide growth factors bind to and activate their receptors, many of which possess intrinsic kinase activity. They subsequently phosphorylate a number of substrates involved in signal transduction and the generation of second messengers. The resultant kinase cascade leads to the activation of nuclear transcription factors, initiates DNA synthesis, and ultimately culminates in cell division. The process of cell proliferation is directed by a family of proteins called cyclins that, when complexed with CDKs, control the phosphorylation of proteins involved in cell cycle progression.

Extracellular Matrix and Cell-Matrix Interactions

ECM is a *dynamic*, *constantly remodeling* macromolecular complex synthesized locally and constituting a significant proportion of any tissue. Besides providing turgor to soft

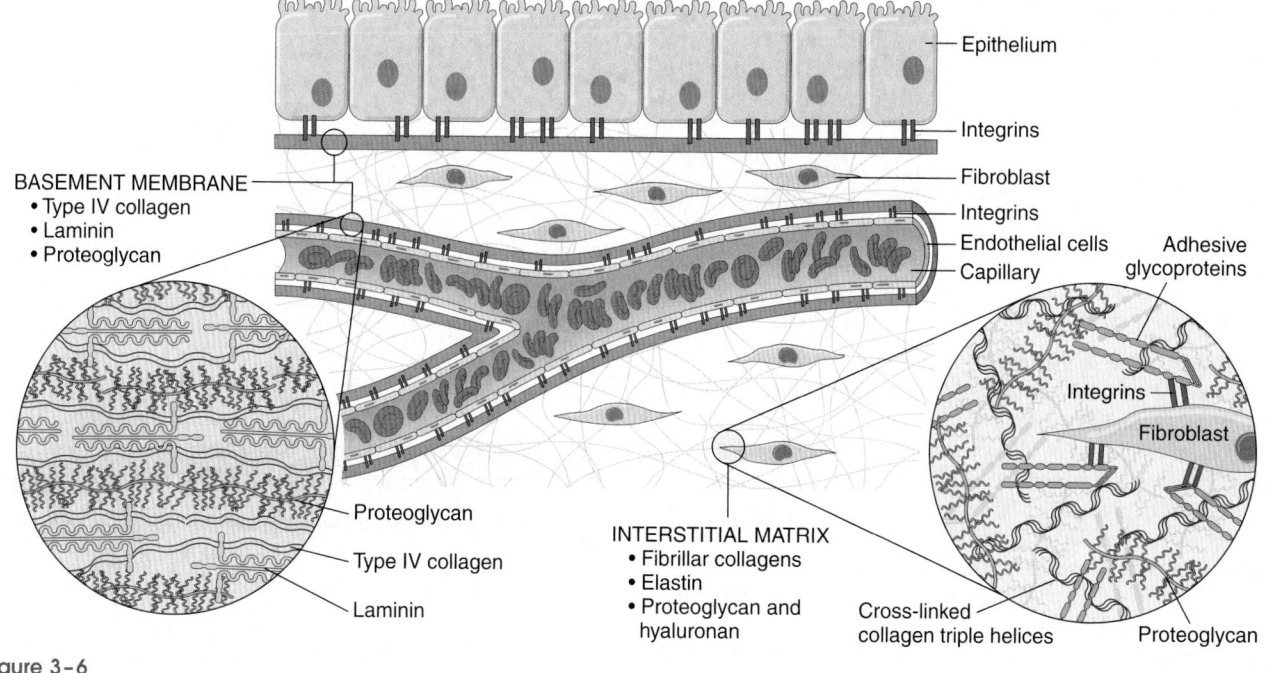

Figure 3-6   ■

Schematic of the major components of the extracellular matrix (ECM), including collagens, proteoglycans, and adhesive glycoproteins. Note that although there are some overlaps in their constituents, basement membrane and interstitial ECM have different general compositions and architecture. Both epithelial and mesenchymal cells (e.g., fibroblasts) interact with ECM via integrins. For the sake of simplifying the diagram, many ECM components have been left out (e.g., elastin, fibrillin, hyaluronan, syndecan).

tissues and rigidity to bone, ECM supplies a substratum for cell adhesion and critically regulates the growth, movement, and differentiation of the cells living within it. ECM occurs in two basic forms: *interstitial matrix* and *basement membrane (BM)* (Fig. 3–6).

■ *Interstitial matrix.* This is present in the spaces between cells in connective tissue, and between epithelium and supportive vascular and smooth muscle structures; it is synthesized by mesenchymal cells (e.g., fibroblasts) and tends to form a three-dimensional amorphous gel. Its major constituents are fibrillar and nonfibrillar collagens, as well as the other proteoglycan and glycoprotein elements described later.
■ *Basement membrane.* The seemingly random array of interstitial matrix in connective tissues becomes highly organized around epithelial cells, endothelial cells, and smooth muscle cells, forming the specialized *basement membrane.* The BM sits beneath epithelium and is synthesized by overlying epithelium and underlying mesenchymal cells; it tends to form a platelike "chicken wire" mesh. Its major constituents are amorphous nonfibrillar type IV collagen and adhesive glycoproteins (see later).

Roles of Extracellular Matrix. The ECM is much more than a space filler around cells; its various roles include

■ Mechanical support for cell anchorage. In the absence of adhesion, most cell types die.
■ Determination of cell orientation *(polarity).* Basolateral (bottom side) versus *apical* (top) are important distinctions for most cells in terms of function (e.g., absorption of

nutrients from the gastrointestinal tract or release of digestive enzymes in the pancreas).
■ Control of cell growth. Growth and differentiation are regulated by cell adhesion and cell shape. Generally, the more adherent a cell is, the more proliferative (and less synthetic) it will be.
■ Maintenance of cell differentiation. The type of ECM proteins also affects the degree of differentiation. Interestingly, the same ECM may have different effects depending on the *mechanical context* in which it is presented (i.e., malleable vs. rigid).
■ Scaffolding for tissue renewal. All tissues are dynamic renewing structures, and maintaining normal structure requires a BM scaffold. It is particularly noteworthy that although labile and stable cells are capable of regeneration, injury to these tissues does not always result in restitution of the normal structure. The integrity of the underlying stroma of the parenchymal cells, and *in particular the basement membrane*, is critical for the organized regeneration of tissues. When basement membrane is disrupted, cells proliferate in haphazard ways, resulting in disorganized and nonfunctional tissues; extensive injury in labile or stable tissues culminates predominantly in scar formation due to the expansion of fibroblast (mesenchymal) populations.
■ Establishment of tissue microenvironments. BM acts as a boundary between epithelium and underlying connective tissue and also forms part of the filtration apparatus in the kidney. The ECM is also the scaffolding that inflammatory cells use for dragging themselves around in search of infectious agents.

■ Storage and presentation of regulatory molecules. For example, fibroblast growth factor (FGF) is excreted and stored in the BM in normal tissues. This allows its rapid deployment to turn on cell growth in situations of local injury.

Components of the Extracellular Matrix. *There are three basic components of ECM: fibrous structural proteins that confer tensile strength and recoil, water-hydrated gels that permit resilience and lubrication, and adhesive glycoproteins that connect the matrix elements one to another and to cells (see Fig. 3–6).*

■ *Collagen.* The *collagens* are fibrous structural proteins conferring tensile strength. These proteins are composed of three separate peptide chains braided into a ropelike triple helix; the individual chains are able to tightly intertwine because the peptide chains have glycines present at every third position. Mutations changing the glycines to other amino acids, or any other abnormalities leading to poor collagen braiding, result in defective ECM synthesis with catastrophic consequences to bone, skin, aorta, and other tissues. More than 30 distinct peptide chains form approximately 18 different collagen types, some of which are unique to specific cells and tissues. Some collagen types (e.g., types I, III, and V) form *fibrils* by virtue of lateral cross-linking of the triple helices; other collagens (e.g., type IV) are *nonfibrillar* and are components of BMs. The tensile strength of the fibrillar collagens derives from their cross-linking, a process dependent on vitamin C; thus, children with ascorbate deficiency have skeletal deformities, bleed easily because of weak vascular wall BM, and heal poorly. The fibrillar collagens form a major proportion of the connective tissue in healing wounds and particularly in scars, and are discussed further later.

■ *Elastin.* Although tensile strength is derived from the fibrillar collagens, the ability of tissues to recoil and return to a baseline structure after physical stress is conferred by elastic tissue. This is especially important in the walls of large vessels (which must accommodate recurrent pulsatile flow), as well as in the uterus, skin, and ligaments. Morphologically, elastic fibers consist of a central core of *elastin* protein, surrounded by a meshlike network of *fibrillin* glycoprotein. Like collagens, elastins require a glycine in every third position, but they differ from collagen by having fewer cross-links. The fibrillin meshwork serves as a scaffold for the deposition of elastin and assembly of elastic fibers; defects in fibrillin synthesis lead to skeletal abnormalities and weakened aortic walls (*Marfan syndrome*; Chapter 7).

■ *Proteoglycans and hyaluronan.* These molecules form highly hydrated compressible gels conferring resilience and lubrication (such as in the cartilage in joints). They consist of long polysaccharides called *glycosaminoglycans* (examples are *dermatan sulfate* and *heparan sulfate*) linked to a protein backbone much like bristles on a test tube brush. *Hyaluronan*, a huge molecule composed of multiple disaccharide repeats without a protein core, is also an important constituent of the ECM, principally because of its ability to bind volumes of water into a viscous, gelatin-like matrix. Besides providing compressibility to a tissue, proteoglycans also serve as

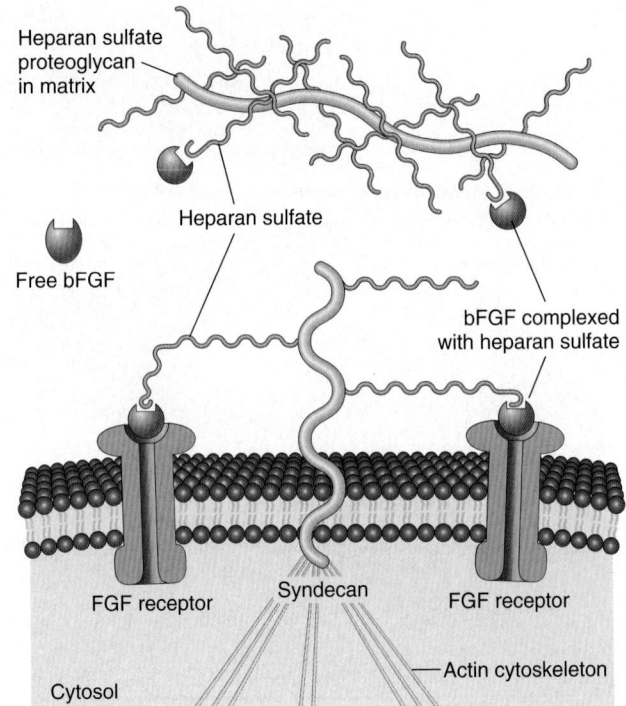

Figure 3–7 ■

Proteoglycans in the ECM and on cells act as reservoirs for growth factors. Heparan sulfate binds basic fibroblast growth factor (bFGF) secreted into the ECM. Any subsequent injury to the ECM can release bFGF, which can then stimulate recruitment of inflammatory cells, fibroblast activation, and new blood vessel formation. Syndecan is a cell surface proteoglycan with a transmembrane core protein and attached extracellular glycosaminoglycan side chains. The glycosaminoglycan chains can also bind free bFGF from the ECM and thereby mediate improved interactions with cell surface FGF receptors. The cytoplasmic tail of syndecan attaches to the intracellular actin cytoskeleton and helps maintain the morphology of epithelial sheets. (Modified from Lodish H, et al [eds]: Molecular Cell Biology, 3rd ed. New York, WH Freeman, 1995.)

reservoirs for growth factors secreted into the ECM (e.g., bFGF) (Fig. 3–7). Any damage to the ECM then releases the bound growth factor, which can initiate the healing process. Proteoglycans can also be integral cell membrane proteins and in that capacity modulate cell growth and differentiation. For example, the transmembrane proteoglycan *syndecan* has attached hyaluronan chains that can bind matrix growth factors like bFGF; this binding facilitates the interactions of bFGF with appropriate cell surface receptors (see Fig. 3–7). *Syndecan* also associates with the intracellular actin cytoskeleton and thereby helps to maintain normal epithelial sheet morphology.

■ Adhesive glycoproteins and integrins. Adhesive glycoproteins are structurally diverse molecules whose major role is to link ECM components to one another and to link ECM to cells via cell surface integrins. The adhesive glycoproteins include (among many) fibronectin (major component of the interstitial ECM) and laminin (major constituent of BM), described here as prototypical of the overall group (Fig. 3–8).

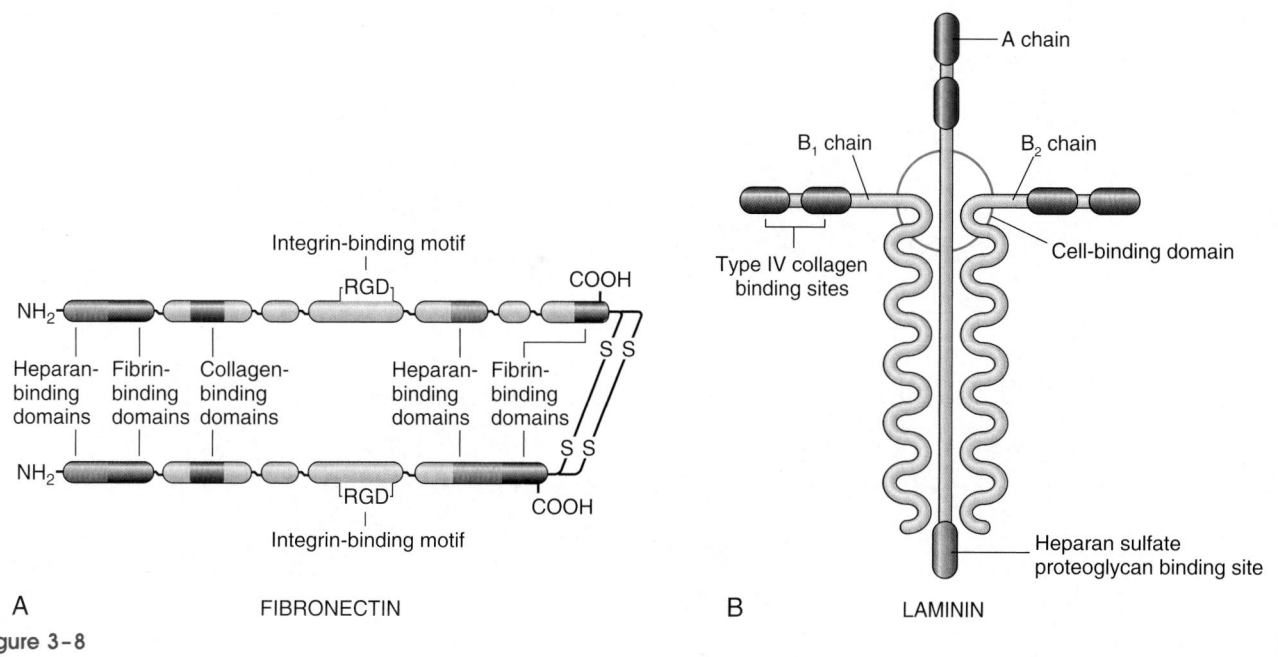

Figure 3-8 ■

Adhesive glycoproteins of the ECM. *A*, The fibronectin molecule consists of a disulfide-linked dimer with various domains that bind to ECM components, as well as the integrin-binding domain containing the Arg-Gly-Asp (RGD) motif. *B*, Laminin is a roughly cross-shaped molecule with domains that allow it to link between components of the ECM and cell surfaces.

■ Fibronectin is a large (450-kD) disulfide-linked heterodimer (see Fig. 3–8A) synthesized by a variety of cells, including fibroblasts, monocytes, and endothelium, and associated with cell surfaces, BMs, and pericellular matrix. It has specific domains that bind to a wide spectrum of ECM components (e.g., collagen, fibrin, heparin, and proteoglycans) and can also attach to cell integrins via a tripeptide arginine-glycine-aspartic acid (abbreviated RGD) motif. This RGD recognition sequence plays a key role in cell-ECM adhesion.

■ Laminin is the most abundant glycoprotein in BM; it is a 820-kD cross-shaped heterotrimer that connects cells to underlying ECM components such as type IV collagen and heparan sulfate (see Fig. 3–8B). Besides mediating attachment to BM, laminin also modulates cell survival, proliferation, differentiation, and motility.

■ Integrins are a family of transmembrane (α- and β-chain) heterodimeric glycoproteins whose intracellular domains associate with cytoskeletal elements (e.g., vinculin and actin at focal adhesion complexes). Recall that in Chapter 2 we encountered some of the integrins as leukocyte surface molecules that mediate firm adhesion and transmigration across endothelium at sites of inflammation, and we will meet them again when we discuss platelet aggregation in Chapter 4. Integrins on epithelial or mesenchymal cells also bind to ECM via RGD motifs; these interactions signal cell attachment and can affect cell locomotion, proliferation, or differentiation. Integrin-ECM interactions can utilize the same intracellular signaling pathways used by growth factor receptors; for example, integrin-mediated adhesion to fibronectin can trigger elements of the MAP kinase, phos-

phatidylinositol 3-kinase, and protein kinase C pathways. In this manner, extracellular mechanical forces can be coupled to intracellular synthetic and transcriptional pathways (Fig. 3–9).

Thus, adhesive matrix proteins such as fibronectin and laminin can directly mediate the attachment, spread, and migration of cells. By activating intracellular signaling pathways, fibronectin also enhances the sensitivity of certain cells (e.g., endothelium) to the proliferative effects of growth factors. In the early stages of healing skin wounds, large quantities of plasma-derived fibronectin accumulate in the ECM and act as a provisional scaffolding for the ingrowth of endothelium and fibroblasts. After 2 or 3 days, the fibronectin in the healing wound is actively synthesized by proliferating endothelial cells (see later).

To summarize, cell growth and differentiation involve at least two types of signals acting in concert. One derives from soluble molecules such as polypeptide growth factors and growth inhibitors. The other involves insoluble elements of the ECM interacting with cellular integrins (see Fig. 3–9).

REPAIR BY CONNECTIVE TISSUE (FIBROSIS)

Overview. Severe or persistent tissue injury with damage both to parenchymal cells and to the stromal framework leads to a situation in which repair cannot be accomplished by parenchymal regeneration alone. Under these conditions, repair occurs by replacement of the nonregenerated

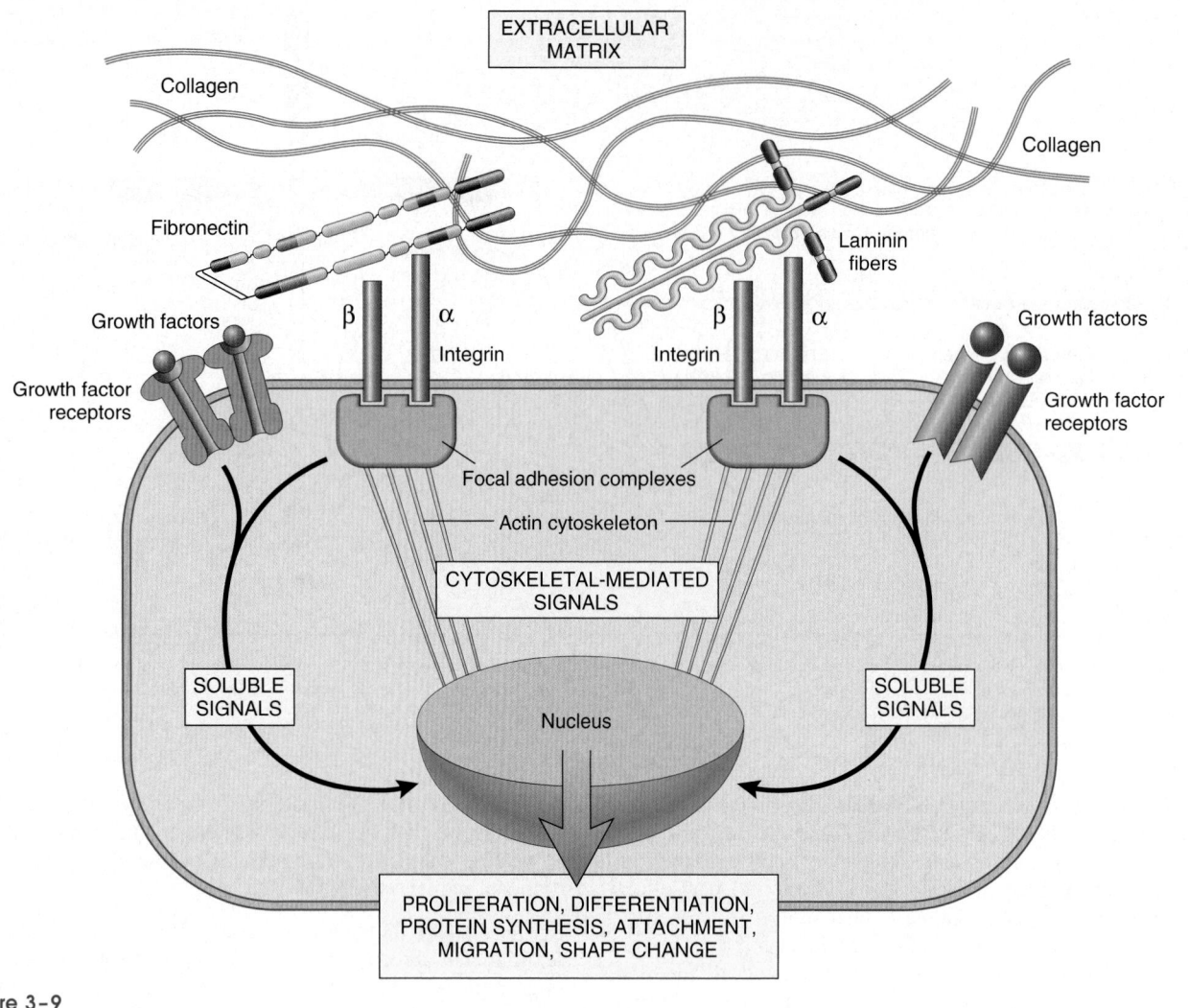

Figure 3-9 ■

Schematic showing mechanisms by which ECM interactions and growth factors can influence cell growth, motility differentiation, and protein synthesis. Integrins bind ECM and interact with the cytoskeleton at focal adhesion complexes (protein aggregates that include vinculin, α-actinin, and talin). This can initiate the production of intracellular second messengers or can directly mediate nuclear signals. Cell surface receptors for growth factors also initiate second signals. Together, these are integrated by the cell to yield various responses, including changes in cell growth, locomotion, and differentiation.

parenchymal cells with connective tissue. There are four general components of this process:

■ Formation of new blood vessels (*angiogenesis*)
■ Migration and proliferation of fibroblasts
■ Deposition of ECM
■ Maturation and reorganization of the fibrous tissue *(remodeling)*

Repair begins within 24 hours of injury by the emigration of fibroblasts and the induction of fibroblast and endothelial cell proliferation. By 3 to 5 days, a specialized type of tissue that is characteristic of healing, called *granulation tissue*, is apparent. The term *granulation tissue* derives from the pink, soft, granular gross appearance, such as that seen beneath the scab of a skin wound. Its histologic appearance is characterized by proliferation of fibroblasts and new thin-walled, delicate capillaries, in a loose ECM (Fig. 3–10A). Granulation tissue then progressively accumulates connective tissue matrix, eventually resulting

in dense fibrosis (scarring; Fig. 3–10B), which may further remodel over time. We next discuss the mechanisms underlying the stages of scar formation.

Angiogenesis

Blood vessels are assembled by two processes: *vasculogenesis*, in which the primitive vascular network is assembled from *angioblasts* (endothelial cell precursors) during embryonic development; and *angiogenesis*, or *neovascularization*, by which preexisting vessels send out capillary sprouts to produce new vessels. Angiogenesis is a critical process in the healing at sites of injury, in the development of collateral circulations at sites of ischemia, and in allowing tumors to increase in size beyond the constraints of their original blood supply. Thus, much work has been done in understanding the mechanisms underlying such neovascularization, and therapies to either augment the process (for example to

Figure 3-10 ■

A, Granulation tissue showing numerous blood vessels, edema, and a loose ECM containing occasional inflammatory cells. This is a trichrome stain that stains collagen blue; minimal mature collagen can be seen at this point. *B,* Trichrome stain of mature scar, showing dense collagen, with only scattered vascular channels.

improve blood flow to a heart ravaged by atherosclerosis) or inhibit it (to frustrate tumor growth) are beginning to come on-line.

Four general steps occur in the development of a new capillary vessel (Fig. 3–11):

■ Proteolytic degradation of the parent vessel BM, allowing formation of a capillary sprout
■ Migration of endothelial cells from the original capillary toward an angiogenic stimulus

■ Proliferation of the endothelial cells behind the leading edge of migrating cells
■ Maturation of endothelial cells with inhibition of growth and organization into capillary tubes; this includes recruitment and proliferation of *pericytes* (for capillaries) and *smooth muscle cells* (for larger vessels) to support the endothelial tube and provide accessory functions

These new vessels are leaky because of incompletely formed interendothelial junctions and increased transcytosis

Figure 3-11 ■

Steps in the process of angiogenesis. The parent mature blood vessel is on the left. (1) Basement membrane and extracellular matrix (ECM) degradation; (2) endothelial migration; (3) endothelial proliferation (mitosis); (4) organization and maturation including the recruitment of vascular pericytes or smooth muscle cells. The number *5* indicates the increased permeability due to intercellular gaps and increased transcytosis. This increased permeability allows deposition of plasma proteins (e.g., fibrinogen) in the extracellular matrix and provides a provisional stroma for fibroblast and endothelial cell ingrowth; it also leads to the edema that occurs in granulation tissue. (Modified from Motamed K, Sage EH: Regulation of vascular morphogenesis by SPARC. Kidney Int 51:1383, 1997.)

(Chapter 2). Indeed, this leakiness explains why granulation tissue is often edematous and accounts in part for edema that may persist in healing wounds long after the acute inflammatory response has resolved.

Several factors induce angiogenesis, but most important are *basic fibroblast growth factor* (bFGF) and *vascular endothelial growth factor* (VEGF) (see later). Both are secreted by a variety of stromal cells, and bFGF can bind to proteoglycans in the BM, presumably to be released when such structures are damaged. Although the angiogenic factors are produced by multiple cell types, the receptors (all with intrinsic kinase activity; see Fig. 3–5) are largely restricted to endothelial cells. Besides causing proliferation, they induce endothelial cells to secrete proteinases to degrade the basement membrane, promote endothelial cell migration, and direct (in conjunction with laminin) vascular tube formation from the expanding endothelial cell population.

Structural ECM proteins also regulate vessel sprouting in angiogenesis, largely by interactions with integrins on the migrating endothelial cells. *Nonstructural ECM proteins* contribute to the process by destabilizing cell-ECM interactions to facilitate continued cell migration (e.g., *thrombospondin* and *tenascin C*), or degrade the ECM to permit remodeling (e.g., *plasminogen activator* and *matrix metalloproteinases*).

Fibrosis (Scar Formation)

Fibrosis, or *scar formation*, builds on the granulation tissue framework of new vessels and loose ECM that develop early at the repair site. The process of fibrosis occurs in two steps: *(1) emigration and proliferation of fibroblasts into the site of injury, and (2) deposition of ECM by these cells.* The recruitment and stimulation of fibroblasts is driven by many of the growth factors described later, *including platelet-derived growth factor (PDGF), bFGF*, and *TGF-β*. One source of these factors is the activated endothelium. However, and perhaps more importantly, growth factors are also elaborated by inflammatory cells. Macrophages, in particular, are important cellular constituents of granulation tissue, and besides clearing extracellular debris and fibrin at the site of injury, they elaborate a host of mediators that induce fibroblast proliferation and ECM production. Sites of inflammation are also rich with mast cells, and with the appropriate chemotactic milieu, lymphocytes may also be present. Each of these can contribute directly or indirectly to fibroblast proliferation and activation.

As healing progresses, the number of proliferating fibroblasts and new vessels decreases; however, the fibroblasts progressively assume a more synthetic phenotype, and hence there is increased deposition of ECM. Collagen synthesis, in particular, is critical to the development of strength in a healing wound site. As described later, collagen synthesis by fibroblasts begins early in wound healing (days 3 to 5) and continues for several weeks, depending on the size of the wound. Many of the same growth factors that regulate fibroblast proliferation also participate in stimulating ECM synthesis. Collagen synthesis, for example, is induced by a number of the molecules, including growth factors (PDGF, bFGF, and TGF-β) and cytokines (inter-

leukin 1 [IL-1] and tumor necrosis factor [TNF]) secreted by leukocytes and fibroblasts. *Net collagen accumulation, however, depends not only on increased synthesis but also on diminished collagen degradation* (discussed later). Ultimately, the granulation tissue scaffolding evolves into a scar composed of largely inactive, spindle-shaped fibroblasts, dense collagen, fragments of elastic tissue, and other ECM components (see Fig. 3–10B). As the scar matures, vascular regression eventually transforms the highly vascularized granulation tissue into a pale, largely avascular scar.

Scar Remodeling

The transition from granulation tissue to scar involves shifts in the composition of the ECM; even after its synthesis and deposition, scar ECM continues to be modified and remodeled. *The outcome at each stage is a balance between ECM synthesis and degradation.* We have already discussed the cells and factors that regulate ECM synthesis. The *degradation* of collagens and other ECM components is accomplished by a family of *metalloproteinases* (so called because they are dependent on *zinc ions* for their activity); these should be distinguished from neutrophil elastase, cathepsin G, plasmin, and other *serine proteinases* that can also degrade ECM but are not metalloenzymes. Metalloproteinases include *interstitial collagenases*, which cleave the fibrillar collagen types I, II, and III; *gelatinases* (or *type IV collagenases*), which degrade amorphous collagen and fibronectin; and *stromelysins*, which catabolize a variety of ECM constituents, including proteoglycans, laminin, fibronectin, and amorphous collagen.

These enzymes are produced by a variety of cell types (fibroblasts, macrophages, neutrophils, synovial cells, and some epithelial cells), and their synthesis and secretion are regulated by growth factors, cytokines, phagocytosis, and even physical stress (Fig. 3–12). Their synthesis is inhibited by TGF-β and may be suppressed pharmacologically with steroids. Given the potential to wreak havoc in tissues, *the activity of the metalloproteinases is tightly controlled.* Thus, they are typically elaborated as inactive (*zymogen*) precursors that must be first activated; this is accomplished by certain chemicals (e.g., $HOCl^-$) or proteases (e.g., plasmin) likely to be present only at sites of injury. In addition, activated collagenases can be rapidly inhibited by specific *tissue inhibitors of metalloproteinase (TIMPs),* produced by most mesenchymal cells (see Fig. 3–12). Collagenases and their inhibitors are spatially and temporally regulated in healing wounds. They are essential in the debridement of injured sites and in the remodeling of the ECM necessary to repair any tissue defects.

GROWTH FACTORS IN CELL REGENERATION AND FIBROSIS

Although there is an impressive array of growth factors (and new ones are constantly being discovered), we review here only those that have a broad target action or are

Figure 3–12   ■

Matrix metalloproteinase regulation. The four mechanisms shown include (1) regulation of synthesis by a variety of growth factors or cytokines, (2) inhibition of synthesis by corticosteroids or transforming growth factor β (TGF-β), (3) regulation of the activation of the secreted but inactive precursors, and (4) blockade of the enzymes by specific tissue inhibitors of metalloproteinases (TIMPs). ECM, extracellular matrix; EGF, epidermal growth factor; IL-1, interleukin 1; PDGF, platelet-derived growth factor; TNF, tumor necrosis factor. (Modified from Matrisian LM: Metalloproteinases and their inhibitors in matrix remodeling. Trends Genet 6:122, 1990.)

specifically involved in directing the healing at a site of injury. Table 3–1 summarizes the most important factors in angiogenesis, recruitment of cells to sites of injury, fibroblast proliferation, and collagen deposition or remodeling. Note that although there are frequently multiple sources for these growth factors at sites of injury, *activated macrophages are usually the most important.*

- *EGF is mitogenic for a variety of epithelial cells and fibroblasts.* It stimulates cell division by binding to a tyrosine kinase receptor on the cell membrane (ERB B-1), followed by phosphorylation and other activation events, as described earlier. TGF-α is homologous to EGF, binds to the EGF receptor, and exhibits biologic activities similar to those of EGF.

- *PDGF* is a cationic A- and B-chain heterodimer (all three possible combinations—AA, AB, and BB—are secreted and are biologically active). While it is released from platelet α granules after activation (hence its name), it is also produced by activated macrophages, endothelial and smooth muscle cells, and a variety of tumors. PDGF induces fibroblast, smooth muscle cell, and monocyte migration and proliferation, but it has other proinflammatory properties as well. It binds to two types of receptors with different ligand specificities (α and β) that have intrinsic protein kinase activity.

- *FGFs* are a family of polypeptides that bind tightly to heparin and other anionic molecules (and thus have a strong affinity for BM); they exhibit a number of activities in addition to growth stimulation. In particular, bFGF recruits macrophages and fibroblasts to wound sites and has the ability to induce all the steps necessary for angiogenesis (see earlier); it is elaborated by activated macrophages and other cells.

- *TGF-β* has pleiotropic and often conflicting effects. It is produced in an inactive form by a variety of cell types, including platelets, endothelium, T cells, and activated macrophages, and it must be proteolytically cleaved (e.g., by plasmin) to become functional.

■

Table 3–1.   MAJOR GROWTH FACTORS IN WOUND HEALING

	EGF OR TGF-α	PDGF	bFGF	TGF-α	VEGF	IL-1 or TNF
Angiogenesis	+	0	++	+	++	+
Chemotaxis						
Monocytes	0	+	+	+	0	+
Fibroblasts	0	+	+	+	0	0
Endothelial cells	+	0	+	−	+	0
Proliferation						
Fibroblasts	+	+	+	±	0	+
Endothelial cells	+	0	++	−	++	0 or −
Collagen Synthesis	+	+	+	++	0	+
Collagenase Secretion	+	+	+	+	0	+

++, major role; +, stimulates; −, inhibits; ±, variable (dose-dependent) effect; 0, no effect; bFGF, basic fibroblast growth factor; EGF, epidermal growth factor; IL-1, interleukin 1; PDGF, platelet-derived growth factor; TGF-α, transforming growth factor α; TNF, tumor necrosis factor; VEGF, vascular endothelial growth factor.

Although TGF-β is a growth inhibitor for most epithelial cell types in culture, it has variable effects on the proliferation of mesenchymal cells. In low concentrations, it induces the synthesis and secretion of PDGF and is therefore indirectly mitogenic. However, at high concentrations, it is growth inhibitory because it blocks the expression of PDGF receptors. TGF-β also stimulates fibroblast chemotaxis and the production of collagen and fibronectin by cells, while at the same time inhibiting degradation of the extracellular matrix by metalloproteinases. All these effects tend to favor fibrogenesis, and *TGF-β is increasingly implicated in the fibrosis elicited in chronic inflammatory states.*

■ *VEGF* is actually a series of dimeric glycoprotein isoforms with partial homology to PDGF. VEGF activity was originally isolated from tumors, where it has a central role in the growth of tumor angiogenesis. It also promotes angiogenesis in normal embryonic development, in healing wounds, and in chronic inflammatory states, and it is responsible for a marked increase in vascular permeability. It is this latter activity that leads to increased deposition of plasma proteins (e.g., fibrinogen) in the extracellular matrix and provides a provisional stroma for fibroblast and endothelial cell ingrowth. The receptors for VEGF are expressed only on endothelial cells, so effects on other cell types are all indirect.

■ *Cytokines* (discussed in Chapter 2 as mediators of inflammation) are also in many cases growth factors. IL-1 and TNF, for example, induce fibroblast proliferation. They are also chemotactic for fibroblasts and stimulate the synthesis of collagen and collagenase by these cells. The net results of their actions tend to be fibrogenic.

WOUND HEALING

Wound healing is a complex but generally orderly process. Sequential waves of specialized cell types first clear the inciting injury and then progressively build the scaffolding to fill in any resulting defect. The events are orchestrated by an interplay of soluble growth factors and ECM; physical factors, including the forces generated by changes in cell shape, also contribute. Wound healing may ultimately be reduced to a sequence of processes (Fig. 3–13) that we have previously discussed:

■ Induction of an acute inflammatory response by the initial injury
■ Parenchymal cell regeneration (where possible)
■ Migration and proliferation of both parenchymal and connective tissue cells
■ Synthesis of ECM proteins
■ Remodeling of parenchymal elements to restore tissue function
■ Remodeling of connective tissue to achieve wound strength

Here, we specifically describe the healing of skin wounds. This is a process involving both epithelial regeneration and

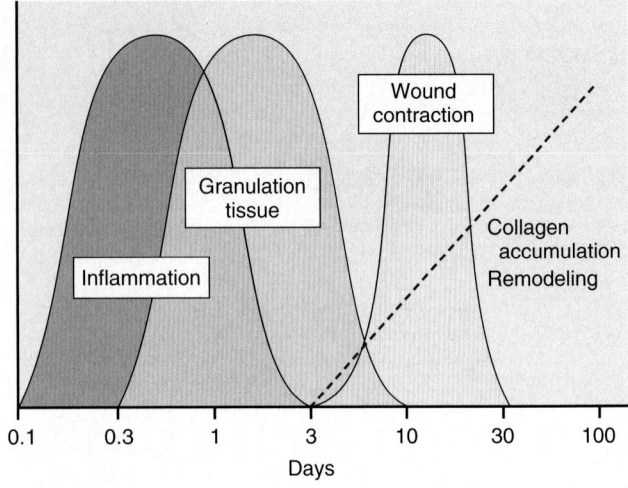

Figure 3–13 ■

The orderly phases of wound healing. (Modified from Clark RA: In Goldsmith LA [ed]: Physiology, Biochemistry, and Molecular Biology of the Skin, 2nd ed, Vol I. New York, Oxford University Press, 1991, p 577.)

the formation of connective tissue scar and is thus illustrative of the general principles that apply to wound healing in all tissues. However, one should be aware that each different tissue in the body has specific cells and features that modify the basic scheme discussed here.

Healing by First Intention

One of the simplest examples of wound repair is the healing of a clean, uninfected surgical incision approximated by surgical sutures (Fig. 3–14). This is referred to as *primary union*, or *healing by first intention.* The incision causes only focal disruption of epithelial basement membrane continuity and death of a relatively few epithelial and connective tissue cells. As a result, epithelial regeneration predominates over fibrosis. The narrow incisional space rapidly fills with fibrin-clotted blood; dehydration at the surface produces a scab to cover and protect the healing repair site.

Within 24 hours, neutrophils are seen at the incision margin, migrating toward the fibrin clot. Basal cells at the cut edge of the epidermis begin to exhibit increased mitotic activity. Within 24 to 48 hours, epithelial cells from both edges have begun to migrate and proliferate along the dermis, depositing basement membrane components as they progress. The cells meet in the midline beneath the surface scab, yielding a thin but continuous epithelial layer.

By day 3, neutrophils have been largely replaced by macrophages, and granulation tissue progressively invades the incision space. Collagen fibers are now evident at the incision margins, but these are vertically oriented and do not bridge the incision. Epithelial cell proliferation continues, yielding a thickened epidermal covering layer.

By day 5, neovascularization reaches its peak as granulation tissue fills the incisional space. Collagen fibrils become more abundant and begin to bridge the incision. The epidermis recovers its normal thickness as differentiation of

HEALING BY FIRST INTENTION   HEALING BY SECOND INTENTION

24 hours
—Scab
—Neutrophils
—Clot

3 to 7 days
—Mitoses
—Granulation tissue
—Macrophage
—Fibroblast
—New capillary

Weeks
—Fibrous union

Wound contraction

Figure 3-14

Steps in wound healing by first intention *(left)* and second intention *(right)*. In the latter, the resultant scar is much smaller than the original wound, owing to wound contraction.

surface cells yields a mature epidermal architecture with surface keratinization.

During the second week, there is continued collagen accumulation and fibroblast proliferation. The leukocyte infiltrate, edema, and increased vascularity are substantially diminished. The long process of "blanching" begins, accomplished by increasing collagen deposition within the incisional scar and the regression of vascular channels.

By the end of the first month, the scar comprises a cellular connective tissue largely devoid of inflammatory cells and covered by an essentially normal epidermis. However, the dermal appendages destroyed in the line of the incision are permanently lost. The tensile strength of the wound increases with time, as described later.

Healing by Second Intention

When cell or tissue loss is more extensive, as in infarction, inflammatory ulceration, abscess formation, or even just large wounds, the reparative process is more complex. In these situations, regeneration of parenchymal cells alone cannot restore the original architecture. As a result, there is extensive ingrowth of granulation tissue from the wound margin, followed in time by accumulation of ECM and scarring. This form of healing is referred to as *secondary union,* or *healing by second intention* (see Fig. 3-14).

Secondary healing differs from primary healing in several respects:

■ *Large tissue defects intrinsically have a greater volume of necrotic debris, exudate, and fibrin that must be removed.* Consequently, the inflammatory reaction is more intense, with greater potential for secondary, inflammation-mediated, injury (Chapter 2).

■ *Much larger amounts of granulation tissue are formed.* Larger defects accrue a greater volume of granulation tissue to fill in the gaps in the stromal architecture and provide the underlying framework for the regrowth of tissue epithelium. A greater volume of granulation tissue generally results in a greater mass of scar tissue.

■ Secondary healing exhibits the phenomenon of *wound contraction.* Within 6 weeks, for example, large skin defects may be reduced to 5% to 10% of their original size, largely by contraction. This process has been ascribed to the presence of *myofibroblasts,* modified fibroblasts exhibiting many of the ultrastructural and functional features of contractile smooth muscle cells.

Wound Strength

Carefully sutured wounds have approximately 70% of the strength of unwounded skin, largely because of the placement of the sutures. When sutures are removed, usually at 1 week, wound strength is approximately 10% of that of unwounded skin, but this increases rapidly over the next 4 weeks. The recovery of tensile strength results from collagen synthesis exceeding degradation during the first 2 months, and from structural modifications of collagen (e.g., cross-linking and increased fiber size) when synthesis declines at later times. Wound strength reaches approximately 70% to 80% of normal by 3 months but usually does not substantially improve beyond that point.

PATHOLOGIC ASPECTS OF REPAIR

In wound healing, normal cell growth and fibrosis may be altered by a variety of influences, frequently reducing the quality or adequacy of the reparative process. These factors may be extrinsic (e.g., infection) or intrinsic to the injured tissue:

■ *Infection* is the single most important cause of delay in healing, by prolonging the inflammation phase of the process and potentially increasing the local tissue injury. *Nutrition* has profound effects on wound healing; protein deficiency, for example, and particularly vitamin C deficiency, inhibit collagen synthesis and retard healing. *Glucocorticoids* (steroids) have well-documented anti-inflammatory effects, and their administration may result in poor wound strength owing to diminished fibrosis. In some instances, however, the anti-inflammatory effects of glucocorticoids are desirable. For example, in corneal infections, glucocorticoids are sometimes prescribed (along with antibiotics) to reduce the likelihood of opacity that may result from collagen deposition. *Mechanical factors* such as increased local pressure or torsion may cause wounds to pull apart, or *dehisce. Poor perfusion,*

due either to arteriosclerosis or to obstructed venous drainage, also impairs healing. Finally, *foreign bodies* such as fragments of steel, glass, or even bone impede healing.

■ *The type (and volume) of tissue injured* is a critical factor. *Complete repair can occur only in tissues composed of stable and labile cells;* even then, extensive injury will likely result in incomplete tissue regeneration and at least partial loss of function. *Injury to tissues composed of permanent cells must inevitably result in scarring* with, at most, attempts at functional compensation by the remaining viable elements. Such is the case with healing of a myocardial infarction.

■ *The location of the injury,* or the character of the tissue in which the injury occurs, is also important. For example, *inflammations arising in tissue spaces (e.g., pleural, peritoneal, synovial cavities) develop extensive exudates.* Subsequent repair may occur by digestion of the exudate, initiated by the proteolytic enzymes of leukocytes and resorption of the liquefied exudate. This is called *resolution,* and in the absence of cellular necrosis, the normal tissue architecture is generally restored. However, in the setting of larger accumulations, the exudate undergoes *organization*—granulation tissue grows into the exudate, followed ultimately by fibrous scar.

■ *Aberrations of cell growth and ECM production may occur even in what begins as normal wound healing.* For example, the accumulation of exuberant amounts of collagen can give rise to prominent, raised scars known as *keloids* (Fig. 3–15). There appears to be a heritable predisposition to keloid formation, and the condition is more common in blacks. Healing wounds may also generate excessive granulation tissue that protrudes above the level of the surrounding skin and in fact hinders re-epithelialization. This is called *exuberant granulation,* or *proud flesh,* and restoration of epithelial continuity requires cautery or surgical resection of the granulation tissue.

Figure 3–15 ■

Keloid. (From Murphy GF, Herzberg AJ: Atlas of Dermatology. Philadelphia, WB Saunders, 1996.)

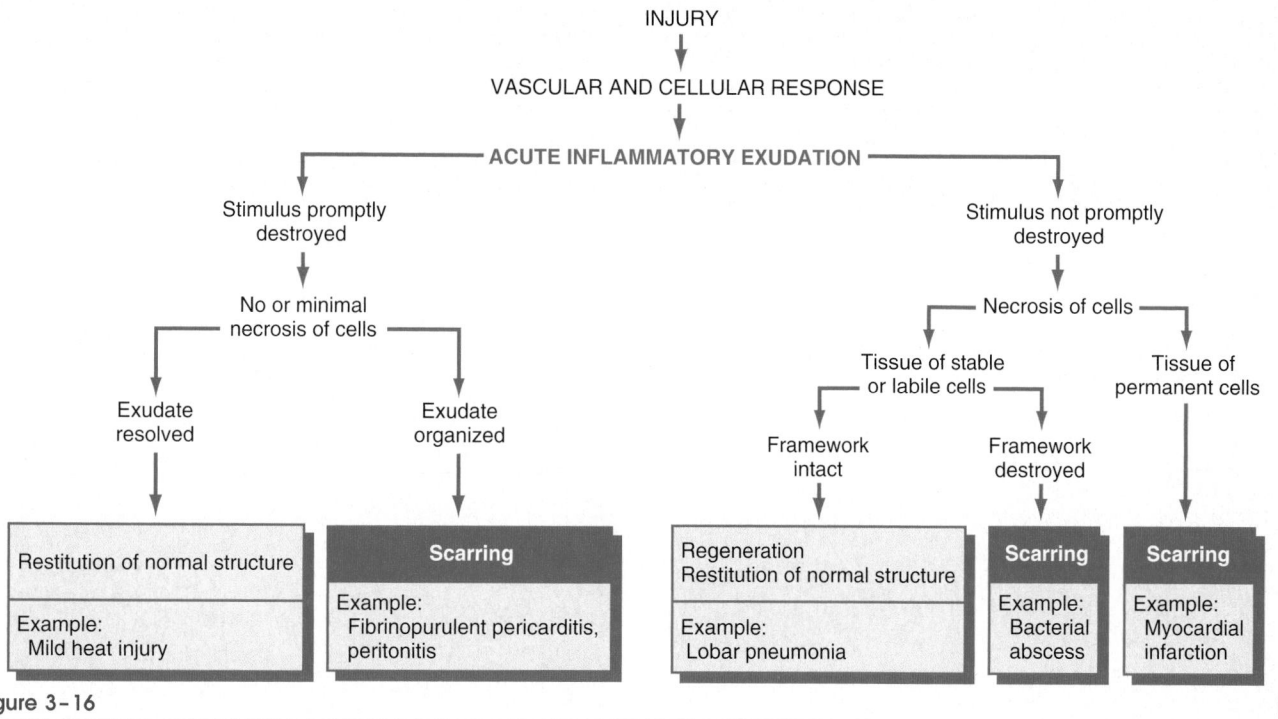

Figure 3–16

Pathways of reparative responses after acute injury.

■ The mechanisms underlying the disabling fibrosis associated with chronic inflammatory diseases such as rheumatoid arthritis, pulmonary fibrosis, and cirrhosis are essentially identical to those that are involved in normal wound healing. However, in these diseases, persistent stimulation of fibrogenesis results from chronic immune/autoimmune reactions that sustain the synthesis and secretion of growth factors, fibrogenic cytokines, and proteases. For example, collagen degradation by collagenases, normally important in wound remodeling, is responsible for much of the joint destruction seen in rheumatoid arthritis (Chapter 5).

OVERVIEW OF THE INFLAMMATORY-REPARATIVE RESPONSE

Figure 3–16 is an overview of the processes that we have covered in the first three chapters (injury, inflammation, and repair) and re-emphasizes certain important concepts. Not all injuries result in permanent damage; some are resolved with almost perfect restoration of structure and function. More often—depending on the type and extent of injury, the nature of the injured tissue, and persistence of inflammatory stimuli—injury results in some degree of residual scarring. Although it is functionally imperfect, scar provides a resilient permanent patch that allows the remaining intact parenchyma to continue functioning. Occasionally, however, the scarring may be so large or so situated that it causes permanent dysfunction. In a healed myocardial infarct, for example, the fibrous tissue not only represents a loss of functioning muscle but also may serve as a nidus for arrhythmias or a focus for thrombus formation.

BIBLIOGRAPHY

Baramova E, Foidart JM: Matrix metalloproteinase family. Cell Biol Int 19:239, 1995. (The chemistry and biology of collagen degradation pathways.)

Birchmeier C, et al: Factors controlling growth, motility, and morphogenesis of normal and malignant epithelial cells. Int Rev Cytol 160:221, 1995. (A detailed overview of growth factors and their down-stream effects.)

Clark RAF, Henson PM (eds): The Molecular and Cellular Biology of Wound Repair. New York, Plenum, 1996. (A comprehensive volume on wound repair.)

Cross MJ, Claesson-Welsh L: FGF and VEGF function in angiogenesis; signaling pathways, biologic responses and therapeutic inhibition. Trends Pharmacol Sci 22:201, 2001. (Reviews of molecular control of angiogenesis.)

Dvorak HF, et al: Vascular permeability factor/vascular endothelial growth factor and the significance of microvascular hyperpermeability in angiogenesis. Curr Top Microbiol Immunol 237:97, 1999. (A good summary of the chemistry and biology of VPF/VEGF.)

Elicieri BP: Integrin and growth factor receptor cross-talk. Circ Res 89:1104, 2001. (A review that emphasizes the role of integrins in cell growth.)

Hanahan D: Signaling vascular morphogenesis and maintenance. Science 277:48, 1997. (Summary of the understanding of how matrix and soluble mediators shape vascular form and function.)

Lania L, et al: Transcriptional control by cell-cycle regulators: a review. J Cell Physiol 179:134, 1999. (A succinct review of cell cycle regulation.)

O'Toole EA: Extracellular matrix and keratinocyte migration. Clin Exp Dermatol 26:525, 2001. (A review of the interplay between ECM and epithelium.)

Prockop DJ, Kivirikko KI: Collagens: molecular biology, diseases and potentials for therapy. Annu Rev Biochem 64:403, 1995. (A detailed description of the chemistry and biology of ECM.)

Rane SG, Reddy EP: Janus kinases: components of multiple signaling pathways. Oncogene 19:5662, 2000. (A good review of the JAK-STAT signaling pathways.)

Ravanti L, Kahari VM: Matrix metalloproteinases in wound repair. Int J Mol Med 6:391, 2000. (An up-to-date review of the role of MMPs in ECM remodeling as well as in cellular activation.)

Schlessinger J: Cell signaling by receptor tyrosine kinases. Cell 103: 211, 2000. (An excellent review of receptor kinase signaling in an issue devoted to multiple facets of intracellular signaling.)

Schwartz MA, Assoian RK: Integrins and cell proliferation: regulation of cyclin-dependent kinases via cytoplasmic signaling pathways. J Cell Sci 114:2553, 2001. (Another review of integrin signaling and cell cycle control.)

Singer AJ, Clark RA: Cutaneous wound healing. N Engl J Med 341:738, 1999. (An excellent and beautifully illustrated review on wound healing in the skin.)

Slavin J: Fibroblast growth factors: at the heart of angiogenesis. Cell Biol Int 19:431, 1995. (A good review of the biology and chemistry of the FGFs.)

Yamaguchi Y, Yoshikawa K: Cutaneous wound healing: an update, J Dermatol 28:521, 2001. (A modern view of wound healing.)

4

Hemodynamic Disorders, Thrombosis, and Shock

RICHARD N. MITCHELL, MD, PhD
RAMZI S. COTRAN, MD*

The health of cells and tissue depends not only on an *intact circulation* to deliver oxygen and remove wastes but also on *normal fluid homeostasis*; the major causes of morbidity and mortality in developed countries are associated, in one way or another, with failure to maintain normal fluid status. *Normal homeostasis encompasses maintenance of vessel wall integrity as well as intravascular pressure and osmolarity within certain physiologic ranges.* Changes in vascular volume, pressure, or protein content or alterations in endothelial function affect the net movement of water across the vascular wall. Such water extravasation into the interstitial spaces is called *edema* and has different import depending on its location. In the lower extremities, edema mainly causes swelling; in the lungs, edema causes water to fill

alveoli, leading to difficulty breathing. *Normal fluid homeostasis also means maintaining blood as a liquid until such time as injury necessitates clot formation.* Clotting that is inappropriate *(thrombosis)* or migration of clots *(embolism)* obstructs blood flow to tissues and leads to cell death *(infarction)*. Conversely, inability to clot after vascular injury results in *hemorrhage*; local bleeding can compromise regional tissue perfusion, while more extensive hemorrhage can result in hypotension *(shock)* and death. Abnormal fluid homeostasis underlies three of the most important causes of pathologic lesions in Western society, that is, myocardial infarction, pulmonary embolism, and cerebrovascular accident (stroke). Thus, the hemodynamic disorders described in this chapter are major factors in much of human disease.

*Deceased

EDEMA

Approximately 60% of lean body weight is water, with two thirds intracellular and the remainder in extracellular compartments, mostly as interstitial fluid (only some 5% of total body water is in blood plasma). The term *edema* signifies increased fluid in the interstitial tissue spaces. In addition, depending on the site, collections of fluid in the different body cavities are variously designated *hydrothorax*, *hydropericardium*, or *hydroperitoneum* (the last is more commonly called *ascites*). *Anasarca* is a severe and generalized edema with profound subcutaneous tissue swelling.

Table 4–1 lists the pathophysiologic categories of edema. The mechanisms of inflammatory edema are largely related to increased vascular permeability and are discussed in Chapter 2; the *noninflammatory causes of edema* are described in further detail later.

In general, the opposing effects of vascular hydrostatic pressure and plasma colloid osmotic pressure are the major factors that govern movement of fluid between vascular and interstitial spaces. Normally, the exit of fluid into the interstitium from the arteriolar end of the microcirculation is nearly balanced by inflow at the venular end; a small residual amount of excess interstitial fluid is drained by the lym-

Figure 4–1

Factors affecting fluid transit across capillary walls (see also Fig. 2–3). Capillary hydrostatic and osmotic forces are normally balanced so that there is no *net* loss or gain of fluid across the capillary bed. However, *increased* hydrostatic pressure or *diminished* plasma osmotic pressure leads to a net accumulation of extravascular fluid (edema). As the interstitial fluid pressure increases, tissue lymphatics remove much of the excess volume, eventually returning it to the circulation via the thoracic duct. If the ability of the lymphatics to drain tissue is exceeded, persistent tissue edema results.

phatics. Either increased capillary pressure or diminished colloid osmotic pressure can result in increased interstitial fluid (Fig. 4–1). As extravascular fluid accumulates in either case, the increased tissue hydrostatic and plasma colloid osmotic pressures eventually achieve a new equilibrium, and water re-enters the venules. Excess interstitial edema fluid is removed by lymphatic drainage, ultimately returning to the bloodstream via the thoracic duct (see Fig. 4–1); clearly, lymphatic obstruction (e.g., due to scarring or tumor) can also impair fluid drainage and cause edema. Finally, a primary retention of sodium (and its obligatory associated water) in renal disease also results in edema.

The edema fluid occurring in hydrodynamic derangements is typically a protein-poor *transudate*, with a specific gravity below 1.012. Conversely, because of the increased vascular permeability, inflammatory edema is a protein-rich *exudate* with a specific gravity that is usually over 1.020.

Increased Hydrostatic Pressure. *Localized increase in intravascular pressure* may result from impaired venous return—for example, secondary to deep venous thrombosis in the lower extremities with edema restricted to the affected leg. *Generalized increases in venous pressure*, with resultant systemic edema, occur most commonly in *congestive heart failure* (Chapter 11) affecting right ventricular cardiac function. Although increased venous hydrostatic pressure is important, the pathogenesis of cardiac edema is more complex (Fig. 4–2). Congestive heart failure is associated with reduced cardiac output and therefore reduced renal perfusion. Renal hypoperfusion in turn triggers the renin-angiotensin-aldosterone axis, inducing sodium and water retention by the kidneys (*secondary aldosteronism*). This is intended to increase intravascular volume and thereby improve cardiac output with restoration of normal renal perfusion. However, if the failing heart cannot

Table 4–1. PATHOPHYSIOLOGIC CATEGORIES OF EDEMA

Increased Hydrostatic Pressure
Impaired venous return
  Congestive heart failure
  Constrictive pericarditis
  Ascites (liver cirrhosis)
  Venous obstruction or compression
    Thrombosis
    External pressure (e.g., mass)
    Lower extremity inactivity with prolonged dependency
Arteriolar dilation
  Heat
  Neurohumoral dysregulation

Reduced Plasma Osmotic Pressure (Hypoproteinemia)
Protein-losing glomerulopathies (nephrotic syndrome)
Liver cirrhosis (ascites)
Malnutrition
Protein-losing gastroenteropathy

Lymphatic Obstruction
Inflammatory
Neoplastic
Postsurgical
Postirradiation

Sodium Retention
Excessive salt intake with renal insufficiency
Increased tubular reabsorption of sodium
  Renal hypoperfusion
  Increased renin-angiotensin-aldosterone secretion

Inflammation
Acute inflammation
Chronic inflammation
Angiogenesis

Modified from Leaf A, Cotran RS: Renal Pathophysiology, 3rd ed. New York, Oxford University Press, 1985, p 146.

Figure 4–2

Sequence of events leading to systemic edema either due to primary heart failure or due to reduced plasma osmotic pressure (as in malnutrition, diminished hepatic protein synthesis, or loss of protein due to the nephrotic syndrome). ADH, antidiuretic hormone; GFR, glomerular filtration rate.

increase cardiac output, the extra fluid load results in increased venous pressure and, eventually, edema. Unless cardiac output is restored or renal water retention reduced (e.g., by salt restriction, diuretics, or aldosterone antagonists), a cycle of renal fluid retention and worsening edema ensues. Although discussed here in the context of edema in congestive heart failure, it should be understood that salt restriction, diuretics, and aldosterone antagonists are also of value in the management of generalized edema resulting from a variety of other causes.

Reduced Plasma Osmotic Pressure. This can result from excessive loss or reduced synthesis of albumin, the serum protein most responsible for maintaining colloid osmotic pressure. An important cause of albumin loss is the *nephrotic syndrome* (Chapter 14), characterized by a leaky glomerular capillary wall and generalized edema. Reduced albumin synthesis occurs in the setting of diffuse liver diseases (e.g., cirrhosis; Chapter 16) or as a consequence of protein malnutrition (Chapter 8). In each case, reduced plasma osmotic pressure leads to a net movement of fluid into the interstitial tissues and a resultant plasma volume contraction. Predictably, with reduced intravascular volume, renal hypoperfusion with secondary

aldosteronism follows. Unfortunately, the retained salt and water cannot correct the plasma volume deficit, because the primary defect of low serum proteins persists. As with congestive heart failure, edema precipitated by low protein is exacerbated by secondary salt and fluid retention.

Lymphatic Obstruction. Impaired lymphatic drainage and consequent *lymphedema* is usually localized; it can result from inflammatory or neoplastic obstruction. For example, the parasitic infection *filariasis* often causes massive lymphatic and lymph node fibrosis in the inguinal region. The resultant edema of the external genitalia and lower limbs is so extreme that it is called *elephantiasis*. Cancer of the breast may be treated by removal and/or irradiation of the breast and the associated axillary lymph nodes. Resection of the lymphatic channels as well as scarring related to the surgery and radiation can result in severe edema of the arm. In carcinoma of the breast, infiltration and obstruction of superficial lymphatics can cause edema of the overlying skin, giving rise to the so-called peau d'orange (orange peel) appearance. Such a finely pitted appearance results from an accentuation of depressions in the skin at the site of hair follicles.

Sodium and Water Retention. These are clearly contributory factors in several forms of edema; however, salt retention may also be a primary cause of edema. Increased salt, with the obligate accompanying water, causes both increased hydrostatic pressure (due to expansion of the intravascular fluid volume) and diminished vascular colloid osmotic pressure. Salt retention may occur with any acute reduction of renal function, including *poststreptococcal glomerulonephritis* and *acute renal failure* (Chapter 14).

MORPHOLOGY

Edema is most easily recognized grossly; microscopically, edema fluid generally is manifest only as subtle cell swelling, with clearing and separation of the extracellular matrix elements. Although any organ or tissue in the body may be involved, edema is most commonly encountered in subcutaneous tissues, lungs, and brain. Severe, generalized edema is also called **anasarca.**

Subcutaneous edema may have different distributions depending on the cause. It can be diffuse, or it may be more prominent in the regions with the highest hydrostatic pressures. In the latter case, the edema distribution is influenced by gravity and is termed **dependent. Edema of the dependent parts of the body** (e.g., the legs when standing, the sacrum when recumbent) **is a prominent feature of cardiac failure, particularly of the right ventricle.** Edema due to **renal dysfunction** or **nephrotic syndrome** is generally more severe than cardiac edema **and affects all parts of the body equally.** However, it may be initially manifest in tissues with a loose connective tissue matrix, such as the eyelids, causing **periorbital edema.** Finger pressure over significantly edematous subcutaneous tissue displaces the interstitial fluid and leaves a finger-shaped depression, so-called **pitting edema.**

Pulmonary edema is a common clinical problem (Chapter 11) most frequently seen in the setting of left ventricular failure (where it often has a dependent distribution in the lungs) but also occurring in renal failure, adult respiratory distress syndrome (ARDS; Chapter 13), pulmonary infections, and hypersensitivity reactions. The lungs are typically two to three times their normal weight, and sectioning reveals frothy, sometimes blood-tinged fluid representing a mixture of air, edema fluid, and extravasated red cells.

Edema of the brain may be localized to sites of focal injury (e.g., abscesses or neoplasm) or may be generalized, as in encephalitis, hypertensive crises, or obstruction to the brain's venous outflow. Trauma may result in local or generalized edema, depending on the nature and extent of the injury. With generalized edema, the brain is grossly swollen with narrowed sulci and distended gyri showing signs of flattening against the unyielding skull (Chapter 23).

Clinical Correlation. The effects of edema may range from merely annoying to fatal. Subcutaneous tissue edema in cardiac or renal failure is important primarily because it points to underlying disease; however, when significant, it can impair wound healing or the clearance of infection. On the other hand, pulmonary edema can cause death by interfering with normal ventilatory function. Not only does fluid collect in the alveolar septa around capillaries and impede oxygen diffusion, but edema fluid in the alveolar spaces also creates a favorable environment for bacterial infection. Brain edema is serious and can be rapidly fatal; if severe, brain substance can *herniate* (be pushed out) through, for example, the foramen magnum, or the brain stem vascular supply can be compressed. Either condition can injure the medullary centers and cause death (Chapter 23).

HYPEREMIA AND CONGESTION

Both the terms *hyperemia* and *congestion* indicate a local increased volume of blood in a particular tissue. Hyperemia is an *active process* resulting from augmented blood flow due to arteriolar dilation—for example, at sites of inflammation or in skeletal muscle during exercise. The affected tissue is redder because of engorgement with oxygenated blood. Congestion is a *passive process* resulting from impaired venous return from a tissue. It may occur systemically, as in cardiac failure, or it may be local, resulting from an isolated venous obstruction. The tissue has a blue-red color (*cyanosis*), especially as worsening congestion leads to accumulation of deoxygenated hemoglobin in the affected tissues.

Congestion of capillary beds is closely related to the development of edema, so that congestion and edema commonly occur together. In long-standing congestion, called *chronic passive congestion*, the stasis of poorly oxygenated blood causes chronic hypoxia, which can result in parenchymal cell degeneration or death, sometimes with microscopic scarring. Capillary rupture at these sites of chronic congestion may also cause small foci of hemorrhage; breakdown and phagocytosis of the red cell debris can eventually result in small clusters of hemosiderin-laden macrophages.

MORPHOLOGY

Cut surfaces of hyperemic or congested tissues are hemorrhagic and wet. Microscopically, **acute pulmonary congestion** is characterized by alveolar capillaries engorged with blood; there may also be associated alveolar septal edema and/or focal minute intra-alveolar hemorrhage. In **chronic pulmonary congestion,** the septa become thickened and fibrotic, and the alveolar spaces may contain numerous hemosiderin-laden macrophages ("heart failure cells"). In **acute hepatic congestion,** the central vein and sinusoids are distended with blood, and there may even be central hepatocyte degeneration; the periportal hepatocytes, better

Figure 4-3   ■

Liver with chronic passive congestion and hemorrhagic necrosis. *A*, Central areas are red and slightly depressed compared with the surrounding tan viable parenchyma, forming a "nutmeg liver" pattern (so called because it resembles the alternating pattern of light and dark seen when a whole nutmeg is cut). *B*, Centrilobular necrosis with degenerating hepatocytes and hemorrhage. (Courtesy of Dr. James Crawford, Department of Pathology, Brigham and Women's Hospital, Boston.)

oxygenated because of their proximity to hepatic arterioles, experience less severe hypoxia and may develop only fatty change. In **chronic passive congestion of the liver,** the central regions of the hepatic lobules are grossly red-brown and slightly depressed (owing to a loss of cells) and are accentuated against the surrounding zones of uncongested tan, sometimes fatty, liver ("nutmeg liver"; Fig. 4-3A). Microscopically, there is evidence of centrilobular necrosis with hepatocyte drop-out and hemorrhage, including hemosiderin-laden macrophages (Fig. 4-3B). In severe and long-standing hepatic congestion (most commonly associated with heart failure), there may even be grossly evident hepatic fibrosis ("cardiac cirrhosis"). It is important to note that because the central portion of the hepatic lobule is the last to receive blood, centrilobular necrosis can also occur whenever there is reduced hepatic blood flow (including shock from any cause); there need not be previous hepatic congestion.

HEMORRHAGE

Hemorrhage generally indicates extravasation of blood due to rupture of blood vessels. As described previously, capillary bleeding can occur under conditions of chronic congestion, and an increased tendency to hemorrhage from usually insignificant injury is seen in a wide variety of clinical disorders collectively called *hemorrhagic diatheses* (Chapter 12). However, rupture of a large artery or vein is almost always due to vascular injury, including trauma, atherosclerosis, or inflammatory or neoplastic erosion of the vessel wall.

■ Hemorrhage may be external or may be enclosed within a tissue; the accumulation is referred to as a *hematoma*. Hematomas may be relatively insignificant (as in a

bruise) or may accumulate sufficient blood to cause death (e.g., a massive retroperitoneal hematoma resulting from rupture of a dissecting aortic aneurysm; Chapter 10).
■ Minute (1- to 2-mm) hemorrhages into skin, mucous membranes, or serosal surfaces are called *petechiae* (Fig. 4-4A) and are typically associated with locally increased intravascular pressure, low platelet counts *(thrombocytopenia),* defective platelet function, or clotting factor deficiencies.
■ Slightly larger (3- to 5-mm) hemorrhages, called *purpuras,* may be associated with many of the same disorders that cause petechiae, as well as in the settings of trauma, vascular inflammation *(vasculitis),* or increased vascular fragility.
■ Larger (1- to 2-cm) subcutaneous hematomas (bruises) are called *ecchymoses.* The erythrocytes in these local hemorrhages are degraded and phagocytosed by macrophages; the hemoglobin (red-blue color) is then enzymatically converted into bilirubin (blue-green color) and eventually into hemosiderin (golden-brown), accounting for the characteristic color changes in a hematoma.
■ Large accumulations of blood in one or another of the body cavities are called *hemothorax, hemopericardium, hemoperitoneum,* or *hemarthrosis* (in joints). Patients with extensive hemorrhages occasionally develop jaundice from the massive breakdown of red cells and systemic release of bilirubin.

The clinical significance of hemorrhage depends on the volume and rate of blood loss. Rapid removal of up to 20% of the blood volume or slow losses of even larger amounts may have little impact in healthy adults; greater losses, however, may result in *hemorrhagic (hypovolemic) shock* (discussed later). The site of hemorrhage is also important; bleeding that would be trivial in the subcutaneous tissues may cause death if located in the brain stem (Fig. 4-4B). Finally, loss of iron, and subsequent iron deficiency anemia, occurs in the setting of chronic or recurrent external blood loss (e.g., a peptic ulcer or menstrual bleeding). In contrast, when red cells are retained, as in hemorrhage into body

Figure 4-4 ■

A, Punctate petechial hemorrhages of the colonic mucosa, seen here as a consequence of thrombocytopenia. *B,* Fatal intracerebral bleed. Even relatively inconsequential volumes of hemorrhage in a critical location, or into a closed space (such as the cranium), can have fatal outcomes.

cavities or tissues, the iron can be reutilized for hemoglobin synthesis.

HEMOSTASIS AND THROMBOSIS

Normal hemostasis results from well-regulated processes that maintain blood in a fluid, clot-free state in normal vessels while inducing the rapid formation of a localized *hemostatic plug* at the site of vascular injury. The pathologic converse to hemostasis is *thrombosis*; it can be thought of as the formation of a blood clot *(thrombus)* in uninjured vessels, or thrombotic occlusion of a vessel after relatively minor injury. Both hemostasis and thrombosis are dependent on three general components: *the vascular wall, platelets, and the coagulation cascade.* We begin our discussion with the process of normal hemostasis and a description of how it is regulated.

Normal Hemostasis

The general sequence of events in hemostasis at a site of vascular injury is shown in Figure 4–5.

■ After initial injury, there is a brief period of *arteriolar vasoconstriction*, largely attributable to reflex neurogenic mechanisms and augmented by the local secretion of factors such as *endothelin* (a potent endothelium-derived vasoconstrictor) (see Fig. 4–5*A*). The effect is transient, however, and bleeding would resume were it not for activation of the platelet and coagulation systems.
■ *Endothelial injury* also exposes highly thrombogenic subendothelial extracellular matrix (ECM), which allows platelets to adhere and become activated, that is, undergo a shape change and release secretory granules. Within minutes, the secreted products have recruited additional platelets *(aggregation)* to form a hemostatic plug; this is the process of *primary hemostasis* (see Fig. 4–5*B*).

■ *Tissue factor*, a membrane-bound procoagulant factor synthesized by endothelium, is also released at the site of injury. It acts in conjunction with the secreted platelet factors to activate the coagulation cascade, culminating in *activation of thrombin*. In turn, thrombin cleaves circulating fibrinogen into insoluble *fibrin*, creating a fibrin meshwork deposition. Thrombin also induces further platelet recruitment and granule release. This *secondary hemostasis* sequence (see Fig. 4–5*C*) takes longer than the formation of the initial platelet plug.
■ Polymerized fibrin and platelet aggregates form a solid, *permanent plug* to prevent any further hemorrhage. At this stage, counter-regulatory mechanisms (e.g., *tissue plasminogen activator* [*t-PA*]) are set into motion to limit the hemostatic plug to the site of injury (see Fig. 4–5*D*).

The following sections discuss these events in greater detail.

ENDOTHELIUM

Endothelial cells modulate several (and frequently opposing) aspects of normal hemostasis. On the one hand, at baseline they exhibit antiplatelet, anticoagulant, and fibrinolytic properties; on the other hand, they are capable (after injury or activation) of exerting procoagulant functions (Fig. 4–6). Recall that endothelium may be activated by infectious agents, by hemodynamic factors, by plasma mediators, and (most significantly) by cytokines (Chapter 2). The balance between endothelial anti- and prothrombotic activities determines whether thrombus formation, propagation, or dissolution occurs.

Antithrombotic Properties

■ *Antiplatelet effects.* An intact endothelium prevents platelets from meeting the highly thrombogenic subendothelial ECM. Nonactivated platelets do not adhere to the endothelium, a property intrinsic to the plasma membrane of endothelium. Moreover, if platelets are activated (e.g., after focal endothelial injury), they are inhibited from adhering to the surrounding uninjured endothelium

A. VASOCONSTRICTION

B. PRIMARY HEMOSTASIS

C. SECONDARY HEMOSTASIS

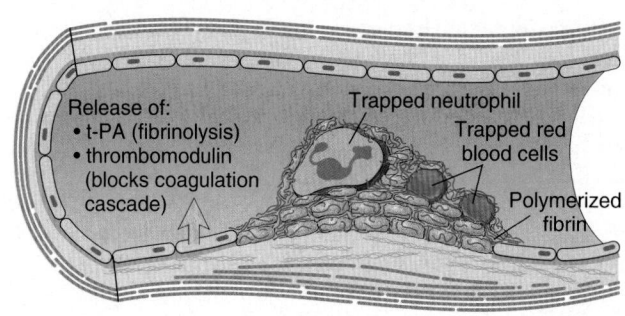

D. ANTITHROMBOTIC COUNTER-REGULATION

Figure 4–5 ■

Diagrammatic representation of the normal hemostatic process. *A,* After vascular injury, local neurohumoral factors induce a transient vasoconstriction. *B,* Platelets adhere to exposed extracellular matrix (ECM) via von Willebrand factor (vWF) and are activated, undergoing a shape change and granule release; released adenosine diphosphate (ADP) and thromboxane A_2 (TXA$_2$) lead to further platelet aggregation, to form the primary hemostatic plug. *C,* Local activation of the coagulation cascade (involving tissue factor and platelet phospholipids) results in fibrin polymerization, "cementing" the platelets into a definitive secondary hemostatic plug. *D,* Counter-regulatory mechanisms, such as release of t-PA (tissue plasminogen activator, a fibrinolytic product) and thrombomodulin (interfering with the coagulation cascade), limit the hemostatic process to the site of injury.

by endothelial prostacyclin (PGI$_2$) and nitric oxide (Chapter 2). Both mediators are potent vasodilators and inhibitors of platelet aggregation; their synthesis by endothelial cells is stimulated by a number of factors (e.g., thrombin and cytokines) produced during coagulation.

Endothelial cells also elaborate adenosine diphosphatase, which degrades adenosine diphosphate (ADP) and further inhibits platelet aggregation (see later).

■ *Anticoagulant properties.* These are mediated by membrane-associated, heparin-like molecules and

Figure 4-6 ■

Schematic illustration of some of the pro- and anticoagulant activities of endothelial cells. Not shown are the pro- and antifibrinolytic properties (see text). NO, nitric oxide; PGI$_2$, prostacyclin; t-PA, tissue plasminogen activator; vWF, von Willebrand factor.

thrombomodulin, a specific thrombin receptor (see Fig. 4–6). *The heparin-like molecules* act indirectly; they are cofactors that allow *antithrombin III* to inactivate thrombin, factor Xa, and several other coagulation factors (see later). *Thrombomodulin* also acts indirectly; it binds to thrombin, converting it from a procoagulant to an anticoagulant capable of activating the anticoagulant protein C. Activated protein C, in turn, inhibits clotting by proteolytic cleavage of factors Va and VIIIa; it requires protein S, synthesized by endothelial cells, as a cofactor.

■ *Fibrinolytic properties.* Endothelial cells synthesize *t-PA*, promoting fibrinolytic activity to clear fibrin deposits from endothelial surfaces (see Fig. 4–5D).

Prothrombotic Properties. While endothelial cells exhibit properties that can limit blood clotting, they are also prothrombotic, affecting platelets, coagulation proteins, and the fibrinolytic system. Recall that endothelial injury leads to adhesion of platelets to subendothelial collagen; this is facilitated by *von Willebrand factor (vWF)*, an essential cofactor for binding platelets to collagen and other surfaces. It should be noted that vWF is a product of normal endothelium, found in the plasma; it is not specifically synthesized after endothelial injury. Endothelial cells are also induced by cytokines (e.g., tumor necrosis factor [TNF] or interleukin 1 [IL-1]) or bacterial endotoxin to secrete *tissue factor*, which, as we shall see, activates the extrinsic clotting pathway. By binding to activated coagulation factors IXa and Xa (see later), endothelial cells further augment the catalytic activities of these proteins. Finally, endothelial cells also secrete inhibitors of *plasminogen activator (PAIs),* which depress fibrinolysis.

In summary, intact endothelial cells serve primarily to inhibit platelet adherence and blood clotting. However, injury or activation of endothelial cells results in a procoagulant phenotype that contributes to localized clot formation.

PLATELETS

Platelets play a central role in normal hemostasis. When circulating, they are membrane-bound smooth discs expressing a number of glycoprotein receptors of the integrin family. Platelets contain two specific types of granules. *α-Granules* express the adhesion molecule P-selectin on their membranes (Chapter 2) and contain fibrinogen, fibronectin, factors V and VIII, platelet factor 4 (a heparin-binding chemokine), platelet-derived growth factor (PDGF), and transforming growth factor α (TGF-α). The other granules are *dense* bodies, or δ granules, which contain adenine nucleotides (ADP and ATP), ionized calcium, histamine, serotonin, and epinephrine.

After vascular injury, platelets encounter ECM constituents that are normally sequestered beneath an intact endothelium; these include collagen (most important), proteoglycans, fibronectin, and other adhesive glycoproteins. *On contact with ECM, platelets undergo three general reactions: (1) adhesion and shape change, (2) secretion (release reaction), and (3) aggregation (see Fig. 4–5B).*

■ *Platelet adhesion* to ECM is mediated largely via interactions with vWF, which acts as a bridge between platelet surface receptors (e.g., glycoprotein Ib [GpIb]) and exposed collagen (Fig. 4–7). Although platelets can

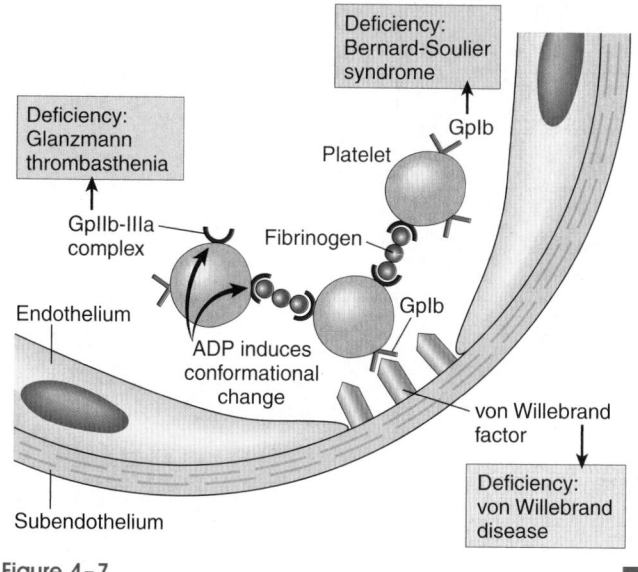

Figure 4–7 ■

Platelet adhesion and aggregation. Von Willebrand factor functions as an adhesion bridge between subendothelial collagen and the glycoprotein Ib (GpIb) platelet receptor. Aggregation is accomplished by fibrinogen's binding to platelet GpIIb-IIIa receptors and bridging many platelets together. Congenital deficiencies in the various receptors or bridging molecules lead to the diseases indicated in the colored boxes. ADP, adenosine diphosphate.

adhere directly to ECM, vWF–glycoprotein Ib associations are the only interactions sufficiently strong to overcome the high shear forces of flowing blood. Genetic deficiencies of vWF (von Willebrand disease; Chapter 12) or its receptors result in serious bleeding disorders, highlighting the importance of these interactions.

■ *Secretion (release reaction)* of the contents of both types of granules occurs soon after adhesion. The process is initiated by the binding of agonists to platelet surface receptors followed by an intracellular phosphorylation cascade. The release of the dense body contents is especially important because calcium is required in the coagulation cascade, and ADP is a potent mediator of *platelet aggregation* (platelets adhering to other platelets; see later). ADP also augments further ADP release from other platelets, leading to amplification of the aggregation. Finally, platelet activation results in surface expression of a *phospholipid complex* that provides a critical nucleation and binding site for calcium and coagulation factors in the *intrinsic clotting pathway* (see later).

■ *Platelet aggregation* follows adhesion and secretion. Besides ADP, the vasoconstrictor thromboxane A_2 (TXA$_2$; Chapter 2), secreted by platelets, is also an important stimulus for platelet aggregation. ADP and TXA$_2$ set up an autocatalytic reaction leading to build-up of an enlarging platelet aggregate, the *primary hemostatic plug*. This primary aggregation is reversible, but with activation of the coagulation cascade, *thrombin* is generated. Thrombin binds to a platelet surface receptor, and with ADP and TXA$_2$ causes further aggregation. This is followed by *platelet contraction*, creating an irreversibly fused mass of platelets ("viscous metamorphosis") con-

stituting the definitive *secondary hemostatic plug*. At the same time, thrombin converts fibrinogen to *fibrin* within and about the platelet plug, essentially cementing the platelets in place (see later).

Fibrinogen is also important in platelet aggregation. ADP activation of platelets induces a conformational change of the platelet surface GpIIb-IIIa receptors so that they can bind fibrinogen. Fibrinogen then acts to connect multiple platelets together to form large aggregates (see Fig. 4–7). The importance of these interactions is demonstrated by the bleeding disorders of patients with congenitally deficient or inactive GpIIb-IIIa proteins. GpIIb-IIIa receptor antagonists are also therapeutically useful in inhibiting platelet aggregation after vascular interventions such as angioplasty.

It is worth emphasizing that the prostaglandin PGI$_2$ (synthesized by endothelium) is a vasodilator and inhibits platelet aggregation, whereas TXA$_2$ is a platelet-derived prostaglandin that activates platelet aggregation and is a potent vasoconstrictor. The interplay of PGI$_2$ and TXA$_2$ constitutes an exquisitely balanced mechanism for modulating human platelet function: in the normal state, it prevents intravascular platelet aggregation, but after endothelial injury it favors the formation of hemostatic plugs. The clinical use of aspirin (a cyclooxygenase inhibitor) in patients at risk for coronary thrombosis is related to its ability to inhibit the synthesis of TXA$_2$. In a manner similar to that of PGI$_2$, nitric oxide also acts as a vasodilator and inhibitor of platelet aggregation (see Fig. 4–6).

Both erythrocytes and leukocytes are also found in hemostatic plugs; leukocytes adhere to platelets and endothelium via adhesion molecules (Chapter 2) and contribute to the inflammatory response that accompanies thrombosis. Thrombin also contributes by directly stimulating neutrophil and monocyte adhesion, and by generating chemotactic *fibrin split products* from the cleavage of fibrinogen.

The series of platelet events can be summarized as follows (see Fig. 4–5):

■ *Platelets adhere to the ECM at sites of endothelial injury and become activated.*

■ *Upon activation, platelets secrete granule products (e.g., ADP) and synthesize TXA$_2$.*

■ *Platelets also expose phospholipid complexes important in the intrinsic coagulation pathway.*

■ *Injured or activated endothelial cells release tissue factor to activate the extrinsic coagulation cascade.*

■ *Released ADP stimulates formation of a primary hemostatic plug, which is eventually converted (via ADP, thrombin, and TXA$_2$) into a larger definitive secondary plug.*

■ *Fibrin deposition stabilizes and anchors the aggregated platelets.*

COAGULATION CASCADE

This constitutes the third component of the hemostatic process and is a major contributor to thrombosis. The pathways are schematically presented in Figure 4–8; only general principles are discussed here.

■ The coagulation cascade is essentially a series of enzymatic conversions, turning inactive proenzymes into activated enzymes and culminating in the formation of

Figure 4–8 ■

The coagulation cascade. Note the common link between the intrinsic and extrinsic pathways at the level of factor IX activation. Factors in red boxes represent inactive molecules; activated factors are indicated with a lower-case *a* and a green box. HMWK, high-molecular-weight kininogen. Not shown are the inhibitory anticoagulant pathways (see Figs. 4–6 and 4–10).

thrombin. Thrombin then converts the soluble plasma protein *fibrinogen* into the insoluble fibrous protein *fibrin.*

■ Each reaction in the pathway results from the assembly of a complex composed of an *enzyme* (activated coagulation factor), a *substrate* (proenzyme form of coagulation factor), and a *cofactor* (reaction accelerator). These components are assembled on a *phospholipid complex* and held together by *calcium ions.* Thus, clotting tends to remain localized to sites where such an assembly can occur, for example, on the surface of activated platelets. Two such reactions—the sequential conversion of factor X to Xa and then factor II (prothrombin) to IIa (thrombin)—are illustrated in Figure 4–9.

■ Traditionally, the blood coagulation scheme has been divided into *extrinsic* and *intrinsic* pathways, converging where factor X is activated (see Fig. 4–8). The intrinsic pathway may be initiated in the clinical laboratory by activation of Hageman factor (factor XII), while the extrinsic pathway is activated by *tissue factor*, a cellular lipoprotein present at sites of tissue injury. However, such a division is only an artifact of in vitro testing; there are, in fact, several interconnections between the two pathways. For example, tissue factor is also involved in the "intrinsic pathway" activation of factor IX (see Fig. 4–8).

■ In addition to catalyzing the final steps in the coagulation cascade, thrombin also exerts a wide variety of effects on the local vasculature and inflammation; it even actively participates in limiting the extent of the hemostatic process (see Fig. 4–6). Most of these thrombin-mediated effects occur via *thrombin receptors*—seven-transmembrane-spanner proteins coupled to G proteins. The mechanism of receptor activation is extremely interesting and involves clipping the end of the thrombin receptor by the proteolytic action of thrombin. This

Figure 4-9   ■

Schematic illustration of the conversion of factor X to factor Xa, which in turn converts factor II (prothrombin) to factor IIa (thrombin). The initial reaction complex consists of an enzyme (factor IXa), a substrate (factor X), and a reaction accelerator (factor VIIIa), which are assembled on the phospholipid surface of platelets. Calcium ions hold the assembled components together and are essential for the reaction. Activated factor Xa then becomes the enzyme part of the second adjacent complex in the coagulation cascade, converting the prothrombin substrate to IIa with the cooperation of the reaction accelerator factor Va. (Modified from Mann KG: The biochemistry of coagulation. Clin Lab Med 4:217, 1984.)

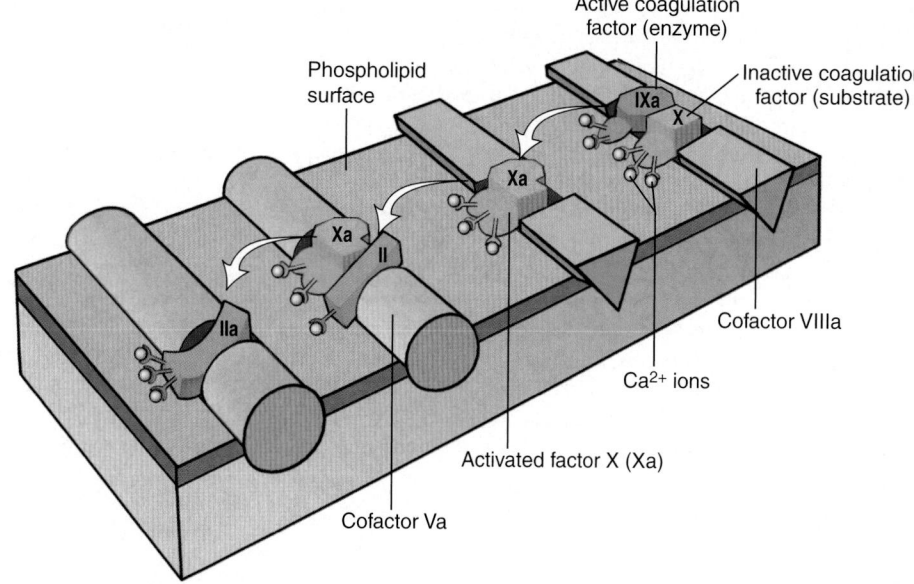

generates a tethered peptide that binds to the rest of the receptor and causes the conformational changes necessary to activate the associated G protein. Thus, the interaction of thrombin and its receptor is essentially a catalytic process, which explains the impressive potency of even relatively small numbers of activated thrombin molecules in eliciting down-stream effects.

■ Once activated, the coagulation cascade must be restricted to the local site of vascular injury to prevent clotting of the entire vascular tree. Besides restricting factor activation to sites of exposed phospholipids, clotting is also controlled by two natural anticoagulants:

   ■ *Antithrombins* (e.g., antithrombin III) inhibit the activity of thrombin and other serine proteases—factors IXa, Xa, XIa, and XIIa. Antithrombin III is activated by binding to heparin-like molecules on endothelial cells; hence, the usefulness of administering heparin in clinical situations to minimize thrombosis (see Fig. 4–6).

   ■ *Proteins C and S* are two vitamin K–dependent proteins that inactivate the cofactors Va and VIIIa. The activation of protein C by thrombomodulin was described earlier (see Fig. 4–6).

■ Besides inducing coagulation, activation of the clotting cascade also sets into motion a *fibrinolytic cascade* that will limit the size of the final clot. This is primarily accomplished by the activation of *plasmin*. Plasmin is derived from enzymatic breakdown of its inactive circulating precursor *plasminogen* either by a factor XII–dependent pathway (Chapter 2) or by plasminogen activators (PAs; Fig. 4–10). The most important of these PAs is the *tissue-type PA (t-PA)*; t-PA is synthesized principally by endothelial cells and is most active when attached to fibrin. The affinity for fibrin makes t-PA a useful therapeutic reagent, since it targets the fibrinolytic enzymatic activity to sites of recent clotting. Plasmin breaks down fibrin and interferes with its polymerization

Figure 4-10   ■

The fibrinolytic system, illustrating the various plasminogen activators and inhibitors (see text).

(see Fig. 4–10). The resulting *fibrin split products* (*FSPs*, or so-called *fibrin degradation products*) can also act as weak anticoagulants. As a clinical correlate, elevated levels of these FSPs are helpful in diagnosing abnormal thrombotic states such as disseminated intravascular coagulation, deep venous thrombosis, or pulmonary thromboembolism (described in detail later). Any free plasmin rapidly complexes with circulating α_2-antiplasmin and is inactivated so that excess plasmin does not lyse clots elsewhere in the body (see Fig. 4–10).

■ Endothelial cells further modulate the coagulation/anticoagulation balance by releasing *plasminogen activator inhibitors (PAIs);* these block fibrinolysis and confer an overall procoagulation effect (see Fig. 4–10). The PAIs are increased by certain cytokines and probably play a role in the intravascular thrombosis accompanying severe inflammations.

Thrombosis

Having discussed the process of normal hemostasis, we can now turn our attention to the dysregulation that underlies pathologic thrombus formation.

Pathogenesis. Three primary influences predispose to thrombus formation, the so-called *Virchow triad*: (1) endothelial injury, (2) stasis *or* turbulence of blood flow, and (3) blood hypercoagulability (Fig. 4–11).

■ *Endothelial injury* is the dominant influence and by itself can lead to thrombosis. It is particularly important in thrombus formation in the heart and arterial circulation, for example, within the cardiac chambers when there has been endocardial injury (e.g., myocardial infarction or valvulitis), over ulcerated plaques in severely atherosclerotic arteries, or at sites of traumatic or inflammatory vascular injury. *It is important to note that endothelium does not need to be denuded or physically disrupted to contribute to the development of thrombosis; any pertur-*

bation in the dynamic balance of prothrombotic and antithrombotic effects can influence local clotting events (see Fig. 4–6). Thus, significant endothelial dysfunction may occur from the hemodynamic stresses of hypertension, turbulent flow over scarred valves, or bacterial endotoxins. Even relatively subtle influences such as homocystinuria, hypercholesterolemia, radiation, or products absorbed from cigarette smoke may be sources of endothelial injury and dysregulation. Regardless of the cause, physical loss of endothelium leads to exposure of subendothelial collagen (and other platelet activators), adherence of platelets, release of tissue factor, and local depletion of PGI_2 and PA (see Fig. 4–6). Dysfunctional endothelium may elaborate greater amounts of procoagulant factors (e.g., adhesion molecules to bind platelets, tissue factor, PAI, etc.) and smaller amounts of anticoagulant effectors (e.g., thrombomodulin, PGI_2, t-PA).

■ *Alterations in normal blood flow. Turbulence* contributes to arterial and cardiac thrombosis by causing endothelial injury or dysfunction, as well as by forming countercurrents and local pockets of stasis; *stasis* is a major factor in the development of venous thrombi. Normal blood flow is *laminar* such that the platelet elements flow centrally in the vessel lumen, separated from the endothelium by a slower-moving clear zone of plasma. Stasis and turbulence therefore (1) disrupt laminar flow and bring platelets into contact with the endothelium, (2) prevent dilution of activated clotting factors by fresh-flowing blood, (3) retard the inflow of clotting factor inhibitors and permit the build-up of thrombi, and (4) promote endothelial cell activation, predisposing to local thrombosis, leukocyte adhesion, and a variety of other endothelial cell effects.

Turbulence and stasis contribute to thrombosis in a number of clinical settings. Ulcerated atherosclerotic plaques not only expose subendothelial ECM but also generate local turbulence. Abnormal aortic and arterial dilations called *aneurysms* cause local stasis and are favored sites of thrombosis (Chapter 10). Myocardial infarctions not only have associated endothelial injury but also have regions of noncontractile myocardium, adding an element of stasis in the formation of mural thrombi. Mitral valve stenosis (e.g., after rheumatic heart disease) results in left atrial dilation. In conjunction with atrial fibrillation, a dilated atrium is a site of profound stasis and a prime location for development of thrombi. *Hyperviscosity syndromes* (such as *polycythemia*; Chapter 12) increase resistance to flow and cause small vessel stasis; the deformed red cells in sickle cell anemia (Chapter 12) cause vascular occlusions, with the resultant stasis predisposing to thrombosis.

■ *Hypercoagulability* generally contributes less frequently to thrombotic states but is nevertheless an important (and interesting) component in the equation. It is loosely defined as any alteration of the coagulation pathways that predisposes to thrombosis, and it can be divided into *primary* (genetic) and *secondary* (acquired) disorders (Table 4–2).

Of the inherited causes of hypercoagulability, mutations in the factor V gene and prothrombin gene are the most common. The characteristic alteration is a mutant factor Va that cannot be inactivated by protein C; as a result, an important antithrombotic counter-regulatory pathway is lost (see Fig. 4–6). Approximately 2% to

Figure 4–11 ■

Virchow triad in thrombosis. Endothelial integrity is the single most important factor. Injury to endothelial cells can also alter local blood flow and affect coagulability. Abnormal blood flow (stasis or turbulence), in turn, can cause endothelial injury. The factors may act independently or may combine to cause thrombus formation.

Table 4-2. CONDITIONS ASSOCIATED WITH AN INCREASED RISK OF THROMBOSIS

Primary (Genetic)
Factor V mutations
Prothrombin mutation
Antithrombin III deficiency
Protein C or S deficiency

Secondary (Acquired)
High risk for thrombosis
  Prolonged bed rest or immobilization
  Myocardial infarction
  Tissue damage (surgery, fracture, burns)
  Cancer
  Prosthetic cardiac valves
  Disseminated intravascular coagulation
  Lupus anticoagulant
Low risk for thrombosis
  Atrial fibrillation
  Cardiomyopathy
  Nephrotic syndrome
  Hyperestrogenic states
  Oral contraceptive use
  Sickle cell anemia
  Smoking

15% of the white population carries a specific factor V mutation (referred to as the Leiden mutation, after the Dutch city in which it was first discovered); among patients with recurrent deep vein thrombosis, the frequency is much higher, approaching 60% in some studies. A mutation in the 3' untranslated region of prothrombin gene (so-called G20210A mutation) is associated with an increased level of prothrombin and hence susceptibility to venous thrombosis. Less common primary hypercoagulable states include inherited deficiencies of anticoagulants such as antithrombin III, protein C, or protein S; affected patients typically present with venous thrombosis and recurrent thromboembolism in adolescence or early adult life. Congenitally elevated levels of homocysteine contribute to arterial and venous thromboses (and indeed to the development of atherosclerosis; Chapter 10), likely via inhibitory effects on antithrombin III and endothelial thrombomodulin.

Although these hereditary disorders are uncommon, the basis of the thrombotic tendencies is reasonably well understood. However, the pathogenesis of *acquired thrombotic diatheses* in a number of common clinical settings is more complicated and multifactorial. In some of the acquired conditions (e.g., cardiac failure or trauma), factors such as stasis or vascular injury may be most important. Even inactivity for the duration of an overseas plane flight may be sufficient to induce deep leg vein thromboses; in such cases, heterozygosity for factor V Leiden or the G20210A prothrombin gene may be synergistic with each other and with acquired causes of hypercoagulability listed in Table 4–2. Among acquired causes (oral contraceptive use and the hyperestrogenic state of pregnancy), hypercoagulability may be related to increased hepatic synthesis of coagulation factors and reduced syn-

thesis of antithrombin III. In disseminated cancers, release of procoagulant tumor products predisposes to thrombosis. The hypercoagulability seen with advancing age may be due to increasing platelet aggregation and reduced PGI$_2$ release by endothelium. Smoking and obesity promote hypercoagulability by unknown mechanisms.

Among the acquired causes of thrombotic diathesis, the so-called *heparin-induced thrombocytopenia (HIT) syndrome* and *antiphospholipid antibody syndrome* (APS; previously called the *lupus anticoagulant syndrome*) deserve special mention.

■ *HIT syndrome.* This syndrome is estimated to affect 3% to 5% of the population; it occurs when administration of unfractionated heparin (for purposes of therapeutic anticoagulation) induces circulating antibodies that can bind to molecular complexes of heparin and a platelet membrane protein (platelet factor 4) (Chapter 12). This antibody can then attach to similar complexes present on platelet and endothelial surfaces; the result is platelet activation and endothelial cell injury, and *a prothrombotic state.* To circumvent this problem, specially manufactured low-molecular-weight heparin preparations that retain anticoagulant activity but do not interact with platelets (and have the additional advantage of a prolonged serum half-life) are used.

■ *APS.* This syndrome refers to a number of heterogeneous clinical manifestations—including recurrent thrombosis—associated with high titers of antibodies directed against anionic phospholipids (e.g., cardiolipin) or, more accurately, plasma protein antigens that are unveiled by binding to such phospholipids. In vitro, these antibodies interfere with the assembly of phospholipid complexes and inhibit coagulation (hence the designation *lupus anticoagulant*). In contrast, the antibodies in vivo induce a hypercoagulable state. The exact incidence of the syndrome is unknown, although it is being increasingly recognized as a possible culprit in a number of thrombotic states; for example, approximately 20% of patients with a recent stroke were found to have anticardiolipin antibodies, versus none in age-matched controls without stroke.

MORPHOLOGY

Thrombi may develop anywhere in the cardiovascular system: within the cardiac chambers, on valve cusps, or in arteries, veins, or capillaries. They are of variable size and shape, depending on the site of origin and the circumstances leading to their development. Arterial or cardiac thrombi usually begin at a site of endothelial injury (e.g., atherosclerotic plaque) or turbulence (vessel bifurcation); venous thrombi characteristically occur in sites of stasis. An area of attachment to the underlying vessel or heart wall, frequently firmest at the point of origin, is characteristic of all thrombi. Arterial thrombi tend to grow in a retrograde direction from the point of attachment; venous thrombi extend in the direction of blood flow, that is, toward the heart. The propagating tail may not be well attached and, particularly in veins, is prone to fragment, creating an **embolus.**

When formed in the heart or aorta, thrombi may have grossly (and microscopically) apparent laminations called **lines of Zahn;** these are produced by pale layers of platelets and fibrin that alternate with darker layers containing more red cells. Lines of Zahn are significant only in that they imply thrombosis at a site of blood flow; in veins or in smaller arteries, the laminations are typically not as apparent, and, in fact, thrombi formed in the sluggish venous flow usually resemble statically coagulated blood (much like blood clotted in a test tube). Nevertheless, careful evaluation generally reveals irregular, somewhat ill-defined laminations.

When arterial thrombi arise in heart chambers or in the aortic lumen, they are usually applied to the wall of the underlying structure and are termed **mural thrombi.** Abnormal myocardial contraction (arrhythmias, dilated cardiomyopathy, or myocardial infarction) or injury to the endomyocardial surface (myocarditis, catheter trauma) leads to the formation of cardiac mural thrombi (Fig. 4–12A), while ulcerated atherosclerotic plaques and aneurysmal dilation are the precursors of aortic thrombus formation (Fig. 4–12B).

Arterial thrombi are usually **occlusive;** the most common sites, in descending order, are coronary, cerebral, and femoral arteries. The thrombus is usually superimposed on an atherosclerotic plaque, although other forms of vascular injury (vasculitis, trauma) may be involved. The thrombi typically are firmly adherent to the injured arterial wall and are gray-white and friable, composed of a tangled mesh of platelets, fibrin, erythrocytes, and degenerating leukocytes.

Venous thrombosis, or **phlebothrombosis,** is almost invariably occlusive; the thrombus often creates a long cast of the vein lumen. Because these thrombi form in the slowly moving venous blood, they tend to contain more enmeshed erythrocytes and are therefore known as **red,** or **stasis, thrombi. Phlebothrombosis most commonly (90% of cases) affects the veins of the lower extremities.** Less commonly, venous thrombi may develop in the upper extremities, periprostatic plexus, or ovarian and periuterine veins; under special circumstances they may be found in the dural sinuses, portal vein, or hepatic vein (Chapter 16). At autopsy, postmortem clots may be mistaken for venous thrombi. Postmortem clots are gelatinous with a dark red dependent portion where red cells have settled by gravity, and a yellow "chicken fat" supernatant; they are usually not attached to the underlying wall. In contrast, red thrombi are firmer, almost always have a point of attachment, and on transection reveal vague strands of pale gray fibrin.

Under special circumstances, thrombi may form on heart valves. Bacterial or fungal blood-borne infections may lead to valve damage and the development of large thrombotic masses, or **vegetations (infective endocarditis,** Chapter 11). Sterile vegetations can also develop on noninfected valves in patients with hypercoagulable states, so-called **nonbacterial thrombotic endocarditis** (Chapter 11). Less commonly, noninfective, **verrucous (Libman-Sacks) endocarditis** may occur in patients who have systemic lupus erythematosus (Chapter 5).

Fate of the Thrombus. If a patient survives the immediate effects of a thrombotic vascular obstruction, thrombi undergo some combination of the following four events in the ensuing days or weeks (Fig. 4–13):

■ *Propagation.* The thrombus may accumulate more platelets and fibrin (propagate), eventually obstructing some critical vessel.
■ *Embolization.* Thrombi may dislodge and be transported to other sites in the vasculature.
■ *Dissolution.* Thrombi may be removed by fibrinolytic activity.

Figure 4–12

Mural thrombi. *A,* Thrombus in the left and right ventricular apices, overlying a white fibrous scar. *B,* Laminated thrombus in a dilated abdominal aortic aneurysm. Numerous friable mural thrombi are also superimposed on advanced atherosclerotic lesions of the more proximal aorta *(left side of picture).*

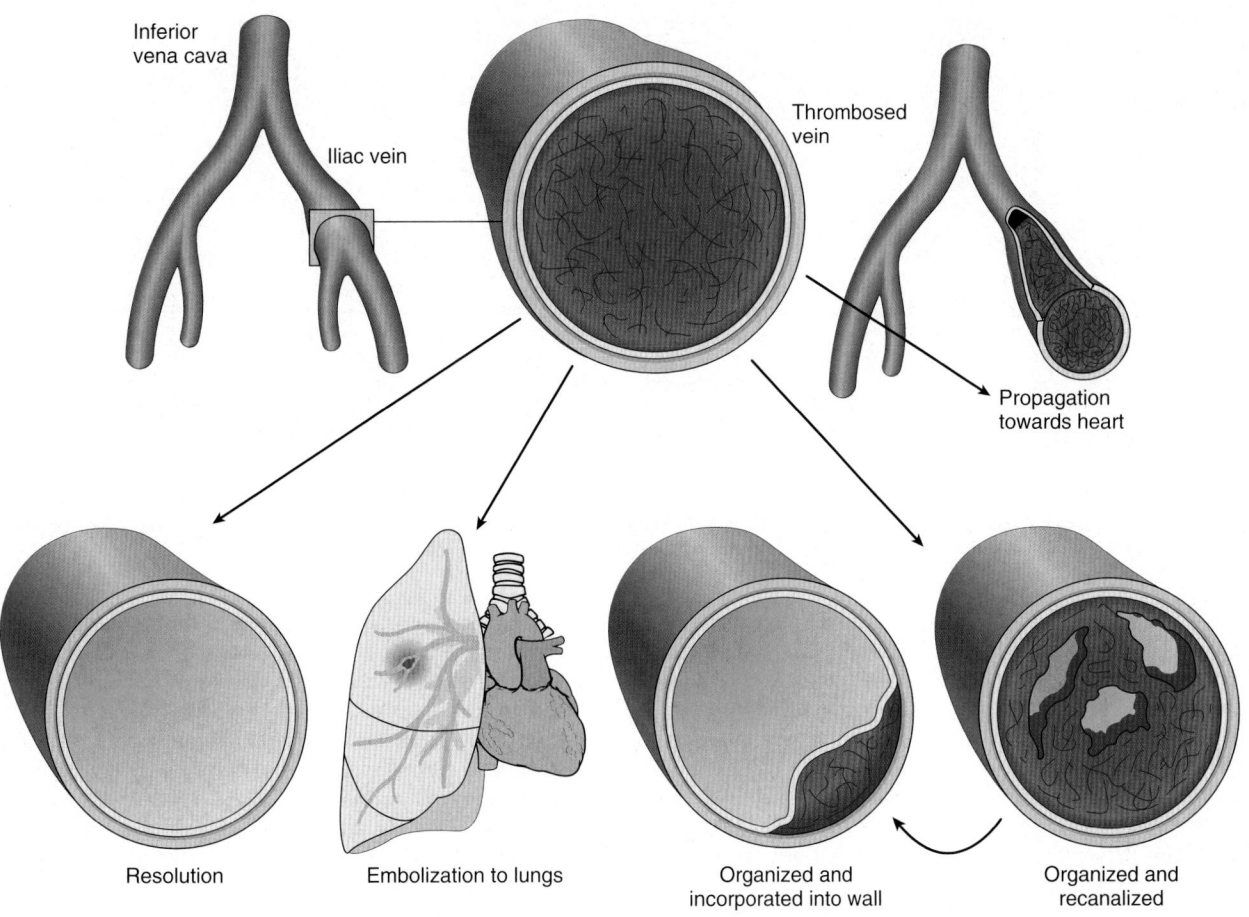

Figure 4–13

Potential outcomes of venous thrombosis (see text).

■ *Organization and recanalization.* Thrombi may induce inflammation and fibrosis *(organization)* and may eventually become *recanalized* (re-establish vascular flow), or they may be incorporated into a thickened vascular wall.

Embolization is discussed in greater detail later. As for dissolution, activation of the fibrinolytic pathways can lead to rapid shrinkage and even total lysis of *recent* thrombi. With older thrombi, extensive fibrin polymerization renders the thrombus substantially more resistant to proteolysis, and lysis is ineffectual. This is important, because therapeutic infusions of fibrinolytic agents such as t-PA (e.g., for pulmonary thromboemboli or coronary thrombosis) are likely to be effective only for a short time after thrombi form.

Older thrombi tend to become *organized.* This refers to the ingrowth of endothelial cells, smooth muscle cells, and fibroblasts into the fibrin-rich thrombus. In time, capillary channels are formed that may anastomose to create conduits from one end of the thrombus to the other, re-establishing to a limited extent the continuity of the original lumen (Fig. 4–14). Although the channels may not successfully restore significant flow to many obstructed vessels, such *recanalization* can potentially convert the thrombus into a vascularized mass of connective tissue that is eventually incorporated as a subendothelial swelling into the vessel wall. With time and contraction of the mesenchy-mal cells, only a fibrous lump may remain to mark the original thrombus site. Occasionally, instead of organizing, the center of a thrombus undergoes enzymatic digestion, presumably because of the release of lysosomal enzymes from trapped leukocytes and platelets. This is particularly likely in large thrombi within aneurysmal dilations or the cardiac chambers. If bacterial seeding occurs, such degraded thrombus is an ideal culture medium, resulting in a so-called *mycotic aneurysm* (Chapter 10).

Clinical Correlations: Venous versus Arterial Thrombosis. Thrombi are significant because (1) they cause obstruction of arteries and veins and (2) they are possible sources of emboli. The importance of each is dependent on where the thrombus occurs. Thus, while venous thrombi may cause congestion and edema in vascular beds distal to an obstruction, a far graver consequence is that they may embolize to the lungs, causing death (p 95). Conversely, although arterial thrombi can embolize, their role in vascular obstruction at critical sites, such as coronary or cerebral vessels, is much more important.

■ *Venous thrombosis (phlebothrombosis).* Most venous thrombi occur in either the superficial or the deep veins of the leg. Superficial venous thrombi usually occur in the saphenous system, particularly when there are varicosities. Such thrombi may cause local conges-

Figure 4-14

Low-power view of a thrombosed artery. *A,* H & E–stained section. *B,* Stain for elastic tissue. The original lumen is delineated by the internal elastic lamina *(arrows)* and is totally filled with organized thrombus, now punctuated by a number of recanalized channels.

tion and cause swelling, pain, and tenderness along the course of the involved vein, but they rarely embolize. However, the local edema and impaired venous drainage do predispose the overlying skin to infections from slight trauma and to the development of *varicose ulcers.* Deep thrombi in the *larger leg veins at or above the knee joint* (e.g., popliteal, femoral, and iliac veins) are more serious because they may embolize. Although they may cause local pain and edema, the venous obstruction may be rapidly offset by collateral bypass channels. Consequently, deep venous thromboses are entirely asymptomatic in *approximately 50% of patients* and are recognized in retrospect only after they have embolized.

Deep venous thrombosis may occur with stasis and in a variety of hypercoagulable states, as described earlier (see Table 4–2). Cardiac failure is an obvious reason for stasis in the venous circulation. Trauma, surgery, and burns usually result in reduced physical activity, injury to vessels, release of procoagulant substances from tissues, and/or reduced t-PA activity. Even relatively minimal stasis such as during long plane flights or car travel may result in deep venous thrombosis when an individual is otherwise genetically predisposed to hypercoagulability (e.g., heterozygosity for factor V Leiden). Clearly, many factors act in concert to predispose to thrombosis in the puerperal and postpartum states. Besides the potential for amniotic fluid infusion into the circulation at the time of delivery (p 96), late pregnancy and the postpartum period are associated with hypercoagulability. Tumor-associated procoagulant release is largely responsible for the increased risk of thromboembolic phenomena seen in disseminated cancers, so-called *migratory thrombophlebitis or Trousseau syndrome.* Regardless of the specific clinical setting, advanced age, bed rest, and immobilization increase the risk of deep venous thrombosis; reduced physical activity diminishes the milking action of muscles in the lower leg and so slows venous return.

■ *Cardiac and arterial thrombosis. Myocardial infarction* may be associated with dyskinetic contraction of the myocardium as well as damage to the adjacent endocardium, providing a site for the origin of a mural thrombus. *Rheumatic heart disease* (Chapter 11) may result in mitral valve stenosis, followed by left atrial dilation; concurrent atrial fibrillation augments atrial blood stasis and formation of mural thrombi. *Atherosclerosis* is a prime initiator of thromboses, related to loss of endothelial integrity and abnormal vascular flow (see Fig. 4–12B). In addition to the obstructive consequences, cardiac and aortic mural thrombi can also embolize peripherally. Virtually any tissue may be affected, but the brain, kidneys, and spleen are prime targets because of their large flow volume.

As a final note, while we clearly understand a number of conditions that predispose to thrombosis, the phenomenon remains somewhat unpredictable. It continues to occur at a distressingly high frequency in otherwise healthy and ambulatory individuals without apparent provocation or underlying abnormality. Equally important is that asymptomatic thrombosis (and presumably subsequent resolution) occurs considerably more frequently than we generally appreciate.

Disseminated Intravascular Coagulation

A variety of disorders ranging from obstetric complications to advanced malignancy may be complicated by disseminated intravascular coagulation (DIC) (Chapter 12), the sudden or insidious onset of widespread fibrin thrombi in the microcirculation. While these thrombi are not usually visible on gross inspection, they are readily apparent microscopically and can cause diffuse circulatory insufficiency, particularly in the brain, lungs, heart, and kidneys. With the development of the multiple thrombi, there is a rapid concurrent consumption of platelets and coagulation proteins (hence the synonym *consumption coagulopathy*); at the same time, fibrinolytic mechanisms are activated, and as a result an initially thrombotic disorder can evolve into a serious bleeding disorder. *It should be emphasized that DIC is not a primary disease but rather is a potential complication of any condition associated with widespread activation of thrombin.* It is discussed in greater detail along with other bleeding diatheses in Chapter 12.

EMBOLISM

An embolus is a detached intravascular solid, liquid, or gaseous mass that is carried by the blood to a site distant from its point of origin. Virtually 99% of all emboli represent some part of a dislodged thrombus, hence the commonly used term *thromboembolism.* Rare forms of emboli include droplets of fat, bubbles of air or nitrogen, atherosclerotic debris *(cholesterol emboli),* tumor fragments, bits of bone marrow, or foreign bodies such as bullets. However, unless otherwise specified, an embolism should be considered to be thrombotic in origin. Inevitably, emboli lodge in vessels too small to permit further passage, resulting in partial or complete vascular occlusion. The potential consequence of such thromboembolic events is the ischemic necrosis of down-stream tissue, known as *infarction.* Depending on the site of origin, emboli may lodge anywhere in the vascular tree; the clinical outcomes are best understood from the standpoint of whether emboli lodge in the pulmonary or systemic circulations.

Pulmonary Thromboembolism

Pulmonary embolism has an incidence of 20 to 25 per 100,000 hospitalized patients. Although the rate of fatal pulmonary emboli (as assessed at autopsy) has declined from 6% to 2% over the last quarter century, pulmonary embolism still causes about 200,000 deaths per year in the United States. In more than 95% of instances, venous emboli originate from deep leg vein thrombi above the level of the knee as described previously (p 94). They are carried through progressively larger channels and usually pass through the right side of the heart into the pulmonary vasculature. Depending on the size of the embolus, it may occlude the main pulmonary artery, impact across the bifurcation *(saddle embolus),* or pass out into the smaller, branching arterioles (Fig. 4–15). Frequently, there are multiple emboli, perhaps sequentially, or as a shower of smaller emboli from a single large mass; in general, *the patient who has had one pulmonary embolus is at high risk of having more.* Rarely, an embolus may pass through an interatrial or interventricular defect to gain access to the systemic circulation *(paradoxical embolism).* A more complete discussion of pulmonary emboli is presented in Chapter 13; only an overview is offered here.

■ Most pulmonary emboli (60% to 80%) are clinically silent because they are small. With time, they undergo organization and become incorporated into the vascular wall; in some cases, organization of the thromboembolus leaves behind a delicate, bridging fibrous *web.*

■ Sudden death, right ventricular failure *(cor pulmonale),* or cardiovascular collapse occur when 60%

Figure 4–15   ■

Large embolus derived from a lower extremity deep venous thrombosis and now impacted in a pulmonary artery branch.

or more of the pulmonary circulation is obstructed with emboli.

■ Embolic obstruction of medium-sized arteries may result in pulmonary hemorrhage but usually does not cause pulmonary infarction because of blood flow into the area from an intact bronchial circulation. However, a similar embolus in the setting of left-sided cardiac failure (and resultant sluggish bronchial artery blood flow) may result in a large infarct.

■ Embolic obstruction of small end-arteriolar pulmonary branches usually does result in associated infarction.

■ Multiple emboli over time may cause pulmonary hypertension with right ventricular failure.

Systemic Thromboembolism

Systemic thromboembolism refers to emboli traveling within the arterial circulation. Most (80%) arise from intracardiac mural thrombi, two thirds of which are associated with left ventricular wall infarcts and another quarter with dilated left atria (e.g., secondary to mitral valve disease). The remainder largely originate from thrombi associated with ulcerated atherosclerotic plaques or aortic aneurysms, or from fragmentation of a valvular vegetation (Chapter 11); only a very small fraction are due to *paradoxical emboli.* In contrast to venous emboli, which tend to lodge primarily in one vascular bed (the lung), arterial emboli can travel to a wide variety of sites; the site of arrest depends on the point of origin of the thromboembolus and the relative blood flow through the down-stream tissues. The major sites for arteriolar embolization are the lower extremities (75%) and the brain (10%), with the intestines, kidneys, and spleen involved to a lesser extent. The consequences of systemic emboli depend on the extent of collateral vascular supply in the affected tissue, the tissue's vulnerability to ischemia, and the caliber of the vessel occluded; in general, however, arterial emboli cause infarction of tissues in the distribution of the obstructed vessel.

Fat Embolism

Microscopic fat globules may be found in the circulation after fractures of long bones (which have fatty marrows) or, rarely, in the setting of soft tissue trauma and burns. Presumably, the fat is released by marrow or adipose tissue injury and enters the circulation by rupture of the marrow vascular sinusoids or rupture of venules. Although traumatic fat embolism occurs in some 90% of individuals with severe skeletal injuries (Fig. 4–16), fewer than 10% of such patients show any clinical findings. *Fat embolism syndrome is characterized by pulmonary insufficiency, neurologic symptoms, anemia, and thrombocytopenia and is fatal in about 10% of cases.* Typically, the symptoms appear 1 to 3 days after injury, with sudden onset of tachypnea, dyspnea, and tachycardia. Neurologic symptoms include irritability and restlessness, with progression to delirium or coma.

The pathogenesis of this syndrome probably involves both mechanical obstruction and chemical injury. While microemboli of neutral fat cause occlusion of pulmonary or cerebral microvasculature, free fatty acids released from fat globules also cause local toxic injury to endothelium. A characteristic petechial skin rash is related to rapid onset of thrombocytopenia, presumably caused by platelets adhering to the myriad fat globules and being removed from the circulation.

Air Embolism

Gas bubbles within the circulation can obstruct vascular flow (and cause distal ischemic injury) almost as readily as thrombotic masses. Air may enter the circulation during ob-

Figure 4–16 ■

Bone marrow embolus in the pulmonary circulation. The cleared vacuoles represent marrow fat that is now impacted in a distal vessel along with the cellular hematopoietic precursors.

stetric procedures or as a consequence of chest wall injury. Generally, in excess of 100 mL of air is required to produce a clinical effect; the bubbles act like physical obstructions and may coalesce to form frothy masses sufficiently large to occlude major vessels.

A particular form of gas embolism called *decompression sickness* occurs when individuals are exposed to sudden changes in atmospheric pressure. Scuba and deep sea divers, underwater construction workers, and individuals in unpressurized aircraft in rapid ascent are at risk. When air is breathed at high pressure (e.g., during a deep sea dive), increased amounts of gas (particularly nitrogen) become dissolved in the blood and tissues. If the diver then ascends (depressurizes) too rapidly, the nitrogen expands in the tissues and bubbles out of solution in the blood to form gas emboli.

The rapid formation of gas bubbles within skeletal muscles and supporting tissues in and about joints is responsible for the painful condition called *the bends* (originally so named in the 1880s because afflicted individuals characteristically arched their backs in a manner reminiscent of a then-popular woman's fashion called the *Grecian Bend*). Gas emboli may also induce focal ischemia in a number of tissues, including brain and heart. In the lungs, edema, hemorrhages, and focal atelectasis or emphysema may appear, leading to respiratory distress, the *chokes*. Treatment of gas embolism consists of placing the individual in a compression chamber where the barometric pressure may be raised, thus forcing the gas bubbles back into solution. Subsequent slow decompression theoretically permits gradual resorption and exhalation of the gases so that obstructive bubbles do not reform.

A more chronic form of decompression sickness is called *caisson disease*, in which persistence of gas emboli in the bones leads to multiple foci of ischemic necrosis; the more common sites are the heads of the femurs, tibiae, and humeri.

Amniotic Fluid Embolism

Amniotic fluid embolism is a grave but fortunately uncommon complication of labor and the immediate postpartum period (1 in 50,000 deliveries). It has a mortality rate in excess of 80%, and as other obstetric complications (e.g., eclampsia, pulmonary embolism) have been better controlled, amniotic fluid embolism has become an important cause of maternal mortality. The onset is characterized by sudden severe dyspnea, cyanosis, and hypotensive shock, followed by seizures and coma. If the patient survives the initial crisis, pulmonary edema typically develops, along with (in half the patients) DIC, due to release of thrombogenic substances from amniotic fluid.

The underlying cause is the infusion of amniotic fluid (and its contents) into the maternal circulation via a tear in the placental membranes and rupture of uterine veins. The classic findings are therefore the presence in the pulmonary microcirculation of squamous cells shed from fetal skin, lanugo hair, fat from vernix caseosa, and mucin derived from the fetal respiratory or gastrointestinal tracts. There is also marked pulmonary edema and changes of diffuse alveolar damage (Chapter 13), as well as systemic fibrin thrombi, indicative of DIC.

INFARCTION

An infarct is an area of ischemic necrosis caused by occlusion of either the arterial supply or the venous drainage in a particular tissue. Tissue infarction is a common and extremely important cause of clinical illness. More than half of all deaths in the United States are caused by cardiovascular disease, and most of these are attributable to myocardial or cerebral infarction. Pulmonary infarction is a common complication in a number of clinical settings, bowel infarction is frequently fatal, and ischemic necrosis of the extremities (gangrene) is a serious problem in the diabetic population.

Nearly 99% of all infarcts result from thrombotic or embolic events, and almost all result from arterial occlusion. Occasionally, infarction may also be caused by other mechanisms, such as local vasospasm, swelling of an atheroma secondary to hemorrhage within a plaque, or extrinsic compression of a vessel, for example, by tumor. Other uncommon causes include twisting of the vessels (e.g., in testicular torsion or bowel volvulus), compression of the blood supply by edema or by entrapment in a hernia sac, or traumatic rupture of the blood supply. Although venous thrombosis may cause infarction, it more often merely induces venous obstruction and congestion. Usually, bypass channels then rapidly open, providing some outflow from the area, which in turn improves the arterial inflow. Infarcts caused by venous thrombosis are more likely in organs with a single venous outflow channel, such as the testis and ovary.

MORPHOLOGY

Infarcts can be classified on the basis of their color (really reflecting the amount of hemorrhage) and the presence or absence of microbial infection. Therefore, infarcts may be either **red (hemorrhagic)** or **white (anemic)** and may be either **septic** or **bland.**

■ **Red infarcts** (Fig. 4–17A) occur (1) with venous occlusions (such as in ovarian torsion); (2) in loose tissues (such as lung) that allow blood to collect in the infarcted zone; (3) in tissues with dual circulations such as lung and small intestine, permitting flow of blood from the unobstructed vascular channel into the necrotic area (obviously such perfusion is not sufficient to rescue the ischemic tissues); (4) in tissues that were previously congested because of sluggish venous outflow; and (5) when flow is re-established to a site of previous arterial occlusion and necrosis (e.g., fragmentation of an occlusive embolus or angioplasty of a thrombotic lesion) (Fig. 4–17B).

■ **White infarcts** occur with arterial occlusions, or in solid organs (such as heart, spleen, and kidney), where the solidity of the tissue limits the amount of hemorrhage that can seep into the area of ischemic necrosis from adjoining capillary beds.

All infarcts tend to be wedge shaped, with the occluded vessel at the apex and the periphery of the organ forming the base (see Fig. 4–17); when the base is a serosal surface, there is often an overlying fibrinous exudate. The lateral margins may be irregular, reflecting the pattern of vascular supply from adjacent vessels. At the outset, all infarcts are poorly defined and slightly hemorrhagic. The margins of both types of infarcts tend to become better defined with time by a narrow rim of hyperemia attributable to inflammation at the edge of the lesion.

In solid organs, the relatively few extravasated red cells are lysed, with the released hemoglobin remaining in the form of hemosiderin. Thus, infarcts resulting from arterial occlusions typically become progressively more pale and sharply defined with time (see Fig. 4–17B). In spongy organs, by comparison, the hemorrhage is too extensive to permit the lesion ever to become pale (see Fig. 4–17A). Over the course of a few days, however, it does become firmer and browner, reflecting the development of hemosiderin pigment.

The dominant histologic characteristic of infarction is **ischemic coagulative necrosis** (Chapter 1). It

Figure 4–17   ■

Examples of infarcts. *A,* Hemorrhagic, roughly wedge-shaped pulmonary infarct. *B,* Sharply demarcated pale infarct in the spleen.

is important to recall that if the vascular occlusion has occurred shortly (minutes to hours) before the death of the patient, no demonstrable histologic changes may be evident; even if the patient survives 12 to 18 hours, the only change present may be a hemorrhagic suffusion.

An inflammatory response begins to develop along the margins of infarcts within a few hours and is usually well defined within 1 or 2 days. Inflammation at these sites is incited by the necrotic tissue, and ultimately, in all forms of infarcts, there is gradual degradation of the dead tissue with phagocytosis of the tissue debris by recruited inflammatory cells. Eventually, the inflammatory response is followed by a reparative response beginning in the preserved margins. In stable or labile tissues, some parenchymal regeneration may occur at the periphery where the underlying stromal architecture has been spared. However, most infarcts are ultimately replaced by scar tissue (Fig. 4–18)). The brain is an exception to these generalizations; like other causes of necrosis, ischemic tissue injury in the central nervous system results in **liquefactive necrosis** (Chapter 1).

Septic infarctions may arise when embolization occurs by a fragment of a bacterial vegetation from a heart valve, or when microbes seed an area of necrotic tissue. In these cases, the infarct is converted into an **abscess**, with a correspondingly greater inflammatory response (Chapter 2). The eventual sequence of organization, however, follows the pattern previously described.

Factors That Influence Development of an Infarct. The consequences of a vascular occlusion can range from no or minimal effect, all the way up to death of a tissue or even the individual. *The major determinants are*

- *Nature of the vascular supply.* The availability of an alternative blood supply is the most important factor in determining whether occlusion of a vessel will cause damage. For example, lungs have a dual pulmonary and bronchial artery blood supply; thus, obstruction of small pulmonary arterioles does not cause infarction in an otherwise healthy individual with an intact bronchial circulation. Similarly, the liver, with its dual hepatic artery and portal vein circulation, and the hand and forearm, with their dual radial and ulnar arterial supply, are all relatively resistant to infarction. In contrast, renal and splenic circulations are end-arterial, and obstruction of such vessels generally causes infarction.
- *Rate of development of occlusion.* Slowly developing occlusions are less likely to cause infarction because they provide time for the development of alternative pathways of flow. For example, small interarteriolar anastomoses, normally with minimal functional flow, interconnect the three major coronary arteries in the heart. If one of the coronaries is only slowly occluded (e.g., by

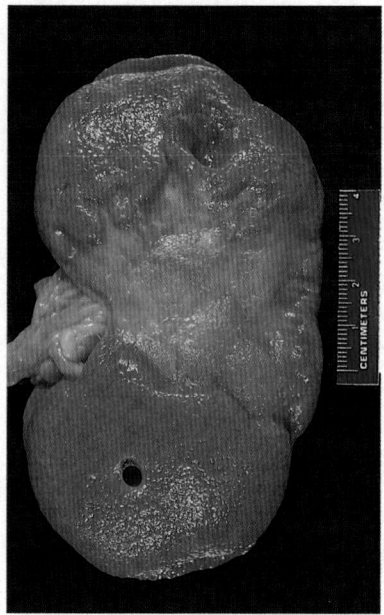

Figure 4–18 ■

An old kidney infarct, now represented by a large depressed fibrotic cortical scar.

an encroaching atherosclerotic plaque), flow within this collateral circulation may increase sufficiently to prevent infarction, even though the major coronary artery is eventually occluded.
- *Vulnerability to hypoxia.* The susceptibility of a tissue to hypoxia influences the likelihood of infarction. Neurons undergo irreversible damage when deprived of their blood supply for only 3 to 4 minutes. Myocardial cells, although hardier than neurons, are also quite sensitive and die after only 20 to 30 minutes of ischemia. In contrast, fibroblasts within myocardium remain viable after many hours of ischemia.
- *Oxygen content of blood.* The partial pressure of oxygen in blood also determines the outcome of vascular occlusion. Partial flow obstruction of a small vessel in an anemic or cyanotic patient might lead to tissue infarction, whereas it would be without effect under conditions of normal oxygen tension. In this way, congestive heart failure, with compromised flow and ventilation, could cause infarction in the setting of an otherwise inconsequential blockage.

SHOCK

Shock, or "cardiovascular collapse," is the final common pathway for a number of potentially lethal clinical events, including severe hemorrhage, extensive trauma or burns, large myocardial infarction, massive pulmonary embolism, and microbial sepsis. Regardless of the underlying pathologic lesion, *shock constitutes systemic hypoperfusion due to a reduction either in cardiac output or in the effective circulating blood volume. Hypotension ensues, followed by impaired tissue perfusion and cellular hypoxia. Although*

Table 4-3. THE THREE MAJOR TYPES OF SHOCK

Type of Shock	Clinical Examples	Principal Mechanisms
Cardiogenic	Myocardial infarction Ventricular rupture Arrhythmia Cardiac tamponade Pulmonary embolism	Failure of myocardial pump due to intrinsic myocardial damage or extrinsic pressure or obstruction to outflow
Hypovolemic	Hemorrhage Fluid loss, e,g., vomiting, diarrhea, burns, or trauma	Inadequate blood or plasma volume
Septic	Overwhelming microbial infections; endotoxic shock, gram-positive septicemia, or fungal sepsis	Peripheral vasodilation and pooling of blood; endothelial activation/injury; leukocyte-induced damage; disseminated intravascular coagulation

the hypoxic and metabolic effects of hypoperfusion initially cause only reversible cellular injury, persistence of the shock eventually causes irreversible tissue injury and can culminate in the death of the patient.

Shock may be grouped into three general categories: cardiogenic, hypovolemic, and septic (Table 4–3). The mechanisms underlying cardiogenic and hypovolemic shock are fairly straightforward; essentially they involve *low cardiac output*. Septic shock, by comparison, is substantially more complicated and is discussed in further detail later.

■ *Cardiogenic shock* results from myocardial pump failure. This may be caused by intrinsic myocardial damage (infarction), ventricular arrhythmias, extrinsic compression (cardiac tamponade, Chapter 11), or outflow obstruction (pulmonary embolism).

■ *Hypovolemic shock* results from loss of blood or plasma volume. This may be caused by hemorrhage, fluid loss from severe burns, or trauma.

■ *Septic shock* is caused by systemic microbial infection. Most commonly, this occurs in the setting of gram-negative infections *(endotoxic shock),* but it can also occur with gram-positive and fungal infections.

Less commonly, shock may occur in the setting of an anesthetic accident or a spinal cord injury *(neurogenic shock),* due to loss of vascular tone and peripheral pooling of blood. *Anaphylactic shock,* initiated by a generalized immunoglobulin E-mediated hypersensitivity response, is associated with systemic vasodilation and increased vascular permeability (Chapter 5). In these instances, widespread vasodilation causes a sudden increase in the capacity of the vascular bed, which cannot be filled adequately by the normal circulating blood volume. Thus, tissue hypoperfusion and cellular anoxia result.

Pathogenesis of Septic Shock

Septic shock, with a 25% to 50% mortality rate, ranks first among the causes of death in intensive care units and accounts for over 200,000 deaths annually in the United States. Moreover, the reported incidence of sepsis syndromes is increasing dramatically, in part due to improved life support for high-risk patients, increasing invasive procedures, and the growing numbers of immunocompromised

hosts (secondary to chemotherapy, immunosuppression, or HIV infection). Septic shock results from spread and expansion of an initially localized infection (e.g., abscess, peritonitis, pneumonia) into the bloodstream.

Most cases of septic shock (approximately 70%) are caused by endotoxin-producing gram-negative bacilli (Chapter 9), hence the term *endotoxic shock.* Endotoxins are bacterial wall lipopolysaccharides (LPSs) released when the cell walls are degraded (e.g., in an inflammatory response); LPS consists of a toxic fatty acid core common to all gram-negative bacteria *(lipid A),* and a complex polysaccharide coat that is unique for each species *(O antigens).* Analogous molecules in the walls of gram-positive bacteria and fungi can also elicit septic shock.

All of the cellular and resultant hemodynamic effects of septic shock may be reproduced by injection of LPS alone. Free LPS attaches to a circulating LPS-binding protein, and the complex then binds to a specific receptor (called CD14) on monocytes, macrophages, and neutrophils. Engagement of CD14 (even at doses as minute as *10 pg/mL*) results in intracellular signaling via an associated "Toll-like receptor," and subsequent profound mononuclear cell activation with production of potent effector cytokines such as IL-1 and TNF (Chapter 2). The Toll-like receptor gets its name because it shares structural homology with a *Drosophila* protein called Toll. In the fruit fly, Toll plays an important role in development; related *Drosophila* molecules are also important in innate defense against infectious organisms, much as they are in mammals (yet another beautiful example of phylogenetically conserved structures and functions!). Presumably, at low doses of LPS in humans, Toll-mediated activation helps to trigger the elements of the innate immune system to efficiently eradicate invading microbes. Unfortunately, depending on the dosage and the number of macrophages that are activated, the secondary effects of LPS release can also cause severe pathologic changes including fatal shock.

At low doses, LPS predominantly serves to activate monocytes, macrophages, and neutrophils, with effects presumably intended to enhance their ability to eliminate invading bacteria. LPS can also directly activate complement, which likewise contributes to local bacterial eradication. The mononuclear phagocytes respond to LPS by producing TNF, which in turn induces IL-1 synthesis. Both TNF and IL-1 act on endothelial cells (and other cell types) to produce further cytokines (e.g., IL-6 and IL-8) and induce

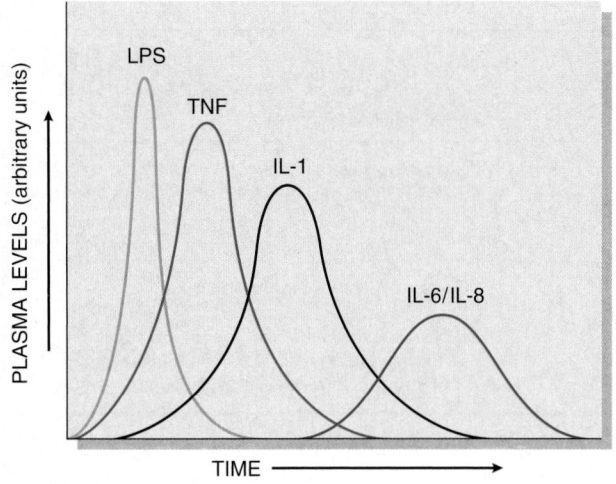

Figure 4–19 ■

Cytokine cascade in sepsis. After release of lipopolysaccharide (LPS), there are successive waves of tumor necrosis factor (TNF), interleukin 1 (IL-1), and IL-6/IL-8 secretion. (Modified from Abbas AK, et al: Cellular and Molecular Immunology, 3rd ed. Philadelphia, WB Saunders, 1997.)

adhesion molecules (Chapter 2). Thus, the initial release of LPS results in a circumscribed cytokine cascade (Fig. 4–19) that enhances the *local* acute inflammatory response and improves clearance of the infection.

With moderately severe infections, and therefore with higher levels of LPS (and a consequent augmentation of the cytokine cascade), cytokine-induced secondary effectors (e.g., nitric oxide and platelet-activating factor; Chapter 2) become significant. In addition, systemic effects of TNF and IL-1 may begin to be seen, including fever, increased synthesis of acute-phase reactants, and increased production of circulating neutrophils (Fig. 4–20 and Chapter 2).

Finally, at still higher levels of LPS, the syndrome of septic shock supervenes (see Fig. 4–20); the same cytokine and secondary mediators now at high levels result in

■ Systemic vasodilation (hypotension)
■ Diminished myocardial contractility
■ Widespread endothelial injury and activation, causing systemic leukocyte adhesion and diffuse alveolar capillary damage in the lung (Chapter 13)
■ Activation of the coagulation system, culminating in DIC (Chapter 12)

The hypoperfusion resulting from the combined effects of widespread vasodilation, myocardial pump failure, and DIC causes *multiorgan system failure* that affects the liver, kidneys, and central nervous system, among others. Unless the underlying infection (and LPS overload) is rapidly brought under control, the patient usually dies. In some experimental models, antibodies to IL-1 or TNF (or their receptors), or pharmacologic inhibitors of the secondary mediators (e.g., nitric oxide synthesis), have demonstrated some efficacy in protecting against septic shock. Unfortunately, these reagents have not yet proved of significant clinical benefit in patients, probably because multiple different pathways and mediators are activated by LPS.

An interesting group of bacterial proteins called *super-antigens* also causes a syndrome similar to septic shock

(e.g., *toxic shock syndrome toxin 1,* responsible for the *toxic shock syndrome*). Superantigens are polyclonal T-lymphocyte activators that induce systemic inflammatory cytokine cascades similar to those that occur down-stream in septic shock (Chapter 5). Their actions can result in a variety of clinical manifestations ranging from a diffuse rash to vasodilation, hypotension, and death.

Stages of Shock

Shock is a progressive disorder that if uncorrected leads to death. Unless the insult is massive and rapidly lethal (e.g., a massive hemorrhage from a ruptured aortic aneurysm), shock tends to evolve through three general (albeit somewhat artificial) stages. These stages have been documented most clearly in hypovolemic shock but are common to other forms as well:

■ An initial *nonprogressive stage* during which reflex compensatory mechanisms are activated and perfusion of vital organs is maintained
■ A *progressive stage* characterized by tissue hypoperfusion and onset of worsening circulatory and metabolic imbalances
■ An *irreversible stage* that sets in after the body has incurred cellular and tissue injury so severe that even if the hemodynamic defects are corrected, survival is not possible.

In the early nonprogressive phase of shock, various *neurohumoral mechanisms* help maintain cardiac output and blood pressure. These include baroreceptor reflexes, release of catecholamines, activation of the renin-angiotensin axis, antidiuretic hormone release, and generalized sympathetic stimulation. The net effect is *tachycardia, peripheral vasoconstriction,* and *renal conservation of fluid.* Cutaneous vasoconstriction, for example, is responsible for the characteristic coolness and pallor of skin in shock (although septic shock may initially cause cutaneous *vasodilation* and thus present with *warm, flushed skin*). Coronary and cerebral vessels are less sensitive to the sympathetic response and thus maintain relatively normal caliber, blood flow, and oxygen delivery to their respective vital organs.

If the underlying causes are not corrected, shock passes imperceptibly to the progressive phase, during which there is widespread tissue hypoxia. In the setting of persistent oxygen deficit, intracellular aerobic respiration is replaced by anaerobic glycolysis with excessive production of lactic acid. The resultant metabolic *lactic acidosis lowers the tissue pH and blunts the vasomotor response*; arterioles dilate, and blood begins to pool in the microcirculation. Peripheral pooling not only worsens the cardiac output but also puts endothelial cells at risk of developing anoxic injury with subsequent DIC. With widespread tissue hypoxia, vital organs are affected and begin to fail; clinically, *the patient may become confused, and the urinary output declines.*

Unless there is intervention, the process eventually enters an irreversible stage. Widespread cell injury is reflected in lysosomal enzyme leakage, further aggravating the shock state. Myocardial contractile function worsens, in part because of nitric oxide synthesis. If ischemic bowel allows in-

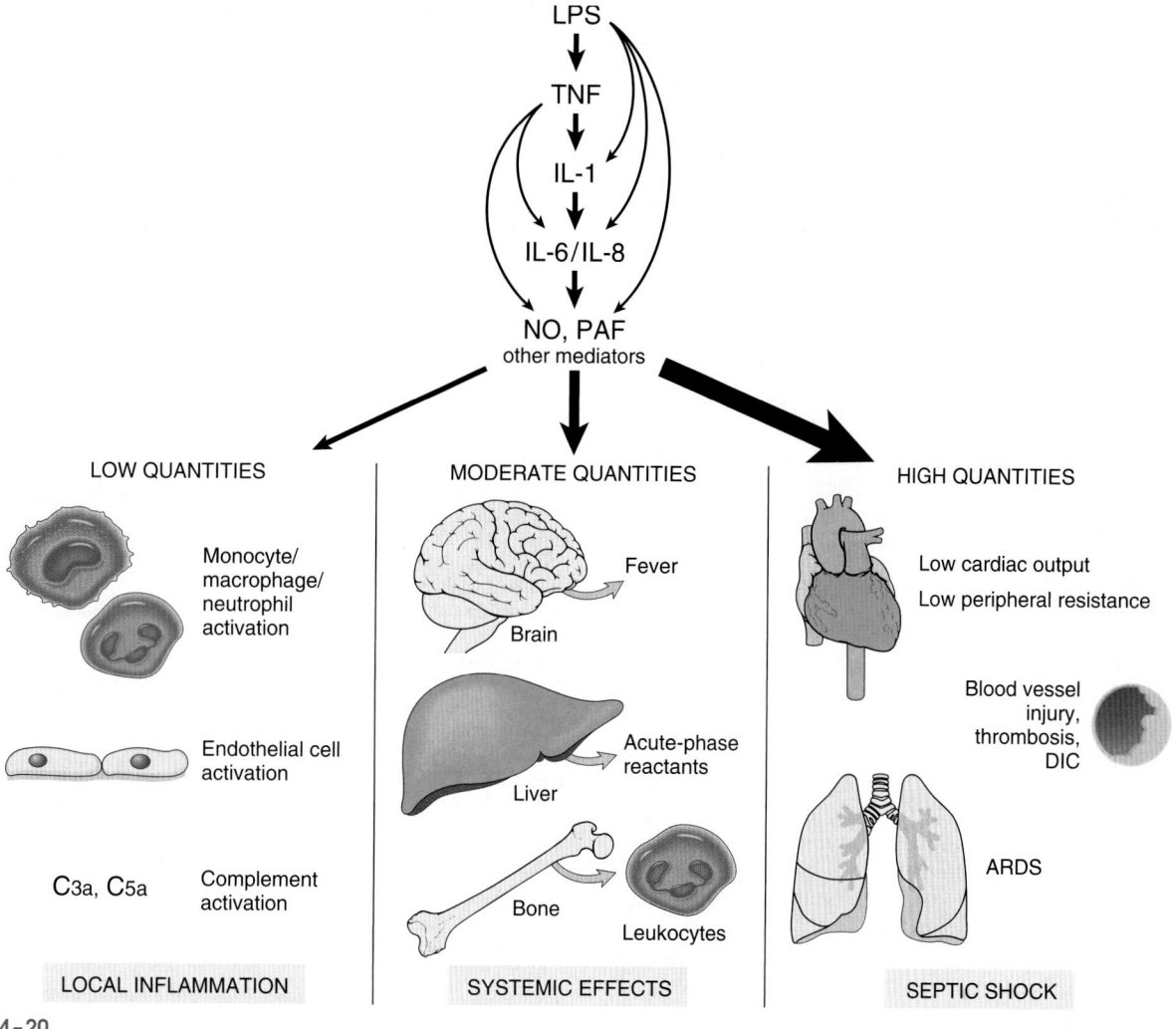

Figure 4-20

Effects of lipopolysaccharide (LPS) and secondarily induced effector molecules. LPS initiates the cytokine cascade described in Figure 4–19; in addition, LPS and the various factors can also directly stimulate down-stream cytokine production, as indicated. Secondary effectors that become important include nitric oxide (NO) and platelet-activating factor (PAF). At low levels, only local inflammatory effects are seen. With moderate levels, more systemic events occur in addition to the local vascular effects. At high concentrations, the syndrome of septic shock is seen. ARDS, adult respiratory distress syndrome; DIC, disseminated intravascular coagulation; IL-1, interleukin 1; IL-6, interleukin 6; IL-8, interleukin 8; TNF, tumor necrosis factor. (Modified from Abbas AK, et al: Cellular and Molecular Immunology, 4th ed. Philadelphia, WB Saunders, 2000.)

testinal flora to enter the circulation, endotoxic shock may also be superimposed. At this point, the patient has complete renal shutdown due to acute tubular necrosis (Chapter 14), and, despite heroic measures, the downward clinical spiral almost inevitably culminates in death.

MORPHOLOGY

The cellular and tissue changes induced by shock are essentially those of hypoxic injury (Chapter 1); since shock is characterized by **failure of multiple organ systems,** the cellular changes may appear in any tissue. Nevertheless, they are particularly evident in the brain, heart, lungs, kidneys, adrenals, and gastrointestinal tract.

The **brain** may develop so-called ischemic encephalopathy, discussed in Chapter 23. The **heart** may undergo focal and widespread coagulation necrosis, or it may exhibit subendocardial hemorrhage and/or contraction band necrosis (Chapter 11). While these changes are not diagnostic of shock (they may also be seen in the setting of cardiac reperfusion after irreversible injury, or after catecholamine administration), they are usually much more extensive in the setting of shock. The **kidneys** typically exhibit extensive tubular ischemic injury (acute tubular necrosis, Chapter 14), so that oliguria, anuria, and electrolyte disturbances constitute major clinical problems. The **lungs** are seldom affected in pure hypovolemic shock because they are somewhat resistant to hypoxic injury. However, when shock is caused by bacterial sepsis or trauma, changes of diffuse alveolar damage (Chapter 13) may appear, the so-called **shock lung**. The **adrenal** changes in shock are those seen in all forms of stress; essentially there is cortical cell lipid depletion. This does not reflect adrenal exhaustion but rather conversion of the relatively inactive vacuolated cells to metabolically active cells that utilize stored lipids for the synthesis of steroids. The **gastrointestinal tract** may suffer patchy mucosal hemorrhage and necrosis, referred to as **hemorrhagic enteropathy**. The **liver** may develop fatty change and, with severe perfusion deficits, central hemorrhagic necrosis (Chapter 16).

With the exception of neuronal and myocyte loss, virtually all of these tissues may revert to normal if the patient survives. Unfortunately, most patients with irreversible changes due to severe shock die before the tissues can recover.

Clinical Course. The clinical manifestations depend on the precipitating insult. In hypovolemic and cardiogenic shock, the patient presents with *hypotension*; a weak, rapid pulse; tachypnea; and cool, clammy, cyanotic skin. In septic shock, however, the skin may be warm and flushed owing to peripheral vasodilation. The initial threat to life stems from the underlying catastrophe that precipitated the shock state (e.g., a myocardial infarct, severe hemorrhage, or uncontrolled bacterial infection). Rapidly, however, the cardiac, cerebral, and pulmonary changes secondary to the shock state materially worsen the problem. Eventually, electrolyte disturbances and metabolic acidosis also exacerbate the situation. If the patients survive the initial complications, they enter a second phase, dominated by renal insufficiency and marked by a progressive fall in urine output as well as severe fluid and electrolyte imbalances.

The prognosis varies with the origin of shock and its duration. Thus, 80% of young, otherwise healthy patients with hypovolemic shock survive with appropriate management, whereas cardiogenic shock associated with extensive myocardial infarction or gram-negative shock carry mortality rates of 75%, even with state-of-the-art care.

BIBLIOGRAPHY

Aquila AM: Deep vein thrombosis. J Caridovasc Nurs 15:25, 2001. (A clinical overview of this common disorder.)

Collen D, Lijnen HR: Molecular basis of fibrinolysis, as relevant for thrombolytic therapy. Thromb Haemost 74:167, 1995. (A brief review of the pathways of fibrinolysis and their clinical applications.)

Dahlbeck B: Blood coagulation. Lancet 355:1627, 2000. (A nice and concise overview.)

Davis S: Amniotic fluid embolism: a review of literature. Can J Anesth 48:88, 2001. (A literature review of this condition.)

Dudney TM, Elliott CG: Pulmonary embolism from amniotic fluid, fat, and air. Prog Cardiovasc Dis 36:447, 1994. (A comprehensive review of nonthrombotic pulmonary emboli, including the mechanisms of injury.)

Goldhaber SZ: Pulmonary embolism. N Engl J Med 339:93, 1998. (An excellent and thorough review of the pathophysiologic and clinical issues regarding pulmonary embolism.)

Jarrar D, et al: Organ dysfunction following hemorrhage and sepsis: mechanisms and therapeutic approaches. Int J Mol Med 4:575, 1999. (Good overview, with emphasis on molecular mechanisms, of the mediators and physiologic effects of shock.)

Mellor A, Soni N: Fat embolism. Anesthesia 56:692, 2001. (A good review of this uncommon condition.)

Ognibene FO: Pathogenesis and innovative treatment of septic shock. Adv Intern Med 42:213, 1997. (Well-written, reasonably up-to-date overview of the interventional strategies in septic shock.)

Parrillo, JE: Mechanisms of disease: pathogenetic mechanisms of septic shock. N Engl J Med 328:1471, 1993. (Well-written review of the pathophysiology of septic shock.)

Pearson JD: Endothelial cell function and thrombosis. Baillieres Best Pract Res Clin Haematol 12:329, 1999. (A concise review of the roles played by endothelium in hemostasis and thrombosis.)

Rosendaal FR: Risk factors for venous thrombosis: Prevalence, risk, and interactions. Semin Hematol 34:171, 1997. (Good clinical discussion of the various elements that contribute to the risk of deep venous thromboses.)

Scurr JH, et al: Frequency and prevention of symptomless deep-vein thrombosis in long-haul flights: a randomised trial. Lancet 357:1485, 2001. (An interesting and provocative clinical trial looking at the incidence of DVT during typical long-distance travel; the incidence is more than might be expected, with increased risks attributed to genetic polymorphisms in factor V and prothrombin.)

Seligsohn U, Lubetsky A: Genetic susceptibility to venous thrombosis. New Engl J Med 344:1222, 2001. (An excellent discussion of inherited hypercoagulability.)

Shapiro SS: The lupus anticoagulant/antiphospholipid syndrome. Ann Rev Med 47:533, 1996. (Good summary of a relatively newly recognized clinical syndrome.)

Sriskandan S, Cohen J: The pathogenesis of septic shock. J Infect 30:201, 1995. (A nice review describing the pathologic mechanisms underlying septic shock; additional articles in the same volume cover management and other therapeutic issues.)

Ten Cate H: Pathophysiology of disseminated intravascular coagulation in sepsis. Crit Care Med 28:S9, 2000. (Succinct review of the interplay between inflammation and coagulation in DIC.)

Triplett DA: Coagulation and bleeding disorders: a review and update. Clin Chem 46:1260, 2000. (A clinically oriented review of hemostasis.)

5

Diseases of Immunity

RICHARD N. MITCHELL, MD, PhD
VINAY KUMAR, MD

The immune system is like the proverbial two-edged sword. On the one hand, we critically depend on intact immunity; defects in immune defenses resulting from immunodeficiency states render the human body easy prey to infections and several kinds of tumors. On the other hand, the immune system is the culprit behind the rejection of transplanted tissues, and hyperactive immunity or immunity against one's own tissues (*autoimmunity*) may cause debilitation and even fatal disease. Thus, diseases of immunity range from those caused by "too little" to those caused by "too much or inappropriate" immune activity. In this chapter, our knowledge of basic lymphocyte biology is reviewed, with an overview of histocompatibility molecules, a discussion of which is relevant to an understanding of several immune-mediated diseases and transplant rejection. Following this the mechanisms of *immunologic tolerance* (why we do not routinely reject our own bodies) and a sample of the autoimmune diseases that arise when tolerance fails are discussed. The chapter will conclude with discussions of primary and acquired immunodeficiency diseases and of *amyloidosis*, a disease caused by the abnormal extracellular deposition of certain proteins (some produced in the setting of immune responses).

The immune system is classically composed of two distinct but interrelated components designed to protect against extracellular and intracellular pathogens: *humoral immunity*, mediated by soluble *antibody* proteins, and *cellular immunity*, mediated by *lymphocytes* (Fig. 5–1). *B lymphocytes* (also called B cells) are the source of antibodies, which participate in immunity either by directly neutralizing extracellular microbes or by activating complement and certain effector cells (neutrophils and macrophages) to kill microorganisms. *T lymphocytes* (also called T cells) can either directly lyse targets (accomplished by *cytotoxic T cells*) or orchestrate the antimicrobial immune response of other cells by producing soluble protein mediators called *cytokines* (made by *helper T cells*). It is important to note that while B cells and their respective antibodies can recognize and bind to intact antigens, T cells can only "see" antigen that has been *processed* (proteolytically fragmented into smaller pieces) and *presented* by other cells in the context of *major histocompatibility complex (MHC)* molecules (see later). Thus, the engagement of T cells in immune responses requires both *antigen-presenting cells* (APCs, including macrophages and *dendritic cells*) to display processed antigen and a variety of effector cells (including macrophages) to eliminate the inciting stimulus. *Natural Killer (NK) cells* are a distinct subset of lymphocytes that act as a first line of defense.

CELLS OF THE IMMUNE SYSTEM

T Lymphocytes

Thymus-derived, or "T," cells direct the diverse elements of cellular immunity and are also essential for inducing the B cell–derived humoral immunity to many antigens. T cells constitute 60% to 70% of the lymphocytes in circulating blood and are also the major lymphocyte type in splenic periarteriolar sheaths and lymph node interfollicular zones. Each T cell is genetically programmed to recognize a unique processed peptide fragment by means of a specific T-cell receptor (TCR). TCR diversity for the billions of potential peptides is generated by somatic rearrangement of the genes that encode individual chains of the TCR. As might be expected, every somatic cell has TCR genes from the germ line. During ontogeny, somatic rearrangements of these genes occur only in T cells; hence, the *demonstration of TCR gene rearrangements by molecular methods (e.g., polymerase chain reaction [PCR]) is a definitive marker of T-lineage cells.* Such analyses are used in classification of lymphoid malignancies (Chapter 12). Furthermore, because each T cell has a unique DNA rearrangement (and hence a unique TCR), *it is possible to distinguish polyclonal (nonneoplastic) T-cell proliferations from monoclonal (neoplastic) T-cell proliferations.*

In the vast majority (>95%) of T cells, the TCR is a protein heterodimer composed of disulfide-linked α and β chains (Fig. 5–2); each chain has a variable region that binds a specific target peptide and a constant region that interacts with associated signaling molecules. In a minority of peripheral blood T cells and in many of the T cells associated with mucosal surfaces (e.g., lung and gastrointestinal tract), TCRs are composed of $\gamma\delta$ heterodimers. Such TCRs recognize nonprotein molecules (e.g., bacterial lipoglycans), and these so-called $\gamma\delta$ T cells may have a unique role in maintaining immunity at interfaces where there is a constant assault by extracellular pathogens. The focus here is on the better characterized $\alpha\beta$ T cells that recognize peptides in the context of MHC molecules.

TCRs are noncovalently linked to a cluster of five invariant polypeptide chains, composed of the γ, δ, and ε proteins of the CD3 (cluster of differentiation-3) molecular complex and two *zeta* (ζ) chains (see Fig. 5–2A). The CD3 proteins and ζ chains do not themselves bind antigenic peptides; instead, they interact with the constant region of the TCR to transduce intracellular signals after TCR ligation. In addition to these signaling proteins, T cells express a variety of other invariant function associated molecules, including CD4 and

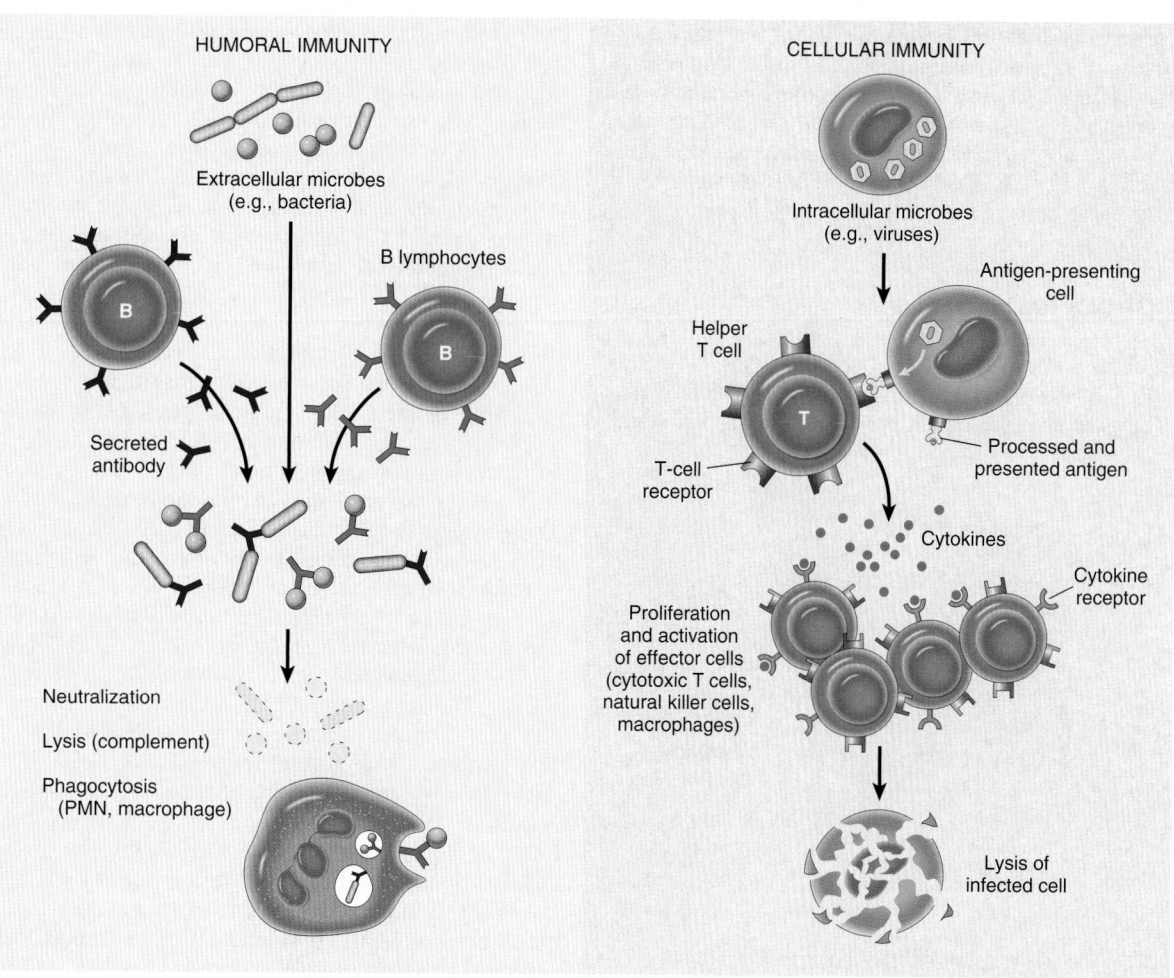

HUMORAL IMMUNITY

Extracellular microbes
(e.g., bacteria)

B lymphocytes

Secreted
antibody

Neutralization

Lysis (complement)

Phagocytosis
(PMN, macrophage)

CELLULAR IMMUNITY

Intracellular microbes
(e.g., viruses)

Antigen-presenting
cell

Helper
T cell

T-cell
receptor

Processed and
presented antigen

Cytokines

Cytokine
receptor

Proliferation
and activation
of effector cells
(cytotoxic T cells,
natural killer cells,
macrophages)

Lysis of
infected cell

Figure 5-1 ■

Schematic of the two arms of the immune system: humoral immunity *(left)*, mediated by soluble antibody proteins produced by B lymphocytes, and cellular immunity *(right)*, mediated by T lymphocytes. Antibodies participate in immunity either by directly neutralizing extracellular microbes or by activating complement and certain effector cells (polymorphonuclear neutrophils [PMNs] and macrophages) to kill microorganisms. T cells can either directly lyse targets (cytotoxic T cells) or orchestrate the immune response of other cells to clear invading microbes by producing soluble protein mediators called cytokines (helper T cells).

CD8 (see Fig. 5–2B). These two molecules are expressed on distinct T-cell subsets and serve as coreceptors for T-cell stimulation. During antigen recognition, CD4 molecules on T cells bind to invariant portions of class II MHC molecules (see later) on selected APCs; in an analogous fashion, CD8 binds to class I MHC molecules. It is noteworthy that T cells require two signals for complete activation. *Signal 1* is provided by engagement of TCR by the appropriate MHC-peptide antigen complex, and the CD4 and CD8 coreceptors enhance this signal. *Signal 2* is delivered by the interaction of CD28 molecules on T cells with costimulatory CD80 or CD86 molecules (also called B7-1 and B7-2, respectively) on APCs (see Fig. 5–2B). CD28 costimulation is critical, because in the absence of signal 2 the T cells undergo apoptosis or become unreactive *(anergic);* in fact, this two-signal fail-safe may be a way that the normal individual prevents autoreactivity.

CD4 is expressed on approximately 60% of mature T cells, whereas CD8 is expressed on about 30% of T cells; in normal healthy individuals, the CD4/CD8 ratio is therefore about 2:1. The CD4- and CD8-expressing T cells (called CD4+ and CD8+, respectively) perform different but overlapping

functions. CD4+ T cells are "helper" T cells because they secrete soluble molecules *(cytokines)* that influence virtually all other cells of the immune system. The central role of CD4+ helper cells in immunity is highlighted by the severe compromise that results from the destruction of this subset by human immunodeficiency virus (HIV) infection. The CD8+ T cells can also secrete cytokines, but they play a more important role in directly killing virus-infected or tumor cells ("cytotoxic" T cells). Because of the role played by the CD4 and CD8 coreceptors, CD4+ helper T cells respond to peptide antigens only in the context of class II MHC, whereas the CD8+ cytotoxic T cells respond only to antigens associated with class I MHC.

CD4+ T cells are further divided into two clinically relevant subsets with different functions defined by their cytokine profiles. The so-called T_H1 (helper T 1) CD4+ cells characteristically secrete cytokines that help direct cell-mediated immune responses, including macrophage and natural killer cell activation; these T_H1 cytokines include interleukin 2 (IL-2) and interferon-γ (IFN-γ). In contrast, T_H2 (helper T 2) CD4+ cells secrete cytokines (e.g., IL-4, IL-5, and IL-10) that antagonize T_H1 effects and/or promote certain aspects of humoral immunity. These include inducing synthesis of IgE, an immunoglobulin type that is pivotal in the pathogenesis of type I hypersensitivity reactions, including bronchial asthma. CD8+ T cells are also divided into analogous subsets that secrete comparable cytokine profiles (called T_C1 and T_C2 cells); nevertheless, the cytotoxic potential of these cells is their most important aspect.

B Lymphocytes

Bone marrow–derived, or "B," lymphocytes comprise 10% to 20% of the circulating peripheral lymphocyte population. They are also present in bone marrow, in peripheral lymphoid tissues (lymph nodes, spleen, and tonsils), and in nonlymphoid organs such as the gastrointestinal tract. B cells are localized to lymphoid follicles in the lymph node cortex and to splenic white pulp. Stimulation (e.g., by local infection) leads to the formation of a central zone of large, activated B cells in follicles, called a *germinal center*.

After stimulation, B cells form *plasma cells* that secrete immunoglobulins, which in turn are the mediators of humoral immunity. There are five basic immunoglobulin isotypes; IgG, IgM, and IgA constitute more than 95% of circulating antibodies with relatively minimal contributions from IgE and IgD. Each isotype has characteristic abilities to activate complement or recruit inflammatory cells, as well as having defined roles; for example, IgA is an important mediator of mucosal immunity, whereas IgE has special importance for helminth infections (and in allergic responses).

B cells recognize antigen via monomeric surface IgM, the so-called B-cell receptor (BCR). As with T cells, each BCR has a unique antigen specificity, derived in part from somatic rearrangements of immunoglobulin genes. *Thus, the presence of rearranged immunoglobulin genes in a lymphoid cell is used as a molecular marker of B-lineage cells; such rearrangements can also be used to identify polyclonal (non-neoplastic) versus monoclonal (neoplastic) B-cell proliferations.* Analogous to the TCR-CD3 complex, BCRs interact with several invariant molecules that are responsible for signal transduction and for complete B-cell activation (Fig. 5–3). One such example is the B-cell CD40 molecule that binds to CD154 on activated T cells and is critical for B-cell maturation and secretion of IgG, IgA, or IgE antibodies. Patients with mutations of CD154 make predominantly IgM and have an immunodeficiency called *X-linked hyper-IgM syndrome* (p 146). CD21 (also known as the CR2 complement receptor) is another important B cell–associated costimulatory molecule; it is also noteworthy as the receptor by which Epstein-Barr virus (EBV) gains access to human B cells.

Macrophages

The origin, differentiation, and role of macrophages in chronic inflammation are discussed extensively in Chapter 2. Here, focus is placed briefly on the roles that macrophages play in the induction and the effector phase of immune response.

Figure 5–2 ■

The T-cell receptor (TCR) complex and its interaction with major histocompatibility complex (MHC) molecules on antigen-presenting cells. *A,* Schematic illustration of TCRα and TCRβ polypeptide chains linked to the CD3 and ζ chain molecular complex. *B,* Schematic representation of antigen recognition by CD4+ T cells. Note that the αβ TCR heterodimer recognizes a peptide fragment of antigen bound to the MHC class II molecule. The CD4 molecule binds to the nonpolymorphic portion of the class II molecule. The interaction between the TCR and the MHC-bound antigen provides signal 1 for T-cell activation. Signal 2 is provided by the interaction of the CD28 molecule with the costimulatory molecules (CD80 or CD86) expressed on antigen-presenting cells. Analogous interactions occur between MHC I molecules and TCR on CD8+ T cells; in that instance, the CD8 molecule binds to the nonpolymorphic portion of the class I molecule.

Figure 5-3   ■

The B-cell receptor (BCR) complex and its interaction with antigen and costimulatory molecules. Membrane-bound immunoglobulin (here shown as IgM) binds to exogenous antigen; intracellular signal 1 for B-cell activation is then provided by interaction with BCR-associated Igα and Igβ heterodimers. Signal 2 is provided by activated complement interacting with B-cell CD21 or by interaction of B-cell surface CD40 with CD154 on activated T cells.

- Macrophages (along with *dendritic cells,* below) express class II MHC (p 109) and are therefore central players in the processing and presentation of antigen to CD4+ helper T cells. Because T cells (unlike B cells) cannot be triggered by free antigen, presentation by macrophages or other APCs is obligatory for induction of cell-mediated immunity.
- Macrophages produce a plethora of cytokines and are therefore important effector cells in certain forms of cell-mediated immunity (e.g., delayed-type hypersensitivity; p 119). These cytokines not only influence T- and B-cell function but also affect other cell types, including endothelium and fibroblasts.
- Macrophages phagocytose (and ultimately kill) microbes coated by antibody and/or complement (*opsonized;* Chapter 2); consequently, they are important effector elements in humoral immunity.

Dendritic Cells

Cells with dendritic morphology (i.e., with fine dendritic cytoplasmic processes) occur as two functionally distinct types.

- *Interdigitating dendritic cells* (or more simply, *dendritic cells*). These are nonphagocytic cells that express high levels of MHC class II and costimulatory molecules. They are widely distributed, occurring in lymphoid tissues and in the interstitium of many nonlymphoid organs, such as the heart and lungs; similar cells within the epidermis are also called *Langerhans cells.* The distribution and surface molecule expression of dendritic cells makes them ideally suited for presenting antigens to CD4+ T cells; they are probably the most potent APC for naive T cells.
- *Follicular dendritic cells.* As suggested by their name, follicular dendritic cells are primarily localized to the germinal centers of lymphoid follicles in the spleen and lymph nodes. These cells bear *Fc receptors* for IgG (receptors that bind the constant, or Fc, portion of antibodies) and hence efficiently trap antigen bound to antibodies. Consequently, after an initial antibody response, antigens can persist in this form in lymphoid tissues and facilitate the maintenance of immunologic memory. Obviously, such cells are important in ongoing immune responses and are discussed in more detail (p 150 and Fig. 5-39) with the acquired immunodeficiency syndrome (AIDS).

Natural Killer (NK) Cells

NK cells are somewhat larger than small lymphocytes and comprise 10% to 15% of peripheral blood lymphocytes. These cells contain abundant azurophilic granules and are able to lyse a variety of tumor cells, virally infected cells, and some normal cells, *without previous sensitization.* These cells are classified as part of the *innate* (as opposed to adaptive) immune system that is the first line of defense against a variety of assaults. Although they share some surface markers with T cells, NK cells do not express TCR and are CD3 negative. NK cells instead express two types of surface receptors that facilitate their ability to kill neoplastic or virus-infected cells. One receptor type is an activating receptor that recognizes as yet ill-defined molecules on target cells. The other receptor type (so-called *killer inhibitor receptor [KIR]*) inhibits NK cytolysis by recognition of self class I MHC molecules. NK cells do not normally lyse healthy nucleated cells because they all express class I MHC molecules. If virus infection or neoplastic transformation reduces normal MHC I expression, inhibitory KIR signals are interrupted and lysis occurs (Fig. 5-4). NK cells may be identified by the presence of two cell-surface molecules, CD16 and CD56; CD16 is of particular functional significance. It is an Fc receptor for IgG and endows NK cells with the additional ability to lyse IgG-opsonized target cells. Called *antibody-dependent cell-mediated cytotoxicity (ADCC),* this process is described in greater detail later in this chapter (p 115). NK cells also secrete cytokines and are an important source of IFN-γ.

HISTOCOMPATIBILITY MOLECULES

General Properties of Histocompatibility Molecules. Although originally characterized as the antigens responsible for the rejection of organs (hence the name *histo-* or tissue

Figure 5–4 ■

Schematic representation of NK cell receptors and killing. Normal cells are not killed because inhibitory signals from MHC class I molecules override activating signals. In tumor cells or virus-infected cells, reduced expression or alteration of MHC molecules interrupts the inhibitory signals, allowing activation of NK cells and lysis of target cells.

compatibility), histocompatibility molecules are now recognized as a critical element in inducing and regulating normal immune function. Recall that T cells (unlike B cells) can recognize only membrane-bound antigens, and only in the context of "self" histocompatibility molecules; this phenomenon is referred to as *MHC restriction. Thus, the principal role of histocompatibility molecules is to bind peptide fragments of foreign proteins for presentation to appropriate antigen-specific T cells.* In addition, by engaging KIRs on NK cells, MHC class I molecules prevent lysis of normal cells by NK cells. Here only the salient features of human histocompatibility molecules will be summarized, primarily to facilitate understanding of their role in transplant rejection and in disease susceptibility. Several genes code for histocompatibility molecules, but the most important are clustered on a small segment of chromosome 6. This cluster constitutes the human major histocompatibility complex (MHC) and is also known as the *HLA (human leukocyte antigen) complex* (Fig. 5–5). The HLA system is highly polymorphic; that is, there are several alternative forms *(alleles)* of a gene at each locus (for example, there are over 400 different HLA-B alleles thus far described). As we shall see, this constitutes a formidable barrier to organ transplantation.

On the basis of their chemical structure, tissue distribution, and function, MHC gene products fall into three categories:

■ Class I MHC molecules are coded by three closely linked loci designated HLA-A, HLA-B, and HLA-C (see Fig. 5–5). Each of these molecules is a heterodimer,

Figure 5–5 ■

Schematic representation of the HLA complex and the HLA molecules. *A,* The relative distances between various genes and regions on chromosome 6 are not drawn to scale. *B,* MHC I and MHC II have homologous structures, although the subunit organization and origin of the peptide in the antigen cleft are different (see text). LT, lymphotoxin; TNF, tumor necrosis factor.

consisting of a polymorphic 44-kD α chain noncovalently associated with a 12-kD nonpolymorphic β-microglobulin (encoded by a separate gene on chromosome 15). The extracellular portion of the α chain contains a cleft where foreign peptides bind to MHC molecules for presentation to CD8+ T cells (see Fig. 5–5). In general, MHC I molecules bind to peptides derived from proteins (e.g., viral antigens) synthesized within the cell. Because MHC I molecules are present on virtually all nucleated cells, virally infected cells can be detected and lysed by cytotoxic T cells.

■ Class II MHC molecules are coded by genes in the HLA-D region, where there are at least three subregions, DP, DQ, and DR. MHC II molecules differ from MHC I molecules in several respects. MHC II molecules are heterodimers of noncovalently linked polymorphic α and β subunits (see Fig. 5–5). Like in MHC I, the extracellular portion of the MHC II heterodimer contains a cleft for the binding of antigenic peptides. Unlike in MHC I, the tissue distribution of MHC II–expressing cells is quite restricted; they are constitutively expressed mainly on APC (monocytes, macrophages, and dendritic cells) and B cells. In addition, other cell types, such as vascular endothelial cells, fibroblasts, and renal tubular epithelial cells, are induced to express MHC II by interferon-α (IFN-α). In general, MHC II molecules bind to peptides derived from proteins (e.g., those derived from extracellular bacteria) synthesized outside the cell. This allows CD4+ T cells to recognize the presence of extracellular pathogens and to orchestrate a protective cytokine-mediated response (see Fig. 5–1).

■ Class III proteins include some of the complement components (C2, C3, and Bf); genes for tumor necrosis factor (TNF) and lymphotoxin (TNF-β) are also encoded within the MHC. Although genetically linked to class I and II antigens, class III molecules and the cytokine genes do not act as histocompatibility (transplantation) antigens and will not be discussed further.

Significance of Histocompatibility Molecules. Any given individual inherits one HLA allele from each parent and thus typically expresses two different molecules for every locus. Cells of a heterozygous individual therefore express six different class I HLA molecules, three of maternal origin and three of paternal origin. Similarly, a given individual will express maternal and paternal alleles of the MHC II loci; because of an ability of the different HLA-D α and β chains to mix-and-match with each other, each MHC II–expressing cell can also have over 20 different MHC II molecules. *Different MHC alleles bind to different peptide fragments depending on the particular amino acid sequence of a given peptide*; the multiplicity of MHC expression therefore allows each cell to present a wide array of peptide antigens. However, owing to the polymorphism at the major HLA loci over the population at large, virtually innumerable combinations of molecules exist, and each individual expresses a unique MHC antigenic profile on his or her cell surface.

The significance of this polymorphism is obvious in the context of transplantation. In fact, HLA molecules were originally discovered in the course of early attempts at tissue transplantation. HLA molecules of the graft evoke both humoral and cell-mediated responses, eventually leading to graft destruction (discussed later in this chapter). Because the severity of the rejection reaction is in large part related to the degree of donor and recipient HLA disparity, HLA typing is of clinical significance in the selection of appropriate donor-recipient combinations.

The role of MHC in T-cell stimulation also has important implications on the genetic regulation of the immune response. Theoretically, the ability of any given MHC allele to bind the peptide antigens generated from a particular pathogen may critically regulate whether an individual's T-cell repertoire can actually "see" and respond to that pathogen. Stated differently, an individual will recognize and mount an immune response against a given antigen only if he or she inherits those MHC molecules that can bind the antigenic peptide and present it to T cells. The consequence of inheriting specific genes also depends on the nature of the antigen and the type of immune response generated. For example, if the antigen is ragweed pollen and the response is production of IgE antibody, the individual will be genetically prone to type I hypersensitivity disease (allergy) to that antigen. On the other hand, good responsiveness to a viral antigen may be beneficial for the host.

HLA and Disease Association. Many diseases are associated with selected HLA types (Table 5–1). The best known is the association between ankylosing spondylitis and HLA-B27; individuals who possess this antigen have a 90-fold greater chance (relative risk) of developing the disease than do those who are negative for HLA-B27. The diseases that are linked to HLA can be broadly grouped into the following categories: (1) *inflammatory diseases*, including ankylosing spondylitis and several postinfectious arthropathies, all associated with HLA-B27; (2) *inherited errors of metabolism*, such as 21-hydroxylase deficiency (HLA-Bw47); and (3) *autoimmune diseases*, including autoimmune endocrinopathies, associated with certain DR alleles. The mechanisms underlying all these associations are not understood at present. In some cases, the linkage results from the fact that the relevant disease-associated gene (e.g., 21-hydroxylase) maps within the HLA complex. In the case of immunologically mediated disorders, it seems likely that the role of MHC II molecules in regulating the immunore-

Table 5-1. ASSOCIATION OF HLA WITH DISEASE

Disease	HLA Allele	Relative Risk
Ankylosing spondylitis	B27	87.4
Postgonococcal arthritis	B27	14.0
Acute anterior uveitis	B27	14.6
Rheumatoid arthritis	DR4	5.8
Chronic active hepatitis	DR3	13.9
Primary Sjögren syndrome	DR3	9.7
Insulin-dependent diabetes	DR3	5.0
	DR4	6.8
	DR3/DR4	14.3
21-Hydroxylase deficiency	Bw47	15.0

sponsiveness may be relevant. For example, it can be speculated that an association between certain autoimmune diseases and HLA-DR may result from an exaggerated or inappropriate immune response to autoantigens.

CYTOKINES: SOLUBLE MEDIATORS OF THE IMMUNE SYSTEM

The induction and regulation of immune responses involve orchestrating the interactions of multiple cell types, including lymphocytes, monocytes, other inflammatory cells (e.g., neutrophils), and endothelium. Many interactions require intimate cell-cell contact; others are mediated by short-acting soluble mediators called *cytokines*.

General Properties of Cytokines. Cytokines are low molecular weight polypeptides (typically 10 to 40 kD) that are secreted by lymphocytes as well as by effector cells and APCs; in certain circumstances, epithelial and mesenchymal cells are also important sources. Although originally classified as *lymphokines* (produced by lymphocytes) and *monokines* (produced by monocytes/macrophages), they are now all generically referred to as cytokines.

■ Cytokines mediate their effects by binding to specific high-affinity receptors on their target cells. For example, IL-2 activates T cells by binding to high-affinity IL-2 receptors (IL-2R). Blockade of the IL-2R by specific antireceptor monoclonal antibodies (e.g., to treat rejection of a transplanted organ) prevents T-cell activation.
■ Cytokines induce their effects in three ways: (1) they act on the same cell that produces them (*autocrine* effect), such as occurs when IL-2 produced by activated T cells promotes T-cell growth; (2) they affect other cells in their vicinity (*paracrine* effect), as occurs when IL-7 produced by marrow stromal cells promotes the differentiation of B-cell progenitors in the marrow; and (3) they affect cells systemically (*endocrine* effect), the best examples in this category being IL-1 and TNF which produce the *acute-phase response* during inflammation.
■ Cytokines can act in amplifying cascades. Thus, TNF induces IL-1 production, which in turn drives IL-6 synthesis.
■ Many individual cytokines are produced by several different cell types. For example, IL-1 and TNF can be produced by virtually any cell.
■ The effects of cytokines are *pleiotropic*: that is, they act on many cell types, causing many different effects. For example, IL-2 was originally described as a T-cell growth factor; however, it was subsequently also found to regulate the growth and differentiation of B cells and NK cells.
■ Multiple cytokines may induce similar effects, that is, they are *redundant*. For example, IL-1 and TNF have very similar effector profiles.
■ Cytokines may be *antagonistic*, and in that fashion they can finely regulate the intensity and type of an immune response. For example, IFN-γ activates macrophages while IL-10 prevents macrophage activation.

General Classes of Cytokines. Although most cytokines have a wide spectrum of effector functions, the currently known cytokines can be organized into five categories on the basis of their general properties. In addition, although these cytokines are also typically produced by multiple cell types, the predominant sources can be identified.

■ *Cytokines that mediate innate immunity.* Included in this group are IL-1, TNF, IL-6, and type 1 interferons. Certain of these cytokines (e.g., interferons) protect against viral infections, while others (e.g., IL-1, TNF, IL-6) initiate nonspecific proinflammatory responses, such as the activation of endothelium and mononuclear inflammatory cells and induction of acute-phase reactant synthesis by the liver. Macrophages are the major source of these cytokines.
■ *Cytokines that regulate lymphocyte growth, activation, and differentiation.* Within this category are IL-2, IL-4, IL-5, IL-12, IL-15, and transforming growth factor α (TGF-α). Some, such as IL-2 and IL-4, usually favor lymphocyte growth and differentiation; others, such as IL-10 and TGF-α, down-regulate immune responses. Note also that some of these cytokines (e.g., IL-2) fall under the rubric of T_H1 cytokines, which direct cell-mediated responses, whereas others (e.g., IL-4, IL-10) are considered to be T_H2 cytokines, which antagonize T_H1 effects and/or promote certain aspects of humoral immunity.
■ *Cytokines that activate inflammatory cells.* In this category are IFN-γ (considered to be a T_H1 cytokine), TNF, lymphotoxin (TNF-β), and migration inhibitory factor. Most of these cytokines are derived from T cells and serve to activate the functions of antigen-nonspecific effector cells.
■ *Chemokines are cytokines that act to recruit inflammatory cells to sites of injury* (Chapter 2). These occur in structurally distinct subfamilies, with the two main groups designated as *C-C* and *C-X-C* chemokines based on the arrangement of certain cysteine (C) residues. The C-X-C chemokines, which include IL-8, are produced by activated macrophages and tissue cells (e.g., endothelium). C-C chemokines are produced largely by T cells and include monocyte chemoattractant protein 1 (MCP-1) and monocyte inflammatory protein 1α (MIP-1α).
■ *Cytokines that stimulate hematopoiesis.* Several members of this family are called *colony-stimulating factors (CSFs)* because their original characterization was based on their ability to promote the growth of hematopoietic cell colonies from bone marrow precursors. Lymphocytes and bone marrow stromal cells are the major sources of these cytokines. Examples include granulocyte-macrophage (GM)-CSF and granulocyte (G)-CSF, which act on committed progenitor cells, and stem cell factor (also called c-*kit* ligand), which acts on pluripotent stem cells.

Although an understanding of cytokine biology may appear daunting, it has many practical therapeutic applications. By regulating cytokine production or action, it is likely that we will be able to control the harmful effects of inflammation or tissue-damaging immune reactions. Moreover, recombinant cytokines can be administered to enhance immunity against cancer or microbial infections *(immunotherapy)*. Both of these avenues are currently in development.

Disease Due to Cytokine Overproduction: Superantigens. *Superantigens* are a class of microbial proteins that bind to class II MHC molecules outside the antigen-binding cleft. These superantigens then stimulate a multitude of CD4+ T cells in an antigen-nonspecific manner by interacting with all TCRs that display a particular variable region on the β chain (Vβ subunit) (Fig. 5–6). Because the same Vβ region may be used by a large number of TCRs (as many as one in five T cells carries the same Vβ subunit), superantigens are functionally *polyclonal T-cell activators*. Thus, when present, superantigens can activate a large percentage of T cells and will result in widespread cytokine-mediated (TNF and IL-2) pathology analogous to shock induced by lipopolysaccharides from gram-negative bacteria (Chapters 4 and 9). Superantigens are typified by the staphylococcal exotoxins, and the pathologic processes associated with staphylococcal enterotoxins (food poisoning), exfoliative toxins *(staphylococcal scalded skin syndrome),* and the exotoxin associated with *toxic shock syndrome* (toxin 1) are all caused by polyclonal T-cell activation, with subsequent supranormal TNF and IL-2 release.

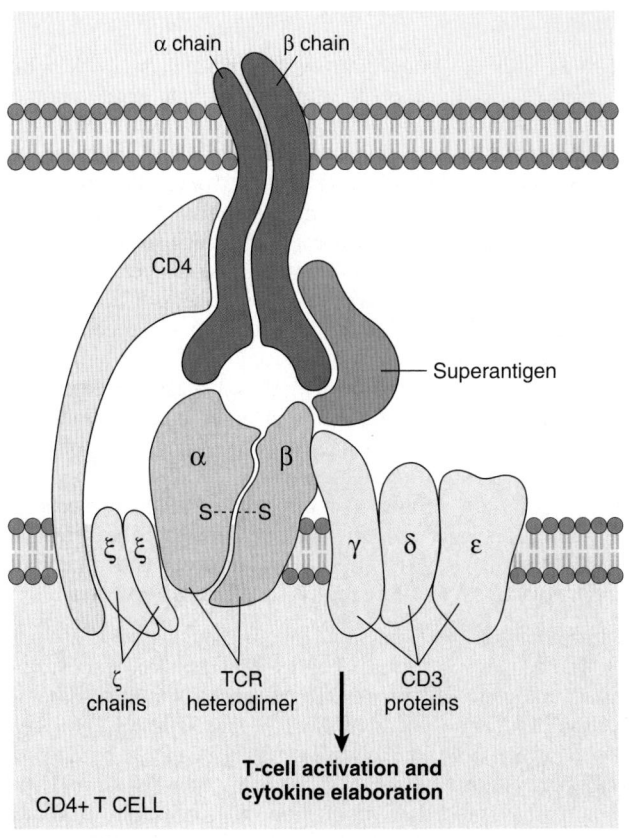

Figure 5-6 ■

Schematic representation of superantigen binding to the β subunit of the TCR and outside the antigen-binding cleft of MHC II molecules. The result is polyclonal activation with cytokine production of any T cell with the appropriate β subunit.

MECHANISMS OF IMMUNE-MEDIATED INJURY (HYPERSENSITIVITY REACTIONS)

Although immune activation leads to the production of antibody and T-cell responses that are generally protective against infections (and to some extent tumors), such responses may also potentially damage host tissues. Normally, an exquisite system of checks and balances optimizes the antigen-specific eradication of infecting organisms with only trivial innocent bystander injury. However, as has been mentioned, certain types of infections (e.g., viruses) may require destroying host tissues to eliminate the disease. Still other types of infections (e.g., tuberculosis) may be controlled only by a cellular response that walls off the offending agent with activated macrophages and scar, often at the expense of adjacent normal parenchyma. It is also noteworthy that certain bacterial products can stimulate macrophages (e.g., endotoxin [Chapters 4 and 9]) or induce a polyclonal activation of T lymphocytes (e.g., superantigens [see earlier]), resulting in systemic pathology from excessive cytokine elaboration. Even when the host response to an infectious agent is specific antibody, that antibody can occasionally cross-react with self-antigens (e.g., anticardiac antibodies following certain streptococcal infections, causing *rheumatic heart disease* [Chapter 11]). Immune complexes composed of specific antibody and circulating antigens may also precipitate at inappropriate sites and cause injury by activation of the complement cascade or by facilitating binding of neutrophils and macrophages (e.g., *poststreptococcal glomerulonephritis* [Chapter 14]). If the antibody made in response to a particular antigen happens to be IgE, any subsequent response to that antigen will be so-called immediate hypersensitivity, potentially culminating in *anaphylaxis*. Finally, not all antigens that attract the attention of lymphocytes are *exogenous*. The immune system occasionally (fortunately, rarely) loses tolerance for *endogenous* antigens, which results in autoimmune disease.

All of these forms of immune-mediated injury are collectively denoted *hypersensitivity reactions*. The term *hypersensitivity* is somewhat misleading because it implies abnormal or excessive sensitivity to an antigen. As indicated earlier, hypersensitivity disease may result from a perfectly normal immune response to an antigen (e.g., the rejection of tissue grafts from antigenically dissimilar donors). Hypersensitivity diseases are best classified on the basis of the immunologic mechanism initiating the disease (Table 5–2). However, this classification of immune-mediated disease is somewhat arbitrary. As will be seen, all types may coexist in one disease; frequently, there is a substantial contribution of cellular injury in "humoral" pathologic states and vice versa. Nevertheless, this approach is of value, because it clarifies the manner in which the immune responses ultimately cause tissue injury and disease.

The hypersensitivity reactions are traditionally subdivided into four types; three are variations on antibody-mediated injury, whereas the fourth is cell mediated:

■ *Type I* disease results from IgE antibodies adsorbed on mast cells or basophils; when these IgE molecules bind their specific antigen (allergen), they are triggered to release vasoactive amines and other mediators that in turn

Table 5–2. MECHANISMS OF IMMUNOLOGICALLY MEDIATED DISORDERS

Type	Immune Mechanism	Prototype Disorder
I Anaphylactic Type	Allergen cross-links IgE antibody → release of vasoactive amines and other mediators from basophils and mast cells → recruitment of other inflammatory cells	Anaphylaxis, some forms of bronchial asthma
II Antibody to Fixed Tissue Antigen	IgG or IgM binds to antigen on cell surface → phagocytosis of target cell or lysis of target cell by complement or antibody-dependent cell-mediated cytotoxicity	Autoimmune hemolytic anemia, erythroblastosis fetalis, Goodpasture disease, pemphigus vulgaris
III Immune Complex Disease	Antigen-antibody complexes → activate complement → attract neutrophils → release of lysosomal enzymes, oxygen free radicals, etc.	Arthus reaction, serum sickness, systemic lupus erythematosus, certain forms of acute glomerulonephritis
IV Cell-Mediated (Delayed) Hypersensitivity	Sensitized T lymphocytes → release of cytokines and T cell–mediated cytotoxicity	Tuberculosis, contact dermatitis, transplant rejection

affect vascular permeability and smooth muscle contraction in various organs.

■ *Type II* disorders are caused by humoral antibodies that bind to fixed tissue or cell surface antigen and cause a pathologic process by predisposing cells to phagocytosis or to complement-mediated lysis.

■ *Type III* disorders are best thought of as "immune complex diseases"; antibodies bind antigens to form large antigen-antibody complexes that precipitate in various vascular beds and activate complement. The immune complexes and complement activation fragments also attract neutrophils. Ultimately, it is the activated complement and the release of neutrophilic enzymes and other toxic molecules (e.g., oxygen metabolites) that cause the tissue damage in immune complex disease.

■ *Type IV* disorders (also called "delayed-type hypersensitivity") are cell-mediated immune responses where antigen-specific T lymphocytes are the ultimate cause of the cellular and tissue injury.

Type I Hypersensitivity (Allergy and Anaphylaxis)

Type I hypersensitivity is a tissue response that occurs rapidly (typically within minutes) after the interaction of allergen with IgE antibody previously bound to the surface of mast cells and basophils in a sensitized host. Depending on the portal of entry, type I hypersensitivity may occur as a local reaction that is merely annoying (e.g., seasonal rhinitis, or hay fever) or severely debilitating (asthma) or may culminate in a fatal systemic disorder (anaphylaxis).

Many localized type I reactions have two well-defined phases: (1) the initial response, characterized by vasodilation, vascular leakage, and smooth muscle spasm, usually evident within 5 to 30 minutes after exposure to an allergen and subsiding by 60 minutes; and (2) a second, late-phase reaction that sets in 2 to 8 hours later and lasts for several days. The late-phase reaction is characterized by more intense infiltration of tissues with eosinophils and other

acute and chronic inflammatory cells as well as by tissue destruction in the form of mucosal epithelial cell damage.

Because mast cells and basophils are central to the development of type I hypersensitivity, some of their salient characteristics are reviewed first and then the immune mechanisms that underlie this form of hypersensitivity are discussed.

■ Mast cells are bone marrow derived and are widely distributed in the tissues; they are found predominantly near blood vessels and nerves and in subepithelial sites. Their cytoplasm contains membrane-bound granules that possess a variety of biologically active mediators. As described later, mast cells (and basophils) are activated by cross-linking IgE bound to their surface by high-affinity Fc receptors; mast cells may also be triggered by other stimuli, such as complement components C5a and C3a (anaphylatoxins [Chapter 2]) binding to specific mast cell membrane receptors. Mast cells can also be induced to disgorge their granules by certain macrophage-derived cytokines (e.g., IL-8), drugs such as codeine and morphine, mellitin (present in bee venom), and physical stimuli (e.g., heat, cold, sunlight).

■ Basophils are similar to mast cells in many respects but are not normally present in tissues. Instead, they circulate in the blood in extremely small numbers and, like other granulocytes, can be recruited to inflammatory sites.

In humans, type I reactions are mediated by IgE antibodies. The sequence of events begins with an initial exposure to certain antigens (allergens). The allergen stimulates the induction of CD4+ T cells of the T$_H$2 type. These CD4+ cells play a pivotal role in the pathogenesis of type I hypersensitivity because the cytokines secreted by them (IL-4 and IL-5 in particular) cause IgE production by B cells, act as growth factors for mast cells, and recruit and activate eosinophils. IgE antibodies bind to high-affinity Fc receptors expressed on mast cells and basophils; once the mast cells and basophils are thus "armed," the individual is primed to develop type I hypersensitivity (Fig. 5–7). Re-exposure to the same antigen results in cross-linking of the cell-bound IgE and

Figure 5–7   ■

Sequence of events leading to type I hypersensitivity. APC, antigen-presenting cell; GM-CSF, granulocyte-macrophage colony-stimulating factor; TCR, T-cell receptor; T_H2 cell, CD4+ helper T cell.

triggers a cascade of intracellular signals leading to the release of several powerful mediators (Fig. 5–8). One set of signals leads to mast cell degranulation with discharge of preformed or primary mediators; another parallel set of signals induces de novo synthesis and release of secondary mediators such as arachidonic acid metabolites and cytokines.

PRIMARY MEDIATORS

After IgE triggering, primary (preformed) mediators within mast cell granules are released to initiate the early events in type I hypersensitivity reactions. Histamine, the most important of these preformed mediators, causes increased vascular permeability, vasodilation, bronchoconstriction, and increased secretion of mucus. Other rapidly released mediators include adenosine (causes bronchoconstriction and inhibits platelet aggregation) and chemotactic factors for neutrophils and eosinophils. Other mediators are found in the granule matrix and include heparin and neutral proteases (e.g., tryptase). The latter generate kinins and cleave complement components to produce additional chemotactic and inflammatory factors (e.g., C3a [Chapter 2]).

SECONDARY MEDIATORS

These include two classes of compounds: lipid mediators and cytokines. The lipid mediators are generated by activation of phospholipase A_2, which cleaves mast cell membrane phospholipids to produce arachidonic acid. In turn, arachidonic acid is the parent compound from which leukotrienes and prostaglandins are synthesized (Chapter 2).

■ Leukotrienes result from the action of 5-lipoxygenase on the arachidonic acid precursor and are extremely

Figure 5–8   ■

Activation of mast cells in type I hypersensitivity and release of their mediators. ECF, eosinophil chemotactic factor; NCF, neutrophil chemotactic factor; PAF, platelet-activating factor.

important in the pathogenesis of type I hypersensitivity. Leukotrienes C_4 and D_4 are the most potent vasoactive and spasmogenic agents known; on a molar basis, they are several thousand times more active than histamine in increasing vascular permeability and causing bronchial smooth muscle contraction. Leukotriene B_4 is highly chemotactic for neutrophils, eosinophils, and monocytes.

■ Prostaglandin D_2 is the most abundant mediator generated by the cyclooxygenase pathway in mast cells. It causes intense bronchospasm as well as increased mucus secretion.

■ Platelet-activating factor (Chapter 2) is another secondary mediator, resulting in platelet aggregation, histamine release, and bronchospasm. It is also chemotactic for neutrophils and eosinophils. Although its production is initiated by the activation of phospholipase A_2, it is not a product of arachidonic acid metabolism.

■ Mast cell–produced cytokines (TNF, IL-1, IL-4, IL-5, and IL-6) and chemokines play an important role in type I hypersensitivity reactions through their ability to recruit and activate a variety of inflammatory cells. TNF is an extremely potent mediator in leukocyte adhesion, emigration, and activation. IL-4 is also a mast cell growth factor and is required to drive IgE synthesis by B cells.

In summary, a variety of chemotactic, vasoactive, and bronchospasmic compounds (Table 5–3) mediate type I hypersensitivity reactions. Some of these compounds are released rapidly from sensitized mast cells and are responsible for the intense immediate reactions associated with conditions such as systemic anaphylaxis. Others, such as cytokines, are responsible for the late-phase reactions, including inflammatory cell recruitment. Not only do the secondarily recruited inflammatory cells release additional mediators, but they also cause local epithelial damage.

Eosinophils are recruited by eotaxin and other chemokines released from TNF-activated epithelium and are important effectors of tissue injury in the late-phase response in type I hypersensitivity. For example, eosinophils produce major basic protein and eosinophil cationic protein, which are toxic to epithelial cells. Similarly, leukotriene C_4 and platelet-activating factor produced by eosinophils directly activate mast cell mediator release. As a result, the recruited cells amplify and sustain the inflammatory response in the absence of any additional allergen exposure. Because inflammation is a major component of the late-phase reaction in type I hypersensitivity, its control usually requires broad-spectrum anti-inflammatory drugs such as corticosteroids.

CLINICAL MANIFESTATIONS

A type I reaction may occur as a systemic disorder or as a local reaction. Often this is determined by the route of antigen exposure. Systemic (parenteral) administration of protein antigens or drugs (e.g., bee venom or penicillin) results in *systemic anaphylaxis*. Within minutes of an exposure in a sensitized host, itching, *urticaria* (hives), and skin erythema appear, followed in short order by profound respiratory difficulty caused by pulmonary bronchoconstriction and accentuated by hypersecretion of mucus. Laryngeal edema may exacerbate matters by causing upper airway obstruction. In addition, the musculature of the entire gastrointestinal tract may be affected, with resultant vomiting, abdominal cramps, and diarrhea. Without immediate intervention, there may be systemic vasodilation *(anaphylactic shock),* and the patient may progress to circulatory collapse and death within minutes.

Local reactions generally occur when the antigen is confined to a particular site by virtue of the route of exposure, such as skin (contact, causing urticaria), gastrointestinal tract (ingestion, causing diarrhea), or lung (inhalation, causing bronchoconstriction). The common forms of skin and food allergies, hay fever, and certain forms of asthma are examples of localized anaphylactic reactions. Susceptibility to localized type I reactions appears to be genetically controlled, and the term *atopy* is used to imply familial predisposition to such localized reactions. Patients who suffer from nasobronchial allergy (including hay fever and some forms of asthma) often have a family history of similar conditions. The genetic basis of atopy is not clearly understood; however, linkage studies suggest an association with cytokine genes on chromosome 5q that regulate the expression of circulating IgE.

Before this discussion of type I hypersensitivity is closed, it is worth noting that these reactions clearly did not evolve to engender human discomfort and disease. Type I hypersensitivity, in particular the late-phase inflammatory reactions, plays an important protective role in parasitic infections. IgE antibodies are produced in response to many helminthic infections, and Figure 5–9 provides a schematic illustration of the process by which these IgE antibodies may serve to direct damage to schistosome larvae by recruiting inflammatory cells and causing antibody-dependent cell-mediated cytotoxicity.

Type II Hypersensitivity (Antibody Dependent)

Type II hypersensitivity is mediated by antibodies directed against target antigens on the surface of cells or

Table 5–3. SUMMARY OF THE ACTION OF MAST CELL MEDIATORS IN TYPE I HYPERSENSITIVITY

Action	Mediator
Cellular infiltration	Cytokines (e.g., TNF)
	Leukotriene B_4
	Eosinophil chemotactic factor of anaphylaxis
	Neutrophil chemotactic factor of anaphylaxis
	Platelet-activating factor
Vasoactive (vasodilation, increased vascular permeability)	Histamine
	Platelet-activating factor
	Leukotrienes C_4, D_4, E_4
	Neutral proteases that activate complement and kinins
	Prostaglandin D_2
Smooth muscle spasm	Leukotrienes C_4, D_4, E_4
	Histamine
	Prostaglandins
	Platelet-activating factor

Figure 5-9   ■

IgE-mediated destruction of parasites.

other tissue components. The antigens may be normal molecules intrinsic to cell membranes or extracellular matrix, or they may be adsorbed exogenous antigens (e.g., a drug metabolite). In either case, the hypersensitivity response results from antibody binding followed by one of three different antibody-dependent mechanisms (Fig. 5–10):

COMPLEMENT-DEPENDENT REACTIONS

Complement can mediate type II hypersensitivity via two mechanisms: *direct lysis* and *opsonization* (see Fig. 5–10*A*). In complement-mediated cytotoxicity, antibody bound to a cell surface antigen causes fixation of complement to the cell surface with subsequent lysis via the membrane attack complex (Chapter 2). Cells coated with antibodies and complement C3b fragments (opsonized) are also susceptible to

phagocytosis. Circulating blood cells are the ones most commonly damaged by this mechanism, although antibody bound to nonphagocytosable tissue can lead to *frustrated phagocytosis* and injury, owing to exogenous release of lysosomal enzymes and/or toxic metabolites (e.g., Goodpasture syndrome [see later]). Clinically, antibody-mediated reactions occur in the following situations:

■ *Transfusion reactions*, where red cells from an incompatible donor are destroyed after being coated with recipient antibodies directed against the donor's blood group antigens.
■ *Erythroblastosis fetalis* due to rhesus antigen incompatibility; maternal antibodies against Rh in a sensitized Rh negative mother cross the placenta and cause destruction of Rh-positive fetal red cells (Chapter 7).
■ *Autoimmune hemolytic anemia, agranulocytosis,* or *thrombocytopenia* resulting from an individual's generating antibodies to his or her own blood cells (Chapter 12).
■ *Drug reactions*, where antibody is directed against a particular drug (or its metabolite) that is nonspecifically adsorbed to a cell surface (an example is the hemolysis that can occur after penicillin administration).
■ *Pemphigus vulgaris* caused by antibodies against desmosomal proteins that lead to disruption of epidermal intercellular junctions (Chapter 22).

ANTIBODY-DEPENDENT CELL-MEDIATED CYTOTOXICITY (ADCC)

This form of antibody-mediated injury involves killing via cell types that bear receptors for the Fc portion of IgG; targets coated by antibody are lysed without phagocytosis or complement fixation (see Fig. 5–10*B*). ADCC may be mediated by a variety of leukocytes, including neutrophils, eosinophils, macrophages, and NK cells. Although ADCC is typically mediated by IgG antibodies, in certain instances (e.g., eosinophil-mediated killing of parasites; see Fig. 5–9) IgE antibodies are used.

ANTIBODY-MEDIATED CELLULAR DYSFUNCTION

In some cases, antibodies directed against cell surface receptors impair or dysregulate function without causing cell injury or inflammation (see Fig. 5–10*C*). Thus, in myasthenia gravis, antibodies against acetylcholine receptors in the motor end-plates of skeletal muscles impair neuromuscular transmission with resultant muscle weakness. Conversely, antibodies can stimulate cell function. In Graves disease, antibodies against the thyroid-stimulating hormone receptor stimulate thyroid epithelial cells and result in hyperthyroidism.

Type III Hypersensitivity (Immune Complex–Mediated)

Type III hypersensitivity is mediated by the deposition of antigen-antibody (immune) complexes, followed by complement activation and accumulation of polymorphonuclear leukocytes. Immune complexes can involve exogenous

A. COMPLEMENT-DEPENDENT

B. ADCC

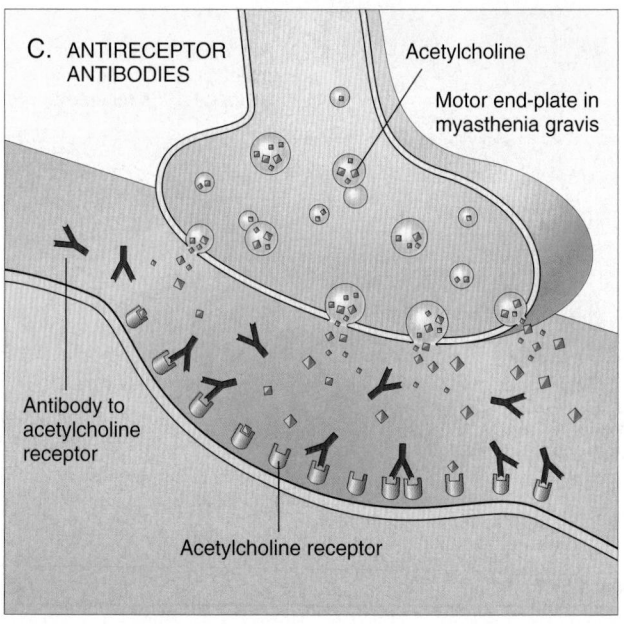

C. ANTIRECEPTOR ANTIBODIES

Figure 5-10

Schematic illustration of three different mechanisms of antibody-mediated injury in type II hypersensitivity. *A,* Complement-dependent reactions. These lead to lysis of cells or render them susceptible to phagocytosis (opsonization). *B,* Antibody-dependent cell-mediated cytotoxicity (ADCC). IgG-coated target cells are killed by cells that bear Fc receptors for IgG (e.g., NK cells). *C,* Antireceptor antibodies. These disturb the normal function of receptors. In this example, acetylcholine receptor antibodies impair neuromuscular transmission in myasthenia gravis. Ab, antibody.

antigens such as bacteria and viruses or endogenous antigens such as DNA. It is important to note that the mere formation of immune complexes does not equate with type III hypersensitivity; antigen-antibody complexes form during many immune responses and represent a normal mechanism of antigen removal. Pathogenic immune complexes either form in the circulation and subsequently deposit in the tissues or form at extravascular sites where antigen has been planted (in situ immune complexes).

Immune complex–mediated injury can be *systemic* when complexes are formed in the circulation and are deposited in multiple organs or *localized* to particular organs (e.g., kidneys, joints, or skin) if the complexes are formed and deposited in a specific site. The mechanism of tissue injury is the same regardless of the pattern of distribution; however, the sequence of events and the conditions leading to the formation of the immune complexes are different and will be considered separately.

SYSTEMIC IMMUNE COMPLEX DISEASE

The pathogenesis of systemic immune complex disease can be divided into three phases: (1) formation of antigen-antibody complexes in the circulation and (2) deposition of the immune complexes in various tissues, thus initiating (3) an inflammatory reaction in various sites throughout the body (Fig. 5–11).

Acute serum sickness is the prototype of a systemic immune complex disease. It was first described in humans when large amounts of foreign serum were administered for passive immunization (e.g., horse antitetanus serum); it is now seen only infrequently (e.g., patients injected with horse antithymocyte globulin for treatment of aplastic anemia). Approximately 5 days after a foreign protein is injected, specific antibodies are produced; these react with the antigen still present in the circulation to form antigen-antibody complexes *(first phase)*. In the *second phase*, antigen-antibody complexes formed in the circulation deposit in various tissue beds. Two important factors determine whether immune complex formation leads to tissue deposition and disease:

■ *Size of the immune complex.* Very large complexes formed in antibody excess are rapidly removed from the circulation by the mononuclear phagocytic cells and are therefore relatively harmless. The most pathogenic complexes are formed during antigen excess and are small or of intermediate size, are cleared less avidly by phagocytic cells, and therefore circulate longer.
■ *Status of the mononuclear phagocyte system.* Because macrophages normally filter out circulating immune complexes, their overload or dysfunction leads to persistence of immune complexes in the circulation and increases the probability of tissue deposition.

In addition, several other factors influence whether and where immune complexes deposit. These include charge of the complex (anionic vs. cationic), valency of the antigen, avidity of the antibody, affinity of the antigen for various tissues, three-dimensional architecture of the complexes, and the hemodynamics of a given vascular bed (Chapter 14). The favored sites of immune complex deposition are kidney, joints, skin, heart, serosal surfaces, and small blood vessels. Localization in the kidney is explained in part by the filtration function of the glomerulus, with trapping of the circulating complexes in the glomeruli. No similar satisfactory explanation exists for the localization of immune complexes in the other sites of predilection.

For complexes to leave the circulation and deposit within or outside the vessel wall, an increase in vascular permeability must occur. This is probably mediated when immune complexes bind to inflammatory cells via Fc and C3b receptors and trigger release of vasoactive mediators and/or permeability-increasing cytokines. Once complexes are deposited in the tissue, the *third phase,* inflammatory reaction, ensues. During this phase (approximately 10 days after antigen administration)*,* clinical features such as fever, urticaria, arthralgias, lymph node enlargement, and proteinuria appear.

Wherever immune complexes deposit, the tissue damage is similar. Complement activation by immune complexes is central to the pathogenesis of injury, releasing biologically

Figure 5–11 ■

Schematic illustration of the three sequential phases in the induction of systemic type III (immune complex) hypersensitivity.

active fragments such as the anaphylatoxins (C3a and C5a), which increase vascular permeability and are chemotactic for polymorphonuclear leukocytes (Chapter 2). Phagocytosis of immune complexes by the accumulated neutrophils

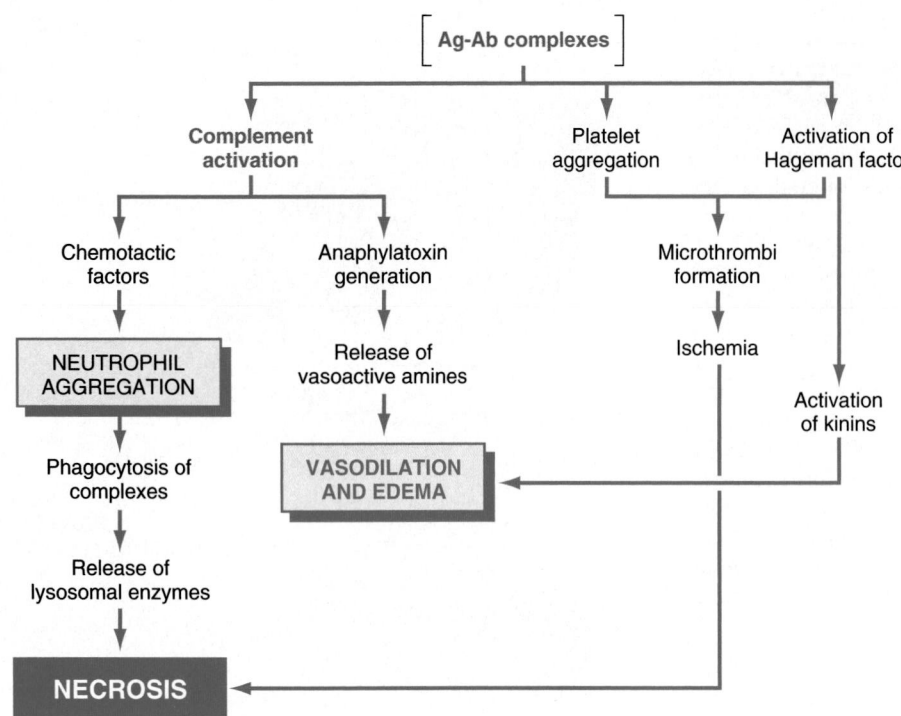

Figure 5-12 ■

Schematic representation of the pathogenesis of immune complex–mediated tissue injury. The morphologic consequences are shown as boxed areas.

results in the release or generation of a variety of additional proinflammatory substances, including prostaglandins, vasodilator peptides, and chemotactic substances, as well as lysosomal enzymes capable of digesting basement membrane, collagen, elastin, and cartilage. Tissue damage is also mediated by oxygen free radicals produced by activated neutrophils. Immune complexes can also cause platelet aggregation and activate Hageman factor; both of these reactions augment the inflammatory process and initiate microthrombi formation that contribute to the tissue injury by producing local ischemia (Fig. 5–12). The resultant pathologic lesion is termed *vasculitis* if it occurs in blood vessels, *glomerulonephritis* if it occurs in renal glomeruli, *arthritis* if it occurs in the joints, and so on.

Obviously, only complement-fixing antibodies (i.e., IgG and IgM) can induce such lesions. Because IgA can also activate complement by the alternative pathway, IgA-containing complexes may also induce tissue injury. The important role of complement in the pathogenesis of the tissue injury is supported by the observation that experimental depletion of serum complement levels greatly reduces the severity of the lesions, as does depletion of neutrophils. *During the active phase of the disease, consumption of complement decreases the serum levels.*

MORPHOLOGY

The morphologic consequences of immune complex injury are dominated by acute **necrotizing vasculitis,** microthrombi, and superimposed ischemic necrosis accompanied by acute inflammation of the affected organs. The necrotic vessel wall takes on a smudgy eosinophilic

appearance called **fibrinoid necrosis** caused by protein deposition (Fig. 5-13). Immune complexes can be visualized in the tissues, usually in the vascular wall, by both electron microscopy (Fig. 5-14A) and immunofluorescence (Fig. 5-14B). In due course the lesions tend to resolve, especially when they were brought about by a single exposure to antigen (e.g., acute serum sickness and acute poststreptococcal glomerulonephritis (Chapter 14)). However, chronic

Figure 5-13 ■

Immune complex vasculitis. The necrotic vessel wall is replaced by smudgy, pink "fibrinoid" material. (Courtesy of Dr. Trace Worrell, Department of Pathology, University of Texas Southwestern Medical School, Dallas.)

Figure 5-14 ■

Immune complex deposition in the glomerulus. *A,* Membranous glomerulonephritis. Electron micrograph showing electron-dense deposits *(arrow)* along the epithelial side of the basement membrane (B). *B,* Immunofluorescence micrograph stained with fluorescent anti-IgG from a patient with diffuse proliferative lupus nephritis. One complete glomerulus and part of another one are seen. Note the mesangial and capillary wall deposits of IgG. CL, capillary lumen; End, endothelium; Ep, epithelium. (*B,* Courtesy of Dr. Helmut Rennke, Department of Pathology, Brigham and Women's Hospital, Boston.)

immune complex disease develops when there is persistent antigenemia or repeated exposure to an antigen. This occurs in some human diseases, such as systemic lupus erythematosus (SLE). Most often, despite the fact that the morphologic changes and other findings strongly implicate immune complex disease, the inciting antigens are unknown. Included in this category are polyarteritis nodosa, membranous glomerulonephritis, and several of the vasculitides.

LOCAL IMMUNE COMPLEX DISEASE (ARTHUS REACTION)

The Arthus reaction may be defined as a localized area of tissue necrosis resulting from acute immune complex vasculitis. The reaction is produced experimentally by injecting an antigen into the skin of a previously immunized animal (i.e., preformed antibodies against the antigen are already present in the circulation). Because of the initial antibody excess, immune complexes are formed as the antigen diffuses into the vascular wall; these are precipitated at the site of injection and trigger the same inflammatory reaction and histologic appearance already discussed for systemic immune complex disease. Arthus lesions evolve over a few hours and reach a peak 4 to 10 hours after injection, when the injection site develops visible edema with severe hemorrhage occasionally followed by ulceration.

Type IV Hypersensitivity (Cell-Mediated)

Cell-mediated immunity is the principal mechanism of response to a variety of microbes, including intracellular pathogens such as *Mycobacterium tuberculosis* and viruses, as well as extracellular agents such as fungi, protozoa, and parasites. However, these processes can also lead to cell death and tissue injury, either as a consequence of the normal clearance of infection or in response to self-antigens (in autoimmune disease). So-called *contact skin sensitivity* to chemical agents (e.g., poison ivy) and graft rejection are other instances of cell-mediated hypersensitivity reactions. Thus, *type IV hypersensitivity is mediated by specifically sensitized T cells* rather than by antibodies and is subdivided into two basic types: (1) *delayed-type hypersensitivity, initiated by CD4+ T cells,* and (2) *direct cell cytotoxicity, mediated by CD8+ T cells.* In delayed hypersensitivity, T$_H$1-type CD4+ T cells secrete cytokines, leading to recruitment of other cells, especially macrophages, which are the major effector cells. In cell-mediated cytotoxicity, cytotoxic CD8+ T cells assume the effector function.

DELAYED-TYPE HYPERSENSITIVITY (DTH)

A classic example of delayed hypersensitivity (DTH) is the tuberculin reaction, elicited in an individual already sensitized to the tubercle bacillus by a previous infection (Chapter 13). Eight to 12 hours after intracutaneous injection of tuberculin (a protein-lipopolysaccharide extract of the tubercle bacillus), a local area of erythema and induration appears, reaching a peak (typically 1 to 2 cm diameter) in 24 to 72 hours (hence the adjective, *delayed*) and thereafter slowly subsiding. Histologically, the DTH reaction is characterized by the perivascular accumulation ("cuffing") of CD4+ helper T cells and, to a lesser extent, macrophages (Fig. 5–15). Local secretion of cytokines by these mononuclear inflammatory cells leads to an associated increased microvascular permeability, giving rise to dermal edema and fibrin deposition; the latter is the main cause of the tissue induration in these responses. The tuberculin response is used to screen populations for individuals who

Figure 5–15   ■

Delayed hypersensitivity in the skin. *A,* Perivascular accumulation ("cuffing") of mononuclear inflammatory cells (lymphocytes and macrophages), with associated dermal edema and fibrin deposition. *B,* Immunoperoxidase staining reveals a predominantly perivascular cellular infiltrate that marks positively with anti-CD4 antibodies. (*B,* Courtesy of Dr. Louis Picker, Department of Pathology, University of Texas Southwestern Medical School, Dallas.)

have had prior exposure to tuberculosis and therefore have circulating memory T cells. Notably, immunosuppression or loss of CD4+ T cells (e.g., owing to HIV) may lead to a negative tuberculin response even in the presence of a severe infection.

The sequence of events in DTH (as exemplified by the tuberculin reaction) begins with the first exposure of the individual to tubercle bacilli. CD4+ lymphocytes recognize peptide antigens of tubercle bacilli in association with class II antigens on the surface of monocytes or dendritic cells that have processed the mycobacterial antigens. This process leads to the formation of sensitized CD4+ cells of the T_H1 type that remain in the circulation for years. Why certain antigens preferentially induce a T_H1 response is not clear, although the cytokine milieu in which naïve T cells are activated seems to be relevant. On subsequent cutaneous injection of tuberculin into such an individual, the memory cells respond to processed antigen on APCs and are activated (undergo blast transformation and proliferation), accompanied by the secretion of T_H1 cytokines. It is these T_H1 cytokines that are ultimately responsible for driving the development of the DTH response. Overall, the most relevant cytokines in the process include the following:

■ *IL-12* is a cytokine produced by macrophages after initial interaction with the tubercle bacillus. It is critical for the induction of DTH in that it is the major cytokine that drives the differentiation of T_H1 cells; in turn, T_H1 cells are the source of other cytokines listed below. IL-12 is also a potent inducer of IFN-γ secretion by T cells and NK cells.

■ *IFN-γ* has a variety of effects and is the most important mediator of DTH. It is an extremely potent activator of macrophages, increasing macrophage production of IL-12. Activated macrophages express more class II molecules on the surface, leading to augmented antigen presentation capacity. They also have increased phagocytic and microbicidal activity, and their capacity to kill tumor cells is enhanced. Activated macrophages secrete several polypeptide growth factors, including platelet-derived growth factor (PDGF) and TGF-α, which stimu-

late fibroblast proliferation and augment collagen synthesis. In short, IFN-γ activation enhances the ability of macrophages to eliminate offending agents; if macrophage activation is sustained, fibrosis ensues.

■ *IL-2* causes the proliferation of the T cells that have accumulated at sites of DTH. Included in this infiltrate are approximately 10% antigen-specific CD4+ cells, although the majority are bystander T cells not specific for the original inciting agent.

■ *TNF* and *lymphotoxin* are cytokines that exert important effects on endothelial cells: (1) increased secretion of nitric oxide and prostacyclin, favoring increased blood flow via local vasodilation; (2) increased expression of E-selectin (Chapter 2), an adhesion molecule promoting mononuclear cell attachment; and (3) induction and secretion of chemotactic factors such as IL-8. Together, these changes facilitate the egress of lymphocytes and monocytes at the site of the DTH responses.

GRANULOMATOUS INFLAMMATION

A *granuloma* is a special form of DTH occurring in the setting of persistent and/or nondegradable antigens. The initial perivascular CD4+ T-cell infiltrate is progressively replaced by macrophages over a period of 2 to 3 weeks; these accumulated macrophages typically exhibit morphologic evidence of activation, that is, they become large, flat, and eosinophilic (denoted as *epithelioid cells*). The epithelioid cells occasionally fuse under the influence of certain cytokines (e.g., IFN-γ) to form multinucleated *giant cells*. A microscopic aggregate of epithelioid cells, typically surrounded by a collar of lymphocytes, is called a *granuloma* (Fig. 5–16*A*), and the pattern is referred to as *granulomatous inflammation*. The process is essentially the same as that described for other DTH responses (Fig. 5–16*B*). Older granulomas develop an enclosing rim of fibroblasts and connective tissue. Recognition of a granuloma is of diagnostic importance because of the limited number of conditions that can cause it (Chapter 2).

DTH is a major mechanism of defense against a variety of intracellular pathogens, including mycobacteria, fungi, and

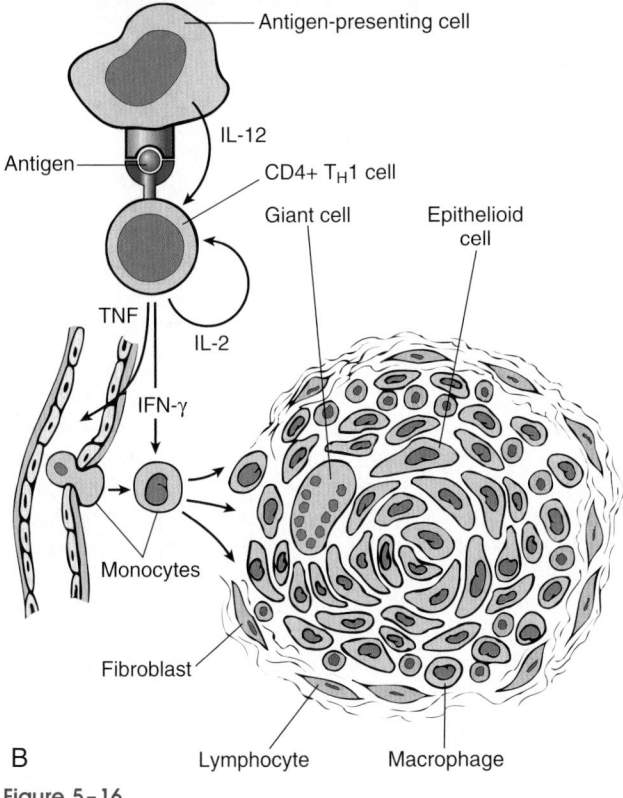

Antigen-presenting cell

IL-12

Antigen

CD4+ T$_H$1 cell

Giant cell

Epithelioid cell

TNF

IL-2

IFN-γ

Monocytes

Fibroblast

Lymphocyte

Macrophage

B

Figure 5-16   ■

Granuloma formation. *A,* A section of a lymph node shows several granulomas, each made up of an aggregate of epithelioid cells and surrounded by lymphocytes. The granuloma in the center shows several multinucleate giant cells. *B,* Schematic illustration of the events that give rise to the formation of granulomas in type IV hypersensitivity reactions. Note the role played by T cell–derived cytokines. (*A,* Courtesy of Dr. Trace Worrell, Department of Pathology, University of Texas Southwestern Medical School, Dallas.)

certain parasites, and it may also be involved in transplant rejection and tumor immunity. The central role of CD4+ T cells in delayed hypersensitivity is evident in patients with AIDS. Because of the loss of CD4+ cells, the host response against intracellular pathogens such as *Mycobacterium tuberculosis* is markedly impaired. The bacteria are engulfed by macrophages but are not killed, and instead of granuloma formation, there is accumulation of unactivated macrophages poorly adapted to deal with the invading microbe.

In addition to its beneficial, protective role, DTH can also be a cause of disease. *Contact dermatitis* is one such example of tissue injury resulting from delayed hypersensitivity. It is evoked by contact with pentadecylcatechol (also known as urushiol, the active component of poison ivy or poison oak) in a sensitized host and manifests as a vesicular dermatitis. The basic mechanism is similar to that described for tuberculin sensitivity. On re-exposure to the plants, sensitized T$_H$1 CD4+ cells accumulate in the dermis and migrate toward the antigen within the epidermis. Here they release cytokines that damage keratinocytes, causing separation of these cells and formation of an intraepidermal vesicle.

T-CELL–MEDIATED CYTOTOXICITY

In this form of type IV hypersensitivity, sensitized CD8+ T cells kill antigen-bearing target cells. As discussed earlier, class I MHC molecules bind to intracellular viral peptides and present them to CD8+ T lymphocytes. The CD8+ effector cells, called cytotoxic T lymphocytes (CTLs), play a critical role in resistance to virus infections. The lysis of infected cells before viral replication is completed leads ultimately to elimination of the infection. It is believed that many tumor-associated peptides (Chapter 6) are also presented on tumor cell surfaces, and hence CTLs may also be involved in tumor immunity.

Two principal mechanisms of CTL killing have been demonstrated: (1) perforin-granzyme–dependent killing and (2) Fas–Fas ligand–dependent killing. Perforins and granzymes are soluble mediators contained in the lysosome-like granules of CTLs. As its name suggests, perforin punches holes in the plasma membrane of target cells; it does so by insertion and polymerization of perforin molecules to form a pore. These pores allow water to enter the cells, eventually resulting in osmotic lysis. The lymphocyte granules also contain a variety of proteases called *granzymes*, which are delivered into the target cells via the perforin pores. Once inside the cell, granzymes activate target cell apoptosis (Chapter 1). Activated CTLs also express Fas ligand (a molecule with homology to TNF), which binds to Fas on target cells. This interaction leads to apoptosis. In addition to viral and tumor immunity, CTLs directed against cell surface histocompatibility antigens also play an important role in graft rejection, to be discussed next.

Transplant Rejection

Rejection of organ transplants is a complex immunologic phenomenon involving both cell- and antibody-mediated hypersensitivity responses of the *host* directed against histocompatibility molecules on the *donor* allograft.

T-CELL–MEDIATED REJECTION

Classic acute rejection in a nonimmunosuppressed host occurs within 10 to 14 days; it is largely the consequence of cell-mediated immunity, involving both DTH and CTL mechanisms. Because the only major antigenic difference between host and donor tissue is their histocompatibility molecules, rejection occurs as a response to MHC. The host recognition and response to the donor MHC occurs by two mechanisms:

■ *Indirect recognition.* In this instance, host CD4+ T cells recognize donor HLA after they are processed and presented by the *host's* own APCs. This involves host APC uptake and processing of HLA shed from donor cells and is similar to the physiologic processing and presentation of other foreign (e.g., microbial) antigens. Clearly, this form of recognition mainly activates DTH pathways.

■ *Direct recognition.* In this instance, the host responds to donor HLA expressed directly on *donor cells.* Direct recognition is paradoxical in that it appears to violate the rules of MHC restriction (p 108); this has been explained by assuming that allogeneic MHC and bound peptides in some manner structurally mimic self-MHC and foreign antigen. Because donor *dendritic cells* express high levels of both MHC I and MHC II, as well as important costimulatory molecules, they are the most likely APCs in direct recognition (macrophages and endothelial cells are also potentially involved). Host CD4+ helper T cells are triggered into proliferation and cytokine production by recognition of donor MHC II (HLA-D) molecules and drive the DTH response. CD8+ T cells can potentially recognize MHC I (HLA-A, -B, -C) on any cell type, but naïve CD8+ T cells also probably require the costimulation provided by "professional" APCs; with the cytokine help of CD4+ T cells, these CD8+ T cells will differentiate into CTL.

Once the donor allograft has been recognized as foreign, rejection proceeds via the effector mechanisms already discussed (Fig. 5–17). Mature CTLs lyse targets in the grafted tissue, causing parenchymal and, perhaps more importantly, endothelial cell death (resulting in thrombosis and graft ischemia). Cytokine-secreting CD4+ T cells cause increased vascular permeability and local accumulation of mononuclear cells (lymphocytes and macrophages). The DTH response with its attendant microvascular injury also results in tissue ischemia, which, along with the destruction mediated by accumulated macrophages, is an important mechanism of graft destruction.

ANTIBODY-MEDIATED REJECTION

Although T cells are of preeminent importance in allograft rejection, antibodies also mediate some forms of rejection:

■ Anti-HLA humoral antibodies develop concurrently with T-cell–mediated rejection (see Fig. 5–17). The major target of antibody-mediated damage in this setting is the vascular endothelium, with bound antibody causing injury (and secondary thrombosis) via complement-, immune complex–, or ADCC-mediated pathways. Superimposed on the immunologic vascular damage are platelet aggregation and coagulation (caused by complement activation), adding further ischemic insult to the injury. Histologically, this form of

rejection resembles the vasculitis described earlier for type III hypersensitivity.

■ *Hyperacute rejection* is a special form of rejection occurring in the setting where *preformed* antidonor antibodies are present in the circulation of the host *before transplant.* This may occur in multiparous women who have anti-HLA antibodies against paternal antigens shed from a fetus or from exposure to foreign HLA (on platelets or leukocytes) from prior blood transfusions. Obviously, such antibodies may also be present in a host who has already rejected an organ transplant. In any event, transplantation in this setting results in immediate (minutes to hours) rejection because the circulating antibodies rapidly bind to the endothelium of the grafted organ, with subsequent complement fixation and vascular thrombosis.

MORPHOLOGY

On the basis of the mechanisms involved, the resulting morphology, and the tempo of the various processes, rejection reactions have been roughly classified as **hyperacute, acute,** and **chronic.** The morphology of these patterns is described in the context of renal transplants; however, similar changes are encountered in any other vascularized organ transplant.

HYPERACUTE REJECTION. Hyperacute rejection occurs within minutes to a few hours after transplantation in a presensitized host and is typically recognized grossly by the surgeon just after the vascular anastomosis is completed. In contrast to a nonrejecting kidney graft that regains a normal pink coloration and tissue turgor and promptly excretes urine, a hyperacutely rejecting kidney rapidly becomes cyanotic, mottled, and flaccid and may excrete only a few drops of bloody fluid. The histology is characterized by widespread acute arteritis and arteriolitis, vessel thrombosis, and ischemic necrosis, all resulting from the binding of preformed humoral antibodies. Virtually all arterioles and arteries exhibit characteristic acute fibrinoid necrosis of their walls, with narrowing or complete occlusion of the lumina by precipitated fibrin and cellular debris. It should be noted that with the current practice of screening potential hosts for preformed anti-HLA antibodies and crossmatching (testing recipients for the presence of antibodies directed against a specific donor's lymphocytes), hyperacute rejection occurs in less than 0.4% of transplants.

ACUTE REJECTION. Acute rejection may occur within days to weeks of transplantation in a nonimmunosuppressed host or may appear months or even years later, even in the presence of adequate immunosuppression. As described earlier, acute rejection is a combined process to which both cellular and humoral mechanisms contribute

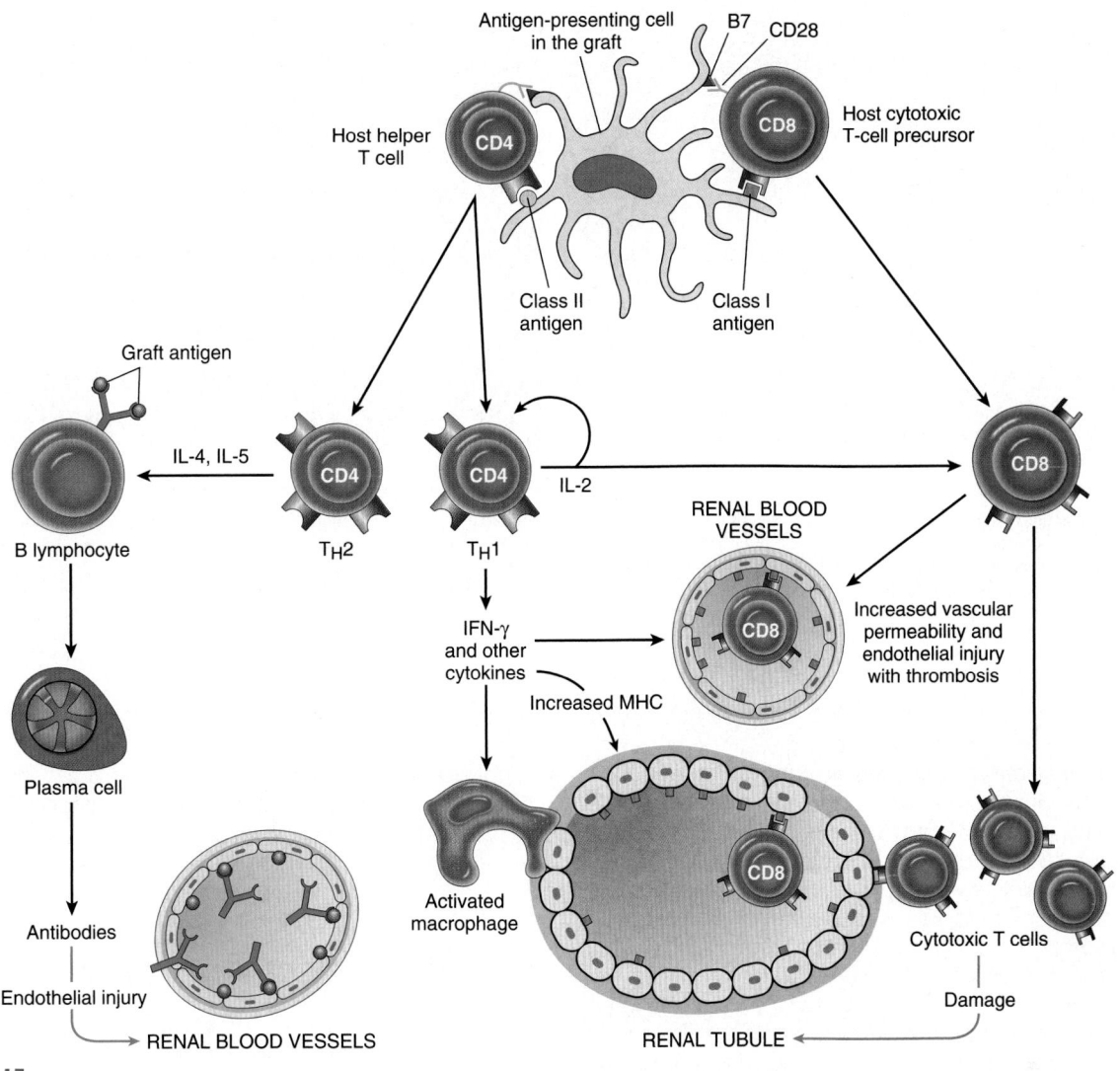

Figure 5–17   ■

Schematic representation of the events that lead to the destruction of histoincompatible grafts. Donor class I and class II antigens along with B7 molecules (CD80, CD86) are recognized by CD8+ cytotoxic T cells and CD4+ helper T cells, respectively, of the host. The interaction of the CD4+ T cells with peptides presented by class II antigens leads to proliferation of T$_H$1-type CD4+ cells and the release of interleukin 2 (IL-2) from the cells. IL-2 further augments the proliferation of CD4+ cells and also provides helper signals for the differentiation of class I–specific CD8+ cytotoxic T cells. In addition, activation of T$_H$2-type CD4+ T cells generates a variety of other soluble mediators (cytokines) that promote B-cell differentiation. The T$_H$1 cells also participate in the induction of a local delayed hypersensitivity reaction. Eventually, several mechanisms converge to destroy the graft: (1) lysis of cells that bear class I antigens by CD8+ cytotoxic T cells, (2) antigraft antibodies produced by sensitized B cells, and (3) nonspecific damage inflicted by macrophages and other cells that accumulate as a result of the delayed hypersensitivity reaction.

and in any one patient one or the other may predominate. Histologically, humoral rejection is associated with vasculitis, whereas cellular rejection is marked by an interstitial mononuclear cell infiltrate, with associated edema and parenchymal injury.

Acute cellular rejection is most commonly seen within the first months after transplantation and is typically accompanied by clinical signs of renal failure. Histologically, there is usually extensive interstitial CD4+ and CD8+ T-cell infiltration with edema and mild interstitial hemorrhage (Fig. 5–18A).

Glomerular and peritubular capillaries contain large numbers of mononuclear cells, which may also invade the tubules and cause focal tubular necrosis. In addition to tubular injury, CD8+ T cells may also injure the endothelium, causing an endotheliitis. Cyclosporine (a widely used immunosuppressive agent) is also nephrotoxic and causes so-called arteriolar hyaline deposits. Consequently, renal biopsy samples taken to assess for rejection may also exhibit superimposed changes from cyclosporine use. Accurate recognition of cellular rejection is important because in the absence of an accompanying

Figure 5–18 ■

Morphology of acute rejection. *A*, Acute cellular rejection of renal allograft manifested by a diffuse mononuclear cell infiltrate and interstitial edema. *B*, Antibody-mediated damage to the blood vessel in a renal allograft. The blood vessel is markedly thickened, and the lumen is obstructed by proliferating fibroblasts and foamy macrophages. (*A*, Courtesy of Dr. Helmut Rennke, Department of Pathology, Brigham and Women's Hospital, Boston; *B*, courtesy of Dr. Ihsan Housini, Department of Pathology, University of Texas Southwestern Medical School, Dallas.)

arteritis patients typically respond promptly to augmented immunosuppressive therapy.

Acute rejection vasculitis (humoral rejection) caused by antidonor antibodies may also be present in acute graft rejection. The histologic lesions may take the form of necrotizing vasculitis with endothelial cell necrosis; neutrophilic infiltration; deposition of antibody, complement, and fibrin; and thrombosis. Such lesions are associated with extensive necrosis of the renal parenchyma. In many cases, the vasculitis is less acute and is characterized by marked thickening of the intima by proliferating fibroblasts, myocytes, and foamy macrophages (Fig. 5–18*B*). The resultant narrowing of the arterioles may cause infarction or renal cortical atrophy. The proliferative vascular lesions mimic arteriosclerotic thickening and are believed to be caused by cytokines that cause growth of vascular smooth muscles.

CHRONIC REJECTION. Patients with chronic rejection clinically present late after transplantation (months to years) with a progressive rise in serum creatinine levels (an index of renal dysfunction) over a period of 4 to 6 months. Chronic rejection is dominated by vascular changes, interstitial fibrosis, and loss of renal parenchyma; there is typically only mild or even no ongoing cellular parenchymal infiltrates. The vascular changes occur predominantly in the arteries and arterioles, which exhibit intimal smooth muscle cell proliferation and extracellular matrix synthesis, potentially occurring as an end stage of the proliferative arteritis described previously. Rather than considering it a low-grade, smoldering, chronic inflammation, it may be more appropriate to characterize chronic rejection as an ongoing healing response; it does

not respond to standard immunosuppression regimens. These lesions ultimately compromise vascular perfusion and result in renal ischemia manifested by loss or hyalinization of glomeruli, interstitial fibrosis, and tubular atrophy.

METHODS OF INCREASING GRAFT SURVIVAL

Because HLA molecules are the major targets in transplant rejection, better matching of the donor and the recipient improves graft survival. The benefits of HLA matching are most dramatic in living, related donor kidney transplants, with MHC II matches giving a better outcome than MHC I matches alone. This effect is probably because MHC II–reactive CD4+ T cells, which are important in both humoral and cellular rejection pathways, are not triggered. By contrast, the beneficial effects of HLA matching on graft survival in renal transplants from nonrelated cadavers are less dramatic, possibly because of differences at other *minor* histocompatibility antigens (polymorphic proteins other than those coded by the HLA complex).

Immunosuppression of the recipient is therefore a practical necessity in all organ transplantation except in the case of identical twins. At present, drugs such as azathioprine, corticosteroids, cyclosporine, antilymphocyte globulins, and monoclonal antibodies (e.g., monoclonal anti-CD3) are employed. Cyclosporine suppresses T-cell–mediated immunity by inhibiting activation of cytokine genes, in particular, the gene for IL-2; its efficacy is limited, however, by its nephrotoxicity. Moreover, although immunosuppression has produced significant gains in graft survival, it is not without a price. Global immunosuppression results in increased susceptibility to opportunistic fungal, viral, and other infections. These patients are also at increased risk for developing EBV-induced lymphomas, human papillomavirus–induced squamous cell carcinomas, and Kaposi sarcoma (KS) (Chapter 13). To circumvent the untoward effects of immunosuppression, much effort is devoted to inducing donor-specific tolerance in host T cells. One strategy being pursued in experimental animals is to prevent host T cells from receiving costimulatory signals from donor dendritic cells during the initial phase of sensitization. This can be accomplished by administration of antibodies to interrupt the interaction between the B7 molecules on the dendritic cells of the graft donor with the CD28 receptors on host T cells. As discussed earlier, this will interrupt the second signal for T-cell activation and either induce apoptosis or render the T cells anergic.

TRANSPLANTATION OF OTHER SOLID ORGANS

Although the kidney is the most frequently transplanted solid organ, transplantation of liver, heart, lungs, and pancreas is also commonly performed. However, unlike living, related kidney transplants, most other solid organs are transplanted without regard for histocompatibility typing. The window of time during which the harvested liver or heart retains viability is too short to allow tissue typing by currently used methods. Thus, in these settings, the only considerations are ABO blood group typing, absence of preformed circulating antibody, and body habitus (e.g., a child cannot receive a heart transplant from an adult).

TRANSPLANTATION OF ALLOGENEIC HEMATOPOIETIC CELLS

Transplantation of bone marrow is a form of therapy increasingly employed for hematopoietic and some nonhematopoietic malignancies, aplastic anemias, and certain immune deficiency states. Hematopoietic stem cells are usually obtained from donor bone marrow but may also be harvested from peripheral blood after mobilization by administration of hematopoietic growth factors. The host receives massive doses of toxic chemotherapy and/or irradiation either to destroy malignant cells (e.g., as in leukemia) or to create a graft bed (as in aplastic anemia), followed by stem cell infusion. *Two major problems complicate this form of transplantation: bone marrow transplant rejection and graft-versus-host disease (GVHD).*

■ *Rejection of allogeneic bone marrow transplants* appears mediated by some combination of host T cells and NK cells that are resistant to radiation therapy and chemotherapy. T-cell–mediated rejection occurs by the same general mechanisms that were described earlier for solid organ transplants. NK cells, by contrast, are triggered to destroy the grafted cells because the allogeneic cells fail to engage the NK inhibitory receptors (see Fig. 5–4).
■ *GVHD* occurs when immunologically competent cells (or their precursors) are transplanted into recipients who are immunologically compromised. Although GVHD happens most commonly in the setting of allogeneic bone marrow transplantation, it may also follow transplantation of solid organs rich in lymphoid cells

(e.g., the liver) or follow transfusion of nonirradiated blood. When immunologically compromised hosts receive normal allogeneic bone marrow cells, immunocompetent T cells derived from the donor marrow recognize the recipient's tissue as "foreign" and react against it. This results in the activation of both CD4+ and CD8+ T cells, ultimately generating DTH and CTL responses.

Acute GVHD (occurring days to weeks after transplant) causes *epithelial cell necrosis in three principal target organs: liver, skin, and gut*. Destruction of small bile ducts gives rise to jaundice, and mucosal ulceration of the gut results in bloody diarrhea. Cutaneous involvement is manifested by a generalized rash. In addition, the host is immunosuppressed and susceptible to a variety of infections (mostly viral). *Chronic GVHD* may follow the acute syndrome or may occur insidiously. These patients are profoundly immunocompromised, but they develop skin lesions resembling those of systemic sclerosis (discussed later) and manifestations mimicking other autoimmune disorders.

GVHD is a potentially lethal complication that can be minimized but not eliminated by HLA matching. As another potential solution, donor T cells can be depleted before marrow transplant. This protocol has proved to be a mixed blessing: the risk of GVHD is reduced, but the incidence of graft failures and the recurrence of leukemia increase. It seems that the multifunctional T cells not only mediate GVHD but also are required for the efficient engraftment of the transplanted bone marrow stem cells and elimination of leukemia cells (so-called *graft-versus-leukemia* effect).

AUTOIMMUNE DISEASES

The evidence is compelling that an immune reaction to *self-antigens* (i.e., *autoimmunity*) is the cause of certain human diseases; a growing number of entities have been attributed to this process (Table 5–4). However, in many of these, the proof is not absolute, and an important caveat is that the simple presence of autoreactive antibodies or T cells does *not* equate to autoimmune disease. For example, apparently nonpathologic antibodies to self-antigens can be readily demonstrated in most otherwise healthy individuals. Moreover, similar innocuous autoantibodies to self-antigens are frequently generated following other forms of injury (e.g., ischemia), presumably serving a physiologic role in the removal of tissue breakdown products. The evidence that the diseases listed in Table 5–4 are indeed the result of autoimmune reactions is more persuasive for some than for others. Thus, for SLE, the presence of a multiplicity of autoantibodies logically explains many of the observed changes. Moreover, those same autoantibodies can be identified within pathologic lesions by immunofluorescence and electron microscopic techniques. In many other disorders, such as polyarteritis nodosa, an autoimmune etiology is suspected but is unproven. Indeed, in some cases of polyarteritis nodosa an exogenous antigen (e.g., hepatitis B virus proteins) may be responsible for the resulting vasculitis.

■

Table 5-4. AUTOIMMUNE DISEASES

Single Organ or Cell Type	Systemic
Probable	*Probable*
Hashimoto thyroiditis	Systemic lupus ery-
Autoimmune hemolytic anemia	thematosus
Autoimmune atrophic gastritis of	Rheumatoid arthritis
pernicious anemia	Sjögren syndrome
Autoimmune encephalomyelitis	Reiter syndrome
Autoimmune orchitis	
Goodpasture syndrome*	*Possible*
Autoimmune thrombocytopenia	Inflammatory myopathy
Type1 (insulin-dependent) diabetes mellitus	Systemic sclerosis
Myasthenia gravis	(scleroderma)
Graves disease	Polyarteritis nodosa
Possible	
Primary biliary cirrhosis	
Chronic active hepatitis	
Ulcerative colitis	
Membranous glomerulonephritis	

*Target is basement membrane of glomeruli and alveolar walls.

Presumed autoimmune diseases range from those in which specific immune responses are directed against one particular organ or cell type and result in localized tissue damage to multisystem diseases characterized by lesions in many organs and associated with a multiplicity of autoantibodies or cell-mediated reactions. In the latter, the pathologic changes occur principally within the connective tissue and blood vessels of the various organs involved. Thus, despite the fact that the reactions in these systemic diseases are not specifically directed against the constituents of connective tissue or blood vessels, they are often referred to as "collagen vascular" or "connective tissue" disorders.

It is obvious that autoimmunity implies loss of self-tolerance, and the question arises as to how this happens. To understand this, it will be important to first familiarize ourselves with the mechanisms of normal immunologic tolerance.

Immunologic Tolerance

Immunologic tolerance is a state in which an individual is incapable of developing an immune response against a specific antigen. Self-tolerance specifically refers to a lack of immune responsiveness to one's own tissue antigens. Obviously, such self-tolerance is necessary if our tissues are to live harmoniously with a marauding army of lymphocytes.

Two broad groups of mechanisms have been forwarded to explain the tolerant state: *central tolerance* and *peripheral tolerance* (Fig. 5–19)

■ *Central tolerance.* This refers to deletion of self-reactive T and B lymphocytes during their maturation in central lymphoid organs (i.e., in the thymus for T cells and in the bone marrow for B cells). It is proposed (with

experimental confirmation in mice) that many autologous (self-) protein antigens are processed and presented by thymic APCs in association with self-MHC. Any developing T cell that expresses a receptor for such self-antigen is negatively selected (deleted by apoptosis), and the resulting peripheral T-cell pool is thereby depleted of self-reactive cells (see Fig. 5–19). As with T cells, deletion of self-reactive B cells also occurs. When developing B cells encounter a membrane-bound antigen during their development in the bone marrow, they undergo apoptosis. Unfortunately, the process of deletion of self-reactive lymphocytes is far from perfect. Many self-antigens are not present in the thymus, and hence T cells bearing receptors for such autoantigens escape into the periphery. There is similar "slippage" in the B-cell system as well, and B cells that bear receptors for a variety of self-antigens, including thyroglobulin, collagen, and DNA, can be readily found in the peripheral blood of healthy individuals.

■ *Peripheral tolerance.* Self-reactive T cells that escape negative selection in the thymus can potentially wreak havoc unless they are deleted or effectively muzzled. Several back-up mechanisms in the *peripheral* tissues that silence such potentially autoreactive T cells have been identified:

■ *Anergy:* This refers to prolonged or irreversible inactivation (rather than apoptosis) of lymphocytes induced by encounter with antigens under certain conditions. Recall that activation of T cells requires two signals: recognition of peptide antigen in association with self-MHC molecules on APCs and a set of second costimulatory signals (e.g., via B7 molecules) provided by the APCs. If the second costimulatory signals are not delivered, the T cell becomes anergic (see Fig. 5–19). Such a cell will be unresponsive even if the relevant antigen is presented again by competent APCs that can deliver costimulation. Because costimulatory molecules are not strongly expressed on most normal tissues, the encounter between autoreactive T cells and their specific self-antigens frequently results in anergy. B cells can also become anergic if they encounter antigen in the absence of specific helper T cells.

■ *Activation-induced cell death:* Another mechanism to prevent uncontrolled T-cell activation during a normal immune response involves apoptosis of activated T cells by the Fas–Fas ligand system. Fas ligand is a membrane protein that is structurally homologous to the cytokine TNF and is expressed chiefly on activated T lymphocytes; its role in CTL-mediated killing (p 121) has already been discussed. Lymphocytes (among many cell types) also express Fas, and, notably, Fas expression is markedly increased on activated T cells. Consequently, engagement of Fas by Fas ligand, coexpressed on the same cohort of activated T cells, may function to suppress the immune response by inducing apoptosis of these cells. Theoretically, such activation-induced cell death can also cause the peripheral deletion of autoreactive T cells. Thus, abundant self-antigens would be expected to

Figure 5–19   ■

Schematic illustration of the mechanisms involved in central and peripheral tolerance of T cells. Similar pathways occur for B cells (see text). APC, antigen-presenting cell; MHC, major histocompatibility complex.

cause repeated and persistent stimulation of autoreactive T cells in the periphery, leading eventually to their elimination via Fas-mediated apoptosis (see Fig. 5–19).

■ *Peripheral suppression by T cells:* Although activation-induced cell death and anergy are the primary mechanisms of peripheral self-tolerance, additional fail-safe mechanisms exist. Much interest has focused on so-called *regulatory T cells*, which can modulate the function of other T cells. Although the mechanisms underlying their effects remain elusive, it is known that certain cytokines elaborated by these cells (e.g., IL-10 and transforming growth factor β [TGF-β]) can dampen a variety of T-cell responses; regulatory T cells also modulate T-cell activity by pathways involving direct cell-cell contact.

Mechanisms of Autoimmune Disease

Breakdown of one or more of the mechanisms of self-tolerance can unleash an immunologic attack on tissues that leads to the development of autoimmune diseases. Immunocompetent cells are undoubtedly involved in mediating the tissue injury, but the precise influences that initiate their reactions against self are not known. Although it would be attractive to explain all autoimmune diseases by a single mechanism, it is now clear that tolerance can be bypassed in a number of ways. More than one defect might be present in each disease, and the defects vary from one disorder to the other. Furthermore, the breakdown of tolerance and initiation of autoimmunity involves the interaction of complicated immunologic, genetic, and microbial factors. Here the initiating immunologic mechanisms (mostly attributable to failure of peripheral tolerance) are discussed, followed by a brief overview of the role of genetic and microbial factors.

FAILURE OF TOLERANCE

Failure of Activation-Induced Cell Death. Persistent activation of potentially autoreactive T cells may lead to their apoptosis via the Fas–Fas ligand system. It therefore follows that defects in this pathway may allow persistence and proliferation of autoreactive T cells in peripheral tissues. In support of this hypothesis, mice with genetic defects in Fas or Fas ligand develop chronic autoimmune diseases resembling SLE. While no patients with SLE have thus far been found to have mutations in the Fas or Fas ligand genes, other subtle defects in activation-induced cell death may well contribute to human autoimmune disease.

Breakdown of T-Cell Anergy. Recall that potentially autoreactive T cells that escape central deletion are rendered anergic when they encounter self-antigens in the absence of costimulation. It follows that such anergy may be broken if normal cells that do not usually express costimulatory molecules can be induced to do so. In fact, such induction may occur after infections, or in other circumstances where

there is tissue necrosis and local inflammation. Up-regulation of the costimulator molecule B7-1 has been noted in the central nervous system of patients with multiple sclerosis, a presumed autoimmune disease in which T cells react to myelin. Similar induction of B7-1 expression has been described in the synovium of patients with rheumatoid arthritis and in the skin of patients with psoriasis. These observations open the exciting possibility of immunologic manipulations in autoimmune disease aimed at interrupting the costimulatory pathways.

Bypass of B-Cell Requirement for T-Cell Help. Many self-antigens have multiple determinants, some recognized by B cells, others by T cells. Antibody response to such antigens occurs only when potentially self-reactive B cells receive help from T cells, and tolerance to such antigens may be associated with deletion or anergy of helper T cells in the presence of fully competent specific B cells. Therefore, this form of tolerance may be overcome if the need for tolerant helper T cells is bypassed or substituted. One way to accomplish this is if the T-cell epitope of a self-antigen is modified, allowing recognition by helper T cells that were not deleted (Fig. 5–20). These could then cooperate with the B cells, leading to the formation of autoantibodies. Such modification of the T-cell determinants of an autoantigen may result from complexing with drugs or microorganisms. For example, autoimmune hemolytic anemia, which occurs after the administration of certain drugs, may result from drug-induced alterations in the red cell surface that create antigens that can be recognized by helper T cells (Chapter 12).

Failure of T-Cell–Mediated Suppression. The possibility that diminished *regulatory* (suppressor) T-cell function might result in autoimmunity is quite attractive. Studies have demonstrated a special type of antigen-specific CD4+ T cell that secretes IL-10; this CD4+ T cell can suppress antigen-specific proliferation of other T cells and, more importantly, prevents autoimmune colitis in a mouse model. Whether loss of such regulatory T cells contributes to human autoimmunity is under investigation.

Molecular Mimicry. Some infectious agents share epitopes with self-antigens, and an immune response against

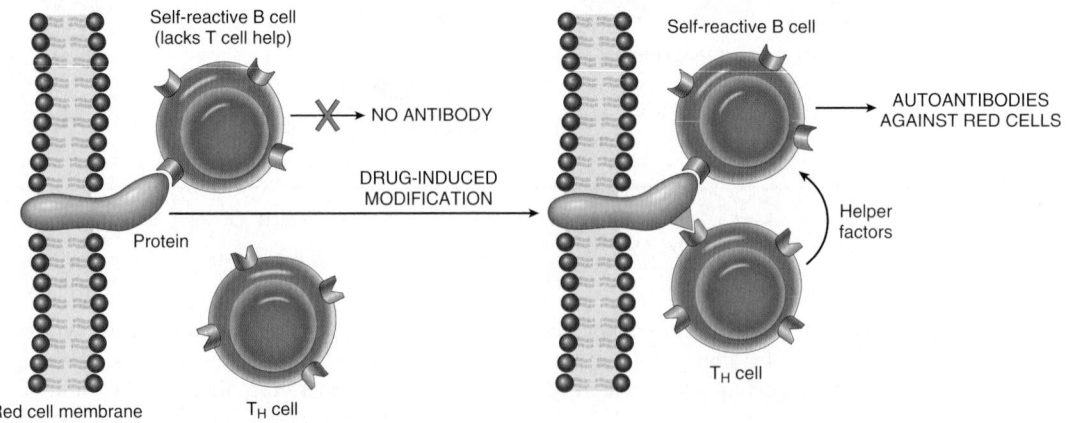

Figure 5–20

Schematic representation of how drug-induced modification of a red cell membrane protein may be recognized by helper T cells and lead to formation of antierythrocyte antibodies.

such microbes will elicit similar responses to the cross-reacting self-antigen. For example, rheumatic heart disease sometimes follows streptococcal infection because antibodies to streptococcal M protein cross-react with cardiac glycoproteins. Molecular mimicry may also apply to T-cell epitopes. The most compelling evidence in support of this has come from myelin basic protein–reactive T-cell clones derived from patients with multiple sclerosis; these clones also react with peptides derived from a variety of non-self proteins, including many derived from viruses.

Polyclonal Lymphocyte Activation. As mentioned earlier, tolerance in some cases is maintained by anergy. Autoimmunity may nevertheless occur if such self-reactive but anergic clones are stimulated by antigen-independent mechanisms. Several microorganisms and their products are capable of causing polyclonal (i.e., antigen-nonspecific) activation of B cells. The best investigated among these is bacterial lipopolysaccharide (endotoxin), which induces mouse lymphocytes to form anti-DNA, antithymocyte, and anti–red cell antibodies in vitro. In addition, certain superantigens can bind to and activate a large pool of CD4+ T cells in an antigen-independent manner (p 111). Thus, in the setting of T-cell superantigen activation, some autoreactive T cells may be stimulated, and autoimmunity can result.

Release of Sequestered Antigens. Regardless of the exact mechanism by which self-tolerance is achieved (deletion or anergy), it is clear that induction of tolerance requires interaction between a given antigen and the immune system. Thus, any self-antigen that is completely sequestered during development is likely to be viewed as foreign if subsequently introduced to the immune system. Spermatozoa and ocular antigens fall into this category. Post-traumatic uveitis and orchitis after vasectomy probably result from immune responses against antigens normally sequestered in the eye and the testis. The mere release of antigens is not sufficient to cause autoimmunity; the inflammation associated with the tissue injury is also essential for the up-regulation of costimulatory pathways that are critical for the induction of an immune response.

Exposure of Cryptic Self and Epitope Spreading. It has been recently appreciated that "molecular sequestration" of antigens is much more common than is anatomic sequestration. Thus, each self-protein has relatively few antigenic determinants (epitopes) that are effectively processed and presented to T cells. During development, most T cells capable of reacting to such dominant epitopes are either deleted in the thymus or rendered anergic in the periphery. By contrast, a large number of self-determinants are not processed and therefore are not recognized by the immune system; thus, T cells specific for such "cryptic" self-epitopes are not deleted. It follows that such T cells could cause autoimmune diseases if the cryptic epitopes are somehow subsequently presented to them in an immunogenic form. The molecular basis of epitope crypticity and the unmasking of such epitopes is not fully understood, although it probably has much to do with the ability of antigens to be processed by APCs. Partial proteolytic degradation of an antigen at a site of tissue injury is only one mechanism by which cryptic epitopes could be generated.

In any event, it is postulated that regardless of the initial trigger of an autoimmune response (e.g., infection with a cross-reacting microbe, release of a sequestered antigen, failure of suppressor T cells), the progression and chronicity of the autoimmune response is maintained by recruitment of autoreactive T cells that recognize normally cryptic self-determinants. The induction of such autoreactive T cells is sometimes referred to as *epitope spreading* because the immune response "spreads" to determinants that were initially not recognized.

GENETIC FACTORS IN AUTOIMMUNITY

There is little doubt that genetic factors play a significant role in the predisposition to autoimmune diseases, as suggested by these observations:

■ Familial clustering of several human autoimmune diseases such as SLE, autoimmune hemolytic anemia, and autoimmune thyroiditis.
■ Linkage of several autoimmune diseases with HLA, especially class II antigens.
■ Induction of autoimmune diseases in transgenic rats. In humans, HLA-B27 is strongly associated with the occurrence of certain autoimmune diseases such as *ankylosing spondylitis*. When cloned human HLA-B27 gene is introduced into the germ line of rats, the transgenic rats also develop ankylosing spondylitis. This model provides direct evidence for genetic regulation of autoimmunity.

The precise role of MHC genes in autoimmunity is not entirely clear. As discussed earlier, it is likely that the MHC class II alleles influence the presentation of autoantigenic peptides to T cells. It should also be noted that many patients with the susceptibility-related MHC gene never develop any disease, and, conversely, individuals without the relevant MHC gene can develop the disease. Expression of a particular MHC gene is therefore but one factor that can facilitate induction of autoimmunity, and genes outside the MHC also clearly influence predisposition to autoimmunity (e.g., cytokine production, proteases).

INFECTION IN AUTOIMMUNITY

A variety of microbes, including bacteria, mycoplasmas, and viruses, have been implicated in the triggering of autoimmunity. Microbes may potentially trigger autoimmune reactions in several ways:

■ Viruses and other microbes, particularly certain bacteria such as streptococci and *Klebsiella* organisms, may share cross-reacting epitopes with self-antigens.
■ Microbial antigens and autoantigens may become associated to form immunogenic units and bypass T-cell tolerance, as described earlier.
■ Some viruses (e.g., EBV) and bacterial products are nonspecific polyclonal B-cell or T-cell mitogens and thus may induce formation of autoantibodies and/or break T-cell anergy.
■ Microbial infections with resultant tissue necrosis and inflammation can cause up-regulation of costimulatory molecules on resting APCs in tissue, thus favoring a breakdown of T-cell anergy.

■ Local inflammatory response may facilitate presentation of cryptic antigens and thus induce epitope spreading.

Clearly, there is no lack of possible mechanisms to explain how infectious agents might participate in the pathogenesis of autoimmunity. At present, however, there is no evidence that clearly implicates any microbe in the causation of human autoimmune diseases.

Against this general background the individual systemic autoimmune diseases will be discussed. Although each disease is discussed separately, it will be apparent that there is considerable overlap in clinical, serologic, and morphologic features. Only the systemic autoimmune diseases are considered in this chapter; the autoimmune diseases that affect single targets are more appropriately discussed in the chapters that deal with the relevant specific organs.

Systemic Lupus Erythematosus

SLE is an autoimmune, multisystem disease of protean manifestations and variable behavior. Clinically, it is an unpredictable, remitting, relapsing disease of acute or insidious onset that may involve virtually any organ in the body; however, it principally affects the skin, kidneys, serosal membranes, joints, and heart. Immunologically, the disease involves a bewildering array of autoantibodies, classically including *antinuclear antibodies (ANA)*. The clinical pre-sentation of SLE is so variable and bears so many similarities to other autoimmune connective tissue diseases (rheumatoid arthritis, polymyositis, and others) that it has been necessary to develop diagnostic criteria (Table 5–5). If a patient demonstrates four or more of the criteria during any interval of observation, the diagnosis of SLE is established.

SLE is a fairly common disease; its prevalence may be as high as 1 case per 2500 persons in certain populations. Like most autoimmune diseases, there is a strong (approximately 9:1) female preponderance, affecting 1 in 700 women of child-bearing age. The disease is more common and severe in black Americans, affecting 1 in 245 women in that group. Its usual onset is in the second or third decade of life, but it may manifest at any age, including early childhood.

Etiology and Pathogenesis. *The fundamental defect in SLE is a failure to maintain self-tolerance.* Consequently, there is generation of a wide array of autoantibodies that can damage tissue either directly or in the form of immune complex deposits. Antibodies have been identified against a host of nuclear and cytoplasmic components of the cell that are neither organ- nor species-specific. Another group of antibodies is directed against cell surface antigens of blood elements, while yet another is directed against proteins complexed to phospholipids (antiphospholipid antibodies [Chapter 4]). The spectrum of autoantibodies will be described first, followed by a brief review of the theories that attempt to explain their origins.

Table 5–5. 1997 REVISED CRITERIA FOR CLASSIFICATION OF SYSTEMIC LUPUS ERYTHEMATOSUS*

Criterion	Definition
1. Malar rash	Fixed erythema, flat or raised, over the malar eminences, tending to spare the nasolabial folds
2. Discoid rash	Erythematous raised patches with adherent keratotic scaling and follicular plugging; atrophic scarring may occur in older lesions
3. Photosensitivity	Rash as a result of unusual reaction to sunlight, by patient history or physician observation
4. Oral ulcers	Oral or nasopharyngeal ulceration, usually painless, observed by a physician
5. Arthritis	Nonerosive arthritis involving two or more peripheral joints, characterized by tenderness, swelling, or effusion
6. Serositis	Pleuritis—convincing history of pleuritic pain or rub heard by a physician or evidence of pleural effusion *or* Pericarditis—documented by electrocardiogram or rub or evidence of pericardial effusion
7. Renal disorder	Persistent proteinuria >0.5 g/dL or >3+ if quantitation not performed *or* Cellular casts—may be red blood cell, hemoglobin, granular, tubular, or mixed
8. Neurologic disorder	Seizures—in the absence of offending drugs or known metabolic derangements, (e.g., uremia, ketoacidosis, or electrolyte imbalance) *or* Psychosis—in the absence of offending drugs or known metabolic derangements, (e.g., uremia, ketoacidosis, or electrolyte imbalance)
9. Hematologic disorder	Hemolytic anemia—with reticulocytosis, *or* Leukopenia—<4.0 × 10⁹/L (4000/mm³) total on two or more occasions *or* Lymphopenia—<1.5 × 10⁹/L (1500/mm³) on two or more occasions *or* Thrombocytopenia—<100 × 10⁹/L (100 × 10³/mm³) in the absence of offending drugs
10. Immunologic disorder	Anti-DNA antibody to native DNA in abnormal titer *or* Anti-Sm—presence of antibody to Sm nuclear antigen *or* Positive finding of antiphospholipid antibodies based on (1) an abnormal serum level of IgG or IgM anticardiolipin antibodies, (2) a positive test for lupus anticoagulant using a standard test, or (3) a false-positive serologic test for syphilis known to be positive for at least 6 months and confirmed by negative *Treponema pallidum* immobilization or fluorescent treponemal antibody absorption test
11. Antinuclear antibody	An abnormal titer of antinuclear antibody by immunofluorescence or an equivalent assay at any point in time and in the absence of drugs known to be associated with drug-induced lupus syndrome

*The proposed classification is based on 11 criteria. For the purpose of identifying patients in clinical studies, a person is said to have systemic lupus erythematosus if any 4 or more of the 11 criteria are present, serially or simultaneously, during any interval of observation.

From Tan EM, et al: The revised criteria for the classification of systemic lupus erythematosus. Arthritis Rheum 25:1271, 1982; and Hochberg MC: Updating the American College of Rheumatology revised criteria for the classification of systemic lupus erythematosus. Arthritis Rheum 40:1725, 1997.

Antinuclear Antibodies (ANAs). ANAs are directed against several nuclear antigens and can be grouped into four categories: (1) antibodies to DNA, (2) antibodies to histones, (3) antibodies to nonhistone proteins bound to RNA, and (4) antibodies to nucleolar antigens. Table 5-6 lists several ANAs and their association with SLE as well as with other autoimmune diseases to be discussed later. Several techniques are used to detect ANAs. Clinically, the most commonly used method is indirect immunofluorescence, which detects a variety of nuclear antigens, including DNA, RNA, and proteins *(generic ANA)*. The pattern of nuclear fluorescence suggests the type of antibody present in the patient's serum, and four basic patterns are recognized:

■ Homogeneous or diffuse staining usually reflects antibodies to chromatin, histones, and double-stranded DNA.
■ Rim or peripheral staining patterns are most commonly indicative of antibodies to double-stranded DNA.
■ Speckled pattern is the most common pattern and refers to the presence of uniform or variable-sized speckles. It reflects the presence of antibodies to non-DNA nuclear constituents such as antibodies to histones and ribonucleoproteins. Examples include Sm antigen, ribonucleoprotein (RNP), and SS-A and SS-B antigens (see Table 5-6).
■ Nucleolar pattern refers to the presence of a few discrete spots of fluorescence within the nucleus that represent antibodies to nucleolar RNA. This pattern is reported most often in patients with systemic sclerosis.

The immunofluorescence test for ANA is positive in virtually every patient with SLE, so that the test is quite *sensitive*. However, it is not *specific*, because patients with other autoimmune diseases (and 5% to 15% of normal persons) also score positive (see Table 5-6). Moreover, the fluorescence patterns are not absolutely specific for the type of antibody, and because of the plethora of antibodies, multiple combinations frequently exist. Some of the clinically useful ANAs are listed in Table 5-6. It should be noted that the presence of antibodies to double-stranded DNA, or to the so-called Smith (Sm) antigen, is virtually diagnostic of SLE.

Antibodies against blood cells, including red cells, platelets, and lymphocytes, are found in many patients. Antiphospholipid antibodies are present in 40% to 50% of lupus patients and react with a wide variety of proteins complexed to phospholipids. Some bind to cardiolipin antigen, used in serologic tests for syphilis, and therefore lupus patients may have a false-positive test result for syphilis. Because phospholipids are required for blood clotting, patients with antiphospholipid antibodies may also display prolongation of in vitro clotting tests, such as the partial thromboplastin time (Chapter 12). Therefore, these antibodies are referred to as "lupus anticoagulants" despite the fact that the patients who have them actually have a prothrombotic state (the *antiphospholipid antibody syndrome* [Chapter 4]). They tend to have venous and arterial thromboses, thrombocytopenia, and recurrent spontaneous miscarriages.

Genetic Factors. The evidence supporting a genetic predisposition to SLE takes many forms.

■ There is a high rate of concordance (25%) in monozygotic twins versus dizygotic twins (1% to 3%).
■ Family members have an increased risk of developing SLE, and up to 20% of clinically unaffected first-degree relatives may reveal autoantibodies.
■ In North American white populations there is a positive association between SLE and class II HLA genes, particularly at the HLA-DQ locus.

Table 5-6. ANTINUCLEAR ANTIBODIES IN VARIOUS AUTOIMMUNE DISEASES

Nature of Antigen	Antibody System	Disease, % Positive					
		SLE	Drug-Induced LE	Systemic Sclerosis —Diffuse	Limited Scleroderma —CREST	Sjögren Syndrome	Inflammatory Myopathies
Many nuclear antigens (DNA, RNA, proteins)	Generic ANA (indirect IF)	>95	>95	70–90	70–90	50–80	40–60
Native DNA	Anti–double-stranded DNA	40–60	<5	<5	<5	<5	<5
Histones	Antihistone	50–70	>95	<5	<5	<5	<5
Core proteins of small nuclear ribonucleoprotein particles (Smith antigen)	Anti-Sm	20–30	<5	<5	<5	<5	<5
Ribonucleoprotein (U1RNP)	Nuclear RNP	30–40	<5	15	10	<5	<5
RNP	SS-A(Ro)	30–50	<5	<5	<5	70–95	10
RNP	SS-B(La)	10–15	<5	<5	<5	60–90	<5
DNA topoisomerase I	Scl-70	<5	<5	28–70	10–18	<5	<5
Centromeric proteins	Anticentromere	<5	<5	22–36	90	<5	<5
Histidyl-tRNA synthetase	Jo-1	<5	<5	<5	<5	<5	25

Boxed entries indicate high correlation.
ANA, antinuclear antibodies; IF, immunofluorescence; LE, lupus erythematosus; RNP, ribonucleoprotein; SLE, systemic lupus erythematosus.

■ Some lupus patients (about 6%) have inherited deficiencies of complement components. Lack of complement presumably impairs removal of immune complexes from the circulation and favors tissue deposition, giving rise to tissue injury.

Nongenetic Factors. The clearest example of nongenetic (e.g., environmental) factors in initiating SLE is the occurrence of a lupus-like syndrome in patients receiving certain drugs, including procainamide and hydralazine. Thus, most patients treated with procainamide for more than 6 months develop ANAs, with clinical features of SLE appearing in 15% to 20% of them. *Sex hormones* also seem to exert an important influence on the occurrence of SLE; witness the overwhelming female preponderance of the disease. This has been attributed to the salutary effects of estrogens on antibody synthesis. Exposure to ultraviolet light is another environmental factor that exacerbates the disease in many individuals. Ultraviolet light may damage DNA and promote cell injury that will release cellular contents and augment the formation of DNA/anti-DNA immune complexes; alternatively, it may modulate local immune responses by increasing keratinocyte production of IL-1.

Immunologic Factors. All the immunologic findings in SLE patients clearly suggest that some fundamental derangement of the immune system is at work in its pathogenesis. However, despite a variety of both T- and B-cell immunologic abnormalities in SLE patients, it is difficult to identify any one of them as causal. For years, intrinsic B-cell hyperactivity was considered a central feature of SLE pathogenesis; in fact, polyclonal B-cell activation can be readily demonstrated in SLE patients as well as in murine SLE models. However, the molecular analyses of anti–double-stranded DNA antibodies strongly suggested that they are not produced by a random polyclonal array of activated B cells but rather derive from a more selective oligoclonal B-cell response to self-antigens. For example, the pathogenic anti-DNA antibodies in SLE patients are cationic (a feature associated with deposition in renal glomeruli), whereas the anti-DNA antibodies produced by polyclonally activated B cells are anionic and nonpathogenic.

The onus of autoimmunity in SLE has therefore shifted to CD4+ helper T cells, creating a model for the pathogenesis as shown in Figure 5–21. It should nevertheless be kept in mind that SLE is a heterogeneous disease; the production of different autoantibodies is regulated by distinct genetic factors, and it should not be surprising that distinct immunoregulatory disturbances are found in patients with different genetic backgrounds and/or autoantibody profiles.

Mechanisms of Tissue Injury. Regardless of the exact sequence by which autoantibodies are formed, they are clearly the mediators of tissue injury. Most of the visceral lesions are mediated by immune complexes (type III hypersensitivity). For example, DNA/anti-DNA complexes can be detected in the glomeruli and low serum levels of complement with granular complement deposits in the glomeruli further support the immune complex nature of the disease. In addition, autoantibodies against red cells, white cells, and platelets mediate effects via type II hypersensitivity. There is no evidence that the ANAs involved in immune complex formation can permeate intact cells. However, if cell nuclei are exposed, the ANAs can bind to them. In tissues, nuclei

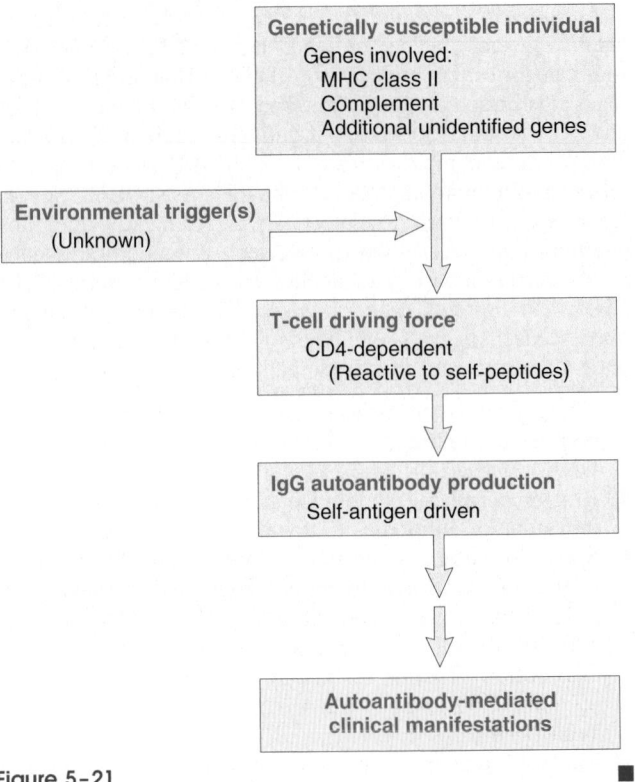

Figure 5–21 ■

Model for the pathogenesis of systemic lupus erythematosus. (Modified from Kotzin BL: Systemic lupus erythematosus. Cell 65:303, 1996. Copyright 1996, Cell Press.)

of damaged cells react with ANAs, lose their chromatin pattern, and become homogeneous, to produce so-called *LE bodies* or *hematoxylin bodies*. An in vitro correlate of this is the *LE cell*—a neutrophil or macrophage that has engulfed the denatured nucleus of another injured cell. When blood is withdrawn and agitated, a number of leukocytes are sufficiently damaged to expose their nuclei to ANAs, with secondary complement activation; these antibody- and complement-opsonized nuclei are then readily phagocytized. Although the LE cell test is positive in up to 70% of patients with SLE, it is now largely of historical interest.

To summarize, SLE is a complex disease of multifactorial origin (including genetic, hormonal, and environmental factors), resulting in a T- and B-cell activation that culminates in the production of several species of autoantibodies.

MORPHOLOGY

SLE is a systemic disease with protean manifestations (see Table 5–5); the frequency of individual organ involvement is shown in Table 5–7. The morphologic changes in SLE are therefore extremely variable and depend on the nature of the autoantibodies, the tissue in which immune complexes deposit, and the course and duration of disease. The most characteristic morphologic changes result from the deposition of immune complexes in a variety of tissues.

Table 5–7. CLINICAL MANIFESTATIONS OF SYSTEMIC LUPUS ERYTHEMATOSUS

Clinical Manifestation	Prevalence in Patients (%)
Hematologic	100
Arthritis	90
Skin	85
Fever	83
Fatigue	81
Weight loss	63
Renal	50
Central nervous system	50
Pleuritis	46
Myalgia	33
Pericarditis	25
Gastrointestinal	21
Raynaud phenomenon	20
Ocular	15
Peripheral neuropathy	14

Figure 5–22   ■

Systemic lupus erythematosus involving the skin. *A,* An H & E–stained section shows liquefactive degeneration of the basal layer of the epidermis and edema at the dermoepidermal junction. *B,* An immunofluorescence micrograph stained for IgG reveals deposits of immunoglobulin along the dermoepidermal junction. (*A,* Courtesy of Dr. Jag Bhawan, Boston University School of Medicine, Boston; *B,* courtesy of Dr. Richard Sontheimer, Department of Dermatology, University of Texas Southwestern Medical School, Dallas.)

An **acute necrotizing vasculitis** affecting small arteries and arterioles may be present in any tissue. The arteritis is characterized by necrosis and by fibrinoid deposits within vessel walls containing antibody, DNA, complement fragments, and fibrinogen; a transmural and perivascular leukocytic infiltrate is also frequently present. In chronic stages, vessels exhibit fibrous thickening with luminal narrowing.

The **skin** is involved in a vast majority of patients; a characteristic erythematous or maculopapular eruption over the malar eminences and bridge of the nose ("butterfly pattern") is observed in about half. **Exposure to sunlight (ultraviolet light) exacerbates the erythema** (so-called **photosensitivity),** and a similar rash may be present elsewhere on the extremities and trunk, frequently in sun-exposed areas. Histologically, there is liquefactive degeneration of the basal layer of the epidermis, edema at the dermoepidermal junction, and mononuclear infiltrates around blood vessels and skin appendages (Fig. 5–22*A*). Immunofluorescence microscopy reveals deposition of immunoglobulin and complement at the dermoepidermal junction (Fig. 5–22*B*); similar immunoglobulin and complement deposits may also be present in apparently uninvolved skin.

Joint involvement is frequent but is usually not associated with striking anatomic changes nor with joint deformity. When present, it consists of swelling and a nonspecific mononuclear cell infiltration in the synovial membranes. Erosion of the membranes and destruction of articular cartilage, such as occurs with rheumatoid arthritis, is exceedingly rare.

CNS involvement is also very common, with focal neurologic deficit and/or neuropsychiatric symptoms. However, the mechanisms remain incompletely understood. CNS injury is often ascribed to acute CNS vasculitis giving rise to multifocal cerebral microinfarcts, but histologic evaluations fail to reveal any significant vascular inflammation. Rather, there appears to be noninflammatory intimal proliferation in small vessels attributable to endothelial injury from antiphospholipid antibodies. Antibodies to a synaptic membrane protein have also been implicated in causing CNS symptoms.

The **spleen** may be moderately enlarged. Capsular fibrous thickening is common, as is follicular hyperplasia with numerous plasma cells in the red pulp. Central penicilliary arteries characteristically show thickening and perivascular fibrosis, producing **onion-skin lesions.**

Pericardium and pleura, in particular, are **serosal membranes** that exhibit a variety of inflammatory changes in SLE ranging (in the acute phase) from serous effusions to fibrinous exudates and progressing to fibrous opacification in the chronic stage.

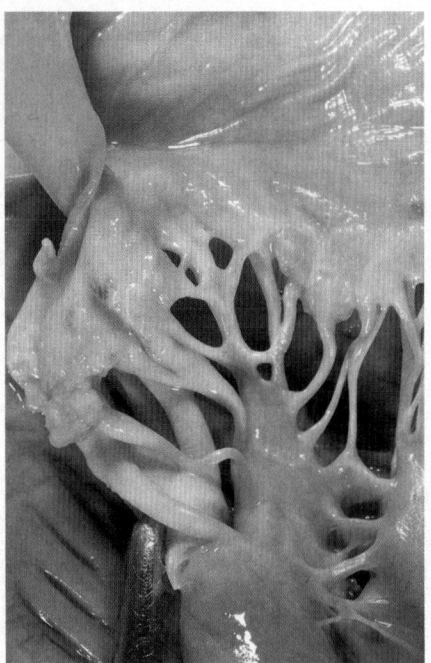

Figure 5-23 ■

Libman-Sacks endocarditis of the mitral valve in systemic lupus erythematosus. The small vegetations attached to the margin of the valve leaflet are easily seen. (Courtesy of Dr. Fred Schoen, Department of Pathology, Brigham and Women's Hospital, Boston.)

Involvement of the heart is manifested primarily in the form of pericarditis; myocarditis, in the form of a nonspecific mononuclear cell infiltrate, may also be present but is less common. Valvular lesions, called **Libman-Sacks endocarditis,** also occur but are less common in the current era of aggressive corticosteroid therapy. This **nonbacterial verrucous endocarditis** takes the form of irregular, 1- to 3-mm warty deposits, distinctively on **either surface of the leaflets** (i.e., on the surface exposed to the forward flow of the blood or on the underside of the leaflet) (Fig. 5-23). An increasing number of patients also show clinical and anatomic manifestations of coronary artery disease. The basis of accelerated atherosclerosis is not fully understood, but it seems to be multifactorial; certainly, immune complexes can deposit in the coronary vasculature and lead to endothelial damage by that pathway. Moreover, glucocorticoid treatment causes alterations in lipid metabolism, and renal disease (common in SLE (see later)) causes hypertension; both of these are risk factors for atherosclerosis (Chapter 10).

Kidney involvement is one of the most important clinical features of SLE, with renal failure being the most common cause of death. The focus here is on glomerular pathology, although interstitial and tubular lesions are also seen in SLE.

The pathogenesis of all forms of **glomerulonephritis** in SLE involves deposition of DNA/anti-DNA complexes within the glomeruli. These evoke an inflammatory response that may cause proliferation of the endothelial, mesangial, and/or epithelial cells and, in severe cases, necrosis of the glomeruli. Although the kidney appears normal by light microscopy in 25% to 30% of cases, almost all cases of SLE show some renal abnormality if examined by immunofluorescence and electron microscopy. According to the World Health Organization morphologic classification, five patterns are recognized (none of which is specific to SLE): **class I**—normal by light, electron, and immunofluorescent microscopy (rare); **class II**—mesangial lupus glomerulonephritis; **class III**—focal glomerulonephritis; **class IV**—diffuse proliferative glomerulonephritis; and **class V**—membranous glomerulonephritis.

Mesangial lupus glomerulonephritis (class II) is seen in 20% of cases and is associated with mild clinical symptoms. Immune complexes deposit in the mesangium, with a slight increase in the mesangial matrix and cellularity.

Focal proliferative glomerulonephritis (class III) is seen in approximately 25% of cases, and, as the name suggests, lesions are visualized in only portions of fewer than half the glomeruli. Typically, one or two foci within an otherwise normal glomerulus exhibit swelling and proliferation of endothelial and mesangial cells, infiltration by neutrophils, and/or fibrinoid deposits with capillary thrombi (Fig. 5-24). Focal glomerulonephritis is usually associated with only mild microscopic hematuria and proteinuria; a transition to a more diffuse form of renal involvement is associated with more severe disease.

Diffuse proliferative glomerulonephritis (class IV) is the most serious form of renal lesions in SLE and is also the most common, occurring in roughly half of patients. Most of the glomeruli show endothelial and mesangial proliferation affecting the entire

Figure 5-24 ■

Lupus nephritis. There are two focal necrotizing lesions at 11 and 2 o'-clock. (H & E stain.) (Courtesy of Dr. Helmut Rennke, Department of Pathology, Brigham and Women's Hospital, Boston.)

Figure 5-25

Lupus nephritis. *A,* Diffuse proliferative type. Note the marked increase in cellularity throughout the glomerulus. (H & E stain.) *B,* Lupus nephritis show-ing a glomerulus with several "wire loop" lesions representing extensive subendothelial deposits of immune complexes. (Periodic acid–Schiff stain.) (Courtesy of Dr. Helmut Rennke, Department of Pathology, Brigham and Women's Hospital, Boston.)

glomerulus. Thus, there is diffuse hypercellularity of the glomeruli (Fig. 5-25A), producing in some cases epithelial crescents that fill Bowman's space. Immune complexes can be visualized by staining with fluorescent antibodies directed against im-munoglobulins or complement, resulting in a granu-lar fluorescent staining pattern (see Fig. 5-14B). When extensive, immune complexes create an overall thickening of the capillary wall, resembling rigid "wire loops" on routine light microscopy (Fig. 5-25B). Electron microscopy reveals electron-dense subendothelial immune complexes (be-tween endothelium and basement membrane; Fig. 5-26). In due course, glomerular injury gives rise

to scarring (glomerulosclerosis). These patients are overtly symptomatic; most have hematuria with moderate to severe proteinuria, hypertension, and renal insufficiency.

Membranous glomerulonephritis (class V) occurs in 15% of cases and is the designation for glomerular disease characterized by widespread thickening of the capillary wall. Membranous glomerulonephritis associated with SLE is very similar to that encoun-tered in idiopathic membranous glomerulopathy (Chapter 14). Thickening of capillary walls occurs by increased deposition of basement membrane–like material, as well as accumulation of immune com-plexes. Patients with this histologic change almost

Figure 5-26

Electron micrograph of a renal glomerular capillary loop from a patient with systemic lupus erythematosus nephritis. Subendothelial dense deposits correspond to "wire loops" seen by light microscopy (see Fig. 5-25B). B, basement membrane; End, endothelium; Ep, epithelial cell with foot processes; Mes, mesangium; RBC, red blood cell in capillary lumen; US, urinary space; *, electron-dense deposits in subendothelial location. (Courtesy of Dr. Edwin Eigenbrodt, Department of Pathology, University of Texas Southwestern Medical School, Dallas.)

always have severe proteinuria with overt nephrotic syndrome (Chapter 14).

Many **other organs and tissues** may be involved. The changes consist essentially of acute vasculitis of the small vessels, foci of mononuclear infiltrations, and fibrinoid deposits. In addition, lungs may reveal interstitial fibrosis, along with pleural inflammation; the liver shows nonspecific inflammation of the portal tracts.

Clinical Manifestations. The diagnosis of SLE may be obvious in a young woman with a classic butterfly rash over the face, fever, arthritis, pleuritic chest pain, and photosensitivity. However, in many patients the presentation of SLE is subtle and puzzling, taking forms such as a febrile illness of unknown origin, abnormal urinary findings, or neuropsychiatric manifestations, including psychosis. A variety of clinical findings may point toward renal involvement, including hematuria, red cell casts, proteinuria, and, in some cases, the classic nephrotic syndrome (Chapter 14). Renal failure may occur, especially in patients with diffuse proliferative or membranous glomerulonephritis, or both. The hematologic derangements mentioned (see Table 5–5) may in some cases be the presenting manifestation as well as the dominant clinical problem. ANAs can be found in virtually 100% of patients, but they can also be found in patients with other autoimmune disorders; nevertheless, anti–double-stranded DNA antibodies are considered highly diagnostic of SLE. Serum complement levels are low, typically as a result of deposition in immune complexes.

The course of SLE is extremely variable. Even without therapy, some patients follow a relatively benign course with only skin manifestations and/or mild hematuria. Rare cases rapidly progress to death within months. Most often, the disease is characterized by remissions and relapses spanning years to decades. Acute flare-ups are usually controlled by steroids or other immunosuppressive drugs. Overall, with current therapies, 90% 5-year and 80% 10-year survivals can be expected. Renal failure, intercurrent infections, and diffuse central nervous system involvement are the major causes of death.

Rheumatoid Arthritis

Rheumatoid arthritis (RA) is a systemic, chronic inflammatory disease affecting multiple tissues but principally attacking the joints to produce a *nonsuppurative proliferative synovitis that frequently progresses to destroy articular cartilage and underlying bone with resulting disabling arthritis.* When extra-articular involvement develops—for example, of the skin, heart, blood vessels, muscles, and lungs—RA may resemble SLE or scleroderma.

RA is a very common condition, with a prevalence of approximately 1%; it is three to five times more common in women than in men. The peak incidence is in the second to fourth decades of life, but no age is immune. Morphology will be considered first, as a background to a discussion of pathogenesis.

MORPHOLOGY

Rheumatoid arthritis causes a broad spectrum of morphologic alterations; the most severe occur in the joints. RA typically presents as **symmetric arthritis, principally affecting the small joints** of the hands and feet, ankles, knees, wrists, elbows, and shoulders. Classically, the proximal interphalangeal and metacarpophalangeal joints are affected, but distal interphalangeal joints are spared. Axial involvement, when it occurs, is limited to the upper cervical spine; similarly, hip joint involvement is extremely uncommon. Histologically, the affected joints show **chronic synovitis,** characterized by (1) synovial cell hyperplasia and proliferation; (2) dense perivascular inflammatory cell infiltrates (frequently forming lymphoid follicles) in the synovium composed of CD4+ T cells, plasma cells, and macrophages; (3) increased vascularity due to angiogenesis; (4) neutrophils and aggregates of organizing fibrin on the synovial surface and in the joint space; and (5) increased osteoclast activity in the underlying bone leading to synovial penetration and bone erosion. The classic appearance is that of a **pannus,** formed by proliferating synovial lining cells admixed with inflammatory cells, granulation tissue, and fibrous connective tissue; the overgrowth of this tissue is so exuberant that the usually thin, smooth synovial membrane is transformed into lush, edematous, frondlike (villous) projections (Fig. 5–27). With full-blown inflammatory joint involvement, periarticular soft tissue edema usually develops, classically manifested first by fusiform swelling of the proximal interphalangeal joints. With progression of the disease, the articular cartilage subjacent to the pannus is eroded and, in time, virtually destroyed. The subarticular bone may also be attacked and eroded. Eventually the pannus fills the joint space, and subsequent **fibrosis and calcification** may cause **permanent ankylosis.** The radiographic hallmarks are joint effusions and juxta-articular osteopenia with erosions and narrowing of the joint space and loss of articular cartilage (Fig. 5–28). Destruction of tendons, ligaments, and joint capsules produces the characteristic deformities, including radial deviation of the wrist, ulnar deviation of the fingers, and flexion-hyperextension abnormalities of the fingers (swan-neck deformity, boutonnière deformity).

Rheumatoid subcutaneous nodules develop in about one fourth of patients, occurring along the extensor surface of the forearm or other areas subjected to mechanical pressure; rarely, they can form in the lungs, spleen, heart, aorta, and other viscera. Rheumatoid nodules are firm, nontender, oval or rounded masses up to 2 cm in diameter. Microscopically, they are characterized by a central focus of fibrinoid necrosis surrounded by a palisade of macrophages, which in turn is rimmed by granulation tissue (Fig. 5–29).

Figure 5-27

Rheumatoid arthritis. *A,* Low magnification reveals marked synovial hypertrophy and hyperplasia with formation of villi. *B,* At higher magnification, sub-synovial tissue containing a dense lymphoid aggregate is seen.

Patients with severe erosive disease, rheumatoid nodules, and high titers of **rheumatoid factor** (circulating IgM that binds IgG (see later)) are at risk of developing vasculitic syndromes; acute necrotizing vasculitis may involve small or large arteries. Serosal involvement may manifest as fibrinous pleuritis or pericarditis or both. Lung parenchyma may be damaged by progressive interstitial fibrosis.

Ocular changes such as uveitis and keratoconjunctivitis (similar to those seen in Sjögren syndrome (see later)) may be prominent in some cases.

Pathogenesis. There is little doubt that there is a genetic predisposition to RA and that the joint inflammation is immunologically mediated; however, the initiating agent or

Figure 5-28   ■

Rheumatoid arthritis. *A,* Early disease, most marked in the second metacarpophalangeal joint, where there is narrowing of the joint space and marginal erosions on both radial and ulnar aspects of the proximal phalanx *(inset). B,* More advanced disease with loss of articular cartilage, narrowing of joint spaces of virtually all the small joints, and ulnar deviation of the fingers. There is dislocation of the second, third, and fourth proximal phalanges produced by advanced articular disease. (Courtesy of Dr. John O'Connor, Boston University Medical Center, Boston.)

Figure 5–29 ■

Subcutaneous rheumatoid nodule with an area of necrosis *(top)* surrounded by a palisade of macrophages and scattered chronic inflammatory cells.

agents and the precise interplay between genetic and environmental factors are not yet understood.

It is proposed that the disease is initiated—in a genetically predisposed individual—by activation of helper T cells responding to some arthritogenic agent, possibly microbial. In turn, the activated CD4+ cells produce cytokines that will (1) activate macrophages and other cells in the joint space, releasing degradative enzymes and other factors that perpetuate inflammation and (2) activate B cells, resulting in the production of antibodies, some of which are directed against self-constituents. The rheumatoid synovium is rich in both lymphocyte- and macrophage-derived cytokines. The activity of these cytokines accounts for many features of rheumatoid synovitis; not only are they proinflammatory, some, such as IL-1 and TGF-α, cause synovial cell and fibroblast proliferation. They also stimulate synovial cell and chondrocyte secretion of proteolytic and matrix-degrading enzymes. More recently, activated T cells in RA lesions have also been shown to express impressive amounts of RANK ligand (Chapter 21). As discussed elsewhere, RANK ligand induces osteoclast differentiation and activation and may play a key role in the bone resorption seen in destructive lesions of RA. In the context of this general scheme, the contributions of genetic factors, T cells, cytokines, B cells, and infectious agents can now be discussed (Fig. 5–30).

Genetic factors in the pathogenesis of RA are suggested by the increased frequency of this disease among first-degree relatives and a high concordance rate in monozygotic twins; there is also a strong association of HLA-DR4 and/or HLA-DR1 with RA. It is of interest that the susceptibility-associated DR alleles share a common stretch of four amino acids, located in the antigen-binding cleft of the DR molecule. Thus, certain DR molecules may predispose to

Antigen (? microbe)

MHC class II (genetic susceptibility)

CD4+ T cells

Cytokines

B-cell activation

Macrophage activation

Endothelial activation

Formation of rheumatoid factor

Cytokines

Immune complex formation and deposition

Fibroblasts Chondrocytes Synovial cells

Proliferation

Expression of adhesion molecules

Joint injury

Release of collagenase, stromelysin, elastase, PGE$_2$, and other enzymes

Accumulation of inflammatory cells

Pannus formation; destruction of bone, cartilage; fibrosis; ankylosis

Figure 5–30

Immunopathogenesis of rheumatoid arthritis.

RA by their capacity to bind selected arthritogenic antigens, which in turn activate helper T cells and initiate disease.

T cells play a primary role in the pathogenesis of RA, including driving the secondary activation of endothelium (to facilitate inflammatory cell recruitment), macrophages, and osteoclasts (as already discussed). B cells (activated by T cells) are also important. In approximately 80% of patients, rheumatoid factors (RFs)—IgM (and to a lesser extent, IgG) autoantibodies directed against the Fc portion of IgG—are present in serum and synovial fluid. Why antibodies against autologous IgG are formed remains unclear. Circulating RFs are putatively involved in many of the extra-articular manifestations of RA, and joint RFs also contribute to the inflammatory reaction in that site. RFs and IgG form immune complexes that fix complement, attract neutrophils, and lead to tissue injury by a type III hypersensitivity reaction. It is noteworthy that RF is not always present (absent in 20% of RA), is occasionally found in other disease states (and even healthy people), and is probably not essential for the causation of RA.

Finally, there are the elusive infectious agent or agents whose antigens activate T cells. Many candidates have been considered, but none has been conclusively proved. Suspects include EBV, *Borrelia* species, *Mycoplasma* species, parvoviruses, and mycobacteria. *Although joint damage in RA is of immune origin and appears to occur in genetically predisposed individuals, the precise trigger that initiates these reactions is still unknown.*

Clinical Course. Although RA is basically a symmetric polyarticular arthritis, there may also be constitutional symptoms such as weakness, malaise, and low-grade fever. Many of the systemic manifestations result from the same mediators that cause joint inflammation (e.g., IL-1 and TNF). The arthritis first appears insidiously, with aching and stiffness of the joints, particularly in the morning. As the disease advances, the joints become enlarged, motion is limited, and in time complete ankylosis may appear. Vasculitic involvement of the extremities may give rise to *Raynaud phenomenon* (p 143) and chronic leg ulcers. Such multisystem involvement must be distinguished from SLE, scleroderma, polymyositis, dermatomyositis, and Lyme disease, as well as other forms of arthritis. Helpful in making the correct diagnosis are (1) characteristic radiographic findings (see Fig. 5–28); (2) sterile, turbid synovial fluid with decreased viscosity, poor mucin clot formation, and inclusion-bearing neutrophils; and (3) RF (80% of patients).

The clinical course of RA is highly variable. In a minority of patients the disease may become stabilized or may even regress; most of the remainder pursue a chronic, remitting-relapsing course. After 15 to 20 years, the majority of patients develop such deforming and destructive arthritis that surgical joint replacement is required. Life expectancy is reduced by a mean of 3 to 7 years. RA is an important cause of reactive amyloidosis (discussed later), which develops in 5% to 10% of these patients, particularly those with long-standing severe disease.

JUVENILE RHEUMATOID ARTHRITIS

Juvenile RA (JRA) refers to chronic idiopathic arthritis that occurs in children. It is not a single disease but a heterogeneous group of disorders, most of which differ significantly from the adult form of RA except for the destructive nature of the arthritis. RF is typically absent, as are rheumatoid nodules. Extra-articular inflammatory manifestations such as uveitis may be present. Some variants involve relatively few larger joints such as knees, elbows, and ankles and are thus called *pauciarticular*. Some cases of JRA are associated with HLA-B27, and their clinical features overlap with the spondyloarthropathies described next. One variant, previously called Still disease, has an acute febrile onset and systemic manifestations, including leukocytosis (15,000 to 25,000 cells/μL), hepatosplenomegaly, lymphadenopathy, and rash.

Seronegative Spondyloarthropathies

For years, several entities in this group of disorders were considered variants of RA; however, careful clinical, morphologic, and genetic studies have distinguished these disorders from RA. The spondyloarthropathies are characterized by the following features:

■ Pathologic changes that begin in the ligamentous attachments to bone rather than in the synovium
■ Involvement of the sacroiliac joints, plus/minus arthritis in other peripheral joints
■ Absence of RFs (hence the name "seronegative" spondyloarthropathies)
■ Association with HLA-B27

This group of disorders includes several clinical subsets, of which *ankylosing spondylitis* is the prototype (Table 5–8). Others include Reiter syndrome, psoriatic arthritis, spondylitis associated with inflammatory bowel diseases, and reactive arthropathies after infections (e.g., with *Yersinia* spp., *Shigella* spp., *Salmonella* spp., *Helicobacter* spp., or *Campylobacter* spp.). Sacroiliitis is a common manifestation in all of these disorders; they are distinguished by the particular peripheral joints involved, as well as by associated extraskeletal manifestations (e.g., urethritis, conjunctivitis, and uveitis are characteristic of Reiter syndrome). Although a triggering infection and immune mechanisms are thought to underlie most of the seronegative spondyloarthropathies, their pathogenesis remains obscure.

Sjögren Syndrome

Sjögren syndrome is a clinicopathologic entity characterized by dry eyes (*keratoconjunctivitis sicca*) and dry mouth (*xerostomia*) resulting from immune-mediated destruction of the lacrimal and salivary glands. It occurs as an isolated disorder (primary form), also known as the *sicca syndrome*, or more often in association with another autoimmune disease (secondary form). Among the associated disorders, RA is the most common, but some patients have SLE, polymyositis, systemic sclerosis, vasculitis, or thyroiditis.

Etiology and Pathogenesis. Several lines of evidence suggest that Sjögren syndrome is an autoimmune disease

Table 5-8. SOME FEATURES OF SPONDYLOARTHROPATHIES

Feature	Ankylosing Spondylitis	Reiter Syndrome	Psoriatic Arthritis	Spondylitis With Inflammatory Bowel Disease	Reactive Arthropathy
HLA-B27	95%	80%	20%–50%	50%	80%
Sacroiliitis	Always	Often	Often	Often	Often
Peripheral joints	Lower > upper (often)	Lower usually	Upper > lower	Lower > upper	Lower > upper
Uveitis	++	++	+	+	+
Conjunctivitis	−	+	−	−	−
Urethritis	−	+	−	−	±
Skin involvement	−	+	++	−	−
Mucosal involvement	−	+	−	+	+

Modified from Wyngaarden J, et al: Cecil Textbook of Medicine, 19th ed. Philadelphia, WB Saunders, 1992, p 1517.

in which the ductal epithelial cells of the exocrine glands are the primary target. Nevertheless, there is also systemic B-cell hyperactivity, as is evidenced by the presence of antinuclear antibodies and RF (even in the absence of associated RA). Most patients with primary Sjögren syndrome have autoantibodies to the ribonucleoprotein (RNP) antigens SS-A (Ro) and SS-B (La); note that these antibodies are also present in some SLE patients and are therefore not diagnostic for Sjögren syndrome (see Table 5-6). Although patients with high titer anti–SS-A antibodies are more likely to have systemic (extraglandular) manifestations, there is no evidence that the autoantibodies cause primary tissue injury.

Genetic factors play a role in the pathogenesis of Sjögren syndrome. As with SLE, inheritance of certain MHC II molecules predisposes to the development of specific RNP autoantibodies. Analogous to SLE as well, the disease is probably initiated by a loss of tolerance in the CD4+ T-cell population, although the nature of the recognized autoantigen or autoantigens is elusive.

MORPHOLOGY

Lacrimal and salivary glands are the primary targets, but other secretory glands, including those in the nasopharynx, upper airway, and vagina, may also be involved. Involved tissues exhibit an intense lymphocyte (primarily activated CD4+ T cells) and plasma cell infiltrate, occasionally forming lymphoid follicles with germinal centers. There is associated destruction of the native architecture (Fig. 5-31).

Lacrimal gland destruction results in a lack of tears, leading to drying of the corneal epithelium, with subsequent inflammation, erosion, and ulceration **(keratoconjunctivitis).** Similar events in the oral mucosa may occur owing to loss of salivary gland output, giving rise mucosal atrophy, with inflammatory fissuring and ulceration **(xerostomia).** Dryness and crusting of the nose may lead to ulcerations and even perforation of the nasal

Figure 5-31

Sjögren syndrome. *A,* Enlargement of the salivary gland. *B,* The histologic view shows intense lymphocytic and plasma cell infiltration with ductal epithelial hyperplasia. (*A,* Courtesy of Dr. Richard Sontheimer, Department of Dermatology, University of Texas Southwestern Medical School, Dallas; *B,* courtesy of Dr. Dennis Burns, Department of Pathology, University of Texas Southwestern Medical School, Dallas.)

septum. When the respiratory passages are involved, secondary laryngitis, bronchitis, and pneumonitis may appear. Approximately 25% of the
patients (especially those with anti–SS-A antibodies) develop extraglandular disease affecting the
central nervous system, skin, kidneys, and muscles.
Renal lesions take the form of mild interstitial
nephritis associated with tubular transport defects;
unlike SLE, glomerulonephritis is rare.

Clinical Course. Approximately 90% of Sjögren syndrome cases occur in women between the ages of 35 and 45
years. Patients present with dry mouth, lack of tears, and the
resultant complications just described. Salivary glands are
often enlarged, owing to lymphocytic infiltrates (see Fig.
5–31). Extraglandular manifestations include synovitis, pulmonary fibrosis, and peripheral neuropathy. About 60% of
Sjögren patients have *another* accompanying autoimmune
disorder such as RA. Interestingly, there is a 40-fold increased risk of developing a non-Hodgkin B-cell lymphoma,
arising in the setting of the initial robust polyclonal B-cell
proliferation. These so-called marginal zone lymphomas
(MALT lymphomas) are discussed in Chapter 12.

Systemic Sclerosis (Scleroderma)

Although commonly called *scleroderma*, this disorder is
better labeled systemic sclerosis (SS) because it is characterized by excessive fibrosis throughout the body and not
just the skin. Although cutaneous involvement is the usual
presenting symptom and eventually appears in approximately 95% of cases, it is the visceral involvement—of the
gastrointestinal tract, lungs, kidneys, heart, and skeletal
muscles—that produces the major morbidity and mortality.
SS occurs most frequently in the third to fifth decades and
affects women three times more often than men.

SS can be classified into two groups on the basis of its
clinical course:

■ Diffuse scleroderma, characterized by initial widespread
skin involvement, with rapid progression and early visceral involvement.
■ Limited scleroderma, with relatively minimal skin involvement, often confined to the fingers and face.
Involvement of the viscera occurs late, and hence the disease in these patients generally has a fairly benign course.
This is also called the CREST syndrome because of its
frequent features of *c*alcinosis, *R*aynaud phenomenon,
*e*sophageal dysmotility, *s*clerodactyly, and *t*elangiectasia.

Etiology and Pathogenesis. Fibroblast activation with
excessive fibrosis is the hallmark of SS. The cause is unknown, although it is attributed to abnormal activation of
the immune system and microvascular injury and not to any
intrinsic defect in fibroblasts or in collagen synthesis. The
interaction of T cells, endothelial injury, and fibroblast activation is schematized in Figure 5–32.

It is proposed that CD4+ cells responding to an as yet
unidentified antigen accumulate in the skin and release

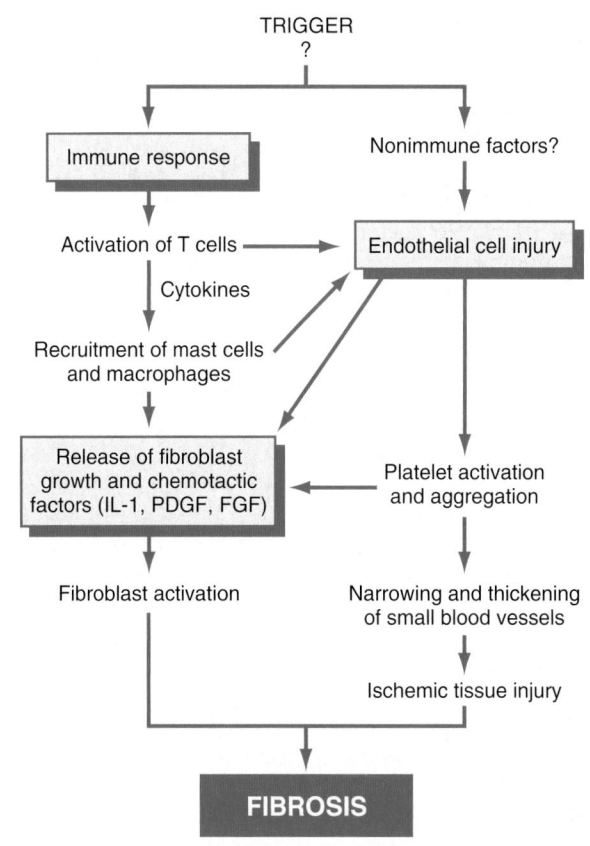

Figure 5–32   ■

Schematic illustration of the possible mechanisms leading to systemic
sclerosis. FGF, fibroblast growth factor; PDGF, platelet-derived growth
factor.

cytokines that activate mast cells and macrophages; in turn,
these cells release fibrogenic cytokines such as IL-1, TNF,
PDGF, TGF-β, and fibroblast growth factors. The possibility that activated T cells play a role in the pathogenesis of
SS is supported by the observation that several features of
this disease (including the cutaneous sclerosis) are seen in
chronic GVHD, a disorder resulting from sustained activation of T cells in recipients of allogeneic bone marrow
transplants. B-cell activation also occurs, as indicated by
the presence of hypergammaglobulinemia and ANAs. Although humoral immunity does not play any significant role
in the pathogenesis of SS, two of the ANAs are more or
less unique to SS and are therefore useful in diagnosis (see
Table 5–6). One of these, directed against *DNA topoiso-
merase I (anti-Scl 70),* is highly specific; it is present in up
to 70% of patients with diffuse scleroderma (and in less
than 1% of patients with other connective tissue diseases)
and is a marker for patients likely to develop more aggressive disease with pulmonary fibrosis and peripheral vascular
pathology. The other ANA is an *anticentromere antibody,*
found in up to 90% of patients with limited scleroderma
(i.e., the CREST syndrome); it indicates a relatively benign
course.

Microvascular disease is also consistently present early
in the course of SS, although the factor or factors that incite endothelial injury remain mysterious. It is also possible

that endothelial injury is not the primary event; rather, endothelial cells are induced to release PDGF and fibroblast chemotactic factors in the setting of T-cell activation. Thus, a primary immunologic abnormality may be the proximate cause of both vascular damage and fibrosis. Regardless of the cause of injury, it is proposed that repeated cycles of endothelial damage followed by platelet aggregation lead to release of platelet factors (e.g., PDGF, TGF-α) that trigger periadventitial fibrosis and eventual ischemic injury caused by widespread narrowing of the microvasculature.

MORPHOLOGY

Virtually any organ may be affected in SS, but the most prominent changes are found in the skin, musculoskeletal system, gastrointestinal tract, lungs, kidneys, and heart.

SKIN. The vast majority of patients have diffuse, sclerotic atrophy of the skin, usually beginning in the fingers and distal regions of the upper extremities and extending proximally to involve the upper arms, shoulders, neck, and face. In the early stages, affected skin areas are somewhat edematous and have a doughy consistency. Histologically, there are edema and perivascular infiltrates containing CD4+ T cells. Capillaries and small arteries (up to 500 μm in diameter) may show thickening of the basal lamina, endothelial cell damage, and partial occlusion. With progression, the edematous phase is replaced by progressive fibrosis of the dermis, which becomes tightly bound to the subcutaneous structures. There is marked increase of compact collagen in the dermis along with thinning of the epidermis, atrophy of the dermal appendages, and hyaline thickening of the walls of dermal arterioles and capillaries (Fig. 5–33A). Focal and sometimes diffuse subcutaneous calcifications may develop, especially in patients with the CREST syndrome. In advanced stages, the fingers take on a tapered, clawlike appearance with limitation of motion in the joints (Fig. 5–33B), and the face becomes a drawn mask. Loss of blood supply may lead to cutaneous ulcerations and to atrophic changes in the terminal phalanges, including autoamputation.

GASTROINTESTINAL TRACT. The gastrointestinal tract is affected in approximately 90% of patients. Progressive atrophy and collagenous fibrous replacement of the muscularis may develop at any level of the gut but are most severe in the esophagus, with the lower two thirds often developing a rubber-hose–like inflexibility. The associated dysfunction of the lower esophageal sphincter gives rise to gastroesophageal reflux and its complications, including Barrett metaplasia (Chapter 15) and strictures. The mucosa is thinned and may be ulcerated, and there is excessive collagenization of the lamina propria and submucosa. Loss of villi and microvilli in the small bowel is the anatomic basis for the malabsorption syndrome sometimes encountered.

Figure 5–33 ■

Systemic sclerosis. *A*, Microscopic appearance in the skin. Note the extensive deposition of dense collagen in the dermis with virtual absence of appendages and thinning of epidermis. *B*, Advanced systemic sclerosis. The extensive subcutaneous fibrosis has virtually immobilized the fingers, creating a clawlike flexion deformity. Loss of blood supply has led to cutaneous ulcerations. (*A*, Courtesy of Dr. Trace Worrell, Department of Pathology, University of Texas Southwestern Medical School, Dallas; *B*, courtesy of Dr. Richard Sontheimer, Department of Dermatology, University of Texas Southwestern Medical School, Dallas.)

MUSCULOSKELETAL SYSTEM. Synovial hyperplasia and inflammation is common in the early stages; fibrosis later ensues. Although these changes are reminiscent of RA, joint destruction is not common in SS. In a small subset of patients (approximately 10%), inflammatory myositis indistinguishable from polymyositis may develop.

LUNGS. SS affects the lungs in more than 50% of patients; this may manifest as pulmonary hypertension and/or interstitial fibrosis. Pulmonary vasospasm from pulmonary vascular endothelial dysfunction is considered important in the pathogenesis of pulmonary hypertension. Pulmonary fibrosis, when present, is indistinguishable from that seen in idiopathic pulmonary fibrosis (Chapter 13).

KIDNEYS. Renal abnormalities occur in two thirds of patients with SS, most typically associated with thickening of the vessel walls of interlobular arteries (150 to 500 μm in diameter). These show intimal cell proliferation with deposition of various glycoproteins and acid mucopolysaccharides. Although similar to the changes seen in malignant hypertension, the alterations in SS are restricted to vessels 150 to 500 μm in diameter and are not always associated with hypertension. Hypertension does occur in 30% of patients with SS, and in 20% of those patients takes an ominously malignant course (**malignant hypertension**). In hypertensive patients, vascular alterations are more pronounced and are often associated with fibrinoid necrosis involving the arterioles together with thrombosis and infarction. Such patients often die of renal failure, accounting for about half the deaths in patients with SS. There are no specific glomerular changes.

HEART. Patchy myocardial fibrosis, along with thickening of intramyocardial arterioles, occurs in one third of the patients; this is putatively caused by microvascular injury and resultant ischemia (so-called cardiac Raynaud). Because of the changes in the lung, right ventricular hypertrophy and failure (cor pulmonale) are frequent.

Clinical Course. SS affects women threefold more often than men, with a peak incidence in the 50- to 60-year age group. Clearly, there is a substantial overlap in presentation between SS and RA, SLE, and dermatomyositis (see later). SS is distinctive, however, because of the striking cutaneous changes. Almost all patients develop *Raynaud phenomenon*, a vascular disorder characterized by reversible vasospasm of the arteries. Typically the hands turn white on exposure to cold, reflecting vasospasm, followed by a blue color as capillaries and venules dilate and blood stagnates. Finally, the color changes to red as reactive vasodilation occurs. Progressive collagenization of the skin leads to atrophy of the hands, with increasing stiffness and eventually complete immobilization of the joints. Difficulty in swallowing results from esophageal fibrosis and resultant hypomotility. Eventually, destruction of the esophageal wall leads to atony and dilation. Malabsorption may appear if the submucosal and muscular atrophy and fibrosis involve the small intestine. Dyspnea and chronic cough reflect the pulmonary changes; with advanced lung involvement, secondary pulmonary hypertension may develop, leading to right-sided cardiac dysfunction. Renal functional impairment secondary to both the advance of SS and the concomitant malignant hypertension is frequently marked.

The course of diffuse SS is difficult to predict. In most patients, the disease pursues a steady, slow, downhill course over the span of many years, although in the absence of renal involvement, life span may be normal. The overall 10-year survival rate ranges from 35% to 70%. The chances of survival are significantly better for patients with localized scleroderma than for those with the usual diffuse progressive disease. *Limited scleroderma*, or CREST syndrome, frequently has Raynaud phenomenon as its presenting feature. It is associated with limited skin involvement confined to the fingers and face, and these two features may be present for decades before the appearance of visceral lesions.

Inflammatory Myopathies

Inflammatory myopathies make up a heterogeneous group of rare disorders characterized by immune-mediated muscle injury and inflammation. Depending on the clinical, morphologic, and immunologic features, three relatively distinct disorders—*polymyositis, dermatomyositis*, and *inclusion body myositis*—have been described. These may occur alone or in conjunction with other autoimmune diseases, such as SS. Women with dermatomyositis have a slightly increased risk of developing visceral cancers (lung, ovary, stomach). Because these disorders are uncommon, only a few salient features will be summarized.

■ Clinically, they are characterized by usually symmetric muscle weakness initially affecting large muscles of the trunk, neck, and limbs. Thus, tasks such as getting up from a chair or climbing steps become increasingly difficult. In dermatomyositis an associated rash (classically described as a *lilac* or *heliotrope* discoloration) affects the upper eyelids and causes periorbital edema (Fig. 5–34A)

■ Histologically, there is infiltration by lymphocytes, and both degenerating and regenerating muscle fibers are seen. The pattern of muscle injury and the location of the inflammatory infiltrates are somewhat distinctive for each subtype (Fig. 5–34B, C).

■ Immunologically, evidence supports antibody-mediated tissue injury in dermatomyositis, whereas polymyositis and inclusion body myositis appear to be mediated by cytotoxic T cells. Antinuclear antibodies are present in most patients. Of these, only Jo-1 antibodies, directed against tRNA synthetase, are specific for this group of disorders (see Table 5–6).

■ The diagnosis of these myopathies is based on clinical features, laboratory evidence of muscle injury (e.g., increased blood levels of creatine kinase), electromyography, and biopsy.

Mixed Connective Tissue Disease

The term *mixed connective tissue disease* is used to connote a spectrum of pathologic processes in patients who clinically present with multiple features suggestive of SLE, polymyositis, and systemic sclerosis; they also have *high titers of antibodies to an RNP antigen called U1RNP*. Two other factors lend distinctiveness to mixed connective tissue disease—the paucity of renal disease and an extremely good response to corticosteroids—both of which suggest a favorable long-term prognosis.

Mixed connective tissue disease may present as arthritis, swelling of the hands, Raynaud phenomenon, esophageal dysmotility, myositis, leukopenia and anemia, fever, lymphadenopathy, and/or hypergammaglobulinemia. Because of these overlapping features, it is not entirely clear whether mixed connective tissue disease constitutes a distinct disease or is a heterogeneous mixture of subsets of SLE, SS, and polymyositis; most authorities do not consider it a specific entity.

Figure 5–34 ■

Dermatomyositis. *A*, Rash affecting the eyelids. *B*, Histologic appearance of muscle shows perifascicular inflammation and atrophy. *C*, Inclusion body myositis shows a vacuole within a myocyte. (Courtesy of Dr. Dennis Burns, Department of Pathology, University of Texas Southwestern Medical School, Dallas.)

Polyarteritis Nodosa and Other Vasculitides

Polyarteritis nodosa belongs to a group of diseases characterized by necrotizing inflammation of the walls of blood vessels, most likely of an immune pathogenesis. The general term *noninfectious necrotizing vasculitis* differentiates these conditions from those attributable to direct vessel infection (e.g., an abscess) and serves to emphasize that any type of vessel may be involved—arteries, arterioles, veins, or capillaries. A detailed classification and description of vasculitides is presented in Chapter 10.

IMMUNODEFICIENCY DISEASES

Immunodeficiency diseases may be caused by inherited defects affecting immune system development, or they may result from secondary effects of other diseases (e.g., infection, malnutrition, aging, immunosuppression, autoimmunity, or chemotherapy). Clinically, patients with immunodeficiency present with increased susceptibility to infections as well as to certain forms of cancer. The type of infections in a given patient depends largely on the component of the immune system that is affected. Patients with defects in immunoglobulin, complement, or phagocytic cells typically suffer from recurrent infections with pyogenic bacteria; on the other hand, those with defects in cell-mediated immunity are prone to infections caused by viruses, fungi, and intracellular bacteria. Here a brief discussion is presented of some of the more important primary immunodeficiencies, followed by a detailed description of the acquired immuno-

deficiency syndrome (AIDS), the most devastating example of secondary immunodeficiency.

Primary Immunodeficiencies

Primary immunodeficiency states are (fortunately) rare but have nevertheless contributed greatly to our understanding of the ontogeny and regulation of the immune system (Fig. 5–35). Most primary immunodeficiency diseases are genetically determined and affect either specific immunity (i.e., humoral or cellular) or nonspecific host defense mechanisms mediated by complement proteins and cells such as phagocytes or NK cells. Defects in specific immunity are often subclassified on the basis of the primary component involved (i.e., B cells or T cells); however, in view of the extensive interactions between T and B lymphocytes, these distinctions are not clear-cut (see Fig. 5–35). In particular, T-cell defects almost always lead to impaired antibody synthesis, and hence isolated deficiencies of T cells are usually indistinguishable from combined deficiencies of T and B cells. Most primary immunodeficiencies come to attention early in life (between 6 months and 2 years of life), usually because of the susceptibility of infants to recurrent infections.

X-LINKED AGAMMAGLOBULINEMIA: BRUTON DISEASE

Bruton disease is one of the more common forms of primary immunodeficiency. It is *characterized by the failure of pre-B cells to differentiate into B cells*; as a consequence, and as the name implies, there is a resultant absence of gamma globulin in the blood. During normal B-cell differentiation, immunoglobulin heavy-chain genes are rearranged first,

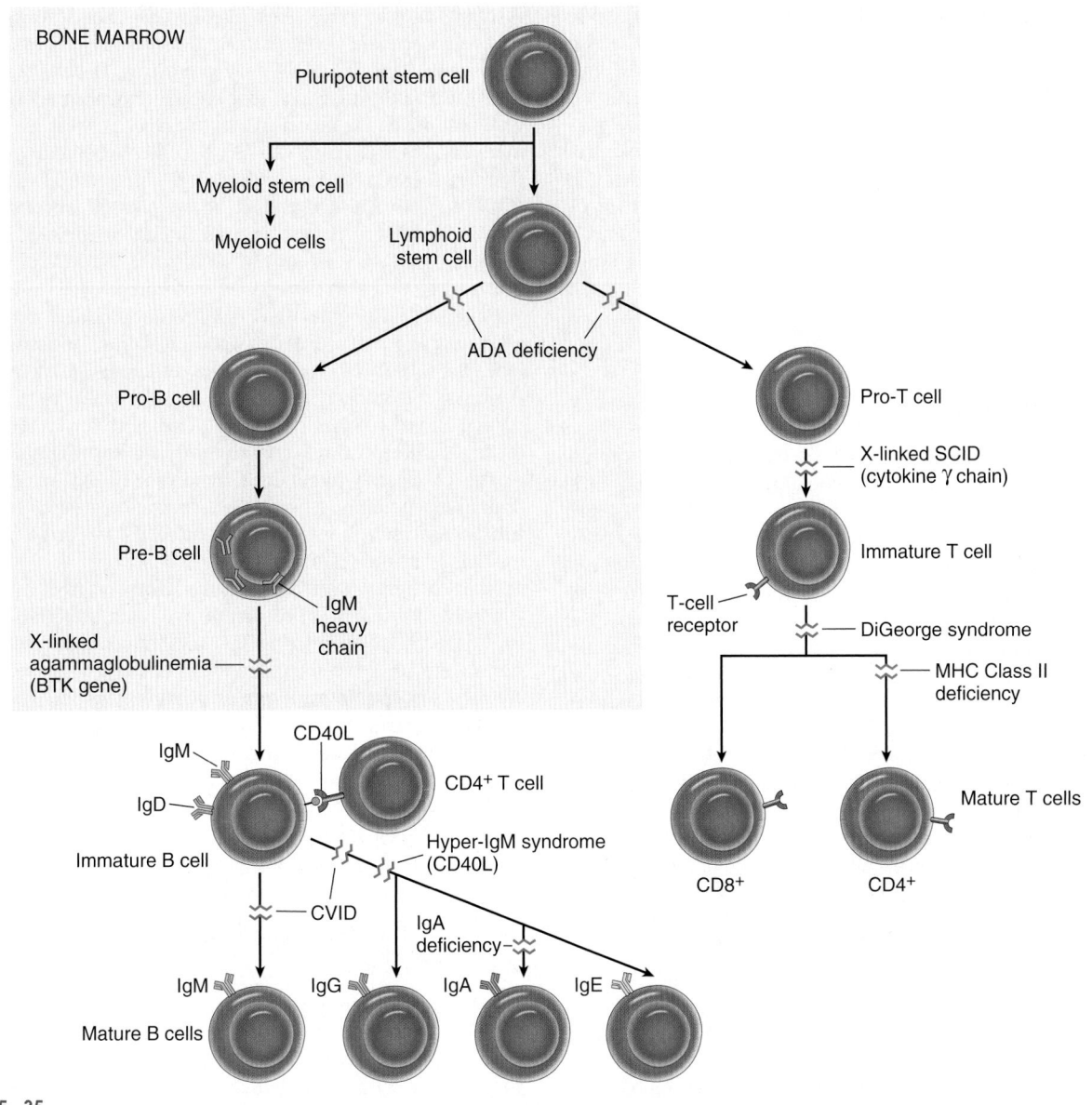

Figure 5–35 ■

Simplified scheme of lymphocyte development and sites of block in primary immunodeficiency diseases. The affected genes are indicated in parentheses for some of the disorders. ADA, adenosine deaminase; CD40L, CD40 ligand (also known as CD154); CVID, common variable immunodeficiency; SCID, severe combined immunodeficiency.

followed by light-chain rearrangement. In Bruton agamma-globulinemia, B-cell maturation stops after the initial heavy-chain gene rearrangement because of mutations in a tyrosine kinase involved in pre-B cell signal transduction. Called *Bruton tyrosine kinase (BTK)*, it is responsible for continued B-cell maturation. Because light chains are not produced, the complete immunoglobulin molecule containing heavy and light chains cannot be assembled and transported to the cell membrane, although free heavy chains can be found in the cytoplasm. Because *BTK* maps to the X chromosome, the disorder is seen primarily in males; nevertheless, sporadic cases have been described in females.

Classically, this disease is characterized by

■ Absent or markedly decreased numbers of B cells in the circulation, with depressed serum levels of all classes of

immunoglobulins. Pre-B cells are found in normal numbers in bone marrow.
■ Underdeveloped or rudimentary germinal centers in peripheral lymphoid tissues, including lymph nodes, Peyer patches, the appendix, and tonsils.
■ Absence of plasma cells throughout the body.
■ Normal T-cell–mediated responses.

Bruton disease does not become apparent until approximately 6 months of age, when maternal immunoglobulins are depleted. In most cases, recurrent bacterial infections such as acute and chronic pharyngitis, sinusitis, otitis media, bronchitis, and pneumonia suggest an underlying immune defect. The causal organisms are typically those bacterial pathogens that are cleared by antibody opsonization (e.g., *Haemophilus influenzae*, *Streptococcus pneumoniae*, or *Staphylococcus aureus*). Because antibodies are important for neutralizing viruses, these patients are also susceptible to certain viral infections, especially those caused by the enteroviruses. Similarly, *Giardia lamblia*, an intestinal protozoan usually resisted by secreted IgA, cannot be efficiently cleared and causes persistent infections. Fortunately, replacement therapy with intravenous immunoglobulin from pooled human serum allows the majority of patients to adequately circumvent bacterial infections. Patients with Bruton disease clear most viral, fungal, and protozoal infections because their T-cell–mediated immunity is intact. For unclear reasons, autoimmune diseases (such as SLE and dermatomyositis) also occur in up to 20% patients with Bruton disease.

COMMON VARIABLE IMMUNODEFICIENCY

This is a heterogeneous group of congenital or acquired disorders characterized by hypogammaglobulinemia, impaired antibody responses to infection (or vaccine), and increased numbers of infections; the clinical manifestations are superficially similar to those of Bruton agammaglobulinemia. However, in contrast to Bruton disease, the sexes are affected equally and the onset of symptoms is much later, in the second or third decade of life. The diagnosis is usually one of exclusion (after other causes of immunodeficiency are ruled out); the basis of the immunoglobulin deficiency is variable (hence the name). Although most patients have normal numbers of mature B cells, plasma cells are absent, suggesting a block in B-cell development. The defective antibody production has been variably attributed to intrinsic B-cell defects, deficient T-cell help, or excessive T-cell suppressor activity. Paradoxically, these patients are prone to develop a variety of autoimmune disorders (hemolytic anemia, pernicious anemia), as well as lymphoid tumors.

ISOLATED IgA DEFICIENCY

The most common of all the primary immunodeficiency diseases, IgA deficiency affects about 1 in 700 white individuals. Recall that IgA is the major immunoglobulin in mucosal secretions and is thus involved in airway and gastrointestinal defense. Although most individuals with this condition are asymptomatic, weakened mucosal defenses predispose patients to recurrent sinopulmonary infections and diarrhea. There is also a significant (but unexplained) association with autoimmune diseases. The pathogenesis of IgA deficiency appears to involve a block in the terminal differentiation of IgA-secreting B cells to plasma cells; IgM and IgG subclasses of antibodies are present in normal or even supranormal levels. Although the molecular basis of this defect is not understood, intrinsic B-cell defects or altered T-cell production of cytokines that drive IgA responses (e.g., TGF-β and IL-5) have been implicated.

HYPER-IgM SYNDROME

In a normal immune response to protein antigen, IgM and IgD antibodies are produced first, followed by the sequential elaboration of IgG, IgA, and IgE antibodies. This orderly appearance of antibody types is called *isotype switching* and is important for generating classes of antibody that can effectively activate complement and/or opsonize bacterial pathogens. The ability of IgM-producing B cells to turn on the transcription of genes that encode other immunoglobulin isotypes depends on certain cytokines, as well as contact-mediated signals from CD4+ T cells. Specifically, interaction between CD40 molecules on B cells and CD40 ligands (CD40L, also known as CD154) expressed on activated T cells is necessary for isotype switching; mutations in either CD40L or CD40 prevent the requisite T- and B-cell interaction and give rise to hyper-IgM syndrome.

Patients with hyper-IgM syndrome produce normal (or even supranormal) levels of IgM antibodies to antigens but lack the ability to produce the other IgG, IgA, or IgE isotypes; the underlying defect is an inability of T cells to induce B-cell isotype switching. The gene for CD40L maps to the X chromosome; consequently, in approximately 70% of the cases, the hyper-IgM syndrome is X-linked. In the remaining patients, the precise mutations have not been fully characterized but probably affect CD40 or other B-cell molecules in the CD40 signaling pathway.

Male patients with the X-linked form of the hyper-IgM syndrome present with recurrent pyogenic infections, owing to low levels of opsonizing IgG antibodies. Because CD40L signals are involved in macrophage activation, these patients are also susceptible to a variety of pathogens that require intact DTH responses, including *Pneumocystis carinii*. Several of the IgM antibodies can react with elements of blood, resulting in autoimmune hemolytic anemia, thrombocytopenia, or neutropenia. In older patients, there may be uncontrolled proliferation of IgM-producing plasma cells with clinically significant infiltration of the gastrointestinal tract.

THYMIC HYPOPLASIA: DiGEORGE SYNDROME

DiGeorge syndrome results from a congenital defect in thymic development with deficient T-cell maturation. T cells are absent in the lymph nodes, spleen, and peripheral blood, and infants with this defect are extremely vulnerable to viral, fungal, and protozoal infections. Susceptibility to intracellular bacteria is also increased, because T-cell activation of the phagocytic cells that eliminate them is absent. B cells and serum immunoglobulins are generally unaffected.

The disorder is a consequence of a developmental malformation affecting the third and fourth pharyngeal pouches—structures that give rise to the thymus, parathyroid glands, and portions of the face and aortic arch. Thus, in addition to the thymic and T-cell defects, there may be parathyroid gland hypoplasia resulting in hypocalcemic tetany, as well as additional midline developmental abnormalities. In 90% of cases of DiGeorge syndrome there is a deletion affecting chromosome 22q11, as discussed in Chapter 7. Transplantation of thymic tissue has successfully treated some of these infants. In others (with partial defects), immunity may improve spontaneously with age.

SEVERE COMBINED IMMUNODEFICIENCY

Severe combined immunodeficiency (SCID) represents a constellation of genetically distinct syndromes all exhibiting defects in both humoral and cell-mediated immune responses. Affected infants are susceptible to severe recurrent infections by a wide array of pathogens, including bacteria, viruses, fungi, and protozoans; opportunistic infections by *Candida, Pneumocystis,* cytomegalovirus, and *Pseudomonas* also cause serious (and occasionally lethal) disease. Despite common clinical features, the underlying defects in individual patients are quite different. Although some forms are caused by a single defect affecting both T and B cells, SCID may also result from a primary T-cell deficit, with secondary impairment of humoral immunity.

Approximately half of the cases are X-linked, resulting from mutations in the gene encoding the common γ chain shared by the cytokine receptors for IL-2, IL-4, IL-7, IL-9, and IL-15. Of these cytokines, IL-7 is the most important because it is the factor responsible for stimulating the survival and expansion of immature B- and T-cell precursors in the bone marrow.

Another 40% to 50% of SCID cases are inherited in an autosomal recessive fashion, with approximately half of those caused by mutations in *adenosine deaminase (ADA)*, an enzyme involved in purine metabolism. ADA deficiency results in accumulation of adenosine and deoxyadenosine triphosphate metabolites, which inhibit DNA synthesis and are toxic to lymphocytes. The other autosomal recessive causes of SCID are attributed to defects in another purine metabolic pathway, primary failure of class II MHC expression, or mutations in the recombinase genes responsible for the effective rearrangement of lymphocyte antigen-receptor molecules. Most of these defects primarily affect the function of CD4+ helper T cells; as noted earlier, both cell-mediated immunity and T-cell–dependent antibody responses are thereby impaired.

In the two most common forms of SCID (cytokine receptor mutation and ADA deficiency), the thymus is hypoplastic. Lymph nodes and lymphoid tissues (e.g., in the tonsils, gut, and appendix) are atrophic and lack B-cell germinal centers as well as paracortical T cells. Affected patients may have marked lymphopenia, with both T- and B-cell deficiency; others may have increased numbers of immature T cells and/or large numbers of non-functional B cells, owing to a lack of T-cell help. Patients with SCID are currently treated by bone marrow transplantation, although gene therapy to replace mutated genes is also being investigated.

IMMUNODEFICIENCY WITH THROMBOCYTOPENIA AND ECZEMA: WISKOTT-ALDRICH SYNDROME

Wiskott-Aldrich syndrome is an X-linked recessive disease characterized by thrombocytopenia, eczema, and a marked vulnerability to recurrent infection, ending in early death; the only treatment is bone marrow transplantation. This is a curious syndrome, in that the clinical presentation and immunologic deficits are difficult to cogently rationalize based on the known underlying genetic defect. The thymus is initially normal, but there is progressive age-related depletion of T lymphocytes in the peripheral blood and lymph nodes, with concurrent loss of cellular immunity. Additionally, patients do not effectively synthesize antibodies to polysaccharide antigens, and affected patients are thereby particularly susceptible to encapsulated,

pyogenic bacteria. (However, B-cell synthesis of antibodies against polysaccharide antigens does not require T-cell help!) Affected patients are also prone to developing malignant lymphomas. The responsible gene maps to the X chromosome and encodes a protein *(Wiskott-Aldrich syndrome protein)* that links intracellular signaling and the cytoskeleton. Although the mechanism is not known, absent or defective protein could mediate its effects by abnormal modulation of cellular morphology (including platelet shape changes?) or by defective targeting of leukocytes to peripheral lymphoid tissues.

GENETIC DEFICIENCIES OF COMPLEMENT COMPONENTS

As discussed earlier in this chapter and in Chapter 2, complement components play important roles in inflammatory and immunologic responses. Consequently, hereditary deficiency of complement components, especially C3 (critical for both the classic and alternative pathways), results in an increased susceptibility to infection with pyogenic bacteria. Inherited deficiencies of C1q, C2, and C4 also increase the risk of immune complex–mediated disease (e.g., SLE), possibly by impairing the clearance of antigen-antibody complexes from the circulation. Conversely, lack of C1 esterase inhibitor allows unfettered C1 esterase activation with the generation of down-stream vasoactive complement mediators; the result is *hereditary angioedema,* characterized by recurrent episodes of localized edema affecting skin and/or mucous membranes. Deficiencies of the other components of the classic complement pathway (C5 to C8) result in recurrent *neisserial* (gonococcal, meningococcal) infections.

Secondary Immunodeficiencies

Secondary immunodeficiencies may be encountered in patients with malnutrition, infection, cancer, renal disease, or sarcoidosis. They also occur in patients receiving chemotherapy or radiation therapy for malignancy or immunosuppressive drugs to prevent graft rejection or treat autoimmune diseases. Some of these secondary immunodeficiency states can be caused by loss of immunoglobulins (as in proteinuric renal diseases), inadequate immunoglobulin synthesis (as in malnutrition), or lymphocyte depletion (from drugs or severe infections). *As a group, the secondary immunodeficiencies are more common than the disorders of primary genetic origin.* Here only AIDS, the most widespread and important of the secondary immunodeficiency states, is discussed.

ACQUIRED IMMUNODEFICIENCY SYNDROME

AIDS is a *retroviral disease caused by the human immunodeficiency virus (HIV) and is characterized by profound immunosuppression leading to opportunistic infections, secondary neoplasms, and neurologic manifestations.* Although AIDS was first described in the United States, it has now been reported in virtually every country in the world. Worldwide, an estimated 22 million people have died of AIDS since the epidemic was recognized some 20 years ago; 3 million people died in the year 2000 alone. The numbers are destined only to get worse, at least in the immediate future. On the basis of serologic data, an estimated 35 million people (roughly 1 in every 100) globally are infected with HIV. This sobering statistic includes approximately 1.4 million children and 17 million women. Ninety-five percent of worldwide HIV infections are in developing countries, with Africa alone carrying over 50% of the HIV burden. Although the largest number of infections are in Africa, the most rapid increases in HIV infection in the past decade are in Southeast Asian countries, including Thailand, India, and Indonesia. The statistics are only slightly better in the industrialized nations; for example, approximately 1 million US citizens are infected (roughly 1 in 300). Moreover, more Americans (almost 500,000) have died of AIDS than in both World Wars combined. Although AIDS-related death rates continue a progressive decline from a 1995 peak, AIDS still represents the fifth most common cause of death in adults between the ages of 25 and 44.

No less imposing is the explosion of new knowledge relating to this modern plague. So rapid is the pace of research on the biology of HIV that any text covering the topic will almost certainly be out of date by the time it goes to press. Nevertheless, the following will attempt to summarize the currently available data on HIV epidemiology, etiology, pathogenesis, and clinical features.

Epidemiology. Since the statistics from the United States are the most current and complete, the focus will be on American data; these are also reasonably representative of most developed countries. Nevertheless, trends in the developing countries are occasionally significantly (and importantly) different, and these will be highlighted where appropriate. Epidemiologic studies in the United States have identified five groups at risk for developing AIDS, with case distributions as noted. In the remaining 9% to 10% of cases, risk factors are either unknown or not reported. It should be apparent from the epidemiologic and subsequent laboratory investigations that transmission of HIV occurs under conditions that facilitate the exchange of blood or body fluids that contain the virus *or virus-infected cells*. Thus, the three major routes are *sexual contact*, *parenteral inoculation*, and *passage of the virus from infected mothers to their newborns*.

- Homosexual or bisexual males still constitute the largest group of infected individuals (approximately 14% also inject drugs), accounting for 46% of reported cases overall and 56% of infected men. However, transmission of AIDS in this category continues to decline, with less than 50% of new cases attributable to male homosexual contacts.
- Intravenous drug abusers with no history of homosexuality compose the next largest group, representing about 25% of all patients. They represent the majority of all cases among heterosexuals.
- Recipients of blood and blood components (but not hemophiliacs) who received transfusions of HIV-infected whole blood or components (e.g., platelets, plasma) account for 1% of patients.
- Hemophiliacs, especially those who received large amounts of factor VIII or IX concentrates before 1985, make up less than 1% of all cases.
- Heterosexual contacts of members of other high-risk groups (chiefly intravenous drug abusers) constitute about 11% of the patient population.

The epidemiology of HIV infection and AIDS is quite different in children (diagnosed when younger than 13 years of age). About 1% of all AIDS cases occur in this population, and the vast majority (about 90%) result from transmission of virus from mother to infant. Approximately 10% of children with AIDS are hemophiliacs and others who received blood or blood products before 1985.

Sexual Transmission. Sexual transmission is clearly the predominant mode of infection worldwide, accounting for greater than 75% of all cases of HIV transmission. Although most sexually transmitted cases in the United States are still due to homosexual or bisexual male contacts, the vast majority of sexually transmitted HIV infections globally are due to heterosexual activity. Even in the United States, *the rate of increase of heterosexual transmission has outpaced transmission by other means*; such spread accounts for the dramatic increase in HIV infection in female sex partners of male intravenous drug abusers.

The virus is present in semen, both extracellularly and within mononuclear inflammatory cells, and enters the recipient's body through tears or abrasions in mucosa. Viral transmission can occur either by direct entry of virus or infected cells into blood vessels breached by trauma or by uptake into mucosal dendritic cells. Clearly, all forms of sexual transmission are aided and abetted by the concomitant presence of other sexually transmitted diseases that cause genital ulcerations, including syphilis, chancroid, and herpes simplex virus. Gonorrhea and chlamydia also act as cofactors to HIV transmission primarily by increasing the seminal fluid content of inflammatory cells (presumably carrying HIV). In addition to male-to-male and male-to-female transmission, HIV is present in the vaginal and cervical cells of infected women and can also be spread from females to males, albeit about 8-fold less efficiently.

Parenteral Transmission. Parenteral transmission of HIV is well documented in three different groups: intravenous drug abusers (the largest group), hemophiliacs receiving factor VIII or IX concentrates, and random recipients of blood transfusion. Among intravenous drug abusers, transmission occurs through shared needles, syringes, or other paraphernalia contaminated with HIV-containing blood. This group occupies a pivotal position in the AIDS epidemic because it represents the principal link in the transmission of HIV to other adult populations through heterosexual activity.

Transmission of HIV by transfusion of blood or blood products such as lyophilized factor VIII concentrates has been virtually eliminated since 1985. Four public health measures are responsible: screening of donated blood and plasma for antibody to HIV, screening for HIV-associated p24 antigen (detectable before the development of humoral antibodies), heat treatment of clotting factor concentrates, and screening of donors on the basis of history. With all these measures, the risk of HIV infection in the United States has been reduced to roughly 1 in 676,000 donations. This translates into approximately 18 (out of 12 million) donations that may transmit HIV. With the advent of nucleic acid testing, this already small risk will show further decline.

Mother-to-Infant Transmission. As noted earlier, mother-to-infant *vertical transmission* is the major cause of pediatric AIDS. Three routes are involved: in utero, by transplacental spread; intrapartum, during delivery; and via ingestion of HIV-contaminated breast milk. Of these, the transplacental and intrapartum routes account for most cases. Vertical transmission rates worldwide vary from 25% to 35%, with a 15% to 25% rate reported in the United States; higher rates of infection occur with high maternal viral load and/or the presence of chorioamnionitis, presumably by increasing placental accumulation of inflammatory cells.

Because of the uniformly fatal outcome of AIDS, the lay public is justifiably concerned about the spread of HIV infection outside recognized high-risk groups. Many of these anxieties can be laid to rest, as extensive studies indicate that *HIV infection cannot be transmitted by casual personal contact in the home, workplace, or school, and no convincing evidence for spread by insect bites has been obtained.* There is an extremely small but definite risk for transmission of HIV infection to health care workers. Seroconversion has been documented after accidental needle-stick injury or exposure of nonintact skin to infected blood in laboratory accidents with a rate about 0.3% per accidental exposure. By comparison, the rate of seroconversion after accidental exposure to hepatitis B–infected blood is about 6% to 30%. Transmission of HIV from an infected health care worker to a patient is extremely rare.

Etiology. AIDS is caused by HIV, a human retrovirus belonging to the lentivirus family (which also includes feline immunodeficiency virus, simian immunodeficiency virus, visna virus of sheep, and the equine infectious anemia virus). Two genetically different but antigenically related forms of HIV, called *HIV-1* and *HIV-2*, have been isolated from patients with AIDS. HIV-1 is the more common type associated with AIDS in the United States, Europe, and Central Africa, whereas HIV-2 causes a similar disease principally in West Africa. Specific tests for HIV-2 are now available, and blood collected for transfusion is also routinely screened for HIV-2 seropositivity. The ensuing discussion relates primarily to HIV-1 and diseases caused by it, but it is generally applicable to HIV-2 as well.

Like most retroviruses, the HIV-1 virion is spherical and contains an electron-dense, cone-shaped core surrounded by

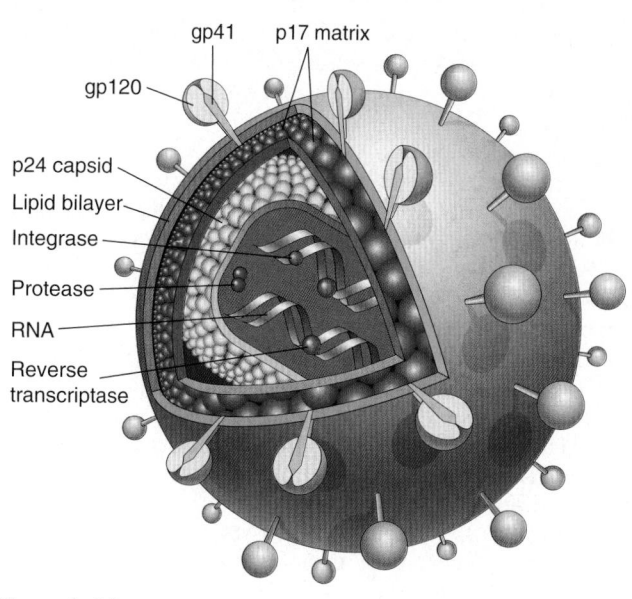

Figure 5-36 ■

Schematic illustration of the human immunodeficiency virus (HIV)-1 virion. The viral particle is covered by a lipid bilayer derived from the host cell and studded with viral glycoproteins gp41 and gp120.

a lipid envelope derived from the host cell membrane (Fig. 5–36). The virus core contains (1) the major capsid protein p24, (2) nucleocapsid protein p7/p9, (3) two copies of genomic RNA, and (4) the three viral enzymes (protease, reverse transcriptase, and integrase). p24 is the most readily detected viral antigen and is therefore the target for the antibodies used to diagnose HIV infection in blood screening. The viral core is surrounded by a matrix protein called *p17*, lying beneath the virion envelope. The viral envelope itself is studded by two viral glycoproteins (gp120 and gp41) critical for HIV infection of cells. The HIV-1 proviral genome contains the *gag*, *pol*, and *env* genes, which code for various viral proteins (Fig. 5–37). The products of the *gag* and *pol* genes are translated initially into large precursor proteins that must be cleaved by the

Figure 5-37 ■

HIV proviral genome. Several viral genes and their recognized functions are illustrated. The genes outlined in red are unique to HIV; others are shared by all retroviruses.

viral protease to yield the mature proteins. The highly effective anti–HIV-1 protease inhibitor drugs thus prevent viral assembly by inhibiting the formation of mature viral proteins.

In addition to these three standard retroviral genes, HIV contains several other genes (given three-letter names such as *tat, rev, vif, nef, vpr,* and *vpu*) that regulate the synthesis and assembly of infectious viral particles. The product of the *tat* (transactivator) gene, for example, is critical for virus replication, causing a 1000-fold increase in the transcription of viral genes. The *nef* protein in particular activates intracellular kinase activity (affecting T-cell activation, viral replication, and viral infectivity) and is essential for the progression of HIV infection in vivo. Thus, strains of simian immunodeficiency virus with mutated *nef* genes cause AIDS in monkeys at a markedly decreased rate, and humans infected with a *nef*-defective HIV-1 strain display exceptionally low viral burden, with AIDS onset at a substantially slower pace than for nonmutant strains. The products of regulatory genes are clearly important for HIV pathogenicity, and a number of therapeutic approaches are being developed to block their actions.

Molecular analysis of different viral isolates reveals considerable variability in many parts of the HIV genome. This is due to the relatively low fidelity of the viral polymerase, with estimates of one mistake for each 10^5 replicated nucleotides. Most variations cluster in certain regions of the envelope glycoproteins. Because the immune response against HIV-1 is targeted against its envelope, such extreme variability in antigen structure poses a formidable barrier for vaccine development.

On the basis of the molecular analysis, HIV-1 can be divided into two broader groups, designated *M* (major) and *O* (outlier). Group M viruses, the more common form worldwide, are further divided into subtypes (also called *clades*), designated A through J. The clades differ in their geographic distribution, with B being the most common form in western Europe and the United States and E being the most common in Thailand. Beyond molecular homologies, the clades also exhibit differences in modes of transmission. Thus, E clade is spread predominantly by heterosexual contact (male-to-female), presumably because of its ability to infect vaginal subepithelial dendritic cells. By contrast, B clade virus grows poorly in dendritic cells and is probably best transmitted by introduction of infected monocytes and lymphocytes.

Pathogenesis. The two major targets of HIV infection—the immune system and the central nervous system—are discussed separately.

Immunopathogenesis of HIV Disease. Profound immunosuppression, primarily affecting cell-mediated immunity, is the hallmark of AIDS. This results chiefly from infection and subsequent loss of CD4+ T cells as well as an impairment in the function of surviving helper T cells; as discussed in subsequent paragraphs, macrophages and dendritic cells (important in CD4+ T-cell activation) are also targets of HIV infection. First described are the mechanisms involved in viral entry into T cells and macrophages and the life cycle of the virus within cells. This is followed by a more detailed review of the interaction between HIV and its cellular targets.

The CD4 molecule is a high-affinity receptor for HIV. This explains the selective tropism of the virus for CD4+ T cells and its ability to infect other CD4+ cells, particularly macrophages and dendritic cells. However, binding to CD4 is not sufficient for infection; the HIV envelope gp120 must also bind to other cell surface molecules (*coreceptors*) to facilitate cell entry. Two cell surface chemokine receptor molecules, CCR5 and CXCR4 (Chapter 2), serve this role. As shown in Figure 5–38, HIV envelope gp120 (noncovalently attached to transmembrane gp41) binds initially to CD4 molecules. This binding leads to a conformational change exposing a new recognition site on gp120 for the

Figure 5–38

Molecular basis of HIV entry into host cells. Interactions with CD4 and CCR5 coreceptors are illustrated. (Adapted with permission from Wain-Hobson S: HIV. One on one meets two. Nature 384:117, 1996. Copyright 1996, Macmillan Magazines Limited.)

CXCR4 (mostly on T cells) or CCR5 (mostly on macrophages) coreceptors. The gp41 then undergoes a conformational change allowing insertion of a gp41 peptide sequence into the target membrane that facilitates cell-viral fusion. After fusion, the virus core containing the HIV genome enters the cytoplasm of the cell. The coreceptors are critical components of the HIV infection process. Thus, chemokines may compete with virus for binding to their receptors, and the level of chemokines in the microenvironment surrounding HIV and its target cells may influence the efficiency of viral infection in vivo. Moreover, individuals with defective CCR5 receptors (in American whites, 20% are heterozygous and 1% are homozygous for the mutant CCR5) are relatively resistant to developing AIDS, despite repeated HIV exposure in vivo.

The discovery of coreceptors for HIV infection also solved some previously unexplained observations regarding HIV tropism. It had been observed that HIV strains could be classified based on their relative ability to infect macrophages and/or CD4+ T cells. Macrophage-tropic (R5 virus) strains infect both monocytes/macrophages and freshly isolated peripheral blood T cells, whereas T-cell tropic (X4 virus) strains infect only T cells. This selectivity is now explained by selective coreceptor usage; R5 strains use CCR5 as their coreceptor, and, because CCR5 is expressed on both monocytes and T cells, these cells succumb to infection by R5 strains. Conversely, X4 strains bind to the CXCR4 expressed on T cells (and not on monocytes/macrophages), so that only T cells are susceptible. Interestingly, approximately 90% of HIV infections are initially transmitted by R5 strains. However, over the course of infection, X4 viruses gradually accumulate; these are especially virulent, deplete T cells, and are responsible for the final rapid phase of disease progression. It is thought that during the course of HIV infection, R5 strains evolve into X4 strains, owing to mutations in genes that encode gp120. Because of the significance of HIV-coreceptor interaction in the pathogenesis of AIDS, preventing this interaction may be of significant therapeutic importance.

Once internalized, the viral genome undergoes reverse transcription, leading to formation of complementary DNA (cDNA). In quiescent T cells, HIV proviral cDNA may remain in the cytoplasm in a linear episomal form. However, in dividing T cells, the cDNA enters the nucleus, and becomes integrated into the host genome. After integration, the provirus may remain nontranscribed for months or years and the infection becomes *latent*; alternatively, proviral DNA may be transcribed to form complete viral particles that bud from the cell membrane. Such productive infections, associated with extensive viral budding, lead to cell death (Fig. 5–39). It is important to note that although HIV-1 can infect resting T cells, the initiation of proviral DNA transcription (and hence productive infection) occurs only when the infected cell is activated by an exposure to antigens or cytokines. Clearly, physiologic stimuli that promote activation and growth of normal T cells (e.g., intercurrent infections with other microbial agents) promote the death of HIV-infected T cells.

T Cells in HIV Infection. HIV infections are marked by a relentless, and eventually profound, loss of CD4+ cells from the peripheral blood. It has been determined that approximately 100 billion new viral particles are produced every day, and 1 to 2 billion CD4+ T cells die each day. Consequently, one might surmise that productive infection of T cells is the mechanism by which HIV causes CD4+ T cell depletion. However, patients with HIV have remarkably few productively infected T cells, and at least early in the disease, the rate of CD4+ cell loss appears low. These apparent contradictions are partially explained by the following observations:

■ HIV colonizes the lymphoid organs (spleen, lymph nodes, tonsils) and infects T cells, macrophages, and dendritic cells (see Fig. 5–39). These, and not the peripheral blood T cells, are reservoirs of infected cells.
■ Initially, the immune system can vigorously proliferate to replace the dying T cells, thus masking the massive cell death occurring primarily in the lymphoid tissues.
■ In addition to direct cell lysis from productive HIV infection, T-cell loss may occur through other mechanisms:

  ■ Loss of immature precursors of CD4+ T cells, either by direct infection of thymic progenitor cells or by infection of accessory cells that secrete cytokines essential for CD4+ T-cell differentiation.
  ■ Fusion of infected and uninfected cells, with formation of syncytia (giant cells) (Fig. 5–40). In tissue culture, the gp120 expressed on productively infected cells binds to CD4 molecules on uninfected T cells, followed by cell fusion, *ballooning*, and death within a few hours. This property of syncytia formation is confined to the X4 HIV.
  ■ Uninfected CD4+ T cells may bind soluble gp120 to the CD4 molecule, followed by concurrent antigen activation through the T-cell receptor; such cross-linking of CD4 molecules and T-cell activation leads to aberrant signaling and apoptosis.
  ■ Cytotoxic CD8+ T-cell killing of infected CD4+ T cells

Thus, loss of CD4+ cells occurs by both increased destruction and reduced production. This leads to an inversion of the CD4-CD8 ratio in the peripheral blood. Thus, while the normal CD4-CD8 ratio is close to 2, patients with AIDS have a ratio ≤ 0.5. Although such inversion is a common finding in AIDS, it may also occur in other viral infections and is therefore not diagnostic.

Although marked reduction in CD4+ T cells is a hallmark of AIDS and can account for much of the immunodeficiency late in the course of HIV infection, there is also compelling evidence for *qualitative defects in T-cell function that can be detected even in asymptomatic HIV-infected persons.* Such defects include reduced antigen-induced T-cell proliferation, impaired T_H1 cytokine production, and abnormal intracellular signaling. There is also a selective loss of memory CD4+ helper T cells early in the course of the disease, possibly related to the higher level of CCR5 expression in this T-cell subset. This latter observation also explains the inability of peripheral blood T cells to be activated when challenged with common recall antigens.

Monocytes/Macrophages in HIV Infection. In addition to infection and loss of CD4+ T cells, *infection of monocytes*

Figure 5–39

Pathogenesis of HIV-1 infection. HIV-1 initially infects T cells and macrophages directly or is carried to these cells by dendritic cells. Viral replication in the regional lymph nodes leads to viremia and widespread seeding of lymphoid tissue. The viremia is controlled by the host immune response *(not shown)*, and the patient then enters a phase of clinical latency. During this phase, viral replication in both T cells and macrophages continues unabated, but there is some immune containment of virus *(not illustrated)*. There continues a gradual erosion of CD4+ cells by productive infection (or other mechanisms; see text). When the CD4+ cells that are destroyed cannot be replenished, CD4+ cell numbers decline and the patient develops clinical symptoms of full-blown AIDS. Macrophages are also parasitized by the virus early; they are not lysed by HIV-1, and they can transport the virus to various tissues, particularly the brain.

and macrophages is also extremely important in the pathogenesis of HIV. Similar to T cells, *most of the HIV-infected macrophages are found in the tissues and not in peripheral blood.* A relatively high frequency (10% to 50%) of infected macrophages is detected in certain tissues such as brain and lungs. Several additional aspects of macrophage HIV infection warrant emphasis:

■ Although cell division is requisite for replication of most retroviruses, HIV-1 can infect and multiply in terminally differentiated nondividing macrophages, a property conferred by the HIV-1 *vpr* gene.

■ Infected macrophages bud relatively small amounts of virus from the cell surface but contain large numbers of virus particles located in intracellular vacuoles.

■ In contrast to CD4+ T cells, macrophages are quite resistant to the cytopathic effects of HIV.

■ In more than 90% of cases, HIV infection is transmitted by R5 strains. The more virulent X4 strains that evolve

Figure 5-40   ■

HIV infection. Formation of giant cells in the brain. (Courtesy of Dr. Dennis Burns, Department of Pathology, University of Texas Southwestern Medical School, Dallas.)

later in the course of HIV infection are inefficient in transmitting HIV. This suggests that the initial infection of macrophages (or dendritic cells) is critical for HIV transmission.

Thus, in all likelihood, macrophages are the gatekeepers of HIV infection. Besides providing a portal for initial transmission, monocytes and macrophages are viral reservoirs and factories, whose output remains largely protected from host defenses. Macrophages also provide a vehicle for HIV transport to various parts of the body, particularly the nervous system. Finally, in late stages of HIV infection, when the CD4+ T cell numbers are massively depleted, macrophages remain a major site of continued viral replication. Although the number of HIV-infected monocytes in the circulation is low, their functional deficits (e.g., impaired microbicidal activity, decreased chemotaxis, abnormal cytokine production, and diminished antigen presentation capacity) have important bearing on host defenses.

Dendritic Cells in HIV Infection. In addition to macrophages, two types of *dendritic cells* are also important targets for the initiation and maintenance of HIV infection: mucosal and follicular dendritic cells. It is thought that mucosal dendritic cells, also called *Langerhans cells, capture the virus and transport it to regional lymph nodes*, where CD4+ T cells are infected. Some virus is carried on the dendritic processes, and other virus is carried within infected dendritic cells. *Follicular dendritic cells in the germinal centers of lymph nodes are important reservoirs* of HIV. Although some follicular dendritic cells are infected by HIV, most virus particles are found on the surface of their

dendritic processes, including bound to Fc receptors via HIV/anti-HIV antibody complexes. The antibody-coated virions localized to follicular dendritic cells retain the ability to infect CD4+ T cells. *To summarize, CD4+ T cells, macrophages, and follicular dendritic cells contained in peripheral lymphoid tissues are the major sites of HIV infection and persistence.*

Low-level chronic or latent infection of T cells and macrophages is an important feature of HIV infection. Although only rare CD4+ T cells express *infectious virus* early in the course of infection, up to 30% of lymph node T cells can be demonstrated to actually harbor the HIV genome. It is widely believed that integrated provirus, without virus expression *(latent infection),* can persist within cells for months to years. Even with potent antiviral therapy (which practically sterilizes the peripheral blood), latent virus lurks in lymph node CD4+ cells (up to 0.05% of resting, long-lived CD4+ T cells are infected). Completion of the viral life cycle in latently infected cells requires cell activation. Thus, latently infected CD4+ cells that encounter their appropriate environmental antigen undergo intracellular activation pathways that unfortunately also drive HIV proviral DNA transcription. This leads to virion production and, in the case of T cells, also results in cell lysis. In addition, TNF, IL-1, and IL-6 produced by activated macrophages during normal immune responses can also lead to transcriptional activation of HIV mRNA. (see Fig. 5–39). Thus, it seems that HIV thrives when the host macrophages and T cells are physiologically activated (e.g., via intercurrent infection by other microbial agents). The life styles of most HIV-infected patients in the United States place them at increased risk for recurrent exposure to other sexually transmitted diseases; in Africa, socioeconomic conditions probably impose a higher burden of chronic microbial infections. Thus, it is easy to understand how AIDS patients develop a vicious cycle of T-cell destruction: infections to which these patients are prone because of diminished helper T-cell function lead to increased production of proinflammatory cytokines, which, in turn, stimulate more HIV production, followed by infection and loss of additional CD4+ T cells.

B Cells and Other Lymphocytes in HIV Infection. Although much attention has been focused on T cells and macrophages, patients with AIDS also display profound abnormalities of B-cell function. Paradoxically, these patients have hypergammaglobulinemia and circulating immune complexes owing to polyclonal B-cell activation. This may result from multiple factors, including infection with cytomegalovirus or EBV, both of which are polyclonal B-cell activators. The gp41 itself can promote B-cell growth and differentiation, and HIV-infected macrophages produce increased amounts of IL-6, which drives B-cell activation. *Despite the presence of spontaneously activated B cells, patients with AIDS are unable to mount an antibody response to a new antigen.* Not only is this attributable to deficient T-cell help, but antibody responses against T-independent antigens are also suppressed, suggesting additional B-cell defects. Impaired humoral immunity renders these patients susceptible to encapsulated bacteria (e.g., *S. pneumoniae* and *H. influenzae*) that require antibodies for effective opsonization.

Decreased response to soluble antigens

Decreased cytokine secretion

HIV

CD4

CD4

Diminished cytotoxic ability, decreased chemotaxis, reduced IL-1 secretion, poor antigen presentation

Macrophage

Decreased specific cytotoxicity

CD8

B

NK

Decreased killing of tumor cells

Depressed Ig production in response to new antigens

Figure 5-41 ■

The multiple effects of CD4+ T-cell loss after HIV infection.

CD4+ T cells play a pivotal role in regulating the immune response: they produce a plethora of cytokines, chemotactic factors, and hematopoietic growth factors (e.g., GM-CSF). Therefore, loss of this "master cell" has ripple effects on virtually every other cell of the immune system, as illustrated in Figure 5–41 and summarized in Table 5–9.

Pathogenesis of Central Nervous System Involvement. The pathogenesis of the neurologic manifestations in AIDS deserves special mention because, in addition to the lymphoid system, the nervous system is a major target of HIV infection. Macrophages and cells belonging to the monocyte and macrophage lineage (microglia) are the predominant cell types in the brain that are infected with HIV. The virus is most likely carried into the brain by infected monocytes (thus, brain HIV isolates are almost exclusively R5 type). The mechanism of HIV-induced damage of the brain, however, remains obscure. Because neurons are not infected by HIV, and the extent of neuropathologic changes is often less than might be expected from the severity of neurologic symptoms, most workers believe that neurologic deficit is caused indirectly by viral products and soluble factors (e.g., cytokines such as TNF) produced by macrophages/microglia. In addition, nitric oxide induced in neuronal cells by gp41 and direct damage of neurons by soluble HIV gp120 have been postulated.

Natural History of HIV Infection. The course of HIV infection can best be understood in terms of an interplay between HIV and the immune system. Three phases reflecting the dynamics of virus-host interaction can be recognized: (1) an early, *acute phase*; (2) a middle, *chronic phase*; and (3) a final, *crisis phase* (Fig. 5–42).

The *acute phase* represents the initial response of an immunocompetent adult to HIV infection. Clinically, this is

■

Table 5-9. MAJOR ABNORMALITIES OF IMMUNE FUNCTION IN AIDS

Lymphopenia

Predominantly caused by selective loss of the CD4+ helper T-cell subset; inversion of CD4-CD8 ratio

Decreased T-Cell Function In Vivo

Preferential loss of memory T cells
Susceptibility to opportunistic infections
Susceptibility to neoplasms
Decreased delayed-type hypersensitivity

Altered T-Cell Function In Vitro

Decreased proliferative response to mitogens, alloantigens, and soluble antigens
Decreased specific cytotoxicity
Decreased helper function for B-cell immunoglobulin production
Decreased interleukin 2 and inteferon-γ production

Polyclonal B-Cell Activation

Hypergammaglobulinemia and circulating immune complexes
Inability to mount de novo antibody response to a new antigen
Refractoriness to the normal signals for B-cell activation in vitro

Altered Monocyte or Macrophage Functions

Decreased chemotaxis and phagocytosis
Decreased HLA class II antigen expression
Diminished capacity to present antigen to T cells
Increased spontaneous secretion of interleukin 1, tumor necrosis factor, interleukin 6

Figure 5-42 ■

Typical course of HIV infection. During the early period after primary infection there is widespread dissemination of virus and a sharp decrease in the number of CD4+ T cells in peripheral blood. An immune response to HIV ensues, with a decrease in viremia followed by a prolonged period of clinical latency. During this period, viral replication continues. The CD4+ T-cell count gradually decreases during the following years, until it reaches a critical level below which there is a substantial risk of opportunistic diseases. (Redrawn from Fauci AS, Lane HC: Human immunodeficiency virus disease: AIDS and related conditions. In Fauci AS, et al [eds]: Harrison's Principles of Internal Medicine, 14th ed. New York, McGraw-Hill, 1997, p 1791.)

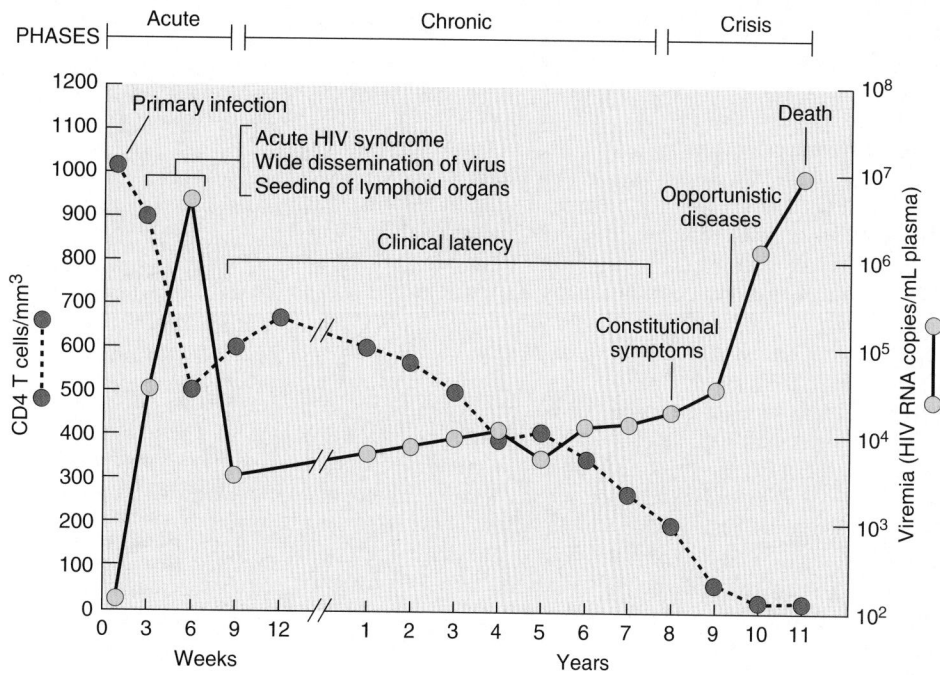

typically a self-limited illness that develops in 50% to 70% of adults 3 to 6 weeks after infection; it is characterized by nonspecific symptoms including sore throat, myalgia, fever, rash, and sometimes aseptic meningitis. This phase is also characterized by high levels of virus production, viremia, and widespread seeding of the peripheral lymphoid tissues, typically with a reduction in CD4+ T cells. Soon, however, a virus-specific immune response develops, evidenced by seroconversion (usually within 3 to 17 weeks of exposure) and by the development of virus-specific CD8+ cytotoxic T cells. As viremia abates, CD4+ T cells return to nearly normal numbers. However, the reduction in plasma virus does not signal the end of viral replication, which continues within tissue macrophages and CD4+ T cells.

The middle, *chronic phase* represents a stage of relative containment of the virus. The immune system is largely intact at this point, but there is *continued HIV replication lasting for several years*. Patients either are asymptomatic or develop persistent lymphadenopathy, and many patients have "minor" opportunistic infections such as thrush (*Candida*) or herpes zoster. During this phase, viral replication in the lymphoid tissues continues unabated. The extensive viral turnover is associated with continued loss of CD4+ cells. However, because of the immense regenerative capacity of the immune system, a large proportion of the CD4+ cells is replenished. Thus, the decline of CD4+ cells in the peripheral blood is modest. After an extended and variable period, host defense begins to wane, the number of CD4+ cells begins to decline, and the proportion of the surviving CD4+ cells infected with HIV increases. Persistent lymphadenopathy with significant constitutional symptoms (fever, rash, fatigue) reflects the onset of immune system decompensation, escalation of viral replication, and the onset of the "crisis" phase.

The final, *crisis phase* is characterized by a catastrophic breakdown of host defenses, a marked increase in viremia, and clinical disease. Typically, patients present with fever

of more than 1 month's duration, fatigue, weight loss, and diarrhea; the CD4+ cell count is reduced below 500 cells/μL. After a variable interval, patients develop serious opportunistic infections, secondary neoplasms, and/or neurologic manifestations (so-called *AIDS-defining conditions*), and the patient is said to have developed full-blown AIDS. Even if the usual AIDS-defining conditions are not manifest, current CDC guidelines define any HIV-infected individual with CD4+ cell counts less than or equal to 200/μL as having AIDS.

In the absence of treatment, most patients with HIV infection develop AIDS after a chronic phase lasting 7 to 10 years. Exceptions to this include *rapid progressors* and long-term *nonprogressors*. In rapid progressors, the middle, chronic phase is telescoped to 2 to 3 years after primary infection. Nonprogressors (fewer than 5% of infected persons) are defined as HIV-infected individuals who remain asymptomatic for 10 years or more, with stable CD4+ counts and low levels of plasma viremia; notably, AIDS eventually develops in the majority of these patients, albeit after a much prolonged clinical latency. Patients with such an uncommon clinical course have attracted great attention in the hope that their study may shed light on host and viral factors that influence disease progression. This group is heterogeneous with respect to the factors that influence the course of the disease; for example, a small subset of nonprogressors is infected with HIV containing deletions or mutations in the *nef* gene. In most cases, the viral isolates do not show any qualitative abnormalities. In all cases, there is evidence of vigorous anti-HIV immune response. These patients have high levels of HIV-specific cytotoxic CD8+ cells, and these levels are maintained over the course of infection. It is not clear whether the robust CD8+ response is the cause or consequence of the slow progression.

Because the loss of immune containment is associated with declining CD4+ cell counts, the CDC classification of HIV infection stratifies patients into three categories on the basis of CD4+ cell counts: CD4+ T cells more than 500 cells/μL, between 200 and 500 cells/μL, and less than 200 cells/μL. Patients in the first group are generally asymptomatic; counts below 500/μL are associated with early symptoms, and a decline of CD4+ levels below 200/μL is associated with severe immunosuppression. For clinical management, CD4+ counts are an important adjunct to HIV viral load measurements. The significance of these two measurements, however, is slightly different: whereas CD4+ cell counts indicate the status of the patient's disease at the time of measurement, the viral load provides information regarding the direction in which the disease is headed.

It should be evident from our discussion that in each of the three phases of HIV infection viral replication continues to occur at a fairly brisk rate. Even in the middle, chronic phase, before the severe decline in the CD4+ cell count, there is extensive viral production. In other words, *HIV infection lacks a phase of true microbiologic latency*, that is, a phase during which *all* the HIV is in the form of proviral DNA and no cell is productively infected. Thus, antiretroviral therapy must commence early in the course of HIV infection, before clinical symptoms appear.

Clinical Features. The clinical manifestations of HIV infection can be readily surmised from the foregoing discussion. They range from a mild acute illness to severe disease. Because the salient clinical features of the acute, early and chronic, middle phases of HIV infection were described earlier, only the clinical manifestations of the terminal phase, commonly known as AIDS, are summarized here.

In the United States, the typical adult patient with AIDS presents with fever, weight loss, diarrhea, generalized lymphadenopathy, multiple opportunistic infections, neurologic disease, and (in many cases) secondary neoplasms. The infections and neoplasms listed in Table 5–10 are included in the surveillance definition of AIDS.

Opportunistic Infections. Opportunistic infections account for approximately 80% of deaths in patients with AIDS. Their spectrum is constantly changing, as a result of improvements in prophylaxis and the increasing life span of HIV-infected individuals. A brief summary of selected opportunistic infections is provided here.

Pneumonia caused by the opportunistic fungus *Pneumocystis carinii* (representing reactivation of a previous latent infection) is the presenting feature in many cases, although its incidence is declining thanks to effective prophylactic regimens. The risk of developing this infection is extremely high in individuals with fewer than 200 CD4+ T cells/μL. Approximately 12% of patients present with an opportunistic infection other than *P. carinii* pneumonia (see Table 5–10). Among the most common are recurrent mucosal candidiasis, disseminated cytomegalovirus infection (particularly enteritis and retinitis), severe ulcerating oral and perianal herpes simplex, and disseminated infection with *M. tuberculosis* and atypical mycobacteria (*Mycobacterium avium-intracellulare*). The AIDS epidemic has caused a resurgence of active tuberculosis in the United States. Although in most cases it represents reactivation, the frequency of new infections is also increasing. Whereas *M. tuberculosis* manifests itself early in the course of AIDS,

Table 5–10. AIDS-DEFINING OPPORTUNISTIC INFECTIONS AND NEOPLASMS FOUND IN PATIENTS WITH HIV INFECTION

Infections

Protozoal and Helminthic Infections

Cryptosporidiosis or isosporidiosis (enteritis)
Pneumocystosis (pneumonia or disseminated infection)
Toxoplasmosis (pneumonia or CNS infection)

Fungal Infections

Candidiasis (esophageal, tracheal, or pulmonary)
Cryptococcosis (CNS infection)
Coccidioidomycosis (disseminated)
Histoplasmosis (disseminated)

Bacterial Infections

Mycobacteriosis ("atypical," e.g., *Mycobacterium avium-intracellulare*, disseminated or extrapulmonary; *M. tuberculosis*, pulmonary or extrapulmonary)
Nocardiosis (pneumonia, meningitis, disseminated)
Salmonella infections, disseminated

Viral Infections

Cytomegalovirus (pulmonary, intestinal, retinitis, or CNS infections)
Herpes simplex virus (localized or disseminated)
Varicella-zoster virus (localized or disseminated)
Progressive multifocal leukoencephalopathy

Neoplasms

Kaposi sarcoma
Non-Hodgkin lymphomas (Burkitt, immunoblastic)
Primary lymphoma of brain
Invasive cancer of uterine cervix

CNS, central nervous system.

infections with atypical mycobacteria are seen late in the course of HIV disease, usually occurring in patients with fewer than 100 CD4+ cells/μL. Toxoplasmosis is the most common secondary infection of the central nervous system. Cryptococcal meningitis is also quite frequent. Persistent diarrhea, so common in patients with AIDS, is often caused by *Cryptosporidium* or *Isospora belli* infections, but bacterial pathogens such as *Salmonella* species and *Shigella* species may also be involved. Because of depressed humoral immunity, AIDS patients are susceptible to infections with *S. pneumoniae* and *H. influenzae*.

Neoplasms. Patients with AIDS have a high incidence of certain tumors, particularly Kaposi sarcoma, non-Hodgkin lymphomas, and cervical cancer in women. The basis of the increased risk of malignancy is multifactorial: profound defects in T-cell immunity, dysregulated B-cell and monocyte functions, and multiple infections with known (e.g., human herpesvirus type 8, EBV, human papillomavirus) and unknown viruses.

Kaposi sarcoma (KS), a vascular tumor that is otherwise rare in the United States (Chapter 10), is the most common neoplasm in AIDS patients. Several features are peculiar to this tumor in the setting of AIDS; it is far more common among homosexual or bisexual males than in intravenous drug abusers or patients belonging to other risk groups. The lesions can arise early, before the immune system is compromised, or in advanced stages of HIV infection.

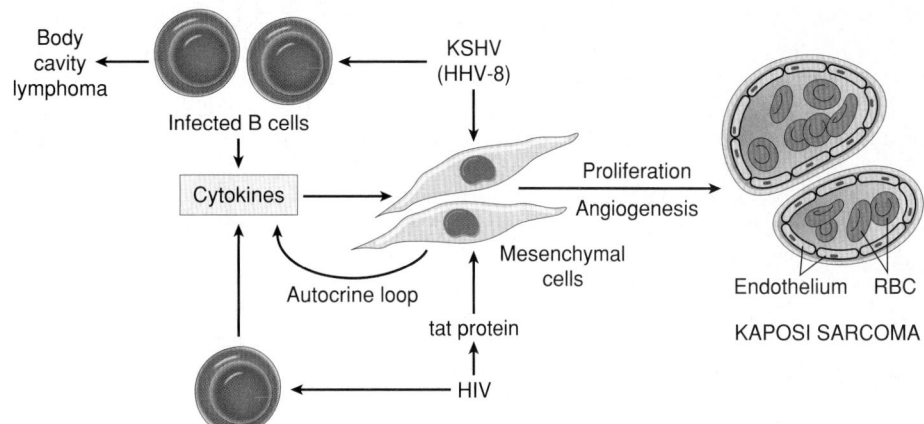

Figure 5–43   ■

Proposed role of HIV, Kaposi sarcoma herpesvirus (KSHV; HHV-8), and cytokines in the pathogenesis of Kaposi sarcoma. Cytokines are produced by the mesenchymal cells infected by KSHV, by B cells infected by KSHV, or by HIV-infected CD4+ cells.

Unlike the lesions in sporadic cases of Kaposi sarcoma, those that occur in AIDS patients are multicentric and tend to be more aggressive; they can affect the skin, mucous membranes, gastrointestinal tract, lymph nodes, and lungs. The lesions contain spindle cells that share features with endothelial cells and smooth muscle cells and are in all likelihood primitive mesenchymal cells that can form vascular channels. Studies indicate that these cells are monoclonal in origin, even in patients with multicentric lesions, indicating that KS is a neoplasm.

Although the cause and pathogenesis of KS are still not clear, a model that favors *a complex web of interaction between human herpesvirus 8 (HHV-8), altered expression and response to cytokines, and modulation of cell growth by HIV gene products is currently favored* (Fig. 5–43).

The high rate of KS in homosexual men relative to patients with parenterally acquired HIV infection points to a sexually transmitted agent, and a novel human herpesvirus (originally named human herpesvirus type 8 [HHV-8]) has been demonstrated in KS lesions. The genomic sequences of this herpesvirus, aptly labeled *KS herpesvirus* (KSHV), are found in virtually all KS lesions, including those that occur in HIV-negative populations. KSHV DNA is also found in a rare type of body cavity–based B-cell lymphoma that occurs in HIV-infected patients. Although the association of this virus with KS is firmly established, its precise role in tumor pathogenesis is much less clear. The KSHV genome encodes homologues of several human genes that can regulate cell proliferation, including IL-6, chemokines and chemokine receptors, cyclin D, and *BCL2* (Chapter 3). There is also evidence that HIV-encoded transactivating protein (tat) plays a role in spindle cell proliferation. Although there is no HIV in KS cells, HIV-infected CD4+ cells produce soluble tat that can stimulate KS cell proliferation, as well as proinflammatory and angiogenic cytokine production. It should be remembered that KS can develop in HIV-negative individuals (Chapter 10), hence HIV or its products are not obligatory for the development of all forms of KS.

Non-Hodgkin lymphomas constitute the second most common type of AIDS-associated tumors. These tumors are highly aggressive, occur most frequently in severely immunosuppressed patients, and involve many extranodal sites. The brain is the most common extranodal site, and hence primary lymphoma of the brain is considered an AIDS-defining condition. In keeping with their aggressive clinical course, most such lymphomas have a diffuse large cell histologic picture (Chapter 12). As with the majority of other diffuse large cell lymphomas, those that occur in the setting of AIDS are primarily of B-cell origin. At least in some cases (30% to 40%), these lymphomas are associated with EBV and progress from polyclonal to monoclonal B-cell lesions. Another, rarer AIDS-related lymphoma is the body-cavity lymphoma associated with KSHV infection as mentioned earlier; it grows exclusively in body cavities in the form of pleural, peritoneal, and pericardial effusions.

Cervical carcinoma is also increased in patients with AIDS. This is attributable to a high prevalence of human papillomavirus infection in patients with AIDS and the AIDS-related immunocompromise. This virus is believed to be intimately associated with squamous cell carcinoma of the cervix and its precursor lesions, cervical dysplasia and carcinoma in situ (Chapter 19). Hence, gynecologic examination should be part of the routine evaluation of HIV-infected women.

Central Nervous System Involvement. Involvement of the central nervous system is a common and important manifestation of AIDS. Ninety percent of patients demonstrate some form of neurologic involvement at autopsy, and 40% to 60% have clinically evident neurologic dysfunction. Significantly, in some patients, neurologic manifestations may be the sole or earliest presenting feature of HIV infection. In addition to opportunistic infections and neoplasms, several virally determined neuropathologic changes occur. These include an aseptic meningitis occurring at the time of seroconversion, vacuolar myelopathy, peripheral neuropathies, and (most commonly) a progressive encephalopathy clinically designated the *AIDS-dementia complex* (Chapter 23).

MORPHOLOGY

The anatomic changes in the tissues (with the exception of lesions in the brain) are neither specific nor diagnostic. In general, the pathologic features of AIDS are those characteristic of widespread op-portunistic infections, Kaposi sarcoma, and lymphoid tumors. Most of these lesions are discussed elsewhere, because they also occur in patients who do not have HIV infection. To appreciate the distinctive nature of lesions in the central nervous system, they are discussed in the context of other disorders affecting the brain (Chapter 23). Here the focus is on changes in the lymphoid organs.

Biopsy specimens from enlarged lymph nodes in the early stages of HIV infection reveal a **marked follicular hyperplasia** (Chapter 12). The medulla shows intense plasmacytosis. These changes, affecting primarily the B-cell areas of the node, are the morphologic counterparts of the polyclonal B-cell activation and hypergammaglobulinemia seen in AIDS patients. In addition to changes in the follicles, the sinuses show increased cellularity, owing primarily to increased numbers of macrophages but also contributed to by B-cell lymphoblasts and plasma cells. HIV particles can be readily demonstrated within the germinal centers, concentrated on the villous processes of the follicular dendritic cells. Viral DNA can also be detected in macrophages and CD4+ T cells.

With disease progression, the frenzy of B-cell proliferation gives way to a pattern of severe follicular involution and generalized lymphocyte depletion. The organized network of follicular dendritic cells is disrupted, and the follicles may even become hyalinized. These "burnt-out" lymph nodes are atrophic and small and may harbor numerous opportunistic pathogens. Because of profound immunosuppression, the inflammatory response to infections both in the lymph nodes and at extranodal sites may be sparse or atypical. For example, with severe immunosuppression, mycobacteria do not evoke granuloma formation because CD4+ T cells are lacking. In the empty-looking lymph nodes and in other organs, the presence of infectious agents may not be readily apparent without the application of special stains. As might be expected, lymphoid depletion is not confined to the nodes; in the later stages of AIDS, the spleen and thymus also appear to be "wastelands."

Non-Hodgkin lymphomas, involving the nodes as well as extranodal sites such as liver, gastrointestinal tract, and bone marrow, are primarily high-grade diffuse B-cell neoplasms (Chapter 12).

Since the emergence of AIDS in 1981, the concerted efforts of epidemiologists, immunologists, and molecular biologists have resulted in spectacular advances in our understanding of this disorder. Despite all this progress, however, the prognosis of patients with AIDS remains dismal. To date, over 22 million people have died from the disease worldwide. Although the mortality rate has begun to decline in the United States as a result of the use of potent combinations of antiretroviral drugs, including protease

inhibitors, all treated patients still carry viral DNA in their lymphoid tissues. Can there be a cure with persistent virus? Although a considerable effort has been mounted to develop a vaccine, many hurdles remain to be crossed before vaccine-based prophylaxis or treatment becomes a reality. Molecular analyses have revealed an alarming degree of polymorphism in viral isolates from different patients, thus rendering vaccine development even more difficult. This task is further complicated by the fact that the nature of the protective immune response is not yet fully understood. Consequently, at present, prevention and effective public health measures remain the mainstays in the fight against AIDS.

AMYLOIDOSIS

Amyloid is the generic term for a variety of proteinaceous materials that are abnormally deposited in tissue interstitium in a spectrum of clinical disorders. Because amyloid deposition appears so insidiously, its clinical recognition ultimately depends on morphologic identification by light microscopy of the material in appropriate biopsy specimens. With usual hematoxylin and eosin tissue stains, *amyloid appears as an amorphous, eosinophilic, hyaline extracellular substance; with progressive accumulation, it encroaches on and produces pressure atrophy of adjacent cells.* At one time it was thought to be starchlike, hence the designation "amyloid"; however, it is now known to be composed primarily of protein.

Despite the striking morphologic uniformity of amyloid in all cases, *amyloid is not a single chemical entity.* Three major and several minor biochemical forms exist, all deposited by several different pathogenic mechanisms. Consequently, amyloidosis should not be considered a single disease; rather, it is a group of diseases that share in common the deposition of similar appearing proteins. At the heart of the morphologic uniformity is the remarkably constant physical organization of amyloid protein, which is considered first. This is followed by a discussion of the chemical nature of amyloid.

Physical Nature of Amyloid. By electron microscopy, amyloid is composed largely of nonbranching fibrils 7.5 to 10 nm in width. X-ray crystallography and infrared spectroscopy demonstrate a characteristic crossed β-pleated sheet conformation (Fig. 5–44); this structural organization is seen regardless of the clinical setting or the chemical composition and is responsible for the distinctive staining and optical properties of amyloid (discussed later). In other words, any fibrillar protein deposited in tissues that yields a β-pleated sheet will be recognized as amyloid. In addition to the fibrils, a nonfibrillar pentagonal glycoprotein (P component) and proteoglycans are minor components of all amyloid deposits. Approximately 95% of any amyloid deposition consists of fibril proteins, with the remaining 5% being the P component and other glycoproteins.

Chemical Nature of Amyloid. *Of the 15 biochemically distinct forms of amyloid proteins that have been identified, three are most common:* (1) *AL (amyloid light chain) is derived from plasma cells and contains immunoglobulin*

Amyloid protein chains

Congo red molecules

Fibril composed of paired filaments

β-pleated sheet

Figure 5-44   ■

Structure of an amyloid fibril, depicting the β-pleated sheet structure and binding sites for the Congo red dye, which is used for diagnosis of amyloidosis. (After Glenner GD: Amyloid deposit and amyloidosis. The β-fibrilloses. N Engl J Med 302:1283, 1980. Reprinted by permission of The New England Journal of Medicine. Copyright 1980, Massachusetts Medical Society.)

light chains, (2) *AA (amyloid-associated) is a unique non-immunoglobulin protein synthesized by the liver*; and (3) *Aβ amyloid is found in the cerebral lesion of Alzheimer disease* (discussed in greater detail in Chapter 23). The two noncerebral amyloid proteins are deposited in distinct clinicopathologic settings:

- The *AL protein* is made up of complete immunoglobulin light chains, the NH_2-terminal fragments of light chains, or both. As might be expected, the amyloid fibril protein of the AL type is produced by immunoglobulin-secreting cells, and its deposition is associated with some form of monoclonal B-cell proliferation.
- The *AA amyloid fibril* is composed of a protein of 8.5-kD molecular mass (76 amino acid residues) that does not have structural homology to immunoglobulins. AA proteins are typically deposited in the setting of chronic inflammatory states; they derive from a larger (12-kD) serum precursor synthesized in the liver called *SAA (serum amyloid-associated) protein.*

Several other biochemically distinct proteins have been found in amyloid deposits in a variety of clinical settings:

- Transthyretin (TTR) is a normal serum protein that binds and *trans*ports *thy*roxine and *retin*ol, hence the name. A mutant form of transthyretin (and its fragments) is deposited in a group of genetic disorders called familial amyloid polyneuropathies. Amyloid transthyretin (ATTR) deposited in the tissues differs from its normal counterpart by a single amino acid. Transthyretin is also deposited in the heart of aged individuals (senile systemic amyloidosis), but in such cases the transthyretin molecule is structurally normal.
- $β_2$-*microglobulin*, a component of the MHC class I molecules and a normal serum protein, has been identified as the amyloid fibril subunit ($Aβ_2m$) in amyloidosis that complicates the course of patients on *long-term*

hemodialysis. $Aβ_2m$ fibers are structurally similar to normal $β_2m$ protein. This protein is present in high concentrations in the serum of patients with renal disease and is retained in circulation because it cannot be filtered through the cuprophane dialysis membranes. In some series, as many as 60% to 80% of the patients on long-term dialysis developed amyloid deposits in the synovium, joints, and tendon sheaths.

- *β-amyloid protein* (Aβ), not to be confused with $β_2$-microglobulin, is a 4-kD peptide that constitutes the core of cerebral plaques found in Alzheimer disease as well as the amyloid deposited in walls of cerebral blood vessels in patients with Alzheimer disease. The Aβ protein is derived from a much larger transmembrane glycoprotein, called *amyloid precursor protein* (APP) (Chapter 23).
- Amyloid deposits derived from diverse precursors such as hormones (procalcitonin) and keratin have also been reported.

Classification of Amyloidosis. Because a given biochemical form of amyloid (e.g., AA) may be associated with amyloid deposition in diverse clinical settings, a combined biochemical-clinical classification is followed for this discussion (Table 5-11). Amyloid may be *systemic* (generalized), involving several organ systems, or it may be *localized*, when deposits are limited to a single organ, such as the heart. On clinical grounds, the systemic, or generalized, pattern is subclassified into *primary amyloidosis* when associated with some immunocyte dyscrasia, or *secondary amyloidosis* when it occurs as a complication of an underlying chronic inflammatory or tissue destructive process. *Hereditary* or familial amyloidosis constitutes a separate, albeit heterogeneous group, with several distinctive patterns of organ involvement.

Immunocyte Dyscrasias With Amyloidosis (Primary Amyloidosis). Amyloid in this category is usually systemic in distribution and is of the AL type. With approximately 3000 new cases each year in the United States, this is the most common form of amyloidosis. The best example in this category is amyloidosis associated with *multiple myeloma*, a malignant neoplasm of plasma cells (Chapter 12). The malignant B cells characteristically synthesize abnormal amounts of a single specific immunoglobulin (monoclonal gammopathy), producing an M (myeloma) protein spike on serum electrophoresis. In addition to the synthesis of whole immunoglobulin molecules, plasma cells may also synthesize and secrete only the λ or κ light chains, also known as *Bence Jones proteins* (by virtue of the small molecular size of the Bence Jones protein, it is also frequently excreted in the urine). These are present in the serum of up to 70% of patients with multiple myeloma, and almost all the patients with myeloma who develop amyloidosis have Bence Jones proteins in the serum or urine, or both. However, only 6% to 15% of myeloma patients who have free light chains develop amyloidosis. Clearly, *the presence of Bence Jones proteins, although necessary, is by itself not enough to produce amyloidosis.* Other factors, such as the type of light chain produced *(amyloidogenic potential)* and the subsequent handling (e.g., degradation), influence the deposition of Bence Jones proteins.

■

Table 5-11. CLASSIFICATION OF AMYLOIDOSIS

Clinicopathologic Category	Associated Diseases	Major Fibril Protein	Chemically Related Precursor Protein
Systemic (Generalized) Amyloidosis			
Immunocyte dyscrasias with amyloidosis (primary amyloidosis)	Multiple myeloma and other monoclonal B-cell proliferations	AL	Immunoglobulin light chains, chiefly λ type
Reactive systemic amyloidosis (secondary amyloidosis	Chronic inflammatory conditions	AA	SAA
Hemodialysis-associated amyloidosis	Chronic renal failure	$A\beta_2m$	β_2-microglobulin
Hereditary amyloidosis			
Familial Mediterranean fever		AA	SAA
Familial amyloidotic neuropathies (several types)		ATTR	Transthyretin
Systemic senile amyloidosis		ATTR	Transthyretin
Localized Amyloidosis			
Senile cerebral	Alzheimer disease	$A\beta$	APP
Endocrine			
Medullary carcinoma of thyroid		A Cal	Calcitonin
Islet of Langerhans	Type 2 diabetes	AIAPP	Islet amyloid peptide
Isolated atrial amyloidosis		AANF	Atrial natriuretic factor

The great majority of patients with AL amyloid do not have classic multiple myeloma or any other overt B-cell neoplasm; such cases are nevertheless classified as primary amyloidosis because their clinical features derive from the effects of amyloid deposition without any other associated disease. In virtually all such cases, patients have a modest increase in the number of plasma cells in the bone marrow and monoclonal immunoglobulins or free light chains can be found in the serum or urine. Clearly, these patients have an underlying B-cell dyscrasia in which production of an abnormal protein, rather than production of tumor masses, is the predominant manifestation.

Reactive Systemic Amyloidosis. The amyloid deposits in this pattern are systemic in distribution and are composed of AA protein. This category was previously referred to as *secondary amyloidosis* because it is secondary to an associated inflammatory condition. The feature common to most cases of reactive systemic amyloidosis is protracted cell injury occurring in a spectrum of infectious and noninfectious chronic inflammatory conditions. Classically, tuberculosis, bronchiectasis, and chronic osteomyelitis were the most common causes; with the advent of effective antimicrobial therapies, reactive systemic amyloidosis is seen most frequently in the setting of chronic inflammation caused by autoimmune states (e.g., rheumatoid arthritis, ankylosing spondylitis, and inflammatory bowel disease). Rheumatoid arthritis is particularly amyloidogenic, with amyloid deposition seen in up to 3% of such patients. Chronic skin infections associated with "skin-popping" of narcotics is also associated with amyloid deposition. Finally, reactive systemic amyloidosis may also occur in association with non–immunocyte-derived tumors, the two most common being renal cell carcinoma and Hodgkin disease.

Heredofamilial Amyloidosis. A variety of familial forms of amyloidosis have been described; most are rare and occur in limited geographic areas. The best characterized is an autosomal recessive condition called *familial*

Mediterranean fever. This is a febrile disorder of unknown cause characterized by attacks of fever accompanied by inflammation of serosal surfaces, including peritoneum, pleura, and synovial membrane. This disorder is encountered largely in individuals of Armenian, Sephardic Jewish, and Arabic origins. It is associated with widespread tissue involvement indistinguishable from reactive systemic amyloidosis. The amyloid fibril proteins are made up of AA proteins, suggesting that this form of amyloidosis is related to the recurrent bouts of inflammation that characterize this disease. The gene for familial Mediterranean fever has been cloned, and its product is called *pyrin;* although its exact function is not known, it has been suggested that pyrin is responsible for regulating acute inflammation, presumably by inhibiting the function of neutrophils. With a mutation in this gene, minor traumas unleash a vigorous, tissue-damaging inflammatory response.

In contrast to familial Mediterranean fever, a group of autosomal dominant familial disorders is characterized by deposition of amyloid predominantly in the peripheral and autonomic nerves. These familial amyloidotic polyneuropathies have been described in kindreds in different parts of the world, for example, in Portugal, Japan, Sweden, and the United States. As mentioned previously, the fibrils in these familial polyneuropathies are made up of mutant transthyretins (ATTR).

Localized Amyloidosis. Sometimes amyloid deposits are limited to a single organ or tissue without involvement of any other site in the body. The deposits may produce grossly detectable nodular masses or be evident only on microscopic examination. Nodular (tumor-forming) deposits of amyloid are most often encountered in the lung, larynx, skin, urinary bladder, tongue, and the region about the eye. Frequently, there are infiltrates of lymphocytes and plasma cells in the periphery of these amyloid masses, raising the question of whether the mononuclear infiltrate is a response to the deposition of amyloid or instead is responsible for it.

At least in some cases, the amyloid consists of AL protein and may therefore represent a localized form of immunocyte-derived amyloid.

Endocrine Amyloid. Microscopic deposits of localized amyloid may be found in certain endocrine tumors, such as medullary carcinoma of the thyroid gland, islet tumors of the pancreas, pheochromocytomas, and undifferentiated carcinomas of the stomach, as well as in the islets of Langerhans in patients with type 2 diabetes mellitus. In these settings, the amyloidogenic proteins seem to be derived either from polypeptide hormones (medullary carcinoma) or from unique proteins (e.g., islet amyloid polypeptide [IAPP]).

Amyloid of Aging. Several well-documented forms of amyloid deposition occur with aging. *Senile systemic amyloidosis* refers to the systemic deposition of amyloid in elderly patients (usually in their 70s and 80s). Because of the dominant involvement and related dysfunction of the heart (typically presenting as a restrictive cardiomyopathy and arrhythmias), this form is also called *senile cardiac amyloidosis.* The amyloid in this form is composed of the normal transthyretin molecule. In addition, another form predominantly affecting only the heart results from the deposition of *a mutant form of transthyretin.* Approximately 4% of the black population in the United States is a carrier of the mutant allele, and cardiomyopathy has been identified in both homozygous and heterozygous patients.

Pathogenesis. Although the precursors of the two major amyloid proteins have been identified, several aspects of their origins are still not clear. In reactive systemic amyloidosis, it appears that long-standing tissue injury and inflammation lead to elevated SAA levels (Fig. 5–45). SAA is synthesized by the liver cells under the influence of cytokines such as IL-6 and IL-1; however, increased production of SAA by itself is not sufficient for the deposition of amyloid. Elevation of serum SAA levels is common to inflammatory states but in most instances does not lead to amyloidosis. It is believed that SAA is normally degraded to soluble end products by the action of monocyte-derived enzymes. Conceivably, individuals who develop amyloidosis have an enzyme defect that results in the incomplete breakdown of SAA, thus generating insoluble AA molecules. In the case of immunocyte dyscrasias, the source of the precursor proteins is well defined, and amyloid material can be derived in vitro by proteolysis of immunoglobulin light chains. However, it is still not known why only a fraction of persons who have circulating Bence Jones proteins develop amyloidosis. Again, defective proteolytic degradation has been invoked, but firm evidence is lacking. The pathogenesis of β-amyloid deposition in Alzheimer disease is discussed in Chapter 23.

MORPHOLOGY

There are no consistent or distinctive patterns of organ or tissue distribution of amyloid deposits in any of the categories cited. Nonetheless, a few generalizations can be made. In amyloidosis secondary to chronic inflammatory disorders, kidneys, liver, spleen, lymph nodes, adrenals, and thyroid, as well as many other tissues, are typically affected. Although immunocyte-associated amyloidosis cannot reliably be distinguished from the secondary form by its organ distribution, it more often involves the heart, gastrointestinal tract, respiratory tract, peripheral nerves, skin, and tongue. However, the same organs affected by reactive systemic amyloidosis (secondary amyloidosis), including kidneys, liver, and spleen, may also contain deposits in the immunocyte-associated form of the disease.

The localization of amyloid deposits in the **heredofamilial syndromes** is varied. In familial Mediterranean fever the amyloidosis may be widespread, involving the kidneys, blood vessels, spleen, respiratory tract, and (rarely) liver. The localization of amyloid in the remaining hereditary syndromes can be inferred

Figure 5–45 ■

Proposed scheme of the pathogenesis of two major forms of amyloid fibrils.

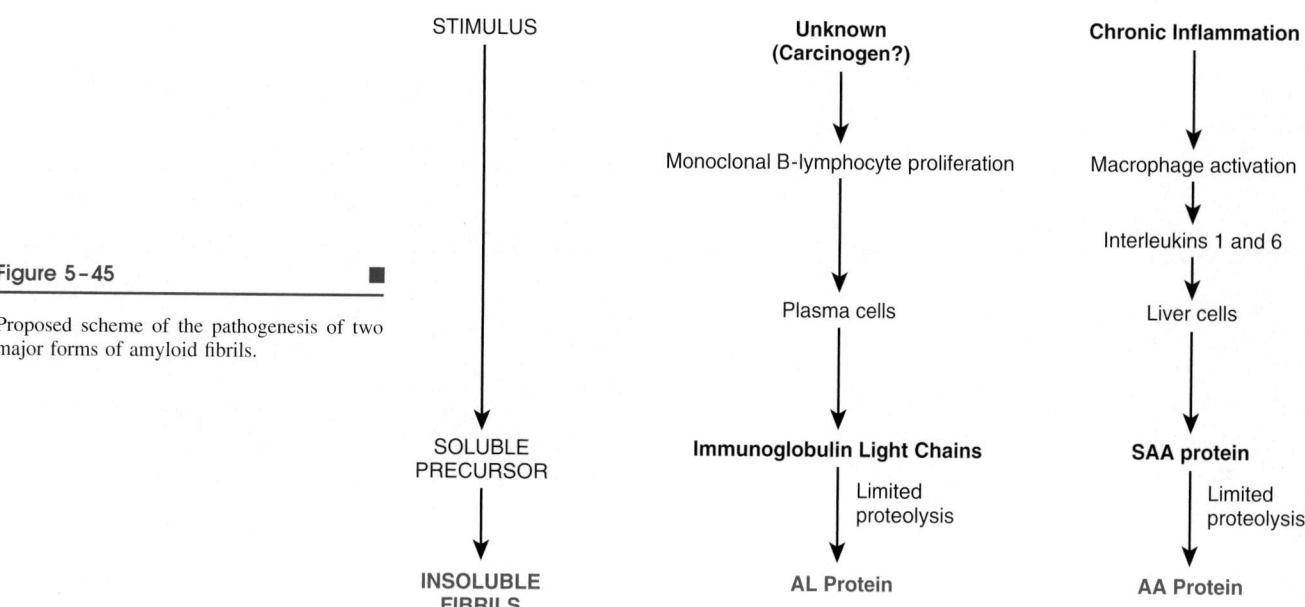

from the designation of these entities. **Localized organ amyloidosis** has already been discussed.

Whatever the clinical disorder, the amyloidosis may or may not be apparent on macroscopic examination. Often, small amounts are not recognized until the surface of the cut organ is painted with iodine and sulfuric acid. This yields mahogany brown staining of the amyloid deposits. When amyloid accumulates in larger amounts, the organ is frequently enlarged and the tissue appears gray with a waxy, firm consistency. **Histologically, the deposition always begins between cells,** often closely adjacent to basement membranes. As the amyloid accumulates, it encroaches on the cells, in time surrounding and destroying them. In the immunocyte-associated form, perivascular and vascular localizations are common.

The histologic diagnosis of amyloid is based almost entirely on its staining characteristics. The most commonly used staining technique utilizes the dye Congo red, which under ordinary light imparts a pink or red color to amyloid deposits. Under polarized light, the Congo red–stained amyloid shows so-called apple green birefringence (Fig. 5–46). This reaction is shared by all forms of amyloid and is caused by the crossed β-pleated configuration of amyloid fibrils. Confirmation can be obtained by electron microscopy, which reveals amorphous nonoriented thin fibrils. AA, AL, and transthyretin amyloid can also be distinguished by specific immunohistochemical staining.

Because the pattern of organ involvement in different clinical forms of amyloidosis is variable, each of the major organ involvements is described separately.

KIDNEY. Amyloidosis of the kidney is the most common and most serious involvement in the disease. Grossly, the kidney may appear unchanged, or it may be abnormally large, pale, gray, and firm; in long-standing cases, the kidney may be reduced in size. Microscopically, the amyloid deposits are found principally in the glomeruli, but they are also present in the interstitial peritubular tissue as well as in the walls of the blood vessels. The glomerulus first develops focal deposits within the mesangial matrix and diffuse or nodular thickenings of the basement membranes of the capillary loops. With progression, the deposition encroaches on the capillary lumina and eventually leads to total obliteration of the vascular tuft (Fig. 5–47A). The interstitial peritubular deposits are frequently associated with the appearance of amorphous pink casts within the tubular lumina, presumably of a proteinaceous nature. Amyloid deposits may develop in the walls of blood vessels of all sizes, often causing marked vascular narrowing.

SPLEEN. Amyloidosis of the spleen often causes moderate or even marked enlargement (200 to 800 g). For obscure reasons, one of two patterns may develop. The deposits may be virtually limited to the splenic follicles, producing tapioca-like granules on gross examination ("sago spleen"), or the involvement may affect principally the splenic sinuses and eventually extend to the splenic pulp, forming large, sheetlike deposits ("lardaceous spleen"). In both patterns, the spleen is firm in consistency and cut surfaces reveal pale, gray, waxy deposits.

LIVER. Amyloidosis of the liver may cause massive enlargement, up to such extraordinary weights as 9000 g. In such advanced cases the liver is extremely pale, grayish, and waxy on both the external surface and the cut section. Histologically, amyloid deposits first appear in the space of Disse and then progressively enlarge to encroach on the adjacent hepatic parenchyma and sinusoids.

Figure 5–46 ■

Amyloidosis. *A,* A section of the liver stained with Congo red reveals pink-red deposits of amyloid in the walls of blood vessels and along sinusoids. *B,* Note the yellow-green birefringence of the deposits when observed by polarizing microscope. (Courtesy of Dr. Trace Worrell and Sandy Hinton, Department of Pathology, University of Texas Southwestern Medical School, Dallas.)

Figure 5-47   ■

Amyloidosis. *A*, Amyloidosis of the kidney. The glomerular architecture is almost totally obliterated by the massive accumulation of amyloid. *B*, Cardiac amyloidosis. The atrophic myocardial fibers are separated by structureless, pink-staining amyloid.

The trapped liver cells undergo compression atrophy and are eventually replaced by sheets of amyloid; remarkably, normal liver function may be preserved even in the setting of severe involvement.

HEART. Amyloidosis of the heart may occur either as isolated organ involvement or as part of a systemic distribution. When accompanied by systemic involvement, it is usually associated with immunocyte dyscrasias. The isolated form **(senile amyloidosis)** is usually confined to older individuals. The deposits may not be evident on gross examination, or they may cause minimal to moderate cardiac enlargement. The most characteristic gross findings are gray-pink, dewdrop-like subendocardial elevations, particularly evident in the atrial chambers. On histologic examination, deposits are typically found throughout the myocardium, beginning between myocardial fibers and eventually causing their pressure atrophy (Fig. 5-47*B*).

OTHER ORGANS. Amyloidosis of other organs is generally encountered in systemic disease. The adrenals, thyroid, and pituitary are common sites of involvement. In this case also the amyloid deposition begins in relation to stromal and endothelial cells and progressively encroaches on the parenchymal cells. Surprisingly, large amounts of amyloid may be present in any of these endocrine glands without apparent disturbance of function. In the gastrointestinal tract, a relatively favored site, amyloid may be found at all levels, sometimes producing tumorous masses that must be distinguished from neoplasms. Nodular depositions in the tongue may produce macroglossia. On the basis of the frequent involvement of the gastrointestinal tract in systemic cases, gingival, intestinal, and rectal biopsies are employed in the diagnosis of suspected cases. Deposition of β_2-microglobulin amyloid in patients receiving long-term dialysis occurs most commonly in the carpal ligaments of the wrist, resulting in compression of the median nerve (carpal tunnel syndrome).

Clinical Correlation. Amyloidosis may be an unsuspected finding at autopsy in a patient who has no apparent related clinical manifestations, or it may be responsible for serious clinical dysfunction and even death. All depends on the particular sites or organs affected and the severity of the involvement. Nonspecific complaints such as weakness, fatigue, and weight loss are the most common initial symptoms. Later in the course, amyloidosis tends to manifest in one of several ways: by renal disease, hepatomegaly, splenomegaly, or cardiac abnormalities. Renal involvement giving rise to severe proteinuria (*nephrotic syndrome*; Chapter 14) is often the major cause of symptoms in reactive systemic amyloidosis. Progression of the renal disease may lead to renal failure, which is an important cause of death in amyloidosis. The hepatosplenomegaly rarely causes significant clinical dysfunction, but it may be the presenting finding. Cardiac amyloidosis may manifest as conduction disturbances or as restrictive cardiomyopathy (Chapter 11). Cardiac arrhythmias are an important cause of death in cardiac amyloidosis. In one large series, 40% of the patients with AL amyloid died of cardiac disease.

The diagnosis of amyloidosis may be suspected from the clinical signs and symptoms and from some of the findings mentioned; however, more specific tests must often be employed for definitive diagnosis. *Biopsy followed by Congo red staining is the most important tool in the diagnosis of amyloidosis.* In general, biopsy is taken from the organ suspected to be involved. For example, renal biopsy is useful in the presence of urinary abnormalities. Rectal and gingival biopsy specimens contain amyloid in up to 75% of cases with generalized amyloidosis. Examination of abdominal fat aspirates stained with Congo red is a simple, low-risk method that is finding widespread use. In suspected cases of AL amyloidosis, serum and urinary protein electrophoresis and immunoelectrophoresis should be performed. Bone marrow aspirate in such cases usually shows plasmacytosis, even if skeletal lesions of multiple myeloma are not present.

The outlook for patients with generalized amyloidosis is poor, with the mean survival time after diagnosis ranging from 1 to 3 years. In AA amyloidosis, the prognosis depends to some extent on the control of the underlying condition. Patients with myeloma-associated amyloidosis have a poorer prognosis, although they may respond to cytotoxic drugs used to treat the underlying disorder. Resorption of amyloid after treatment of the associated condition has been reported, but this is a rare occurrence.

BIBLIOGRAPHY

Abbas AK, et al: Functional diversity of helper T lymphocytes. Nature 383:787, 1996. (An excellent review of T_H1 and T_H2 lymphocytes and the implications of this dichotomy.)

Bellotti V, Merlini G: Current concepts on the pathogenesis of systemic amyloidosis. Nephrol Dial Transplant 11(Suppl 9):53, 1996. (Good review of the general pathogenic mechanisms in various forms of systemic amyloid.)

Callen JP: Collagen vascular diseases. Med Clin North Am 82:1217, 1998. (Extensive review of the autoimmune diseases with cutaneous manifestations, including SLE, dermatomyositis, and scleroderma.)

Dalakas MC: Molecular immunology and genetics of inflammatory muscle diseases. Arch Neurol 55:1509, 1998. (An excellent review of the current thinking on the etiology, pathogenesis, and clinical aspects of inflammatory myopathies.)

Davidson A, Diamond B: Autoimmune diseases. N Engl J Med 345:340, 2001. (A readable and current overview of the etiology, pathogenesis, and therapy for autoimmune diseases.)

Ensoli B, et al: Biology of Kaposi's sarcoma. Eur J Cancer 37:1251, 2001. (A thorough treatment of the biology and pathogenesis of Kaposi sarcoma.)

Friman C, Pettersson T: Amyloidosis. Curr Opin Rheumatol 8:62, 1996. (A more clinically oriented review of the features and therapy for various systemic amyloidoses.)

Gravallese EM, Goldring SR: Cellular mechanisms and the role of cytokines in bone erosions in rheumatoid arthritis. Arthritis Rheum 43:2143, 2000. (A concise and authoritative review of the mechanisms underlying the destructive bone lesions in rheumatoid arthritis.)

Hogan CM, Hammer SM: Host determinants in HIV infection and disease. Ann Intern Med 134:761 Part 1 and 978 Part 2.

Hunter CA, Reiner SL: Cytokines and T cells in host defense. Curr Opin Immunol 12:413, 2000. (Good overview of the role of cytokines and costimulatory signals in regulating T-cell responses.)

Kamradt T, Mitchison NA: Tolerance and autoimmunity. N Engl J Med 344:655, 2001. (Excellent review of the mechanisms of tolerance maintenance and loss in autoimmune disease.)

Kay AB: Allergy and allergic diseases. N Engl J Med 344:30 and 344:109, 2001. (Superb two-part review of the mechanisms and manifestations of type I hypersensitivity.)

Kotzin BL: Systemic lupus erythematosus. Cell 85:303, 1996. (An in-depth discussion of the immunologic derangements in SLE.)

Kumar V, et al: Role of murine NK cells and their receptors in hybrid resistance. Curr Opin Immunol 9:52, 1997. (Good summary of the mechanisms of NK target recognition and cytolysis.)

Lee DM, Weinblatt ME: Rheumatoid arthritis. Lancet 358:903, 2001. (An authoritative article summarizing clinical aspects of rheumatoid arthritis.)

Lewis EJ, et al: Severe lupus nephritis: importance of re-evaluating the histologic classification and the approach to patient care. J Nephrol 14:223, 2001. (A scholarly and detailed discussion of the renal disease in lupus.)

Luster AD: Chemokines—chemotactic cytokines that mediate inflammation. N Engl J Med 338:436, 1998. (Superb review of the biology of chemokines.)

Mascola JR, Nabel GJ: Vaccines for the prevention of HIV-1 disease. Curr Opin Immunol 13:489, 2001. (Review of the current status of vaccine development in HIV prophylaxis.)

McCune J: The dynamics of CD4+ T-cell depletion in HIV disease. Nature 410:974, 2001. (An excellent discussion of factors that cause loss of CD4+ T cells.)

Moder KG, Mason TG: The current use and interpretation of rheumatologic tests. Adolesc Med 9:25, 1998. (Readable contemporary summary of the various serologic assays for rheumatologic disease and their use.)

Morison L: The global epidemiology of HIV/AIDS. Br Med Bull 58:7, 2001. (A current review of the changing patterns of the epidemiology of HIV infection.)

O'Brien SJ, Moore JP: The effect of genetic variation in chemokines and their receptors on HIV transmission and progression to AIDS. Immunol Rev 177:99, 2000. (Up-to-date discussion of the role played by chemokine receptors in HIV transmission and resistance.)

Levine JS, Branch DW, Rauch J: The antiphospholipid syndrome. N Engl J Med 346:752, 2002. (An excellent discussion of this not uncommon syndrome.)

Libby P, Pober JS: Chronic rejection. Immunity 14:387, 2001. (Extremely well-written summary of the mechanisms of allograft arteriopathy.)

Rosen FS, et al: The primary immunodeficiencies. N Engl J Med 333:431, 1995. (An extremely lucid review of the molecular basis of primary immunodeficiency.)

Ruiz-Irastorza G, et al: Systemic lupus erythematosus. Lancet 357:1027, 2001. (Update on clinical issues related to the pathogenesis and therapy for SLE.)

Saloojee H, Violari A: Regular review: HIV infection in children. BMJ 323:670, 2001. (A review covering various aspects of AIDS in children.)

Sapadin AN, et al: Immunopathogenesis of scleroderma—evolving concepts. Mt Sinai J Med 68:233, 2001. (A current summary of the pathology and pathogenesis of scleroderma.)

Sayegh MH, Turka LA: The role of T-cell costimulatory activation pathways in transplant rejection. N Engl J Med 338:1813, 1998. (Excellent discussion of the mechanisms involved in allograft recognition and rejection).

Sepkowitz KA: AIDS—The first 20 years. N Engl J Med 344:1764, 2001. (Excellent historical review of the AIDS epidemic and insights gleaned from the long-term perspective.)

Sparano JA: Clinical aspects and management of AIDS-related lymphoma. Eur J Cancer 37:1296, 2001. (Overview of the pathogenesis and therapy for AIDS-associated lymphomas.)

Suthanthiran M, Strom TB: Renal transplantation. N Engl J Med 331:365, 1994. (A very readable review of the modern view of the immunobiology and clinical aspects of renal transplantation.)

Vanderborght A, et al: The autoimmune pathogenesis of rheumatoid arthritis: role of autoreactive T cells and new immunotherapies. Semin Arthritis Rheum 31:160, 2001. (An up-to-date summary of the role for autoimmunity in the pathogenesis of rheumatoid arthritis.)

Wesselingh SL, Thompson KA: Immunopathogenesis of HIV-associated dementia. Curr Opin Neurol 14:375, 2001. (Brief summary regarding the pathogenesis of CNS disease in AIDS.)

Neoplasia

CLINICAL FEATURES OF NEOPLASIA
Effects of Tumor on Host
Cancer Cachexia
Paraneoplastic Syndromes
Grading and Staging of Cancer

Laboratory Diagnosis of Cancer
Morphologic Methods
Biochemical Assays
Molecular Diagnosis
Molecular Profiling of Tumors

Cancer is the second leading cause of death in the United States; only cardiovascular diseases exact a higher toll. Even more agonizing than the mortality rate is the emotional and physical suffering inflicted by neoplasms. Patients and the public often ask, "When will there be a cure for cancer?" The answer to this simple question is difficult because cancer is not one disease but many disorders that share a profound growth dysregulation. Some cancers, such as Hodgkin lymphomas, are curable, whereas others, such as cancer of the pancreas, have a high mortality. The only hope for controlling cancer lies in learning more about its cause and pathogenesis, and great strides have been made in understanding the cause and molecular basis of cancer. This chapter deals with the basic biology of neoplasia—the nature of benign and malignant neoplasms and the molecular basis of neoplastic transformation. The host response to tumors and the clinical features of neoplasia are also discussed.

DEFINITIONS

Neoplasia literally means "new growth." A neoplasm, as defined by Willis, is "an abnormal mass of tissue the growth of which exceeds and is uncoordinated with that of the normal tissues and persists in the same excessive manner after the cessation of the stimuli which evoked the change." *Fundamental to the origin of all neoplasms is loss of responsiveness to normal growth controls.* Neoplastic cells are said to be transformed because they continue to replicate, apparently oblivious to the regulatory influences that control normal cell growth. In addition, neoplasms seem to behave as parasites and compete with normal cells and tissues for their metabolic needs. Tumors may flourish in patients who are otherwise wasting. Neoplasms also enjoy a certain degree of autonomy and more or less steadily increase in size regardless of their local environment and the nutritional status of the host. Their autonomy is by no means complete, however. Some neoplasms require endocrine support, and such dependencies sometimes can be exploited to the disadvantage of the neoplasm. All neoplasms depend on the host for their nutrition and blood supply.

In common medical usage, a neoplasm is often referred to as a *tumor*, and the study of tumors is called *oncology* (from *oncos*, "tumor," and *logos*, "study of"). In oncology, the division of neoplasms into benign and malignant categories is important. This categorization is based on a judgment of a neoplasm's potential clinical behavior.

A tumor is said to be *benign* when its microscopic and gross characteristics are considered relatively innocent, implying that it will remain localized, it cannot spread to other sites, and it is generally amenable to local surgical removal; the patient generally survives. It should be noted, however, that benign tumors can produce more than localized lumps, and sometimes they are responsible for serious disease, as pointed out later.

Malignant tumors are collectively referred to as *cancers*, derived from the Latin word for *crab*—they adhere to any part that they seize on in an obstinate manner, similar to a crab. *Malignant*, as applied to a neoplasm, implies that the lesion can invade and destroy adjacent structures and spread to distant sites (metastasize) to cause death. Not all cancers pursue so deadly a course. Some are discovered early and are treated successfully, but the designation *malignant* constitutes a red flag.

NOMENCLATURE

All tumors, benign and malignant, have two basic components: (1) the parenchyma, made up of transformed or neoplastic cells, and (2) the supporting, host-derived, non-neoplastic stroma, made up of connective tissue and blood vessels. The parenchyma of the neoplasm determines its biologic behavior, and it is this component from which the tumor derives its name. The stroma carries the blood supply and provides support for the growth of parenchymal cells and is crucial to the growth of the neoplasm.

Benign Tumors. In general, benign tumors are designated by attaching the suffix *-oma* to the cell type from which the tumor arises. A benign tumor arising in fibrous tissue is a *fibroma*; a benign cartilaginous tumor is a *chondroma*. The nomenclature of benign epithelial tumors is more complex. They are classified sometimes on the basis of their microscopic pattern and sometimes on the basis of their macroscopic pattern. Others are classified by their cells of origin. Some examples follow.

The term *adenoma* is applied to benign epithelial neoplasms producing gland patterns and to neoplasms derived from glands but not necessarily exhibiting gland patterns. A benign epithelial neoplasm arising from renal tubule cells and growing in glandlike patterns would be termed an adenoma, as would a mass of benign epithelial cells that produces no glandular patterns but has its origin in the adrenal cortex.

Papillomas are benign epithelial neoplasms, growing on any surface, that produce microscopic or macroscopic finger-like fronds (Fig. 6–1).

Figure 6-1 ■

Papilloma of the colon with finger-like projections into the lumen. (Courtesy of Dr. Trace Worrell, Department of Pathology, University of Texas Southwestern Medical School, Dallas.)

A *polyp* is a mass that projects above a mucosal surface, as in the gut, to form a macroscopically visible structure. Although this term commonly is used for benign tumors, some malignant tumors also may appear as polyps. Sometimes, especially in the colon, the term is applied to non-neoplastic growths that form polypoid masses.

Cystadenomas are hollow cystic masses; typically they are seen in the ovary.

Malignant Tumors. The nomenclature of malignant tumors essentially follows that of benign tumors, with certain additions and exceptions.

Malignant neoplasms arising in mesenchymal tissue or its derivatives are called *sarcomas*. A cancer of fibrous tissue origin is a *fibrosarcoma*, and a malignant neoplasm composed of chondrocytes is a *chondrosarcoma*. Sarcomas are designated by their histogenesis (i.e., the cell type of which they are composed). Malignant neoplasms of epithelial cell origin are called *carcinomas*. It must be remembered that the epithelia of the body are derived from all three germ-cell layers; a malignant neoplasm arising in the renal tubular epithelium (mesoderm) is a carcinoma, as are the cancers arising in the skin (ectoderm) and lining epithelium of the gut (endoderm). It is evident that mesoderm may give rise to carcinomas (epithelial) and sarcomas (mesenchymal). Carcinomas may be qualified further. *Squamous cell carcinoma* would denote a cancer in which the tumor cells resemble stratified squamous epithelium, and *adenocarcinoma* denotes a lesion in which the neoplastic epithelial cells grow in gland patterns. Sometimes the tissue or organ of origin can be identified, as in the designation of renal cell adenocarcinoma or in cholangiocarcinoma, which implies an origin from bile ducts. Sometimes the tumor grows in an undifferentiated pattern and must be called *poorly differentiated carcinoma*.

The parenchymal cells in a neoplasm, whether benign or malignant, resemble each other, as though all had been derived from a single progenitor. Indeed, neoplasms are of monoclonal origin, as is documented later. In some

instances, however, the stem cell may undergo *divergent differentiation*, creating so-called *mixed tumors*. The best example is mixed tumor of salivary gland origin. These tumors have obvious epithelial components dispersed throughout an apparent fibromyxoid stroma, sometimes harboring islands of cartilage or bone (Fig. 6-2). All of these diverse elements are thought to derive from epithelial cells, myoepithelial cells, or both in the salivary glands, and the preferred designation of these neoplasms is *pleomorphic adenoma*. Fibroadenoma of the female breast is another common mixed tumor. This benign tumor contains a mixture of proliferated ductal elements (adenoma) embedded in a loose fibrous tissue (fibroma). Although studies suggest that only the fibrous component is neoplastic, the term *fibroadenoma* remains in common usage.

The multifaceted mixed tumors should not be confused with a *teratoma*, which contains recognizable mature or immature cells or tissues representative of more than one germ-cell layer and sometimes all three. Teratomas originate from totipotential cells such as those normally present in the ovary and testis and sometimes abnormally present in sequestered midline embryonic rests. Such cells have the capacity to differentiate into any of the cell types found in the adult body and so, not surprisingly, may give rise to neoplasms that mimic, in a helter-skelter fashion, bits of bone, epithelium, muscle, fat, nerve, and other tissues. When all the component parts are well differentiated, it is a *benign (mature) teratoma*; when less well differentiated, it is an immature, potentially or overtly *malignant teratoma*.

The specific names of the more common forms of neoplasms are presented in Table 6-1. Some glaring inconsistencies may be noted. For example, the terms *lymphoma*, *mesothelioma*, *melanoma*, and *seminoma* are used for malignant neoplasms. These inappropriate usages are firmly entrenched in medical terminology.

There are other instances of confusing terminology. *Hamartoma* is a malformation that presents as a mass of

Figure 6-2 ■

Mixed tumor of the parotid gland contains epithelial cells forming ducts and myxoid stroma that resembles cartilage. (Courtesy of Dr. Trace Worrell, Department of Pathology, University of Texas Southwestern Medical School, Dallas.)

Table 6-1. NOMENCLATURE OF TUMORS

Tissue of Origin	Benign	Malignant
Composed of One Parenchymal Cell Type		
Tumors of mesenchymal origin		
Connective tissue and derivatives	Fibroma	Fibrosarcoma
	Lipoma	Liposarcoma
	Chondroma	Chondrosarcoma
	Osteoma	Osteogenic sarcoma
Endothelial and related tissues		
Blood vessels	Hemangioma	Angiosarcoma
Lymph vessels	Lymphangioma	Lymphangiosarcoma
Synovium		Synovial sarcoma
Mesothelium		Mesothelioma
Brain coverings	Meningioma	Invasive meningioma
Blood cells and related cells		
Hematopoietic cells		Leukemias
Lymphoid tissue		Lymphomas
Muscle		
Smooth	Leiomyoma	Leiomyosarcoma
Striated	Rhabdomyoma	Rhabdomyosarcoma
Tumors of epithelial origin		
Stratified squamous	Squamous cell papilloma	Squamous cell or epidermoid carcinoma
Basal cells of skin or adnexa		Basal cell carcinoma
Epithelial lining of glands or ducts	Adenoma	Adenocarcinoma
	Papilloma	Papillary carcinomas
	Cystadenoma	Cystadenocarcinoma
Respiratory passages	Bronchial adenoma	Bronchogenic carcinoma
Renal epithelium	Renal tubular adenoma	Renal cell carcinoma
Liver cells	Liver cell adenoma	Hepatocellular carcinoma
Urinary tract epithelium (transitional)	Transitional cell papilloma	Transitional cell carcinoma
Placental epithelium	Hydatidiform mole	Choriocarcinoma
Testicular epithelium (germ cells)		Seminoma
		Embryonal carcinoma
Tumors of melanocytes	Nevus	Malignant melanoma
More than One Neoplastic Cell Type—Mixed Tumors, Usually Derived from One Germ-Cell Layer		
Salivary glands	Pleomorphic adenoma (mixed tumor of salivary origin)	Malignant mixed tumor of salivary gland origin
Renal anlage		Wilms tumor
More than One Neoplastic Cell Type Derived from More than One Germ-Cell Layer—Teratogenous		
Totipotential cells in gonads or in embryonic rests	Mature teratoma, dermoid cyst	Immature teratoma, teratocarcinoma

disorganized tissue indigenous to the particular site. One may see a mass of mature but disorganized hepatic cells, blood vessels, and possibly bile ducts within the liver, or there may be a hamartomatous nodule in the lung containing islands of cartilage, bronchi, and blood vessels. Another misnomer is the term *choristoma*. This congenital anomaly is better described as a *heterotopic rest* of cells. For example, a small nodule of well-developed and normally organized pancreatic substance may be found in the submucosa of the stomach, duodenum, or small intestine. This heterotopic rest may be replete with islets of Langerhans and exocrine glands. The term *choristoma*, connoting a neoplasm, imparts to the heterotopic rest a gravity far beyond its usual trivial significance. Although regrettably the terminology of neoplasms is not simple, it is important because it is the language by which the nature and significance of tumors are categorized.

CHARACTERISTICS OF BENIGN AND MALIGNANT NEOPLASMS

Nothing is more important to the patient with a tumor than being told "It is benign." In most instances such a prediction can be made with remarkable accuracy based on long-established clinical and anatomic criteria, but some neoplasms defy easy characterization. Certain features may indicate innocence, and others may indicate malignancy. In a few instances, there is not perfect concordance between the appearance of a neoplasm and its biologic behavior. In some instances, molecular profiling may be needed (see p 208). These problems are not the rule, however, and there are generally reliable criteria by which benign and malignant tumors can be distinguished. Tumors can be distinguished on the basis of differentiation and anaplasia, rate of growth, local invasion, and metastasis.

Differentiation and Anaplasia

Differentiation and anaplasia refer only to the parenchymal cells that constitute the transformed elements of neoplasms. The stroma carrying the blood supply is crucial to the growth of tumors but does not aid in the separation of benign from malignant ones. The amount of stromal connective tissue does determine, however, the consistency of a neoplasm. Certain cancers induce a dense, abundant fibrous stroma (desmoplasia), making them hard, so-called scirrhous tumors. *The differentiation of parenchymal cells refers to the extent to which they resemble their normal forebears morphologically and functionally.*

Benign neoplasms are composed of well-differentiated cells that closely resemble their normal counterparts. A lipoma is made up of mature fat cells laden with cytoplasmic lipid vacuoles, and a chondroma is made up of mature cartilage cells that synthesize their usual cartilaginous matrix, evidence of morphologic and functional differentiation. In well-differentiated benign tumors, mitoses are extremely scant in number and are of normal configuration.

Malignant neoplasms are characterized by a wide range of parenchymal cell differentiation, from surprisingly well differentiated (Fig. 6–3) to completely undifferentiated. Malignant neoplasms that are composed of undifferentiated cells are said to be *anaplastic*. Lack of differentiation, or anaplasia, is considered a hallmark of malignancy. The term *anaplasia* literally means "to form backward." It implies dedifferentiation, or loss of the structural and functional differentiation of

Figure 6–4   ■

Anaplastic tumor of the skeletal muscle (rhabdomyosarcoma). Note the marked cellular and nuclear pleomorphism, hyperchromatic nuclei, and tumor giant cells. (Courtesy of Dr. Trace Worrell, Department of Pathology, University of Texas Southwestern Medical School, Dallas.)

normal cells. It is now known, however, that cancers arise from stem cells in tissues, so that failure of differentiation, rather than dedifferentiation of specialized cells, accounts for undifferentiated tumors.

Anaplastic cells display marked *pleomorphism* (i.e., marked variation in size and shape) (Fig. 6–4). Characteristically the *nuclei are extremely hyperchromatic* and large. The nuclear-cytoplasmic ratio may approach 1:1 instead of the normal 1:4 or 1:6. *Giant cells* that are considerably larger than their neighbors may be formed and possess either one enormous nucleus or several nuclei. *Anaplastic nuclei are variable and bizarre in size and shape.* The chromatin is coarse and clumped, and nucleoli may be of astounding size. More important, *mitoses are often numerous and distinctly atypical*; anarchic multiple spindles may be seen and sometimes can be resolved as tripolar or quadripolar forms (Fig. 6–5). Also, anaplastic

Figure 6–3   ■

Well-differentiated squamous cell carcinoma of the skin. The tumor cells are strikingly similar to normal squamous epithelial cells, with intercellular bridges and nests of keratin pearls *(arrow).* (Courtesy of Dr. Trace Worrell, Department of Pathology, University of Texas Southwestern Medical School, Dallas.)

Figure 6–5   ■

High-power detail view of anaplastic tumor cells shows cellular and nuclear variation in size and shape. The prominent cell in the center field has an abnormal tripolar spindle.

cells usually fail to develop recognizable patterns of orientation to each other (i.e., they lose normal polarity). They may grow in sheets, with total loss of communal structures, such as gland formations or stratified squamous architecture. Anaplasia is the most extreme disturbance in cell growth encountered in the spectrum of cellular proliferations. As mentioned, malignant tumors differ widely with respect to differentiation. At one extreme are extremely undifferentiated, anaplastic tumors, and at the other extreme are cancers that bear striking resemblance to their tissue of origin. For example, well-differentiated adenocarcinomas of the prostate may contain normal-looking glands. Such tumors sometimes may be difficult to distinguish from benign proliferations. Between the two extremes lie tumors loosely referred to as *moderately well differentiated*.

The better the differentiation of the cell, the more completely it retains the functional capabilities found in its normal counterparts. Benign neoplasms and even well-differentiated cancers of endocrine glands frequently elaborate the hormones characteristic of their origin. Well-differentiated squamous cell carcinomas elaborate keratin (see Fig. 6–3), just as well-differentiated hepatocellular carcinomas elaborate bile. In some instances unanticipated functions emerge, however. Some cancers may elaborate fetal proteins (antigens) not produced by comparable cells in the adult. Cancers of nonendocrine origin may assume hormone synthesis to produce so-called ectopic hormones. For example, bronchogenic carcinomas may produce adrenocorticotropic hormone (ACTH), parathyroid-like hormone, insulin, glucagon, and others. More is said about these phenomena later. Despite exceptions, *the more rapidly growing and the more anaplastic a tumor, the less likely it is to have specialized functional activity.*

Before we leave the subject of differentiation and anaplasia, we should discuss *dysplasia*, a term used to describe disorderly but non-neoplastic proliferation. Dysplasia is encountered principally in the epithelia. It is a *loss in the uniformity of the individual cells and a loss in their architectural orientation.* Dysplastic cells exhibit considerable pleomorphism (variation in size and shape) and often possess deeply stained (hyperchromatic) nuclei that are abnormally large for the size of the cell. Mitotic figures are more abundant than usual. Frequently the mitoses appear in abnormal locations within the epithelium. In dysplastic stratified squamous epithelium, mitoses are not confined to the basal layers, where they normally occur, but may appear at all levels and even in surface cells. There is considerable architectural anarchy. For example, the usual progressive maturation of tall cells in the basal layer to flattened squames on the surface may be lost and replaced by a disordered scrambling of dark basal-appearing cells (Fig. 6–6). When dysplastic changes are marked and involve the entire thickness of the epithelium, the lesion is referred to as *carcinoma in situ*, a preinvasive stage of cancer (Chapter 19). Although dysplastic changes are often found adjacent to foci of cancerous transformation, and although long-term studies of cigarette smokers show that epithelial dysplasia almost invariably antedates the appearance of cancer, *the term dysplasia without qualifications does not indicate cancer, and dysplasias do not necessarily progress to cancer.* Mild-to-moderate changes that do not involve the entire thickness of epithelium may be reversible, and with removal of the putative inciting causes, the epithelium may revert to normal.

In summary, the cells in benign tumors almost always are well differentiated and resemble their normal cells of origin. The cells in cancers are more or less differentiated, but some loss of differentiation is always present.

Rate of Growth

Most benign tumors grow slowly, and most cancers grow much faster, eventually spreading locally and to distant sites (metastasizing) and causing death. There are

Figure 6–6 ■

A, Carcinoma in situ. Low-power view shows the entire thickness of the epithelium is replaced by atypical dysplastic cells. There is no orderly differentiation of squamous cells. The basement membrane is intact, and there is no tumor in the subepithelial stroma. *B,* High-power view of another region shows failure of normal differentiation, marked nuclear and cellular pleomorphism, and numerous mitotic figures extending toward the surface. The basement membrane (below) is not seen in this section.

Figure 6-7 ■

Fibroadenoma of the breast. The tan-colored, encapsulated small tumor is sharply demarcated from the whiter breast tissue.

many exceptions to this generalization, however, and some benign tumors grow more rapidly than some cancers. For example, the rate of growth of leiomyomas (benign smooth muscle tumors) of the uterus is influenced by the circulating levels of estrogens. They may increase rapidly in size during pregnancy and cease growing or atrophy and become largely fibrocalcific after menopause. Other influences, such as adequacy of blood supply and possibly pressure constraints, also may affect the growth rate of benign tumors. Adenomas of the pituitary gland locked into the sella turcica have been observed to shrink suddenly. Presumably, they undergo a wave of necrosis as progressive enlargement compresses their blood supply. Noting these variables, it is nonetheless true that most benign tumors under clinical observation for long periods increase in size slowly over the span of months to years, but there is some variation in rate of growth from one neoplasm to another.

The rate of growth of malignant tumors correlates in general with their level of differentiation. There is wide variation. Some grow slowly for years, then enter a phase of rapid growth, signifying the emergence of an aggressive subclone of transformed cells. Others grow relatively slowly, and there are exceptional instances when growth comes almost to a standstill. Even more exceptionally, cancers (particularly choriocarcinomas) have disappeared spontaneously as they have become totally necrotic, leaving only secondary metastatic implants. With the exception of these rarities, most cancers progressively enlarge over time, some slowly, others rapidly, but the notion that they "emerge out of the blue" is not true. Many lines of experimental and clinical evidence document that most if not all cancers take years and sometimes decades to

evolve into clinically overt lesions. Rapidly growing malignant tumors often contain central areas of ischemic necrosis because the tumor blood supply, derived from the host, fails to keep pace with the oxygen needs of the expanding mass of cells.

Local Invasion

A benign neoplasm remains localized at its site of origin. It does not have the capacity to infiltrate, invade, or metastasize to distant sites, as do cancers. For example, as fibromas and adenomas slowly expand, *most develop an enclosing fibrous capsule* that separates them from the host tissue. This capsule probably is derived from the stroma of the native tissue as the parenchymal cells atrophy under the pressure of the expanding tumor. The stroma of the tumor itself also may contribute to the capsule (Figs. 6-7 and 6-8). It should be emphasized, however, that *not all benign neoplasms are encapsulated.* For example, the leiomyoma of the uterus is discretely demarcated from the surrounding smooth muscle by a zone of compressed and attenuated normal myometrium, but there is no well-developed capsule. Nonetheless, a well-defined cleavage plane exists around these lesions. A few benign tumors are neither encapsulated nor discretely defined; this is particularly true of some vascular benign neoplasms of the dermis. These exceptions are pointed out only to emphasize that although encapsulation is the rule in benign tumors, the lack of a capsule does not imply that a tumor is malignant.

Figure 6-8 ■

Microscopic view of fibroadenoma of the breast seen in Figure 6-7. The fibrous capsule *(below)* sharply delimits the tumor from the surrounding tissue. (Courtesy of Dr. Trace Worrell, Department of Pathology, University of Texas Southwestern Medical School, Dallas.)

Figure 6-9 ■

Cut section of invasive ductal carcinoma of the breast. The lesion is retracted, infiltrating the surrounding breast substance, and would be stony-hard on palpation.

Cancers grow by progressive infiltration, invasion, destruction, and penetration of the surrounding tissue (Figs. 6-9 and 6-10). They do not develop well-defined capsules. There are, however, occasional instances in which a slowly growing malignant tumor deceptively appears to be encased by the stroma of the surrounding native tissue, but usually microscopic examination reveals tiny, crablike feet penetrating the margin and infiltrating adjacent structures. The infiltrative mode of growth makes it necessary to remove a wide margin of surrounding normal tissue when surgical excision of a malignant tumor is attempted. Surgical pathologists carefully examine the margins of resected tumors to ensure that they are devoid of cancer cells *(clean margins). Next to the development of metastases, local invasiveness is the most reliable feature that distinguishes malignant from benign tumors.*

Figure 6-10 ■

Microscopic view of breast carcinoma seen in Figure 6-9 illustrates the invasion of breast stroma and fat by nests and cords of tumor cells (compare with Fig. 6-8). Note the absence of a well-defined capsule. (Courtesy of Dr. Trace Worrell, Department of Pathology, University of Texas Southwestern Medical School, Dallas.)

Figure 6-11 ■

A liver studded with metastatic cancer.

Metastasis

The term *metastasis* connotes the development of secondary implants (metastases) discontinuous with the primary tumor, possibly in remote tissues (Fig. 6-11). *The properties of invasiveness and, even more so, metastasis more unequivocally identify a neoplasm as malignant than any of the other neoplastic attributes.* Not all cancers have equivalent ability to metastasize, however. At one extreme are basal cell carcinomas of the skin and most primary tumors of the central nervous system that are highly invasive in their primary sites of origin but rarely metastasize. At the other extreme are osteogenic (bone) sarcomas, which usually have metastasized to the lungs at the time of initial discovery.

Approximately 30% of newly diagnosed patients with solid tumors (excluding skin cancers other than melanomas) present with clinically evident metastases. An additional 20% have occult metastases at the time of diagnosis.

In general, the more anaplastic and the larger the primary neoplasm, the more likely is metastatic spread; however, exceptions abound. Extremely small cancers have been known to metastasize, and, conversely, some large, ugly lesions may not spread. Dissemination strongly prejudices, if it does not preclude, the possibility of cure of the disease, so it is obvious that, short of prevention of cancer, no achievement would confer greater benefit on patients than methods to prevent metastasis.

Malignant neoplasms disseminate by one of three pathways: (1) seeding within body cavities, (2) lymphatic spread, or (3) hematogenous spread. Although direct transplantation of tumor cells (e.g., on surgical instruments or on the surgeon's gloves) theoretically may occur, in clinical practice it is exceedingly rare and in any event is an artificial mode of dissemination.

Seeding of cancers occurs when neoplasms invade a natural body cavity. Carcinoma of the colon may penetrate the wall of the gut and reimplant at distant sites in the peritoneal cavity. A similar sequence may occur with lung cancers in the pleural cavities. This mode of dissemination is particularly characteristic of cancers of the ovary, which often cover the peritoneal surfaces widely. The implants literally may

Table 6–2.   COMPARISON OF BENIGN AND MALIGNANT TUMORS

Characteristics	Benign	Malignant
Differentiation/anaplasia	Well differentiated; structure may be typical of tissue of origin	Some lack of differentiation with anaplasia; structure is often atypical
Rate of growth	Usually progressive and slow; may come to a standstill or regress; mitotic figures are rare and normal	Erratic and may be slow to rapid; mitotic figures may be numerous and abnormal
Local invasion	Usually cohesive and expansile, well-demarcated masses that do not invade or infiltrate the surrounding normal tissues	Locally invasive, infiltrating the surrounding normal tissues; sometimes may seem cohesive and expansile but with microscopic invasion
Metastasis	Absent	Frequently present; the larger and less differentiated the primary, the more likely are metastases

glaze all peritoneal surfaces and yet not invade the underlying parenchyma of the abdominal organs. Here is an instance of the ability to reimplant elsewhere that seems to be separable from the capacity to invade. Neoplasms of the central nervous system, such as a medulloblastoma or ependymoma, may penetrate the cerebral ventricles and be carried by the cerebrospinal fluid to reimplant on the meningeal surfaces, either within the brain or in the spinal cord.

Lymphatic spread is more typical of carcinomas, whereas the hematogenous route is favored by sarcomas. There are numerous interconnections, however, between the lymphatic and vascular systems, and so all forms of cancer may disseminate through either or both systems. The pattern of lymph node involvement depends principally on the site of the primary neoplasm and the natural lymphatic pathways of drainage of the site. Lung carcinomas arising in the respiratory passages metastasize first to the regional bronchial lymph nodes, then to the tracheobronchial and hilar nodes. Carcinoma of the breast usually arises in the upper outer quadrant and first spreads to the axillary nodes. Medial lesions may drain through the chest wall to the nodes along the internal mammary artery. Thereafter, in both instances, the supraclavicular and infraclavicular nodes may be seeded. In some cases, the cancer cells seem to traverse the lymphatic channels within

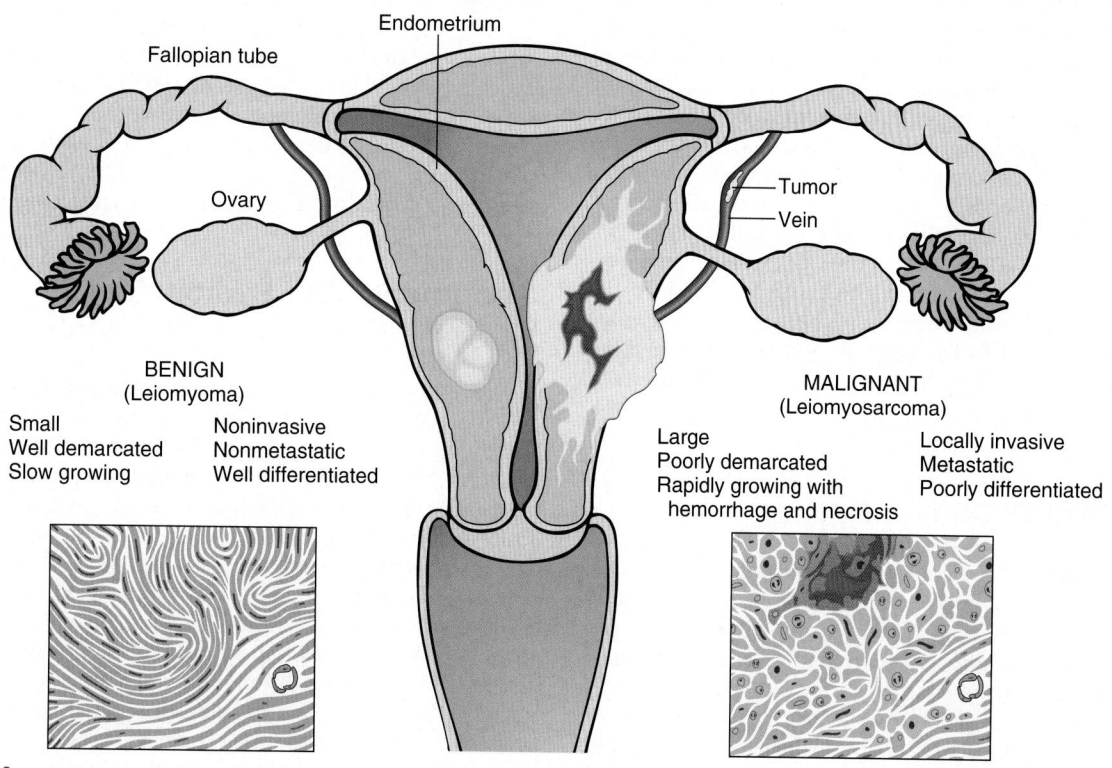

Figure 6–12

Comparison between a benign tumor of the myometrium (leiomyoma) and a malignant tumor of similar origin (leiomyosarcoma).

the immediately proximate nodes to be trapped in subsequent lymph nodes, producing so-called skip metastases. The cells may traverse all of the lymph nodes ultimately to reach the vascular compartment via the thoracic duct.

It should be noted that although enlargement of nodes near a primary neoplasm should arouse strong suspicions of metastatic spread, it does not always imply cancerous involvement. The necrotic products of the neoplasm and tumor antigens often evoke reactive changes in the nodes, such as enlargement and hyperplasia of the follicles (lymphadenitis) and proliferation of macrophages in the subcapsular sinuses (sinus histiocytosis).

Hematogenous spread is the most feared consequence of a cancer. It is the favored pathway for sarcomas, but carcinomas use it as well. As might be expected, arteries are penetrated less readily than are veins. With venous invasion, the bloodborne cells follow the venous flow draining the site of the neoplasm. *The liver and lungs are the most frequently involved secondary sites in such hematogenous dissemination.* All portal area drainage flows to the liver, and all caval blood flows to the lungs. Cancers arising near the vertebral column often embolize through the paravertebral plexus; this pathway probably is involved in the frequent vertebral metastases of carcinomas of the thyroid and prostate.

Certain carcinomas have a propensity for invasion of veins. Renal cell carcinoma often invades the renal vein to grow in a snakelike fashion up the inferior vena cava, sometimes reaching the right side of the heart. Hepatocellular carcinomas often penetrate portal and hepatic radicles to grow within them into the main venous channels. Remarkably, such intravenous growth may not be accompanied by widespread dissemination.

Many observations suggest that mere anatomic localization of the neoplasm and natural pathways of venous drainage do not wholly explain the systemic distributions of metastases. For example, prostatic carcinoma preferentially spreads to bone, bronchogenic carcinomas tend to involve the adrenals and the brain, and neuroblastomas spread to the liver and bones. Conversely, skeletal muscles are rarely the site of secondary deposits. The probable basis of such tissue-specific homing of tumor cells is discussed later.

In conclusion, the various features discussed in the preceding sections, as summarized in Table 6–2 and Figure 6–12, permit the differentiation of benign and malignant neoplasms. Against this background of the structure and behavior of neoplasms, we can turn to some considerations of their nature and origins.

EPIDEMIOLOGY

Because cancer is a disorder of cell growth and behavior, its ultimate cause has to be defined at the cellular and molecular levels. Cancer epidemiology can contribute substantially to knowledge about the origin of cancer. The now well-established concept that cigarette smoking is causally associated with lung cancer arose primarily from epidemiologic studies. A comparison of the incidence of colon cancer and dietary patterns in the Western world and Africa led to the recognition that dietary fat and fiber content may be important factors in the causation of this cancer. Major insights into the causes of cancer can be obtained by epidemiologic studies that relate particular environmental, racial (possibly hereditary), and cultural influences to the occurrence of specific neoplasms. Certain diseases associated with an increased risk of developing cancer (preneoplastic disorders) also provide clues to the pathogenesis of cancer. In the following discussion, we first summarize the overall incidence of cancer to gain an insight into the magnitude of the cancer problem, then we review some factors relating to the patient and environment that influence the predisposition to cancer.

Cancer Incidence

Some perspective on the likelihood of developing a specific form of cancer can be gained from national incidence and mortality data. Overall, it is estimated that about *1.3 million* new cancer cases will occur in 2002, and 555,500 people will die of cancer in the United States. The incidence of the most common forms of cancer and the major killers is presented in Figure 6–13.

The death rates of many forms of malignant neoplasia have changed (Fig. 6–14). Particularly notable is the significant increase in the overall cancer death rate among men that was attributable largely to lung cancer, but this has finally begun to drop. In contrast, the overall death rate among women has fallen slightly, owing mostly to the decline in death rates from cancers of the uterus, stomach, and large bowel. These welcome trends have more than counterbalanced the striking climb in the rate of lung cancer among women, which not long ago was a relatively uncommon form of neoplasia in this sex. The declining death rate from uterine cancer can reasonably be attributed to the control of cervical carcinoma, made possible by the widespread use of cytologic smear studies for early detection of carcinoma while it is still curable. The causes of decline in death rates for cancers of the large bowel and stomach are obscure; however, there have been speculations about decreasing exposure to dietary carcinogens.

Geographic and Environmental Factors

Notwithstanding the impressive advances in understanding the molecular pathogenesis of cancer by analysis of hereditary cancers, it is fair to state that environmental factors are the predominant determinant of the most common sporadic cancers. In one large study, the proportion of risk from environmental causes was found to be 65%, whereas heritable factors contributed 26% to 42% of cancer risk. These estimates are supported by the geographic differences in deaths from specific forms of cancer. For example, death rates from breast cancer are about fourfold to fivefold higher in the United States and Europe compared with Japan. Conversely, the death rate for stomach carcinoma in men and women is about seven times higher in Japan than in the United States. Liver cell carcinoma is relatively infrequent in the United States but is the most lethal cancer among

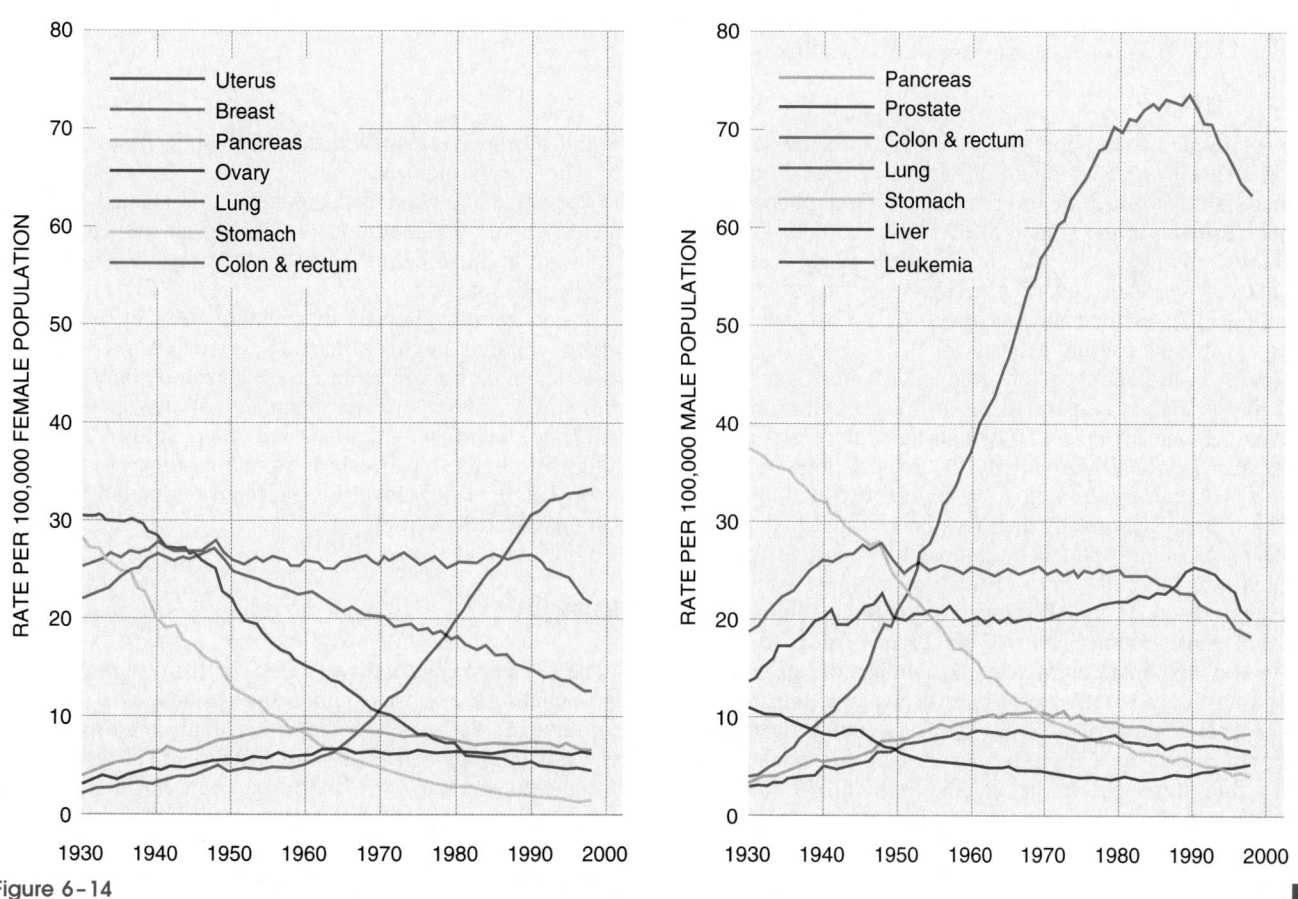

Figure 6-13

Cancer incidence and mortality by site and sex. (Adapted from Jemal A, et al: Cancer statistics, 2002. CA Cancer J Clin 52:23, 2002.)

Figure 6-14

Age-adjusted cancer death rates for selected sites in the United States. (Adapted from Jemal A, et al: Cancer statistics, 2002. CA Cancer J Clin 52:23, 2002.)

■

Table 6-3. OCCUPATIONAL CANCERS

Agents or Groups of Agents	Human Cancer Site for Which Reasonable Evidence Is Available	Typical Use or Occurrence
Arsenic and arsenic compounds	Lung, skin, hemangiosarcoma	Byproduct of metal smelting. Component of alloys, electrical and semiconductor devices, medications and herbicides, fungicides, and animal dips.
Asbestos	Lung, mesothelioma; gastrointestinal tract (esophagus, stomach, large intestine)	Formerly used for many applications because of fire, heat, and friction resistance; still found in existing construction and fire-resistant textiles, friction materials (i.e., brake linings), underlayment and roofing papers, and floor tiles.
Benzene	Leukemia, Hodgkin lymphoma	Principal component of light oil. Although use as solvent is discouraged, many applications exist in printing and lithography, paint rubber, dry cleaning, adhesives and coatings, and detergents. Formerly widely used as solvent and fumigant.
Beryllium and beryllium compounds	Lung	Missile fuel and space vehicles. Hardener for lightweight metal alloys, particularly in aerospace applications and nuclear reactors.
Cadmium and cadmium compounds	Prostate	Uses include yellow pigments and phosphors. Found in solders. Used in batteries and as alloy and in metal platings and coatings.
Chromium compounds	Lung	Component of metal alloys, paints, pigments, and preservatives.
Ethylene oxide	Leukemia	Ripening agent for fruits and nuts. Used in rocket propellant and chemical synthesis, in fumigants for foodstuffs and textiles, and in sterilants for hospital equipment.
Nickel compounds	Nose, lung	Nickel plating. Component of ferrous alloys, ceramics, and batteries. Byproduct of stainless steel arc welding.
Radon and its decay products	Lung	From decay of minerals containing uranium. Can be serious hazard in quarries and underground mines.
Vinyl chloride	Liver, angiosarcoma	Refrigerant. Monomer for vinyl polymers. Adhesive for plastics. Formerly inert aerosol propellant in pressurized containers.

Modified from Stellman JM, Stellman SD: Cancer and workplace. CA Cancer J Clin 46:70, 1996.

many African native populations. Nearly all the evidence indicates that these geographic differences are environmental rather than genetic in origin. Nisei (second-generation Japanese living in the United States) have mortality rates for certain forms of cancer that are intermediate between those of natives of Japan and of Americans who haved lived in the United States for many genarations. The two rates come closer with each passing generation.

There is no paucity of environmental carcinogens. They lurk in the ambient environment, in the workplace, in food, and in personal practices. They can be as universal as sunlight, can be found particularly in urban settings (e.g., asbestos), or can be limited to a certain occupation (Table 6–3). Certain features of diet have been implicated as possible predisposing influences. Among the possible environmental influences, the most distressing are those incurred in personal practices, notably cigarette smoking and chronic alcohol consumption. The risk of cervical cancer is linked to age at first intercourse and the number of sex partners (pointing to a possible causal role for venereal transmission of an oncogenic virus). There is no escape: It seems that everything one does to earn a livelihood, to subsist, or to enjoy life turns out to be illegal, immoral, or fattening, or—most disturbing—possibly carcinogenic.

Age

In general, the frequency of cancer increases with age. Most cancer mortality occurs between ages 55 and 75 years;

the rate declines, along with the population base, after age 75. The rising incidence with age may be explained by the accumulation of somatic mutations associated with the emergence of malignant neoplasms (discussed later). The decline in immune competence that accompanies aging also may be a factor.

Cancer causes slightly more than 10% of all deaths among children younger than 15 years (Chapter 7). The major lethal cancers in children are leukemia, tumors of the central nervous system, lymphomas, soft tissue sarcomas, and bone sarcomas. As discussed later, study of several childhood tumors, particularly retinoblastoma and Wilms tumor, has provided novel insights into the pathogenesis of malignant transformation.

Heredity

The evidence now indicates that for many types of cancer, including the most common forms, there exist not only environmental influences but also hereditary predispositions. For example, lung cancer in most instances is clearly related to cigarette smoking, yet mortality from lung cancer has been shown to be four times greater among nonsmoking relatives (parents and siblings) of lung cancer patients than among nonsmoking relatives of controls. Hereditary forms of cancer can be divided into three categories (Table 6–4).

Inherited Cancer Syndromes. Inherited cancer syndromes include several well-defined cancers in which inheritance of a single mutant gene greatly increases the risk of

■

Table 6-4.   INHERITED PREDISPOSITION TO CANCER

Inherited Cancer Syndromes (Autosomal Dominant)

Inherited predisposition indicated by strong family history of uncommon
    cancer and/or associated marker phenotype
    Familial retinoblastoma
    Familial adenomatous polyposis (FAP) of the colon
    Multiple endocrine neoplasia (MEN) syndromes
    Neurofibromatosis types 1 and 2
    von Hippel–Lindau (VHL) syndrome

Familial Cancers

Evident familial clustering of cancer but role of inherited predisposition
    may not be clear in an individual case
    Breast cancer
    Ovarian cancer
    Colon cancers other than familial adenomatous polyposis

Autosomal Recessive Syndromes of Defective DNA Repair

Xeroderma pigmentosum
Ataxia telangiectasia
Bloom syndrome
Fanconi anemia

---

a person's developing a tumor. The predisposition to these tumors shows an autosomal dominant pattern of inheritance. Childhood retinoblastoma is the most striking example of this category. Approximately 40% of retinoblastomas are familial. Carriers of this gene have a 10,000-fold increased risk of developing retinoblastoma, usually bilaterally. They also have a greatly increased risk of developing a second cancer, particularly osteogenic sarcoma. As is discussed later, a *cancer suppressor gene* has been implicated in the pathogenesis of this tumor. Familial adenomatous polyposis is another hereditary disorder marked by an extraordinarily high risk of cancer. Individuals who inherit the autosomal dominant mutation have, at birth or soon thereafter, innumerable polypoid adenomas of the colon, and virtually 100% of patients develop a carcinoma of the colon by age 50 (see Table 6–4).

Tumors within this group often are associated with a specific marker phenotype. There may be multiple benign tumors in the affected tissue, as occurs in familial polyposis of the colon and in multiple endocrine neoplasia. Sometimes, there are abnormalities in tissue that are not the target of transformation (e.g., Lisch nodules and café-au-lait spots in neurofibromatosis type 1; Chapter 7).

Familial Cancers. Virtually all the common types of cancers that occur sporadically have been reported to occur in familial forms. Examples include carcinomas of colon, breast, ovary, and brain. *Features that characterize familial cancers include early age at onset, tumors arising in two or more close relatives of the index case, and sometimes multiple or bilateral tumors.* Familial cancers are not associated with specific marker phenotypes. For example, in contrast to the familial adenomatous polyposis syndrome, familial colonic cancers do not arise in preexisting benign polyps. The transmission pattern of familial cancers is not clear. In general, sibs have a relative risk between 2 and 3. Segregation analysis of large families usually reveals that predisposition to the tumors is dominant, but multifactorial inheritance cannot be easily ruled out. As discussed later,

certain familial cancers can be linked to the inheritance of mutant genes. Examples include linkage of *BRCA1* and *BRCA2* genes to familial breast and ovarian cancers.

Autosomal Recessive Syndromes of Defective DNA Repair. Besides the dominantly inherited precancerous conditions, a small group of autosomal recessive disorders is collectively characterized by chromosomal or DNA instability. One of the best-studied examples is xeroderma pigmentosum, in which DNA repair is defective. This and other familial disorders of DNA instability are described later.

In summary, no more than 5% to 10% of all human cancers fall into one of the three aforementioned categories. What can be said about the influence of heredity in the large preponderance of malignant tumors? There is emerging evidence that the influence of hereditary factors is subtle and indirect. The genotype may influence the likelihood of one's developing environmentally induced cancers. As discussed later in the section on chemical carcinogenesis, for example, polymorphisms in drug-metabolizing enzymes confer genetic predisposition to lung cancers in cigarette smokers. A striking genetic predisposition to developing mesotheliomas (an asbestos-associated tumor) also has been noted, but the relevant gene is not yet known.

Acquired Preneoplastic Disorders

In addition to the genetic influences described earlier, certain clinical conditions are well-recognized predispositions to the development of malignant neoplasia and are referred to as *preneoplastic disorders*. This designation is unfortunate because it implies a certain inevitability, but in fact, although such conditions may increase the likelihood, in most instances cancer does not develop. A brief listing of the chief conditions follows:

■ Persistent regenerative cell replication (e.g., squamous cell carcinoma in the margins of a chronic skin fistula or in a long-unhealed skin wound; hepatocellular carcinoma in cirrhosis of the liver)
■ Hyperplastic and dysplastic proliferations (e.g., endometrial carcinoma in atypical endometrial hyperplasia; bronchogenic carcinoma in the dysplastic bronchial mucosa of habitual cigarette smokers)
■ Chronic atrophic gastritis (e.g., gastric carcinoma in pernicious anemia)
■ Chronic ulcerative colitis (e.g., an increased incidence of colorectal carcinoma in long-standing disease)
■ Leukoplakia of the oral cavity, vulva, or penis (e.g., increased risk of squamous cell carcinoma)
■ Villous adenomas of the colon (e.g., high risk of transformation to colorectal carcinoma)

In this context, it may be asked, "What is the risk of malignant change in a benign neoplasm?" or, stated differently, "Are benign tumors precancerous?" In general, the answer is no, but inevitably there are exceptions, and perhaps it is better to say that each type of benign tumor is associated with a particular level of risk, ranging from high to virtually nonexistent. For example, adenomas of the colon as they enlarge can undergo malignant transformation in 50% of cases; in contrast, malignant change is extremely rare in leiomyomas of the uterus.

CARCINOGENESIS: THE MOLECULAR BASIS OF CANCER

It could be argued that the proliferation of literature on the molecular basis of cancer has outpaced the growth of even the most malignant of tumors. It is easy to get lost in the growing forest of information. First, we list some fundamental principles before delving into the details of the genetic basis of cancer.

■ *Nonlethal genetic damage lies at the heart of carcinogenesis.* Such genetic damage (or mutation) may be acquired by the action of environmental agents, such as chemicals, radiation, or viruses, or it may be inherited in the germ line. The genetic hypothesis of cancer implies that a tumor mass results from the clonal expansion of a single progenitor cell that has incurred the genetic damage (i.e., tumors are monoclonal). This expectation has been realized in most tumors that have been analyzed. Clonality of tumors is assessed readily in women who are heterozygous for polymorphic X-linked markers, such as the enzyme glucose-6-phosphate dehydrogenase or X-linked restriction fragment length polymorphisms. The principle underlying such an analysis is illustrated in Figure 6–15.

■ *Three classes of normal regulatory genes—growth-promoting protooncogenes; growth-inhibiting cancer suppressor genes (antioncogenes); and genes that regulate programmed cell death, or apoptosis—are the principal targets of genetic damage.* Mutant alleles of protooncogenes are called *oncogenes.* They are considered dominant because they transform cells despite the presence of their normal counterpart. In contrast, both normal alleles of tumor suppressor genes must be damaged for transformation to occur, so this family of genes sometimes is referred to as *recessive oncogenes.* Genes that regulate apoptosis may be dominant, as are protooncogenes, or they may behave as cancer suppressor genes.

■ In addition to the three classes of genes mentioned earlier, a fourth category of genes, those that regulate repair of damaged DNA, is pertinent in carcinogenesis. DNA repair genes affect cell proliferation or survival indirectly by influencing the ability of the organism to repair nonlethal damage in other genes, including protooncogenes, tumor suppressor genes, and genes that regulate apoptosis. A disability in the DNA repair genes can predispose to widespread mutations in the genome and to neoplastic transformation.

■ *Carcinogenesis is a multistep process at both the phenotypic and the genetic levels.* A malignant neoplasm has several phenotypic attributes, such as excessive growth, local invasiveness, and the ability to form distant metastases. These characteristics are acquired in a stepwise fashion, a phenomenon called *tumor progression.* At the molecular level, progression results from the accumulation of genetic lesions that in some instances are favored by defects in

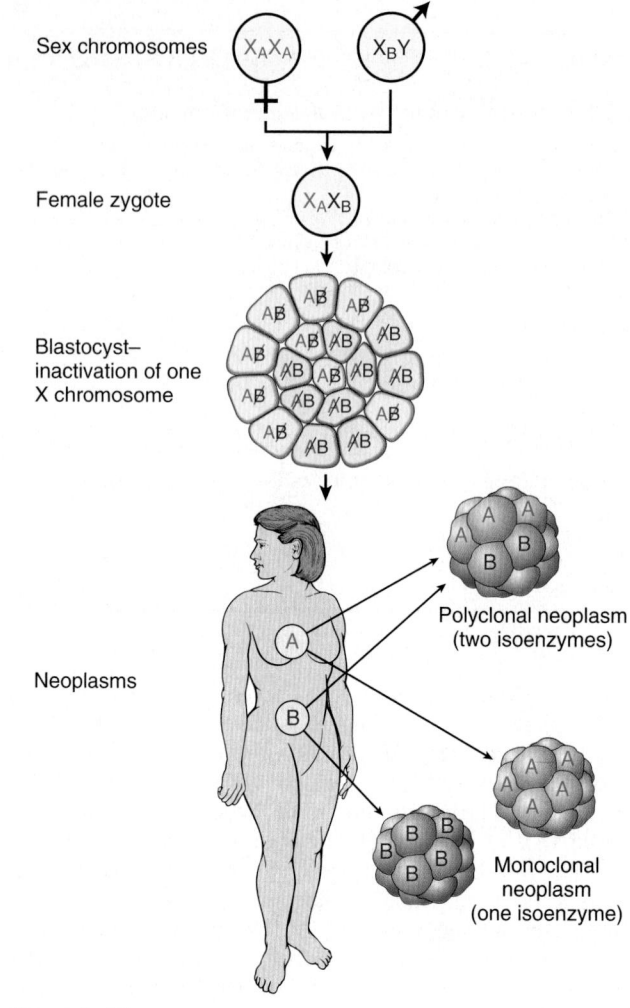

Figure 6–15

Diagram depicting the use of X-linked isoenzyme cell markers as evidence of the monoclonality of neoplasms. Because of random X inactivation, all females are mosaics with two cell populations (with glucose-6-phosphate dehydrogenase isoenzyme A or B in this case). When neoplasms that arise in women who are heterozygous for X-linked markers are analyzed, they are made up of cells that contain the active maternal (X_A) or the paternal (X_B) X chromosome, but not both.

DNA repair. The genetic changes that fuel tumor progression involve not only growth-regulatory genes but also genes that regulate angiogenesis, invasion, and metastases. Cancer cells also must bypass the normal process of aging that limits cell division.

With this overview (Fig. 6–16), we can now address in detail the molecular pathogenesis of cancer and discuss the carcinogenic agents that inflict genetic damage. In the 1980s and 1990s, hundreds of cancer-associated genes were discovered. Some, such as *TP53* (formerly *p53*), are commonly mutated; others, such as *c-ABL*, are affected only in certain leukemias. Each of the cancer genes has a specific function, the dysregulation of which contributes to the origin or progression of malignancy. It is traditional to describe cancer-causing genes on the basis of their presumed function. It is beneficial, however, to consider cancer-related genes in the context of six fundamental changes in cell physiology that together dictate malignant phenotype (Fig. 6–17):

Figure 6–16 ■

Flow chart depicting a simplified scheme of the molecular basis of cancer.

1. Self-sufficiency in growth signals
2. Insensitivity to growth-inhibitory signals
3. Evasion of apoptosis
4. Limitless replicative potential (i.e., overcoming cellular senescence)
5. Sustained angiogenesis
6. Ability to invade and metastasize

Mutations in genes that regulate these cellular traits are seen in every cancer. However, the precise genetic pathways that give rise to these attributes differ between cancers, even within the same organ. It is widely believed that the occurrence of mutations in cancer-causing genes is conditioned by the robustness of the DNA repair machinery of the cell. When genes that normally sense and repair DNA damage are impaired or lost, the resultant genomic instability favors mutations in genes that regulate the six acquired capabilities of cancer cells. This group of *enabler* genes is considered last because it affects the genes in all other pathways. In the ensuing discussion it should be noted that gene symbols are italicized but their protein products are not (e.g., *RB* gene and RB protein).

Self-Sufficiency in Growth Signals

Genes that promote autonomous cell growth in cancer cells are called *oncogenes*. They are derived by mutations in pro-tooncogenes and are characterized by the ability to promote cell growth in the absence of normal growth-promoting signals. Their products, called *oncoproteins*, resemble the normal products of protooncogenes except that oncoproteins are devoid of important regulatory elements, and their production in the transformed cells does not depend on growth factors or other external signals. To aid in the understanding of the nature and functions of oncoproteins, it is necessary to review briefly the sequence of events that characterize normal cell proliferation; these are discussed in Chapter 3. Under physiologic conditions, cell proliferation can be readily resolved into the following steps:

■ The binding of a growth factor to its specific receptor on the cell membrane
■ Transient and limited activation of the growth factor receptor, which in turn activates several signal-transducing proteins on the inner leaflet of the plasma membrane
■ Transmission of the transduced signal across the cytosol to the nucleus via second messengers
■ Induction and activation of nuclear regulatory factors that initiate DNA transcription
■ Entry and progression of the cell into the cell cycle, resulting ultimately in cell division

With this background, we can identify the strategies used by cancer cells to acquire self-sufficiency in growth signals. They can be grouped on the basis of their role in the signal transduction cascade and cell cycle regulation.

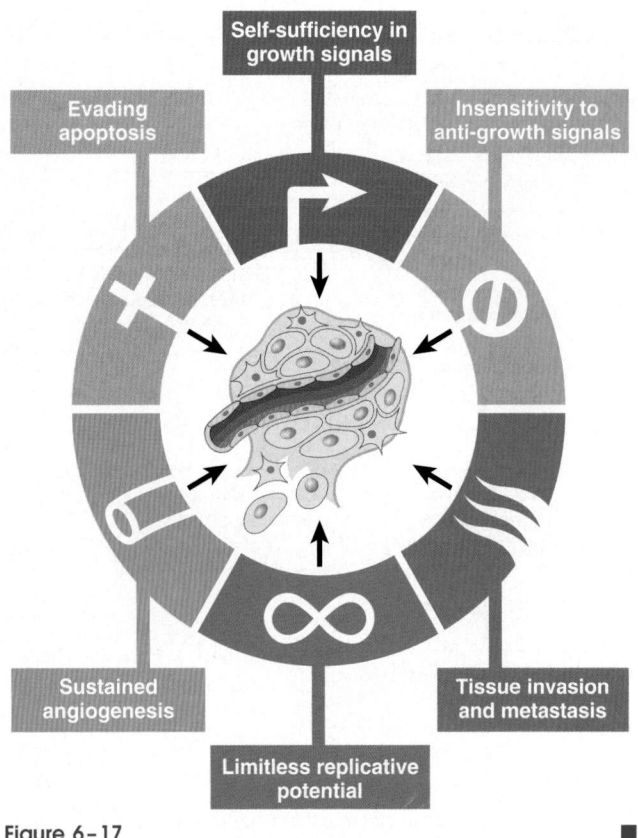

Figure 6-17 ■

Six hallmarks of cancer. Most cancer cells acquire these properties during their development, typically by mutations in the relevant genes. (From Hanahan D, Weinberg RA: The hallmarks of cancer. Cell 100:57, 2000.)

GROWTH FACTORS

All normal cells require stimulation by growth factors to undergo proliferation. Most soluble growth factors are made by one cell type and act on a neighboring cell to stimulate proliferation (paracrine action). Many cancer cells acquire growth self-sufficiency, however, by acquiring the ability to synthesize the same growth factors to which they are responsive. Such is the case with platelet-derived growth factor (PDGF) and transforming growth factor α (TGF-α). Many glioblastomas secrete PDGF, and sarcomas make TGF-α. Similar autocrine loops are fairly common in many types of cancer. In many instances, the growth factor gene itself is not altered or mutated, but the products of other oncogenes (e.g., *RAS*) cause overexpression of growth factor genes. Consequently the cell may be forced to secrete large amounts of growth factors such as TGF-α. In addition to PDGF, genes that encode homologues of fibroblast growth factors (e.g., *hst-1* and *FGF3*) have been detected in several gastrointestinal and breast tumors.

GROWTH FACTOR RECEPTORS

The next group in the sequence of signal transduction involves growth factor receptors, and several oncogenes that encode growth factor receptors have been found. Mutations and pathologic overexpression of normal forms of growth factor receptors have been detected in several tumors. Mutant receptor proteins deliver continuous mitogenic signals to cells, even in the absence of the growth factor in the environment. More common than mutations is overexpression of growth factor receptors. This overexpression can render cancer cells hyperresponsive to normal levels of the growth factor, a level that would not normally trigger proliferation. The best-documented examples of overexpression involve the epidermal growth factor (EGF) receptor family. *ERBB1*, the EGF receptor, is overexpressed in 80% of squamous cell carcinomas of the lung. A related receptor, called *HER2* (*ERBB2*), is amplified in 25% to 30% of breast cancers and adenocarcinomas of the lung, ovary, and salivary glands. These tumors are exquisitely sensitive to the mitogenic effects of small amounts of growth factors, and a high level of HER2 protein in breast cancer cells is a harbinger of poor prognosis. The significance of *HER2* in the pathogenesis of breast cancers is illustrated dramatically by the clinical benefit derived from blocking the extracellular domain of this receptor with anti-*HER2* antibodies. Treatment of breast cancer with anti-HER2 antibody is an elegant example of "bench to bedside" medicine.

SIGNAL-TRANSDUCING PROTEINS

A relatively common mechanism by which cancer cells acquire growth autonomy is by mutations in genes that encode various components of the signaling pathways. These signaling molecules couple growth factor receptors to their nuclear targets. Many such signaling proteins are associated with the inner leaflet of the plasma membrane, where they receive signals from activated growth factor receptors and transmit them to the nucleus. Two important members in this category are *RAS* and *ABL*. Each of these is discussed briefly.

Approximately 30% of all human tumors contain mutated versions of the *RAS* gene. In some tumors, such as colon and pancreatic cancers, the incidence of *RAS* mutations is even higher. Mutation of the *RAS* gene is the most common oncogene abnormality in human tumors. The RAS family of proteins binds guanosine nucleotides (guanosine triphosphate [GTP] and guanosine diphosphate [GDP]), as do the well-known G proteins. Normal RAS proteins flip back and forth between an excited signal-transmitting state and a quiescent state. In the inactive state, RAS proteins bind GDP; when cells are stimulated by growth factors, inactive RAS becomes activated by exchanging GDP for GTP (Fig. 6–18). The activated RAS in turn activates downstream regulators of proliferation, including the *RAF-MAP* kinase mitogenic cascade, which flood the nucleus with signals for cell proliferation. The excited signal-emitting stage of the normal RAS protein is short lived, however, because its intrinsic guanosine triphosphatase (GTPase) activity hydrolyzes GTP to GDP, releasing a phosphate group and returning the protein to its quiescent ground state. The GTPase activity of the activated RAS protein is magnified dramatically by a family of GTPase-activating proteins (GAPs). GAPs act as molecular brakes that prevent uncontrolled RAS activation by favoring hydrolysis of GTP to GDP. Mutant RAS proteins can bind GAPs, but their GTPase activity fails to be augmented. Thus, mutant RAS is trapped in its activated GTP-bound form, and the cell

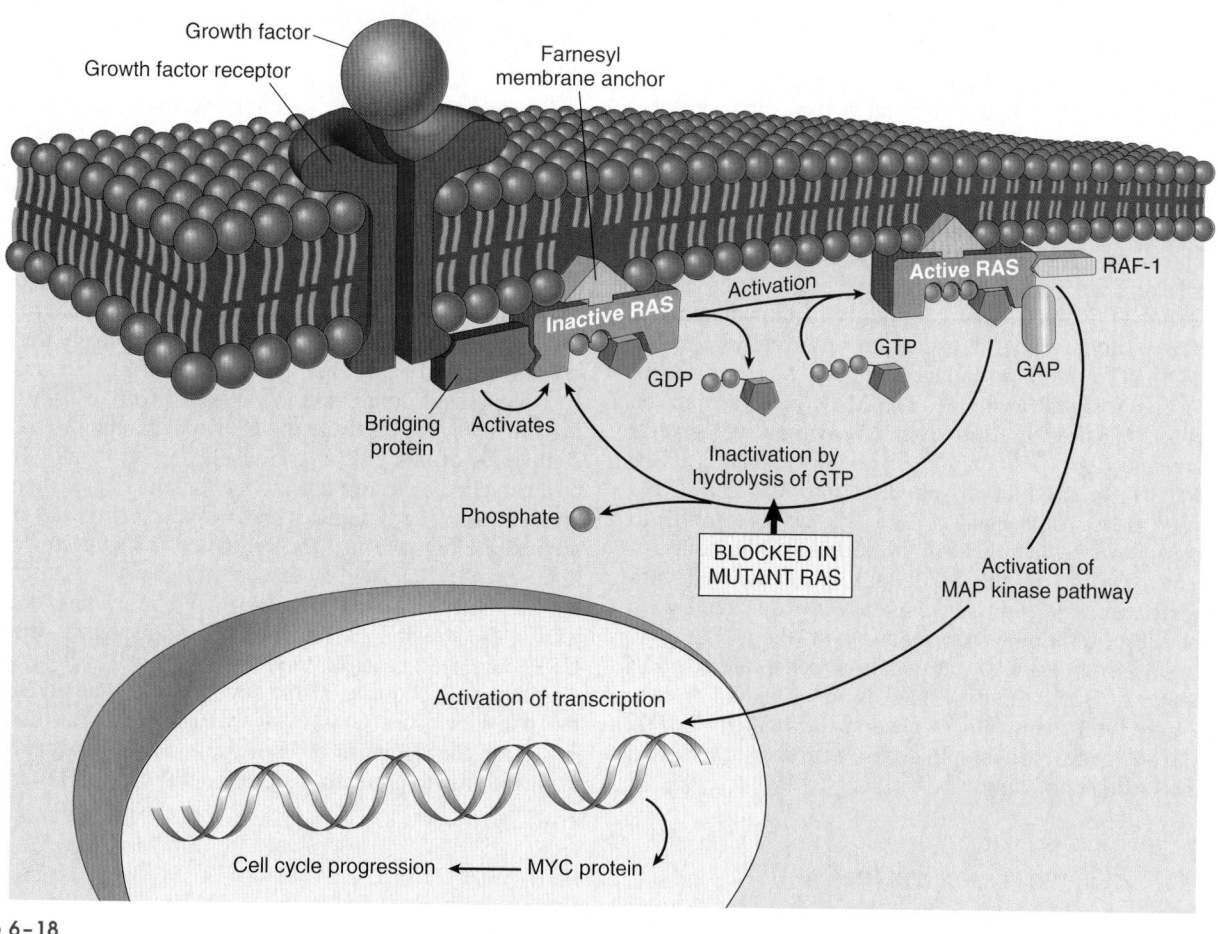

Figure 6–18

Model for action of *RAS* genes. When a normal cell is stimulated through a growth factor receptor, inactive (GDP-bound) RAS is activated to a GTP-bound state. Activated RAS recruits RAF-1 and stimulates the MAP-kinase pathway to transmit growth-promoting signals to the nucleus. The mutant RAS protein is permanently activated because of inability to hydrolyze GTP, leading to continuous stimulation of cells without any external trigger. The anchoring of RAS to the cell membrane by the farnesyl moiety is essential for its action, and drugs that inhibit farnesylation can inhibit RAS action.

is led to believe that it must continue to proliferate. It follows from this scenario that the consequences of mutations in the RAS protein would be mimicked by mutations in the GAPs that fail to restrain normal RAS proteins. Indeed, disabling mutation of neurofibromin 1 (NF-1), a GTPase-activating protein, is associated with familial neurofibromatosis type 1 (Chapter 7).

The *RAS* gene is commonly activated by point mutations. Molecular analyses of *RAS* mutations have revealed three hot spots centered around codons 12, 13, and 61. The molecular basis for the hot spots has been revealed by the crystal structure of RAS protein. Amino acids coded by codons 12 and 13 occur in the binding pocket for GTP, and codon 61 encodes the region essential for hydrolysis of GTP. Mutations at these locations interfere with GTP hydrolysis that is essential to convert RAS into an inactive stage.

In addition to *RAS*, several non–receptor-associated tyrosine kinases also function in signal transduction pathways. In this group, *ABL* is the most well defined with respect to carcinogenesis. The *ABL* protooncogene has tyrosine kinase activity that is dampened by negative regulatory domains. In chronic myeloid leukemia and certain acute leukemias, this activity is unleashed because the *ABL* gene is translocated

from its normal abode on chromosome 9 to chromosome 22, where it fuses with part of the breakpoint cluster region (*BCR*) gene. The *BCR-ABL* hybrid gene has potent tyrosine kinase activity, and it activates several pathways, including the *RAS-RAF* cascade just described. The crucial role of *BCR-ABL* in transformation has been confirmed by the dramatic clinical response of patients with chronic myeloid leukemia after therapy with an inhibitor of *ABL* kinase called STI 571 (Gleevec); this is another example of rational drug design emerging from an understanding of the molecular basis of cancer.

Other studies have revealed a completely novel function of *ABL* in oncogenesis. Normal ABL protein localizes in the nucleus, where its role is to promote apoptosis of cells that suffer DNA damage. This is analogous to the role of the *TP53* gene (discussed later). The *BCR-ABL* gene cannot perform this function because it is retained in the cytoplasm. Thus, a cell with *BCR-ABL* fusion gene is dysregulated in two ways. There is inappropriate tyrosine kinase activity leading to growth autonomy, and at the same time, apoptosis is impaired. The drug STI 571 acts on both fronts: it inhibits growth by neutralizing the kinase activity, and it promotes apoptosis by nuclear localization of *ABL*.

NUCLEAR TRANSCRIPTION FACTORS

Ultimately, all signal transduction pathways enter the nucleus and have an impact on a large bank of responder genes that orchestrate the cells' orderly advance through the mitotic cycle. Growth autonomy may occur as a consequence of mutations affecting genes that regulate transcription of DNA. A host of oncoproteins, including products of the *MYC, MYB, JUN, FOS,* and *REL* oncogenes, have been localized to the nucleus. Of these, the *MYC* gene is involved most commonly in human tumors. The *MYC* protooncogene is expressed in virtually all cells, and the MYC protein is induced rapidly when quiescent cells receive a signal to divide. The MYC protein binds to the DNA, causing transcriptional activation of several growth-related genes, including cyclin-dependent kinases (CDKs), whose product drives cells into the cell cycle (discussed next). In normal cells, MYC levels decline to near basal level when the cell cycle begins. In contrast, oncogenic versions of the *MYC* gene are associated with persistent expression or overexpression, contributing to sustained proliferation. Dysregulation of the *MYC* gene resulting from a t(8;14) translocation occurs in Burkitt lymphoma, a B-cell tumor; *MYC* is amplified in breast, colon, lung, and many other cancers; the related *N-MYC* and *L-MYC* genes are amplified in neuroblastomas and small cell cancers of lung.

CYCLINS AND CYCLIN-DEPENDENT KINASES

The ultimate outcome of all growth-promoting stimuli is the entry of quiescent cells into the cell cycle. Cancers may become autonomous if the genes that drive the cell cycle become dysregulated by mutations or amplification. As alluded to in Chapter 3, the orderly progression of cells through the various phases of the cell cycle is orchestrated by CDKs after they are activated by binding with another family of proteins called *cyclins* (see Fig. 3–2). The CDKs phosphorylate crucial target proteins and are expressed constitutively during the cell cycle but in an inactive form. By contrast, various cyclins are synthesized during specific phases of the cell cycle, and their function is to activate the CDKs by binding to them. On completion of this task, cyclin levels decline rapidly. Because of the cyclic nature of their production and degradation, these proteins have been termed *cyclins*. The cell cycle may be seen as a relay race in which each lap is regulated by a distinct set of cyclins, and as one set of cyclins leaves the track, the next set takes over (Fig. 6–19). While cyclins arouse the CDKs, their inhibitors, of which there are many, silence the CDKs and exert negative control over the cell cycle.

Although each phase of the circuitry is monitored carefully, the transition from G_1 to S is believed to be an extremely important checkpoint in the cell cycle clock. When a cell encounters growth-promoting signals, levels of the D family of

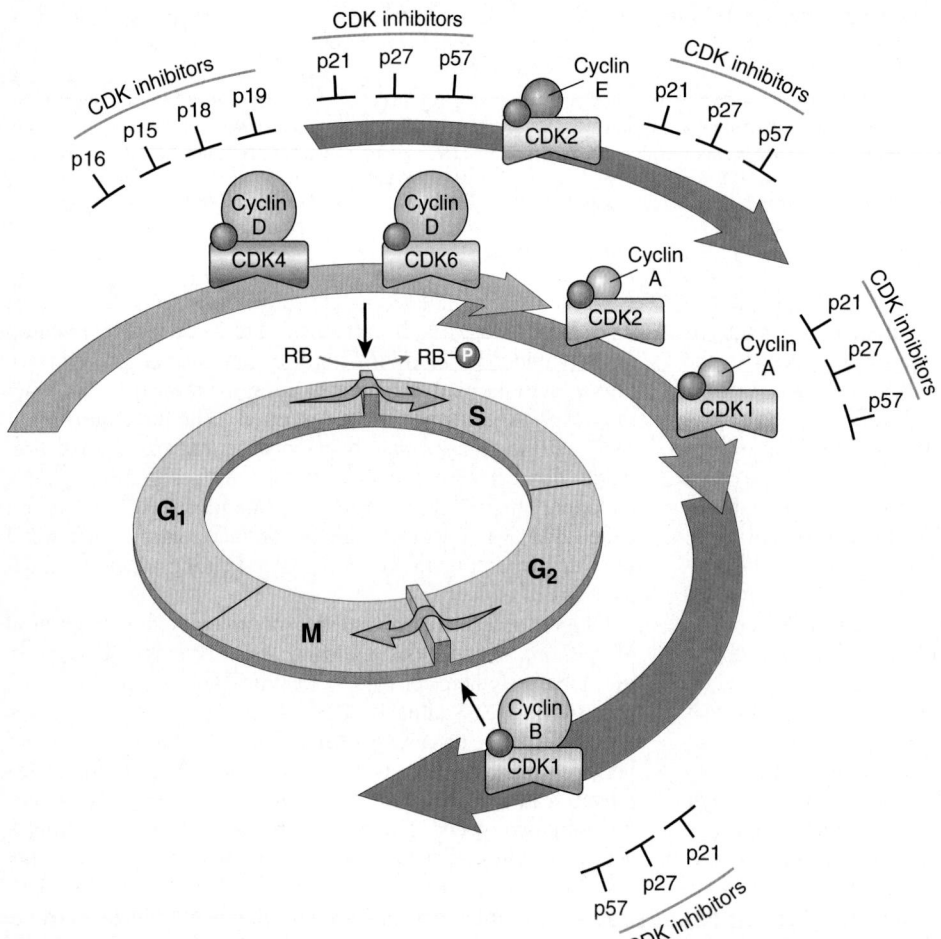

Figure 6–19 ■

Schematic illustration of the role of cyclins, cyclin-dependent kinases (CDKs), and cyclin-dependent kinase inhibitors (CDKIs) in regulating the cell cycle. The shaded arrows represent the phases of the cell cycle during which specific cyclin/CDK complexes are active. As illustrated, cyclin D/CDK4, cyclin D/CDK6, and cyclin E/CDK2 regulate the $G_1 \rightarrow S$ transition by phosphorylation of the RB protein (pRB). Cyclin A/CDK2 and cyclin A/CDK1 are active in the S phase. Cyclin B/CDK1 is essential for the $G_2 \rightarrow M$ transition. Two families of CDK inhibitors, so-called INK4 inhibitors composed of p16, p15, p18, and p19, act on cyclin D/CDK4 and cyclin D/CDK6. The other family of three inhibitors, p21, p27, and p57, can inhibit all CDKs.

cyclins go up, and CDK4 and CDK6 are activated. This checkpoint, as we see later, is guarded by the product of the retinoblastoma protein (pRB). Phosphorylation of pRB brought about by CDKs overcomes the $G_1 \rightarrow S$ hurdle and allows entry of cells into the DNA synthetic phase. Further progress from the S phase to the G_2 phase is facilitated by up-regulation of cyclin A, which binds to CDK2 and to CDK1. Early in the G_2 phase, B cyclin takes over. By forming complexes with CDK1, it helps to move the cell from G_2 to M.

The activity of CDKs is regulated by two families of CDK inhibitors (CDKIs). One family of CDKIs, composed of three proteins, called CDKN1A (p21), p27, and p57, inhibits the CDKs broadly, whereas the other family of CDKIs has selective effects on cyclin D/CDK4 and cyclin D/CDK6. The four members of this family (p15, CDKN2A [p16], p18, p19) are sometimes called INK4 proteins (because they are inhibitors of CDK4 and CDK6).

With this background, it is easy to appreciate that mutations that dysregulate the activity of cyclins and CDKs would favor cell proliferation. Mishaps affecting the expression of cyclin D or CDK4 seem to be a common event in neoplastic transformation. The cyclin D genes are overexpressed in many cancers, including those affecting the breast, esophagus, and liver and in a subset of lymphomas. Amplification of the CDK4 gene occurs in melanomas, sarcomas, and glioblastomas. Mutations affecting cyclin B and cyclin E and other CDKs also occur in certain malignant neoplasms, but they are much less frequent than those affecting cyclin D/CDK4.

Insensitivity to Growth-Inhibitory Signals

Isaac Newton predicted that every action has an equal and opposite reaction. Although Newton was not a cancer biologist, his formulation holds true for cell growth. Although oncogenes encode proteins that promote cell growth, the products of tumor suppressor genes apply brakes to cell proliferation. Disruption of such genes renders cells refractory to growth inhibition and mimics the growth-promoting effects of oncogenes. In this section, we describe cancer suppressor genes, their products, and possible mechanisms by which loss of their function contributes to unregulated cell growth.

We begin our discussion with the retinoblastoma *(RB)* gene, the first and prototypic cancer suppressor gene to be discovered. Similar to many advances in medicine, the discovery of cancer suppressor genes was accomplished by the study of a rare disease, in this case retinoblastoma, an uncommon childhood tumor. Approximately 60% of retinoblastomas are sporadic, and the remaining ones are familial, the predisposition to tumor being transmitted as an autosomal dominant trait. To account for the sporadic and familial occurrence of an identical tumor, Knudson, in 1974, proposed his now famous *two-hit hypothesis*, which in molecular terms can be stated as follows:

■ Two mutations *(hits)* are required to produce retinoblastoma. These involve the *RB* gene, located on chromosome 13q14. Both of the normal alleles of the *RB* locus must be inactivated (two hits) for the development of retinoblastoma (Fig. 6–20).

■ In familial cases, children inherit one defective copy of the *RB* gene in the germ line; the other copy is normal. Retinoblastoma develops when the normal *RB* gene is lost in the retinoblasts as a result of somatic mutation. Because in retinoblastoma families only a single somatic mutation is required for expression of the disease, the familial transmission follows an autosomal dominant inheritance pattern.

■ In sporadic cases, both normal *RB* alleles are lost by somatic mutation in one of the retinoblasts. The end result is the same: A retinal cell that has lost both of the normal copies of the *RB* gene becomes cancerous.

Although the loss of normal *RB* genes was discovered initially in retinoblastomas, it is now evident that homozygous loss of this gene is a fairly common event in several tumors, including breast cancer, small cell cancer of the lung, and bladder cancer. Patients with familial retinoblastoma also are at greatly increased risk of developing osteosarcomas and some soft tissue sarcomas.

At this point, we should clarify some terminology. A cell heterozygous at the *RB* locus is not malignant. Cancer develops when the cell becomes *homozygous* for the mutant allele or, in other words, *loses heterozygosity* of the normal *RB* gene. Because neoplastic transformation is associated with loss of both of the normal copies of the *RB* gene, this and other cancer suppressor genes also are often called *recessive cancer genes*.

The signals and signal-transducing pathways for growth inhibition are much less well understood than are those for growth promotion. Nevertheless, it is reasonable to assume that, similar to mitogenic signals, growth-inhibitory signals may originate outside the cell and use receptors, signal transducers, and nuclear transcription regulators to accomplish their effects. The tumor suppressor genes seem to encode various components of this growth-inhibitory pathway.

In principle, antigrowth signals can prevent cell proliferation by two complementary mechanisms. The antigrowth signal may cause dividing cells to go into G_0 (quiescence), where they remain until external cues prod their reentry into the proliferative pool. Alternatively the cells may enter a postmitotic, differentiated pool and lose replicative potential. It is now clear that at the molecular level antigrowth signals exert their effects on the $G_1 \rightarrow S$ checkpoint of the cell cycle. As alluded to earlier, this transition is controlled by the RB protein, and it is useful to begin our discussion of growth-inhibitory mechanisms and their evasion by focusing initially on the *RB* gene.

RB GENE AND CELL CYCLE

Much is known about the *RB* gene because this was the first tumor suppressor gene discovered. The *RB* gene product is a DNA-binding protein that is expressed in every cell type examined, where it *exists in an active hypophosphorylated and an inactive hyperphosphorylated state*. In its active state, *RB* serves as a brake in the advancement of cells from G_1 to the S phase of the cell cycle. When the cells are stimulated by growth factors, the RB protein is inactivated by phosphorylation, the brake is released, and the cells transverse the $G_1 \rightarrow S$ checkpoint. When the cells enter S phase, they are committed to divide without additional

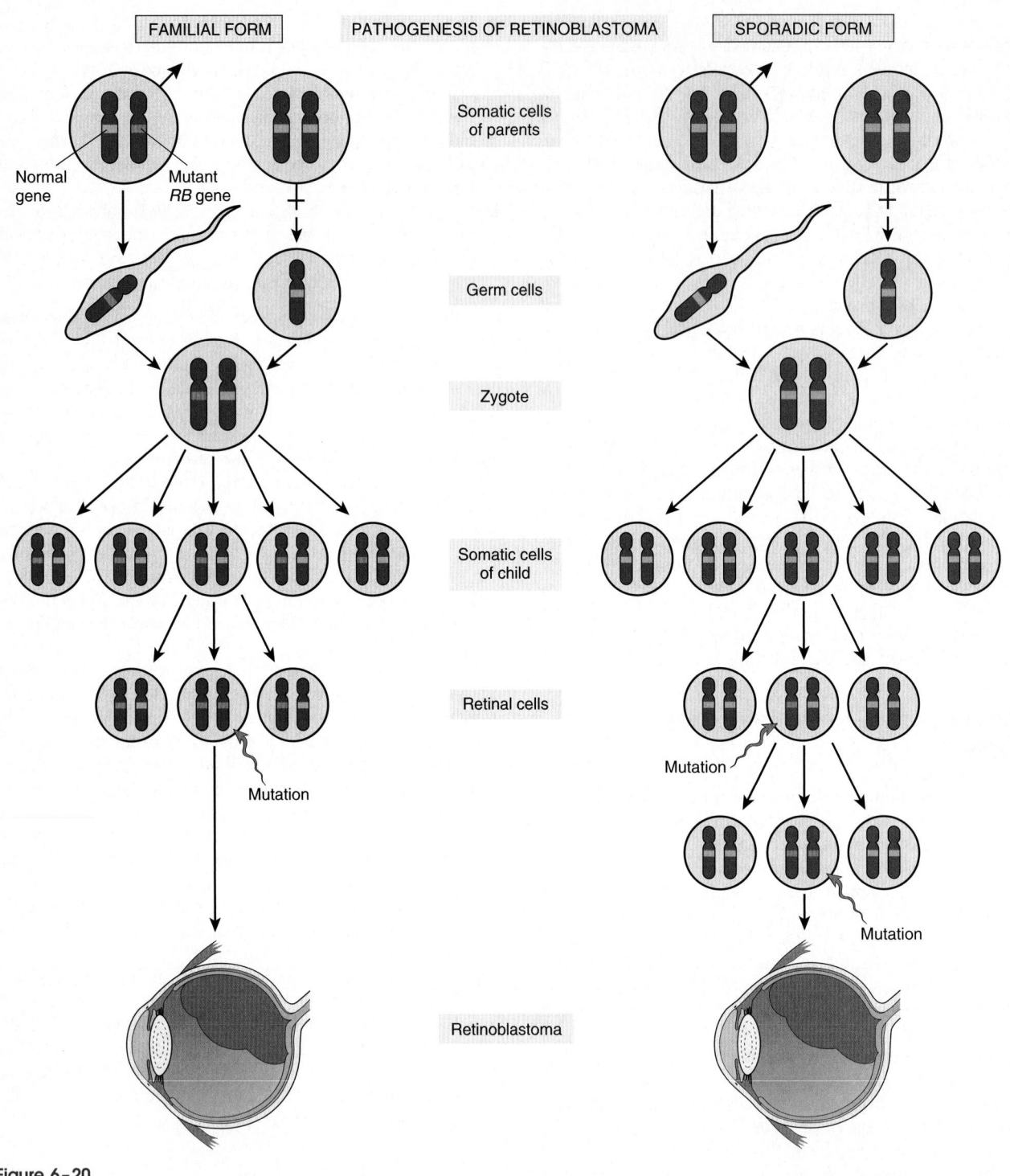

Figure 6-20 ■

Pathogenesis of retinoblastoma. Two mutations of the *RB* locus on chromosome 13q14 lead to neoplastic proliferation of the retinal cells. In the familial form, all somatic cells inherit one mutant *RB* gene from a carrier parent. The second mutation affects the *RB* locus in one of the retinal cells after birth. In the sporadic form, both mutations at the *RB* locus are acquired by the retinal cells after birth.

growth factor stimulation. During the ensuing M phase, the phosphate groups are removed from RB by cellular phosphates, regenerating the dephosphorylated form of RB.

The molecular basis of this braking action has been unraveled in elegant detail. *Quiescent cells (in G_0 or G_1)* *contain the active hypophosphorylated form of RB. In this state, RB prevents cell replication by binding, and possibly sequestering, the E2F family of transcription factors.* When the quiescent cells are stimulated by growth factors, the concentrations of the D and E cyclins (see earlier) go up,

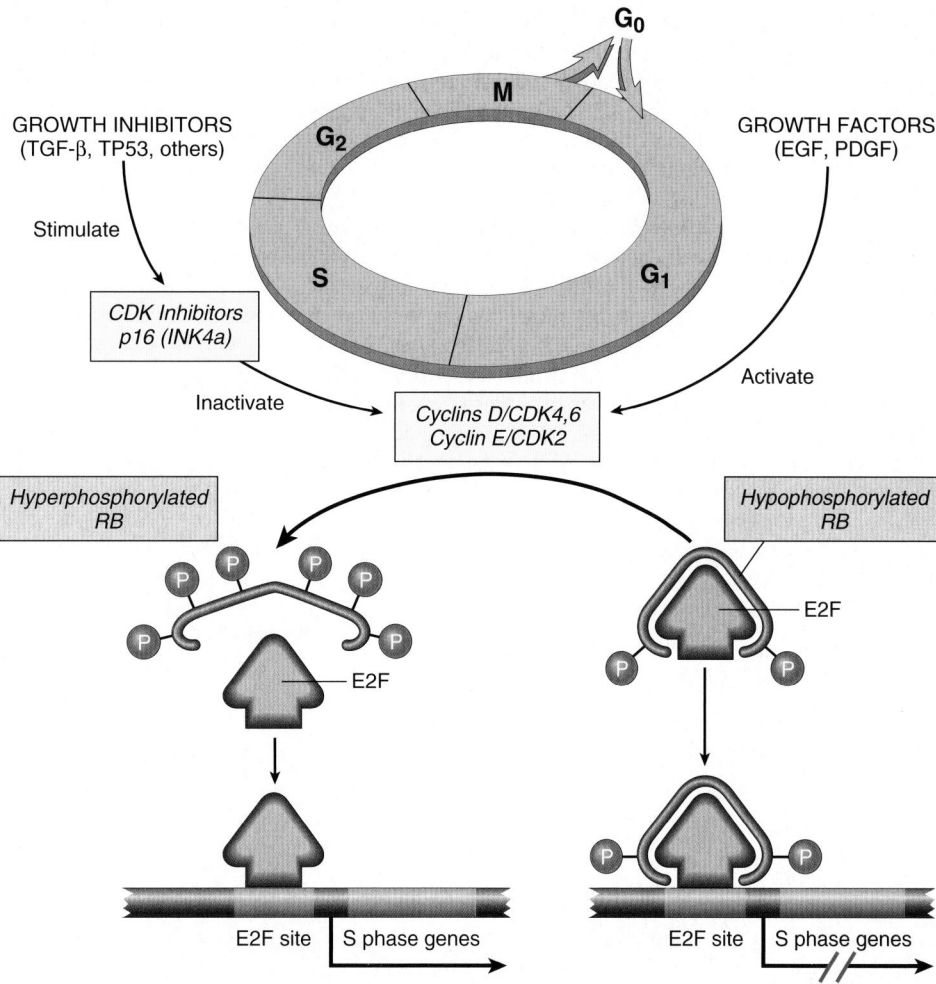

Figure 6-21 ■

The role of RB in regulating the $G_1 \rightarrow S$ checkpoint of the cell cycle. Hypophosphorylated RB complexed to the E2F transcription factors binds to DNA and inhibits transcription of genes whose products are required for the S phase of the cell cycle. When RB is phosphorylated by the cyclin D/CDK4, cyclin D/CDK6, and cyclin E/CDK2 complexes, it releases E2F. The latter then activates transcription of S-phase genes. The phosphorylation of RB is inhibited by CDK inhibitors because they inactivate cyclin/CDK complexes. Virtually all cancer cells show dysregulation of the $G_1 \rightarrow S$ checkpoint owing to mutation in one of four genes that regulate the phosphorylation of RB; these genes (*RB*, *CDK4*, *cyclin D*, and *CDKN2A* [*p16*]) are boxed. EGF, epidermal growth factor; PDGF, platelet-derived growth factor.

and the resultant activation of cyclin D/CDK4, cyclin D/CDK6, and cyclin E/CDK2 leads to phosphorylation of RB (Fig. 6–21). The hyperphosphorylated form of RB releases the E2F transcription factors and activates the transcription of several target genes. If the RB protein is absent, or its ability to sequester transcription factors is derailed by mutations, the molecular brakes on the cell cycle are released, and the cells move blithely into the S phase.

Mutations in other genes that control RB phosphorylation can mimic the effect of RB loss; such genes are mutated in many cancers that seem to have normal *RB* genes. For example, mutational activation of cyclin D or CDK4 would favor cell proliferation by facilitating RB phosphorylation. Cyclin D is overexpressed in many tumors because of gene amplification or translocation. Mutational inactivation of CDKIs also would drive the cell cycle by unregulated activation of cyclins and CDKs. One such inhibitor, encoded by the *CDKN2A* gene (also called inhibitor of kinase 4 [*INK4a*]), is an extremely common target of deletion or mutational inactivation in human tumors. Germ-line mutations of *CDKN2A* are associated with 25% of melanoma-prone kindreds. Somatically acquired deletion or inactivation of *CDKN2A* is seen in 75% of pancreatic carcinomas; 40% to 70% of glioblastomas; 50% of esophageal cancers; and 20% of non–small cell lung carcinomas, soft tissue sarcomas, and bladder cancers. *The*

emerging paradigm is that loss of normal cell cycle control is central to malignant transformation and that at least one of the four key regulators of cell cycle (CDKN2A, *cyclin D,* CDK4, RB) *is mutated in most human cancers.* In cells that harbor mutations in *CDKN2A*, cyclin D, or CDK4, the function of the *RB* gene is disrupted even if the *RB* gene itself is not mutated. The transforming proteins of several oncogenic animal and human DNA viruses seem to act, in part, by neutralizing the growth-inhibitory activities of RB. SV40 and polyomavirus large T antigens, adenoviruses EIA protein, and human papillomavirus (HPV) E7 protein all bind to the hypophosphorylated form of RB. The RB protein, unable to bind to the E2F transcription factors, is functionally deleted, and the cells lose the ability to be inhibited by antigrowth signals that funnel through the *RB* nexus.

TRANSFORMING GROWTH FACTOR β PATHWAY

Although much is known about the circuitry that applies brakes to the cell cycle, the molecules that transmit antiproliferative signals to cells are less well characterized. Best known is TGF-β, a member of a family of dimeric growth factors that includes bone morphogenetic proteins and activins. In most normal epithelial, endothelial, and hematopoietic cells,

TGF-β is a potent inhibitor of proliferation. It regulates cellular processes by binding to three receptors, called *types I, II,* and *III*. The antiproliferative effects of TGF-β are mediated in large part by regulating the RB pathways. TGF-β arrests cells in the G_1 phase of the cell cycle by stimulating production of the CDKI p15 and by inhibiting the transcription of CDK2, CDK4, and cyclins A and E. As can be inferred from our earlier discussion, these changes result in decreased phosphorylation of RB and cell cycle arrest.

In many forms of cancer, the growth-inhibiting effects of TGF-β pathways are impaired by mutations in the TGF-β signaling pathway. These mutations may affect the type II TGF-β receptor or SMAD molecules that serve to transduce antiproliferative signals from the receptor to the nucleus. Mutations affecting the type II receptor are seen in cancers of the colon, stomach, and endometrium. Mutational inactivation of SMAD4, one of 10 proteins involved in TGF-β signaling, is common in pancreatic cancers. *In 100% of pancreatic cancers and 83% of colon cancers, at least one component of the TGF-β pathway is mutated.*

ADENOMATOUS POLYPOSIS COLI– β-CATENIN PATHWAY

The *APC* gene, the loss of which is common in colon cancer, exerts antiproliferative effects in an unusual manner.

It is a cytoplasmic protein whose dominant function is to regulate the intracellular levels of β-catenin, a protein with many functions. On the one hand, β-catenin binds to the cytoplasmic portion E-cadherin, a cell surface protein that maintains intercellular adhesiveness; on the other hand, it can translocate to the nucleus and activate cell proliferation. The focus is on the latter function in this section. β-Catenin is an important component of the so-called WNT signaling pathway illustrated in Figure 6–22. WNT is a soluble factor that can induce cellular proliferation. It does so by binding to its receptor and transmitting signals that prevent the degradation of β-catenin, allowing it to translocate to the nucleus, where it acts as a transcriptional activator in conjunction with another molecule, called TcF (see Fig. 6–22B). In quiescent cells, which are not exposed to WNT, cytoplasmic β-catenin is degraded by a *destruction complex,* of which APC is an integral part. In resting normal cells, APC prevents β-catenin signaling by favoring its destruction (see Fig. 6–22A). With loss of APC (in malignant cells), β-catenin degradation is prevented, and the WNT signaling response is continually activated (see Fig. 6–22C). This leads to transcription of growth-promoting genes, such as cyclin D1 and *MYC*.

APC behaves as a typical tumor suppressor gene. Individuals born with one mutant allele develop hundreds to thousands of adenomatous polyps in the colon during

NO proliferation   **Proliferation**   **Proliferation**

Figure 6–22   ■

A–C, The role of APC in regulating the stability and function of β-catenin. APC and β-catenin are components of the WNT signaling pathway. In resting cells (not exposed to WNT), β-catenin forms a macromolecular complex containing the APC protein. This complex leads to the destruction of β-catenin, and intracellular levels of β-catenin are low. When cells are stimulated by secreted WNT molecules, the *destruction complex* is deactivated, β-catenin degradation does not occur, and cytoplasmic levels increase. β-catenin translocates to the nucleus, where it binds to TcF, a transcription factor that activates several genes involved in the cell cycle. When APC is mutated or absent, the destruction of β-catenin cannot occur. β-Catenin translocates to the nucleus and coactivates genes that promote the cell cycle, and cells behave as if they are under constant stimulation by the WNT pathway.

their teens or 20s. Almost invariably, one or more polyps undergo malignant transformation. As with other tumor suppressor genes, both copies of the *APC* gene must be lost for tumor development. When this occurs, adenomas form. As discussed later, additional mutations must occur for colonic cancers to develop. *APC* mutations are seen in 70% to 80% of sporadic colon cancers. Colonic cancers that have normal *APC* genes show activating mutations of β-catenin that render them refractory to the degrading action of APC.

TP53 GENE: GUARDIAN OF THE GENOME

The *TP53* (previously *p53*) tumor suppressor gene is one of the most commonly mutated genes in human cancers. It has multiple functions and cannot be classified conveniently into any specific functional group similar to other genes described in this section. TP53 *can exert antiproliferative effects, but equally important, it regulates apoptosis.* Fundamentally, *TP53* can be viewed as a central monitor of stress, directing the cell toward an appropriate response, be it cell cycle arrest or apoptosis. A variety of stresses can trigger the *TP53* response pathways, including anoxia, inappropriate oncogene expression (e.g., *MYC*), and damage to the integrity of DNA. By managing the DNA-damage response, *TP53* plays a central role in maintaining the integrity of the genome, as is evident from the following discussion.

Normal TP53 in nonstressed cells has a short half-life (20 minutes). This short half-life is due to an association with MDM2, a protein that targets it for destruction. When the cell is stressed, such as by an assault on its DNA, *TP53* undergoes post-transcriptional modifications that release it from MDM2 and increase its half-life. During the process of being unshackled from MDM2, TP53 also becomes activated as a transcription factor. Dozens of genes whose transcription is triggered by *TP53* have been found. They can be grouped into two broad categories—those that cause cell cycle arrest and those that cause apoptosis.

TP53-*mediated cell cycle arrest may be considered the primordial response to DNA damage* (Fig. 6–23). It occurs late in the G_1 phase and is caused mainly by *TP53*-dependent transcription of the CDKI *CDKN1A (p21)*. The

Figure 6–23   ■

The role of *TP53* in maintaining the integrity of the genome. Activation of normal *TP53* by DNA-damaging agents or by hypoxia leads to cell cycle arrest in G_1 and induction of DNA repair, by transcriptional up-regulation of the cyclin-dependent kinase inhibitor *CDKN1A (p21)* and the *GADD45* genes. Successful repair of DNA allows cells to proceed with the cell cycle; if DNA repair fails, *TP53*-induced activation of the *BAX* gene promotes apoptosis. In cells with loss or mutations of *TP53*, DNA damage does not induce cell cycle arrest or DNA repair, and genetically damaged cells proliferate, giving rise eventually to malignant neoplasms.

CDKN1A gene, as described earlier, inhibits cyclic/CDK complexes and prevents phosphorylation of RB essential for cells to enter G_1 phase. Such a pause in cell cycling is welcome because it gives the cells "breathing time" to repair DNA damage. *TP53* also helps the process by inducing certain proteins, such as GADD45 (growth arrest and DNA damage), that help in DNA repair. If DNA damage is repaired successfully, *TP53* up-regulates transcription of MDM2, which then down-regulates *TP53*, relieving cell cycle block. If during the pause *DNA damage cannot be successfully repaired, normal* TP53 *directs the cell to the graveyard by triggering apoptosis*. It does so by inducing apoptosis-inducing genes such as *BAX* (described later). How *TP53* senses DNA damage and how it determines the adequacy of DNA repair are not completely understood. One such DNA damage sensor may be the ATM protein that is mutated in the human disease ataxia-telangiectasia. Patients with ataxia-telangiectasia are unable to repair x-ray damage. The ATM protein can bind to damaged DNA and phosphorylate TP53. It could be speculated that patients with ataxia-telangiectasia cannot repair DNA damage because the ATM sensor cannot trigger the *TP53* pathway. In addition to sensors of initial damage, *TP53* must have other allies to inform it whether apoptosis is to be triggered.

To summarize, TP53 *senses DNA damage by unknown mechanisms and assists in DNA repair by causing G_1 arrest and inducing DNA repair genes. A cell with damaged DNA that cannot be repaired is directed by* TP53 *to undergo apoptosis (see Fig. 6–23). In view of these activities,* TP53 *has been rightfully called a "guardian of the genome." With homozygous loss of* TP53, *DNA damage goes unrepaired, mutations become fixed in dividing cells, and the cell turns onto a one-way street leading to malignant transformation.*

The importance of *TP53* in controlling carcinogenesis is attested to by the fact that more than 70% of human cancers have a defect in this gene, and the remaining have defects in genes up-stream or down-stream of *TP53*. Homozygous loss of the *TP53* gene is found in virtually every type of cancer, including carcinomas of the lung, colon, and breast—the three leading causes of cancer deaths. In most cases, the inactivating mutations affecting both *TP53* alleles are acquired in somatic cells. Less commonly, some individuals inherit a mutant *TP53* allele. As with the *RB* gene, inheritance of one mutant allele predisposes individuals to develop malignant tumors because only one additional *hit* is needed to inactivate the second, normal allele. Such individuals, said to have the *Li-Fraumeni syndrome,* have a 25-fold greater chance of developing a malignant tumor by age 50 compared with the general population. In contrast to patients who inherit a mutant *RB* allele, the spectrum of tumors that develop in patients with Li-Fraumeni syndrome is varied; the most common types of tumors are sarcomas, breast cancer, leukemia, brain tumors, and carcinomas of the adrenal cortex. Compared with sporadic tumors, those that affect patients with Li-Fraumeni syndrome occur at a younger age, and the affected individual may develop multiple primary tumors.

As with RB protein, normal TP53 also can be rendered nonfunctional by certain DNA viruses. Proteins encoded by oncogenic HPVs, hepatitis B virus (HBV), and possibly Epstein-Barr virus (EBV) can bind to normal TP53 proteins and nullify their protective functions. Thus, DNA viruses can subvert two of the best-understood tumor suppressor genes, *RB* and *TP53*.

Evasion of Apoptosis

Accumulation of neoplastic cells may result not only from activation of growth-promoting oncogenes or inactivation of growth-suppressing tumor suppressor genes, but also from mutations in the genes that regulate apoptosis. Just as cell growth is regulated by growth-promoting and growth-inhibiting genes, cell survival is conditioned by genes that promote and inhibit apoptosis. A large family of genes that regulate apoptosis has been identified. Before we can understand how tumor cells evade apoptosis, it is essential to review (Chapter 1) briefly the biochemical pathways to apoptosis. Figure 6–24 shows, in simplified form, the sequence of events that lead to apoptosis by signaling through the death receptor CD95 (Fas) and by DNA damage. When CD95 is bound to its ligand, CD95L, it trimerizes, and its cytoplasmic *death domains* attract the intracellular adaptor protein FADD. This protein recruits procaspase 8 to form the death-inducing signaling complex. Procaspase 8 is activated by cleavage into smaller subunits. Caspase 8 activates down-stream caspases such as caspase 3, a typical *executioner caspase* that cleaves DNA and other substrates to cause cell death. The other pathway of apoptosis is initiated by DNA damage (and other causes, such as growth factor deprivation). Mitochondria play a central role in this pathway by releasing cytochrome *c*, which in turn forms a complex with apoptosis-inducing factor 1 (APAF-1), procaspase 9, and ATP. Within this complex, procaspase 9 is activated to caspase 9, which then triggers caspase 3 (where the two pathways join). The release of cytochrome *c* is believed to be a key event in apoptosis, and it is regulated by genes of the *BCL2* family. Some members of this family (e.g., *BCL2, BCL-X_L*) inhibit apoptosis by preventing release of cytochrome *c*, whereas others, such as *BAD, BAX,* and *BID,* promote apoptosis by favoring cytochrome *c* release. The proapoptotic effects of *TP53* triggered by DNA damage seem to be mediated by up-regulation of BAX synthesis. Similarly, caspase 8 activates the proapoptotic protein BID.

Within this framework, it is possible to illustrate the multiple sites at which apoptosis is frustrated by cancer cells (see Fig. 6–24). Starting from the surface, reduced levels of CD95 in hepatocellular carcinomas render the tumor cells less susceptible to apoptosis by FasL. CD95 levels are regulated by TP53, and loss of TP53 may be responsible for reduced CD95. Some tumors have high levels of FLIP, a protein that can bind death-inducing signaling complex and prevent activation of caspase 8. Of all the genes, perhaps *best established is the role of* BCL2 *in protecting tumor cells from apoptosis.* As discussed later, approximately 85% of B-cell lymphomas of the follicular type (Chapter 12) carry a characteristic t(14;18) (q32;q21) translocation. Recall that 14q32, the site where immunoglobulin heavy-chain genes are found, also is involved in Burkitt lymphoma. Juxtaposition of this transcriptionally active locus with *BCL2* (located at 18q21) causes overexpression of the BCL2 protein. Overexpression of BCL2 protects lymphocytes from apoptosis and allows them to survive for long periods; there is a steady

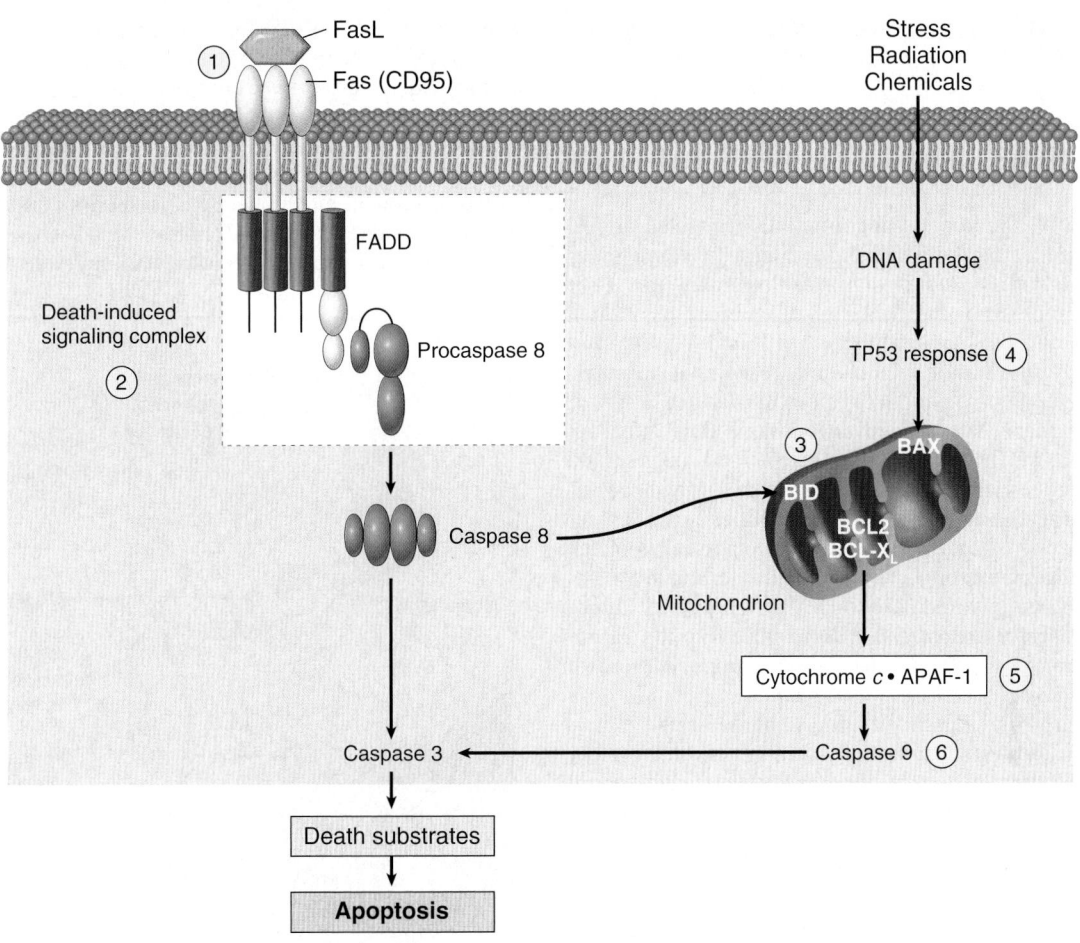

Figure 6–24 ■

Simplified schema of CD95 receptor–induced and DNA damage–triggered pathways of apoptosis and mechanisms used by tumor cells to evade cell death. (1) Reduced CD95 level. (2) Inactivation of death-induced signaling complex by FLICE protein. (3) Reduced egress of cytochrome *c* from mitochondrion owing to up-regulaion of BCL2. (4) Reduced levels of proapoptotic BAX owing to loss of TP53. (5) Loss of APAF-1. (6) Up-regulation of inhibitors of apoptosis (IAP).

accumulation of B lymphocytes, resulting in lymphadenopathy and marrow infiltration. Because BCL2-overexpressing lymphomas arise in large part from reduced cell death rather than explosive cell proliferation, they tend to be indolent (slow growing) compared with most other lymphomas.

As mentioned previously, TP53 *is an important proapoptotic gene that induces apoptosis in cells that are unable to repair DNA damage.* The actions of *TP53* are mediated in part by transcriptional activation of *BAX.* Two novel mechanisms by which tumor cells evade apoptosis have recently been discovered. Certain melanoma cells show loss of APAF-1, blocking the mitochondrial–cytochrome *c* pathway. These cells are resistant to *TP53*-induced apoptosis. Finally, in some tumors, there is transcriptional up-regulation of inhibitors of apoptosis that inactivate caspases. This up-regulation occurs in certain lymphomas of mucosal lymphoid tissue (so-called MALT lymphomas) as a result of the t(11;18) translocation.

Limitless Replicative Potential

As was discussed in the section on cellular aging (Chapter 1), most normal human cells have a capacity of 60 to 70

doublings. After this, the cells lose the capacity to divide and enter a nonreplicative senescence. This phenomenon has been ascribed to progressive shortening of *telomeres* at the ends of chromosomes. With each cell division, telomeres are shortened, and beyond a certain point, loss of telomeres leads to massive chromosomal abnormalities and death. The senescence of cultured human fibroblasts can be partially circumvented by disabling their *RB* and *TP53* genes. These cells also eventually undergo a *crisis,* however, characterized by massive cell death. It follows that for tumors to grow indefinitely, as they often do, loss of growth restraint is not sufficient. *Tumor cells also must develop ways to avoid cellular senescence*; this is acquired by activation of the enzyme telomerase, which can maintain normal telomere length. Telomerase is active in normal stem cells but is absent from most somatic cells. By contrast, telomere maintenance is seen in virtually all types of cancers. In 85% to 95% of cancers, this is due to up-regulation of the enzyme telomerase. A few use other mechanisms. The relevance of telomerase activation in vivo is attested to by experiments in mice. Mice with homozygous loss of *CDKN2A (p16, INK4A)* develop tumors when exposed to carcinogens. When *CDKN2A* "knockout" mice were crossed with telomerase "knockout" mice, tumor incidence was reduced greatly, and the resulting tumors exhibited severe karyotypic disarray.

Development of Sustained Angiogenesis

Even with all the genetic abnormalities discussed above, tumors cannot enlarge beyond 1 to 2 mm in diameter or thickness unless they are vascularized. Presumably the 1- to 2-mm zone represents the maximal distance across which oxygen and nutrients can diffuse from blood vessels. Beyond this size, the tumor fails to enlarge without vascularization because hypoxia induces apoptosis by activation of *TP53* (see earlier). Neovascularization has a dual effect on tumor growth: Perfusion supplies nutrients and oxygen, and newly formed endothelial cells stimulate the growth of adjacent tumor cells by secreting polypeptides, such as insulin-like growth factors, PDGF, granulocyte-macrophage colony-stimulating factor (GM-CSF), and interleukin (IL)-1. Angiogenesis is required not only for continued tumor growth but also for metastasis. Without access to the vasculature, the tumor cells cannot metastasize. *Angiogenesis is a necessary biologic correlate of malignancy.*

How do growing tumors develop a blood supply? Several studies indicate that tumors contain factors that are capable of affecting the entire series of events involved in the formation of new capillaries (Chapter 3). Tumor-associated angiogenic factors may be produced by tumor cells or may be derived from inflammatory cells (e.g., macrophages) that infiltrate tumors. Of the dozen or so tumor-associated angiogenic factors, the two most important are vascular endothelial growth factor (VEGF) and basic fibroblast growth factor. It is now clear that tumor cells not only produce angiogenic factors but also induce antiangiogenesis molecules. *The emerging paradigm is that tumor growth is controlled by the balance between angiogenic factors and factors that inhibit angiogenesis.* Antiangiogenesis factors, such as thrombospondin-1, may be produced by the tumor cells themselves, or their production may be induced by tumor cells. To the latter category belong angiostatin, endostatin, and vasculostatin. These three potent angiogenesis inhibitors are derived by proteolytic cleavage of plasminogen, collagen, and transthyretin, respectively.

Early in their growth, most human tumors do not induce angiogenesis. They remain small or in situ for years until the *angiogenic switch* terminates the stage of vascular quiescence. The molecular basis of the angiogenic switch is not entirely clear but may involve increased production of angiogenic factors or loss of angiogenesis inhibitors. The wild-type *TP53* gene seems to inhibit angiogenesis by inducing the synthesis of the antiangiogenic molecule thrombospondin-1. With mutational inactivation of both *TP53* alleles (a common event in many cancers), the levels of thrombospondin-1 drop precipitously, tilting the balance in favor of angiogenic factors.

Hypoxia within the growing tumor favors angiogenesis by release of hypoxia-inducible factor-1 (HIF-1). HIF-1 controls transcription of VEGF. The transcription of VEGF also is under the control of *RAS* oncogene, and *RAS* activation up-regulates the production of VEGF. Proteases are also involved in regulating the balance between angiogenic and antiangiogenic factors. Many proteases can release basic fibroblast growth factor stored in the extracellular matrix (ECM); conversely, cleavage of plasmin gives rise to angiostatin, a potent angiogenesis inhibitor. Because of the crucial role of angiogenesis in tumor growth, much interest is focused on antiangiogenesis therapy. Results of ongoing clinical trials with several angiogenesis inhibitors seem promising, and more are awaited.

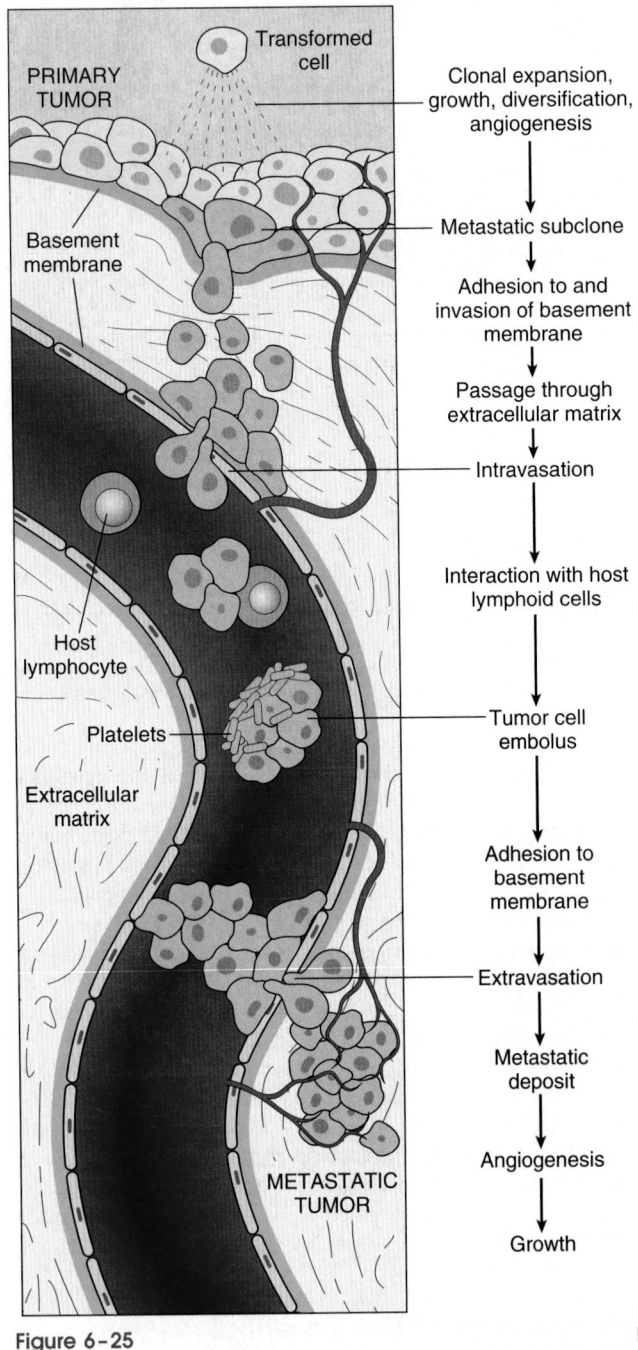

Figure 6-25

The metastatic cascade. Schematic illustration of the sequential steps involved in the hematogenous spread of a tumor.

Ability to Invade and Metastasize

The spread of tumors is a complex process involving a series of sequential steps, diagrammed in Figure 6–25. Predictably, this sequence of steps may be interrupted at any stage by either host-related or tumor-related factors. As is discussed later, cells within a tumor are heterogeneous with respect to metastatic potential. Only certain subclones possess the right combination of gene products to complete all the steps outlined in Figure 6–25. For the purpose of discussion, the metastatic cascade can be subdivided into two phases: invasion of extracellular matrix and vascular dissemination and homing of tumor cells.

INVASION OF EXTRACELLULAR MATRIX

As is well known, human tissues are organized into a series of compartments separated from each other by two types of ECM: basement membranes and interstitial connective tissue. Although organized differently, each of these components of ECM is composed of collagens, glycoproteins, and proteoglycans. A review of Figure 6–26 reveals that tumor cells must interact with the ECM at several stages in the metastatic cascade. A carcinoma first must breach the underlying basement membrane, then traverse the interstitial connective tissue, and ultimately gain access to the circulation by penetrating the vascular basement membrane. This cycle is repeated when tumor cell emboli extravasate at a distant site. Invasion of the ECM is an active process that is accomplished in four steps (see Fig. 6–26):

1. Detachment of tumor cells from each other
2. Attachment of tumor cells to matrix components
3. Degradation of ECM
4. Migration of tumor cells

The first step in the metastatic cascade is a *loosening* of tumor cells. As mentioned earlier, E-cadherins act as intercellular glues, and their cytoplasmic portions bind to β-catenin (see Fig. 6–22). Not only do adjacent E-cadherin molecules keep the cells together, but also homotypic adhesions mediated by E-cadherin transmit antigrowth signals via β-catenin. Free β-catenin can activate transcription of growth-promoting genes. *E-cadherin function is lost in almost all epithelial cancers, either by mutational inactivation of E-cadherin genes or by activation of β-catenin genes.* Changes in the pattern of expression of other cell-adhesion molecules of the immunoglobulin superfamily (Chapter 2) also contribute to invasion. For example, in neuroblastomas and small cell lung cancer, there is a switch from a highly adhesive isoform to a poorly adhesive isoform of the neural cell adhesion molecule (N-CAM).

Figure 6–26   ■

A–D, Schematic illustration of the sequence of events in the invasion of epithelial basement membranes by tumor cells. Tumor cells detach from each other because of reduced adhesiveness, then attach to the basement membrane via the laminin receptors and secrete proteolytic enzymes, including type IV collagenase and plasminogen activator. Degradation of the basement membrane and tumor cell migration follow.

A. LOOSENING OF INTERCELLULAR JUNCTIONS

Type IV collagen   Laminin
Cadherins   Basement membrane

B. ATTACHMENT

Type IV collagen   Fibronectin receptor   Laminin
Laminin receptor

C. DEGRADATION   Type IV collagenase   Plasminogen activator

Type IV collagen cleavage

D. MIGRATION

Autocrine motility factor
Fibronectin

The second step, attachment of tumor cells to ECM proteins such as laminin and fibronectin, is important for invasion and metastasis. Normal epithelial cells have receptors for basement membrane laminin that are polarized at their basal surface. In contrast, carcinoma cells have many more receptors, and these are distributed all around the cell membrane. There is a correlation between the density of laminin receptors on breast carcinoma cells and lymph node metastases. A change in the pattern of integrin expression also favors invasion. In many carcinoma cells, attachment to stroma is facilitated by a loss of the integrins that bind to normal ECM and their replacement by integrins that bind to ECM degraded by proteases.

The third step in invasion is local degradation of the basement membrane and interstitial connective tissue. Tumor cells secrete proteolytic enzymes themselves or induce the host cells (e.g., fibroblasts) to elaborate proteases. Several matrix-degrading enzymes termed *metalloproteinases*, including gelatinases, collagenases, and stromelysins, are involved. Type IV collagenase is a gelatinase that cleaves type IV collagen of the epithelial and vascular basement membranes. Benign tumors of the breast, colon, and stomach show little type IV collagenase activity, whereas their malignant counterparts overexpress this enzyme. Concurrently the levels of metalloproteinase inhibitors are reduced so that the balance is tilted greatly toward tissue degradation. Similar correlations have been noted with other proteases, including cathepsin D. Overexpression of cathepsin D occurs in invasive breast cancers. Because of these observations, attempts are being made to use protease inhibitors as therapeutic agents.

Locomotion is the final step of invasion, propelling tumor cells through the degraded basement membranes and zones of matrix proteolysis. Migration seems to be mediated by tumor cell–derived cytokines, such as autocrine motility factors. In addition, cleavage products of matrix components (e.g., collagen, laminin) and some growth factors (e.g., insulin-like growth factors I and II) have chemotactic activity for tumor cells. Stromal cells also produce paracrine effectors of cell motility, such as hepatocyte growth factor/scatter factor (HGF/SCF), which bind to receptors on tumor cells. Concentrations of HGF/SCF are elevated at the advancing edges of the highly invasive brain tumor glioblastoma multiforme, supporting their role in motility.

VASCULAR DISSEMINATION AND HOMING OF TUMOR CELLS

When in the circulation, tumor cells are vulnerable to destruction by the host immune cells (discussed later). In the bloodstream, some tumor cells form emboli by aggregating and adhering to circulating leukocytes, particularly platelets; aggregated tumor cells are thus afforded some protection from the antitumor host effector cells. Most tumor cells circulate, however, as single cells. Extravasation of free tumor cells or tumor emboli involves adhesion to the vascular endothelium, followed by egress through the basement membrane by mechanisms similar to those involved in invasion.

The site of extravasation and the organ distribution of metastases generally can be predicted by the location of the primary tumor and its vascular or lymphatic drainage. However, in many cases, the natural pathways of drainage do not readily explain the distribution of metastases. As pointed out earlier, some tumors (e.g., lung cancers) tend to involve the adrenals with some regularity but almost never spread to skeletal muscle. Such organ tropism may be related to the expression of adhesion molecules by tumor cells whose ligands are expressed preferentially on the endothelium of target organs. Another novel mechanism of site-specific homing involves chemokines and their receptors. Chemokines are involved in directed movement (chemotaxis) of leukocytes (Chapter 2). It appears that cancer cells have also read that chapter and use similar tricks to home in on specific tissues. Human breast cancer cells express high levels of the chemokine receptor genes *CXCR4* and *CCR7*. The ligands for these receptors (i.e., chemokines CCL21 and CXCL12) are highly expressed only in those organs where breast cancer cells metastasize. On the basis of this fact, it is speculated that blockade of chemokine receptors may limit metastases. Despite the foregoing considerations, the precise localization of metastases cannot be predicted with any form of cancer. Evidently many tumors have not read all chapters of the pathology textbooks!

Genomic Instability—Enabler of Malignancy

The preceding section discussed the six defining features of malignancy and the genetic alterations that are responsible for the phenotypic attributes of cancer cells. How do these mutations arise? Although humans literally swim in environmental agents that are mutagenic (e.g., chemicals, radiation, sunlight), cancers are relatively rare outcomes of these encounters. This state of affairs results from the ability of normal cells to repair DNA damage. Although definitive answers to the origin and accumulation of cancer-causing mutations are still not available, it does seem that the propensity to develop mutations results from subtle or overt defects in DNA repair. The importance of DNA repair in maintaining the integrity of the genome is highlighted by several inherited disorders in which genes that encode proteins involved in DNA repair are defective. *Individuals born with such inherited mutations of DNA repair proteins are at a greatly increased risk of developing cancer.* Examples are as follows:

■ The role of DNA repair genes in predisposition to cancer is illustrated dramatically by hereditary nonpolyposis colon carcinoma (HNPCC) syndrome. This disorder, characterized by familial carcinomas of the colon affecting predominantly the cecum and proximal colon (Chapter 15), results from defects in genes involved in DNA mismatch repair. When a strand of DNA is being repaired, these genes act as "spell checkers." For example, if there is an erroneous pairing of G with T rather than the normal A with T, the mismatch repair genes correct the defect. Without these "proofreaders," errors slowly accumulate in several genes, including protooncogenes and cancer suppressor genes. Mutations in at least five mismatch repair genes have been found to underlie HNPCC (Chapter 15). Each affected individual inherits one defective copy of one of several DNA mismatch repair genes and acquires the second hit in colonic epithelial cells. Thus, DNA repair genes behave similarly to tumor suppressor genes in their mode of inheritance, but in contrast to tumor suppressor genes (and oncogenes), they affect cell growth only indirectly—by allowing mutations in other genes during the process of normal cell division. In HNPCC, type II TGF-β receptor and *BAX* genes, which control cell growth and apoptosis, are mutated.

■ Patients with another inherited disorder, xeroderma pigmentosum, are at increased risk for the development of cancers of the skin exposed to the ultraviolet (UV) light contained in sun rays. The basis of this disorder also is defective DNA repair. UV light causes cross-linking of pyrimidine residues, preventing normal DNA replication. Such DNA damage is repaired by the nucleotide excision repair system. Several proteins and genes are involved in nucleotide excision repair, and an inherited loss of any one can give rise to xeroderma pigmentosum.

■ In addition to the examples mentioned earlier, a group of autosomal recessive disorders comprising Bloom syndrome, ataxia-telangiectasia, and Fanconi anemia is characterized by hypersensitivity to other DNA-damaging agents, such as ionizing radiation (Bloom syndrome and ataxia-telangiectasia), or DNA cross-linking agents, such as nitrogen mustard (Fanconi anemia). Their phenotype is complex and includes, in addition to predisposition to cancer, features such as neural symptoms (ataxia-telangiectasia), anemia (Fanconi anemia), and developmental defects (Bloom syndrome). The ataxia-telangiectasia gene seems to control several processes, including the normal functioning of the *TP53* gene. As discussed earlier, ATM is required for sensing DNA damage and the consequent activation of *TP53*.

■ Evidence for the role of DNA repair genes in the origin of cancer also comes from the study of hereditary breast cancer. Mutations in two genes, *BRCA1* and *BRCA2*, account for 80% of cases of familial breast cancer. In addition to breast cancer, women with *BRCA1* mutation have a substantially higher risk of epithelial ovarian cancers, and men have a slightly higher risk of prostate cancer. Likewise, mutations in the *BRCA2* gene increase the risk of breast cancer in men and women and cancer of the ovary, prostate, pancreas, bile ducts, stomach, and melanocytes. Although the functions of these genes have not been elucidated fully, there is increasing evidence that they regulate DNA repair. Cells that lack these genes develop chromosomal breaks and severe aneuploidy. BRCA1 interacts with several proteins in the DNA repair pathway, including the ATM protein mentioned earlier. Current evidence indicates that BRCA1 is a part of a multiprotein complex that is crucial for repair of double-stranded breaks in chromosomes. Similar to other tumor suppressor genes, both copies of *BRCA1* and *BRCA2* must be inactivated for cancer to develop. Although linkage of *BRCA1* and *BRCA2* to familial breast cancers is established, these genes are rarely inactivated in sporadic cases of breast cancer. In this regard, *BRCA1* and *BRCA2* are different from other tumor suppressor genes, such as *APC* and *TP53*, which are inactivated in familial and in sporadic cancers.

Molecular Basis of Multistep Carcinogenesis

Given that malignant tumors must develop the six fundamental abnormalities discussed earlier, it follows that *each cancer must result from accumulation of multiple mutations*. Several epidemiologic, morphologic, and molecular observations are consistent with this hypothesis.

■ Even before the discovery of oncogenes and cancer suppressor genes, cancer epidemiologists suggested that the age-associated increase in cancers could be explained best by postulating that five or six independent steps are required for tumorigenesis.

■ Every human cancer that has been analyzed reveals multiple genetic alterations involving activation of several oncogenes and the loss of two or more cancer suppressor genes. Each of these alterations represents crucial steps in the progression from a normal cell to a malignant tumor. A dramatic example of incremental acquisition of the malignant phenotype is documented by the study of colon carcinoma. These lesions are believed to evolve through a series of morphologically identifiable stages: colon epithelial hyperplasia followed by formation of adenomas that progressively enlarge and ultimately undergo malignant transformation (Chapter 15). The proposed molecular correlates of this adenoma-carcinoma sequence are illustrated in Figure 6–27. According to this scheme, inactivation of the *APC* tumor suppressor gene occurs first, followed by activation of

Figure 6–27 ■

Molecular model for the evolution of colorectal cancers through the adenoma-carcinoma sequence. (Based on studies of Fearon ER, Vogelstein B: A genetic model of colorectal carcinogenesis. Cell 61:759, 1990. Copyright 1990, Cell Press.)

Component   Acquired Capability

↱   Self-sufficiency in growth signals

⊘   Insensitivity to anti-growth signals

†   Evading apoptosis

∞   Limitless replicative potential

⬚   Sustained angiogenesis

〰   Tissue invasion and metastasis

Figure 6–28   ■

Multiple pathways of carcinogenesis. All cancers must acquire the same six hallmark traits, but their means of doing so vary mechanistically and chronologically. As shown, the order in which these capabilities are acquired is variable across different cancers. In some tumors, a particular mutation may confer several capabilities simultaneously, decreasing the number of intermediate mutational steps required for full development. Loss of the *TP53* tumor suppressor gene may facilitate resistance to apoptosis and angiogenesis (e.g., in the five-step pathway shown *[bottom pathway]*). In other tumors, by comparison, a collaboration of two or more distinct genetic changes may be needed to acquire a given trait. In the eight-step model *(top pathway)*, invasion metastasis and resistance to apoptosis are each acquired in two steps. (Modified from Hanahan D, Weinberg RA: The hallmarks of cancer. Cell 100:576, 2000.)

RAS and, ultimately, loss of a tumor suppressor gene on 18q and *TP53* genes. The precise temporal sequence of mutations is different in each organ. Figure 6–28 illustrates that tumors may arise by several distinct and parallel pathways.

TUMOR PROGRESSION AND HETEROGENEITY

It is well established that over a period of time, many tumors become more aggressive and acquire greater malignant potential. This phenomenon is referred to as *tumor progression* and must be distinguished from an increase in tumor size. Careful clinical and experimental studies reveal that increasing malignancy (e.g., accelerated growth, invasiveness, and ability to form distant metastases) is often acquired in an incremental fashion. This biologic phenomenon is related to the sequential appearance of subpopulations of cells that differ with respect to several phenotypic attributes, such as invasiveness, rate of growth, metastatic ability, karyotype, hormonal responsiveness, and susceptibility to antineoplastic drugs. *Despite the fact that most malignant tumors are monoclonal in origin, by the time they become clinically evident, their constituent cells are extremely heterogeneous.* At the molecular level, tumor progression and associated heterogeneity most likely result from multiple mutations that accumulate independently in different cells, generating subclones with different characteristics (Fig. 6–29). Some of these mutations may be lethal; others may spur cell growth by affecting other protooncogenes or cancer suppressor genes. The subclones so

generated are subjected to immune and nonimmune selection pressures. For example, cells that are highly antigenic are destroyed by host defenses, whereas those with reduced growth factor requirements are positively selected. A growing tumor, therefore, tends to be enriched for those subclones that "beat the odds" and are adept at survival, growth, invasion, and metastasis.

The rate at which mutant subclones are generated is variable. In some tumors, such as osteosarcomas, metastatic subclones already are present when the patient walks into the physician's office. In others, typified by mixed salivary gland tumors, aggressive subclones develop late and infrequently. Knowledge of such biologic differences is important to understanding the clinical potential of cancers and to the management of cancer patients. Figure 6–30 summarizes the possible functions and subcellular location of several genes that are altered during multistep carcinogenesis.

Karyotypic Changes in Tumors

The genetic damage that activates oncogenes or inactivates tumor suppressor genes may be subtle (e.g., point mutations) or large enough to be detected in a karyotype. The *RAS* oncogene represents the best example of activation by point mutation. As discussed earlier, there are several mutational hot spots in the *RAS* gene, all of which cluster around the binding pocket for GTP and influence the GTPase activity. In certain neoplasms, karyotypic abnormalities are nonrandom and common. Specific abnormalities have been identified in most leukemias and lymphomas and in an increasing number of nonhematopoietic

Figure 6-29 ■

Tumor progression and generation of heterogeneity. New subclones arise from the descendants of the original transformed cell by multiple mutations, as illustrated in Figure 6-27. With progression the tumor mass becomes enriched for variants that are more adept at evading host defenses and are likely to be more aggressive.

tumors. The common types of nonrandom structural abnormalities in tumor cells are (1) balanced translocations, (2) deletions, and (3) cytogenetic manifestations of gene amplification. In addition, whole chromosomes may be gained or lost.

Balanced Translocations. Balanced translocations are extremely common, especially in hematopoietic neoplasms. Most notable is the Philadelphia (Ph) chromosome in chronic myelogenous leukemia, comprising a reciprocal and balanced translocation between chromosomes 22 and, usually, 9 (Fig. 6–31). As a consequence, chromosome 22 appears abbreviated. *This cytogenetic change, seen in more than 90% of cases of chronic myelogenous leukemia, is a reliable marker of the disease. The few Ph chromosome–negative cases of chronic myelogenous leukemia show molecular evidence of the* BCR-ABL *rearrangement,* the crucial consequence of Ph translocation. In more than 90% of cases of Burkitt lymphoma, the cells have a translocation, usually between chromosomes 8 and 14. In follicular B-cell lymphomas, a reciprocal translocation between chromosomes 14 and 18 is extremely common.

Deletions. Chromosome deletions are the second most prevalent structural abnormality in tumor cells. *Compared with translocations, deletions are more common in non-hematopoietic solid tumors.* As discussed, deletions of

chromosome 13q band 14 are associated with retinoblastoma. Deletions of 17p, 5q, and 18q, all noted in colorectal cancers, harbor three tumor suppressor genes. Deletion of 3p, noted in several tumors, is extremely common in small cell lung carcinomas, and the hunt is on for one or more cancer suppressor genes at this locale.

Gene Amplifications. There are two karyotypic manifestations of gene amplification: homogeneously staining regions on single chromosomes and double minutes (Fig. 6–32), which are seen as small paired fragments of chromatin. Neuroblastomas and breast cancers are the best-studied examples of gene amplification involving the *N-MYC* and *HER-2* genes.

ETIOLOGY OF CANCER: CARCINOGENIC AGENTS

Genetic damage lies at the heart of carcinogenesis. What agents inflict such damage? Three classes of carcinogenic agents can be identified: (1) chemicals, (2) radiant energy, and (3) microbial agents. Chemicals and radiant energy are documented causes of cancer in humans, and oncogenic viruses are involved in the pathogenesis of tumors in several animal models and at least some human tumors. In the

Figure 6-30 ■

Subcellular localization and functions of major classes of proteins encoded by cancer-associated genes. The products of protooncogenes are colored red; cancer suppressor genes, blue; DNA repair genes, green; and proteins that regulate apoptosis, purple.

following discussion, each class of agents is considered separately, but it is important to note that several may act in concert or sequentially to produce the multiple genetic abnormalities characteristic of neoplastic cells.

Chemical Carcinogens

It has been over 200 years since the London surgeon Sir Percival Pott correctly attributed scrotal skin cancer in chimney sweeps to chronic exposure to soot. A few years later, based on this observation, the Danish Chimney Sweeps Guild ruled that its members must bathe daily. No public health measure since that time has achieved so much in the control of a form of cancer. Since that time, hundreds of chemicals have been shown to be carcinogenic in animals. The following pertinent observations have emerged from the study of chemical carcinogens:

■ They are of extremely diverse structure and include natural and synthetic products.
■ Some are direct reacting and require no chemical transformation to induce carcinogenicity, but most are indirect reacting and become active only after metabolic

conversion. Such agents are referred to as *procarcinogens*, and their active end products are called *ultimate carcinogens*.
■ All direct-reacting and ultimate chemical carcinogens are highly reactive electrophiles (i.e., have electron-deficient atoms) that react with the electron-rich atoms in RNA, cellular proteins, and, mainly, DNA.
■ The carcinogenicity of some chemicals is augmented by agents that by themselves have little, if any, transforming activity. Such augmenting agents traditionally have been called *promoters*; however, many carcinogens have no requirement for promoting agents.
■ Several chemical carcinogens may act in concert with other types of carcinogenic influences (e.g., viruses or radiation) to induce neoplasia.

Some of the major agents are presented in Table 6–5. Only a few comments are offered on some.

DIRECT-ACTING AGENTS

Direct-acting agents, as already noted, require no metabolic conversion to become carcinogenic. They are in general weak carcinogens but are important because some of

Figure 6-31 ■

The chromosomal translocations and associated oncogenes in Burkitt lymphoma and chronic myelogenous leukemia.

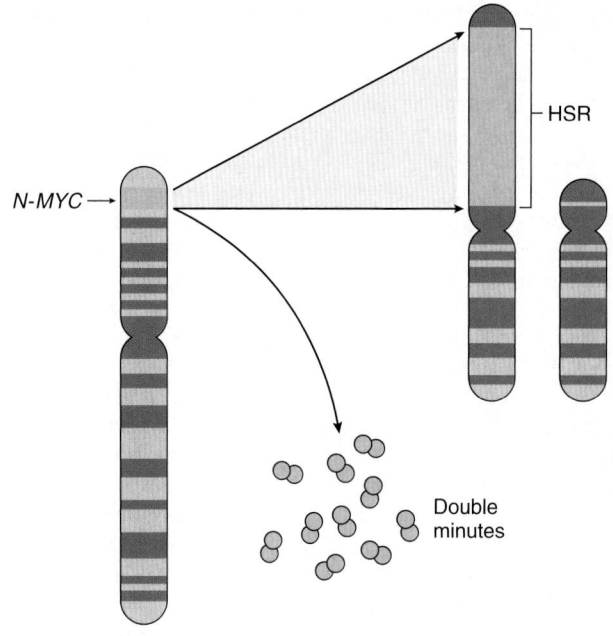

Figure 6-32 ■

Amplification of the *N-MYC* gene in human neuroblastomas. The *N-MYC* gene, present normally on chromosome 2p, becomes amplified and is seen either as extra chromosomal double minutes or as a chromosomally integrated homogeneous-staining region (HSR). The integration involves other autosomes, such as 4, 9, or 13. (Modified from Brodeur GM, et al: Clinical implication of oncogene activation in human neuroblastomas. Cancer 58:541, 1986. Copyright © 1986 American Cancer Society. Reprinted by permission of Wiley-Liss, Inc, a subsidiary of John Wiley & Sons, Inc.)

Table 6-5. MAJOR CHEMICAL CARCINOGENS

Direct-Acting Carcinogens

Alkylating agents
    Anticancer drugs (cyclophosphamide, chlorambucil, nitrosoureas, and others)
Acylating agents
    1-Acetyl-imidazole
    Dimethylcarbamyl chloride

Procarcinogens That Require Metabolic Activation

Polycyclic and heterocyclic aromatic hydrocarbons
    Benz[a]anthracene
    Benzo[a]pyrene
    Dibenz[a,h] anthracene
    3-Methylcholanthrene
    7,12-Dimethylbenz[a]anthracene
Aromatic amines, amides, azo dyes
    2-Naphthylamine (β-naphthylamine)
    2-Acetylaminofluorene
    Dimethylaminoazobenzene (butter yellow)
Natural plant and microbial products
    Aflatoxin B1
    Griseofulvin
    Betel nuts
Others
    Nitrosamine and amides
    Vinyl chloride, nickel, chromium
    Insecticides, fungicides
    Polychlorinated biphenyls (PCBs)
    Arsenic
    Asbestos

them are cancer chemotherapeutic drugs (e.g., alkylating agents) that have successfully cured, controlled, or delayed recurrence of certain types of cancer (e.g., leukemia, lymphoma, Hodgkin disease, and ovarian carcinoma), only to evoke later a second form of cancer, usually leukemia. This situation is even more tragic when their initial use has been for non-neoplastic disorders, such as rheumatoid arthritis or Wegener granulomatosis. The risk of induced cancer is low, but the fact that it exists dictates judicious use of such agents.

INDIRECT-ACTING AGENTS

The designation *indirect-acting agent* refers to chemicals that require metabolic conversion before they become active. Some of the most potent indirect chemical carcinogens—the polycyclic hydrocarbons—are present in fossil fuels. Benz[a]anthracene produces cancer wherever it is applied:

When painted on the skin, it induces skin cancers; when injected subcutaneously, it induces fibrosarcomas. Polycyclic agents also are produced in the combustion of organic substances. For example, benzo[a]pyrene and other carcinogens are formed in the high-temperature combustion of tobacco in cigarette smoking. *These products are implicated in the causation of lung cancer in cigarette smokers.* Polycyclic hydrocarbons also may be produced from animal fats during the process of broiling meats and are present in smoked meats and fish. The principal active products in many hydrocarbons are epoxides, which form covalent adducts (addition products) with molecules in the cell, principally DNA, but also with RNA and proteins.

The aromatic amines and azo dyes are another class of indirect agents. Before its carcinogenicity was recognized, β-naphthylamine was responsible for a 50-fold increased incidence of bladder cancers in heavily exposed workers in the aniline dye and rubber industries. Many other occupational carcinogens are listed in Table 6–3. Some of the azo dyes were developed to color food (e.g., butter-yellow to make margarine more enticing and scarlet-red for maraschino cherries). What price aesthetics? Because many chemical carcinogens require metabolic activation for their conversion to DNA-damaging agents, much interest is focused on the enzymatic pathways that are involved. In particular, the cytochrome P-450–dependent monooxygenases are involved in generating mutagenic intermediates from many carcinogens. The genes that encode these enzymes are polymorphic, and enzyme activity varies among different individuals. It is suspected that the susceptibility to chemical carcinogenesis depends at least in part on the specific allelic form of the enzyme inherited. This and similar observations suggest that it may be possible in the future to assess cancer risk in a given individual by genetic analysis of such enzyme polymorphisms.

A few other agents merit brief mention. Nitrosamines and nitrosamides have aroused great concern because of the evidence that they can be formed endogenously in the acidic environment of the stomach. Various amines derived from food may undergo nitrosylation with nitrites that have been added to food as preservatives or derived from nitrates by bacterial action. Nitroso compounds also are present in tobacco smoke and after absorption could lead to cancers in a variety of organs. Aflatoxin B_1 is of interest because it is a naturally occurring agent produced by some strains of *Aspergillus*, a mold that grows on improperly stored grains and nuts. There is a *strong correlation between the dietary level of this food contaminant and the incidence of hepatocellular carcinoma in some parts of Africa and the Far East.* There also is a correlation between the prevalence of infection with HBV and hepatocellular carcinoma. Aflatoxin and HBV may act in concert to produce hepatic cancers (Chapter 16). Saccharin and cyclamates have been incriminated as carcinogens in experimental animals, but because induction of cancer with these artificial sweeteners requires extremely large doses, their role in human carcinogenesis remains in doubt. Finally, vinyl chloride, arsenic, nickel, chromium, insecticides, fungicides, and polychlorinated biphenyls (PCBs) are potential carcinogens in the workplace and about the house.

MECHANISMS OF ACTION OF CHEMICAL CARCINOGENS

Because malignant transformation results from mutations that affect protooncogenes and cancer suppressor genes, it should come as no surprise that most chemical carcinogens are mutagenic. Although any gene may be the target of chemical carcinogens, *RAS* gene mutations are particularly common in several chemically induced cancers in rodents. Among tumor suppressor genes, *TP53* is an important target. Specific chemical carcinogens, such as aflatoxin B_1, produce characteristic mutations in the *TP53* gene. The association is sufficiently strong to incriminate aflatoxin, if the analysis of the *TP53* gene reveals the *signature* mutation. These associations are proving useful tools in epidemiologic studies of chemical carcinogenesis.

It was mentioned earlier that carcinogenicity of some chemicals is augmented by subsequent administration of *promoters* (e.g., phorbol esters, hormones, phenols, and drugs) that by themselves are nontumorigenic. To be effective, repeated or sustained exposure to the promoter must *follow* the application of the mutagenic chemical, or *initiator.* The initiation-promotion sequence of chemical carcinogenesis raises an important question: Since promoters are not mutagenic, how do they contribute to tumorigenesis? Although the effects of tumor promoters are pleiotropic, *induction of cell proliferation is a sine qua non of tumor promotion.* Tetra-decanoylphorbol-acetate (TPA), a phorbol ester and the best-studied tumor promoter, is a powerful activator of protein kinase C, an enzyme that is a crucial component of several signal transduction pathways, including those activated by growth factors. TPA also causes growth factor secretion by some cells. It seems most likely that while the application of an initiator may cause the mutational activation of an oncogene such as *RAS*, subsequent application of promoters leads to clonal expansion of initiated (mutated) cells. Such cells (especially after *RAS* activation) have reduced growth factor requirements and may be less responsive to growth-inhibitory signals in their extracellular milieu. Forced to proliferate, the initiated clone of cells suffers additional mutations, developing eventually into a malignant tumor.

The concept that sustained cell proliferation increases the risk of mutagenesis, and hence neoplastic transformation, is also applicable to human carcinogenesis. For example, pathologic hyperplasia of the endometrium (Chapter 19) and increased regenerative activity that accompanies chronic liver cell injury are associated with the development of cancer in these organs. The influence of estrogens on the occurrence of breast cancers may relate in part to the proliferative effects of estrogen on mammary ductal epithelium. The fact that many breast cancers express estrogen receptors and benefit from estrogen receptor antagonists supports a role for estrogen in breast cancer (Chapter 19).

It must be emphasized that carcinogen-induced damage to DNA does not necessarily lead to initiation of cancer. Several forms of DNA damage (incurred spontaneously or through the action of carcinogens) can be repaired by cellular enzymes. Were this not the case, the incidence of environmentally induced cancer in all likelihood would be much higher. This is best exemplified by the rare hereditary disorders of

DNA repair, including xeroderma pigmentosum, which is associated with defective DNA repair and a greatly increased risk of cancers induced by UV light and certain chemicals.

Radiation Carcinogenesis

Radiation, whatever its source—UV rays of sunlight, x-rays, nuclear fission, radionuclides—is an established carcinogen. The evidence is so voluminous that only a few examples are given. Many of the pioneers in the development of roentgen rays developed skin cancers. Miners of radioactive elements have suffered a ten-fold increased incidence of lung cancers. Follow-up of survivors of the atomic bombs dropped on Hiroshima and Nagasaki disclosed a markedly increased incidence of leukemia—principally acute and chronic myelocytic leukemia—after an average latent period of about 7 years. Decades later, the leukemia risk for individuals heavily exposed is still above the level for control populations, as is the mortality rate from thyroid, breast, colon, and pulmonary carcinomas and others. The nuclear power accident at Chernobyl in the former Soviet Union continues to exact its toll in the form of high cancer incidence in the surrounding areas. Even therapeutic irradiation has been documented to be carcinogenic. Papillary thyroid cancers have developed in approximately 9% of individuals exposed during infancy and childhood to head and neck irradiation (Chapter 20).

It is abundantly clear that radiation is strongly oncogenic. This effect of ionizing radiation is related to its mutagenic effects; it causes chromosome breakage, translocations, and, less frequently, point mutations. Biologically, double-stranded DNA breaks seem to be the most important for radiation carcinogenesis. There also is some evidence that nonlethal doses of radiation may induce genomic instability, favoring carcinogenesis. Because the latent period of irradiation-associated cancers is extremely long, it seems that cancers emerge only after the progeny of initially damaged cells accumulate additional mutations, induced possibly by other environmental factors.

The oncogenic effect of UV rays merits special mention because it highlights the importance of DNA repair in carcinogenesis. Natural UV radiation derived from the sun can cause skin cancers (melanomas, squamous cell carcinomas, and basal cell carcinomas). At greatest risk are fair-skinned people who live in locales that receive a great deal of sunlight. Cancers of the exposed skin are particularly common in Australia and New Zealand. Nonmelanoma skin cancers are associated with total cumulative exposure to UV radiation, whereas melanomas are associated with intense intermittent exposure—as occurs with sunbathing. UV light has several biologic effects on cells. Of particular relevance to carcinogenesis is the ability to damage DNA by forming pyrimidine dimers. This type of DNA damage is repaired by a complex set of proteins that effect nucleotide excision repair. With extensive exposure to UV light, the repair systems may be overwhelmed, and skin cancer results. The importance of nucleotide excision repair is illustrated dramatically in an inherited disease called *xeroderma pigmentosum*. In these individuals, *the nucleotide excision repair mechanism is defective or deficient*, and there is a greatly increased predisposition to skin cancers. UV light charac-

teristically causes mutations in the *TP53* gene. Three other disorders of DNA repair and genomic instability—ataxia-telangiectasia, Fanconi anemia, and Bloom syndrome—also are characterized by an increased risk of cancer, related to some inability to repair environmentally induced DNA damage. These disorders were discussed earlier.

Viral and Microbial Oncogenesis

Many DNA and RNA viruses have proved to be oncogenic in animals as disparate as frogs and primates. Despite intense scrutiny, however, only a few viruses have been linked with human cancer. Our discussion focuses on human oncogenic viruses. Also discussed is the emerging role of *Helicobacter pylori* in gastric cancer.

RNA ONCOGENIC VIRUSES

The study of oncogenic retroviruses in animals has provided spectacular insights into the genetic basis of cancer. Animal retroviruses transform cells by two mechanisms. Some, called *acute transforming viruses*, contain a transforming viral oncogene (v-onc), such as V-SRC, V-ABL, or V-MYB. Others, called *slow transforming viruses* (e.g., mouse mammary tumor virus), do not contain a v-onc, but the proviral DNA is always found inserted near a cellular oncogene. Under the influence of a strong retroviral promoter, the adjacent normal or mutated cellular oncogene is overexpressed. This mechanism of transformation is called *insertional mutagenesis*. With this brief summary of retroviral oncogenesis in animals, we can turn to the only known human retrovirus that is associated with cancer.

Human T-Cell Leukemia Virus Type 1. Human T-cell leukemia virus-1 (HTLV-1) is associated with a form of T-cell leukemia/lymphoma that is endemic in certain parts of Japan and the Caribbean basin but is found sporadically elsewhere, including the United States. Similar to the acquired immunodeficiency syndrome (AIDS) virus, HTLV-1 has tropism for CD4+ T cells, and this subset of T cells is the major target for neoplastic transformation. Human infection requires transmission of infected T cells via sexual intercourse, blood products, or breast-feeding. Leukemia develops in only about 1% of infected individuals after a long latent period of 20 to 30 years.

There is little doubt that HTLV-1 infection of T lymphocytes is necessary for leukemogenesis, but the molecular mechanisms of transformation are not clear. In contrast to acute transforming retroviruses, HTLV-1 does not contain a v-onc, and in contrast to slow transforming retroviruses, no consistent integration next to a cellular oncogene has been discovered. The genome of HTLV-1 contains, in addition to the usual retroviral genes, a unique region called *pX*. This region encodes several proteins, including one called TAX. It seems that the secrets of its transforming activity are locked in the *TAX* gene. The TAX protein can activate the transcription of several host cell genes, including genes encoding the cytokine IL-2 and its receptor and the gene for GM-CSF. In addition, TAX can repress the function of several tumor suppressor genes that control the cell cycle. These include the CDKIs *CDKN2A/p16* and *TP53*. From these and other observations the following scenario is

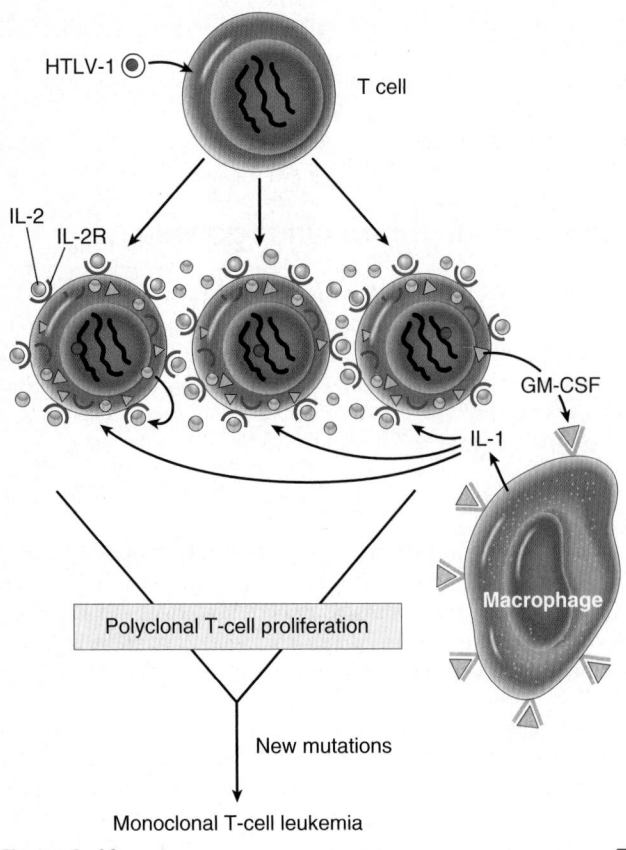

Figure 6–33 ■

Pathogenesis of human T-cell lymphotropic virus (HTLV-1)–induced T-cell leukemia/lymphoma. HTLV-1 infects many T cells and initially causes polyclonal proliferation by autocrine and paracrine pathways triggered by the *TAX* gene. Simultaneously, TAX neutralizes growth inhibitory signals by affecting *TP53* and *CDKN2A/p16* genes. Ultimately, a monoclonal T-cell leukemia/lymphoma results when one proliferating T cell suffers additional mutations.

emerging (Fig. 6–33): HTLV-1 infection stimulates proliferation of T cells. This stimulation is brought about by the *TAX* gene, which turns on genes that encode IL-2 and its receptor, setting up an autocrine system for proliferation. At the same time, a paracrine pathway is activated by the increased production of GM-CSF. By acting on neighboring macrophages, this myeloid growth factor induces increased secretion of other T-cell mitogens, such as IL-1. Acting in concert with these growth-promoting activities are inhibition of growth-suppressive pathways. Initially the T-cell proliferation is polyclonal because the virus infects many cells. The proliferating T cells are at increased risk of secondary transforming events (mutations), which lead ultimately to the outgrowth of a monoclonal neoplastic T-cell population.

DNA ONCOGENIC VIRUSES

As with RNA viruses, several oncogenic DNA viruses that cause tumors in animals have been identified. Four DNA viruses—HPV, Epstein-Barr virus (EBV) human herpesvirus 8 (HHV-8), and HBV—are of special interest because they are strongly associated with human cancer. HHV-8, also called Kaposi sarcoma herpesvirus, is discussed in Chapter 5. The others are presented here.

Human Papillomavirus (HPV)

Scores of genetically distinct types of HPV have been identified. Some types (e.g., 1, 2, 4, and 7) definitely cause benign squamous papillomas (warts) in humans (Chapters 19 and 22). HPVs also have been implicated in the genesis of several cancers, particularly squamous cell carcinoma of the cervix and anal, perianal, vulvar, and penile cancers. Emerging evidence indicates that about 20% of oropharyngeal cancers are HPV-associated. Epidemiologic studies suggest that carcinoma of the cervix is caused by a sexually transmitted agent, and HPV is strongly linked to this cancer. DNA sequences of HPV types 16 and 18 are found in 75% to 100% of invasive squamous cell cancers and their presumed precursors (i.e., severe dysplasias and carcinoma in situ). In contrast to cervical cancers, genital warts with low malignant potential are associated with distinct HPV types, predominantly HPV-6 and HPV-11.

The oncogenic potential of HPV can be related to products of two early viral genes, E6 and E7. Together, they interact with a variety of growth-regulating proteins encoded by oncogenes and tumor suppressor genes. The E7 protein binds to the retinoblastoma protein and displaces the E2F transcription factors that are normally sequestered by RB. It also inactivates the CDKIs CDKN1A/p21 and p27. E7 proteins from high-risk HPV types (types 16, 18, and 31) bind and presumably activate cyclins E and A. The E6 protein also has multiple effects. It binds to and inactivates the TP53 protein; it mediates degradation of BAX, a proapoptotic member of the *BCL2* family; and it activates telomerase.

To summarize, infection with high-risk HPV types simulates the loss of tumor suppressor genes, activates cyclins, inhibits apoptosis, and combats cellular senescence. Thus, it is evident that many of the hallmarks of cancer discussed earlier are driven by HPV proteins. Infection with HPV itself is not sufficient for carcinogenesis, however. For example, when human keratinocytes are transfected with DNA from HPV 16, 18, or 31 in vitro, they are immortalized, but they do not form tumors in experimental animals. Cotransfection with a mutated *RAS* gene results in full malignant transformation. These data strongly suggest that HPV in all likelihood acts in concert with other environmental factors (Chapter 19).

Epstein-Barr Virus (EBV)

EBV has been implicated in the pathogenesis of several human tumors: Burkitt lymphoma, post-transplant lymphoproliferative disease, primary central nervous system lymphoma in AIDS patients, a subset of other AIDS-related lymphomas, a subset of Hodgkin lymphoma, and nasopharyngeal carcinoma. Except for nasopharyngeal carcinoma, all others are B-cell tumors. A subset of T-cell lymphomas and the rare natural killer (NK) cell lymphomas also may be EBV-related.

Burkitt lymphoma is endemic in certain parts of Africa and is sporadic elsewhere. In endemic areas, tumor cells in virtually all patients carry the EBV genome. EBV exhibits strong tropism for B cells and infects many B cells, causing them to proliferate. In vitro, such infection leads to immortalization of B cells, producing lymphoblastoid cell lines. These cell lines express several EBV-encoded antigens.

The molecular basis of B-cell proliferations induced by EBV is complex. One of the EBV-encoded genes, called

LMP-1, acts as an oncogene, and its expression in transgenic mice induces B-cell lymphomas. *LMP-1* promotes B-cell proliferation by activating signaling pathways that mimic B-cell activation via the B-cell surface molecule CD40. Concurrently, *LMP-1* prevents apoptosis by activating BCL2. Another EBV-encoded gene, *EBNA-2*, transactivates several host genes, including cyclin D and the *src* family.

In immunologically normal individuals, EBV-driven polyclonal B-cell proliferation in vivo is readily controlled, and the individual either remains asymptomatic or develops a self-limited episode of infectious mononucleosis (Chapter 12). In regions of the world where Burkitt lymphoma is endemic, concomitant (endemic) malaria (or other infections) impairs immune competence, allowing sustained B-cell proliferation. In addition, the B cells do not express cell surface antigens that can be recognized by host T cells. Relieved from immunoregulation, such B cells are at increased risk of acquiring mutations, such as the t(8;14) translocation, which activates the *MYC* oncogene and is a consistent feature of this tumor. The activation of *MYC* causes further loss of growth control, and the stage is set for additional gene damage, which ultimately leads to the emergence of a monoclonal neoplasm. It should be noted that in nonendemic areas, 80% of tumors do not harbor the EBV genome, but all tumors possess the specific translocation. This fact suggests that B cells triggered by other mechanisms also may suffer similar mutations and give rise to non-African Burkitt lymphoma.

In immunosuppressed patients, including those with human immunodeficiency virus (HIV) disease and organ transplant recipients, EBV-infected B cells undergo polyclonal expansion, producing in vivo counterparts of lymphoblastoid cell lines. In contrast to tumor B cells in Burkitt lymphoma, the B lymphoblasts in immunosuppressed patients do express cell surface antigens recognized by T cells. These potentially lethal proliferations can be subdued if the immunologic status of the host improves, as may occur with withdrawal of immunosuppressive drugs in transplant recipients.

Nasopharyngeal carcinoma is endemic in southern China and some other locales, and the EBV genome is found in all tumors. As in Burkitt lymphoma, EBV acts in concert with other unidentified factors (Chapter 13).

Hepatitis B Virus (HBV)

The epidemiologic evidence linking chronic HBV infection with hepatocellular carcinoma is strong (Chapter 16), but the mode of action of the virus in tumor production is not fully elucidated. The HBV genome does not encode any transforming proteins, and there is no consistent pattern of integration in liver cells. HBV DNA is integrated, however, in 90% of patients with liver cancer who are positive for hepatitis surface B antigen, and the tumors are clonal with respect to these insertions. The oncogenic effect of HBV seems to be multifactorial. First, by causing chronic liver cell injury and accompanying regeneration, HBV predis-poses the cells to mutations, caused possibly by environmental agents (e.g., dietary toxins). Second, an HBV-encoded regulatory element called *HBx* disrupts normal growth of infected liver cells by transcriptional activation of several growth-controlling genes via the NF-κB pathway. Third, cytosolic signal transduction pathways (e.g., RAS-MAP kinase) are turned on (recall TAX proteins of HTLV-1). Whether HBx also causes inactivation of *TP53* is controversial. The role of the *HBx* gene in hepatic curcinogenesis is supported by the development of hepatocellular carcinomas in mice that are transgenic for this gene. Finally, in some patients, viral integration seems to cause secondary rearrangements of chromosomes, including multiple deletions that may harbor unknown tumor suppressor genes. Thus, it seems that virus-induced gene damage in regenerating liver cells may set the stage for multistep carcinogenesis.

Although not a DNA virus, hepatitis C virus (HCV) also is strongly linked to hepatocellular carcinoma. In general, the mechanism of HCV-related liver cancer is similar to that described for HBV. Extensive death of liver cells with their regeneration, and disruption of growth regulation are important factors. Unlike HBV, HCV does not contain the X-protein.

HELICOBACTER PYLORI

First incriminated as a cause of peptic ulcers, *H. pylori* now has acquired the dubious distinction of being blamed for causation of gastric carcinoma and gastric lymphoma. The gastric lymphomas are of B-cell origin, and because the transformed B cells normally reside in the marginal zones of lymphoid follicles, these tumors also are called MALTomas (marginal zone–associated lymphomas; Chapter 12). Their pathogenesis involves initial chronic gastritis that causes lymphoid follicles to develop in the gastric mucosa. It is thought that *H. pylori* infection leads to the formation of *H. pylori*–reactive T cells, which in turn cause polyclonal B-cell proliferations. In time, a monoclonal B-cell tumor emerges in the proliferating B cells, perhaps as a result of accumulation of mutations in growth-regulatory genes. In keeping with this, early in the course of disease, eradication of *H. pylori* "cures" the lymphoma by removing antigenic stimulus for T cells.

In addition to B-cell lymphomas, *H. pylori* has now been linked strongly to the pathogenesis of gastric epithelial cancers. Here the scenario seems to be an initial development of chronic gastritis, followed by gastric atrophy, intestinal metaplasia of the lining cells, dysplasia, and cancer. This sequence takes decades to complete and occurs in only 3% of infected patients.

Although *H. pylori* causes three diseases (peptic ulcer, gastric lymphoma, and gastric carcinoma), these conditions do not occur often in the same patient. For unknown reasons, patients who have duodenal ulcers (not gastric ulcers) almost never develop gastric carcinoma. Such exclusions are even more puzzling than the pathogenesis of *H. pylori*–linked diseases.

HOST DEFENSE AGAINST TUMORS: TUMOR IMMUNITY

Malignant transformation, as has been discussed, is associated with complex genetic alterations, some of which may result in the expression of proteins that are seen as non-self by the immune system. The idea that tumors are not entirely self was conceived by Ehrlich, who proposed that immune-mediated recognition of autologous tumor cells may be a "positive mechanism" capable of eliminating transformed cells. Subsequently, Lewis Thomas and McFarlane Burnet formalized this concept by coining the term *immune surveillance* to refer to recognition and destruction of non-self tumor cells on their appearance. The fact that cancers occur suggests that immune surveillance is imperfect; however, the fact that some tumors escape such policing does not preclude the possibility that others may have been aborted. It is necessary to explore certain questions about tumor immunity: What is the nature of tumor antigens? What host effector systems may recognize tumor cells? Is tumor immunity effective against spontaneous neoplasms?

Tumor Antigens

Antigens that elicit an immune response have been shown in many experimentally induced tumors and in human cancers. They can be classified broadly into two categories: tumor-specific antigens, which are present only on tumor cells and not on any normal cells, and tumor-associated antigens, which are present on tumor cells and on some normal cells. Experimental studies in murine models and the study of tumor-infiltrating lymphocytes in humans have revealed an important role for CD8+ cytotoxic T cells (CTLs) in tumor immunity. As is well known, CTLs recognize peptide antigens presented on the cell surface by major histocompatibility complex (MHC) class I molecules. The nature of tumor antigens recognized by CTLs is illustrated in Figure 6–34 and described next.

Cancer-Testis Antigens. These antigens are encoded by genes that are silent in all adult tissues except the testis—hence their name. Although the protein is present in the testis, it is not expressed on the cell surface because sperms do not express MHC I antigens. Thus, for all practical purposes, these antigens are tumor specific. Prototypic of this group is the MAGE family of genes. Although they are tumor specific, MAGE antigens are not unique for individual tumors. MAGE-1 is expressed on 37% of melanomas and a variable number of lung, liver, stomach, and esophageal carcinomas. Similar antigens called GAGE, BAGE, and RAGE have been detected in other tumors.

Tissue-Specific Antigens. Antigens in this category are best considered differentiation-specific antigens, and they are expressed on tumor cells and their untransformed counterparts. Such antigens include melanocyte-specific proteins such as MART-1, gp100, and tyrosinase. Peptides derived from these are expressed on normal melanocytes and melanomas. Thus, cytotoxic T cells directed against these antigens would destroy not only melanoma cells but also normal melanin-containing cells. Because melanin is present in retina and brain, such immunization has to be considered carefully.

Antigens Resulting From Mutational Change in Proteins. Antigens in this category are derived from mutant oncoproteins and cancer suppressor proteins. Unique tumor antigens arise from products of β-catenin, RAS, TP53, and CDK4 genes, which frequently are mutated in tumors. Because the mutant proteins are present only in tumors, their peptides are expressed only in tumor cells. Because many tumors may carry the same mutation, however, such antigens are shared by different tumors. Although cytotoxic T cells can be induced against such antigens, they do not give rise to spontaneous responses in vivo.

Overexpressed Antigens. These tumor antigens are products of normal genes that are overexpressed because of gene amplification or other mechanisms. To this category belongs the HER-2 (neu) protein, which is overexpressed in 30% of breast and ovarian cancers. Although present in normal ovarian and breast cells, its level is generally too low for T-cell recognition.

Viral Antigens. Antigens derived from oncogenic viruses such as HPV and EBV can be targeted by CD8+ T cells. Such tumor antigens are shared between all tumors of similar type in different patients. They can be effective targets for immunotherapy because they are not expressed in normal cells.

Other Tumor Antigens. *Mucins* can give rise to tumor-specific antigens. In some cancers, such as those derived from pancreas, ovary, and breast, underglycosylation of mucins generates epitopes that previously were masked by carbohydrates. Therefore, these antigens, for all practical purposes, are tumor specific. To this group belongs the MUC-1 antigen.

Oncofetal Antigens. Oncofetal antigens or embryonic antigens, such as carcinoembryonic antigen (CEA) and α-fetoprotein, are expressed during embryogenesis but not in normal adult tissues. Derepression of the genes that encode these causes their reexpression in colon and liver cancers. Antibodies can be raised against these, and they are useful for detection of oncofetal antigens. These antigens serve as serum markers for cancer.

Differentiation-Specific Antigens. Differentiation-specific antigens, such as CD10 and prostate-specific antigen (PSA), are expressed on neoplastic and normal B cells and on benign and malignant prostatic epithelium, respectively. These serve mainly as diagnostic markers for the type of cell involved in transformation.

Antitumor Effector Mechanisms

Cell-mediated and humoral immunity can have antitumor activity. The cellular effectors that mediate immunity were described in Chapter 5, so it is necessary here only to characterize them briefly (Fig. 6–35).

■ *Cytotoxic T lymphocytes.* The role of specifically sensitized cytotoxic T cells in experimentally induced tumors is well established. In humans, they seem to play a protective role, chiefly against virus-associated neoplasms (e.g., EBV-induced Burkitt lymphoma and HPV-induced tumors). The presence of MHC-restricted CD8+ cells that can kill autologous tumor cells within human tumors suggests that the role of T cells in immunity against human tumors may be broader than previously suspected. They recognize antigens described earlier. In some cases, such CD8+ T cells do not develop spontaneously in vivo but can be generated by immunization with tumor antigen–pulsed dendritic cells.

■ *Natural killer cells.* NK cells are lymphocytes that are capable of destroying tumor cells without prior sensitization; they may provide the first line of defense against tu-

NORMAL CELL　　　　　**TUMOR CELL**

Figure 6–34   ■

A–E, Molecular mechanisms underlying formation of tumor antigens recognized by CD8+ T cells.

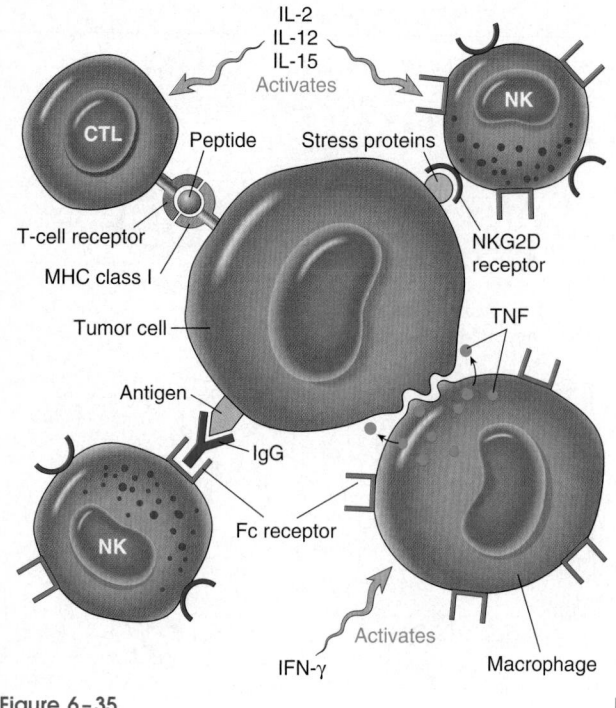

Figure 6-35 ■

Cellular effectors of antitumor immunity and some cytokines that modulate antitumor activities. The nature of antigen recognized by T cells is depicted in Figure 6–34. CTL, cytotoxic T cell; IFN, interferon; MHC, major histocompatibility complex; NK, natural killer; TNF, tumor necrosis factor.

mor cells. After activation with IL-2, NK cells can lyse a wide range of human tumors, including many that seem to be nonimmunogenic for T cells. T cells and NK cells seem to provide complementary antitumor mechanisms. Tumors that fail to express MHC class I antigens cannot be recognized by T cells, but these tumors may trigger NK cells because the latter are inhibited by recognition of normal autologous class I molecules (see Fig. 5–4). The triggering receptors on NK cells are extremely diverse and belong to several gene families. NKG2D proteins expressed on NK cells and some T cells are important triggering receptors. They recognize stress-induced antigens that are expressed mainly on tumor cells. There is some evidence in mice that blocking the NKG2D receptors renders animals more susceptible to carcinogens. In addition to direct lysis of tumor cells, NK cells can also participate in antibody-dependent cellular cytotoxicity, as described in Chapter 5.

■ *Macrophages.* Activated macrophages exhibit selective cytotoxicity against tumor cells in vitro. T cells, NK cells, and macrophages may collaborate in antitumor reactivity because interferon-γ, a cytokine secreted by T cells and NK cells, is a potent activator of macrophages. These cells may kill tumors by mechanisms similar to those used to kill microbes (e.g., production of reactive oxygen metabolites; Chapter 2) or by secretion of tumor necrosis factor (TNF). In addition to its many other effects, this cytokine is lytic for several tumor cells.

■ *Humoral mechanisms.* These may participate in tumor cell destruction by two mechanisms: (1) activation of

complement and (2) induction of antibody-dependent cellular cytotoxicity by NK cells.

Immunosurveillance

Given the host of possible and potential antitumor mechanisms, is there any evidence that they operate in vivo to prevent the emergence of neoplasms? The strongest argument for the existence of immunosurveillance is the increased frequency of cancers in immunodeficient hosts. About 5% of individuals with congenital immunodeficiencies develop cancers, a rate that is about 200 times that for individuals without such immunodeficiencies. Analogously, immunosuppressed transplant recipients and patients with AIDS have increased numbers of malignancies. It should be noted that most (but not all) of these neoplasms are lymphomas, often lymphomas of activated B cells. Particularly illustrative is X-linked lymphoproliferative disorder. When affected boys develop an EBV infection, such infection does not take the usual self-limited form of infectious mononucleosis but instead evolves into a chronic or sometimes fatal form of infectious mononucleosis or, even worse, malignant lymphoma.

Most cancers occur in individuals who do not suffer from any overt immunodeficiency. If immunosurveillance exists, how do cancers evade the immune system in immunocompetent hosts? Several escape mechanisms have been proposed:

■ *Selective outgrowth of antigen-negative variants.* During tumor progression, strongly immunogenic subclones may be eliminated.

■ *Loss or reduced expression of histocompatibility antigens.* Tumor cells may fail to express normal levels of human leukocyte antigen (HLA) class I, escaping attack by cytotoxic T cells. Such cells, however, may trigger NK cells.

■ *Lack of costimulation.* Sensitization of T cells requires two signals, one by foreign peptide presented by MHC and the other by costimulatory molecules (Chapter 5); although tumor cells may express peptide antigens with class I molecules, they often do not express costimulatory molecules, such as B7-1. This not only prevents sensitization but also may render T cells anergic or cause them to undergo apoptosis. To bypass this problem, attempts are being made to immunize cancer patients with autologous tumor cells transfected with B7-1. In another approach, dendritic cells, known to express high levels of costimulatory molecules, are pulsed with tumor peptides and infused into the patient.

■ *Immunosuppression.* Many oncogenic agents (e.g., chemicals and ionizing radiation) suppress host immune responses. Tumors or tumor products also may be immunosuppressive. For example, transforming growth factor (TGF)-β, secreted in large quantities by many tumors, is a potent immunosuppressant. In some cases, the immune response induced by the tumor (e.g., activation of regulatory T cells) may inhibit tumor immunity. Another clever mechanism used by tumors is to express Fas ligand, which engages Fas on the surface of T cells and sends a death signal to the immune cells.

CLINICAL FEATURES OF NEOPLASIA

Ultimately the importance of neoplasms lies in their effects on people. Any tumor, even a benign one, may cause morbidity and mortality. Every new growth requires careful appraisal as to whether it is cancerous. This differentiation comes into sharpest focus with lumps in the female breast. Cancers and many benign disorders of the female breast present as palpable masses. Benign lesions are more common than cancers. Although clinical evaluation may suggest one or the other, "the only unequivocally benign breast mass is the excised and anatomically diagnosed one"; this is equally true of all neoplasms. There are, however, instances when adherence to this dictum must be tempered by clinical judgment. Subcutaneous lipomas, for example, are quite common and are readily recognized by their soft, yielding consistency. Unless they are uncomfortable, subject to trauma, or aesthetically disturbing, small lesions often are merely observed for significant increase in size. A few other examples might be cited, but it suffices to say that *with a few exceptions, all masses require anatomic evaluation*. In addition to the concern malignant neoplasms arouse, even benign lesions may have many adverse effects. The following discussion considers (1) the effects of a tumor on the host, (2) the grading and clinical staging of cancer, and (3) the laboratory diagnosis of neoplasms.

Effects of Tumor on Host

Cancers are far more threatening to the host than benign tumors are. Nonetheless, both types of neoplasia may cause problems because of location and impingement on adjacent structures, effects on functional activity such as hormone synthesis, and production of bleeding and secondary infections when the lesion ulcerates through adjacent natural surfaces. Cancers also may be responsible for cachexia (wasting) or paraneoplastic syndromes.

Location is crucial in benign and malignant tumors. A small (1-cm) pituitary adenoma can compress and destroy the surrounding normal gland and give rise to hypopituitarism. A 0.5-cm leiomyoma in the wall of the renal artery may lead to renal ischemia and serious hypertension. A comparably small carcinoma within the common bile duct may induce fatal biliary tract obstruction.

Hormone production is seen with benign and malignant neoplasms arising in endocrine glands. Adenomas and carcinomas arising in the β cells of the islets of the pancreas often produce hyperinsulinism, sometimes fatal. Analogously, some adenomas and carcinomas of the adrenal cortex elaborate corticosteroids that affect the patient (e.g., aldosterone, which induces sodium retention, hypertension,

and hypokalemia). Such hormonal activity is more likely with a well-differentiated benign tumor than with a corresponding carcinoma.

Ulceration through a surface with consequent bleeding or secondary infection needs no further comment, but a few less obvious ramifications can be mentioned. The benign or malignant neoplasm that protrudes into the gut lumen may get caught in the peristaltic pull to telescope the neoplasm and its site of origin into the down-stream segment of gut—intussusception (Chapter 15)—leading to ulceration of the mucosa or, even worse, intestinal obstruction or infarction.

CANCER CACHEXIA

Many cancer patients suffer progressive loss of body fat and lean body mass, accompanied by profound weakness, anorexia, and anemia. This wasting syndrome is referred to as *cachexia*. Usually an intercurrent infection brings an end to the slow deterioration. There is in general some correlation between the size and extent of spread of the cancer and the severity of the cachexia. Small, localized cancers are generally silent and produce no cachexia, but there are many exceptions.

The origins of cancer cachexia are multifactorial. Anorexia is a common problem in patients who have cancer, even those who do not have tumors of the gastrointestinal tract. Reduced food intake has been related to abnormalities in taste and in the central control of appetite, but reduced calorie intake is not sufficient to explain the cachexia of malignancy. In patients with cancer, calorie expenditure remains high, and basal metabolic rate is increased, despite reduced food intake. This is in contrast to the lower metabolic rate that occurs as an adaptational response in starvation. The basis of these metabolic abnormalities is not fully understood. Perhaps circulating factors such as TNF and IL-1, released from activated macrophages, are involved. TNF suppresses appetite and inhibits the action of lipoprotein lipase, inhibiting the release of free fatty acids from lipoproteins. A protein-mobilizing factor that causes breakdown of skeletal muscle proteins by the ubiquitin-proteosome pathway has been detected in the serum of cancer patients. In healthy animals, injection of this material causes acute weight loss without causing anorexia. Other molecules with lipolytic action also have been found. There is no satisfactory treatment for cancer cachexia other than removal of the underlying cause, the tumor.

PARANEOPLASTIC SYNDROMES

Symptom complexes other than cachexia that occur in patients with cancer and that cannot be readily explained by local or distant spread of the tumor or by the elaboration of hormones indigenous to the tissue of origin of the tumor are referred to as *paraneoplastic syndromes*. They appear in 10% to 15% of patients with cancer, and it is important to recognize them for several reasons:

- They may represent the earliest manifestation of an occult neoplasm.
- In affected patients, they may represent significant clinical problems and may be lethal.

■

Table 6–6. SOME PARANEOPLASTIC SYNDROMES

Clinical Syndromes	Major Forms of Underlying Cancer	Causal Mechanisms
Endocrinopathies		
Cushing syndrome	Small cell cancer of the lung Pancreatic carcinoma Neural tumors	ACTH or ACTH-like substance
Syndrome of inappropriate ADH secretion	Small cell carcinoma of lung Intracranial neoplasms	ADH or atrial natriuretic factor
Hypercalcemia	Squamous cell carcinoma of lung Breast carcinoma Renal carcinoma	PTHrP, TGF-α, vitamin D
Carcinoid syndrome	Bronchial carcinoid Pancreatic carcinoma Gastric carcinoma	Serotonin, bradykinin, histamine (?)
Polycythemia	Renal carcinoma Cerebellar hemangioma Hepatocellular carcinoma	Erythropoietin
Nerve and Muscle Syndromes		
Disorders of the central and peripheral nervous systems	Small cell carcinoma of lung Breast carcinoma	Immunologic (?), toxic (?)
Myasthenia gravis	Thymoma	Immunologic (?)
Osseous, Articular, and Soft Tissue Changes		
Hypertrophic osteoarthropathy and clubbing of the fingers	Carcinoma of lung	Unknown
Vascular and Hematologic Changes		
Venous thrombosis (Trousseau phenomenon)	Pancreatic carcinoma Lung carcinoma Other cancers	Hypercoagulability
Nonbacterial thrombotic endocarditis	Advanced cancers	Hypercoagulability

ACTH, adrenocorticotropic hormone; ADH, antidiuretic hormone; PTHrP, parathyroid hormone–related protein; TGF-α, transforming growth factor α.

■ They may mimic metastatic disease and confound treatment.

The paraneoplastic syndromes are diverse and are associated with many different tumors (Table 6–6). The most common syndromes are hypercalcemia, Cushing syndrome, and nonbacterial thrombotic endocarditis; the neoplasms most often associated with these and other syndromes are bronchogenic and breast cancers and hematologic malignancies. Cushing syndrome as a paraneoplastic phenomenon is usually related to ectopic production by the cancer of ACTH or ACTH-like polypeptides. The mediation of hypercalcemia, another common paraneoplastic syndrome, is multifactorial. Perhaps the most important factor is the synthesis of a parathyroid hormone–related protein (PTHrP) by tumor cells, especially squamous cell carcinomas of the lung. Although structurally PTHrP resembles parathyroid hormone, it can be distinguished from it by specific assays. Also implicated are other tumor-derived factors, such as TGF-α, a polypeptide factor that activates osteoclasts, and the active form of vitamin D. Another possible mechanism for hypercalcemia is widespread osteolytic metastatic disease of bone, but *it should be noted that hypercalcemia resulting from skeletal metastases is not a paraneoplastic syndrome.* Sometimes one tumor induces several syndromes concurrently. For example, bronchogenic carcinomas may elaborate products identical to or having the effects of ACTH, antidiuretic hormone, parathyroid hormone, serotonin, human chorionic gonadotropin, and other bioactive substances.

Paraneoplastic syndromes may take many other forms, such as hypercoagulability leading to venous thrombosis and nonbacterial thrombotic endocarditis (Chapter 11) or the development of clubbing of the fingers and hypertrophic osteoarthropathy in patients with lung carcinomas (Chapter 13). Still others are discussed in the consideration of cancers of the various organs of the body.

Grading and Staging of Cancer

Methods to quantify the probable clinical aggressiveness of a given neoplasm and to express its apparent extent and spread in the individual patient are necessary for comparisons of end results of various forms of treatment. For instance, the results of treating extremely small, highly differentiated thyroid adenocarcinomas that are localized to the thyroid gland are likely to be different from those obtained from treating highly anaplastic thyroid cancers that have invaded the neck organs.

The *grading* of a cancer attempts to establish some estimate of its aggressiveness or level of malignancy based on the cytologic differentiation of tumor cells and the number of mitoses within the tumor. The cancer may be classified as grade I, II, III, or IV, in order of increasing anaplasia. Criteria for the individual grades vary with each form of neoplasia and so are not detailed here. Difficulties in establishing clear-cut criteria have led in some instances to descriptive characterizations (e.g., "well-differentiated adenocarcinoma with no evidence of vascular or lymphatic invasion" or "highly anaplastic sarcoma with extensive vascular invasion").

Staging of cancers is based on the size of the primary lesion, its extent of spread to regional lymph nodes, and the presence or absence of metastases. This assessment is usually based on clinical and radiographic examination (computed tomography and magnetic resonance imaging) and in some cases surgical exploration. Two methods of staging are currently in use: the TNM system (*T*, primary tumor; *N*, regional lymph node involvement; *M*, metastases) and the AJC (American Joint Committee) system. In the TNM system, T1, T2, T3, and T4 describe the increasing size of the primary lesion; N0, N1, N2, and N3 indicate progressively advancing node involvement; and M0 and M1 reflect the absence or presence of distant metastases. In the AJC method, the cancers are divided into stages 0 to IV, incorporating the size of primary lesions and the presence of nodal spread and of distant metastases. Examples of the application of these two staging systems are cited in subsequent chapters. It is worth noting that *when compared with grading, staging has proved to be of greater clinical value.*

Laboratory Diagnosis of Cancer

MORPHOLOGIC METHODS

In most instances, the laboratory diagnosis of cancer is not difficult. The two ends of the benign-malignant spectrum pose no problems; however, in the middle lies a "no man's land" where the wise tread cautiously. Clinicians tend to underestimate the contributions they make to the diagnosis of a neoplasm. Clinical data are invaluable for optimal pathologic diagnosis. Radiation-induced changes in the skin or mucosa can be similar to those of cancer. Sections taken from a healing fracture can mimic an osteosarcoma. The laboratory evaluation of a lesion can be only as good as the specimen submitted for examination. The specimen must be adequate, representative, and properly preserved.

Several sampling approaches are available, including excision or biopsy, fine-needle aspiration, and cytologic smears. When excision of a lesion is not possible, selection of an appropriate site for biopsy of a large mass requires awareness that the margins may not be representative and the center may be largely necrotic. Analogously with disseminated lymphoma (i.e., involving many nodes), nodes in the inguinal region that drain large areas of the body often undergo reactive changes that may mask neoplastic involvement. Requesting *frozen-section* diagnosis is sometimes desirable, as, for example, in determining the nature of a breast lesion or in evaluating the margins of an excised cancer to ascertain that the entire neoplasm has been removed. This method, in which a sample is quick-frozen and sectioned, permits histologic evaluation within minutes. With a breast biopsy, for example, frozen-section diagnosis allows determination of whether the

lesion is malignant and may require wider excision or sampling of axillary nodes for possible spread. The patient is spared the expense and trauma of a subsequent operation. In experienced, competent hands, frozen-section diagnosis is accurate, but there are particular instances in which the better histologic detail provided by the more time-consuming routine methods is needed. In such instances, it is better to wait a few days, despite the drawbacks, than to perform inadequate or unnecessary surgery.

Fine-needle aspiration of tumors is another approach that is growing in popularity. It involves aspiration of cells from a mass, followed by cytologic examination of the smear. This procedure is employed most commonly with readily palpable lesions affecting the breast, thyroid, lymph nodes, and salivary glands. Modern imaging techniques enable the method to be extended to deeper structures, such as the liver, pancreas, and pelvic lymph nodes. It obviates surgery and its attendant risks. Although it entails some difficulties, such as small sample size and sampling errors, in experienced hands it can be extremely reliable, rapid, and useful.

Cytologic (Papanicolaou) smears provide another method for the detection of cancer. This approach is used widely for the discovery of carcinoma of the cervix, often at an in situ stage, but it also is used with many other forms of suspected malignancy, such as endometrial carcinoma, bronchogenic carcinoma, bladder and prostate tumors, and gastric carcinomas; for the identification of tumor cells in abdominal, pleural, joint, and cerebrospinal fluids; and, less commonly, with other forms of neoplasia. Neoplastic cells are less cohesive than others and so are shed into fluids or secretions (Fig. 6–36). The shed cells are evaluated for features of anaplasia indicative of their origin in cancer. The gratifying control of cervical cancer is the best testament to the value of the cytologic method.

Immunocytochemistry offers a powerful adjunct to routine histology. Detection of cytokeratin by specific monoclonal antibodies labeled with peroxidase points to a diagnosis of undifferentiated carcinoma rather than large cell lymphoma. Similarly, detection of prostate-specific antigen (PSA) in metastatic deposits by immunohistochemistry allows definitive diagnosis of a primary tumor in the prostate. Immunocytochemical detection of estrogen receptors and HER-2 (neu) allows prognostication and directs therapeutic intervention in breast cancers.

Flow cytometry now is used routinely in the classification of leukemias and lymphomas. In this method, fluorescent antibodies against cell surface molecules and differentiation antigens are employed to obtain the phenotype of malignant cells. Flow cytometry also is useful in assessing DNA content of the tumor cells. In many tumors, DNA content (ploidy) has a bearing on prognosis.

BIOCHEMICAL ASSAYS

Biochemical assays for tumor-associated enzymes, hormones, and other tumor markers in the blood cannot be construed as modalities for the diagnosis of cancer; however, they contribute to finding cases and in some instances are useful in determining the effectiveness of therapy. The application of these assays is considered with many of the specific forms of neoplasia discussed in other chapters, so

Figure 6-36 ■

A, Normal Papanicolaou smear from the uterine cervix. Large, flat cells with small nuclei. *B,* Abnormal smear containing a sheet of malignant cells with large, hyperchromatic nuclei. There is nuclear pleomorphism, and one cell is in mitosis. There are few interspersed neutrophils with compact lobated nuclei and much smaller size. (Courtesy of Dr. Richard M. DeMay, Department of Pathology, University of Chicago, Chicago.)

only a few examples suffice here. Prostatic carcinoma can be suspected when elevated levels of PSA are found in the blood. The levels also may be elevated in benign prostatic hyperplasia, and elevations in PSA are not diagnostic of an underlying cancer (Chapter 18). Radioimmunoassays for circulating hormones may point to the presence of tumors in the endocrine system and in some instances to the ectopic production of hormones by nonendocrine tumors.

A host of circulating tumor markers have been described, and new ones are identified every year. Only a few have stood the test of time and proved to be clinically useful. The two best established are CEA and α-fetoprotein. CEA, normally produced in embryonic tissue of the gut, pancreas, and liver, is a complex glycoprotein that is elaborated by many different neoplasms. Depending on the serum level adopted as representative of a significant elevation, CEA is variously reported to be positive in 60% to 90% of colorectal carcinomas, 50% to 80% of pancreatic cancers, and 25% to 50% of gastric and breast tumors. Much less consistently, elevated CEA levels have been described in other forms of cancer. In almost all types of neoplasia, the level of elevation is correlated with the body burden of tumor so

that the highest levels are found in patients with advanced metastatic disease. CEA elevations also have been reported in many benign disorders, however, such as alcoholic cirrhosis, hepatitis, ulcerative colitis, and Crohn disease. Occasionally, levels of this antigen are elevated in apparently healthy smokers. *Thus, CEA assays lack specificity and sensitivity required for the detection of early cancers.* They are still useful, however, in providing presumptive evidence of the possibility of colorectal carcinoma because this tumor yields the highest CEA levels; these assays are particularly useful in the detection of recurrences after excision. With successful resection of the tumor, CEA disappears from the serum; its reappearance almost always signifies the beginning of the end (Chapter 15).

The other well-established tumor marker is α-fetoprotein. Elevated circulating levels are encountered in adults with cancers arising principally in the liver and from yolk sac remnants in the gonads. Less regularly, it is elevated in teratocarcinomas and embryonal cell carcinomas of the testis, ovary, and extragonadal sites and occasionally in cancers of the stomach and pancreas. As with CEA, benign conditions, including cirrhosis, hepatitis, and pregnancy (especially with fetal distress or death), may cause modest elevations of α-fetoprotein. There is then a problem with specificity and sensitivity, but the marker still may provide presumptive evidence of, for example, a hepatocellular carcinoma and is of value in the follow-up of therapeutic interventions. More details are found in Chapter 16. This cursory overview suffices to indicate the many laboratory approaches in use for the detection and diagnosis of tumors.

MOLECULAR DIAGNOSIS

An increasing number of molecular techniques are being used for the diagnosis of tumors and for predicting their behavior. Because each T and B cell has unique rearrangement of its antigen receptor genes, polymerase chain reaction (PCR)-based detection of T-cell receptor or immunoglobulin genes allows distinction between monoclonal (neoplastic) and polyclonal (reactive) proliferations. PCR-based detection of *BCR-ABL* transcripts provides a molecular signature of chronic myeloid leukemia. Fluorescent in situ hybridization (FISH) technique (Chapter 7) is useful in detecting translocations characteristic of many tumors, including Ewing sarcoma and several leukemias and lymphomas. FISH and PCR methods can also be used for showing amplification of oncogenes such as *HER-2* and *N-MYC*. These oncogenes, as discussed earlier, provide prognostic information for breast cancers and neuroblastomas. Another emerging use of molecular techniques is detection of minimal residual disease after treatment. For example, detection of *BCR-ABL* transcripts by PCR gives a measure of residual leukemia in patients treated for chronic myeloid leukemia.

MOLECULAR PROFILING OF TUMORS

One of the most exciting advances in the molecular analysis of tumors has been made possible by DNA-microarray analysis. This technique allows simultaneous measurements of the expression levels of several thousand

Figure 6-37   ■

Schematic illustration of cDNA microarray analysis. mRNA is extracted from the samples, reverse transcribed to cDNA, and labeled with fluorescent molecules. In the case illustrated, red fluorescent molecules were used for normal cDNA, and green molecules were used for tumor cDNA. The labeled cDNAs are mixed and applied to a gene chip, which contains thousands of DNA probes representing known genes. The labeled cDNAs hybridize to spots that contain complementary sequences. The hybridization is detected by laser scanning of the chip, and the results are read in units of red or green fluorescence intensity. In the example shown, spot A has high red fluorescence, indicating that a greater number of cDNAs from neoplastic cells hybridized to gene A. Thus, gene A seems to be up-regulated in tumor cells. (Courtesy of Robert Anders, MD, PhD, Chief Resident, Department of Pathology, University of Chicago, Chicago.)

genes. The principle of this so-called gene chip technology is illustrated in Figure 6–37 and described briefly here.

As can be seen, the process begins by extraction of mRNA from any two sources (e.g., normal and malignant, normal and preneoplastic, or two tumors of the same histologic type). cDNA copies of the mRNA are synthesized in vitro with fluorescently labeled nucleotides. The fluorescent-labeled cDNA strands are hybridized to sequence specific DNA probes

linked to a solid support, such as a silicon chip. A 1-cm² chip can contain thousands of probes arranged in an array of columns and rows. After hybridization, high-resolution laser scanning detects fluorescent signals from each of the spots. The fluorescence intensity of each spot is proportional to the level of expression of the original mRNA used to synthesize the CDNA hybridized to that spot. For each sample, therefore, the expression level of thousands of genes is obtained, and by using bioinformatic tools, the relative levels of gene expression in different samples can be compared. In essence, a molecular profile is generated for each tissue analyzed.

Such analysis has revealed that phenotypically identical large B-cell lymphomas (Chapter 12) from different patients are heterogeneous with respect to their gene expression. Nevertheless, clusters of gene expression patterns can be detected that allow segregation of phenotypically similar tumors into distinct subcategories with dramatically different survival rates. This type of molecular profiling indicates that the currently available morphologic and molecular tools are insufficient for stratification of tumors into prognostically different subgroups. Similar analyses have been performed on breast cancers and melanomas. Although the data currently available have to be validated by analysis of a larger cohort of patients, the proof of principle has been obtained. It is extremely likely that, in the not too distant future, molecular profiling will become an adjunct in the diagnosis, classification, and management of cancer. This type of analysis also may reveal novel gene targets for tumors and development of new drugs. Therapy may be tailored to the specific genes dysregulated in a given patient. Who knows, advertisements for "designer genes" may appear side by side with ads for "designer jeans"!

BIBLIOGRAPHY

Adams JM, Cory S: Life-or-death decisions by Bcl-2 protein family. Trends Biochem Sci 26:61, 2001. (A detailed review of the role of BCL-2 family in apoptosis.)

Ahr A, et al: Identification of high risk breast cancer patients by gene expression profiling. Lancet 359:131, 2002. (A report on the power of gene chip technology to subdivide prognostically distinct subgroups of breast cancer. Also contains references to earlier reports.)

Bertram JS: The molecular biology of cancer. Mol Aspects Med 21:167, 2001. (A comprehensive, well-written review of the molecular basis of cancer with possible clinical applications of basic science.)

Brechot C, et al: Molecular basis for development of hepatitis B virus (HBV)–related hepatocellular carcinoma. Semin Cancer Biol 10:211, 2000. (An exhaustive review of molecular pathogenesis of HBV-associated liver cancer.)

Butel JS: Viral carcinogenesis: revelation of molecular mechanisms and etiology of human disease. Carcinogenesis 21:405, 2000. (An excellent and exhaustive review of the mechanisms of viral carcinogenesis and virus-associated human cancers.)

Cleaver JE: Common pathways for ultraviolet skin carcinogenesis in the repair and replication defective groups of xeroderma pigmentosum. J Dermatol Sci 23:1, 2000. (A biochemically oriented review of UV light carcinogenesis.)

Clemons M, Goss P: Estrogen and the risk of breast cancer. N Engl J Med 344:276, 2001. (A review of estrogen–breast cancer links.)

Cohen JI: Epstein-Barr virus infections. N Engl J Med 343:481, 2000. (A good molecular and clinical review of EBV-associated tumors.)

Derynck R, Akhurst RJ, Balmain A: TGFβ signalling in tumor suppression and cancer progression. Nat Genet 29:117, 2001. (A detailed discussion of the TGF-β pathway and its involvement in cancer.)

Eichhorst ST, Krammer PH: Derangement of apoptosis in cancer. Lancet 358:345, 2001. (A succinct discussion of mechanisms by which cancer cells evade apoptosis.)

Eisenhauer EA: From the molecule to the clinic—inhibiting HER-2 to beat breast cancer. N Engl J Med 344:841, 2001. (An editorial that summarizes the clinical trials with anti-*HER-2* antibody.)

Fearnhead NS, Britton MP, Bodmer WF: The ABC of APC. Hum Mol Genet 10:721, 2001. (A detailed review of the molecular basis of the *APC* tumor suppressor gene.)

Fox JG, Wang TC: *Helicobacter pylori*—not a good bug after all. N Engl J Med 345:829, 2001. (An editorial that summarizes evidence linking *H. pylori* to gastric cancer.)

Haber D: Roads leading to breast cancer. N Engl J Med 343:1566, 2000. (A succinct account of the role of DNA repair and *BRCA1* in breast cancer.)

Hanahan D, Weinberg RA: The hallmarks of cancer. Cell 100:57, 2000. (An excellent, brief account of the fundamental properties of cancer and their molecular basis. The organization of genetic changes in cancer is based on this article.)

Harari D, Yarden Y: Molecular mechanisms underlying ERBB2/HER-2 action in breast cancer. Oncogene 19:6102, 2000. (A detailed discussion of the molecular basis of *HER-2* gene actions.)

Kerbel RS: Tumor angiogenesis: past, present and the near future. Carcinogenesis 21:505, 2000. (An excellent review of angiogenesis and antiangiogenic factors with clinical implications.)

Lichtenstein P, et al: Environmental and heritable factors in causation of cancers. N Engl J Med 343:78, 2000. (A large study of twins and cancer risk from Sweden.)

Little JB: Radiation carcinogenesis. Carcinogenesis 21:397, 2000. (An update written by a pioneer in the field of radiation injury.)

Lui Y, Kulesz-Martin M: TP53 protein at the hub of cellular DNA damage response pathways through sequence-specific and non–sequence specific DNA binding. Carcinogenesis 22:851, 2001. (A biochemically oriented review of *TP53* functions.)

Murphy PM: Chemokines and the molecular basis of metastasis. N Engl J Med 345:833, 2001. (A succinct discussion of breast cancer metastasis regulation by chemokines and their receptors.)

Nevins JR: The RB/E2F pathway and cancer. Hum Mol Genet 10:699, 2001. (An update on the role of the *RB* gene in regulating the cell cycle.)

Polakis P: More than one way to skin a catenin. Cell 105:563, 2001. (An article for the brave—it describes various mechanisms by which catenin can become oncogenic.)

Renkvist N, et al: A listing of human tumor antigens recognized by T cells. Cancer Immunol Immunother 50:3, 2001. (A comprehensive listing of human tumor antigens of various types.)

Shay JW, et al: Telomerase and cancer. Hum Mol Genet 10:677, 2001. (A discussion of telomerase, cell sequence, and cancer.)

Tisdale MJ: Cancer anorexia and cachexia. Nutrition 17:438, 2001. (An excellent review of an enigmatic problem.)

Walker GJ, Hayward NK: p16INK4A and p14ARF tumor suppressors in melanoma: lessons from the mouse. Lancet 359:7, 2002. (A commentary on the role of CDK inhibitors in melanoma.)

Webb CP, Van de Woude GF: Genes that regulate metastases and angiogenesis. J Neurooncol 50:71, 2000. (An excellent review of genes involved in angiogenesis, invasion, and distant spread.)

Welcsh PL, King M-C: BRCA1 and BRCA2 and the genetics of breast and ovarian cancer. Hum Mol Genet 10:705, 2001. (A detailed discussion of the function of *BRCA1* and *BRCA2* in cancer causation.)

Williams GM: Mechanisms of chemical carcinogenesis and application to human cancer risk assessment. Toxicology 166:3, 2001. (A brief overview of chemical carcinogenesis.)

Yoshida M: Multiple viral strategies of HTLV-1 for dysregulation of cell growth control. Annu Rev Immunol 19:475, 2001. (A review of the molecular mechanisms that underline HTLV-1-induced leukemia/lymphoma.)

Young LS, Dawson CW, Eliopoulos AG: The expression and function of Epstein-Barr virus encoded latent proteins. J Clin Pathol Mol Pathol 53:238, 2000. (A detailed discussion of EBV genes and their transforming activities.)

Zheng L, Lee W-H: The retinoblastoma gene: a prototypic and multifunctional tumor suppressor. Exp Cell Res 264:2, 2001. (A detailed review of the multiple roles of the *RB* gene.)

Zur Hausen H: Papillomaviruses causing cancer: evasion from host cell control in early events in carcinogenesis. J Natl Cancer Inst 92:690, 2000. (A summary of the transforming properties of human papillomavirus.)

7

Genetic and Pediatric Diseases

ANIRBAN MAITRA, MD
VINAY KUMAR, MD

Genetic Diseases

Pediatric Diseases

211

Genetic Diseases

The completion of the human genome project has been a landmark event in the study of human diseases. We now know that humans have only about 30,000 genes, far less than the 100,000 previously estimated. The unraveling of our "genetic architecture" promises to unlock secrets of genetic as well as acquired human disease, since ultimately all diseases involve changes in gene structure or expression. Powerful new technologies now allow applications of the human gene sequences to the analysis of human diseases. For example, DNA chips can be used to simultaneously screen for the expression of thousands of genes in diseased tissues. Such "molecular profiling" has become an important tool in the study of malignant diseases (Chapter 6).

With this background of developments in human genetics, we can turn to the time-honored classification of human diseases into three categories: (1) those that are genetically determined, (2) those that are almost entirely environmentally determined, and (3) those to which both nature and nurture contribute. However, progress in understanding the molecular basis of many so-called environmental disorders has tended to blur these distinctions. At one time, microbial infections were cited as examples of disorders arising wholly from environmental influences, but it is now clear that to a considerable extent, an individual's genetic makeup influences his or her immune response and susceptibility to microbiologic infections. Despite the complexities of this nature-nurture interplay, there is little doubt that nature (i.e., the genetic component) plays a major, if not the determining, role in the occurrence and severity of many human diseases. Such disorders are far more frequent than is commonly appreciated.

Surveys indicate that as much as 20% of the pediatric inpatients in university hospital populations suffer from disorders of genetic origin. These data describe only the tip of the iceberg. Chromosomal aberrations have been identified in up to 50% of spontaneous abortuses during the first trimester, and many more abortuses likely had gene mutations. Only those mutations compatible with independent existence constitute the reservoir of genetic disease in the population at large.

Because several pediatric disorders are of genetic origin, we discuss developmental and pediatric diseases along with genetic diseases in this chapter. However, *it must be borne in mind that not all genetic disorders present in infancy and childhood, and conversely, many pediatric diseases are not of genetic origin.* To the latter category belong diseases resulting from immaturity of organ systems. In this context, it is helpful to clarify three commonly used terms: hereditary, familial, and congenital. *Hereditary* disorders, by definition, are derived from one's parents, are transmitted in the gametes through the generations, and therefore are *familial.* The term *congenital* simply implies "present at birth." It should be noted that some congenital diseases are not genetic (e.g., congenital syphilis). On the other hand, not all genetic diseases are congenital; Huntington disease, for example, begins to be expressed only after the third or fourth decade of life.

It is beyond the scope of this book to review normal human genetics, but it is beneficial to recall some fundamental concepts that have a bearing on the understanding of genetic diseases.

Figure 7–1   ■

Schematic illustration of a point mutation resulting from a single–base pair change in the DNA. In the example shown, a CTC to CAC change alters the meaning of the genetic code (GAG to GUG in the opposite strand), leading to replacement of glutamic acid by valine in the polypeptide chain. This change, affecting the sixth amino acid of the normal β-globin (β_A) chain, converts it to sickle β-globin (β_S). mRNA, messenger RNA.

MUTATIONS

As is well known, the term *mutation* refers to permanent changes in the DNA. Those that affect germ cells are transmitted to the progeny and may give rise to inherited diseases. Mutations in somatic cells are not transmitted to the progeny but are important in the causation of cancers and some congenital malformations.

Details of specific mutations and their effects are discussed along with the relevant disorders throughout this text. Here we cite only some common examples of gene mutations and their effects.

Point mutations result from the substitution of a single nucleotide base by a different base, resulting in the replacement of one amino acid by another in the protein product. The mutation giving rise to sickle cell anemia is an excellent example of a point mutation that alters the meaning of the genetic code (Fig. 7–1). Such mutations are sometimes called *missense mutations*.

In contrast, certain point mutations may change an amino acid codon to a chain termination codon, or *stop codon*. Such "nonsense" mutations interrupt translation, and the resultant truncated proteins are rapidly degraded. The effect of a nonsense mutation in the messenger RNA (mRNA) of β-globin is illustrated in Figure 7–2.

Frameshift mutations occur when the insertion or deletion of one or two base pairs alters the reading frame of the DNA strand (Fig. 7–3). If the number of base pairs involved in a deletion is three or a multiple of three, frameshift does not occur; instead, a protein missing one or more amino acids is synthesized (Fig. 7–4).

Trinucleotide repeat mutations belong to a special category because these mutations are characterized by amplification of a sequence of three nucleotides. Although the specific nucleotide sequence that undergoes amplification differs in various disorders, all affected sequences share the nucleotides guanine (G) and cytosine (C). For example, in fragile X syndrome, prototypical of this category of disorders, there are

Figure 7–2   ■

Point mutation leading to premature chain termination. Partial mRNA sequence of the β-globin chain of hemoglobin shows codons for amino acids 38 through 40. A point mutation (C → U) in codon 39 changes a glutamine (Gln) codon to a stop codon, and hence protein synthesis stops at the 38th amino acid.

Figure 7–3   ■

Single-base deletion at the ABO (glycosyltransferase) locus, leading to a frameshift mutation responsible for the O allele. (From Thompson MW, et al: Thompson and Thompson Genetics in Medicine, 5th ed. Philadelphia, WB Saunders, 1991, p 134.)

```
               — Ile — Ile — Phe — Gly — Val —
 Normal DNA    ...T ATC ATC TTT GGT GTT...
```

```
                            ΔF508
                         ┌──────┐
 CF DNA        ...T ATC AT─ ──T GGT GTT...
               — Ile — Ile ──────── Gly — Val —
```

Figure 7–4   ■

Three-base deletion in the common cystic fibrosis (CF) allele results in synthesis of a protein that is missing amino acid 508 (phenylalanine). Because the deletion is a multiple of three, this is not a frameshift mutation. (From Thompson MW, et al: Thompson and Thompson Genetics in Medicine, 5th ed. Philadelphia, WB Saunders, 1991, p 135.)

250 to 4000 tandem repeats of the sequence CGG within a gene called *FMR1*. In normal populations, the number of repeats is small, averaging 29. It is believed that expansions of the trinucleotide sequences prevent normal expression of the *FMR1* gene, thus giving rise to mental retardation. Another distinguishing feature of trinucleotide repeat mutations is that they are dynamic (i.e., the degree of amplification increases during gametogenesis). These features, discussed in greater detail later in this chapter, influence the pattern of inheritance and the phenotypic manifestations of the diseases caused by this class of mutations.

With this brief review of the nature of mutations, we can turn our attention to the three major categories of genetic disorders: (1) those related to mutant genes of large effect, (2) diseases with multifactorial (polygenic) inheritance, and (3) those arising from chromosomal aberrations. The first category, sometimes referred to as *mendelian disorders*, includes many uncommon conditions, such as the storage diseases and inborn errors of metabolism, all resulting from single-gene mutations of large effect. Most of these conditions are hereditary and familial. The second category includes some of the most common disorders of humans, such as hypertension and diabetes mellitus. Multifactorial, or polygenic, inheritance implies that both genetic and environmental influences condition the expression of a phenotypic characteristic or disease. The third category includes disorders that have been shown to be the consequence of numeric or structural abnormalities in the chromosomes.

To these well-known categories, it is necessary to add a heterogeneous group of genetic disorders that, like mendelian disorders, involve single genes but do not follow simple mendelian rules of inheritance. These single-gene disorders with nonclassic inheritance include those resulting from triplet repeat mutations, those arising from mutations in mitochondrial DNA, and those in which the transmission is influenced by an epigenetic phenomenon called *genomic imprinting*. Each of these four categories is discussed separately.

MENDELIAN DISORDERS (DISEASES CAUSED BY SINGLE-GENE DEFECTS)

Single-gene defects (mutations) follow the well-known mendelian patterns of inheritance. Thus, the conditions they

Table 7–1.   PREVALENCE OF SELECTED MONOGENIC DISORDERS AMONG LIVEBORN INFANTS

Disorder	Estimated Prevalence
Autosomal Dominant	
Familial hypercholesterolemia	1 in 500
Polycystic kidney disease	1 in 1250
Huntington disease	1 in 2500
Hereditary spherocytosis	1 in 5000
Marfan syndrome	1 in 20,000
Autosomal Recessive	
Sickle cell anemia	1 in 625 (US blacks)
Cystic fibrosis	1 in 2000 (Caucasians)
Tay-Sachs disease	1 in 3000 (US Jews)
Phenylketonuria	1 in 12,000
Mucopolysaccharidoses (all types)	1 in 25,000
Glycogen storage diseases (all types)	1 in 50,000
Galactosemia	1 in 57,000
X-Linked	
Duchenne muscular dystrophy	1 in 7000
Hemophilia	1 in 10,000

From Wyngaarden JB, et al: Cecil Textbook of Medicine, 19th ed. Philadelphia, WB Saunders, 1992, p 121.

produce are often called *mendelian disorders*. The number of known mendelian disorders has grown to more than 5000. Although individually each is rare, altogether they account for approximately 1% of all adult admissions to hospitals and about 6% to 8% of all pediatric hospital admissions. Table 7–1 lists some of the more common mendelian disorders and their prevalence. Many of these are discussed in this chapter; most of the remaining ones are described elsewhere in the text.

Mutations involving single genes follow one of three patterns of inheritance: autosomal dominant, autosomal recessive, or X-linked. Although gene expression is usually described as dominant or recessive, it should be remembered that in some cases both alleles of a gene pair may be fully expressed in the heterozygote, a condition called *codominance*. Histocompatibility and blood group antigens are good examples of codominant inheritance, as well as of *polymorphism* (i.e., the presence of multiple allelic forms of a single gene).

A single-gene mutation may lead to many phenotypic effects *(pleiotropy)*, and conversely, mutations at several genetic loci may produce the same trait *(genetic heterogeneity)*. For example, Marfan syndrome, which results from a basic defect in connective tissue, is associated with widespread effects involving the skeleton, eye, and cardiovascular system, all of which stem from a mutation in fibrillin, a component of connective tissues. On the other hand, retinitis pigmentosa, an inherited cause of abnormal retinal pigmentation and consequent visual impairment, can be caused by several different types of mutations. Recognition of genetic heterogeneity not only is important in genetic counseling but also facilitates the understanding of the pathogenesis of common disorders such as diabetes mellitus (Chapter 17).

Transmission Patterns of Single-Gene Disorders

AUTOSOMAL DOMINANT DISORDERS

Autosomal dominant disorders are manifested in the heterozygous state, so at least one parent of an index case is usually affected; both males and females are affected, and both can transmit the condition. When an affected person marries an unaffected one, every child has one chance in two of having the disease. The following features also pertain to autosomal dominant diseases:

■ With any autosomal dominant disorder, some patients do not have affected parents. Such patients owe their disorder to new mutations involving either the egg or the sperm from which they were derived. Their siblings are neither affected nor at increased risk of developing the disease.
■ Clinical features can be modified by reduced penetrance and variable expressivity. Some individuals inherit the mutant gene but are phenotypically normal. This is referred to as *reduced penetrance.* The factors that affect penetrance are not clearly understood. In contrast to penetrance, if a trait is seen in all individuals carrying the mutant gene but is expressed differently among individuals, the phenomenon is called *variable expressivity.* For example, manifestations of neurofibromatosis type I range from brownish spots on the skin to multiple tumors and skeletal deformities.
■ In many conditions, the age at onset is delayed: symptoms and signs do not appear until adulthood (as in Huntington disease).
■ In autosomal dominant disorders, a 50% reduction in the normal gene product is associated with clinical symptoms. Because a 50% loss of enzyme activity can usually be compensated for, involved genes usually do not encode enzyme proteins. Two major categories of nonenzyme proteins are usually affected in autosomal dominant disorders:

■ Those involved in regulation of complex metabolic pathways, often subject to feedback control (examples are membrane receptors and transport proteins). One example of this is familial hypercholesterolemia, which results from mutation in the low-density lipoprotein (LDL) receptor gene. Heterozygotes have elevated serum cholesterol levels because of lack of feedback inhibition through the LDL receptor (discussed later).
■ Key structural proteins, such as collagen and cytoskeletal components of the red cell membrane (e.g., spectrin).

The biochemical mechanisms by which a 50% reduction in the levels of such proteins results in an abnormal phenotype are not fully understood. In some cases, especially when the gene encodes one subunit of a multimeric protein, the product of the mutant allele can interfere with the assembly of a functionally normal multimer. For example, the collagen molecule is a trimer in which the three collagen chains are arranged in a helical configuration. Each of the three collagen chains in the helix must be normal for the assembly and stability of the collagen molecule. Even with a single mutant collagen chain, normal collagen trimers cannot be formed, and hence there is

Table 7-2. AUTOSOMAL DOMINANT DISORDERS

System	Disorder
Nervous	Huntington disease Neurofibromatosis Myotonic dystrophy Tuberous sclerosis
Urinary	Polycystic kidney disease
Gastrointestinal	Familial polyposis coli
Hematopoietic	Hereditary spherocytosis Von Willebrand disease
Skeletal	Marfan syndrome* Ehlers-Danlos syndrome (some variants)* Osteogenesis imperfecta Achondroplasia
Metabolic	Familial hypercholesterolemia* Acute intermittent porphyria

*Discussed in this chapter. Other disorders listed are discussed in appropriate chapters of this book.

a marked deficiency of collagen. In this instance, the mutant allele is called *dominant negative* because it impairs the function of a normal allele. This effect is illustrated by some forms of osteogenesis imperfecta (Chapter 21). Table 7–2 lists the more common autosomal dominant disorders. Most are discussed elsewhere in the text. Selected prototypical diseases are described later in this chapter.

AUTOSOMAL RECESSIVE DISORDERS

Autosomal recessive diseases make up the largest group of mendelian disorders. They occur when both of the alleles at a given gene locus are mutants; therefore, such disorders are characterized by the following features: (1) the trait does not usually affect the parents, but siblings may show the disease; (2) siblings have one chance in four of being affected (i.e., the recurrence risk is 25% for each birth); and (3) if the mutant gene occurs with a low frequency in the population, there is a strong likelihood that the proband is the product of a consanguineous marriage.

In contrast to the features of autosomal dominant diseases, the following features generally apply to most autosomal recessive disorders.

■ The expression of the defect tends to be more uniform than in autosomal dominant disorders.
■ Complete penetrance is common.
■ Onset is frequently early in life.
■ Although new mutations for recessive disorders do occur, they are rarely detected clinically. Because the affected individual is an asymptomatic heterozygote, several generations may pass before the descendants of such a person mate with other heterozygotes and produce affected offspring.
■ In many cases, enzyme proteins are affected by the mutation. In heterozygotes, equal amounts of normal and defective enzyme are synthesized. Usually the natural "margin of safety" ensures that cells with half of their usual complement of the enzyme function normally.

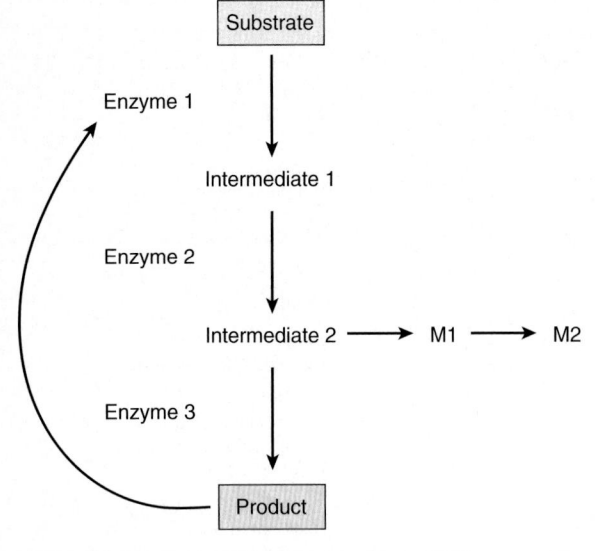

Figure 7–5 ■

Scheme of a possible metabolic pathway in which a substrate is converted to an end product by a series of enzyme reactions. Ml, M2, products of a minor pathway.

To illustrate possible mechanisms by which an enzyme deficiency may give rise to an autosomal recessive disorder, Figure 7–5 provides an example of an enzyme reaction in which the substrate is converted by intracellular enzymes through intermediates into an end product. In this example, the final product exerts feedback control on enzyme 1. A minor pathway producing small quantities of M1 and M2 also exists. The biochemical consequences of an enzyme defect in such a reaction have two major implications:

1. Depending on the site of the block, accumulation of the substrate may be accompanied by build-up of one or both intermediates. Moreover, an *i*ncreased concentration of intermediate 2 may stimulate the minor pathway and thus lead to an excess of M1 and M2. Under these conditions, tissue injury may result if the precursor, the intermediates, or the products of the minor pathways are toxic in high concentrations. For example, in galactosemia, a deficiency of galactose-1-phosphate uridylyltransferase leads to the accumulation of galactose, with consequent tissue damage. Similarly, a deficiency of phenylalanine hydroxylase (officially, phenylalanine 4-monooxygenase) results in the accumulation of phenylalanine. Excessive accumulation of complex substrates within the lysosomes occurring as a result of a deficiency of degradative enzymes is responsible for a group of diseases generally referred to as *lysosomal storage diseases* (p 222).
2. The enzyme defect can lead to a metabolic block and a decreased amount of an end product that may be necessary for normal function. For example, a deficiency of melanin may result from lack of tyrosinase, which is necessary for the biosynthesis of melanin from its precursor, tyrosine. This results in a clinical condition called *albinism.* If the end product is a feedback inhibitor of the enzymes involved in the early reactions (for example, in Figure 7–5 it is shown that the final product inhibits enzyme 1), the deficiency of the end product may permit overproduction of intermediates and their catabolic products, some of which may be injurious at high concentrations. A prime example of a disease with such an underlying mechanism is the Lesch-Nyhan syndrome (Chapter 21).

Enzyme deficiencies may act in other ways as well. For example, α_1-antitrypsin is a protease inhibitor whose chief function is to inactivate neutrophil elastase. In patients with α_1-antitrypsin deficiency, the elastic tissue in the walls of pulmonary alveoli falls prey to the unopposed destructive activity of neutrophil elastase, leading eventually to emphysema (Chapter 13).

Table 7–3 provides a list of the more common examples of autosomal recessive disorders. Some of these are discussed in this chapter, but most are described elsewhere, along with other diseases of the affected organ system.

X-LINKED DISORDERS

All sex-linked disorders are X-linked. To date, no Y-linked diseases are known. Save for determinants that dictate male differentiation, the only characteristic that may be located on the Y chromosome is the not-altogether-devastating attribute of hairy ears. Most X-linked disorders are X-linked recessive and are characterized by the following features:

■ They are transmitted by heterozygous female carriers virtually only to sons, who of course are hemizygous for the X chromosome.
■ Heterozygous females rarely express the full phenotypic change, owing to the presence of the paired normal allele; however, because of the inactivation of one of the X chromosomes in females (discussed later), it is remotely possible for the normal allele to be inactivated

■

Table 7-3. AUTOSOMAL RECESSIVE DISORDERS

System	Disorder
Metabolic*	Cystic fibrosis*
	Phenylketonuria*
	Galactosemia*
	Homocystinuria
	Lysosomal storage diseases*
	α_1-Antitrypsin deficiency
	Wilson disease
	Hemochromatosis
	Glycogen storage diseases*
Hematopoietic	Sickle cell anemia
	Thalassemias
Endocrine	Congenital adrenal hyperplasia
Skeletal	Ehlers-Danlos syndrome (some variants)*
	Alkaptonuria
Nervous	Neurogenic muscular atrophies
	Friedreich ataxia
	Spinal muscular atrophy

*Discussed in this chapter. Many others are discussed throughout the text.

Table 7–4. X-LINKED RECESSIVE DISORDERS

System	Disease
Musculoskeletal	Duchenne muscular dystrophy
Blood	Hemophilias A and B Chronic granulomatous disease Glucose-6-phosphate dehydrogenase deficiency
Immune	Agammaglobulinemia Wiskott-Aldrich syndrome
Metabolic	Diabetes insipidus Lesch-Nyhan syndrome
Nervous	Fragile X syndrome*

*Discussed in this chapter.

in most cells, permitting full expression of the disease in heterozygous females.

■ An affected male does not transmit the disorder to sons, but all daughters are carriers. Sons of heterozygous women have one chance in two of receiving the mutant gene.

There are a very few X-linked dominant diseases. Their inheritance pattern is characterized by transmission of the disease to 50% of the sons and daughters of an affected heterozygous female. An affected male cannot transmit the disease to his sons, but all daughters are affected. One example of such a disease is vitamin D–resistant rickets.

X-linked recessive disorders are much less common than disorders arising from autosomal mutations. Some of the more important conditions having this mode of transmission are listed in Table 7–4.

Although mendelian disorders are often grouped according to their patterns of transmission, it is perhaps more appropriate to categorize them on the basis of the nature of the protein that is affected, because in large part the type of protein affected determines the pattern of inheritance. Hence, in Table 7–5, selected single-gene disorders are classified into broad groupings on the basis of the protein abnormality.

Diseases Caused by Mutations in Structural Proteins

MARFAN SYNDROME

In this autosomal dominant disorder of connective tissues, the basic biochemical abnormality affects *fibrillin 1*. This glycoprotein, secreted by fibroblasts, is the major component of microfibrils found in the extracellular matrix. These serve as scaffolding for the deposition of elastin and are considered integral components of elastic fibers. Fibrillin 1 is encoded by the *FBN1* gene, which maps to chromosome 15q21. Mutations in the *FBN1* gene are found in all patients with Marfan syndrome. However, molecular diagnosis of Marfan syndrome is not feasible because over 100 distinct mutations affecting the *FBN1* gene have been found. Since heterozygotes have clinical symptoms, it follows that the mutant fibrillin 1 protein must act as a dominant negative by preventing the assembly of normal microfibrils. The prevalence of Marfan syndrome is estimated to be 2 to 3 per 10,000. Approximately 75% of cases are familial, and the rest are sporadic, arising from new mutations in the germ cells of parents.

Table 7–5. BIOCHEMICAL BASIS AND INHERITANCE PATTERN OF SOME MENDELIAN DISORDERS

Protein Type/Function	Example	Pattern of Inheritance	Disease
Enzyme	Phenylalanine hydroxylase Hexosaminidase Adenosine deaminase	Autosomal recessive	Phenylketonuria Tay-Sachs disease Severe combined immunodeficiency
Enzyme Inhibitor	α_1-Antitrypsin	Autosomal recessive	Emphysema and liver disease
Receptor	Low-density lipoprotein receptor	Autosomal dominant	Familial hypercholesterolemia
Transport Oxygen	Hemoglobin	Autosomal codominant*	α-Thalassemia β-Thalassemia Sickle cell anemia
Ions	Cystic fibrosis transmembrane conductance regulator	Autosomal recessive	Cystic fibrosis
Structural Extracellular	Collagen	Autosomal dominant	Osteogenesis imperfecta; Ehlers-Danlos syndromes†
	Fibrillin	Autosomal dominant	Marfan syndrome
Cell membrane	Dystrophin	X-linked recessive	Duchenne/Becker muscular dystrophy
	Spectrin, ankyrin, or protein 4.1	Autosomal dominant	Hereditary spherocytosis
Hemostasis	Factor VIII	X-linked recessive	Hemophilia A
Growth Regulation	RB protein	Autosomal dominant	Hereditary retinoblastoma
	NF-1 protein	Autosomal dominant	Neurofibromatosis type 1

*Heterozygotes either are asymptomatic or have mild disease.
†Some variants of Ehlers-Danlos syndrome are autosomal recessive or X-linked recessive.

Although connective tissue throughout the body is affected, the principal clinical manifestations relate to three systems: the skeleton, the eyes, and the cardiovascular system.

MORPHOLOGY

Skeletal abnormalities are the most obvious feature of Marfan syndrome. Patients have a slender, elongated habitus with abnormally long legs, arms, and fingers (arachnodactyly); a high-arched palate; and hyperextensibility of joints. A variety of spinal deformities, such as severe kyphoscoliosis, may appear. The chest is classically deformed, exhibiting either pectus excavatum (i.e., deeply depressed sternum) or a pigeon-breast deformity. President Lincoln is thought to have had features suggestive of Marfan syndrome. The most characteristic **ocular change** is bilateral dislocation, or subluxation, of the lens owing to weakness of its suspensory ligaments. It should be noted that the ciliary zonules that support the lens are devoid of elastin and are made up exclusively of fibrillin. Most serious, however, is the involvement of the **cardiovascular system.** Fragmentation of the elastic fibers in the tunica media of the aorta predisposes to aneurysmal dilation and aortic dissection (Chapter 10). These changes are not specific for Marfan syndrome. Similar lesions occur in patients with hypertension and in aging. Loss of medial support causes dilation of the aortic valve ring, giving rise to aortic incompetence. The cardiac valves, especially the mitral and, less commonly, the tricuspid valve, may be excessively distensible and regurgitant (floppy valve syndrome), giving rise to congestive cardiac failure (Chapter 11). Death from aortic rupture may occur at any age and is the most common cause of death. Less commonly, cardiac failure is the terminal event.

In addition to these features, Marfan patients have defects in the skin, skeletal muscles, and lungs. "Stretch marks" occur in areas of flexural stress; muscle appears myopathic with loss of bulk and hypotonia; damage to the connective tissue in lungs may manifest as spontaneous pneumothorax. Although the lesions described are typical of Marfan syndrome, they are not seen in all cases. There is much variation in clinical expression, and some patients may exhibit predominantly cardiovascular lesions with minimal skeletal and ocular changes. The variable expressivity is believed to be related to different allelic mutations in the fibrillin gene. Because of such variations, it is not feasible to develop a simple screening test that can detect all mutations that underlie Marfan syndrome.

EHLERS-DANLOS SYNDROMES

Ehlers-Danlos syndromes (EDSs) are characterized by defects in collagen synthesis or structure. All are single-gene disorders, but the mode of inheritance encompasses all three of the mendelian patterns. This should not be surprising, because biosynthesis of collagen is a complex process that may be disturbed by genetic errors affecting any one of the numerous structural collagen genes or the genes that code for the enzymes necessary for post-transcriptional events, such as cross-linking of collagen fibers. It should be recalled that there are at least 18 distinct types of collagen, and all of them have characteristic tissue distributions and are the products of different genes. To some extent, the clinical heterogeneity of EDS can be explained on the basis of mutations in different collagen genes.

At least 10 clinical and genetic variants of EDS are recognized. Because defective collagen is present in all the variants, certain clinical features are common to all.

As might be expected, tissues rich in collagen, such as skin, ligaments, and joints, are frequently involved in most variants of EDS. Because the abnormal collagen fibers lack adequate tensile strength, *skin is hyperextensible and joints are hypermobile.* These features permit grotesque contortions, such as bending the thumb backward to touch the forearm and bending the knee upward to create almost a right angle. Indeed, it is believed that most contortionists have one of the EDSs; however, a predisposition to joint dislocation is one of the prices paid for this virtuosity. *The skin is extraordinarily stretchable, extremely fragile, and vulnerable to trauma.* Minor injuries produce gaping defects, and surgical repair or any surgical intervention is accomplished only with great difficulty because of the lack of normal tensile strength. The basic defect in connective tissue may lead to serious internal complications, including rupture of the colon and large arteries (EDS type IV); ocular fragility, with rupture of the cornea and retinal detachment (EDS type VI); and diaphragmatic hernias (EDS type I), among others.

The molecular bases of EDS are varied and include the following:

■ *Deficiency of the enzyme lysyl hydroxylase.* Decreased hydroxylation of lysyl residues in types I and III collagen interferes with the normal cross-links among collagen molecules. As might be expected, this variant (type VI), resulting from an enzyme deficiency, is inherited as an autosomal recessive disorder.
■ *Deficient synthesis of type III collagen owing to mutations in the pro-α_1 (III) gene.* This variant (type IV) is inherited as an autosomal dominant disorder and is characterized by weakness of tissues rich in type III collagen (e.g., blood vessels, bowel wall).
■ *Defective conversion of procollagen type I to collagen,* resulting from a mutation in the type I collagen gene in EDS type VII.

Diseases Caused by Mutations in Receptor Proteins

FAMILIAL HYPERCHOLESTEROLEMIA

Familial hypercholesterolemia is among the most common mendelian disorders; the frequency of heterozygotes is 1 in 500 in the general population. It is caused by a mutation in

NORMAL

FAMILIAL HYPERCHOLESTEROLEMIA (FH)

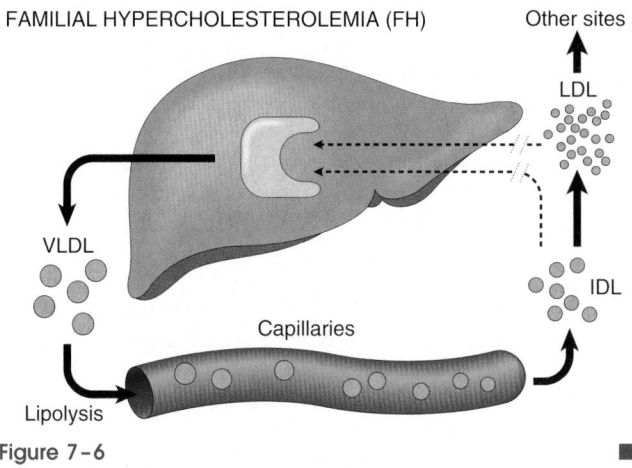

Figure 7–6 ■

Schematic illustration of low-density lipoprotein (LDL) metabolism and the role of the liver in its synthesis and catabolism, in normal persons and those with familial hypercholesterolemia. IDL, intermediate-density lipoprotein; VLDL, very-low-density lipoprotein.

the gene that specifies the receptor for low-density lipoprotein (LDL), the form in which 70% of total plasma cholesterol is transported. As you know, cholesterol may be derived from the diet or from endogenous synthesis. Dietary triglycerides and cholesterol are incorporated into chylomicrons in the intestinal mucosa, which drain via the gut lymphatics into the blood. These chylomicrons are hydrolyzed by an endothelial lipoprotein lipase in the capillaries of muscle and fat. The chylomicron remnants, rich in cholesterol, are then delivered to the liver. Some of the cholesterol enters the metabolic pool (to be described), and some is excreted as free cholesterol or bile acids into the biliary tract. The endogenous synthesis of cholesterol and LDL begins in the liver (Fig. 7–6). The first step in the synthesis of LDL is the secretion of triglyceride-rich very-low-density lipoprotein (VLDL) by the liver into the blood. In the capillaries of adipose tissue and muscle, the VLDL particle undergoes lipolysis and is converted to intermediate-density lipoprotein (IDL). Compared with VLDL, the content of triglyceride is reduced and that of cholesteryl esters enriched in IDL, but IDL retains on its surface two of the three VLDL-associated apoproteins, B-100 and E. Further metabolism of IDL occurs along two pathways: most of the IDL particles are taken up by the liver through the LDL receptor described later; others are converted to cholesterol-rich LDL by a further loss of triglycerides and apoprotein E. Two thirds of the resultant LDL particles are metabolized by the LDL receptor pathway, and the rest is metabolized by a receptor for oxidized LDL (scavenger receptor), to be described later. The LDL receptor binds to apoproteins B-100 and E and hence is involved in the transport of both LDL and IDL. Although the LDL receptors are widely distributed, approximately 75% are located on hepatocytes, so the liver plays an extremely important role in LDL metabolism.

The first step in the receptor-mediated transport of LDL involves binding to the cell surface receptor, followed by endocytotic internalization (Fig. 7–7). Within the cell, the endocytic vesicles fuse with the lysosomes, and the LDL molecule is enzymatically degraded, resulting ultimately in the release of free cholesterol into the cytoplasm. The cho-

Figure 7–7 ■

Sequential steps in low-density lipoprotein (LDL) pathway in cultured mammalian cells. ACAT, acyl-CoA:cholesterol acyltransferase; HMG-CoA reductase, 3-hydroxy-3-methylglutaryl coenzyme A reductase. (From Goldstein JL, Brown MS: The LDL receptor defect in familial hypercholesterolemia. Implications for pathogenesis and therapy. Med Clin North Am 66:335, 1982.)

lesterol not only is utilized by the cell for membrane synthesis but also takes part in intracellular cholesterol homeostasis by a sophisticated system of feedback control:

- It suppresses cholesterol synthesis by inhibiting the activity of the enzyme 3-hydroxy-3-methylglutaryl (3-HMG) coenzyme A reductase (HMG-CoA reductase), which is the rate-limiting enzyme in the synthetic pathway.
- It activates the enzyme acyl-CoA:cholesterol acyltransferase (ACAT), which favors esterification and storage of excess cholesterol.
- It down-regulates the synthesis of cell surface LDL receptors, thus protecting cells from excessive accumulation of cholesterol.

The transport of LDL by the scavenger receptors, alluded to earlier, appears to take place in cells of the mononuclear phagocyte system and possibly in other cells as well. Monocytes and macrophages have receptors for chemically modified (e.g., acetylated or oxidized) LDL. The amount catabolized by this "scavenger receptor" pathway is directly related to the plasma cholesterol level.

In familial hypercholesterolemia, mutations in the LDL receptor gene impair the intracellular transport and catabolism of LDL, resulting in accumulation of LDL cholesterol in the plasma. In addition, the absence of LDL receptors on liver cells also impairs the transport of IDL into the liver, and hence a greater proportion of plasma IDL is converted into LDL. Thus, patients with familial hypercholesterolemia develop excessive levels of serum cholesterol owing to the combined effects of reduced catabolism and excessive biosynthesis (see Fig. 7-6). In the presence of such hypercholesterolemia, there is a marked increase of cholesterol traffic into the monocyte macrophages and vascular walls via the scavenger receptor. This accounts for the appearance of skin xanthomas and premature atherosclerosis.

Familial hypercholesterolemia is an autosomal dominant disease. Heterozygotes have a two- to threefold elevation of plasma cholesterol levels, whereas homozygotes may have in excess of a fivefold elevation. Although their cholesterol levels are elevated from birth, heterozygotes remain asymptomatic until adult life, when they develop cholesterol deposits (xanthomas) along tendon sheaths and premature atherosclerosis resulting in coronary artery disease. Homozygous persons are much more severely affected, developing cutaneous xanthomas in childhood and often dying of myocardial infarction by the age of 15 years.

Analysis of the cloned LDL receptor gene has revealed that more than 150 different mutations can give rise to familial hypercholesterolemia. These can be grouped in five categories. Class I mutations are associated with loss of receptor synthesis; with class II mutations, the most prevalent form, the receptor protein is synthesized, but its transport from the endoplasmic reticulum to the Golgi apparatus is impaired; class III mutations produce receptors that are transported to the cell surface but fail to bind LDL normally; class IV mutations give rise to receptors that fail to internalize after binding to LDL; class V mutations encode receptors that can bind LDL and are internalized but are trapped in endosomes because dissociation of receptor and bound LDL does not occur.

The discovery of the critical role of LDL receptors in cholesterol homeostasis yielded the Nobel Prize for Brown and Goldstein; more importantly, these studies led to the rational design of the statin family of drugs. These agents, now widely used, lower plasma cholesterol by inhibiting the enzyme HMG-CoA reductase and thus promoting greater synthesis of LDL receptor (see Fig. 7-7).

Diseases Caused by Mutations in Enzyme Proteins

PHENYLKETONURIA

There are several variants of this inborn error of metabolism. The most common form, referred to as *classic phenylketonuria* (PKU), is quite common in persons of Scandinavian descent and is distinctly uncommon in blacks and Jews.

Homozygotes with this autosomal recessive disorder classically have a severe lack of phenylalanine hydroxylase, leading to hyperphenylalaninemia and PKU. Affected infants are normal at birth but within a few weeks develop a rising plasma phenylalanine level, which in some way impairs brain development. Usually by 6 months of life *severe mental retardation* becomes all too evident; fewer than 4% of untreated phenylketonuric children have IQs greater than 50 or 60. About one third of these children are never able to walk, and two thirds cannot talk. *Seizures,* other neurologic abnormalities, *decreased pigmentation of hair and skin,* and *eczema* often accompany the *mental retardation* in untreated children. Hyperphenylalaninemia and the resultant mental retardation can be avoided by restriction of phenylalanine intake early in life. Hence, a number of screening procedures, including the Guthrie test, are routinely performed to detect PKU in the immediate postnatal period.

Many clinically normal female PKU patients, treated with diet early in life, reach childbearing age. Most of them have marked hyperphenylalaninemia because dietary treatment is discontinued after they reach adulthood. Children born to such women are profoundly mentally retarded and have multiple congenital anomalies, even though the infants themselves are heterozygotes. This syndrome, termed *maternal PKU,* results from the teratogenic effects of phenylalanine that crosses the placenta and affects the developing fetus. Hence, *it is imperative that maternal phenylalanine levels be lowered by dietary means before conception.* Maternal hyperphenylalaninemia also increases the risk of spontaneous abortions.

The biochemical abnormality in PKU is an inability to convert phenylalanine into tyrosine. In normal children, less than 50% of the dietary intake of phenylalanine is necessary for protein synthesis. The rest is converted to tyrosine by the phenylalanine hydroxylase system (Fig. 7-8). When phenylalanine metabolism is blocked because of a lack of phenylalanine hydroxylase, minor shunt pathways come into play, yielding several intermediates that are excreted in large amounts in the urine and in the sweat. These impart a *strong musty or mousy odor* to affected infants. It is believed that excess phenylalanine or its metabolites contribute to the brain damage in PKU. Concomitant lack of tyrosine (see Fig. 7-8), a precursor of melanin, is responsible for the light color of hair and skin.

Figure 7–8 ■

The phenylalanine hydroxylase system.

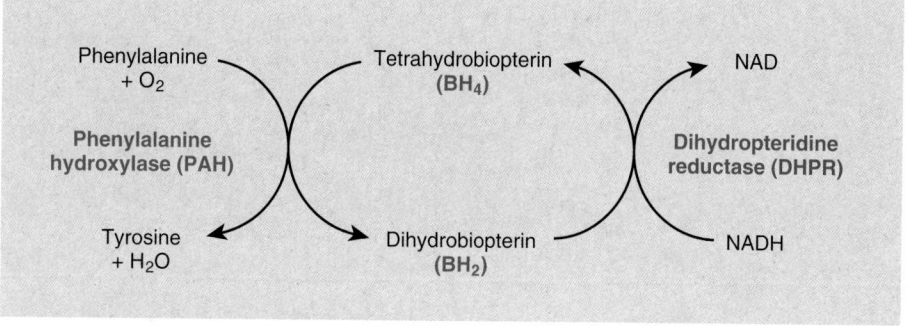

At the molecular level, approximately 100 mutant alleles of the phenylalanine hydroxylase gene have been identified, only some of which cause a severe deficiency of the enzyme and thus result in classic PKU. In those with a partial deficiency of phenylalanine hydroxylase, only modest elevations of phenylalanine levels occur, and there is no neurologic damage. This condition, referred to as *benign hyperphenylalaninemia*, is important to recognize because affected individuals may test positive in the widely utilized Guthrie screening test but do not develop the stigmata of classic PKU. Measurement of serum phenylalanine levels is necessary to differentiate benign hyperphenylalaninemia from PKU.

As alluded to earlier, a number of variant forms of PKU have been identified. These account for 2% to 3% of all cases of PKU and result from deficiencies of enzymes other than phenylalanine hydroxylase, such as dihydropteridine reductase (DHPR) (see Fig. 7–8). *It is clinically important to recognize these variant forms of PKU, because they cannot be treated by dietary restriction of phenylalanine.*

GALACTOSEMIA

Galactosemia is an autosomal recessive disorder of galactose metabolism. Normally, lactase splits lactose, the major carbohydrate of mammalian milk, into glucose and galactose in the intestinal microvilli. Galactose is then converted to glucose in several steps, in one of which the enzyme galactose-1-phosphate uridyltransferase is required. Lack of this enzyme is responsible for galactosemia. As a result of this lack of transferase, galactose 1-phosphate and other metabolites, including galactitol, accumulate in many locations, including the liver, spleen, lens of the eye, kidney, and cerebral cortex.

The liver, eyes, and brain bear the brunt of the damage. The early-developing hepatomegaly is due largely to fatty change, but in time widespread scarring that closely resembles the cirrhosis of alcohol abuse may supervene (Chapter 16). Opacification of the lens (cataracts) develops, probably because the lens absorbs water and swells as galactitol, produced by alternative metabolic pathways, accumulates and increases its tonicity. Nonspecific alterations appear in the central nervous system, including loss of nerve cells, gliosis, and edema. There is still no clear understanding of the mechanism of injury to the liver and brain.

Almost from birth, these infants fail to thrive. *Vomiting and diarrhea* appear within a few days of milk ingestion. *Jaundice* and *hepatomegaly* usually become evident during the first week of life. *Cataracts* develop within a few weeks, and within the first 6 to 12 months of life, *mental retardation* may be detected. Accumulation of galactose and galactose 1-phosphate in the kidney impairs amino acid transport, resulting in aminoaciduria. There is an increased frequency of fulminant *Escherichia coli* septicemia.

Most of the clinical and morphologic changes can be prevented by early removal of galactose from the diet for at least the first 2 years of life. The diagnosis can be suspected by the presence in the urine of a reducing sugar other than glucose, but tests that directly identify the deficiency of the transferase in leukocytes and erythrocytes are more reliable. Antenatal diagnosis is possible by enzyme assays or DNA-based testing of cultured amniocytes or chorionic villi. In the white population of the United States, 70% of cases are caused by a single missense mutation. The mutations are more heterogeneous in blacks.

LYSOSOMAL STORAGE DISEASES

Lysosomes, as is well known, contain a variety of hydrolytic enzymes that are involved in the breakdown of complex substrates, such as sphingolipids and mucopolysaccharides, into soluble end products. These large molecules may be derived from the turnover of intracellular organelles that enter the lysosomes by autophagocytosis, or they may be acquired from outside the cells by phagocytosis. With an inherited lack of a lysosomal enzyme, catabolism of its substrate remains incomplete, leading to accumulation of the partially degraded insoluble metabolites within the lysosomes (Fig. 7–9). As might be expected, these missing-enzyme syndromes are inherited as autosomal recessive disorders, and the storage of insoluble intermediates occurs mainly in cells of the mononuclear phagocyte system, because they ingest and degrade senescent red cells, leukocytes, and other tissue breakdown products.

Approximately 35 lysosomal storage diseases have been identified, each resulting from the functional absence of a specific lysosomal enzyme. The numerous lysosomal storage diseases can be divided into broad categories based on the biochemical nature of the substrates and the accumulated metabolites (Table 7–6). Within each group are several entities, each resulting from the deficiency of a specific enzyme. Fortunately for both medical students and the potential victims of the diseases, most of these conditions are very rare, and their detailed description is better relegated to specialized texts and reviews. Only a few of the more

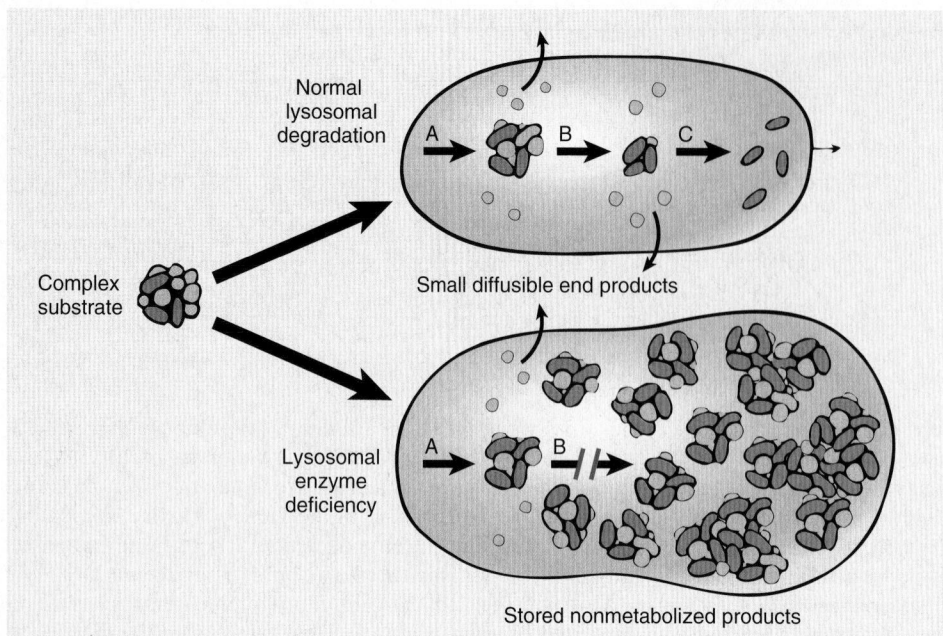

Figure 7-9 ■

Schematic diagram illustrating the pathogenesis of lysosomal storage diseases. In the example illustrated, a complex substrate is normally degraded by a series of lysosomal enzymes (A, B, and C) into soluble end products. If there is a deficiency or malfunction of one of the enzymes (e.g., B), catabolism is incomplete, and insoluble intermediates accumulate in the lysosomes.

common conditions (see Table 7–6) are considered here. Type II glycogen storage disease (Pompe disease), also a lysosomal disorder, is discussed later.

Tay-Sachs Disease (G_{M2} Gangliosidosis: Hexosaminidase *a*-Subunit Deficiency). Gangliosidoses are characterized by accumulation of gangliosides, principally in the brain, as a result of a deficiency of a catabolic lysosomal enzyme. Depending on the ganglioside involved, these disorders are subclassified into G_{M1} and G_{M2} categories. Tay-Sachs disease, by far the most common of all gangliosidoses, is characterized by a mutation in and consequent deficiency of the α subunit of the enzyme hexosaminidase A, which is necessary for the degradation of G_{M2}. Over 85 mutations have been described; most affect protein folding or intracellular transport. The brain is principally affected, because it is most involved in ganglioside metabolism. *The storage of G_{M2} occurs within neurons, axon cylinders of nerves, and glial cells throughout the central nervous system.* Affected cells appear swollen, possibly foamy (Fig. 7–10A). Electron microscopy reveals a whorled configuration within lysosomes (Fig. 7–10B). These anatomic changes are found throughout the central nervous system (including the spinal cord), peripheral nerves, and autonomic nervous system. The retina is usually involved as well.

Tay-Sachs disease, like other lipidoses, is most common among Ashkenazi Jews, among whom the frequency of heterozygous carriers is estimated to be 1 in 30. Heterozygotes can be reliably detected by estimating the level of

■

Table 7-6. LYSOSOMAL STORAGE DISORDERS

Disease	Enzyme Deficiency	Major Accumulating Metabolite
Glycogenoses		
Type II (Pompe disease)	Lysosomal glucosidase	Glycogen
Sphingolipidoses		
G_{M1} (gangliosidoses)	G_{M1} ganglioside β-galactosidase	G_{M1} ganglioside, galactose-containing oligosaccharides
G_{M2} (gangliosidoses)	Hexosaminidase A	G_{M2} ganglioside
Tay-Sachs disease		
Sulfatidoses		
Gaucher disease	Glucocerebrosidase	Glucocerebroside
Niemann-Pick disease, types A and B	Sphingomyelinase	Sphingomyelin
Mucopolysaccharidoses		
MPS I H (Hurler)	L-Iduronidase	Heparan sulfate
		Dermatan sulfate
MPS II (Hunter)	L-Iduronosulfate sulfatase	Heparan sulfate
(X-linked recessive)		Dermatan sulfate
Glycoproteinoses	Enzymes involved in degradation of oligosaccharide side chains of glycoproteins (several)	Several, depending on specific enzyme

Figure 7-10 ■

A, Ganglion cells in Tay-Sachs disease. Under the light microscope, a large neuron has obvious lipid vacuolation. *B*, Tay-Sachs disease. A portion of a neuron under the electron microscope shows prominent lysosomes with whorled configurations. Part of the nucleus is shown above. (*A*, Courtesy of Dr. Arthur Weinberg, Department of Pathology, University of Texas, Southwestern Medical Center, Dallas; *B*, courtesy of Dr. Joe Rutledge, University of Texas Southwestern Medical School, Dallas.)

hexosaminidase in the serum or by DNA analysis. Antenatal diagnosis is possible, and detection of Tay-Sachs disease in the fetus is considered a possible indication for therapeutic abortion. Infants who are born suffer from mental retardation, blindness, and severe neurologic dysfunctions that lead to certain death within 2 or 3 years.

Niemann-Pick Disease. This designation refers to a group of three disorders that can be segregated into two categories on the basis of biochemical and molecular criteria. One category, including types A and B, is characterized by a primary deficiency of acid sphingomyelinase and the resultant accumulation of sphingomyelin. The other category, typified by Niemann-Pick disease (type C), results from mutation in the NPC1 protein. This protein is involved in intracellular processing and transport of LDL-derived cholesterol. All types are rare, so remarks are confined to the sphingomyelinase-deficient (type A) variant. With a deficiency of sphingomyelinase, the breakdown of sphingomyelin into ceramide and phosphorylcholine is impaired, and excess sphingomyelin accumulates in all phagocytic cells and in the neurons. The phagocytic cells become stuffed with droplets or particles of the complex lipid, imparting a fine vacuolation or foaminess to the cytoplasm (Fig. 7–11). Because of their high content of phagocytic cells, *the organs most severely affected are the spleen, liver, bone marrow, lymph nodes, and lungs.* The splenic enlargement may be striking. In addition, the entire central nervous system, including the spinal cord and ganglia, is involved in this tragic, inexorable process. The affected neurons are enlarged and vacuolated owing to the storage of lipids. This variant manifests itself in infancy with *massive visceromegaly and severe neurologic deterioration.* Death usually occurs within the first 3 years of life. Estimation of

sphingomyelinase activity in the leukocytes or cultured fibroblasts can be used for diagnosis of suspected cases, as well as for detection of carriers. Antenatal diagnosis is possible by enzyme assays or DNA-probe analysis.

Gaucher Disease. This disease results from mutation in the gene that encodes glucocerebrosidase. There are three autosomal recessive variants of Gaucher disease resulting from distinct allelic mutations. Common to all three is variably deficient activity of a glucocerebrosidase that normally cleaves the glucose residue from ceramide. This leads to an accumulation of glucocerebrosides in the

Figure 7-11 ■

Niemann-Pick disease in liver. The hepatocytes and Kupffer cells have a foamy, vacuolated appearance owing to deposition of lipids. (Courtesy of Dr. Arthur Weinberg, Department of Pathology, University of Texas Southwestern Medical Center, Dallas.)

Figure 7-12 ■

Gaucher disease involving the bone marrow. *A,* Gaucher cells with abundant lipid-laden granular cytoplasm. *B,* Electron micrograph of Gaucher cells with elongated distended lysosomes. (*A* and *B,* Courtesy of Dr. Mathew Fries, Department of Pathology, University of Texas Southwestern Medical Center, Dallas.)

mononuclear phagocytic cells and the formation of so-called Gaucher cells. Normally the glycolipids derived from the breakdown of senescent blood cells, particularly erythrocytes, are sequentially degraded. In Gaucher disease, the degradation stops at the level of glucocerebrosides, which, in transit through the blood as macromolecules, are engulfed by the phagocytic cells of the body, especially those in the liver, spleen, and bone marrow. These phagocytes (Gaucher cells) become enlarged, sometimes up to 100 μm, because of the accumulation of distended lysosomes, and develop a pathognomonic cytoplasmic appearance characterized as "wrinkled tissue paper" (Fig. 7-12). No distinct vacuolation is present.

One variant, type I, also called the *chronic non-neuronopathic form,* accounts for 99% of cases of Gaucher disease. It is characterized by hepatosplenomegaly and the absence of central nervous system involvement. The spleen often enlarges massively, filling the entire abdomen. Gaucher cells are found in the liver, spleen, lymph nodes, and bone marrow. Marrow replacement and cortical erosion may produce radiographically visible skeletal lesions, as well as a reduction in the formed elements of blood. Hypersplenism (Chapter 12) also contributes to the anemia and leukopenia. Type I is most common in Ashkenazi Jews and, unlike other variants, Iis compatible with long life. The type II variant is highly lethal, affects children by 6 months of age, and is characterized by severe central nervous system involvement. Although the liver and spleen are also involved, the clinical features are dominated by neurologic disturbances.

The type III (juvenile) variant involves the brain as well as viscera, but the course is intermediate between that of types I and II. The three variants result from distinct mutations that affect the glucocerebrosidase gene.

The level of glucocerebrosidase in leukocytes or cultured fibroblasts is helpful in diagnosis and in the detection of heterozygotes. Current therapy is aimed at enzyme replacement by infusion of purified glucocerebrosidase. On the horizon is somatic gene therapy involving infusion of autologous hematopoietic stem cells transfected with the normal glucocerebrosidase gene in vitro.

Mucopolysaccharidoses. Mucopolysaccharidoses (MPSs) are characterized by defective degradation (and therefore storage) of mucopolysaccharides in various tissues. Recall that mucopolysaccharides form a part of ground substance and are synthesized in the connective tissues by fibroblasts. Most of the mucopolysaccharide is secreted into the ground substance, but a certain fraction is degraded within lysosomes. Several enzymes are involved in this catabolic pathway; it is the lack of these enzymes that leads to accumulation of mucopolysaccharides within the lysosomes. Several clinical variants of MPS, classified numerically from MPS I to MPS VII, have been described, each resulting from the deficiency of one specific enzyme. The mucopolysaccharides that accumulate within the tissues include dermatan sulfate, heparan sulfate, keratan sulfate, and (in some cases) chondroitin sulfate.

In general, the MPSs are progressive disorders characterized by involvement of multiple organs, including the liver, spleen, heart, and blood vessels. Most are associated with *coarse facial features, clouding of the cornea, joint stiffness, and mental retardation.* Urinary excretion of the accumulated mucopolysaccharides is often increased. All of these disorders except one are inherited as autosomal recessive conditions; the exception, Hunter syndrome, is an X-linked recessive disease. Of the seven recognized variants, only two well-characterized syndromes are discussed briefly here.

Hurler syndrome, also called *MPS I H,* results from a deficiency of L-iduronidase. Affected children have a life expectancy of 6 to 10 years. Like patients with most other forms of MPS, they develop coarse facial features associated with skeletal deformities, which creates an appearance referred to as *gargoylism.* Death is often due to cardiac complications resulting from the formation of raised endothelial and endocardial lesions by the deposition of mucopolysaccharides in the coronary arteries and heart valves. Accumulation of dermatan sulfate and heparan sulfate is seen in cells of the mononuclear phagocyte system, in fibroblasts, and within endothelium and smooth muscle cells of the vascular wall. The affected cells are swollen and have clear cytoplasm, resulting from the accumulation of periodic acid–Schiff (PAS)–positive material within engorged, vacuolated lysosomes. Lysosomal inclusions are also found in neurons, accounting for the mental retardation. Although most of the clinical features can be explained on the basis of excessive storage of mucopolysaccharides, joint stiffness, for example, probably results from disturbances in collagen synthesis, which occur secondary to the derangement in the ground substance.

The other variant of MPS, called *Hunter syndrome*, differs from Hurler syndrome in its mode of inheritance (X-linked), the absence of corneal clouding, and often its milder clinical course. As in Hurler syndrome, the accumulated mucopolysaccharides in Hunter syndrome are heparan sulfate and dermatan sulfate, but this results from a deficiency of L-iduronate sulfatase. Despite the difference in enzyme deficiency, an accumulation of identical substrates occurs because breakdown of heparan sulfate and dermatan sulfate requires both L-iduronidase and the sulfatase; if either one is missing, further degradation is blocked.

GLYCOGEN STORAGE DISEASES (GLYCOGENOSES)

An inherited deficiency of any one of the enzymes involved in glycogen synthesis or degradation can result in excessive accumulation of glycogen or some abnormal form of glycogen in various tissues. The type of glycogen stored, its intracellular location, and the tissue distribution of the affected cells vary depending on the specific enzyme deficiency. Regardless of the tissue or cells affected, the glycogen is most often stored within the cytoplasm, or sometimes within nuclei. One variant, Pompe disease, is a form of lysosomal storage disease, because the missing enzyme is localized to lysosomes. Most glycogenoses are inherited as autosomal recessive diseases, as is common with "missing enzyme" syndromes.

Approximately a dozen forms of glycogenoses have been described on the basis of specific enzyme deficiencies. On the basis of pathophysiology, they can be grouped into three categories:

■ *Hepatic forms.* Liver contains several enzymes that synthesize glycogen for storage and also break it down into free glucose. Hence, a deficiency of the hepatic enzymes involved in glycogen metabolism is associated with two major clinical effects: *enlargement of the liver owing to storage of glycogen* and *hypoglycemia owing to a failure of glucose production* (Fig. 7–13). Von Gierke disease (type I glycogenosis), resulting from a lack of glucose-6-phosphatase, is the most important example of the hepatic form of glycogenosis (Table 7–7).

■ *Myopathic forms.* In striated muscle, glycogen is an important source of energy. When enzymes that are involved in glycolysis are deficient, glycogen storage occurs in muscles, and there is an associated muscle weakness due to impaired energy production. Typically, *the myopathic forms of glycogen storage diseases are marked by muscle cramps after exercise and failure of exercise to induce an elevation in blood lactate levels owing to a block in glycolysis.* McArdle disease (type V glycogenosis), resulting from a deficiency of muscle phosphorylase, is the prototype of myopathic glycogenoses.

Figure 7–13   ■

Top, A simplified scheme of normal glycogen metabolism in the liver and skeletal muscles. *Middle,* The effects of an inherited deficiency of hepatic enzymes involved in glycogen metabolism. *Bottom,* The consequences of a genetic deficiency in the enzymes that metabolize glycogen in skeletal muscles.

■ Two other forms of glycogenoses do not fit into either of the two categories described. Type II glycogenosis *(Pompe disease)* is caused by a deficiency of lysosomal acid maltase and so is associated with deposition of glycogen in virtually every organ, but cardiomegaly is most prominent. Brancher glycogenosis (type IV) is caused by deposition of an abnormal form of glycogen, with detrimental effects on the liver, heart, and muscles.

The principal subgroups of glycogen storage diseases are summarized in Table 7–7.

Diseases Caused by Mutations in Proteins That Regulate Cell Growth

As detailed in Chapter 6, two classes of genes, protooncogenes and cancer suppressor genes, regulate normal cell growth and differentiation. Mutations affecting these genes, most often in the somatic cells, are involved in the pathogenesis of tumors. In approximately 5% of all cancers, however, mutations affecting certain tumor suppressor genes are present in all cells of the body, including germ cells, and hence can be transmitted to the offspring. These mutant genes predispose the offspring to hereditary tumors, a topic discussed in greater detail in Chapter 6. Here, two

Table 7-7. PRINCIPAL SUBGROUPS OF GLYCOGENOSES

Clinicopathologic Category	Specific Type	Enzyme Deficiency	Morphologic Changes	Clinical Features
Hepatic type	Hepatorenal (von Gierke disease, type I)	Glucose-6-phosphatase	Hepatomegaly: intracytoplasmic accumulations of glycogen and small amounts of lipid; intranuclear glycogen. Renomegaly: intracytoplasmic accumulations of glycogen in cortical tubular epithelial cells	In untreated patients, failure to thrive, stunted growth, hepatomegaly, and renomegaly. Hypoglycemia due to failure of glucose mobilization, often leading to convulsions. Hyperlipidemia and hyperuricemia resulting from deranged glucose metabolism; many patients develop gout and skin xanthomas. Bleeding tendency due to platelet dysfunction. With treatment (providing continuous source of glucose), most patients survive and develop late complications (e.g., hepatic adenomas).
Myopathic type	McArdle syndrome (type V)	Muscle phosphorylase	Skeletal muscle only— accumulations of glycogen predominant in subsarcolemmal location	Painful cramps associated with strenuous exercise. Myoglobinuria occurs in 50% of cases. Onset in adulthood (>20 yr). Muscular exercise fails to raise lactate level in venous blood. Compatible with normal longevity.
Miscellaneous type	Generalized glycogenosis (Pompe disease, type II)	Lysosomal glucosidase (acid maltase)	Mild hepatomegaly: ballooning of lysosomes with glycogen creating lacy cytoplasmic pattern. Cardiomegaly: glycogen within sarcoplasm as well as membrane-bound. Skeletal muscle: similar to heart (see Cardiomegaly)	Massive cardiomegaly, muscle hypotonia, and cardiorespiratory failure within 2 yr. Milder adult form with only skeletal muscle involvement presents with chronic myopathy.

prototypic familial tumors resulting from inherited mutations in growth-regulating genes are described.

NEUROFIBROMATOSIS: TYPES 1 AND 2

The neurofibromatoses consist of at least two autosomal dominant disorders affecting approximately 100,000 persons in the United States. They are referred to as *neurofibromatosis type 1* (NF-1; previously known as *von Recklinghausen disease*) and *neurofibromatosis type 2* (previously called *bilateral acoustic or central neurofibromatosis*). Although the occurrence of neurogenic tumors is common to both, the two entities are clinically and genetically distinct. Neurofibromatosis type 1, which accounts for more than 90% of cases, has three major features:

1. Multiple neurofibromas develop, usually in the form of pedunculated nodules protruding from the skin. The neurofibromas are discrete, generally unencapsulated, soft nodules. In some cases, the tumors, so-called plexiform neurofibromas, diffusely involve subcutaneous tissue and contain numerous tortuous thickened nerves; the under-

lying skin is often hyperpigmented. Microscopically, neurofibromas reveal proliferation of all elements of peripheral nerve, including Schwann cells, neurites, and fibroblasts. These components are dispersed in a disorderly pattern within a loose myxoid stroma. Similar tumors, ranging from microscopic to monstrous masses, may occur in every conceivable site (e.g., along nerve trunks, the cauda equina, and cranial nerves; in the retroperitoneum, orbit, tongue, and gastrointestinal tract).

2. Pigmented skin lesions known as café-au-lait spots sometimes overlie a neurofibroma. Infrequently, patients with neurofibromatosis type 1 have only the café-au-lait spots, an example of variable expressivity of a genetic defect.

3. Pigmented iris hamartomas, called *Lisch nodules*, do not present any clinical problem but are helpful in establishing the diagnosis.

In addition to being a disfiguring condition, neurofibromatosis may be extremely serious, either by virtue of the location of a lesion (e.g., within the spinal canal) or because one or more of the benign neurofibromas have transformed into a malignant neoplasm (in approximately 3% of patients).

Usually, the neurogenic sarcomas arise in the plexiform tumors attached to large nerve trunks of the neck or extremities. These patients also are at greater risk of developing other tumors, particularly optic gliomas, meningiomas, and pheochromocytomas. In addition, approximately 30% to 50% of patients have a wide variety of associated skeletal lesions. These include scoliosis, erosive bone defects, and bone cysts.

The *NF1* gene has been mapped to chromosome 17, and it encodes a protein *(neurofibromin)* that acts as a negative regulator of the RAS oncoprotein. As detailed in Chapter 6, overactivity of the RAS protein can contribute to tumorigenesis.

Type 2 neurofibromatosis is much rarer than is type 1. Although most patients have café-au-lait spots, the defining feature of this variant is the presence of bilateral acoustic schwannomas and multiple meningiomas. Lisch nodules are absent. The gene for type 2 neurofibromatosis, located on 22q12, encodes *merlin*, which resembles cytoskeletal proteins. Like neurofibromin, it is also a tumor suppressor protein. Its mode of action is unknown.

DISORDERS WITH MULTIFACTORIAL INHERITANCE

Multifactorial (also called *polygenic*) inheritance is involved in many of the physiologic characteristics of humans (e.g., height, weight, blood pressure, hair color). A multifactorial physiologic or pathologic trait may be defined as one governed by the additive effect of two or more genes of small effect but conditioned by environmental, nongenetic influences. Even monozygous twins reared separately may achieve different heights because of nutritional or other environmental influences. When surveyed in a large population, phenotypic attributes governed by multifactorial inheritance fall on a continuous Gaussian distribution (Fig. 7–14). Presumably, there is some threshold effect, so that a disorder becomes manifest only when a certain number of effector genes, as well as conditioning environmental

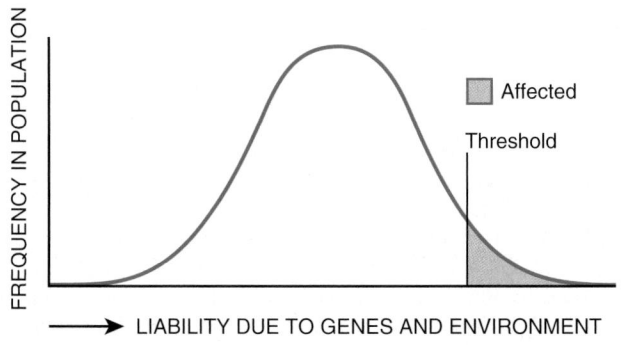

Figure 7–14 ■

Multifactorial inheritance. The continuous distribution of the liability to develop a multifactorial disease is determined by many genes and the environment. A threshold of liability indicates the limit beyond which disease is expressed. (From Elsas LJ II, Priest JH: Medical genetics. In Sodeman WA, Sodeman TM [eds]: Pathologic Physiology: Mechanisms of Disease, 7th ed. Philadelphia, WB Saunders, 1985, p 59.)

influences, are involved. The threshold effect also explains why parents of a child with a polygenic disorder may themselves be normal. Once the threshold value is exceeded, the severity of the disease is directly proportional to the number and the degree of influence of the pathologic genes.

The following features characterize multifactorial inheritance. These have been established for the multifactorial inheritance of congenital malformations and, in all likelihood, obtain for other multifactorial diseases.

■ The risk of expressing a multifactorial disorder is conditioned by the number of mutant genes inherited. Thus, the risk is greater in siblings of patients having severe expressions of the disorder.
■ The rate of recurrence of the disorder (in the range of 2% to 7%) is the same for all first-degree relatives (i.e., parents, siblings, and offspring) of the affected individual. Thus, if parents have had one affected child, the risk that the next child will be affected is between 2% and 7%. Similarly, there is the same chance that one of the parents will be affected.
■ The likelihood that both identical twins will be affected is significantly less than 100% but is much greater than the chance that both nonidentical twins will be affected. Experience has proved, for example, that the frequency of concordance for identical twins is in the range of 20% to 40%.
■ The risk of recurrence of the phenotypic abnormality in subsequent pregnancies depends on the outcome in previous pregnancies. When one child is affected, there is up to a 7% chance that the next child will be affected, but after two affected siblings, the risk rises to about 9%.

This form of inheritance is believed to underlie such common diseases as diabetes mellitus, hypertension, gout, schizophrenia, bipolar diorder, and certain forms of congenital heart disease, as well as some skeletal abnormalities. Hypertension provides an excellent example of multifactorial inheritance. There is good evidence that the level of blood pressure of an individual, at least in some part, is under genetic control, apparently governed by multiple genes of small effect. The pressure levels of the population at large fall along a continuous Gaussian curve of distribution. At some arbitrary level of blood pressure, hypertension is said to exist, because pressures above this level are associated with a significant disadvantage to the individual. (Hypertension is described in Chapter 10.)

CYTOGENETIC DISORDERS

Before we embark on a discussion of chromosomal aberrations, it should be recalled that karyotyping is the basic tool of the cytogeneticist. A karyotype is a photographic representation of a stained metaphase spread in which the chromosomes are arranged in order of decreasing length. A variety of techniques for staining chromosomes have been developed. With the widely used Giemsa stain (G banding) technique, each chromosome set can be seen to possess a distinctive pattern of alternating light and dark bands of variable widths (Fig. 7–15). The use of banding techniques allows certain identification of each chromosome, as well

Figure 7–15

Normal male karyotype with G banding. (Courtesy of Dr. Nancy R. Schneider, Department of Pathology, University of Texas Southwestern Medical School, Dallas.)

as precise localization of structural changes in the chromosomes (described later).

Chromosomal abnormalities occur much more frequently than is generally appreciated. It is estimated that approximately 1 of 200 newborn infants has some form of chromosomal abnormality. The figure is much higher in fetuses that do not survive to term. It is estimated that in 50% of first-trimester abortions, the fetus has a chromosomal abnormality. Cytogenetic disorders may result from alterations in the number or structure of chromosomes and may affect autosomes or sex chromosomes.

Numeric Abnormalities. In humans, the normal chromosome count is 46 (i.e., $2n = 46$). Any exact multiple of the haploid number *(n)* is called *euploid*. Chromosome numbers such as $3n$ and $4n$ are called *polyploid*. Polyploidy generally results in a spontaneous abortion. Any number that is not an exact multiple of *n* is called *aneuploid*. The chief cause of aneuploidy is nondisjunction of a homologous pair of chromosomes at the first meiotic division or a failure of sister chromatids to separate during the second meiotic division. The latter may also occur during somatic cell division, leading to the production of two aneuploid cells. Failure of pairing of homologous chromosomes followed by random assortment (anaphase lag) can also lead to aneuploidy. When nondisjunction occurs at the time of meiosis, the gametes formed have either an extra chromosome $(n + 1)$ or one less

chromosome $(n - 1)$. Fertilization of such gametes by normal gametes would result in two types of zygotes: trisomic, with an extra chromosome $(2n + 1)$, or monosomic $(2n - 1)$. Monosomy involving an autosome is incompatible with life, whereas trisomies of certain autosomes and monosomy involving sex chromosomes are compatible with life. These, as we shall see, are usually associated with variable degrees of phenotypic abnormality. *Mosaicism* is a term used to describe the presence of two or more populations of cells in the same individual. In the context of chromosome numbers, postzygotic mitotic nondisjunction would result in the production of a trisomic and a monosomic daughter cell; the descendants of these cells would then produce a mosaic. As discussed later, mosaicism affecting sex chromosomes is common, whereas autosomal mosaicism is not.

Structural Abnormalities. Structural changes in the chromosomes usually result from chromosomal breakage followed by loss or rearrangement of material. Such changes are usually designated using a cytogenetic shorthand in which *p* (petit) denotes the short arm of a chromosome, and *q*, the long arm. Each arm is then divided into numbered regions (1, 2, 3, and so on) from centromere outward, and within each region the bands are numerically ordered (Fig. 7–16). Thus, 2q34 indicates chromosome 2, long arm, region 3, band 4. The patterns of chromosomal rearrangement after breakage (diagrammed in Fig. 7–17) are as follows:

■ Negative or pale-staining G bands
■ Positive G bands
■ Variable bands

Figure 7–16 ■

Diagrammatic representation of midmetaphase chromosome bands to indicate the nomenclature of arms, regions, and bands. (After Yunis JJ, Chandler MS: The chromosomes of man—clinical and biologic significance. A review. Am J Pathol 8:466, 1977.)

■ *Translocation* implies transfer of a part of one chromosome to another chromosome. The process is usually reciprocal (i.e., fragments are exchanged between two chromosomes). In genetic shorthand, translocations are indicated by *t* followed by the involved chromosomes in numeric order, for example, 46,XX,t(2;5)(q31;p14). This would indicate a reciprocal translocation involving the long arm (q) of chromosome 2 at region 3, band 1, and the short arm of chromosome 5, region 1, band 4. When the entire broken fragments are exchanged, the resulting balanced reciprocal translocation (see Fig. 7–17) is not harmful to the carrier, who has the normal number of chromosomes and the full complement of genetic mater-

ial. However, during gametogenesis, abnormal (unbalanced) gametes are formed, resulting in abnormal zygotes. A special pattern of translocation involving two acrocentric chromosomes is called *centric fusion–type*, or *robertsonian*, translocation. Typically, the breaks occur close to the centromere, affecting the short arms of both chromosomes. Transfer of the segments leads to one very large chromosome and one extremely small one (see Fig. 7–17). The short fragments are lost, and the carrier has 45 chromosomes. Because the short arms of all acrocentric chromosomes have multiple copies of genes for ribosomal RNA, such loss is compatible with survival. However, difficulties arise during gametogene-

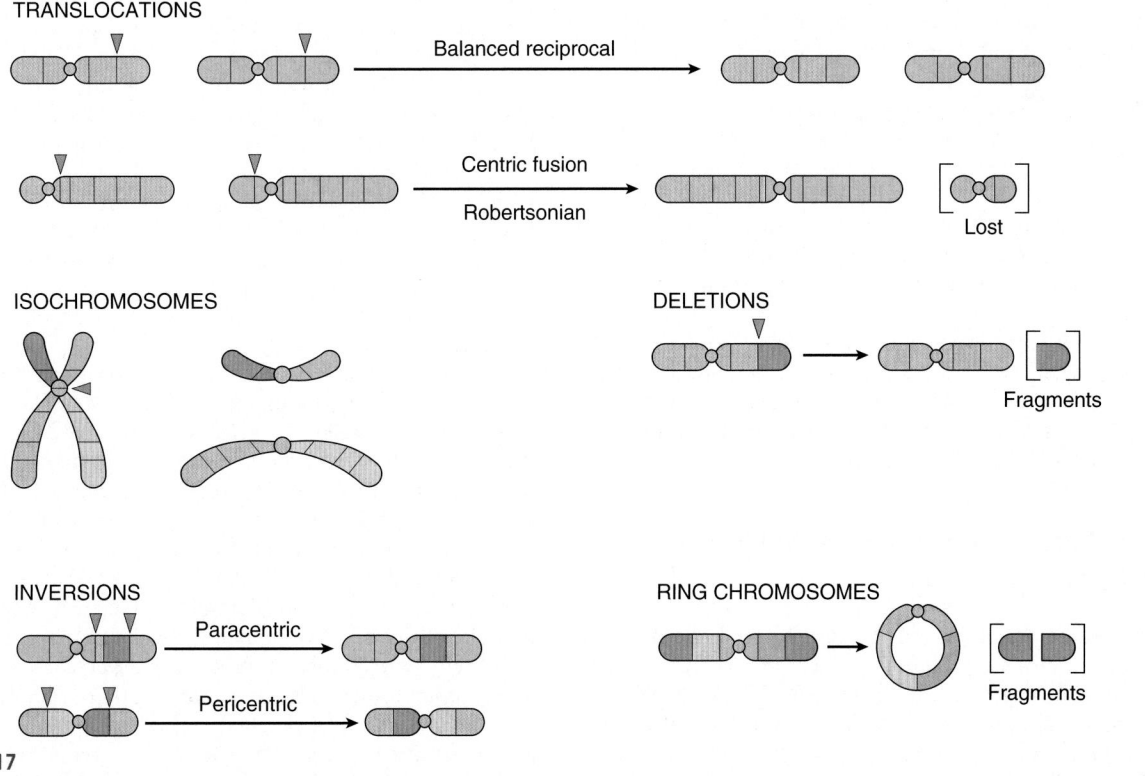

Figure 7–17 ■

Types of chromosomal rearrangements.

sis, resulting in the formation of unbalanced gametes that could lead to abnormal offspring.

■ *Isochromosomes* result when the centromere divides horizontally rather than vertically. One of the two arms of the chromosome is then lost, and the remaining arm is duplicated, resulting in a chromosome with two short arms only or two long arms only. The most common isochromosome present in live births involves the long arm of the X chromosome and is designated i(Xq). When fertilized by a gamete that contains a normal X chromosome, there is monosomy for genes on Xp and trisomy for genes on Xq.

■ *Deletion* involves loss of a portion of a chromosome. A single break may delete a terminal segment. Two interstitial breaks, with reunion of the proximal and distal segments, may result in loss of an intermediate segment. The isolated fragment, which lacks a centromere, almost never survives, and thus many genes are lost.

■ *Inversions* occur when there are two interstitial breaks in a chromosome, and the segment reunites after a complete turnaround.

■ A *ring chromosome* is a variant of a deletion. After loss of segments from each end of the chromosome, the arms unite to form a ring.

Against this background, we can turn first to some general features of chromosomal disorders, followed by some specific examples of diseases involving changes in the karyotype.

■ Chromosomal disorders may be associated with absence (deletion, monosomy), excess (trisomy), or abnormal rearrangements (translocations) of chromosomes.

■ In general, loss of chromosomal material produces more severe defects than does gain of chromosomal material.

■ Excess chromosomal material may result from a complete chromosome (as in trisomy) or from part of a chromosome (as in robertsonian translocation).

■ Imbalances of sex chromosomes (excess or loss) are tolerated much better than are similar imbalances of autosomes.

■ Sex chromosomal disorders often produce subtle abnormalities, sometimes not detected at birth. Infertility, a common manifestation, cannot be diagnosed until adolescence.

■ In most cases, chromosomal disorders result from de novo changes (i.e., parents are normal, and risk of recurrence in siblings is low). An uncommon but important exception to this principle is exhibited by the translocation form of Down syndrome.

Cytogenetic Disorders Involving Autosomes

Three autosomal trisomies (21, 18, and 13) and one deletion syndrome (cri du chat syndrome), which results from partial deletion of the short arm of chromosome 5, were the first chromosomal abnormalities identified. More recently, several additional trisomies and deletion syndromes (such as that affecting 22q) have been described. Most of these disorders are quite uncommon, but their clinical features should

permit ready recognition. Some of the features of the three most common entities are presented in Figure 7–18.

Only trisomy 21 and 22q11 deletion occur with sufficient frequency to merit further consideration.

TRISOMY 21 (DOWN SYNDROME)

Down syndrome is the most common of the chromosomal disorders. About 95% of affected persons have trisomy 21, so their chromosome count is 47. As mentioned earlier, the most common cause of trisomy, and therefore of Down syndrome, is meiotic nondisjunction. The parents of such children have a normal karyotype and are normal in all respects. *Maternal age has a strong influence on the incidence of Down syndrome.* It occurs in 1 in 1550 live births in women younger than 20 years, in contrast to 1 in 25 live births in women older than 45 years. The correlation with maternal age suggests that in most cases the meiotic nondisjunction of chromosome 21 occurs in the ovum. Indeed, in 95% of cases the extra chromosome is of maternal origin. The reason for the increased susceptibility of the ovum to nondisjunction is not fully understood. No effect of paternal age has been found in those cases in which the extra chromosome is derived from the father.

In about 4% of all patients with trisomy 21, the extra chromosomal material is present not as an extra chromosome but as a translocation of the long arm of chromosome 21 to chromosome 22 or 14. Such cases are usually familial, and the translocated chromosome is inherited from one of the parents, who is most frequently a carrier of a robertsonian translocation. The consequences of the mating of a 14;21 translocation carrier (who may be phenotypically normal, with a chromosome count of 45) and a normal individual are depicted in Figure 7–19. Although theoretically the carrier has one chance in three of bearing a live child with Down syndrome, the observed frequency of affected children in such cases is much lower. The reasons for this discrepancy are not well understood. Approximately 1% of trisomy 21 patients are mosaics, usually having a mixture of 46- and 47-chromosome cells. These result from mitotic nondisjunction of chromosome 21 during an early stage of embryogenesis. Symptoms in such cases are variable and milder, depending on the proportion of abnormal cells.

The clinical features of Down syndrome are illustrated in Figure 7–18. The combination of *epicanthic folds* and *flat facial profile* is quite characteristic. Trisomy 21 is a leading cause of *mental retardation*. The degree of mental retardation is severe: IQ varies from 25 to 50. Congenital malformations are common and quite disabling. Approximately 40% of patients with trisomy 21 have *cardiac malformations*, which are responsible for most of the deaths in early childhood. *Serious infections* are another important cause of morbidity and mortality. As with most other clinical features, the basis of increased susceptibility to infection is not clearly understood. The chromosomal imbalance, in some undefined manner, also *increases the person's risk of developing acute leukemias*, particularly acute megakaryocytic leukemia.

The overall prognosis for individuals with Down syndrome has improved remarkably in the recent past owing to

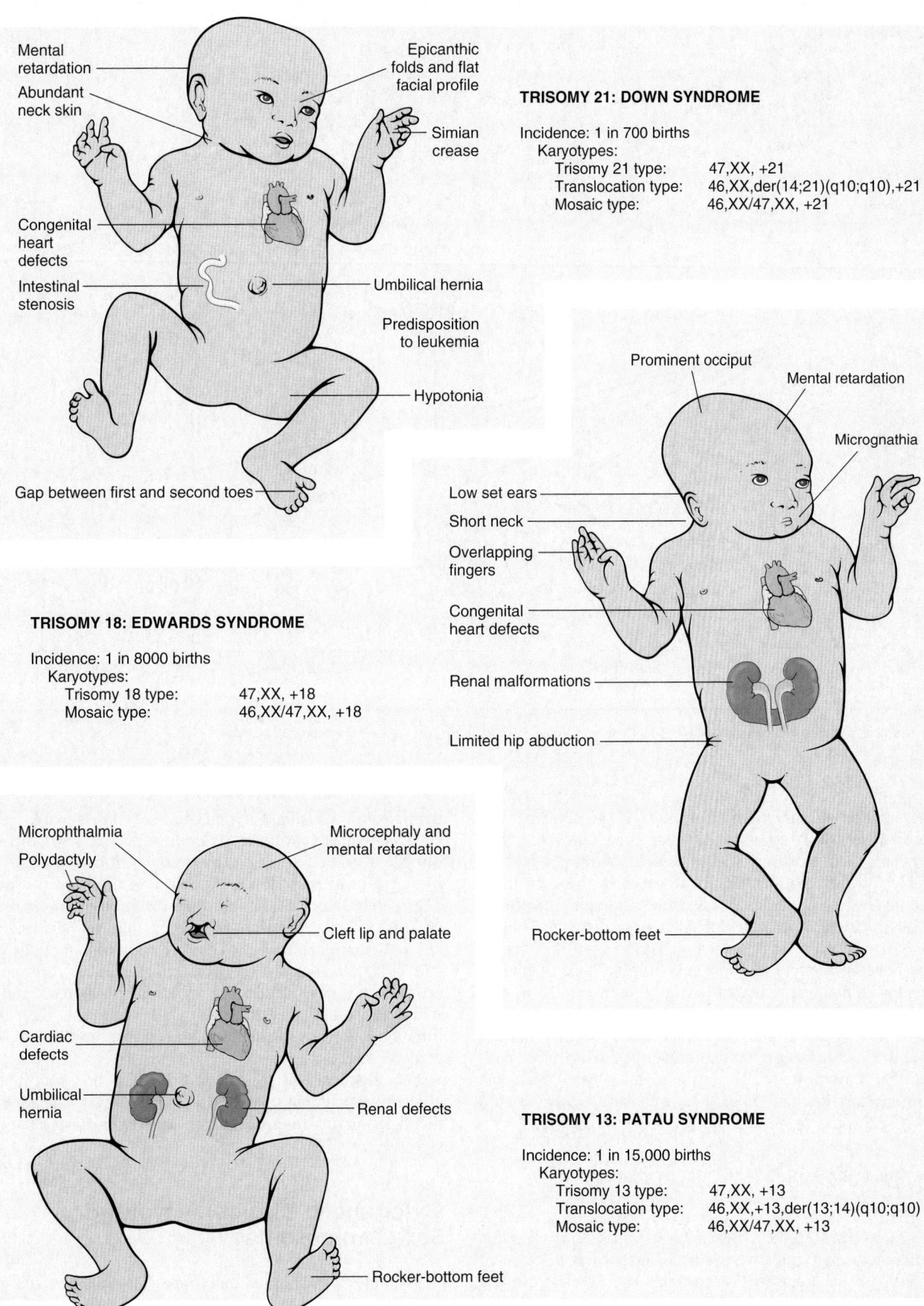

TRISOMY 21: DOWN SYNDROME

Incidence: 1 in 700 births
Karyotypes:
    Trisomy 21 type: 47,XX, +21
    Translocation type: 46,XX,der(14;21)(q10;q10),+21
    Mosaic type: 46,XX/47,XX, +21

TRISOMY 18: EDWARDS SYNDROME

Incidence: 1 in 8000 births
Karyotypes:
    Trisomy 18 type: 47,XX, +18
    Mosaic type: 46,XX/47,XX, +18

TRISOMY 13: PATAU SYNDROME

Incidence: 1 in 15,000 births
Karyotypes:
    Trisomy 13 type: 47,XX, +13
    Translocation type: 46,XX,+13,der(13;14)(q10;q10)
    Mosaic type: 46,XX/47,XX, +13

Figure 7–18

Clinical features and karyotypes of selected autosomal trisomies.

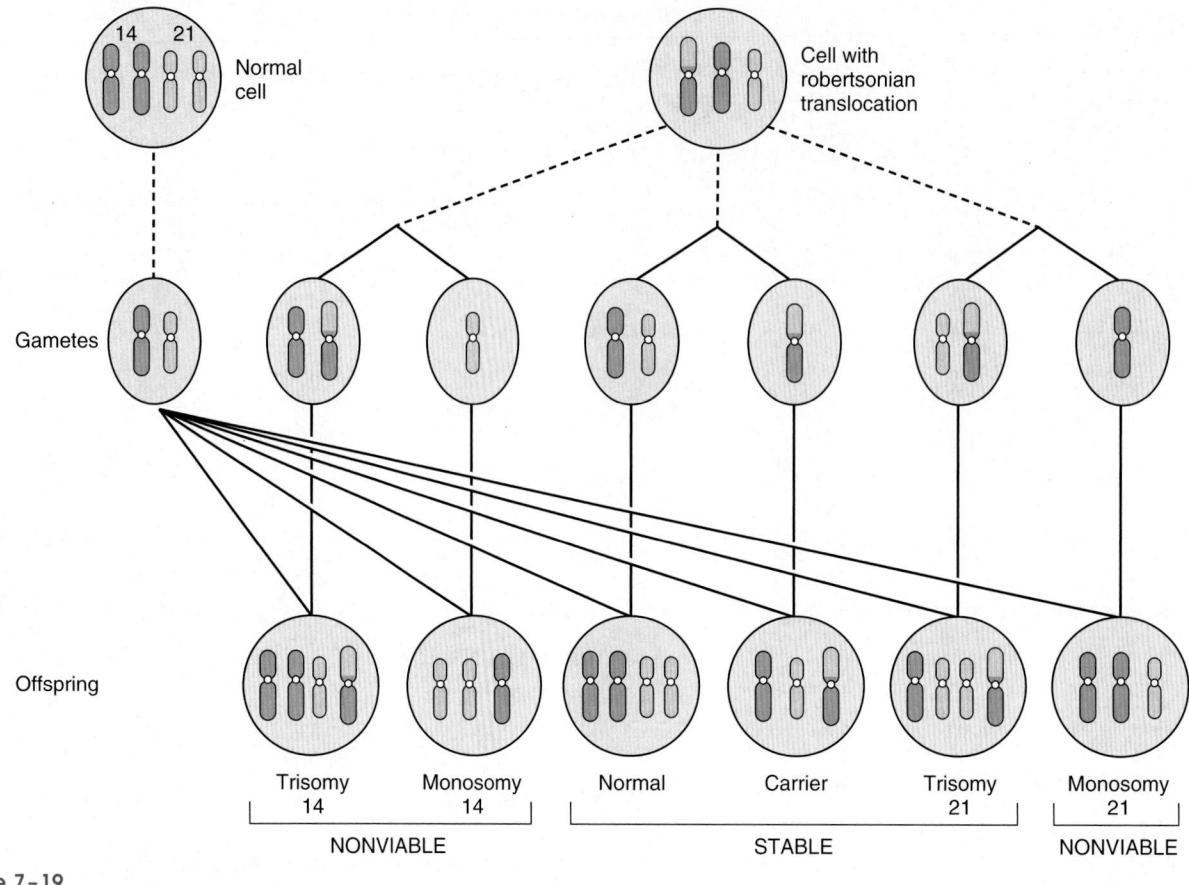

Figure 7-19

Consequences of robertsonian translocation (14;21) for gametogenesis and production of Down syndrome.

better control of infections. Currently, it is estimated that approximately 80% of those without congenital heart disease can expect to survive 30 years. The outlook is less favorable for those with cardiac malformations. Most of those who survive into middle age develop histologic, metabolic, and neurochemical changes of Alzheimer disease (Chapter 23). Many develop frank dementia. The basis of this association is being actively investigated, with the hope of finding clues to the pathogenesis of Alzheimer disease.

Although the karyotype of Down syndrome has been known for decades, the molecular basis of this disease remains elusive. Data from the human genome project indicate that chromosome 21 carries 225 genes. What the critical genes are and how their imbalance gives rise to Down syndrome are now under active investigation.

CHROMOSOME 22q11 DELETION SYNDROME

Chromosome 22q11 syndrome encompasses a spectrum of disorders that result from a small interstitial deletion of band 11 on the long arm of chromosome 22. The clinical features of this deletion include congenital heart disease affecting the outflow tracts, abnormalities of the palate, facial dysmorphism, developmental delay, thymic hypoplasia with impaired T-cell immunity, and parathyroid

hypoplasia causing hypocalcemia. Previously, these clinical features were believed to represent two different disorders—*DiGeorge syndrome* and *velocardiofacial syndrome*. However, it is now known that both are caused by 22q11 deletion. It is thought that variations in the size and position of the deletion is responsible for the variable clinical manifestations. When T-cell immunodeficiency and hypocalcemia are the dominant features, the patients are said to have DiGeorge syndrome, whereas patients with the so-called velocardiofacial syndrome have mild immunodeficiency with pronounced dysmorphology and cardiac defects.

The diagnosis of this condition may be suspected on clinical grounds but can be established only by detection of the deletion by fluorescence in situ hybridization (FISH) (see Fig. 7–43*B*).

Cytogenetic Disorders Involving Sex Chromosomes

A number of abnormal karyotypes involving the sex chromosomes, ranging from 45,X to 49,XXXXY, are compatible with life. Indeed, males who are phenotypically normal have been identified as having two and even three Y chromosomes. Such extreme karyotypic deviations are not encountered with the autosomes. In large part this latitude relates to two factors: (1) lyonization of X chromosomes and (2) the scant amount of genetic information carried by the Y chromosome. The consideration of lyonization must begin with the Barr body, or sex chromatin, a prominent clump of chromatin attached to the nuclear membrane in the interphase nuclei of all somatic cells of females. In 1962, Mary Lyon proposed that the *Barr body represents one genetically inactivated X chromosome.* This inactivation occurs early in fetal life, about 16 days after conception, and randomly inactivates either the paternal or the maternal X chromosome in each of the primitive cells representing the developing embryo. Once inactivated, the same X chromosome remains genetically neutralized in all of the progeny of these cells. Moreover, all but one X chromosome is inactivated, and so a 48,XXXX female has only one active X chromosome and three Barr bodies. This phenomenon explains why normal females do not have a double dose (compared with males) of phenotypic attributes coded by the X chromosome. The Lyon hypothesis also explains why normal females are in reality mosaics, containing two cell populations—one with an active maternal X, the other with an active paternal X. Although essentially accurate, the Lyon hypothesis has been somewhat modified, as we shall discuss under Turner syndrome.

Extra Y chromosomes are readily tolerated because the only information known to be carried on the Y chromosome appears to relate to male differentiation. It should be noted that whatever the number of X chromosomes, the presence of a Y invariably dictates the male phenotype. The Y body appears as a small, brightly fluorescing spot in interphase nuclei stained with fluorescent dyes and examined with the ultraviolet microscope. The genes for male differentiation are located on the short arm of the Y.

Two disorders—Klinefelter syndrome and Turner syndrome—arising in aberrations of sex chromosomes are described briefly.

KLINEFELTER SYNDROME

This syndrome is best defined as male hypogonadism that develops when there are at least two X chromosomes and one or more Y chromosomes. Most patients are 47,XXY. This karyotype results from nondisjunction of sex chromosomes during meiosis. The extra X chromosome may be of either maternal or paternal origin. Advanced maternal age and a history of irradiation of either parent may contribute to the meiotic error resulting in this condition. Approximately 15% of patients show mosaic patterns, including 46,XY/47,XXY,47,XXY/48,XXXX, and variations on this theme. The presence of a 46,XY line in mosaics is usually associated with a milder clinical condition.

Although the following description applies to most patients, it should be noted that Klinefelter syndrome is associated with a wide range of clinical manifestations. In some it may be expressed only as hypogonadism, but most patients have a distinctive body habitus with an *increase in length between the soles and the pubic bone,* which creates the appearance of an elongated body. Also characteristic is eunuchoid body habitus. *Reduced facial, body, and pubic hair* and *gynecomastia* are also frequently noted. The testes

are markedly reduced in size, sometimes to only 2 cm in greatest dimension. Along with the *testicular atrophy,* the serum testosterone levels are lower than normal, and urinary gonadotropin levels are elevated.

The principal clinical effect of this syndrome is sterility. Only rarely are patients fertile, and these are presumably mosaics with a large proportion of 46,XY cells. The sterility is due to impaired spermatogenesis, sometimes to the extent of total azoospermia. Histologically, there is hyalinization of tubules, which appear as ghostlike structures in tissue section. By contrast, Leydig cells are prominent, owing to either hyperplasia or an apparent increase related to loss of tubules. Although Klinefelter syndrome may be associated with mental retardation, the degree of intellectual impairment is typically mild and in some cases is undetectable. The reduction in intelligence is correlated with the number of extra X chromosomes. Thus, in patients with the most common variant (XXY), intelligence is nearly normal, but in those with rare variant forms involving additional X chromosomes, significantly subnormal levels of intelligence, as well as more severe physical abnormalities, are found.

TURNER SYNDROME

Turner syndrome, characterized by primary hypogonadism in phenotypic females, results from partial or complete monosomy of the short arm of the X chromosome. In approximately 57% of patients, the entire X chromosome is missing, resulting in a 45,X karyotype. These patients are the most severely affected, and the diagnosis can often be made at birth or early in childhood. Typical clinical features associated with 45,X Turner syndrome include significant growth retardation, leading to abnormally short stature (below third percentile); swelling of the nape of the neck due to distended lymphatic channels (in infancy) that is seen as webbing of the neck in older children; low posterior hairline; cubitus valgus (an increase in the carrying angle of the arms); shieldlike chest with widely spaced nipples; high-arched palate; lymphedema of the hands and feet; and a variety of congenital malformations such as horseshoe kidney, bicuspid aortic valve, and coarctation of the aorta (Fig. 7–20). Affected girls fail to develop normal secondary sex characteristics; the genitalia remain infantile, breast development is minimal, and little pubic hair appears. Most have primary amenorrhea, and morphologic examination reveals transformation of the ovaries into white streaks of fibrous stroma devoid of follicles. The mental status of these patients is usually normal, but subtle defects in nonverbal, visual-spatial information processing have been noted. Curiously, hypothyroidism caused by autoantibodies is noted in 25% to 30% of patients, especially in women with isochromosome Xp (see below). In adult patients, *a combination of short stature and primary amenorrhea should prompt strong suspicion of Turner syndrome.* The diagnosis is established by karyotyping.

Approximately 43% of patients with Turner syndrome either are mosaics (one of the cell lines being 45,X) or have structural abnormalities of the X chromosome. These are listed in Figure 7–20. The most common is deletion of the small arm, resulting in the formation of an isochromosome of the long arm, 46,X,i(X)(q10). The net effect

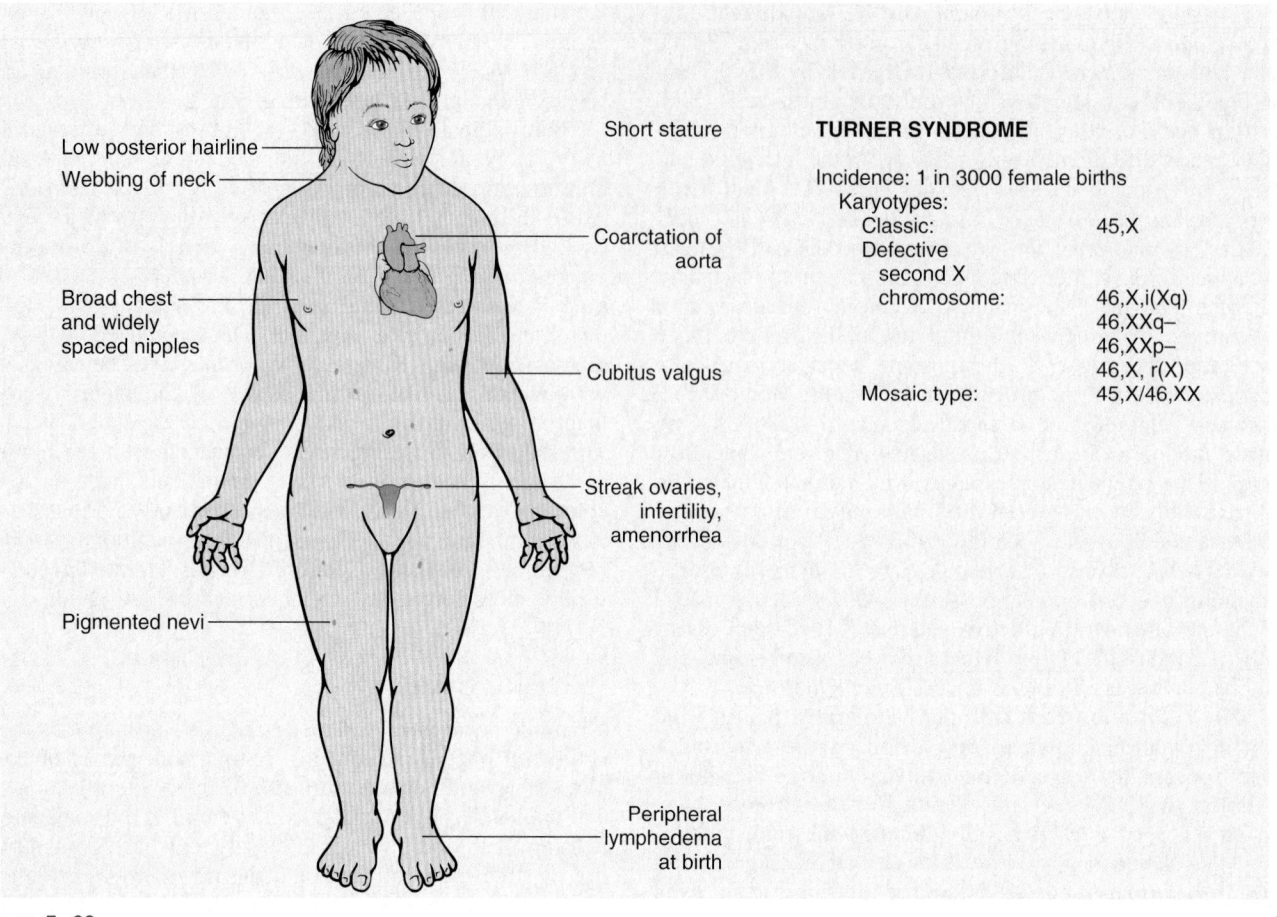

Figure 7-20   ■

Clinical features and karyotypes of Turner syndrome.

of the associated structural abnormalities is to produce partial monosomy of the X chromosome. Combinations of deletions and mosaicism are reported. It is important to appreciate the karyotypic heterogeneity associated with Turner syndrome because it is responsible for significant variations in the phenotype. In contrast to the patients with monosomy X, those who are *mosaics or have dele-tion variants may have an almost normal appearance and may present only with primary amenorrhea.*

It is pertinent to recall the Lyon hypothesis in the context of Turner syndrome. If only one active X chromosome were necessary for the development of normal females (as proposed in the Lyon hypothesis), patients with partial or complete loss of one X chromosome would not be expected to display the stigmata of Turner syndrome. In view of this inconsistency and other observations, the Lyon hypothesis has been modified. It is now known that although one X chromosome is inactivated in all cells during embryogenesis, it is selectively reactivated in germ cells before first meiotic division. Furthermore, it seems that certain X chromosome genes remain active on both X chromosomes in many somatic cells of normal females. Thus, it seems that two copies of some X-linked genes are essential for normal gametogenesis and female development. Some of these genes are beginning to be identified. For example, a homeobox gene aptly called short-stature homeobox *(SHOX),* located

on Xp22.32, seems to be involved in vertical growth. This is one of those genes that remain active on both copies of the X chromosome. Homologues of the *SHOX* gene are also found on the Y chromosome, ensuring that males with only one copy of the X chromosome develop normally.

SINGLE-GENE DISORDERS WITH ATYPICAL PATTERNS OF INHERITANCE

Three groups of diseases resulting from mutations affecting single genes do not follow the mendelian rules of inheritance:

■ Diseases caused by triplet repeat mutations
■ Diseases caused by mutations in mitochondrial genes
■ Diseases associated with genomic imprinting

TRIPLET REPEAT MUTATIONS: FRAGILE X SYNDROME

Fragile X syndrome is the prototype of diseases in which the mutation is characterized by a long repeating sequence of three nucleotides. Other examples of diseases associated with trinucleotide repeat mutations include Huntington disease and myotonic dystrophy. The origins of over a dozen diseases have now been assigned to pathologic expansions of trinucleotide repeats, and all disorders discovered so far are associated with neurodegenerative changes. In each of these conditions, *amplification of specific sets of three nucleotides within the gene disrupts its function.* Certain unique features of trinucleotide repeat mutations, described later, are responsible for the atypical pattern of inheritance of the associated diseases.

Fragile X syndrome is characterized by mental retardation and an abnormality in the X chromosome (Fig. 7–21). It is one of the most common causes of familial mental retardation. The cytogenetic alteration is induced by certain culture conditions and is seen as a *discontinuity of staining or constriction in the long arm of the X chromosome.* Clinically affected males have moderate to severe mental retardation. They express a characteristic physical phenotype that includes a long face with a large mandible, large everted ears, and large testicles *(macro-orchidism).* Although characteristic of fragile X syndrome, these abnormalities are not always present or may be quite subtle. The only distinctive physical abnormality that can be detected in at least 90% of postpubertal males with fragile X syndrome is macro-orchidism.

Fragile X syndrome results from a mutation in the *FMR1* gene that maps to Xq27.3. Like all X-linked recessive disorders, this disease affects males. However, unlike patients with other X-linked recessive disorders, approximately 20% of males who are known to carry the fragile X mutation are clinically and cytogenetically normal. These "carrier males" can transmit the disease to their grandsons through their phenotypically normal daughters. Another peculiarity is the presence of mental retardation in 50% of carrier females. These unusual features have been related to the dynamic nature of the mutation (Fig. 7–22). In the normal population, the number of CGG repeats in the

FMR1 gene is small, averaging around 29, whereas affected individuals have 230 to 4000 repeats. These so called full mutations are believed to arise through an intermediate stage of *premutations* characterized by 52 to 230 CGG repeats. Carrier males and females have premutations. During oogenesis (but not spermatogenesis) the premutations can be converted to full mutations by further amplification of the CGG repeats, which can then be transmitted to both the sons and the daughters of the carrier female. These observations provide an explanation for why some carrier males are unaffected (they have premutations) and certain carrier females are affected (they inherit full mutations).

The molecular basis of fragile X syndrome is beginning to be understood. The CGG repeats are located in the 5' untranslated region of the *FMR1* gene (Fig. 7–23). In patients with this disease, the expanded CGG repeats are hypermethylated. Methylation then extends up stream into the promoter region, resulting in transcriptional silencing of the *FMR1* gene. The product of the *FMR1* gene, called FMR protein (FMRP), is widely expressed in normal tissues, but higher levels of transcripts are found in the brain and the testis. Current evidence suggests that FMRP is an RNA-binding protein that regulates protein translation. Thus, it is speculated that loss of FMRP in fragile X syndrome dysregulates the production of some critical target proteins that are involved in normal neuronal functions.

Before closing this discussion, it is appropriate to offer some general comments on other diseases related to trinucleotide repeat expansions.

■ In all cases, gene functions are altered by an expansion of the repeats, but the precise threshold at which premutations are converted to full mutations differs with each disorder.

■ While the expansion in fragile X syndrome occurs during oogenesis, in other disorders, such as Huntington disease, premutations are converted to full mutations during spermatogenesis.

■ The expansion may involve any part of the gene, including untranslated regions, exons, and introns (see Fig. 7–23). In some cases, as in fragile X syndrome, there is suppression of protein synthesis, whereas in others, typified by Huntington disease, abnormal gene products interfere with the function of normal proteins (Chapter 23).

DISEASES CAUSED BY MUTATIONS IN MITOCHONDRIAL GENES

Mitochondria contain several genes that encode enzymes involved in oxidative phosphorylation. Inheritance of mitochondrial DNA differs from that of nuclear DNA in that the former is associated with *maternal inheritance.* This peculiarity results from the fact that ova contain mitochondria within their abundant cytoplasm, whereas spermatozoa contain few, if any, mitochondria. Hence, the mitochondrial DNA complement of the zygote is derived entirely from the ovum. Thus, mothers transmit mitochondrial genes to all of their offspring, both male and female; however, daughters but not sons transmit the DNA further to their progeny.

Figure 7–21   ■

Fragile X, seen as discontinuity of staining. (Courtesy of Dr. Patricia Howard-Peebles, University of Texas Southwestern Medical School, Dallas.)

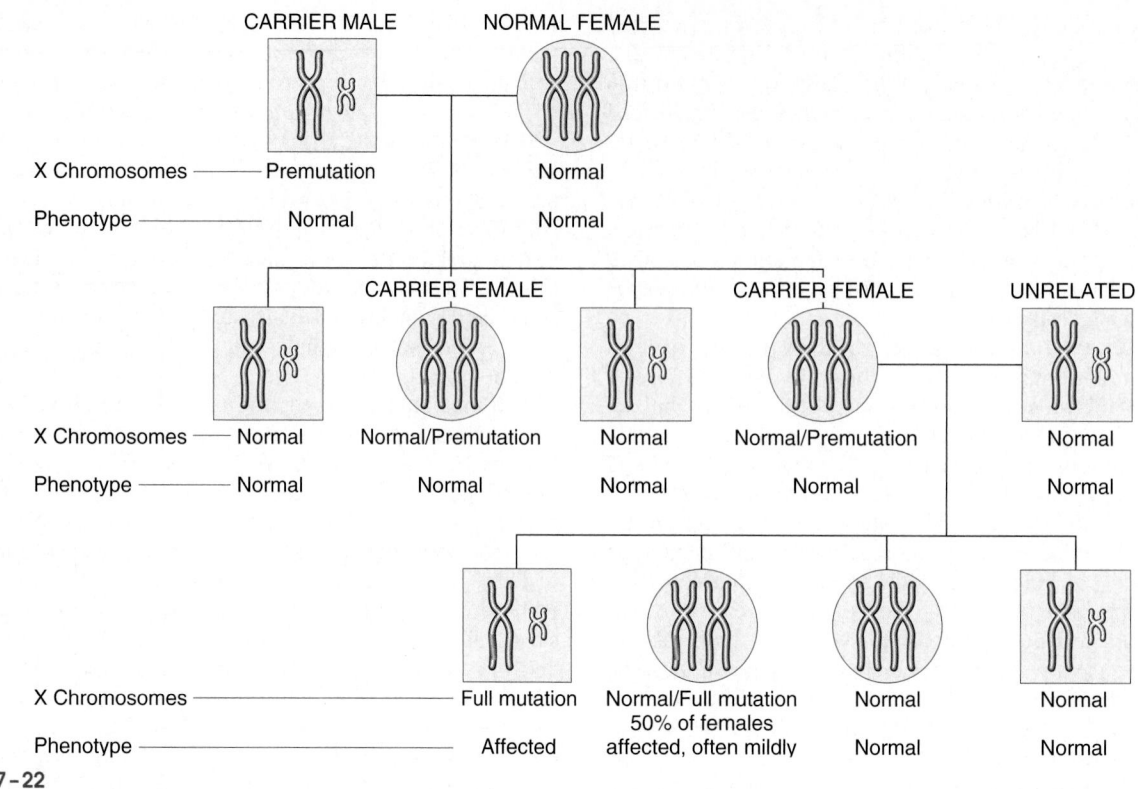

Figure 7-22 ■

Fragile X pedigree. Note that in the first generation, all sons are normal and all females are carriers. During oogenesis in the carrier female, premutation expands to full mutation; hence in the next generation, all males who inherit the X with full mutation are affected. However, only 50% of females who inherit the full mutation are affected, and often only mildly. (Original sketch courtesy of Dr. Nancy Schneider, Department of Pathology, University of Texas Southwestern Medical School, Dallas.)

Diseases caused by mutations in mitochondrial genes are rare. Leber hereditary optic neuropathy is the prototypical disorder in this group. This neurodegenerative disease manifests itself as progressive bilateral loss of central vision that leads in due course to blindness.

GENOMIC IMPRINTING: PRADER-WILLI AND ANGELMAN SYNDROMES

All humans inherit two copies of each gene, carried on homologous maternal and paternal chromosomes. It has usually been assumed that there is no difference between normal homologous genes derived from the mother or the father. Indeed, this is true for many genes. However, it has now been established that with respect to several genes, functional differences exist between the paternal and the maternal genes. These differences arise from an epigenetic process called *genomic imprinting*, whereby certain genes are differentially "inactivated" during paternal and maternal gametogenesis. Thus, *maternal imprinting* refers to transcriptional silencing of the maternal allele, whereas *paternal imprinting* implies that the paternal allele is inactivated. Imprinting occurs in ovum or sperm and is then stably transmitted to all somatic cells derived from the zygote.

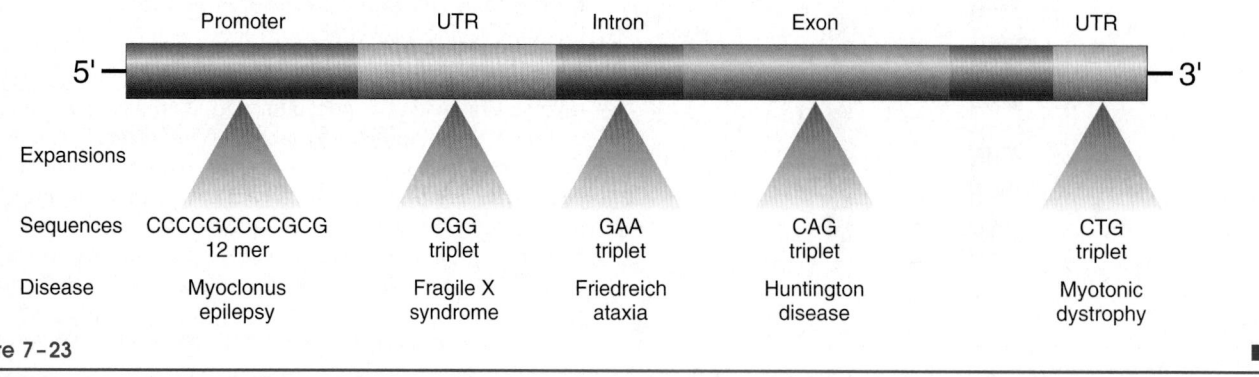

Figure 7-23 ■

Sites of expansion and the affected sequence in selected diseases caused by nucleotide repeat mutations. UTR, untranslated region.

Genomic imprinting is best illustrated by considering two uncommon genetic disorders: Prader-Willi syndrome and Angelman syndrome.

Prader-Willi syndrome is characterized by mental retardation, short stature, hypotonia, obesity, small hands and feet, and hypogonadism. In 50% to 60% of cases, an interstitial deletion of band q12 in the long arm of chromosome 15 [i.e., del(15)(q11;q13)] can be detected. In many patients without a detectable cytogenetic abnormality, FISH analysis reveals smaller deletions within the same region. *It is striking that in all cases the deletion affects the paternally derived chromosome 15.* In contrast with Prader-Willi syndrome, patients with the phenotypically distinct *Angelman syndrome* are born with a deletion of the same chromosomal region derived from their mothers. Patients with Angelman syndrome are also mentally retarded, but in addition they present with ataxic gait, seizures, and inappropriate laughter. Because of the laughter and ataxia, this syndrome is also called the *happy puppet syndrome.* A comparison of these two syndromes clearly demonstrates the "parent-of-origin" effects on gene function. If all the paternal and maternal genes contained within chromosome 15 were expressed in an identical fashion, clinical features resulting from these deletions would be expected to be identical regardless of the parental origin of chromosome 15.

The molecular basis of these two syndromes can be understood in the context of imprinting (Fig. 7–24). It is believed that a set of genes on maternal chromosome 15q12 is imprinted (and hence silenced), and thus the only functional alleles are provided by the paternal chromosome. When these are lost as a result of a deletion (in the paternal chromosome), the patient develops Prader-Willi syndrome. Conversely, a distinct gene that also maps to the same region of chromosome 15 is imprinted on the paternal chromosome. Only the maternally derived allele of the gene is normally active. Deletion of this maternal gene on chromosome 15 gives rise to the Angelman syndrome. Molecular studies of cytogenetically normal patients with Prader-Willi syndrome have revealed that in some cases both of the structurally normal chromosome 15s are derived from the mother. Inheritance of both chromosomes of a pair from one parent is called uniparental disomy. The net effect is the same (i.e., the patient does not have a functional set of genes from the [nonimprinted] paternal chromosome 15). Angelman syndrome, as might be expected, can also result from uniparental disomy of parental chromosome 15.

The Angelman syndrome gene (imprinted on paternal chromosome) is now known to encode a ligase that has a role in the ubiquitin-proteasome proteolytic pathway (Chapter 1). This gene, called, somewhat laboriously, *UBE3A,* is expressed primarily from the maternal allele in specific regions of *the* normal brain. In Angelman syndrome, *UBE3A* is not expressed in these areas of the brain— hence the neurologic disorder. Prader-Willi syndrome, unlike Angelman syndrome, is most likely caused by the loss of several genes located between 15q11 and q13. These genes are still being fully characterized.

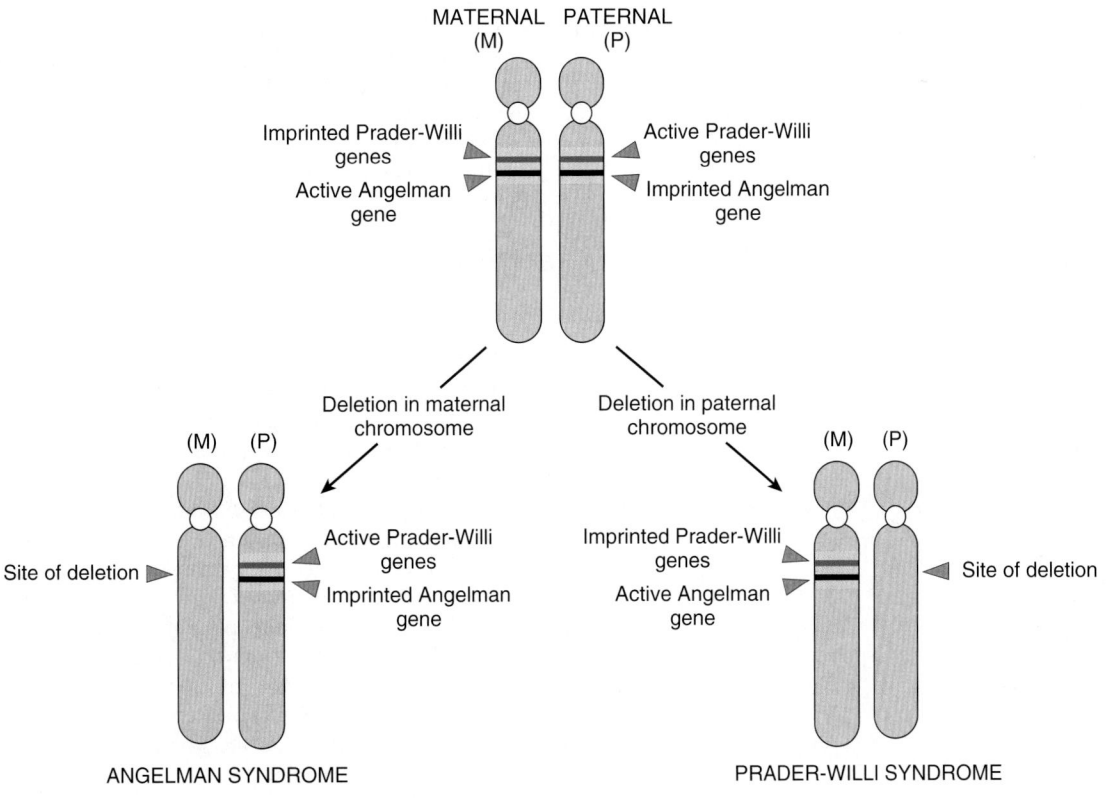

Figure 7–24   ■

Diagrammatic representation of the genetics of Angelman and Prader-Willi syndromes.

■ Pediatric Diseases

As mentioned earlier and illustrated by several examples, many diseases of infancy and childhood are of genetic origin. Others, although not genetic, either are unique to children or take distinctive forms in this stage of life and so merit the designation *pediatric diseases.*

During each stage of development, infants and children are prey to a somewhat different group of diseases (Table 7–8). Clearly, diseases of infancy (i.e., the first year of life) pose the highest risk of mortality. During this phase, the neonatal period (the first 4 weeks of life) is unquestionably the most hazardous time.

Once the infant survives the first year of life, the outlook brightens considerably. However, it is sobering to note that between 1 year and 15 years of age, injuries resulting from accidents are the leading cause of death. Not all conditions

■

Table 7–8. CAUSES OF DEATH BY AGE

Causes	Rate*
Under 1 Yr: All Causes	692
Perinatal conditions	
Intrauterine growth retardation/low birth weight	
Respiratory distress syndrome	
Intrauterine hypoxia/birth asphyxia	
Birth trauma	
Others	
Congenital anomalies	
Sudden infant death syndrome	
Pneumonia	
Gastointestinal disorders	
1–4 Yr: All Causes	43.3
Injuries	
Congenital anomalies	
Malignant neoplasms	
Homicide	
Diseases of the heart	
5–9 Yr: All Causes	18.5
Injuries	
Malignant neoplasms	
Congenital anomalies	
Homicide	
Diseases of the heart	
10–14 Yr: All Causes	18.5
Injuries	
Malignant neoplasms	
Suicide	
Homicide	
Congenital anomalies	

*Number of deaths per 100,000 population.

listed in Table 7–8 are described in this chapter, but only a select few that are most common. Although general principles of neoplastic disease and specific tumors are discussed elsewhere, a few tumors of children are described in this chapter to highlight the differences between pediatric and adult neoplasms.

CONGENITAL ANOMALIES

Congenital anomalies are structural defects that are present at birth, although some, such as cardiac defects and renal anomalies, may not become clinically apparent until years later. As will be evident from the ensuing discussion, the term *congenital* does not imply or exclude a genetic basis for birth defects. It is estimated that about 3% of newborns have a major anomaly, defined as a birth defect having either cosmetic or functional significance. As indicated in Table 7–8, congenital anomalies are an important cause of infant mortality. Moreover, they continue to be a significant cause of illness, disability, and death throughout the early years of life.

Before the etiology and pathogenesis of congenital anomalies are described, it is essential to define some of the terms used to describe errors in morphogenesis.

■ *Malformations* represent primary errors of morphogenesis. In other words, there is an *intrinsically abnormal developmental process.* Malformations are usually multifactorial rather than the result of a single gene or chromosomal defect. They may present in several patterns. In some, such as congenital heart diseases, single body systems may be involved, whereas in other cases, multiple malformations involving many organs and tissues may coexist (Fig. 7–25).

■ *Disruptions* result from secondary destruction of an organ or body region that was previously normal in development; thus, in contrast to malformations, disruptions arise from an *extrinsic disturbance in morphogenesis. Amniotic bands,* denoting rupture of amnion with resultant formation of "bands" that encircle, compress, or attach to parts of the developing fetus, are the classic example of a disruption (Fig. 7–26). A variety of environmental agents may cause disruptions (see later). Understandably, disruptions are not heritable and hence are not associated with risk of recurrence in subsequent pregnancies.

■ *Deformations,* like disruptions, also represent an *extrinsic disturbance of development* rather than an intrinsic error of

Figure 7–25   ■

Human malformations can range in severity from the incidental to the lethal. *Polydactyly* (one or more extra digits) and *syndactyly* (fusion of digits), both of which are illustrated in *A,* have little functional consequence when they occur in isolation. Similarly, *cleft lip (B),* with or without associated *cleft palate,* is compatible with life when it occurs as an isolated anomaly; in this case, however, the child had an underlying *malformation syndrome* (trisomy 13) and expired because of severe cardiac defects. The stillbirth illustrated in *C* represents a severe and essentially lethal malformation, in which the mid-face structures are fused or ill-formed; in almost all cases, this degree of external dysmorphogenesis is associated with severe internal anomalies such as maldevelopment of the brain and cardiac defects. *A* and *C,* Courtesy of Dr. Reade Quinton; *B,* courtesy of Dr. Beverly Rogers, Department of Pathology, University of Texas Southwestern Medical Center, Dallas.)

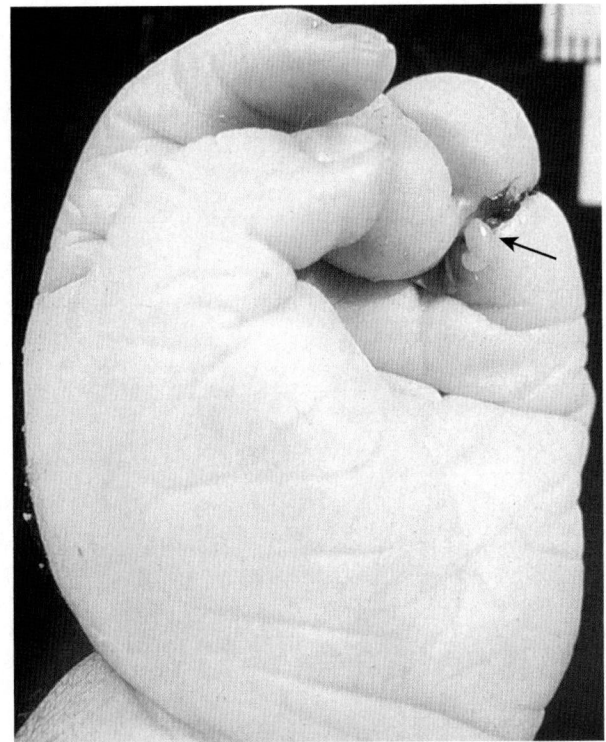

Figure 7–26   ■

Disruptions occur in a normally developing organ or structure because of an extrinsic abnormality that interferes with normal morphogenesis. Amniotic bands *(arrow)* are a frequent cause of disruptions and in the illustrated example resulted in maldevelopment of the fingers.

morphogenesis. Deformations are common problems, affecting approximately 2% of newborn infants to various degrees. Fundamental to the pathogenesis of deformations is localized or generalized compression of the growing fetus by abnormal biomechanical forces, leading eventually to a variety of structural abnormalities. The most common underlying factor responsible for deformations is uterine constraint. Between the 35th and 38th weeks of gestation, rapid increase in the size of the fetus outpaces the growth of the uterus, and the relative amount of amniotic fluid (which normally acts as a cushion) also decreases. Thus, even the normal fetus is subjected to some form of uterine constraint. However, several factors increase the likelihood of excessive compression of the fetus, including maternal conditions such as first pregnancy, small uterus, malformed (bicornuate) uterus, and leiomyomas. Factors relating to the fetus, such as multiple fetuses, oligohydramnios, and abnormal fetal presentation, may also be involved.

■ *Sequence* refers to multiple congenital anomalies that result from *secondary effects of a single localized aberration in organogenesis.* The initiating event may be a malformation, deformation, or disruption. An excellent example is the oligohydramnios (or Potter) sequence (Fig. 7–27A). Oligohydramnios, denoting decreased amniotic fluid, may be caused by a variety of unrelated maternal, placental, or fetal abnormalities. Chronic leakage of amniotic fluid owing to rupture of the amnion; uteroplacental insufficiency resulting from maternal hypertension or severe toxemia; and renal agenesis in the fetus (as fetal urine is a major constituent of amniotic fluid) all are causes of oligohydramnios. The fetal compression associ-

Figure 7–27

A, Infant with oligohydramnios (Potter) sequence. Note flattened facial features and deformed foot (talipes equinovarus). *B,* Schematic diagram of the pathogenesis of the oligohydramnios (Potter) sequence.

ated with significant oligohydramnios in turn results in a classic phenotype in the newborn infant, including flattened facies and positional abnormalities of the hands and feet (Fig. 7–27*B*). The hips may be dislocated. Growth of the chest wall and the contained lungs is also compromised, sometimes to such an extent that survival is not possible. If the embryologic connection between these defects and the initiating event is not recognized, a sequence may be mistaken for a malformation syndrome.

■ *Malformation syndrome* refers to the presence of several defects that cannot be explained on the basis of a single localizing initiating error in morphogenesis. Syndromes are most often caused by a single causative factor (e.g., viral infection or a specific chromosomal abnormality) that simultaneously affects several tissues.

■ In addition to the global definitions listed previously, some general terms are applied to organ-specific malformations. *Agenesis* refers to the complete absence of an organ or its anlage whereas *aplasia* and *hypoplasia* are used to indicate incomplete development or underdevelopment of an organ. *Atresia* describes the absence of an opening, usually of a hollow visceral organ or duct such as intestines and bile ducts.

Etiology. Known causes of errors in human malformations can be grouped into two major categories: *genetic* and *environmental* (Table 7–9). *Almost half have no recognized cause.*

Genetic causes of malformations include all of the previously discussed mechanisms of genetic disease. Virtually all chromosomal syndromes are associated with congenital malformations. Examples include Down syndrome and other trisomies, Turner syndrome, and Klinefelter syndrome. Most

Table 7–9.   CAUSES OF CONGENITAL MALFORMATIONS IN HUMANS

Cause	Malformed Live Births (%)
Genetic	
Chromosomal aberrations	10–15
Mendelian inheritance	2–10
Multifactorial	20–25
Environmental	
Maternal/placental infections	2–3
Rubella	
Toxoplasmosis	
Syphilis	
Cytomegalovirus infection	
Human immunodeficiency virus infection	
Maternal disease states	6–8
Diabetes	
Phenylketonuria	
Endocrinopathies	
Drugs and chemicals	~1
Alcohol	
Folic acid antagonists	
Androgens	
Phenytoin	
Thalidomide	
Warfarin	
13-*cis*-Retinoic acid	
Others	
Irradiation	~1
Unknown	40–60

Adapted from Stevenson RE, et al (eds): Human Malformations and Related Anomalies. New York, Oxford University Press, 1993, p 115.

chromosomal disorders arise during gametogenesis and hence are not familial. Single-gene mutations, characterized by mendelian inheritance, may underlie major malformations. For example, holoprosencephaly is the most common developmental defect of the forebrain and midface in humans (Chapter 23); mutations of the *SHH (sonic hedgehog homologue)* gene have been implicated in the pathogenesis of a subset of these cases. Similarly, mutations of the *PAX6* gene are seen in a proportion of patients with congenital absence of the iris (aniridia). *Multifactorial inheritance*, which implies the interaction of environmental factors with two or more genes of small effect, is the most common genetic cause of congenital malformations. Included in this category are some relatively common malformations such as cleft lip and palate and neural tube defects. The importance of environmental contributions to multifactorial inheritance is underscored by the dramatic reduction of the incidence of neural tube defects by periconceptional intake of folic acid in the diet. The recurrence risks and mode of transmission of multifactorial disorders were described earlier in this chapter (p 227).

Environmental influences, such as viral infections, drugs, and irradiation to which the mother was exposed during pregnancy, may cause fetal malformations (the appellation of "malformation" is loosely used in this context, since technically, these anomalies represent *disruptions*). Among the viral infections listed in Table 7–9, the effects of rubella and cytomegalovirus infection have been studied most extensively. Although maternal rubella and the resultant rubella syndrome have been virtually eliminated as a result of immunization with rubella vaccine, this viral infection serves as an important model of environmental teratogenesis and hence is discussed briefly.

As with all environmental teratogens, the *gestational age at which fetal exposure* to rubella occurs is critically important. The frequency of embryonic rubella infection following symptomatic maternal infection is greater than 80% during the first 12 weeks of gestation and drops to 25% at the end of the second trimester. Malformations attributable to rubella, however, almost always occur before the 16th week of development. The tetrad of congenital heart defects, cataracts, deafness, and mental retardation represents the classic manifestations of *rubella embryopathy*. Congenital cytomegalovirus infection is discussed in Chapter 13.

A variety of drugs and chemicals have been suspected to be teratogenic, but perhaps less than 1% of congenital malformations are caused by these agents. The list includes thalidomide; folate antagonists; androgenic hormones; alcohol; anticonvulsants; warfarin (oral anticoagulant); and 13-*cis*-retinoic acid, which is used in the treatment of severe acne. For example, *thalidomide*, once used as a tranquilizer in Europe and currently being considered for its anti-angiogenic properties, causes an extremely high incidence (50% to 80%) of limb malformations. *Alcohol*, perhaps the most widely used agent today, is an important environmental teratogen. Affected infants show prenatal and postnatal growth retardation, facial anomalies (microcephaly, short palpebral fissures, maxillary hypoplasia), and psychomotor disturbances. These together are labeled the *fetal alcohol syndrome*. While cigarette smoke–derived nicotine has not been convincingly demonstrated to be a teratogen, there is a high incidence of

spontaneous abortions, premature labor, and placental abnormalities in pregnant smokers; babies born to mothers who smoke often have a low birth weight and may be prone to the sudden infant death syndrome. *In light of these findings, it is best to avoid nicotine exposure altogether during pregnancy.*

Among maternal conditions listed in Table 7–9, diabetes mellitus is a common entity, and despite advances in antenatal obstetric monitoring and glucose control, the incidence of major malformations in infants of diabetic mothers stands between 6% to 10% in most series. Maternal hyperglycemia–induced fetal hyperinsulinemia results in fetal macrosomia (organomegaly and increased body fat and muscle mass); cardiac anomalies, neural tube defects, and other central nervous system malformations are some of the major anomalies seen in *diabetic embryopathy*.

Pathogenesis. The pathogenesis of congenital malformations is complex and still poorly understood, but two important general principles of developmental pathology are relevant regardless of the etiologic agent:

■ *The timing of the prenatal insult has an important impact on both the occurrence and the type of malformation produced.* The intrauterine development of humans can be divided into two phases: the embryonic period, occupying the first 9 weeks of pregnancy, and the fetal period, which terminates at birth. In the early embryonic period (the first 3 weeks after fertilization), an injurious agent damages either enough cells to cause death and abortion, or only a few cells, presumably allowing the embryo to recover without developing defects. Between the third and ninth weeks, the embryo is extremely susceptible to teratogenesis; the peak sensitivity during this period is between the fourth and fifth weeks. It is during this period that organs are being crafted out of the germ cell layers. The fetal period that follows organogenesis is marked chiefly by further growth and maturation of the organs, with greatly reduced susceptibility to teratogenic agents. Instead, the fetus is susceptible to growth retardation or injury to already-formed organs. It is therefore possible for the same teratogenic agent to produce different effects if exposure occurs at different times of gestation. As previously described, viral infections such as rubella produce disruption of the developmental program in the first trimester, but later during pregnancy the result of viral infection is usually tissue injury accompanied by inflammation (e.g., congenital encephalitis). The approximate timing of the insult can be gauged from the pattern of disruption that is present at birth or in the abortus. For example, a ventricular septal defect resulting from exposure to a teratogen must have occurred before 6 weeks of gestation, because the ventricular septum closes at this time.

■ *Genes that regulate morphogenesis may be the target of teratogens.* The role of single-gene mutations in causing human malformations is becoming increasingly evident. It is not surprising, therefore, that the function of genes controlling developmental events is likely to be affected by teratogens as well. One such class of genes, called *HOX* genes, regulates transcription of several other genes, and in experimental animals, agents that alter *HOX* gene expression are known to produce malformations. Infants born to mothers treated with retinoic acid for severe acne develop *retinoic acid embryopathy*, characterized by defects in the central nervous system, heart, and facies. At least some of the teratogenic effects of retinoic acid are mediated by *HOX* gene modulation; recent evidence has also shown the involvement of other developmental genes, such as sonic hedgehog homologue *(SHH)*, in retinoic acid embryopathy.

PERINATAL INFECTIONS

Infections of the fetus and neonate may be acquired transcervically (ascending infections) or transplacentally (hematologic infections).

Transcervical, or *ascending*, *infections* involve spread of infection from the cervicovaginal canal and may be acquired in utero or during birth. Most bacterial infections (e.g., β-hemolytic streptococcal infection) and a few viral infections (e.g., herpes simplex) are acquired in this manner. In general, the fetus acquires the infection by "inhaling" infected amniotic fluid into the lungs or by passing through an infected birth canal during delivery. Fetal infection is usually associated with inflammation of the placental membranes (chorioamnionitis) and inflammation of the umbilical cord (funisitis). This mode of spread usually gives rise to pneumonia and, in severe cases, to sepsis and meningitis.

Transplacental infections are usually caused by viruses, parasites (e.g., *Plasmodium* species, the cause of malaria), and some bacteria (e.g., *Treponema pallidum*). The infecting microbes gain access to the fetal bloodstream through chorionic villi. The effects of transplacental infections are more widespread than those of ascending infections. The most important transplacental infections can be conveniently remembered by the acronym *TORCH*. The elements of the TORCH complex are the following: *Toxoplasma* (T), rubella virus (R), cytomegalovirus (C), herpesvirus (H), and any of a number of other (O) microbes such as *T. pallidum*. These agents are grouped together because they may evoke similar clinical and pathologic manifestations, including fever, encephalitis, chorioretinitis, hepatosplenomegaly, pneumonia, myocarditis, and hemolytic anemia. Rubella embryopathy has been discussed; congenital cytomegalovirus infection and syphilis are described in Chapters 13 and 18, respectively.

PREMATURITY AND INTRAUTERINE GROWTH RETARDATION

Prematurity is the most common cause of neonatal mortality and morbidity and is defined by a gestational age less than 37 weeks. As might be expected, infants born before completion of gestation also weigh less than normal (<2500 g). The *major risk factors for prematurity* include premature rupture of membranes (PROM), chorioamnionitis, placental abnormalities, and twin pregnancy. It is well established that children born before completion of the full period of gestation have higher morbidity and mortality rates than do full-term infants. The immaturity of organ

systems in preterm infants makes them especially vulnerable to several complications, including

■ Hyaline membrane disease (respiratory distress syndrome)
■ Necrotizing enterocolitis
■ Intraventricular and germinal matrix hemorrhage (Chapter 23)

Although preterm infants have low birth weights, it is usually appropriate once adjusted for their gestational age. In contrast, up to one third of infants who weigh less than 2500 g are born at term and are therefore undergrown rather than immature. These *small-for-gestational-age (SGA) infants suffer from intrauterine growth retardation (IUGR)*. IUGR may result from fetal, maternal, or placental abnormalities, although in many cases the specific cause is unknown.

■ Among *fetal causes* are those that impair growth despite an adequate uteroplacental axis. These include chromosomal disorders, congenital malformations, and congenital infections. When caused by factors intrinsic to the fetus, growth retardation is *symmetric* (i.e., affects all organ systems equally).
■ *Placental causes* include any factor that compromises the uteroplacental supply line. This may result from placenta previa (low implantation of the placenta), placental abruption (separation of placenta from the decidua by a retroplacental clot), or placental infarction. With placental (and maternal) causes of IUGR, the growth retardation is *asymmetric* (i.e., the brain is spared relative to visceral organs such as the liver).
■ *Maternal factors are by far the most common cause of the growth deficit in SGA infants.* These include vascular diseases such as preeclampsia ("toxemia of pregnancy") (Chapter 19) and chronic hypertension. In addition, maternal narcotic abuse, alcoholism, and heavy cigarette smoking adversely affect fetal growth.

The SGA infant is handicapped not only in the perinatal period but also in childhood and adult life. These individuals are at increased risk for cerebral dysfunction, learning disabilities, and sensory (i.e., visual, hearing) impairment.

RESPIRATORY DISTRESS SYNDROME OF THE NEWBORN

There are many causes of respiratory distress in the newborn, including excessive sedation of the mother, fetal head injury during delivery, aspiration of blood or amniotic fluid, and intrauterine hypoxia brought about by coiling of the umbilical cord about the neck. However, the most common cause is respiratory distress syndrome (RDS), also known as *hyaline membrane disease* because of the formation of "membranes" in the peripheral airspaces of infants who succumb to this condition. Approximately 60,000 cases of RDS are reported each year in the United States, with annual deaths totaling 5000.

Pathogenesis. *RDS is basically a disease of premature infants.* It affects 15% to 20% of those born between 32

and 36 weeks' gestation, and the prevalence increases to 60% for infants delivered before 28 weeks. Other contributing influences are *maternal diabetes*, *cesarean section before the onset of labor*, and *twin gestation. Males* are at greater risk than are females.

The fundamental defect in RDS is the inability of the immature lung to synthesize sufficient surfactant. Surfactant is a complex of surface-active phospholipids, principally dipalmitoylphosphatidylcholine (lecithin) and at least two proteins thought to be essential to the normal function and metabolism of the lipid. Surfactant is synthesized by type II pneumocytes and, with the healthy newborn's first breath, rapidly coats the surface of alveoli, reducing surface tension and thus decreasing the pressure required to keep alveoli open. In a lung deficient in surfactant, alveoli tend to collapse, and a relatively greater inspiratory effort is required with each breath to open the alveoli. The infant rapidly tires from breathing, and generalized atelectasis sets in. The resulting hypoxia sets into motion a sequence of events that lead to epithelial and endothelial damage and eventually to the formation of hyaline membranes (Fig. 7–28).

Surfactant synthesis is regulated by hormones. Corticosteroids stimulate the formation of surfactant lipids and associated apoproteins. Therefore, conditions associated with intrauterine stress and fetal growth restriction that increase corticosteroid release lower the risk of developing RDS. Thyroxine acts synergistically with corticosteroids, but insulin antagonizes this effect. Uncontrolled diabetes in a pregnant woman gives rise to compensatory hyperinsulinism in the fetus, which in turn can suppress surfactant synthesis. This may explain the higher risk of RDS in infants born to diabetic mothers. Labor is known to increase surfactant synthesis; hence, cesarean section before the onset of labor may increase the risk of RDS.

MORPHOLOGY

The lungs in RDS infants are of normal size but are heavy and relatively airless. They have a mottled purple color, and microscopically the tissue appears solid, with poorly developed, generally collapsed (atelectatic) alveoli. If the infant dies within the first several hours of life, only necrotic cellular debris is present in the terminal bronchioles and alveolar ducts. Later in the course, characteristic eosinophilic hyaline membranes line the respiratory bronchioles, alveolar ducts, and random alveoli (Fig. 7–29). These "membranes" contain necrotic epithelial cells admixed with extravasated plasma proteins. In addition to the formation of membranes, there is intense vascular congestion. If the infant dies after several days, evidence of reparative changes, including proliferation of type II pneumocytes and interstitial fibrosis, is seen.

Clinical Features. Although with other causes of respiratory distress the newborn may be apneic or hypoxic from the moment of birth, infants with RDS usually appear normal at birth but within minutes to a few hours develop a labored, grunting respiration that progressively worsens and, unless controlled by therapy, causes death.

PREMATURITY

Reduced surfactant synthesis, storage, and release → Decreased alveolar surfactant → Increased alveolar surface tension → Atelectasis → Uneven perfusion / Hypoventilation → **Hypoxemia + CO₂ retention** → Acidosis → Pulmonary vasoconstriction → Pulmonary hypoperfusion → Endothelial damage / Epithelial damage → Plasma leak into alveoli → Fibrin + necrotic cells (hyaline membrane); Increased diffusion gradient

Figure 7–28

Schematic outline of the pathophysiology of respiratory distress syndrome (see text).

Figure 7–29

Hyaline membrane disease (H & E stain). There is alternating atelectasis and dilation of the alveoli. Note the eosinophilic thick hyaline membranes lining the dilated alveoli.

Indeed, RDS is the major cause of death in the neonatal period.

Treatment is designed to support ventilation until the infant is able to breathe on his or her own, which in milder cases can be expected by the third or fourth day of life. Therapy with aerosolized natural or recombinant surfactant is widely used for both prophylaxis and treatment of RDS. The greater the birth weight and gestational age, the better the outlook. Death and morbidity may result not only from hypoxemia but also from other complications of a premature birth (intraventricular hemorrhage, necrotizing enterocolitis).

A minority of infants who survive RDS suffer long-term sequelae related to neurodevelopmental defects and chronic lung disease. The neurologic abnormalities result from the effects of hypoxia on neurons or from intracerebral hemorrhage. The chronic lung disease, manifested as *bronchopulmonary dysplasia*, has a multifactorial etiology. It results from the primary anoxic injury, as well as from exposure to the high concentrations of oxygen and positive-pressure ventilation required for the treatment of this disease. Pathologic findings in bronchopulmonary dysplasia include hyperplasia and squamous metaplasia of bronchial epithelium, peribronchial fibrosis, fibrotic obliteration of bronchioles, and overdistended alveoli. Several months after the acute injury, extensive interstitial fibrosis and "honeycombing," analogous to the changes following diffuse alveolar damage in adults (Chapter 13), may be seen.

The most effective method of reducing the morbidity and mortality from RDS is prevention—notably, prevention of premature delivery until the maturing lung is capable of adequate surfactant synthesis. Reasonably reli-

able estimates of fetal pulmonary maturity can be achieved by measuring the concentration of surfactant phospholipids (e.g., lecithin) in amniotic fluid obtained by amniocentesis. Other, noninvasive, measurements of fetal maturity (e.g., by ultrasonography) are commonly employed. When the test indicates pulmonary immaturity, efforts are made to delay delivery until the lung matures. If early delivery is unavoidable, administration of corticosteroids to the mother may decrease the risk of RDS by increasing surfactant synthesis.

NECROTIZING ENTEROCOLITIS

Necrotizing enterocolitis (NEC) is predominantly a complication of premature infants and is associated with a high perinatal morbidity and mortality. The cause of NEC is controversial, but in all likelihood it is multifactorial. *Intestinal ischemia* is a prerequisite and may result from either generalized hypoperfusion or selective reduction of blood flow to the intestines in order to divert oxygen to vital organs such as the brain. Other predisposing conditions include *bacterial colonization* of the gut and administration of *formula feeds*, both of which aggravate mucosal injury in the immature bowel.

NEC typically involves the terminal ileum, cecum, and right colon, although any part of the small or large intestine may be involved. The involved segment is distended, friable, and congested (Fig. 7–30), or it can be frankly gangrenous; intestinal perforation with accompanying peritonitis may be seen. Microscopically, mucosal or transmural coagulative necrosis, ulceration, bacterial coloniza-

Figure 7–30 ■

Necrotizing enterocolitis. *A,* Postmortem examination in a severe case shows that the entire small bowel is markedly distended with a perilously thin wall (usually this implies impending perforation). *B,* The congested portion of the ileum corresponds to areas of hemorrhagic infarction and transmural necrosis seen on microscopy. Submucosal gas bubbles *(pneumatosis intestinalis)* can be seen in several areas *(arrows).*

tion, and submucosal gas bubbles are all features associated with NEC. Reparative changes, such as granulation tissue and fibrosis, may be seen shortly after the acute episode.

The clinical course is fairly typical, with the onset of bloody stools, abdominal distention, and development of circulatory collapse. Abdominal radiographs often demonstrate gas within the intestinal wall *(pneumatosis intestinalis)*. When detected early on, NEC can often be managed conservatively, but many cases require operative intervention and resection of the necrotic segments of bowel. NEC is associated with high perinatal mortality; infants who survive often develop *post-NEC strictures* from fibrosis caused by the healing process.

SUDDEN INFANT DEATH SYNDROME

The definition of sudden infant death syndrome (SIDS) is "the sudden and unexpected death of an infant less than 1 year of age whose death remains unexplained after the performance of a complete autopsy, examination of the scene of death, and review of the case history."

SIDS accounts for approximately 3000 deaths in the United States annually. It is the leading cause of death during the first year of life in developed countries. In 90% of cases, the infant is younger than 6 months; most are between the ages of 2 and 4 months. The diagnosis of SIDS in children younger than 1 month or older than 6 months should be made with caution. Usually, death occurs during sleep and without any apparent struggle; hence the former names "crib death" and "cot death." Although the cause of SIDS is unknown, several factors related to both the mother and the infant are associated with an increased risk of SIDS (Table 7–10). For reasons not quite clear, there is an increased risk of SIDS in infants who sleep in a prone position, prompting the American Academy of Pediatrics to recommend placing infants in the supine position when laying them down to sleep. This simple "back to sleep" strategy has reduced the incidence of SIDS by 40% in the past 10 years.

Anatomic studies of victims have yielded inconsistent histologic findings, such as the presence of thymic petechiae or congestion of pulmonary vessels. These features are usually subtle, of uncertain significance, and not present in all cases. The importance of a postmortem examination rests in identifying other causes of sudden death in infancy, such as unsuspected myocarditis, congenital heart disease, or bronchopneumonia (the presence of any of which would *exclude* a diagnosis of SIDS), and in ruling out the possibility of child abuse. A variety of microscopic alterations have been found in certain regions of the brain, most importantly the brain stem. In this locale are structures that control respiratory and cardiac rhythm or coordinate the body's response to hypoxemia and hypercarbia (e.g., the arcuate nucleus). It should be noted, however, that the microscopic changes observed in these structures could either lead to or result from chronic hypoxia, so the possibility exists that they are not of themselves the basic defects.

Most authorities believe that SIDS is not a single entity but a disorder with multiple origins. In some infants, it may be a manifestation of an inborn error of fatty acid metabolism, such as a deficiency of medium-chain acyl coenzyme A (acyl-CoA) dehydrogenase. In others, it may result from a neural developmental delay that may manifest as a respiratory dysfunction. In still others, it may be an unusual manifestation of a microbial infection. The litany of hypotheses could be continued, but suffice it to say that none of these theories, alone or in combination, can at present explain these tragic deaths.

HYDROPS FETALIS

Hydrops fetalis (HF) is the term used for *generalized edema of the fetus*, a severe manifestation of progressive fluid accumulation during intrauterine growth that is frequently lethal. The causes of HF are manifold; the most important causes are listed in Table 7–11. In the past, hemolytic anemia caused by Rh blood group incompatibility between mother and fetus *(immune hydrops)* was the most common cause of HF, but with the successful prophylaxis of this disorder during pregnancy, causes of *nonimmune hydrops* have become the principal culprits. Notably, the causes listed in Table 7–11 do not always result in hydrops fetalis, which represents the most severe manifestation in the spectrum of intrauterine fluid accumulation (Fig. 7–31); it is not uncommon to have more localized degrees of edema, such as isolated pleural and peritoneal effusions, or postnuchal fluid accumulation *(cystic hygroma;* see later). The mechanism of immune hydrops is discussed first, followed by other important causes of HF.

Table 7-10.   FACTORS ASSOCIATED WITH SUDDEN INFANT DEATH SYNDROME

Maternal	Infant
Youth (<20 yr of age)	Prematurity
Unmarried	Low birth weight
Short intergestational intervals	Male sex
Low socioeconomic status	Product of multiple birth
Smoking	Not first sibling
Drug abuse	SIDS in prior sibling
Black race (? socioeconomic)	

SIDS, sudden infant death syndrome.

Table 7-11.   MAJOR CAUSES OF HYDROPS FETALIS

Chromosomal abnormality
   Turner syndrome
   Trisomies (21, 13, 18)
Fetal anemia
   Immune-mediated: Rh and ABO hemolysis
   Nonimmune: homozygous α-thalassemia, parvovirus B19 infection
Cardiovascular (cardiac anomalies, arrhythmias)
Twin pregnancy (twin-twin transfusion syndrome)

Figure 7-31 ■

Hydrops fetalis. *A,* Generalized accumulation of fluid in the fetus. *B,* Fluid accumulation particularly prominent in the soft tissues of the neck. This condition has been termed *cystic hygroma.* Cystic hygromas are characteristically seen with, but not limited to, constitutional chromosomal anomalies such as 45,X0 karyotypes. (Courtesy of Dr. Beverly Rogers, Department of Pathology, University of Texas Southwestern Medical Center, Dallas.)

Immune Hydrops

Immune hydrops fetalis results from an antibody-induced hemolytic disease in the newborn that is caused by blood group incompatibility between mother and fetus. Such an incompatibility occurs only when the fetus inherits red cell antigenic determinants from the father that are foreign to the mother. The most common antigens to result in clinically significant hemolysis are the Rh and ABO blood group antigens. Of the numerous antigens included in the Rh system, only the D antigen is a major cause of Rh incompatibility. Fetal red cells may reach the maternal circulation during the last trimester of pregnancy, when the cytotrophoblast is no longer present as a barrier, or during childbirth itself (*fetomaternal bleed*). The mother thus becomes sensitized to the foreign antigen and develops antibodies that can freely traverse the placenta to the fetus and cause red cell destruction. Once immune hemolysis is initiated, there is progressive anemia in the fetus, with resultant tissue ischemia, intrauterine cardiac failure, and peripheral pooling of fluid (edema). As discussed later, *cardiac failure may be the final pathway* by which edema occurs in many cases of nonimmune HF as well.

Several factors influence the immune response to Rh-positive fetal red cells that reach the maternal circulation.

■ Concurrent ABO incompatibility protects the mother against Rh immunization because the fetal red cells are promptly coated by isohemagglutinins and removed from the maternal circulation.
■ The antibody response depends on the dose of immunizing antigen; hence, hemolytic disease develops only when the mother has experienced a significant transplacental bleed (more than 1 mL of Rh-positive red cells).

■ The isotype of the antibody is important because immunoglobulin G (IgG) (but not IgM) antibodies can cross the placenta. The initial exposure to Rh antigen evokes the formation of IgM antibodies, *so Rh disease is very uncommon with the first pregnancy.* Subsequent exposure during the second or third pregnancy generally leads to a brisk IgG antibody response.

Appreciation of the role of prior sensitization in the pathogenesis of Rh-hemolytic disease of the newborn has led to its remarkable control. Currently, Rh-negative mothers are administered anti-D globulin soon after the delivery of an Rh-positive baby. The anti-D antibodies mask the antigenic sites on the fetal red cells that may have leaked into the maternal circulation during childbirth, thus preventing long-lasting sensitization to Rh antigens.

Owing to the remarkable success achieved in prevention of Rh hemolysis, fetomaternal ABO incompatibility is currently the most common cause of immune hemolytic disease of the newborn. Although ABO incompatibility occurs in approximately 20% to 25% of pregnancies, only a small fraction of infants subsequently born develop hemolysis, and in general the disease is much milder than is Rh incompatibility. ABO hemolytic disease occurs almost exclusively in infants of group A or B who are born to group O mothers. The normal anti-A and anti-B isohemagglutinins in group O mothers are usually of the IgM type and so do not cross the placenta. However, for reasons not well understood, certain group O women possess IgG antibodies directed against group A or B antigens (or both) even without prior sensitization. Therefore, the firstborn may be affected. Fortunately, even with transplacentally acquired antibodies, lysis of the infant's red cells is minimal. There is no effective method of preventing hemolytic disease resulting from ABO incompatibility.

Nonimmune Hydrops

The major causes of nonimmune hydrops include those associated with *cardiovascular defects*, *chromosomal anomalies*, and *fetal anemia*. Both structural and functional (i.e., arrhythmias) cardiovascular defects may result in intrauterine cardiac failure and hydrops. Among the chromosomal anomalies, 45,X karyotype (Turner syndrome) and trisomies 21 and 18 are associated with fetal hydrops; most often, the basis for this is the presence of underlying structural cardiac anomalies, although in Turner syndrome, there may be an abnormality of lymphatic drainage from the neck leading to postnuchal fluid accumulation (*cystic hygromas*). Fetal anemias due to causes other than Rh or ABO incompatibility also result in hydrops fetalis (HF). In fact, in some parts of the world (e.g., Southeast Asia), severe fetal anemia caused by homozygous α-thalassemia is probably the most common cause of HF. Transplacental infection by parvovirus B19 is increasingly recognized as an important cause of HF. The virus gains entry into erythroid precursors (normoblasts), where it replicates. This leads to erythrocyte maturation arrest and aplastic anemia. Parvoviral intranuclear inclusions can be seen within circulating and marrow erythroid precursors (Fig. 7–32A). The basis for HF in fetal anemia of both immune and nonimmune cause is tissue ischemia with secondary myocardial dysfunction and circulatory failure. Additionally, secondary liver failure may ensue, with loss of synthetic function contributing to hypoalbuminemia, reduced oncotic pressure, and edema.

MORPHOLOGY

The anatomic findings in fetuses with intrauterine fluid accumulation vary with both the severity of the disease and the underlying etiology. As previously noted, HF represents the most severe and generalized manifestation (see Fig. 7–31), and lesser degrees of edema such as isolated pleural, peritoneal, or postnuchal fluid collections can occur. Accordingly, infants may be stillborn, die within the first few days, or recover completely. The presence of dysmorphic features suggests underlying constitutional chromosomal abnormalities; postmortem examination may reveal a cardiac anomaly. In HF associated with fetal anemia, both fetus and placenta are characteristically pale; in most cases, the liver and spleen are enlarged from cardiac failure and congestion. Additionally, the bone marrow shows compensatory hyperplasia of erythroid precursors (parvovirus-associated aplastic anemia being a notable exception), and extramedullary hematopoiesis is present in the liver, the spleen, and possibly other tissues such as the kidneys, the lungs, and even the heart. The increased hematopoietic activity accounts for the presence in the peripheral circulation of large numbers of immature red cells, including reticulocytes, normoblasts, and erythroblasts **(erythroblastosis fetalis)** (Fig. 7–32B).

The presence of hemolysis in Rh or ABO incompatibility is associated with the added complication of increased circulating bilirubin from the red cell breakdown. When hyperbilirubinemia is marked (usually above 20 mg/dL in full-term infants, often less in

Figure 7–32   ■

A, Nuclear parvoviral inclusions in erythroid precursors *(normoblasts);* these inclusions may be seen within red cell precursors in the bone marrow, or within circulating normoblasts. *B,* In severe anemia with immune or nonimmune causes, there is marked compensatory extramedullary hematopoiesis, with circulating erythroid precursors seen in the peripheral blood. In this section of fetal lung, clusters of normoblasts with darkly staining nuclei are seen in the tissue as well as blood vessels (erythroblastosis fetalis). (Courtesy of Dr. Beverly Rogers, Department of Pathology, University of Texas Southwestern Medical Center, Dallas.)

premature infants), the central nervous system may be damaged **(kernicterus).** The circulating unconjugated bilirubin is taken up by the brain tissue, on which it apparently exerts a toxic effect. The basal ganglia and brain stem are particularly prone to deposition of bilirubin pigment, which imparts a characteristic yellow hue to the parenchyma (Fig. 7–33). It is interesting that adults are protected from this effect of hyperbilirubinemia by the blood-brain barrier.

Clinical Course. Early recognition of HF is imperative, since even severe cases can sometimes be salvaged with currently available therapy. HF that results from Rh incompatibility may be more or less accurately predicted, because it correlates well with rapidly rising Rh antibody titers in the mother during pregnancy. Amniotic fluid obtained by amniocentesis may show high levels of bilirubin. The human antiglobulin test (Coombs test, Chapter 12) is positive on fetal cord blood if the red cells have been coated by maternal antibody. Antenatal exchange transfusion is an effective form of therapy. Postnatally, phototherapy is helpful because visible light converts bilirubin to readily excreted dipyrroles. As already discussed, in an overwhelming majority of cases, administration of anti-D globulins to the mother can prevent the occurrence of Rh erythroblastosis. Group ABO hemolytic disease is more difficult to predict but is readily anticipated by awareness of the blood incompatibility between mother and father and by hemoglobin and bilirubin determinations in the vulnerable newborn infant. Needless to say, in fatal instances of HF, a thorough postmortem examination is imperative to determine the cause of

Figure 7–33 ■

Kernicterus. Severe hyperbilirubinemia in the neonatal period—for example, secondary to immune hydrolysis—results in deposition of bilirubin pigment *(arrows)* in the brain parenchyma. This occurs because the blood-brain barrier is less well developed in the neonatal period than it is in adulthood. Infants who survive develop long-term neurologic sequelae.

hydrops and to exclude a potentially recurring cause such as a chromosomal abnormality.

CYSTIC FIBROSIS

With an incidence of 1 in 2500 live births and a carrier frequency of 1 in 25 to 30, cystic fibrosis (CF) is the most common lethal autosomal recessive disorder that affects whites. It is distinctly uncommon among Asians and blacks. CF is associated with a widespread defect in the secretory process of all exocrine glands. Indeed, abnormally viscid mucus secretions that block the airways and the pancreatic ducts are responsible for the two most important clinical manifestations: recurrent and chronic pulmonary infections and pancreatic insufficiency. In addition, although the exocrine sweat glands are structurally normal (and remain so throughout the course of this disease), *a high level of sodium chloride in the sweat is a consistent and characteristic biochemical abnormality in CF.*

Pathogenesis. Although a large number of abnormalities have been described in CF, *the primary defect is in the transport of chloride (Cl^-) ions across epithelia.* The changes in mucus are considered secondary to the disturbance in transport of Cl^- ions. In normal epithelia, the transport of Cl^- ions across the cell membrane occurs through transmembrane proteins that form chloride channels. These channels are like gates through which Cl^- ions enter or leave the cell. There are two types of Cl^- channels: those that are opened by a cyclic adenosine monophosphate (cAMP)–dependent pathway, and others that are regulated by Ca^{++} ions. In CF, the cAMP-dependent Cl^- channels, also called *cystic fibrosis transmembrane conductance regulators (CFTRs),* are defective. Mutations in the *CFTR* gene render the epithelial membranes relatively impermeable to Cl^- ions (Fig. 7–34). However, the impact of this defect on transport function is tissue-specific. In sweat glands, for example, the concentrations of Na^+ and Cl^- secreted into the gland lumen are normal, but the epithelium that lines the sweat ducts is impermeable to Cl^-. Hence, as the sweat moves toward the surface, the normal reabsorption of Cl^- through CFTR, and the accompanying cation Na^+, fails to occur. This is responsible for the high concentration of NaCl in the sweat of CF patients. In the respiratory tract, the flow of Cl^- ions and the consequences of *CFTR* mutation are quite different. In the normal airway epithelium, Cl^- is secreted into the airways through cAMP-dependent chloride channels. The impaired transport of Cl^- from the epithelium into the lumen of the airways causes a series of secondary effects, which lead ultimately to increased absorption of Na^+ and water from the airspace to the blood. This lowers the water content of the mucus blanket coating the respiratory epithelium. The resulting dehydration of the mucus layer leads to defective mucociliary action and the accumulation of viscid secretions that obstruct the air passages and predispose to recurrent pulmonary infections (Fig. 7–35).

However, obstruction alone seems insufficient to explain the pathogenesis of pulmonary disease, and it is believed that many other factors contribute. The lung in cystic fibrosis is characterized by an exaggerated yet ineffective inflammatory response. The excessive neutrophilic inflammatory reaction

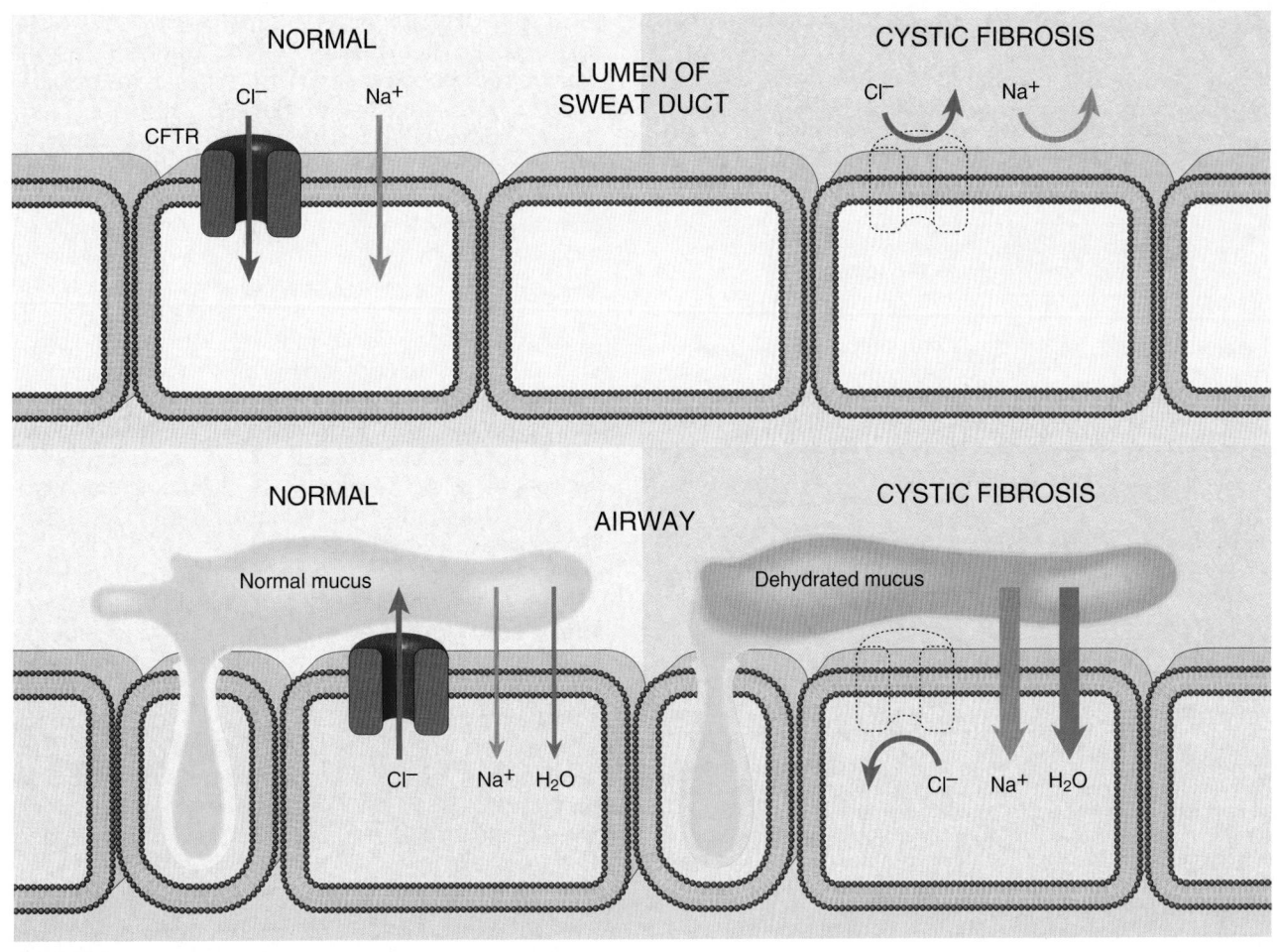

NORMAL

CYSTIC FIBROSIS

LUMEN OF
SWEAT DUCT

Cl^- Na^+

CFTR

Cl^- Na^+

NORMAL

CYSTIC FIBROSIS

AIRWAY

Normal mucus

Dehydrated mucus

Cl^- Na^+ H_2O

Cl^- Na^+ H_2O

Figure 7–34   ■

Ion transport in normal sweat duct and airway epithelium, compared with corresponding tissues from a patient with cystic fibrosis. In cystic fibrosis, absence of the Cl^- channel, cystic fibrosis transmembrane conductance regulator (CFTR), prevents reabsorption of Cl^- and therefore Na^+ in the sweat duct, thus accounting for the high salt content of sweat. In the airways, failure of Cl^- secretion from the cells to the airspaces indirectly causes increased reabsorption of Na^+ ions and water, rendering the mucus dehydrated.

seems to occur independently of infection; for example, the bronchoalveolar fluid of lungs from infants contains high levels of interleukin 8 (IL-8), a major chemoattractant for neutrophils, in the absence of infection. With infection, such a response is even more pronounced. In addition, the concentration of the antimicrobial peptide *defensin* is reduced in lung fluids. Recent studies indicate that due to the Cl^- channel defect, the epithelium in CF consumes more oxygen than normal epithelium, thus creating an anaerobic environment. The normally aerobic *Pseudomonas aeruginosa* responds to this change by asssuming a mucoid phenotype that is resistant to phagocytosis by neutrophils. Thus, the exuberant neutrophil response damages tissues while the bacteria seem to go home free.

The pathogenesis of pancreatic dysfunction is even less clear. As described later, obstruction of pancreatic ducts may cause total loss of exocrine pancreatic function. Interestingly, isolated chronic pancreatitis (Chapter 17) has been related to mutations in the CF gene (*CFTR*).

The *CFTR* gene is located on chromosome 7 (7q31-32), and to date more than 300 mutations have been identified in this gene. Approximately 70% of patients have a common

mutation characterized by a three–base pair deletion leading to the deletion of phenylalanine at amino acid position 508 (ΔF508). The remaining 30% of cases are due to a variety of other genetic lesions, including frameshifts, missense, and nonsense mutations. To some extent, the severity of clinical manifestations and the organ systems involved are related to the nature of the mutation. The ΔF508 mutation, the most common form, leads to a virtual absence of CFTR in the cell membrane and hence extreme impermeability to Cl^- ions. These patients have severe disease with early pancreatic insufficiency and variable degrees of respiratory disease. By contrast, some of the other, much less common mutations give rise to Cl^- channels that allow relatively normal chloride transport; in patients with such mutations, sweat chloride is normal, and male infertility may be the only manifestation of the disease (see later).

MORPHOLOGY

The anatomic changes in CF are highly variable and depend on the type of mutation and hence

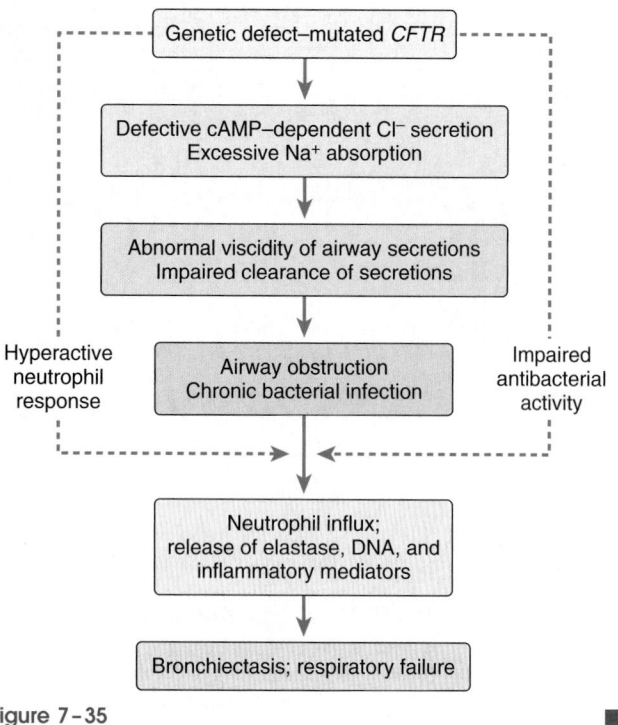

Figure 7–35 ■

Pathophysiologic sequelae of mutation in the cystic fibrosis transmembrane conductance regulator *(CFTR)* gene, leading to bronchiectasis and respiratory failure. How the *CFTR* mutation gives rise to a hyperactive neutrophil response and decreased antibacterial activity is not known. cAMP, cyclic AMP. (Modified from Knowles MR, et al: Pharmacologic modulation of salt and water in the airway epithelium of cystic fibrosis. Am J Respir Crit Care Med 151[Suppl 3]:S65, 1995.)

the severity of expression of this genetic disorder. **Pancreatic abnormalities** are present in approximately 85% of patients. These abnormalities may consist only of accumulations of characteristic hypereosinophilic secretions, representing viscid mucin, within dilated ducts (Fig. 7–36A). In more advanced cases, the ducts become totally plugged, causing atrophy of the exocrine glands; the islets of Langerhans are usually, but not always, spared. The ducts may be converted into cysts separated only by islets of Langerhans and an abundant fibrous stroma, a picture that gave rise to the designation **fibrocystic disease of the pancreas.** Loss of pancreatic secretion may lead to severe malabsorption, particularly of fats. A resultant lack of vitamin A, a fat-soluble vitamin, may then contribute to squamous metaplasia of the linings of the ducts. Hypereosinophilic secretions similar to those in the pancreas may be present within ileal, colonic, appendiceal, and salivary glands. **Pulmonary lesions** are seen in almost every case and, with adequate treatment of the pancreatic problems, are the most serious aspect of this disease. Retention of abnormally viscid mucin within the small airways leads to dilation of bronchioles and bronchi with secondary infection, so that severe chronic bronchitis, bronchiectasis, and lung abscesses (Chapter 13) are frequent sequelae. *Staphylococcus aureus* and *P. aeruginosa* are the two pathogens most commonly isolated in CF patients. As explained earlier, the mucoid form of *P. aeruginosa,* rarely found in persons who do not have CF, is found in more than 50% of those who have the disease. There is increasing frequency of infections with another microbe, *Burkholderia cepacia,* an opportunistic bacterium that is particularly difficult to eradicate. The

Figure 7–36 ■

A, Cystic fibrosis of the pancreas. Dilated ducts plugged with inspissated eosinophilic material are seen. Note the background fibrosis and atrophy of the pancreatic acini. *B,* Cirrhosis of the liver is an uncommon complication of cystic fibrosis and is usually seen in older individuals (*A* and *B,* Courtesy of Dr. Linda Margraf, Department of Pathology, University of Texas Southwestern Medical School, Dallas.)

subtended pulmonary parenchyma may undergo emphysema or atelectasis (Chapter 13). Obstruction of the small bowel secondary to impacted viscid mucin **(meconium ileus)** is not an uncommon complication in newborns with CF; intestinal obstruction may be severe enough to cause rupture in utero, resulting in meconium peritonitis. In approximately 25% of patients, inspissation of mucus within the bile ducts impairs excretion of bile, adding to the malabsorption problems; over time, **biliary cirrhosis** (Chapter 16) may develop in a proportion of these patients (Fig. 7–36B). The ducts and glands of the male reproductive tract are commonly affected; obstruction of vas deferens, epididymis, and seminal vesicles results in azoospermia and **infertility** in more than 95% of CF males. Bilateral absence of the vas deferens is a rare manifestation of CF, but in some males, it may be the only feature suggesting an underlying *CFTR* mutation.

Clinical Features. The clinical manifestations of this condition are extremely varied and range from mild to severe and from onset at birth to onset years later. Approximately 5% to 10% of cases come to clinical attention at birth or soon after because of an attack of *meconium ileus.* More commonly, manifestations of *malabsorption* (e.g., large, foul-smelling stools; abdominal distention; and poor weight gain) appear during the first year of life. The faulty fat absorption may induce deficiency of the fat-soluble vitamins, resulting in manifestations of avitaminosis A, D, E, or K. If the child survives these hazards, *pulmonary problems* such as chronic cough, persistent lung infections, obstructive pulmonary disease, and cor pulmonale may make their appearance. Some patients also develop *upper respiratory tract manifestations* (chronic sinusitis, recurrent nasal polyps). Persistent pulmonary infections are responsible for 80% to 90% of the deaths. With improved control of infections, more patients are currently surviving to adulthood; median life expectancy is approximately 30 years.

The diagnosis of CF is based on clinical findings and the biochemical abnormalities in sweat. A properly administered and interpreted sweat chloride test is crucial to the diagnosis. An increase in sweat electrolytes is common (often the mother makes the diagnosis because her infant "tastes salty"). Biochemical analysis of sweat is not useful for detection of heterozygotes (who have normal sweat chloride levels) or for prenatal diagnosis; however, because the CF gene has been cloned and more than two thirds of patients owe their disease to a single mutation, detection of carriers with the most common mutation is now possible. Genetic analysis is also invaluable in establishing the diagnosis of CF in patients with atypical symptoms, or in cases in which the sweat test is difficult to administer (or, rarely, normal). In couples with a previously affected offspring, or who have been identified as CF carriers, direct mutation analysis in the antenatal period provides reliable results with regard to *CFTR* status in the unborn child. The number of mutations that can give rise to CF is very large, however, and therefore population-based screening studies are not feasible.

The treatment of CF is largely symptomatic, but gene therapy is on the horizon. Transfer of the *CFTR* gene into cells of CF patients corrects the Cl^- transport defect in vitro, and with suitable vectors it may be possible to devise effective strategies for transferring the gene in vivo.

TUMORS AND TUMOR-LIKE LESIONS OF INFANCY AND CHILDHOOD

Malignant neoplasms are the second most common cause of death in children between the ages of 4 and 14 years; only accidents exact a higher toll. Benign tumors are even more common than are cancers.

It is difficult to segregate, on morphologic grounds, true tumors from tumor-like lesions in the infant and child. In this context, two special categories of tumor-like lesions should be recognized.

■ *Heterotopia* or *choristoma* refers to microscopically normal cells or tissues that are present in abnormal locations. Examples include a rest of pancreatic tissue found in the wall of the stomach or small intestine, or a small mass of adrenal cells found in the kidney, lungs, ovaries, or elsewhere. Heterotopic rests are usually of little significance, but they can be confused clinically with neoplasms.

■ *Hamartoma* refers to an excessive but focal overgrowth of cells and tissues native to the organ in which it occurs. Although the cellular elements are mature and identical to those found in the remainder of the organ, they do not reproduce the normal architecture of the surrounding tissue. Hamartomas can be thought of as the linkage between malformations and neoplasms. The line of demarcation between a hamartoma and a benign neoplasm is frequently tenuous and is variously interpreted. Hemangiomas, lymphangiomas, rhabdomyomas of the heart, and adenomas of the liver are considered by some to be hamartomas and by others to be true neoplasms.

Benign Tumors

Virtually any tumor may be encountered in the pediatric age group, but three—hemangiomas, lymphangiomas, and sacrococcygeal teratomas—deserve special mention here because they occur commonly in childhood.

Hemangiomas are the most common tumors of infancy. Both cavernous and capillary hemangiomas may be encountered (Chapter 10), although the latter are often more cellular than in adults, and hence are deceptively worrisome. In children, most hemangiomas are located in the skin, particularly on the face and scalp, where they produce flat to elevated, irregular, red-blue masses; the flat, larger lesions are referred to as *port wine stains*. Hemangiomas may enlarge as the child gets older, but in many instances they spontaneously regress (Fig. 7–37). The vast majority of superficial hemangiomas have no more than a cosmetic significance; rarely, they may be the manifestation of a hereditary disorder associated with disease within internal organs, such as the von Hippel–Lindau and Sturge-Weber syndromes (Chapter 23).

Figure 7-37 ■

Congenital capillary hemangioma at birth (A) and at 2 years of age (B) after the lesion had undergone spontaneous regression. (Courtesy of Dr. Eduardo Yunis, Children's Hospital of Pittsburgh.)

Lymphangiomas represent the lymphatic counterpart of hemangiomas. They are characterized by cystic and cavernous spaces lined by endothelial cells and surrounded by lymphoid aggregates; the spaces usually contain pale fluid. They may occur on the skin but, more importantly, are also encountered in the deeper regions of the neck, axilla, mediastinum, and retroperitoneum. Although histologically benign, they tend to increase in size after birth and may encroach on mediastinal structures or nerve trunks in axilla. *Cystic hygromas* are postnuchal collections of lymphatic fluid that are commonly seen in aborted fetuses with a 45,X karyotype (Turner syndrome); unlike lymphangiomas, dilated endothelium-lined spaces are not seen.

Sacrococcygeal teratomas are the most common germ cell tumors of childhood, accounting for 40% or more of cases (Fig. 7–38). In view of the overlap in the mechanisms underlying teratogenesis and oncogenesis, it is interesting that approximately 10% of sacrococcygeal teratomas are associated with congenital anomalies, primarily defects of the hindgut and cloacal region and other midline defects (e.g., meningocele, spina bifida) not believed to result from local effects of the tumor. Approximately 75% of these tumors are histologically mature with a benign course, and about 12% are unmistakably malignant and lethal (Chapter 18). The remainder are designated immature teratomas, and their malignant potential correlates with the amount of immature tissue elements present. Most of the benign teratomas are encountered in younger infants (<4 months), whereas children with malignant lesions tend to be somewhat older.

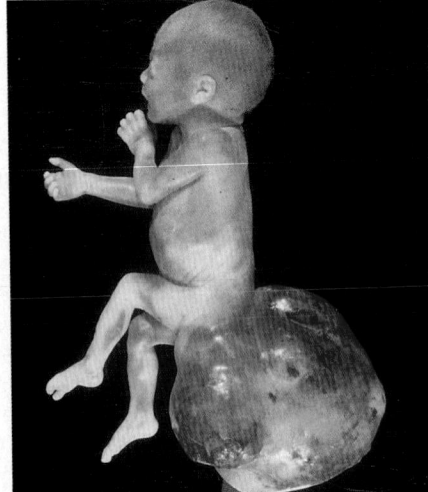

Figure 7-38 ■

Sacrococcygeal teratoma. Note the size of the lesion compared with that of the infant.

Malignant Tumors

The organ systems involved most commonly by malignant neoplasms in infancy and childhood include the hematopoietic system, neural tissue, and soft tissues (Table 7–12). This is in sharp contrast to adults, in whom tumors of the lung, heart, prostate, and colon are the most common forms. Malignant tumors of infancy and childhood differ biologically and histologically from those in adults. The main differences are as follows:

- Relatively frequent demonstration of a close relationship between abnormal development (teratogenesis) and tumor induction (oncogenesis)
- Prevalence of constitutional genetic abnormalities or syndromes that predispose to cancer
- Tendency of fetal and neonatal malignancies to spontaneously regress or undergo "differentiation" into mature elements
- Improved survival or cure of many childhood tumors, so that more attention is now being paid to minimizing the adverse delayed effects of chemotherapy and radiotherapy in survivors, including the development of second malignancies

Table 7-12.   COMMON MALIGNANT NEOPLASMS OF INFANCY AND CHILDHOOD

0-4 Yr	5-9 Yr	10-14 Yr
Leukemia	Leukemia	
Retinoblastoma	Retinoblastoma	
Neuroblastoma	Neuroblastoma	
Wilms tumor		
Hepatoblastoma	Hepatocarcinoma	Hepatocarcinoma
Soft tissue sarcoma (especially rhabdomyosarcoma)	Soft tissue sarcoma	Soft tissue sarcoma
Teratomas		
Central nervous system tumors	Central nervous system tumors	
	Ewing tumor	
	Lymphoma	Osteogenic sarcoma
		Thyroid carcinoma
		Hodgkin disease

Histologically, many malignant pediatric neoplasms are unique. In general, they tend to have a primitive (*embryonal*) rather than pleomorphic-anaplastic microscopic appearance, and frequently they exhibit features of organogenesis specific to the site of tumor origin. Because of their primitive histologic appearance, many childhood tumors have been collectively referred to as *small, round, blue cell tumors*. These are characterized by sheets of cells with small, round nuclei. The tumors in this category include neuroblastoma, lymphoma, rhabdomyosarcoma, Ewing sarcoma (peripheral neuroectodermal tumor), and some cases of Wilms tumor. There are usually sufficient distinctive features to render a definitive diagnosis on the basis of histologic examination alone, but when necessary, clinical and radiographic findings, combined with ancillary studies (e.g., chromosome analysis, immunoperoxidase stains, and electron microscopy) are used. Three common tumors—neuroblastoma, retinoblastoma, and Wilms tumor—are described here to highlight the differences between pediatric tumors and those in adults.

NEUROBLASTOMA

Neuroblastoma, the most common solid tumor of childhood other than central nervous system neoplasms, accounts for about 15% of all childhood cancer deaths. Most (80% to 90%) are found in children younger than 5 years, many in the first year of life. Neuroblastomas demonstrate several unique features in their natural history, including *spontaneous regression* and *spontaneous- or therapy-induced maturation*.

Of neural crest origin, *neuroblastomas may arise anywhere in the sympathetic nervous system* from the head to the pelvis. About 75% arise within the abdomen: about half in the adrenal glands and the other half in the abdominal paravertebral autonomic ganglia. Similar neoplasms rarely arise in the brain. Most occur sporadically, but a few are familial with autosomal dominant transmission, and in such cases the neoplasms may involve both of the adrenals or multiple primary autonomic sites.

MORPHOLOGY

These tumors range from microscopic nodules (usually in infants) to masses that virtually fill the abdomen. Smaller tumors may appear to be circumscribed or even encapsulated, but larger masses often grow into nearby organs (kidney, liver, pancreas). Advanced disease frequently invades the renal vein, often extending into the inferior vena cava. On cross-section they are gray-white, soft, and friable, and larger tumors often have areas of hemorrhage, necrosis, cystic degeneration, and calcification.

Histologically, the cells, which grow in solid sheets, are round to ovoid and primitive-looking with large, hyperchromatic nuclei surrounded by scant cytoplasm (Fig. 7-39A). It is evident that such total lack of differentiation makes it difficult to distinguish these neoplasms from other small, round, blue cell tumors. However, more characteristic features can often be identified in neuroblastomas: for example, rosettes **(Homer-Wright pseudorosettes),** in which the tumor cells are arranged about the periphery of a central space filled with fibrillar extensions of the cells. Other helpful features include immunochemical detection of neuron-specific enolase and ultrastructural demonstration of small, membrane-bound, cytoplasmic catecholamine-containing secretory granules.

Some neoplasms show signs of maturation, either spontaneous or therapy-induced. Larger cells having more abundant cytoplasm with large vesicular nuclei and a prominent nucleolus, representing **ganglion cells** in various stages of maturation, may be found in tumors admixed with primitive neuroblasts **(ganglioneuroblastoma).** Even better-differentiated lesions contain many more large cells resembling mature ganglion cells in the absence of residual neuroblasts; such neoplasms merit the designation **ganglioneuroma** (Fig. 7-39B). Maturation of neuroblasts into ganglion cells is usually accompanied by the appearance of spindle-shaped

Figure 7-39

A, Neuroblastomas are composed of sheets of primitive cells, with hyperchromatic nuclei and little cytoplasm, qualifying for the designation *small blue cell tumor.* Nuclear karyorrhexis and mitoses, both features of rapid turnover, are easily seen. *B,* Ganglioneuromas, arising from spontaneous or therapy-induced maturation of neuroblastomas, are characterized by clusters of large cells with vesicular nuclei and abundant eosinophilic cytoplasm *(arrow),* representing neoplastic ganglion cells. Spindle-shaped Schwann cells are present in the background stroma.

Schwann cells; it is believed the latter do not arise through neuroblastic maturation but represent a reactive population recruited from the surrounding non-neoplastic tissues by the tumor cells. The presence of ganglion cells and schwannian stroma is associated with a favorable prognosis (see later).

Clinical Course. Children younger than 2 years with neuroblastomas generally present with protuberant abdomen owing to an abdominal mass, fever, and weight loss. In older children, the neuroblastomas may remain unnoticed until metastases cause hepatomegaly, ascites, and bone pain. Neuroblastomas may metastasize widely through the hematogenous and lymphatic systems, particularly to liver, lungs, and bones, in addition to the bone marrow. About 90% of neuroblastomas, regardless of location, produce catecholamines (similar to the catecholamines associated with pheochromocytomas), which are an important diagnostic feature (i.e., elevated blood levels of catecholamines and elevated urine levels of catecholamine metabolites such as vanillylmandelic acid [VMA] and homovanillic acid [HVA]). Despite the elaboration of catecholamines, hypertension is much less frequent with these neoplasms than with pheochromocytomas (Chapter 20).

Many factors influence prognosis, but the most important are the stage of the tumor and the age of the patient. Staging of neuroblastomas (Table 7–13) assumes great importance in establishing a prognosis. Special note should be taken of stage IV-S (*S* stands for special), because the outlook for these patients is excellent, despite the spread of disease. As noted in Table 7–13, the primary tumor would be classified as being in stage I or II but for the presence of metastases, which are limited to liver, skin, and bone marrow, without bone involvement. Such infants have an excellent prognosis with minimal therapy, and it is not uncommon for the primary or metastatic tumors to undergo spontaneous regression. The biologic basis of this welcome behavior is not clear. Age is the other important determinant of outcome, and children younger than 1 year have a much more favorable outlook than do older children at a comparable stage of disease. Most neoplasms in the infant years are stage I or II, or stage IV-S.

Molecular and genetic analysis of these tumors also provides prognostic information. Deletion of the short arm of chromosome 1 (1p36) is usually associated with aggressive disease; presumably some of these deletions involve the *TP73* (formerly *p73*) gene, belonging to the *TP53* (formerly *p53*) family of tumor suppressor genes. Amplification of the *MYCN* (formerly *N-myc*) oncogene

Table 7–13. STAGING OF NEUROBLASTOMAS

Stage	
I	Tumor confined to organ of origin.
II	Tumor extends in continuity beyond organ of origin but does not cross midline. Ipsilateral lymph nodes may or may not be involved.
III	Tumor extends in continuity beyond midline. Ipsilateral lymph nodes may or may not be involved.
IV	Metastatic disease to viscera, distant lymph nodes, soft tissue, and skeleton.
IV-S	Patients whose tumors would be stage I or II but who have distant disease of liver, skin, or bone marrow (without evidence of bone involvement).

From Silverman ML, Lee AK: Anatomy and pathology of the adrenal glands. Urol Clin North Am 16:417, 1989.

is also a harbinger of poor prognosis. There is a high degree of concordance between 1p36 deletion and increase in *MYCN* copy numbers, and tumors with this genetic profile have an extremely aggressive phenotype.

RETINOBLASTOMA

Retinoblastoma is the most common malignant eye tumor of childhood. From a pathologic as well as a clinical standpoint, retinoblastoma is unusual in several aspects when compared with most other solid tumors. Retinoblastoma frequently occurs as a *congenital tumor*, it can be *multifocal* and *bilateral*, it undergoes *spontaneous regression*, and patients have a high incidence of *second primary tumors*. The incidence decreases with age, most cases being diagnosed before the age of 4 years.

Retinoblastomas occur in both familial and sporadic patterns. *Familial cases typically develop multiple tumors that are bilateral*, although they may be unifocal and unilateral. All of the sporadic nonheritable tumors are unilateral and unifocal. Patients with familial retinoblastoma are also at increased risk for developing *osteosarcoma* and other soft tissue tumors.

As detailed in Chapter 6, retinoblastoma serves as a prototype of a diverse group of human cancers associated with recessive, loss-of-function mutations at distinct genetic loci harboring cancer suppressor genes.

MORPHOLOGY

Retinoblastoma is believed to arise from a cell of neuroepithelial origin, usually in the posterior retina (Fig.7–40A). The tumors tend to be nodular masses, often with satellite seedings. On light microscopic examination, undifferentiated areas of these tumors are found to be composed of small, round cells with large hyperchromatic nuclei and scant cytoplasm, resembling undifferentiated retinoblasts.

Differentiated structures are found within many retinoblastomas, the most characteristic of these being the rosettes described by Flexner and Wintersteiner **(Flexner-Wintersteiner rosettes;** Fig. 7–40B). These structures consist of clusters of cuboidal or short columnar cells arranged around a central lumen (contrast with the **pseudorosettes** of neuroblastoma, which lack a central lumen). The nuclei are displaced away from the lumen, which by light microscopy appears to have a limiting membrane resembling the external limiting membrane of the retina.

Tumor cells may disseminate beyond the eye through the optic nerve or subarachnoid space. The most common sites of distant metastases are the central nervous system, skull, distal bones, and lymph nodes.

Clinical Features. The median age at presentation is 2 years, although the tumor may be present at birth. The presenting findings include poor vision, strabismus, a whitish hue to the pupil ("cat's eye reflex"), and pain and tenderness in the eye. Approximately 60% to 70% of the tumors are associated with a germ-line mutation in the *RB1* gene and are hence heritable. The remaining 30% to 40% of the tumors develop sporadically, and these have somatic *RB1* gene mutations. Untreated, the tumors are usually fatal, but after early treatment with enucleation, chemotherapy, and radiotherapy, survival is the rule. As noted earlier, some tumors spontaneously regress, and patients with familial retinoblastoma are at increased risk for developing osteosarcoma and other soft tissue tumors.

Figure 7–40

Retinoblastoma. *A*, Note poorly cohesive tumor in retina abutting optic nerve. *B*, Higher-power view showing Flexner-Wintersteiner rosettes *(arrows)* and numerous mitotic figures. (H & E × 40.)

WILMS TUMOR

Wilms tumor, or *nephroblastoma*, is the most common primary tumor of the kidney in children. Most cases occur in children between 2 and 5 years of age. This tumor illustrates several important concepts of childhood tumors: the relationship between congenital malformation and increased risk of tumors, the histologic similarity between tumor and developing organ, and finally, the remarkable success in the treatment of childhood tumors. Each of these will be evident from the following discussion.

Three groups of congenital malformations are associated with an increased risk of developing Wilms tumor. Patients with the *WAGR syndrome*, characterized by *a*niridia, *g*enital abnormalities, and mental *r*etardation, have a 33% chance of developing Wilms tumor. Another group of patients, those with the so-called *Denys-Drash syndrome*, also has an extremely high risk of developing Wilms tumor. This syndrome is characterized by gonadal dysgenesis and renal abnormalities. Both of these conditions are associated with loss of genetic material on chromosome 11p13, where the tumor suppressor gene Wilms tumor 1 *(WT1)* has been mapped. A third group of patients, those with the *Beckwith-Wiedemann syndrome*, also has an increased risk of developing Wilms tumor. These patients have enlargement of individual body organs (e.g., tongue, kidneys, or liver), or entire body segments (hemihypertrophy); enlargement of adrenal cortical cells (adrenal cytomegaly) is a characteristic microscopic feature. The genetic locus involved in these patients is also on chromosome 11, but at 11p15.5. There are several candidate genes at this locus (putatively designated *WT2*), but the precise identity of the gene implicated in tumorigenesis remains unknown. *Beckwith-Wiedemann syndrome is an example of a disorder of genomic imprinting* (see earlier), and aberrant expression of normally repressed growth-promoting genes such as insulin-like growth factor 2 ("loss of imprinting") is postulated to result in both organ enlargement and tumorigenesis. Thus, these associations suggest that in some cases congenital malformations and tumors represent related manifestations of genetic damage affecting a single gene or closely linked genes.

Figure 7–41 ■

Wilms tumor in the lower pole of the kidney with the characteristic tan to gray color and well-circumscribed margins.

Epithelial "differentiation" usually takes the form of abortive tubules or glomeruli. Stromal cells are usually fibrocytic or myxoid in nature, although skeletal muscle "differentiation" is not uncommon. Rarely, other heterologous elements are identified, including squamous or mucinous epithelium, smooth muscle, adipose tissue, cartilage, and osteoid and neurogenic tissue. Approximately 5% of tumors contain foci of **anaplasia** (cells with large, hyperchromatic, pleomorphic nuclei and abnormal mitoses) (see Fig. 7–42). The pattern of distribution of anaplastic cells within the primary tumor (focal vs.

MORPHOLOGY

Grossly, Wilms tumor tends to present as a large, solitary, well-circumscribed mass, although 10% are either bilateral or multicentric at the time of diagnosis. On cut section, the tumor is soft, homogeneous, and tan to gray, with occasional foci of hemorrhage, cystic degeneration, and necrosis (Fig. 7–41).

Microscopically, Wilms tumors are characterized by recognizable attempts to recapitulate different stages of nephrogenesis. The classic triphasic combination of blastemal, stromal, and epithelial cell types is observed in most lesions, although the percentage of each component is variable (Fig. 7–42). Sheets of small blue cells, with few distinctive features, characterize the blastemal component.

Figure 7–42 ■

Triphasic histologic appearance of Wilms tumor with a stromal, less cellular area on the left, spindle-shaped cells, and epithelial (one clear tubule in the center) and blastemic (tightly packed blue cells) elements. (Courtesy of Dr. Charles Timmons, Department of Pathology, University of Texas Southwestern Medical School, Dallas.)

diffuse) has important implications in therapy and prognosis (see later).

Nephrogenic rests are putative precursor lesions of Wilms tumors and are sometimes present in the renal parenchyma adjacent to the tumor. Nephrogenic rests have a spectrum of histologic appearances, from expansile masses that resemble Wilms tumors (hyperplastic rests) to sclerotic rests consisting predominantly of fibrous tissue with occasional admixed immature tubules or glomeruli. It is important to document the presence of nephrogenic rests in the resected specimen, since these patients are at an increased risk of developing Wilms tumors in the **contralateral** kidney.

Clinical Course. Patients' complaints are usually referable to the tumor's enormous size. Commonly, there is a readily palpable abdominal mass, which may extend across the midline and down into the pelvis. Less often, the patient presents with fever and abdominal pain, with hematuria, or, occasionally, with intestinal obstruction as a result of pressure from the tumor. The prognosis for Wilms tumor is generally very good, and excellent results are obtained with a combination of nephrectomy and chemotherapy. Two-year survival rates are as high as 90%, even for tumors that have spread beyond the kidney, and survival for 2 years usually implies a cure. Tumors with diffuse anaplasia, especially those with extrarenal spread, have the least favorable outcome, underscoring the need for correctly identifying this histologic pattern.

DIAGNOSIS OF GENETIC DISEASES

The human genome is composed of 23 pairs of chromosomes, which contain approximately 30,000 genes, in addition to large tracts of noncoding DNA sequences. Therefore, the examination of genetic material can involve examination of entire chromosomes (conventional cytogenetic analysis), specific chromosomal regions using DNA probes (FISH), or specific DNA sequences themselves (molecular analysis). Conventional cytogenetic analysis involves karyotyping (p 228). FISH and molecular analysis are briefly discussed in the following sections.

Fluorescence in Situ Hybridization (FISH)

FISH has become an important adjunct to routine karyotyping. A major limitation of karyotyping is that it is applicable only to cells that are dividing or can be induced to divide in vitro. This problem can be overcome with DNA probes that recognize chromosome-specific sequences.

Such probes are labeled with fluorescent dyes and applied to metaphase spreads or interphase nuclei. The probe binds to its complementary sequence on the chromosome and thus labels the specific chromosomal region that can be visualized under a fluorescent microscope. The ability of FISH to circumvent the need for dividing cells is invaluable when a rapid diagnosis is warranted (e.g., in a critically ill infant suspected of having an underlying genetic disorder). Such analysis can be performed on prenatal samples (e.g., cells obtained by amniocentesis, chorionic villus biopsy, or umbilical cord blood), peripheral blood lymphocytes, and even archival tissue sections. FISH has been used for detection of numeric abnormalities of chromosomes (aneuploidy) (Fig. 7–43A); for the demonstration of subtle microdeletions (Fig. 7–43B) or complex translocations not detectable by routine karyotyping; for analysis of gene amplification (e.g., *ERBB2* [*HER2/NEU*] amplification in breast cancers or *MYCN* amplification in neuroblastomas); and for mapping newly isolated genes of interest to their chromosomal loci.

Molecular Detection of Genetic Disorders

Many genetic diseases are caused by subtle changes in individual genes that cannot be detected by routine karyotyping, or even FISH. Traditionally, the diagnosis of single-gene disorders has depended on the identification of abnormal gene products (e.g., in mutant hemoglobin or enzymes) or their clinical effects, such as anemia or mental retardation (e.g., in phenylketonuria). Now, it is possible to identify mutations at the level of DNA and offer genetic diagnosis for several mendelian disorders. The molecular detection of inherited diseases has distinct advantages over other techniques:

- It is remarkably sensitive. The amount of DNA required for diagnosis by molecular hybridization techniques can be readily obtained from 100,000 cells. Furthermore, the use of polymerase chain reaction (PCR) allows several million–fold amplification of DNA or RNA, making it possible to utilize as few as 1 or 100 cells for analysis. Tiny amounts of whole blood or even dried blood can supply sufficient DNA for PCR amplification.
- DNA-based tests are not dependent on a gene product that may be produced only in certain specialized cells (e.g., brain) or expression of a gene that may occur late in life. Because virtually all normal cells of the body contain the same DNA in inherited genetic disorders, each postzygotic cell carries the mutant gene.

These two features have profound implications for the prenatal diagnosis of genetic diseases, because a sufficient number of cells can be obtained from a few milliliters of amniotic fluid or from a biopsy of chorionic villus that can be performed as early as the first trimester.

There are two distinct approaches to the molecular diagnosis of single-gene diseases: direct detection of mutations, and indirect detection based on linkage of the disease gene with surrogate markers in the genome. These two methods are described in the following sections.

Figure 7-43 ■

Fluorescence in situ hybridization (FISH). *A,* Interphase nucleus from a male patient with suspected trisomy 18. Three different fluorescent probes have been used in a "FISH cocktail"—the green probe hybridizes to the X chromosome centromere (one copy), the red probe to the Y chromosome centromere (one copy), and the aqua probe to the chromosome 18 centromere (three copies). *B,* A metaphase spread in which two fluorescent probes have been used, one hybridizing to chromosome 22q13 region *(green)* and the other hybridizing to chromosome 22q11.2 region *(red)*. There are two 22q13 signals. One of the two chromosomes does not stain with the probe for 22q11.2, indicating a microdeletion in this region. This deletion gives rise to the 22q11.2 deletion syndrome (DiGeorge syndrome). *(A* and *B,* Courtesy of Dr. Nancy R. Schneider and Jeff Doolittle, Cytogenetics Laboratory, University of Texas Southwestern Medical Center, Dallas.)

DIRECT GENE DIAGNOSIS

Victor McKusick, an eminent geneticist, has appropriately called direct gene diagnosis the *diagnostic biopsy of the human genome.* Such diagnosis depends on the detection of an important qualitative change in the DNA. There are two variations of direct gene diagnosis.

One technique relies on the fact that some mutations alter or destroy certain restriction sites on the normal DNA (restriction sites are short, specific DNA sequences recognized by *restriction enzymes,* which have the ability to cleave DNA at these sites). For example, in the normal β-globin gene, there are three sites that are recognized by the restriction enzyme *Mst*II (Fig. 7-44). The sickle mutation responsible for sickle cell anemia (Chapter 12) involves a single–base pair change (A → T) that abolishes one of the three *Mst*II sites. When DNA from a normal individual is digested with *Mst*II, subjected to electrophoresis on a gel, and hybridized with the radioactive DNA probe specific for the β-globin gene (Southern blot hybridization), a single 1.15-kb band that reacts with the probe is detected. Such a band results from the formation of identical 1.15-kb fragments from each of the two normal chromosomes. On the other hand, similar analysis of DNA from the cells of a patient homozygous for the sickle cell hemoglobin (HbS) gene leads to the formation of a single larger (1.35-kb) fragment, owing to the loss of the *Mst*II sites from both chromosomes. In heterozygotes, the normal chromosome yields a 1.15-kb band, whereas the chromosome carrying the mutation gives rise to the 1.35-kb band. Thus, Southern blot analysis reveals two different-sized bands, allowing detection of a heterozygote carrier.

If the mutation does not alter any known restriction site, an alternative approach based on the use of *allele-specific oligonucleotides* can be utilized (Fig. 7-45). For example, many cases of α_1-antitrypsin (α_1-AT) deficiency are due to a single G → A change in the α_1-antitrypsin gene, producing the so-called Z allele (Chapter 13). Two oligonucleotides, having at their center the single base by which the normal and mutant genes differ, are synthesized. Such allele-specific oligonucleotides can then be used as radiolabeled probes in a Southern blot analysis. The oligonucleotide containing the sequence of the normal gene hybridizes with both the normal and the mutant DNA, but hybridization to the mutant DNA is unstable, owing to the single–base pair mismatch. Thus, under stringent conditions of hybridization, the labeled normal probe produces a strong autoradiographic signal with DNA from a normal individual, no signal in the DNA extracted from a patient homozygous for the mutant gene, and a faint signal with DNA from a hererozygote. With the probe containing the mutant sequence, the pattern of hybridization is reversed. Of course, heterozygotes react with both probes because they carry one normal and one mutant gene.

PCR Analysis. Techniques such as Southern blot hybridization require large quantities of genomic DNA. In contrast, PCR analysis, which involves exponential amplification of DNA, requires much smaller quantities of starting material. PCR analysis is now widely used in molecular diagnosis. If RNA is used as the substrate, it is first reverse transcribed *to* obtain cDNA and then amplified by PCR. This method is often abbreviated as RT-PCR.

As with the other methods of direct gene diagnosis, the sequence of the normal gene must be known. To detect

Figure 7-44 ■

Direct gene diagnosis: detection of the sickle mutation by Southern blot analysis. An A → T substitution in the sixth codon of the β_A globin gene yields the β_S allele. This substitution eliminates an MstII recognition site in the β-globin DNA. Thus, when digested with MstII and probed with an appropriate complementary DNA (cDNA), the β_S allele generates a 1.35-kb fragment rather than the normal 1.15-kb fragment. Hb, hemoglobin.

the mutant gene, two primers that bind to the 3′ and 5′ ends of the normal sequence are designed. By utilizing appropriate DNA polymerases and thermal cycling, the target DNA is greatly amplified, producing millions of copies of the DNA sequence between the two primer sites. If the specific mutation is known to affect a restriction site, then the amplified DNA can be digested. Because the mutation affects a restriction site, the mutant and normal alleles give rise to products of different sizes. These would appear as different bands on agarose gel electrophoresis. If, on the other hand, the sequence of the normal gene is known but that of the mutant allele is unknown, the vastly amplified DNA obtained from the patient can be sequenced by conventional methods. By comparison with the sequence of the normal gene, the disease-causing mutation can be pinpointed.

PCR analysis is also very useful when a mutation is associated with deletions or expansions. As discussed earlier, several diseases, such as the fragile X syndrome, are associated with trinucleotide repeats. Figure 7–46 reveals how PCR analysis can be used to detect this mutation. Two primers that bind to a sequence at the 5′ end of the FMR1 gene, which is affected by trinucleotide repeats, are used to amplify the intervening sequences. Because there are large differences in the number of repeats, the size of the PCR products obtained from the DNA of normal

individuals and those with premutation is quite different. These size differences are revealed by differential migration of the amplified DNA products on a gel. The full mutation cannot be detected by PCR analysis because the affected segment of DNA is too large for conventional PCR analysis. In such cases, a Southern blot analysis of genomic DNA has to be performed (see Fig. 7–46).

A variety of PCR-based technologies that use fluorophore indicators to detect the presence or absence of mutations in "real time" (i.e., during the exponential phase of DNA amplification) have become available. This has significantly reduced the time required for mutation detection by removing the restriction digestion and electrophoresis steps used in conventional PCR assays. One example of high-throughput mutation analysis is the molecular beacon technology. Molecular beacons are hairpin-shaped fluorescent oligonucleotide probes that fluoresce only on hybridization to target sequences (wild-type DNA). In the presence of nucleotide mismatch because of mutations, effective pairing does not occur and there is no fluorescence.

LINKAGE ANALYSIS

Direct gene diagnosis is possible only if the mutant gene and its normal counterpart have been identified and cloned

SOUTHERN BLOT ANALYSIS

Figure 7-45 ■

Direct gene diagnosis using an oligonucleotide probe and Southern blot analysis. *A,* A G → A change converts a normal α_1-antitrypsin allele (allele M) to a mutant Z allele. This change involves exon V of the α_1-antitrypsin gene, which lies between restriction sites for the enzymes *Xba*I and *Hind*III. *B,* The principle of oligonucleotide probe analysis. Two synthetic oligonucleotide probes, one corresponding in sequence to the normal allele (M-allele probe) and the other corresponding to the mutant allele (Z-allele probe), are lined up against normal and mutant genes, and the expected pattern of hybridization with different combinations is indicated on the right. *C,* The results of Southern blot analysis when DNA from normal individuals or those heterozygous or homozygous for the mutant Z allele is digested (with *Xba*I and *Hind*III) and probed with the normal (M) or Z oligonucleotide probe.

and their nucleotide sequences are known. In several diseases that have a genetic basis, including some common disorders, direct gene diagnosis is not feasible, because either the sequence of the implicated gene is unknown or the disease is multifactorial (polygenic) and no single gene is involved. In such cases, surrogate markers in the genome, also known as marker loci, must be used to localize the chromosomal regions of interest, based on their linkage to one or more putative disease-causing genes. *Linkage analysis* deals with assessing these marker loci in family members exhibiting the disease or trait of interest, based on the assumption that marker loci very close to the disease allele are transmitted through pedigrees. Over time, it becomes possible to define a "disease haplotype" based on a panel of marker loci all of which cosegregate with the putative disease allele. Eventually, linkage analysis facilitates localization and cloning of the disease allele. The marker loci utilized in linkage studies are naturally occurring variations in DNA sequences known as *polymorphisms*. DNA polymorphisms occur at a frequency of approximately one nucleotide in every 300- to 1000-base pair stretch. Two common types of single-base pair variations—restriction fragment length polymorphism and single-nucleotide polymorphism—are discussed in this section.

Certain DNA polymorphisms may abolish or create recognition sites for restriction enzymes, thereby altering the length of DNA fragments produced after digestion. The term *restriction fragment length polymorphism* (RFLP) refers to variation in fragment length between individuals that results from DNA-sequence polymorphisms. With the use of appropriate DNA probes that hybridize with sequences in the vicinity of the polymorphic sites, it becomes possible to detect the DNA fragments of different lengths by Southern blot analysis. Although RFLPs are usually restricted to noncoding regions of the genome, they can prove invaluable in genetic diagnosis by virtue of their linkage to disease-causing genes. Figure 7–47 illustrates the principle of RFLP analysis. In this example of an autosomal recessive disease, both of the parents are heterozygote carriers and the children are normal, are carriers, or are affected. In the illustrated example, the normal chromosome (A) has two restriction sites, 7.6 kb apart, whereas

Figure 7-46   ■

Diagnostic application of Southern blot and polymerase chain reaction (PCR) in fragile X syndrome. With PCR, the differences in the size of CGG repeat between normal and premutation give rise to products of different sizes and mobility. With a full mutation, the region between the primers is too large to be amplified by conventional PCR. In Southern blot analysis, the DNA is cut by enzymes that flank the CGG repeat region and is then probed with a DNA that binds to the affected part of the gene. A single small band is seen in normal males, a higher-molecular-weight band in males with premutation, and a very large (usually diffuse) band in those with the full mutation.

chromosome B, which carries the mutant gene, has a cosegregating DNA-sequence polymorphism resulting in the creation of an additional (third) restriction site for the same enzyme. Note that the additional restriction site has not resulted from the mutation. When DNA from such an individual is digested with the appropriate restriction enzyme and probed with a cloned DNA fragment that hybridizes with a stretch of sequences between the restriction sites, the normal chromosome yields a 7.6-kb band, whereas the other chromosome (carrying the mutant gene) produces a smaller, 6.8-kb band. Thus, on Southern blot analysis two bands are noted. It is possible by this technique to distinguish family members who have inherited both normal chromosomes from those who are heterozygous or homozygous for the mutant gene. RFLPs have been useful in the antenatal diagnosis of CF, Huntington disease, and adult polycystic kidney disease, among others. It is obvious that when a disease gene is identified and cloned, direct gene diagnosis becomes the preferred method.

The second type of polymorphism, by far more common than RFLPs, is known as single-nucleotide polymorphism (SNP). SNPs are found throughout the genome (e.g., in exons and introns and in regulatory sequences); technically, RFLPs can also be considered a type of SNP. SNPs serve both as a physical landmark within the genome and as a genetic marker whose transmission can be followed from parent to child. Because of their prevalence throughout the genome and relative stability, SNPs can be used in linkage analysis for identifying haplotypes associated with disease, leading to gene discovery and mapping. In the last decade, SNPs have become the genetic marker of choice for the study of complex genetic

Figure 7-47   ■

Schematic illustration of the principles underlying restriction fragment length polymorphism analysis in the diagnosis of genetic diseases.

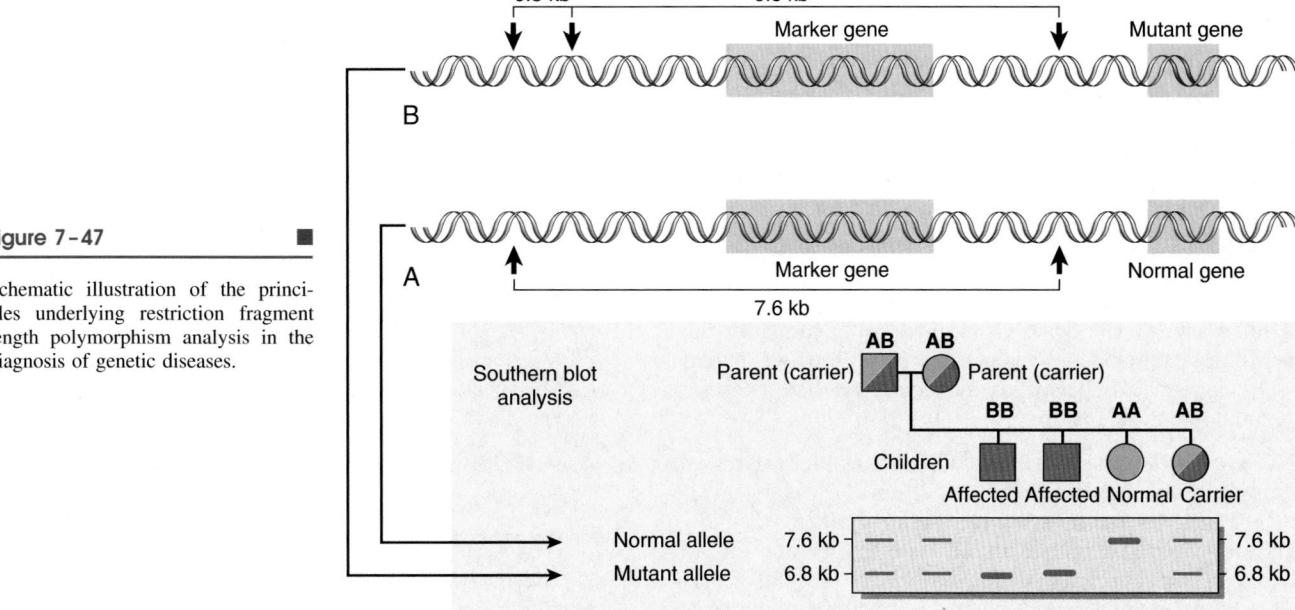

traits. Population studies have found associations between specific SNPs and multifactorial diseases such as hypertension, heart disease, or diabetes. For example, certain polymorphisms within the *angiotensinogen* gene are associated with variations in resting blood pressures and a predisposition to hypertension. A move is under way to map all SNPs in the human genome, which would facilitate the eventual construction of "SNP chips" for genetic risk profiling of individuals.

Indications for Genetic Analysis

In the preceding discussion, we described some of the many techniques available today for the diagnosis of genetic diseases. In order to judiciously utilize these methods, it is important to recognize which individuals require genetic testing. In general, genetic testing can be divided into prenatal and postnatal analysis. It may involve conventional cytogenetics, FISH, molecular diagnostics, or a combination of these techniques.

Prenatal genetic analysis should be offered to all patients who are at risk of having cytogenetically abnormal progeny. It can be performed on cells obtained by amniocentesis, on chorionic villus biopsy material, or on umbilical cord blood. Some important indications are the following:

■ A mother of advanced age (>34 years), because of greater risk of trisomies
■ A parent who is a carrier of a balanced reciprocal translocation, robertsonian translocation, or inversion (in these cases the gametes may be unbalanced, and hence the progeny would be at risk for chromosomal disorders)
■ A parent with a previous child with a chromosomal abnormality
■ A parent who is a carrier of an X-linked genetic disorder (to determine fetal sex)

Postnatal genetic analysis is usually performed on peripheral blood lymphocytes. Indications are as follows:

■ Multiple congenital anomalies
■ Unexplained mental retardation and/or developmental delay
■ Suspected aneuploidy (e.g., features of Down syndrome)
■ Suspected unbalanced autosome (e.g., Prader-Willi syndrome)
■ Suspected sex chromosomal abnormality (e.g., Turner syndrome)
■ Suspected fragile X syndrome
■ Infertility (to rule out sex chromosomal abnormality)
■ Multiple spontaneous abortions (to rule out the parents as carriers of balanced translocation; both partners should be evaluated)

In closing, it should be pointed out that the progress in unraveling the genetic basis of disease is likely to be breathtaking for the next decade. Perhaps genetic diagnosis will allow disease genes to be detected before clinical manifestations appear, thus allowing either preventive measures to be instituted or "genetic" corrections to be made before irreversible tissue damage occurs. We all wait in anticipation.

BIBLIOGRAPHY

Barkin RM, Gausche-Hill M : Sudden infant death syndrome. In Marx: Rosen's Emergency Medicine: Concepts and Clinical Practice, 5th edition. Baltimore, Mosby, 2002, p 2392. (An up-to-date discussion of the pathogenesis and prevention of SIDS.)

Beckwith JB: Nephrogenic rests and the pathogenesis of Wilms tumors: developmental and clinical considerations. Am J Med Genet 79:268, 1998. (An authoritative review on the association between Wilms tumors and their precursor lesions, nephrogenic rests.)

Cassidy SB, et al: Prader-Willi and Angelman syndromes: sister imprinted disorders. Am J Med Genet 97:136, 2000. (A detailed discussion of these two syndromes including clinical and molecular features.)

Doull IJM: Recent advances in cystic fibrosis. Arch Dis Child 85:62, 2001. (An excellent article addressing the complexity of pathogenesis, and genotype-phenotype correlations.)

Goldstein JL, Brown MS: The cholesterol quartet. Science 292:1310, 2001. (A succinct and well-written review of genetic defects that affect the function of LDL receptors.)

Grundy P, Coppes M: An overview of the clinical and molecular genetics of Wilms tumor. Med Pediatr Oncol 27:394, 1996. (A concise review of syndromes and genetic associations of Wilms tumor.)

Guntheroth WG, Spiers PS: Sleeping prone and the risk of sudden infant death syndrome. JAMA 267:2359, 1992. (One of the earliest epidemiologic studies that focused on the role of prone sleeping position in sudden infant death syndrome.)

Hanel ML, Wevrick R: The role of genomic imprinting in human developmental disorders: lessons from Prader-Willi syndrome. Clin Genet 59:156, 2001. (An excellent discussion of genomic imprinting.)

Hsueh W, et al: Necrotizing enterocolitis of the newborn: pathogenic concepts in perspective. Pediatr Dev Pathol 1:2, 1998. (A review of the pathogenic mechanisms of NEC, including experimental animal models.)

Jin P, Warren ST: Understanding the molecular basis of fragile X syndrome. Hum Mol Genet 9:901, 2000. (An excellent summary of the function of FMR-1 protein.)

Johns DR: Mitochondrial DNA and disease. N Engl J Med 333:638, 1995. (An excellent review of diseases caused by inheritance of mitochondrial DNA.)

Kalousek D: Clinical significance of morphologic and genetic examination of spontaneously aborted embryos. Am J Reprod Immunol 39:108, 1998. (An excellent commentary on the importance of performing a thorough postmortem examination in aborted fetuses.)

Kolodny EH: Niemann-Pick disease. Curr Opin Hematol 7:48, 2000. (A short but succinct review of the various forms of this rare disease.)

Mahuran DJ: Biochemical consequences of mutations causing the GM2 gangliosidoses. Biochim Biophys Acta 1455:105, 1999. (A detailed review of the biochemistry of GM2 gangliosidoses—only for the brave!)

Pyeritz RE: The Marfan syndrome. Ann Rev Med 51:481, 2001. (An excellent discussion of the causation and clinical features by an expert.)

Ranke MB, Saenger P: Turner syndrome. Lancet 358:309, 2001. (An excellent basic and clinical review of Turner syndrome.)

Reeves RH, et al: Too much of a good thing: mechanisms of gene action in Down syndrome. Trends Genet 17:83, 2001. (A listing of genes that may be involved in Down syndrome and attempts at correlating phenotype with genetic changes.)

Rogers BB: Parvovirus B19: twenty-five years in perspective. Pediatr Dev Pathol 2:296, 1999. (A comprehensive review of the epidemiology, clinical features and perinatal consequences of parvovirus B19 infections.)

Scambler PJ: The 22q11 deletion syndromes. Hum Mol Genet 9:2421, 2000. (An update on the clinical and molecular features of the syndrome.)

Schork NJ, Chakravarti A: A nonmathematical overview of modern gene mapping techniques applied to human diseases. In Mockrin S (ed): Molecular Genetics and Gene Therapy of Cardiovascular Disease. New York, Dekker, 1996, p 79. (A nontechnical overview of linkage analysis and related methods.)

Schork NJ, et al: Single nucleotide polymorphisms and the future of genetic epidemiology. Clin Genet 58:250, 2000. (A review on the importance and potential applications of SNPs.)

Sheppard DN, Ostegaard LS: Understanding how cystic fibrosis mutations cause a loss of Cl⁻ channel function. Mol Med Today 2:290, 1996. (A lucid description of the molecular mechanisms underlying cystic fibrosis.)

Shimada H, et al: Terminology and morphologic criteria of neuroblastic tumors. Cancer 86:349, 1999. (A update on the consensus diagnostic criteria and classification of neuroblastomas and other neuroblastic tumors.)

Smyth Cm, Bremmer WJ: Kleinfelter syndrome. Arch Intern Med 158:1309, 1998. (An excellent clinical review.)

Usdin K, Grabczyk E: DNA repeat expansions and human disease. Cell Mol Life Sci 57:914, 2000. (A detailed overview of the currently recognized trinucleotide repeat disorders.)

Wolfsdorf JI, et al: Glycogen storage diseases. Endocrinol Metab Clin North Am 28:801, 1999. (An exhaustive discussion of glycogen storage diseases.)

Worlitzsch D, et al: Effects of reduced mucus oxygen concentrations in airway *Pseudomonas* infections of cystic fibrosis patients. J Clin Invest 109:317, 2002. (This paper provides novel insights into the pathogenesis of *Pseudomonas* infection in CF.)

8

Environmental Diseases

The term *environmental diseases* as used here refers to lesions and diseases caused by chemical or physical injuries, including those encountered in the workplace, as well as to diseases of nutritional origin. Environmental diseases are surprisingly common. Although there are no precise data on how many individuals are affected by environmental hazards of all kinds, there are some reasonable estimates of the frequency of work-related deaths and injuries. The International Labor Organization has estimated that work-related injuries and illnesses kill 1.1 million people per year globally—more deaths than are caused by road accidents and wars combined (500,000). Most of these

*The section on Pneumoconioses was revised by Anirban Maitra, MD work-related problems were caused by illnesses rather than by accidents. Whatever the precise numbers, it is clear that environmental (including nutritional) diseases constitute an enormous burden financially and in disability and suffering.

Four US agencies are charged with overseeing and regulating hazards of environmental origin:

■ The Environmental Protection Agency
■ The Food and Drug Administration
■ The Occupational Safety and Health Administration
■ The Consumer Products Safety Commission

These agencies attempt to set limits on the permissible levels of exposure to the known environmental hazards (e.g., the maximum level of carbon monoxide in air that is noninjurious or the tolerable levels of radiation that are harmless or "safe"). But a host of factors (such as the complex interaction of various pollutants having multiplicative effects; age; and level of physical activity) create wide variations in individual sensitivity, rendering the concept of "safe levels" of limited value. With this brief overview of the nature and magnitude of the problem, we can turn to a consideration of some of the more important hazards.

ENVIRONMENTAL POLLUTION

Air Pollution

Precious as air is—especially to those deprived of it—it is often laden (sometimes loaded) with many potential causes of disease. Airborne microorganisms contaminating food and water have long been major causes of morbidity and mortality, especially in third world countries. More widespread are the chemical and particulate pollutants found in the air,

especially in industrialized nations. Here, we consider these hazards first in outdoor air and then in indoor air.

OUTDOOR AIR POLLUTION

The ambient air in industrialized nations is contaminated with an unsavory mixture of gaseous and particulate pollutants, more heavily in cities and in proximity to heavy industry than in undeveloped areas where people are few and nature is relatively unspoiled. In the United States, the Environmental Protection Agency (EPA) monitors and sets allowable upper limits for six pollutants. Table 8–1 lists them, along with their origins and potential consequences. Collectively, these agents produce the well-known smog that sometimes stifles large cities such as London, Los Angeles, Houston, and Mexico City. In addition, the air may be locally polluted in the vicinity of industries by all manner of industrial waste, such as polycyclic hydrocarbons (potential carcinogens) and the metal isocyanate released into the air by the industrial explosion at Bhopal, India, and by accidental pollutants such as the volcanic dust spewed into the atmosphere by the eruption of Mount Saint Helens.

Several points require emphasis:

■ Ozone is probably the most intractable air pollutant. Levels found in some cities frequently exceed the EPA upper limits. Its toxicity in part relates to its initiation of free radicals, which in turn injure respiratory passages with the release of inflammatory mediators. After exposures, healthy subjects experience mild respiratory symptoms (decreased lung function and pain), but it is particularly harmful to people with asthma or emphysema.
■ The air particles that constitute the greatest hazard are less than 10 μm in diameter whatever their composition. Larger particles are filtered out in the nares or trapped and evacuated by the mucociliary "escalator." The

Table 8-1. MAJOR OUTDOOR AIR POLLUTANTS

	Origins(s)	Consequences
Ozone (O_3)	Interactions of oxygen with various pollutants such as oxide of nitrogen, sulfur, and hydrocarbons	Is highly reactive and oxidizes polyunsaturated lipids that become irritants and induce release of inflammatory mediators affecting all airways down to bronchoalveolar junctions
Nitrogen dioxide	Combustion of fossil fuels such as coal, gasoline, and wood	Dissolves in secretions in airways to form nitric and nitrous acids, which irritate and damage linings of airways
Sulfur dioxide	Combustion of fossil fuels such as coal, gasoline, and wood	Yields sufuric acid, bisulfites, and sulfites, which irritate and damage linings of airways; together with nitric acid, contributes to acid rain
Carbon monoxide	Incomplete combustion of gasoline, oil, wood, and natural gas	Combines with hemoglobin to displace oxyhemoglobin and thus induce systemic asphyxia (see later)
Lead	Discussed in a subsequent section	
Particulates	Great variety of finely divided (and therefore airborne) pollutants ranging from relatively innocuous plaster dust to highly dangerous asbestos dust (discussed later with pneumoconioses) May include lead, ash, hydrocarbon residues (some may be carcinogenic), and other industrial and nuclear wastes	Major contributor to smog and a major cause of respiratory disease; see Pneumoconioses.

Table 8-2. PATTERNS OF LUNG INJURY RELATED TO AIR POLLUTION

Lung Response	Pathogenic Mechanism(s)
Acute or chronic inflammation (e.g., chronic bronchitis)	Direct cell injury
Emphysema	Enhanced proteolysis
Asthma	Allergic or irritant effect
Hypersensitivity pneumonitis	Immunologic injury
Pneumoconiosis	Fibrotic reactions caused by cytokines released from macrophages and other recruited leukocytes
Neoplasia	Mutagenic and promoting effects

smaller particles remain in the airstream to reach the vulnerable airspaces, where they are phagocytosed by macrophages and neutrophils that then release mediators (such as macrophage inflammatory protein 1α [MIP-1α] and endothelin 1), inciting a respiratory inflammatory reaction. It is these same fine particles that contribute significantly to the creation of smog.

■ While single pollutants have the capacity to impair lung function, combinations amplify their effect. For example, low levels of ozone may be well tolerated but are injurious to lung function when combined with particulate pollution. Because rarely are pollutants found singly, the combinations truly constitute a "witch's brew."

The lungs bear the brunt of the adverse consequences (Table 8–2), although air pollutants can affect many organ systems (e.g., lead absorbed through the lungs affects the brain, bone marrow, and other organs). Except for the pneumoconioses and some general comments on smoking, pollutant-caused lung diseases are discussed in Chapter 13.

INDOOR AIR POLLUTION

As we increasingly "button up" our homes to exclude the environment, the potential for pollution of the indoor air increases. The commonest pollutant is tobacco smoke (discussed separately later), but additional offenders are cited in Table 8–3. Some, such as carbon monoxide and nitrogen dioxide, were briefly mentioned as outdoor pollutants; asbestos is a major hazard and is discussed separately (p 272). Only a few comments about some of remaining ones will be made.

Wood smoke, containing various oxides of nitrogen and carbon particulates, may be only an irritant, but it also predisposes to lung infections and may contain the far more dangerous carcinogenic polycyclic hydrocarbons. *Radon,* a radioactive gas derived from uranium, is widely present in soil. Very low levels of radon are present in homes, particularly those near nuclear plants and waste disposal sites. Exposure to even low levels of radon over time has been suspected in the etiology of lung cancer. *Bioaerosols* range from microbiologic agents capable of causing infectious diseases such as legionnaire's disease, viral pneumonia, and the common cold, and also less threatening but nonetheless distressing allergens derived from pet dander, dust mites,

and fungi and molds responsible for rhinitis, eye irritation, and even asthma. We might mention here the so-called sick building syndrome. It remains an elusive problem of uncertain origin and quite conceivably may be secondary to any one of the indoor pollutants mentioned or, alternatively, may be only a reaction to poor ventilation.

Industrial Exposures

Industrial exposures are as varied as the industries themselves. The spectrum of diseases is surveyed in Table 8–4. As can be seen, they range from mere irritation of the mucosa of the airways caused by fumes of formaldehyde or ammonia; to lung cancer secondary to exposure to asbestos, volatilized nickel, arsenic, or chromium; to leukemia after prolonged exposure to benzene or uranium. A few categories of industrial pollutants are worthy of comment.

Organic compounds are widely used in huge quantities worldwide. Some, such as chloroform and carbon tetrachloride, are found in degreasing and dry cleaning agents and paint removers. Acute exposure to high levels of vapors can cause dizziness and confusion, leading to central nervous system depression and even coma. Lower levels have toxicity for the liver and kidneys. Polycyclic hydrocarbons may be released from the combustion of fossil fuels, particularly at the high-temperature burning of coal and gas in steel foundries. As was pointed out in the discussion of neoplasia (Chapter 6), polycyclic hydrocarbons are among the most potent carcinogens and have been implicated in industrial exposures in the production of lung and bladder cancer. Other organic compounds are widely used in the production of plastics. In the past, exposure to vinyl chloride monomers used in the synthesis of polyvinyl resins was found to lead to angiosarcoma of the liver. Rubber

Table 8-3. HEALTH EFFECTS OF INDOOR AIR POLLUTANTS

Pollutant	Population at Risk	Effects
Carbon monoxide	Adults and children	Acute poisoning
Nitrogen dioxide	Children	Increased respiratory infections
Wood smoke	Children	Increased respiratory infections
Formaldehyde	Adults and children	Eye and nose irritation, asthma
Radon	Adults and children	Lung cancer
Asbestos fibers	Maintenance and abatement workers	Lung cancer; mesothelioma
Manufactured mineral fibers	Maintenance and construction workers	Skin and airway irritation
Bioaerosols	Adults and children	Allergic rhinitis, asthma

Data from Lambert WE, Samet JM: Indoor air pollution. In Harber P, et al (eds): Occupational and Environmental Respiratory Disease. St. Louis, Mosby–Year Book, 1996, p 784; and Menzies D, Bourbeau J: Building-related illnesses. N Engl J Med 337:1524, 1997.

■

Table 8-4. HUMAN DISEASES ASSOCIATED WITH OCCUPATIONAL EXPOSURES

Organ/System	Effect	Toxicant
Cardiovascular system	Heart disease	Carbon monoxide, lead, solvents, cobalt, cadmium
Respiratory system	Nasal cancer	Isopropyl alcohol, wood dust
	Lung cancer	Radon, asbestos, silica, bis(chloromethyl)ether, nickel, arsenic, chromium, mustard gas
	Chronic obstructive lung disease	Grain dust, coal dust, cadmium
	Hypersensitivity	Beryllium, isocyanates
	Irritation	Ammonia, sulfur oxides, formaldehyde
	Fibrosis	Silica, asbestos, cobalt
Nervous system	Peripheral neuropathies	Solvents, acrylamide, methyl chloride, mercury, lead, arsenic, DDT
	Ataxic gait	Chlordane, toluene, acrylamide, mercury
	Central nervous system depression	Alcohols, ketones, aldehydes, solvents
	Cataracts	Ultraviolet radiation
Urinary system	Toxicity	Mercury, lead, glycol ethers, solvents
	Bladder cancer	Naphthylamines, 4-aminobiphenyl, benzidine, rubber products
Reproductive system	Male infertility	Lead, phthalate plasticizers
	Female infertility	Cadmium, lead
	Teratogenesis	Mercury, polychlorinated biphenyls
Hematopoietic system	Leukemia	Benzene, radon, uranium
Skin	Folliculitis and acneiform dermatosis	Polychlorinated biphenyls, dioxins, herbicides
	Cancer	Ultraviolet radiation
Gastrointestinal tract	Liver angiosarcoma	Vinyl chloride

Adapted from Leigh JP, et al: Occupational injury and illness in the United States. Estimates of costs, morbidity, and mortality. Arch Intern Med 157:1557, 1997; Mitchell FL: Hazardous waste. In Rom WN (ed): Environmental and Occupational Medicine, 2nd ed. Boston, Little, Brown, 1992, p 1275; and Levi PE: Classes of toxic chemicals. In Hodgson E, Levi PE (eds): A Textbook of Modern Toxicology. Stamford, CT, Appleton & Lange, 1997, p 229.

workers using 1,3-butadiene have developed leukemia, and the doleful litany could be extended.

Metals are another form of occupational hazard. Lead poisoning is not restricted to workers in particular industries; it is a potential household and domestic danger, as discussed later. When volatilized, as occurs in the mining industries and smelters, arsenic, chromium, and nickel may lead to lung cancer. Other exposures to metals are cited in Table 8–5.

Another important category of occupational disease is the pneumoconioses, discussed next.

PNEUMOCONIOSES

Pneumoconiosis is a term originally coined to describe the non-neoplastic lung reaction to inhalation of mineral dusts. The term has been broadened to include diseases

■

Table 8-5. TOXIC AND CARCINOGENIC METALS

Metal	Disease	Occupation
Lead	Renal toxicity	Battery and ammunition workers, foundry workers, spray painters, radiator repairers
	Anemia, colic	
	Peripheral neuropathy	
	Insomnia, fatigue	
	Cognitive deficits	
Mercury	Renal toxicity	Chlorine-alkali industry workers
	Muscle tremors, dementia	
	Cerebral palsy	
	Mental retardation	
Arsenic	Cancer of skin, lung, liver	Miners, smelters, oil refinery workers, farm workers
Beryllium	Acute lung irritant	Beryllium refinery workers, aerospace manufacturing workers, ceramics workers
	Chronic lung hypersensitivity	
	? Lung cancer	
Cobalt and tungsten carbide	Lung fibrosis	Toolmakers, grinders, diamond polishers
	Asthma	
Cadmium	Renal toxicity	Battery workers, smelters, welders, soldering workers
	? Prostate cancer	
Chromium	Cancer of lung and nasal cavity	Pigment workers, smelters, steel workers
Nickel	Cancer of lung and nasal sinuses	Smelters, steel workers, electroplating workers

Adapted from Levi PE: Classes of toxic chemicals. In Hodgson E, Levi PE (eds): A Textbook of Modern Toxicology. Stamford, CT. Appleton & Lange, 1997, p 229; and Sprince NL: Hard metal disease. In Rom WN (ed): Environmental and Occupational Medicine, 2nd ed. Boston, Little, Brown, 1992, p 791.

Table 8–6.   MINERAL DUST–INDUCED LUNG DISEASE

Agent	Disease	Exposure
Coal dust	Simple coal workers' pneumoconiosis: macules and nodules Complicated coal workers' pneumoconiosis: PMF, Caplan syndrome	Coal mining
Silica	Acute silicosis, chronic silicosis, PMF, Caplan syndrome	Sandblasting, quarrying, mining, stone cutting, foundry work, ceramics
Asbestos	Asbestosis, Caplan syndrome, pleural effusions, pleural plaques or diffuse fibrosis, mesothelioma, carcinoma of the lung, larynx, stomach, colon	Mining, milling, and fabrication of ores and materials; installation and removal of insulation
Beryllium	Acute berylliosis, beryllium granulomatosis	Nuclear energy and aircraft industries

PMF, progressive massive fibrosis.

induced by organic as well as inorganic particulates, and some experts also regard chemical fume- and vapor-induced non-neoplastic lung diseases as pneumoconioses.

The mineral dust pneumoconioses—the four most common of which result from exposure to coal dust, silica, asbestos, and beryllium—nearly always result from exposure in the workplace. However, the increased risk of cancer as a result of asbestos exposure extends to family members of asbestos workers and to other individuals exposed to asbestos outside the workplace. Table 8–6 indicates the pathologic conditions associated with each mineral dust and the major industries in which the dust exposure is sufficient to produce disease.

Pathogenesis. The reaction of the lung to mineral dusts depends on many factors, including the size, shape, solubility, and reactivity of the particles. For example, particles greater than 5 to 10 μm are unlikely to reach distal airways, whereas particles smaller than 0.5 μm tend to act like gases and move into and out of alveoli, often without substantial deposition and injury. Particles that are 1 to 5 μm are the most dangerous because they impact on the bifurcation of the distal airways. Coal dust is relatively inert, and large amounts must be deposited in the lungs before lung disease is clinically detectable. Silica, asbestos, and beryllium are more reactive than coal dust, resulting in fibrotic reactions at lower concentrations. A unifying concept for the development of lesions in all pneumoconioses is depicted in Figure 8–1. Most inhaled dust is entrapped in the mucus blanket and rapidly removed from the lung by ciliary movement. However, some of the particles become impacted at alveolar duct bifurcations, where macrophages accumulate and endocytose the impacted particulates. The more reactive particulates trigger the macrophages to release a number of products that are toxic to the lung, mediating an inflammatory response and initiating fibroblast proliferation and collagen deposition. *The pulmonary*

alveolar macrophage is a key cellular element in the initiation and perpetuation of lung injury and fibrosis. Important mediators released by macrophages into the local milieu include (1) *free radicals*: reactive oxygen and reactive nitrogen species that induce lipid peroxidation and tissue damage; (2) *chemotactic factors*: leukotriene B$_4$ (LTB$_4$), interleukin 8 (IL-8), IL-6, and tumor necrosis factor (TNF), which recruit and activate inflammatory cells, which in turn release damaging oxidants and proteases; and (3) *fibrogenic cytokines*: IL-1, TNF, fibronectin, platelet-derived growth factor (PDGF), and insulin-like growth factor 1 (IGF-1), which recruit fibroblasts. Some of the inhaled particles may reach the lymphatics either by direct drainage or within migrating macrophages and thereby initiate an immune response to components of the particulates and/or to self-proteins, modified by the particles. This then leads to an amplification and extension of the local reaction. *Tobacco smoking worsens the effects of all inhaled mineral dusts,* more so with asbestos than with any other particle.

Coal Workers' Pneumoconiosis

A number of British novels, including D. H. Lawrence's *Sons and Lovers,* poignantly describe the tragedy of the coal miners at the turn of the 20th century who toiled lifelong underground, only to die of "black lung" complicated by tuberculosis. Dust reduction in the coal mines has drastically reduced the incidence of coal dust–induced disease. The spectrum of lung findings in coal workers is wide, ranging from *asymptomatic anthracosis,* in which pigment accumulates without a perceptible cellular reaction, to *simple coal workers' pneumoconiosis* (CWP), in which cellular accumulations of macrophages occur with little to no pulmonary dysfunction, and *complicated CWP* or *progressive massive fibrosis* (PMF), in which fibrosis is extensive and lung function is compromised (see Table 8–6). Although statistics vary, it appears that fewer than 10% of cases of simple CWP progress to PMF. It should be noted that PMF is a generic term that applies to a confluent fibrosing reaction in the lung; this can be a complication of any one of the four pneumoconioses discussed here.

Although coal is mainly carbon, coal mine dust contains a variety of trace metals, inorganic minerals, and crystalline silica. The ratio of carbon to contaminating chemicals and minerals ("coal rank") increases from bituminous to anthracite coal; in general, anthracite mining has been associated with a higher risk of CWP.

MORPHOLOGY

Pulmonary anthracosis is the most innocuous coal-induced pulmonary lesion in coal miners and is also commonly seen in all urban dwellers and tobacco smokers. Inhaled carbon pigment is engulfed by alveolar or interstitial macrophages, which then accumulate in the connective tissue along the lymphatics, including the pleural lymphatics, or in organized lymphoid tissue along the bronchi or in the lung hilus. At autopsy, linear streaks and aggregates of anthracotic pigment readily identify pulmonary lymphatics and mark the pulmonary lymph nodes.

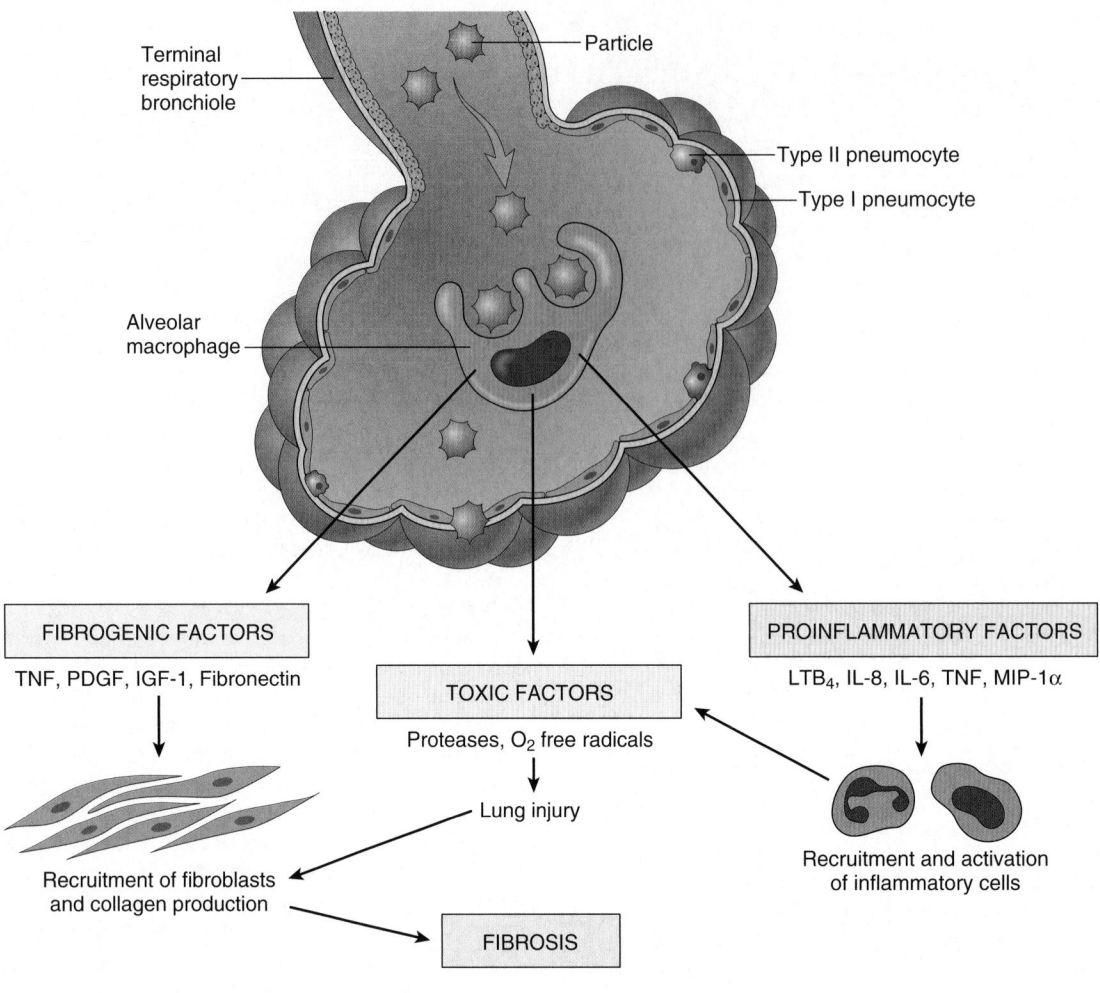

Figure 8-1 ■

Pathogenesis of pneumoconiosis. Inhaled particulates usually impact at the bifurcations of terminal respiratory bronchioles, where they are engulfed by alveolar macrophages, which are then stimulated to secrete (1) various fibrogenic factors that recruit fibroblasts and induce collagen synthesis, (2) toxic factors that initiate lung injury directly, and (3) proinflammatory factors that recruit additional inflammatory cells. IGF-1, insulin-like growth factor 1; IL, interleukin; LTB_4, leukotriene B_4; MIP-1α, macrophage inflammatory protein 1α; PDGF, platelet-derived growth factor; TNF, tumor necrosis factor.

Simple CWP is characterized by **coal macules** and the somewhat larger **coal nodule.** The coal macule consists of dust-laden macrophages; the nodule in addition contains small amounts of a delicate network of collagen fibers. Although these lesions are scattered throughout the lung, the upper lobes and upper zones of the lower lobes are more heavily involved. They are primarily located adjacent to respiratory bronchioles, the site of initial coal dust accumulation. In due course, dilation of adjacent alveoli occurs, a condition sometimes referred to as **centrilobular emphysema** (Chapter 13). Functionally significant emphysema is more common in the United Kingdom and Europe, probably because the coal rank is higher than in the United States, where disabling emphysema is no more common than in the general population once cigarette smoking has been taken into consideration.

Complicated CWP (PMF) occurs on a background of simple CWP by coalescence of coal nodules and generally requires many years to develop. It is characterized by intensely blackened scars larger than 2 cm, sometimes up to 10 cm in greatest diameter. They are usually multiple (Fig. 8-2). Microscopically the lesions consist of dense collagen and pigment. The center of the lesion is often necrotic, resulting most likely from ischemia.

Caplan syndrome is defined as the coexistence of rheumatoid arthritis with a pneumoconiosis, leading to the development of distinctive nodular pulmonary lesions that develop fairly rapidly. There is no evidence that coal mining per se predisposes to rheumatoid arthritis. Like rheumatoid nodules (Chapter 5), the nodular lesions in Caplan syndrome exhibit central necrosis surrounded by palisading fibroblasts, plasma cells, macrophages containing coal dust, and collagen. This syndrome also occurs in asbestosis and silicosis.

Figure 8-2 ■

Progressive massive fibrosis superimposed on coal workers' pneumoconiosis. The large blackened scars are principally in the upper lobe. Note the extensions of scars into surrounding parenchyma and retraction of adjacent pleura. (Courtesy of Dr. Werner Laquer, Dr. Jerome Kleinerman, and the National Institute of Occupational Safety and Health.)

Clinical Course. CWP is usually a benign disease that produces little decrement in lung function. Even mild forms of complicated CWP fail to demonstrate abnormalities of lung function. However, in a minority of cases PMF develops, leading to increasing pulmonary dysfunction, pulmonary hypertension, and cor pulmonale. Progression from CWP to PMF has been linked to a variety of factors including coal dust exposure level and total dust burden. Unfortunately, PMF has a tendency to progress even in the absence of further exposure. Unlike with silicosis (see later), there is no convincing evidence that coal dust increases susceptibility to contracting tuberculosis. Similarly, once smoking-related risk has been factored into consideration, there is no increased frequency of bronchogenic carcinoma in coal miners, a feature that distinguishes CWP from both silica and asbestos exposures (see later).

Silicosis

Silicosis is caused by inhalation of crystalline silica, mostly in occupational settings. The occupations most commonly associated with the development of silicosis include quarry mining, sandblasting, drilling, tunneling, and stone cutting. Approximately 1500 cases of silicosis are diagnosed each year in the United States, and far greater numbers are detected in countries where workplace restrictions on silica exposure are less stringent. Silica occurs in both crystalline and amorphous forms, but crystalline forms (including quartz, cristobalite, and tridymite) are by far biologically the most toxic and fibrogenic. Of these, quartz is most commonly implicated in silicosis. After inhalation, particles of quartz smaller than 5 μm may reach the terminal airways, and those approximately 1 μm in size are particularly apt to be retained and to cause fibrosis.

Based on the intensity of silica exposure and the time course of appearance of symptoms, silicosis can be classified into several different forms:

■ *Acute silicosis.* This results from exposure to very high levels of silica and develops fairly quickly after the environmental insult. Patients often present with rapid-onset tachypnea, cough, cyanosis, and respiratory failure. Histologic examination of tissue sections reveals interstitial inflammation and the accumulation of proteinaceous fluid rich in surfactants within the alveolar spaces (hence, this disease is also known as *silicoproteinosis*).
■ *Chronic (or nodular) silicosis.* This results from the inhalation of crystalline silica over prolonged periods of time, with the formation of characteristic fibrotic nodules of silicosis (see later). Nodules are predominantly present in the upper zones of the lung and in subpleural spaces and are visible radiologically as fairly well demarcated rounded opacities. The latency period for chronic silicosis is inversely proportional to the dose of exposure and is usually quite long.
■ *Complicated (or conglomerate silicosis).* This results from progression of chronic silicosis, with expansion and coalescence of individual silicotic nodules and destruction of lung parenchyma (progressive massive fibrosis). The size of silicotic nodules in complicated disease is usually greater than 2 cm.
■ *Other pulmonary diseases.* Silicosis is associated with an increased susceptibility to *tuberculosis.* It is postulated that silicosis results in a depression of cell-mediated immunity, and crystalline silica may inhibit the ability of pulmonary macrophages to kill phagocytosed mycobacteria. Nodules of silicotuberculosis often display a central zone of caseation. Caplan syndrome (see earlier) may also occur in patients with silicosis but is uncommon. The relationship between silica and *lung cancer* has been a contentious issue, but in 1997, based on evidence from several epidemiologic studies, the International Agency for Research on Cancer (IARC) concluded that *crystalline silica from occupational sources is carcinogenic in humans.* Silica-induced carcinogenesis may be related to its ability to generate reactive oxygen species in tissues.

MORPHOLOGY

Silicotic nodules are characterized grossly in their early stages by tiny, barely palpable, discrete, pale-to-blackened (if coal dust is also present) nodules in the upper zones of the lungs (Fig. 8-3). Microscopically, the silicotic nodule demonstrates concentrically arranged hyalinized collagen fibers surrounding an amorphous center. The "whorled" appearance of the collagen fibers is quite distinctive for silicosis (Fig. 8-4). Examination of the nodules by polarized microscopy reveals weakly birefringent silica particles, primarily in the center of the nodules. As the disease progresses, the individual nodules may coalesce into hard, collagenous scars, with eventual progression to PMF. The intervening lung parenchyma may be compressed or overexpanded, and a honeycomb pattern may develop. Fibrotic lesions may also occur in the hilar lymph nodes and pleura. Sometimes, thin sheets of calcification occur in the lymph nodes and are appreciated radiographically as "eggshell" calcification (e.g., calcium surrounding a zone lacking calcification).

Figure 8-4 ■

Several coalescent collagenous silicotic nodules. (Courtesy of Dr. John Godleski, Brigham and Women's Hospital, Boston.)

Clinical Course. Chronic silicosis is usually detected in routine chest radiographs performed on asymptomatic workers. The radiographs typically show a fine nodularity in the upper zones of the lung, but pulmonary function is either normal or only moderately affected. Most patients do not develop shortness of breath until late in the course, after PMF is present. At this time, the disease may be progressive, even if the patient is no longer exposed. Many patients with PMF develop pulmonary hypertension and cor pulmonale, as a result of chronic hypoxia-induced vasoconstriction and parenchymal destruction. The disease is slow to kill, but impaired pulmonary function may severely limit activity.

Asbestosis and Asbestos-Related Diseases

Asbestos is a family of crystalline hydrated silicates with a fibrous geometry. On the basis of epidemiologic studies, occupational exposure to asbestos is linked to (1) parenchymal interstitial fibrosis *(asbestosis);* (2) bronchogenic carcinoma; (3) pleural effusions; (4) localized fibrous plaques or, rarely, diffuse pleural fibrosis; (5) malignant pleural and peritoneal mesotheliomas; and (6) possibly laryngeal carcinoma. An increased incidence of asbestos-related cancer in family members of asbestos workers has alerted the general public to the potential hazards of asbestos in the environment. For instance, asbestos is widely present in insulation and is detectable in water and air.

Pathogenesis. Concentration, size, shape, and solubility of the different forms of asbestos dictate whether disease will occur. There are two distinct forms of asbestos: *serpentine* (in which the fiber is curly and flexible) and *amphibole* (in which the fiber is straight, stiff, and brittle). There are several subtypes of curly and straight asbestos fibers. The serpentine *chrysotile* accounts for most of the asbestos used in industry. It is important to make the distinction among various forms of amphiboles and serpentines, because amphiboles, even though less prevalent, are more pathogenic than the serpentine chrysotile, particularly with respect to induction of malignant mesotheliomas. Indeed, some studies of mesotheliomas have shown the link is almost invariably to amphibole exposure. The greater pathogenicity of straight and stiff amphiboles is apparently related to several factors:

Figure 8-3 ■

Advanced silicosis seen on transection of lung. Scarring has contracted the upper lobe into a small dark mass *(arrow).* Note the dense pleural thickening. (Courtesy of Dr. John Godleski, Brigham and Women's Hospital, Boston.)

- The serpentine chrysotiles, with their more flexible, curled structure, are likely to become impacted in the upper respiratory passages and removed by the mucociliary elevator. Those that are trapped in the lungs are gradually leached from the tissues because they are more soluble than amphiboles.
- The straight, stiff amphiboles align themselves in the airstream and are hence delivered deeper into the lungs, where they may penetrate epithelial cells and reach the interstitium.

Despite these differences, both asbestos forms are fibrogenic, and increasing exposure is associated with a higher incidence of all asbestos-related diseases except mesothelioma. In addition to cellular and fibrotic lung reactions, asbestos probably also functions as both a tumor initiator and a promoter. Some of the oncogenic effects of asbestos on the mesothelium are mediated by reactive free radicals generated by asbestos fibers, which preferentially localize in the distal lung close to the mesothelial layer. However, potentially toxic chemicals adsorbed onto the asbestos fibers undoubtedly contribute to the pathogenicity of the fibers as well. For example, *the adsorption of carcinogens in tobacco smoke onto asbestos fibers may well be important to the remarkable synergy between tobacco smoking and the development of bronchogenic carcinoma in asbestos workers.*

Asbestosis, like other pneumoconioses, causes fibrosis by interacting with lung macrophages. It is not completely understood, however, why some inorganic dusts, exemplified by silicosis, cause nodular fibrosis, whereas others, such as asbestos, cause diffuse interstitial fibrosis. The more diffuse distribution may be related to the ability of asbestos to reach alveoli more consistently, its ability to penetrate epithelial cells, or both.

MORPHOLOGY

Asbestosis is marked by diffuse pulmonary interstitial fibrosis. These changes are indistinguishable from those resulting from other causes of diffuse interstitial fibrosis such as idiopathic pulmonary fibrosis (Chapter 13), except for the presence of asbestos bodies, which are seen as **golden brown, fusiform or beaded rods with a translucent center. They consist of asbestos fibers coated with an iron-containing proteinaceous material** (Fig. 8–5). Asbestos bodies apparently arise when macrophages attempt to phagocytose asbestos fibers; the iron is presumably derived from phagocyte ferritin. Asbestos bodies can sometimes be found in the lungs of normal persons, but usually in much lower concentrations and without an accompanying interstitial fibrosis.

Asbestosis begins as fibrosis around respiratory bronchioles and alveolar ducts and extends to involve adjacent alveolar sacs and alveoli. Contraction of the fibrous tissue distorts the native architecture, creating enlarged airspaces enclosed within thick fibrous walls. In this way the affected regions become honeycombed. In contrast to CWP and silicosis, asbestosis begins in the lower lobes and subpleurally, but the middle and upper lobes of the lungs become affected as fibrosis progresses. Simultaneously, the visceral pleura undergoes fibrous thickening and sometimes binds the lungs to the chest wall. Large parenchymal nodules typical of Caplan syndrome may appear in a few patients who have concurrent rheumatoid arthritis. The scarring may trap and narrow pulmonary arteries and arterioles, causing pulmonary hypertension and cor pulmonale.

Pleural plaques are the most common manifestation of asbestos exposure and are well-circumscribed plaques of dense collagen (Fig. 8–6), often containing calcium. They develop most frequently on the anterior and posterolateral aspects of the **parietal** pleura and over the domes of the diaphragm. They do not contain asbestos bodies, and only rarely do they occur in persons who have no history or evidence of asbestos exposure. Uncommonly, asbestos exposure induces pleural effusions, which are usually serous but may be bloody. Rarely, diffuse visceral pleural fibrosis may occur and, in advanced cases, bind the lung to the thoracic cavity wall.

Both bronchogenic carcinomas and malignant mesotheliomas develop in workers exposed to asbestos. The risk of bronchogenic carcinoma is increased about fivefold for asbestos workers; the relative risk for mesotheliomas, normally a very rare tumor (2 to 17 cases per 1 million persons), is more than 1000-fold greater. Both pleural and peritoneal mesotheliomas have an association with asbestos exposure. Concomitant cigarette smoking greatly increases the risk of bronchogenic carcinoma but not that of mesothelioma. These asbestos-related tumors are morphologically indistinguishable from cancers of other causes and are described in Chapter 13.

Figure 8–5 ■

High-power detail of an asbestos body, revealing the typical beading and knobbed ends *(arrow)*.

Figure 8-6

■

Asbestosis. Markedly thickened visceral pleura covers the lateral and diaphragmatic surface of lung. Note also severe interstitial fibrosis diffusely affecting the lower lobe of the lung.

Clinical Course. The clinical findings in asbestosis are indistinguishable from those of any other diffuse interstitial lung disease (Chapter 13). Typically, progressively worsening dyspnea appears 10 to 20 years after exposure. The dyspnea is usually accompanied by a cough associated with production of sputum. The disease may remain static or progress to congestive heart failure, cor pulmonale (Chapter 11), and death. The development of Caplan syndrome may accelerate the clinical course. Pleural plaques are usually asymptomatic and are detected on radiographs as circumscribed densities. Lung or pleural cancer associated with asbestos exposure has a particularly grim prognosis.

Berylliosis

Heavy exposure to airborne dusts or to fumes of metallic beryllium or its oxides, alloys, or salts may induce acute pneumonitis; more protracted low-dose exposure may cause pulmonary and systemic granulomatous lesions that closely mimic those of sarcoidosis (Chapter 13). Limitations on worker exposure to beryllium have resulted in the disappearance of acute berylliosis and a marked reduction in the incidence of chronic disease. Currently, workers in the nuclear and aerospace industries who work with beryllium alloys are at highest risk for exposure.

Chronic berylliosis is caused by induction of T-cell–mediated immunity in genetically susceptible individuals. Indeed, linkage to specific alleles of major histocompatibility complex (MHC) class II genes has been demonstrated. It appears that beryllium acts as a hapten that binds to proteins and renders them immunogenic for CD4+ helper T cells. The resultant delayed hypersensitivity leads to the formation of noncaseating granulomas in the lungs and hilar nodes or, less commonly, in spleen, liver, kidneys, adrenals, and distant lymph nodes. In addition, beryllium itself can induce TNF and other proinflammatory cytokines from alveolar macrophages. The pulmonary granulomas become progressively fibrotic, giving rise to irregular, fine nodular densities detected on chest radiographs. Hilar adenopathy is present in about half of the cases.

Chronic berylliosis may not result in clinical manifestations until many years after exposure, when the patient presents with dyspnea, cough, weight loss, and arthralgias. Some cases stabilize, others remit and relapse, and still others progress to pulmonary failure. Epidemiologic evidence links heavy beryllium exposure to an increased incidence of cancer.

TOBACCO SMOKE

In contrast to the pneumoconioses, which are largely occupational diseases, tobacco smoking is a self-inflicted major health hazard worldwide.

Although all forms of tobacco are implicated—cigars, pipes, snuff—the principal offender is cigarettes. The World Health Organization reported that in 1998 there were about 1235 billion adult smokers in a world population of 5926 billion and that the number of smokers can be expected to increase to 1671 billion in 2020. In the United States alone, tobacco is responsible for over 400,000 deaths annually, one third of these attributable to lung cancer. With all of the effort devoted in the United States to discourage smoking, the harsh facts are that the number of smokers held steady during the 1990s, and the number of deaths increased, particularly in women (by 147% between 1974 and 1994). It appears that young people are starting to smoke at an earlier age. The following discussion summarizes (1) the detrimental effects of cigarette smoking, (2) the reversal of these effects with cessation of smoking, and (3) the evidence that passive smoke inhalation is also injurious to health.

The number of potentially noxious chemicals in tobacco smoke is extraordinary. Table 8–7 provides only a partial list and includes the likely mechanism by which each of these agents produces injury. This injury translates into a

■

Table 8-7. EFFECTS OF SELECTED TOBACCO SMOKE CONSTITUENTS

Substance	Effect
Tar	Carcinogenesis
Polycyclic aromatic hydrocarbons	Carcinogenesis
Nicotine	Ganglionic stimulation and depression, tumor promotion
Phenol	Tumor promotion and irritation
Benzopyrene	Carcinogenesis
Carbon monoxide	Impaired oxygen transport and utilization
Formaldehyde	Toxicity to cilia and irritation
Oxides of nitrogen	Toxicity to cilia and irritation
Nitrosamine	Carcinogenesis

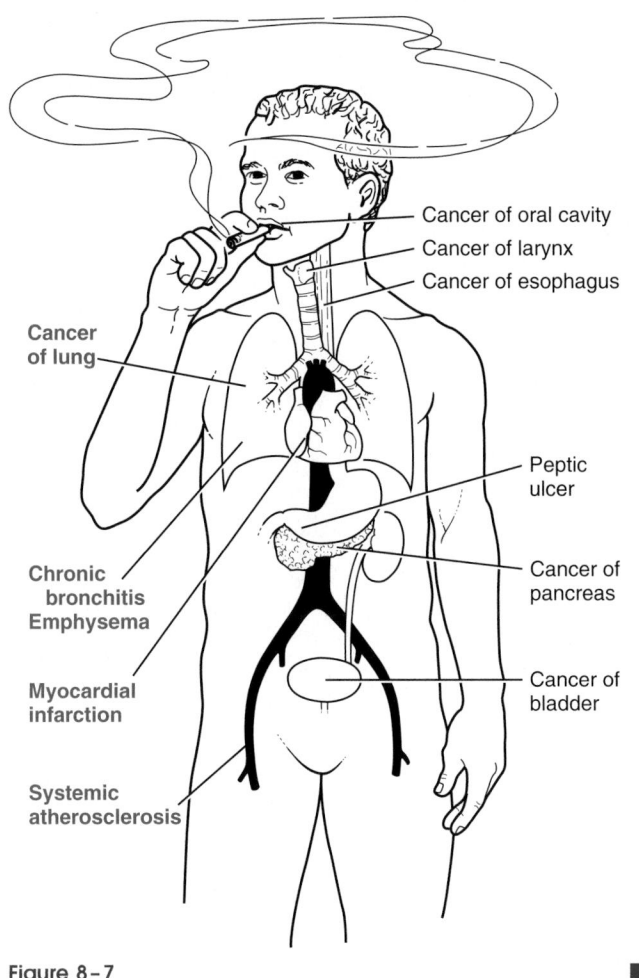

Figure 8–7 ■

Adverse effects of smoking: the more common on the left and the somewhat less common on the right.

number of important diseases (Fig. 8–7), the most common being emphysema, chronic bronchitis, and lung cancer, discussed in detail in later chapters. However, we should point out here some of the mechanisms for these diseases. Agents in smoke have a direct irritant effect on the tracheobronchial mucosa, producing inflammation and increased mucus production (bronchitis). Cigarette smoke also results in the recruitment of leukocytes to the lung, with increased local elastase production and subsequent injury to lung tissue, leading to emphysema. Components of cigarette smoke, particularly tars with their polycyclic hydrocarbons, are potent experimental carcinogens and cancer promoters and are likely involved in the origins of cancers in the lung arising from the bronchial epithelium (bronchogenic carcinoma). The risk of development of these diseases is related to the intensity of exposure, frequently expressed in terms of "pack years" (e.g., one pack daily for 20 years equals 20 pack years). Moreover, smoking multiplies the risk of other carcinogenic influences; witness the 10-fold increased incidence of bronchogenic carcinoma in asbestos workers who smoke over those who do not smoke.

In addition to lung disease, atherosclerosis and its major complication, myocardial infarction, have also been strongly

linked to cigarette smoking; causal mechanisms likely relate to several factors, including increased platelet aggregation, decreased myocardial oxygen supply (because of significant lung disease coupled with the hypoxia related to the carbon monoxide content of cigarette smoke) accompanied by an increased oxygen demand, and a decreased threshold for ventricular fibrillation. Almost one third of all heart attacks are attributed to cigarette smoking. Smoking has a multiplicative effect when combined with hypertension and hypercholesterolemia.

As might be expected, cessation of smoking leads to substantial benefits. The 1990 US Surgeon General's report summarized the data on this issue. The overall risk of dying in individuals of all ages is increased if the individuals smoke but is reduced somewhat within a year after quitting. The risk of lung cancer continues to decrease for at least 15 years but does not disappear. Not shown in Figure 8–7 is the effect of smoking on the unborn fetus. Maternal smoking increases the risk of spontaneous abortions and preterm births and results in intrauterine growth retardation (Chapter 7); birth weights of infants born to mothers who stopped smoking before pregnancy are normal.

Breathing sidestream smoke (passive smoke inhalation) is also associated with some of the same detrimental effects that result from active smoking. It is estimated that the relative risk of lung cancer in nonsmokers exposed to environmental smoke is about 1.3 times that of nonsmokers who are not exposed to smoke. The US Environmental Protection Agency estimates that in the United States, approximately 3000 lung cancer deaths in nonsmokers over the age of 35 years can be attributed each year to environmental tobacco smoke. Even more striking is the increased risk of coronary atherosclerosis and fatal myocardial infarction. Studies report that every year 30,000 to 60,000 cardiac deaths in the United States are associated with exposure to passive smoke. Children living in a household with an adult who smokes have an increased incidence of respiratory illnesses and asthma. It is clear that the transient pleasure a puff may give comes with a heavy long-term price.

INJURY BY CHEMICAL AGENTS

There is a nearly endless list of chemical agents that can be injurious when inhaled, ingested, injected, or absorbed through the skin. Some may produce injury in the course of therapy for another disease (therapeutic agents); others (nontherapeutic agents) are introduced accidentally or intentionally into the body. Some of the latter agents (e.g., alcohol and drugs of abuse) are used principally because of their psychotropic or mind-altering effects. Poison control center data indicate that about 2 million potentially hazardous exposures occur annually in the United States. Of these, about 90% were unintentional and 10% were intentional poisonings, 73% involved oral intake, and 61% of the victims were children younger than 6 years. Only about 2% were adverse drug reactions (see later). As might be expected, the most frequent offending agents were substances commonly available in the home, such as cleaning agents, analgesics, cosmetics, plants, or cold preparations. The great majority had either minor or no toxic effects, but a significant number—on the order of 500—were fatal.

The following principles are important in understanding the mechanisms of chemical injury:

■ *Dose.* In general, the higher the dose, the greater the toxicity, although small doses may cause serious sequelae, particularly over a protracted period. An example is impairment of mental development in children chronically exposed to low levels of lead.

■ *Requirement for metabolic conversion.* Some agents (e.g., certain alkaline cleaning materials) are directly toxic to cells and hence injure the mucosa of the oral cavity, esophagus, and stomach when swallowed. In contrast, many drugs, including alcohol, are converted in the liver to compounds that are more toxic than the parent compound. Thus, there may be little or no injury to the site of entry, and the liver may bear the brunt of injury.

■ *Sites of absorption, accumulation, or excretion.* These may be the targets of maximal injury. For chemicals that are direct cell toxins, the site of entry is obviously important in determining the type of injury. The site of accumulation is also important. The aminoglycoside antibiotics, for instance, are particularly prone to accumulate in the endolymph and perilymph of the ear and in the renal cortex, thus explaining the propensity of these drugs (e.g., tetracycline) to cause ototoxicity and nephrotoxicity.

■ *Individual variation.* An important determinant of the rate of drug metabolism is inherited polymorphisms in the enzymes that metabolize the drugs. For example, acetylation of the antihypertensive drug hydralazine is genetically determined. Individuals who are slow acetylators are more likely to develop drug-induced lupus (Chapter 5).

■ *The capacity of the chemical to induce an immune response.* Many chemicals are not directly toxic but inflict injury by inducing an immune response. For example, penicillin may induce an immunoglobulin E (IgE)-mediated anaphylactic response or an IgG-mediated hemolytic anemia in those who are genetically prone to develop type I or type II hypersensitivity reactions to this drug (Chapter 5).

■ *Unintentional transmission of infections.* Another mechanism of drug injury (discussed later) is the unintentional transmission of infections (e.g., hepatitis B or C or AIDS) when the drug is taken parenterally.

Injury by Therapeutic Agents (Adverse Drug Reactions)

Adverse drug reactions (ADRs) refer to untoward effects of drugs that are given in conventional therapeutic settings. These reactions are extremely common in the practice of medicine and are believed to affect 7% to 8% of patients admitted to a hospital. About 10% of these prove fatal. Several examples of ADRs were given in the previous discussion of general principles; Table 8–8 lists common pathologic findings in ADRs and the drugs most frequently involved. As can be seen in the table, many of the drugs involved in

Table 8–8. SOME COMMON ADVERSE DRUG REACTIONS AND THEIR AGENTS

Reaction	Major Offenders
Blood Dyscrasias (feature of almost half of all drug-related deaths)	
Granulocytopenia, aplastic anemia, pancytopenia	Antineoplastic agents, immuno-suppressives, and chloramphenicol
Hemolytic anemia, thrombo-cytopenia	Penicillin, methyldopa, quinidine
Cutaneous	
Urticaria, macules, papules, vesicles, petechiae, exfoliative dermatitis, fixed drug eruptions	Antineoplastic agents, sulfonamides, hydantoins, many others
Cardiac	
Arrhythmias	Theophylline, hydantoins
Cardiomyopathy	Doxorubicin, daunorubicin
Renal	
Glomerulonephritis	Penicillamine
Acute tubular necrosis	Aminoglycoside antibiotics, cyclosporin, amphotericin B
Tubulointerstitial disease with papillary necrosis	Phenacetin, salicylates
Pulmonary	
Asthma	Salicylates
Acute pneumonitis	Nitrofurantoin
Interstitial fibrosis	Busulfan, nitrofurantoin, bleomycin
Hepatic	
Fatty change	Tetracycline
Diffuse hepatocellular damage	Halothane, isoniazid, acetominophen
Cholestasis	Chlorpromazine, estrogens, contraceptive agents
Systemic	
Anaphylaxis	Penicillin
Lupus erythematosus syndrome (drug-induced lupus)	Hydralazine, procainamide
Central Nervous System	
Tinnitus and dizziness	Salicylates
Acute dystonic reactions and parkinsonian syndrome	Phenothiazine antipsychotics
Respiratory depression	Sedatives

ADRs, such as the antineoplastic agents, are highly potent, and the ADR is a calculated risk of the dosage assumed to achieve the maximal antineoplastic effect. Because they are widely used, estrogens and oral contraceptives (OCs) are discussed next in more detail. In addition, acetaminophen and aspirin are so commonly used as nonprescription drugs that they are important causes of accidental or intentional overdose and so merit additional comment, as do sedative, hypnotic, and anxiolytic agents in the context of drug abuse.

EXOGENOUS ESTROGENS AND ORAL CONTRACEPTIVES

Estrogens and OCs are discussed separately because (1) estrogens for the postmenopausal syndrome may be given alone and are usually natural estrogens, and (2) OCs contain synthetic estrogens, always with some form of progestin.

Exogenous Estrogens. Estrogen therapy, once used primarily for distressing menopausal symptoms (e.g., hot flashes), is currently widely used in postmenopausal women, with or without added progestins, to prevent or slow the progression of osteoporosis (Chapter 21) and to reduce the likelihood of a "heart attack." Such therapy is referred to as *hormone replacement therapy* (HRT). Given the fact that endogenous hyperestrinism increases the risk of developing endometrial carcinoma and, probably, breast carcinoma, there is understandable concern about the use of HRT. Current data support the following adverse effects of estrogen therapy:

■ *Endometrial carcinoma.* Unopposed estrogen therapy increases the risk of endometrial carcinoma three- to six-fold after 5 years of use and more than 10-fold after 10 years. This risk is drastically reduced or even eliminated when progestins are added to the therapeutic regimen.
■ *Breast carcinoma.* Studies continue to point to an increased risk of this form of cancer with the use of HRT. This increased risk, while small, is *not* eliminated by the combination of estrogen and progestins; quite the contrary, the combination therapy *increased* the risk over that for women taking estrogen alone in a recent large-scale study.
■ *Thromboembolism.* Whereas high doses of estrogen definitely increase the risk of venous thromboembolism, the effect of lower doses used for HRT is less certain. Overall, it appears that there is a small but significant increase in risk of thromboembolic disease. This is particularly true for those who have other risk factors such as immobilization or underlying mutations in factor V or prothrombin.
■ *Cardiovascular disease.* Myocardial infarction and stroke are among the leading causes of death in postmenopausal women. Estrogens tend to elevate the level of high-density lipoprotein (HDL) and reduce the level of low-density lipoprotein (LDL). This lipid profile is protective against the development of atherosclerosis. Progestins, on the other hand, tend to lower HDL and elevate LDL, which counters to some extent the estrogen effect. Several epidemiologic studies suggest a 40% to 50% decrease in the risk of ischemic heart disease in women who received HRT beginning at or near the onset of menopause, compared with those who did not. However, it should be pointed out that definitive data from a large placebo-controlled clinical trial are still lacking. One such study, the Women's Health Initiative, is ongoing, and results are expected in 2005.

Oral Contraceptives. Although OCs have been in use for over 30 years, and despite innumerable analyses of their risks and benefits, disagreement continues about their safety and adverse effects. They nearly always contain a synthetic estradiol and a variable amount of a progestin (combined OCs), but a few preparations contain only progestins. Currently prescribed OCs contain a smaller amount of estrogens (<50 μg/day) and are clearly associated with fewer side effects than were earlier formulations. Hence, the results of epidemiologic studies must be interpreted in the context of the dosage. Nevertheless, there is reasonable evidence to support the following conclusions:

■ *Breast carcinoma.* Despite the disagreements, the prevailing opinion is that there is a slight or no increase in breast cancer risk when combined OCs are used by women younger than 45 years, particularly nulliparous women younger than 25 years. For women older than 45 years, the risk, if any, is negligible. However the risk is significantly increased if women have a family history of breast cancer or are known to carry mutations of either *BRCA1* or *BRCA2* (Chapter 6).
■ *Endometrial cancer.* There is no increased risk, and very likely OCs exert a protective effect.
■ *Cervical cancer.* OCs carry some increased risk, which is correlated with duration of use. More recent studies suggest that the increased risk may be more strongly correlated with life style than with the drug (Chapter 19).
■ *Ovarian cancer.* OCs protect against ovarian cancer. The longer they are used, the greater the protection, and this protection persists for some time after OC use stops. This benefit may outweigh the increased risks of other forms of cancer.
■ *Thromboembolism.* Most studies indicate that OCs, including the newer low-dose (<50 μg of estrogen) preparations, are clearly associated with a three- to sixfold increased risk of venous thrombosis and pulmonary thromboembolism because of increased hepatic synthesis of coagulation factors and reduced activity of protein C. This risk may be even higher with newer "third-generation" OCs that contain synthetic progestins, particularly in women who are carriers of factor V Leiden mutation.
■ *Hypertension.* Even the newer low-estrogen formulations of OCs cause a slight increase in blood pressure. The effect is more marked in older women with a family history of hypertension.
■ *Cardiovascular disease.* As discussed, estrogens and progestins have opposing effects on HDL and LDL levels. The overall effect on the levels of these lipoproteins seems to depend on the preparations used, particularly the dose of progestin in the formulation. There is considerable uncertainty regarding the risk of atherosclerosis and myocardial infarction in users of OCs. It appears that OCs do not increase the risk of coronary artery disease in women younger than 30 years or in older women who are nonsmokers, especially if they use the newer, low-estrogen formulations.
■ *Hepatic adenoma.* There is a well-defined association between the use of OCs and this rare benign hepatic tumor, especially in older women who have used OCs for prolonged periods.
■ *Gallbladder disease.* The slightly increased risk found with older formulations is not seen with the newer ones.

Obviously, the pros and cons of OCs must be viewed in the context of their wide applicability and acceptance as a form of contraception that protects against unwanted pregnancies with their attendant hazards.

ACETAMINOPHEN

When taken in very large doses, this widely used nonprescription analgesic and antipyretic causes hepatic necrosis. The window between the usual therapeutic dose (0.5 g) and the toxic dose (15 to 25 g) is large, however, and the drug is ordinarily very safe. Toxicity begins with nausea, vomiting, diarrhea, and sometimes shock, followed in a few days by evidence of jaundice. With serious overdose, liver failure ensues, with centrilobular necros0is that may extend to the entire lobule. Some patients show evidence of concurrent renal and myocardial damage.

ASPIRIN (ACETYLSALICYLIC ACID)

Overdose may result from accidental ingestion of a large number of 325-mg tablets by young children; in adults, overdose is frequently suicidal. The major untoward consequences are metabolic with few morphologic changes. At first, respiratory alkalosis develops, followed by metabolic acidosis that often proves fatal before anatomic changes can appear. Ingestion of as little as 2 to 4 g by children or 10 to 30 g by adults may be fatal, but survival has been reported after doses five times larger.

Chronic aspirin toxicity (salicylism) may develop in persons who take 3 g or more daily (the dose required to treat chronic inflammatory conditions). Chronic salicylism is manifested by headaches, dizziness, ringing in the ears (tinnitus), difficulty hearing, mental confusion, drowsiness, nausea, vomiting, and diarrhea. The central nervous system changes may progress to convulsions and coma. The morphologic consequences of chronic salicylism are varied. Most often, there is an acute erosive gastritis (Chapter 15), which may produce overt or covert gastrointestinal bleeding and lead to gastric ulceration. A bleeding tendency may appear concurrently with chronic toxicity, because aspirin acetylates platelet cyclooxygenase and blocks the ability to make thromboxane A_2, an activator of platelet aggregation. Petechial hemorrhages may appear in the skin and internal viscera, and bleeding from gastric ulcerations may be exaggerated.

Proprietary analgesic mixtures of aspirin and phenacetin or its active metabolite, acetaminophen, when taken over a span of years, have caused renal papillary necrosis, referred to as *analgesic nephropathy* (Chapter 14).

Injury by Nontherapeutic Toxic Agents

Table 8–9 lists some of the more common agents involved in acute poisoning, along with their major pathologic effects. This list emphasizes both the diversity of agents that cause injury and the variety of responses that they can produce. A more detailed discussion of lead and carbon monoxide (CO) follows. Alcohol and drugs of abuse are considered in a subsequent section.

LEAD

Acute lead poisoning may occur under unusual circumstances (e.g., battery burning). More commonly, lead compounds accumulate slowly over weeks and months until they reach toxic levels. Adults usually present with colicky abdominal pain, fatigue, and perhaps headache, but in infants and children, lead poisoning may remain unsuspected until it erupts in a catastrophic encephalopathic crisis.

Table 8–9. SOME COMMON NONTHERAPEUTIC TOXIC AGENTS AND THE MAJOR ASSOCIATED PATHOLOGIC EFFECTS

Agent	Pathologic Effects
Carbon monoxide	Binds to hemoglobin with high affinity, causing systemic hypoxia
Cleaning compounds	
Bleach (sodium hypochlorite)	Local irritant, unlikely to scar
Caustic (acid or basic) agents	Local erosions with scarring
Chloroform, carbon tetrachloride	Central nervous system (CNS) depression, liver necrosis
Cyanide	Blocking of cytochrome oxidase activity, resulting in rapid death owing to severe hypoxia
Ethylene glycol (antifreeze)	CNS depression, metabolic acidosis, acute tubular necrosis
Insecticides	
Chlorinated hydrocarbon (e.g., DDT)	CNS stimulant, accumulates in fat stores for long periods ? Carcinogenic
Organophosphates	Acetylcholinesterase inhibition (muscle weakness, cardiac arrhythmias, respiratory depression)
Isopropanol (rubbing alcohol)	Similar to those of ethanol (gastritis, CNS depression)
Mercurials	
High-dose mercury vapors	Pneumonitis
Low-dose exposure	Intention tremor, memory loss, gingivitis, skin rashes, nephrotic syndrome
Methanol (Sterno, antifreeze)	CNS depression, acidosis, blindness
Mushrooms	
Amanita muscaria	Parasympathomimetic symptoms, including bradycardia, hypotension
Amanita phalloides	Gastrointestinal symptoms with shock, convulsions, coma
Petroleum distillates (kerosene, benzene, gasoline)	Respiratory depression, gastrointestinal inflammation, severe pneumonitis
Polychlorinated biphenyls (PCBs)	Insidious development of chloracne, visual loss, impotence

There are innumerable sources of lead in the environment (Fig. 8–8). Indeed, it is hard to avoid exposure to lead. Environmental lead is absorbed either through the gastrointestinal tract or through the lungs. Which of the potential sources of lead is most important remains controversial, but most experts agree that urban air, soil, water, and food are the major culprits. Despite the reduction in the use of leaded gasoline, the lead content of urban air remains significant. Volatilized lead is particularly hazardous, because almost all is readily absorbed in the lungs. By contrast, only a fraction of ingested lead is absorbed. Urban adults average a daily intake of 100 to 150 μg of lead in water and food, only about 10% of which is absorbed. Although children on average have a lower intake, they unfortunately absorb about 50%. Flaking lead paint in older houses and soil contamination pose major hazards to youngsters, and ingestion of up to 200 μg/day may occur. Indeed, a single chip of lead

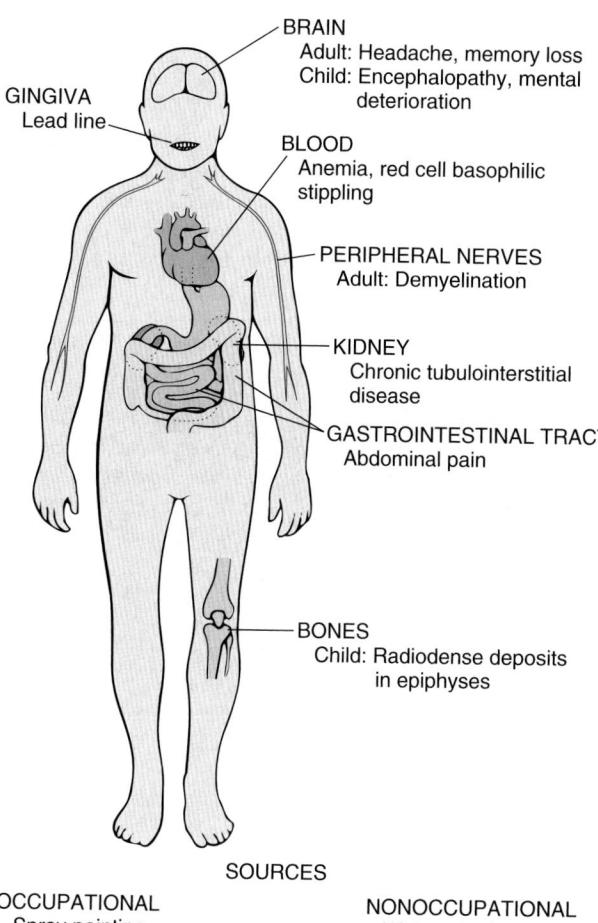

GINGIVA
Lead line

BRAIN
Adult: Headache, memory loss
Child: Encephalopathy, mental
deterioration

BLOOD
Anemia, red cell basophilic
stippling

PERIPHERAL NERVES
Adult: Demyelination

KIDNEY
Chronic tubulointerstitial
disease

GASTROINTESTINAL TRACT
Abdominal pain

BONES
Child: Radiodense deposits
in epiphyses

SOURCES

OCCUPATIONAL
Spray painting
Foundry work
Mining and extracting lead
Battery burning

NONOCCUPATIONAL
Water supply
Paint dust and flakes
House dust
Urban soil
Newsprint
Automotive exhaust

Figure 8–8 ■

Clinical and pathologic features of lead poisoning.

Figure 8–9 ■

Lead poisoning. Impaired remodeling of calcified cartilage in the epiphyses (arrows) of the wrist has caused a marked increase in their radiodensity, so that they are as radiopaque as the cortical bone. (Courtesy of Dr. G. W. Dietz, Department of Radiology, University of Texas Southwestern Medical School, Dallas.)

paint the size of a thumbnail may contain 500,000 μg of lead, enough to produce highly toxic levels if completely absorbed. According to one national survey, 2.3% of white American children had blood lead levels in excess of 10 μg/dL (the maximal allowable level), but 11.2% of black children exceeded that limit, a reflection of older homes, peeling paint, and other socioeconomic factors.

Most of the absorbed lead (80% to 85%) is taken up by bone and developing teeth; the blood accumulates about 5% to 10%, and the remainder is distributed throughout the soft tissues. In children, excess lead interferes with the normal remodeling of calcified cartilage and primary bone trabeculae in the epiphyses, leading to increased bone density, which is detected as radiodense "lead lines" on radiographs (Fig. 8–9). Lead lines of a different sort may also occur in the gums, where excess lead stimulates hyperpigmentation of the gum tissue adjacent to the teeth. Excretion of lead occurs via the kidneys, thereby exposing these organs to potential damage.

Lead causes injury by its multiple metabolic effects:

■ It has a high affinity for sulfhydryl groups and interferes with enzymes involved in heme synthesis—aminolevulinic acid dehydratase and delta ferrochelatase; thus, iron incorporation into heme is hindered or blocked, leading to a hypochromic anemia.
■ It competes with calcium and is stored in bone.
■ It interferes with nerve transmission and brain development in infants.
■ It interferes with membrane-associated enzymes and so hampers the action of sodium-potassium ion pumps, leading to shortened red cell survival and a hemolytic anemia.
■ Its membrane effects damage the kidneys as absorbed lead is excreted.

MORPHOLOGY

The major anatomic targets of lead toxicity are the blood, nervous system, gastrointestinal tract, and kidneys (see Fig. 8–8).

Blood changes resulting from lead accumulation occur fairly early and are characteristic. Lead interferes with normal heme biosynthesis, as indicated. As a consequence, zinc-protoporphyrin is formed instead of heme. Thus, the elevated blood level of zinc-protoporphyrin or its product, free erythrocyte protoporphyrin, is an important indicator of lead poisoning. Typically, a **microcytic, hypochromic, mild hemolytic anemia appears.** Even more distinctive is a **punctate basophilic stippling of the erythrocytes.**

Brain damage is prone to occur in children. It may be very subtle, producing mild dysfunction, or it may be massive and lethal. In young children, sensory, motor, intellectual, and psychologic impairments have been described, including reduced IQ; learning disabilities; retarded psychomotor development; blindness; and, in more severe cases, psychoses, seizures, and coma. Lead toxicity in the mother may impair brain development in the prenatal infant. The anatomic changes underlying the more subtle functional deficits are ill defined, but there is concern that some of the defects may be permanent. At the more severe end of the spectrum are marked brain edema, demyelination of the cerebral and cerebellar white matter, and necrosis of cortical neurons accompanied by diffuse astrocytic proliferation. In adults, the central nervous system is less often affected, but frequently a peripheral demyelinating neuropathy appears, typically involving the motor innervation of the most commonly used muscles. Thus, the extensor muscles of the wrist and fingers are often the first to be affected, followed by paralysis of the peroneal muscles (wristdrop and footdrop).

The **gastrointestinal** tract is also a major source of clinical manifestations. Lead "colic" is characterized by extremely severe, poorly localized abdominal pain.

Kidneys may develop proximal tubular damage with intranuclear lead inclusions. Chronic renal damage leads eventually to interstitial fibrosis and possibly renal failure and findings suggestive of gout ("saturnine gout"). Other findings are shown in Figure 8–8.

The diagnosis of lead poisoning requires constant awareness of its prevalence. It may be suspected on the basis of neurologic changes in children or unexplained anemia with basophilic stippling in red cells. Elevated blood lead and free erythrocyte protoporphyrin levels (above 50 μg/dL) or, alternatively, zinc-protoporphyrin levels are required for definitive diagnosis.

CARBON MONOXIDE

This nonirritating, colorless, tasteless, odorless gas produced by the imperfect oxidation of carbonaceous materials continues to be a cause of accidental and suicidal death. Its sources include automotive engines, industrial processes using fossil fuels, home heating with oil (not natural gas), and cigarette smoke. The low levels often found in ambient air may contribute to impaired respiratory function, but of themselves they are not life-threatening. In a small, closed garage, the average car exhaust can induce lethal coma within 5 minutes. CO kills by inducing central nervous system depression, which appears so insidiously that victims

may not be aware of their plight and indeed may be unable to help themselves.

CO acts as a systemic asphyxiant. Hemoglobin has 200-fold greater affinity for CO than for oxygen. The resultant carboxyhemoglobin is incapable of carrying oxygen. Systemic hypoxia appears when the hemoglobin is 20% to 30% saturated with CO, and unconsciousness and death are likely with 60% to 70% saturation. Depending on the rate of conversion to carboxyhemoglobin and the ultimate severity, one of two patterns can be recognized.

MORPHOLOGY

In light-skinned patients, acute poisoning is marked by a characteristic **generalized cherry-red color of the skin and mucous membranes, resulting from the carboxyhemoglobin.** If death occurs, depending on the rapidity of onset, morphologic changes may not be present; with longer survival, the brain may be slightly edematous, with punctate hemorrhages and hypoxia-induced neuronal changes. The morphologic changes are not specific; they simply imply systemic hypoxia. When exposure has not been prolonged, complete recovery is possible; however, sometimes impairments of memory, vision, hearing, and speech remain.

Chronic poisoning may appear because the carboxyhemoglobin, once formed, is remarkably stable and, with low-level persistent exposure, may accumulate to a life-threatening concentration in the blood. The slowly developing hypoxia can insidiously evoke widespread ischemic changes in the central nervous system; these are particularly marked in the basal ganglia and lenticular nuclei. With cessation of exposure to CO, the victim usually recovers, but often there are permanent neurologic sequelae. The diagnosis of CO poisoning is critically dependent on the identification of significant levels of carboxyhemoglobin in the blood.

ALCOHOL AND DRUGS OF ABUSE

Drug abuse may be defined as the use of mind-altering substances in a way that differs from generally approved medical or social practices. Ethanol is imbibed, at least partly, for its mood-altering properties but when used in moderation is socially acceptable and not injurious. When excessive amounts are used, alcohol can cause marked physical and psychologic damage. Table 8–10 provides a classification of drugs that are abused, with examples of each. Our purpose here is to describe the lesions directly associated with the abuse of alcohol and with illicit drug use.

Ethanol. Despite all the attention given to cocaine and heroin addiction, alcohol use and abuse are a more widespread hazard and claim many more lives. Fifty percent of adults in the Western world drink alcohol, and about 5% to 10% have chronic alcoholism. It is broadly estimated that alcohol is responsible for 100,000 deaths annually in the United States, most often caused by cirrhosis of the liver, which is the fourth most frequent cause of death among

Table 8-10.   CLASSIFICATION OF DRUGS OF ABUSE

Class	Examples
Sedatives and hypnotics	Alcohol, barbiturates, benzodiazepines
CNS sympathomimetics or stimulants	Cocaine, amphetamines, methylphenidate (Ritalin), weight loss products
Opioids	Heroin, morphine, methadone, and almost all prescription analgesics
Cannabinols	Marijuana, hashish
Hallucinogens or psychedelics	Lysergic acid diethylamide (LSD), mescaline, psilocybin, phencyclidine (PCP)
Inhalants	Aerosol sprays, glues, toluene, gasoline, paint thinner, amyl nitrite, nitrous oxide
Nonprescription drugs	Ingredients: Atropine, scopolamine, weak stimulants, antihistamines, weak analgesics

Modified from Schuckit MA (ed): Drug and Alchohol Abuse: A Clinical Guide to Diagnosis and Treatment, 3rd ed. New York, Plenum, 1989.

people 25 to 64 years of age. After consumption, ethanol is absorbed unaltered in the stomach and small intestine. It is then distributed to all the tissues and fluids of the body in direct proportion to the blood level. Less than 10% is excreted unchanged in the urine, sweat, and breath. The amount exhaled is proportional to the blood level and forms the basis of the breath test employed by law enforcement agencies.

Most of the alcohol in the blood is biotransformed to acetaldehyde by alcohol dehydrogenase in the cytosol of cells in the liver and gastric mucosa and with rising blood levels also by cytochrome P-450 (CYP2E1) and catalase in the liver. In the course of these reactions, nicotinamide adenine dinucleotide (NAD) is reduced to NADH. The acetaldehyde is then converted to acetic acid (Fig. 8–10). A number of metabolic consequences follow from the biotransformations:

■ The ethanol is a substantial source of energy (empty calories), and this leads to malnutrition and deficiencies, particularly of the B vitamins.
■ Excess NADH contributes to acidosis, reduces excretion of uric acid, opposes gluconeogenesis, and inhibits fatty acid oxidation, having secondary effects on the liver.
■ Acetaldehyde has many adverse effects and may in fact be responsible for the damage wreaked on many organs (especially the liver and brain) by chronic alcoholism.

The blood alcohol level is determined by the amount and rate of ethanol consumed and the rate of metabolism. Approximately 3 ounces of ethanol (12 ounces of fortified wine, 8 bottles of beer, 6 ounces of 100-proof whiskey) produce a blood alcohol level of 100 mg/dL when consumed by a 70-kg man in a few hours; this is the legal upper limit for sobriety. Drowsiness occurs at 200 mg/dL, stupor at 300 mg/dL, and coma, with possible respiratory arrest, at higher levels. The rate of metabolism obviously affects the blood alcohol level. Persons with chronic alcoholism can tolerate levels of up to 700 mg/dL, partially explained by a five- to tenfold increased induction of the

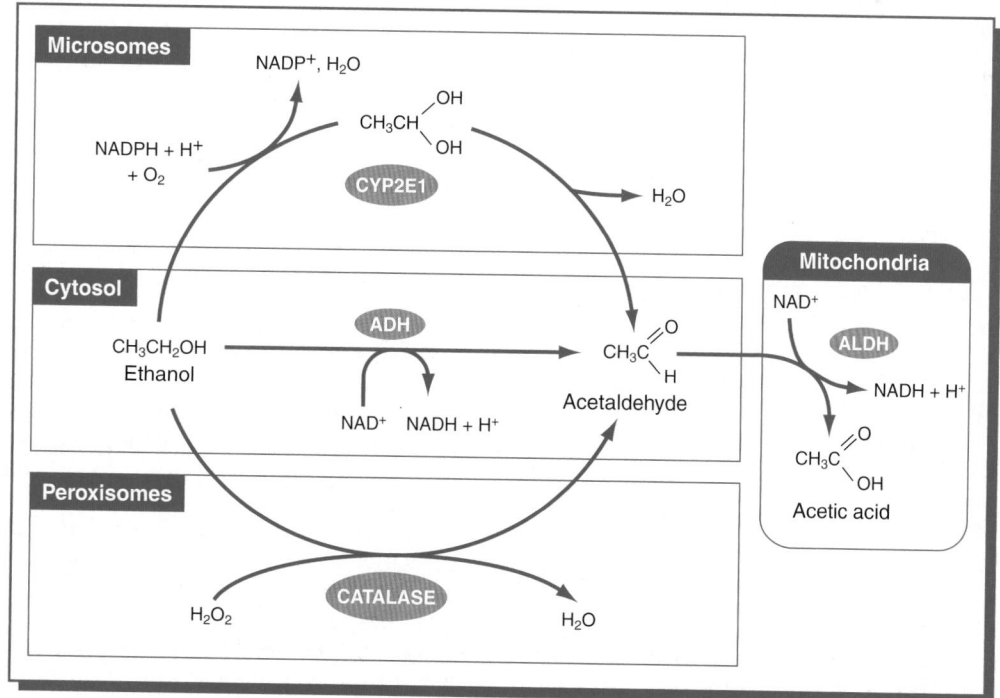

Figure 8-10

Metabolism of ethanol. ADH, alcohol dehydrogenase; ALDH, aldehyde dehydrogenase. (From Parkinson A: Biotransformation of xenobiotics. In Klassen CD [ed]: Casarett and Doull's Toxicology: The Basic Science of Poisons, 5th ed. New York, McGraw-Hill, 1996, p 128.)

cytochrome P-450 enzyme system in the liver. The elevated enzyme levels increase the metabolism of other drugs as well, such as cocaine and acetaminophen. Conversely, there are genetic polymorphisms involving these enzymes that lower their metabolic rate of function (e.g., women have lower levels of gastric alcohol dehydrogenase than men, accounting for the fact that they tend to get "drunk" more readily).

The adverse effects of ethanol must be divided into its acute actions and the consequences of chronic alcoholism.

Acute alcoholism exerts its effects mainly on the central nervous system, but it may induce hepatic and gastric changes that are reversible in the absence of continued alcohol consumption. The hepatic changes are described in Chapter 16. The gastric changes constitute acute gastritis and ulceration (Chapter 15). In the central nervous system, alcohol is a depressant, first affecting subcortical structures (probably the high brain stem reticular formation) that modulate cerebral cortical activity. Consequently, there is stimulation and disordered cortical, motor, and intellectual behavior. At progressively higher blood levels, cortical neurons and then lower medullary centers are depressed, including those that regulate respiration. Respiratory arrest may follow.

Chronic alcoholism is responsible for morphologic alterations in virtually all organs and tissues in the body, particularly the liver and stomach. Only the gastric lesions that appear immediately after exposure can be related to the direct effects of ethanol on the mucosal vasculature. The origin of the other chronic changes is less clear. Acetaldehyde, the major metabolite of ethanol, is a very reactive compound and has been proposed as the mediator of the widespread tissue and organ damage. Although the catabolism of acetaldehyde is more rapid than that of alcohol, chronic ethanol consumption reduces the oxidative capacity of the liver, raising the blood level of acetaldehyde; this increase is further augmented by the increased rate of ethanol metabolism in the habituated drinker. Other suggested mechanisms of injury include increased free radical activity and, possibly, immune reactions against hepatic neoantigens generated by acetaldehyde or free radical–induced alteration of proteins. Dependence on alcohol seems to be genetically regulated. This is supported by studies in twins; the concordance rate for chronic alcoholism is significantly higher in monozygotic twins than in dizygotic twins. Family studies also support this notion. It is believed that multiple genes contribute to the genetic vulnerability. This is an area of active investigation.

Whatever the basis, people with chronic alcoholism suffer significant morbidity and a shortened life span, related principally to damage to the liver, gastrointestinal tract, central nervous system, cardiovascular system, and pancreas.

- *Liver.* Alcohol, the most common cause of hepatic injury, may lead to cirrhosis (Chapter 16).
- *Gastrointestinal tract.* Massive bleeding from gastritis, gastric ulcer, or esophageal varices (associated with cirrhosis) may prove fatal.
- *Central nervous system.* A deficiency of thiamine is common in chronic alcoholic patients; the principal lesions of this deficiency are peripheral neuropathies and

the Wernicke-Korsakoff syndrome (discussed later in this chapter and in Chapter 23). Cerebral atrophy, cerebellar degeneration, and optic neuropathy may also occur, possibly directly related to alcohol or its products.
- *Cardiovascular system.* Alcohol has diverse effects on the heart. Direct injury to the myocardium may produce dilated congestive cardiomyopathy (Chapter 11). On the other hand, moderate amounts of alcohol (one drink/day) have been observed to increase levels of HDL and inhibit platelet aggregation, lowering the incidence of coronary heart disease. But heavy consumption, with attendant liver injury, results in decreased levels of HDL, increasing the likelihood of coronary heart disease. Chronic alcoholism is also associated with an increased incidence of hypertension.
- *Pancreas.* Excess alcohol intake increases the risk of acute and chronic pancreatitis (Chapter 17).
- *Other effects.* The use of ethanol during pregnancy—as little as one drink per day—can cause fetal alcohol syndrome (i.e., growth retardation and some reduction in mental functions in the newborn). Chronic alcohol consumption is associated, on epidemiologic grounds, with an *increased incidence of cancer* of the oral cavity, esophagus, liver, and, possibly, breast in females. How it acts is uncertain, but it is believed that ethanol itself, or the metabolite acetaldehyde, acts as a tumor promoter rather than a direct carcinogen.

It is evident that alcohol has wide-ranging unpleasant consequences.

Cocaine. There has been a major escalation in the use of cocaine, along with its derivative "crack"; currently, there are an estimated 2 to 6 million cocaine abusers in the United States. Extracted from the leaves of the coca plant, cocaine is usually prepared as a water-soluble powder, cocaine hydrochloride, but when sold on the street, it is liberally diluted with talcum powder, lactose, or other lookalikes. Crystallization of the pure alkaloid from cocaine hydrochloride yields nuggets of crack (so called because of the cracking or popping sound it makes when heated). The pharmacologic actions of cocaine and crack are identical, but crack is far more potent. Both forms of the drug are absorbed from all sites and so can be snorted, smoked after mixing with tobacco, ingested, or injected subcutaneously or intravenously.

Cocaine produces an intense euphoria with so-called reinforcing qualities, making it one of the most addictive of all drugs. Experimental animals will press a lever more than 1000 times and forgo food and drink to obtain the drug. In the cocaine abuser, although physical dependence appears not to occur, the psychologic withdrawal is profound and can be extremely difficult to treat. Recurrent intense cravings to re-experience drug-associated "highs" are particularly severe in the first several months after abstinence, but they can recur for years.

The most serious physical effects of cocaine relate to its acute action on the cardiovascular system, where it behaves as a sympathomimetic (Fig. 8–11). It facilitates neurotransmission both in the central nervous system, where it blocks the reuptake of dopamine, and at adrenergic nerve endings, where it blocks the reuptake of both epinephrine and norepinephrine while stimulating the

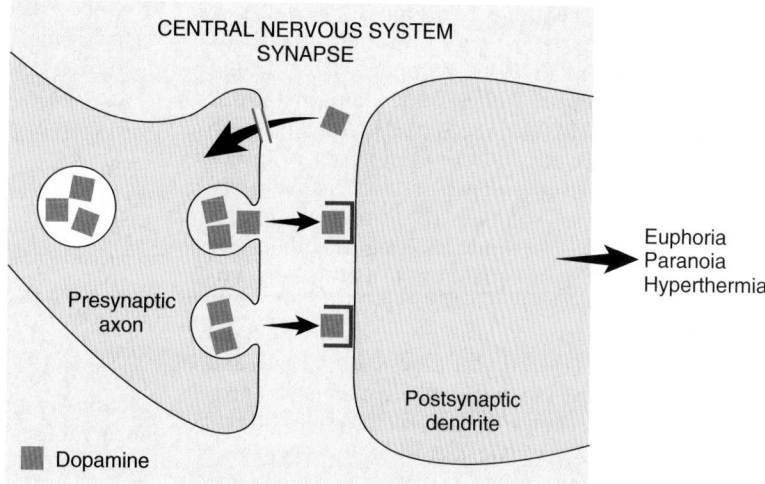

CENTRAL NERVOUS SYSTEM
SYNAPSE

Presynaptic
axon

Postsynaptic
dendrite

Euphoria
Paranoia
Hyperthermia

■ Dopamine

Figure 8-11 ■

The effect of cocaine on neurotransmission. The
drug inhibits reuptake of the neurotransmitters
dopamine and norepinephrine by presynaptic neurons, leading to excess stimulation of postsynaptic
fibers or effector cells.

SYMPATHETIC NEURON–TARGET CELL
INTERFACE

Hypertension
Cardiac arrhythmia
Myocardial infarct
Cerebral hemorrhage
and infarct

● Norepinephrine

presynaptic release of norepinephrine. The net effect is
the accumulation of these two neurotransmitters in
synapses, resulting in excess stimulation, manifested by
tachycardia and hypertension. Cocaine also induces
myocardial ischemia, the basis for which is multifactorial. It causes coronary artery vasoconstriction, promotes
thrombus formation by facilitating platelet aggregation,
and induces premature atherosclerosis in long-term users.
Cocaine-induced coronary vasospasm is potentiated by
cigarette smoking. Thus, on the one hand, cocaine induces increased myocardial oxygen demand by its sympathomimetic action; on the other hand, it reduces
coronary blood flow, thus setting the stage for myocardial
ischemia that may lead to myocardial infarction. In addition to its detrimental effects on myocardial oxygenation,
cocaine can also precipitate *lethal arrhythmias* by enhanced sympathetic activity as well as by disrupting normal ion (K^+, Ca^{++}, Na^+) transport in the myocardium.
These toxic effects are not necessarily dose-related, and a
fatal event may occur in a first-time abuser with what is a
typical mood-altering dose. The following are some manifestations of acute cocaine toxicity.

■ Sympathetic nervous system stimulation, resulting in dilated pupils, vasoconstriction, an increase in arterial
blood pressure, and tachycardia.

■ Lethal arrhythmias and myocardial infarction.
■ Cerebral infarction and intracranial hemorrhage, the latter in persons who have preexisting vascular malformations and probably related to the sudden acute elevations
in blood pressure. The most common central nervous
system findings are hyperpyrexia (thought to be caused
by aberrations of the dopaminergic pathways that control
body temperature) and seizures.
■ Rhabdomyolysis, sometimes accompanied by renal failure. The mechanism is not understood but may relate to
intense vasoconstriction together with a direct effect of
the drug on muscle.
■ In pregnant women, decreased blood flow to the placenta, causing fetal hypoxia and spontaneous abortion.
In chronic users of the drug, fetal neurologic development may be impaired.

In contrast to acute toxicity, chronic cocaine use may result in (1) perforation of the nasal septum in cocaine
snorters, (2) decreased lung diffusing capacity in those who
inhale the smoke from cocaine, and (3) rarely, the development of dilated cardiomyopathy.

When combined with alcohol, cocaine has been shown
to be teratogenic in mice, and there are suggestions that
the combination may have the same consequences in
humans.

Heroin. Heroin is even more hazardous than cocaine. In one survey, it was found that over 3 million Americans use or have used heroin. In 1993, heroin was implicated in almost 4000 deaths in the United States, and in 1996 it was responsible for 10,000 emergency department visits (a number that had doubled since 1990). Heroin is an addictive opioid derived from the poppy plant and closely related to morphine. As sold on the street, it is cut (diluted) with an agent (often talc or quinine); thus, the size of the dose is not only variable but also usually unknown to the buyer. The heroin, along with any contaminating substances, is usually self-administered intravenously or subcutaneously. Effects are varied and include euphoria, hallucinations, somnolence, and sedation. Heroin has a wide range of adverse physical effects related to (1) the pharmacologic action of the agent, (2) reactions to the cutting agents or contaminants, (3) hypersensitivity reactions to the drug or its adulterants (quinine itself has neurologic, renal, and auditory toxicity), and (4) diseases contracted incident to the use of the needle.

■ Sudden death, usually related to overdose, is an ever-present risk because drug purity is generally unknown and may range from 2% to 90%. The yearly mortality is estimated to be between 1% and 3%. Sudden death can also occur if tolerance for the drug, built up over time, is lost (as during a period of incarceration). The mechanisms of death include profound respiratory depression, arrhythmia and cardiac arrest, and severe pulmonary edema.

■ Pulmonary complications include moderate to severe edema, septic embolism, lung abscess, opportunistic infections, and foreign body granulomas from talc and other adulterants. Although granulomas occur principally in the lung, they are sometimes found in the mononuclear phagocyte system, particularly in the spleen, liver, and lymph nodes that drain the upper extremities. Examination under polarized light often highlights trapped talc crystals, sometimes enclosed within foreign body giant cells.

■ Infectious complications are common. The four sites most commonly affected are the skin and its subcutaneous tissue, heart valves, liver, and lungs. In a series of addicted patients admitted to the hospital, more than 10% had endocarditis, which often takes a distinctive form involving right-sided heart valves, particularly the tricuspid. Most cases are caused by *Staphylococcus aureus*, but fungi and a multitude of other organisms have also been implicated. Viral hepatitis is the most common infection among addicted persons and is acquired by the casual sharing of dirty needles. In the United States, this practice has also led to a very high incidence of AIDS in intravenous drug abusers.

■ Cutaneous lesions are probably the most frequent telltale sign of heroin addiction. Acute changes include abscesses, cellulitis, and ulcerations owing to subcutaneous injections. Scarring at injection sites, hyperpigmentation over commonly used veins, and thrombosed veins are the usual sequelae of repeated intravenous inoculations.

■ Kidney disease is a relatively common hazard. The two forms most frequently encountered are amyloidosis and focal glomerulosclerosis; both induce heavy proteinuria and the nephrotic syndrome. Amyloidosis is secondary to chronic skin infections (Chapter 5).

Marijuana. Marijuana, or "pot," is the most widely used illegal drug. It is made from the leaves of the *Cannabis sativa* plant, which contain the psychoactive substance Δ^9-tetrahydrocannabinol (THC). When it is smoked, about 5% to 10% is absorbed. Despite numerous studies, the central question of whether the drug has persistent adverse physical and functional effects remains unresolved. Some of the untoward anecdotal effects may be allergic or idiosyncratic reactions or may possibly be related to contaminants in the preparations rather than to marijuana's pharmacologic effects. On the other hand, two beneficial effects of THC are its capacity to decrease intraocular pressure in glaucoma and to combat intractable nausea secondary to cancer chemotherapy.

■ The functional and organic central nervous system consequences of marijuana have received greatest scrutiny. Clearly, the use of pot distorts sensory perception and impairs motor coordination, but these acute effects generally clear in 4 to 5 hours. With continued use, these changes may progress to cognitive and psychomotor impairments, such as inability to judge time, speed, and distance. Among adolescents, such changes often lead to automobile accidents.

■ Not unexpectedly, the lungs are affected by chronic pot smoking; laryngitis, pharyngitis, bronchitis, cough and hoarseness, and asthma-like symptoms have all been described, along with mild but significant airway obstruction. Smoking a marijuana cigarette, compared with a tobacco cigarette, is associated with a threefold increase in the amount of tar inhaled and retained in the lungs. Presumably, the larger puff volume, deeper inhalation, and longer breath holding are responsible. Long-term smokers of marijuana may also be at increased risk for lung cancer.

■ Marijuana increases the heart rate and sometimes blood pressure and in a person with a fixed coronary artery narrowing may cause angina.

■ Marijuana may induce chromosomal damage in somatic and germ cells, but the evidence is not incontrovertible. A large study involving many thousands of female marijuana users revealed lower infant birth weights, shorter gestational periods, and an increased number of malformations among the offspring. Because the peak use of marijuana is among teenagers and young adults, these provocative findings require further study.

Other Illicit Drugs. The variety of drugs that have been tried by those seeking "new experiences" defies belief. They range from various stimulants (e.g., amphetamines) to depressants (e.g., benzodiazepines) to hallucinogens (e.g., phenylcyclohexyl piperidine [PCP], "ecstasy"). Because they are used haphazardly and in various combinations, little is known of their long-time deleterious effects, but this much is clear—they are a dangerous combination with alcohol and driving!

INJURY BY PHYSICAL AGENTS

Injury induced by physical agents is divided into the following categories: mechanical trauma, thermal injury, electrical injury, and injury produced by ionizing radiation.

Mechanical Trauma

Mechanical forces may inflict a variety of forms of damage. The type of injury depends on the shape of the colliding object, the amount of energy discharged at impact, and the tissues or organs that bear the impact. Bone and head injuries result in unique damage and are discussed elsewhere (Chapter 23). All soft tissues react similarly to mechanical forces, and the patterns of injury can be divided into abrasions, contusions, lacerations, incised wounds, and puncture wounds.

MORPHOLOGY

ABRASION. An abrasion is a wound produced by scraping or rubbing, resulting in removal of the superficial layer. Skin abrasions may remove only the epidermal layer.

CONTUSION. A contusion, or bruise, is a wound usually produced by a blunt object and is characterized by damage to blood vessels and extravasation of blood into tissues.

LACERATION. A laceration is a tear or disruptive stretching of tissue caused by the application of force by a blunt object. In contrast to an incision, most lacerations have intact bridging blood vessels and jagged, irregular edges.

INCISED WOUND. An incised wound is one inflicted by a sharp instrument. The bridging blood vessels are severed.

PUNCTURE WOUND. A puncture wound is caused by a long narrow instrument and is termed **penetrating** when the instrument pierces the tissue and **perforating** when it traverses a tissue to also create an exit wound. Gunshot wounds are special forms of puncture wounds that demonstrate distinctive features important to the forensic pathologist. For example, a wound from a bullet fired at close range leaves powder burns, whereas one fired from more than 4 or 5 feet away does not.

One of the most common causes of mechanical injury is vehicular accidents. Injuries typically sustained result from (1) hitting a part of the interior of the vehicle or being hit by an object that enters the passenger compartment during the crash, such as the motor; (2) being thrown from the vehicle; or (3) being trapped in a burning vehicle. The pattern of injury relates to whether one or all three of these mechanisms are operative. For example, in a head-on collision, a common pattern of injury sustained by a driver who is not wearing a

Figure 8-12   ■

Transverse rupture of the descending thoracic aorta incurred in an automobile accident. (Courtesy of Dr. Charles Petty, Department of Pathology and Forensic Medicine, University of Texas Southwestern Medical School, Dallas.)

seat belt includes trauma to the head (windshield impact), chest (steering column impact), and knees (dashboard impact). Under these conditions, common chest injuries include sternal and rib fractures, heart contusions, aortic lacerations (Fig. 8–12), and (less commonly) lacerations of the spleen and liver. Thus, in caring for an automobile injury victim, it is essential to remember that superficial abrasions, contusions, and lacerations are often accompanied by internal wounds. Indeed, in many cases, external evidence of serious internal damage is completely absent.

Thermal Injury

Both excess heat and excess cold are important causes of injury. Burns are all too common and are discussed first; a brief discussion of hyperthermia and hypothermia follows.

THERMAL BURNS

In the United States, burns cause 5000 deaths per year and result in the hospitalization of more than 10 times that many persons. Many victims are children, who are often scalded by hot liquids. Fortunately, since the 1970s, marked decreases have been seen in both mortality rates and the length of hospitalizations. These improvements have been achieved by a better understanding of the systemic effects of massive burns and discoveries of better ways to prevent wound infection and facilitate the healing of skin surfaces.

The clinical significance of burns depends on the following important factors:

- Depth of the burn
- Percentage of body surface involved
- Possible presence of internal injuries from inhalation of hot and toxic fumes
- Promptness and efficacy of therapy, especially fluid and electrolyte management and prevention or control of wound infections

A *full-thickness* burn involves total destruction of the epidermis and dermis, with loss of the dermal appendages that would have provided cells for epithelial regeneration. Both third- and fourth-degree burns are in this category. In *partial-thickness* burns, at least the deeper portions of the dermal appendages are spared. Partial-thickness burns include first-degree burns (epithelial involvement only) and second-degree burns (involving both epidermis and superficial dermis).

MORPHOLOGY

Grossly, full-thickness burns are white or charred, dry, and anesthetic (because of nerve ending destruction), whereas, depending on the depth, partial-thickness burns are pink or mottled with blisters and are painful. Histologically, devitalized tissue reveals coagulative necrosis, adjacent to vital tissue that quickly accumulates inflammatory cells and marked exudation.

Despite continuous improvement in therapy, any burn exceeding 50% of the total body surface, whether superficial or deep, is grave and potentially fatal. With burns of more than 20% of the body surface, there is a rapid shift of body fluids into the interstitial compartments, both at the burn site and systemically, which can result in hypovolemic shock (Chapter 4). Because protein from the blood is lost into interstitial tissue, generalized edema, including pulmonary edema, may become severe.

Another important consideration in patients with burns is the degree of injury to the airways and lungs. Inhalation injury is frequent in persons trapped in burning buildings and may result from the direct effect of heat on the mouth, nose, and upper airways or from the inhalation of heated air and gases in the smoke. Water-soluble gases, such as chlorine, sulfur oxides, and ammonia, may react with water to form acids or alkalis, particularly in the upper airways, and so produce inflammation and swelling, which may lead to partial or complete airway obstruction. Lipid-soluble gases, such as nitrous oxide and products of burning plastics, are more likely to reach deeper airways, producing pneumonitis. Unlike shock, which develops within hours, pulmonary manifestations may not develop for 24 to 48 hours.

Organ system failure resulting from burn sepsis continues to be the leading cause of death in burned patients. The burn site is ideal for growth of microorganisms; the serum and debris provide nutrients, and the burn injury compromises blood flow, blocking effective inflammatory responses. The most common offender is the opportunist *Pseudomonas aeruginosa*, but antibiotic-resistant strains of other common hospital-acquired bacteria, such as *S. aureus*, and fungi, particularly *Candida* species, may also be involved. Furthermore, cellular and humoral defenses against infections are compromised, and both lymphocyte and phagocyte functions are impaired. Direct bacteremic spread and release of toxic substances such as endotoxin from the local site have dire consequences. Pneumonia or septic shock with renal failure and/or the acute respiratory distress syndrome (ARDS) (Chapter 13) are the most common serious sequelae.

Another very important pathophysiologic effect of burns is the development of a hypermetabolic state with excess heat loss and an increased need for nutritional support. It is estimated that when more than 40% of the body surface is burned, the resting metabolic rate may approach twice normal.

HYPERTHERMIA

Prolonged exposure to elevated ambient temperatures can result in heat cramps, heat exhaustion, and heat stroke.

- *Heat cramps* result from loss of electrolytes via sweating. Cramping of voluntary muscles, usually in association with vigorous exercise, is the hallmark. Heat-dissipating mechanisms are able to maintain normal core body temperature.
- *Heat exhaustion* is probably the most common hyperthermic syndrome. Its onset is sudden, with prostration and collapse, and it results from a failure of the cardiovascular system to compensate for hypovolemia, secondary to water depletion. After a period of collapse, which is usually brief, equilibrium is spontaneously re-established.
- *Heat stroke* is associated with high ambient temperatures and high humidity. Thermoregulatory mechanisms fail, sweating ceases, and core body temperature rises. Body temperatures of 112° to 113°F have been recorded in some terminal cases. Clinically, a rectal temperature of 106°F or higher is considered a grave prognostic sign, and the mortality rate for such patients exceeds 50%. The underlying mechanism is marked generalized peripheral vasodilation with peripheral pooling of blood and a decreased effective circulating blood volume. Necrosis of the muscles and myocardium may occur. Arrhythmias, disseminated intravascular coagulation, and other systemic effects are common. Elderly persons, individuals undergoing intense physical stress (including young athletes and military recruits), and persons with cardiovascular disease are prime candidates for heat stroke.

HYPOTHERMIA

Prolonged exposure to low ambient temperature leads to hypothermia, a condition seen all too frequently in homeless persons. Lowering of body temperature is hastened by high humidity, wet clothing, and dilation of superficial blood vessels occurring as a result of the ingestion of alcohol. At about 90°F, loss of consciousness occurs, followed by bradycardia and atrial fibrillation at lower core temperatures.

Local Reactions. Chilling or freezing of cells and tissues causes injury in two ways.

■ Direct effects are probably mediated by physical dislocations within cells and high salt concentrations incident to the crystallization of the intra- and extracellular water.
■ Indirect effects are exerted by circulatory changes. Depending on the rate at which the temperature drops and the duration of the drop, slowly developing chilling may induce vasoconstriction and increased permeability, leading to edematous changes. Such changes are typical of "trench foot." Atrophy and fibrosis may follow. Alternatively, with sudden sharp drops in temperature that are persistent, the vasoconstriction and increased viscosity of the blood in the local area may cause ischemic injury and degenerative changes in peripheral nerves. In this situation, only after the temperature begins to return to normal do the vascular injury and increased permeability with exudation become evident. However, during the period of ischemia, hypoxic changes and infarction of the affected tissues may develop (e.g., gangrene of toes or feet).

ELECTRICAL INJURY

Electrical injuries, which may result in death, can arise from low-voltage currents (i.e., in the home and workplace) or from high-voltage currents from high-power lines or lightning. Injuries are of two types: (1) burns and (2) ventricular fibrillation or cardiac and respiratory center standstill resulting from disruption of normal electrical impulses. The type of injury and the severity and extent of burning depend on the amperage and path of the electric current within the body.

Current flow (amperes) equals voltage (volts) divided by resistance (ohms). Voltage in the household and workplace (120 or 220 V) is high enough that with low resistance at the site of contact (as when the skin is wet), sufficient current can pass through the body to cause serious injury, including ventricular fibrillation. If current flow continues long enough, it generates enough heat to produce burns at the site of entry and exit as well as in internal organs. An important characteristic of alternating current, the type available in most homes, is that it induces tetanic muscle spasm, so that when a live wire or switch is grasped, irreversible clutching is likely to occur, prolonging the period of current flow. This results in a greater likelihood of developing extensive electrical burns and, in some cases, spasm of the chest wall muscles, producing death from asphyxia. Currents generated from high-voltage sources cause similar damage; however, because of the large current flows generated, these are more likely to produce paralysis of medullary centers and extensive burns. Lightning is a classic cause of high-voltage electrical injury.

Before leaving the subject of electrical injury, a word about the health risk of exposure to electromagnetic fields (EMFs). Some studies linked exposure to EMFs to an increased risk of cancer, particularly leukemias among electrical workers (especially those who worked on high-power lines) and children living near high-power lines. *Further analyses failed to confirm these findings.* However, EMF, as well as microwave radiation, when sufficiently intense may produce burns, usually of the skin and subjacent connective tissue. Both forms of radiation can interfere with cardiac pacemakers.

INJURY PRODUCED BY IONIZING RADIATION

Ionizing radiation is a double-edged sword: it provides an invaluable means of clinical diagnosis and for some tumors a curative mode of therapy, but at the same time it is a potent mutagen and destroyer of cells. It occurs in two forms: (1) electromagnetic waves (x-rays and gamma rays) and (2) high-energy neutrons and charged particles (alpha and beta particles and protons as well as smaller forms). All types of ionizing radiation exert their effects on cells by displacing electrons from molecules and atoms with which they collide, causing ionization and inducing a cascade of events that may alter the cell transiently or permanently. The most important target in living cells is DNA. Ionizing radiation may directly damage DNA (direct target theory), but more often it indirectly damages DNA by inducing the formation of free radicals, particularly those that form from the radiolysis of water (indirect target theory). Other cell molecules that may also be direct or indirect targets of radiant injury include lipids in cell membranes and proteins that function as critical enzymes. The transfer of energy to a target atom or molecule from the incident source of radiant energy occurs within microfractions of a second, yet its biologic effect may not become apparent for minutes or, if the effect is on DNA, even decades.

The following terms are used to express radiation dose:

■ Roentgen (R) is a unit of x- or gamma radiation that ionizes a specific volume of air. Thus, it is a measure of exposure.
■ Radiation absorbed dose (rad) and grays (Gy) are units that express the energy absorbed by target tissue from gamma rays and x-rays. A rad or its equivalent, the centigray (cGy), is the dose that results in absorption of 100 erg of energy per gram of tissue.
■ Rem is the dose of radiation that produces the biologic effect equivalent to 1 rad of x-rays or gamma rays.
■ Curie (Ci) defines the disintegrations per second of a spontaneously disintegrating radionuclide (radioisotope). One Ci is equal to 3.7×10^{10} disintegrations per second.

These measurements do not directly quantify energy transferred per unit of tissue and therefore do not predict the biologic effects of radiation. The following terms provide a better approximation of such values:

■ Linear energy transfer (LET) expresses energy loss per unit of distance traveled as electron volts per micrometer. This value depends on the type of ionizing radiation. LET is very high for alpha particles, less for beta particles, and even less for gamma rays and x-rays. Thus, alpha and beta particles penetrate short distances and interact with many molecules within these short distances. Gamma rays and x-rays penetrate deeply but interact with relatively few molecules per unit distance. It should be evident that if equivalent amounts of energy entered the body in the form of alpha and gamma radiation, the alpha particles would induce heavy damage in a more or less superficial restricted area, whereas gamma rays would dissipate energy over a longer, deeper course and produce considerably less damage per unit of tissue.

■ Relative biologic effectiveness (RBE) is simply a ratio that represents the relationship of the LETs of various forms of radiation to cobalt gamma rays and megavolt x-rays, both of which have an RBE of unity.

In addition to the physical properties of the radiation, its biologic effects depend heavily on the following factors:

1. Since the primary target of ionizing radiation is DNA, rapidly dividing cells are more vulnerable to injury than are intermitotic cells. Except at extremely high doses that impair DNA transcription, DNA damage is compatible with survival if the cell remains in the intermitotic phase; however, during mitosis, cells that have incurred irreparable DNA damage die, because chromosome abnormalities prevent normal division. Understandably, therefore, *tissues with a high rate of cell turnover, such as bone marrow, lymphoid tissue, and the mucosa of the gastrointestinal tract, are extremely vulnerable to radiation*, and the injury is manifested early after exposure. Tissues with slower turnover rates, such as liver and endothelium, are not affected immediately after irradiation but are depopulated slowly, because cell division is slowed or interrupted. Tissues with nondividing cells, such as brain and myocardium, do not demonstrate radiation effects except at doses that are so high that DNA transcription or some other molecule vital to the normal functioning of the cell is affected.

2. Because tissues are made up of many cell types, the effects of radiation are complex. For example, vascular injury can result in changes that interfere with repair, and therefore parenchymal cells may reveal manifestations of radiation injury months to years later. Endothelial cells, which are moderately sensitive to radiation, may be damaged, and the resultant narrowing or occlusion of the blood vessels may lead to impaired healing of parenchymal cells or chronic ischemic atrophy. Vascular changes in the central nervous system after irradiation can lead to late manifestations of radiation damage, although nerve cells were not directly affected by the ionizing radiation.

3. The rate of delivery significantly modifies the biologic effect. Although the effect of radiant energy is cumulative, delivery in divided doses may allow cells to repair some of the damage in the intervals. Thus, fractional doses of radiant energy have a cumulative effect only to the extent that repair during the intervals is incomplete. Radiotherapy of tumors exploits the fact that in general, normal cells are capable of more rapid repair and recovery than tumor cells and so do not sustain as much cumulative radiation damage.

4. Radiant energy may interact with molecular oxygen to induce free radicals, such as superoxide, which can then interact with atoms and molecules to compound the cellular injury. The *oxygen effect* is significant in the radiotherapy of neoplasms. The center of rapidly growing tumors may be poorly vascularized and therefore somewhat hypoxic, making radiotherapy less effective.

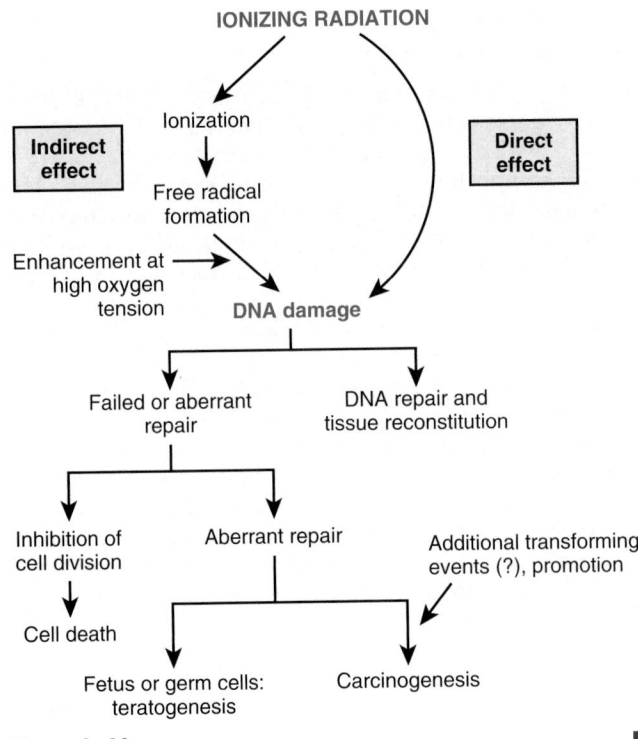

Figure 8–13 ■

Effects of ionizing radiation on DNA. The major effect is indirect, via free radical formation.

5. The size of the field exposed to radiation has a great effect on its consequences. The body can sustain relatively high doses of radiation when delivered to small, carefully shielded fields, whereas smaller doses delivered to larger fields may prove lethal.

6. Even at low doses, radiation can alter gene expression (e.g., increased expression of protooncogenes such as *MYC* [formerly c-*myc*] or *FOS* [formerly c-*fos*]; induction of cytokines such as TNF; or activation of the tumor suppressor gene *TP53* [formerly *p53*] causes cell cycle arrest and possibly apoptosis). In brief, radiation deranges the entire panoply of intracellular homeostatic mechanisms. A summary of the biologic effects of ionizing radiation is provided in Figure 8–13.

MORPHOLOGY

At the **molecular level**, DNA reveals a variety of alterations. These include the formation of pyrimidine dimers, cross-links, single-strand or double-strand breaks, and various rearrangements. Most single-strand breaks are rapidly repaired, often within minutes; double-strand breaks are more often irreparable. As discussed in Chapter 6, cells with unrepaired DNA damage are induced to undergo apoptosis by the activation of the *TP53* gene. Surviving cells show a wide range of structural changes in chromosomes, including deletions, breaks, translocations, and fragmentation. The mitotic spindle often becomes disorderly, and polyploidy and aneuploidy may be encountered. At the **cellular level,** nuclear swelling and condensation and clumping of chromatin may appear; sometimes the nuclear membrane breaks. Apoptosis may occur. All forms of abnormal nuclear morphology may be produced. Giant cells with pleomorphic nuclei or more than one nucleus may appear and persist for years after exposure. At extremely high dose levels of radiant energy, nuclear pyknosis, or lysis appears quickly as a marker of cell death.

In addition to affecting DNA and nuclei, radiant energy may induce a variety of **cytoplasmic changes,** including cytoplasmic swelling, mitochondrial distortion, and degeneration of the endoplasmic reticulum. Plasma membrane breaks and focal defects may appear. The histologic constellation of cellular pleomorphism, giant cell formation, conformational changes in nuclei, and mitotic figures creates a more than passing similarity between radiation-injured cells and cancer cells, a problem that plagues the pathologist when evaluating postirradiation tissues for the possible persistence of tumor cells.

At the light microscopic level, vascular changes and interstitial fibrosis are prominent in irradiated tissues (Fig. 8–14). During the immediate postirradiation period, vessels may show only dilation. Later, or with higher doses, a variety of degenerative changes appear, including endothelial cell swelling and vacuolation, or even dissolution with total necrosis of the walls of small vessels such as capillaries and venules. Affected vessels may rupture or thrombose. Still later, endothelial cell proliferation and collagenous hyalinization with thickening of the media are seen in irradiated vessels, resulting in marked narrowing or even obliteration of the vascular lumina. At this time, an increase in interstitial collagen in the irradiated field usually becomes evident, leading to scarring and contractions.

Effects on Organ Systems. Figure 8–15 depicts the organs that are particularly radiosensitive, together with common early and late manifestations.

The *hematopoietic* and *lymphoid* systems are extremely susceptible to radiant injury and deserve special mention here. With high dose levels and large exposure fields, severe lymphopenia may appear within hours of irradiation, along with shrinkage of the lymph nodes and spleen. Radiation directly destroys lymphocytes, both in the circulating blood and in tissues (nodes, spleen, thymus, gut). With sublethal doses of radiation, regeneration from viable precursors is prompt, leading to restoration of a normal lymphocyte count in the blood within weeks to months. The circulating *granulocyte count* may first rise but begins to fall toward the end of the first week. Levels near zero may be reached during the second week. If the patient survives, recovery of the

Figure 8–14 ■

A, Chronic vascular injury with subintimal fibrosis occluding the lumen. *B*, Radiation fibrosis of the breast stroma after radiotherapy for infiltrating ductal carcinoma. The nests of remaining tumor cells are pleomorphic and multinucleated. (*A* and *B*, Courtesy of American Registry of Pathology © 1990.)

normal granulocyte count may require 2 to 3 months. *Platelets* are similarly affected, with the nadir of the count occurring somewhat later than that of granulocytes; recovery is similarly delayed. *Hematopoietic cells in the bone marrow*, including red cell precursors, are also quite sensitive to radiant energy. Erythrocytes are radioresistant, but anemia may nonetheless appear after 2 to 3 weeks and persist for months because of marrow damage.

Another effect of irradiation on organ systems that deserves special mention relates to malignant transformation (see Fig. 8–13 and Chapter 6). Any cell capable of division that has sustained a mutation has the potential to become cancerous. Thus, an increased incidence of neoplasms may occur in any organ after radiation. The level of radiation required to increase the risk of cancer development is difficult if not impossible to determine. Radiation in very large doses kills cells and therefore is not associated with occurrence of tumors. Sublethal but relatively high doses are clearly associated with an increased risk. This is documented by the increased incidence of neoplasms in survivors of the atomic bombings of Hiroshima and Nagasaki, in radiologists, and in the survivors of nuclear accidents such as occurred at Chernobyl. Prolonged exposure to low-dose radiation may impose risks as well, as will be evident

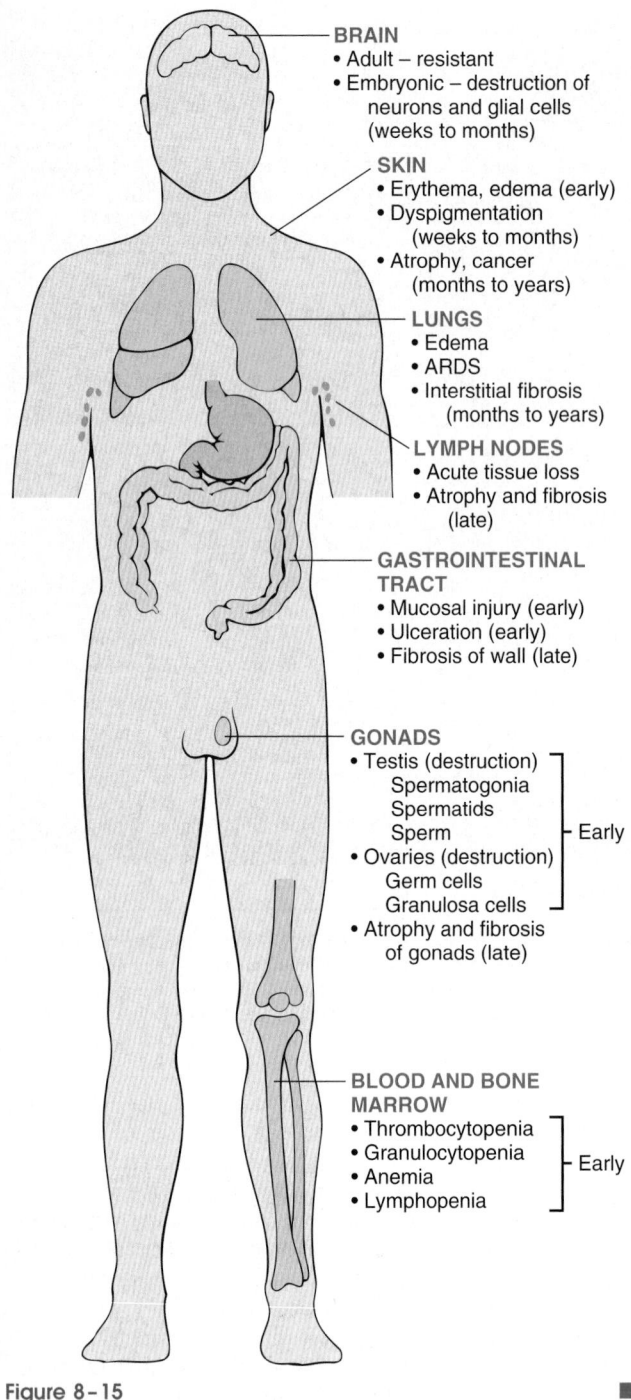

BRAIN
• Adult – resistant
• Embryonic – destruction of
  neurons and glial cells
  (weeks to months)

SKIN
• Erythema, edema (early)
• Dyspigmentation
  (weeks to months)
• Atrophy, cancer
  (months to years)

LUNGS
• Edema
• ARDS
• Interstitial fibrosis
  (months to years)

LYMPH NODES
• Acute tissue loss
• Atrophy and fibrosis
  (late)

GASTROINTESTINAL TRACT
• Mucosal injury (early)
• Ulceration (early)
• Fibrosis of wall (late)

GONADS
• Testis (destruction)
  Spermatogonia
  Spermatids
  Sperm
• Ovaries (destruction)   ⎫ Early
  Germ cells
  Granulosa cells
• Atrophy and fibrosis
  of gonads (late)

BLOOD AND BONE MARROW
• Thrombocytopenia
• Granulocytopenia   ⎫ Early
• Anemia
• Lymphopenia

Figure 8–15   ■

Overview of the major morphologic consequences of radiation injury. Early changes occur in hours to weeks; late changes occur in months to years. ARDS, acute respiratory distress syndrome.

Table 8–11. SYNDROMES ASSOCIATED WITH VARIOUS LEVELS OF TOTAL-BODY IRRADIATION

Syndrome	Dose (rad)	Clinical Manifestations
Hematopoietic	200–500	Nausea and vomiting, lymphopenia, thrombocytopenia, neutropenia, later anemia
Gastrointestinal	500–1000	Severe gastrointestinal symptoms, including diarrhea, hemorrhage, emaciation; at higher doses, death within days; at lower doses, hematopoietic system manifestations
Cerebral	>5000	Listlessness and drowsiness, followed by convulsions, coma, and death within hours

(or radon "daughters") are alpha particle–emitting particulates. These particulates are more readily deposited in lung tissue and can accumulate, producing short-range DNA damage. Over a period of time, cells that suffer sufficient unrepaired DNA damage could become neoplastic and give rise to lung carcinomas. However, despite numerous studies, it is not yet certain that the levels of radiation in most households are sufficient to cause lung cancer, except in those regions of the United States where uranium is closer to the surface and home construction practices facilitate leakage and entrapment of gases from the soil in basements. In these particular settings, it is suspected that radon has contributed to the origin of lung cancer.

Total-Body Irradiation. Exposure of large areas of the body to even very small doses of radiation may have devastating effects, as was pointed out earlier. Although 10 to 50 rad of gamma or x-ray exposure may exert no discernible effects when delivered to limited areas, 50 to 100 rad of whole-body irradiation may cause as many as 10% of exposed individuals to manifest nausea and vomiting, fatigue, and transient decreases in lymphocytes and granulocytes. As little as 100 to 300 rad of radiant energy in total-body exposure delivered in one dose may induce an "acute radiation syndrome." To place this radiation level in context, it must be appreciated that doses of 4000 rad or more are often used in carefully shielded patients for radiotherapy of tumors. The lethal range in humans for total-body irradiation begins at about 200 rad, and at 700 rad, death is certain without medical intervention. Three often fatal acute radiation syndromes have been identified: (1) hematopoietic, (2) gastrointestinal, and (3) cerebral—defined briefly in Table 8–11.

NUTRITIONAL DISEASES

Millions of people in undeveloped or developing nations starve or live on the cruel edge of starvation, while those in the industrial world struggle to avoid calories and the attendant obesity or fear that what they eat may

from the following discussion of the relationship of radon to bronchogenic carcinoma.

Radon is a ubiquitous alpha particle–emitting product of the spontaneous decay of uranium. Because radon is a gas, it moves freely into and out of the lungs and generally does not accumulate in tissues, nor does it cause damage because, as previously discussed, alpha emitters penetrate tissues very poorly. In contrast, two radon decay byproducts contribute to atherosclerosis and hypertension. So overnutrition or the lack of it continues to be a major concern to most humans.

An appropriate diet should provide (1) sufficient energy, in the form of carbohydrates, fats, and proteins, for the body's daily metabolic needs; (2) essential (as well as nonessential) amino acids and fatty acids to be used as building blocks for synthesis of structural and functional proteins and lipids; and (3) vitamins and minerals, which function as coenzymes or hormones in vital metabolic pathways or, as in the case of calcium and phosphate, as important structural components. In primary malnutrition, one or all of these components are missing from the diet. By contrast, in secondary, or conditioned, malnutrition, the supply of nutrients is adequate, but malnutrition results from nutrient malabsorption, impaired nutrient utilization or storage, excess nutrient losses, or increased need for nutrients. Ignorance about the nutritional content of foods may also contribute to malnutrition. Iron deficiency is often seen in infants fed exclusively artificial milk diets. Polished rice as the mainstay of the diet may lack adequate amounts of thiamine, and iodine is often lacking from food and water in regions removed from the oceans when supplementation is not instituted. Many other examples might be offered, but it suffices to state that malnutrition is widespread and may be gross or subtle.

Common causes of dietary insufficiencies are

■ Ignorance and poverty. Homeless persons, aged individuals, and children of the poor often suffer from protein-energy malnutrition (PEM) as well as trace nutrient deficiencies. Even the affluent may fail to recognize that infants, adolescents, and pregnant women have increased nutritional needs.
■ Chronic alcoholism. Alcoholic persons may sometimes suffer PEM but are more frequently lacking in several vitamins, especially thiamine, pyridoxine, folate, and vitamin A, owing to a combination of dietary deficiency, defective gastrointestinal absorption, abnormal nutrient utilization and storage, increased metabolic needs, and an increased rate of loss. A failure to recognize the likelihood of thiamine deficiency in patients with chronic alcoholism may result in irreversible brain damage (e.g., Korsakoff psychosis, discussed in Chapter 23).
■ Acute and chronic illnesses. The basal metabolic rate (BMR) becomes accelerated in many illnesses (in patients with extensive burns, it may double), resulting in an increased daily requirement for all nutrients. Failure to appreciate this fact can compromise recovery.
■ Self-imposed dietary restriction. Anorexia nervosa, bulimia nervosa, and less overt eating disorders affect a large population of individuals who are concerned about body image or suffer from an unreasonable fear of cardiovascular disease.
■ Other, less common causes of malnutrition include the malabsorption syndromes, genetic diseases, specific drug therapies (which block uptake or utilization of particular nutrients), and total parenteral nutrition (TPN).

The sections that follow barely skim the surface of nutritional disorders. Particular attention is devoted to PEM, deficiencies of most of the vitamins and trace minerals,

obesity, and a brief overview of the relationships of diet to atherosclerosis and cancer. Other nutrients and nutritional issues are discussed in the context of specific disorders throughout the text.

Protein-Energy Malnutrition

Severe PEM is a serious, often lethal disease. It is common in third world countries, where up to 25% of children may be affected, and where it is a major factor in the high death rates among children younger than 5 years. It presents as a range of clinical syndromes, all characterized by a dietary intake of protein and calories inadequate to meet the body's needs. The two ends of the spectrum are known as *marasmus* and *kwashiorkor*. In considering these conditions, it is important to remember that from a functional standpoint, there are two protein compartments in the body: the somatic protein compartment, represented by skeletal muscles, and the visceral protein compartment, represented by protein stores in the visceral organs, primarily the liver. These two compartments are regulated differently, and, as we shall see, the somatic compartment is affected more severely in marasmus, and the visceral compartment is depleted more severely in kwashiorkor. Before discussing the clinical presentations of marasmus and kwashiorkor, some comments will be made on the clinical assessment of undernutrition and some of its general metabolic characteristics.

The diagnosis of PEM is obvious in its most severe forms; in mild to moderate forms, the usual approach is to compare the body weight for a given height with standard tables; other parameters are also helpful, including evaluation of fat stores, muscle mass, and serum proteins. With a loss of fat, the thickness of skinfolds (which includes skin and subcutaneous tissue) is reduced. If the somatic protein compartment is catabolized, the resultant reduction in muscle mass is reflected by reduced circumference of the midarm. Measurement of levels of serum proteins (albumin, transferrin, and others) provides a measure of the adequacy of the visceral protein compartment.

The most common victims of PEM worldwide are children. A child whose weight falls to less than 80% of normal is considered malnourished. When the level falls to 60% of normal weight for sex, height, and age, the child is considered to have *marasmus*. A marasmic child suffers growth retardation and loss of muscle. The loss of muscle mass results from catabolism and depletion of the somatic protein compartment. This seems to be an adaptational response that serves to provide the body with amino acids as a source of energy. Interestingly, the visceral protein compartment, which is presumably more precious and critical for survival, is depleted only marginally, and hence *serum albumin levels are either normal or only slightly reduced*. In addition to muscle proteins, subcutaneous fat is also mobilized and used as fuel. With such losses of muscle and subcutaneous fat, the *extremities are emaciated*; by comparison, the head appears too large for the body. Anemia and manifestations of multivitamin deficiencies are present, and there is evidence of *immune deficiency*, particularly T-cell–mediated immunity. Hence, concurrent infections are usually present, and they impose an additional stress on an already weakened body.

Kwashiorkor occurs when protein deprivation is relatively greater than the reduction in total calories. This is the most common form of PEM seen in African children who have been weaned (often too early, owing to the arrival of another child) and subsequently fed an exclusively carbohydrate diet. The prevalence of kwashiorkor is also high in impoverished countries of Southeast Asia. Less severe forms may occur worldwide in persons with chronic diarrheal states in which protein is not absorbed or in those with conditions in which chronic protein loss occurs (e.g., protein-losing enteropathies, the nephrotic syndrome, or after extensive burns).

Kwashiorkor is a more severe form of malnutrition than marasmus. Unlike in marasmus, marked protein deprivation is associated with severe loss of the visceral protein compartment, and the resultant hypoalbuminemia gives rise to generalized or dependent edema (Fig. 8–16). The weight of children with severe kwashiorkor is typically 60% to 80% of normal. However, the true loss of weight is masked by the increased fluid retention (edema). In further contrast to marasmus, there is relative sparing of subcutaneous fat and muscle mass. The modest loss of these compartments may also be masked by edema. Children with kwashiorkor have characteristic *skin lesions*, with alternating zones of hyperpigmentation, areas of desquamation, and hypopigmentation, giving a "flaky paint" appearance. *Hair changes* include overall loss of color or alternating bands of pale and darker hair; straightening; fine texture; and loss of firm attachment to the scalp. Other features that differentiate kwashiorkor from marasmus include an enlarged, *fatty liver* (resulting from reduced synthesis of carrier proteins) and a tendency

to develop apathy, listlessness, and loss of appetite. As in marasmus, other vitamin deficiencies are likely to be present, as are *defects in immunity* and *secondary infections*. The latter add to the catabolic state, thus setting up a vicious circle. It should be emphasized that marasmus and kwashiorkor are two ends of a spectrum, and considerable overlap exists.

Secondary PEM is not uncommon in chronically ill or hospitalized patients within the United States. Table 8–12 summarizes the secondary forms of these two syndromes. A particularly severe form of secondary PEM, called *cachexia*, is seen with advanced cancer (Chapter 6). The wasting is all too apparent and often presages death. Although loss of appetite may partly explain it, cachexia may appear before a decrease in appetite. A number of explanations have been offered, including an elevated resting metabolic rate and the production of catabolic cytokines by the tumor, including IL-1, TNF, and IL-6.

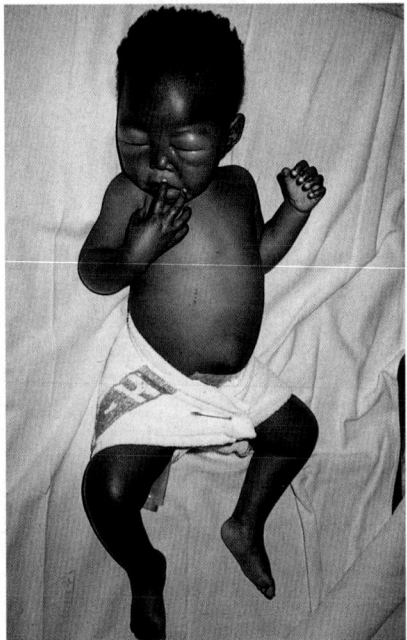

Figure 8-16 ■

Kwashiorkor. The infant shows generalized edema, seen in the form of puffiness of the face, arms, and legs.

MORPHOLOGY

The central anatomic changes in PEM are (1) growth failure; (2) peripheral edema in kwashiorkor; and (3) loss of body fat and atrophy of muscle, more marked in marasmus.

The **liver** in kwashiorkor, but not in marasmus, is enlarged and fatty; superimposed cirrhosis is rare.

In kwashiorkor (rarely in marasmus) the **small bowel** shows a decrease in the mitotic index in the crypts of the glands, associated with mucosal atrophy and loss of villi and microvilli. In such cases, concurrent loss of small intestinal enzymes occurs, most often manifested as disaccharidase deficiency. Hence, infants with kwashiorkor initially may not respond well to full-strength, milk-based diets. With treatment, the mucosal changes are reversible.

The **bone marrow** in both kwashiorkor and marasmus may be hypoplastic, owing mainly to decreased numbers of red cell precursors. How much of this derangement is due to a deficiency of protein and folates and how much to reduced synthesis of transferrin and ceruloplasmin is uncertain. Thus, anemia is usually present, most often hypochromic microcytic anemia, but a concurrent deficiency of folates may lead to a mixed microcytic-macrocytic anemia.

The **brain** in infants who are born to malnourished mothers and who suffer PEM during the first 1 or 2 years of life has been reported by some to show cerebral atrophy, a reduced number of neurons, and impaired myelinization of white matter.

Many **other changes** may be present, including (1) thymic and lymphoid atrophy (more marked in kwashiorkor than in marasmus), (2) anatomic alterations induced by intercurrent infections, particularly with all manner of endemic worms and other parasites, and (3) deficiencies of other required nutrients such as iodine and vitamins.

Table 8-12.   COMPARISON OF SEVERE MARASMUS-LIKE AND KWASHIORKOR-LIKE SECONDARY PROTEIN-ENERGY MALNUTRITION SYNDROMES

Syndromes	Clinical Setting	Time Course	Clinical Features	Laboratory Findings	Prognosis
Marasmus-like PEM	Chronic illness (e.g., chronic obstructive lung disease, cancer)	Months	History of weight loss Muscle wasting Absent subcutaneous fat	Normal or mildly reduced serum proteins	Variable; depends on underlying disease
Kwashiorkor-like PEM	Acute, catabolic illness (e.g., severe trauma, burns, sepsis)	Weeks	Normal fat and muscle Edema Easily pluckable hair	Serum albumin <2.8 gm/dL	Poor

Modified from Bennett JC, Plum F (eds): Cecil Textbook of Medicine, 20th ed. Philadelphia, WB Saunders, 1996, p 1156.
Original table adapted from Weinsier RL, et al: Handbook of Clinical Nutrition, 2nd ed. St. Louis, CV Mosby, 1989.
PEM, protein-energy malnutrition.

Anorexia Nervosa and Bulimia

Anorexia nervosa is self-induced starvation, resulting in marked weight loss; bulimia is a condition in which the patient binges on food and then induces vomiting. These eating disorders occur primarily in previously healthy young women who have developed an obsession with attaining thinness.

The clinical findings in anorexia nervosa are generally similar to those in severe PEM. In addition, effects on the endocrine system are prominent. *Amenorrhea*, resulting from decreased secretion of gonadotropin-releasing hormone (GnRH) (and subsequent decreased secretion of luteinizing hormone [LH] and follicle-stimulating hormone [FSH]), is so common that its presence is a diagnostic feature for the disorder. Other common findings, related to decreased thyroid hormone release, include cold intolerance, bradycardia, constipation, and changes in the skin and hair. The skin becomes dry and scaly and may be yellow owing to excess carotene in the blood. Body hair may be increased but is usually fine and pale (lanugo). Bone density is decreased, most likely owing to low estrogen levels, which mimics the postmenopausal acceleration of osteoporosis. As expected with severe PEM, anemia, lymphopenia, and hypoalbuminemia may be present. A major complication of anorexia nervosa is an increased susceptibility to cardiac arrhythmia and sudden death, resulting in all likelihood from hypokalemia.

In bulimia, binge eating is the norm. Huge amounts of food, principally carbohydrates, are ingested, only to be followed by induced vomiting. Although menstrual irregularities are common, amenorrhea occurs in less than 50% of bulimic patients, probably because weight and gonadotropin levels are maintained near normal. The major medical complications relate to continual induced vomiting and include (1) electrolyte imbalances (hypokalemia), which predispose the patient to cardiac arrhythmias; (2) pulmonary aspiration of gastric contents; and (3) esophageal and stomach cardiac rupture.

Vitamin Deficiencies

Thirteen vitamins are necessary for health; four—A, D, E, and K—are fat-soluble, and the remainder are water-soluble. The distinction between fat- and water-soluble vitamins is important; although the former are more readily stored in the body, they are likely to be poorly absorbed in gastrointestinal disorders of fat malabsorption (Chapter 15). Certain vitamins can be synthesized endogenously—vitamin D from precursor steroids, vitamin K and biotin by the intestinal microflora, and niacin from tryptophan, an essential amino acid. Notwithstanding this endogenous synthesis, a dietary supply of all vitamins is essential for health.

A deficiency of vitamins may be primary (dietary in origin) or secondary (because of disturbances in intestinal absorption, transport in the blood, tissue storage, or metabolic conversion). In the following sections, deficiency states of vitamins A, D, and C are presented in some detail because of their wide-ranging morphologic consequences, followed by brief characterizations in tabular form of the remaining vitamins (E, K, and the B complex) and some essential minerals, because the morphologic consequences seen in deficiency states of these elements are less complex. However, it should be emphasized that deficiencies of a single vitamin are uncommon, and a deficiency of a combination of vitamins may be submerged in concurrent PEM.

VITAMIN A

The fat-soluble vitamin A is actually a group of related natural and synthetic chemicals that exert a hormone-like activity or function. The relationship among some major members of this group is presented in Figure 8-17.

Figure 8-17   ■

Interrelationships of retinoids and their major functions.

Retinol is perhaps the most important form of vitamin A; it is the transport form and, as the retinol ester, also the storage form. It is oxidized in vivo to the aldehyde retinal (the form used in visual pigment) and retinoic acid. Important dietary sources of vitamin A are animal-derived (e.g., liver, fish, eggs, milk, butter). Yellow and leafy green vegetables such as carrots, squash, and spinach supply large amounts of carotenoids, many of which are provitamins that can be metabolized to active vitamin A in vivo; the most important of these is β-carotene. A widely used term, *retinoids*, refers to both natural and synthetic chemicals that are structurally related to vitamin A but do not necessarily have vitamin A activity. As with all fats, the digestion and absorption of carotenes and retinoids require bile, pancreatic enzymes, and some level of antioxidant activity in the food. Retinol, whether derived from ingested esters or from β-carotene (through an intermediate oxidation step involving retinal), is transported in chylomicrons to the liver for esterification and storage. More than 90% of the body's vitamin A reserves are stored in the liver, predominantly in the perisinusoidal stellate (Ito) cells. In healthy persons who consume an adequate diet, these reserves are sufficient for at least 6 months' deprivation. Retinoic acid, on the other hand, can be absorbed unchanged; it represents a small fraction of vitamin A in the blood and is active in epithelial differentiation and growth but not in the maintenance of vision.

When dietary intake of vitamin A is inadequate, the retinol esters in the liver are mobilized, and released retinol is then bound to a specific retinol-binding protein (RBP), synthesized in the liver. The uptake of retinol by the various cells of the body is dependent on surface receptors specific for RBP, rather than for the retinol. Retinol is transported across the cell membrane, where it binds to a cellular retinol-binding protein, and the RBP is released back into the blood.

Function. In humans, the best-defined functions of vitamin A are

■ Maintaining normal vision in reduced light
■ Potentiating the differentiation of specialized epithelial cells, mainly mucus-secreting cells
■ Enhancing immunity to infections, particularly in children and particularly measles

In addition, the retinoids, β-carotene, and some related carotenoids have been shown to function as photoprotective and antioxidant agents.

The visual process involves four forms of vitamin A–containing pigments: rhodopsin in the rods, the most light-sensitive pigment and therefore important in reduced light, and three iodopsins in cone cells, each responsive to specific colors in bright light. The synthesis of rhodopsin from retinol involves (1) oxidation to all-*trans*-retinal, (2) isomerization to 11-*cis*-retinal, and (3) interaction with the rod protein, opsin, to form rhodopsin. When a photon of light impinges on the dark-adapted retina, rhodopsin undergoes a sequence of configurational changes to ultimately yield all-*trans*-retinal and opsin. In the process, a nerve impulse is generated (by changes in membrane potential) that is transmitted via neurons from the retina to the brain. During dark adaptation, some of the all-*trans*-retinal is reconverted to 11-*cis*-retinal,

but most is reduced to retinol and lost to the retina, dictating the need for continuous input of retinol.

Vitamin A plays an important role in the orderly differentiation of mucus-secreting epithelium; when a deficiency state exists, the epithelium undergoes squamous metaplasia and differentiation to a keratinizing epithelium. The mechanism is not precisely understood, but in cell culture systems, retinoic acid (retinol is much less potent) regulates the gene expression of a number of cell receptors and secreted proteins, including receptors for growth factors. *Trans*-retinoic acid has been shown to induce temporary remission of promyelocytic leukemia (PML). In this leukemia, the t(15:17) translocation (Chapter 12) results in the fusion of a truncated retinoic acid receptor α gene *(RARA)* on chromosome 17 with the *PML* gene on chromosome 15. The fusion gene encodes an abnormal retinoic acid receptor that blocks myeloid cell differentiation. Pharmacologic doses of all-*trans*-retinoic acid overcome the block, causing neoplastic myelocytes to differentiate into neutrophils. Although this "differentiation therapy" induces remission in most patients with acute promyelocytic leukemia, all patients ultimately relapse because production of abnormal myeloid progenitor cells outpaces the differentiation induced by retinoic acid.

Vitamin A plays some role in host resistance to infections. This beneficial effect of vitamin A seems to derive in part from its ability to stimulate the immune system, possibly through the formation of a metabolite called 14-hydroxyretinol. In addition, it appears that during infections, the bioavailability of vitamin A is reduced. The acute-phase response that accompanies many infections reduces the formation of RBP in the liver, resulting in depression of circulating retinol levels, which in turn leads to reduced tissue availability of vitamin A. In keeping with this, supplements of the vitamin during the course of infections such as measles dramatically improve the clinical outcome.

Deficiency State. Vitamin A deficiency occurs worldwide either on the basis of general undernutrition or as a conditioned deficiency among individuals having some cause for malabsorption of fats. One of the earliest manifestations of vitamin A deficiency is impaired vision, particularly in reduced light (night blindness). Because vitamin A and retinoids are involved in maintaining the differentiation of epithelial cells, persistent deficiency gives rise to a series of changes, the most devastating of which occur in the eyes. Collectively, the ocular changes are referred to as *xerophthalmia* (dry eye). First, there is dryness of the conjunctiva (xerosis conjunctivae) as the normal lachrymal and mucus-secreting epithelium is replaced by keratinized epithelium. This is followed by the build-up of keratin debris in small opaque plaques *(Bitot spots)* and, eventually, erosion of the roughened corneal surface with softening and destruction of the cornea (keratomalacia) and total blindness.

In addition to the ocular epithelium, the epithelium lining the upper respiratory passage and urinary tract is replaced by keratinizing squamous cells (squamous metaplasia). Loss of the mucociliary epithelium of the airways predisposes to secondary pulmonary infections, and desquamation of keratin debris in the urinary tract predisposes to renal

Figure 8-18

Vitamin A deficiency: its major consequences in the eye and in the production of keratinizing metaplasia of specialized epithelial surfaces, and its possible role in potentiating neoplasia.

and urinary bladder stones. Hyperplasia and hyperkeratinization of the epidermis with plugging of the ducts of the adnexal glands may produce follicular or papular dermatosis. The pathologic effects of vitamin A deficiency are summarized in Figure 8-18.

Another very serious consequence of avitaminosis A is immune deficiency. This impairment of immunity leads to higher mortality rates from common infections such as measles, pneumonia, and infectious diarrhea. In parts of the world where a deficiency of vitamin A is prevalent, dietary supplements reduce mortality by 20% to 30%.

In passing, we should note that despite past enthusiasms for megadoses, current evidence indicates that vitamin A offers no protection from lung cancer.

Vitamin A Toxicity. Both short- and long-term excesses of vitamin A may produce toxic manifestations, a point of some concern because of the megadoses being popularized by certain sellers of supplements. The clinical consequences of acute hypervitaminosis A include headache, vomiting, stupor, and papilledema, symptoms suggestive of brain tumor. Chronic toxicity is associated with weight loss, nausea, and vomiting, as well as possible damaging effects on cell membranes and the DNA during embryogenesis. Although synthetic retinoids used for the treatment of acne are not associated with the complications listed, their use in pregnancy should be avoided owing to a well-established increase in the incidence of congenital malformations.

VITAMIN D

The major function of the fat-soluble vitamin D is the maintenance of normal plasma levels of calcium and phosphorus. In this capacity, it is required for the prevention of bone diseases (rickets in growing children whose epiphyses have not already closed and osteomalacia in adults) and the prevention of hypocalcemic tetany. With respect to tetany, vitamin D maintains the correct concentration of ionized calcium in the extracellular fluid compartment required for normal neural excitation and relaxation of muscle. Insufficient ionized calcium in the extracellular fluid results in continuous excitation of muscle, leading to the convulsive state, hypocalcemic tetany. Our attention here will be focused on the function of vitamin D in the regulation of serum calcium levels.

Metabolism of Vitamin D. The major source of vitamin D for humans is endogenous synthesis in the skin by photochemical conversion of a precursor, 7-dehydrocholesterol, via the energy of solar or artificial ultraviolet (UV) light. Depending on the skin's level of melanin pigmentation, which absorbs UV light, and the amount of exposure to sunlight, about 90% of the vitamin D needed is endogenously derived. Only the small remainder must be obtained from dietary sources, such as deep-sea fish, plants, and grains; this requires normal fat absorption. In plant sources, vitamin D is present in its precursor form (ergosterol), which is converted to vitamin D in the body.

The metabolism of vitamin D can be outlined as follows:

1. Absorption of vitamin D along with other fats in the gut or synthesis from precursors in the skin.
2. Binding to plasma α_1-globulin (D-binding protein) and transport to liver.
3. Conversion to 25-hydroxyvitamin D (25-OH-D) by 25-hydroxylase in the liver.
4. Conversion of 25-OH-D to 1,25-dihydroxyvitamin D [1,25(OH)$_2$-D] by α_1-hydroxylase in the kidney; biologically this is the most active form of vitamin D.

NORMAL VITAMIN D METABOLISM

A

VITAMIN D DEFICIENCY

B

Figure 8–19 ■

A, Schema of normal vitamin D metabolism. *B,* Vitamin D deficiency. There is inadequate substrate for the renal hydroxylase (1), yielding a deficiency of $1,25(OH)_2$-D (2), and deficient absorption of calcium and phosphorus from the gut (3), with consequent depressed serum levels of both (4). The hypocalcemia activates the parathyroid glands (5), causing mobilization of calcium and phosphorus from bone (6a). Simultaneously, the parathyroid hormone (PTH) induces wasting of phosphate in the urine (6b) and calcium retention. Consequently, the serum levels of calcium are normal or nearly normal but the phosphate is low; hence, mineralization is impaired (7).

The production of 1,25(OH)$_2$-D by the kidney is regulated by three mechanisms:

1. In a feedback loop, increased levels of 1,25(OH)$_2$-D down-regulate synthesis of this metabolite by inhibiting the action of α_1-hydroxylase, and decreased levels have the opposite effect.
2. Hypocalcemia stimulates secretion of parathyroid hormone (PTH), which in turn augments the conversion of 25-OH-D to 1,25(OH)$_2$-D by activating α_1-hydroxylase.
3. Hypophosphatemia directly activates α_1-hydroxylase and thus increases formation of 1,25(OH)$_2$-D.

Functions of Vitamin D. 1,25(OH)$_2$-D, the biologically active form of vitamin D, is best regarded as a steroid hormone. Like other steroid hormones, it acts by binding to a high-affinity nuclear receptor that in turn binds to regulatory DNA sequences, which induce transcription of messenger RNA coding for specific proteins that carry out the functions of vitamin D. These receptors for 1,25-(OH)$_2$-D are now known to be present in most nucleated cells of the body, and they transduce the signals that promote the differentiated function of the cells. Best understood are the functions that involve the maintenance of normal plasma levels of calcium and phosphorus, involving actions on the intestines, bones, and kidneys.

The active form of vitamin D

■ Stimulates intestinal absorption of calcium and phosphorus
■ Collaborates with PTH in the mobilization of calcium from bone
■ Stimulates the PTH-dependent reabsorption of calcium in the distal renal tubules

How 1,25(OH)$_2$-D stimulates intestinal absorption of calcium and phosphorus is still somewhat unclear. The weight of evidence favors the view that it binds to mucosal epithelial receptors, activating the synthesis of calcium transport proteins. The increased absorption of phosphorus is independent of calcium transport.

The effects of vitamin D on bone depend on the plasma levels of calcium. On the one hand, with hypocalcemia, 1,25(OH)$_2$-D collaborates with PTH in the resorption of calcium and phosphorus from bone to support blood levels. On the other hand, vitamin D is required for normal mineralization of epiphyseal cartilage and osteoid matrix. It is still not clear how the resorptive function is mediated, but direct activation of osteoclasts is ruled out. It is more likely that vitamin D favors the formation of osteoclasts from their precursors (monocytes), possibly by influencing the production of RANK ligand (Chapter 21). The precise details of mineralization of bone when vitamin D levels are adequate are also uncertain. The main function of vitamin D may be to maintain calcium and phosphorus at supersaturated levels in the plasma. However, vitamin D clearly activates osteoblasts to synthesize the calcium-binding protein, osteocalcin, involved in the deposition of calcium into osteoid matrix and may thus contribute to bone mineralization.

Equally unclear is the role of vitamin D in renal reabsorption of calcium. PTH is clearly necessary, but so is

Table 8-13. CAUSES OF RICKETS OR OSTEOMALACIA

1. Decreased endogenous synthesis of vitamin D
   a. Inadequate exposure to sunlight
   b. Heavy melanin pigmentation of skin (blacks)
2. Decreased absorption of fat-soluble vitamin D in the intestine
   a. Dietary lack
   b. Biliary tract, pancreatic, or intestinal dysfunction
3. Enhanced degradation of vitamin D and 25-OH-D
   a. Phenytoin, phenobarbital, rifampin induction of cytochrome P-450 enzymes
4. Impaired synthesis of 25-OH-D
   a. Diffuse liver disease
5. Decreased synthesis of 1,25(OH)$_2$-D
   a. Advanced renal disease with failure
   b. Vitamin D–dependent rickets type I (inherited deficiency of renal α_1-hydroxylase)
6. Target organ resistance to 1,25(OH)$_2$-D
   a. Vitamin D–dependent rickets type II (congenital lack of or defective receptors for active metabolite)
7. Phosphate depletion
   a. Poor absorption—long-term use of antacids, which bind phosphates and render them insoluble
   b. Renal tubular disorders, acquired or genetic, causing increased excretion

vitamin D. There is no substantial evidence that vitamin D participates in renal reabsorption of phosphorus. An overview of the normal metabolism of vitamin D and the consequences of a deficiency are depicted in Figure 8–19.

Deficiency States. Rickets in growing children and osteomalacia in adults are worldwide skeletal diseases. They may result from deficient diets, but probably more important is limited exposure to sunlight (heavily veiled women, children born to vitamin D–deficient mothers, northern climates with scant sunlight). Other, less common causes of rickets and osteomalacia are given in Table 8–13. Whatever the basis, a deficiency of vitamin D tends to cause hypocalcemia. When hypocalcemia occurs, PTH production is increased, which (1) activates renal α_1-hydroxylase, thus increasing the amount of active vitamin D and calcium absorption; (2) mobilizes calcium from bone; (3) decreases renal calcium excretion; and (4) increases renal excretion of phosphate. Thus, the serum level of calcium is restored to near normal, but hypophosphatemia persists, and so mineralization of bone is impaired.

An understanding of the morphologic changes in rickets and osteomalacia is facilitated by a brief summary of normal bone development and maintenance. The development of flat bones in the skeleton involves intramembranous ossification, while the formation of long tubular bones reflects endochondral ossification. With intramembranous bone formation, mesenchymal cells differentiate directly into osteoblasts, which synthesize the collagenous osteoid matrix on which calcium is deposited. In contrast, with endochondral ossification, growing cartilage at the epiphyseal plates is provisionally mineralized and then progressively resorbed and replaced by osteoid matrix, which undergoes mineralization to create bone (Fig. 8–20B).

MORPHOLOGY

The basic derangement in both rickets and osteomalacia is an excess of unmineralized matrix. The changes that occur in the growing bones of children with rickets, however, are complicated by inadequate provisional calcification of epiphyseal cartilage, deranging endochondral bone growth. The following sequence ensues in rickets:

■ Overgrowth of epiphyseal cartilage due to inadequate provisional calcification and failure of the cartilage cells to mature and disintegrate
■ Persistence of distorted, irregular masses of cartilage, many of which project into the marrow cavity
■ Deposition of osteoid matrix on inadequately mineralized cartilaginous remnants
■ Disruption of the orderly replacement of cartilage by osteoid matrix, with enlargement and lateral expansion of the osteochondral junction (Fig. 8–20A)
■ Abnormal overgrowth of capillaries and fibroblasts in the disorganized zone resulting from microfractures and stresses on the inadequately mineralized, weak, poorly formed bone
■ Deformation of the skeleton due to the loss of structural rigidity of the developing bones

The gross skeletal changes depend on the severity of the rachitic process; its duration; and, in particular, the stresses to which individual bones are subjected. During the nonambulatory stage of infancy, the head and chest sustain the greatest stresses. The softened occipital bones may become flattened, and the parietal bones can be buckled inward by pressure; with the release of the pressure, elastic recoil snaps the bones back into their original positions **(craniotabes).** An excess of osteoid produces **frontal bossing** and a **squared appearance to the head.** Deformation of the chest results from overgrowth of cartilage or osteoid tissue at the costochondral junction, producing the **"rachitic rosary."** The weakened metaphyseal areas of the ribs are subject to the pull of the respiratory muscles and thus bend inward, creating anterior protrusion of the sternum **(pigeon breast deformity).** The inward pull at the margin of the diaphragm creates the **Harrison groove,** girdling the thoracic cavity at the lower margin of the rib cage. The pelvis may become deformed. When an ambulating child develops rickets, deformities are likely to affect the spine, pelvis, and long bones (e.g., tibia), causing, most notably, **lumbar lordosis** and **bowing of the legs** (Fig. 8–21).

In adults, the lack of vitamin D deranges the normal bone remodeling that occurs throughout life. The newly formed osteoid matrix laid down by osteoblasts is inadequately mineralized, thus producing the excess of persistent osteoid that is characteristic of osteomalacia. Although the contours of the bone are not affected, the bone is weak and vulnerable to gross fractures or microfractures, which are most likely to affect vertebral bodies and femoral necks.

Histologically, the unmineralized osteoid can be visualized as a thickened layer of matrix (which stains pink in hematoxylin and eosin preparations) arranged about the more basophilic, normally mineralized trabeculae.

Persistent failure of mineralization in adults leads eventually to loss of skeletal mass, referred to as *osteopenia*. It is then difficult to differentiate osteomalacia from other osteopenias such as osteoporosis (Chapter 21). Osteoporosis, unlike osteomalacia, results from reduced production of osteoid, the protein matrix of the bone. Studies suggest that vitamin D may also be essential for preventing demineralization of bones. In certain familial forms of osteoporosis, the defect has been localized to the vitamin D receptor. It appears that certain genetically determined variants of the vitamin D receptor are associated with an accelerated loss of bone minerals with aging.

Toxicity. Prolonged exposure to sunlight does not produce an excess of vitamin D. Only the orally administered vitamin has that potential; such an excess may take the form of metastatic calcifications of soft tissues. In passing, we might point out that the toxic potential of this vitamin is so great that in sufficiently large doses it is a potent rodenticide.

VITAMIN C (ASCORBIC ACID)

A deficiency of water-soluble vitamin C leads to the development of *scurvy*, characterized principally by bone disease in growing children and by hemorrhages and healing defects in both children and adults. Ascorbic acid cannot be synthesized endogenously, and therefore humans are entirely dependent on the diet for this nutrient. Ascorbic acid is present in milk and some animal products (liver, fish) and is abundant in a variety of fruits and vegetables. All but the most restricted diets provide adequate amounts of vitamin C.

Because of the abundance of ascorbic acid in so many foods, scurvy has ceased to be a global problem, although it is sometimes encountered even in affluent populations as a conditioned deficiency, particularly among elderly individuals, persons who live alone, and those with alcoholism—groups that often have erratic and inadequate eating patterns. Occasionally, scurvy appears in patients undergoing peritoneal dialysis and hemodialysis and among food faddists. Tragically, the condition sometimes appears in infants who are maintained on formulas of evaporated milk without supplementation of vitamin C.

Ascorbic acid functions in a variety of biosynthetic pathways by accelerating hydroxylation and amidation reactions. The most clearly established function of vitamin C is the activation of prolyl and lysyl hydroxylases from inactive precursors, providing for hydroxylation of procollagen.

Figure 8-20

A, Detail of a rachitic costochondral junction. The palisade of cartilage is lost. Some of the trabeculae are old, well-formed bone, but the paler ones consist of uncalcified osteoid. *B,* For comparison, normal costochondral junction in a young child demonstrates the orderly transition from cartilage to new bone formation.

Figure 8-21

Rickets. The bowing of legs in a toddler due to the formation of poorly mineralized bones is evident.

Inadequately hydroxylated procollagen cannot acquire a stable helical configuration and cannot be adequately cross-linked, so it is poorly secreted from the fibroblast. Those molecules that are secreted lack tensile strength, are more soluble, and are more vulnerable to enzymatic degradation. Collagen, which normally has the highest content of hydroxyproline, is most affected, particularly in blood vessels, accounting for the predisposition to hemorrhages in scurvy. In addition, it appears that a deficiency of vitamin C leads to suppression of the rate of synthesis of collagen peptides, independent of an effect on proline hydroxylation.

While the role of vitamin C in collagen synthesis has been known for many decades, it is only in relatively recent years that its antioxidant properties have been recognized. Vitamin C can scavenge free radicals directly in aqueous phases of the cell and can act indirectly by regenerating the antioxidant form of vitamin E. Thus, vitamins E and C act in concert. It is because of these synergistic actions that both of these vitamins have attracted interest as agents that may retard atherosclerosis by reducing the oxidation of LDL (Chapter 10).

MORPHOLOGY

Scurvy in a growing child is far more dramatic than in an adult. **Hemorrhages** constitute one of the most striking features. Because the defect in collagen synthesis results in inadequate support of the walls of capillaries and venules, purpura and ecchymoses often appear in the skin and in the gingival mucosa. Furthermore, the loose attachment of the periosteum to bone, together with the vascular wall defects, leads to extensive subperiosteal hematomas and **bleeding into joint spaces** after minimal trauma. Retrobulbar, subarachnoid, and intracerebral hemorrhages may prove fatal.

Skeletal changes may also develop in infants and children. The primary disturbance is in the formation of osteoid matrix, rather than in mineralization or calcification, such as occurs in rickets. In scurvy, the palisade of cartilage cells is formed as usual and is provisionally calcified. However, there is insufficient production of osteoid matrix by osteoblasts. Resorption of the cartilaginous matrix then fails or slows, and as a consequence there is cartilaginous overgrowth, with long spicules and plates projecting into the metaphyseal region of the marrow cavity and, sometimes, widening of the epiphysis (Fig. 8-22). The scorbutic bone yields to the stresses of weight bearing and muscle tension, with bowing of the long bones of the lower legs and abnormal depression of the sternum with outward projection of the ends of the ribs. The bone changes in adults are similar to those in children, with decreased formation of osteoid matrix, but deformation does not occur.

In severely scorbutic children and adults, **gingival swelling, hemorrhages,** and **secondary bacterial periodontal infection** are common. A distinctive **perifollicular, hyperkeratotic, papular rash** that may be ringed by hemorrhage often appears. **Wound healing and localization of focal infections are impaired** because of the derangement in collagen synthesis.

Anemia is common, resulting from bleeding and from a secondary decrease in iron absorption (Chapter 12). The major features of scurvy are summarized in Figure 8-23.

Toxicity. The popular notion that megadoses of vitamin C will protect against the common cold, or at least allay the symptoms, has not been borne out by controlled clinical studies. Such slight relief as may be experienced is likely owed to the mild antihistamine action of ascorbic acid. The large excesses are promptly excreted in the urine but have sometimes caused uricosuria and have increased absorption of iron with the potential of iron overload.

Other vitamins and some of the essential minerals are briefly characterized in Table 8-14 and Table 8-15. Folic acid and vitamin B_{12} are discussed in Chapter 12.

Figure 8-22 ■

A, Longitudinal section of a scorbutic costochondral junction with widening of the epiphyseal cartilage and projection of masses of cartilage into the adjacent bone. *B*, Detail of a scorbutic costochondral junction. The orderly palisade is totally destroyed. There is dense mineralization of the spicules but no evidence of newly formed osteoid.

Figure 8-23

The major consequences of vitamin C deficiency.

Table 8-14. OTHER VITAMINS

Function	Basis of Deficiency	Changes in Deficiency	Toxicity

Vitamin E (fat-soluble)
Encompasses eight tocopherols and tocotrienols, α-tocopherol most active
Antioxidants and free radical scavengers
Acts along with selenium in maintenance of cell (neuronal) membranes
	Abundant in vegetables, grains, and nuts
	Primary deficiency rare
	Secondary deficiency
	  In premature infants
	  With fat malabsorption
	  With abetalipoproteinemia
		Increased RBC fragility and hemolytic anemia
		Peripheral neuropathy
		Degeneration of spinal cord posterior columns spinocerebellar tracts
		May favor oxidation of LDL and development of atherosclerosis and cardiovascular disease
			Depresses vitamin K procoagulant levels

Vitamin K (fat-soluble)
Required cofactor for liver carboxylation of glutamic acid residues in many proteins (e.g., clotting factors VII, IX, and X; prothrombin; and anticoagulant proteins C and S)
Required cofactor for osteocalcin (in bone matrix) and for renal epithelium
	Derived from endogenous bacteria and green vegetables
	Deficiency uncommon except
	  In breast-fed newborns (lacking endogenous flora)
	  With fat malabsorption
	  With broad-spectrum antibiotics
	  With large doses of vitamin E or anticoagulants
		Bleeding diathesis (e.g., hemorrhagic disease of newborn)	In infants: hemolytic anemia

Table continued on following page

Table 8-14. OTHER VITAMINS *Continued*

Function	Basis of Deficiency	Changes in Deficiency	Toxicity
Vitamin B₁—Thiamine (water-soluble) Becomes phosphorylated to form thiamine pyrophosphate, involved in many α-ketoacid decarboxylation and transketolation reactions such as in synthesis of ATP May also have role in neuronal conduction	Widely available except in refined foods (e.g., polished rice, white flour) Deficiency syndrome With diets largely of polished rice In chronic alcoholism With renal dialysis	Classic deficiency syndrome is beri-beri "Wet" beri-beri with cardiac failure and edema "Dry" beri-beri with peripheral neuropathy Focal hemorrhages into mamillary bodies, periventricular thalamus (Wernicke-Korsakoff syndrome described in Chapter 23) Various combinations of above	Rare Fleeting lethargy, ataxia
Vitamin B₂—Riboflavin (water-soluble) Component of coenzymes flavin mononucleotide and flavin adenine dinucleotide in various redox reactions	Widely available in meat, dairy products, and vegetables Deficiency syndrome In economically deprived Frequently in conjunction with lack of other B vitamins Rare as secondary deficiency in alcoholic patients, and in debilitated (e.g., cancer) patients	Ariboflavinosis characterized by Cheilosis—fissures at angles of mouth Glossitis—tongue atrophy Eye changes—interstitial keratosis Dermatitis—naso-labial folds Sometimes anemia	Unreported in humans
Niacin—Vitamin B₃ (water-soluble) Generic term nicotinic acid and nicotinamide Latter component of nicotinamide adenine dinucleotide (NAD) and its phosphate (NADP) Widely involved as electron acceptors and hydrogenases	Widely available in grains, beans, and seed oils Can be endogenously synthesized from tryptophan Deficiency can occur from lack of B₃ or lack of tryptophan Deficiency seen usually: In chronic alcoholism In chronic diarrhea In debilitating illnesses With diets largely of corn (maize), in which niacin is tightly bound Deficiency also seen in carcinoid syndrome where tryptophan is diverted to synthesis of serotonin and other products Prolonged use of antituberculosis drug isoniazid	Deficiency state is known as *pellagra* (three D's): Diarrhea Dementia owing to loss of neurons in brain Dermatitis symmetric on exposed skin	Formerly seen with pharmacologic doses as hypolipidemic agent Flushing, hyperglycemia, and possible liver damage
Vitamin B₆ (water-soluble) Three substances—pyridoxine, pyridoxal, and pyridoxamine—together with phosphates are all called pyridoxine Phosphate forms serve as coenzymes in metabolism of lipids and amino acids (e.g., synthesis of niacin from tryptophan)	Deficiency rare in primary form because B₆ is present in all natural foods, but destroyed in processing Bottle-fed babies at risk Deficiency usually in combination with other vitamin B deficiencies, and in chronic alcoholism because acetaldehyde enhances degradation	Usually combined with lack of other B vitamins Changes are indistinguishable from those related to other B deficiencies (e.g., angular cheilitis, stomatitis, glossitis)	Peripheral neuropathies with chronic use of large doses

LDL, low-density lipoprotein; RBC, red blood cell.

Table 8-15. SELECTED TRACE ELEMENTS AND DEFICIENCY SYNDROMES

Element	Function	Basis of Deficiency	Clinical Features
Zinc	Component of enzymes, principally oxidases	Inadequate supplementation in artificial diets Interference with absorption by other dietary constituents Inborn error of metabolism	Rash around eyes, mouth, nose, and anus called acrodermatitis enteropathica Anorexia and diarrhea Growth retardation in children Depressed mental function Depressed wound healing and immune response Impaired night vision Infertility
Iron	Essential component of hemoglobin as well as a number of iron-containing metalloenzymes	Inadequate diet Chronic blood loss	Hypochromic microcytic anemia
Iodine	Component of thyroid hormone	Inadequate supply in food and water	Goiter and hypothyroidism
Copper	Component of cytochrome C oxidase, dopamine β-hydroxylase, tyrosinase, lysyl oxidase, and unknown enzyme involved in cross-linking collagen	Inadequate supplementation in artificial diet Interference with absorption	Muscle weakness Neurologic defects Abnormal collagen cross-linking
Fluoride	Mechanism unknown	Inadequate supply in soil and water Inadequate supplementation	Dental caries
Selenium	Component of glutathione peroxidase Antioxidant with vitamin E	Inadequate amounts in soil and water	Myopathy Cardiomyopathy (Keshan disease)

Obesity

Over half of Americans between 20 and 75 years of age are overweight. Because obesity is highly correlated with an increased incidence of several diseases (e.g., diabetes, hypertension), it is important to define and recognize it, to understand its causes, and to be able to initiate appropriate measures to prevent it or to treat it.

Obesity is defined as a state of increased body weight, due to adipose tissue accumulation, that is of sufficient magnitude to produce adverse health effects. How does one measure fat accumulation? There are several highly technical ways to approximate the measurement, but for practical purposes the following ones are commonly used:

■ Some expression of weight in relation to height, such as the measurement referred to as the body mass index (BMI) = (weight in kilograms)/(height in meters)^2
■ Skinfold measurements
■ Various body circumferences, particularly the ratio of the waist-hip circumference

The BMI, expressed in kilograms per square meter, is closely correlated with body fat. A BMI of approximately 25 kg/m^2 is considered normal. It is generally agreed that a 20% excess in body weight (BMI greater than 27 kg/m^2) imparts a health risk. A BMI below 20 kg/m^2 is also associated with an increased mortality rate. This may be related to smoking and its attendant risks, because smoking is known to decrease appetite and, subsequently, the BMI.

The untoward effects of obesity are related not only to the total body weight but also to the distribution of the stored fat. Central, or visceral, obesity, in which fat accumulates in the trunk and in the abdominal cavity (in the mesentery and around viscera), is associated with a much higher risk for several diseases than is excess accumulation of fat diffusely in subcutaneous tissue.

The etiology of obesity is complex and incompletely understood. Involved are genetic, environmental, and psychologic factors. However, simply put, obesity is a disorder of energy balance. The two sides of the energy equation, intake and expenditure, are finely regulated by neural and hormonal mechanisms, and thus, body weight is maintained within a narrow range for many years. Apparently, this fine balance is maintained by an internal set point, or "lipostat," that can sense the quantity of the energy stores (adipose tissue) and appropriately regulate the food intake as well as the energy expenditure. In recent years, several "obesity genes" have been identified. As might be expected, they encode the molecular components of the physiologic system that regulates energy balance. A key player in energy homeostasis is the *Ob* gene and its product, *leptin*. This unique member of the cytokine family, secreted by adipocytes, regulates both sides of the energy equation—intake of food and expenditure of energy. Leptin exerts its actions through a complex cascade of signaling pathways referred to as the *leptin-regulated central melanocortin circuit*. The major components of this circuit are illustrated in Figure 8–24. Leptin actions are initiated by binding to specific receptors on two classes of neurons in the hypothalamus. One class of leptin-sensitive neurons produces the feeding-inducing (orexigenic) neuropeptides, neuropeptide Y (NPY) and agouti-related protein (AgRP). The other class of leptin receptor–bearing neurons produces anorexigenic peptides, α-melanocyte–stimulating hormone (α-MSH) and cocaine- and amphetamine-related transcript (CART). These two molecules reduce food intake. The actions of the orexigenic and anorexigenic neuropeptides are exerted by binding to another set of receptors, the two

Figure 8–24

The neurohumoral circuits that regulate body weight. See text for details.

most important being the NPY receptor and the melanocortin 4 receptor (MC4R), to which latter receptor α-MSH and AgRP bind. The pathways down-stream of these receptors have not been fully characterized.

By mechanisms not clearly understood, the output of leptin is regulated by the adequacy of fat stores. With abundant adipose tissue, leptin secretion is stimulated, and the hormone travels to the hypothalamus, where it binds to leptin receptors (see Fig. 8–24). This interaction reduces food intake by stimulating the production of α-MSH and CART (anorexigenic) and inhibiting the synthesis of NPY and AgRP (orexigenic). The opposite sequence of events occurs when there are inadequate stores of body fat—leptin secretion is diminished and food intake is increased. In individuals with stable weight, the activities of these pathways are balanced.

As indicated earlier, leptin regulates not only energy intake (appetite) but also energy expenditure, through a distinct set of pathways. Thus, abundance of leptin increases physical activity, production of heat, and energy expenditure. The neurohumoral mediators of leptin-induced energy expenditure are less well defined. Thermogenesis seems to be controlled in part by leptin receptor–mediated hypothalamic signals that increase the release of norepinephrine from sympathetic nerve endings in adipose tissue. The fat cells express β_3-adrenergic receptors that when stimulated by norepinephrine cause fatty acid hydrolysis and also uncouple energy production from storage. Thus, the fats are

literally burned, and the energy so produced is dissipated as heat. There are other catabolic effects mediated by leptin, all transduced through its hypothalamic receptor, which in turn communicates with other endocrine glands via the hypothalamic pituitary axis.

This schema is buttressed by the observation that in rodents and humans, mutations that affect the leptin-regulated melanocortin circuit give rise to massive obesity. Mice with mutations that disable the leptin gene or its receptor continue to eat and gain weight. Mice with a mutant leptin gene fail to sense the adequacy of fat stores, and hence they behave as if they are undernourished. In keeping with this, in mice with mutations of the leptin receptor, the afferent signals impinging on the hypothalamus fail to affect appetite and energy expenditure. As in mice, mutations of the leptin gene or receptor cause massive obesity in humans. However, such patients are rare. More commonly, mutations of the MC4R give rise to obesity, as is the case in 4% to 5% of patients with massive obesity. While these monogenic forms of human obesity are uncommon, they underscore the importance of the leptin-melanocortin circuit in the control of body weight. Furthermore, they suggest that other acquired defects in these pathways may be pathogenetic in the more common forms of obesity. For example, in many obese individuals, blood leptin levels are high, suggesting that leptin resistance rather than leptin deficiency may be more prevalent in humans.

There is little doubt but that genetic influences play an important role in weight control. However, as with all complex traits, obesity is not merely a genetic disease. There are definite environmental factors; the prevalence of obesity in Asians who immigrate to the United States is much higher than in those who remain in their native land. These changes in all likelihood result from changes in the type and amount of dietary intake. After all, regardless of genetic makeup, obesity would not occur without intake of food!

Obesity, *particularly central obesity, increases the risk for a number of conditions*, including diabetes, hypertension, hypertriglyceridemia, low HDL cholesterol (Chapter 10), and possibly coronary artery disease. The mechanisms underlying these associations are complex and likely to be interrelated. Obesity, for instance, is associated with *insulin resistance* and hyperinsulinemia, important features of type 2 (formerly called non–insulin-dependent) diabetes, and weight loss is associated with improvement (Chapter 17). It has been speculated that excess insulin, in turn, may play a role in the retention of sodium, expansion of blood volume, production of excess norepinephrine, and smooth muscle proliferation that are the hallmarks of hypertension. Regardless of whether these pathogenic mechanisms are actually operative, *the risk of developing hypertension among previously normotensive persons increases proportionately with weight.*

Obese persons are likely to have hypertriglyceridemia and a low HDL cholesterol value, and these factors may increase the risk of *coronary artery disease* in the very obese. It should be emphasized that the association between obesity and heart disease is not straightforward, and such linkage as there may be relates more to the associated diabetes and hypertension than to weight per se.

Cholelithiasis (gallstones) is six times more common in obese than in lean subjects. The mechanism is mainly an increase in total body cholesterol, increased cholesterol turnover, and augmented biliary excretion of cholesterol in the bile, which in turn predisposes to the formation of cholesterol-rich gallstones (Chapter 16).

Hypoventilation syndrome is a constellation of respiratory abnormalities in very obese persons. It has been called the *pickwickian syndrome*, after the fat lad who was constantly falling asleep in Charles Dickens' *Pickwick Papers*. Hypersomnolence, both at night and during the day, is characteristic and is often associated with apneic pauses during sleep, polycythemia, and eventual right-sided heart failure.

Marked adiposity predisposes to the development of degenerative joint disease (*osteoarthritis*). This form of arthritis, which typically appears in older persons, is attributed in large part to the cumulative effects of wear and tear on joints. The greater the body burden of fat, the greater the trauma to joints with passage of time.

The relationship between *obesity and stroke* is unclear, and opposing views can be found in the literature. According to some, the true relationship is between stroke and hypertension, not between stroke and obesity per se (i.e., obese patients who are not hypertensive are not at higher risk for stroke).

Equally controversial is the relationship between *obesity and cancer*, particularly cancers arising in the endometrium and breast. Here, the problem is complicated by the role of particular foods, such as animal fats, which may be independently associated with cancer and obesity.

Nevertheless, it seems that obese women are at a higher risk of developing endometrial cancer than are lean women in the same age group. This relationship may be indirect; high estrogen levels are associated with increased risk of endometrial cancer (Chapter 19), and obesity is known to raise estrogen levels. With breast cancer, the data are controversial. It seems that in postmenopausal women who live in countries with a moderate or low risk of breast cancer (e.g., Japan), central obesity is associated with an increased risk of breast cancer. Again, the role of sex hormones is a confounding factor.

Diet and Systemic Diseases

The problems of under- and overnutrition, as well as specific nutrient deficiencies, have been discussed; however, the composition of the diet, even in the absence of any of these problems, may make a significant contribution to the causation and progression of a number of diseases. A few examples suffice here.

Currently, one of the most important and controversial issues is the contribution of diet to atherogenesis. The central question is "Can dietary modification—specifically, reduction in the consumption of cholesterol and saturated animal fats (e.g., eggs, butter, beef)—reduce serum cholesterol levels and prevent or retard the development of atherosclerosis (most importantly, coronary heart disease)?" The average adult in the United States consumes an inordinate amount of fat and cholesterol daily, with a ratio of saturated fatty acids to polyunsaturated fatty acids of about 3:1. Lowering the level of saturates to the level of the polyunsaturates effects a 10% to 15% reduction in serum cholesterol level within a few weeks. Vegetable oils (e.g., corn and safflower oils) and fish oil contain polyunsaturated fatty acids and are good sources of such cholesterol-lowering lipids. Fish oil fatty acids belonging to the omega-3, or n-3, family have more double bonds than do the omega-6, or n-6, fatty acids found in vegetable oils. A study of Dutch men whose usual daily diet contained 30 mg of fish revealed a substantially lower frequency of death from coronary heart disease than that among comparable controls. Although dietary modification can affect heart disease, currently there are insufficient data to suggest that long-term supplementation of food with omega-3 fatty acids is of benefit in reducing coronary artery disease.

There are other examples of the effect of diet on disease:

■ Hypertension is beneficially affected by restricting sodium intake.

■ Dietary fiber, or roughage, resulting in increased fecal bulk, is thought by some to have a preventive effect against diverticulosis of the colon.

■ Caloric restriction has been convincingly demonstrated to increase life span in experimental animals. The basis of this striking observation is not clear. It seems, however, that in such animals, the age-related decline in immunologic functions is modest, and the animals are more resistant to experimental carcinogenesis.

■ Even lowly garlic has been touted to protect against heart disease (and also, alas, kisses), although research has yet to prove this effect unequivocally.

Diet and Cancer

With respect to carcinogenesis, three aspects of the diet are of concern: (1) the possible content of exogenous carcinogens, (2) the potential that carcinogens might be endogenously synthesized from dietary components, and (3) a possible lack of protective factors. Relative to exogenous carcinogens, aflatoxins are clearly carcinogenic. Debate continues about the carcinogenicity of food additives, artificial sweeteners, and contaminating pesticides. Some artificial sweeteners (cyclamates and saccharin) have been implicated in bladder cancers, but convincing evidence is lacking.

The concern about endogenous synthesis of carcinogens or promoters from components of the diet relates principally to gastric carcinomas. With gastric carcinoma, nitrosamines and nitrosamides are believed by some to be carcinogens because they have been clearly shown to induce gastric cancer in animals. These compounds can be formed in the body from nitrites and amines or amides derived from digested proteins. Sources of nitrites include sodium nitrite added to foods as a preservative, and nitrates, present in common vegetables, which are reduced in the gut by bacterial flora. There is, then, the potential for endogenous production of carcinogenic agents from dietary components, which might well have an effect on the stomach exposed to high concentrations.

High animal fat intake combined with low fiber intake has been implicated in the causation of colon cancer. The most convincing explanation of these associations is as follows: High fat intake increases the level of bile acids in the gut, which in turn modifies intestinal flora, favoring the growth of microaerophilic bacteria. The bile acids or bile acid metabolites produced by these bacteria might serve as carcinogens or promoters. The protective effect of a high-fiber diet might relate to (1) increased stool bulk and decreased transit time, which decreases the exposure of mucosa to putative offenders, and (2) the capacity of certain fibers to bind carcinogens and thereby protect the mucosa. Attempts to document these theories in clinical and experimental studies have, on the whole, led to contradictory results.

Finally, some dietary components have been considered anticarcinogenic. As mentioned earlier, vitamins C and E, β-carotenes, and selenium could be protective because of their antioxidant properties. Oxidants can cause mutations, the first step in carcinogenesis. However, to date there is no convincing evidence that these antioxidants do in fact act as chemopreventive agents.

Thus, we must conclude that despite many tantalizing trends and proclamations by "diet gurus," to date there is no definite proof that diet can cause or protect against cancer. Nonetheless, concern persists that carcinogens lurk in things as pleasurable as a juicy steak and rich ice cream.

BIBLIOGRAPHY

Al Jared N: Asbestos-related disease. J R Coll Physicians Lond 33:532, 1999. (An overview of the various manifestations of the disease.)

Bates CJ: Vitamin A. Lancet 345:31, 1995. (A succinct survey of this vitamin.)

Billings CH, Howard P: Asbestos exposure, lung cancer and asbestosis. Monaldi Arch Chest Dis 55:151, 2000. (A study of the carcinogenicity of asbestos.)

Burke W: Oral contraceptives and breast cancer. JAMA 284:1837, 2000. (A balanced view of a controversial subject.)

Castranova V, Vallyathan V: Silicosis and coal workers' pneumoconiosis. Environ Health Perspect 108(4S):675, 2000. (An excellent review article discussing the pathogenesis and histologic features of these two pneumoconioses.)

Chyka PA: Role of US poison centers in adverse drug reactions monitoring. Vet Human Toxicol 41:400, 1999. (A survey of the magnitude of the problem.)

Fraser DR: Vitamin D. Lancet 345:104, 1995. (A brief summary of the major causes and consequences of a deficiency of this vitamin.)

Greenberg ER, Sporn MB: Antioxidant vitamins, cancer and cardiovascular disease. N Engl J Med 334:1189, 1996.

Herbert R, Landrigan PJ: Work related death: a continuing epidemic. Am J Public Health 90:541, 2000.

Kamp DW, Weitzman SA: The molecular basis of asbestos induced lung injury. Thorax 54:638, 1999. (A topical review summarizing the proposed mechanisms of asbestos-related lung injury, especially the free radical pathway.)

Kelleher P, et al: Organic dust pneumonias: the metal-related parenchymal disorders. Environ Health Perspect 108(4S):685, 2000. (An excellent review of metal-induced lung disease, especially berylliosis.)

Kopelman PG: Obesity as a medical problem. Nature 404:635, 2000. (A discussion of epidemiology and associated morbidity of obesity.)

Markowitz M: Lead poisoning: a disease for the next millennium. Curr Probl Pediatr 30:62, 2000. (An overview of the magnitude of the problem.)

McDonald C: Silica and lung cancer: hazard or risk. Ann Occup Hyg 44:1, 2000 (A thought-provoking and balanced editorial in light of the elevation of silica to the status of a human carcinogen.)

Moerman CJ, et al: Postmenopausal hormone therapy: less favorable risk-benefits ratios in healthy Dutch women. J Intern Med 248:143, 2000. (An important review on this vexed issue.)

Mossman BT, Churg A: Mechanisms in the pathogenesis of asbestosis and silicosis. Am J Respir Crit Care Med 157:1666, 1998. (Another excellent review on pathogenesis of pneumoconiosis.)

Samet JM: Indoor radon exposure and lung cancer: risky or not—all over again. J Natl Cancer Inst 89:4, 1997. (Another evaluation of this controversial question.)

Samet JM, et al: Fine particulate air pollution and mortality in 20 US cities 1987–1994. N Engl J Med 343:1742, 2000. (A substantial study of the problem.)

Sesso JD, et al: Seven year changes in alcohol consumption and subsequent risk of cardiovascular disease in men. Arch Intern Med 160:2605, 2000. (A useful comment on alcohol and ischemic heart disease.)

Spiegelman B, Flier JS: Obesity and regulation of energy balance. Cell 104:531, 2001. (An excellent discussion of the genes and pathways that regulate energy balance.)

Sporer KA: Acute heroin overdose. Ann Intern Med 130:584, 1999. (A good survey of a major problem.)

Taylor R, et al: Passive smoking and lung cancer: a cumulative meta-analysis. Aust N Z J Public Health 25:203, 2001. (An exhaustive analysis of the subject.)

Triadale MJ: Biology of cachexia. J Natl Cancer Inst 89:1763, 1997. (An in-depth study of this common but poorly understood syndrome.)

Vandenbroucke JP, et al: Oral contraceptives and the risk of venous thrombosis. N Engl J Med 344:1527, 2001. (An up-to-date review of this important problem.)

General Pathology of Infectious Diseases

JOHN SAMUELSON, MD, PhD

Despite improved living conditions, widespread vaccination, and the availability of effective antibiotics, infectious diseases continue to take a heavy toll in the United States among persons debilitated with chronic disease, treated with immunosuppressive drugs, or suffering from acquired immunodeficiency syndrome (AIDS) in the absence of effective antiretroviral therapies. In developing countries, unsanitary living conditions and malnutrition contribute to a massive burden of infectious disease that kills more than 10 million persons each year. Most of these deaths are among children who suffer respiratory and diarrheal infections caused by viruses and bacteria. In addition, an increasing number of deaths in Africa and Asia occur among adults who are infected with human immunodeficiency virus (HIV) and cannot afford even the least expensive antiviral drugs.

HISTORY

Table 9–1 presents, in chronological sequence, 12 major breakthroughs in our understanding of infectious diseases and their causes, selected with the intent of providing a historical perspective for the concepts of microbial pathogenesis to be discussed here. Jenner's discovery in 1796 that milkmaids working with cows were resistant to smallpox paved the way to an understanding of cross-reactive immunity. Vaccinia virus (cowpox) induces immune reactions that neutralize subsequent infection with the much more virulent variola virus of smallpox. Because of a heroic vaccination campaign by the World Health Organization and others, smallpox is the first and only disease of humans that has been eradicated from the

Table 9-1. TWELVE MAJOR DISCOVERIES IN MICROBIAL PATHOGENESIS

Year	Investigator	Discovery
1796	Jenner	Vaccination against smallpox
1865	Pasteur	Proof of germ theory and beginning of modern biology
1882	Koch	Criteria for proof of causality in infectious disease
1884	Metchnikoff	Description of phagocytosis by macrophages
1902	Ross	Identification of mosquito vector for *Plasmodium falciparum* malaria
1906	Ehrlich	Description of chemotherapeutic agents
1908	Ellerman and Bang	Viral oncogenesis in chickens
1933	Lancefield	Serotyping of organisms and association of bacterial clones with disease
1945	Avery	Identification of DNA as genetic material and start of molecular biology revolution
1949	Enders	Culture of viruses and production of polio vaccine
1984	Montagnier and Gallo	Identification of HIV as cause of AIDS
1997	Venter	Sequence of genome of *Haemophilus influenzae*

earth. Metchnikoff's 1884 discovery of the process of phagocytosis, whereby leukocytes ingest foreign particles, initiated the study of white cells and cell-mediated immunity in the protection against infection.

Koch established the criteria for linking a specific microorganism to a specific disease: (1) the organism is regularly found in the lesions of the disease, (2) the organism can be isolated as single colonies on solid medium, (3) inoculation of this culture causes disease in an experimental animal, and (4) the organism can be recovered from lesions in the animal. A molecular version of Koch's postulates, suggested by Falkow, attempts to link a particular trait of an organism to a particular disease process. To this end, bacterial surface antigens defined by Lancefield's serotypes have been used to link particular bacterial strains with particular diseases (e.g., group A streptococci with scarlet fever, rheumatic heart disease, and glomerulonephritis). Avery identified DNA as the genetic material that encoded the pneumococcal capsule, an important virulence factor. The successful culture of polioviruses by Enders and Weller led to the development of a formalin-killed and attenuated live vaccine to prevent crippling infections by polio. Culture of HIV led to the development of tests for diagnosis and for screening blood and to antiviral therapies based on understanding the structure of particular HIV enzymes, although there is as yet no effective vaccine to prevent the pandemic.

Whole-genome sequencing of *Haemophilus influenzae* was made possible by Venter's use of numerous sequencing machines in parallel and large computers to assemble the data. Since 1996, the genomes of all the major bacterial pathogens have been sequenced, as have those of a number of fungi and parasites (e.g., *Candida albicans*, which causes systemic infections in immunosuppressed persons, and *Plasmodium falciparum*, which causes malaria). As expected, intracellular bacteria, which depend on the host for numerous metabolic functions, have the smallest genomes (~1000 genes), while extracellular bacteria have 3000 to 5000 genes. What was not expected was the exchange of hundreds of genes, particularly those involved in virulence, from one bacterium to another. For example, the enteroinvasive *Escherichia coli* serotype

0157:H7 has over 1300 genes more than the noninvasive K12 strain *E. coli*, which is used to make recombinant proteins. These extra genes are clustered together on bacterial chromosomes in so-called pathogenicity islands, which are often expressed together in response to particular host stimuli. Some of these virulence-associated genes have also been laterally transferred from bacteria to parasites (e.g., genes encoding fermentation enzymes of luminal protozoans, including *Entamoeba histolytica*, *Giardia lamblia*, and *Trichomonas vaginalis*). In contrast, *Mycobacterium leprae*, which causes leprosy, has lost more than 2000 protein-encoding genes in comparison with *Mycobacterium tuberculosis*.

Whole-genome sequencing of the human genome has revealed an orchestra of chemokines, cytokines, immunoglobulins, complement proteins, and antimicrobial peptides, which determine the host response to infectious agents. For example, granulomas in response to *M. tuberculosis* infection involve all types of T cells, including CD4+, CD8+, and double-negative cells. These antimicrobial responses are studied using microarray technologies, which reveal the activity of thousands of host cell genes in response to a particular infection, and by using "knockout" mice, in which the gene encoding the effector protein of interest has been deleted. These studies promise to produce a much richer description of the host response to infectious agents than the morphologic descriptions of inflammation at the end of this chapter.

NEW AND EMERGING INFECTIOUS DISEASES

Although infectious diseases such as leprosy have been known since biblical times and parasitic schistosomes have been demonstrated in Egyptian mummies, a surprising number of new infectious agents are described each year Table 9–2). The cause of some infections with significant morbidity and mortality (e.g., *Helicobacter* gastritis, hepatitis virus B and C (HBV and HCV) hepatitis, rotavirus diarrhea, and legionnaire's pneumonia) were previously unrecognized, because the infectious agent was difficult to culture. Some new infectious agents (e.g., Ebola virus, Hantaan virus, and

Table 9-2. SOME RECENTLY RECOGNIZED INFECTIOUS AGENTS

Year	Agent	Disease
1973	Rotavirus	Infantile diarrhea
1975	*Cryptosporidium parvum*	Acute and chronic diarrhea
1977	Ebola virus	Epidemic hemorrhagic fever
	Hantaan virus	Hemorrhagic fever with renal disease
	Legionella pneumophila	Legionnaire's pneumonia
	Campylobacter jejuni	Enteritis
1980	HTLV-I	T-cell lymphoma or leukemia
1981	*Staphylococcus aureus*	Toxic shock syndrome
1982	HTLV-II	Hairy cell leukemia
	Escherichia coli 0157:H7	Hemorrhagic colitis and hemolytic-uremic syndrome
	Borrelia burgdorferi	Lyme disease
1983	HIV	AIDS
	Helicobacter pylori	Chronic gastritis
1985	*Enterocytozoon bieneusi*	Chronic diarrhea
1988	HHV-6	Roseola exanthema subitum
	Hepatitis E	Enterically transmitted hepatitis
1989	Hepatitis C	Non-A, non-B hepatitis
	Ehrlichia chaffeensis	Human ehrlichiosis
1992	*Vibrio cholerae* 0139	New epidemic cholera strain
	Bartonella henselae	Cat-scratch disease
1993	*Encephalitozoon cuniculi*	Opportunistic infections
1995	HHV-8	Kaposi sarcoma in AIDS

HHV, human herpesvirus; HIV, human immunodeficiency virus; HTLV, human T-cell lymphotropic virus.
Adapted from Lederberg J: Infectious disease: An evolutionary paradigm. Emerg Infect Dis 3:417, 1997.

"flesh-eating bacteria" that cause streptococcal toxic shock syndrome) are newsworthy for their lethality, even though they are rare or infect persons in faraway places. Other infections may genuinely be new to humans (e.g., HIV, causing AIDS, and *Borrelia burgdorferi*, causing Lyme disease) or may be secondary to severe immunosuppression caused by AIDS (e.g., cytomegalovirus [CMV], human herpesvirus 8 [HHV-8], *Mycobacterium avium-intracellulare*, *Pneumocystis carinii*, and *Cryptosporidium parvum*).

Changes in the environment may increase the rates of infectious diseases: reforestation of the eastern part of the United States has led to massive increases in deer and mice, which carry the ticks that transmit Lyme disease, babesiosis, and ehrlichiosis. Failure of DDT to control mosquitoes that transmit malaria, in association with the development of drug-resistant parasites, has dramatically increased the morbidity and mortality of *P. falciparum* infection in Asia, Africa, and Latin America. Similarly, the development of new drug-resistant *M. tuberculosis*, *Neisseria gonorrhoeae*, *Staphylococcus aureus*, and *Enterococcus faecium* has had a significant impact on the treatment of these infections.

The goal of this chapter is to discuss mechanisms by which infectious organisms cause disease. In discussing these mechanisms, two separate but inter-related aspects must be considered: (1) the specific properties of the organisms causing the infection, and (2) the host response to infectious agents. Only a few of the many human infections are used to illustrate the concepts of microbial pathogenesis; greater coverage of particular organisms is found in the chapters that describe diseases by organ system (e.g., HBV in Chapter 16 and *M. tuberculosis* in Chapter 13). In addition, the roles of the immune system and immunodeficiencies (including AIDS) in microbial infection are discussed in Chapter 5.

CATEGORIES OF INFECTIOUS AGENTS

Organisms that cause infectious diseases range in size from the 20-nm poliovirus to the 10-m tapeworm *Taenia saginata* (Table 9–3).

Prions. Prions, which are apparently composed only of a modified host protein and so are not included in Table 9–3, cause spongiform encephalopathies including kuru (associated with human cannibalism) and Creutzfeldt-Jakob disease (CJD; associated with corneal transplants) (Chapter 23). Several cases of atypical CJD have occurred in England, where more than 100,000 cattle have died of prion-associated bovine spongiform encephalopathy, better known as "mad cow" disease. Infectious prion proteins (PrP^{sc}) are not viruses, because they lack RNA or DNA. PrP^{sc} proteins are protease resistant and combine with normal protease-sensitive host proteins (PrP^c) that are present on the surface of neurons. Infectious PrP^{sc} proteins then induce a conformational change on the normal PrP^c proteins, and abnormal complexes are internalized into neurons, damaging the cells and causing the spongiform encephalopathy.

Viruses. Animal viruses are obligate intracellular agents that depend on the host's metabolic machinery for their replication. Viruses are classified by the type of nucleic acid they contain—either DNA or RNA, but not both—and by the shape of their protein coat, or capsid. Viral pathogens account for a major share of all human infections, many of which cause acute illness (e.g., colds or influenza epidemics). Other viruses are not eliminated from the body but persist for years, continuing to multiply and remaining demonstrable (e.g., chronic infection with hepatitis B virus) or surviving in some latent noninfectious form with the potential to be reactivated later. For example, the herpes zoster virus, the cause of

Table 9-3. CATEGORIES OF HUMAN MICROBIAL PATHOGENS

Taxonomic Class	Size	Site of Propagation	Sample Species	Related Disease
Viruses	20–30 nm	Obligate intracellular	Poliovirus	Poliomyelitis
Chlamydiae	200–1000 nm	Obligate intracellular	Chlamydia trachomatis	Trachoma
Rickettsiae	300–1200 nm	Obligate intracellular	Rickettsia prowazekii	Typhus fever
Mycoplasmas	125–350 nm	Extracellular	Mycoplasma pneumoniae	Atypical pneumonia
Bacteria, spirochetes, mycobacteria	0.8–15 μm	Cutaneous	Staphylococcus epidermidis	Wound infection
		Mucosal	Vibrio cholerae	Cholera
		Extracellular	Streptococcus pneumoniae	Pneumonia
		Facultative intracellular	Mycobacterium tuberculosis	Tuberculosis
Fungi imperfecti	2–200 μm	Cutaneous	Trichophyton spp.	Tinea pedis ("athlete's foot")
		Mucosal	Candida albicans	Thrush
		Extracellular	Sporothrix schenckii	Sporotrichosis
		Facultative intracellular	Histoplasma capsulatum	Histoplasmosis
Protozoans	1–50 mm	Mucosal	Giardia lamblia	Giardiasis
		Extracellular	Trypanosoma gambiense	Sleeping sickness
		Facultative intracellular	Trypanosoma cruzi	Chagas disease
		Obligate intracellular	Leishmania donovani	Kala-azar
Helminths	3 mm–10 m	Mucosal	Enterobius vermicularis	Pinworm
		Extracellular	Wuchereria bancrofti	Filariasis
		Intracellular	Trichinella spiralis	Trichinosis

chickenpox, may persist in the dorsal root ganglia and be periodically activated to cause the painful skin condition called *shingles*. Different species of viruses can produce the same pathologic features (e.g., upper respiratory tract infections), and a single virus (e.g., CMV) can produce different clinical manifestations depending on the host's resistance and age (Chapter 13).

Because viruses are only 20 to 300 nm in size, individual viruses are best visualized with the electron microscope, where they may appear spherical if capsid proteins form an icosahedron or cylindrical if they form a helix. Some viral particles aggregate within the cells they infect and form characteristic *inclusion bodies*, which may be diagnostic with the light microscope. For example, CMV-infected cells are enlarged and show a large eosinophilic nuclear inclusion and smaller basophilic cytoplasmic inclusions (Fig. 9–1); herpesviruses form a large nuclear inclusion surrounded by a clear halo; and both smallpox and rabies viruses form characteristic cytoplasmic inclusions. Often viral inclusions are difficult to find (e.g., HBV), and many viruses do not give rise to inclusions (e.g., HIV, Epstein-Barr virus [EBV]).

Bacteriophages, Plasmids, and Transposons. Bacteriophages, plasmids, and transposons are mobile genetic elements that infect bacteria and indirectly cause human diseases by encoding bacterial virulence factors, including adhesins, toxins, and enzymes, that confer drug resistance. The addition of a bacteriophage or plasmid converts nonpathogenic bacteria into virulent ones, and plasmids encoding antibiotic resistance frequently make therapy difficult and expensive (e.g., therapy for vancomycin-resistant enterococci and methicillin-resistant staphylococci, both of which are endemic in many hospitals).

Bacteria. Bacteria are prokaryotes, which lack nuclei and endoplasmic reticulum. Bacteria have cell walls composed of two phospholipid bilayer membranes separated by a peptidoglycan layer (gram-negative organisms) or an inner membrane surrounded by a peptidoglycan layer (gram-positive organisms) (see Fig. 9–9).

A normal healthy person is colonized by as many as 10^{12} bacteria on the skin, 10^{10} bacteria in the mouth, and 10^{14} bacteria in the alimentary tract. Bacteria colonizing the skin include *Staphylococcus epidermidis*, *Corynebacterium* spp., and *Propionibacterium acnes* (the cause of acne among adolescents). Aerobic and anaerobic bacteria, particularly *Streptococcus mutans*, contribute to a dense microbial mass called *dental plaque*, a major cause of tooth decay. In the colon, more than 99.9% of bacteria are anaerobic, including *Bacteroides* spp. Many bacteria remain extracellular when they invade the body, whereas *facultative intracellular* bacteria (e.g., *Mycobacterium* spp.) can survive and replicate either outside of host cells or within host cells.

Chlamydiae, Rickettsias, and Mycoplasmas. These infectious agents are grouped together because they are

Figure 9-1

Cytomegalovirus. Distinct nuclear and ill-defined cytoplasmic inclusions in the lung.

similar to bacteria (they divide by binary fusion and are susceptible to antibiotics) but lack certain structures (e.g., *Mycoplasma* organisms do not have a rigid cell wall) or metabolic capabilities (e.g., *Chlamydia* spp. cannot synthesize ATP). Chlamydiae and rickettsiae are obligate intracellular agents that replicate in phagosomes of epithelial cells and in the cytoplasm of endothelial cells, respectively. *Chlamydia trachomatis* is the leading infectious cause of female sterility (by scarring and narrowing the fallopian tubes) and blindness (by trachoma, a chronic inflammation of the conjunctiva that eventually scars and opacifies the cornea).

Rickettsiae are transmitted by arthropod vectors, including lice (epidemic typhus), ticks (Q fever, Rocky Mountain spotted fever [RMSF]), and mites (scrub typhus). By injuring the endothelial cells, rickettsiae cause a hemorrhagic vasculitis that is often visible as a skin rash (Fig. 9–2), but they may also cause a transient pneumonia or hepatitis (Q fever) or injure the central nervous system and cause death (RMSF and epidemic typhus).

Mycoplasma organisms and the closely related *Ureaplasma* organisms are the tiniest free-living organisms known (125 to 300 nm). Infections with *Mycoplasma* spread from person to person in aerosols. The organisms bind to the surface of epithelial cells in the airways and cause an atypical pneumonia characterized by peribronchiolar infiltrates of lymphocytes and plasma cells (Chapter 13). *Ureaplasma* infections are transmitted venereally and may cause nongonococcal urethritis (NGU) (Chapter 18).

Fungi. Fungi possess thick, ergosterol-containing cell walls and grow as perfect, sexually reproducing forms in vitro and as imperfect forms in vivo; the latter include budding yeast cells and slender tubes (hyphae). Some yeast forms produce spores, which are resistant to extreme environmental conditions, while hyphae may produce fruiting bodies called *conidia*. Some fungal species (e.g., those of the *Tinea* group, which cause "athlete's foot") are confined to the superficial layers of the human skin; other "dermatophytes" preferentially damage the hair shafts or nails. Certain fungal species invade the subcutaneous tissue, causing abscesses or granulomas, as happens in sporotrichosis and in tropical mycoses.

Figure 9-3 ■

Mucicarmine stain of cryptococci in a Virchow-Robin perivascular space of the brain (soap-bubble lesion).

Deep fungal infections can spread systemically to destroy vital organs in immunocompromised hosts but heal spontaneously or remain latent in otherwise normal hosts. Some deep fungal species are limited to a particular geographic region (e.g., *Coccidioides* in the Far West and *Histoplasma* in the Ohio River Valley). Opportunistic fungi (e.g., *Candida, Aspergillus, Mucor,* and *Cryptococcus*; Fig. 9–3), by contrast, are ubiquitous contaminants colonizing the normal human skin or gut without causing illness. Only in immunosuppressed individuals do opportunistic fungi give rise to life-threatening infections, characterized by tissue necrosis, hemorrhage, and vascular occlusion, with minimal or no inflammatory response. In addition, AIDS patients are frequent victims of the opportunistic fungus-like organism *Pneumocystis carinii.*

Protozoal Parasites. Parasitic protozoans are motile, single-celled eukaryotes that are among the foremost causes of disease and death in developing countries (e.g., 1 million deaths per year caused by *P. falciparum* malaria). The simplest protozoal parasites are *Trichomonas* spp., which have a single flagellated form, are sexually transmitted, and colonize the vagina and the male urethra. The most prevalent intestinal protozoans are *E. histolytica* and *G. lamblia*, each of which has two forms: (1) motile trophozoites that attach to the intestinal epithelial wall and may invade *(E. histolytica)* and (2) immobile cysts that are infectious when eaten because they have a chitin wall that is resistant to stomach acids.

Protozoans that reside in plasma (e.g., *Trypanosoma brucei,* cause of African sleeping sickness), in red blood cells (e.g., *Plasmodium* spp.), and in macrophages (e.g., *Leishmania* spp.) are transmitted by insect vectors, in which they replicate extracellularly and are motile. *Toxoplasma,*

Figure 9-2 ■

Rocky Mountain spotted fever with thrombosed vessel and vasculitis.

an intracellular parasite that causes severe infections in individuals lacking cellular immunity (e.g., fetuses or AIDS patients), is acquired when humans ingest intramuscular cysts in undercooked meat.

Helminths. Parasitic worms are highly differentiated multicellular organisms. Their life cycles are complex; most alternate between sexual reproduction in the definitive host and asexual multiplication in an intermediary host or vector. Thus, depending on parasite species, humans may harbor adult worms (e.g., *Ascaris* spp.), immature forms (e.g., *Toxocara canis*), or asexual larval forms (e.g., *Echinococcus* spp.). Once adult worms become resident in humans they do not multiply, but they generate eggs or larvae destined for the next phase of the cycle. An exception is *Strongyloides*, the larvae of which can become infective inside the gut and cause overwhelming autoinfection in immunosuppressed persons. There are two important consequences of the lack of replication of adult worms: (1) disease is often caused by inflammatory responses to the eggs rather than to the adults (e.g., schistosomiasis; Fig. 9–4), and (2) the severity of disease is proportional to the number of organisms that have infected the host (e.g., 10 hookworms have little effect, whereas 1000 hookworms cause severe anemia by consuming 100 mL of blood per day).

Parasitic worms are of three classes. A collagenous tegument and a nonsegmented structure characterize the first class, *roundworms* (nematodes). These include *Ascaris* spp., hookworms, and *Strongyloides* spp. among the intestinal worms and the filariae and *Trichinella* spp. among the tissue invaders. The second class, *flatworms* (cestodes), comprises gutless worms, whose head (scolex) sprouts a ribbon of flat segments (proglottids) covered by an absorptive tegument. This class includes the pork, beef, and fish tapeworms and the cystic tapeworm larvae (cysticerci and hydatid cysts). The third class, *flukes* (trematodes), which are primitive leaflike worms with a syncytial integument, includes the Asian liver and lung flukes and the blood-dwelling schistosomes.

Ectoparasites. Ectoparasites are insects (lice, bedbugs, fleas) or arachnids (mites, ticks) that attach and live on or in the skin. These arthropods may cause itching and excori-

ations (e.g., pediculosis caused by lice attached to hair shafts, or scabies caused by mites burrowing into the stratum corneum). At the site of the bite, mouthparts may be found in association with a mixed infiltrate of lymphocytes, macrophages, and eosinophils. In addition, attached arthropods can be vectors for other pathogens that produce characteristic skin lesions (e.g., the expanding erythematous plaque caused by the Lyme disease spirochete *B. burgdorferi*, which is transmitted by deer ticks).

We now discuss the pathogenesis of infection, beginning with the normal host defenses against the entry and establishment of infectious agents and how these defenses can be overwhelmed.

HOST BARRIERS TO INFECTION AND HOW THEY BREAK DOWN

Host barriers to infection prevent access of microbes to the body and their subsequent spread throughout the tissues. The first barriers are intact skin and mucosal surfaces and the secretions that these surfaces produce (e.g., lysozyme in tears degrades the peptidoglycan wall of bacteria). These are formidable defenses against most infections. Only four of every 10 exposures to gonococci result in gonorrhea, and it takes 10^{11} vibrios to produce cholera in human volunteers with normal gastric juices. Still, some infectious agents are able to overcome these barriers, so that as few as 100 *Shigella* organisms, *Giardia* cysts, or *M. tuberculosis* organisms are sufficient to cause illness. In general, respiratory, gastrointestinal, and genitourinary tract infections occur in healthy persons and are caused by relatively virulent organisms that are able to damage intact epithelial barriers. In contrast, most skin infections are caused by less virulent organisms entering the skin through cuts or insect bites.

Skin

The human skin is normally inhabited by a variety of bacterial and fungal species, including some potential opportunists such as *S. epidermidis* and *C. albicans*. The dense, keratinized outer skin layer bearing resident microbes is constantly shed and renewed. The low pH of the skin (about 5.5) and the presence of fatty acids also inhibit microbial growth, but wet skin is more permeable to microorganisms. Human papillomavirus (HPV), the cause of venereal warts, and *Treponema pallidum*, the agent of syphilis, both penetrate warm, moist skin during sexual intercourse. Superficial infections of the stratum corneum of the epidermis by *S. aureus* (impetigo) or by cutaneous fungi are all aggravated by heat and humidity. Schistosome larvae released from freshwater snails penetrate swimmers' skin by releasing collagenase, elastase, and other enzymes that dissolve the extracellular matrix. Most other microorganisms penetrate through lesions in skin, including superficial pricks (fungal infections), deep wounds (staphylococci), burns (*Pseudomonas aeruginosa*), and diabetic and pressure-related foot sores (multibacterial infections). Intravenous catheters in hospitalized patients

Figure 9–4 ■

Schistosoma mansoni granuloma with a miracidium-containing egg *(center)* and numerous scattered eosinophils.

frequently cause bacteremia with *Staphylococcus* spp. or gram-negative organisms. Needle sticks, whether intentional (by needle-sharing drug abusers) or unintentional (accidental sticks by health care workers), expose the recipient to potentially infected blood and may transmit HBV, HCV, and HIV. Bites by fleas, ticks, mosquitoes, mites, and lice break the skin and transmit diverse infectious organisms, including arboviruses (causes of yellow fever and encephalitis), rickettsiae, bacteria (plague, Lyme disease), protozoans (malaria, leishmaniasis), and helminths (filariasis). Animal bites may cause infections with anaerobic bacteria or with the deadly rabies virus.

Urogenital Tract

Even though urine can support the growth of many bacteria, the urinary tract is normally sterile because it is flushed many times per day. Women have more than 10 times as many urinary tract infections (UTIs) as men, because the distance between the urinary bladder and the bacteria-laden skin (i.e., the length of the urethra) is 5 cm in women, compared with 20 cm in men. In addition, girls and boys with obstruction of urinary flow and/or reflux of urine into the ureters are much more susceptible to UTIs. When UTI spreads retrogradely from the bladder to the kidney, it causes acute and chronic pyelonephritis (Chapter 14), which is the major preventable cause of renal failure. The pathogens that infect the urinary tract (mostly bacteria from the perianal area or from an infected sexual partner [e.g., with *Gonococcus*]) are those that adhere best to the epithelium of the urinary tract. Most acute UTIs are caused by a few strains of *E. coli* that have adherent fimbriae, while chronic infections are caused by *Proteus*, *Pseudomonas*, *Klebsiella*, or *Enterococcus* spp., which are often drug resistant.

Respiratory Tract

Some 10,000 microorganisms, including viruses, bacteria, and fungi, are inhaled daily by every city inhabitant. The distance these microorganisms travel into the respiratory system is inversely proportional to their size. Large microbes are trapped in the mucociliary blanket that lines the nose and the upper respiratory tract. Microorganisms are trapped in the mucus secreted by goblet cells and are then transported by ciliary action to the back of the throat, where they are swallowed and cleared. Organisms smaller than 5 μm travel directly to the alveoli, where they are phagocytosed by alveolar macrophages or by neutrophils recruited to the lung by cytokines.

Damage to the mucociliary defense results from repeated insults in smokers and patients with cystic fibrosis, whereas acute injury occurs in intubated patients and in those who aspirate gastric acid. Virulent respiratory pathogens escape the intact mucociliary defense by attaching via hemagglutinins to carbohydrates on epithelial cells in the lower respiratory tract and pharynx (e.g., influenzavirus). Furthermore, influenza, parainfluenza, and mumps viruses use viral neuraminidase to lower the viscosity of mucus and free themselves from entrapment. Certain organisms (e.g., *H. influenzae*) release

factors that inhibit ciliary motion. Secondary respiratory infections with *Streptococcus pneumoniae* or *Staphylococcus* spp., which lack specific adherence factors, occur after viral damage to epithelial cells. *M. tuberculosis* causes respiratory infection, because it is able to escape phagocytotic killing by the macrophage. Finally, opportunistic fungi infect the lungs when cellular immunity is depressed or when leukocytes are deficient in number (e.g., *P. carinii* in AIDS patients and *Aspergillus* spp. in patients receiving chemotherapy).

Intestinal Tract

Most gastrointestinal pathogens are transmitted by food or drink contaminated with fecal material. Sanitary disposal of waste and vermin, clean drinking water, hand washing, and thorough cooking of food can therefore reduce exposure. Where hygiene fails, diarrheal disease becomes rampant.

Normal defenses against ingested pathogens include (1) acid gastric juice, (2) the viscous mucus layer covering the gut, (3) lytic pancreatic enzymes and bile detergents, and (4) secreted immunoglobulin A (IgA) antibodies. IgA antibodies are made by B cells located in mucosa-associated lymphoid tissues (MALTs), which are covered by a single layer of specialized epithelial cells called M cells. M cells are important for transport of antigen to MALT and for binding and/or uptake of numerous gut pathogens, including poliovirus, enteropathic *E. coli*, *Vibrio cholerae*, *Salmonella typhi*, and *Shigella flexneri*.

Pathogenic organisms must compete for nutrients with abundant commensal bacteria resident in the lower gut, and all gut microbes are intermittently expelled by defecation. Host defenses are weakened by low gastric acidity, by antibiotics that unbalance the normal bacterial flora (e.g., pseudomembranous colitis [Chapter 15]), or when there is stalled peristalsis or mechanical obstruction (e.g., blind loop syndrome). Most enveloped viruses are killed by the digestive juices, but nonenveloped ones may be resistant (e.g., the hepatitis A virus, rotaviruses, reoviruses, and Norwalk agents). Rotaviruses directly damage the intestinal epithelial cells they infect, whereas reoviruses pass through mucosal M cells into the bloodstream without any detectable local cell injury.

Enteropathogenic bacteria elicit gastrointestinal disease by a variety of mechanisms. (1) While growing on contaminated food, certain staphylococcal strains release powerful enterotoxins that, on ingestion, cause food-poisoning symptoms without any bacterial multiplication in the gut. (2) *V. cholerae* and toxigenic *E. coli* multiply inside the mucus layer overlying the gut epithelium and release exotoxins that cause the gut epithelium to secrete excessive volumes of watery diarrhea. (3) By contrast, *Shigella*, *Salmonella*, and *Campylobacter* organisms invade and damage the intestinal mucosa and lamina propria and so cause ulceration, inflammation, and hemorrhage, clinically manifested as dysentery (Fig. 9–5). (4) *S. typhi* passes from the damaged mucosa through Peyer patches and mesenteric lymph nodes and into the bloodstream, resulting in a systemic infection.

Fungal infection of the gastrointestinal tract occurs mainly in immunologically compromised patients. *Candida* organisms show a predilection for stratified squamous epithelium, causing oral thrush or membranous esophagitis,

Figure 9–5 ■

Close-up of colonic mucosa in *Shigella* colitis with erythema, ulceration, and pseudomembrane formation (white plaques).

but they may also disseminate to the stomach, lower gastrointestinal tract, and systemic organs.

The cyst forms of intestinal protozoans are essential for their transmission because cysts resist stomach acid. In the gut, cysts convert to motile trophozoites and attach to sugars on the intestinal epithelia via surface lectins. Thereafter, there is wide species variation: *G. lamblia* attaches to the epithelial brush border, whereas *Cryptosporidium* organisms are taken up by enterocytes, in which they form gametes and spores. *E. histolytica* causes contact-mediated cytolysis analogous to that of cytotoxic T lymphocytes by releasing a channel-forming pore protein that depolarizes and kills its cellular prey (Fig. 9–6). In this manner, the colonic mucosa is ulcerated and invaded. Intestinal helminths, as a rule, cause disease only when present in large numbers or in ectopic sites, for example, by obstructing the gut or invading and damaging the bile ducts *(Ascaris)*. Hookworms may cause iron deficiency anemia by chronic loss of blood, sucked from intestinal villi; the fish tapeworm, *Diphyllobothrium*, competes with and can deplete its host of vitamin B_{12}, giving rise to an illness resembling pernicious anemia. Finally, the larvae of several helminth parasites pass through the gut briefly on their way toward another organ habitat; for example, *Trichinella* larvae preferentially encyst in muscle, and *Echinococcus* larvae in the liver or lung.

Figure 9–6 ■

Amebiasis of the colon with three *Entamoeba histolytica* trophozoites.

Spread of Microbes Throughout the Body

Microbes spread rapidly along the wet epithelial surfaces of the intestines, lungs, and genitourinary tract and slowly, if at all, on the dry surface of the skin (Fig. 9–7). Many microbes do not travel beyond the epithelium because they proliferate only in superficial layers of epithelia (e.g., HPV organisms), but others are able to penetrate (e.g., streptococci and staphylococci, which secrete hyaluronidase, which degrades the extracellular matrix between host cells). The routes of microbial spread initially follow tissue planes of least resistance and the regional lymphatic and vascular anatomy. For example, staphylococci cause a locally expanding skin abscess (furuncle), followed by a regional lymphadenitis that sometimes leads to bacteremia (bloodborne infection) and colonization of distant organs deep to the body's surfaces (heart, liver, brain, spleen, bones). Once in the blood, organisms are transported by a variety of means. HBV and polioviruses, most bacteria and fungi, occasional protozoal parasites (e.g., African trypanosomes), and all helminths are transported free in the plasma. Herpesviruses, HIV, CMV, and *Mycobacterium*, *Leishmania*, and *Toxoplasma* organisms are carried by leukocytes. Certain viruses (e.g., Colorado tick fever virus) and parasites (e.g., *Plasmodium* and *Babesia* organisms) are carried by red cells.

Dissemination of pathogens in the blood can lead to systemic signs of infection, including fever, which is caused by host cytokines released in response to bacterial endotoxin (Chapter 2). Massive sustained bloodstream invasion by pyogenic bacteria and certain parasites (e.g., *Plasmodium* species, causing malaria) may be fatal. Infectious foci disseminated by blood are called *secondary foci* and usually have a widespread distribution, either in a single organ (e.g., miliary, or seedlike, distribution of progressive tuberculosis within the lung) or through many tissues (e.g., microabscesses throughout the kidneys, intestines, and skin caused by septic emboli shed from a staphylococcal aortic valve infection). Invasive microbes quickly spread within serosalined cavities such as the pleura, peritoneum, and meninges.

Frequently, organisms cause major disease manifestations at sites distant from the point of entry. For example, the chickenpox virus enters through the lungs but causes rashes in the skin; polioviruses enter through the intestine but selectively cause damage to motor neurons; and *Schistosoma*

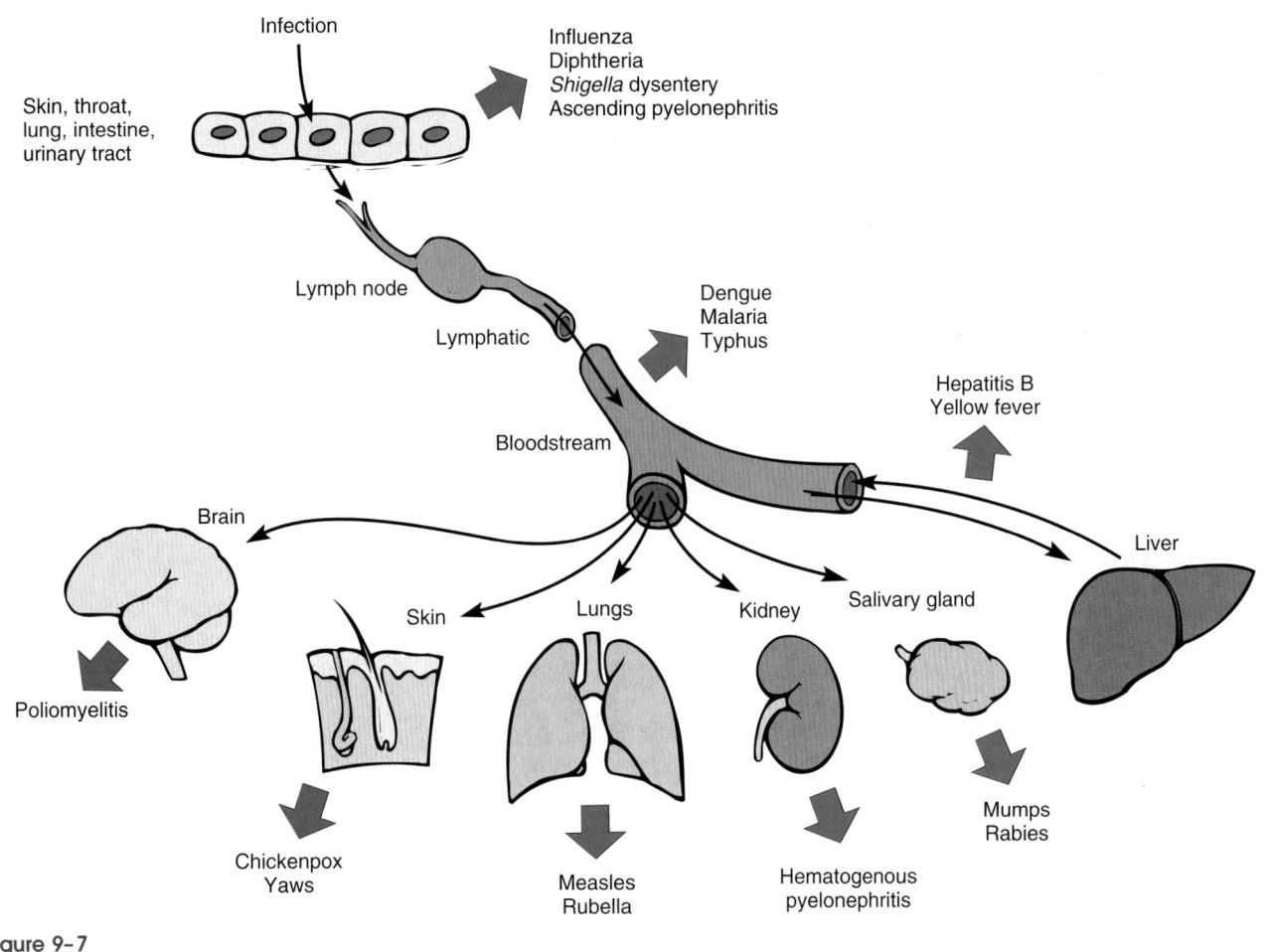

Infection

Skin, throat,
lung, intestine,
urinary tract

Influenza
Diphtheria
Shigella dysentery
Ascending pyelonephritis

Lymph node

Lymphatic

Dengue
Malaria
Typhus

Bloodstream

Hepatitis B
Yellow fever

Brain

Liver

Skin

Lungs

Kidney

Salivary gland

Poliomyelitis

Mumps
Rabies

Chickenpox
Yaws

Measles
Rubella

Hematogenous
pyelonephritis

Figure 9–7 ■

Routes of entry, dissemination, and release of microbes from the body. (Adapted from Mims CA: The Pathogenesis of Infectious Disease. Orlando, FL, Academic, 1987.)

mansoni organisms penetrate the skin but eventually localize in blood vessels of the portal system and the mesentery, causing damage to the liver and intestines. *Rhabdovirus* organisms, causing rabies, track to the brain in a retrograde fashion along nerves, while the varicella-zoster virus, after its viremic phase, hides in dorsal root ganglia, whence it may travel along the nerves and cause shingles.

Severe damage to the developing fetus occurs when infectious organisms circulate in the mother's blood or reach the uterus from the vagina to infect the placenta and the fetus. Placental or fetal infections with bacteria frequently cause premature birth or stillbirth, while viral infections can also cause maldevelopment of the fetus, depending on the time of infection (Chapter 7). Rubella infection in the first trimester may cause congenital heart disease, mental retardation, cataracts, or deafness in the infant, whereas little damage is caused by rubella infection in the third trimester. In contrast, transmission of treponemes gives rise to syphilis only when the organisms invade the fetus late in the second trimester, but then they cause a severe fetal osteochondritis and periostitis that leads to multiple bony lesions (Chapter 18).

Because the fetus receives antibodies but not sensitized T cells from the mother, opportunistic pathogens common to AIDS patients (e.g., CMV, herpesviruses, and *Toxoplasma* spp.) may cause severe damage to the fetus. During

the birth process, infants can also become infected with the mother's viruses and bacteria, which may subsequently cause AIDS (HIV), chronic hepatitis or liver cancer (HBV), blindness (*Chlamydia* spp.), and multisystem organ failure (herpesviruses).

Release of Microbes from the Body

For transmission of disease, the exit of infectious agents from the host's body is as important as their entry into it. Many of the mechanisms by which infectious organisms are cleared from the infected individual are responsible for their spread from one person to another, including skin shedding, coughing, sneezing, urination, and defecation. Stool pathogens that are resistant to drying (e.g., bacterial spores, protozoal cysts, nematode eggs) survive in the environment for a long time, whereas certain viruses must be quickly passed from person to person, often by direct contact. Stool-contaminated food and water are important vehicles for spread of epidemic and endemic pathogens. Viruses that infect the salivary glands (e.g., herpesvirus, mumps virus) are released during talking, singing, spitting, and kissing. All classes of organisms may be transmitted by intimate mucosal or venereal contact, including viruses (e.g., herpesvirus,

HPV, HBV, HIV), *Chlamydia*, bacteria *(T. pallidum* and *N. gonorrhoeae)*, fungi *(Candida* spp.), protozoans *(Trichomonas* spp.*)*, and arthropods *(Phthirus pubis,* or crab lice). Microorganisms transmitted by blood-sucking arthropods must be in the blood to infect the next insect that feeds, even when the major lesions caused by them are in the brain (viral encephalitis), liver, spleen *(Leishmania donovani),* or heart *(Trypanosoma cruzi* in Chagas disease).

HOW INFECTIOUS AGENTS CAUSE DISEASE

Having reviewed the manner by which infectious agents break host barriers, we next examine how they injure cells and cause tissue damage. There are three general mechanisms:

1. Infectious agents can contact or enter host cells and directly cause cell death.
2. Pathogens can release endotoxins or exotoxins that kill cells at a distance, release enzymes that degrade tissue components, or damage blood vessels and cause ischemic injury.
3. Pathogens can induce host cell responses that may cause additional tissue damage, usually by immune-mediated mechanisms.

Immune-mediated injury is discussed in Chapter 5. Here we describe some of the specific mechanisms whereby viruses and certain bacteria cause cell and tissue injury.

Mechanisms of Virus-Induced Injury

Viruses damage host cells by entering the cell and replicating at the host's expense. They have specific surface viral proteins (ligands) that bind to particular host proteins (receptors), many of which have known functions. For example, HIV binds to CD4, which is involved in T-cell activation, and to chemokine receptors; EBV binds to the complement receptor on macrophages; and rhinoviruses bind to intercellular adhesion molecule 1 (ICAM-1) on mucosal cells. For several viruses, x-ray crystallographic studies have identified the specific part of the viral attachment protein that binds to a particular segment of the host cell receptor.

The presence or absence of host cell proteins that allow the virus to attach is one reason for *viral tropism,* or the tendency of certain viruses to infect specific cells but not others. For example, influenzaviruses replicate in respiratory epithelial cells, which express a protease necessary for cleaving and activating the hemagglutinin on the surface of the virus. A second major cause of viral tropism is the ability of the virus to replicate inside some cells but not in others. For example, JC papovavirus, which causes leukoencephalopathy, is restricted to oligodendroglia in the central nervous system because JC virus promoter and enhancer DNA sequences up-stream from the viral genes are active in glial cells but not in neurons or endothelial cells.

Once attached, the entire virion, or a portion containing the genome and essential polymerases, penetrates the cell cytoplasm by (1) translocation of the entire virus across the plasma membrane, (2) fusion of the viral envelope with the cell membrane, or (3) receptor-mediated endocytosis and fusion with endosomal membranes. Within the cell, the virus uncoats, separating its genome from its structural components and losing its infectivity. Viruses then replicate, using enzymes that are distinct for each virus family. For example, RNA polymerase is used by negative-sense RNA viruses to generate positive-sense messenger RNA (mRNA), while reverse transcriptase is used by retroviruses to generate DNA from their RNA template. These virus-specific enzymes provide points at which drugs may be used to inhibit viral replication. The subgroup of HIV that is present in southern Africa is particularly virulent because its transcription is markedly increased by inflammatory cytokines, such as tumor necrosis factor (TNF), that are induced by concurrent infection with other microbes. Viruses also use host enzymes for viral synthesis, and such enzymes may be present in some but not all tissues. Newly synthesized viral genomes and capsid proteins are assembled into progeny virions in the nucleus or cytoplasm and are either released directly (unencapsulated viruses) or bud through the plasma membrane (encapsulated viruses).

Viruses kill host cells and cause tissue damage in a number of ways (Fig. 9–8):

■ Viruses may inhibit host cell DNA, RNA, or protein synthesis. For example, the poliovirus inactivates "cap-binding protein," which is essential for translation of host cell mRNAs, but leaves translation of poliovirus mRNAs unaffected.
■ Viral proteins may insert into the host cell's plasma membrane and directly damage its integrity or promote cell fusion (HIV, measles, and herpesviruses).
■ Viruses replicate efficiently and lyse host cells. For example, respiratory epithelial cells are killed by explosive rhinovirus or influenzavirus multiplication, liver cells by yellow fever virus, and neurons by poliovirus or rabies viruses.
■ Viral proteins on the surface of the host cells may be recognized by the immune system, and the host lymphocytes may attack the virus-infected cells. For example, acute liver failure during HBV infection may be accelerated by Fas ligands on cytotoxic T lymphocytes, which bind to Fas receptors on the surface of hepatocytes and induce apoptosis (programmed cell death) in target cells. Respiratory syncytial virus, a major cause of lower respiratory infections in infants, causes release of cytokines interleukin 4 (IL-4) and IL-5 from T_H2-type helper T cells, which cause mast cell and eosinophil activation, respectively, inducing wheezing and asthma.
■ Viruses may also damage cells involved in host antimicrobial defense, leading to secondary infections. For example, viral damage to respiratory epithelium predisposes to the subsequent development of pneumonia caused by pneumococci or *Haemophilus* organisms, while HIV depletes CD4+ helper lymphocytes and opens the floodgates for many opportunistic infections.
■ Viral killing of cells of one type may cause damage to other cells that are dependent on their integrity. Denervation by the attack of poliovirus on motor neurons causes atrophy, and sometimes death, of distal skeletal muscle cells.

Figure 9–8

Mechanisms by which viruses cause injury to cells.

■ Slow viral infections (e.g., subacute sclerosing panencephalitis caused by measles virus) culminate in severe, progressive disease after a long latency period.

In addition to all the potential mechanisms of killing cells, viruses (e.g., EBV, HPV, HBV, and human T-cell lymphotropic virus I [HTLV-I]) can cause cell proliferation and transformation, resulting in cancer (Chapter 6).

Mechanisms of Bacteria-Induced Injury: Bacterial Adhesins and Toxins

Bacterial damage to host tissues depends on the ability of the bacteria to adhere to and enter host cells or to deliver toxins. *The coordination of bacterial adherence and toxin delivery is so important to bacterial virulence that the genes encoding adherence proteins and toxins are frequently coregulated by specific environmental signals.* For example, changes in temperature, osmolarity, or pH trigger the synthesis by *Bordetella pertussis* of some 20 different proteins, including the filamentous hemagglutinin, fimbrial proteins, and pertussis toxin. Similarly, the virulence of enterotoxic *E. coli* depends on the expression of adherence proteins that allow the bacteria to bind to the intestinal epithelial cells and coordinate synthesis and release of heat-labile or heat-stable toxins that cause intestinal cells to secrete isotonic fluids.

Bacterial Adhesins. Bacterial adhesins are molecules that bind bacteria to host cells. They are limited in type but have a broad range of host cell specificity. The surface of gram-positive cocci such as streptococci is covered with two molecules that may mediate adherence of the bacteria to host cells (Fig. 9–9). First, *lipoteichoic acids* are hydrophobic molecules that bind to the surface of all eukaryotic cells but have a higher affinity to particular receptors on blood cells and oral epithelial cells. Second, a nonfibrillar adhesin called *protein F* binds to fibronectin, an extracellular matrix protein also found on most host cells. M proteins, which form fibrillae on the surface of gram-positive bacteria and their carbohydrate capsules prevent phagocytosis by host macrophages. In the case of pneumococci, a transparent form, which has a narrow capsule, is adapted to bind to nasopharyngeal epithelium, while an opaque form, which has a thick capsule, is adapted to survive in the blood.

Fimbriae, or *pili*, on the surface of gram-negative rods and cocci are nonflagellar filamentous structures composed of repeating subunits. While sex pili are used to exchange genes carried on plasmids or transposons from one bacterium to another, most pili mediate adherence of bacteria to host cells. The base of the subunit that anchors the pilus to the bacterial cell wall is similar for widely divergent bacteria (e.g., *Mycobacterium, Pseudomonas, Neisseria*). At the tips of the pili are minor protein components that determine to which host cells the microbes will attach (bacterial tropism). In *E. coli*, these minor proteins are antigenically distinct and are associated with particular infections (e.g., type I proteins bind mannose and cause lower urinary tract infections, type P proteins bind galactose and cause pyelonephritis, type S proteins bind sialic acid and cause meningitis). A single bacterium can express more than one type of pilus, as well as adhesins not located in pili (e.g., proteins I and II of gonococci). Other molecules on the surface of gram-negative bacteria important for virulence are lipopolysaccharides and a carbohydrate capsule (discussed later).

Figure 9-9

Some molecules on the surface of gram-negative and gram-positive bacteria involved in pathogenesis of bacterial diseases.

Unlike viruses, which infect a broad range of host cells, facultative intracellular bacteria are more restricted and infect epithelial cells (*Shigella* and enteroinvasive *E. coli*), macrophages (*M. tuberculosis, M. leprae*), or both (*S. typhi*). Bacterial proteins involved in attachment and invasion are often coregulated and exported by a type III secretory machine, which transports proteins across the bacterial envelope and injects them into the cytosol of the target cell. Most of these bacteria attach to host cell integrins, plasma membrane proteins that bind complement, or extracellular matrix proteins, including fibronectin, laminin, and collagen (Chapter 3). For example, *Legionella* organisms, *M. tuberculosis*, and the protozoan *Leishmania* all bind to CR3, the cell receptor for complement C3bi. Enteropathic *E. coli* secretes a protein that inserts into the target cell plasma membrane and is used by the bacterium as an additional attachment site for the bacterium. *Shigella* secretes proteins that reorganize the cytoskeleton of target epithelial cells and enclose the bacterium. Once in the cytoplasm, *Shigella* and *E. coli* inhibit host protein synthesis, rapidly replicate, and within 6 hours lyse the host cells. In contrast, *Salmonella* and *Yersinia* organisms replicate within the phagolysosomes of the macrophage, while *Mycobacterium* and *Legionella* organisms inhibit the acidification that normally occurs after endosome fusion with the lysosome. Within the phagolysosome, *Salmonella* organisms secrete a second set of proteins by the type III apparatus, while *Legionella* organisms use a type IV secretory apparatus to disrupt the endocytic process. In the absence of a host cellular immune response, many replicating organisms persist within the macrophages (e.g., lepromatous leprosy, *M. avium-intracellulare* infection in AIDS patients), but activated macrophages can kill these organisms or limit their growth.

Bacterial Endotoxin. Bacterial endotoxin is a lipopolysaccharide (LPS) that is a structural component of the outer cell wall of gram-negative bacteria. Lipopolysaccharide is composed of a long-chain fatty acid anchor (lipid A) connected to a core sugar chain, both of which are the same in all gram-negative bacteria. Attached to the core sugar is a variable carbohydrate chain (O antigen), which is used to serotype and distinguish different bacteria. The many biologic activities of endotoxins are discussed elsewhere in this book and include induction of fever (Chapter 2), septic shock (Chapter 4), disseminated intravascular coagulation (Chapter 12), the acute respiratory distress syndrome (Chapter 13), and a variety of effects on cells of the immune system. All the biologic activities of endotoxin come from lipid A and the core sugars. They are mediated both by direct effects of endotoxin and by the induction of host cytokines such as IL-1, TNF, and others.

Bacterial superantigens (e.g., *Staphylococcus* enterotoxins and toxic shock syndrome toxin [TSST]) cause fever, shock, and multisystem organ failure by a mechanism distinct from that of endotoxin. Bacterial superantigens bind to the major histocompatibility complex (MHC) class II molecules on the surface of many antigen-presenting cells (APCs), without the usual internal processing or discrimination (Chapter 5). These superantigen-containing APCs then indiscriminately stimulate numerous T cells to secrete excess IL-2, which in turn causes overproduction of TNF and other cytokines responsible for the systemic disturbances.

Bacterial Exotoxins. Bacterial exotoxins are secreted proteins that directly cause cellular injury and determine disease manifestations. For example, lethal factor, which is the exotoxin of *Bacillus anthracis*, was likely responsible for the fifth and sixth plagues of Egypt. Because anthrax forms spores, which are heat resistant and infect by aerosols, this bacterium has great potential as a biologic weapon. Diphtheria toxin is composed of fragment B (the carboxyl end) and fragment A (the amino end), which are held together by a disulfide bridge (Fig. 9–10). The toxin binds to glycoproteins on the surface of target cells via its carboxyl end and enters the acidic endosome, where it fuses with the endosomal membrane and enters the cell cytoplasm. Within the cytoplasm, the disulfide bond of diphtheria toxin is reduced and broken, releasing the enzymatically active amino fragment A of the toxin, which catalyzes the covalent transfer of adenosine diphosphate (ADP)–ribose from nicotinamide adenine dinucleotide (NAD) to EF-2 (an elongation factor in polypeptide synthesis), inactivating it. One toxin molecule can kill a cell by ADP-ribosylating more than 10^6 EF-2 molecules. The effect of the toxin is to create a layer of dead cells in the throat, on which *Corynebacterium diphtheriae* bacteria

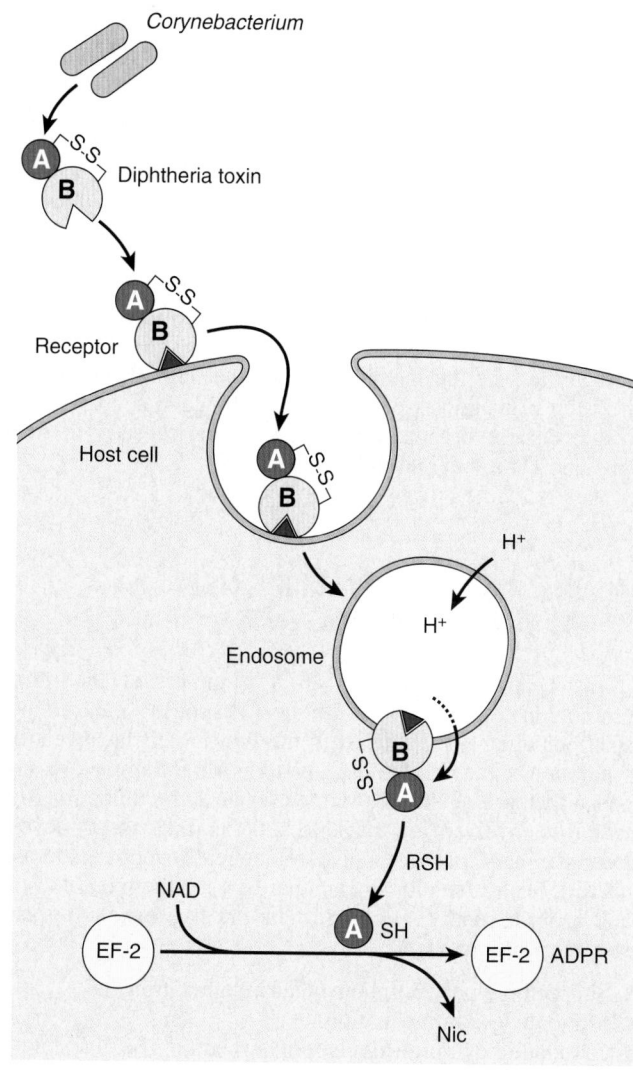

Figure 9–10

Inhibition of cellular protein synthesis by diphtheria toxin. See text for abbreviations. (Adapted from Collier RJ: Corynebacteria. In Davis BD, et al [eds]: Microbiology. New York, Harper & Row, 1990.)

the spinal interneurons. This results in violent muscle contractions that characterize tetanic spasm. *Clostridium botulinum* toxins block the release of cholinergic neurotransmitters, particularly at the neuromuscular junctions, resulting in progressive paralysis of the limbs, respiratory muscles, and cranial motor nerves. Remarkably, both botulinum and tetanus toxins are endopeptidases that cleave synaptobrevins, which are proteins involved in synaptic vesicle formation.

IMMUNE EVASION BY MICROBES

Humoral and cellular immune responses that protect the host from most infections and the mechanisms of immune-mediated damage to host tissues induced by microbes (e.g., anaphylactic reactions, immune complex reactions) were discussed in Chapter 5. Here, we focus on the ways in which microorganisms escape the host immune system by (1) remaining inaccessible; (2) cleaving antibody, resisting complement-mediated lysis, or surviving in phagocytotic cells; (3) varying or shedding antigens; and (4) causing specific or nonspecific immunosuppression.

Microbes that propagate in the lumen of the intestine (e.g., toxin-producing *Clostridium difficile*) or gallbladder (e.g., *S. typhi*) are inaccessible to the host immune defenses, including secretory IgA. Viruses shed from the luminal surface of epithelial cells (e.g., CMV in urine or milk and poliovirus in stool) or those that infect the keratinized epithelium (poxviruses that cause molluscum contagiosum) are also inaccessible to the host humoral immune system. Some organisms establish infections by rapidly invading host cells before the host humoral response becomes effective (e.g., malaria sporozoites entering liver cells; *Trichinella* and *T. cruzi* entering skeletal and cardiac muscles, respectively). Some larger parasites (e.g., the larvae of tapeworms) form cysts in host tissues that are covered by a dense fibrous capsule that walls them off from host immune responses.

The carbohydrate capsule on the surface of all the major pathogens that cause pneumonia or meningitis (*Streptococcus pneumoniae*, *Neisseria meningitides*, *Haemophilus*, *Klebsiella*, and *E. coli*) makes them more virulent by covering bacterial antigens and preventing phagocytosis of the organisms by neutrophils. *Pseudomonas* bacteria secrete a leukotoxin that kills neutrophils. Some *E. coli* have K antigens that prevent activation of complement by the alternative pathway and lysis of the cells. Conversely, some gram-negative bacteria have very long polysaccharide O antigens that bind host antibody and activate complement at such a distance from the bacterial cells that the organisms fail to lyse. Staphylococci are covered by protein A molecules that bind the Fc portion of the antibody and so inhibit phagocytosis. *Neisseria*, *Haemophilus*, and *Streptococcus* spp. all secrete proteases that degrade antibodies.

Viral infection evokes neutralizing antibodies, which prevent viral attachment, penetration, or uncoating. This highly specific immunity is the basis of antiviral

outgrow competing bacteria. Subsequently, wide dissemination of diphtheria toxin causes neural and myocardial dysfunction. The heat-labile enterotoxins of *V. cholerae* and of *E. coli* also have an A-B structure and are ADP-ribosyl transferases, but these enzymes catalyze transfer from NAD to the guanyl nucleotide–dependent regulatory component of adenylate cyclase. This generates excess cyclic adenosine monophosphate (cAMP), which causes intestinal epithelial cells to secrete isosmotic fluid, resulting in voluminous diarrhea and loss of water and electrolytes.

The gram-positive anaerobic *Clostridium perfringens*, the agent of gas gangrene, literally digests host tissues, including the relatively resistant collagens. Its α toxin is a lecithinase that disrupts plasma membranes, including those of red and white blood cells. *Clostridium tetani*, a wound contaminant, secretes an exotoxin called *tetanospasmin* that interferes with release of inhibitory transmitter substances such as γ-aminobutyric acid from presynaptic terminals of vaccination, but it cannot protect against viruses with many antigenic variants (e.g., rhinoviruses or influenzaviruses). Pneumococci are capable of more than 80 permutations of their capsular polysaccharides, so that in repeated infections the host is unlikely to recognize the new serotype. *N. gonorrhoeae* have pilar (attachment) proteins composed of a constant region and a hypervariable region. One species of *Neisseria* can take up DNA from another *Neisseria* species and so is able to change its repertoire of attachment proteins in the absence of mutation. The spirochete *Borrelia recurrentis* causes a relapsing fever by repeatedly switching its surface antigens before the host exterminates each successive clone. Successive clones of African trypanosomes also vary their major surface antigen to escape host antibody responses. Cercariae of *S. mansoni* shed and so get rid of parasite antigens, which are recognized by host antibodies within minutes of penetrating the skin. Finally, viruses that infect lymphocytes (HIV and EBV) directly damage the host immune system and cause opportunistic infections (e.g., AIDS).

SPECIAL TECHNIQUES FOR DIAGNOSIS OF INFECTIOUS AGENTS

Some infectious agents or their products can be directly observed in H & E–stained sections (e.g., the inclusion bodies formed by CMV and herpesvirus; bacterial clumps, which usually stain blue; *Candida* and *Mucor*, among the fungi; most protozoans; and all helminths). However, many infectious agents are best visualized after staining with special stains that identify organisms based on particular characteristics of their cell walls or coat (Gram, acid-fast, silver, mucicarmine, and Giemsa stains) or after labeling with specific antibody probes (Table 9–4). Regardless of the staining technique, organisms are usually best visualized at the advancing edge of a lesion rather than at its center, particularly if there is necrosis. Because these morphologic techniques cannot speciate organisms, determine drug sensitivity, or identify virulence characteristics, cultures of lesional tissue must be performed. Poly-

merase chain reaction (PCR)–based methods are used to identify microbes that grow slowly in culture (*Mycobacterium* or CMV organisms) or cannot be cultured at all (HBV and HCV). DNA sequence analysis has been used to classify bacteria that have never been cultured, including those that cause Whipple disease (a gram-positive actinobacterium called *Tropheryma whippelii*) and hepatic peliosis and bacillary angiomatosis (a rickettsia). In addition, PCR-based methods have been used to characterize the influenzavirus, which caused the 1918 influenza pandemic that killed 20 to 40 million persons worldwide.

Regardless of the method of microbial identification, the final step in diagnosis of infectious pathogens is correlation of the suspect organism with the lesion caused and the signs and symptoms produced.

INFLAMMATORY RESPONSE TO INFECTIOUS AGENTS

This chapter concludes with a summary of the most common histologic patterns of host responses induced by infectious agents. In contrast to the vast molecular diversity of parasites, the morphologic patterns of inflammatory response to these agents are limited, even if the inflammatory mediators involved are variable. At the microscopic level, therefore, many pathogens evoke identical reaction patterns, and few of the features are unique to or pathognomonic of each agent. Broadly speaking, there are five histologic patterns of tissue reaction:

■ Suppurative polymorphonuclear inflammation
■ Mononuclear inflammation
■ Cytopathic-cytoproliferative inflammation
■ Necrotizing inflammation
■ Chronic inflammation and scarring

Suppurative Polymorphonuclear Inflammation. This is the familiar reaction to acute tissue damage described in Chapter 2, marked by increased vascular permeability and neutrophilic exudation. The neutrophils are attracted to the site of infection by release of chemoattractants from *the rapidly dividing "pyogenic" bacteria that evoke this response, mostly extracellular gram-positive cocci and gram-negative rods.* The bacterial chemoattractants include secreted bacterial peptides, all of which contain *N*-formyl methionine residues at their amino terminals that are recognized by specific receptors on neutrophils. Alternatively, bacteria attract neutrophils indirectly by releasing endotoxin, which stimulates macrophages to secrete IL-1 or TNF, or by cleaving complement into the chemoattractant peptide C5a. Massing of neutrophils results in the formation of pus. The size of exudative lesions may vary tremendously, from tiny microabscesses formed in multiple organs during sepsis secondary to a colonized heart valve, to distended, pus-filled fallopian tubes caused by *N. gonorrhoeae* (the gonococcus), to diffuse involvement of the meninges during *H. influenzae* infection, or to pneumonia, in which multiple lobes of the lung are involved. How destructive the lesions are depends on their location and the organism involved. For example,

Table 9–4. SPECIAL TECHNIQUES FOR DIAGNOSIS OF INFECTIOUS AGENTS

Technique	Agent(s) Detected
Gram stain	Most bacteria
Acid-fast stain	*Mycobacterium, Nocardia* (modified)
Silver stains	Fungi, *Legionella, Pneumocystis*
Periodic acid–Schiff	Fungi, amebae
Mucicarmine	Cryptococci
Giemsa	*Campylobacter, Leishmania*, malaria plasmodium
Antibody probes	Viruses, rickettsiae
Culture	All classes
DNA probes	Viruses, bacteria, protozoans

Figure 9-11   ■

Pneumococcal pneumonia. Note the intra-alveolar polymorphonuclear exudate and intact alveolar septa.

Figure 9-13   ■

Leprosy. High-power view of acid-fast bacilli proliferating in foamy macrophages.

pneumococci usually spare pulmonary alveolar walls and cause lobar pneumonia, permitting resolution (Fig. 9–11), while staphylococci and *Klebsiella* spp. destroy alveolar walls and form abscesses, which can only be followed by scarring (Chapter 13). Bacterial pharyngitis heals without sequelae, whereas untreated acute bacterial inflammation can destroy a joint in a matter of days.

Mononuclear Inflammation. Diffuse, predominantly mononuclear interstitial infiltrates are a common feature of all chronic inflammatory processes, but when they occur acutely, they are *often a response to viruses, intracellular bacteria, or intracellular parasites. In addition, spirochetes and helminths cause chronic inflammation.* Which mononuclear cell predominates within the inflammatory lesion depends on the host immune response to the organism. For example, many plasma cells are seen in the primary and secondary lesions of syphilis (Fig. 9–12), while lymphocytes predominate in HBV or in viral infections of the brain. These lymphocytes represent cell-mediated immunity against

the pathogen or the pathogen-infected cells. At the other extreme, macrophages filled with *M. avium-intracellulare* are present in many tissues of AIDS patients, who have no helper T cells left and can mount no immune response to the organisms. In *M. leprae* infection and cutaneous leishmaniasis, some persons mount a strong immune response, so that their lesions contain few organisms, few macrophages, and many lymphocytes; others, with a weak immune response, have lesions that contain many organisms, many macrophages, and few lymphocytes (Fig. 9–13). Granulomatous inflammation (described in detail in Chapter 2) is a distinctive form of mononuclear inflammation usually evoked by relatively slowly dividing infectious agents (e.g., *M. tuberculosis*) and by agents of relatively large size (e.g., schistosome eggs). Granulomatous inflammation almost always reflects a cell-mediated immune reaction (Chapter 5).

Cytopathic-Cytoproliferative Inflammation. These reactions, usually produced by viruses, are characterized by damage to individual host cells, with little or no host inflammatory response. Some viruses replicate within cells and make viral aggregates that are visible as inclusion bodies (e.g., CMV, adenovirus) or induce cells to fuse and form polykaryons (e.g., measles, herpesviruses). Focal cell damage may cause epithelial cells to become discohesive and form blisters (e.g., chickenpox virus). Viruses can also cause epithelial cells to proliferate and take unusual forms (e.g., venereal warts by HPV or the umbilicated papules of molluscum contagiosum by poxviruses). Finally, viruses can cause dysplastic changes and cancers in epithelial cells and lymphocytes (Chapter 6).

Necrotizing Inflammation. *C. perfringens* and other organisms that secrete very strong toxins cause such rapid and severe tissue damage that cell death is the dominant feature. Because so few inflammatory cells are involved, these lesions resemble infarcts, with disruption or loss of basophilic nuclear staining and preservation of cellular outlines. Often clostridia are opportunistic pathogens introduced into muscle tissue by penetrating trauma or by infection of the bowel in a neutropenic host. Similarly, the parasite *E. histolytica* causes colonic ulcers and liver abscesses characterized by extensive tissue destruction with

Figure 9-12   ■

Secondary syphilis in the dermis with perivascular lymphoplasmacytic infiltrate and endothelial proliferation.

liquefactive necrosis in the absence of an inflammatory infiltrate. Occasionally, viruses can cause necrotizing inflammation when host cell damage is particularly widespread and severe; for example, there may be total destruction of the temporal lobes of the brain by herpesvirus or of the liver by HBV.

Chronic Inflammation and Scarring. The final common pathway of many infections is chronic inflammation, which may lead to extensive scarring (e.g., chronic gonococcal salpingitis). Chronic HBV infection may cause cirrhosis of the liver, in which dense, fibrous septa surround nodules of regenerating hepatocytes. For some organisms that are relatively inert, the exuberant host scarring response is the major cause of disease (e.g., the "pipe-stem" fibrosis of the liver caused by schistosomal eggs or gummas of tertiary syphilis in the liver, central nervous system, and bones).

These patterns of tissue reaction are useful for analyzing the infective processes, but they frequently overlap. For example, a cutaneous lesion of leishmaniasis may contain two separate histopathologic regions: a central ulcerated area filled with neutrophils and a peripheral region containing a mixed infiltrate of lymphocytes and mononuclear cells, where the leishmanial parasites are located. The lung of an AIDS patient may be infected with CMV, which causes cytolytic changes, and at the same time by *Pneumocystis*, which causes interstitial inflammation. Similar patterns of inflammation can also be seen in tissue responses to physical or chemical agents and in inflammatory diseases of unknown cause (e.g., sarcoidosis).

It is evident that many factors that relate to the invader and the host modify the development and nature of the microbe-induced disease and its outcome. This chapter has emphasized the structural and molecular mechanisms relevant to the interaction between microbe and host. However, it should also be remembered that considering the multiplicity of potential invaders, most infectious diseases are caused by a relatively small number of agents that differ in geographic locales and are determined largely by environmental, socioeconomic, and public health factors.

BIBLIOGRAPHY

Anderson DM, Scheewind O: Type III machines of gram-negative pathogens: injecting virulence factors into host cell. Curr Opin Microbiol 2:18, 1999.

Baillie L, Read TD: *Bacillus anthracis*, a bug with an attitude! Curr Opin Microbiol 4:78, 2001.

Cole ST, et al: Massive gene decay in the leprosy bacillus. Nature 409:1007, 2001.

Diehn M, Relman DA: Comparing functional genomic datasets: lessons from DNA microarray of host-pathogen interactions. Curr Opin Microbiol 4;95, 2001.

Falkow S: Molecular Koch's postulates applied to microbial pathogenicity. Rev Infect Dis 10:S274, 1988.

Linz B, et al: Frequent interspecific genetic exchange between commensal neisseriae and *Neisseria meningitidis*. Mol Microbiol 36:1049, 2000.

Lucas RL, Lee CA: Unraveling the mysteries of virulence gene regulation in *Salmonella typhimurium*. Mol Microbiol 36:1024, 2000.

Mims CA: The Pathogenesis of Infectious Disease, 4th ed. San Diego, CA, Academic, 1996. (An extensive discussion of the mechanisms of microbial pathogenesis.)

Murray CJ, Lopez AD: Global mortality, disability, and the contribution of risk factors: Global Burden of Disease Study. Lancet 349:1436, 1997.

O'Connor DH, et al: Pathology of Infectious Diseases. Stamford, CT, Appleton & Lang, 1996. (Extensive descriptions and illustrations of the histopathology of infectious diseases.)

Sayers AA, Whitt DD: Bacterial Pathogenesis: A Molecular Approach. Washington, DC, ASM, 1994. (A well-selected set of examples of the molecular basis of bacterial diseases.)

Swartz MN: Recognition and management of anthrax—an update. N Engl J Med 345:1621, 2001. (A useful review of this new weapon of bioterrorism.)

Taubenberger JK, Reid AH, Fanning TG: The 1918 influenza virus: a killer comes into view. Virology 274:241, 2000.

Tuomanen E: Molecular and cellular biology of pneumococcal infection. Curr Opin Microbiol 2:35, 1999.

Von Lichtenberg F: Pathology of Infectious Disease. New York, Raven, 1991. (An authoritative and concise presentation of the broad gamut of microbial diseases, with excellent coverage of the resultant morphologic lesions.)

2

DISEASES OF ORGAN SYSTEMS

10

The Blood Vessels

FREDERICK J. SCHOEN, MD, PhD
RAMZI S. COTRAN, MD*

---

*Deceased

325

Diseases of arteries are responsible for more morbidity and mortality than any other category of human disease. However, disorders of veins can also be significant. Vascular abnormalities cause clinical disease by two principal mechanisms:

■ *Narrowing* or *completely obstructing* the lumina, either progressively (e.g., by atherosclerosis [ATH]) or precipitously (e.g., by thrombosis or embolism), often inducing downstream deficiency of blood flow to the tissue perfused by that vessel.
■ *Weakening* of the walls, leading to dilation or rupture.

To facilitate the understanding of the diseases that affect blood vessels, we first consider some of the anatomic and functional characteristics of these highly specialized and dynamic tissues.

NORMAL VESSELS

The basic constituents of the walls of blood vessels are cells, predominantly endothelial cells (ECs) and smooth muscle cells (SMCs), and extracellular matrix, including elastin, collagen, and glycosaminoglycans. The three concentric layers—*intima, media,* and *adventitia*—are most clearly defined in the larger vessels (Fig. 10–1). In normal arteries, the intima consists of a single layer of ECs with minimal underlying subendothelial connective tissue and is separated from the media by a dense elastic membrane called the *internal elastic lamina.* The smooth muscle cell layers of the media near the vessel lumen receive oxygen and nutrients by direct diffusion from the vessel lumen, facilitated by holes *(fenestrations)* in the internal elastic membrane. However, diffusion from the lumen is inadequate for the outer portion of the media in large and medium-sized vessels, which are nourished by small arterioles arising from outside the vessel (termed *vasa vasorum,* literally "vessels of the vessels") and coursing into the outer one half to two thirds of the media. The outer limit of the media of most arteries is defined by the *external elastic lamina.* External to the media is the adventitia, consisting

Endothelium — Intima
Internal elastic lamina
Media
External elastic lamina
Adventitia

Figure 10–1 ■

Diagrammatic representation of the main components of the vascular wall, seen here in a muscular artery. (Redrawn with permission from Ross R, Glomset JA: The pathogenesis of atherosclerosis. N Engl J Med 295:369, 1976.)

of investing connective tissue with nerve fibers and the vasa vasorum.

Based on their size and structural features, *arteries* are divided into three types: (1) large, or *elastic, arteries,* including the aorta, its large branches (particularly the innominate, subclavian, common carotid, and iliac), and pulmonary arteries; (2) medium-sized, or *muscular, arteries,* including other branches of the aorta (e.g., coronary and renal arteries); and (3) small arteries (less than approximately 2 mm in diameter) and *arterioles* (20 to 100 μm in diameter), which lie within the substance of tissues and organs.

In elastic arteries, an elastic, fiber-rich media expands during systole; elastic recoil of the vascular wall during diastole propels blood through the peripheral vascular system. In muscular arteries, smaller arteries, and arterioles, the media is composed predominantly of SMCs. In these vessels (see later), regional blood flow and blood pressure are regulated by changes in lumen size through smooth muscle cell contraction *(vasoconstriction)* or relaxation *(vasodilation).*

In arterioles, medial smooth muscle cell contraction causes dramatic changes in the lumen diameter that regulate systemic arterial blood pressure and significantly influence blood flow distribution among various capillary beds. Because the resistance of a tube to fluid flow is inversely proportional to the fourth power of the diameter (i.e., halving the diameter increases resistance 16-fold), small changes in the lumen size of small arteries by structural change or vasoconstriction can have a profound flow-limiting effect. Thus, *arterioles are the principal points of physiologic resistance to blood flow, inducing a sharp reduction in pressure and velocity and a change from pulsatile to steady flow.*

Some pathologic lesions involve arteries of a characteristic size range. For example, ATH affects elastic and muscular arteries, hypertension affects small muscular arteries and arterioles, and specific types of vasculitis characteristically involve only certain vessels.

Capillaries, which are approximately the diameter of a red blood cell (7 to 8 μm), have an endothelial cell lining but no media. Collectively, capillaries have very large total cross-sectional area. With thin walls only one cell thick, and with slow flow, capillaries are ideally suited to the rapid exchange of diffusible substances between blood and tissue.

Blood returning to the heart from capillary beds flows initially into the *postcapillary venules* and then sequentially through collecting venules and small, medium, and large veins. In many types of inflammation, vascular leakage and leukocytic exudation occur preferentially in postcapillary venules (Chapter 2).

Relative to corresponding arteries, veins have larger diameters, larger lumina, and thinner and less well organized walls. Thus, with poor support, *veins are predisposed to irregular dilation, compression, and easy penetration by tumors and to inflammatory processes.* The venous system collectively has a large capacity; approximately two thirds of all systemic blood is in veins. Reversed flow is prevented by venous valves in the extremities, where blood flows against gravity.

Lymphatics are thin-walled, endothelium-lined channels that serve as a drainage system for returning interstitial tissue fluid to the blood. *Lymphatics constitute an important pathway for disease dissemination through transport of bacteria and tumor cells to distant sites.*

VASCULAR WALL CELLS AND THEIR RESPONSE TO INJURY

As the main cellular components of the blood vessel walls, *endothelial cells (ECs)* and *smooth muscle cells (SMCs)* play an important role in vascular pathology.

Endothelial Cells: Function and Dysfunction

ECs form a monolayer (the *endothelium*) that lines the entire vascular system. Their structural and functional integrity is fundamental to the maintenance of vessel wall homeostasis and circulatory function. They uniquely contain *Weibel-Palade bodies*, the 0.1-μm wide, 0.3-μm long membrane-bound storage organelle for von Willebrand factor. ECs can be identified immunohistochemically with antibody to von Willebrand factor and CD31.

Vascular endothelium is a versatile multifunctional tissue that has many synthetic and metabolic properties (Table 10–1) and that is an active participant in blood-tissue

■

Table 10–1.   ENDOTHELIAL CELL PROPERTIES AND FUNCTIONS

Maintenance of Permeability Barrier

Elaboration of Anticoagulant and Antithrombotic Molecules

Prostacyclin
Thrombomodulin
Plasminogen activator
Heparin-like molecules

Elaboration of Prothrombotic Molecules

von Willebrand factor (factor VIII-vWF)
Tissue factor
Plasminogen activator inhibitor

Extracellular Matrix Production (Collagen, Proteoglycans)

Modulation of Blood Flow and Vascular Reactivity

Vasoconstrictors: endothelin, ACE
Vasodilators: NO, prostacyclin

Regulation of Inflammation and Immunity

IL-1, IL-6, IL-8
Adhesion molecules
Histocompatibility antigens

Regulation of Cell Growth

Growth stimulators: PDGF, CSF, FGF
Growth inhibitors: heparin, TGF-β

Oxidation of Low-Density Lipoprotein

ACE, angiotensin-converting enzyme (angiotensin I → angiotensin II); CSF, colony-stimulating factor; FGF, fibroblast growth factor; IL, interleukin; NO, nitric oxide; PDGF, platelet-derived growth factor; TGF-β, transforming growth factor beta.

interaction. As a semipermeable membrane, endothelium controls the transfer of small and large molecules into the vascular wall. In most regions, the intercellular junctions are normally largely impermeable; however, the relatively tight junctions between ECs may widen under the influence of hemodynamic factors (e.g., high blood pressure) and vasoactive agents (e.g., histamine in inflammation) (Chapter 2). Moreover, ECs play a role in the maintenance of a nonthrombogenic blood-tissue interface (Chapter 4), the modulation of blood flow and vascular resistance, the metabolism of hormones, the regulation of immune and inflammatory reactions, and the growth regulation of other cell types, particularly SMCs.

Endothelial injury may be responsible, at least in part, for the initiation of thrombus formation, ATH and the vascular lesions of hypertension, and other disorders. Frank loss (denudation) of ECs stimulates thrombosis (Chapter 4) and SMC proliferation (see later). However, structurally intact ECs can respond to various abnormal stimuli by adjusting their usual (constitutive) functions and by expressing newly acquired (induced) properties. The term *endothelial dysfunction* describes several types of potentially reversible changes in the functional state of ECs that occur in response to environmental stimuli. Some of these changes are rapid (within minutes), reversible, and independent of new protein synthesis (e.g., EC contraction induced by histamine and other vasoactive mediators that causes gaps in venules, depressed release of the EC-derived relaxing factor nitric oxide) (Chapter 4). Other changes involve alterations in gene expression and protein synthesis and may require hours or even days to occur. Endothelial dysfunction may be manifested as impaired endothelium-dependent vasodilation, reduced synthesis of nitric oxide, elevated levels of endothelin, and production of oxygen free radicals.

Endothelial dysfunction is very important in the pathogenesis of vascular disease. *Inducers* of endothelial dysfunction include cytokines and bacterial products, which also cause inflammatory injury and septic shock (Chapter 4); hemodynamic stresses and lipid products, critical to the pathogenesis of ATH (see later); and other injuries. Dysfunctional ECs, in turn, elaborate adhesion and prothrombotic molecules, growth factors, and other products (Chapter 4).

Vascular Smooth Muscle Cells

As the predominant cellular element of the vascular media, SMCs cause vasoconstriction or dilation in response to normal or pharmacologic stimuli; synthesize collagen, elastin, and proteoglycans; elaborate growth factors and cytokines; and migrate to the intima and proliferate after vascular injury. Thus, SMCs comprise an important element of both normal vascular repair and pathologic processes such as ATH.

The migratory and proliferative activity of SMCs is physiologically regulated by growth promoters and inhibitors. Promoters include platelet-derived growth factor derived from platelets (and ECs and macrophages), basic fibroblast growth factor, and interleukin 1. Inhibitors include heparan sulfates, nitric oxide, interferon γ, and transforming growth factor β.

1. Migration of smooth muscle cells to the intima
2. Smooth muscle cell mitosis
3. Elaboration of extracellular matrix

Endothelium

Internal elastic lamina

Smooth muscle cells

Intima

Media

Figure 10-2 ■

Schematic mechanism for intimal thickening, emphasizing smooth muscle cell migration to, and proliferation and extracellular matrix elaboration in, the intima. (Modified and redrawn from Schoen FJ: Interventional and Surgical Cardiovascular Pathology: Clinical Correlations and Basic Principles. Philadelphia, WB Saunders, 1989, p 254.)

Intimal Thickening—A Response to Vascular Intimal Injury

Vascular injury (constituting acute EC loss or chronic endothelial injury/dysfunction) stimulates SMC growth by disrupting the physiologic balance between inhibition and stimulation. Reconstitution of the damaged vascular wall represents a physiologic healing response with the formation of a *neointima*, in which SMCs (1) migrate from the media to the intima, (2) multiply as intimal SMCs, and (3) synthesize and deposit extracellular matrix (Fig. 10–2).

During the healing response, SMCs undergo changes that resemble dedifferentiation. In the intima they lose the capacity to contract and gain the capacity to divide. Intimal SMCs may return to a nonproliferative state when either the overlying endothelial layer is re-established after acute injury or the chronic stimulation ceases. However, an exaggerated healing response leads to *intimal thickening*, which can cause stenosis or occlusion of small and medium-sized blood vessels.

VASCULAR DISEASES

Congenital Anomalies

Although rarely symptomatic, aberrations of the usual anatomic pattern of branching and anastomosing are important to recognize to prevent unexpected vascular injury during surgery. Among the diverse congenital vascular anomalies, two have importance: *developmental* or *berry aneurysms* and *arteriovenous fistulas*. Berry aneurysms involve cerebral vessels and are discussed in Chapter 23.

ARTERIOVENOUS FISTULA

Arteriovenous fistulas are rare and usually small abnormal communications between arteries and veins that may arise as developmental defects; from rupture of an arterial aneurysm into the adjacent vein; from penetrating injuries that pierce the walls of artery and vein; or secondary to inflammatory necrosis of adjacent vessels. When arteriovenous connections are large or extensive, they may be of clinical significance because they short-circuit blood from the arterial to the venous side, thereby causing the heart to pump additional volume; sometimes high-output cardiac failure ensues. Moreover, they can rupture and cause hemorrhage, especially in the brain. In contrast, intentionally created arteriovenous fistulas are used to provide vascular access for chronic hemodialysis.

ARTERIOSCLEROSIS

Arteriosclerosis (literally, "hardening of the arteries") is a generic term for thickening and loss of elasticity of arterial walls. It occurs in three forms:

■ As the most frequent and important pattern, *ATH* will be discussed in this section.

■ Of much less clinical importance is *Mönckeberg medial calcific sclerosis*, characterized by calcific deposits in muscular arteries in persons older than 50 years. These radiographically visible, often palpable calcifications do not encroach on the vessel lumen.

■ Disease of small arteries and arterioles *(arteriolosclerosis)* is the third pattern. Two anatomic variants, hyaline and hyperplastic arteriolosclerosis, cause thickening of vessel walls with luminal narrowing that may induce downstream ischemic injury. Most often associated with hypertension and diabetes mellitus, arteriolosclerosis will be described later in this chapter in the section on hypertension.

Atherosclerosis (ATH)

Atherosclerosis is characterized by intimal lesions called *atheromas*, or *atheromatous* or *fibrofatty plaques*, that protrude into and obstruct vascular lumina, weaken the underlying media, and may undergo serious complications. Global in distribution, ATH overwhelmingly contributes to more mortality—approximately half of all deaths—and serious morbidity in the Western world than any other disorder. Because coronary artery disease is an important manifestation of ATH, *epidemiologic data on ATH are ex-*

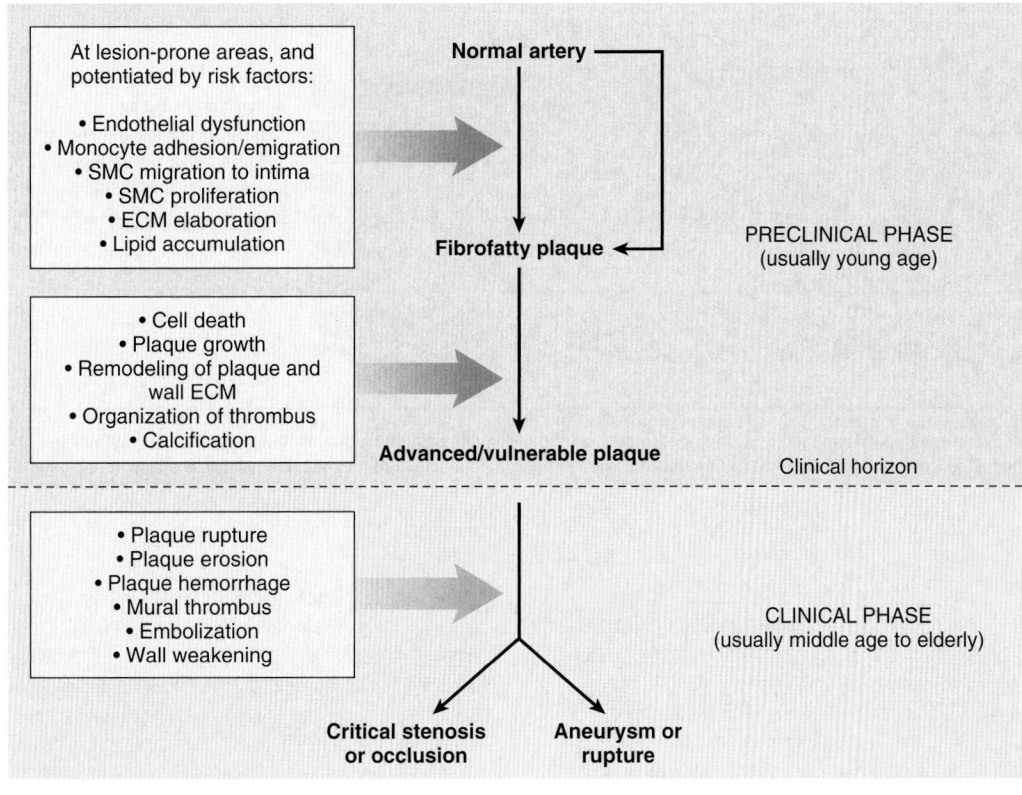

Figure 10-3

Summary of the pathology, pathogenesis, complications, and natural history of atherosclerosis. Plaques usually develop slowly and insidiously over many years, beginning in childhood or shortly thereafter and exerting their clinical effect in middle age or later. As described in the text, they may progress from a fatty streak to a fibrous plaque and then to plaque complications that lead to disease. The schematic diagram interrelates the morphology, pathogenesis, and complications of atherosclerosis and provides a unified approach to this serious disease process. ECM, extracellular matrix; SMC, smooth muscle cell.

pressed largely in terms of the incidence of the number of deaths caused by ischemic heart disease (IHD) (Chapter 11). Indeed, myocardial infarction alone is responsible for 20% to 25% of all deaths in the United States.

Clinical Significance. ATH primarily affects elastic arteries (e.g., aorta, carotid, and iliac arteries) and large and medium-sized muscular arteries (e.g., coronary and popliteal arteries). *Symptomatic atherosclerotic disease most often involves the arteries supplying the heart, brain, kidneys, and lower extremities. Myocardial infarction (heart attack), cerebral infarction (stroke), aortic aneurysms, and peripheral vascular disease (gangrene of the legs) are the major consequences of ATH.* ATH also takes a toll through other consequences of acutely or chronically diminished arterial perfusion, *such as mesenteric occlusion, sudden cardiac death, chronic IHD, and ischemic encephalopathy.* The interactions of morphology, mechanisms, and clinical consequences are summarized in Figure 10–3, which provides a blueprint for the discussion of ATH that follows.

In small arteries, atheromas can occlude lumina, compromise blood flow to distal organs, and cause ischemic injury. Moreover, atherosclerotic plaques can undergo disruption and precipitate thrombi that further obstruct blood flow. In large arteries, plaques are destructive, encroaching on the subjacent media and weakening the affected vessel wall, causing aneurysms that may rupture. Moreover, exten-

sive atheromas are friable, often yielding emboli into the distal circulation.

Considerable progress on the health impact of ATH-related disease has been made over the past decades in the United States and elsewhere. Between 1963 (the peak year) and 2000 there has been an approximately 50% decrease in the death rate from IHD and a 70% decrease in death from strokes, a reduction in mortality that increased the average life expectancy in the United States by 5 years. Three factors have contributed to this impressive improvement: (1) prevention of ATH through changes in life style, including reduced cigarette smoking, altered dietary habits with reduced consumption of cholesterol and saturated animal fats, and control of hypertension; (2) improved methods of treatment of myocardial infarction and other complications of IHD; and (3) prevention of recurrences in patients who have previously suffered serious ATH-related clinical events.

MORPHOLOGY

The key processes in ATH are intimal thickening and lipid accumulation giving rise to atheroma. These are described first; discussed subsequently is fatty streak, the presumed precursor lesion for atheromas. An **atheroma** (derived from the Greek word for gruel) or

FIBROUS CAP
(smooth muscle cells, macrophages,
foam cells, lymphocytes, collagen,
elastin, proteoglycans, neovascularization)

NECROTIC CENTER
(cell debris, cholesterol crystals,
foam cells, calcium)

MEDIA

Figure 10–4 ■

Schematic depiction of the major components of well-developed atheromatous plaque: fibrous cap composed of proliferating smooth muscle cells, macrophages, lymphocytes, foam cells, and extracellular matrix. The necrotic core consists of cellular debris, extracellular lipid with cholesterol crystals, and foamy macrophages.

atheromatous plaque consists of a raised focal lesion initiating within the intima, having a soft, yellow, grumous core of lipid (mainly cholesterol and cholesterol esters) and covered by a firm, white fibrous cap (Fig. 10–4). Also called fibrous, fibrofatty, lipid, or fibrolipid plaques, atheromatous plaques appear white to whitish yellow and impinge on the lumen of the artery. They vary in size from 0.3 to 1.5 cm in diameter but sometimes coalesce to form larger masses (Fig. 10–5). Atherosclerotic lesions usually involve the arterial wall only partially around its circumference ("eccentric" lesions) and are patchy and variable along the vessel length. Focal and sparsely distributed at first, atherosclerotic lesions become more and more numerous and diffuse as the disease advances.

In the characteristic distribution of atherosclerotic plaques in humans, the abdominal aorta is usually much more involved than is the thoracic aorta, and lesions tend to be much more prominent around the origins (ostia) of major branches. In descending order (after the lower abdominal aorta), the most extensively involved vessels are the coronary arteries, the popliteal arteries, the internal carotid arteries, and the vessels of the circle of Willis. Vessels of the upper extremities are usually spared, as are the mesenteric and renal arteries, except at their ostia. Nevertheless, in an individual case, the severity of AS in one artery does not predict its severity in another.

Atherosclerotic plaques have three principal components: (1) cells, including SMCs, macrophages, and other leukocytes; (2) extracellular matrix, in-

Figure 10–5 ■

Gross views of atherosclerosis in the aorta. *A,* Mild atherosclerosis composed of fibrous plaques, one of which is denoted by the arrow. *B,* Severe disease with diffuse and complicated lesions.

cluding collagen, elastic fibers, and proteoglycans; and (3) intracellular and extracellular lipid (see Fig. 10–4). These components occur in varying proportions and configurations in different lesions. Typically, the superficial fibrous cap is composed of SMCs and relatively dense collagen. Beneath and to the side of the cap (the "shoulder") is a cellular area consisting of macrophages, SMCs, and T lymphocytes. Deep to the fibrous cap is a necrotic core, containing a disorganized mass of lipid (primarily cholesterol and cholesterol esters), clefts containing cholesterol, debris from dead cells, foam cells, fibrin, variably organized thrombus, and other plasma proteins. **Foam cells** are large lipid-laden cells that derive predominantly from blood monocytes (tissue macrophages), but SMCs can also imbibe lipid to become foam cells. Finally, particularly around the periphery of the lesions, there is usually evidence of **neovascularization** (proliferating small blood vessels). Typical atheromas contain relatively abundant lipid, but many so-called fibrous plaques are composed mostly of SMCs and fibrous tissue.

Plaques generally continue to change and progressively enlarge through cell death and degeneration, synthesis and degradation (remodeling) of extracellular matrix, and organization of thrombus. Moreover, atheromas often undergo calcification. Patients with advanced coronary calcification (as determined by computed tomography) appear to be at increased risk for coronary events. Figure 10–6 shows the typical features of advanced plaque.

The advanced lesion of ATH is the most vulnerable to the following pathologic changes that have clinical significance:

■ Focal **rupture, ulceration, or erosion** of the luminal surface of atheromatous plaques may result in exposure of highly thrombogenic substances that induce thrombus formation (Fig. 10–7) or discharge of debris into the bloodstream, producing microemboli composed of lesion contents **(cholesterol emboli or atheroemboli).**

■ **Hemorrhage** into a plaque may occur, especially in the coronary arteries, initiated by rupture of either the overlying fibrous cap or the thin-walled capillaries that vascularize the plaque. A contained hematoma may expand the plaque or induce plaque rupture.

■ Superimposed **thrombosis**, the most feared complication, usually occurs on disrupted lesions (those with rupture, ulceration, erosion, or hemorrhage) and may partially or completely occlude the lumen. Thrombi may become incorporated into and thereby enlarge the intimal plaque by subsequent organization.

■ **Aneurysmal dilation** may result from ATH-induced pressure or ischemic atrophy of the underlying media, with loss of elastic tissue, causing weakness and potential rupture, discussed later.

Fatty streaks, composed of lipid-filled foam cells, are not significantly raised and thus do not cause any disturbance in blood flow. They begin as multiple yellow, flat spots (fatty dots) less than 1 mm in diameter that coalesce into elongated streaks, 1 cm long or longer (Fig. 10–8). Fatty streaks appear in the aortas of some children younger than 1 year of age and all children older than 10 years, regardless of geography, race, sex, or environment. Coronary fatty streaks begin to form in adolescence, at the same anatomic sites that later tend to develop plaques. The relationship of fatty streaks to atherosclerotic plaques is uncertain; although they may evolve into precursors of plaques, not all fatty streaks are destined to become advanced atherosclerotic lesions.

Epidemiology and Risk Factors. Virtually ubiquitous among most developed nations, ATH is much less prevalent in Central and South America, Africa, and Asia. The mortality rate for IHD in the United States is among the highest in the world and is six times higher than that in Japan. Interestingly, Japanese who emigrate to the United States and adopt the life styles and dietary customs of their new home acquire the predisposition to ATH typical of the American population.

The prevalence and severity of the disease among individuals and groups are related to a number of factors, some constitutional and therefore immutable but others acquired and potentially capable of control (Table 10–2). The constitutional factors include age, sex, and genetics.

Age is a dominant influence. Death rates from IHD rise with each decade even into advanced age. ATH is not usually clinically evident until middle age or later, when the arterial lesions precipitate organ injury. Between ages 40 and 60 the incidence of myocardial infarction increases five-fold.

Other factors being equal, men are much more prone to ATH and its consequences than are women. Myocardial infarction and other complications of ATH are uncommon in premenopausal women unless they are predisposed by diabetes, hyperlipidemia, or severe hypertension. After menopause, however, the incidence of ATH-related diseases increases, probably owing to a decrease in natural estrogen levels. Indeed, the frequency of myocardial infarction in the two sexes equalizes by the seventh to eighth decade of life. Some protection against ATH is afforded by postmenopausal hormone replacement therapy (Chapter 8).

The well-established familial predisposition to ATH and IHD is most likely polygenic. In some instances it relates to familial clustering of other risk factors, such as hypertension or diabetes, whereas in others it involves well-defined hereditary genetic derangements in lipoprotein metabolism that result in excessively high blood lipid levels, such as familial hypercholesterolemia (Chapter 7).

Although the aforementioned factors are unchangeable in an individual, *other risk factors, particularly diet, life*

Figure 10-6 ■

Histologic features of atheromatous plaque in the coronary artery. *A,* Overall architecture demonstrating fibrous cap (F) and a central lipid core (C) with typical cholesterol clefts. The lumen (L) has been moderately narrowed. Note the plaque-free segment of the wall *(arrow).* In this section, collagen has been stained blue (Masson's trichrome stain). *B,* Higher-power photograph of a section of the plaque shown in *A,* stained for elastin *(black)* demonstrating that the internal and external elastic membranes are destroyed and the media of the artery is thinned under the most advanced plaque *(arrow).* C, Higher-magnification photomicrograph at the junction of the fibrous cap and core showing scattered inflammatory cells, calcification *(broad arrow),* and neovascularization *(small arrows).*

style, and personal habits, are to a large extent amenable to control. The four major risk factors that can be modified are hyperlipidemia, hypertension, cigarette smoking, and diabetes.

Hyperlipidemia is a major risk factor for ATH. Most of the evidence specifically implicates *hypercholesterolemia.* The major component of the total serum cholesterol associated with increased risk is low-density lipoprotein (LDL) cholesterol. In contrast, the higher the level of high-density lipoprotein (HDL), the lower is the risk. HDL is believed to mobilize cholesterol from developing an existing atheroma and transport it to the liver for excretion in the bile, thereby earning its designation as the "good cholesterol." There is thus great interest in dietary, pharmacologic, and behavioral methods of lowering serum LDL and raising serum HDL. Both exercise

and moderate consumption of ethanol raise the HDL level, whereas obesity and smoking lower it.

High dietary intake of cholesterol and saturated fats, such as those present in egg yolk, animal fats, and butter, raises the plasma cholesterol level. Conversely, a diet low in cholesterol and low in the ratio of saturated to polyunsaturated fats lowers plasma cholesterol levels. Moreover, omega-3 fatty acids, abundant in fish oils, are likely beneficial, whereas hardened *(trans)* unsaturated fats produced by artificial hydrogenation of polyunsaturated vegetable fats and used in commercially baked goods and margarine may adversely affect cholesterol profiles and contribute to ATH.

Hypertension is a major risk factor for ATH at all ages. Men ages 45 to 62 whose blood pressure exceeds 169/95

Figure 10–7

Atherosclerotic plaque rupture. *A,* Plaque rupture without superimposed thrombus, in patient who died suddenly. *B,* Acute coronary thrombosis superimposed on an atherosclerotic plaque with focal disruption of the fibrous cap, triggering fatal myocardial infarction. *C,* Massive plaque rupture with superimposed thrombus, also triggering a fatal myocardial infarction *(special stain highlighting fibrin in red).* In both *A* and *B,* an arrow points to the site of plaque rupture. (*B,* Reproduced from Schoen FJ: Interventional and Surgical Cardiovascular Pathology: Clinical Correlations and Basic Principles. Philadelphia, WB Saunders, 1989, p 61.)

Figure 10–8

Fatty streak—a collection of foam cells in the intima. *A,* Aorta with fatty streaks *(arrows),* associated largely with the ostia of branch vessels. *B,* Close-up of fatty streaks from aorta of an experimental hypercholesterolemic rabbit after staining with Sudan red, a lipid-soluble dye. Note again the proximity to ostia of branch vessels. *C,* Photomicrograph of fatty streak in an experimental hypercholesterolemic rabbit, demonstrating intimal macrophage-derived foam cells *(arrow).* (*B* and *C,* Courtesy of Myron I. Cybulsky, MD, University of Toronto, Toronto, Ontario, Canada.)

■

Table 10-2. RISK FACTORS FOR ATHEROSCLEROSIS

Major Risks	Lesser, Uncertain, or Nonquantitated Risks
Nonmodifiable	Obesity
	Physical inactivity
Increasing age	Stress ("type A" personality)
Male gender	Postmenopausal estrogen deficiency
Family history	High carbohydrate intake
Genetic abnormalities	Lipoprotein(a)
Potentially Controllable	Hardened *(trans)* unsaturated
	fat intake
Hyperlipidemia	*Chlamydia pneumoniae*
Hypertension	
Cigarette smoking	
Diabetes	

mm Hg have a more than five-fold greater risk of IHD than those with blood pressures of 140/90 mm Hg or lower. Both systolic and diastolic levels are important in increasing risk. Antihypertensive therapy reduces the incidence of ATH-related diseases, particularly strokes and IHD.

Cigarette smoking is a well-established risk factor in men and is thought to account for the relatively recent increase in the incidence and severity of ATH in women. When one or more packs of cigarettes are smoked per day for several years, the death rate from IHD increases by up to 200%. Cessation of smoking reduces the increased risk substantially.

Diabetes mellitus induces hypercholesterolemia and a markedly increased predisposition to ATH. Other factors being equal, the incidence of myocardial infarction is twice as high in diabetics as in nondiabetics. There is also an increased risk of strokes and, even more striking, perhaps a 100-fold increased risk of ATH-induced gangrene of the lower extremities.

Patients with *homocystinuria*, rare inborn errors of metabolism resulting in high levels of circulating homocysteine (>100 μmol/L), have premature vascular disease. Beyond these unfortunate individuals, clinical and epidemiologic studies have shown a more general relationship between total serum homocysteine levels and coronary artery disease, peripheral vascular disease, stroke, or venous thrombosis.

Hyperhomocystinemia can be caused by low folate and vitamin B intake, and some evidence (obtained in women) suggests that ingestion of folate and vitamins B_6 and B_{12} beyond conventional dietary recommendations may reduce the incidence of cardiovascular disease. However, firm data on the benefit of dietary supplementations to reduce homocysteine levels are lacking.

Additional Factors Affecting Hemostasis/Thrombosis. Epidemiologic evidence also indicates that several markers of hemostatic and thrombotic function are potent predictors of risk for major atherosclerotic events, including myocardial infarction and stroke. Such markers include those related to fibrinolysis (e.g., elevated plasminogen activator inhibitor 1) and inflammation (e.g., C-reactive protein).

Lipoprotein a [Lp(a)] is an altered form of LDL that contains the apolipoprotein B-100 portion of the LDL linked to apolipoprotein A (apo A). Epidemiologic studies suggest a correlation between increased blood levels of lipoprotein Lp(a) and coronary and cerebrovascular disease, independent of the level of total cholesterol or LDL.

Other Factors. Factors associated with a less pronounced and/or difficult-to-quantitate risk include lack of exercise; competitive, stressful life style with "type A" personality behavior; and unrestrained weight gain (largely because obesity induces hypertension, diabetes, hypertriglyceridemia, and decreased HDL). Epidemiologic data also indicate a protective role for moderate intake of alcohol.

Multiple risk factors have a multiplicative effect; two risk factors increase the risk approximately fourfold. When three risk factors are present (e.g., hyperlipidemia, hypertension, and smoking), the rate of myocardial infarction is increased seven times. However, ATH and its consequences may develop in the absence of any apparent risk factors, so that even those who live "the prudent life" and have no apparent genetic predispositions are not immune to this killer disease.

Pathogenesis. Understandably, the overwhelming clinical importance of ATH has stimulated enormous efforts to discover its cause. Historically, two hypotheses for atherogenesis were dominant: one emphasized cellular proliferation in the intima, whereas the other emphasized organization and repetitive growth of thrombi. The contemporary view of the pathogenesis of ATH incorporates elements of both older theories and accommodates the risk factors previously discussed. This concept, called *the response to injury hypothesis, considers ATH to be a chronic inflammatory response of the arterial wall initiated by injury to the endothelium* (Fig. 10–9). Central to this thesis are the following:

■ *Chronic endothelial injury*, usually subtle, with resultant endothelial dysfunction, yielding increased permeability, leukocyte adhesion, and thrombotic potential.
■ Insudation of *lipoproteins* into the vessel wall, mainly LDL with its high cholesterol content.
■ Modification of lesional lipoproteins by *oxidation* (see later).
■ Adhesion of *blood monocytes* (and other leukocytes) to the endothelium, followed by their migration into the intima and their transformation into *macrophages* and *foam cells.*
■ Adhesion of *platelets.*
■ Release of factors from activated platelets, macrophages, or vascular cells that cause *migration of SMCs* from media into the intima.
■ *Proliferation of SMCs* in the intima, and elaboration of extracellular matrix, leading to *accumulation of collagen and proteoglycans.*
■ *Enhanced accumulation of lipids* both within cells (macrophages and SMCs) and extracellularly.

Several aspects of the atherogenic process will now be considered in detail.

1. Chronic endothelial "injury":
   - Hyperlipidemia
   - Hypertension
   - Smoking
   - Homocysteine
   - Hemodynamic factors
   - Toxins
   - Viruses
   - Immune reactions

Response to injury

2. Endothelial dysfunction (e.g., increased permeability, leukocyte adhesion) Monocyte adhesion and emigration.

3. Smooth muscle emigration from media to intima. Macrophage activation.

Fatty streak

4. Macrophages and smooth muscle cells engulf lipid

Lymphocyte

Fibrofatty atheroma

5. Smooth muscle proliferation, collagen and other ECM deposition, extracellular lipid

Lymphocyte   Collagen   Lipid debris

The Role of Endothelial Injury. Chronic or repetitive endothelial injury is the cornerstone of the response to injury hypothesis. Endothelial injury induced in experimental animals by mechanical denudation, hemodynamic forces, immune complex deposition, irradiation, and chemicals causes intimal thickening and, in the presence of high-lipid diets, typical atheromas. However, *early human lesions begin at sites of morphologically intact endothelium.* Thus, nondenuding endothelial dysfunction causing increased endothelial permeability, enhanced leukocyte adhesion, and alterations in expression of EC gene products is critical to the human disease.

The specific cause of endothelial dysfunction in early ATH is unknown: potential culprits include circulating derivatives of cigarette smoke, homocysteine, and possibly viruses and other infectious agents. However, the two most important determinants of endothelial alterations, perhaps acting in concert, are thought to be hemodynamic disturbances that accompany normal circulatory function and adverse effects of hypercholesterolemia.

In support of a hemodynamic effect is the well-defined tendency for plaques to occur at ostia of exiting vessels, branch points, and along the posterior wall of the abdominal aorta, where there are disturbed flow patterns. Additionally, in vitro studies suggest that the normal laminar flow typically encountered in *lesion-protected areas* of the arterial vasculature induces endothelial genes whose products (e.g., the antioxidant superoxide dismutase) actually *protect* from the development of lesions. These "atheroprotective" genes could explain the nonrandom localization of early atherosclerotic lesions.

The Role of Lipids. It should be recalled that the various classes of blood lipids are transported as lipoproteins complexed to specific apoproteins. Dyslipoproteinemias result either from mutations that yield defective apolipoproteins or from some other underlying disorder, such as the nephrotic syndrome, alcoholism, hypothyroidism, or diabetes mellitus. Examples of lipoprotein abnormalities frequently found in the population (and, indeed, present in many myocardial infarction survivors) are (1) increased LDL cholesterol levels, (2) decreased HDL cholesterol levels, and (3) increased levels of the abnormal Lp(a) (see earlier).

The major evidence implicating hypercholesterolemia in the genesis of AS includes the following:

■ Genetic defects in lipoprotein metabolism causing hyperlipoproteinemia are associated with accelerated ATH. For example, homozygous familial hypercholesterolemia, which often results in myocardial infarction before age 20 years, is caused by defects in the LDL receptor, leading to

---

Figure 10–9   ■

Processes in the response to injury hypothesis. *1* and *2,* Endothelial injury with adhesion of monocytes and platelets (latter to denuded endothelium) and monocyte emigration (from the lumen) into the intima. *3,* Migration of smooth muscle cells (from the media) into the intima. *4,* Accumulation of lipid in smooth muscles and macrophages in the intima. *5,* Fully developed plaque with smooth muscle proliferation and formation of a lipid core.

inadequate hepatic uptake of LDL and markedly increased circulating LDL (Chapter 7).

■ Other genetic or acquired disorders (e.g., diabetes mellitus, hypothyroidism) that cause hypercholesterolemia lead to premature and severe ATH.

■ The major lipids in atheromas (plaques) are plasma-derived cholesterol and cholesterol esters.

■ Epidemiologic analyses demonstrate a significant correlation between the severity of ATH and the levels of total plasma cholesterol or LDL cholesterol.

■ Lowering levels of serum cholesterol by diet or drugs slows the rate of progression of ATH, causes regression of some plaques, and reduces the risk of cardiovascular events. Indeed, lowering cholesterol increases overall survival and reduces risk of ATH-related events in patients with established coronary heart disease with elevated or average cholesterol levels, as well as in patients with hypercholesterolemia but without overt ATH-related disease.

The mechanisms by which hyperlipidemia contributes to atherogenesis include the following:

■ Chronic hyperlipidemia, particularly hypercholesterolemia, may directly impair EC function through increased production of oxygen free radicals that deactivate nitric oxide, the major endothelial-relaxing factor.

■ With chronic hyperlipidemia, lipoproteins accumulate within the intima at sites of increased endothelial permeability.

■ Chemical changes of lipid induced by free radicals generated in macrophages or EC in the arterial wall yield *oxidized (modified) LDL.* Oxidized LDL (1) is ingested by macrophages through the *scavenger receptor,* distinct from the LDL receptor (Chapter 7), thus forming foam cells; (2) increases monocyte accumulation in lesions; (3) stimulates release of growth factors and cytokines; (4) is cytotoxic to ECs and SMCs; and (5) can induce endothelial cell dysfunction.

Consistent with the role of oxidant stress is the finding that coronary arterial ATH may be decreased by antioxidant vitamins (β-carotene and vitamin E). It should be noted, however, that data are insufficient to recommend dietary supplementation with antioxidants for the prevention of ATH.

The Role of Macrophages. Monocytes and macrophages play a key role in ATH. These cells

■ Adhere to endothelium early in ATH by means of specific endothelial adhesion molecules induced on the surface of dysfunctional ECs.

■ Migrate between ECs to localize in the intima.

■ Transform into macrophages and avidly engulf lipoproteins, largely oxidized LDL, to become foam cells.

Macrophages also produce interleukin 1 and tumor necrosis factor, which increase adhesion of leukocytes; several chemokines generated by macrophages (e.g., monocyte chemoattractant protein 1) may further recruit leukocytes into the plaque. Macrophages produce toxic oxygen species that also cause oxidation of the LDL in

the lesions, and they elaborate growth factors that may contribute to SMC proliferation. T lymphocytes (both CD4+ and CD8+) are also present in atheromas, but their role is uncertain.

The Role of Smooth Muscle Cell Proliferation. *SMC proliferation and the extracellular matrix that SMCs deposit in the intima convert a fatty streak into a mature fibrofatty atheroma and contribute to the progressive growth of atherosclerotic lesions.* Several growth factors have been implicated in the proliferation of SMCs, including platelet-derived growth factor (released by platelets adherent to a focus of endothelial injury, and macrophages, ECs, and SMCs), fibroblast growth factor, and transforming growth factor α.

The development of the atheromatous plaque could also be explained if SMC proliferation were in fact the primary event. The *monoclonal hypothesis* of atherogenesis, put forth in 1977, was based on the observation that some human plaques are monoclonal or, at most, oligoclonal. One interpretation of oligoclonality is that plaques may be equivalent to benign neoplastic growths, perhaps induced by an exogenous chemical (e.g., cholesterol or some of its oxidized products) or an oncogenic virus.

Infection. Infectious processes could contribute to ATH, but this thesis has not been proved. Microbiologic organisms, including herpesvirus, cytomegalovirus, and *Chlamydia pneumoniae,* have been detected in atherosclerotic plaque but not in normal arteries. It has been suggested that the infectious organism incites a chronic inflammatory process that contributes to atheroma formation. Evidence for participation of *C. pneumoniae* is strongest; studies suggest that antibiotic therapy appropriate for this organism reduces recurrent clinical events in patients with IHD.

The previous discussion emphasizes that the evolving atheroma is a dynamic and complex lesion containing chronic inflammatory cells (macrophages, lymphocytes), ECs, and SMCs, all expressing or contributing a variety of factors that could play roles in the pathogenesis of these lesions. At an early stage, the intimal plaque is an aggregation of foam cells of macrophage and SMC origin, some of which have died and released lipid and debris, surrounded by SMCs. With progression, the atheroma is modified by SMC-synthesized collagen and proteoglycans. Connective tissue is particularly prominent on the intimal aspect, producing the fibrous cap, but many lesions retain a central core of lipid-laden cells and fatty debris. Disruption of the fibrous cap with superimposed thrombus is often associated with catastrophic clinical events (Fig. 10–3; see later).

Figure 10–10 summarizes the major proposed cellular mechanisms of atherogenesis. This schema considers ATH a chronic inflammatory response of the vascular wall to a variety of events that are initiated early in life. Multiple mechanisms contribute to plaque formation and progression, including endothelial dysfunction, monocyte adhesion and infiltration, lipid accumulation and oxidation, SMC proliferation, extracellular matrix deposition, and thrombosis.

Prevention. Efforts to reduce the consequences and impact of ATH include *primary prevention* programs aimed at

Figure 10-10   ■

Schematic diagram of hypothetical sequence of cellular events and cellular interactions in atherosclerosis. Hyperlipidemia and other risk factors are thought to cause endothelial injury, resulting in adhesion of platelets and monocytes and release of growth factors, including platelet-derived growth factor (PDGF), which lead to smooth muscle cell migration and proliferation. Smooth muscle cells produce large amounts of extracellular matrix, including collagen and proteoglycans. Foam cells of atheromatous plaques are derived from both macrophages and smooth muscle cells—from macrophages via the very-low-density lipoprotein (VLDL) receptor and the scavenger receptor recognizing modified low-density lipoprotein (LDL) (e.g., oxidized LDL), and from smooth muscle cells by less certain mechanisms. Extracellular lipid is derived from insudation from the vessel lumen, particularly in the presence of hypercholesterolemia, and also from degenerating foam cells. Cholesterol accumulation in the plaque should be viewed as reflecting an imbalance between influx and efflux, and it is possible that high-density lipoprotein (HDL) helps clear cholesterol from these accumulations.

either delaying atheroma formation or causing regression of established lesions in persons who have never suffered a serious complication of atherosclerotic coronary heart disease, and *secondary prevention* programs intended to prevent recurrence of events such as myocardial infarction in patients with symptomatic disease.

As detailed earlier, there is ample justification for the following recommendations for primary prevention of ATH-related complications in adults by virtue of risk factor modification: abstention from or cessation of cigarette smoking; control of hypertension; weight reduction and increased exercise; and, most importantly, lowering total and LDL blood cholesterol levels while increasing HDL.

Moreover, several lines of evidence suggest that risk factor examination and prevention directed at modification of risk should begin in childhood:

■ Morphologic studies have established that atherosclerotic coronary artery disease begins in childhood.
■ Cardiovascular risk factors in children predict the adult profile and have distinct ethnic and sex differences that relate to adult heart disease.
■ Serum cholesterol concentrations and smoking are important determinants of the early stages of ATH noted at autopsy in adolescents and young adults.

Secondary prevention involves use of lipid-lowering drugs (statins) and use of antiplatelet drugs. These can successfully reduce recurrent myocardial infarctions.

Clinicopathologic Effects of Atherosclerotic Coronary Artery Disease.   *The down-stream complications of atherosclerotic coronary artery disease* (Chapter 11) *occur through impaired coronary perfusion relative to* *myocardial demand (myocardial ischemia). The vascular changes comprise a complex dynamic interaction among fixed atherosclerotic narrowing of the epicardial coronary arteries, intraluminal thrombosis overlying a disrupted atherosclerotic plaque, platelet aggregation, and vasospasm.*

HYPERTENSIVE VASCULAR DISEASE

Elevated blood pressure (*hypertension*) affects both the function and the structure of blood vessels. Hypertension as a risk factor for ATH was discussed earlier. In this section, we discuss first the mechanisms of normal blood pressure control, next the possible mechanisms of hypertension, and finally the pathologic changes in the small blood vessels associated with the disorder.

Hypertension

Although hypertension is a common health problem with sometimes devastating consequences, it often remains asymptomatic until late in its course. It is one of the most important risk factors in both coronary heart disease and cerebrovascular accidents; in addition, hypertension may also lead to cardiac hypertrophy and heart failure *(hypertensive heart disease),* aortic dissection, and renal failure. The detrimental effects of blood pressure increase continuously as the pressure rises; no rigidly defined threshold level of blood pressure distinguishes risk from safety. Nevertheless, a sustained diastolic pressure greater than 90 mm Hg, or a sustained systolic pressure in excess of 140 mm Hg, is considered to constitute hypertension. By either of these criteria, screening programs reveal that 25% of persons in the general population are hypertensive. The prevalence and vulnerability to complications increase with age and for unknown reasons are high in blacks. Reduction of blood pressure dramatically reduces the incidence and death rates from IHD, heart failure, and stroke.

Table 10–3 lists the major causes of hypertension. *Ninety percent to 95% of hypertension is idiopathic (essential hypertension), which is compatible with long life, unless a myocardial infarction, cerebrovascular accident, or other complication supervenes.* Most of the remainder of "benign hypertension" is secondary to renal disease or, less often, to narrowing of the renal artery, usually by an atheromatous plaque (renovascular hypertension). Infrequently, hypertension is secondary to diseases of the adrenal glands, such as primary aldosteronism, Cushing syndrome, pheochromocytoma, or other disorders.

About 5% of hypertensive persons show a rapidly rising blood pressure that if untreated leads to death within 1 or 2 years. Termed *accelerated* or *malignant hypertension*, the clinical syndrome is characterized by severe hypertension (diastolic pressure over 120 mm Hg), renal failure, and retinal hemorrhages and exudates, with or without papilledema. It may develop in previously normotensive persons but more

Table 10–3. TYPES AND CAUSES OF HYPERTENSION (SYSTOLIC AND DIASTOLIC)

Essential Hypertension (90%–95% of cases)
Secondary Hypertension
Renal

Acute glomerulonephritis
Chronic renal disease
Polycystic disease
Renal artery stenosis
Renal vasculitis
Renin-producing tumors

Endocrine

Adrenocortical hyperfunction (Cushing syndrome, primary aldosteronism, congenital adrenal hyperplasia, licorice ingestion)
Exogenous hormones (glucocorticoids, estrogen [including pregnancy-induced and oral contraceptives], sympathomimetics and tyramine-containing foods, monoamine oxidase inhibitors)
Pheochromocytoma
Acromegaly
Hypothyroidism (myxedema)
Hyperthyroidism (thyrotoxicosis)
Pregnancy-induced

Cardiovascular

Coarctation of aorta
Polyarteritis nodosa
Increased intravascular volume
Increased cardiac output
Rigidity of the aorta

Neurologic

Psychogenic
Increased intracranial pressure
Sleep apnea
Acute stress, including surgery

often is superimposed on preexisting benign hypertension, either essential or secondary.

PATHOGENESIS OF HYPERTENSION

The multiple mechanisms of hypertension constitute aberrations of the normal physiologic regulation of blood pressure.

Regulation of Normal Blood Pressure. *The blood pressure level is a complex trait that is determined by the interaction of multiple genetic, environmental, and demographic factors that influence two hemodynamic variables: cardiac output and total peripheral resistance.* Cardiac output is affected by blood volume, itself greatly dependent on body sodium homeostasis. Total peripheral resistance is predominantly determined at the level of the arterioles and depends on the effects of neural and hormonal influences. Normal vascular tone reflects the balance between humoral vasoconstricting influences (including angiotensin II and catecholamines) and vasodilators (including kinins, prostaglandins, and nitric oxide). Resistance vessels also exhibit *autoregulation,* whereby increased blood flow induces vasoconstriction to protect against tissue hyperperfusion. Other local factors such as pH and hypoxia, as well as neural interactions (α- and β-adrenergic systems), may be important.

The kidneys play an important role in blood pressure regulation, as follows:

■ Through the renin-angiotensin system, the kidney influences both peripheral resistance and sodium homeostasis. Renin elaborated by the juxtaglomerular cells of the kidney transforms *plasma angiotensinogen* to *angiotensin I,* which is then converted to *angiotensin II* by angiotensin-converting enzyme (ACE) (Fig. 10–11). Angiotensin II raises blood pressure by increasing both peripheral resistance (direct action on vascular SMCs) and blood volume (stimulation of aldosterone secretion, increase in distal tubular reabsorption of sodium).

■ The kidney also produces a variety of vasodepressor or antihypertensive substances (including prostaglandins and nitric oxide) that presumably counterbalance the vasopressor effects of angiotensin.

■ When blood volume is reduced, the *glomerular filtration rate* falls, leading to increased reabsorption of sodium by proximal tubules and thereby conserving sodium and expanding blood volume.

■ *Glomerular filtration rate–independent natriuretic factors* including atrial natriuretic peptide, secreted by heart atria in response to volume expansion, inhibit sodium reabsorption in distal tubules and cause vasodilation.

■ When renal excretory function is impaired, increased arterial pressure is a compensatory mechanism that helps restore fluid and electrolyte balance.

MECHANISMS OF ESSENTIAL HYPERTENSION

Arterial hypertension occurs when the relationship between blood volume and total peripheral resistance is altered. For many of the secondary forms of hypertension, these factors are reasonably well understood. For example, in *renovascular hypertension,* renal artery stenosis causes decreased glomerular flow and decreased pressure in the afferent arteriole of the glomerulus. This (1) induces renin secretion, initiating angiotensin II–induced vasoconstriction and increasing peripheral resistance and (2) through the aldosterone mechanism, increases sodium reabsorption and, therefore, blood volume. In pheochromocytoma, a tumor of the adrenal medulla (Chapter 20), catecholamines produced by tumor cells cause episodic vasoconstriction and thus induce hypertension.

Figure 10–11

Blood pressure variation and the renin-angiotensin system. Components of the systemic renin-angiotensin system are shown in black. Genetic disorders that affect blood pressure by altering activity of this pathway are indicated in red; arrows indicate sites in the pathway altered by mutation. Genes that are mutated in these disorders are indicated in parentheses. Acquired disorders that alter blood pressure through effects on this pathway are indicated in blue. AME, apparent mineralocorticoid excess; ENaC, epithelial sodium channel; GRA, glucocorticoid remediable aldosteronism; HSD, hydroxysteroid dehydrogenase. (Modified with permission from Lifton RP, et al: Molecular genetics of human blood pressure variation. Science 272:676, 1996. Copyright 1996, American Association for the Advancement of Science.)

Blood pressure, like height and weight, is believed to be a continuously distributed variable, and essential hypertension is one extreme of this distribution rather than a distinct disease. *Genetic factors* clearly play a role in determining pressure levels, as is evidenced by studies comparing blood pressure in monozygotic and dizygotic twins and by studies of familial aggregation of hypertension. Moreover, several single-gene disorders that affect specific pathways that control normal blood pressure cause relatively rare forms of hypertension (see Fig. 10–11). In addition, mutations in some genes not directly involved in regulating blood pressure have also been documented in patients with essential hypertension. These include mutations in the gene for cytoskeletal protein α-adducin and a polymorphism in the β_3 subunit of a heterotrimeric G protein. It is postulated that α-adducin may regulate transport of sodium in the renal tubules and that the G protein could be in a signaling pathway that maintains sodium homeostasis. However, it is unlikely that a mutation at a single gene locus will emerge as a major cause of essential hypertension. More likely, the combined effect of mutations or polymorphisms at several gene loci influences blood pressure. Thus, essential hypertension seems to be caused by different combinations of genetic variations that are individually of little consequence. Current efforts, therefore, are focused on genome scans to identify candidate genes and uncover disease-associated polymorphisms. It should be noted, however, that although genetic effects are important, environmental factors *that affect cardiac output, and/or peripheral resistance, are likely also to be important.*

Several factors may then be postulated to contribute to the primary defect(s) in essential hypertension, encompassing both subtle genetic and environmental influences (Fig. 10–12):

■ Reduced renal sodium excretion in the presence of normal arterial pressure may well be the initiating event in essential hypertension. Decreased sodium excretion might lead sequentially to an increase in fluid volume, increased cardiac output, and peripheral vasoconstriction, thereby elevating blood pressure. At the higher setting of blood pressure, enough additional sodium could be excreted by the kidneys to equal intake and prevent fluid retention. Thus, an altered but steady state of sodium excretion would be achieved ("resetting of pressure natriuresis"), but at the expense of stable increases in blood pressure.

■ An alternative hypothesis implicates vasoconstrictive influences (either factors that induce functional vasoconstriction or stimuli that induce direct structural changes in the vessel wall causing increased peripheral resistance) as the primary cause of hypertension. Moreover, chronic or repeated vasoconstrictive influences could cause structural thickening of the resistance vessels. In this model, the structural changes in the vessel wall may then occur early in hypertension, preceding rather than being strictly secondary to the vasoconstriction.

■ Environmental factors could modify expression of the genetic determinants of increased pressure. Stress, obesity, smoking, physical inactivity, and heavy consumption of salt have all been implicated as exogenous factors in hypertension. Indeed, evidence linking the level of dietary sodium intake with the prevalence of hypertension in different population groups is particularly impressive. Moreover, in both essential and secondary hypertension, heavy sodium intake augments the condition.

To summarize, essential hypertension is a complex multifactorial disorder. Environmental factors (e.g., stress, salt intake) affect the variables that control blood pressure in the genetically predisposed individual. Susceptibility genes for essential hypertension are currently unknown but may

Figure 10–12 ■

Hypothetical scheme for the pathogenesis of essential hypertension, implicating genetic defects in renal excretion of sodium, functional regulation of vascular tone, and structural regulation of vascular caliber. Environmental factors, especially increased salt intake, potentiate the effects of genetic factors. The resultant increase in cardiac output and peripheral resistance contributes to hypertension. ECF, extracellular fluid.

Figure 10–13   ■

Vascular pathology in hypertension. *A*, Hyaline arteriolosclerosis. The arteriolar wall is hyalinized and the lumen is markedly narrowed. *B*, Hyperplastic arteriolosclerosis (onion-skinning) causing luminal obliteration *(arrow)*, with secondary ischemic changes, manifest by wrinkling of the glomerular capillary vessels at the upper left (periodic acid-Schiff [PAS] stain). (Courtesy of Helmut Rennke, MD, Brigham and Women's Hospital, Boston.)

well include genes that govern responses to an increased renal sodium load, levels of pressor substances, reactivity of vascular SMCs to pressor agents, or SMC growth. In established hypertension, both increased blood volume and increased peripheral resistance contribute to the increased pressure.

VASCULAR PATHOLOGY IN HYPERTENSION

Hypertension not only accelerates atherogenesis but also causes degenerative changes in the walls of large and medium arteries that potentiate both aortic dissection and cerebrovascular hemorrhage. Hypertension is also associated with two forms of small blood vessel disease: hyaline arteriolosclerosis and hyperplastic arteriolosclerosis (Fig. 10–13).

MORPHOLOGY

HYALINE ARTERIOLOSCLEROSIS. This vascular lesion consists of a homogeneous, pink hyaline thickening of the walls of arterioles with loss of underlying structural detail and with narrowing of the lumen (see Fig. 10-13A). Encountered frequently in elderly patients, whether normotensive or hypertensive, hyaline arteriosclerosis is more generalized and more severe in patients with hypertension. It is also common in diabetes as part of the characteristic microangiography (Chapter 17).

The lesions reflect leakage of plasma components across vascular endothelium and excessive extracellular matrix production by SMCs secondary to the chronic hemodynamic stress of hypertension or a metabolic stress in diabetes that accentuates EC injury. **Hyaline arteriolosclerosis is a major morphologic characteristic of benign nephrosclerosis,** in which the arteriolar narrowing

causes diffuse impairment of renal blood supply, loss of nephrons, and symmetric contraction of the kidneys (Chapter 14).

HYPERPLASTIC ARTERIOLOSCLEROSIS. Related to more acute or severe elevations of blood pressure, hyperplastic arteriolosclerosis is characteristic of, but not limited to, malignant hypertension (diastolic pressures usually over 120 mm Hg). Hyperplastic arteriolosclerosis has onion-skin, concentric, laminated thickening of the walls of arterioles with progressive narrowing of the lumina (see Fig. 10–13B). With the electron microscope, the laminations are seen to consist of SMCs and thickened and reduplicated basement membrane. In malignant hypertension, these hyperplastic changes are accompanied by fibrinoid deposits and acute necrosis of the vessel walls, referred to as **necrotizing arteriolitis,** particularly in the kidney (Chapter 14).

ANEURYSMS AND DISSECTIONS

An *aneurysm* is a *localized abnormal dilation of a blood vessel or the heart.* When a bulging aneurysm is bounded by arterial wall components or the attenuated wall of the heart, it is called a "true" aneurysm. Atherosclerotic, syphilitic, and congenital vascular aneurysms and the left ventricular aneurysm that can follow a myocardial infarction are of this type. In contrast, a *false aneurysm* (also called *pseudoaneurysm*) is a breach in the vascular wall leading to an extravascular hematoma that freely communicates with the intravascular space ("pulsating hematoma"), most commonly a post–myocardial infarction rupture that has been contained by a pericardial adhesion or a leak at the junction *(anastomosis)* of a vascular graft with a natural artery. An arterial *dissection* arises when blood enters the wall of the artery, as a hematoma dissecting between its layers. Dissections are often but not always aneurysmal.

The two most important causes of aortic aneurysms are ATH and cystic medial degeneration of the arterial media. However, any vessel may be affected by a wide variety of disorders that weaken the wall, including trauma (traumatic aneurysms or arteriovenous aneurysms), congenital defects such as that producing *berry* aneurysms (small, spherical dilatations, most frequently in the brain) (Chapter 23), infections (*mycotic aneurysms;* see later) or syphilis. Arterial aneurysms can also be caused by systemic diseases, as in some vasculitides (see later).

Infection of a major artery that weakens its wall is called a *mycotic aneurysm.* Thrombosis and rupture are possible complications. Mycotic aneurysms may originate (1) from embolization and arrest of a septic embolus at some point within a vessel, usually as a complication of infective endocarditis; (2) as an extension of an adjacent suppurative process; or (3) by circulating organisms directly infecting the arterial wall.

For descriptive purposes, aneurysms can be classified by macroscopic shape and size. *Saccular* aneurysms are essentially spherical (involving only a portion of the vessel wall) and vary in size from 5 to 20 cm in diameter, often partially or completely filled by thrombus. Alternatively, aneurysms may be *fusiform* (involving a long segment). Fusiform aneurysms vary in diameter (up to 20 cm) and in length; many involve the entire ascending and transverse portions of the aortic arch, whereas others may involve large segments of the abdominal aorta or even the iliacs. However, these shapes are not specific for any disease or clinical manifestations.

Abdominal Aortic Aneurysms

Atherosclerosis, the most frequent etiology of aneurysms, causes arterial wall thinning through medial destruction secondary to plaque that originates in the intima. *Atherosclerotic aneurysms most frequently occur in the abdominal aorta (abdominal aortic aneurysm,* often abbreviated AAA), but the common iliac arteries, the arch, and descending parts of the thoracic aorta can be involved.

Figure 10–14   ■

Gross photographs of an abdominal aortic aneurysm that ruptured. *A,* External view of the large aneurysm; the rupture site is indicated by an arrow. *B,* Opened view, with the location of the rupture tract indicated by a probe. The wall of the aneurysm is exceedingly thin, and the lumen is filled by a large quantity of layered but largely unorganized thrombus.

MORPHOLOGY

Usually positioned below the renal arteries and above the bifurcation of the aorta (Fig. 10–14), AAAs are saccular or fusiform, sometimes up to 15 cm in greatest diameter, and of variable length (up to 25 cm). In these areas of severe complicated ATH, there is destruction and thinning of the underlying aortic media that has weakened the wall. The aneurysm and the nearby aorta often contain atheromatous ulcers covered by granular mural thrombi, prime sites for the formation of atheroemboli that may lodge in the vessels of the kidneys or lower extremities. Additionally, a thrombus frequently fills at least part of the dilated segment. Occasionally, the aneurysm may affect the origins of the renal and superior or inferior mesenteric arteries, either by producing direct pressure on these vessels or by narrowing or occluding their ostia with mural thrombi. Not infrequently, AAAs are accompanied by smaller fusiform or saccular dilations of the iliac arteries.

Two variants of AAAs merit special mention. **Inflammatory AAAs** are characterized by dense periaortic fibrosis containing an abundant lymphoplasmacytic inflammatory reaction with many macrophages and often giant cells. Their cause is uncertain. **Mycotic AAAs** are atherosclerotic lesions that have become infected by lodgment of circulating organisms in the wall, particularly in bacteremia from a primary *Salmonella* gastroenteritis. In such cases, suppuration further destroys the media, potentiating rapid dilation and rupture.

Pathogenesis. ATH is a major cause of AAAs, but other factors contribute. AAAs rarely develop before the age of 50 and are more common in men. They have been shown to be familial, and this association is independent of the familial/genetic predisposition to ATH or hypertension. For example, as discussed subsequently in the section on Marfan syndrome and aortic dissection, genetic defects in structural components of the aorta can themselves produce aneurysms and dissections. Moreover, it has been postulated that subtle defects in a connective tissue component responsible for the strength of blood vessels or in the balance of collagen degradation and synthesis could provide a particularly susceptible substrate on which ATH or hypertension, or both, could act to weaken the aortic wall.

Clinical Course. The clinical consequences of AAAs depend primarily on location and size, including

■ Rupture into the peritoneal cavity or retroperitoneal tissues with massive, potentially fatal hemorrhage
■ Obstruction of a vessel, particularly of the iliac, renal, mesenteric, or vertebral branches that supply the spinal cord
■ Embolism from atheroma or mural thrombus
■ Impingement on an adjacent structure, such as compression of a ureter or erosion of vertebrae
■ Presentation of an abdominal mass (often palpably pulsating) that simulates a tumor

The risk of rupture is directly related to the size of the aneurysm, varying from about 2% for a small AAAs (less than approximately 4 cm in diameter) to 5% to 10% per year for aneurysms larger than 5 cm in diameter. Thus, large aneurysms are usually surgically replaced or bypassed by prosthetic grafts. Timely surgery is critical; operative mortality for unruptured aneurysms is approximately 5%, whereas emergency surgery after rupture carries a mortality rate of more than 50%.

Because ATH, the underlying cause of abdominal aortic aneurysm, is a systemic disease, patients with AAAs are also at significantly increased risk for IHD and stroke.

Syphilitic (Luetic) Aneurysms

The obliterative endarteritis characteristic of the tertiary stage of syphilis (lues) may involve small vessels in any part of the body, but it is clinically most devastating when it involves the vasa vasorum of the aorta. Such a complication gives rise to thoracic aortitis, which in turn can lead to aneurysmal dilation affecting the aorta and the aortic annulus. Fortunately, better control and treatment of syphilis in its early stages has decreased the frequency of these complications.

MORPHOLOGY

Inflammatory involvement begins in the aortic adventitia, particularly involving the vasa vasorum, inducing **obliterative endarteritis** rimmed by an infiltrate of lymphocytes and plasma cells **(syphilitic aortitis).** The narrowing of the lumina of the vasa vasorum causes ischemic injury of the aortic media, with patchy loss of the medial elastic fibers and muscle cells, followed by inflammation and scarring. With destruction of the media, the aorta loses its elastic recoil and may become dilated, producing a syphilitic aneurysm. Contraction of fibrous scars may lead to wrinkling of intervening segments of aortic intima, noted grossly as "tree-barking." Luetic involvement of the aorta favors the development of superimposed atherosclerosis of the aortic root (an unusual location for "garden

variety" ATH), which can envelop and occlude the coronary ostia. **Even when these aneurysms are complicated by ATH, the thoracic location distinguishes them from typical atherosclerotic aneurysms, which rarely affect the aortic arch and never involve the root of the aorta.**

Luetic aortitis may also cause aortic valve ring dilation, resulting in valvular insufficiency through circumferential stretching of the valve cusps, widening of the commissures between the cusps, and turbulence-induced thickening and rolling of the free margins. Owing to aortic insufficiency, the left ventricular wall can undergo massive volume overload hypertrophy, sometimes to 1000 g (about three times normal weight), descriptively referred to as "cor bovinum" (cow's heart).

Whatever the etiology, thoracic aortic aneurysms can give rise to signs and symptoms referable to (1) encroachment on mediastinal structures, (2) respiratory difficulties caused by encroachment on the lungs and airways, (3) difficulty in swallowing caused by compression of the esophagus, (4) persistent cough from irritation of or pressure on the recurrent laryngeal nerves, (5) pain caused by erosion of bone (i.e., ribs and vertebral bodies), (6) cardiac disease as the aortic aneurysm leads to aortic valve dilation with valvular insufficiency or narrowing of the coronary ostia causing myocardial ischemia, and (7) rupture. Most patients with syphilitic aneurysms die of heart failure induced by aortic valvular incompetence.

Aortic Dissection (Dissecting Hematoma)

Aortic dissection is a catastrophic illness characterized by dissection of blood between and along the laminar planes of the media, with the formation of a blood-filled channel within the aortic wall (Fig. 10–15) that often ruptures outward, causing massive hemorrhage. In contrast to atherosclerotic and syphilitic aneurysms, aortic dissection may or may not be associated with marked dilatation of the aorta. For this reason, the older term dissecting aneurysm is discouraged.

Aortic dissection occurs principally in two groups of patients. The first group includes men 40 to 60 years of age with antecedent hypertension (more than 90% of cases of dissection). The second major group of patients, usually younger, has a systemic or localized abnormality of connective tissue that affects the aorta (e.g., Marfan syndrome, discussed in Chapter 7). Dissection can also be iatrogenic, as a complication of arterial cannulation (e.g., during diagnostic catheterization or cardiopulmonary bypass). Rarely, for unknown reasons, dissection of the aorta or other branches, including the coronary arteries, occurs during or after pregnancy. Dissection is unusual in the presence of substantial ATH or other cause of medial scarring such as syphilis. Presumably, the scarring obstructs the advancement of a dissecting hematoma.

Figure 10-15 ■

A, Gross photograph of proximal aortic dissection demonstrating a small, oblique intimal tear *(demarcated by probe),* allowing blood to enter the media, creating an intramural hematoma *(narrow arrows).* Note that the intimal tear has occurred in a region largely free of atherosclerotic plaque and that propagation of the intramural hematoma is arrested at a site more distally where atherosclerosis begins *(broad arrow). B,* Histologic view of the dissection demonstrating an aortic intramural hematoma *(asterisk).* Aortic elastic layers are black and blood is red in this section, stained with the Movat stain.

MORPHOLOGY

In spontaneous dissection, an intimal tear marking the point of origin usually extends into but not through the media of the ascending aorta, usually within 10 cm of the aortic valve (see Fig. 10-15A). Such tears are usually transverse or oblique and 1 to 5 cm in length, with sharp but jagged edges. The dissection can extend along the aorta proximally toward the heart as well as distally, sometimes all the way into the iliac and femoral arteries. The dissecting hematoma spreads characteristically along the laminar planes of the aorta, usually approximately between the middle and outer thirds (see Fig. 10-15B). It often ruptures out, causing massive hemorrhage. In some instances, the blood reruptures into the lumen of the aorta, producing a second or distal intimal tear and a new vascular channel within the media of the aortic wall (to produce a "double-barreled aorta" with "false channel"). This averts a fatal extra-aortic hemorrhage. In the course of time, false channels may become endothelialized ("chronic dissection").

In most cases, no specific underlying preexisting and causal pathology is seen in the aortic wall. The most frequent preexisting histologically detectable lesion is **cystic medial degeneration** (CMD). CMD is sometimes called "cystic medial necrosis," an inac-

curate term because necrosis is not usually present. CMD is characterized by elastic tissue fragmentation and separation of the elastic and fibromuscular elements of the tunica media by small cleftlike or cystic spaces filled with the amorphous extracellular matrix of connective tissue. Ultimately, there may be large-scale loss of elastic laminae (Fig. 10-16). Inflammation is absent. CMD of the aorta frequently accompanies Marfan syndrome, but patients with dissection caused by hypertension have variable nonspecific changes in aortic wall histology ranging from mild fragmentation of elastic tissue (most commonly) to overt CMD.

Pathogenesis. Hypertension is clearly the major risk factor overall, but its contribution to aortic medial damage is uncertain. Severe degenerative changes in some cases are also frequently found incidentally at autopsy of patients who are free from dissection. Thus, *medial structural lesions do not always lead to dissection, and abnormal medial histology is not prerequisite to dissection.* Some dissections are related to the inherited connective tissue disorders that cause abnormal vascular structure, most prominently Marfan syndrome, an autosomal dominant disease of connective tissue fibrillin characterized by skeletal, cardiovascular, and ocular manifestations (Chapter 7). The cause of spontaneous dissections not associated with hypertension or genetic disorders is unknown.

Figure 10–16

Cystic medial degeneration. *A,* Cross-section of aortic media with marked elastin fragmentation and formation of areas devoid of elastin that resemble cystic spaces *(asterisks),* from a patient with Marfan syndrome. *B,* Normal media for comparison, showing the regular layered pattern of elastic tissue. In both *A* and *B,* the tissue section is stained to highlight elastin as black.

Regardless of the underlying cause, the trigger for the intimal tear and intramural aortic hemorrhage is unknown in most cases. Nevertheless, once the tear has occurred, increased systemic blood pressure fosters progression of the medial hematoma. Indeed, aggressive antihypertensive therapy is often effective in limiting an evolving dissection.

Clinical Course. The risk and nature of serious complications of dissection depend strongly on the level of the aorta affected, with the most serious complications occurring from the aortic valve to the arch. Thus, aortic dissections are generally classified into two types:

■ The more common (and dangerous) *proximal* lesions, involving either the ascending portion only or both the ascending and the descending aorta (types I and II of the DeBakey classification, often collectively called type A)
■ *Distal lesions not involving the ascending part* and usually beginning distal to the subclavian artery (DeBakey type III, often called type B)

The classic clinical symptoms of aortic dissection are the sudden onset of excruciating pain, usually beginning in the anterior chest, radiating to the back, and moving downward as the dissection progresses. This intense pain can be readily confused with that of acute myocardial infarction.

The most common cause of death is rupture of the dissection outward into any of the three body cavities (i.e., pericardial, pleural, or peritoneal). Retrograde dissection into the aortic root can cause disruption of the aortic valvular apparatus. Thus, common clinical manifestations include cardiac tamponade, aortic insufficiency, and myocardial infarction or extension of the dissection into the great arteries of the neck or into the coronary, renal, mesenteric, or iliac arteries, causing critical vascular obstruction; compression of spinal arteries may cause transverse myelitis.

At one time, aortic dissection was usually fatal, but the prognosis has markedly improved. The development of surgical procedures involving plication of the aortic wall and the early institution of intensive antihypertensive therapy permit salvage of 65% to 75% of patients with dissections.

INFLAMMATORY DISEASE—THE VASCULITIDES

Inflammation of the walls of vessels, called *vasculitis,* is encountered in diverse clinical settings. Vessels of any type in virtually any organ can be affected; clinical manifestations often include constitutional signs and symptoms such as fever, myalgia, arthralgias, and malaise. The two most common mechanisms of vasculitis are immune-mediated inflammation and direct invasion of vascular walls by infectious pathogens (Table 10–4). Nevertheless, infections can indirectly induce a noninfectious vasculitis, for example, by generating immune complexes or triggering cross-reactivity. In a particular patient, it is critical to distinguish between direct infectious and immunologic mechanisms, because immunosuppressive therapy is appropriate for immune-mediated vasculitis but would be potentially harmful for infectious vasculitis. Physical and chemical injury, such as from irradiation, mechanical trauma, and toxins, can also cause vascular damage.

Pathogenesis of Noninfectious Vasculitis. Noninfectious vasculitis appears to be initiated by one of several immunologic mechanisms. Of these so-called *systemic necrotizing vasculitides,* several types affect the aorta and medium-sized vessels, but most affect small vessels, such as arterioles, venules, and capillaries (designated *small vessel vasculitis*).

Immune Complexes. The evidence for involvement of immune complexes in vasculitides can be summarized as follows:

Table 10-4. CLASSIFICATION OF VASCULITIS BASED ON PATHOGENESIS

Direct Infection

Bacterial (e.g., *Neisseria*)
Rickettsial (e.g., Rocky Mountain spotted fever)
Spirochetal (e.g., syphilis)
Fungal (e.g., aspergillosis, mucormycosis)
Viral (e.g., herpes zoster-varicella)

Immunologic

Immune complex–mediated
    Infection–induced (e.g., hepatitis B and C virus)
    Henoch-Schönlein purpura
    Systemic lupus erythematosus and rheumatoid arthritis
    Drug-induced
    Cryoglobulinemia
    Serum sickness
Antineutrophil cytoplasmic autoantibody–mediated
    Wegener granulomatosis
    Microscopic polyangiitis (microscopic polyarteritis)
    Churg-Strauss syndrome
Direct antibody attack–mediated
    Goodpasture syndrome (anti–glomerular basement membrane antibodies)
    Kawasaki disease (antiendothelial antibodies)
Cell-mediated
    Allograft organ rejection
Inflammatory bowel disease
Paraneoplastic vasculitis

Unknown

Giant cell (temporal) arteritis
Takayasu arteritis
Polyarteritis nodosa (classic polyarteritis nodosa)

Data from Jennette JC, Falk RJ: Update of the pathobiology of vasculitis. In Schoen FJ, Gimbrone MA (eds): Cardiovascular Pathology: Clinicopathologic Correlations and Pathogenetic Mechanisms. Baltimore, Williams & Wilkins, 1995, p 156; and Jennette JC, Falk RJ: Small-vessel vasculitis. N Engl J Med 1337:1512, 1997.

■ The vascular lesions resemble those found in experimental immune complex–mediated conditions, such as the local Arthus phenomenon and serum sickness. Immune reactants and complement can be detected in the serum or vessels of patients with vasculitis (e.g., DNA/anti-DNA complexes are present in the vascular lesions of systemic lupus erythematosus–associated vasculitis; IgG, IgM, and complement in cryoglobulinemic vasculitis).

■ Hypersensitivity to drugs causes approximately 10% of vasculitic skin lesions through vascular deposits of immune complexes. Some, such as penicillin, conjugate serum proteins, whereas others (e.g., streptokinase) are foreign proteins. In both cases, antigen-antibody complexes are deposited in vessel walls.

■ The most impressive evidence comes from vasculitis associated with viral infections, particularly hepatitis. There is a high incidence of hepatitis B antigen (HBsAg) and HbsAg/anti-HBsAg immune complexes in the serum and, with complement, in the vascular lesions of some patients with vasculitis, most frequently with polyarteritis nodosa (PAN). Chronic hepatitis C (HCV) infection can give rise to glomerulonephritis, and in such cases HCV antigens and anti-HCV immunoglobulin antibodies can be seen in glomeruli.

Whether complexes accrue in vessel walls by deposition from the circulation, by in situ formation, or by a combination of these mechanisms is not known (Chapter 5). However, many small vessel vasculitides show a paucity of vascular immune deposits, and therefore other mechanisms have been sought for these so-called *pauci-immune* vasculitides.

Antineutrophil Cytoplasmic Antibodies. Serum from many patients with vasculitis reacts with cytoplasmic antigens in neutrophils, indicating the presence of *antineutrophil cytoplasmic autoantibodies (ANCAs)*. ANCAs comprise a heterogeneous group of autoantibodies directed against enzymes mainly found within the azurophil or primary granules in neutrophils, in the lysosomes of monocytes, and in ECs. There are two main immunofluorescent patterns of staining of ethanol-fixed neutrophils. One shows cytoplasmic localization of the staining (c-ANCA); the most common target antigen is proteinase 3 (PR-3), a neutrophil granule constituent. The second shows perinuclear staining (p-ANCA) and is usually specific for myeloperoxidase. It should be noted that this localization of staining represents an artifact of fixation. Myeloperoxidase is contained in neutrophil granules. Either ANCA specificity may occur in a patient with ANCA-associated small vessel vasculitis, but c-ANCA is typically found in Wegener granulomatosis and p-ANCA is found in most cases of microscopic polyangiitis and Churg-Strauss syndrome. However, approximately 10% of patients with these disorders are ANCA negative.

ANCAs serve as useful quantitative diagnostic markers for these disorders, and their discovery has led to segregation of a group of these disorders as the *ANCA-associated vasculitides*. The close association between ANCA titers and disease activity, particularly c-ANCA in Wegener granulomatosis, suggests that they may be important in the pathogenesis of this disease, but the precise mechanisms are unknown.

Whether ANCAs are mere markers of vasculitides or play a role in tissue injury is not entirely clear. In vitro studies have revealed that when neutrophils are activated by cytokines, ANCA-related cytoplasmic proteins (PR-3 and myeloperoxidase) are displayed on the cell surface, and this is followed by degranulation. This, in turn, releases chemoattractants and toxic free radicals. When ANCAs bind to their target antigen on the activated neutrophils, the process of degranulation and consequent tissue injury is exacerbated. In addition, activated neutrophils bind to ECs and cause vascular injury. Why ANCAs are generated in the first place remains entirely mysterious, as does the origin of most other autoantibodies.

Antiendothelial Cell Antibodies. Antibodies to ECs, perhaps induced by defects in immune regulation, may predispose to certain vasculitides, such as those associated with systemic lupus erythematosus and Kawasaki disease.

Classification. The systemic vasculitides are classified on the basis of the size and anatomic site of the involved blood vessels (Fig. 10–17), histologic characteristics of the lesion, and clinical manifestations. There is considerable clinical and pathologic overlap among these disorders, as noted in Figures 10–18, 10–19, and 10–20.

Figure 10–17 ■

Diagrammatic representation of the sites of the vasculature involved by the major forms of vasculitis. The widths of the trapezoids indicate the frequencies of involvement of various portions. Note that large-, medium- and small-vessel vasculitis affect arteries but only small-vessel vasculitis involves vessels smaller than arteries. LCA, leukocytoclastic angiitis. (Reproduced with permission from Jennette JC, Falk RJ: Small-vessel vasculitis. N Engl J Med 337:1512, 1997. Copyright © 1997, Massachusetts Medical Society. All rights reserved.)

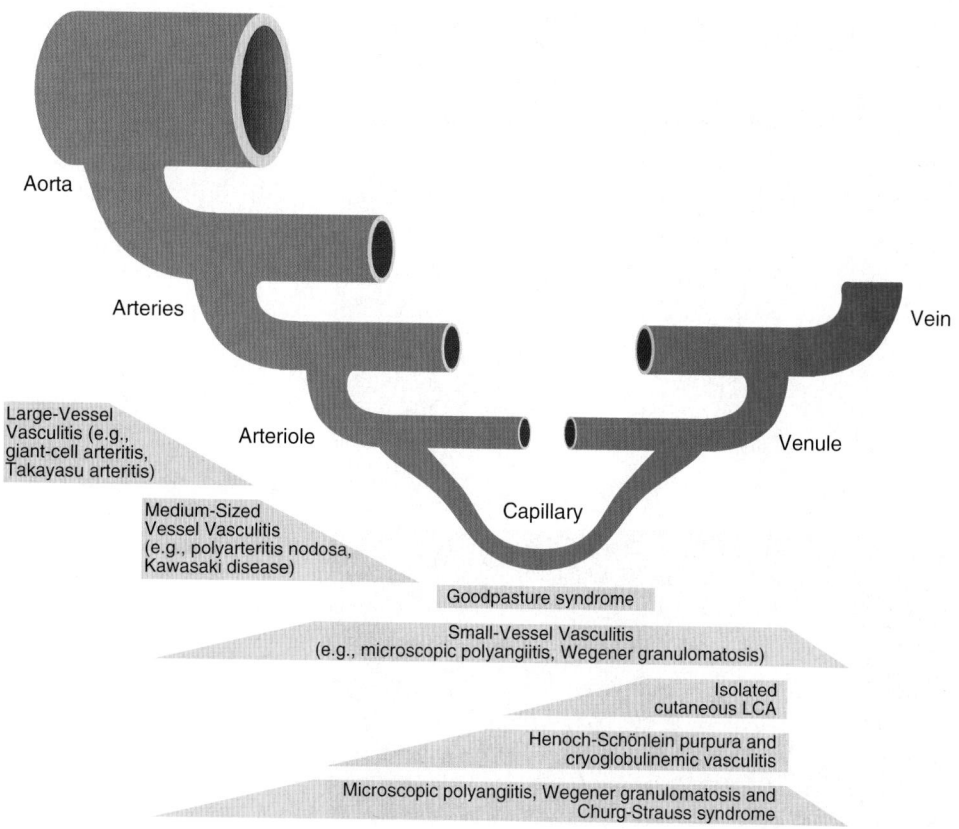

Giant Cell (Temporal) Arteritis

Giant cell (temporal) arteritis, the most common of the vasculitides, is an acute and chronic, often granulomatous, inflammation of arteries of large to small size. It affects principally the arteries in the head—especially the temporal arteries but also the vertebral and ophthalmic arteries. Blindness may occur if the ophthalmic artery is involved. Lesions have also been found in other arteries throughout the body, including the aorta *(giant cell aortitis).*

MORPHOLOGY

Characteristically, segments of affected arteries develop **nodular thickenings with reduction of the lumen** and may become thrombosed. In the more common variant there is **granulomatous inflammation** of the inner half of the media centered on the internal elastic membrane marked by a lymphocytic infiltrate, multinucleate giant cells, and

Figure 10–18 ■

Temporal (giant cell) arteritis. *A,* H & E stain of giant cells at the degenerated internal elastic membrane in active arteritis. *B,* Elastic tissue stain demonstrating focal destruction of internal elastic membrane *(arrow)* and intimal thickening (IT) characteristic of long-standing or healed arteritis.

Figure 10-19 ■

Takayasu arteritis. *A,* Aortic arch angiogram showing narrowing of brachio-cephalic, carotid, and subclavian arteries *(arrows). B,* Gross photograph of two cross-sections of the right carotid artery taken at autopsy of the patient shown in *A,* demonstrating marked intimal thickening with minimal residual lumen. *C,* Histologic view of active Takayasu aortitis, illustrating destruction of the arterial media by mononuclear inflammation with giant cells.

fragmentation of the internal elastic lamina (see Fig. 10-18). Macrophages are frequently seen in close proximity to the damaged elastic lamina. Both CD4+ and CD8+ lymphocytes are found, although the CD4+ T cells predominate. In the less common pattern, granulomas and giant cells are rare or absent and there is a nonspecific panarteritis with a

mixed inflammatory infiltrate composed largely of lymphocytes and macrophages admixed with neutrophils and eosinophils. The later healed stage of both of these patterns reveals collagenous thickening of the vessel wall; organization of the luminal thrombus sometimes transforms the artery into a fibrous cord. However, the scarring may be difficult to distinguish from changes associated with aging.

Pathogenesis. The cause of this relatively common disease remains elusive. However, much evidence points to a T-cell–mediated immune response to an unknown, possibly vessel wall, antigen. Supporting this hypothesis are a granulomatous inflammatory response with the presence of CD4+ red T cells in the lesions; an association with certain HLA-DR antigens; and the presence of a clonal T-cell population at multiple affected sites, suggesting a response to a specific antigen. In addition, studies have revealed that giant cell arteritis is associated with the inheritance of a particular polymorphism of the gene that encodes intercellular adhesion molecule 1. This molecule mediates cellular interaction between cells of the immune system and EC.

Clinical Features. Temporal arteritis is most common in older individuals and is rare before the age of 50. Symptoms either are only vague and constitutional—fever, fatigue, weight loss—without localizing signs or symptoms or are facial pain or headache, often most intense along the course of the superficial temporal artery, which may be painful to palpation. More serious are ocular symptoms (associated with involvement of the ophthalmic artery), which appear quite abruptly in about half of patients and range from diplopia to transient or complete vision loss. The diagnosis depends on biopsy and histologic confirmation, but because of the segmental nature of the involvement, adequate biopsy requires at least a 2- to 3-cm length of artery, and a negative biopsy result does not rule out the condition. Treatment with anti-inflammatory agents is remarkably effective.

Takayasu Arteritis

This granulomatous vasculitis of medium and larger arteries was described in 1908 by Takayasu and is *characterized principally by ocular disturbances and marked weakening of the pulses in the upper extremities (pulseless disease), related to fibrous thickening of the aorta, particularly the aortic arch and its branches, with narrowing or virtual obliteration of the origins or more distal portions* (see Fig. 10-19). The illness is seen predominantly in females younger than 40 years old. The cause and pathogenesis are unknown, although immune mechanisms are suspected.

MORPHOLOGY

Takayasu arteritis classically involves the aortic arch, but in one third of cases it also affects the remainder of the aorta and its branches (often for some distance), and in half of the cases the pulmonary

Figure 10-20   ■

Representative forms of medium to small vessel vasculitis. *A*, Polyarteritis nodosa. *B*, Wegener granulomatosis. *C*, Thromboangiitis obliterans (Buerger disease). In polyarteritis nodosa *(A)*, there is segmental
fibrinoid necrosis and thrombotic occlusion of the lumen of this small
artery. Note that part of the vessel wall at the upper right *(arrow)* is uninvolved. In Wegener granulomatosis *(B)*, there is inflammation (vasculitis) of a small artery along with adjacent granulomatous inflammation,
in which epithelioid cells and giant cells *(arrows)* are seen. In a typical
case of Buerger disease *(C)*, the lumen is occluded by a thrombus containing two abscesses *(arrows)*. The vessel wall is infiltrated with
leukocytes. (*A* and *B*, Courtesy of Sid Murphree, MD, Department of
Pathology, University of Texas Southwestern Medical School, Dallas.)

arteries are involved. The gross morphologic changes
include, in most cases, irregular thickening of the
aortic or branch vessel wall with intimal wrinkling
(see Fig. 10-19*A*). When the aortic arch is involved,
the orifices of the major arteries to the upper portion
of the body may be markedly narrowed or even
obliterated by intimal thickening (see Fig. 10-19*B*).
This lesion is responsible for weakness of the pulses,
accounting for the older designation of **pulseless
disease.** The coronary and renal arteries may be
similarly affected. Histologically, the changes range
from an adventitial mononuclear infiltrate with
perivascular cuffing of the vasa vasorum, to intense
mononuclear inflammation in the media, to granulomatous inflammation, replete with giant cells and
patchy necrosis of the media. Some cases (see Fig.
10-19*C*) may be indistinguishable from giant cell
(temporal) arteritis. **Thus, distinctions among active
giant cell lesions of the aorta are based largely on
the age of the patient, and most giant cell lesions of
the aorta in young patients are designated Takayasu
arteritis.** Later, as the disease runs its course, or after
treatment with corticosteroids, there is collagenous fibrosis involving all layers of the vessel wall but, particularly, the intima, accompanied by lymphocytic infiltration. Involvement of the root of the aorta may
cause dilation, producing aortic valve insufficiency.

Narrowing of the coronary ostia may lead to myocardial infarction.

Clinical Features. Early in the course of disease, the
symptoms are nonspecific, including fatigue, weight loss, and
fever. With progression, vascular symptoms appear and dominate the clinical picture. These include markedly lower blood
pressure and weaker pulses in the upper extremities than in
the lower extremities with coldness or numbness of the fingers; ocular disturbances, including visual defects, retinal
hemorrhages, and total blindness; and neurologic deficits. Involvement of the more distal aorta may lead to claudication
of the legs; that of the pulmonary arteries may lead to pulmonary hypertension. Renal artery narrowing gives rise to
systemic hypertension in about 50% of cases. The course of
the disease is variable. In some persons there is rapid progression, but in others a quiescent stage is reached in 1 or 2
years, permitting long-term survival, albeit sometimes with
visual or neurologic deficits.

Polyarteritis Nodosa

Polyarteritis nodosa (PAN) is a systemic vasculitis of small
or medium-sized muscular arteries (but not arterioles, capillaries, or venules), typically involving renal and visceral vessels but sparing the pulmonary circulation.

MORPHOLOGY

Classic PAN is characterized by segmental transmural necrotizing inflammation of **arteries of medium to small size, in any organ** (with the exception of the lung). The distribution of lesions in descending order of frequency is kidneys, heart, liver, and gastrointestinal tract, followed by pancreas, testis, skeletal muscles, nervous system, and skin. Individual lesions may involve only a portion of the vessel circumference and have a predilection for branching points and bifurcations. Segmental erosion with **weakening of the arterial wall** caused by the inflammatory process may cause aneurysmal dilation or localized rupture. **Impairment of perfusion,** causing ulcerations, infarcts, ischemic atrophy, or hemorrhages in the area supplied by these vessels, may provide the first clue to the existence of the underlying disorder. Sometimes the lesions are exclusively microscopic with no gross changes.

The histologic picture during the acute phase is characterized by **transmural inflammation of the arterial wall** demonstrating neutrophils, eosinophils, and mononuclear cells and is frequently accompanied by fibrinoid necrosis (see Fig. 10–20A). The lumen may become thrombosed. Later, the acute inflammatory infiltrate disappears and is replaced by **fibrous thickening of the vessel wall** that may extend into the adventitia. Firm nodularity sometimes marks the lesions. **Particularly characteristic of PAN is that all stages of activity may coexist in different vessels or even within the same vessel.**

Clinical Course. Although a disease of young adults, classic PAN may occur in children and older individuals. The course may be acute, subacute, or chronic and is frequently remittent and episodic, with long symptom-free intervals. Because the vascular involvement is widely scattered, the clinical signs and symptoms of PAN may be varied and puzzling. The most common manifestations are malaise, fever of unknown cause, and weight loss; hypertension, usually developing rapidly; abdominal pain and melena (bloody stool) caused by vascular lesions in the gastrointestinal tract; diffuse muscular aches and pains; and peripheral neuritis, which is predominantly motor. Renal involvement is often prominent and a major cause of death. Because small vessel involvement is absent, however, there is no glomerulonephritis. About 30% of patients with PAN have hepatitis B antigen in their serum. There is no association with ANCA. If untreated, the disease is fatal in most cases, either during an acute fulminant attack or after a protracted course, but therapy with corticosteroids and cyclophosphamide results in remissions or cures in 90%. The presentations are so diverse that clinical diagnosis often needs to be established by biopsy of the suspected area of involvement.

Kawasaki Disease (Mucocutaneous Lymph Node Syndrome)

Kawasaki disease is an acute febrile illness of infancy and childhood that is associated with an arteritis affecting large, medium-sized, and small vessels. Its clinical significance stems from the involvement of coronary arteries. It usually affects young children, with 80% of those affected being younger than age 4 years. It is the leading cause of acquired heart disease in children. Kawasaki disease is sometimes called *mucocutaneous lymph node syndrome.* It presents as an acute but usually self-limited illness manifested by fever, conjunctival and oral erythema and erosion, edema of the hands and feet, erythema of the palms and soles, a rash often with desquamation, and enlargement of cervical lymph nodes. Epidemic in Japan, the disease has also been reported in Hawaii and increasingly in the continental United States. Approximately 20% of untreated patients develop cardiovascular sequelae, ranging in severity from asymptomatic vasculitis of the coronary arteries, coronary artery ectasia, or aneurysm formation to giant coronary artery aneurysms (7 to 8 mm) with rupture or thrombosis, myocardial infarction, or sudden death. With intravenous immunoglobulin therapy the rate of coronary artery disease is reduced to about 4%. Pathologic changes outside the cardiovascular system are rarely significant.

MORPHOLOGY

The vasculitis is PAN-like, with necrosis and pronounced inflammation affecting the entire thickness of the vessel wall, but fibrinoid necrosis is usually less prominent in Kawasaki disease than in PAN. Although the acute vasculitis subsides spontaneously or in response to treatment, aneurysm formation, or thrombosis and myocardial infarction, can supervene. As with other causes of arteritis, healed lesions may have obstructive intimal thickening.

The cause of the condition is uncertain, but there is evidence that the vasculitis is characterized by T-cell and macrophage activation in response to an unknown antigen. This leads to the secretion of cytokines, polyclonal B-cell hyperactivity, and the formation of autoantibodies to ECs and SMCs. These antibodies precipitate an acute vasculitis. It is currently speculated that in genetically susceptible persons, a variety of common infectious agents (most likely viral) may trigger the disease.

Microscopic Polyangiitis (Microscopic Polyarteritis, Hypersensitivity, or Leukocytoclastic Angiitis)

This type of necrotizing vasculitis generally affects arterioles, capillaries, and venules—vessels smaller than those involved in PAN. In unusual cases, larger arteries may be involved. Furthermore, unlike PAN, all lesions tend to be of the same age in a single patient. It typically involves the skin, mucous membranes, lungs, brain, heart, gastrointestinal tract, kidneys, and muscle. *In contrast to PAN, necrotizing glomerulonephritis (90% of patients) and pulmonary capillaritis are particularly common.* The major clinical features are hemoptysis, hematuria, and proteinuria; bowel pain or bleeding; muscle pain or weakness; and palpable cutaneous purpura. In many cases, an immunologic reaction to an antigen such as drugs (e.g., penicillin), microorganisms (e.g., streptococci), heterologous proteins, and tumor antigens is the precipitating cause. Nevertheless, although immunoglobulins and complement components may be present in early lesions of the skin, *there is generally little or no immunoglobulin demonstrable by immunofluorescence microscopy ("pauci-immune injury").*

MORPHOLOGY

The transmural necrotizing lesions of microscopic polyangiitis often resemble those of PAN with segmental fibrinoid necrosis of the media. However, in contrast to PAN, medium-sized and larger arteries are usually spared; thus, macroscopic infarcts similar to those seen in PAN are uncommon. Although microscopic polyangiitis has the same spectrum of manifestations as Wegener granulomatosis (see later), the granulomatous inflammation typical of Wegener granulomatosis is absent. In some lesions the change is limited to infiltration with neutrophils, which become fragmented as they follow the vessel wall, giving rise to the term **leukocytoclastic angiitis,** most commonly found in postcapillary venules.

With the exception of those who develop widespread renal or brain involvement, most patients respond well simply to removal of the offending agent. p-ANCAs are present in over 80% of patients. Disseminated vascular lesions of hypersensitivity angiitis may also appear in Henoch-Schönlein purpura, essential mixed cryoglobulinemia, vasculitis associated with some of the connective tissue disorders, and vasculitis associated with malignancy. ANCAs are not present in these conditions.

In *allergic granulomatosis and angiitis* (Churg-Strauss syndrome), vascular lesions may be histologically similar to those of classic PAN or microscopic polyangiitis. *There is a strong association, however, with allergic rhinitis, bronchial asthma, and eosinophilia.* Vessels in the lung, heart, spleen, peripheral nerves, and skin are frequently involved by intravascular and extravascular granulomas, and infiltration of vessels and perivascular tissues by eosinophils is striking. However, unlike in Wegener granulomatosis, severe renal disease is infrequent. Coronary arteritis and myocarditis are the principal causes of morbidity and mortality. p-ANCAs are present in 70% of patients.

Wegener Granulomatosis

Wegener granulomatosis is a necrotizing vasculitis characterized by the triad of (1) *acute necrotizing granulomas* of the upper respiratory tract (ear, nose, sinuses, throat) or the lower respiratory tract (lung) or both; (2) *necrotizing or granulomatous vasculitis* affecting small to medium-sized vessels (e.g., capillaries, venules, arterioles, and arteries), most prominent in the lungs and upper airways but affecting other sites as well; and (3) renal disease in the form of *focal necrotizing, often crescentic, glomerulonephritis.* Some patients who do not manifest the full triad are said to have "limited" Wegener granulomatosis, in which the involvement is restricted to the respiratory tract. Conversely, widespread Wegener granulomatosis affects the eye, skin, and (rarely) other organs, notably the heart, and the clinical syndromes may be very similar to PAN with the addition of respiratory involvement.

MORPHOLOGY

The upper respiratory tract lesions range from inflammatory sinusitis resulting from mucosal granulomas to ulcerative lesions of the nose, palate, or pharynx, rimmed by **necrotizing granulomas and accompanying vasculitis.** Microscopically, the granulomas reveal a geographic pattern of necrosis. They are rimmed by lymphocytes, plasma cells, macrophages, and variable numbers of giant cells. In association with such lesions there is a necrotizing or granulomatous vasculitis of small and sometimes larger arteries and veins (see Fig. 10–20B). These areas are generally surrounded by a zone of fibroblastic proliferation with giant cells and leukocytic infiltrate in the lungs. Dispersed focal necrotizing granulomas may coalesce to produce radiographically visible nodules that may undergo cavitation, creating a more than superficial resemblance to a tubercle. Thus, the major pathologic differential is mycobacterial or fungal infection. Lesions may ultimately undergo progressive fibrosis and organization. With lung lesions, alveolar hemorrhage may be prominent.

The **renal lesions** are of two types (Chapter 14). In milder or early forms, there is acute focal proliferation and necrosis in the glomeruli, with thrombosis of isolated glomerular capillary loops (focal necrotizing glomerulonephritis). More advanced glomerular lesions are characterized by diffuse necrosis, proliferation, and crescent formation (**crescentic glomerulonephritis).** Patients with focal lesions may have only hematuria and proteinuria responsive to therapy, whereas those with diffuse disease can develop rapidly progressive renal failure.

Pathogenesis. The resemblance to PAN and serum sickness suggests that Wegener granulomatosis may represent some form of hypersensitivity, possibly to an inhaled infectious or other environmental agent, but this is unproved. The presence of granulomas and dramatic response to immunosuppressive therapy also strongly support an immunologic mechanism, perhaps of the cell-mediated type. c-ANCAs are present in the serum in up to 95% of these cases, and perhaps, as discussed earlier, they also participate in disease pathogenesis.

Clinical Features. Males are affected more often than females, at an average age of about 40 years, with peak incidence in the fifth decade. Typical clinical features include persistent pneumonitis with bilateral nodular and cavitary infiltrates (95%), chronic sinusitis (90%), mucosal ulcerations of the nasopharynx (75%), and evidence of renal disease (80%). Other features include rashes, muscle pains, articular involvement, mononeuritis or polyneuritis, and fever. If untreated, the course of the disease is malignant; 80% of patients die within 1 year. c-ANCAs are present in the serum in up to 95% of patients with active generalized disease, and this appears to be a useful marker for disease activity. Following treatment, a rising titer of c-ANCA suggests a relapse; most patients in remission have a negative test, or the titer falls significantly.

It should be apparent from the foregoing discussion that Wegener granulomatosis, microscopic polyangiitis, and Churg-Strauss syndrome are characterized by the presence of ANCAs, and hence they are often referred to as *ANCA-associated small vessel vasculitides.* Although they share this serologic feature, each has certain distinctive characteristics. Wegener granulomatosis is differentiated from the other two by the presence of necrotizing granulomas in the absence of asthma; Churg-Strauss syndrome, like Wegener granulomatosis, has necrotizing granulomatous inflammation but is distinguished by asthma and eosinophilia; by contrast, microscopic polyangiitis does not show asthma, eosinophilia, or granulomas. It should also be recalled that although any type of ANCA may occur in a patient with ANCA-associated vasculitis, in general, c-ANCA is seen in Wegener granulomatosis and the other two entities are typically associated with p-ANCA.

Thromboangiitis Obliterans (Buerger Disease)

Thromboangiitis obliterans (Buerger disease), a distinctive disease that often leads to vascular insufficiency, is characterized by segmental, thrombosing, acute and chronic inflammation of medium-sized and small arteries, principally the tibial and radial arteries and sometimes secondarily extending to veins and nerves of the extremities. Previously a condition that occurred almost exclusively in men who were heavy smokers of cigarettes, Buerger disease has been increasingly reported in women, probably reflecting recently increased smoking by women. The disease begins before the age of 35 years in most cases.

The relationship to cigarette smoking is one of the most consistent aspects of this disorder. Several possibilities have been postulated for this association, including direct endothelial cell toxicity by some tobacco products or hypersensitivity to them. In support of this, endothelial dysfunction can be demonstrated in many patients. This is manifested as impaired endothelium-dependent vasodilation when challenged with acetylcholine. Anti-endothelial cell antibodies have also been found. There is an increased prevalence of HLA-A9 and HLA-B5 in these patients, and the condition is far more common in Israel, Japan, and India than in the United States and Europe, all of which hints at genetic influences.

MORPHOLOGY

Thromboangiitis obliterans is characterized by a **sharply segmental acute and chronic vasculitis of medium-sized and small arteries,** predominantly of the upper and lower extremities. Microscopically, acute and chronic inflammation permeates the arterial walls, accompanied by thrombosis of the lumen, which may undergo organization and recanalization. Typically, the thrombus contains small **microabscesses** with a central focus of neutrophils surrounded by granulomatous inflammation (see Fig. 10-20C). The inflammatory process extends into contiguous veins and nerves (rare with other forms of vasculitis), and in time all three structures become encased in fibrous tissue.

Clinical Features. The early manifestations are a superficial nodular phlebitis, cold sensitivity of the Raynaud type (see later) in the hands, and pain in the instep of the foot induced by exercise (so-called *instep claudication*). In contrast to the insufficiency caused by ATH, in Buerger disease the insufficiency tends to be accompanied by severe pain, even at rest, related undoubtedly to the neural involvement. Chronic ulcerations of the toes, feet, or fingers may appear, perhaps followed in time by frank gangrene. Abstinence from cigarette smoking in the early stages of the disease often brings dramatic relief from further attacks.

Vasculitis Associated With Other Disorders

Vasculitis resembling hypersensitivity angiitis or classic PAN may sometimes be associated with an underlying disorder, such as rheumatoid arthritis, systemic lupus erythematosus, malignancy, or systemic illnesses such as mixed cryoglobulinemia and Henoch-Schönlein purpura. *Rheumatoid vasculitis* occurs predominantly after long-standing, severe rheumatoid arthritis and usually affects small and medium-sized arteries leading to visceral infarction; it may also cause a clinically significant aortitis.

Infectious Arteritis

Localized arteritis may be caused by the direct invasion of infectious agents, usually bacteria or fungi, particularly *Aspergillus* and members of the order Mucorales. Vascular lesions frequently accompany bacterial pneumonia or occur adjacent to caseous tuberculosis, adjacent to abscesses, or in the superficial cerebral vessels in cases of meningitis. Much less commonly, they arise from the hematogenous spread of bacteria, in cases of septicemia or embolization from infective endocarditis.

Vascular infections may weaken the arterial wall to result in a *mycotic aneurysm* (see earlier) or induce thrombosis and infarction. For example, inflammation of the superficial vessels of the brain in bacterial meningitis may predispose to thrombosis, with subsequent infarction of and extension of a subarachnoid infection into brain parenchyma.

RAYNAUD DISEASE

Raynaud disease refers to paroxysmal pallor or cyanosis of the digits of the hands or feet and, infrequently, the tips of the nose or ears (acral parts). Characteristically, the fingers change color in the sequence white-blue-red. Raynaud disease is caused by intense vasospasm of small arteries or arterioles, principally of young, otherwise healthy women. *Structural changes in the arterial walls are absent except late in the course, when intimal thickening can appear.* Raynaud disease reflects an exaggeration of normal central and local vasomotor responses to cold or emotion. The course of Raynaud disease is usually benign, but long-standing, chronic cases can result in atrophy of the skin, subcutaneous tissues, and muscles. Ulceration and ischemic gangrene are rare.

In contrast, *Raynaud phenomenon* refers to arterial insufficiency of the extremities *secondary to the arterial narrowing induced by various conditions, including systemic lupus erythematosus, systemic sclerosis (scleroderma), ATH, or Buerger disease* (see earlier). Indeed, Raynaud phenomenon may be the first manifestation of such conditions.

VEINS AND LYMPHATICS

Varicose veins and phlebothrombosis/thrombophlebitis together account for at least 90% of clinical venous disease.

Varicose Veins

Varicose veins are abnormally dilated, tortuous veins produced by prolonged, increased intraluminal pressure and loss of vessel wall support. The *superficial veins* of the upper and lower leg are the predominant sites of involvement (Fig. 10–21). When the legs are dependent for long periods of time, venous pressures in these sites are markedly elevated (up to 10 times normal). Therefore, occupations that require long periods of standing and long automobile or airplane rides frequently lead to marked venous stasis and pedal edema, even in individuals with essentially normal veins *(simple orthostatic edema)*. It is estimated that 15% to 20% of the general population eventually develop varicose veins in the lower legs. The condition is much more common in those older than the age of 50, in obese persons, and in women, a reflection of the elevated venous pressure in lower legs caused by pregnancy. A *familial tendency* toward premature varicosities is postulated to be caused by defective venous wall development.

Figure 10–21   ■

Varicose veins of the leg. (Courtesy of Magruder C. Donaldson, MD, Brigham and Women's Hospital, Boston.)

MORPHOLOGY

Veins with varicosities are dilated, tortuous, elongated, and scarred, with thinning at the points of maximal dilatation. Intraluminal thrombosis and valvular deformities (thickening, rolling, and shortening of the cusps) are frequently discovered when these vessels are opened. Microscopically, the changes consist of variations in the thickness of the vein wall caused by dilation in some areas and by compensatory hypertrophy of the smooth muscle and subintimal fibrosis in others. Frequently, there are elastic tissue degeneration and spotty calcifications within the media **(phlebosclerosis)**.

Clinical Course. Varicose dilation of veins renders the valves incompetent and leads to venous stasis, congestion, edema, pain, and thrombosis. The most disabling sequelae include persistent edema in the extremity and trophic changes in the skin that lead to stasis dermatitis, ulcerations, vulnerability to injury, and poorly healing wounds and infections that may become chronic *varicose ulcers. However, embolism or other serious complications are very rare. This is in sharp contrast to the relatively frequent thromboembolism that arises from thrombosed deep veins* (see later).

Varicosities also occur in two other sites that deserve mention. *Esophageal varices* form in patients who have cirrhosis of the liver and its attendant portal hypertension (Chapter 16); rupture of esophageal varices can lead to massive upper gastrointestinal hemorrhage. *Hemorrhoids* result from varicose dilation of the hemorrhoidal plexus of veins at the anorectal junction. Presumed to be caused by prolonged pelvic congestion resulting from repeated pregnancies or straining at stools, hemorrhoids are uncomfortable and may be a source of bleeding. They sometimes thrombose; in this distended state, they are prone to painful ulceration.

Thrombophlebitis and Phlebothrombosis

The deep leg veins account for more than 90% of cases of thrombophlebitis and phlebothrombosis, two designations for venous thrombosis and inflammation. Cardiac failure, neoplasia, pregnancy, obesity, the postoperative state, and prolonged bed rest or immobilization are the most important clinical predispositions. Genetic hypercoagulability syndromes (Chapter 4) can also be associated with venous thrombosis.

In patients with cancer, particularly adenocarcinomas of the pancreas, colon, or lung, hypercoagulability occurs as a paraneoplastic syndrome (Chapter 6). The resultant venous thromboses have a tendency to appear in one site, only to disappear and be followed by thromboses in other veins, giving rise to so-called *migratory thrombophlebitis (Trousseau sign)*. The periprostatic venous plexus in the male and the pelvic veins in the female are additional sites, as are the large veins in the skull and the dural sinuses when these channels become inflamed by bacterial infections of the meninges, middle ears, or mastoids. Similarly, infections in the abdominal cavity, such as peritonitis, acute appendicitis, acute salpingitis, and pelvic abscesses, may lead to inflammation and thrombosis of the portal vein.

Thrombi in the legs tend to produce few, if any, signs or symptoms in the early stages. Indeed, local manifestations, including edema distal to the occluded vein, dusky cyanosis, dilatation of superficial veins, heat, tenderness, redness, swelling, and pain may be absent in a bedridden patient. In some cases, however, pain can be elicited by pressure over affected veins, squeezing the calf muscles, or forced dorsiflexion of the foot (Homan sign).

Pulmonary embolism is a common and serious clinical sequel to deep leg vein thrombosis (Chapter 4). The contraction of surrounding muscles tends to "milk" the contents loose from their attachments to the vein walls. *Not infrequently, the first manifestation of thrombophlebitis is the development of an embolic episode*; in a very ill patient, pulmonary embolization often constitutes the "final blow."

A special variant of primary phlebothrombosis is *phlegmasia alba dolens* (painful white leg), referring to iliofemoral venous thrombosis occurring in pregnant women before or after delivery (aptly also called "milk leg"). It is postulated that the thrombus (predisposed by stasis caused by the pressure of the gravid uterus and to a hypercoagulable state during pregnancy) initiates a phlebitis and that the perivenous inflammatory response induces lymphatic blockage with painful swelling.

Superior and Inferior Vena Caval Syndromes

The superior vena caval syndrome is usually caused by neoplasms that compress or invade the superior vena cava, most commonly a bronchogenic carcinoma or mediastinal lymphoma. The consequent obstruction produces a distinctive clinical complex manifested by dusky cyanosis and marked dilation of the veins of the head, neck, and arms. Commonly, the pulmonary vessels are also compressed, inducing respiratory distress.

The inferior vena caval syndrome may be caused by neoplasms that either compress or penetrate the walls of the inferior vena cava or a thrombus from the femoral or iliac vein that propagates upward. Moreover, certain neoplasms, particularly hepatocellular carcinoma and renal cell carcinoma, show a striking tendency to grow within veins, which ultimately may include the inferior vena cava. Obstruction to the inferior vena cava induces marked edema of the legs, distention of the superficial collateral veins of the lower abdomen, and, when the renal veins are involved, massive proteinuria.

Lymphangitis and Lymphedema

Primary disorders of the lymphatic vessels are extremely uncommon; secondary processes develop in association with inflammation or cancer.

Bacterial infections may spread into and through the lymphatics to create acute inflammatory involvement in these channels *(lymphangitis)*. The most common etiologic agents are the group A β-hemolytic streptococci, although any virulent pathogen may cause acute lymphangitis. Anatomically, the affected lymphatics are dilated and filled with an exudate, chiefly of neutrophils and monocytes, that usually extends through the wall into the perilymphatic tissues and, in severe cases, produces cellulitis or focal abscesses. Clinically, lymphangitis is recognized by painful subcutaneous red streaks that extend along the course of lymphatics, with painful enlargement of the regional lymph nodes *(acute lymphadenitis)*. If the lymph nodes fail to block the spread of bacteria, spillage into the venous system can initiate a bacteremia or septicemia.

Occlusion of lymphatic drainage is followed by the abnormal accumulation of interstitial fluid in the affected part, called *obstructive lymphedema*. Lymphatic blockage is most commonly secondary to (1) spread of malignant tumors obstructing either the lymphatic channels or the regional lymph nodes, (2) radical surgical procedures with removal of regional groups of lymph nodes (e.g., the axillary dissection of lymph nodes in radical mastectomy), (3) postirradiation fibrosis, (4) filariasis, and (5) postinflammatory thrombosis and scarring. *Chylous ascites, chylothorax,* and *chylopericardium* are caused by rupture of obstructed, dilated lymphatics into the peritoneum, pleural cavity, or pericardium, usually caused by obstruction of lymphatics by an infiltrating tumor mass.

In contrast, *primary lymphedema* may occur as an isolated congenital defect (simple congenital lymphedema) or as the familial *Milroy disease (heredofamilial congenital lymphedema)*. A third form of primary lymphedema, known as *lymphedema praecox*, appears between the ages of 10 and 25 years, usually in females. Of unknown cause, edema begins in the feet and slowly accumulates throughout life. The involved extremity may swell to many times its normal size, and the process may extend upward to affect the trunk. Potential consequences are disability from the size of the limb, superimposed infection, or chronic ulcerations.

Regardless of its cause, lymphedema gives rise to dilatation of lymphatics distal to the points of obstruction. The resultant increase in hydrostatic pressure causes an increase of interstitial fluid. Persistence of the edema leads to increased subcutaneous interstitial fibrous tissue, with consequent enlargement of the affected part and brawny induration. The thickened skin assumes the texture of orange peel (because hair follicles appear to be pitted), giving rise to the so-called *peau d'orange* appearance of the skin, often seen in patients with lymphatic dissemination of breast cancer. Chronic lymphedema gives rise to ulcers in the overlying skin, because adequate perfusion is impaired.

TUMORS

Tumors of the blood and lymphatic vessels constitute a spectrum from benign hemangiomas (some of which are regarded as hamartomatous) to intermediate lesions that are locally aggressive but infrequently metastasize, to relatively rare, highly malignant angiosarcomas (Table 10–5). In addition, congenital or developmental malformations may present as tumor-like lesions, as do some non-neoplastic reactive vascular proliferations, such as *bacillary angiomatosis*. For these reasons, vascular neoplasms are difficult to categorize clinically and histologically. Neoplasms of this group display endothelial cell differentiation (e.g., hemangioma, lymphangioma, angiosarcoma) or appear to be derived from cells that support and/or invest blood vessels (e.g., glomus tumor, hemangiopericytoma). Most such lesions occur outside the vascular system per se, in soft tissues and viscera. Primary tumors of the large vessels, such as aorta, pulmonary artery, and vena cava, are extremely rare, most being connective tissue sarcomas.

Although in most cases a well-differentiated benign hemangioma can be readily distinguished from an anaplastic high-grade angiosarcoma, the line dividing benign from

■

Table 10–5.　CLASSIFICATION OF VASCULAR TUMORS AND TUMOR-LIKE CONDITIONS

Benign Neoplasms, Developmental and Acquired Conditions

Hemangioma
　Capillary hemangioma
　Cavernous hemangioma
　Pyogenic granuloma (lobular capillary hemangioma)
Lymphangioma
　Simple (capillary) lymphangioma
　Cavernous lymphangioma (cystic hygroma)
Glomus tumor
Vascular ectasias
　Nevus flammeus
　Spider telangiectasia (arterial spider)
　Hereditary hemorrhagic telangiectasis (Osler-Weber-Rendu disease)
Reactive vascular proliferations
　Bacillary angiomatosis

Intermediate-Grade Neoplasms

Kaposi sarcoma
Hemangioendothelioma

Malignant Neoplasms

Angiosarcoma
Hemangiopericytoma

malignant is frequently poorly defined. However, the following criteria are helpful:

- Benign tumors produce readily recognized vascular channels filled with blood cells, or in the case of lymphatics, with lymph. They are lined by a monolayer of normal ECs, without atypia.
- Malignant tumors are more solidly cellular with cytologic anaplasia, including mitotic figures, and usually do not form well-organized vessels.

The endothelial derivation of neoplastic proliferations that do not form distinct vascular lumina can usually be confirmed by immunohistochemical demonstration of endothelial cell–specific markers such as CD31 or von Willebrand factor (see earlier). Because these lesions are caused by unregulated vascular proliferation, the possibility of controlling such growth by agents that inhibit blood vessel formation (antiangiogenic factors) is particularly exciting.

Benign Tumors and Tumor-like Conditions

HEMANGIOMA

Hemangiomas are characterized by increased numbers of normal or abnormal vessels filled with blood. Difficult to distinguish with certainty from malformations or hamartomas (Fig. 10–22), *hemangiomas (angiomas)* are most commonly localized; however, some involve large segments of the body such as an entire extremity (called *angiomatosis*). The majority are superficial lesions, often of the head or neck, but they may occur internally, with nearly one third in the liver. Malignant transformation occurs rarely, if at all.

Common in infancy and childhood, hemangiomas constitute 7% of all benign tumors. Most are present from birth and expand along with the growth of the child. Nevertheless, many of the capillary lesions regress spontaneously at or before puberty. There are several histologic and clinical variants.

Capillary Hemangioma. *Capillary hemangiomas,* the largest single type of vascular tumor, are most common in the skin, subcutaneous tissues, and mucous membranes of the oral cavities and lips, but they may also occur in the liver, spleen, and kidneys. The "strawberry type" of capillary hemangioma (*juvenile hemangioma*) of the skin of newborns is extremely common (1 in 200 births) and may be multiple. It grows rapidly in the first few months, begins to fade when the child is 1 to 3 years old, and regresses by age 7 in 75% to 90% of cases.

MORPHOLOGY

Varying in size from a few millimeters up to several centimeters in diameter, they are bright red to blue and level with the surface of the skin or slightly elevated, with intact covering epithelium (see Fig. 10–22A). Occasionally, they are pedunculated. Histologically, capillary hemangiomas are usually lobulated but unencapsulated aggregates of **closely packed, thin-walled capillaries,** usually blood filled

Figure 10-22 ■

Hemangiomas. *A,* Hemangioma of the tongue. *B,* Histology of juvenile capillary hemangioma. *C,* Histology of cavernous hemangioma. *D,* Pyogenic granuloma of the lip. (*A* and *D,* Courtesy of John Sexton, MD, Beth Israel Hospital, Boston; *B,* courtesy of Christopher D. M. Fletcher, MD, Brigham and Women's Hospital, Boston; and *C,* courtesy of Thomas Rogers, MD, University of Texas Southwestern Medical School, Dallas.)

and lined by a flattened endothelium. The vessels are separated by scant connective tissue stroma (see Fig. 10-22*B*). The lumina may be partially or completely thrombosed and organized. Rupture of vessels causes scarring and accounts for the hemosiderin pigment occasionally found in these lesions.

Cavernous Hemangioma. Less common than the capillary variety, *cavernous hemangiomas* are characterized by the formation of large, dilated vascular channels. As compared with capillary hemangiomas, they are less circumscribed and more frequently involve deep structures.

MORPHOLOGY

Grossly, the usual cavernous hemangioma is a red-blue, soft, spongy mass 1 to 2 cm in diameter. Rarely, giant forms occur that affect large subcutaneous areas of the face, extremities, or other regions of the body. Histologically, the mass is sharply defined, but not encapsulated, and made up of **large, cavernous vascular spaces,** partly or completely filled with blood separated by a scant connective tissue stroma (see Fig. 10-22*C*). Intravascular thrombosis with associated dystrophic calcification is common.

In most situations, the tumors are of little clinical significance; however, they can be a cosmetic disturbance, owing to their vulnerability to traumatic ulceration and bleeding. Moreover, when picked up in internal organs by computed tomography or magnetic resonance imaging, they must be distinguished from more ominous lesions. Those in the brain are most threatening, because they may cause pressure symptoms or rupture. In one rare systemic entity, *von Hippel-Lindau disease* (discussed in Chapter 14), cavernous hemangiomas occur within the cerebellum or brain stem and eye grounds, along with similar angiomatous lesions or cystic neoplasms in the pancreas and liver and renal neoplasms.

Pyogenic Granuloma (Lobular Capillary Hemangioma). This polypoid form of capillary hemangioma occurs as a rapidly growing exophytic red nodule attached by a stalk to the skin and gingival or oral mucosa, which bleeds easily and is often ulcerated (see Fig. 10-22*D*). Approximately one third of lesions develop after trauma, growing rapidly to reach a maximum size of 1 to 2 cm within a few weeks. The proliferating capillaries are often accompanied by extensive edema and an acute and chronic inflammatory infiltrate, especially when ulcerated. This appearance may bear a striking resemblance to exuberant granulation tissue. Recurrence occurs infrequently as a solitary nodule or as satellite nodules. *Pregnancy tumor* (granuloma gravidarum) is a pyogenic granuloma that occurs in the gingiva of 1% of pregnant women and regresses after delivery.

LYMPHANGIOMA

Lymphangiomas are the benign lymphatic analogue of the hemangiomas of blood vessels.

Simple (Capillary) Lymphangioma. These lesions, composed of small lymphatic channels, tend to occur subcutaneously in the head and neck region and in the axilla. Rarely, they are found in other subcutaneous connective tissue or within internal organs. On body surfaces, they are slightly elevated or sometimes pedunculated lesions that are 1 to 2 cm in diameter. Histologically, they are composed of a network of endothelium-lined lymph spaces that can be *distinguished from capillary channels only by the absence of blood cells.*

Cavernous Lymphangioma (Cystic Hygroma). Analogous to cavernous hemangiomas, cavernous lymphangiomas occur in children in the neck or axilla and only rarely retroperitoneally. They occasionally achieve considerable size, up to 15 cm in diameter, and may fill the axilla or produce gross deformities in and about the neck. The tumors are made up of massively dilated, cystic lymphatic spaces lined by ECs and separated by a scant intervening connective tissue stroma that often contains lymphoid aggregates. Because the margins of the tumor are not discrete, and these lesions are not encapsulated, removal can be difficult. For unexplained reasons, cavernous lymphangiomas of the neck are frequently seen in Turner syndrome (Chapter 7).

GLOMUS TUMOR (GLOMANGIOMA)

Glomus tumors are biologically benign but often exquisitely painful tumors that arise from the modified SMCs of the glomus body, a specialized arteriovenous anastomosis that is involved in thermoregulation. They *are most commonly found in the distal portion of the digits*, especially under the fingernails. Excision is curative.

MORPHOLOGY

Grossly, the lesions are usually small (under 1 cm in diameter), slightly elevated, rounded, red-blue, firm nodules that may appear as minute foci of fresh hemorrhage under the nail. Histologically, there are branching vascular channels separated by a connective tissue stroma that contains **aggregates, nests, and masses of the specialized glomus cells, which typically are arranged around vessels.** Individual cells are usually small, regular in size, and round or cuboidal, with scant cytoplasm and features very similar to SMCs on electron microscopy. Glomangiomas comprise a distinct subgroup that resemble cavernous hemangiomas.

VASCULAR ECTASIAS

Vascular ectasias comprise a common group of lesions characterized by localized dilation of preexisting vessels. They are not neoplasms. The term *telangiectasia* designates a congenital anomaly or acquired exaggeration of preformed vessels composed of prominent capillaries, venules, and arterioles that creates a small focal red lesion, usually in the skin or mucous membranes.

Nevus Flammeus. This is the most common form of ectasia; it characteristically forms on the head and neck, is flat, and ranges in color from light pink to deep purple. This lesion is the ordinary "birthmark." Histologically, nevus flammeus shows only dilation of vessels in the dermis. Most ultimately fade and regress.

A special form of nevus flammeus, the *port wine stain*, may grow proportionately with a child, thicken the skin surface, become unsightly, and demonstrate no tendency to fade. Port wine stains in the distribution of the trigeminal nerve may be associated with the *Sturge-Weber syndrome* (also called *encephalotrigeminal angiomatosis*), an extremely uncommon congenital disorder attributed to faulty development of certain mesodermal and ectodermal elements. Sturge-Weber syndrome is characterized by venous angiomatous masses in the leptomeninges over the cortex and by ipsilateral port wine nevi of the face. It is often associated with mental retardation, seizures, hemiplegia, and radiopacities in the skull. Thus, *a large vascular malformation in the face may indicate the presence of more extensive vascular malformation in a child who exhibits some evidence of mental deficiency.*

Spider Telangiectasia (Arterial Spider). Another clearly non-neoplastic vascular lesion is *spider telangiectasia*, a more or less radial and often pulsatile array of dilated subcutaneous arteries or arterioles about a central core that blanches with pressure applied to its center. It tends to be on the face, neck, or upper chest and is most frequent in pregnant women and in patients with cirrhosis. The hyperestrinism found in these two settings is believed to in some way play a role in the development of these telangiectases.

Hereditary Hemorrhagic Telangiectasia (Osler-Weber-Rendu Disease). In the autosomal dominant *Osler-Weber-Rendu disease*, telangiectases are malformations made up of dilated capillaries and veins. They are present from birth and are distributed widely over the skin and mucous membranes of the oral cavity, lips, and respiratory, gastrointestinal, and urinary tracts. Rarely, these lesions rupture, causing serious nosebleeds, bleeding into the gut, or hematuria.

BACILLARY ANGIOMATOSIS

First described in patients with the acquired immunodeficiency syndrome (AIDS), *bacillary angiomatosis* is an opportunistic infection of immunocompromised persons that manifests as vascular proliferations involving skin, bone, brain, and other organs. Along with the closely related vascular lesion of the liver and spleen called *bacillary peliosis*, bacillary angiomatosis is caused by infection with gram-negative bacilli of the *Bartonella* family. Two species are implicated: *Bartonella henselae*, the organism that causes cat-scratch disease in immunocompetent persons, and *B. quintana*, the cause of trench fever that affected soldiers during World War I. The domestic cat is the principal reservoir of *B. henselae*, and the cat flea is its vector, whereas the human body louse plays an important role in infection caused by *B. quintana*. Human infections are initiated by traumatic inoculation of skin. Difficult to cultivate in the laboratory, these organisms can be demonstrated using molecular methods. How these organisms cause the exuberant vessel lesions is unclear.

MORPHOLOGY

Grossly, cutaneous bacillary angiomatosis is marked by one to numerous red papules and nodules or rounded subcutaneous masses. Histologically, there is a tumor-like growth pattern with proliferation of capillaries having protuberant epithelioid ECs, which have nuclear atypia and mitoses. The lesions contain numerous stromal neutrophils, nuclear dust, and purplish granular material that represents the causative bacteria.

Intermediate-Grade (Borderline Low-Grade Malignant) Tumors

KAPOSI SARCOMA

Once thought to be an uncommon neoplasm, Kaposi sarcoma (KS) has come to the forefront because of its frequent occurrence in patients with AIDS. Four forms of the disease are recognized:

■ *Chronic*, also called *classic* or *European KS*, first described by Kaposi in 1872, occurs primarily (90%) in older men of Eastern European (especially Ashkenazic Jews) or Mediterranean descent. It is uncommon in the United States. This form is also associated with a second malignant tumor or altered immune state but is not associated with human immunodeficiency virus (HIV). Clinically, chronic KS commences with multiple red to purple skin plaques or nodules primarily in the distal lower extremities, slowly increasing in size and number and spreading to more proximal sites. The tumors frequently remain asymptomatic and localized to the skin and subcutaneous tissue but are locally persistent, with an erratic course of lapses and remissions.
■ *Lymphadenopathic*, also called *African* or *endemic KS*, is particularly prevalent among young Bantu children of South Africa (same geographic distribution as Burkitt lymphoma), who present with localized or generalized lymphadenopathy and in whom the disease is extremely aggressive. Skin lesions are sparse. The disorder occasionally involves the viscera.
■ *Transplant-associated KS* occurs several months to a few years postoperatively in solid organ transplant recipients who receive high doses of immunosuppressive therapy. Lesions are either localized to the skin or widely metastatic. Skin lesions sometimes regress when immunosuppressive therapy is markedly reduced, but organ or internal involvement is usually fatal.
■ *AIDS-associated (epidemic) KS* is found in approximately one fourth or more of AIDS patients, particularly male homosexuals, compared with 5% of others with AIDS.

Diagnosis of the tumor may precipitate the clinical recognition of the syndrome. AIDS-associated KS lesions have no site of predilection, but involvement of lymph nodes and the gut and wide dissemination tend to occur early in the course. Most patients eventually succumb to the opportunistic infectious complications of AIDS rather than directly to the consequences of KS. However, about one third of patients with KS subsequently develop a second malignancy, most often lymphoma.

MORPHOLOGY

The morphology of KS is illustrated in Figure 10–23. In the relatively indolent, classic disease of older men, and sometimes in the other variants, three stages can be identified: patch, plaque, and nodule. The **patches** are pink to red to purple solitary or multiple macules that in the classic disease are usually confined to the distal lower extremities or feet. Microscopic examination discloses only dilated, perhaps irregular and angulated blood vessels lined by ECs with an interspersed infiltrate of lymphocytes, plasma cells, and macrophages (sometimes containing hemosiderin). These lesions are difficult to distinguish from granulation tissue. Over time, lesions in the classic disease spread proximally and usually convert into larger, violaceous, **raised plaques** that reveal dermal, dilated, jagged vascular channels lined by somewhat plump spindle cells accompanied by perivascular aggregates of similar spindled cells. Scattered between the vascular channels are red blood cells (escaping from leaky vessels), hemosiderin-laden macrophages, lymphocytes, and plasma cells. Pink hyaline globules of uncertain nature may be found in the spindled cells and macrophages. Occasional mitotic figures may be present.

At a still later stage, the lesions may become **nodular** and more distinctly neoplastic and may be composed of sheets of plump, proliferating spindle cells, mostly in the dermis or subcutaneous tissues (see Fig. 10–23*B*). Particularly characteristic in this cellular background are scattered small vessels and slitlike spaces that often contain rows of red cells and hyaline droplets. More marked hemorrhage, hemosiderin pigment, lymphocytes, and occasional macrophages may be admixed with this cellular background. Mitotic figures are common, as are the round, pink, cytoplasmic globules. The nodular stage is often accompanied by involvement of lymph nodes and of viscera, particularly in the African and AIDS-associated diseases.

Pathogenesis. The pathogenesis of KS remains uncertain, as does the nature of the undifferentiated spindle-shaped tumor cells. However, current evidence favors a virus-associated (if not virus-caused) neoplasm of primitive mesenchymal or ECs whose course is greatly influenced by the immune status of the individual. As discussed in Chapter 5, both HIV products and cytokines produced by

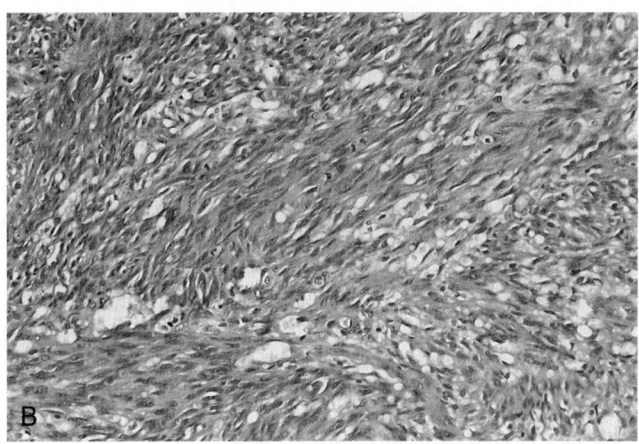

Figure 10–23

Kaposi sarcoma. *A,* Gross photograph, illustrating coalescent red-purple macules and plaques of the skin. *B,* Histologic view of the nodular form demonstrating sheets of plump, proliferating spindle cells and vascular spaces. (Courtesy of Christopher D. M. Fletcher, MD, Brigham and Women's Hospital, Boston.)

infected T cells and human herpesvirus type 8 may play a major role in the etiology of these tumors in AIDS patients. However, since KS can develop in HIV-negative individuals, other pathways must also be involved.

Clinical Course. The presentation and natural course of KS vary widely and are significantly affected by the clinical setting. Whereas the classic form at the outset is largely restricted to the surface of the body, in the endemic and epidemic subsets, visceral involvement may be present when the cutaneous manifestations appear, particularly in persons who have AIDS. Thus, the classic disease is relatively indolent and compatible with long survival, but the endemic and epidemic patterns may be more aggressive.

HEMANGIOENDOTHELIOMA

The term *hemangioendothelioma* is used to denote a wide spectrum of vascular neoplasms showing histologic features and clinical behavior *intermediate between the benign, well-differentiated hemangiomas and the frankly anaplastic angiosarcomas* (see later).

Representative of this group is the *epithelioid hemangioendothelioma*, a unique vascular tumor occurring around medium-sized and large veins in the soft tissue of adults. In such tumors, well-defined vascular channels are inconspicuous and the tumor cells are plump and often cuboidal, thus resembling epithelial cells. The differential diagnosis includes metastatic carcinoma, melanoma, and sarcomas that can assume an epithelioid appearance. Clinical behavior of epithelioid hemangioendothelioma is variable; most are cured by excision, but up to 40% recur, 20% to 30% eventually metastasize, and perhaps 15% of patients die of the tumors.

Malignant Tumors

ANGIOSARCOMA

Angiosarcomas are malignant endothelial neoplasms (Fig. 10–24) with structure varying from highly differenti-

ated tumors that resemble hemangiomas *(hemangiosarcoma)* to those whose anaplasia makes them difficult to distinguish from carcinomas or melanomas. They occur in both sexes and more often affect older adults. They can be found anywhere in the body but most often in the skin, soft tissue, breast, and liver.

The rare *hepatic angiosarcomas* are associated with distinct carcinogens, including arsenic (exposure to arsenical pesticides), Thorotrast (a radioactive contrast medium formerly used for radiologic imaging), and polyvinyl chloride (PVC) (a widely used plastic). The increased frequency of angiosarcomas among workers in the PVC industry is one of the truly well-documented instances of chemical carcinogenesis in humans. With all three agents, there is a very long latent period of many years between exposure and the development of tumors.

Angiosarcomas may also arise in the setting of lymphedema, classically 10 years after radical mastectomy for breast cancer. In such cases, the tumor presumably arises from dilated lymphatic vessels *(lymphangiosarcoma).* Angiosarcomas have been induced by radiation and associated with foreign material introduced into the body either iatrogenically or accidentally.

MORPHOLOGY

Grossly, cutaneous angiosarcomas may begin as deceptively small, sharply demarcated, asymptomatic, often multiple red nodules; but eventually most such tumors become large, fleshy masses of pale gray-white, soft tissue (see Fig. 10–24A). The margins blend imperceptibly with surrounding structures. Central softening and areas of necrosis and hemorrhage are frequent.

Microscopically, **all degrees of differentiation of these tumors may be found,** from those that are largely vascular with plump, anaplastic but recog-

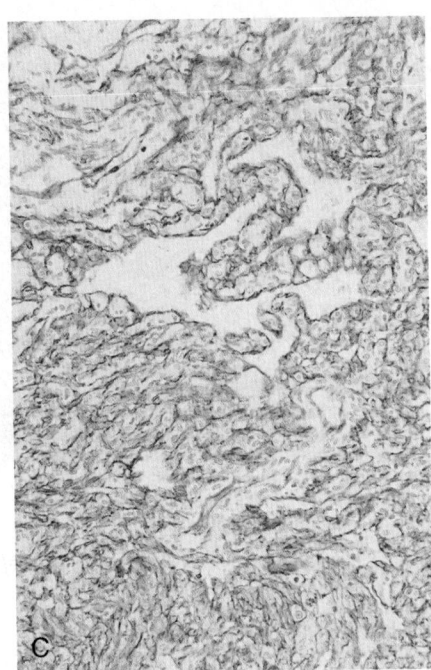

Figure 10-24

Angiosarcoma. *A*, Gross photograph of angiosarcoma of the heart (right ventricle). *B*, Photomicrograph of moderately well differentiated angiosarcoma with dense clumps of irregular, moderate anaplastic cells and distinct vascular lumens. *C*, Positive immunohistochemical staining of angiosarcoma for the endothelial cell marker CD31, proving the endothelial nature of the tumor cells.

nizable ECs producing vascular channels (see Fig. 10–24*B*) to tumors that are quite undifferentiated, produce no definite blood vessels, are markedly atypical, and have a solid spindle cell appearance. The derivation of ECs is demonstrated by staining with CD31 or von Willebrand factor (see Fig. 10–24*C*).

Clinically, angiosarcomas show local invasion and distal metastatic spread. The majority of patients have a poor outcome with very few surviving 5 years.

HEMANGIOPERICYTOMA

These tumors are derived from pericytes, which are normally arranged along capillaries and venules. Hemangiopericytomas are rare neoplasms that may occur as slowly enlarging, painless masses at any anatomic site but are most common on the lower extremities (especially the thigh) and in the retroperitoneum. They consist of numerous branching capillary channels and large gaping sinusoidal spaces surrounded by and enclosed within nests and masses of spindle-shaped to round cells. Silver impregnation can be used to confirm that these cells are outside the basement membrane of the endothelium and hence are pericytes. The tumors may recur, and as many as 50% metastasize to lungs, bone, and liver.

BIBLIOGRAPHY

Beckman JA, O'Gara PT: Diseases of the aorta. Adv Intern Med 44:267, 1999. (A broad overview of aortic diseases.)

Coady MA, et al: Natural history, pathogenesis, and etiology of thoracic aortic aneurysms and dissections. Cardiol Clin 17:615; 1999. (A comprehensive discussion of aortic dissection.)

Dammerman M, Breslow JL: Genetic basis of lipoprotein disorders. Circulation 91:505, 1995. (A comprehensive review of inherited dyslipedemias.)

Ernst CB: Abdominal aortic aneurysm. N Engl J Med 328:1167, 1993. (A nice clinical review.)

Frishman WH: Biologic markers as predictors of cardiovascular disease. Am J Med 104(6A):18S, 1998. (A good discussion of metabolic and biochemical markers that confer risk of ischemic heart disease.)

Gimbrone MA Jr, et al: Endothelial dysfunction, hemodynamic forces, and atherogenesis. Ann N Y Acad Sci 902:230, 2000. (An excellent discussion of endothelial dysfunction and vascular disease.)

Kaplan NM: Systemic hypertension: Mechanisms and diagnosis. In Braunwald E, et al (eds): Heart Disease, 6th ed. Philadelphia, WB Saunders, 2001, p 941. (A recent chapter in hypertension, covering all aspects.)

Libby P: The vascular biology of atherosclerosis. In Braunwald E, et al (eds): Heart Disease, 6th ed. Philadelphia, WB Saunders, 2001, p 995. (A good, detailed review of pathogenesis of atherosclerosis.)

Lifton RP: Molecular genetics of human blood pressure variation. Science 272:676, 1996. (A very scholarly review of the genetic factors that underlie hypertension.)

Olin JW: Thromboangiitis obliterans. N Engl J Med 343:864, 2000. (An update on this disorder.)

Ridker PM, Genest J, Libby P: Risk factors for atherosclerotic disease, In Braunwald E, et al (eds): Heart Disease, 6th ed. Philadelphia, WB Saunders, 2001, p 1010. (A detailed discussion of risk factors for atherosclerosis.)

Ross R: Atherosclerosis—an inflammatory disease. N Engl J Med 340:115, 1999. (An elegant and scholarly discussion of the current model of atherogenesis.)

Savige J, et al: Antineutrophil cytoplasmic antibodies and associated diseases: A review of the clinical and laboratory features. Kidney Int 57:846, 2000. (An excellent review of this complicated subject.)

Timberlake DS: Molecular genetics of essential hypertension: recent results and emerging strategies. Curr Opin Nephrol Hypertens 10:71, 2001. (An excellent review of the complex genetics of essential hypertension.)

Whelan P, Scadden DT: New developments in the etiopathogenesis and treatment of HIV-related Kaposi's sarcoma. Clin Dermatol 18:469, 2000. (A review of the possible factors that lead to the Kaposi sarcoma.)

11

The Heart

DENNIS K. BURNS, MD
VINAY KUMAR, MD

In addition to serving as a source of inspiration to poets, the human heart also accomplishes the enormous task of propelling over 6000 liters of blood through the body daily. In most cases, it performs its duties quietly and efficiently, providing the tissues with a steady supply of vital nutrients and facilitating the excretion of waste products. As might be anticipated, cardiac dysfunction can be associated with devastating physiologic consequences. Heart disease remains the leading cause of death and disability in the industrialized nations of the world and currently accounts for nearly 40% of all deaths in the United States. The major categories of cardiac diseases considered in this chapter include coronary artery disease, hypertensive heart disease, heart disease caused by intrinsic pulmonary diseases (cor pulmonale), valvular heart diseases, primary myocardial diseases, and selected congenital heart diseases. A few comments about pericardial diseases and cardiac neoplasms are also offered. Before considering details of specific heart diseases, we will review salient features of congestive heart failure, the common end point of many types of heart disease.

CONGESTIVE HEART FAILURE

Congestive heart failure is a multisystem derangement that occurs when the heart is no longer able to eject the blood delivered to it by the venous system. Excluded from this definition are conditions in which inadequate cardiac output occurs because of blood loss or some other process that impairs the return of blood to the heart. In an additional minority of cases, heart failure may result because of greatly increased demands for blood by the tissues, a process sometimes referred to as *high output failure.* Inadequate cardiac output, also termed *forward failure,* is almost always accompanied by increased congestion of the venous circulation *(backward failure),* because the failing ventricle is unable to eject the normal volume of venous blood delivered to it during diastole. This results in an increase in the volume of blood in the ventricle at the end of diastole, an elevation in end-diastolic pressure within the heart, and, finally, elevated venous pressure. Congestive heart failure may involve the left or right side of the heart or all of the cardiac chambers.

The most common causes of left-sided cardiac failure are systemic hypertension, mitral or aortic valve disease, ischemic heart disease, and primary diseases of the myocardium. The most common cause of right-sided heart failure is left ventricular failure, with its associated pulmonary congestion and elevation in pulmonary arterial pressure. Right-sided failure may also occur in the absence of left-sided heart failure in patients with intrinsic diseases of the lung parenchyma and/or pulmonary vasculature (cor pulmonale) and in patients with pulmonic or tricuspid valve disease. It sometimes follows congenital heart diseases, in which there is a left-to-right shunt.

As the heart begins to fail, a number of local *adaptive responses* are triggered in an attempt to maintain normal cardiac output. These include *neurohumoral reactions* as well as *molecular and morphologic changes* within the heart. One of the earliest neurohumoral responses to decreased cardiac output is an increase in the activity of the sympathetic nervous system. Catecholamines cause both a more forceful contraction of the heart muscle (a positive inotropic effect) and an increase in heart rate. Over time, the overburdened heart may respond to increased demands by undergoing various forms of "remodeling," including hypertrophy and dilatation. Because cardiac muscle fibers in the adult no longer have the ability to proliferate to any significant degree, the major initial structural adaptation to a chronically increased workload is hypertrophy of individual muscle fibers. In the case of a cardiac chamber

subjected to a pure pressure load (e.g., hypertension, valvular stenosis), the hypertrophy is characterized by an increase in the diameter of individual muscle fibers. This pattern of fiber enlargement results in the development of classic *concentric hypertrophy*, in which the thickness of the ventricular wall increases without an increase in the size of the chamber (see Fig. 11–9, under discussion of Hypertensive Heart Disease). However, when the heart is subjected to an *abnormal volume load*, as opposed to a pressure load (e.g., valvular regurgitation or abnormal shunts), the length of individual muscle fibers also increases. This pattern of hypertrophy, sometimes referred to as *eccentric hypertrophy*, is characterized by an increase in heart size as well as an increase in wall thickness.

The development of hypertrophy initially serves as a positive, adaptive response, in much the same way as hypertrophy of skeletal muscle fibers enables a conditioned athlete to accommodate increased workloads. Despite the potential hemodynamic benefits associated with hypertrophy, however, it has become increasingly apparent that the development of hypertrophy comes at a significant cost to the cell. Oxygen requirements of the hypertrophic myocardium are increased, owing to increased myocardial cell mass and increased tension of the ventricular wall. Because the myocardial capillary bed does not always increase sufficiently to meet the increased oxygen demands of the hypertrophic muscle fibers, the myocardium becomes vulnerable to *ischemic* injury. Additional evidence suggests that molecular signals that lead to the development of hypertrophy may also be accompanied by the expression of certain proteins that lead, in turn, to impaired myocyte contractility and even to premature myocyte death.

Increased cardiac workload of any type predisposes to the development of cardiac *dilatation*, or chamber enlargement, when increased sympathetic activity and myocyte hypertrophy prove insufficient to expel all the venous blood that drains into the heart. As cardiac failure progresses, end-diastolic pressure increases, causing individual cardiac muscle fibers to stretch, ultimately increasing the volume of the cardiac chamber. In accordance with the Frank-Starling relationship, these lengthened fibers initially contract more forcibly, thereby increasing cardiac output. If the dilated ventricle is able to maintain cardiac output at a level that meets the needs of the body, the patient is said to be in *compensated heart failure.* However, cardiac dilatation, like hypertrophy, has certain deleterious effects on the heart. Increasing degrees of dilatation result in an increase in wall tension of the affected chamber, which causes, in turn, an increase in the oxygen requirements of an already-compromised myocardium. With time, the failing myocardium is no longer able to propel sufficient blood to meet the needs of the body, even at rest. At this point, patients enter a phase termed *decompensated heart failure.*

Heart failure causes changes in other organs as well. As noted previously, cardiac failure inevitably includes an element of backward failure, the result of which is *congestion of the venous circulation.* In a patient with left-sided failure, this results in passive congestion of the pulmonary circulation. As left ventricular failure progresses, the hydrostatic pressure in the pulmonary vasculature increases sufficiently to cause leakage of fluid and, occasionally, erythrocytes into the interstitial tissue and airspaces of the lungs to produce *pulmonary edema*. Congestion of the pulmonary circulation also causes an increase in pulmonary vascular resistance and, with it, an increased workload on the right side of the heart. This increased burden, if sustained and severe, may ultimately cause the right side of the heart to fail also. Failure of the right side of the heart, in turn, contributes to the development of *systemic venous congestion and soft tissue edema* (Chapter 4).

As the heart fails, a number of *systemic alterations also occur that serve to maintain cardiac output at near-normal levels*. Decreased left ventricular output (forward failure) is associated with decreased perfusion of the kidneys, which in turn causes local activation of the renin-angiotensin system. Aldosterone released in response to activation of the renin-angiotensin system causes the renal tubules to resorb both sodium and water. This sequence of events, sometimes called *secondary hyperaldosteronism*, increases the total plasma volume of extracellular fluid. However, unless the performance of the cardiac pump improves, the failing heart is unable to pump the increased intravascular volume, which remains pooled in the veins, thereby adding further to systemic and pulmonary venous congestion. This ultimately contributes further to both pulmonary and soft tissue edema.

MORPHOLOGY

The failing **cardiac chambers are dilated** and are usually hypertrophied as well. In **left-sided failure,** the **lungs** are boggy and congested and the cut surface exudes a frothy mixture of surfactant-rich fluid and blood. Microscopically, the pulmonary alveolar capillaries are congested. There is transudation of fluid, initially limited to perivascular interstitial spaces, causing widening of the alveolar septa. In time, it overflows into the alveoli **(pulmonary edema)**. The protein-poor edema fluid stains pale pink when viewed under the microscope. With persistent elevation of pulmonary venous pressure, the capillaries may become tortuous and may rupture to produce small hemorrhages into the alveolar spaces. Alveolar macrophages phagocytose red blood cells and eventually become filled with hemosiderin. These pigmented macrophages are called **heart failure cells**. Persistence of septal edema may induce fibrosis within the alveolar walls, which, together with the accumulation of hemosiderin, is characteristic of **chronic venous congestion** of lungs. The lungs thus become dark brown and firm, an appearance that has been referred to as **brown induration of the lungs.**

Long-standing **right-sided heart failure** is associated with congestion of the abdominal viscera, soft tissue edema, and, in some cases, fluid in the pleural, pericardial, and abdominal cavities. Changes in the **liver** include chronic passive congestion, characterized by atrophy of hepatocytes around the central veins that gives rise to a nutmeg-like appearance on the cut surface of the organ (see Fig. 4-3, p 83). Hemorrhagic necrosis of centrilobular hepatocytes is common in severe cases, particularly in patients with concomitant left ventricular failure. With long-standing cardiac failure, the liver may become fibrotic and, in extreme cases, frankly cirrhotic (Chapter 16).

Clinical Features. The most common manifestation of left ventricular failure is *dyspnea*, or a sense of breathlessness. This is caused predominantly by decreased lung compliance resulting from pulmonary edema and congestion and by increased activity of autonomic stretch receptors within the lung. Dyspnea is most noticeable during periods of physical activity *(exertional dyspnea)*. It is also prominent when the person is lying down *(orthopnea)* because of the increased amount of venous blood returned to the thorax from the lower extremities and because the diaphragm is elevated in this position. *Paroxysmal nocturnal dyspnea* is an especially dramatic form of dyspnea that awakens the patient with sudden, severe shortness of breath, accompanied by coughing, a choking sensation, and wheezing. Other manifestations of left ventricular failure include muscle fatigue, an enlarged heart, tachycardia, a third heart sound (S_3), and fine rales at the lung bases, produced by the flow of air through edematous pulmonary alveoli. With progressive ventricular dilation, the papillary muscles are displaced laterally, causing mitral regurgitation and a high-pitched systolic murmur. Chronic dilation of the left atrium may also occur, which is often associated, in turn, with the development of *atrial fibrillation*, manifested by an "irregularly irregular" heartbeat.

As stated earlier, right-sided heart failure is most often caused by left-sided failure. Its major consequences are *systemic venous congestion* and *soft tissue edema*. Systemic venous congestion is manifested clinically by distended neck veins and an enlarged, sometimes tender liver. It is also associated with an increased frequency of deep venous thrombi and pulmonary embolism (Chapter 4). Edema causes weight gain and usually becomes apparent first in the dependent areas of the body, such as the feet and lower legs. With more severe degrees of ventricular failure, the edema may become generalized. Pleural effusions are common, particularly on the right side, and may be accompanied by pericardial effusions and ascites. Unlike inflammatory edema, the edema fluid in congestive heart failure has a low protein content.

As congestive heart failure progresses, patients may become frankly cyanotic and acidotic, owing to decreased tissue perfusion. Ventricular arrhythmias caused by myocardial irritability and overactivity of the sympathetic nervous system are common and are an important cause of sudden death in this setting.

ISCHEMIC HEART DISEASE

Ischemic heart disease refers to a group of closely related syndromes caused by an imbalance between the myocardial oxygen demand and the blood supply. The most common cause of ischemic heart disease is narrowing of the lumina of the coronary arteries by atherosclerosis, and hence ischemic heart disease is often termed *coronary heart disease* or *coronary artery disease.*

Ischemic heart disease is the single most common cause of death in economically developed countries of the world, including the United States and western Europe, where it is responsible for about one third of all deaths. Depending on the rate and severity of coronary artery narrowing and the myocardial response, one of four syndromes may develop: (1) various forms of *angina pectoris* (chest pain), (2) *acute myocardial infarction (MI)*, (3) *sudden cardiac death*, and (4) *chronic ischemic heart disease with congestive heart failure.* These syndromes are all late manifestations of coronary atherosclerosis that probably begins during childhood or early adulthood. The term *acute coronary syndromes* is applied to the spectrum of three acute catastrophic manifestations of ischemic heart disease—unstable angina, acute MI, and sudden cardiac death. As will be discussed later, all three result from acute changes in the morphology of atherosclerotic plaques.

Epidemiology. Clinical manifestations of coronary atherosclerosis may occur at any age but are most common in older adults, with a peak incidence after the age of 60 years in men and 70 years in women. Men are more commonly affected than women until the ninth decade, by which time the frequency of coronary artery disease is similar in both sexes. Factors that contribute to the development of coronary atherosclerosis are similar to those responsible for atherosclerosis in general and include *hypertension, diabetes mellitus, smoking*, and *high levels of low-density lipoprotein cholesterol* (Chapter 10). *Genetic factors* undoubtedly play an important role in the development of coronary atherosclerosis. In some families the genetic influences include inheritance of some of the previously mentioned risk factors (e.g., hypercholesterolemia, diabetes mellitus). In other cases of familial coronary artery disease the specific genetic abnormalities have not been defined.

Much attention has also been given to factors that might reduce the risk of coronary atherosclerosis. *Regular exercise*, by increasing myocardial vascularity, appears to significantly reduce the risk of coronary artery disease and its sequelae. It appears that *moderate consumption of red wine* and perhaps other alcoholic beverages may also reduce the risk of coronary artery disease, possibly by increasing levels of high-density lipoprotein cholesterol. Welcome though these associations may be to connoisseurs of fine wine and the sedentary individuals among us, the beneficial effects of moderate alcohol consumption are probably slight at best. More importantly, they do not compensate for the detrimental effects of smoking, an indiscriminate diet, or a lack of exercise.

Pathogenesis. Severe and chronic atherosclerosis that causes narrowing of the lumen of one or more coronary arteries is the fundamental disorder underlying ischemic heart disease. *With a 75% or greater atherosclerotic reduction in the lumen of one or more major coronary arteries*, any augmented coronary blood flow that may occur as a result of compensatory coronary vasodilation is insufficient to meet even moderate increases in myocardial oxygen de-

mand, giving rise to classic angina pectoris. Hence, a fixed 75% or greater reduction in the lumen of the coronary artery is defined as "critical stenosis." The onset of symptoms and the prognosis of ischemic heart disease, however, depend not only on the extent and severity of fixed, chronic anatomic disease but also critically on dynamic changes in the morphology of the coronary plaque. These include the following:

■ Acute plaque changes
■ Coronary artery thrombosis
■ Coronary artery vasospasm

Acute Plaque Changes. As mentioned earlier, myocardial ischemia underlying the acute coronary syndromes—unstable angina, acute MI, and (in many cases) sudden cardiac death—is precipitated by abrupt changes in plaque followed by thrombosis. Acute changes in the morphology of chronic atherosclerotic plaques include fissuring, hemorrhage into the plaque, and overt plaque rupture with embolization of atheromatous debris into distal coronary vessels. In addition to causing enlargement of the plaque, local disruption of plaque increases the risk of platelet aggregation and thrombosis at that site. Such acute changes often develop in plaques associated with lesser degrees of stenosis than the critical 75% figure mentioned earlier. Acute changes developing in areas of more moderate (50% to 75%) stenosis account for the all-too-frequent development of acute myocardial infarcts (discussed later) that occur in previously asymptomatic individuals.

Because of their catastrophic consequences, there is much interest in understanding the factors that induce dynamic instability in plaques. Disrupted plaques are markedly eccentric (not uniform around the vessel circumference) and have a large, soft core of necrotic debris and lipid covered by a thin, fibrous cap. In addition, such plaques are rich in macrophages and T cells. It is thought that metalloproteinases secreted by macrophages help degrade the collagen cap. T cells presumably activate macrophages via interferon-γ secretion. Hemodynamic trauma also plays a role. Thus, plaques tend to fissure at the junction of the fibrous cap and the adjacent plaque-free vessel wall, a site where the mechanical stresses induced by the blood flow are maximal. Whereas acute coronary syndromes are the most dramatic manifestation of plaque rupture (with superimposed thrombosis), it is now believed that repeated, "silent" ruptures and thrombosis followed by organization may play an important role in the progression of coronary atherosclerosis.

Coronary Artery Thrombosis. Plaque rupture exposes thrombogenic lipids and subendothelial collagen, thus initiating a wave of platelet aggregation, thrombin generation, and, ultimately, thrombus formation (Fig. 11–1). This is a critical event in the pathogenesis of acute coronary syndromes. If the vessel is completely occluded by the thrombus overlying the ruptured plaque, acute MI occurs. In contrast, if the luminal obstruction by the thrombus is incomplete and dynamic, the patient may develop unstable angina or a lethal arrhythmia, giving rise to sudden cardiac death. The nonocclusive mural thrombus can also embolize small fragments of thrombotic material in the distal branches of the coronary artery. This may

Figure 11-1 ■

Photomicrograph of an atherosclerotic coronary artery, with rupture of the atherosclerotic plaque and an overlying occlusive thrombus. The thrombus is deep red and crescentic; it is completely filling the markedly narrowed coronary artery lumen. More than 80% of the lumen is filled by an atherosclerotic plaque, which shows a central soft area in which cholesterol, represented by clear spaces, is present. The left side of the deep red thrombus is hugging the area of plaque rupture *(arrowhead)*. (Courtesy of Sid Murphree, MD, Department of Pathology, University of Texas Southwestern Medical School, Dallas.)

give rise to microinfarcts, which are found in patients who have had unstable angina.

Coronary Artery Vasospasm. This usually occurs in patients with at least some preexisting atherosclerosis. The mechanism for coronary vasospasm is not entirely clear. At the site of plaque disruption, it may be induced by the release of vasospastic mediators such as thromboxane A₂ from platelet aggregates. Endothelial dysfunction may also precipitate vasospasm by reduced elaboration of endothelial cell–derived relaxing factors. Increased adrenergic activity and smoking have also been implicated.

Other Pathologic Processes. Uncommonly, processes other than atherosclerosis or its complications may compromise blood flow through the coronary arteries. These include emboli originating from vegetations on the aortic or mitral valves and coronary vasculitis. Severe systemic hypotension may also be associated with decreased coronary artery flow and myocardial ischemia, particularly in patients with preexisting coronary atherosclerosis. In addition to factors that compromise coronary blood flow, increased myocardial oxygen demand may also contribute to the development of myocardial ischemia. This often occurs because of left ventricular myocardial hypertrophy, as might be encountered in patients with systemic hypertension or diseases of the heart valves.

With this overview of the pathogenesis of myocardial ischemia, we can turn our attention to the specific clinical presentations of ischemic heart disease and the morphologic changes associated with them.

Angina Pectoris

The term *angina pectoris* refers to *intermittent chest pain caused by transient, reversible myocardial ischemia*. Three

major variants of angina pectoris are recognized: typical (stable) angina pectoris, Prinzmetal (variant) angina, and unstable angina pectoris. More than one pattern of angina may be present in a given patient.

■ *Typical or stable angina pectoris* refers to episodic chest pain associated with exertion or some other form of stress. The pain is classically described as a crushing or squeezing substernal sensation, which may radiate down the left arm. Stable angina pectoris is usually associated with a *fixed atherosclerotic narrowing* (usually 75% or greater) of one or more coronary arteries. With this degree of obstruction ("critical stenosis"), the myocardial oxygen demand may be adequate under basal conditions but cannot be augmented sufficiently to meet the increased requirements imposed by exercise or other conditions that stress the heart. The pain is usually relieved by rest (reducing demand) or by administration of nitroglycerin. This vasodilator reduces venous blood delivered to the heart (and hence cardiac work) by causing venous dilation; in larger doses, it may increase blood supply to the myocardium by coronary vasodilation.

■ *Prinzmetal, or variant, angina* refers to angina that occurs at rest or, in some cases, awakens the patient from sleep. Angiographic studies have shown that Prinzmetal angina is associated with coronary artery spasm. Although the spasm usually occurs near an atherosclerotic plaque, it may affect a normal vessel. The cause and mechanism of such spasms is not clear, but they respond to the administration of vasodilators. Variant angina should not be confused with vasospasms that occur at the site of plaque rupture.

■ *Unstable angina pectoris*, sometimes called *crescendo angina*, is characterized by the increased frequency of anginal pain. The attacks tend to be precipitated by progressively less exertion, and they are more intense and often last longer than episodes of stable angina pectoris. Unstable angina is a harbinger of more serious, potentially irreversible myocardial ischemia and hence is sometimes referred to as *preinfarction angina*. In most patients it is induced by acute plaque change with superimposed partial thrombosis, distal embolization of the thrombus, and/or vasospasm. The morphologic changes in the heart are those of coronary atherosclerosis and its associated lesions.

Myocardial Infarction

The term *myocardial infarction* indicates the *development of an area of myocardial necrosis caused by local ischemia*. Acute MI, also known as "heart attack," is the single most common cause of death in industrialized nations. In the United States, an estimated 1.5 million people per year suffer an MI, with roughly 500,000 fatalities. Among fatal cases, nearly half of the patients die before reaching the hospital. The risk of acute MI increases progressively throughout life. Between the ages of 45 and 54, men are four to five times as likely to develop an MI as women. As with ischemic heart disease in general, however, the risk of disease becomes the same in both sexes after 80 years of age. The major risk factors for acute MI are the same as those discussed previously for coronary atherosclerosis (Chapter 10).

Pathogenesis. Although any of the forms of coronary artery disease discussed earlier may cause acute MI, angiographic studies indicate that *most acute MIs are caused by coronary artery thrombosis.* Disruption of an underlying atherosclerotic plaque (e.g., fissure formation) serves as the nidus for the generation of the thrombus in many cases. Vasospasm and platelet aggregation may contribute to coronary artery occlusion, but they are seldom, if ever, the sole cause of the occlusion. Sometimes, particularly in the case of infarcts limited to the subendocardial myocardium, thrombi may be absent. In most such cases there is diffuse, stenosing coronary atherosclerosis but neither plaque disruption nor thrombosis. In such cases, hypoperfusion of coronary vessels compromised by atherosclerosis is presumably sufficient to cause necrosis of subendocardial myocytes.

Myocardial necrosis begins within 20 to 30 minutes of the coronary artery occlusion. Under normal circumstances, the subendocardial region of the myocardium is the most poorly perfused region of the ventricular wall. Not only is it the last area to receive blood from branches of the epicardial coronary arteries, but the relatively high intramural pressures that exist in this area further compromise inflow of blood. *Because of this increased vulnerability to ischemic injury, myocardial infarcts typically begin in the subendocardial region.* The zone of necrosis extends externally over the next several hours to involve the mid- and subepicardial areas of the myocardium. The infarct usually reaches its full size within 3 to 6 hours. During this period of evolution, lysis of the thrombus by the administration of thrombolytic agents (e.g., streptokinase or tissue plasminogen activator) may limit the size of the infarct. The progression of ischemic necrosis in the myocardium is summarized in Figure 11–2. With time, a "wavefront" of cell death moves from the subendocardium to involve the entire thickness of the ventricle. In addition, it should be evident that patchy nontransmural infarction may be seen if an occlusive thrombus is lysed by thrombolytic agents or by angioplasty before the wavefront of necrosis extends fully across the ventricular wall.

The location of an MI is determined by the site of the vascular occlusion and by the anatomy of the coronary circulation. Occlusion of the left anterior descending coronary artery typically causes an infarct in the anterior and apical areas of the left ventricle and adjacent interventricular septum (anteroapical MI). Occlusion of the right coronary artery is responsible for most infarcts involving the posterior and basal portions of the left ventricle. The underlying anatomy of the coronary circulation also has a significant influence on the location of the infarct. For example, occlusion of the right coronary artery would have different consequences in an individual whose posterior ventricle was supplied by branches of the right coronary artery (right dominant circulation) than in a person whose posterior wall was supplied by branches of the circumflex coronary artery (left dominant circulation).

The size of the infarct is influenced by several factors. In general, occlusion of more proximal segments of the coronary arteries produces larger infarcts, involving the full thickness of the myocardium. Conversely, thrombi in more distal arterial branches tend to cause smaller infarcts. The extent of the infarct is also influenced by the degree of collateral circulation that exists at the time of the occlusion. In patients with long-standing coronary atherosclerosis, collateral circulation may develop over time in response to chronic ischemia. Such collateral vessels may limit the size of the infarct, particularly in the epicardial regions of the myocardium.

MORPHOLOGY

The appearance of a myocardial infarct is determined primarily by its age. The essential sequence of events, which is reviewed in more detail later, is that of coagulation necrosis and inflammation, followed by the formation of granulation tissue, resorption of the necrotic myocardium, and, finally, organization of the granulation tissue to form a collagen-rich scar. These events occur in a fairly predictable pattern, allowing one to estimate the age of a given infarct from its gross and microscopic appearances. It should be noted, however, that other factors may modify the appearance of an infarct. Because smaller infarcts tend to heal more rapidly than larger lesions, the morphology of a myocardial infarct at a given point in time is also influenced by its size. Other variables, such as recurrent infarcts in the same territory and reperfusion of necrotic myocardium after thrombolysis or angioplasty, also affect the appearance of a myocardial infarct.

The frequencies of occlusion of various coronary arteries and the distribution of the resultant infarcts are as follows:

Left anterior descending coronary artery (40% to 50%)	Anterior and apical left ventricle; anterior two thirds of the interventricular septum
Right coronary artery (30% to 40%)	Posterior wall of the left ventricle; posterior one third of the interventricular septum (in persons with right-dominant coronary circulation)
Left circumflex coronary artery (15% to 20%)	Lateral wall of left ventricle (may also involve the posterior wall in persons with left-dominant coronary circulation)

Myocardial infarcts may involve most of the thickness of the ventricular wall, in which case they are referred to as **transmural infarcts,** while those restricted to the inner one third of the myocardium are designated **subendocardial infarcts.** Virtually all transmural infarcts involve the left ventricle and/or

Figure 11-2   ■

Schematic representation of the progression of myocardial necrosis after coronary artery occlusion. Necrosis begins in a small zone of the myocardium under the endocardial surface in the center of the ischemic zone that depends on the occluded vessel for perfusion. This entire region *(shaded)* is the area at risk. Note that although necrosis proceeds from the subendocardium to the epicardium, a very narrow zone of myocardium immediately beneath the endocardium is spared from necrosis because it can be oxygenated by diffusion from the ventricle. (Modified from original sketches by Dr. Fred Schoen, Department of Pathology, Brigham and Women's Hospital, Boston.)

interventricular septum. Sometimes those in the posterior wall and septum extend into the adjacent right ventricular wall. Isolated infarction of the right ventricle or the atria is rare.

The morphologic changes associated with MI are listed in Table 11-1. **For the first 12 hours,** no changes are evident on gross examination. Between 18 and 24 hours, a slight pallor or mottling may become apparent. Microscopically, **coagulation necrosis** becomes obvious by 12 to 18 hours, at which time the cytoplasm of the necrotic myocytes becomes increasingly eosinophilic, with a loss of cross-striations, while the nuclei begin to undergo fragmentation (karyorrhexis) or contraction (pyknosis). **Wavy fiber change,** probably caused by stretching of viable but malfunctioning myocytes, is common at the periphery of the infarct. **Neutrophils** are attracted by the necrotic myocardium, and a neutrophilic infiltrate becomes apparent during the initial 18 to 24 hours. Neutrophils are present in all myocardial infarcts by 48 hours, reach a peak on day 3, and subsequently diminish. Some degree of hemorrhage may be present but is usually not extensive unless lysis or angioplasty has permitted reperfusion of the necrotic zone. At the periphery of the infarct, some myocytes may contain brightly eosinophilic, coarse, transverse bands

Table 11-1. SEQUENCE OF CHANGES IN MYOCARDIAL INFARCTION

Time	Gross	Light Microscope	Electron Microscope	Other
0–30 min	No change	No change	*Reversible* changes (mitochondrial swelling, relaxation of myofibrils)	Loss of enzyme activity; glycogen loss
1–2 hr	No change	Few "wavy" fibers at margin of infarct	*Irreversible* changes (sarcolemmal disruption, electron-dense mitochondrial deposits)	
4–12 hr	No change	Early coagulation necrosis; edema; occasional neutrophils; minimal hemorrhage		
18–24 hr	Slight pallor or mottling	Continuing coagulation necrosis (nuclear pyknosis and disintegration; cytoplasmic eosinophilia); "contraction band" necrosis at periphery of infarct; neutrophilic infiltrate		
24–72 hr	Pallor	Complete coagulation necrosis of myofibers; heavy neutrophilic infiltrate with early fragmentation of neutrophil nuclei		
4–7 days	Central pallor with hyperemic border	Macrophages appear; early disintegration and phagocytosis of necrotic fibers; granulation tissue visible at edge of infarct		
10 days	Maximally yellow, soft, shrunken; purple border	Well-developed phagocytosis; prominent granulation tissue in peripheral areas of infarct		
7–8 wk	Firm, gray	Fibrosis		

known as **contraction bands.** These structures, produced by hypercontraction of myofibrils in dying cells, are induced by the influx of calcium ions from the plasma into cells with damaged cell membranes (Fig. 11-3). Hence, contraction bands tend to be more prominent when there is early reperfusion of the ischemic area. Reperfused areas also tend to be hemorrhagic, owing to concomitant microvascular injury. As discussed in Chapter 1, reperfusion injury may also contribute to impaired contractility of residual viable cardiomyocytes in the ischemic area ("stunned" myocardium). A thin zone of residual viable myocytes is usually present immediately beneath the surface of the endocardium, where direct diffusion of nutrients from the ventricular cavity is sufficient to sustain the cells. However, cells in this immediate subendocardial area are not completely normal; they often assume a vacuolated appearance, termed **myocytolysis,** resulting from influx of water across injured cell membranes.

By days 4 to 7, the infarct appears grossly as a pale, firm, fairly well-defined region with a hyperemic border (Fig. 11-4). Macrophages, fibroblasts, and capillaries first appear at the margins of the infarct on about the fourth day, migrating progressively toward the center of the lesion over the next several weeks. During this period, macrophages begin to phagocytize the necrotic myocytes.

By day 10, the necrotic area is yellow, soft, and sunken; the granulation tissue is visible grossly at the edge of the infarct as a red-purple zone. Microscopically, the necrotic myofibers at the periphery of the infarct have been replaced by granulation tissue. Pigmented macrophages, laden with the remnants of necrotic myocytes, are present in large numbers. Early maturation of the granulation tissue is manifested by the appearance of collagen fibers at the periphery of the infarct.

Phagocytosis of necrotic myocytes and maturation of granulation tissue continue over the next several weeks. **By the end of the fourth week,** virtually all of the necrotic myocardium has been resorbed, with only a few residual islands visible microscopically. As the granulation tissue matures, its vascularity diminishes, while the amount of collagen increases. **By approximately the eighth week,** most infarcts have been replaced by dense scar tissue and can be considered healed. The ventricular wall is thinned, firm, and gray at the site of the healed infarct (Fig. 11-5).

Several important complications may be encountered in patients who have suffered myocardial infarcts, particularly if they are **transmural.** These occur at different times during the evolution of the infarct and can be summarized as follows:

Figure 11-3   ■

Photomicrograph of a 48-hour-old myocardial infarct (MI). The cardiac muscle fibers are brightly eosinophilic, owing to coagulative necrosis, and an infiltrate of neutrophils is seen between the fibers. In addition, the myocardial fibers show contraction bands in the form of deeply stained transverse bands. (Courtesy of Dr. Sid Murphree, MD, Department of Pathology, University of Texas Southwestern Medical School, Dallas.)

Figure 11-5   ■

Healed myocardial infarction. By about 2 months, the necrotic myocardium has been completely replaced by dense scar tissue, visible here as a thinned gray area in the left ventricular myocardium.

Figure 11-4   ■

Acute myocardial infarction, 4 to 7 days old. The infarct is visible as a well-demarcated, pale yellow lesion in the posterolateral region of the left ventricle. The border of the infarct is accentuated by a dark red zone of inflammation. The adjacent viable left ventricular wall is hypertrophic, perhaps reflecting the presence of preexisting hypertension.

■ **Papillary muscle dysfunction** occurs frequently in patients with MIs. In most cases, it is caused by local bulging of the injured left ventricular wall at the site of attachment of the papillary muscle, ischemia and impaired contractility of the papillary muscle, or generalized dilation of the left ventricle in the setting of heart failure. Less commonly (less than 1% of cases of MI), **an infarcted papillary muscle may rupture,** with resultant detachment of the chordae tendineae and severe mitral insufficiency. Papillary muscle rupture is most common about 3 days after the development of the infarct. It causes acute left ventricular failure and is associated with a high mortality rate.

■ **External rupture of the infarct** occurs in up to 10% of patients dying in the hospital with an acute MI. This catastrophic event may occur at any time during the first 2 weeks of the infarct, but it is most common between days 4 and 7, when extensive softening of the myocardium has occurred but granulation tissue and fibrosis are poorly developed. The rupture usually develops over the course of several days, during which time blood dissects progressively through the soft, necrotic myocardium (Fig. 11-6). Rupture through the epicardial surface causes massive hemopericardium, with resultant cardiac tamponade. Less commonly (1% to 3% of cases of MI), **rupture of the intraventricular septum** may occur. It causes an acute left-to-right shunt, with resultant congestive heart failure.

■ **Mural thrombi,** which may develop on the endocardial surface overlying an infarct, are potential sources for systemic emboli and their

Figure 11-6 ■

Myocardial rupture 6 days after a myocardial infarction. The patient developed a cardiac tamponade and died. (From the teaching collection of the Pathology Department, University of Texas Southwestern Medical School, Dallas.)

complications, such as brain infarcts. Such thrombi are particularly common in patients who develop a ventricular aneurysm (discussed below). Organization of mural thrombi typically produces an area of dense endocardial fibrosis.

■ Clinically apparent **acute pericarditis** occurs in up to 15% of patients with MI within 2 to 4 days after the development of a transmural infarct. It may cause a significant pericardial effusion.

■ **Ventricular aneurysms** are a late complication of large transmural MIs and are caused by the bulging of the noncontractile fibrous myocardium during systole. They are most common in the anteroapical region of the heart, where they appear as a thin-walled, fibrous outpouching of the ventricular wall (Fig. 11-7). A mural thrombus is often present within the aneurysm. In addition to serving as a source of emboli, ventricular aneurysms may cause congestive heart failure, papillary muscle dysfunction, and recurrent arrhythmias. Surgical resection is beneficial in some cases.

Clinical Features. The onset of MI is usually accompanied by severe, crushing substernal chest pain, which may radiate to the neck, jaw, epigastrium, shoulder, or left arm. In about 50% of patients the MI is preceded by episodes of angina pectoris. In contrast to the pain of angina pectoris, however, the pain associated with an MI typically lasts several hours to days and is not significantly relieved by nitroglycerin. The pulse is generally rapid and weak, and patients are often diaphoretic. Dyspnea is common and is caused by impaired contractility of the ischemic myocardium, with resultant pulmonary

congestion and edema. With massive MIs involving over 40% of the left ventricle, cardiogenic shock develops. In a sizable minority of patients (20% to 30%) the MI does not cause chest pain. Such "silent" MIs are particularly common in patients with underlying diabetes mellitus and hypertension and in elderly patients.

Electrocardiographic abnormalities are an important manifestation of MI. These include changes such as Q waves, ST-segment abnormalities, and T-wave inversion. Arrhythmias caused by electrical abnormalities of the ischemic myocardium and by conduction disturbances are common.

Sudden cardiac death, caused by a lethal arrhythmia, occurs in approximately 25% of patients with MI and accounts for the vast majority of deaths occurring before hospitalization. Of patients who reach the hospital, 10% to 20% experience no complications. The remaining 80% to 90% develop one or more of the following:

■ Cardiac arrhythmias (75% to 95%)
■ Left ventricular failure with mild to severe pulmonary edema (60%)
■ Cardiogenic shock (10%)
■ Rupture of free wall, septum, or papillary muscle (4% to 8%)
■ Thromboembolism (15% to 49%)

Laboratory evaluation is an integral part of the clinical management of a suspected MI. A number of enzymes and other proteins are released into the circulation by dying myocardial cells. Measurement of the level of some of these molecules in the serum is helpful in the diagnosis of an MI. The various myocardial markers used to monitor the evolution of MI, and their patterns of elevation, are summarized below:

■ *Creatine kinase (CK)* is an enzyme that is highly concentrated in brain, myocardium, and skeletal muscle. The enzyme is composed of two dimers designated

Figure 11-7 ■

Healed myocardial infarction with a ventricular aneurysm. The aneurysm is visible as a thin-walled outpouching of the ventricular wall. Such aneurysms are often complicated by thrombosis, arrhythmias, and heart failure.

"M" and "B." CK-MM is derived predominantly from skeletal muscle and heart; CK-BB from brain, lung, and many other tissues; and CK-MB principally from myocardium, although variable amounts of the MB form are also present in skeletal muscle. *Total CK activity* begins to rise within 2 to 4 hours of an MI, peaks at 24 hours, and returns to normal within approximately 72 hours. Although *total CK activity is one of the most sensitive determinants of acute myocardial necrosis, it is not specific,* because CK is also elevated in other conditions, such as skeletal muscle injury. The specificity for the detection of MI is enhanced by measurement of the CK-MB fraction. CK-MB rises within 2 to 4 hours of the onset of an MI, peaks at 18 hours, and usually disappears by 48 hours. Although minor elevations of CK-MB occur in patients with extensive skeletal muscle injury, the amount of CK-MB relative to total CK is much higher in MI than in any other condition in which the CK level is elevated. This is sometimes expressed as a calculated value termed the *CK index.* An absence of a change in the levels of CK and CK-MB during the first 2 days after the development of chest pain essentially excludes the diagnosis of MI.

■ *Troponins* are a group of proteins found in both human skeletal and cardiac muscle. They regulate calcium-mediated contraction of muscles. Different isoforms of these proteins exist in mature skeletal muscle and myocardium. By the use of sensitive immunologic assays, it has been possible to distinguish cardiac troponin T (cTnT) and troponin I (cTnI) from troponins of skeletal muscle origin. Cardiac troponin I is found only in heart muscle and is thus more specific than CK-MB, which is also found in skeletal muscle in small proportion. Cardiac troponin I is not detected in serum after pure skeletal muscle injury and is therefore a reliable marker of myocardial necrosis, even when confounding skeletal muscle injury exists. After an acute MI, both cTnT and cTnI levels rise at about the same time as CK-MB. The diagnostic sensitivity of cardiac troponin measurements is similar to that of CK-MB in the early stages of acute MI. In contrast to CK-MB levels, however, troponin levels remain elevated for 4 to 7 days after the acute event, allowing the diagnosis of an acute MI long after CK-MB levels have returned to normal. Both cTnT and cTnI levels have also been shown to have prognostic value in patients with unstable angina, with elevated levels correlating with the subsequent development of acute MI.

■ *Lactate dehydrogenase (LD)* is another myocardial enzyme that has been used extensively in the past to evaluate suspected MIs. With the introduction of troponin assays, the measurement of LD levels for the diagnosis of MI is largely obsolete.

Chronic Ischemic Heart Disease

The term *chronic ischemic heart disease,* sometimes called *ischemic cardiomyopathy,* is used to describe the development of progressive congestive heart failure as a consequence of long-term ischemic myocardial injury. Many cases are associated with a history of angina pectoris and may be preceded by recognized infarcts. In other cases the condition may develop more insidiously.

MORPHOLOGY

The coronary arteries invariably contain areas of **moderate to severe atherosclerosis.** The heart is **enlarged,** sometimes to a striking degree, secondary to **dilation of all cardiac chambers.** Multiple areas of **myocardial fibrosis,** often including foci of transmural scarring, are usually present. A moderate degree of **hypertrophy** of the remaining myocardium is common. Despite the hypertrophy, however, wall thickness may be normal because of concomitant dilation. The endocardium is thick and opaque, and thrombi in varying stages of organization may be adherent to the endocardial surface. Microscopy reveals extensive myocardial fibrosis, owing to chronic ischemia. Among the remaining myocytes, both atrophic and hypertrophic fibers are present. Vacuolation of the sarcoplasm of some myofibers **(myocytolysis)** is common, particularly in the subendocardial areas.

Clinical Features. Chronic ischemic heart disease is characterized by the development of severe, progressive heart failure, sometimes punctuated by episodes of angina pectoris or MI. Arrhythmias are common and, along with congestive heart failure and intercurrent MI, account for many deaths. This form of ischemic heart disease may be difficult to distinguish clinically from dilated cardiomyopathy (p 385).

Sudden Cardiac Death

Sudden death has been defined in many different ways, ranging from instantaneous death to death occurring within 24 hours of the onset of symptoms. Excluded from most definitions of sudden death are events such as homicide, suicide, accidental trauma, and exposure to lethal toxins. Sudden death can be caused by a wide range of diseases, including heart disease, pulmonary embolism, ruptured aortic aneurysm, disorders of the central nervous system, and infections. *Most cases of sudden death in the Western world are caused by heart disease.* Sudden cardiac death accounts for approximately 300,000 deaths each year in the United States and for about 50% of all deaths caused by cardiovascular disease. The major forms of cardiac diseases associated with sudden death are listed in Table 11–2. *The most common cause of sudden cardiac death is ischemic heart disease.* Chronic ischemia predisposes the myocardium to the development of lethal ventricular arrhythmias, usually in the form of ventricular fibrillation, which is the most common cause of sudden death in these cases. In some cases, sudden death is preceded by other clinical manifestations of myocardial

Table 11-2. CARDIAC CAUSES OF SUDDEN DEATH

Coronary Artery Diseases
Coronary atherosclerosis
Developmental abnormalities (anomalous origin, hypoplasia)
Coronary artery embolism
Other (vasculitis, dissection)

Myocardial Diseases
Cardiomyopathies
Myocarditis and other infiltrative processes
Right ventricular dysplasia

Valvular Diseases
Mitral valve prolapse
Aortic stenosis and other forms of left ventricular outflow obstruction
Endocarditis

Conduction System Abnormalities

Modified from Virmani R, Roberts WC: Sudden cardiac death. Hum Pathol 18:485, 1987.

ischemia. Tragically, however, sudden death is the initial manifestation of ischemic heart disease in about 50% of patients with the disease.

MORPHOLOGY

The most common cardiac lesions in sudden death are those of coronary atherosclerosis and its complications. In most cases the degree of atherosclerosis is marked, with more than 75% reduction in the cross-sectional area of two or more vessels. The proximate cause of sudden cardiac death is not entirely clear in many cases. A number of studies suggest that acute plaque rupture, followed by coronary thrombosis and possibly vasospasm, triggers fatal ventricular arrhythmias. However, occlusive thrombi are absent in over 80% of cases of sudden cardiac death. In such cases, death is attributed to fatal arrhythmia. Morphologic manifestations of ischemic heart disease, such as recent or remote MIs, patchy myocardial fibrosis, wavy fiber change, or contraction band necrosis, are usually present. Other structural cardiac abnormalities have also been associated with sudden death and should be carefully sought in cases of sudden death associated with minimal atherosclerosis. These changes include various primary myocardial disorders (discussed later), conduction system abnormalities, and developmental abnormalities of the coronary arteries.

Summary of Ischemic Heart Disease. *Cardiac ischemia resulting from atherosclerosis of the coronary arteries may present as several well-defined but somewhat overlapping syndromes (Fig. 11–8). Typical angina pectoris results from an increased myocardial oxygen demand that cannot be met because of fixed critical stenosis of the coronary arteries. The three acute coronary syndromes (unstable angina, acute MI, and some cases of sudden cardiac death) seem to result from acute changes in fixed atherosclerotic*

lesions. In unstable angina, a small fissure or rupture of an atherosclerotic plaque triggers platelet aggregation, vasoconstriction, and formation of a mural thrombus that may not be occlusive; thus, there is a severe, but not complete, reduction in myocardial oxygenation. Acute transmural MI occurs when complete thrombotic occlusion is superimposed on acute plaque disruption. Sometimes acute plaque rupture and the resultant mural or occlusive thrombosis and vasospasm induce a rapidly fatal arrhythmia that causes sudden cardiac death. Finally, in some patients, chronic and progressive coronary atherosclerosis causes gradual loss of myocardium that eventuates in congestive heart failure. Patients in this last group are diagnosed as having chronic ischemic heart disease.

HYPERTENSIVE HEART DISEASE

As discussed in Chapter 10, chronic hypertension is a common disorder associated with considerable morbidity. Inadequately controlled hypertension has serious effects on many organs, including the heart, brain, and kidneys. Our comments here will focus on the cardiac complications of this disorder. Other effects of hypertension are discussed elsewhere in the text, along with other diseases of specific organs.

The diagnosis of hypertensive heart disease is based on the presence of *left ventricular hypertrophy in an individual with a history of hypertension* and in whom other causes of ventricular hypertrophy (e.g., aortic stenosis or primary hypertrophic cardiomyopathy) have been excluded. The stimulus to ventricular hypertrophy in patients with hypertension is a sustained pressure load on the left ventricular myocardium. The cellular events leading to myocardial hypertrophy are incompletely understood but appear to involve both local mechanical effects and growth factors, which lead in turn to changes in the genes controlling the expression of myosin, actin, and other cellular constituents. As noted in the earlier discussion of congestive heart failure, the same molecular signals that promote hypertrophy also trigger the expression of gene products that lead to myocyte dysfunction and, in all likelihood, premature cell death.

The *metabolic requirements* of hypertrophic myocardium, understandably, are greater than those of normal myocardium. With increasing degrees of hypertrophy, the metabolic requirements continue to increase but the ability of the heart to meet these demands decreases. This occurs because hypertrophy renders the myocardium stiff, thus increasing wall tension while simultaneously decreasing diastolic filling and stroke volume. Capillary density in the hypertrophic myocardium does not increase sufficiently to meet the metabolic demands of the myocytes. The distance over which oxygen and other nutrients delivered by the capillaries must diffuse is increased. To make matters worse, chronic hypertension also predisposes to atherosclerosis. In concert, these various changes predispose the hypertrophic myocardium to ischemic injury, eventually resulting in the development of congestive heart failure, MIs, and/or arrhythmias.

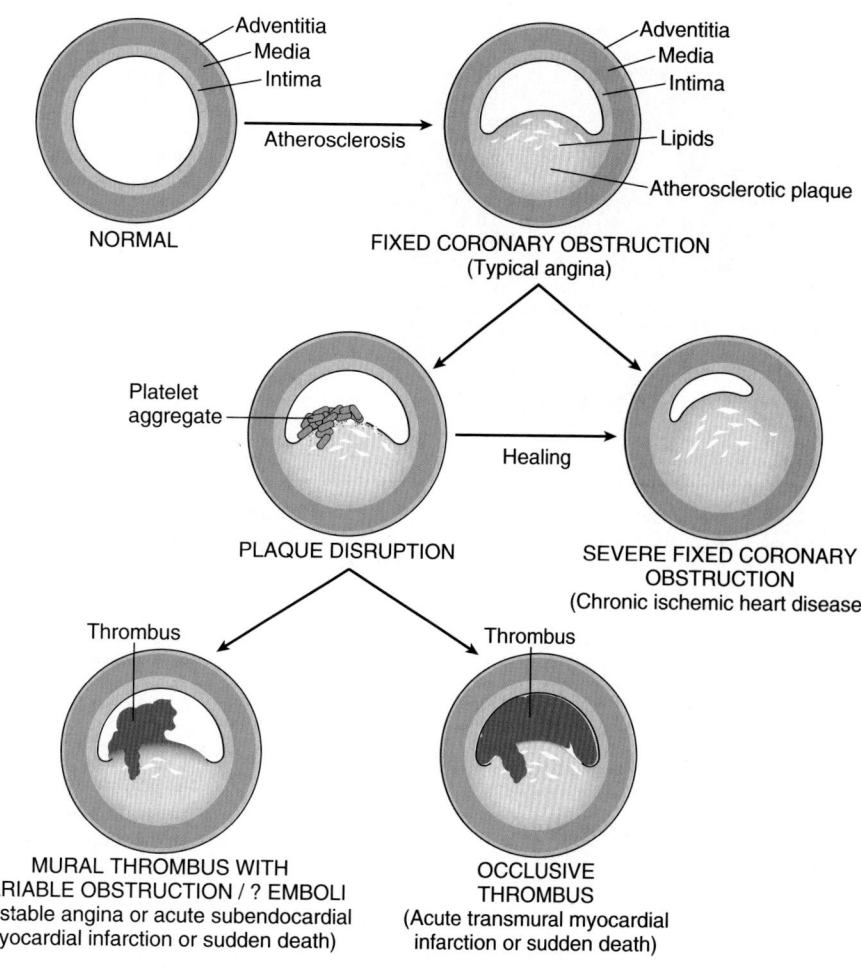

Figure 11–8   ■

Schematic representation of some of the morphologic manifestations of coronary artery atherosclerosis, its complications, and the related coronary syndromes. (Modified and redrawn from Schoen FJ: Interventional and Surgical Cardiovascular Pathology: Clinical Correlations and Basic Principles. Philadelphia, WB Saunders, 1989, p 63.)

MORPHOLOGY

The essential feature of hypertensive heart disease is **left ventricular hypertrophy.** The weight of the heart usually exceeds 450 g. The hypertrophy typically involves the ventricular wall in a symmetric, circumferential pattern termed **concentric hypertrophy** (Fig. 11–9), with free wall thicknesses exceeding 2.0 cm. On occasion, particularly in long-standing cases, hypertrophy may be more pronounced in the septal area, mimicking the appearance of hypertrophic cardiomyopathy (discussed later). The size of the chamber is normal in the early stages of hypertensive heart disease, but in long-standing cases some degree of dilation is common. As left ventricular failure progresses, right ventricular hypertrophy and dilation may also develop. Coronary artery disease is present in most cases, with its associated morphologic effects on the myocardium. Microscopically, the cardiac myocytes are enlarged and contain large, hyperchromatic, rectangular "box-car"-shaped nuclei. The nuclear changes are caused by tetraploidy, presumably reflecting abortive attempts at cell replication. Superimposed ischemic changes, including interstitial fibrosis and recent or remote infarcts, are common.

Clinical Features. In its early stages, while the cardiac output is maintained at normal levels, hypertensive heart disease may cause no symptoms. In these patients, the diagnosis is usually based on the detection of left ventricular enlargement in chest radiographs or echocardiograms or by electrocardiographic evidence of left ventricular hypertrophy. As the left ventricle begins to fail, the clinical manifestations of heart failure appear. Heart failure in the setting of hypertension is associated with a poor prognosis. Signs and symptoms of myocardial ischemia, such as angina pectoris, often punctuate the course of hypertensive cardiac disease. In addition, progressive renal damage or cerebrovascular accidents may occur and contribute to both morbidity and mortality. The risk of sudden cardiac death is also increased. There is substantial

Figure 11-9 ■

Concentric left ventricular hypertrophy in a patient with long-standing hypertension. Any process that imposes a chronic pressure load on the left ventricle, such as systemic hypertension or aortic stenosis, can cause similar changes.

Table 11-3. DISORDERS THAT PREDISPOSE TO COR PULMONALE

Diseases of the Lungs
Chronic obstructive lung disease
Diffuse pulmonary interstitial fibrosis
Extensive, persistent atelectasis
Cystic fibrosis
Diseases of Pulmonary Vessels
Pulmonary embolism
Primary pulmonary vascular sclerosis
Extensive pulmonary arteritis (e.g., Wegener granulomatosis)
Drug-, toxin-, or radiation-induced vascular sclerosis
Disorders Affecting Chest Movement
Kyphoscoliosis
Marked obesity (pickwickian syndrome)
Neuromuscular diseases
Disorders Inducing Pulmonary Arteriolar Constriction
Metabolic acidosis
Hypoxemia
   Chronic altitude sickness
   Obstruction to major airways
   Idiopathic alveolar hypoventilation

evidence that effective control of hypertension can prevent or lead to regression of hypertrophy and its associated risks.

COR PULMONALE

The term *cor pulmonale*, or *pulmonary heart disease*, is used to describe disease of the right-sided cardiac chambers caused by pulmonary hypertension resulting from pulmonary parenchymal or pulmonary vascular disease. Excluded from this definition are cases of pulmonary hypertension caused by left ventricular failure or other primary diseases of the left side of the heart and of pulmonary hypertension caused by congenital heart disease. The condition may be acute or chronic. The major causes of cor pulmonale are listed in Table 11-3, the more common being pulmonary emboli, chronic obstructive and restrictive lung diseases, and pulmonary vascular diseases.

Acute cor pulmonale is most often caused by pulmonary embolism. When emboli acutely obstruct more than 50% of the pulmonary vascular bed, the sudden increase in the burden on the right side of the heart causes right ventricular failure. The right ventricle is typically dilated but is not hypertrophied.

Chronic cor pulmonale can be caused by any of the diseases listed in Table 11-3, all of which cause pulmonary hypertension. Of these, the *most common cause is chronic obstructive lung disease* (Chapter 13). In chronic cor pulmonale, in contrast to acute cor pulmonale, sustained pulmonary hypertension allows sufficient time for the development of compensatory right ventricular hypertrophy. The right ventricle is even less suited to accommodating increased pressure loads than is the left ventricle. Over time, the right ventricle progressively dilates and is ultimately unable to maintain cardiac output at normal levels. When this occurs, symptoms and signs typical of right-sided congestive heart failure

develop. Acute decompensation may occur at any point in a patient with chronic cor pulmonale. Patients with cor pulmonale are also at increased risk for the development of lethal ventricular arrhythmias.

MORPHOLOGY

In isolated **acute cor pulmonale,** the right ventricle is usually dilated. However, if sudden death occurs, for example, after massive pulmonary embolism, the heart may be of normal size. **Chronic cor pulmonale** is characterized by right ventricular, and often right atrial, hypertrophy. In extreme cases, the thickness of the right ventricular wall may exceed that of the left ventricle. When ventricular failure develops, the right ventricle and atrium may also be dilated. Such dilation may mask right ventricular hypertrophy. Because chronic cor pulmonale occurs in the setting of chronically elevated pulmonary arterial pressure, the pulmonary arteries often contain atheromatous plaques and other lesions of pulmonary hypertension (Chapter 13).

VALVULAR HEART DISEASES

Diseases of the heart valves include a diverse group of acquired and congenital lesions. Some of these occur in isolation, and others occur in association with other heart diseases. In this section, we will devote our attention to primary valvular diseases. Valvular lesions that occur in association with congenital cardiac malformations will be considered later, along with other congenital heart

■

TABLE 11–4. MAJOR CAUSES OF ACQUIRED HEART VALVE DISEASE

Mitral Valve Disease	Aortic Valve Disease
Mitral Stenosis	**Aortic Stenosis**
Postinflammatory scarring (rheumatic heart disease)	Postinflammatory scarring (rheumatic heart disease)
	Senile calcific aortic stenosis
	Calcification of congenitally deformed valve
Mitral Regurgitation	**Aortic Regurgitation**
Abnormalities of leaflets and commissures	Intrinsic valvular disease
Postinflammatory scarring	Postinflammatory scarring (rheumatic heart disease)
Infective endocarditis	Infective endocarditis
Mitral valve prolapse	Aortic disease
Abnormalities of tensor apparatus	Degenerative aortic dilation
Rupture of papillary muscle	Syphilitic aortitis
Papillary muscle dysfunction (fibrosis)	Ankylosing spondylitis
Rupture of chordae tendineae	Rheumatoid arthritis
Abnormalities of left ventricular cavity and/or annulus	Marfan syndrome
Left ventricular enlargement (myocarditis, congestive cardiomyopathy)	
Calcification of mitral ring	

Modified from Schoen FJ: Surgical pathology of removed natural and prosthetic valves. Hum Pathol 18:558, 1987.

diseases. Syphilis, an important cause of aortic valve disease, is discussed in Chapter 10 along with other disorders of the aorta.

Deformed cardiac valves may cause disease by two major mechanisms. First, *they impose a major hemodynamic burden on the cardiac chambers* by causing obstruction (stenosis) or regurgitation (incompetence) or sometimes a combination of the two. Second, the *abnormal valves are more susceptible to infection* and thus predispose patients to infective endocarditis and its many complications. The important forms of acquired valvular disease affecting the mitral and aortic valves are listed in Table 11–4. With the possible exception of infective endocarditis and carcinoid heart disease, lesions of the tricuspid and pulmonic valves are much less common; therefore, most of our discussion will focus on diseases of the aortic and mitral valves.

Rheumatic Fever and Heart Disease

Rheumatic fever is an acute, immunologically mediated, multisystem inflammatory disease that follows an episode of group A streptococcal pharyngitis after an interval of a few weeks. The antecedent pharyngitis may sometimes be almost asymptomatic. Certain "rheumatogenic" strains of group A streptococci appear to be particularly associated with an increased risk of rheumatic fever, perhaps caused by the presence of a well-developed, highly antigenic capsule. It is interesting to note that rheumatic fever rarely

follows infections by streptococci at other sites, such as the skin. The incidence and mortality rate of rheumatic fever have declined remarkably in many parts of the world over the past 35 years thanks to improved socioeconomic conditions, rapid diagnosis and treatment of streptococcal pharyngitis, and an unexplained decrease in the virulence of group A streptococci. Nevertheless, in third world countries and in many crowded, economically depressed urban areas in the Western world, rheumatic fever remains an important public health problem. Rheumatic fever may cause heart disease during its acute phase *(acute rheumatic carditis)*, or it may cause *chronic valvular deformities* that may not manifest themselves until many years after the acute disease. Fortunately, rheumatic fever occurs in only about 3% of patients with group A streptococcal pharyngitis. However, after an initial attack, there is increased vulnerability to reactivation of the disease with subsequent pharyngeal infections.

The pathogenesis of acute rheumatic fever and its chronic sequelae is not fully understood. It is strongly suspected that *acute rheumatic fever is a hypersensitivity reaction induced by group A streptococci.* It is proposed that antibodies directed against the M proteins of group A streptococci cross-react with normal proteins present in the heart, joints, and other tissues. The fact that symptoms typically do not develop until 2 to 3 weeks after infection and that streptococci are absent from the lesions supports the concept that rheumatic fever results from an immune response against the offending bacteria. Because the nature of cross-reacting antigens has been difficult to define, it has also been suggested that the streptococcal infection evokes an autoimmune response against self-antigens. The major aspects of the pathogenesis and morphology of rheumatic carditis are summarized in Figure 11–10.

MORPHOLOGY

In **acute rheumatic fever,** inflammatory infiltrates may occur in a wide range of sites, including synovium, joints, skin, and (most importantly) the heart. The initial tissue reaction is that of focal fibrinoid necrosis. This provokes a mixed inflammatory response, which may take the form of either a diffuse cellular infiltrate or a localized aggregation of cells that resembles a granuloma. Areas of fibrosis eventually develop at sites of inflammation. **Fibrosis is particularly common in cardiac tissues,** where it is responsible for the valvular deformities seen in chronic rheumatic heart disease.

Acute rheumatic carditis is characterized by inflammatory changes in all three layers of the heart, and thus it is appropriately designated a pancarditis. The hallmark of acute rheumatic carditis is the presence of multiple foci of inflammation within the connective tissues of the heart, called **Aschoff bodies** (Fig. 11–11). They contain a central focus of fibrinoid necrosis surrounded by a chronic mononuclear inflammatory infiltrate and occasional large macrophages with vesicular nuclei and abundant basophilic cytoplasm, called **Anitschkow cells.**

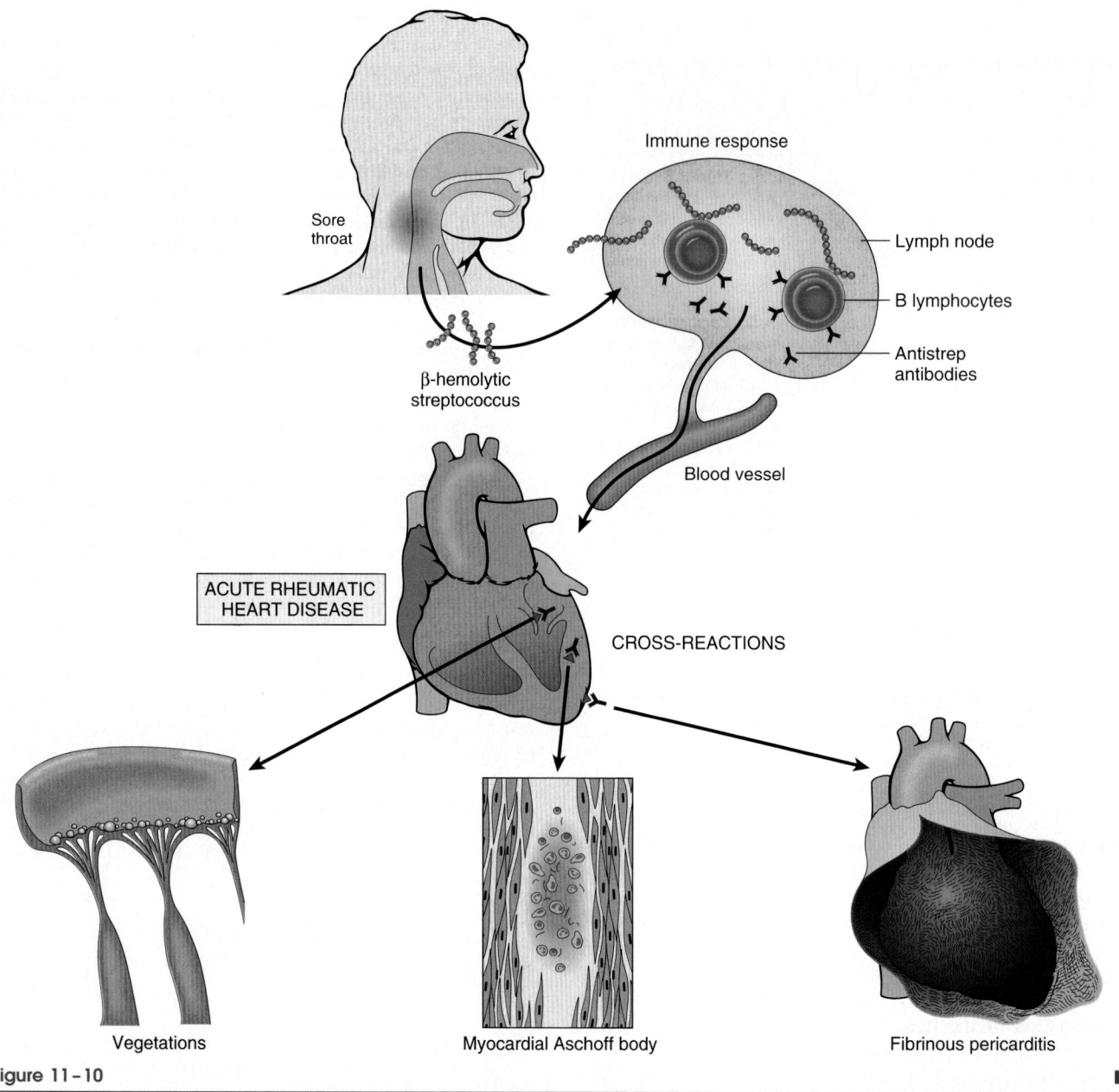

Sore throat

β-hemolytic streptococcus

Immune response

Lymph node

B lymphocytes

Antistrep antibodies

Blood vessel

ACUTE RHEUMATIC HEART DISEASE

CROSS-REACTIONS

Vegetations

Myocardial Aschoff body

Fibrinous pericarditis

Figure 11–10 ■

Pathogenesis and key morphologic changes of acute rheumatic heart disease. Acute rheumatic fever causes changes in the endocardium, myocardium, and epicardium. Chronic rheumatic heart disease is almost always caused by deformity of the heart valves, particularly the mitral and aortic valves.

Aschoff bodies may be found anywhere in the connective tissues of the heart. In the myocardium, they often lie in close proximity to a small vessel and may encroach on its wall. In addition to Aschoff bodies, the myocardium may also contain diffuse interstitial inflammatory infiltrates. In severe cases, the myocarditis may impair myocardial function sufficiently to cause generalized dilation of the cardiac chambers. **Pericardial involvement** is manifested grossly and microscopically by the presence of fibrinous pericarditis, sometimes associated with a serous or serosanguineous pericardial effusion. Involvement of

the **endocardium** is common and may affect any valve. However, valvular inflammation tends to be most pronounced in the mitral and aortic valves. The affected valves are edematous and thickened and show foci of fibrinoid necrosis, but Aschoff nodules are not common. The inflammation of the valve predisposes to the formation of small vegetations, seen as wartlike excrescences, particularly along the lines of valve closure **(verrucous endocarditis)** (Fig. 11–12). The acute changes may resolve without sequelae or may progress to cause significant scarring and chronic valvular deformities, described later.

Figure 11–11   ■

Aschoff body in a patient who died of acute rheumatic carditis. In the interstitium of the myocardium there is a circumscribed (granulomatous) collection of mononuclear inflammatory cells. There are some large histiocytes with prominent nucleoli and also a prominent binucleate histiocyte. The central necrosis seen within these lesions is not prominent in this field. (Courtesy of Sid Murphree, MD, Department of Pathology, University of Texas Southwestern Medical School, Dallas.)

Changes encountered in other organs include nonspecific **arthritis of the large joints,** characterized by chronic inflammatory infiltrates and edema in the involved joints and periarticular soft tissues. In contrast to the cardiac lesions, the arthritis is self-limited and does not cause chronic deformity. **Pulmonary involvement,** manifested by chronic interstitial inflammatory infiltrates and fibrinous inflammation of the pleural surface, is uncommon. **Skin changes** take the form of **subcutaneous nodules** or **erythema marginatum.** Microscopically, the skin nodules contain focal lesions that are essentially large Aschoff bodies. Erythema marginatum presents as a maculopapular rash.

Chronic rheumatic heart disease is characterized by irreversible deformity of one or more cardiac valves, resulting from previous episodes of acute valvulitis. The mitral valve is abnormal in approximately 95% of cases of chronic rheumatic heart disease, and combined aortic and mitral valve disease is present in about 25% of patients. Right-sided valvular disease is relatively uncommon. Scarring of the valve leaflets may cause a reduction in the diameter of the valve orifice **(stenosis),** or it may prevent proper closure of the valve leaflets, resulting in **regurgitation** of blood during diastole. Sometimes stenosis and regurgitation coexist, although one hemodynamic defect usually predominates. Valvular stenosis and regurgitation increase the demands on the myocardium because of increased pressure and/or volume load, which, if severe enough, eventually causes **cardiac failure.** Damage to the valves also predisposes the patients to superimposed **infective endocarditis.**

Chronic rheumatic mitral valvulitis causes stenosis more often than regurgitation, and it is the most common cause of mitral stenosis. It occurs more frequently in females than in males, for reasons that remain unclear. In **mitral stenosis,** the valve leaflets and chordae tendineae are thick, rigid, and interadherent (Fig. 11–13A). The mitral orifice is narrowed to a slitlike channel, sometimes designated a "fish-mouth" deformity (Fig. 11–13B). The left atrium is dilated and hypertrophied, and the endocardial surface is often thickened, particularly above the posterior mitral leaflet. Mural thrombi may be present (see Fig. 11–13B), representing a potential source of systemic emboli. The lungs are firm and heavy as a result of chronic passive congestion, and in longstanding cases the right ventricle and atrium are dilated and hypertrophied as well.

In cases of **mitral regurgitation,** the deformed mitral leaflets are retracted, and the added volume load on the left ventricle causes left ventricular dilation and hypertrophy.

Chronic aortic valvulitis is encountered more often in males than in females. Aortic valve disease is almost invariably associated with an element of mitral valvulitis. In patients with **aortic stenosis,** the valve cusps are thickened, firm, and adherent to each other, and the resultant aortic valve orifice is reduced to a rigid, triangular channel (see Fig. 11–14B). Aortic stenosis places a pressure load on the left ventricle, which undergoes concentric hypertrophy. Subsequent left ventricular failure is associated with dilation of the chamber and other morphologic sequelae of congestive heart failure. Fibrosis of the valve leaflets may also cause them to retract toward the aortic wall, resulting in **aortic regurgitation,** left ventricular hypertrophy, and dilation.

Figure 11–12   ■

Acute rheumatic mitral valvulitis superimposed on chronic rheumatic heart disease. Small vegetations are visible along the line of closure of the mitral valve leaflet *(arrows).* Previous episodes of rheumatic valvulitis have caused fibrous thickening and fusion of valve leaflets and chordae tendineae.

Figure 11–13

Chronic (healed) rheumatic carditis. *A,* The mitral valve leaflets are thickened, opaque, and fused at the commissures. The chordae tendineae are also thickened and shortened as a result of fibrosis. *B,* Seen from the left atrial side, the mitral valve looks markedly stenotic, appearing as a pinhole *(arrowhead).* The opened, dilated left atrium contains a large thrombus resulting from stasis of blood in this chamber.

Clinical Features. *Acute rheumatic fever* occurs anywhere from 10 days to 6 weeks after an episode of pharyngitis caused by group A streptococci. Because only a minority of infected patients develop rheumatic fever, genetic susceptibility that regulates the hypersensitivity reaction is suspected. The peak incidence is between the ages of 5 and 15, although younger children and adults may also develop the disease. Although pharyngeal cultures for streptococci are negative by the time the illness begins, antibodies to one or more streptococcal enzymes, such as streptolysin O and DNAse B, are present in the sera of most patients. Reliable assays, such as the Streptozyme test, are widely available for the detection of these antibodies. The predominant clinical manifestations of acute rheumatic fever are those of arthritis and carditis. The *arthritis,* which is much more common in adults than in children, preferentially occurs in larger joints and tends to involve different joints sequentially (migratory polyarthritis). Clinical features related to *acute carditis* include pericardial friction rubs, weak heart sounds (because of pericardial effusion),

tachycardia, and other arrhythmias. In severe cases, myocarditis may cause overt congestive heart failure. The associated left ventricular dilatation causes the papillary muscles to pull on the chordae tendineae of the mitral valve cusps, which may result, in turn, in the development of functional, potentially reversible mitral insufficiency. Less than 5% of patients with rheumatic fever succumb to the acute disease.

Chronic rheumatic carditis usually does not cause clinical manifestations for years or even decades after the initial episode of rheumatic fever. The signs and symptoms of valvular disease depend on which cardiac valve or valves are involved. In addition to various cardiac murmurs, cardiac hypertrophy and dilation, and congestive heart failure, patients with chronic rheumatic heart disease may suffer from arrhythmias (particularly atrial fibrillation in the setting of mitral stenosis), thromboembolic complications, and infective endocarditis. Timely surgical replacement of diseased valves has greatly improved the outlook for patients with chronic rheumatic heart disease.

Figure 11–14

Degenerative calcific aortic stenosis. *A,* View from the aortic side of an unopened, markedly deformed tricuspid aortic valve. Calcific masses protrude into the sinuses of Valsalva. Note that the valve commissures are not fused. *B,* In contrast, healed rheumatic aortic valvulitis shows aortic stenosis caused by fibrosis and fusion of the valves and the commissures.

Calcific Aortic Stenosis

Degenerative changes in the cardiac valves are an inevitable part of the aging process, given the repetitive mechanical stresses to which they are subjected during life. Some of these changes, which can be thought of as the valvular counterparts of age-related arteriosclerosis, include fibrosis of the valve cusps, usually accompanied by some degree of calcification. Valve sclerosis occurs most frequently in the aortic and mitral valves. In most cases, age-related valve sclerosis is asymptomatic and is discovered incidentally in chest radiographs or at the time of autopsy. In some patients, the sclerosis may be severe enough to cause clinically apparent disease. *Sclerosis and calcification of the aortic valve are the most common causes of isolated aortic stenosis in the United States.* This lesion, sometimes called *degenerative calcific aortic stenosis,* may occur in a congenitally bicuspid or unicuspid aortic valve, or it may develop in previously normal semilunar valve cusps. Calcification of the mitral valve typically involves the valve annulus and is usually asymptomatic, but in some cases it may cause conduction disturbances.

MORPHOLOGY

In degenerative calcific aortic stenosis, the aortic valve leaflets are rigid and deformed by irregular calcified masses. The calcium deposits lie behind the valve cusps and extend into the sinus of Valsalva (Fig. 11–14A). Stigmata of rheumatic valvulitis, such as fusion of aortic valve commissures, are not present; these features help to distinguish degenerative calcific aortic stenosis from chronic rheumatic aortic valvulitis (Fig. 11–14B). Degenerative changes in the mitral valve are restricted to fibrosis and calcification along the lines of closure and within the valve annulus. Concentric hypertrophy of the left ventricle and ventricular dilation are commonly seen with long-standing disease.

Clinical Features. Like aortic stenosis in general, the cardinal manifestations of degenerative calcific aortic stenosis include angina pectoris, syncope, and (in later stages) congestive heart failure. Degenerative calcific aortic stenosis arising in a previously normal valve is usually asymptomatic until the eighth or ninth decade. Calcific aortic stenosis may also occur in *congenitally bicuspid* aortic valves, a common lesion present in up to 2% of the general population. The abnormal configuration of these bicuspid valves exposes them to excessive hemodynamic stresses, resulting in greater wear and tear and earlier degenerative changes. Thus, these lesions become clinically manifested 10 to 20 years earlier than degenerative calcific aortic stenosis. Regardless of the cause of aortic stenosis, physical examination discloses a harsh crescendo-decrescendo systolic murmur and left ventricular hypertrophy. *Angina* occurs because of the increased oxygen requirements of the hypertrophied myocardium coupled with reduced aortic outflow and, in many patients, concomitant coronary artery disease. *Syncope* reflects poor perfusion of the brain, particularly during

episodes of exertion. Untreated aortic stenosis usually causes death within 3 to 4 years of the onset of symptoms, either from congestive heart failure or from a lethal arrhythmia. Degenerative calcific aortic stenosis is an important indication for surgical valve replacement.

Mitral Valve Prolapse

As noted in the preceding sections (and in Table 11–4), mitral regurgitation may occur in patients with rheumatic heart disease, ischemic heart disease, or congestive heart failure of any origin. However, the most common cause of isolated mitral regurgitation is a disorder known as *mitral valve prolapse,* first recognized by Barlow in the 1960s. Mitral valve prolapse is one of the most common cardiac disorders, occurring in 3% to 5% of the general adult population. Most cases are discovered between the ages of 20 and 40; the disease is more common in women than in men. It is characterized by an accumulation of loose ground substance within the leaflets and chordae of the mitral valve, which causes the valve to become "floppy" and incompetent during systole. Mitral valve prolapse may arise as a complication of Marfan syndrome or similar connective tissue disorders, and it has also been reported as an isolated autosomal dominant condition that maps to chromosome 16p. Even less commonly, it is inherited as an X-linked recessive disorder. Most cases occur as isolated, apparently sporadic abnormalities, however.

MORPHOLOGY

The mitral valve cusps, particularly the posterior cusp, are soft and enlarged, causing a characteristic ballooning of the valve leaflets into the left atrium during systole (Fig. 11–15). The chordae tendineae, which are often elongated and fragile, may rupture in severe cases. The mitral annulus may be dilated. Histologic examination reveals excessive amounts of loose, edematous, faintly basophilic tissue within the middle layer (spongiosa) of the valve leaflets and chordae. Similar changes may be seen in the tricuspid and, less commonly, the pulmonic valve.

Clinical Features. Most patients with mitral valve prolapse are asymptomatic. In a minority of cases, however, patients may complain of palpitations, fatigue, or atypical chest pain. Auscultation of the chest discloses a sharp midsystolic click, caused by abrupt tension on the redundant valve leaflets and chordae tendineae, followed by a late systolic murmur. Although the majority of patients with mitral valve prolapse have a relatively benign course, approximately 3% of patients experience one of several complications. These include hemodynamically significant mitral regurgitation and congestive heart failure, particularly if the chordae or valve leaflets rupture. Patients with mitral valve prolapse are also at increased risk for the development of infective endocarditis (discussed later) and sudden death caused by ventricular arrhythmias.

Figure 11–15

Mitral valve prolapse. The opened mitral valve shows ballooning *(arrowheads)* of the valve leaflets into the left atrium. (From the teaching collection of the Pathology Department, University of Texas Southwestern Medical School, Dallas.)

Stroke or other systemic infarction may occur from embolism of thrombi formed in the left atrium.

Nonbacterial Thrombotic Endocarditis

Nonbacterial thrombotic endocarditis (NBTE) is characterized by the deposition of small masses of fibrin, platelets, and other blood components on the leaflets of the cardiac valves. In contrast to the vegetations of infective endocarditis, discussed in the next section, the valvular lesions of NBTE are sterile and do not contain microorganisms. Valvular damage is not a prerequisite for NBTE. Indeed, the condition is usually found on previously normal valves. The pathogenesis of NBTE is incompletely understood; it is thought that subtle endothelial abnormalities and hypercoagulable states predispose to its development. Malignancies, particularly adenocarcinomas, have been identified in up to 50% of patients with NBTE. These patients may also exhibit other features of hypercoagulability, such as deep venous thrombosis. Although NBTE may occur in otherwise healthy individuals, a wide variety of diseases associated with general debility or wasting are associated with an increased risk of NBTE. The term *marantic endocarditis* has also been used to describe this entity, in recognition of the increased frequency of NBTE in cachectic patients.

MORPHOLOGY

Grossly, NBTE is characterized by the presence of multiple small nodules along the lines of valve closure, similar to the valvular lesions of acute rheumatic fever. The nodules usually measure less than 5 mm in diameter but may become fairly

large and friable (Fig. 11–16). The valve leaflets appear normal on gross inspection. Although any valve may be affected, the mitral valve is the most common site, followed by the aortic valve. Microscopically, the nodules are composed of eosinophilic material (fibrin) and a delicate layer of aggregated platelets. The underlying valve is typically free of inflammation or fibrosis, in contrast to the valves in acute rheumatic fever. The lesions of NBTE often resolve spontaneously, leaving in their wake delicate strands of fibrous tissue termed **Lambl excrescences.**

Clinical Features. NBTE is usually asymptomatic. Sometimes, particularly in patients with larger lesions, fragments of the vegetations may embolize and cause infarcts in the brain and other organs. The lesions of NBTE also serve as a potential nidus for bacterial colonization and thus may be complicated by the development of infective endocarditis.

Libman-Sacks Endocarditis

The term *Libman-Sacks endocarditis* refers to sterile vegetations that may develop on the cardiac valves of patients with systemic lupus erythematosus. These lesions occur most frequently on the ventricular surfaces of the mitral and tricuspid valves but can also involve other endocardial surfaces. In contrast to the lesions of typical NBTE (discussed earlier), the small vegetations of Libman-Sacks endocarditis have no special predilection for the lines of valve closure. With increasing use of steroids for treatment of lupus, these lesions have become quite uncommon.

Figure 11–16

Nonbacterial thrombotic endocarditis. Irregular yellow-tan vegetations are present on the mitral valve. Note that unlike the valves in chronic rheumatic carditis (see Fig. 11–13), this valve shows normal, thin leaflets, and the chordae tendineae are thin and glistening. (From the teaching collection of the Pathology Department, University of Texas Southwestern Medical School, Dallas.)

Infective Endocarditis

The term *infective endocarditis* designates infection of the cardiac valves or mural surface of the endocardium, resulting in the formation of an adherent, bulky mass of thrombotic debris and organisms, termed a *vegetation*. Virtually any type of microorganism is capable of causing endocarditis, although most cases are caused by bacteria.

Infective endocarditis has traditionally been subdivided into acute and subacute forms. Cases of *acute endocarditis* are classically associated with infection of the valves by organisms of high virulence, such as *Staphylococcus aureus*. Such organisms are capable of infecting even structurally normal valves and cause rapidly progressive infection, with little accompanying local host reaction. *Subacute endocarditis*, in contrast, is typically associated with infection of previously abnormal valves by organisms of lower virulence, such as α-hemolytic streptococci. The resultant infections tend to progress somewhat more slowly and are often accompanied by the development of a local inflammatory reaction and granulation tissue in the affected valve. In the era of antibiotics, however, therapy often modifies the morphology and clinical progression of disease, thus blurring the distinction between acute and subacute cases.

Etiology and Pathogenesis. Infection occurs when organisms are implanted on the endocardial surface during episodes of bacteremia. In some instances the cause of the hematogenous infection is obvious, as in the case of intravenous drug abusers who inject contaminated material directly into the bloodstream; an infection elsewhere or a previous dental, surgical, or other interventional procedure (e.g., urinary catheterization) may also seed the bloodstream. In other cases, however, the source of bacteremia is occult and presumably related to trivial injuries to the skin or mucosal surfaces, as may be encountered, for example, during brushing the teeth. In some cases, the initial valvular change is that of endothelial injury followed by the development of a localized fibrin-platelet aggregate (see NBTE, discussed earlier). These foci may then serve as attachment sites for circulating microorganisms. In other instances, bacteria may adhere directly to the valve surface in the absence of a preexisting focus of NBTE.

Conditions that increase the risk of infective endocarditis can be segregated into three categories: (1) preexisting cardiac abnormalities, (2) prosthetic heart valves, and (3) intravenous drug abuse.

■ A number of cardiac abnormalities predispose individuals to infective endocarditis. The risk of endocarditis is increased by any condition that causes increased hemodynamic trauma to the endocardial surface, such as high pressure shunts within the heart (e.g., small ventricular septal defects) or chronic valvular diseases (e.g., chronic rheumatic heart disease, degenerative calcific aortic stenosis, mitral valve prolapse). Because of its high prevalence, mitral valve prolapse has emerged as the most common predisposing factor for infective endocarditis.

■ With an increasing number of patients undergoing valve replacement surgery, prosthetic valves now account for 10% to 20% of cases of infective endocarditis. There is no difference in the incidence of endocarditis between mechanical and bioprosthetic valves. The frequency of endocarditis is also increased, as might be expected, in individuals with indwelling intravascular catheters.

■ Intravenous drug abusers are at a high risk for development of infective endocarditis. In this setting, infective endocarditis usually occurs on previously normal valves, often involving the cardiac valves on the right side of the heart.

The causative organisms differ somewhat in the three high-risk groups. Endocarditis of native (not prosthetic) valves is caused most commonly (50% to 60% of cases) by α-hemolytic (viridans) streptococci, which usually attack previously damaged valves. The more virulent *S. aureus* organisms attack healthy or deformed valves and are responsible for 10% to 20% of cases. The roster of the remaining bacteria includes enterococci and the so-called HACEK group (*Haemophilus*, *Actinobacillus*, *Cardiobacterium*, *Eikenella*, and *Kingella*), all commensals in the oral cavity. Prosthetic valve endocarditis is caused most commonly by coagulase-negative staphylococci (e.g., *S. epidermidis*). Other agents include gram-negative bacilli and fungi. In intravenous drug abusers, *S. aureus*, commonly found on the skin, is the major offender; other, less frequent, causes in this population of patients include streptococci, gram-negative rods, and fungi.

Infective endocarditis is a particularly difficult infection to eradicate because of the avascular nature of the heart valves. In view of the paucity of blood vessels, the inflammatory response to the infection is relatively scant, if present at all. Thus, even avirulent organisms can proliferate in an uncontrolled fashion. Before effective antibiotics were available, infective endocarditis was almost always fatal.

MORPHOLOGY

The hallmark of infective endocarditis is the presence of valvular vegetations containing bacteria or other organisms. The aortic (Fig. 11–17A) and mitral valves are the most common sites of infection, although the valves of the right side of the heart may also be involved, particularly in cases of endocarditis occurring in intravenous drug abusers (Fig. 11–17B). The vegetations may be single or multiple and may involve more than one valve. The appearance of the vegetations is influenced by the type of organism responsible for the infection, the degree of host reaction to the infection, and previous antibiotic therapy. Fungal endocarditis, for example, tends to cause larger vegetations than does bacterial infection. Although highly virulent organisms tend to cause acute endocarditis, treatment with antibiotics may curb the infection sufficiently to change the morphology of the vegetations to a more subacute form.

The vegetations in cases of classic **acute endocarditis** begin as small excrescences, which may be grossly indistinguishable from those of NBTE, although they are more commonly solitary than the vegetations in the latter condition. As the organisms proliferate, the vegetations enlarge progressively

Figure 11-17 ■

A, Acute bacterial endocarditis of the aortic valve. Irregular vegetations are attached to the valve, which has been severely damaged and perforated. The metal probe is traversing a hole in the valve leaflet. *B,* Opened right atrium shows large, irregular, friable vegetations causing virtual occlusion of the tricuspid valve. Such vegetations are often noted in intravenous drug abusers.

and eventually form bulky, friable lesions that may obstruct the valve orifice (see Fig. 11-17*B*). The vegetations may cause rapid destruction of the valves, often resulting in rupture of the leaflets, chordae tendineae, or papillary muscles. The infection may eventually extend through the valve into the adjacent myocardium to produce abscesses in the perivalvular tissue known as **ring abscesses.** Microscopic examination of the vegetations reveals large numbers of organisms admixed with fibrin and blood cells. When confined to the valve, the vegetations elicit minimal inflammatory response. A brisk neutrophilic inflammatory response occurs once the infection extends beyond the avascular valves. **Systemic emboli** may occur at any time because of the friable nature of the vegetations, and they may cause infarcts in the brain, kidneys, myocardium, and other tissues. Because the embolic fragments contain large numbers of virulent organisms, **abscesses often develop at the sites of such emboli** (Fig. 11-18).

The vegetations of **subacute endocarditis** tend to be somewhat firmer and are associated with less valvular destruction than those of acute endocarditis, although the distinction between the two forms may be difficult. Subacute infections are less likely to erode into the myocardium, and perivalvular abscesses are uncommon. Microscopically, the vegetations of typical subacute infective endocarditis are distinguished from those of acute disease by the presence of **granulation tissue** at their bases. With the passage of time, fibrosis, calcification, and a chronic inflammatory infiltrate may develop. **Systemic emboli** may also develop in subacute endocarditis. In contrast to those of acute endocarditis, however, **the resultant infarcts are less likely to undergo suppuration** because of the less virulent nature of the offending organisms.

Clinical Features. The onset of infective endocarditis may be gradual or explosive, depending on the organism responsible for the infection. Low-grade fever, malaise, and weight loss are characteristic of cases caused by organisms of low virulence, while more acute cases, in contrast, typically present as high fevers, shaking chills, and other evidence of overt septicemia. *Changing cardiac murmurs* are almost always present, although they may be difficult to detect early in the course of acute endocarditis. The *spleen is often enlarged,* and clubbing of the digits may be seen, particularly in subacute cases. *Systemic emboli* are very common in all forms of infective endocarditis, manifesting as neurologic deficits, retinal

Figure 11-18 ■

Heart from a patient who died of acute bacterial endocarditis of the aortic valve caused by *Staphylococcus aureus*. The left ventricular myocardium contains multiple abscesses, caused by detachment and embolization of vegetations via the coronary arteries. Embolic fragments laden with highly virulent organisms such as *S. aureus* characteristically cause systemic abscesses, whereas those containing less virulent organisms tend to produce bland infarcts. (Courtesy of Eileen Bigio, MD, Department of Pathology, University of Texas Southwestern Medical School, Dallas.)

abnormalities, necrosis of the digits, and infarcts of the myocardium and other viscera. Pulmonary emboli may occur in patients with right-sided endocarditis and large vegetations on the tricuspid or pulmonic valves. Entrapment of infected emboli in the walls of blood vessels may cause local infection and weakening of the vessel wall, with the formation of so-called *mycotic* aneurysms. Petechiae (small hemorrhages) may be seen on the skin or mucosal surfaces. They may be caused by microemboli or deposition of immune complexes formed in response to chronic antigenemia. *Renal lesions* are common and include both renal infarcts and glomerulonephritis, the latter resulting from entrapment of immune complexes in the glomeruli. Over a period of days to months, progressive valvular destruction in untreated cases results in valvular regurgitation and congestive heart failure.

Repeated blood cultures are extremely important in the evaluation of patients with suspected infective endocarditis. Cultures for both aerobic and anaerobic organisms should be obtained the moment the possibility of endocarditis is considered. In a minority of cases of infective endocarditis, blood cultures remain negative because of either the fastidious nature of the organism or the effects of previous antibiotic therapy.

Prosthetic Cardiac Valves

The introduction of effective prosthetic heart valves has radically altered the prognosis of patients with many of the valvular diseases discussed previously. Two types of prosthetic valves are used: those derived from glutaraldehyde-fixed porcine or bovine tissues or cryopreserved human valves (bioprosthetic valves), and synthetic (mechanical) valves. Each type of valve has its advantages and disadvantages. Several complications are common to all prosthetic valves.

Mechanical deterioration is a particularly important complication of bioprosthetic valves. Virtually all biologic valve leaflets undergo some degree of stiffening after implantation. This loss of mobility may be sufficient to cause significant valvular stenosis. Calcification of the leaflets is also common and may contribute to the stenosis. Bioprosthetic valves may perforate or tear, resulting in valvular insufficiency. In general, mechanical valves are less susceptible to structural deterioration than are biologic valves.

Thrombi may develop on any type of prosthetic valve but are especially troublesome with mechanical valves. Such thrombi may cause local obstruction of blood flow or serve as a source of systemic emboli. Although anticoagulants are routinely administered to patients with prosthetic valves, they carry with them the additional risk of hemorrhagic complications.

Infective endocarditis, as noted earlier, occurs with increased frequency in prosthetic valves of all types. In mechanical valves the infection typically involves the valve suture line and adjacent perivalvular tissue and may cause the valve to detach. In bioprosthetic valves the valve leaflets as well as the perivalvular tissues may become infected, causing perforation of the leaflets and valvular regurgitation.

Paravalvular leaks may also develop in either type of prosthetic valve. This may occur in the immediate perioperative period or later in the patient's course. Valvular infection is an important cause of paravalvular leaks.

Significant *hemolysis* occurs in a minority of patients with prosthetic valves, particularly in those with mechanical aortic valves, because of the shearing effect of the mechanical valve on erythrocytes. In rare cases the hemolysis is sufficiently severe to require implantation of a different prosthetic valve.

PRIMARY MYOCARDIAL DISEASES

It should be clear from the previous sections that myocardial dysfunction occurs commonly in a number of different conditions, such as coronary artery disease, chronic hypertension, and valvular heart disease. Far less frequent are diseases that are intrinsic to myocardial fibers. Such primary myocardial diseases are a diverse group that includes inflammatory disorders (*myocarditis*), immunologic diseases (e.g., rheumatic fever), systemic metabolic disorders (e.g., hemochromatosis), muscular dystrophies (e.g., Duchenne muscular dystrophy), and an additional category of idiopathic diseases termed *cardiomyopathies*. Only myocarditis and cardiomyopathies occur with sufficient frequency to warrant further consideration here.

Myocarditis

Under this category are grouped inflammatory processes of the myocardium that result in injury to the cardiac myocytes. However, the presence of inflammation alone is not diagnostic of myocarditis, because inflammatory infiltrates may also be seen as a secondary phenomenon in conditions such as ischemic injury. In myocarditis, by contrast, the inflammatory process plays a primary role in the development of myocardial injury. Some of the causes of myocarditis are listed in Table 11–5.

Table 11–5. MAJOR CAUSES OF MYOCARDITIS

Infections
Viruses (e.g., coxsackievirus, echovirus, influenzavirus, human immunodeficiency virus, cytomegalovirus)
Chlamydia (e.g., *C. psittaci*)
Rickettsia (e.g., *R. typhi* [typhus fever])
Bacteria (e.g., *Corynebacterium* [diphtheria], *Neisseria* [meningococcus], *Borrelia* [Lyme disease])
Fungi (e.g., *Candida*)
Protozoa (e.g., Trypanosoma [Chagas disease], toxoplasmosis)
Helminths (e.g., trichinosis)
Immune-Mediated Reactions
Postviral
Poststreptococcal (rheumatic fever)
Systemic lupus erythematosus
Drug hypersensitivity (e.g., methyldopa, sulfonamides)
Transplant rejection
Unknown
Sarcoidosis
Giant cell myocarditis

Infections are a particularly important cause of myocarditis. In the United States, *viruses* are the most common cause of myocarditis. Coxsackieviruses A and B and other enteroviruses probably account for most of these cases. Studies suggest that adenoviruses may also be common pathogens in myocarditis. Other less common etiologic agents include cytomegalovirus, human immunodeficiency virus, and a host of other agents listed in Table 11–5. Although it is often difficult to isolate the offending virus from the tissues after the onset of clinical symptoms, serologic studies and, more recently, the identification of viral DNA or RNA sequences in the myocardium may help to identify the responsible virus. Whether the viruses are the direct cause of the myocardial injury or they initiate an immune response that cross-reacts with myocardial cells is unclear in most cases. As with hepatitis viruses (Chapter 16), T cells may damage virus-infected myofibers by reacting against viral antigens expressed on the cell membrane. Recent evidence indicates that enteroviral infection may cause cytoskeletal abnormalities within cardiac myocytes. *Parasites* are an important cause of myocarditis. In particular, Chagas disease, caused by infection with *Trypanosoma cruzi*, is the most common cause of myocarditis in South America. Other parasitic diseases associated with myocarditis include toxoplasmosis and trichinosis. Bacterial infections, including Lyme disease and diphtheria, are additional infectious causes of myocarditis. In the case of diphtheritic myocarditis, toxins released by *Corynebacterium diphtheriae* appear to be responsible for the myocardial injury. To this list should be added certain drugs, such as doxorubicin (antitumor agent) and other anthracyclines, especially when given with the anti-HER2/neu antibody (Herceptin) in patients with breast cancer.

In addition to its role in some cases of infectious myocarditis, *immune-mediated injury* appears to play a role in the pathogenesis of other forms of myocarditis. Examples of immunologically mediated, noninfectious myocarditis include cardiac allograft rejection, drug hypersensitivity reactions, and cases of myocarditis associated with systemic lupus erythematosus, inflammatory myopathies, and other autoimmune diseases (Chapter 5). Myocardial inflammation may also occur in sarcoidosis. In many cases, the cause of the myocarditis remains elusive.

Figure 11–19 ■

Histologic section of heart from a patient who died of myocarditis, demonstrating a multifocal, predominantly lymphocytic inflammatory infiltrate around blood vessels and between cardiac myocytes.

MORPHOLOGY

In patients who die early after the onset of myocarditis, the heart may be of normal size, but more commonly it is dilated. The myocardium is flabby and pale and often contains small areas of hemorrhage, imparting a mottled appearance to the cut surface. In cases of myocarditis caused by bacteria, frank abscesses may be visible. The histologic appearance varies considerably, depending on the cause of the myocarditis. In acute **viral myocarditis**, the myocardium is edematous and contains an **inflammatory infiltrate dominated by lymphocytes and other mononuclear cells**

(Fig. 11–19). Some degree of **myocyte degeneration and/or necrosis** is almost always present. Viral inclusions may be seen in some cases (e.g., cytomegaloviral myocarditis) but are not a feature of many of the more common forms of viral myocarditis. In more chronic cases, there is marked ventricular dilation. Histologically, inflammation is less conspicuous, while myocardial fibrosis becomes more prominent as cardiac myocytes are lost. At this late stage, myocarditis may be indistinguishable from idiopathic dilated cardiomyopathy, to be described later. In cases of myocarditis caused by **parasites,** the organism is usually demonstrable histologically, as in the case of Chagas disease, in which trypanosomes directly infect cardiac muscle fibers. In patients with **bacterial myocarditis,** the myocardium contains a neutrophilic infiltrate, sometimes complicated by abscess formation. **Cardiac transplant rejection** is characterized by the presence of interstitial lymphocytes and myocyte degeneration, which in some cases may be difficult to distinguish from infectious myocarditis. Finally, there is a morphologically distinctive myocarditis of unknown cause called **giant cell myocarditis.** As the name indicates, it is characterized by an inflammatory infiltrate in which multinucleated giant cells are prominent. In addition, one may encounter lymphocytes, macrophages, eosinophils, and scattered foci of necrosis.

Clinical Features. The clinical manifestations of myocarditis range from an asymptomatic state to severe congestive heart failure. Arrhythmias are common and may occur in the absence of heart failure; lethal ventricular arrhythmias account for most sudden cardiac deaths occurring in the setting of myocarditis. In most cases, myocarditis appears to be self-limited, although some patients develop chronic congestive heart failure months to years after the initial insult. If seen for the first time at such a late stage, they may be considered to have dilated cardiomyopathy.

Cardiomyopathies

The term *cardiomyopathy* (literally, heart muscle disease) could be applied to almost any heart disease, but by convention it is used to describe *heart disease resulting from a primary abnormality in the myocardium.* This definition is somewhat arbitrary and often frustrating as one attempts to wade through various classification schemes, because some authors exclude any myocardial disorder of known etiology, while others take a more ecumenical view and include any heart disease manifested by primary myocardial dysfunction. Excluded from this definition in almost all classifications, however, are cases of heart failure resulting from hypertension, valvular disease, congenital heart disease, obvious myocarditis, systemic metabolic disturbances, nutritional disorders (e.g., wet beriberi), and hypersensitivity diseases (e.g., acute rheumatic fever). Although chronic myocardial dysfunction caused by ischemia should also probably be excluded from the cardiomyopathy rubric, the term *ischemic cardiomyopathy,* used to describe chronic congestive heart failure caused by coronary artery disease, has gained some popularity among clinicians. We will leave these controversial areas behind and resort to the traditional subdivision of cardiomyopathies into three major clinicopathologic groups: *dilated, hypertrophic,* and *restrictive* cardiomyopathy. While the causes of many cases of cardiomyopathy remain elusive, work conducted over the past decade has provided exciting new insights into the molecular basis of many forms of cardiomyopathy. These developments will be discussed briefly in the paragraphs that follow.

DILATED CARDIOMYOPATHY

This diagnosis is applied to a form of cardiomyopathy characterized by *progressive cardiac hypertrophy, dilation,* and *contractile (systolic) dysfunction.* It is sometimes called congestive cardiomyopathy. This clinicopathologic picture can result from a large number of different myocardial insults. *Viral nucleic acids* from coxsackievirus B and other enteroviruses have been detected in the myocardium of some patients, suggesting that, in at least some cases, dilated cardiomyopathy may represent a late stage of myocarditis. It remains unclear, however, whether such viruses actually cause chronic myocardial injury or simply represent incidental "innocent bystanders." *Alcohol abuse* is also strongly associated with the development of dilated cardiomyopathy, raising the possibility that ethanol toxicity (Chapter 8) or a secondary nutritional disturbance may be the cause of the myocardial injury. In yet other cases, a more clearly defined *toxic insult* is the cause of the myocardial failure. Particularly important in this last group is myocardial injury caused by cobalt and certain chemotherapeutic agents, including doxorubicin and other anthracyclines. A special form of dilated cardiomyopathy, termed *peripartum cardiomyopathy,* occurs late in pregnancy

or several weeks to months post partum. The cause of peripartum cardiomyopathy is poorly understood.

In recent years, it has become clear that *inherited genetic abnormalities* are responsible for a significant percentage (20% to 30%) of cases of dilated cardiomyopathy, including many cases previously consigned to the "idiopathic" category. *Mutations in genes coding for cytoskeletal proteins, in particular, appear to be responsible for many cases of hereditary dilated cardiomyopathy.* A link between inherited cytoskeletal protein abnormalities and cardiomyopathy was first suggested by the association between certain muscular dystrophies, now known to be caused by abnormal cytoskeletal protein expression, and cardiomyopathy. The best known of these are mutations in the *dystrophin gene* on the X chromosome that are responsible for Becker and Duchenne muscular dystrophy (discussed in Chapter 21). Abnormalities in genes encoding other cytoskeletal proteins, including desmin, dystrophin-associated proteins termed sarcoglycans, and merosin, have also been associated with both muscular dystrophy and cardiomyopathy. Abnormalities in non-cytoskeletal proteins, including certain mitochondrial enzymes, appear to be responsible for still other cases of dilated cardiomyopathy. Curiously, mutations in certain sarcomere protein genes (e.g., β-myosin and cardiac troponin T) can also cause dilated cardiomyopathies. As will be noted later, distinct mutations in these genes also cause hypertrophic cardiomyopathy. Thus, many puzzles regarding cardiomyopathies remain to be solved.

Dilated cardiomyopathy may occur at any age but is most common between the ages of 20 and 60 years. Most cases apparently arise sporadically, although familial cases, as noted earlier, are being recognized with increasing frequency. Dilated cardiomyopathy occurs more frequently in men than in women, possibly reflecting the association between chronic alcohol abuse and cardiomyopathy.

> ### MORPHOLOGY
>
> The heart is enlarged and flabby, with weights often exceeding 900 g. The enlargement is caused by a **combination of dilation and hypertrophy of all chambers** (Fig. 11-20). The substantial dilation and poor contractile function cause stasis of blood in the cardiac chambers and predispose to the development of fragile mural thrombi and subsequent emboli. The microscopic features are nonspecific and include myocyte hypertrophy, interstitial fibrosis, wavy fiber change, and (in some cases) a scanty mononuclear inflammatory infiltrate.

Clinical Features. Dilated cardiomyopathy is the most common form of cardiomyopathy, accounting for about 90% of cases. *The fundamental defect in dilated cardiomyopathy is ineffective contraction.* Patients may have an ejection fraction of less than 25% (normal, 50% to 65%). Hence, the clinical picture is that of progressive congestive heart failure, which becomes refractory to therapy. An exception to this dismal prognosis occurs in peripartum cardiomyopathy,

Figure 11-20 ■

Dilated cardiomyopathy with generalized cardiac hypertrophy and dilation. Such changes are usually idiopathic, as in this patient, or the result of a more specific myocardial insult.

in which up to half of the patients recover spontaneously. However, the illness may recur with subsequent pregnancies. Idiopathic cases are usually fatal. Death results from severe and intractable heart failure, embolic complications, or ventricular arrhythmias. Cardiac transplantation is lifesaving in this and other cardiomyopathies. Of note, dilated cardiomyopathy is the most common diagnosis in patients referred for cardiac transplantation.

HYPERTROPHIC CARDIOMYOPATHY

Hypertrophic cardiomyopathy, also referred to as *asymmetric septal hypertrophy and idiopathic hypertrophic subaortic stenosis*, is a cardiac disorder characterized by *myocardial hypertrophy, abnormal diastolic filling*, and (in many cases) *intermittent ventricular outflow obstruction*. In contrast to the feebly contracting heart in patients with dilated cardiomyopathy, hypertrophic cardiomyopathy is characterized by powerful, hyperkinetic contractions that rapidly expel blood from the ventricular cavities. Because the thick-walled ventricle is abnormally stiff, diastolic filling is impaired. In about 50% of cases, the disorder is inherited as an autosomal dominant trait with variable penetrance and expression. In contrast to the situation with dilated cardiomyopathy (discussed earlier), in which abnormalities in cytoskeletal proteins account for a significant number of cases, *abnormalities in genes encoding sarcomeric contractile proteins appear to play a critical role in the development of hypertrophic cardiomyopathies*. Of the nine known disease genes, the best characterized are mutations involving the heavy chain of β-myosin, which account, in aggregate, for about one third of the cases of inherited hypertrophic cardiomyopathy. In addition, mutations in α-

tropomyosin, troponins I and T, and myosin light chains have also been identified in cases of familial hypertrophic cardiomyopathy. In addition to this locus heterogeneity, there is also considerable allelic heterogeneity, since numerous mutations have been found in all these genes. It is important to take note of this because the prognosis varies with the genetic defect, and, hence, molecular diagnosis of hypertrophic cardiomyopathy is likely to be useful in stratifying individuals with differing degrees of risk for mortality, especially sudden cardiac death.

MORPHOLOGY

The essential feature of hypertrophic cardiomyopathy is **myocardial hypertrophy, which is most pronounced in the left ventricle and interventricular septum.** The degree of hypertrophy varies from patient to patient, even in familial cases, but weights in excess of 800 g are common. **In most cases the interventricular septum is substantially thicker than the free (lateral) wall of the left ventricle,** a feature best demonstrated in coronal sections through the chamber (Fig. 11-21A). In other cases, the hypertrophy may be concentric or preferentially involve the more apical portions of the left ventricle. Although disproportionate hypertrophy can involve the entire septum, septal hypertrophy is usually most conspicuous in the subaortic region. Asymmetric septal hypertrophy is often associated with a significant degree of ventricular outflow obstruction during systole, a feature emphasized in the older designation idiopathic **hypertrophic subaortic stenosis.** In this group of patients, the systolic obstruction is caused by abnormal anterior motion of the mitral valve leaflet during systole. Because of this abnormal systolic anterior motion, there is recurrent, forceful contact between the septum and the anterior leaflet of the mitral valve. This in turn leads to **thickening of the anterior mitral leaflet and adjacent septal endocardium.** Ventricular dilation is uncommon, but the left atrium may be dilated because of impaired diastolic filling of the thickened, rigid left ventricle.

Microscopically, hypertrophic cardiomyopathy is characterized by a **haphazard arrangement of hypertrophied, abnormally branching myocytes** surrounded by increased connective tissue (Fig. 11-21B). This change is most pronounced in sections taken from the interventricular septum. In later stages of the disease, considerable myocardial fibrosis may develop.

Clinical Features. The basic physiologic abnormality in hypertrophic cardiomyopathy is an *inability to fill a hypertrophic left ventricle during diastole*. Ejection is forceful but ineffective because the amount of blood in the left ventricle is greatly reduced. In addition, there may be dynamic obstruction to the left ventricular outflow caused by abnormal movement of the anterior mitral leaflet, as explained earlier.

Figure 11-21

Hypertrophic cardiomyopathy. *A,* The ventricular septum is disproportionately thickened and bulges into the lumen of the left ventricle. Contact between the hypertrophic septum and the anterior leaflet of the mitral valve may cause significant left ventricular outflow obstruction. *B,* Microscopic picture shows hypertrophy and extreme disarray of fibers. (Courtesy of Sid Murphree, MD, Department of Pathology, University of Texas Southwestern Medical School, Dallas.)

The limitation of cardiac output and a secondary increase in pulmonary venous pressure cause exertional dyspnea. Auscultation discloses a harsh systolic ejection murmur, caused by anterior motion of the mitral leaflets and by ventricular outflow obstruction. Myocardial ischemia is common, even in the absence of concomitant coronary artery disease, and thus anginal pain is frequent. Hypertrophic cardiomyopathy is associated with an increased incidence of ventricular arrhythmias and sudden death and is one of the most common causes of sudden unexplained death in young athletes. The risk of infective endocarditis is also increased. In the later stages of the disease, progressive myocardial fibrosis may cause congestive heart failure.

RESTRICTIVE CARDIOMYOPATHY

Restrictive cardiomyopathy is a disorder characterized by a *primary decrease in ventricular compliance, resulting in impaired ventricular filling during diastole.* It is considerably less common than either dilated or hypertrophic cardiomyopathy. Restrictive cardiomyopathy can be caused by any process that reduces myocardial compliance. Worldwide, the most common cause of this form of cardiomyopathy is a disease called *endomyocardial fibrosis,* a disorder of unknown etiology that accounts for up to 10% of cases of childhood heart disease in tropical areas of the world. *Eosinophilic endomyocardial fibrosis,* or Löffler syndrome, is a rare cause of restrictive cardiomyopathy that may be related to the tropical form of the disease. In the case of Löffler syndrome, the development of endomyocardial fibrosis has been attributed to proteins released from degranulating eosinophils; whether this process also contributes to the endomyocardial fibrosis in cases seen in the tropics is less clear. Genetic factors are less clearly defined in cases of restrictive cardiomyopathy than in the dilated or hypertrophic cardiomyopathies but likely also account for some cases. In addition to its association with dilated cardiomyopathy, for example, desmin mutations appear to account for some cases of restrictive

cardiomyopathy. Additional important causes of restrictive cardiomyopathy are *cardiac amyloidosis, endocardial fibroelastosis, hemochromatosis,* and *radiation injury* to the heart.

MORPHOLOGY

The appearance of the heart varies with the cause of the restrictive cardiomyopathy. The morphology of cardiac amyloidosis and hemochromatosis is described in detail in Chapters 5 and 16 and will not be repeated here. In patients with **tropical endomyocardial fibrosis** and **Löffler syndrome,** the atria are typically dilated. The ventricles may be of normal size, although some degree of dilation may occur, particularly in the later stages of the disease. **The endocardium is thickened and opaque,** especially in the left ventricle. The cardiac valves are thickened in some cases, and mural or valvular thrombi may be present. Histologic sections reveal dense endocardial fibrosis, which extends into the underlying myocardium. In cases of endomyocardial fibrosis associated with hypereosinophilia, the endocardium and myocardium may be infiltrated by eosinophils, particularly in the early stages of the disease. **Endocardial fibroelastosis** is a relatively uncommon disorder that occurs most frequently in children younger than 2 years of age. It is characterized by the presence of abundant fibroelastic tissue in the endocardium, which imparts a porcelain-like appearance to the endocardial surface. The changes may be localized, or they may involve the entire ventricular cavity. Associated congenital cardiac valvular abnormalities are common. Endocardial fibroelastosis is probably not a single disease entity. An abnormal reaction to ventricular dilation during fetal life has been suggested as a cause in some cases.

Clinical Features. The physiologic problem in restrictive cardiomyopathy is *a stiff and inelastic ventricle that can be filled only with great effort.* In this aspect it resembles hypertrophic cardiomyopathy. However, unlike the latter, the systole is not forceful. As with other cardiomyopathies, the symptoms in patients with restrictive cardiomyopathy include fatigue, exertional dyspnea, and chest pain. In patients with Löffler syndrome, systemic emboli may arise from mural or valvular thrombi. The course is often complicated by arrhythmias and atrioventricular blocks, particularly when the myocardial fibrosis or infiltrative process encroaches on the conduction system. Myocardial contractility, although often normal early in the course of the disease, usually declines, causing congestive heart failure in later stages. The hemodynamic derangements associated with restrictive cardiomyopathy are quite similar to those seen in patients with constrictive pericardial disease (discussed later). Distinction between these two processes is of vital importance because primary pericardial disease may be amenable to surgical treatment.

CONGENITAL HEART DISEASE

Congenital abnormalities of the heart occur in about 8 per 1000 live births, making them one of the most common types of congenital malformations. With the declining incidence of acute rheumatic fever, congenital heart disease is now the most common cause of heart disease in children in the Western world. Congenital heart diseases encompass a broad spectrum of malformations, ranging from mild lesions that produce only minimal symptoms until adult life, to severe anomalies that cause death in the perinatal period. The cause of most cases of congenital heart disease is unknown. The etiology of congenital malformations in general was discussed in Chapter 7. We will therefore confine our remarks to factors of particular relevance to congenital cardiac malformations.

Genetic factors play an obvious role in some cases, as evidenced by the occurrence of familial forms of congenital heart disease and by well-defined associations between certain chromosomal abnormalities (e.g., trisomies 13, 15, 18, and 21 and Turner syndrome) and congenital cardiac malformations. *Environmental factors,* such as congenital rubella infection, are responsible for some additional cases. Overall, however, obvious genetic or environmental influences are identifiable in only about 10% of cases of congenital heart disease. In the remaining 90%, the cause is not clearly defined. Multifactorial genetic and environmental factors probably account for the many cases of congenital heart disease currently classified as idiopathic.

The frequency at birth of major forms of congenital heart disease is listed in Table 11–6. For purposes of discussion, congenital heart diseases can be subdivided into three major groups:

■ Malformations causing a *left-to-right shunt*
■ Malformations causing a *right-to-left shunt* (cyanotic congenital heart diseases)
■ Malformations causing *obstruction*

Table 11–6. RELATIVE FREQUENCIES OF CARDIAC MALFORMATIONS AT BIRTH

Malformation	Congenital Heart Disease (%)
Ventricular septal defect	30.5
Patent ductus arteriosus	9.7
Pulmonary stenosis	6.9
Tetralogy of Fallot	5.8
Aortic stenosis	6.1
Coarctation of the aorta	6.8
Atrial septal defect	9.8
Transposition of the great arteries	4.2
Truncus arteriosus	2.2
Tricuspid atresia	1.3
All others	16.5

Modified from Braunwald E: Heart Disease: A Textbook of Cardiovascular Medicine, 6th ed. Philadelphia, WB Saunders, 2001, p 1506.

Within each of these subdivisions, we will consider the pathogenesis, morphology, and clinical manifestations of some of the more common congenital cardiac malformations. Common to all is the risk of infective endocarditis.

Left-to-Right Shunts

Left-to-right shunts, or abnormal communications permitting blood to flow from the left to the right cardiac chambers, represent the most common type of congenital cardiac malformation. They include *atrial septal defects (ASDs), ventricular septal defects (VSDs),* and *patent (persistent) ductus arteriosus (PDA).* These malformations may be asymptomatic at birth, or they may cause fulminant congestive heart failure. *Cyanosis is not an early feature* of this group of malformations, but it may occur late, after the left-to-right shunt has produced sufficient pulmonary hypertension to cause a reversal of blood flow through the shunt. The term *tardive (late) cyanosis* is often used to describe this phenomenon.

ATRIAL SEPTAL DEFECTS

The atrial septum develops between the fourth and sixth weeks of embryonic life (Fig. 11–22). The initial phase is marked by the growth of a primary septum (*septum primum*) from the dorsal wall of the common atrial chamber toward the developing *endocardial cushions* as the latter begin to separate the atrial and ventricular cavities. A gap, termed the *ostium primum,* initially separates the developing septum primum from the endocardial cushions. Continued growth and fusion of the septum with endocardial cushions ultimately obliterates the ostium primum; however, at this time a second opening, *ostium secundum,* appears in the central area of the primary septum. This allows continued flow of oxygenated blood from the right atrium to the left, essential for fetal life. As the ostium secundum enlarges, a secondary septum (*septum secundum*) makes its appearance just to the right of the septum primum. The

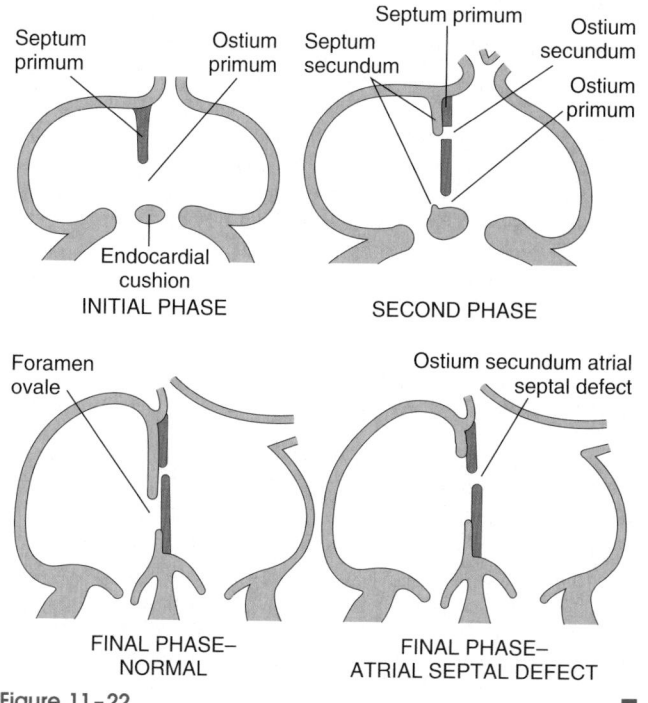

Septum primum | Ostium primum | Septum secundum | Septum primum | Ostium secundum | Ostium primum

Endocardial cushion
INITIAL PHASE

SECOND PHASE

Foramen ovale

Ostium secundum atrial septal defect

FINAL PHASE– NORMAL

FINAL PHASE– ATRIAL SEPTAL DEFECT

Figure 11–22 ■

Embryogenesis of an atrial septal defect, ostium secundum type. The right atrium is to the left of the septum primum.

septum secundum proliferates to form a crescent-shaped structure surrounding a space termed the *foramen ovale*. The foramen ovale is guarded on its left side by a flap of tissue derived from the primary septum, which acts as a one-way valve, allowing blood to keep on flowing from right to left during intrauterine life. At the time of birth, as pulmonary vascular resistance falls and systemic arterial pressure increases, pressure in the left atrium rises above that in the right atrium, resulting in functional closure of the foramen ovale. In most individuals the foramen ovale is permanently sealed by fusion of the primary and secondary septa, although a minor degree of patency persists in about 25% of the general population.

Abnormalities in this sequence of events result in the development of various ASDs, which allow free communication between the left and right atria. Three types of ASD are recognized. The most common (75% of cases) is the *ostium secundum ASD*, which arises if the septum secundum does not enlarge sufficiently to cover the ostium secundum. *Ostium primum ASDs* are less common (15% of cases), and they occur if the septum primum and endocardial cushions fail to fuse. This defect is often associated with abnormalities in other structures derived from the endocardial cushions, such as the mitral and tricuspid valves. The pathogenesis of the least common (10% of cases), *sinus venosus ASD*, is unclear.

MORPHOLOGY

The ostium secundum ASD appears as a smooth-walled defect in the vicinity of the foramen ovale (Fig. 11–23). This may occur as an isolated lesion, or it may be associated with other cardiac

abnormalities. Hemodynamically significant lesions are accompanied by right atrial and ventricular dilation, right ventricular hypertrophy, and dilation of the pulmonary artery, reflecting the effects of a chronically increased volume load on the right side of the heart and (in some cases) pulmonary hypertension. **Ostium primum ASDs** occur in the lowermost part of the atrial septum and extend to the mitral and tricuspid valves (see Fig. 11–23). An abnormality of the atrioventricular valves is usually present, typically in the form of a cleft in the anterior leaflet of the mitral valve or septal leaflet of the tricuspid valve, reflecting the close relationship between development of the septum primum and endocardial cushions. In more severe cases the ostium primum defect is accompanied by a VSD and severe mitral and tricuspid valve deformities, with a resultant **common atrioventricular canal. Sinus venosus ASDs** are located high in the atrial septum and are often accompanied by anomalous drainage of the pulmonary veins into the right atrium or superior vena cava.

Clinical Features. ASDs are the most common congenital cardiac malformations first diagnosed in adults because many VSDs (more common at birth) close spontaneously. ASDs cause left-to-right shunts after birth, owing to the lower pressures in the pulmonary circulation and right side of the heart. Ostium secundum defects are the most common, and in general these defects are well tolerated, especially if they are less than 1 cm in diameter, but even larger lesions do not produce any symptoms in childhood because the flow of blood is from left to right. With time, pulmonary vascular resistance increases,

Figure 11–23 ■

Atrial septal defect. This unusual case shows both the ostium secundum and primum defects and allows comparison of the two. The upper secundum type of atrial septal defect forms an opening in the atrial septal wall in the region of the foramen ovale. The less common ostium primum defect, in contrast, is lower in the atrial septum. (Courtesy of Arthur Weinberg, MD, Department of Pathology, University of Texas Southwestern Medical School, Dallas.)

culminating in the development of pulmonary hypertension in some patients. This, in turn, causes reversal of the left-to-right shunt, manifested by the development of cyanosis and congestive heart failure. Ostium primum defects may be initially asymptomatic, but they are more likely to be associated with evidence of congestive heart failure, in part because of the high frequency of associated mitral insufficiency.

VENTRICULAR SEPTAL DEFECTS

The ventricular septum develops between the fourth and eighth weeks of gestation. It is formed by the fusion of an *intraventricular muscular ridge* that grows upward from the apex of the heart to a thinner membranous partition that grows downward from the endocardial cushions. The basal (membranous) region is the last part of the septum to develop and is the site where approximately 70% of septal defects are located. *VSDs are the most common congenital heart defects at birth*, but because many small VSDs close spontaneously in childhood, the overall incidence of VSDs in adults is lower than that of atrial defects. Like ASDs, they may occur in isolation (around 30% of cases), but they are usually encountered in association with other cardiac malformations.

MORPHOLOGY

The size and location of VSDs are variable, ranging from minute defects in the muscular or membranous portions of the septum to large defects involving virtually the entire septum (Fig. 11-24). In defects associated with a significant left-to-right shunt, the right ventricle is hypertrophied and often dilated. The diameter of the pulmonary artery is increased, owing to the increased volume ejected by the right ventricle. Vascular changes typical of pulmonary hypertension are common (Chapter 13).

Figure 11-24 ■

Ventricular septal defect, membranous type. Ventricular septal defects may involve any part of the interventricular septum. Most are high in the membranous portion of the septum, as in this case. (Courtesy of Arthur Weinberg, MD, Department of Pathology, University of Texas Southwestern Medical School, Dallas.)

Clinical Features. Small VSDs may be asymptomatic, and those in the muscular portion of the septum may close spontaneously during infancy or childhood. Larger defects, however, cause a severe left-to-right shunt, often complicated by pulmonary hypertension and congestive heart failure. Progressive pulmonary hypertension, with resultant reversal of the shunt and cyanosis, occurs earlier and more frequently in patients with VSDs than in those with ASDs; hence, early surgical correction is indicated in the case of larger lesions. A particular risk for those with small or medium-sized defects that produce jet lesions in the right ventricle is superimposed infective endocarditis.

PATENT DUCTUS ARTERIOSUS

The ductus arteriosus is an arterial channel that courses between the pulmonary artery and aorta. During intrauterine life, the ductus arteriosus permits blood to flow freely from the pulmonary artery to the aorta, thereby bypassing the unoxygenated lungs. Shortly after birth, the ductus begins to constrict in response to increased levels of arterial oxygen, decreasing pulmonary vascular resistance, and declining levels of prostaglandin E_2. In healthy term infants, functional closure is usually complete within 1 to 2 days after birth. Complete, irreversible closure occurs within the first few months of extrauterine life to form the *ligamentum arteriosum*. Ductal closure may be significantly delayed in infants with hypoxia caused by respiratory distress or heart disease. Isolated PDA accounts for about 10% of cases of congenital heart disease. This lesion may also occur in combination with other anomalies, particularly VSDs.

MORPHOLOGY

The usual PDA arises from the left pulmonary artery and joins the aorta just distal to the origin of the left subclavian artery. Its lumen is generally uniform and is lined by smooth endothelium. Oxygenated blood flows out from the left ventricle, and some of it is shunted back to the lungs through the patent ductus, eventually returning to the left atrium. Because of volume overload, the left atrium and ventricle are dilated and may be hypertrophied. The proximal pulmonary arteries are also dilated. With the development of pulmonary hypertension, atherosclerosis of the main pulmonary arteries and proliferative changes in more distal pulmonary vessels are seen. These are accompanied by right ventricular hypertrophy and dilation and by right atrial dilation.

Clinical Features. PDA causes a high-pressure left-to right shunt, audible as a harsh waxing and waning murmur sometimes referred to as a "machinery" murmur. A small PDA causes no symptoms; with larger defects, symptoms develop in childhood or adulthood. As with other left-to-right shunts, the development of pulmonary hypertension is announced by the appearance of cyanosis and congestive heart failure. The high-pressure shunt also predisposes affected individuals to the development of infective endocarditis. Early surgical correction of large PDAs may be lifesaving.

Right-to-Left Shunts

Cardiac malformations associated with right-to-left shunts are distinguished by *cyanosis at or near the time of birth.* This occurs because poorly oxygenated blood from the right side of the heart is introduced directly into the arterial circulation. Two of the most important conditions associated with cyanotic congenital heart disease are *tetralogy of Fallot* and *transposition of the great vessels.*

TETRALOGY OF FALLOT

Accounting for about 6% of all congenital cardiac malformations, tetralogy of Fallot is *the most common cause of cyanotic congenital heart disease.* The four components of the tetralogy are (1) a VSD, (2) a "dextraposed" aortic root that overrides the VSD, (3) right ventricular outflow obstruction, and (4) right ventricular hypertrophy (Fig. 11–25). Abnormal division of the truncus arteriosus into a pulmonary trunk and aortic root has been suggested as the primary event in the development of this malformation, although many details of its pathogenesis remain unsettled.

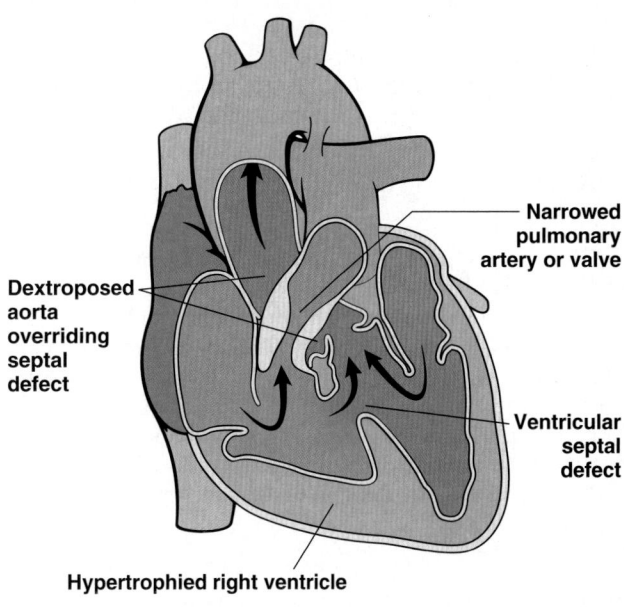

Dextraposed aorta overriding septal defect

Narrowed pulmonary artery or valve

Ventricular septal defect

Hypertrophied right ventricle

Figure 11–25   ■

Tetralogy of Fallot demonstrating ventricular septal defect, pulmonic stenosis, over-riding aorta, and secondary right ventricular hypertrophy. The flow of blood is indicated by arrows.

MORPHOLOGY

The heart is enlarged externally and often boot shaped, owing to right ventricular hypertrophy. The proximal aorta is often larger than normal, and the pulmonary trunk is reduced in diameter. The cardiac chambers on the left side of the heart are of normal size, while the thickness of the right ventricular wall may equal or even exceed that of the left. The VSD lies in the vicinity of the membranous portion of the interventricular septum and may efface all or part of the membranous septum. The aortic valve lies immediately over the VSD. The pulmonary outflow tract is narrowed, and, in a few cases, the pulmonic valve itself may be stenotic. Additional abnormalities are present in a significant minority of cases, including PDA or ASD. These are protective because they allow some blood flow to the lungs.

Clinical Features. The hemodynamic consequences of tetralogy of Fallot are a right-to-left shunt, decreased blood flow to the lungs, and increased blood flow through the aorta. *The extent of shunting is determined by the degree of right ventricular outflow obstruction.* If the pulmonic obstruction is mild, the condition resembles an isolated VSD, because the higher pressure on the left side causes a left-to-right shunt with no cyanosis. More commonly, marked stenosis causes significant cyanosis early in life. Thus, most patients with tetralogy of Fallot are cyanotic from birth or soon thereafter. As patients with tetralogy of Fallot grow, the pulmonic orifice does not

enlarge, despite an overall increase in the size of the heart. Therefore, typically, the degree of stenosis becomes worse with time and is associated with increasing cyanosis. The lungs are protected from excessive hemodynamic load by the pulmonic stenosis, and pulmonary hypertension does not develop. These patients develop complications of chronic cyanosis, such as erythrocytosis with attendant hyperviscosity, and digital clubbing. Because of the right-to-left shunt, patients with tetralogy of Fallot are also at increased risk for infective endocarditis, systemic emboli, and brain abscesses. Surgical correction of this defect is now possible in almost all instances.

TRANSPOSITION OF THE GREAT ARTERIES

Transposition of the great arteries is the second leading cause of cyanotic congenital heart disease, after tetralogy of Fallot. Because of abnormal truncal septation, *the aorta arises from the right ventricle and the pulmonary artery arises from the left ventricle.* In its complete form, the pulmonary and systemic circulations are entirely separate, and there is no shunting of blood. However, such a condition is incompatible with extrauterine life; therefore, those who survive after birth must have some type of shunt, such as an ASD, VSD, or PDA, that allows oxygenated blood to reach the aorta.

MORPHOLOGY

Transposition of the great arteries has many variants, and a detailed review of the morphology of this condition is beyond the scope of this chapter. The fundamental lesion, as noted, is abnormal origin of the pulmonary trunk and aortic root. Some degree of right ventricular hypertrophy is usually present because of the increased (systemic) pressure load placed on that chamber. Varying combinations of ASD, VSD, and PDA are seen in patients surviving beyond the neonatal period.

Clinical Features. The predominant manifestation of transposition of the great arteries is cyanosis. The prognosis depends on the degree of intracardiac or extracardiac shunting and the degree of arterial oxygen saturation. Infusions of prostaglandin E_2 may be used to restore patency of the ductus arteriosus. Maneuvers such as atrial balloon septostomy are sometimes used to create shunts that enhance arterial oxygen saturation and allow the patient to survive until definitive surgical correction can be undertaken.

Congenital Obstructive Lesions

A number of malformations cause obstruction of blood flow. In some cases, these are isolated lesions, as in congenital valvular aortic stenosis. In other instances, they are one component of a more complex malformation, as in pulmonic stenosis associated with tetralogy of Fallot. Here we will discuss coarctation of the aorta, a fairly common obstructive anomaly.

COARCTATION OF THE AORTA

Coarctation of the aorta, defined as an abnormal narrowing of the aortic lumen, is one of the most important forms of obstructive congenital heart disease. *In about 50% of cases, this lesion occurs as an isolated cardiac anomaly.* In the remaining cases, coarctation is associated with other malformations, such as PDA, VSD, and ASD. The malformation has also been associated with saccular aneurysms of the central nervous system, and it occurs with increased frequency in patients with Turner syndrome. Coarctation is somewhat more common in males than in females, particularly when it occurs as an isolated lesion. Most cases of coarctation of the aorta can be placed into one of two major categories: preductal and postductal. The postductal type is the more common.

MORPHOLOGY

Preductal coarctation, formerly referred to as infantile coarctation, is characterized by **narrowing of the so-called aortic isthmus,** the segment of aorta that lies between the left subclavian artery and the point of entry of the ductus arteriosus. In some cases the preductal narrowing takes the form of a fairly distinct ridge; in other cases the entire aortic arch is hypoplastic. The ductus arteriosus is usually patent and is the main source of blood delivered to the distal aorta. Because the right side of the heart is called on to perfuse the body distal to the

site of the coarctation, the right cardiac chambers are often hypertrophic and dilated; the pulmonary trunk is also dilated to accommodate the increased blood flow.

In the more common **postductal,** or **adult-type, coarctation,** the aorta is constricted by a sharply defined ridge of tissue at, or just distal to, the obliterated ductus arteriosus (the ligamentum arteriosum) (Fig. 11–26). The constricted segment is made up of smooth muscle and elastic fibers that are continuous with the aortic media and are lined by a thickened layer of intima. The ductus arteriosus is closed. Proximal to the coarctation, the aortic arch and its branch vessels are dilated and, in older patients, often atherosclerotic. The left ventricle is hypertrophic. Collateral flow through the intercostal, phrenic, and epigastric arteries supplies most of the blood to the distal aorta, and these collateral channels are almost always dilated.

Clinical Features. Patients with *preductal coarctation* usually present in infancy, hence the older designation of *infantile* coarctation. Classic features include congestive heart failure and selective cyanosis of the lower extremities, the latter caused by perfusion of the lower part of the body by poorly oxygenated blood delivered via the ductus arteriosus. The femoral pulses are almost invariably weaker than those of the upper extremities, although narrowing of more proximal segments of the aortic root may cause diminished pulses in the upper extremities as well. These patients do not survive the neonatal period without surgical correction.

Figure 11–26 ■

Coarctation of the aorta, postductal type. The area of coarctation is visible here as a segmental narrowing of the aorta *(arrow)*. Such lesions typically present later in life than do preductal coarctations. Note the dilated ascending aorta and major branch vessels to the left of the coarctation. A large amount of blood reaches the lower extremities via dilated, tortuous collateral channels. (Courtesy of Sid Murphree, MD, Department of Pathology, University of Texas Southwestern Medical School, Dallas.)

Postductal coarctation, in contrast, is more likely to present as signs and symptoms in older children and adults. Because the blood reaching the distal aorta in these cases comes from collateral branches connected to the proximal aorta, the oxygen content is normal and selective cyanosis of the lower extremities is not seen. *Hypertension of the upper extremities is noted in most cases, owing in part to decreased perfusion of the kidneys and activation of the renin-angiotensin system.* By contrast, blood pressure is low and pulses are weak in the lower extremities. In addition, there are often signs and symptoms of arterial insufficiency in the legs, such as intermittent claudication.

PERICARDIAL DISEASES

Diseases of the pericardium include inflammatory conditions and effusions. These are most frequently noted in conjunction with local myocardial or mediastinal diseases and in patients with certain systemic conditions, such as uremia.

Pericarditis

Primary pericarditis is uncommon and usually infectious in origin. *Viruses are responsible for most cases,* although it may also be caused by other organisms, including pyogenic bacteria, mycobacteria, and fungi. An accompanying myocarditis may be present, particularly in the case of viral infections. More often the pericarditis is secondary to acute MI, cardiac surgery, or radiation to the mediastinum. *Uremia* is probably the most common systemic disorder associated with pericarditis. Less common secondary causes include rheumatic fever, systemic lupus erythematosus, and metastatic malignancies. The latter are usually associated with a bloody effusion. Pericarditis may (1) cause immediate hemodynamic complications if a significant effusion is present, (2) resolve without significant sequelae, or (3) progress to a chronic fibrosing process.

MORPHOLOGY

The appearance of **acute pericarditis** varies with its cause. In patients with uremia or acute rheumatic fever, the exudate is typically fibrinous and imparts a shaggy, irregular appearance to the pericardial surface ("bread and butter" pericarditis) (Fig. 11-27). A fibrinous exudate may also be seen in cases of viral pericarditis. In acute bacterial pericarditis the pericardial exudate is fibrinopurulent, while in tuberculosis the pericardium contains caseous material. Pericardial metastases are visible grossly as irregular nodular excrescences, often with a shaggy fibrinous exudate and a bloody effusion. In most cases, acute fibrinous or fibrinopurulent pericarditis resolves without any sequelae. However, when there is extensive suppuration or caseation, healing gives rise to chronic pericarditis.

The appearance of **chronic pericarditis** ranges from delicate adhesions to dense, fibrotic scars that obliterate the pericardial space. In extreme cases the heart is so completely encased by dense scar tissue that it cannot expand normally during diastole, a condition called **constrictive pericarditis.**

Clinical Features. The manifestations of pericarditis include atypical chest pain, which is often worse on reclining, and a high-pitched friction rub. When associated with significant exudate in the pericardial sac, acute pericarditis may cause signs and symptoms of cardiac tamponade, which include faint distant heart sounds, distended neck veins, declining cardiac output, and shock. Chronic constrictive pericarditis produces a combination of venous distention and low cardiac output, which may be difficult to distinguish from restrictive cardiomyopathy, as noted previously.

Pericardial Effusions

Processes besides inflammation may cause fluid to accumulate in the pericardial space. The nature of the fluid varies with the cause of the effusion. The major types of pericardial effusion and some of their more common causes are listed as follows:

- *Serous:* congestive heart failure, hypoalbuminemia of any cause
- *Serosanguineous:* blunt chest trauma, malignancy
- *Chylous:* mediastinal lymphatic obstruction

Pericardial effusions are often symptomatic. Surprisingly large volumes of fluid can be accommodated if the accumulation occurs slowly. Massive or rapidly developing effusions may cause cardiac tamponade.

Hemopericardium, more properly considered separately from hemorrhagic pericardial effusions, indicates the

Figure 11-27 ■

Acute fibrinous pericarditis. The normally smooth, glistening pericardial surface is covered by shaggy fibrinous exudate. In this case, the pericarditis developed because of uremia and caused a fatal cardiac tamponade.

presence of pure (undiluted) blood in the pericardial sac. Important causes include ruptured aortic aneurysms, ruptured myocardial infarcts, and penetrating traumatic injury to the heart. The escaping blood rapidly fills the pericardial space and leads to cardiac tamponade and death.

CARDIAC TUMORS

The heart is usually spared the ugliness of tumors. Those that occur are usually metastatic and will be considered first.

Metastatic Neoplasms

Metastatic neoplasms involving the heart are far more common than primary cardiac tumors. Metastases to the heart occur in up to 10% of patients with disseminated cancer. Most often, they involve the pericardium, where they may cause pericarditis and hemorrhagic pericardial effusions. The most common primary neoplasms that metastasize to the heart are carcinomas of the lung and breast, malignant melanomas, and hematopoietic malignancies (lymphomas and leukemias). Metastases may reach the heart via lymphatic, venous, or arterial channels.

Primary Neoplasms

Primary tumors of the heart are rare. The most common types encountered, in descending order of frequency, are myxomas, lipomas, papillary elastofibromas, rhabdomyomas, angiosarcomas, and rhabdomyosarcomas.

Myxomas are histologically benign neoplasms that arise most frequently in the left atrium near the fossa ovalis. They appear as sessile or pedunculated lesions, usually covered by an intact endocardium. They occur most often in adults but may arise at any age. Microscopically, they are composed of multinucleated stellate cells suspended in an edematous, mucopolysaccharide-rich stroma. Immature and mature smooth muscle cells may also be present. Although histologically benign, myxomas may cause significant problems for the patient, either because of the tendency of some lesions to fragment and embolize or because they may cause a "ball-valve" obstruction of the atrioventricular valves, with resultant syncopal episodes and even sudden death. Surgical resection of such lesions can be lifesaving.

Cardiac rhabdomyomas are the most common primary cardiac tumors of infancy and childhood, often discovered because of obstruction of a valvular orifice. They may occur as apparently isolated lesions, but they are best known for their association with *tuberous sclerosis*, one of the so-called neurocutaneous syndromes. It is likely that these proliferations represent malformations or hamartomas rather than true neoplasms. Grossly, cardiac rhabdomyomas present as myocardial masses that often project into the ventricular lumen. They may be solitary or multifocal. Microscopically, they are composed of eosinophilic, polygonal cells, many of which contain large, glycogen-rich cytoplasmic granules. Myofibrils can be demonstrated in such cells under the electron microscope.

Lipomas may occur anywhere in the heart. They most likely represent malformations rather than true neoplasms. Lipoma-like accumulations in the interatrial septum are relatively common and sometimes glorified with the designation *lipomatous hypertrophy*. Although morphologically benign, they have been implicated in some cases of sudden cardiac death.

BIBLIOGRAPHY

Beggs AH: Dystrophinopathy, the expanding phenotype. Circulation 95:2344, 1997. (A review of the spectrum of clinical disorders linked to mutations in the dystrophin molecule, including a discussion of associated cardiovascular manifestations.)

Bonne G, et al: Familial hypertrophic cardiomyopathy: from mutations to functional defects. Circ Res 83:580, 1998. (An excellent discussion of the mutations that give rise to hypertrophic cardiomyopathy.)

Brickner ME, et al: Congenital heart disease in adults. N Engl J Med 342:256 and 334, 2000. (A nice two-part review of congenital cardiac malformations.)

Feldman AM, McNamara D: Myocarditis. N Engl J Med 343:1388, 2000. (A nice review of etiology, pathogenesis, and clinical features.)

Fuster V, et al: Acute coronary syndromes: biology. Lancet 353 (Suppl II):59, 1999. (An excellent review of the acute coronary syndromes.)

Groves AM: Rheumatic fever and rheumatic heart disease: an overview. Trop Doct 92:129, 1999. (A recent review of the epidemiology of acute rheumatic fever and rheumatic heart disease, with an emphasis on their importance in developing countries.)

Hasdai D, et al: Cardiogenic shock complicating acute coronary syndromes. Lancet 356:749, 2000. (A clinically oriented discussion of cardiogenic shock.)

Katz AM: Heart Failure: Pathophysiology, Molecular Biology, and Clinical Management. Philadelphia, Lippincott Williams & Wilkins, 2000. (A review encompassing the history, clinical features, physiology, and molecular basis of congestive heart failure and the molecular biology of a number of cardiomyopathies.)

Kushwaha SS, et al: Restrictive cardiomyopathy. N Engl J Med 336:267, 1997. (An excellent discussion of these rare disorders.)

Lee G-H, et al: Dissociation of sarcoglycans and the dystrophin carboxyl terminus from the sarcolemma in enteroviral cardiomyopathy. Circ Res 87:489, 2000. (A study addressing one intriguing mechanism for the development of cardiac dysfunction in enteroviral myocarditis.)

Mylonkis E, Calderwood SB: Infective endocarditis in adults. N Engl J Med 345:1318, 2001. (A review of the progress in the previous decade.)

Reimold SC, Rutherford JD: Peripartum cardiomyopathy. N Engl J Med 344:1629, 2001. (A succinct account of this enigmatic entity.)

Schrier RW, Abraham WT: Hormones and hemodynamics in heart failure. N Engl J Med 341:577, 1999. (An excellent review of the neurohumoral pathways that are triggered in heart failure.)

Tegos TJ, et al: The genesis of atherosclerosis and risk factors: a review. Angiology 52:89, 2001. (A detailed, up-to-date review of the epidemiological relationship between coronary artery disease and lipid disorders, hypertension, tobacco use, diabetes mellitus, and other risk factors.)

Towbin JA, Bowles NE: Genetic abnormalities responsible for dilated cardiomyopathy. Curr Cardiol Rep 2:475, 2000.

Van de Wer F: Cardiac troponins in acute coronary syndromes. N Engl J Med 335:1388, 1996. (An editorial that summarizes the results of several clinical studies designed to assess the utility of cardiac troponin measurements in diagnosis of ischemic heart disease.)

Watkins H: Sudden death in hypertrophic cardiomyopathy. N Engl J Med 342:422, 2000. (A clinically oriented discussion of one of the dreaded complications of cardiomyopathies.)

Yeghiazarians Y, et al: Unstable angina pectoris. N Engl J Med 342:101, 2000. (A review of the pathogenesis and management of unstable angina.)

12

The Hematopoietic and Lymphoid Systems

JON ASTER, MD, PhD

Bleeding Disorders

Disorders That Affect the Spleen and Thymus

Disorders of the hematopoietic and lymphoid systems encompass a wide range of diseases. They may affect primarily the red cells, the white cells, or the hemostatic mechanisms. *Red cell disorders* are usually reflected in *anemia. White cell disorders*, in contrast, most often involve overgrowth, which is usually malignant. Hemostatic derangements result in *hemorrhagic diatheses* (bleeding disorders). Finally, splenomegaly, a feature of several hematopoietic diseases, is discussed at the end of the chapter, as are tumors of the thymus.

Unlike many other organ systems, the lymphohematopoietic system is not confined to a single anatomic site, and hence hematopoietic disorders appear puzzling at first because they involve several anatomically distinct locales. Therefore, when considering hematopoietic disorders, it is important to remember that the lymphoid and hematopoietic cells are spread throughout the body and that there is constant "traffic" of cells between various compartments. For example, a patient who on the basis of a lymph node biopsy is diagnosed as having a malignant lymphoma may also have neoplastic lymphocytes in the bone marrow and blood and thus be considered to have a leukemia. The malignant lymphoid cells in the marrow may suppress normal production of red cells and platelets, giving rise to anemia and thrombocytopenia; seeding of liver and spleen may cause their enlargement. These apparently diverse manifestations have the same underlying basis.

Red Cell Disorders

Disorders of the red blood cells (RBCs) usually result in some form of anemia or sometimes in erythrocytosis (i.e., an increase in the number of red cells). *Anemia* is a reduction in the oxygen-transporting capacity of blood, usually because of a reduction of the total circulating RBC mass to below-normal levels. This is reflected in subnormal hematocrit (HCT) and hemoglobin (Hb) concentrations.

Anemia results from bleeding or from increased destruction or decreased production of RBCs. These diverse mechanisms serve as one useful basis for its classification (Table 12–1). With the exception of the anemia of chronic renal failure, in which renal erythropoietin-producing cells are lost, the decrease in tissue O_2 tension that attends anemia triggers increased erythropoietin production. This drives a compensatory hyperplasia of erythroid precursors in the bone marrow and, in severe anemias, the appearance of extramedullary hematopoiesis within the secondary hematopoietic organs (the spleen, liver, and lymph nodes). In well-nourished individuals who become anemic because of acute bleeding or increased destruction (hemolysis), this compensatory response can increase the regeneration of RBCs as much as fivefold to eightfold and is marked by the release of increased numbers of newly formed RBCs (reticulocytes) into the peripheral blood. In contrast, disorders of decreased RBC production (aregenerative anemias) are characterized by reticulocytopenia.

Another classification of anemias is based on the morphology of RBCs, which often correlates with the cause of their deficiency. Specific characteristics that provide etiologic clues include the RBC size (normocytic, microcytic, or macrocytic); degree of hemoglobinization, reflected in the color of RBCs (normochromic or hypochromic); and several other special features, such as RBC shape. These RBC indices are judged subjectively by visual inspection of peripheral smears and are also measured objectively and expressed by various terms, as follows:

- *Mean cell volume* (MCV): the average volume of an RBC, expressed in femtoliters (cubic micrometers)
- *Mean cell hemoglobin* (MCH): the average content (mass) of Hb per RBC, expressed in picograms
- *Mean cell hemoglobin concentration* (MCHC): the average concentration of Hb in a given volume of packed RBCs, expressed in grams per deciliter
- *RBC distribution width* (RDW): the coefficient of variation of RBC volume.

In modern clinical laboratories, specialized instruments directly measure or automatically calculate the RBC indices. Adult reference ranges are shown in Table 12–2.

■

Table 12-1.   CLASSIFICATION OF ANEMIA ACCORDING TO MECHANISM OF PRODUCTION

I. Blood Loss

A. Acute: trauma
B. Chronic: lesions of gastrointestinal tract, gynecologic disturbances

II. Increased Rate of Destruction (Hemolytic Anemias)

A. Intrinsic (intracorpuscular) abnormalities of RBCs
  1. Hereditary
    a. Disorders of RBC membrane cytoskeleton (e.g., spherocytosis, elliptocytosis)
    b. RBC enzyme deficiencies
      1) Glycolytic enzymes: pyruvate kinase, hexokinase
      2) Enzymes of hexose monophosphate shunt: glucose-6-phosphate dehydrogenase, glutathione synthetase
    c. Disorders of hemoglobin synthesis
      1) Deficient globin synthesis: thalassemia syndromes
      2) Structurally abnormal globin synthesis (hemoglobinopathies): sickle cell anemia, unstable hemoglobins
  2. Acquired
    a. Membrane defect: paroxysmal nocturnal hemoglobinuria
B. Extrinsic (extracorpuscular) abnormalities
  1. Antibody mediated
    a. Isohemagglutinins: transfusion reactions, erythroblastosis fetalis (Rh disease of the newborn)
    b. Autoantibodies: idiopathic (primary), drug-associated, systemic lupus erythematosus
  2. Mechanical trauma to RBCs
    a. Microangiopathic hemolytic anemias: thrombotic thrombocytopenic purpura, disseminated intravascular coagulation
  3. Infections: malaria

III. Impaired Red Cell Production

A. Disturbance of proliferation and differentiation of stem cells: aplastic anemia, pure RBC aplasia, anemia of renal failure, anemia of endocrine disorders
B. Disturbance of proliferation and maturation of erythroblasts
  1. Defective DNA synthesis: deficiency or impaired utilization of vitamin B_{12} and folic acid (megaloblastic anemias)
  2. Defective hemoglobin synthesis
    a. Deficient heme synthesis: iron deficiency
    b. Deficient globin synthesis: thalassemias
  3. Unknown or multiple mechanisms: sideroblastic anemia, anemia of chronic inflammation, myelophthisic anemias due to marrow infiltrations

Table 12-2. ADULT REFERENCE RANGES FOR RED BLOOD CELLS*

	Units	Men		Women
Hemoglobin (Hb)	Ag/dL	13.6–17.2		12.0–15.0
Hematocrit (HCT)	%	39–49		33–43
Erythrocyte count (red blood cells [RBCs])	$\times 10^6/mm^3$	4.3–5.9		3.5–5.0
Reticulocyte count	%		0.5–1.5	
Mean cell volume (MCV)	fL		76–100	
Mean cell hemoglobin (MCH)	pg		27–33	
Mean cell hemoglobin concentration (MCHC)	g/dL		33–37	
RBC distribution width (RDW)			11.5–14.5	

*Reference ranges vary among laboratories. The reference ranges for the laboratory providing the result should always be used when interpreting a laboratory test.

HEMORRHAGE: BLOOD LOSS ANEMIA

With acute blood loss, the immediate threat to the patient is hypovolemia (shock) rather than anemia. If the patient survives, hemodilution begins at once and achieves its full effect within 2 to 3 days, unmasking the extent of the RBC loss. *The anemia is normocytic normochromic.* Recovery from blood-loss anemia is enhanced by a rise in the erythropoietin level, which stimulates increased RBC production within several days. The onset of the marrow response is marked by reticulocytosis.

With chronic blood loss, iron stores are gradually depleted. Iron is essential for Hb synthesis and effective erythropoiesis, and its deficiency thus leads to a chronic anemia of underproduction. Because iron deficiency anemia can occur in other clinical settings as well, it is described later in this chapter along with other anemias of diminished erythropoiesis (p 409).

INCREASED RATE OF RED CELL DESTRUCTION: THE HEMOLYTIC ANEMIAS

Normal RBCs have a life span of about 120 days. Anemias that are associated with a decreased RBC life span are termed *hemolytic anemias.* Shortened survival may be caused by either inherent (intracorpuscular) RBC defects, which are usually inherited, or external (extracorpuscular) factors, which are usually acquired. Several examples are listed in Table 12–1.

Before discussing the various disorders individually, we will describe certain general features of hemolytic anemias. All are characterized by (1) an increased rate of RBC destruction; (2) a compensatory increase in erythropoiesis that results in reticulocytosis; and (3) the retention by the body of the products of RBC destruction, including iron. Because the iron is conserved and recycled readily, RBC regeneration can keep pace with the hemolysis. Consequently, these anemias are almost invariably associated with a marked *erythroid hyperplasia within the marrow* and an *increased reticulocyte count in peripheral blood.* If the anemia is severe, extramedullary hematopoiesis may develop in the spleen, liver, and lymph nodes.

Destruction of RBCs may occur within the vascular compartment (intravascular hemolysis) or within the cells of the mononuclear phagocyte, or reticuloendothelial (RE), system (extravascular hemolysis). *Intravascular hemolysis* occurs when RBCs are subjected to mechanical trauma or damaged by a variety of biochemical or physical agents (e.g., fixation of complement, exposure to clostridial toxins, or heat). Regardless of cause, intravascular hemolysis results in hemoglobinemia, hemoglobinuria, and hemosiderinuria. Conversion of the heme pigment to bilirubin may give rise to unconjugated hyperbilirubinemia and jaundice. Massive intravascular hemolysis sometimes leads to acute tubular necrosis (Chapter 14). Levels of *serum haptoglobin,* a protein that binds free Hb, are characteristically low.

Extravascular hemolysis, the more common mode of RBC destruction, takes place largely within the phagocytic cells of the spleen and liver. The mononuclear phagocyte system removes erythrocytes from the circulation whenever RBCs are injured or immunologically altered. Because extreme alterations of shape are necessary for RBCs to successfully navigate the splenic sinusoids, reduced deformability makes this passage difficult and leads to splenic sequestration, followed by phagocytosis (Fig. 12–1). This is believed to be an important factor in the pathogenesis of RBC destruction in a variety of hemolytic anemias. Extravascular hemolysis is not associated with hemoglobinemia and hemoglobinuria, but it may result in jaundice and, if of long standing, in the formation of bilirubin-rich gallstones (so-called pigment stones). *Serum haptoglobin* is always decreased, because some Hb invariably escapes into the plasma. In most forms of hemolytic anemia, there is reactive hyperplasia of the mononuclear system, which results in splenomegaly.

Because the pathways for the excretion of excess iron are limited, there is a tendency in hemolytic anemias for abnormal amounts of iron to accumulate, giving rise to systemic hemosiderosis (Chapter 1) or, in very severe cases, secondary hemochromatosis (Chapter 16).

Hereditary Spherocytosis

This disorder is characterized by an inherited (intrinsic) defect in the RBC membrane that renders the erythrocytes

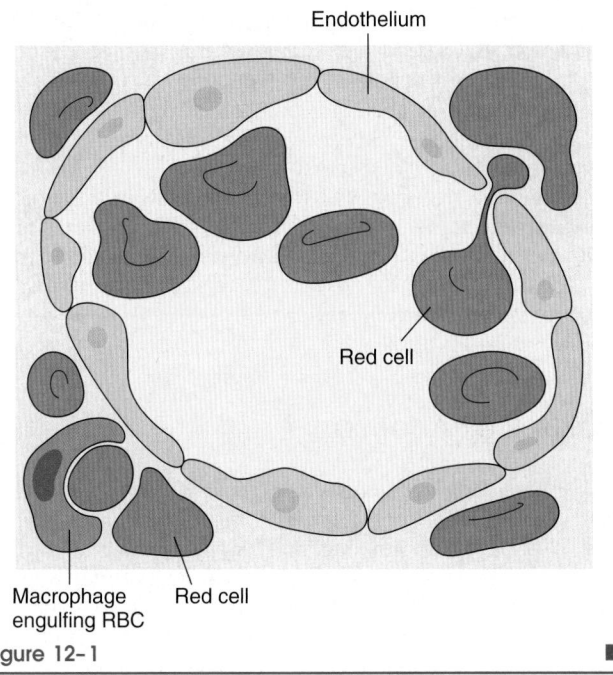

Endothelium

Red cell

Macrophage
engulfing RBC   Red cell

Figure 12–1   ■

Schematic of splenic sinus. An erythrocyte is in the process of squeezing
from the cord into the sinus lumen. Note the degree of deformability required for the RBCs to pass through the wall of the sinus.

*spheroidal, less deformable, and vulnerable to splenic se-
questration and destruction.* Hereditary spherocytosis (HS)
is most commonly transmitted as an autosomal dominant
trait; approximately 25% of patients have an autosomal recessive form of the disease that is much more severe than
the autosomal dominant form.

Pathogenesis. In HS, the *primary abnormality resides in
the proteins that form the skeleton of the RBC membrane.*
Several such proteins (Fig. 12–2) form a meshlike network on the intracellular face of the cell membrane. The
major protein in this network is spectrin, which is a long,
flexible heterodimer. The spectrin network is linked at two
points to the membrane: through ankyrin to the intrinsic
membrane protein band 3 and through band 4.1 to the
intrinsic membrane protein glycophorin. The horizontal
spectrin/spectrin and vertical spectrin/intrinsic membrane
protein interactions serve to stabilize the RBC membrane
and are responsible for the normal shape, strength, and
flexibility of the RBC.

Multiple mutations have been described in HS, but all
serve to disrupt vertical interactions between the spectrin
meshwork and one or the other intrinsic membrane proteins. The most commonly mutated component is ankyrin,
but mutations in spectrin, band 4.1, and band 3 have also
been described (see Fig. 12–2). In all types of HS, the
RBCs have reduced membrane stability and consequently

Figure 12–2   ■

Schematic representation of the RBC membrane cytoskeleton and effects of alterations in the cytoskeletal proteins on the shape of RBCs. With mutations
that affect the integrity of the membrane cytoskeleton, the normal biconcave erythrocyte loses membrane fragments. To accommodate the loss of surface
area, the cell adopts a spherical shape. Such spherocytic cells are less deformable than normal and are therefore trapped in the splenic cords, where they
are phagocytosed by macrophages.

lose membrane fragments after their release into the periphery, while retaining most of their volume. As a result, the surface area–to-volume ratio of HS cells decreases until they assume the smallest possible diameter for a given volume, namely, a sphere (see Fig. 12–2).

The spleen plays a major role in the destruction of spherocytes. RBCs must undergo extreme degrees of deformation to leave the cords of Billroth and enter the splenic sinusoids. The discoid shape of normal RBCs allows considerable latitude for changes in cell shape. In contrast, because of their spheroidal shape and reduced membrane plasticity, spherocytes have great difficulty leaving the splenic cords. The abnormal RBCs are sequestered and eventually destroyed by macrophages, which are plentiful in the splenic cords. *The critical role of the spleen in this process is illustrated by the invariably beneficial effect of splenectomy. The RBC defect and spherocytes persist, but the anemia is corrected.*

MORPHOLOGY

On smears, the RBCs lack the central zone of pallor because of their spheroidal shape. Spherocytosis, although distinctive, is not diagnostic, because it is seen in any condition that leads to loss of the cell membrane, as, for example, in immune hemolytic anemias, discussed later. To compensate for the excessive RBC destruction, erythropoiesis in the marrow is stimulated. As with other hemolytic anemias, RBC regeneration is demonstrated by reticulocytosis in the peripheral blood. Splenomegaly is greater and more common in HS than in any other form of hemolytic anemia. Splenic weight is usually between 500 and 1000 g but may be greater. The enlargement of the spleen results from striking congestion of the cords of Billroth (leaving the splenic sinuses virtually empty) and increased numbers of mononuclear phagocytes. Phagocytosed RBCs are frequently seen within hypertrophic macrophages lining the sinusoids and, in particular, within the cords. In long-standing cases, there is prominent systemic hemosiderosis.

The other general features of hemolytic anemias described earlier are present with this disorder. In particular, cholelithiasis occurs in 40% to 50% of these patients.

Clinical Course. The characteristic clinical features are *anemia*, *splenomegaly*, and *jaundice*. The severity of this disorder is highly variable. Asymptomatic cases occur, as do cases characterized by a profound anemia, but in general the anemia is moderate. Because the RBCs are spheroidal, there is little margin for expansion of volume when cells are exposed to hypotonic salt solution. As a result, *increased osmotic fragility is a characteristic finding that is helpful in diagnosis.*

The more or less stable clinical course may be punctuated by an aplastic crisis. These episodes, often triggered by parvovirus infection of developing erythroblasts in the marrow, are associated with transient cessation of RBC production. Because of the shortened life span of HS cells, the failure of erythropoiesis for even a few days results in a rapid worsening of anemia accompanied by reticulocytopenia. In most cases, such episodes are self-limited, but some patients may need blood transfusions.

There is no treatment for HS. In those who are symptomatic, splenectomy is beneficial because the major site of RBC destruction is removed; however, splenectomy must be weighed against the risk of increased susceptibility to infections, particularly in children.

Sickle Cell Anemia

The hemoglobinopathies are a group of hereditary disorders characterized by the presence of a structurally abnormal Hb. Of the more than 300 variant hemoglobins that have been discovered, one third are associated with significant clinical manifestations. The prototype and most prevalent hemoglobinopathy is caused by a mutation in the gene encoding the β-globin chain that causes the formation of sickle Hb (HbS). The associated disease, sickle cell anemia, is discussed here; other hemoglobinopathies are infrequent and beyond our scope.

HbS, like 90% of other abnormal Hbs, results from a single amino acid substitution in the globin chain. Normal hemoglobins, as may be recalled, are tetramers composed of two pairs of similar chains. On average, the normal adult RBC contains 96% HbA ($\alpha_2\beta_2$), 3% HbA$_2$ ($\alpha_2\delta_2$), and 1% fetal Hb (HbF, $\alpha_2\gamma_2$). Substitution of valine for glutamic acid at the sixth position of the β-chain produces HbS. In homozygotes, all HbA is replaced by HbS, whereas in heterozygotes, only about half is replaced.

Incidence. Approximately 8% of American blacks are heterozygous for HbS. In parts of Africa where malaria is endemic, the gene frequency approaches 30%, attributed to the slight protective effect of HbS against *Plasmodium falciparum* malaria. In the United States, sickle cell anemia affects approximately 1 of every 600 blacks; worldwide, sickle cell anemia is the most common form of familial hemolytic anemia.

Etiology and Pathogenesis. On deoxygenation, HbS molecules undergo polymerization, a process sometimes called *gelation* or *crystallization*. The change in the physical state of HbS distorts the RBCs, which assume an elongated crescentic, or sickle, shape (Fig. 12–3). Sickling of RBCs is initially reversible by oxygenation; however, membrane damage occurs with each episode of sickling, and eventually the cells accumulate calcium, lose potassium and water, and become irreversibly sickled, despite adequate oxygenation.

Many factors influence sickling of RBCs in vivo. The three most important ones are as follows:

■ *The presence of hemoglobins other than HbA.* In heterozygotes, approximately 40% of Hb is HbS; the rest is HbA, which interacts only weakly with HbS during the processes of aggregation. Therefore, the RBCs of heterozygotes have little tendency to sickle, and these individuals are said to have the *sickle cell trait.* HbC,

Figure 12–3 ■

Peripheral blood smear from a patient with sickle cell anemia. *A,* Low magnification shows sickle cells, anisocytosis, poikilocytosis, and target cells. *B,* Higher magnification shows an irreversibly sickled cell in the center. (Courtesy of Dr. Robert W. McKenna, Department of Pathology, University of Texas Southwestern Medical School, Dallas.)

another mutant β-globin, is fairly common. The carrier rate for HbC in American blacks is about 2.3%, giving the likelihood that 1 in 1250 newborns will be a double heterozygote for HbS and HbC (i.e., will have the HbS gene from one parent and HbC from the other). HbC has a greater tendency to aggregate with HbS than does HbA, so those with HbS and HbC (called *Hb SC disease*) have a more severe disease than do those with sickle cell trait. Conversely, HbF interacts poorly with HbS, and therefore newborns with sickle cell anemia do not manifest the disease until they are 5 to 6 months old, when the HbF falls to adult levels. This, as we will see, can be exploited for the treatment of sickle cell anemia.

■ *The concentration of HbS in the cell.* The tendency for deoxygenated HbS to form the insoluble polymers that create sickle cells is strongly dependent on the concentration of HbS. Thus, RBC dehydration, by increasing the MCHC, greatly facilitates sickling and may trigger occlusion of small blood vessels. Conversely, the coexistence of α-thalassemia (described later), characterized by reduced synthesis of globin chains, reduces the MCHC and therefore the severity of sickling. The relatively low concentration of HbS also contributes to the lack of symptomatic sickling in heterozygotes.

■ *The length of time that RBCs are exposed to low O₂ tension.* Normal transit times for RBCs passing through capillaries are not sufficient for significant aggregation of deoxygenated HbS to occur. Hence, sickling of RBCs is confined to microvascular beds where blood flow is sluggish. This is normally the case in the spleen and the bone marrow, which are prominently affected by sickle cell disease. It has been suggested that two factors play particularly important pathogenic roles in other vascular beds: inflammation and increased RBC adhesion. As you will recall, the exodus of blood from inflamed tissues is slowed, owing to the adhesion of leukocytes and RBCs to activated endothelium and the exudation of fluid

through leaky vessels. As a result, RBCs have longer transit times through inflamed vascular beds, making them prone to clinically significant sickling. For reasons that are unclear, sickle RBCs also express increased levels of adhesive surface proteins, such as CD36, even in the absence of overt inflammatory disease. RBC adhesion to endothelium in vitro correlates with clinical severity, presumably because "stickiness" influences RBC transit time in vivo.

Two major consequences stem from the sickling of RBCs (Fig. 12–4). First, repeated episodes of deoxygenation cause membrane damage and dehydration of RBCs, which become rigid and irreversibly sickled. These dysfunctional RBCs are recognized and removed by mononuclear phagocyte cells, producing a chronic extravascular hemolytic anemia. Overall, the mean life span of sickle cell RBCs is reduced from 120 days to approximately 20 days. Second, the sickling of RBCs produces widespread *microvascular obstructions* and resulting ischemic tissue damage. Vaso-occlusion can be triggered and exacerbated by infection, inflammation, dehydration, and acidosis.

MORPHOLOGY

The anatomic alterations stem from the following three aspects of the disease: (1) hemolysis, with resultant anemia; (2) increased breakdown of Hb, with bilirubin formation; and (3) capillary stasis, leading to tissue ischemia and infarction. In peripheral smears, irreversibly sickled RBCs are evident as bizarre, elongated, spindled, or boat-shaped structures (see Fig. 12–3). Both the severe anemia and the vascular stasis lead to fatty changes in the heart, liver, and renal tubules. Erythropoiesis is activated in the bone marrow. Expansion of marrow may lead to resorption of bone with appositional new bone formation on the

Figure 12–4

Pathophysiology and morphologic consequences of sickle cell anemia.

external aspect of the skull, leading to a "crew-cut" appearance on radiographs. Extramedullary hematopoiesis may appear in the spleen and liver.

In children there is moderate splenomegaly (splenic weight up to 500 g), caused by congestion of the red pulp with masses of RBCs sickled and jammed together. Eventually this splenic erythrostasis leads to enough hypoxic tissue damage, sometimes with frank infarction, to create a shrunken, fibrotic spleen. This process, referred to as **autosplenectomy,** is seen in all long-standing adult cases. Ultimately, the spleen is reduced to a small nubbin of fibrous tissue.

Vascular congestion, thrombosis, and infarction may affect any organ, including bones, liver, kidney, retina, and skin. The bone marrow is particularly prone to ischemia, because of the relatively sluggish blood flow and high rate of metabolism. Priapism is another common problem that may lead to fibrosis and eventual erectile dysfunction. As with the other hemolytic anemias, hemosiderosis and gallstones are common.

Clinical Course. Homozygous sickle cell disease usually becomes apparent after the sixth month of life, as HbF is gradually replaced by HbS. The anemia is severe, with HCT values ranging between 18% and 30% (normal range, 35% to 45%). The chronic hemolysis is associated with marked reticulocytosis and hyperbilirubinemia. From the time of onset, the process runs an unremitting course, punctuated by sudden episodes of so-called crises. The most serious of these are the *vaso-occlusive*, or *pain*, *crises*. Pain crises can involve many sites but are most commonly localized to the bone marrow. Such crises may occur without warning, and they often progress to marrow infarction and necrosis.

In some instances, necrotic marrow gives rise to fat emboli that secondarily involve the lung. This complication can lead to the *acute chest syndrome*, which is more commonly triggered by pulmonary infections. The blood flow in the inflamed, ischemic lung becomes sluggish and "spleen-like," leading to sickling within hypoxemic pulmonary beds. This exacerbates the underlying pulmonary dysfunction, creating a vicious cycle of worsening pulmonary and systemic hypoxemia, sickling, and vaso-occlusion. Another major complication is *central nervous system stroke*, which sometimes occurs in the setting of the acute chest syndrome. Although virtually any organ may be damaged by ischemic injury in the course of the disease, *the acute chest syndrome and stroke are the two leading causes of ischemia-related death.*

A second acute event, *aplastic crisis*, represents a sudden but usually temporary cessation of erythropoiesis. Reticulocytes disappear from the blood, and anemia worsens. As in hereditary spherocytosis, the aplastic crisis is usually triggered by parvovirus infection of erythroblasts.

In addition to these crises, patients with sickle cell disease are prone to infections. Both children and adults with sickle cell disease are functionally asplenic, making them susceptible to infections caused by encapsulated bacteria, such as pneumococci. In adults the basis for "hyposplenism" is autoinfarction. In the preceding childhood phase of splenic enlargement, congestion caused by trapped sickle RBCs apparently interferes with bacterial sequestration and killing; hence, even children with enlarged spleens are at risk for fatal septicemia. Defects in the alternative complement pathway that impair the opsonization of encapsulated bacteria are also observed. For reasons that are not entirely clear, patients with sickle cell disease are particularly predisposed to *Salmonella* osteomyelitis.

In full-blown sickle cell disease, at least some irreversibly sickled RBCs can be seen on an ordinary peripheral blood smear. In sickle cell trait, sickling can be induced in vitro by exposing cells to marked hypoxia. Ultimately, the diagnosis depends on the electrophoretic demonstration of HbS. Prenatal diagnosis of sickle cell anemia can be performed by analyzing the DNA in fetal cells obtained by amniocentesis or biopsy of chorionic villi (Chapter 7).

The clinical course of patients with sickle cell anemia is highly variable. As a result of improvements in supportive care, an increasing number of patients are surviving into adulthood and producing offspring. Of particular importance is prophylactic treatment with penicillin to prevent pneumococcal infections. Approximately 50% survive beyond the fifth decade. Sickle cell trait, in contrast, generally remains entirely asymptomatic unless the patient becomes extremely hypoxic.

As mentioned earlier, the presence of HbF in cells retards sickling by inhibiting polymer formation. This observation has been exploited therapeutically. Hydroxyurea, a drug commonly used in cancer chemotherapy, affects erythropoietic stem cells in a manner that results in increased levels of HbF in the newly formed cells. However, the therapeutic response to hydroxyurea may precede the rise in HbF levels, implying that other mechanisms are also important. Of note, hydroxyurea acts as an anti-inflammatory agent by inhibiting the production of white cells, and in doing so may reduce inflammation-related RBC stasis and sickling. It is hypothesized that both actions contribute to a reduction in pain crises.

Thalassemia

The thalassemias are a heterogeneous group of genetic disorders of Hb synthesis characterized by a lack of or decreased synthesis of globin chains. In α-thalassemia, α-globin chain synthesis is reduced, whereas in β-thalassemia, β-globin chain synthesis is either absent (designated β^0 thalassemia) or markedly deficient (β^+ thalassemia). Unlike the hemoglobinopathies, which represent qualitative abnormalities, thalassemias result from quantitative abnormalities of globin chain synthesis. The consequences of reduced synthesis of one globin chain derive not only from the low level of intracellular Hb but also from the relative excess of the other globin chain, as will be discussed later.

Thalassemia is inherited as an autosomal codominant condition. The heterozygous form (*thalassemia minor* or *thalassemia trait*) may be asymptomatic or mildly symptomatic. The homozygous form, *thalassemia major*, is associated with severe hemolytic anemia. The mutant genes are particularly common among Mediterranean, African, and Asian populations.

Molecular Pathogenesis. A complex pattern of molecular defects underlies the thalassemias. Recall that adult Hb, or HbA, is a tetramer composed of two α chains and two β chains. The α chains are encoded by two α-globin genes, which lie in tandem on chromosome 11. In contrast, the β chains are encoded by a single β-globin gene located on chromosome 16.

β-Thalassemia. As mentioned earlier, β-thalassemia syndromes can be classified into two categories: (1) β^0-thalassemia, associated with total absence of β-globin chains in the homozygous state, and (2) β^+-thalassemia, characterized by reduced (but detectable) β-globin synthesis in the homozygous state. Sequencing of cloned β-globin genes obtained from thalassemic patients has revealed more than 100 different mutations responsible for β^0- or β^+-thalassemia. Most of these result from single base changes. In contrast to α-thalassemias, described later, *gene deletions rarely underlie β-thalassemias* (Table 12–3).

Details of these mutations and their effects on β-globin synthesis are beyond our scope, but a few illustrative examples will be cited (Fig. 12–5):

■ The promoter region controls the initiation and rate of transcription, and therefore mutations affecting promoter sequences usually lead to reduced globin gene transcription. Because some β-globin is synthesized, patients develop β^+-thalassemia.

■ Mutations in the coding sequences are usually associated with more serious consequences. For example, in some cases a single nucleotide change in one of the exons leads to the formation of a termination, or "stop," codon, which interrupts translation of β-globin messenger RNA (mRNA). Premature termination generates nonfunctional truncated forms of β-globin, leading to β^0-thalassemia.

■ *Mutations that lead to aberrant mRNA processing are the most common cause of β-thalassemia.* Most of these affect introns, but some have been located within exons. If the mutation alters the normal splice junctions, splicing does not occur, and all of the mRNA formed is abnormal. Unspliced mRNA is degraded within the nucleus, and β^0-thalassemia results. However, some mutations affect the introns at locations away from the normal intron-exon splice junction. These mutations create new sites that are substrates for the action of splicing enzymes at abnormal locations—within an intron, for example. Because normal splice sites remain intact, both normal and abnormal splicing occur, giving rise to normal as well as abnormal β-globin mRNA. These patients develop β^+-thalassemia.

Two factors contribute to the pathogenesis of anemia in β-thalassemia. Reduced synthesis of β-globin leads to inadequate HbA formation, so that the overall Hb concentration (MCHC) per cell is lower, and the cells appear *hypochromic.*

Table 12-3. CLINICAL AND GENETIC CLASSIFICATION OF THALASSEMIAS

Clinical Nomenclature	Genotype	Disease	Molecular Genetics
β-Thalassemias			
Thalassemia major	Homozygous β^0-thalassemia (β^0/β^0); homozygous β^+-thalassemia (β^+/β^+)	Severe, requires blood transfusions regularly	Rare gene deletions in β^0/β^0 Defects in transcription processing, or translation of β-globin messenger RNA
Thalassemia minor	β^0/β β^+/β	Asymptomatic with mild or no anemia; RBC abnormalities seen	
α-Thalassemia			
Silent carrier	$-\alpha/\alpha\alpha$	Asymptomatic; no RBC abnormality	Gene deletions mainly
α-Thalassemia trait	$-\alpha/\alpha\alpha$ (Asian); $-\alpha/-\alpha$ (black African)	Asymptomatic; like thalassemia minor	
HbH disease	$-/-\alpha$	Severe anemia, tetramers of β-globin (HbH) formed in RBCs	
Hydrops fetalis	$-/-$	Lethal in utero	

Much more important is the *hemolytic component* of β-thalassemia. This is caused not by lack of β-globin but by the relative excess of α-globin chains, whose synthesis remains normal. Unpaired α-chains form insoluble aggregates that precipitate within the RBCs (Fig. 12–6). These inclusions damage the cell membranes, reduce their plasticity, and render the RBCs susceptible to phagocytosis by the mononuclear phagocyte system. Not only are mature RBCs susceptible to premature destruction, but also a majority of the erythroblasts within the marrow are destroyed, owing to the presence of the inclusions that damage the membranes. Such intramedullary destruction of RBCs (*ineffective erythropoiesis*) has another untoward effect: it is associated with inappropriately increased absorption of dietary iron, which contributes to iron overload in these patients.

α-Thalassemia. The molecular basis of α-thalassemia is quite different from that of β-thalassemia. Most of the α-thalassemias are caused by deletions of α-globin gene loci. Because there are four functional α-globin genes, there are four possible degrees of α-thalassemia, based on loss of one to four α-globin genes from the chromosomes. These cover a wide spectrum of clinical disorders, the severity of which is related to the number of deleted α-globin genes (see Table 12–3). Loss of a single α-globin gene is associated with a silent carrier state, whereas deletion of all four α-globin genes is associated with fetal death in utero, because the blood has virtually no oxygen-delivering capacity.

With loss of three α-globin genes, there is a relative excess of β-globin or other non–α-globin chains. Excess β-globin (or γ-globin chains early in life) forms relatively stable β_4 and γ_4 tetramers known as HbH and Hb Bart, respectively, that cause less membrane damage than do free α-globin chains. Therefore, the hemolytic anemia and ineffective erythropoiesis tend be less severe in α-thalassemia than in β-thalassemia. Unfortunately, both HbH and Hb Bart have abnormally high affinity for O_2, rendering them ineffective at delivering O_2 to the tissues.

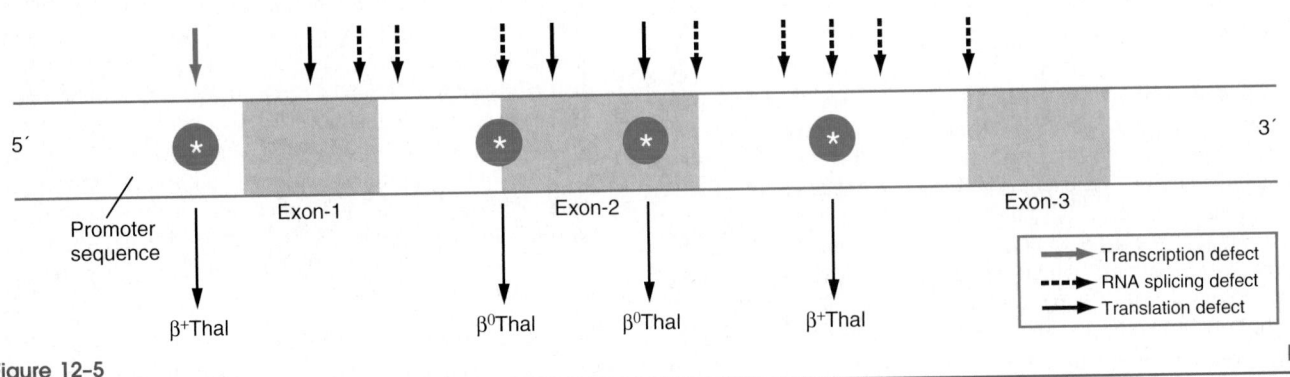

Figure 12–5

Diagrammatic representation of the β-globin gene and some sites where point mutations giving rise to β-thalassemia have been localized. (Modified from Wyngaarden JB, Smith LH, Bennett JC [eds]: Cecil Textbook of Medicine, 19th ed. Philadelphia, WB Saunders, 1992.)

Figure 12–6

Pathogenesis of β-thalassemia major. Note that aggregates of excess α-globin are not visible on routine blood smears. Blood transfusions, on the one hand, correct the anemia and reduce stimulus for erythropoietin secretion and deformities induced by marrow expansion; on the other hand, they add to systemic iron overload.

MORPHOLOGY

Only the morphologic changes in β-thalassemia, which is more common in the United States, will be described. As is true in all disorders that interfere with the synthesis of Hb, the peripheral blood RBCs in thalassemia major are abnormally small (microcytic) and pale (hypochromic). These cells also have a relatively large surface area to volume ratio. This may lead Hb to collect in a central "puddle" when the RBCs are spread on glass slides, giving them a target-like appearance (target cells). In addition, there is **severe poikilocytosis, anisocytosis, and reticulocytosis.** Normoblasts are seen spilling into the peripheral blood, reflecting the marked hyperplasia of erythroid progenitors.

In β-thalassemia major, the anatomic changes are those common to all hemolytic anemias but extreme in degree. The combination of ineffective erythropoiesis and hemolysis results in a striking hyperplasia of erythroid progenitors, with a shift toward primitive forms. The burgeoning erythropoietic marrow may completely fill the intramedullary space of the skeleton, invade the bony cortex, impair bone growth, and produce **skeletal deformities.** Extramedullary hematopoiesis and hyperplasia of the mononuclear phagocytes produces prominent **splenomegaly, hepatomegaly,** and **lymphadenopathy.** The expanded mass of ineffective erythropoietic tissue consumes nutrients, producing **growth retardation** and a degree of **cachexia** reminiscent of that seen in cancer patients. Unless steps are taken to prevent iron overload, over the span of years **severe hemosiderosis** develops (see Fig. 12–6).

Clinical Course. *Thalassemia major* manifests itself postnatally as HbF synthesis diminishes. Affected children fail to develop normally, and their growth is retarded almost from birth. They are sustained only by repeated blood transfusions, which improve the anemia and reduce the skeletal deformities associated with excessive erythropoiesis. With transfusions alone, survival into the second or third decade is possible, but gradually systemic iron overload develops. Both iron present in transfused RBCs and iron inappropriately taken up from the gut (somehow related to ineffective erythropoiesis) contribute to iron overload. Unless patients are treated aggressively with iron chelators, cardiac failure from secondary hemochromatosis commonly occurs and often causes death in the second or third decade of life. When feasible, bone marrow transplantation at an early age is the treatment of choice.

With *thalassemia minor* there is usually only a mild microcytic hypochromic anemia, and in general these patients have a normal life expectancy. Because *iron deficiency anemia is associated with a similar RBC appearance,* it should be excluded by appropriate laboratory tests, described later in this chapter. The diagnosis of β-thalassemia minor is made by Hb electrophoresis. In addition to reduced amounts of HbA ($\alpha_2\beta_2$), the level of HbA$_2$ ($\alpha_2\delta_2$) is increased. The diagnosis of β-thalassemia major can generally be made on clinical grounds. The peripheral blood shows a severe microcytic hypochromic anemia, with marked variation in cell shapes (poikilocytosis). The reticulocyte count is increased. Hb electrophoresis shows profound reduction or absence of HbA and increased levels of HbF. The HbA$_2$ level may be normal or increased. Prenatal diagnosis of both forms of thalassemia can be made by DNA analysis.

Glucose-6-Phosphate Dehydrogenase Deficiency

The erythrocyte and its membrane are vulnerable to injury by endogenous and exogenous oxidants. Normally, intracellular reduced glutathione (GSH) inactivates such oxidants. Abnormalities of enzymes that participate in the hexose

monophosphate shunt or glutathione metabolism reduce the ability of RBCs to protect themselves from oxidative injury and lead to hemolytic anemias. The prototype and most prevalent of these anemias is caused by a deficiency of glucose-6-phosphate dehydrogenase (G6PD). The G6PD gene is on the X chromosome, and there is considerable polymorphism at this locus. More than 400 G6PD genetic variants, most not associated with any disease, have been identified. In the United States, the G6PD A$^-$ variant is associated with hemolytic anemia. It is encountered primarily in blacks. Approximately 10% of black males in the United States are affected. In these individuals, a normal amount of enzyme is synthesized in the RBC precursors, but it decays more rapidly than normal in mature RBCs, which lack the capacity to synthesize proteins. Therefore, older RBCs become progressively more deficient in enzyme activity and are most vulnerable to oxidant stress.

This disorder produces no symptoms unless the RBCs are subjected to oxidant injury by exposure to certain drugs, toxins, or infections. The drugs incriminated include antimalarials (e.g., primaquine), sulfonamides, nitrofurantoin, phenacetin, aspirin (in large doses), and vitamin K derivatives. More important are infections that presumably trigger hemolysis, owing to release of free radicals from phagocytic cells. The effect of these offending agents is to cause oxidation of reduced glutathione (GSH) to oxidized glutathione (GSSG) through the production of hydrogen peroxide. Because regeneration of GSH is impaired in G6PD-deficient cells, hydrogen peroxide accumulates and denatures globin chains by oxidation of sulfhydryl groups. Denatured Hb is precipitated within the RBCs in the form of inclusions called *Heinz bodies.* These precipitates of denatured Hb may damage the cell membrane sufficiently to cause intravascular hemolysis. In addition, the inclusion-bearing RBCs are less deformable, and their cell membranes are further damaged when splenic phagocytes attempt to "pluck out" the

Figure 12–7 ■

Peripheral blood smear from a patient with glucose-6-phosphate dehydrogenase deficiency after exposure to an oxidant drug. *Inset,* RBCs with precipitates of denatured globin (Heinz bodies) revealed by supravital staining. As the splenic macrophages pluck out these inclusions, "bite cells" like the one in this smear are produced. (Courtesy of Dr. Robert W. McKenna, Department of Pathology, University of Texas Southwestern Medical School, Dallas.)

inclusions, creating so-called bite cells (Fig. 12–7). All these changes predispose the RBCs to becoming trapped in the splenic sinuses and destroyed by the phagocytes (extravascular hemolysis).

The drug-induced hemolysis is acute and of variable clinical severity. Typically, patients develop evidence of hemolysis after a lag period of 2 or 3 days. Because the G6PD gene is on the X chromosome, all the erythrocytes of affected males are deficient in enzyme activity. However, because of random inactivation of one X chromosome in women (Chapter 7), heterozygous females have two distinct populations of RBCs: some normal and others deficient in G6PD activity. Thus, affected males are more vulnerable to oxidant injury, whereas most carrier females are asymptomatic, except those with a very large proportion of deficient RBCs (a chance situation known as *unfavorable lyonization*). Because the enzyme deficiency is most marked in older RBCs, these cells are more susceptible to lysis. As the marrow compensates by producing new (young) RBCs, hemolysis tends to abate even if drug exposure continues. In other variants, such as G6PD Mediterranean, found mainly in the Middle East, the enzyme deficiency and the resultant hemolysis are more severe.

Paroxysmal Nocturnal Hemoglobinuria

A rare disorder of unknown etiology, paroxysmal nocturnal hemoglobinuria (PNH) is mentioned here because it is the only form of hemolytic anemia that results from an *acquired membrane defect secondary to a mutation that affects myeloid stem cells*. The mutant gene, called *PIGA*, is required for the synthesis of a specific type of intramembranous glycolipid anchor (phosphatidylinositol glycan [PIG]) that is shared by diverse membrane-associated proteins. Without the membrane anchor, these "PIG-tailed" proteins cannot be expressed on the surface of cells. Those affected include three proteins that limit the spontaneous activation of complement on the surface of cells. As a result, PIGA-deficient precursors give rise to RBCs that are inordinately sensitive to the lytic activity of complement. A number of other "PIG-tailed" proteins are also deficient from the membranes of granulocytes and platelets, possibly explaining the striking susceptibility of these patients to *infections* and intravascular *thromboses*.

PIGA is X-linked, and thus normal cells have only a single active *PIGA* gene, mutation of which is sufficient to give rise to PIGA deficiency. As all myeloid lineages are affected in PNH, the responsible mutations must occur in a multipotent stem cell. Remarkably, it is now appreciated that most, if not all, normal individuals harbor small numbers of PIGA-deficient bone marrow cells that have mutations identical to those that cause clinically manifest PNH. It is believed that these mutant cells come to dominate the marrow (thus producing clinically evident PNH) only in very rare instances in which the PIGA-deficient clone has a survival advantage. Consistent with this view, PNH often arises in the setting of primary bone marrow failure (aplastic anemia), which appears most often to be caused by

immune-mediated destruction or suppression of marrow stem cells. It is hypothesized that in PNH patients, autoreactive T cells specifically recognize PIG-tailed surface antigens on normal bone marrow progenitors. Because PIGA-deficient stem cells do not express these targets, they escape immune attack and eventually replace the normal marrow elements. Based on this scenario, immunosuppression is now being evaluated in the treatment PNH.

Immunohemolytic Anemias

These uncommon forms of hemolytic anemia are caused by antibodies that react against normal or altered RBC membranes. Anti-RBC antibodies may arise spontaneously in autoimmune hemolytic anemias, or they may be induced to form by exogenous agents such as drugs or chemicals. Immunohemolytic anemias are classified on the basis of the nature of the antibody involved and possible associated predisposing conditions, which are presented in simplified form in Table 12–4.

Whatever the cause of antibody formation, the diagnosis of immunohemolytic anemias depends on the demonstration of anti-RBC antibodies. The method most commonly used to detect such antibodies is the *Coombs antiglobulin test*, which is based on the capacity of antibodies raised in animals against human immunoglobulins to agglutinate RBCs. A positive result indicates that the patient's RBCs are coated with human antibodies that can react with the antihuman immunoglobulin serum. This is called the *direct Coombs test*. The *indirect Coombs test* is used to detect antibodies in the patient's serum and involves incubating normal RBCs with the patient's serum, followed by a direct Coombs test on these incubated RBCs.

Warm Antibody Immunohemolytic Anemias. These are characterized by the presence of immunoglobulin G (IgG) (rarely, immunoglobulin A [IgA]) antibodies, which are active at 37°C. Many cases (more than 60%) are idiopathic (primary) and belong to the category of autoimmune diseases. Approximately one fourth of the cases are associated with an underlying disease (e.g., systemic lupus erythematosus [SLE]) affecting the immune system or are induced by drugs. The *pathogenesis of hemolysis in most instances involves opsonization of the RBCs by the IgG antibodies and subsequent phagocytosis by splenic*

Table 12–4. CLASSIFICATION OF IMMUNOHEMOLYTIC ANEMIAS

Warm Antibody Type

Primary (idiopathic)
Secondary: B-cell lymphoid neoplasms (e.g., CLL/SLL), SLE, drugs (e.g., α-methyldopa, penicillin, quinidine)

Cold Antibody Type

Acute: *Mycoplasma* infection, infectious mononucleosis
Chronic: idiopathic, B-cell lymphoid neoplasms (e.g., lymphoplasmacytic lymphoma)

CLL/SLL, chronic lymphocytic leukemia/small lymphocytic lymphoma; SLE, systemic lupus erythematosus.

macrophages. Spheroidal cells resembling those found in hereditary spherocytosis are often found in idiopathic immune hemolytic anemia. Presumably, bits of cell membrane are injured and removed during attempted phagocytosis of antibody-coated cells; this reduces the surface area–to-volume ratio, leading to the formation of *spherocytes.* These are destroyed in the spleen, as described earlier (p 398). The clinical severity of immunohemolytic anemia is quite variable. Most patients have chronic mild anemia with moderate splenomegaly and often require no treatment.

The mechanisms of hemolysis induced by drugs are varied and in some cases poorly understood. Drugs such as α-methyldopa induce an anemia indistinguishable from the primary idiopathic form of hemolytic anemia. Autoantibodies directed against intrinsic RBC antigens, in particular Rh blood group antigens, are formed. Presumably, the drug alters native epitopes and thus allows a bypass of T-cell tolerance to the membrane proteins (see Fig. 5–20). In other cases, drugs such as penicillin act as haptens and induce an antibody response by binding to an RBC membrane protein. Sometimes antibodies bind and form immune complexes with the drug in the circulation. These complexes may be deposited on the surface of RBC membranes, which are then damaged or opsonized following the fixation of complement.

Cold Antibody Immunohemolytic Anemias. These anemias are characterized by the presence of low-affinity immunoglobulin M (IgM) antibodies, which bind to RBC membranes at temperatures below 30°C, as may be encountered in distal body parts (e.g., hands, toes). Fixation of complement may cause intravascular hemolysis. However, most commonly the antibody- and complement-coated cells are not lysed, because complement is most active at 37°C. When such antibody- and complement-coated cells travel to warmer areas, the weakly bound IgM antibody is released, and the cell is left with a coating of C3b. Because the latter is an opsonin (Chapter 2), the cells are phagocytosed by the mononuclear phagocyte system, especially Kupffer cells; hence, the *hemolysis is extravascular.* Cold agglutinins occur acutely during recovery from *Mycoplasma* pneumonia and infectious mononucleosis. The resulting anemia is mild, transient, and of no clinical import. Chronic cold agglutinin formation and associated hemolytic anemia may also occur in association with lymphoid neoplasms or as an idiopathic condition. In addition to anemia, Raynaud phenomenon may occur in these patients, owing to agglutination of RBCs in the capillaries of exposed parts of the body.

Hemolytic Anemias Resulting From Mechanical Trauma to Red Cells

RBCs may be disrupted by physical trauma in a variety of circumstances. *Clinically important hemolytic anemias are sometimes caused by cardiac valve prostheses or by narrowing and partial obstruction of the vasculature.* Traumatic hemolytic anemia is more severe with artificial, mechanical valves than with bioprosthetic, porcine valves. In patients with prosthetic valves of either type, the RBCs are damaged by the shear stresses resulting from the turbulent blood flow and abnormal pressure gradients caused by the

Figure 12–8 ■

Microangiopathic hemolytic anemia. The peripheral blood smear from a patient with hemolytic-uremic syndrome shows several fragmented RBCs. (Courtesy of Dr. Robert W. McKenna, Department of Pathology, University of Texas Southwestern Medical School, Dallas.)

valves. Microangiopathic hemolytic anemia, on the other hand, is characterized by mechanical damage to the RBCs as they squeeze through abnormally narrowed vessels. Most often, the narrowing is caused by widespread deposition of fibrin in the small vessels in association with disseminated intravascular coagulation (DIC) (p 444). Other causes of microangiopathic hemolytic anemia include malignant hypertension, SLE, thrombotic thrombocytopenic purpura, hemolytic-uremic syndrome, and disseminated cancer. Most of these disorders are discussed elsewhere in this book. Common to all of these disorders is the presence of vascular lesions that predispose the circulating RBCs to mechanical injury. The morphologic alterations in the injured RBCs (schistocytes) may be striking. Thus, "burr cells," "helmet cells," and "triangle cells" may be seen in the peripheral blood film (Fig. 12–8). It should be pointed out that, except for thrombotic thrombocytopenic purpura and the related hemolytic uremic syndrome, hemolysis is not a major clinical problem in most instances.

Malaria

It has been estimated that 200 million persons suffer from this infectious disease; it is one of the most widespread afflictions of humans. Malaria is endemic in Asia and Africa, but with widespread jet travel, cases are now reported all over the world. The fact that the eradication of malaria is theoretically feasible makes its prevalence even more unfortunate. Malaria is caused by one of four types of protozoa: *Plasmodium vivax* causes benign tertian malaria;

P. malariae causes quartan malaria, another benign form; *P. ovale* causes ovale malaria, a relatively uncommon and benign form similar to vivax malaria; and *P. falciparum* causes tertian malaria (falciparum malaria), a more serious disorder with a high fatality rate. All forms are transmitted only by the bite of female *Anopheles* mosquitoes, and humans are the only natural reservoir.

Etiology and Pathogenesis. The life cycle of plasmodia is complex. As mosquitoes feed, sporozoites are introduced from the saliva and within a few minutes infect human liver cells. The parasites multiply rapidly within liver cells to form a schizont containing thousands of merozoites. After a period of days to several weeks that varies with the *Plasmodium* species, the infected hepatocytes release the merozoites, which quickly infect RBCs. Here they can either continue asexual reproduction to produce more merozoites or give rise to gametocytes that infect the next hungry mosquito. During asexual reproduction in the erythrocytes, the merozoites first develop into trophozoites that are somewhat distinctive for each of the four forms of malaria. Thus, *the specific form of malaria can be recognized in appropriately stained thick smears of peripheral blood.* The asexual phase is completed when the trophozoites give rise to new merozoites, which escape by destroying the RBCs.

Clinical Features. The distinctive clinical and anatomic features of malaria are related to the following events:

1. Showers of new merozoites are released from the RBCs at intervals of approximately 48 hours for *P. vivax, P. ovale,* and *P. falciparum,* and 72 hours for *P. malariae.* The clinical spikes of shaking, chills, and fever coincide with this release.
2. The parasites destroy large numbers of RBCs and thus cause hemolytic anemia.
3. A characteristic brown malarial pigment, probably a derivative of Hb that is identical to hematin, is released from the ruptured RBCs along with the merozoites, discoloring principally the spleen, but also the liver, lymph nodes, and bone marrow.
4. Activation of the phagocytic defense mechanisms of the host leads to marked hyperplasia of the mononuclear phagocyte system throughout the body, reflected in massive splenomegaly. Less frequently, the liver may also be enlarged.

Fatal falciparum malaria is characterized by prominent involvement of the brain, a complication known as cerebral malaria. Normally, RBCs have negatively charged surfaces that interact poorly with endothelial cell surfaces. Infection of RBCs with *P. falciparum* induces the appearance of positively charged surface knobs containing parasite-encoded proteins that promote binding to adhesion molecules expressed on activated endothelium; of these, platelet endothelial cell adhesion molecule 1 (PECAM-1, CD31) and intercellular adhesion molecule 1 (ICAM-1) appear most important. Infected RBCs also form rosettes about uninfected RBCs. This tendency to aggregate and adhere to endothelium leads to sequestration of RBCs in postcapillary venules. Engorged cerebral vessels are full of parasitized RBCs and are often occluded by microthrombi. Cerebral malaria may begin suddenly or slowly, but it is rapidly

progressive, with the development of high fever, chills, convulsions, coma, and death, usually within days to weeks. In other cases, falciparum malaria pursues a more chronic course that may be punctuated at any time by an uncommon but dramatic complication known as *blackwater fever.* The trigger for this complication is obscure, but it is associated with massive hemolysis, leading to jaundice, hemoglobinemia, and hemoglobinuria.

With appropriate chemotherapy, the prognosis for patients with most forms of malaria is good; however, treatment of falciparum malaria is becoming more difficult, owing to the emergence of drug-resistant strains. Because of the potentially serious consequences of this disease, early diagnosis and treatment are particularly important but are sometimes delayed in nonendemic settings. The ultimate solution is an effective vaccine, which is long sought but still elusive.

ANEMIAS OF DIMINISHED ERYTHROPOIESIS

Included in this category are anemias that are caused by an inadequate supply to the bone marrow of some substance necessary for hematopoiesis. The most common deficiencies are those of iron, folic acid, or vitamin B_{12}. Another important cause of impaired erythropoiesis is suppression of marrow stem cells, such as disorders of bone marrow failure (aplastic anemia) and bone marrow infiltration (myelophthisic anemia). In the following sections, some common examples of anemias resulting from nutritional deficiencies and marrow suppression are discussed individually.

Iron Deficiency Anemia

It is estimated that 10% of the population in developed countries and as much as 25% to 50% in developing countries are anemic. Iron deficiency accounts for most of this prevalence. It is without question *the most common form of nutritional deficiency.* The factors responsible for iron deficiency differ somewhat in various populations and can be best considered in the context of normal iron metabolism.

Total body iron content is about 2 g for women and 6 g for men. Approximately 80% of functional body iron is found in Hb; the remainder is in myoglobin and iron-containing enzymes (e.g., catalase and cytochromes). The iron storage pool, represented by hemosiderin and ferritin-bound iron, contains 15% to 20% of total body iron. Stored iron is found in all tissues but particularly in liver, spleen, bone marrow, and skeletal muscle. Because *serum ferritin* is largely derived from the storage pool of iron, its level is a good indicator of the adequacy of body iron stores. *Staining bone marrow* for iron-containing macrophages is another useful and simple method for estimating body iron content. Iron is transported in the plasma by an iron-binding protein called *transferrin.* In normal persons, transferrin is about 33% saturated with iron, yielding serum iron levels that average 120 μg/dL in men and 100 μg/dL in women.

Thus, the total iron-binding capacity of serum is in the range of 300 to 350 μg.

As might be expected given the very high prevalence of iron deficiency in human populations, evolutionary pressures have yielded iron metabolism pathways that are strongly biased toward the retention of iron. There is no regulated pathway for iron excretion, which is limited to the 1 to 2 mg/day that is lost by shedding of mucosal and skin epithelial cells. *Iron balance, therefore, is maintained largely by regulating the absorption of dietary iron.* The normal daily Western diet contains 10 to 20 mg of iron. Most of this is in the form of heme contained in animal products, with the remainder being inorganic iron in vegetables. About 20% of heme iron (in contrast to 1% to 2% of nonheme iron) is absorbable, so the average Western diet contains sufficient iron to balance fixed daily losses. Iron is absorbed in the duodenum, where it must pass through the apical and basolateral membranes to traverse the villus enterocytes (Fig. 12–9). Nonheme iron uptake is carried across each of these two membranes by distinct transporters. Divalent metal transporter 1 (DMT1) first moves dietary nonheme iron across the apical membrane. At least two proteins are then required for the basolateral transfer of iron to transferrin in the plasma: ferroportin, which acts as a transporter, and hephaestin, a ferrioxidase whose precise role is uncertain. Both DMT1 and ferroportin are widely distributed in the body, suggesting their involvement in iron transport in other tissues as well. Dietary heme iron is absorbed through a different mechanism that is not yet understood. As depicted in Figure 12–9, only a proportion of heme as well as nonheme iron that enters the cell is delivered rapidly to plasma transferrin by the action of various tranporters. The remainder is bound to mucosal ferritin within the cell, some to be transported more slowly to the blood and some to be lost with the exfoliation of mucosal cells. When the body is replete with iron, most of the iron that enters the cell is bound to ferritin and is lost with exfoliation; in iron deficiency, or when there is ineffective erythropoiesis, transfer to plasma transferrin is enhanced. The regulatory mechanisms that allow the body to sense total body iron levels and adjust absorption accordingly also remain to be elucidated.

Negative iron balance and consequent anemia may result from low dietary intake, malabsorption, excessive demand, and chronic blood loss:

■ Low dietary intake alone is rarely the cause of iron deficiency in the United States, because the average daily dietary intake of 10 to 20 mg is more than enough for males and about adequate for females. In other parts of the world, however, low intake and poor bioavailability from predominantly vegetarian diets are an important cause of iron deficiency.

■ Malabsorption may occur with sprue and celiac disease or after gastrectomy (Chapter 15).

■ Increased demands not met by normal dietary intake occur around the world during pregnancy and infancy.

■ Chronic blood loss is the most important cause of iron deficiency anemia in the Western world; this loss may occur from the gastrointestinal tract (e.g., peptic ulcers, colonic cancer, hemorrhoids, hookworm disease) or the female genital tract (e.g., menorrhagia, metrorrhagia, cancers).

Regardless of the cause, iron deficiency develops insidiously. At first there is depletion of stored iron, which is marked by a *decline in serum ferritin and depletion of stainable iron in the bone marrow.* There follows a decrease in circulating iron, with a low level of serum iron and a rise in the serum transferrin iron-binding capacity. Ultimately, the inadequacy makes its impact on Hb, myoglobin, and other iron compounds. With more significant deficits, impaired work performance and brain function and reduced immunocompetence may develop.

MORPHOLOGY

Except in unusual circumstances, iron deficiency anemia is relatively mild. The RBCs are **microcytic** and **hypochromic**, reflecting the reduced MCV and MCHC (Fig. 12–10). For unclear reasons, iron deficiency is often accompanied by an increase in the platelet count. Although there is normoblastic hyperplasia, it is limited by the availability of iron, and thus active marrow is usually only slightly increased. Extramedullary hematopoiesis is uncommon.

Figure 12-9 ■

Diagrammatic representation of iron absorption. Mucosal uptake of heme and nonheme iron is depicted. When the storage sites of the body are replete with iron and erythropoietic activity is normal, most of the absorbed iron is lost into the gut by shedding of the epithelial cells. Conversely, when body iron needs increase or when erythropoiesis is stimulated, a greater fraction of the absorbed iron is transferred into plasma transferrin, with a concomitant decrease in iron loss through mucosal ferritin.

In some cases, atrophic glossitis is present, giving the tongue a smooth, glazed appearance. When this is accompanied by dysphagia and esophageal webs, it constitutes the **Plummer-Vinson syndrome.**

Clinical Course. In most instances, iron deficiency anemia is asymptomatic. Nonspecific manifestations, such as weakness, listlessness, and pallor, may be present in severe cases. With long-standing severe anemia, thinning, flattening, and eventually "spooning" of the fingernails sometimes appears. A curious but characteristic neurobehavioral complication is *pica,* the compunction to consume nonfood-stuffs such as dirt or clay.

Diagnostic criteria include low Hb levels; low HCT; low mean corpuscular volume; hypochromic microcytic RBCs; low serum ferritin; low serum iron levels; low transferrin saturation; increased total iron-binding capacity; and, ultimately, response to iron therapy. Persons frequently die *with* this form of anemia but rarely *of* it. It is important to remember that in reasonably well-nourished persons, microcytic hypochromic anemia is not a disease but rather a symptom of some underlying disorder.

Anemia of Chronic Disease

This is the most common form of anemia in hospitalized patients. It superficially resembles the anemia of iron

Figure 12–10   ■

Hypochromic microcytic anemia of iron deficiency. Note the small RBCs containing a narrow rim of hemoglobin at the periphery. Contrast to the scattered, fully hemoglobinized cells derived from a recent blood transfusion given to the patient. (Courtesy of Dr. Robert W. McKenna, Department of Pathology, University of Texas Southwestern Medical School, Dallas.)

deficiency, but it stems from inflammation-induced sequestration of iron within the cells of the reticuloendothelial system. It occurs in a variety of chronic inflammatory disorders, including the following:

■ Chronic microbial infections such as osteomyelitis, bacterial endocarditis, and lung abscess
■ Chronic immune disorders such as rheumatoid arthritis and regional enteritis
■ Neoplasms such as Hodgkin disease and carcinomas of the lung and breast

The anemia of chronic disease is associated with low serum iron, and the RBCs may be normocytic and normochromic or hypochromic and microcytic, as in anemia of iron deficiency. However, *the presence of increased storage iron in the marrow macrophages, a high serum ferritin level, and reduced total iron-binding capacity readily rule out iron deficiency as the cause of anemia.* This combination of findings results from a block in the transfer of iron from the mononuclear phagocyte storage pool to the erythroid precursors. In addition, the compensatory increase in erythropoietin levels is not adequate for the degree of anemia. The teleologic explanation for iron sequestration in the presence of a wide variety of chronic inflammatory disorders is unclear; it may serve to inhibit the growth of iron-dependent microorganisms or to augment certain aspects of host immunity.

The common feature among the diverse diseases associated with the anemia of chronic disease is that all induce a prolonged state of systemic inflammation. The suppression of erythropoiesis and sequestration of iron in the storage compartment result from the action of a number of the inflammatory mediators, including interleukin 1 (IL-1), tumor necrosis factor (TNF), and interferon-α, which are secreted in response to the underlying chronic inflammatory or neoplastic disease. Administration of erythropoietin may improve the anemia, but only effective treatment of the underlying condition reliably corrects the anemia.

Megaloblastic Anemias

There are two principal types of megaloblastic anemia: one caused by a folate deficiency and another caused by a lack of vitamin B_{12}. These anemias may be caused by a nutritional deficiency (e.g., of folic acid [folate]), or they may result from impaired absorption, as is the case with vitamin B_{12}. Both of these vitamins are required for DNA synthesis, and, hence, the effects of their deficiency on erythropoiesis are quite similar.

Pathogenesis. The morphologic hallmark of megaloblastic anemias is an enlargement of erythroid precursors (termed *megaloblasts*), which gives rise to abnormally large RBCs (macrocytes). The other myeloid lineages are also affected. Most notably, granulocyte precursors are also enlarged (*giant metamyelocytes*), yielding highly characteristic *hypersegmented neutrophils*. Underlying the cellular gigantism is an impairment of DNA synthesis, which results in a delay in nuclear maturation and cell division. Because the synthesis of RNA and cytoplasmic elements proceeds at a normal rate and thus outpaces that of the nucleus, hematopoietic precursors in megaloblastic anemias exhibit *nuclear-cytoplasmic* *asynchrony.* This maturational derangement contributes to anemia in several ways. Some megaloblasts are so defective in DNA synthesis that they undergo apoptosis in the marrow without producing any RBCs (ineffective hematopoiesis). Others succeed in giving rise to some mature RBCs, but because they do so after fewer cell divisions, the total output from these precursors is diminished. Granulocyte and platelet precursors are similarly affected. As a result, most patients with megaloblastic anemia exhibit pancytopenia (anemia, thrombocytopenia, granulocytopenia). Finally, the abnormally large RBCs produced by megaloblasts are prone to premature destruction by the mononuclear phagocyte system. This increased breakdown of RBCs and precursors leads to iron accumulation, mostly in the mononuclear phagocytic cells of the bone marrow.

MORPHOLOGY

Certain morphologic features are common to all forms of megaloblastic anemias. The **bone marrow** is markedly hypercellular, owing to increased numbers of **megaloblasts.** These cells are larger than normoblasts and have a delicate, finely reticulated nuclear chromatin (suggestive of nuclear immaturity) and an abundant, strikingly basophilic cytoplasm (Fig. 12–11). As the megaloblasts differentiate and begin to acquire Hb, the nucleus retains its finely distributed chromatin and fails to undergo the chromatin clumping typical of an orthochromatic normoblast. Similarly, the granulocytic precursors also demonstrate nuclear-cytoplasmic asynchrony, yielding giant metamyelocytes. Megakaryocytes, too, may be abnormally large, with bizarre multilobed nuclei.

In the **peripheral blood,** the earliest change is usually the appearance of **hypersegmented neutrophils.** These appear even before the onset of anemia. Although the normal number of lobes in a neutrophil nucleus is three or four, with megaloblastic anemias this number may be markedly increased, to five, six, or more. **Erythrocytes are typically large and oval (macro-ovalocytes), with mean corpuscular volumes often over 110 fL** (normal, 82 to 92 fL). Large, misshapen platelets may also be seen. Although macrocytes appear hyperchromic because of their large size, in reality the MCHC is normal. Morphologic changes in other systems, especially the gastrointestinal tract, may also occur, giving rise to some of the clinical features.

Figure 12–11 ■

Comparison of normoblasts *(left)* and megaloblasts *(right)*. The megaloblasts are larger, have relatively immature nuclei with finely reticulated chromatin, and have an abundant basophilic cytoplasm. (Courtesy of Dr. José Hernandez, Department of Pathology, University of Texas Southwestern Medical School, Dallas.)

FOLATE (FOLIC ACID) DEFICIENCY ANEMIA

Megaloblastic anemia secondary to a lack of folate is not common, but marginal folate stores are surprisingly common. High risk of clinically significant folate deficiency is associated with poor diet (as in the economically deprived, the indigent, and the elderly) and increased metabolic needs (as in pregnant women and patients with chronic hemolytic anemias).

Ironically, folate is widely prevalent in nearly all foods but is readily destroyed by 10 to 15 minutes of cooking. Thus, the best sources of folate are fresh or fresh-frozen vegetables and fruits eaten either uncooked or lightly cooked. Food folates are predominantly in polyglutamate form, and most must be split into monoglutamates for absorption. Acidic foods and substances found in beans and other legumes hamper absorption by inhibiting intestinal conjugases that catalyze the formation of monoglutamates from polyglutamates. Phenytoin (Dilantin) and a few other drugs also inhibit folate absorption. Others, such as methotrexate, inhibit folate metabolism (see later). The principal site of intestinal absorption is the upper third of the small intestine, so malabsorptive disorders such as celiac disease and tropical sprue, which affect this level of the gut, impair absorption.

The metabolism and physiologic functions of folate are complex. It is sufficient here to note that, after absorption, folate is transported in the blood mainly as a monoglutamate. Within cells it undergoes conversion to several derivatives, but of principal importance is that it must be reduced to tetrahydrofolate by a reductase. (This reductase is sensitive to inhibition by folate analogues such as methotrexate, which deprives cells of folate and the capacity to rapidly divide—a property that is the basis for the use of folate antagonists as antineoplastic agents.) Tetrahydrofolate acts as an acceptor and donor of one-carbon units in a variety of steps involved in the synthesis of purines and thymidylate, the building blocks of DNA, and its deficiency accounts for the inadequate DNA synthesis that is characteristic of megaloblastic anemia.

The onset of the anemia is insidious and is associated with nonspecific symptoms such as weakness and easy fatigability. The clinical picture may be complicated by coexistent deficiency of other vitamins, especially in alcoholics. Because the gastrointestinal tract, like the hematopoietic system, is a site of rapid cell turnover, symptoms referable to the alimentary tract are common and often severe. These include sore tongue and cheilosis. *It should be stressed that unlike in vitamin B_{12} deficiency, neurologic abnormalities do not occur.*

The diagnosis of a megaloblastic anemia is readily made from examination of a smear of peripheral blood and bone marrow. The important differentiation between the anemia of folate deficiency and that of vitamin B_{12} deficiency is best accomplished by assays for serum folate and vitamin B_{12} and determination of RBC folate levels.

VITAMIN B_{12} (COBALAMIN) DEFICIENCY ANEMIA: PERNICIOUS ANEMIA

Inadequate levels of vitamin B_{12}, or cobalamin, in the body result in a megaloblastic macrocytic anemia similar hematologically to that of folate deficiency. However, a deficiency of vitamin B_{12} also causes a demyelinating disorder involving the peripheral nerves and, ultimately and most importantly, the spinal cord. There are many causes of vitamin B_{12} deficiency. The term *pernicious anemia* (PA), a relic of the days when the cause and therapy of this condition were unknown, is used to describe vitamin B_{12} deficiency resulting from inadequate gastric production or defective function of intrinsic factor (IF) necessary to absorb B_{12}. IF plays a critical role in the absorption of vitamin B_{12}, as will be evident from the following sequence of events involved in vitamin B_{12} absorption:

■ Peptic digestion releases dietary vitamin B_{12}, which is then bound to salivary B_{12}-binding proteins called *cobalophilins*, or *R binders.*

■ R-B_{12} complexes, transported to the duodenum, are split by pancreatic proteases, and the released B_{12} attaches to IF secreted by the parietal cells of the gastric fundic mucosa.

■ The IF-B_{12} complex passes to the distal ileum, where it attaches to the epithelial IF receptors, followed by absorption of vitamin B_{12}.

■ The absorbed B_{12} is bound to transport proteins called *transcobalamins*, which then deliver it to the liver and other cells of the body.

Etiology. Among the many potential causes of cobalamin deficiency, malabsorption is the most common and important. A dietary deficiency of cobalamin is virtually limited to strict vegetarians. This nutrient is abundant in all animal foods, including eggs and dairy products. Indeed, bacterial contamination of water and nonanimal foods may provide adequate amounts of vitamin B_{12}; it is stored in the liver and efficiently reabsorbed from the bile, so 5 to 20 years are required to deplete the normal reserves. Moreover, it is resistant to cooking and boiling. A tiny daily supply, therefore, suffices. Thus, a dietary lack of vitamin B_{12} is uncommon; until proved otherwise, *a deficiency of this nutrient (in the Western world) implies PA secondary to inadequate production or function of IF.*

The deranged synthesis of IF appears to be caused by an autoimmune reaction against parietal cells and IF itself, producing gastric mucosal atrophy (Chapter 15). Several findings favor the concept of gastric autoimmunity:

1. Autoantibodies are present in the serum and gastric juice of most patients with PA. Three types of antibodies have

been found: *parietal canalicular antibodies* bind to the mucosal parietal cells; *blocking antibodies* block the binding of vitamin B_{12} to IF; and *binding antibodies* react with IF-B_{12} complex and prevent it from binding to the ileal receptor.

2. The association of PA with other autoimmune diseases such as Hashimoto thyroiditis, Addison disease, and type I diabetes mellitus is well documented.

3. The frequency of serum antibodies to IF is increased in patients with other autoimmune diseases.

In addition to PA, malabsorption of vitamin B_{12} may result from gastrectomy, which leads to loss of IF-producing cells; resection of ileum, the site of absorption of the IF-B_{12} complex; and disorders that involve the distal ileum, such as regional enteritis, tropical sprue, and Whipple disease. In individuals older than 70 years of age, gastric atrophy and achlorhydria interfere with vitamin B_{12} absorption. In the absence of acid-pepsin, the vitamin is not released from its bound form in the diet.

The metabolic defects induced by a vitamin B_{12} deficiency are intertwined with folate metabolism. Vitamin B_{12} is required for recycling of tetrahydrofolate, and hence its deficiency reduces the availability of the form of folate that is required for DNA synthesis. This concept is supported by the fact that the anemia of vitamin B_{12} deficiency improves with administration of folates, whereas the anemia of folate deficiency is unaffected by supplementation of vitamin B_{12}. The biochemical basis of the neuropathy in vitamin B_{12} deficiency is unclear. Although both folate and vitamin B_{12} deficiency give rise to megaloblastic anemia, neurologic disease does not occur in patients with folate deficiency, and administration of folate may actually exacerbate the neurologic disease caused by vitamin B_{12} deficiency. It thus appears that the function of vitamin B_{12} in the nervous system is independent of its effects on folate metabolism. The principal neurologic lesions associated with vitamin B_{12} deficiency are *demyelination of the posterior and lateral columns of the spinal cord*, sometimes beginning in the peripheral nerves. In time, axonal degeneration may supervene. The severity of neurologic manifestations is not related to the degree of anemia. Indeed, uncommonly, the neurologic disease may occur in the absence of overt megaloblastic anemia.

Clinical Features. Manifestations of vitamin B_{12} deficiency are nonspecific; as with any other anemia, there is pallor, easy fatigability, and, in severe cases, dyspnea and even congestive heart failure. Increased destruction of erythroid progenitors may give rise to mild jaundice. Gastrointestinal symptoms similar to those described under folate deficiency may also be present. Neurologic changes, such as symmetric numbness, tingling, and burning in feet or hands, followed by unsteadiness of gait and loss of position sense, particularly in the toes, may also be present. Although the anemia responds dramatically to parenteral vitamin B_{12}, the neurologic manifestations often fail to resolve. As discussed in Chapter 15, patients with PA have an increased risk of gastric carcinoma.

The diagnostic features of PA include (1) low serum vitamin B_{12} levels; (2) normal or elevated serum folate levels; (3) histamine-fast gastric achlorhydria (caused by loss of gastric parietal cells); (4) serum anti-IF antibodies; (5)

inability to absorb an oral dose of cobalamin (the Schilling test); (6) moderate to severe megaloblastic anemia; (7) leukopenia with hypersegmented granulocytes; and (8) dramatic reticulocytic response (within 2 or 3 days) to parenteral administration of vitamin B_{12}.

Aplastic Anemia

Aplastic anemia is a disorder characterized by the *suppression of multipotent myeloid stem cells, with resultant anemia, thrombocytopenia, and neutropenia (pancytopenia)* Notwithstanding its name, aplastic anemia should not be confused with selective suppression of erythroid stem cells (pure red cell aplasia), in which anemia is the only manifestation.

Etiology and Pathogenesis. In more than half of cases, aplastic anemia appears without any apparent cause and so is termed *idiopathic.* In other cases, exposure to a known myelotoxic agent can be identified, such as whole-body irradiation (as may occur in nuclear plant accidents) or use of myelotoxic drugs. Drugs and chemicals are the most common causes of secondary aplastic anemia. With some agents, the marrow damage is predictable, dose related, and usually reversible. Included in this category are antineoplastic drugs (e.g., alkylating agents, antimetabolites), benzene, and chloramphenicol. In other instances, marrow toxicity occurs as an apparent "idiosyncratic" or sensitivity reaction to small doses of known myelotoxic drugs (e.g., chloramphenicol) or after the use of such agents as phenylbutazone, sulfonamides, or methylphenylethylhydantoin, which are not myelotoxic in other persons.

Aplastic anemia sometimes arises after certain viral infections, most often community-acquired viral hepatitis. The specific virus responsible is not known; hepatitis viruses A, B, and C are apparently not the culprits. Marrow aplasia develops insidiously several months after recovery from the hepatitis and follows a relentless course.

The pathogenetic events leading to marrow failure remain vague, but it increasingly appears that autoreactive T cells play an important role. This is supported by a variety of experimental data and clinical experience, which has shown that acquired aplastic anemia responds to immunosuppressive therapy aimed at T cells (e.g., cyclosporine and antithymocyte globulin) in 70% to 80% of cases. Much less clear are the events that trigger the T-cell attack on marrow stem cells; perhaps viral antigens, drug-derived haptens, and/or genetic damage create neoantigens within stem cells that serve as targets for autoreactive T cells.

MORPHOLOGY

The bone marrow typically is markedly hypocellular, with greater than 90% of the intertrabecular space being occupied by fat. These changes are better appreciated in a bone marrow biopsy specimen than in marrow aspirates, which often yield a "dry tap" because of hypocellularity. In marrow biopsy specimens, small foci of lymphocytes and plasma cells may be seen. A number of secondary changes may accompany marrow failure. Hepatic fatty change may result from anemia, and thrombocytopenia and granulocytopenia may give rise to hemorrhages and bacterial infections, respectively. Multiple transfusions may cause hemosiderosis.

Clinical Course. Aplastic anemia affects persons of all ages and both sexes. Slowly progressive anemia causes the insidious development of weakness, pallor, and dyspnea. Thrombocytopenia often presents as the appearance of petechiae and ecchymoses. *Granulocytopenia* may be manifested only by frequent and persistent minor infections or by the sudden onset of chills, fever, and prostration. It is important to distinguish aplastic anemia from anemias caused by marrow infiltration (myelophthisic anemia), "aleukemic leukemia," and granulomatous diseases. Because pancytopenia is common to these conditions, their clinical manifestations may be indistinguishable. However, with aplastic anemia the marrow is hypocellular, owing to stem cell failure, whereas in myelophthisic anemias and other conditions listed above, the marrow is replaced by abnormal neoplastic or inflammatory elements. *Splenomegaly is characteristically absent* in aplastic anemia; if it is present, the diagnosis of aplastic anemia should be seriously questioned. Typically, the RBCs are normocytic and normochromic, although slight macrocytosis is occasionally present; *reticulocytosis is absent.*

The prognosis of marrow aplasia is quite unpredictable. As mentioned earlier, withdrawal of toxic drugs may lead to recovery in some cases. The idiopathic form has a poor prognosis if left untreated. Bone marrow transplantation is an extremely effective form of therapy, especially in patients younger than 40 years, if performed in nontransfused patients. It is hypothesized that transfusion results in a further stimulation of T cells, producing a high engraftment failure rate in transplant recipients. As mentioned earlier, patients who are older, lack a donor, or have been multiply transfused benefit from immunosuppressive therapy.

Myelophthisic Anemia

This form of marrow failure is caused by extensive replacement of the marrow by tumors or other lesions. It is most commonly associated with metastatic cancer arising from a primary lesion in the breast, lung, prostate, or thyroid. Multiple myeloma, lymphomas, leukemias, advanced tuberculosis, lipid storage disorders, and osteosclerosis are less commonly implicated. Myelophthisic anemia is also seen with progressive fibrosis of the bone marrow (myelofibrosis), discussed later (p 440). The manifestations of marrow infiltration include anemia and thrombocytopenia. The white cell series is less affected. Characteristically, misshapen and immature RBCs, which may resemble teardrops, are seen in the peripheral blood, along with a slightly elevated white cell count. Immature granulocytic and erythrocytic precursors may also be seen (leukoerythroblastosis). Treatment obviously involves the management of the underlying condition.

Laboratory Diagnosis of Anemias

The diagnosis of anemia is established by low Hb, reduced HCT, and reduced numbers of RBCs. Examination of peripheral smears allows the categorization of anemias into major morphologic subgroups: normocytic normochromic, microcytic hypochromic, and macrocytic. In addition, abnormalities in RBC shape and size, such as the presence of spherocytes, sickled cells, and fragmented cells, provide additional clues to the etiology of anemia. In suspected hemoglobinopathies, electrophoresis allows detection of abnormal Hbs such as HbS by their pattern of migration. Immunologically mediated hemolysis of RBCs is confirmed by the Coombs test. Reticulocyte counts are extremely useful in the work-up of anemias. This simple measurement indicates whether the anemia is caused by impaired RBC production, in which case the reticulocyte count is low, or by increased RBC destruction. The latter is accompanied by reticulocytosis as the marrow undergoes erythroid hyperplasia. Biochemical tests, such as serum iron, serum iron–binding capacity, transferrin saturation, and serum ferritin levels, are required to distinguish between hypochromic microcytic anemias caused by iron deficiency, anemia of chronic disease, and thalassemia minor. The distinction between the two major causes of megaloblastic anemias is achieved by measurement of serum and RBC folate and vitamin B_{12} levels. Unconjugated hyperbilirubinemia supports the diagnosis of hemolytic anemia but is not useful in distinguishing among various forms. Much more sensitive than serum bilirubin is serum haptoglobin, because its level is markedly reduced in all forms of hemolytic anemia. In isolated anemia, tests performed on the peripheral blood usually suffice to establish a cause. In contrast, when anemia occurs in combination with thrombocytopenia and/or granulocytopenia, it is much more likely to be associated with marrow aplasia or infiltration; and in these instances marrow examination is often critical for diagnosis.

POLYCYTHEMIA

Polycythemia, or *erythrocytosis*, as it is sometimes referred to, denotes an increased concentration of RBCs, usually with a corresponding increase in Hb level. Such an increase may be *relative*, when there is hemoconcentration caused by decreased plasma volume, or *absolute*, when there is an increase in total RBC mass. Relative polycythemia results from any cause of dehydration, such as deprivation of water, prolonged vomiting, diarrhea, or excessive use of diuretics. Absolute polycythemia is said to be *primary* when the increase in RBC mass results from an autonomous proliferation of the myeloid stem cells and *secondary* when the RBC progenitors are normal but proliferate in response to increased levels of erythropoietin. Primary polycythemia (polycythemia vera) is one of several expressions of clonal, neoplastic proliferation of myeloid stem cells and is therefore considered later in this chapter with other myeloproliferative disorders. Secondary polycythemias may be caused by an increase in erythropoietin secretion that is physiologically appropriate or by an inappropriate (pathologic) secretion of erythropoietin (Table 12–5).

■

Table 12-5.   PATHOPHYSIOLOGIC CLASSIFICATION OF POLYCYTHEMIA

Relative

Reduced plasma volume (hemoconcentration)

Absolute

Primary: Abnormal proliferation of myeloid stem cells, normal or low erythropoietin levels (polycythemia vera); inherited activating mutations in the erythropoietin receptor (rare)
Secondary: Increased erythropoietin levels
  Appropriate: lung disease, high-altitude living, cyanotic heart disease
  Inappropriate: erythropoietin-secreting tumors (e.g., renal cell carcinoma, hepatoma, cerebellar hemangioblastoma); surreptitious erythropoietin use (e.g., in endurance athletes)

White Cell Disorders

Disorders of white cells may be associated with a deficiency of leukocytes (leukopenias) or with proliferations that may be reactive or neoplastic. Reactive proliferation in response to an underlying primary, often microbial, disease is fairly common. Neoplastic disorders, although less common, are more ominous; they cause approximately 9% of all cancer deaths in adults and a staggering 40% in children younger than 15 years. In the following discussion we first describe some non-neoplastic conditions and then consider in some detail malignant proliferations of white cells.

NON-NEOPLASTIC DISORDERS OF WHITE CELLS

Under this heading are included leukopenias as well as nonspecific and specific reactive proliferations.

Leukopenia

A decrease in the peripheral white cell count may occur because of decreased numbers of any of the specific types of leukocytes, but most often it involves the neutrophils (neutropenia). Lymphopenias are much less common; they are associated with congenital immunodeficiency diseases or are acquired in association with specific clinical states, such as advanced human immunodeficiency virus (HIV) infection or treatment with corticosteroids. Only the more common leukopenias that affect granulocytes are discussed here.

NEUTROPENIA/AGRANULOCYTOSIS

A reduction in the number of granulocytes in blood is known as *neutropenia* or sometimes, when severe, as *agranulocytosis*. Characteristically, the total white cell count is reduced to 1000/μL and in some instances to as few as 200 to 300/μL. Affected persons are extremely susceptible to infections, which may be severe enough to cause death.

Etiology and Pathogenesis. The mechanisms that cause neutropenia can be broadly divided into two categories:

■ *Inadequate or ineffective granulopoiesis.* Reduced granulopoiesis may be a manifestation of generalized marrow failure, such as occurs in aplastic anemia and a variety of leukemias. Cancer chemotherapy agents also produce neutropenia by inducing transient marrow aplasia. Alternatively, some neutropenias are isolated, with only the differentiation of committed granulocytic precursors being affected. These are most commonly caused by certain drugs, or, more rarely, by neoplastic proliferations of large granular lymphocytes (so-called LGL leukemia).
■ *Accelerated removal or destruction of neutrophils.* This may be encountered with immune-mediated injury to neutrophils, triggered in some cases by drugs such as aminopyrine, or it may be idiopathic. Increased peripheral utilization may occur in overwhelming bacterial, fungal, or rickettsial infections. An enlarged spleen may also lead to accelerated removal of neutrophils by sequestration.

MORPHOLOGY

Anatomic alterations in bone marrow depend on the underlying basis of the neutropenia. **Marrow hypercellularity** caused by increased numbers of immature granulocytic precursors is seen when the neutropenia results from excessive destruction of the mature neutrophils or in ineffective granulopoiesis, such as occurs in megaloblastic anemia. In contrast, agents that suppress granulocytopoiesis are associated with **a marked decrease in maturing granulocytic precursors in the marrow.** Erythropoiesis and megakaryopoiesis may remain at normal levels (if the agent specifically affects granulocytes); but with certain myelotoxic drugs, all marrow elements may be affected.

Clinical Course. The initial symptoms are often malaise, chills, and fever, followed by marked weakness and fatigability. Infections constitute the major problem; they commonly present as ulcerating, necrotizing lesions of the gingiva, floor of the mouth, buccal mucosa, pharynx, or other sites within the oral cavity (agranulocytic angina). All of these lesions often show massive growth of microorganisms, with a relatively poor leukocyte response. In addition to removal of the offending drug and control of infections, current treatment efforts also include administration of recombinant hematopoietic growth factors, such as granulocyte colony-stimulating factor, which stimulate neutrophil production by the bone marrow.

Reactive Leukocytosis

An increase in the number of white cells is a common reaction in a variety of inflammatory states caused by microbial and nonmicrobial stimuli. Leukocytoses are relatively nonspecific and can be classified on the basis of the particular white cell series affected (Table 12–6). As will be discussed later, in some cases reactive leukocytosis may mimic leukemia. Such *leukemoid* reactions must be distinguished from true malignancies of the white cells. Infectious mononucleosis, a form of lymphocytosis

---

■

Table 12-6. CAUSES OF LEUKOCYTOSIS

Neutrophilic Leukocytosis

Acute bacterial infections, especially those caused by pyogenic organisms; sterile inflammation caused by, for example, tissue necrosis (myocardial infarction, burns)

Eosinophilic Leukocytosis (Eosinophilia)

Allergic disorders such as asthma, hay fever, allergic skin diseases (e.g., pemphigus, dermatitis herpetiformis); parasitic infestations; drug reactions; certain malignancies (e.g., Hodgkin disease and some non-Hodgkin lymphomas); collagen vascular disorders and some vasculitides; atheroembolic disease (transient)

Basophilic Leukocytosis (Basophilia)

Rare, often indicative of a myeloproliferative disease (e.g., chronic myelogenous leukemia)

Monocytosis

Chronic infections (e.g., tuberculosis), bacterial endocarditis, rickettsiosis, and malaria; collagen vascular diseases (e.g., systemic lupus erythematosus); and inflammatory bowel diseases (e.g., ulcerative colitis)

Lymphocytosis

Accompanies monocytosis in many disorders associated with chronic immunologic stimulation (e.g., tuberculosis, brucellosis); viral infections (e.g., hepatitis A, cytomegalovirus, Epstein-Barr virus); *Bordetella pertussis* infection caused by Epstein-Barr virus (EBV) infection, merits separate consideration because it gives rise to a distinctive syndrome.

INFECTIOUS MONONUCLEOSIS

In the Western world, infectious mononucleosis (IM) is an acute, self-limited disease of adolescents and young adults (it is common in college students) that is caused by B lymphocytotropic EBV, a member of the herpesvirus family. The infection is characterized mainly by (1) fever, sore throat, and generalized lymphadenitis; (2) an increase of lymphocytes in blood, many of which have an atypical morphology; and (3) a humoral antibody response to EBV. It should be noted that cytomegalovirus may induce a similar syndrome that can be differentiated only by serologic methods.

Epidemiology and Immunology. EBV is ubiquitous in all human populations. Where economic deprivation results in inadequate living standards, EBV infection early in life is nearly universal. At this age, symptomatic disease is uncommon, and despite the fact that infected hosts develop an immune response (described later), more than half of the population continues to be virus shedders, explaining the dissemination of infection. In contrast, in developed countries that enjoy better standards of hygiene, infection is usually delayed until adolescence or young adulthood. Perhaps better standards of health and less underlying intercurrent chronic disease permit a more effective immune response to the EBV, so only about 20% of healthy seropositive persons shed the virus. Concomitantly, only about 50% of those exposed acquire the infection. Transmission to a seronegative "kissing cousin" usually involves direct intimate oral contact. It is hypothesized (but has not been proven formally) that the virus initially infects oropharyngeal epithelial cells and then spreads to underlying lymphoid tissue (tonsils and adenoids) where B lymphocytes, which have receptors for EBV, are infected. Infection of B cells takes one of two forms. In a minority of B cells, a productive infection leads to cellular lysis and release of virions. In most cells, however, the infection is nonproductive, and the viral DNA persists in latent form as an extrachromosomal episome. *B cells that are latently infected with EBV undergo polyclonal activation and proliferation,* owing to the action of several EBV-encoded polypeptides. They disseminate in the circulation and secrete antibodies with several specificities, including the well-known heterophil anti-sheep RBC antibodies used for the diagnosis of IM. During this early acute infection, virus produced in infected cells is shed into the saliva; it is not known if the source of these virions is oropharyngeal epithelial cells or B cells.

A normal immune response is extremely important in controlling the proliferation of EBV-infected B cells and cell-free virus. Early in the course of the infection, IgM, and later IgG, antibodies are formed against viral capsid antigens. The latter persist for life. More important in the control of polyclonal B-cell proliferation are cytotoxic CD8+ T cells and natural killer (NK) cells. *Virus-specific cytotoxic T cells appear as atypical lymphocytes in the circulation,* which is characteristic of this disease. In otherwise healthy persons, the fully developed humoral and cellular responses to EBV act as brakes on viral shedding,

limiting the number of infected B cells rather than eliminating them. Latent EBV remains in a few B cells and possibly oropharyngeal epithelial cells as well. As will be seen, impaired immunity in the host can have disastrous consequences.

MORPHOLOGY

The major alterations involve the blood, lymph nodes, spleen, liver, central nervous system, and, occasionally, other organs. The **peripheral blood** shows absolute lymphocytosis with a total white cell count between 12,000 and 18,000/µL, more than 60% of which are lymphocytes. Many of these are large, **atypical lymphocytes**, 12 to 16 µm in diameter, characterized by an abundant cytoplasm containing multiple clear vacuolations and an oval, indented, or folded nucleus (Fig. 12–12). These atypical lymphocytes bear T-cell markers and are usually sufficiently distinctive to suggest the diagnosis from examination of a peripheral blood smear.

The **lymph nodes** are typically discrete and enlarged throughout the body, principally in the posterior cervical, axillary, and groin regions. Histologically, the lymphoid tissue is flooded by atypical lymphocytes, which occupy the paracortical (T-cell) areas. There is in addition some B-cell reaction, with enlargement of follicles. Occasionally, cells resembling Reed-Sternberg cells (p 432), the hallmark of Hodgkin lymphoma, may also be found in the nodes. Because of these atypical features, special tests are sometimes needed to distinguish the reactive changes of IM from malignant lymphoma.

The **spleen** is enlarged in most cases, weighing between 300 and 500 g. The histologic changes are analogous to those of the lymph nodes,

---

Figure 12–12   ■

Atypical lymphocytes in infectious mononucleosis. The cell on the left is a typical small lymphocyte with a compact nucleus filling the entire cytoplasm. In contrast, an atypical lymphocyte on the right has abundant cytoplasm and a large nucleus with fine chromatin.

showing a heavy infiltration of atypical lymphocytes. The rapid increase in splenic size and the infiltration of the trabeculae and capsule by the lymphocytes together contribute to making such spleens fragile; splenic rupture may occur after even minor trauma.

Liver function is almost always transiently impaired to some degree. Histologically, atypical lymphocytes are seen in the portal areas and sinusoids, and scattered, isolated cells or foci of parenchymal necrosis filled with lymphocytes may be present. This histologic picture may be difficult to distinguish from that of other forms of viral hepatitis.

Clinical Course. Although classically *IM presents as fever, sore throat, lymphadenitis,* and the other features mentioned earlier, quite often it is more aberrant in behavior. It may present (1) with little or no fever and only malaise, fatigue, and lymphadenopathy, raising the specter of leukemia-lymphoma; (2) as a fever of unknown origin without significant lymphadenopathy or other localized findings; (3) as hepatitis that is difficult to differentiate from one of the hepatotropic viral syndromes (Chapter 16); or (4) as a febrile rash resembling rubella. Ultimately, the diagnosis depends on the following findings, in increasing order of specificity: (1) lymphocytosis with the characteristic atypical lymphocytes in the peripheral blood, (2) a positive heterophil reaction (monospot test), and (3) specific antibodies for EBV antigens (viral capsid antigens, early antigens, or Epstein-Barr nuclear antigen). In most patients, IM resolves within 4 to 6 weeks, but sometimes the fatigue lasts longer. Occasionally, one or more complications supervene. These may involve virtually any organ or system in the body. Perhaps most common is marked hepatic dysfunction, with jaundice; elevated hepatic enzyme levels; disturbed appetite; and, rarely, even liver failure. Other complications involve the nervous system, kidneys, bone marrow, lungs, eyes, heart, and spleen (splenic rupture has been fatal).

EBV is a potent transforming virus that plays a role in a number of human malignancies, including several types of B-cell lymphoma (Chapter 6). A serious complication in those lacking T-cell immunity (particularly organ and bone marrow transplant recipients) is that the EBV-driven B-cell proliferation may run amok, leading to death. This process can be initiated by an acute infection or the reactivation of a latent B-cell infection and generally begins as a polyclonal proliferation that progresses to overt monoclonal B-cell lymphoma over time. Reconstitution of immunity (e.g., by cessation of immunosuppressive therapy) is sometimes sufficient to cause complete regression of the B-cell proliferation, which is uniformly fatal if left untreated.

The importance of T cells and NK cells is also driven home by X-linked lymphoproliferative syndrome, a rare inherited immunodeficiency characterized by inability to mount an immune response against EBV. Most affected boys have a mutation in the *SH2D1A* gene, which encodes a signaling protein that is important in the activation of T cells and NK cells. On exposure to EBV, these boys develop an overwhelming infection that is usually fatal.

Reactive Lymphadenitis

Infections and nonmicrobial inflammatory stimuli not only cause leukocytosis but also involve the lymph nodes, which act as defensive barriers. Here an immune response against foreign antigens develops, a process often associated with lymph node enlargement (lymphadenopathy). The infections that cause lymphadenitis are numerous and varied. In most instances the histologic picture in the nodes is entirely nonspecific, designated acute or chronic nonspecific adenitis. A somewhat distinctive form of lymphadenitis that occurs with cat-scratch disease will be described separately.

ACUTE NONSPECIFIC LYMPHADENITIS

This form of lymphadenitis may be confined to a local group of nodes draining a focal infection, or it may be generalized when there is systemic bacterial or viral infection.

MORPHOLOGY

Macroscopically, acutely inflamed nodes are swollen, gray-red, and engorged. Histologically, there are large germinal centers containing numerous mitotic figures. When the condition is caused by pyogenic organisms, a neutrophilic infiltrate is seen about the follicles and within the lymphoid sinuses. With severe infections, the centers of follicles may undergo necrosis, resulting in the formation of an abscess.

Affected nodes are tender and, when abscess formation is extensive, become fluctuant. The overlying skin is frequently red, and penetration of the infection to the skin may produce draining sinuses. With control of the infection, the lymph nodes may revert to their normal appearance, or scarring may follow more destructive disease.

CHRONIC NONSPECIFIC LYMPHADENITIS

This condition may assume one of three patterns, depending on the causative agent: follicular hyperplasia, paracortical lymphoid hyperplasia, or sinus histiocytosis.

MORPHOLOGY

FOLLICULAR HYPERPLASIA. This pattern is associated with infections or inflammatory processes that activate B cells. Proliferating B cells at various stages of differentiation accumulate within large round or oblong germinal centers (secondary follicles). These nodular aggregates also feature scattered phagocytic macrophages containing nuclear debris (tingible body macrophages) and an inconspicuous meshwork of dendritic cells that function in antigen presentation. Some causes of follicular hyperplasia are rheumatoid arthritis, toxoplasmosis, and the early stages of HIV infection. This form of lymphadenitis may be confused morphologically with follicular lymphomas (p 426). Findings that favor a diagnosis of follicular hyperplasia are (1) preservation of the lymph node architecture, with normal lymphoid tissue between germinal centers; (2) marked variation in the shape and size of the lymphoid nodules; (3) a mixed population of lymphocytes at different stages of differentiation; and (4) prominent phagocytic and mitotic activity in germinal centers.

PARACORTICAL LYMPHOID HYPERPLASIA. This pattern is characterized by reactive changes within the T-cell regions of the lymph node. Parafollicular T cells undergo proliferation and transformation to immunoblasts that may efface the germinal follicles. Paracortical lymphoid hyperplasia is encountered, particularly, in viral infections or after smallpox vaccination, and in immune reactions induced by certain drugs (especially phenytoin).

SINUS HISTIOCYTOSIS. This reactive pattern is characterized by distention and prominence of the lymphatic sinusoids, owing to marked hypertrophy of lining endothelial cells and infiltration with histiocytes. Sinus histiocytosis is often encountered in lymph nodes draining cancers and may represent an immune response to the tumor or its products.

CAT-SCRATCH DISEASE

Cat-scratch disease is a self-limited lymphadenitis caused by *Bartonella henselae*. This microbe is related to rickettsiae, but unlike rickettsiae it can be grown in artificial culture. It is primarily a disease of childhood, with 90% of patients being younger than 18 years. It takes the form of regional lymphadenopathy, most frequently in the axilla and neck. The nodal enlargement appears approximately 2 weeks after a feline scratch or, uncommonly, after a splinter or thorn injury. A raised, inflammatory nodule, vesicle, or eschar may or may not be visible at the site of skin injury. In most patients, the lymph node enlargement regresses over the next 2 to 4 months. Rarely, patients develop encephalitis, osteomyelitis, or thrombocytopenia.

MORPHOLOGY

The anatomic changes in the lymph node are quite characteristic; initially, **sarcoid-like granulomas are formed that develop central necrosis with accumulation of neutrophils.** These irregular stellate necrotizing granulomas are similar in appearance to those seen in certain other infections, such as lymphogranuloma venereum. The microbe is extracellular and can be visualized only with silver stains or electron microscopy. Diagnosis is based on a history of exposure to cats, clinical findings, positive skin test to the microbial antigen, and the distinctive morphologic changes in the lymph nodes.

NEOPLASTIC PROLIFERATIONS OF WHITE CELLS

Tumors represent the most important of the white cell disorders. They can be divided into three broad categories based on the origin of the tumor cells:

■ *Lymphoid neoplasms*, which include non-Hodgkin lymphomas (NHLs), Hodgkin lymphomas, lymphocytic leukemias, and plasma cell dyscrasias and related disorders. In many instances, these tumors are composed of cells that appear to be blocked at particular stages of differentiation resembling normal stages of lymphocyte differentiation, a feature that serves as one of the bases for their classification.

■ *Myeloid neoplasms* arise from stem cells that normally give rise to the formed elements of the blood: granulocytes, RBCs, and platelets. The myeloid neoplasms fall into three fairly distinct subcategories: *acute myelogenous leukemias*, in which immature progenitor cells accumulate in the bone marrow; *chronic myeloproliferative disorders*, in which inappropriately increased production of formed blood elements leads to elevated blood cell counts; and *myelodysplastic syndromes*, which are characteristically associated with ineffective hematopoiesis and cytopenias.

■ *Histiocytic neoplasms* represent proliferative lesions of histiocytes. Of special interest are a spectrum of proliferations comprising Langerhans cells (the *Langerhans cell histiocytoses*).

Lymphoid Neoplasms

The lymphoid neoplasms encompass a group of entities that vary widely in terms of their clinical presentation and behavior, thus presenting challenges to students and clinicians alike. Some of these neoplasms characteristically present as *leukemias*, arising in the bone marrow and circulating in the peripheral blood. Others, the *lymphomas*, typically appear as tumor masses within either lymph nodes or other organs. Tumors composed predominantly of plasma cells, the *plasma cell dyscrasias*, usually present as masses within bone and cause systemic symptoms related to the inappropriate production of a complete or partial monoclonal immunoglobulin polypeptide. Despite these tendencies, all lymphoid neoplasms have the potential for spread to lymph nodes and various tissues throughout the body, especially the liver, spleen, and bone marrow. In some cases, lymphomas or plasma cell tumors spill over into the peripheral blood, creating a leukemia-like picture. Conversely, leukemias of lymphoid cells, originating in the bone marrow, may infiltrate lymph nodes and other tissues, creating the histologic picture of lymphoma. Thus, *the distinction among these broad clinical categories of lymphoid neoplasia may be blurred in some cases.*

Two groups of lymphomas are recognized: Hodgkin lymphoma and non-Hodgkin lymphomas. Although both arise in the lymphoid tissue, Hodgkin lymphoma is set apart by the presence in the lesions of the distinctive neoplastic

Reed-Sternberg giant cells (p 432) and by the fact that in the involved nodes, non-neoplastic inflammatory cells usually greatly outnumber the tumor cells. The biologic behavior and clinical treatment of Hodgkin lymphoma are also different from those of most NHLs, making its distinction of practical importance.

Few areas of pathology have evoked as much controversy and confusion as the classification of lymphoid neoplasms, which is perhaps inevitable given the intrinsic complexity of the immune system from which they arise. However, over the course of the past decade, an international working group of pathologists, molecular biologists, and clinicians has formulated a widely accepted classification scheme that relies on a combination of clinical, morphologic, phenotypic, and genotypic features. Before we delve into the classification of lymphoid neoplasia, certain important relevant principles must be emphasized:

■ Most lymphoid neoplasms in Western countries (80% to 85%) are of B-cell origin, with T-cell tumors making up most of the remainder. Tumors of NK cells also occur but are quite uncommon. B- and T-cell tumors are often composed of cells that are arrested at specific stages along their normal differentiation pathways (Fig. 12–13). It will be noted that CD2, CD3, CD4, CD7, and CD8 are useful for identification of T cells and their tumors, and CD10,

CD19, and CD20 and surface Ig are markers of normal and neoplastic B cells. CD16 and CD56 are markers for NK cells. Immature T and B cells (lymphoblasts) express the enzyme terminal deoxytransferase (TdT), which is useful in distinguishing them from immature myeloid cells (myeloblasts) and mature lymphocytes. Other markers, such as CD13, CD14, CD15, and CD64, are specifically expressed on myeloid cells and are thus useful in the distinction of myeloid neoplasms from lymphoid neoplasms, as will be described later. CD34 is expressed on pluripotent stem cells and is retained on the earliest lymphoid and myeloid progenitor cells (see Fig. 12–13).

■ Many tumors of mature B cells arise from and recapitulate the follicular growth pattern of normal B cells. Thus, in certain B-cell tumors, the neoplastic cells are clustered into identifiable nodules resembling normal follicles; these tumors are called *follicular lymphomas.* Other B-cell tumors do not produce nodules, nor do any of the tumors of T cells or histiocytes; instead, they spread diffusely in the lymph nodes. This architecture is referred to as *diffuse lymphoma.* With either pattern, the normal architecture of the lymph nodes is effaced.

■ As tumors of the immune system, lymphoid neoplasms often disrupt normal immune regulatory mechanisms. Both immunodeficiency (as evidenced by susceptibility to infection) and autoimmunity may be seen, sometimes

Figure 12–13

Schematic illustration of the phenotypic and genotypic changes associated with the differentiation of B cells and T cells. Not shown are some CD4+, CD8+ cells (common thymocytes) that also express CD3. Stages between resting B cells and plasma cells are not depicted. CD, cluster of differentiation; DR, HLA-class II antigens; Ig, immunoglobulin; TCR, T-cell receptor; TdT, terminal deoxynucleotidyl transferase.

in the same patient. Ironically, patients with inherited or acquired immunodeficiency are themselves at high risk of developing certain lymphoid neoplasms, particularly those associated with EBV infection.

- All lymphoid neoplasms are derived from a single transformed cell and are therefore monoclonal. As will be recalled from Chapter 5, during the differentiation of precursor B and T cells there is a somatic rearrangement of their antigen receptor genes. This process ensures that each lymphocyte makes a single, unique antigen receptor. Because antigen receptor gene rearrangement precedes transformation, the daughter cells derived from a given malignant progenitor share the same antigen receptor gene configuration and synthesize identical antigen receptor proteins (either immunoglobulins or T-cell receptors). For this reason, *analysis of antigen receptor genes and their protein products is frequently used to differentiate monoclonal neoplasms from polyclonal, reactive processes.*

- Although NHLs often present as involvement of a particular tissue site, sensitive molecular assays usually show that the tumor is widely disseminated at the time of diagnosis. As a result, with few exceptions, only systemic therapies are curative. In contrast, Hodgkin lymphoma often presents at a single site and spreads methodically to contiguous lymph node groups. For this reason, early in its course, Hodgkin lymphoma may be cured with local therapy alone (excision and local radiation).

With this background, we can return to the issue of classification of lymphoid neoplasms. Early classification schemes based on morphology and clinical features failed to take into account immunophenotypic and cytogenetic features, both of which were subsequently shown to be necessary to define certain entities. To address these limitations, in 1994 an International Lymphoma Study Group convened with the goal of creating a list of commonly agreed upon, distinct clinicopathologic entities. Termed the *Revised European, American Classification of Lymphoid Neoplasms* (commonly abbreviated as REAL), the resulting classification scheme considers the morphology, cell of origin (determined in practice by immunophenotyping), clinical features, and genotype (karyotype, presence of viral genomes) of each entity. This classification includes all lymphoid neoplasms, including leukemias and multiple myeloma, and segregates them on the basis of origin into three major categories: (1) tumors of B cells, (2) tumors of T cells and NK cells, and (3) Hodgkin lymphoma.

An updated version of the REAL Classification of lymphoid neoplasms is presented in Table 12–7. As can be seen, the diagnostic entities are numerous. Our focus will be on the subset of neoplasms listed here, which together constitute more than 90% of the lymphoid neoplasms seen in the United States:

- Precursor B- and T-cell lymphoblastic leukemia/lymphoma
- Small lymphocytic lymphoma/chronic lymphocytic leukemia
- Follicular lymphoma
- Mantle cell lymphoma
- Diffuse large B-cell lymphomas
- Burkitt lymphoma
- Multiple myeloma and related plasma cell dyscrasias
- Hodgkin lymphoma

Table 12–7. REAL CLASSIFICATION OF LYMPHOID NEOPLASMS*

IA. Precursor B-Cell Neoplasms
1. Precursor B-cell leukemia/lymphoma

IB. Peripheral B-Cell Neoplasms
1. **B-cell chronic lymphocytic leukemia/small lymphocytic lymphoma**
2. B-cell prolymphocytic leukemia
3. Lymphoplasmacytic lymphoma
4. **Mantle cell lymphoma**
5. **Follicular lymphoma**
6. **Extranodal marginal zone lymphoma (MALT lymphoma)**
7. Splenic marginal zone lymphoma
8. Nodal marginal zone lymphoma
9. Hairy cell leukemia
10. **Plasmacytoma/plasma cell myeloma**
11. **Diffuse large B-cell lymphoma**
12. **Burkitt lymphoma**

IIA. Precursor T-Cell Neoplasms
1. Precursor T-cell leukemia/lymphoma

IIB. Peripheral T-/NK-Cell Neoplasms
1. T-cell prolymphocytic leukemia
2. T-cell granular lymphocytic leukemia
3. Aggressive NK-cell leukemia
4. Adult T-cell lymphoma/leukemia (HTLV1+)
5. Extranodal NK/T-cell lymphoma, nasal type
6. Enteropathy-type T-cell lymphoma
7. Hepatosplenic γδ T-cell lymphoma
8. Subcutaneous panniculitis-like T-cell lymphoma
9. **Mycosis fungoides/Sézary syndrome**
10. Anaplastic large cell lymphoma, primary cutaneous type
11. **Peripheral T-cell lymphoma, not otherwise specified (NOS)**
12. Angioimmunoblastic T-cell lymphoma
13. Anaplastic large cell lymphoma, primary systemic type

III. Hodgkin Lymphoma
1. Lymphocyte predominance, nodular
2. **Nodular sclerosis**
3. **Mixed cellularity**
4. Lymphocyte depletion

*Boldface entries are among the most common lymphoid tumors.

The salient features of the more common lymphoid neoplasms are summarized in Table 12–8. We will also touch on a few of the uncommon entities that have distinctive clinicopathologic features.

PRECURSOR B- AND T-CELL LYMPHOBLASTIC LEUKEMIA/LYMPHOMA

These aggressive tumors, composed of immature lymphocytes (lymphoblasts), occur predominantly in children and young adults. The various lymphoblastic tumors are morphologically indistinguishable and often cause similar signs and symptoms. Because of these overlapping features, we will consider precursor B- and T-cell neoplasms here together.

Just as B-cell precursors normally arise within the bone marrow, pre-B-lymphoblastic tumors characteristically present as leukemias with extensive bone marrow and peripheral blood involvement. Similarly, pre-T-lymphoblastic tumors commonly present as mediastinal masses involving the thymus, the site of normal early T-cell

Table 12-8. SUMMARY OF THE MORE COMMON LYMPHOID NEOPLASMS

Entity	Frequency	Salient Morphology	Immunophenotype	Comments
Precursor B-cell leukemia/lymphoma	80% of childhood leukemia; less frequent in adults	Lymphoblasts with dispersed chromatin, small nucleoli, scant cytoplasm	TdT+ immature B cells (CD19+, CD10+)	Presents as acute leukemia. Prognosis is predicted by karyotype.
Precursor T-cell leukemia/lymphoma	20% of childhood leukemias; 40% of childhood lymphomas	Lymphoblasts with irregular nuclear contours, dispersed chromatin, small nucleoli, scant cytoplasm	TdT+ immature T cells (CD2+, CD7+)	May present as a mediastinal mass or acute leukemia. Most common in adolescent males. Karyotype distinct from pre-B-cell tumors; not clearly correlated with prognosis.
Small lymphocytic lymphoma/chronic lymphocytic leukemia (SLL/CLL)	3%–4% of adult lymphomas, 30% of all leukemias	Small, unstimulated lymphocytes in a diffuse pattern	CD5+ mature B cells expressing surface immunoglobulin	Occurs in old age; generalized lymphadenopathy with marrow and variable peripheral blood involvement; indolent course with prolonged survival.
Follicular lymphomas	40% of adult lymphomas	Germinal center cells arranged in a follicular pattern	CD10+, BCL2+ mature B cells expressing surface immunoglobulin	Occur in older patients; generalized lymphadenopathy; associated with t(14;18); leukemia less common than in SLL; indolent course but difficult to cure.
Mantle cell lymphoma	3%–4% of adult lymphomas	Diffuse or vaguely nodular pattern with small cleaved cells	CD5+ mature B cells expressing surface immunoglobulin and cyclin D1	Occurs predominantly in older males; disseminated disease in nodes, spleen, marrow, and gastrointestinal tract common; t(11;14) is characteristic; aggressive and difficult to cure.
Extranodal marginal zone lymphoma (MALT lymphoma)	~5% of adult lymphomas; more common in parts of Europe (Italy)	Variable; small round to irregular lymphocytes predominate; 40% show plasmacytic differentiation; B cells invade epithelium in small nests (lymphoepithelial lesions)	Mature B cells expressing surface immunoglobulin CD5−, CD10−	Occurs at extranodal sites involved by chronic inflammation. Very indolent; may be cured by local excision.
Diffuse large B-cell lymphomas	40%–50% of adult lymphomas	Various cell types; predominantly large germinal center–like cells; others with immunoblastic morphology	Mature B cells, ± surface immunoglobulin	Occur in older patients as well as pediatric age group; greater frequency of extranodal, visceral disease; marrow involvement and leukemia very uncommon at diagnosis and poor prognostic sign; aggressive tumors, but up to 50% are curable.
Burkitt lymphoma	< 1% of lymphomas in the United States	Cells intermediate in size between small lymphocytes and immunoblasts; prominent nucleoli; high mitotic rate; starry sky appearance caused by high rate of apoptosis	Mature B cells expressing CD10 and surface immunoglobulin	Endemic in Africa; sporadic elsewhere; increased frequency in the immunosuppressed; predominantly affects children; extranodal visceral involvement presenting features; rapidly progressive but responsive to therapy.
Plasmacytoma/plasma cell myeloma	Most common lymphoid neoplasm in older adults	Plasma cells in sheets, sometimes with prominent nucleoli or inclusions containing immunoglobulin	Mature B cells that contain cytoplasmic immunoglobulin	Myeloma presents as disseminated disease with destructive bone lesions. Hypercalcemia, renal insufficiency, pathologic fractures, and

Table 12–8. SUMMARY OF THE MORE COMMON LYMPHOID NEOPLASMS *Continued*

Entity	Frequency	Salient Morphology	Immunophenotype	Comments
				susceptibility to infections typical. Plasmacytomas may present as isolated lesions in aerodigestive mucosa.
Mycosis fungoides/ Sézary syndrome	Most common type of cutaneous lymphoma	Variable; in most cases, small cells with markedly convoluted nuclei predominate; cells often infiltrate the epidermis (Pautrier abscess)	CD4+ mature T cells (CD3+)	Presents with local or more generalized skin involvement. Very indolent course. Sézary syndrome associated with diffuse erythroderma and peripheral blood involvement
Peripheral T-cell lymphoma, not otherwise specified (NOS)	Most comon type of T-cell lymphoma in adults	Variable; usually a spectrum of small to large tumor cells with irregular nuclei	Mature T-cell phenotype (CD3+)	Not clearly a specific entity. Often presents as disseminated disease. Generally poor prognosis.
Hodgkin lymphoma, nodular sclerosis type	Most common form of Hodgkin disease	Lacunar RS cell variants in a mixed inflammatory background; broad sclerotic bands usually present.	CD15+ CD30+ RS cells; B- and T-cell markers not usually expressed on tumor cells	Most common in young women. Often presents as cervical or mediastinal lymphadenopathy. Minority of cases EBV+.
Hodgkin lymphoma, mixed cellularity type	Second most common form of Hodgkin disease	Frequent classic RS cells in a mixed inflammatory background	CD15+ CD30+ RS cells; B- and T-cell markers not usually expressed on tumor cells	Most common in men. May present as advanced stage disease. 70% of cases EBV+.

differentiation. However, most pre-T-cell tumors presenting as mediastinal masses progress rapidly to a leukemic phase, whereas other cases present as marrow involvement only. Hence, *both pre-B- and pre-T-lymphoblastic tumors usually have the clinical appearance of an acute lymphoblastic leukemia (ALL) at some time during their course.* Together, the ALLs constitute 80% of childhood leukemia, peaking in incidence at age 4, with most cases being of the pre-B-cell phenotype. The pre-T-cell tumors are more common in adolescent males, with the peak incidence occurring between 15 and 20 years of age.

The pathophysiology, laboratory findings, and clinical features of ALL closely resemble those of acute myeloblastic leukemia (AML), the other major type of acute leukemia. Because of these similarities, we will first step back to review the features common to the acute leukemias before discussing those that are specific to ALL.

Pathophysiology of Acute Leukemias. Morphologic and cell kinetic studies indicate that in acute leukemias (whether lymphoblastic or myeloblastic) there is a block in differentiation and that the neoplastic blasts have a prolonged rather than shortened generation time. Thus, the accumulation of blasts results from clonal expansion and a failure of maturation of the progeny into functional mature cells. As blasts accumulate in the marrow, they suppress normal hematopoietic stem cells. This has two important clinical implications: (1) the major manifestations of acute leukemia result from the paucity of normal RBCs, white cells, and platelets; and (2) therapeutically, the aim is to reduce the population of the leukemic clone enough to allow reconstitution with the progeny of remaining normal stem cells.

Clinical Features of Acute Leukemias. The acute leukemias have the following characteristics:

■ *Abrupt stormy onset.* Most patients present within 3 months of the onset of symptoms.
■ *Symptoms related to depression of normal marrow function.* These include fatigue, owing mainly to anemia; fever, reflecting an infection resulting from an absence of mature leukocytes; and bleeding (petechiae, ecchymoses, epistaxis, gum bleeding) secondary to thrombocytopenia.
■ *Bone pain and tenderness.* These result from marrow expansion with infiltration of the subperiosteum.
■ *Generalized lymphadenopathy*, *splenomegaly*, and *hepatomegaly*. These reflect dissemination of the leukemic cells; this occurs in all acute leukemias but is more pronounced in ALL.
■ *Central nervous system manifestations.* These include headache, vomiting, and nerve palsies resulting from meningeal spread; these features are more common in children than in adults and are more common in ALL than AML.

Laboratory Findings of Acute Leukemias. Anemia is almost always present. The white cell count is variably elevated, sometimes to more than 100,000/µL, but in about 50% of patients, it is less than 10,000/µL. Much more important is the identification of blast forms in the circulating blood and the bone marrow, where they make up 60% to 100% of all the cells. The platelet count is usually depressed to less than 100,000/µL. Uncommonly, there is pancytopenia with few blast cells in the blood (aleukemic leukemia), but the bone marrow is nonetheless flooded with blasts, ruling out aplastic anemia.

MORPHOLOGY

Because of differing responses to therapy, it is of great practical importance to differentiate ALL from AML. The nuclei of lymphoblasts in Wright-Giemsa–stained preparations have somewhat coarse and clumped chromatin and one or two nucleoli (Fig. 12–14A); myeloblasts tend to have finer chromatin and more cytoplasm, which may contain granules (Fig. 12–14B). Commonly, the cytoplasm of lymphoblasts contains large aggregates of periodic acid–Schiff (PAS)-positive material, whereas myeloblasts are often peroxidase positive.

Having completed our "short course" in acute leukemia, we will return to lymphoblastic leukemia/lymphoma; the acute myelogenous leukemias are discussed later.

Immunophenotyping. Immunophenotyping is of great utility in subtyping lymphoblastic tumors and distinguishing them from AML (Fig. 12–15). TdT, a DNA polymerase, is a useful marker because it is present in more than 95% of cases. Further subtyping into pre-B- and pre-T-cell types requires the staining of cells for lineage-specific markers, such as CD19 (B cell) and CD2 (T cell). Although immunophenotyping has historically proven somewhat useful in predicting clinical outcome, the tumor karyotype provides more robust and specific prognostic information.

Karyotypic Changes. Approximately 90% of patients with lymphoblastic leukemia/lymphoma have nonrandom karyotypic abnormalities. Most common in pre-B-cell tumors is hyperdiploidy (> 50 chromosomes/cell), which is associated with the presence of a cryptic (12;21) chromosomal translocation involving the *TEL1* and *AML1* genes. The presence of these aberrations correlates with a good outcome. Poor outcomes are observed with pre-B-cell tumors having translocations involving the *ML1* gene on chromosome 11q23 or the Philadelphia (Ph) chromosome. Pre-T-cell tumors have rearrangements entirely different from those found in pre-B-cell tumors, indicating that they have a distinct molecular pathogenesis.

Prognosis. Treatment of lymphoblastic tumors of childhood represents one of the great success stories in oncology. Children 2 to 10 years of age with pre-B-cell tumors have the best prognosis, and most can be cured. Other groups of patients do less well, however. Factors correlated with worse outcomes include male sex, age younger than 2 or older than 10, and a high leukocyte count at diagnosis. Age-dependent differences in various karyotypic abnormalities may partially explain the relationship of age to outcome. Tumors with rearrangements of *MLL* or the Ph chromosome (both associated with a poor outcome) are most common in children younger than age 2 and adults, respectively. Tumors with "good prognosis" chromosomal aberrations (such as the t[12;21] and hyperdiploidy) are common in the 2- to 10-year age group.

SMALL LYMPHOCYTIC LYMPHOMA/CHRONIC LYMPHOCYTIC LEUKEMIA

These are virtually identical tumors that differ only in the extent of peripheral blood involvement; those with large numbers of circulating cells are called chronic lymphocytic leukemia (CLL), whereas those without are called small lymphocytic lymphoma (SLL). This can be thought of as an aleukemic form of CLL. Most patients are leukemic at diagnosis and thus classified as having CLL. CLL/SLL constitutes 30% of leukemias in Western countries, but it is quite uncommon in Asia. It typically affects persons older than age 50 years.

Figure 12–14

Morphologic comparison of lymphoblasts and myeloblasts. *A,* Lymphoblastic leukemia/lymphoma. Lymphoblasts have fewer nucleoli than do myeloblasts, and the nuclear chromatin is more condensed. Cytoplasmic granules are absent. *B,* Acute myeloblastic leukemia (M1). Myeloblasts have delicate nuclear chromatin, prominent nucleoli, and fine azurophilic granules in the cytoplasm. (Courtesy of Dr. Robert W. McKenna, Department of Pathology, University of Texas Southwestern Medical School, Dallas.)

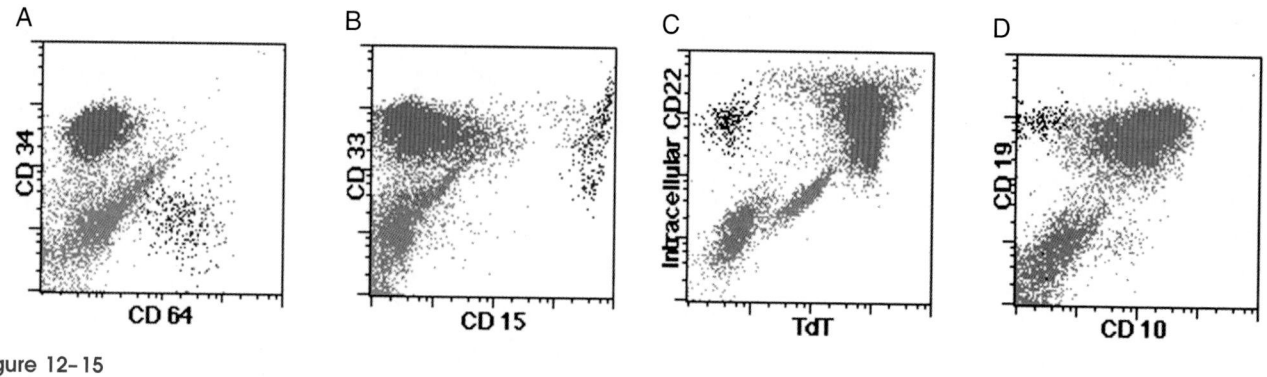

Figure 12–15

Immunophenotypic comparison of acute lymphoblastic leukemia (ALL) and acute myeloblastic leukemia (AML). *A* and *B* represent the phenotype of AML, M1 subtype (shown in Fig. 12–14*B*). The myeloid blasts, represented by the red dots, express CD34, a marker of multipotent stem cells, but do not express CD64, a marker of mature myeloid cells. In *B*, the same myeloid blasts express CD33, a marker expressed by immature myeloid cells, and some cells also express CD15, a marker of more mature myeloid cells. Thus, these blasts are minimally differentiated myeloid cells. *C* and *D* represent the phenotype of a precursor B-cell ALL (shown in Fig. 12–14*A*). Note that the lymphoblasts represented by the red dots express terminal deoxynucleotidyl transferase (TdT) and the B-cell marker CD22 *(C)*. In *D*, the same cells are seen to express two other B-cell markers, CD10 and CD19. Thus, these cells represent pre-B lymphoblasts. (Courtesy of Dr. Louis Picker, Department of Pathology, University of Texas Southwestern Medical School, Dallas.)

MORPHOLOGY

Sheets of small round lymphocytes and scattered ill-defined foci of larger cells termed **prolymphocytes** diffusely efface involved lymph nodes (Fig. 12–16*A*). The predominant cells are compact, small, apparently unstimulated lymphocytes with dark-staining round nuclei, scanty cytoplasm, and little variation in size (Fig. 12–16*B*). The foci of mitotically active prolymphocytes are called **proliferation centers;** their presence is pathognomonic for CLL/SLL. Mitotic figures are rare except in the proliferation centers, and there is little or no cytologic atypia. In addition to the lymph nodes, the bone marrow, spleen, and liver are involved in almost all cases. In most patients, there is an **absolute lymphocytosis** of small, mature-looking lymphocytes.

The neoplastic lymphocytes are fragile and frequently disrupted mechanically during smear preparation, producing characteristic **smudge cells.** Variable numbers of larger prolymphocytes are also usually present in the blood smear.

Immunophenotype. CLL/SLL is a neoplasm of mature (peripheral) B cells expressing the pan-B-cell markers CD19, CD20, and CD23, surface immunoglobulin (e.g., IgM, IgD), and either κ or λ light chains, indicating monoclonality. Unlike most peripheral B cells, the tumor cells also express the T-cell–associated antigen CD5, a tendency that is shared only with mantle cell lymphoma among the B-cell neoplasms.

Pathophysiology. The neoplastic B cells do not respond to antigenic stimulation and, through mechanisms that are

Figure 12–16

Nodal involvement by small lymphocytic lymphoma/chronic lymphocytic leukemia. *A,* Low-power view shows diffuse effacement of nodal architecture. *B,* At high power, the majority of the tumor cells have the appearance of small round lymphocytes. A single "prolymphocyte," a larger cell with a centrally placed nucleolus, is also present in this field. (*A,* Courtesy of Dr. José Hernandez, Department of Pathology, University of Texas Southwestern Medical School, Dallas.)

not understood, suppress normal B-cell function; thus, many of the patients with CLL/SLL have hypogammaglobulinemia. Paradoxically, approximately 15% of patients also have antibodies against autologous RBCs, giving rise to a hemolytic anemia. Approximately 50% of patients have karyotypic abnormalities, the most common of which are trisomy 12 and deletions of chromosomes 11 and 12. Chromosomal translocations, so common in other NHLs, are rare. *To summarize, CLL/SLL is characterized by the accumulation of long-lived, nonfunctional B lymphocytes that infiltrate the bone marrow, blood, lymph nodes, and other tissues.*

Clinical Features. CLL/SLL is often asymptomatic. When symptoms are present, they are nonspecific and include easy fatigability, weight loss, and anorexia. Because of *hypogammaglobulinemia*, there is increased susceptibility to bacterial infections. *Autoimmune hemolytic anemia and/or autoimmune thrombocytopenia* may be present. Generalized *lymphadenopathy* and *hepatosplenomegaly* are present in 50% to 60% of cases. The total leukocyte count may be increased only slightly (in SLL) or may reach 200,000/μL. The course and prognosis of CLL/SLL are extremely variable. Many patients live more than 10 years after diagnosis and die of unrelated causes; the median survival is 4 to 6 years. However, over time CLL/SLL tends to transform to more aggressive tumors that resemble either prolymphocytic leukemia or diffuse large B-cell lymphoma. Once transformation occurs, the median survival is less than 1 year.

FOLLICULAR LYMPHOMA

These tumors, characterized by a nodular or follicular architecture, are extremely common, constituting 40% of adult NHLs in the United States.

MORPHOLOGY

Lymph nodes are effaced by proliferations that usually have a distinctly nodular appearance under low power (Fig 12–17A). The tumor cells resemble normal germinal center B cells. Most commonly, the predominant neoplastic cells are "centrocyte-like." These cells are slightly larger than resting lymphocytes, with an angular "cleaved" nuclear contour characterized by prominent indentations and linear infoldings (see Fig. 12–17B). Nuclear chromatin is coarse and condensed, and nucleoli are indistinct. These small cleaved cells are mixed with variable numbers of larger "centroblast-like" cells that are three to four times the size of resting lymphocytes. This second cell type has vesicular chromatin, several nucleoli, and modest amounts of cytoplasm, and it resembles the mitotically active cells found within normal germinal centers. In most tumors, centroblast-like cells are a minor component of the overall cellularity, mitoses are infrequent, and single necrotic cells (apoptosis) are not seen. These findings help to distinguish neoplastic follicles from reactive germinal centers, in which mitoses and apoptosis are prominent.

Uncommonly, centroblast-like cells make up the predominant cell type, a histology that correlates with more aggressive clinical behavior.

Immunophenotype. As neoplasms of follicular center cells, these tumors express pan-B-cell markers such as CD19 and CD20, and many tumors express the more restricted B-cell marker CD10. In addition, the neoplastic cells express BCL2 protein, a feature that distinguishes them from normal germinal center B cells, which are BCL2 negative.

Clinical Features. The follicular lymphomas have the following distinctive clinical characteristics:

■ They occur predominantly in older persons (rarely before age 20 years).
■ They affect males and females equally.
■ They present as painless lymphadenopathy, which is frequently generalized. Involvement of extranodal (e.g., visceral) sites is uncommon, but bone marrow is almost always involved at the time of diagnosis.
■ Peripheral blood involvement in the form of frank leukemia is uncommon, but small clonal B-cell populations can be detected in most cases by flow cytometry or molecular techniques.
■ In the majority of patients, tumor cells reveal a characteristic translocation t(14;18). The break point on chromosome 18 involves 18q21, where the antiapoptosis gene *BCL2* has been mapped. This translocation causes overexpression of the BCL2 protein (Chapter 6).
■ They have a long natural history (median survival, 7 to 9 years) that appears to be largely unaffected by treatment. Hence, despite their indolent course, *they are not easily curable*, a feature that is common to most of the indolent lymphoid malignancies. Their lack of response to chemotherapy may be caused in part by the antiapoptotic effect of BCL2, which may protect tumor cells from the effects of chemotherapeutic agents.
■ In about 40% of patients the follicular lymphomas progress to a diffuse large B-cell lymphoma, with or without treatment. Such a transition reflects the emergence of an aggressive subclone of neoplastic B cells. Progression is often associated with mutations in the *TP53* gene. Such transformed tumors are much less curable than de novo diffuse large B-cell lymphomas, described later.

MANTLE CELL LYMPHOMA

Mantle cell lymphomas are composed of B cells that resemble the mantle zone of normal lymphoid follicles. They constitute approximately 4% of all NHLs and occur mainly in older males.

MORPHOLOGY

Mantle cell lymphomas show a diffuse or vaguely nodular pattern of lymph node involvement. In

Figure 12-17

Follicular lymphoma, involving a lymph node. *A,* Nodular aggregates of lymphoma cells are present throughout the lymph node. *B,* At high magnification, small lymphoid cells with condensed chromatin and irregular or cleaved nuclear outlines (centrocytes) are mixed with a population of larger cells with nucleoli (centroblasts). (*A,* Courtesy of Dr. Robert W. McKenna, Department of Pathology, University of Texas Southwestern Medical School, Dallas.)

most cases, the tumor cells are slightly larger than normal lymphocytes and have an irregular cleaved nucleus and inconspicuous nucleoli. Less commonly, the cells are larger and morphologically resemble lymphoblasts. The bone marrow is involved in the majority of cases, with about 20% of cases being "leukemic" at presentation. One unexplained but characteristic tendency is the frequent involvement of the gastrointestinal tract, sometimes in the form of multifocal submucosal nodules that grossly resemble polyps (lymphomatoid polyposis).

Immunophenotype. The tumor cells usually coexpress surface IgM and IgD, the pan-B-cell antigens CD19, CD20, CD22, and (like CLL/SLL) CD5. Mantle cell lymphoma is distinguished from CLL/SLL by the absence of proliferation centers and the presence of abnormally high levels of cyclin D1 protein.

Karyotype. Most (and possibly all) tumors have a t(11;14) translocation that fuses the cyclin D1 gene on chromosome 11 to immunoglobulin heavy-chain promoter/enhancer elements on chromosome 14. This translocation dysregulates the expression of cyclin D1, a cell cycle regulator (Chapter 6), and serves as the basis for the characteristic increased cyclin D1 protein levels.

Clinical Features. Most patients present with fatigue and lymphadenopathy and are found to have generalized disease involving the bone marrow, spleen, liver, and (often) the gastrointestinal tract. These tumors are aggressive and incurable, with a median survival of 3 to 5 years.

DIFFUSE LARGE B-CELL LYMPHOMA

This diagnostic category includes several forms of NHL that share certain features, including a B-cell phenotype, a diffuse growth pattern, and an aggressive clinical history.

As a group, this is the most important type of lymphoma in adults, accounting for approximately 50% of all adult NHLs.

MORPHOLOGY

The nuclei of the neoplastic B cells are large (at least three to four times the size of resting lymphocytes) and can take a variety of forms. In many tumors, large cells with round, irregular, or cleaved nuclear contours, dispersed chromatin, and several distinct nucleoli predominate (Fig. 12-18). The cytoplasm in such tumors tends to be pale and modest in volume. Such cells resemble "centroblasts," the large cells seen in reactive germinal centers. In other tumors, the cells have a round or multilobu-

Figure 12-18

Diffuse large B-cell lymphoma. The tumor cells have large nuclei with open chromatin and prominent nucleoli. (Courtesy of Dr. Robert W. McKenna, Department of Pathology, University of Texas Southwestern Medical School, Dallas.)

lated large vesicular nucleus with one or two centrally placed prominent nucleoli. They have abundant cytoplasm that can be either deeply staining and pyroninophilic or clear. These cells resemble "immunoblasts," normal antigen-activated interfollicular lymphoid cells.

Immunophenotype. These are mature B-cell tumors that express pan-B-cell antigens, such as CD19, CD20, and CD79a. Many also express IgM and/or IgG as well as κ or λ light chains. Other antigens (e.g., CD10) are variably expressed.

Distinct Subtypes. Several distinctive clinicopathologic subtypes are included in the general category of diffuse large B-cell lymphoma.

■ *Epstein-Barr virus (EBV)* is implicated in the pathogenesis of diffuse large B-cell lymphomas that arise in the setting of the acquired immunodeficiency syndrome and iatrogenic immunosuppression (e.g., in transplant patients). In the post-transplant setting, these tumors often begin as EBV-driven polyclonal B-cell proliferations that may disappear if immunity can be restored. Otherwise, with time, progression to monoclonal large B-cell lymphoma is observed.

■ *Human herpesvirus type 8 (HHV-8) infection* is associated with a rare group of tumors that present as malignant effusions. The tumor cells are infected with HHV-8, which encodes proteins homologous to several known oncoproteins, including cyclin D1. Patients with these *primary effusion lymphomas* are usually immunosuppressed. Note that this virus is also associated with Kaposi sarcoma in AIDS patients (Chapter 5).

■ *Mediastinal large B-cell lymphoma* usually presents in young females and shows a predilection for spread to abdominal viscera and the central nervous system.

Clinical Features. As a group, these tumors share the following general clinical features:

■ Although they occur mainly in older persons (median age about 60 years), the age range is wide; diffuse large B-cell lymphomas constitute about 15% of childhood lymphomas.

■ Patients with these tumors typically present with a rapidly enlarging, often symptomatic mass at a single nodal or extranodal site. Localized disease and extranodal manifestations are common. Indeed, involvement of the gastrointestinal tract, skin, bone, or brain may be the presenting feature. Unlike more indolent lymphomas (e.g., follicular lymphoma), involvement of liver, spleen, and bone marrow is not common at the time of diagnosis. With progressive disease, however, any site may be involved, and, rarely, a leukemic picture may emerge.

■ Approximately 30% of patients have a t(14;18) translocation, with rearrangement of the *BCL2* gene. These tumors are believed to have arisen by progression of follicular lymphomas. About one third of diffuse large cell lymphomas show rearrangement of the *BCL6* gene, lo-

cated on 3q27, and in many more there is a mutation in this gene without any cytogenetic alterations.

■ Diffuse large cell B-cell lymphomas are aggressive tumors that are rapidly fatal if untreated. With intensive combination chemotherapy, however, complete remission can be achieved in 60% to 80% of the patients; and, of these, approximately 50% remain free of disease for several years and may be considered cured. In contrast, recall that indolent B-cell neoplasms (CLL/SLL and follicular lymphoma) are very difficult to cure. Much work is now being directed at gene microarray–based molecular profiling of these tumors to predict which patients will be cured with conventional chemotherapy (Chapter 6). The others may benefit from more aggressive therapy (e.g., high-dose therapy and bone marrow transplantation).

BURKITT LYMPHOMA

Burkitt lymphoma is endemic in some parts of Africa and sporadic in other areas, including the United States. Histologically, the African and nonendemic diseases are identical, although there are clinical and virologic differences. The relationship of these disorders to EBV is discussed in Chapter 6.

> ### *MORPHOLOGY*
>
> The tumor cells are monotonous, are intermediate in size between small lymphocytes and large noncleaved cells, and have round or oval nuclei containing two to five prominent nucleoli (Fig. 12–19). The nuclear size approximates that of benign macrophages within the tumor. There is a moderate amount of faintly basophilic or amphophilic cytoplasm, which is intensely pyroninophilic and often contains small, lipid-filled vacuoles. A high mitotic rate is very characteristic of this tumor, as is cell death, accounting for the presence of numerous tissue macrophages with ingested nuclear debris. Because these benign macrophages are often surrounded by a clear space, they create a "starry sky" pattern.

Immunophenotype. These are tumors of B cells that express surface IgM and pan-B-cell markers such as CD19, as well as the CD10 antigen.

Karyotype. Burkitt lymphoma is strongly associated with translocations involving the *MYC* gene on chromosome 8. Most translocations fuse *MYC* with the *IgH* gene on chromosome 14, but variant translocations involving the κ or λ light-chain loci on chromosomes 2 and 22, respectively, are also observed. The net result of each is the inappropriate overexpression of the MYC protein, which has potent transforming activity.

Clinical Features. Both the endemic and non-African cases mainly affect children or young adults, accounting for approximately 30% of childhood NHLs in the United States. In both forms, the disease rarely arises in lymph nodes. In African patients, involvement of the maxilla or mandible is the common mode of presentation, whereas abdominal tumors (bowel, retroperitoneum, ovaries) are more

Figure 12-19 ■

Burkitt lymphoma. The tumor cells and their nuclei are fairly uniform, giving a monotonous appearance. Note the high mitotic activity (*arrowheads*) and prominent nucleoli. The "starry sky" pattern produced by interspersed, lightly staining, normal macrophages is better appreciated at a lower magnification. (Courtesy of Dr. Robert W. McKenna, Department of Pathology, University of Texas Southwestern Medical School, Dallas.)

common in North America. Leukemic presentations are uncommon, especially in African cases, but they do occur, and they must be distinguished from ALL, which responds to different drug regimens. Burkitt lymphoma is a high-grade tumor that may be the fastest growing human neoplasm; however, with very aggressive chemotherapy regimens, the majority of patients can be cured.

MULTIPLE MYELOMA AND RELATED PLASMA CELL DYSCRASIAS

The plasma cell dyscrasias are a group of B-cell neoplasms that have in common the *expansion of a single clone of immunoglobulin-secreting cells and a resultant increase in serum levels of a single homogeneous immunoglobulin or its fragments.* The homogeneous immunoglobulin identified in the blood is often referred to as an *M component.* Because a common feature of the various plasma cell dyscrasias is the presence in the serum of excessive amounts of immunoglobulins, these disorders have also been called *monoclonal gammopathies.* Although the presence of an M component may be indicative of a B-cell malignancy, it should be remembered that M components are also seen in otherwise normal elderly persons, a condition called monoclonal gammopathy of undetermined significance. Collectively, these disorders account for about 15% of deaths from malignant white cell disease; they are most common in middle-aged and elderly persons.

The plasma cell dyscrasias can be divided into six major variants: (1) multiple myeloma, (2) localized plasmacytoma (solitary myeloma), (3) lymphoplasmacytic lymphoma, (4) heavy-chain disease, (5) primary or immunocyte-associated amyloidosis, and (6) monoclonal gammopathy of undetermined significance. Each of these disorders will be briefly characterized before the morphologic features of the more common forms are presented.

Multiple Myeloma. Multiple myeloma, by far the most common of the malignant plasma cell dyscrasias, is a *clonal proliferation of neoplastic plasma cells in the bone marrow that is usually associated with multifocal lytic lesions throughout the skeletal system.* The proliferation of neoplastic plasma cells, also called *myeloma cells,* is supported by the cytokine interleukin 6 (IL-6), produced by fibroblasts and macrophages in the bone marrow stroma. As is true of many other B-cell malignancies, it has recently been appreciated that many myelomas have chromosomal translocations involving the *IgG* locus on chromosome 14. One fusion partner is the fibroblast growth factor 3 receptor gene on chromosome 4, which appears to be truncated so as to produce a constitutively active receptor.

In approximately 60% of patients, the M component is IgG; in 20% to 25%, IgA; rarely, it is IgM, IgD, or IgE. In the remaining 15% to 20% of cases, the plasma cells produce *only κ or λ* light chains, which, because of their low molecular weight, are readily excreted in urine, where they are termed *Bence Jones proteins.* In these patients, Bence Jones proteinuria without serum M component is present *(light-chain disease).* However, in up to 80% of patients, the malignant plasma cells synthesize complete immunoglobulin molecules as well as excess light chains; therefore, both Bence Jones proteins and serum M components are present.

Localized Plasmacytoma. This designation refers to the presence of a single lesion in the skeleton or in the soft tissues. Solitary skeletal plasmacytoma tends to occur in the same locations as multiple myeloma, whereas the extraosseous lesions usually form tumorous masses in the upper respiratory tract (sinuses, nasopharynx, larynx). Modest elevations in the levels of M protein are demonstrable in some of these patients. Those with solitary skeletal myelomas usually have occult lesions elsewhere. These patients may remain stable for several years, but, after a lapse of 5 to 10 years, most develop disseminated disease. Extraosseous (soft tissue) plasmacytomas spread less commonly and are often cured by local resection.

Lymphoplasmacytic Lymphoma. This tumor is composed of a mixed proliferation of B cells that range from small round lymphocytes to plasmacytic lymphocytes (so-called plymphocytes) to plasma cells. It is associated with chromosomal translocations involving the *IgH* locus on chromosome 14 and the *PAX5* gene on chromosome 9, which encodes a transcription factor that normally regulates B-cell differentiation. Like myeloma, there is an M component, but in most cases it is caused by the production of monoclonal IgM, with IgA or IgG being observed in a small fraction of cases. Clinically, the disease resembles other indolent B-cell lymphomas (such as SLL), as the neoplastic B lymphocytes diffusely infiltrate the lymphoid organs, including bone marrow, lymph nodes, and spleen. Unlike myeloma, lytic bone lesions are not seen. Usually the neoplastic B cells produce large enough amounts of IgM to give rise to a hyperviscosity syndrome called Waldenström macroglobulinemia.

Heavy-Chain Disease. This is not a specific entity but a group of proliferations in which only heavy chains are produced. These may be of the IgG, IgA, or IgM class. The clinical picture resembles certain other lymphomas. IgG heavy-chain disease often presents as diffuse lymphadenopathy and hepatosplenomegaly, thus resembling lymphoplasmacytic lymphoma. IgA heavy-chain disease shows a predilection for the lymphoid tissues that are normally the site of IgA synthesis, such as the small intestine and respiratory tract, and may represent a variant of MALT lymphoma (discussed later).

Primary or Immunocyte-Associated Amyloidosis. It may be recalled that monoclonal proliferation of plasma cells, with excessive production of light chains, underlies this form of amyloidosis (Chapter 5). The amyloid deposits (AL type) consist of partially degraded light chains.

Monoclonal Gammopathy of Undetermined Significance. M proteins can be detected in the serum of 1% to 3% of asymptomatic, healthy persons older than age 50 years. The term *monoclonal gammopathy of undetermined significance (MGUS)* is applied to this dysproteinosis without any associated disease. This is the most common monoclonal gammopathy. Approximately 20% of patients with MGUS develop a well-defined plasma cell dyscrasia (myeloma, lymphoplasmacytic lymphoma, or amyloidosis) over a period of 10 to 15 years. The diagnosis of MGUS should be made with caution and after careful exclusion of all other specific forms of monoclonal gammopathies. In general, patients with MGUS have less than 3 g/dL of monoclonal protein in the serum and no Bence Jones proteinuria.

MORPHOLOGY

Multiple myeloma presents most often as multifocal destructive bone lesions throughout the skeletal system. Although any bone may be affected, the following distribution was found in a large series of cases: vertebral column, 66%; ribs, 44%; skull, 41%; pelvis, 28%; femur, 24%; clavicle, 10%; and scapula, 10%. These focal lesions generally begin in the medullary cavity, erode the cancellous bone, and progressively destroy the cortical bone. The bone resorption results from the secretion of certain cytokines (e.g., IL-1β, TNF, IL-6) by myeloma cells. These cytokines enhance osteoclast formation and activation by the RANK ligand–RANK pathway (Chapter 21). Plasma cell lesions often produce pathologic fractures; they are most common in the vertebral column but may affect any of the numerous bones suffering erosion and destruction of their cortical substances. Most commonly, the lesions appear radiographically as punched-out defects, usually 1 to 4 cm in diameter (Fig. 12–20A), but in some cases only diffuse demineralization is evident. Microscopic examination of the marrow reveals an increased number of plasma cells, constituting 10% to 90% of all cells in the marrow. The neoplastic plasma cells may resemble normal mature plasma cells but more often show abnormal features, such as prominent nucleoli or abnormal cytoplasmic inclusions containing immunoglobulin (Fig. 12–20B). With progressive disease, plasma cell infiltrations of soft tissues may be encountered in the spleen, liver, kidneys, lungs, and lymph nodes, or, more widely and terminally, a leukemic picture may emerge.

Renal involvement, generally called **myeloma nephrosis,** is one of the more distinctive features of multiple myeloma. Microscopically, interstitial infiltrates of abnormal plasma cells may be encoun-

Figure 12–20 ■

Multiple myeloma. *A*, Radiograph of the skull (lateral view). The sharply punched-out bone defects are most obvious in the calvarium. *B*, Bone marrow aspirate. Normal marrow cells are largely replaced by plasma cells, including atypical forms with multiple nuclei, prominent nucleoli, and cytoplasmic droplets containing immunoglobulin.

tered. Proteinaceous casts are prominent in the distal convoluted tubules and collecting ducts. Most of these casts are made up of Bence Jones proteins, but they may also contain complete immunoglobulins, Tamm-Horsfall protein, and albumin. Some casts have tinctorial properties of amyloid. This is not surprising, in view of the fact that AL amyloid is derived from Bence Jones proteins (Chapter 5). Multinucleate giant cells created by the fusion of infiltrating macrophages usually surround the casts. Very often the cells that line tubules containing casts become necrotic or atrophic because of the toxic actions of free light chains (Bence Jones proteins). Metastatic calcification may be encountered within the kidney because of the **hypercalcemia** caused by bone resorption. When complicated by systemic amyloidosis, nodular glomerular lesions are present. Pyelonephritis may occur, owing to the increased susceptibility of these patients to infections.

In contrast to multiple myeloma, lymphoplasmacytic lymphoma is not associated with lytic skeletal lesions. Instead, the neoplastic cells diffusely infiltrate the bone marrow, lymph nodes, spleen, and sometimes the liver. Infiltrations of other organs also occur, particularly with disease progression. The cellular infiltrate consists of lymphocytes, plasma cells, and "plymphocytes." The remaining forms of plasma cell dyscrasias have either already been described (e.g., primary amyloidosis (Chapter 5)) or are too rare for further description.

Clinical Course. The clinical manifestations of the plasma cell dyscrasias are varied. They result from the destructive or otherwise damaging effect of the infiltrating neoplastic cells in various tissues and from the effects of the abnormal immunoglobulins secreted by the tumors. In multiple myeloma, the pathologic effects of tumorous masses of plasma cells predominate, whereas in lymphoplasmacytic lymphoma most of the signs and symptoms result from the IgM macroglobulins in the serum.

The peak age of incidence of multiple myeloma is between 50 and 60 years. The major clinical features of this disease are as follows:

■ Bone pain, resulting from infiltration by neoplastic plasma cells, is extremely common. Pathologic fractures and hypercalcemia occur, with focal bone destruction and diffuse resorption. Hypercalcemia may cause neurologic manifestations such as confusion and lethargy; it also contributes to renal disease. Anemia results from marrow replacement as well as from inhibition of hematopoiesis by tumor cells.
■ Recurrent infections with bacteria such as *Staphylococcus aureus*, *Streptococcus pneumoniae*, and *Escherichia coli* are serious clinical problems. They result from severe suppression of normal immunoglobulin secretion.
■ Excessive production and aggregation of myeloma proteins may lead to the hyperviscosity syndrome (described later).
■ As many as 50% of patients suffer renal insufficiency. It results from multiple factors, such as recurrent bacterial infections and hypercalcemia, but most importantly from the toxic effects of Bence Jones proteins on cells lining the tubules.
■ Amyloidosis develops in 5% to 10% of patients.

The diagnosis of multiple myeloma can be readily made by the characteristic focal, punched-out radiologic defects in the bone, especially when these are present in the vertebrae or calvarium. Electrophoresis of the serum and urine is an important diagnostic tool in suspected cases. In 99% of cases a monoclonal spike of complete immunoglobulin or

immunoglobulin light chain can be detected in the serum, in the urine, or in both. In the remaining 1% of cases, monoclonal immunoglobulins can be found within the plasma cell masses but not in the serum or urine. Such cases are sometimes called *nonsecretory myelomas*.

Lymphoplasmacytic lymphoma affects somewhat older persons, with the peak incidence being between the sixth and seventh decades. Most clinical symptoms of this disease can be traced to the presence of IgM globulins. Because of their size, the increased macroglobulins greatly enhance blood viscosity, giving rise to the *hyperviscosity syndrome* known as *Waldenström macroglobulinemia*. This is characterized by the following features:

■ Visual impairment, related to the striking tortuosity and distention of retinal veins; retinal hemorrhages and exudates may also contribute to the visual problems.
■ Neurologic problems such as headaches, dizziness, deafness, and stupor, stemming from sluggish blood flow and sludging.
■ Bleeding, related to the formation of complexes between macroglobulins and clotting factors as well as interference with platelet functions.
■ Cryoglobulinemia, related to precipitation of macroglobulins at low temperatures and producing symptoms such as Raynaud phenomenon and cold urticaria.

Multiple myeloma is a progressive disease, with median survival ranging from 2 to 4 years. The median survival in lymphoplasmacytic lymphoma is somewhat longer, in the range of 4 to 5 years. Although aggressive therapies are being tried in both, neither disease is presently curable.

HODGKIN LYMPHOMA

Hodgkin lymphoma, like the NHLs, is a disorder involving primarily the lymphoid tissues. It arises almost invariably in a single node or chain of nodes and spreads characteristically to the anatomically contiguous nodes. It is separated from the NHLs for several reasons. First, it is *characterized morphologically by the presence of distinctive neoplastic giant cells called Reed-Sternberg (RS) cells* admixed with a variable infiltrate of reactive, nonmalignant inflammatory cells. Second, it is often associated with somewhat distinctive clinical features, including systemic manifestations such as fever. Third, its stereotypic pattern of spread allows it to be treated differently than most other lymphoid neoplasms. Despite these distinguishing features, recent molecular studies have clearly shown that it is, in most cases, a tumor of B lymphocytes and therefore best considered an unusual form of lymphoma.

Classification. Four subtypes of Hodgkin lymphoma are recognized: (1) nodular sclerosis, (2) mixed cellularity, (3) lymphocyte predominance, and (4) lymphocyte depletion. The fourth subtype is very rare and is not mentioned further. Before delineating the remaining three, however, we should describe the common denominator among all—RS cells and variants thereof—and the method used to characterize the extent of the disease in a patient, namely, the staging system.

MORPHOLOGY

The sine qua non for the histologic diagnosis of Hodgkin lymphoma is the **RS cell** (Fig. 12–21). The RS cell has abundant, usually slightly eosinophilic, cytoplasm and ranges in diameter from 15 to 45 μm. It is distinguished principally either by having a multilobate nucleus or being multinucleate with large, round, prominent nucleoli. **Particularly characteristic are two mirror-image nuclei or nuclear lobes, each containing a large (inclusion-like) acidophilic nucleolus surrounded by a distinctive clear zone; together they impart an owl-eyed appearance. The nuclear membrane is distinct.** As we will see, such "classic" RS cells are common in the mixed cellularity subtype, uncommon in the nodular sclerosis subtype, and rare in the lymphocyte-predominance subtype; in these latter two subtypes, other characteristic RS cell variants predominate.

The staging of Hodgkin lymphoma (Table 12–9) is of great clinical importance, because the course, choice of therapy, and prognosis are all intimately related to the distribution of the disease. It will become apparent from the ensuing discussion that the more aggressive the variant of the disease, the more likely it is to be in an advanced stage at the time of diagnosis.

With this background, we can turn to the morphologic classification of Hodgkin lymphoma into its subgroups and point out some of the salient clinical features of each. Later the manifestations common to all will be presented. The essential morphologic feature that serves to differentiate the major sub-groups (lymphocyte predominance, nodular sclerosis, and mixed cellularity) is the morphology and frequency of the neoplastic elements (RS cells) relative to the reactive elements, represented by small lymphocytes. The relative frequency of the four histologic subtypes may be gleaned from Table 12–10.

NODULAR SCLEROSIS HODGKIN LYMPHOMA. This is by far the most common histologic form. It is distinct from the other forms both clinically and histologically and is characterized morphologically by two features:

■ The presence of a particular variant of the RS cell, the **lacunar cell** (Fig. 12–22). This cell is large and has a single hyperlobate nucleus with multiple small nucleoli and an abundant,

Table 12-9. CLINICAL STAGES OF HODGKIN AND NON-HODGKIN LYMPHOMAS (ANN ARBOR CLASSIFICATION)*

Stage	Distribution of Disease
I	Involvement of a single lymph node region (I) or involvement of a single extralymphatic organ or tissue (I_E)
II	Involvement of two or more lymph node regions on the same side of the diaphragm alone (II) or with involvement of limited contiguous extralymphatic organs or tissue (II_E)
III	Involvement of lymph node regions on both sides of the diaphragm (III), which may include the spleen (III_S), limited contiguous extralymphatic organ or site (III_E), or both (III_{ES})
IV	Multiple or disseminated foci of involvement of one or more extralymphatic organs or tissues with or without lymphatic involvement

*All stages are further divided on the basis of the absence (A) or presence (B) of the following systemic symptoms: significant fever, night sweats, unexplained loss of more than 10% of normal body weight.

From Carbone PT, et al: Symposium (Ann Arbor): staging in Hodgkin disease. Cancer Res 31:1707, 1971.

Figure 12-21

Hodgkin lymphoma. A binucleate Reed-Sternberg cell with large, inclusion-like nucleoli and abundant cytoplasm is surrounded by lymphocytes, and an eosinophil can be seen below. (Courtesy of Dr. Robert W. McKenna, Department of Pathology, University of Texas Southwestern Medical School, Dallas.)

Table 12-10. PERCENTAGE OF PATIENTS IN EACH PATHOLOGIC STAGE ACCORDING TO HISTOLOGIC SUBTYPE

Histologic Subtype	No. of Patients	Pathologic Stage (%)		
		I and II	III	IV
Lymphocyte predominance	55	76	22	2
Mixed cellularity	215	44	47	9
Lymphocyte depletion	21	19	62	19
Nodular sclerosis	628	60	35	5

From Desforges JF, et al: Hodgkin's disease. N Engl J Med 301:1212, 1979. Reprinted by permission of the New England Journal of Medicine.

Figure 12–22   ■

Hodgkin lymphoma, nodular sclerosis type. A distinctive "lacunar cell" with multilobed nucleus containing many small nucleoli is seen lying within a clear space created by retraction of its cytoplasm. It is surrounded by lymphocytes. (Courtesy of Dr. Robert W. McKenna, Department of Pathology, University of Texas Southwestern Medical School, Dallas.)

Figure 12–24   ■

Hodgkin disease, mixed cellularity type. A diagnostic, binucleate Reed-Sternberg cell is surrounded by multiple cell types, including eosinophils (bright red cytoplasm), lymphocytes, and histiocytes. (Courtesy of Dr. Robert W. McKenna, Department of Pathology, University of Texas Southwestern Medical School, Dallas.)

pale-staining cytoplasm. In formalin-fixed tissue, the cytoplasm often retracts, giving rise to the appearance of cells lying in clear spaces, or lacunae.

■ The presence in most cases of collagen bands that divide the lymphoid tissue into circumscribed nodules (Fig. 12–23). The fibrosis may be scant or abundant, and the cellular infiltrate may show varying proportions of lymphocytes, eosinophils, histiocytes, and lacunar cells. Classic RS cells are infrequent.

The immunophenotype of the lacunar variants is identical to that of classic RS cells. These cells express CD15 and CD30 and usually do not express B- and T-cell–specific antigens.

MIXED-CELLULARITY HODGKIN LYMPHOMA. This is the most common form of Hodgkin lymphoma in patients older than the age of 50 and overall comprises about 25% of cases. There is a male predominance. Typical RS cells are plentiful within a distinctive heterogeneous cellular infiltrate, which includes small lymphocytes, eosinophils, plasma cells, and benign histiocytes (Fig. 12–24). Compared with the other common subtypes, more patients with mixed cellularity present with disseminated disease (Table 12–11), and these patients more often have systemic manifestations.

LYMPHOCYTE PREDOMINANCE HODGKIN LYMPHOMA. This subgroup, comprising about 5% of

Figure 12–23   ■

Hodgkin lymphoma, nodular sclerosis type. A low-power view shows well-defined bands of pink, acellular collagen that have subdivided the tumor cells into nodules. (Courtesy of Dr. Robert W. McKenna, Department of Pathology, University of Texas Southwestern Medical School, Dallas.)

Table 12–11. CLINICAL DIFFERENCES BETWEEN HODGKIN AND NON-HODGKIN LYMPHOMAS

Hodgkin Lymphoma	Non-Hodgkin Lymphoma
More often localized to a single axial group of nodes (cervical, mediastinal, para-aortic)	More frequent involvement of multiple peripheral nodes
Orderly spread by contiguity	Noncontiguous spread
Mesenteric nodes and Waldeyer ring rarely involved	Waldeyer ring and mesenteric nodes commonly involved
Extranodal involvement uncommon	Extranodal involvement common

Figure 12–25 ■

Hodgkin disease, lymphocyte predominance type. Numerous mature-looking lymphocytes surround scattered, large, pale-staining L&H variants ("popcorn" cells). (Courtesy of Dr. Robert W. McKenna, Department of Pathology, University of Texas Southwestern Medical School, Dallas.)

Hodgkin lymphoma, is characterized by a large number of small, mature-looking reactive lymphocytes admixed with a variable number of benign histiocytes (Fig. 12–25), often within large, poorly defined nodules. Other types of reactive cells, such as eosinophils, neutrophils, and plasma cells, are scanty or absent, and typical RS cells are extremely difficult to find. More common are L&H variant cells that have a delicate multilobed, puffy nucleus that has been likened in appearance to popcorn (**"popcorn cell"**). The typical nodular growth pattern of lymphocyte predominance Hodgkin lymphoma has long suggested that this might be a neoplasm of follicular B cells; indeed, phenotypic studies have revealed that the L&H variants in lymphocyte predominance Hodgkin lymphoma express B-cell markers (e.g., CD20). Furthermore, L&H variants have rearranged and somatically mutated *IgH* genes, which strongly supports a follicular B-cell origin. Most patients present with isolated cervical or axillary lymphadenopathy and have an excellent prognosis.

Clinically, nodular sclerosis Hodgkin lymphoma is the only form more common in women, and it has a striking propensity to involve the lower cervical, supraclavicular, and mediastinal lymph nodes. Most of the patients are adolescents or young adults, and they have an excellent prognosis, especially when their disease is in clinical stages I and II.

It is apparent that Hodgkin lymphoma spans a wide range of histologic patterns and that certain forms, with their characteristic fibrosis, eosinophils, neutrophils, and plasma cells, come deceptively close to simulating an inflammatory reactive process. **The histologic diagnosis, then, of Hodgkin lymphoma rests on the unmistakable identification of RS cells or their variants in the appropriate background of reactive cells.** Immunophenotyping plays an important adjunct role in helping to distinguish atypical forms of Hodgkin lymphoma from large cell NHLs.

In all forms, involvement of the spleen, liver, bone marrow, and other organs and tissues may appear in due course and take the form of irregular, tumor-like nodules of tissue resembling that present in the nodes. At times the spleen is much enlarged and the liver moderately enlarged by these nodular masses.

Etiology and Pathogenesis. Determining the origin of the neoplastic RS cells of Hodgkin lymphoma has proved daunting, in part because these cells are rare compared with the surrounding reactive inflammatory infiltrate. It has been recognized for some time that the L&H variants of RS cells found in nodular lymphocyte predominance Hodgkin lymphoma express B-cell markers, supporting a B-cell origin. By contrast, the RS cells in other forms of Hodgkin lymphoma generally do not express lineage-specific lymphoid markers and have thus remained enigmatic. This uncertainty has been largely resolved by elegant studies performed on single micro-dissected RS cells obtained from cases of mixed cellularity and nodular sclerosis Hodgkin lymphoma. Sequence analysis of DNA amplified from such cells has generally shown that all RS cells from individual cases possess the same immunoglobulin gene rearrangements and that the rearranged immunoglobulin genes have undergone somatic hypermutation, an event that is normally confined to germinal center B cells. Although rare tumors of T-cell origin may also exist, it now seems to be settled that, in most cases, Hodgkin lymphoma is a neoplasm of transformed germinal center B cells.

Given that RS cells represent the malignant component, what causes the neoplastic transformation? For years, EBV has been suspected as an etiologic agent on the basis of epidemiologic and serologic studies. This notion has been bolstered recently by molecular studies. The EBV genome can be identified in RS cells in up to 70% of cases of the mixed cellularity type and a smaller fraction of the nodular sclerosis type. More importantly, the EBV genome is present in a clonal pattern, indicating that infection precedes (and therefore may be related to) transformation. Thus, as in Burkitt lymphoma and B-cell lymphomas in immunodeficient patients, EBV infection may be one of several steps in the pathogenesis of Hodgkin lymphoma, particularly the mixed cellularity type.

If EBV is playing a causative role, what then is the pathogenetic basis of EBV-negative forms? A possible clue stems from the observation that RS cells in EBV-positive and EBV-negative forms of Hodgkin lymphoma contain high levels of activated NF-κB, a transcription factor that normally stimulates B-cell proliferation and protects B cells from pro-apoptotic signals. Hence, abnormal activation of

NF-κB may be one common pathway involved in lymphomagenesis. Of interest, several EBV proteins activate NF-κB in latently infected B cells. Presumably, some other pathogenetic event, such as somatic mutations in host genes, underlies the activation of NF-κB in the EBV-negative cases.

The characteristic non-neoplastic, inflammatory cell infiltrate appears to result from a number of cytokines secreted by RS cells, including IL-5 (an attractant and growth factor for eosinophils), transforming growth factor β (a fibrogenic factor), and IL-13 (which may stimulate RS cells through an autocrine mechanism). Conversely, the reactive cells, rather than being innocent bystanders, may produce factors (such as CD30 ligand) that may aid the growth and survival of RS cells.

Clinical Course. Hodgkin lymphomas, like NHLs, usually present as a painless enlargement of the lymph nodes. Although a definitive distinction from NHL can be made only by examination of a lymph node biopsy specimen, several clinical features favor the diagnosis of Hodgkin lymphoma (see Table 12–11). Younger patients with the more favorable histologic types tend to present in clinical stage I or II (see Table 12–10) and are usually free of systemic manifestations. Patients with disseminated disease (stages III and IV) are more likely to present with systemic complaints such as fever, unexplained weight loss, pruritus, and anemia. As mentioned earlier, these patients generally have the histologically less favorable variants. The outlook after aggressive radiotherapy and chemotherapy for patients with this disease, including those with disseminated disease, is generally very good. *With current modalities of therapy, the histologic picture has very little impact on the prognosis; instead, clinical stage appears to be the important prognostic indicator.* The 5-year survival rate of patients with stage I-A or II-A disease is close to 100%. Even with advanced disease (stage IV-A or IV-B), a 50% 5-year disease-free survival rate can be achieved. However, these therapeutic advances have also brought new problems. Long-term survivors of combined chemotherapy-radiotherapy protocols are at much higher risk of developing acute leukemia, lung cancer, melanomas, breast cancer, and some forms of NHLs. As a result, current efforts are aimed at developing less genotoxic therapeutic regimens that decrease therapy-related complications while preserving a high cure rate.

MISCELLANEOUS LYMPHOID NEOPLASMS

Of the many remaining forms of lymphoid neoplasia within the REAL classification, several with distinctive or clinically important features merit brief discussion.

Extranodal Marginal Zone Lymphoma (MALT Lymphoma). This is a special category of low-grade B-cell tumors that arise most commonly in mucosal-associated lymphoid tissue (MALT), such as salivary glands, small and large bowel, and lungs, and some nonmucosal sites such as the orbit and breast. The tumor cells resemble normal memory B cells that home to areas at the margins of B-cell follicles. Most extranodal marginal zone lymphomas develop in the setting of Sjögren syndrome, Hashimoto thyroiditis, or *Helicobacter pylori* infection in the stomach, suggesting that sustained antigenic stimulation contributes to lymphomagenesis. In the case of *H. pylori*–associated gastric MALT lymphoma, eradication of the organism with antibiotic therapy often leads to regression of the tumor, which appears to be dependent on cytokines secreted by *H. pylori*–specific T cells for its growth and survival (Chapter 6). When arising at other sites, MALT tumors can often be cured by local excision or radiotherapy. Two recurrent cytogenetic abnormalities are recognized: t(1;14), involving the *BCL10* and *IgH* genes; and t(11;18), involving the *MALT1* and *IAP2* genes.

Hairy Cell Leukemia. This uncommon, indolent B-cell leukemia is distinguished by the presence of leukemic cells that have fine, hairlike cytoplasmic projections, best recognized under the phase contrast microscope but also visible in routine blood smears. The hairy cells express pan-B-cell markers, including CD19 and CD20, and surface immunoglobulin with a single light chain, confirming clonality. In addition, the tumor cells express CD11c and CD103; these antigens are not present on most other B-cell tumors, making them useful in the diagnosis of hairy cell leukemia.

This tumor occurs mainly in older males, and its *manifestations result largely from infiltration of bone marrow and spleen.* Splenomegaly, which is often massive, is the most common and sometimes the only abnormal physical finding. *Pancytopenia*, resulting from marrow infiltration and splenic sequestration, is seen in more than half the cases. Hepatomegaly is less common and not as marked, and lymphadenopathy is distinctly rare. *Leukocytosis is not a common feature*, being present in only 15% to 20% of patients, but hairy cells can be identified in the peripheral blood smear in most cases. The disease is indolent but progressive if untreated; pancytopenia and infections are major problems. Unlike most other low-grade lymphoid neoplasms, this tumor is extremely sensitive to chemotherapeutic agents, particularly purine nucleosides. Complete durable responses are the rule, and the overall prognosis is excellent.

Mycosis Fungoides and Sézary Syndrome. These tumors of peripheral CD4+ T cells are characterized by involvement of the skin and therefore belong to the group of *cutaneous T-cell lymphomas.*

Mycosis fungoides presents as an inflammatory premycotic phase and progresses through a plaque phase to a tumor phase. Histologically, there is infiltration of the epidermis and upper dermis by neoplastic T cells, which often have a cerebriform nucleus characterized by marked infolding of the nuclear membrane. With progressive disease, both nodal and visceral dissemination appear. Sézary syndrome is a related condition in which skin involvement is manifested clinically as a generalized exfoliative erythroderma along with an associated leukemia of Sézary cells, which also have a cerebriform nucleus. Circulating Sézary cells can also be identified in as many as 25% of cases of mycosis fungoides in the plaque, or tumor, phase. These are incurable, but indolent, tumors with a median survival time of 8 or 9 years.

Adult T-Cell Leukemia/Lymphoma. This T-cell neoplasm, caused by infection with a retrovirus, human T-cell leukemia virus type 1 (HTLV-1), is endemic in southern Japan and the Caribbean basin, but similar cases have been found sporadically elsewhere, including the southeastern

United States. The pathogenesis of this tumor is discussed in Chapter 6. In addition to causing lymphoid malignancies, HTLV-1 infection can also give rise to a progressive demyelinating disease that affects the central nervous system and the spinal cord.

Adult T-cell leukemia/lymphoma is characterized by skin lesions, generalized lymphadenopathy, hepatosplenomegaly, hypercalcemia, and an elevated leukocyte count with multilobed CD4+ lymphocytes. The leukemic cells constitutively express high levels of receptors for IL-2. In most cases this is an extremely aggressive disease, with a median survival time of about 8 months. In 15% to 20% of patients the course of the disease is chronic; their disease is clinically indistinguishable from cutaneous T-cell lymphomas.

Peripheral T-Cell Lymphomas. This is a heterogeneous group of tumors that together make up about 15% of adult NHLs. Although several rare distinctive subtypes fall under this heading, most tumors in this group are unclassifiable. In general, they present as disseminated disease, are aggressive, and respond poorly to therapy.

Myeloid Neoplasms

Myeloid neoplasms arise within hematopoietic stem cells and typically give rise to monoclonal proliferations that diffusely replace normal bone marrow cells. There are three general categories of myeloid neoplasia. *Acute myeloblastic leukemias* are tumors marked by a blockage in the differentiation of early myeloid cells. Immature myeloid cells (myeloblasts) accumulate in the marrow, replacing normal elements, and frequently circulate in the peripheral blood. In *chronic myeloproliferative disorders,* the neoplastic clone retains the capacity to undergo terminal differentiation but exhibits increased or dysregulated growth. Commonly, there is an increase in one or more of the formed elements (RBCs, platelets, and/or granulocytes) of the peripheral blood. *Myelodysplastic syndromes* are disorders in which terminal differentiation occurs but is disordered and ineffective. As a result, these are marked by the presence of dysplastic marrow precursors and peripheral blood cytopenias.

Although these three categories provide a useful starting point when considering the myeloid neoplasms, the divisions between them can blur. Both myelodysplastic syndromes and myeloproliferative disorders often transform to a picture identical to acute myeloblastic leukemia, and some patients may present with disorders that have features of both myelodysplastic and myeloproliferative disorders. Given that all arise from hematopoietic stem cells, the close relationship among these disorders is not surprising.

ACUTE MYELOBLASTIC LEUKEMIA

Acute myeloblastic leukemia (AML) primarily affects adults. Its incidence increases steadily with age, with the median age being 50 years. It is an extremely heterogeneous disorder, as will be discussed below. The clinical signs and symptoms closely resemble those of lymphoblastic leukemia and are usually related to marrow failure caused by the replacement of normal marrow elements by leukemic blasts. Fatigue and pallor, abnormal bleeding, and

infections are common in newly diagnosed patients, who typically present within a few weeks of the onset of symptoms. Splenomegaly and lymphadenopathy are in general less prominent than in lymphoblastic leukemia, but, rarely, AML may present as a discrete tissue mass (so-called granulocytic sarcoma). Ideally, the diagnosis and classification of AML is based on the results of morphologic, histochemical, immunophenotypic, and karyotypic studies. Of these tests, karyotyping is most predictive of outcome.

MORPHOLOGY

In most cases, myeloblasts can be distinguished from lymphoblasts with routine Wright-Giemsa stains. The blasts have delicate nuclear chromatin; three to five nucleoli; and fine, azurophilic granules in the cytoplasm (see Fig. 12–14B). Distinctive red-staining rodlike structures **(Auer rods)** are present in some cases, more often in the promyelocytic variant (Fig. 12–26). Auer rods are found only in neoplastic myeloblasts and are thus a helpful diagnostic clue when present.

Classification. *AMLs are diverse in terms of their predominant line of differentiation and the maturity of cells.* This diversity has served as the basis for one classification scheme, the French-American-British (FAB) classification, which divides AML into eight groups. These are listed in Table 12–12, along with their relative frequency and special features.

Experience has shown, however, that the FAB classification is of limited prognostic value, whereas *a number of recurrent cytogenetic abnormalities correlate well with outcome.* For this reason, it has been proposed that AML

Figure 12–26 ■

Acute promyelocytic leukemia (M3 subtype). Bone marrow aspirate shows neoplastic promyelocytes with abnormally coarse and numerous azurophilic granules. Other characteristic findings include the presence of several cells with bilobed nuclei and a cell in the center of the field that contains multiple needle-like Auer rods. (Courtesy of Dr. Robert W. McKenna, Department of Pathology, University of Texas Southwestern Medical School, Dallas.)

Table 12-12. FAB CLASSIFICATION OF ACUTE MYELOBLASTIC (MYELOCYTIC) LEUKEMIAS (AML)

Class	Morphology	Comments
M0 Minimally differentiated AML	Blasts lack definitive cytologic and cytochemical markers of myeloblasts but express myeloid lineage antigens	2% to 3% of AML
M1 AML without differentiation	Very immature myeloblasts predominate; few granules or Auer rods	20% of AML; Ph chromosome, present in 10% to 15% of cases, worsens prognosis
M2 AML with differentiation	Myeloblasts and promyelocytes predominate; Auer rods commonly present	30% of AML; presence of t(8;21) translocation associated with good prognosis
M3 Acute promyelocytic leukemia	Hypergranular promyelocytes, often with many Auer rods per cell; may have reniform or bilobed nuclei	5% to 10% of AML; disseminated intravascular coagulation common; presence of t(15;17) translocation is characteristic; responds to retinoic acid therapy
M4 Acute myelomonocytic leukemia	Myelocytic and monocytic differentiation evident; myeloid elements resemble M2; peripheral monocytosis	20% to 30% of AML; presence of inv16 or del16q associated with better prognosis
M5 Acute monocytic leukemia	Monoblasts (peroxidase-negative, esterase-positive) and promonocytes predominate	10% of AML; usually in children and young adults; gum infiltration common; associated with abnormalities of chromosome 11q23
M6 Acute erythroleukemia	Bizarre, multinucleated, megaloblastoid erythroblasts predominate; myeloblasts also present	5% of AML; high blood counts and organ infiltration are rare; affected persons are of advanced age
M7 Acute megakaryocytic leukemia	Blasts of megakaryocytic lineage predominate; react with antiplatelet antibodies; myelofibrosis or increased bone marrow reticulin	

be classified as good, intermediate, or bad risk based on the results of karyotyping. Multiple cytogenetic changes have been noted in AML, some of which are correlated with particular FAB groups. The relationships of the various FAB groups to cytogenetic aberrations that influence prognosis are indicated in Table 12–12.

Of particular interest is the t(15;17) translocation in M3, or acute promyelocytic, leukemia. This translocation results in the fusion of the retinoic acid receptor α gene *(RARA)* on chromosome 17 with the *PML* gene on chromosome 15. The chimeric gene(s) produce abnormal PML/RARA fusion proteins that block myeloid differentiation at the promyelocytic stage, probably by inhibiting the function of normal RARA receptors. Remarkably, pharmacologic doses of retinoic acid (Chapter 8), a vitamin A analogue, overcome this block, causing the neoplastic promyelocytes to terminally differentiate into neutrophils and die. Because neutrophils live, on average, for 6 hours, the result is the rapid clearance of tumor cells and remission in a high fraction of patients. The effect is very specific; AMLs without the t(15;17) translocation do not respond to retinoic acid. Patients relapse if treated with retinoic acid alone, possibly because the neoplastic progenitor that gives rise to the promyelocytes is resistant to the pro-differentiative effects of retinoic acid. Nonetheless, this is an important example of an effective therapy that is targeted at a tumor-specific molecular defect.

Histochemistry. Cases with myelocytic differentiation are typically positive for the enzyme myeloperoxidase, which is detected by incubation of cells with peroxidase substrates. Auer rods are intensely peroxidase positive, which can help bring out their presence when they are rare. Monocytic differentiation is demonstrated by staining for lysosomal nonspecific esterases.

Immunophenotype. The expression of immunologic markers is heterogeneous in AML. Most express some combination of myeloid-associated antigens, such as CD13, CD14, CD15, or CD64. CD33 is expressed on pluripotent stem cells but is retained on myeloid progenitor cells. Such markers are helpful in distinguishing AML from ALL (as shown in Fig. 12–15) and identifying primitive AMLs (e.g., the M0 subtype). In addition, monoclonal antibodies reactive with platelet-associated antigens are very helpful in the diagnosis of M7.

Prognosis. AML is a devastating disease. Tumors with "good risk" karyotypic aberrations (t[8;21], inv[16]) are associated with a 50% chance of long-term disease-free survival, but the overall long-term disease-free survival is only 15% to 30% with conventional chemotherapy. An increasing number of patients with AML are being treated with more aggressive approaches, such as allogeneic bone marrow transplantation. Currently, this seems to be the only treatment that can lead to cure of the disease.

MYELODYSPLASTIC SYNDROMES

This term refers to a group of clonal stem cell disorders characterized by maturation defects resulting in ineffective hematopoiesis and an increased risk of transformation to acute myeloblastic leukemias.

In patients with this syndrome, bone marrow is partly or wholly replaced by the clonal progeny of a mutant multipotent stem cell that retains the capacity to differentiate into RBCs, granulocytes, and platelets but in a manner that is both ineffective and disordered. As a result, the bone marrow is usually hypercellular or normocellular but the peripheral blood shows pancytopenia. The abnormal stem cell clone in the bone marrow is genetically unstable, with a tendency to accumulate mutations and give rise to AML. Most cases are idiopathic, but some patients develop the syndrome after chemotherapy with alkylating agents or exposure to ionizing radiation therapy.

Cytogenetic studies reveal that a chromosomally abnormal clone of cells is present in the marrow of up to 70% of patients. Some common karyotypic abnormalities include a loss of chromosomes 5 or 7 or deletions of their long arms. Morphologically, the marrow is populated by aberrant cells, such as megaloblastoid erythroid precursors, bizarre-looking blasts, and micromegakaryocytes, among others.

Most patients are older males between 50 and 70 years of age. Of these patients, 10% to 40% develop AML; the remainder suffer from infections, anemia, and hemorrhages, owing to a lack of differentiated myeloid cells. The response to chemotherapy is usually poor, leading to the suggestion that myelodysplasia arises in a background of stem cell failure. Of interest in this regard, some patients with aplastic anemia eventually develop a myelodysplastic syndrome, and a significant minority of patients with myelodysplasia respond to T-cell immunosuppressants. These relationships suggest that, at least in a subset of patients, the mutant clone may "grow out" because normal stem cells are being attacked by T cells. As discussed earlier, a similar mechanism seems to underlie paroxysmal nocturnal hemoglobinuria. The prognosis is variable; median survival time varies from 9 to 29 months and is worse in those with increased marrow blasts or cytogenetic abnormalities at the time of diagnosis.

CHRONIC MYELOPROLIFERATIVE DISORDERS

These neoplastic proliferations are marked by an increase in the proliferation of neoplastic bone marrow progenitors, which seed secondary hematopoietic organs (the spleen, liver, and lymph nodes) and retain the capacity for terminal differentiation. This combination results in hepatosplenomegaly (caused by neoplastic extramedullary hematopoiesis), mild lymphadenopathy, and an increase in one or more formed elements of the peripheral blood.

Most patients with clinical features typical of the chronic myeloproliferative disorders fall into one of four diagnostic entities: chronic myelogenous leukemia (CML), polycythemia vera, myeloid metaplasia with myelofibrosis, and essential thrombocythemia. Although some overlap exists, CML is clearly separated from the other disorders by being associated with a characteristic cytogenetic abnormality, the Ph chromosome. Only CML, polycythemia vera, and myeloid metaplasia with myelofibrosis are presented here. Essential thrombocythemia occurs too infrequently to merit further discussion.

Chronic Myelogenous Leukemia

CML principally affects adults between 25 and 60 years of age and accounts for 15% to 20% of all cases of leukemia. The peak incidence is in the fourth and fifth decades of life.

Pathophysiology. *CML is associated in all cases with the presence of a unique chromosomal abnormality, the Ph (Philadelphia) chromosome.* In approximately 95% of patients with CML, the Ph chromosome, representing a reciprocal translocation from the long arm of chromosome 22 to the long arm of chromosome 9, can be identified in granulocytic, erythroid, and megakaryocytic precursors, as well as B cells and, in some cases, T cells. This finding is *firm evidence for the clonal origin of CML from pluripotent stem cells.* Recall that the translocation responsible for the appearance of the Ph chromosome gives rise to a *BCR-ABL* fusion gene, which is critical for neoplastic transformation (Chapter 6). Indeed, patients who appear to be Ph negative by cytogenetic studies have cryptic *BCR-ABL* fusion genes that are detectable at the molecular level by Southern blot analysis or polymerase chain reaction (PCR) technique. Although the Ph chromosome is highly characteristic of CML, it should be remembered that by itself it is not diagnostic of this disorder, because it is present in 30% of adult ALL and rare cases of AML.

In all cases of CML, the chimeric *BCR-ABL* gene encodes a fusion protein consisting of portions of BCR and the tyrosine kinase domain of ABL. This fusion protein possesses an increased, dysregulated tyrosine kinase activity that plays a critical role in the pathophysiology of CML.

Although CML originates in the pluripotent stem cells, granulocyte precursors constitute the dominant cell line. *In contrast to acute leukemias, there is no block in the maturation of leukemic stem cells,* as evidenced by the vast number of granulocytes in the bone marrow and peripheral blood. The basis of the increased myeloid stem cell mass in CML seems to lie in a failure of stem cells to respond to physiologic signals that regulate their proliferation.

Clinical Features. The onset of CML is usually slow, and the initial symptoms may be nonspecific (e.g., easy fatigability, weakness, and weight loss). Sometimes the first symptom is a dragging sensation in the abdomen, caused by the *extreme splenomegaly* that is characteristic of this condition. The laboratory findings are critical in making the diagnosis. Usually there is marked elevation of the leukocyte count, commonly exceeding 100,000/μL. *The circulating cells are predominantly neutrophils and myelocytes* (Fig. 12–27), *but basophils and eosinophils are also prominent.* A small proportion of myeloblasts, usually less than 5%, can be detected in the peripheral blood. Because CML originates from stem cells, it is not surprising that as many as 50% of patients have *thrombocytosis.* The bone marrow is hypercellular, with hyperplasia of granulocytic and megakaryocytic lineages. The frequency of myeloblasts is increased only slightly. The red pulp of the enlarged spleen has an appearance similar to that of the marrow, owing to the presence of extensive extramedullary hematopoiesis. This burgeoning mass of hematopoietic cells often compromises the local blood supply, causing splenic infarcts. These may present as acute onset left upper quadrant pain.

It is sometimes necessary to distinguish CML from a leukemoid reaction, which is also associated with a striking elevation of the granulocyte count in response to infection, stress, chronic inflammation, and certain neoplasms. *Most important for differentiating leukemoid reactions from CML is the presence of the Ph chromosome* and increased numbers of basophils in the peripheral blood, both of which are quite typical of CML. In addition, the granulocytes in CML are almost completely devoid of alkaline phosphatase, whereas this enzyme is increased in leukemoid reactions.

The course of CML is one of slow progression. Even without treatment, median survival is 3 years. After a variable (and unpredictable) period, approximately 50% of patients enter an accelerated phase, during which there is gradual failure of response to treatment; increasing anemia and new thrombocytopenia; acquisition of additional cytogenetic abnormalities; and, finally, *transformation into a picture resembling acute leukemia* (i.e., blast crisis). In the remaining 50%, blast crises occur abruptly, without an intermediate accelerated phase. It is of interest to note that in 30% of patients, the blasts contain TdT, a marker of primitive lymphoid cells, and express B-cell–lineage antigens such as CD10 and CD19. They also reveal clonal rearrangement of immunoglobulin genes. The emergence of B-cell blasts further attests to the origin of CML from a pluripotent stem cell. In the remaining 70% of patients, the blasts exhibit features of myeloblasts. CML less commonly progresses to a phase of extensive bone marrow fibrosis resembling that seen in other myeloproliferative disorders, most notably myeloid metaplasia with myelofibrosis.

Treatment of CML is evolving rapidly. Most patients were formerly treated palliatively with "gentle" chemotherapy, which unfortunately did not prevent the development of blast crisis. Bone marrow transplantation was (and remains) a definitive form of therapy, being curative in 70% of patients, but it carries a high risk of death in patients without a matched donor and in the aged. The picture has changed dramatically with the development of STI-571, an adenosine triphosphate analogue that specifically inhibits a subset of tyrosine kinases, including the BCR-ABL fusion protein. Most patients with stable-phase or accelerated-phase CML treated with this single agent achieve a complete remission within several months with little of the toxicity associated with nonspecific chemotherapeutic agents. It is too early to tell whether this response will be long lasting, but the experience with STI-571 (Gleevec) has validated the exciting concept of "designer" drugs that specifically target oncoproteins.

Polycythemia Vera

Polycythemia vera is associated with excessive proliferation of erythroid, granulocytic, and megakaryocytic elements, all derived from a single neoplastic stem cell. Although platelets and granulocytes are increased, the most obvious clinical signs and symptoms are related to the *absolute increase in RBC mass.* This needs to be distinguished from *relative polycythemia,* which results from hemoconcentration. Unlike other forms of absolute polycythemia that result from increased secretion of erythropoietin, polycythemia vera is associated with low levels of erythropoietin in the serum, a reflection of the fact that the neoplastic proliferation of erythroid progenitors is erythropoietin independent. Growth and maturation of granulocytes and megakaryocytes is also growth factor independent, suggesting that the mutation(s) responsible for polycythemia vera likely affect some common signaling event downstream of multiple membrane receptors.

Figure 12-27

Chronic myelogenous leukemia. Peripheral blood smear shows many mature neutrophils, some metamyelocytes, and a myelocyte. (Courtesy of Dr. Robert W. McKenna, Department of Pathology, University of Texas Southwestern Medical School, Dallas.)

MORPHOLOGY

The major anatomic changes stem from the increase in blood volume and viscosity brought about by the erythrocytosis. Plethoric congestion of all tissues and organs is characteristic of polycythemia vera. The liver is enlarged and frequently contains foci of extramedullary hematopoiesis. The spleen is slightly enlarged in about 75% of patients, up to 250 to 300 g, owing to the presence of extramedullary hematopoiesis and vascular congestion. **Consequent to the increased viscosity and vascular stasis, thromboses and infarctions are common; they affect most often the heart, spleen, and kidneys.** Hemorrhages occur in about a third of these patients, probably owing to excessive distention of blood vessels and abnormal platelet function. They usually affect the gastrointestinal tract, oropharynx, or brain. Although these hemorrhages are said on occasion to be spontaneous, more often they follow some minor trauma or surgical procedure. Platelets, which are also produced from the neoplastic clone, may be dysfunctional. Depending on the nature of the platelet defect, it may either exacerbate the tendency for thrombosis or lead to abnormal bleeding. As in CML, the peripheral blood often shows increased basophils.

The bone marrow is hypercellular, with hyperplasia of erythroid, myeloid, and megakaryocytic forms. In addition, some degree of marrow fibrosis is present in 10% of patients at the time of diagnosis. In a subset of patients, the disease progresses to myelofibrosis, where the marrow space is largely replaced by fibroblasts and collagen.

Clinical Course. Polycythemia vera appears insidiously, usually in late middle age (40 to 60 years). Patients with this disorder classically are plethoric and often somewhat cyanotic. There may be an intense pruritus, resulting perhaps from histamine released as a result of an increase in basophils. The excess histamine may also account for the peptic ulceration seen in these patients. Other complaints are referable to the thrombotic and hemorrhagic tendencies and to hypertension. *Headache, dizziness, gastrointestinal symptoms, hematemesis, and melena are common.* Because of the high rate of cell turnover, symptomatic gout is seen in 5% to 10% of cases, and many more patients have asymptomatic hyperuricemia.

The diagnosis is usually made in the laboratory. RBC counts range from 6 to 10 million/μL, and the hematocrit may approach 60%. Because there is hyperproliferation of all myeloid lineages, the white cell count may be as high as 50,000/mm^3, and the platelet count is often greater than 400,000/mm^3. Basophil counts are frequently elevated. The platelets are morphologically and functionally abnormal in most cases. Giant forms and megakaryocytic fragments are seen in the blood. About 30% of patients develop thrombotic complications, usually affecting the brain or heart. Hepatic vein thrombosis, giving rise to the Budd-Chiari syndrome (Chapter 16), is an uncommon but grave complication. Minor hemorrhages (e.g., epistaxis and bleeding from gums) are common; life-threatening hemorrhages occur in 5% to 10% of patients. In patients who receive no treatment, death resulting from these vascular episodes occurs within months after diagnosis; however, if the RBC mass can be maintained near normal by phlebotomies, median survival of 10 years can be achieved.

Prolonged survival with treatment has revealed that the *natural history of polycythemia vera involves a gradual transition to a "spent phase," during which the clinical and anatomic features of myeloid metaplasia with myelofibrosis develop.* Fifteen percent to 20% of patients undergo such a transformation after an average interval of 10 years. This transition is brought about by creeping fibrosis in the bone marrow (myelofibrosis) and a shift of hematopoiesis to the spleen, which enlarges markedly. Transformation to acute leukemia also occurs, but much less frequently than in CML. AML develops in about 2% of patients who are treated with phlebotomy alone and in about 15% of those who receive myelosuppressive treatment with chlorambucil or marrow irradiation with radioactive phosphorus. Presumably, the increase in the latter groups is related to the mutagenic effects of these therapeutic agents.

Myeloid Metaplasia With Myelofibrosis

In this chronic myeloproliferative disorder, the "spent phase" of marrow fibrosis occurs early in the disease course. As hematopoiesis shifts from the fibrotic marrow to the spleen, liver, and lymph nodes, extreme splenomegaly and hepatomegaly develop. Hematopoiesis in these extramedullary sites tends to be disordered and inefficient and, together with the marrow fibrosis, leads to moderate to severe anemia and thrombocytopenia in most patients.

Although marrow fibrosis is characteristic of this condition, the fibroblasts are not clonal descendants of the transformed stem cells. Instead, marrow fibrosis is secondary to derangements in hematopoietic cells, particularly megakaryocytes. It is believed that *marrow fibroblasts are stimulated to proliferate by platelet-derived growth factor and transforming growth factor β* released from neoplastic megakaryocytes. These two growth factors are known to be mitogenic for fibroblasts. As the disease progresses, marrow fibrosis occurs secondary to the elaboration of fibroblast growth factors mentioned earlier. By the time patients come to clinical attention, marrow fibrosis and marked extramedullary hematopoiesis are usually evident. More uncommonly, marrow fibrosis is less advanced at diagnosis; in such patients, the marrow hypercellularity, leukocytosis, and thrombocytosis that are typical of other myeloproliferative disorders is seen.

MORPHOLOGY

The principal site of the extramedullary hematopoiesis is the **spleen,** which is usually markedly enlarged, sometimes up to 4000 g. As with most causes of massive splenomegaly, multiple subcapsular infarcts may be present. Histologically, there is trilineage proliferation affecting normoblasts, granulocyte precursors, and megakaryocytes; however, megakaryocytes are usually prominent, owing to increased numbers and bizarre morphology. Sometimes disproportional activity of any one of the three major cell lines is seen.

The **liver** may be moderately enlarged, with foci of extramedullary hematopoiesis. Microscopically, the **lymph nodes** also contain foci of extramedullary hematopoiesis, but these are insufficient to cause appreciable enlargement.

The **bone marrow** in a typical case is **hypocellular and shows diffuse fibrosis.** However, the marrow is hypercellular in early cases, with equal representation of the three major cell lines. Megakaryocytes are often prominent and may show dysplastic changes.

Clinical Course. Myeloid metaplasia may begin with a blood picture suggestive of polycythemia vera or CML but more commonly has progressed to marrow fibrosis by the time it comes to clinical attention. Most patients have moderate to severe anemia. The white cell count may be normal, reduced, or markedly elevated. Early in the course of the disease, the platelet count is normal or elevated, but eventually patients develop thrombocytopenia. The *peripheral blood smear appears markedly abnormal* (Fig. 12–28).

Figure 12-28 ■

Myelofibrosis with myeloid metaplasia, peripheral blood smear. Two nucleated erythroid precursors and several teardrop-shaped red cells (dacryocytes) are evident. Immature myeloid cells were present in other fields. An identical picture can be seen in other diseases producing marrow distortion and fibrosis.

RBC abnormalities include the presence of nucleated forms and bizarre shapes (poikilocytes, teardrop cells). Immature white cells (myelocytes and metamyelocytes) are also seen, and basophils are usually increased. The presence of nucleated RBC precursors and immature white cells is referred to as *leukoerythrocytosis*. Platelets are often abnormal in size and shape and defective in function. In some cases the clinical and blood picture may resemble CML, but the *Ph chromosome is absent*. Patients with myelophthisic anemia, in which marrow fibrosis results from an identifiable cause of marrow injury, may also present as leukoerythrocytosis; therefore, a careful history must be taken to exclude such causes. Because of a high rate of cell turnover, hyperuricemia and gout may also complicate the picture.

The outcome of myeloid metaplasia is variable. There is constant threat of infections, as well as thrombotic and hemorrhagic episodes stemming from platelet abnormalities. Splenic infarctions are common. As many as 5% to 15% of patients eventually suffer a blast crisis resembling AML. The median survival time is 4 to 5 years.

Histiocytic Neoplasms

LANGERHANS CELL HISTIOCYTOSES

The term *histiocytosis* is an "umbrella" designation for a variety of proliferative disorders of histiocytes or macrophages. Some, such as very rare histiocytic lymphomas, are clearly malignant. Others, such as the reactive histiocytic proliferations in lymph nodes, are clearly benign. Between these two extremes is a small cluster of relatively rare conditions, *the Langerhans cell histiocytoses*, characterized by the clonal proliferation of a special type of cell, the *Langerhans cell* (Chapter 5). These are dendritic antigen-presenting cells that are normally distributed in many organs, most prominently the skin.

In the past, these disorders were referred to as *histiocytosis X* and subdivided into three categories: Letterer-Siwe syndrome, Hand-Schüller-Christian disease, and eosinophilic granuloma. These three conditions are now believed to represent different expressions of the same basic disorder. The proliferating Langerhans cells are human leukocyte antigen DR (HLA-DR) positive and express the CD1 antigen. *Characteristically, these cells have HX bodies (Birbeck granules) in their cytoplasm. Under the electron microscope, these are seen to have a pentalaminar, rodlike, tubular structure, with characteristic periodicity and sometimes a dilated terminal end ("tennis racket" appearance).* Under the light microscope, the proliferating Langerhans cells in these disorders do not resemble their normal dendritic counterparts. Instead, they have abundant, often vacuolated, cytoplasm, with vesicular nuclei. This appearance is more akin to that of tissue histiocytes (macrophages), hence the term *Langerhans cell histiocytosis*.

As mentioned previously, Langerhans cell histiocytosis presents as one of three clinicopathologic entities: acute disseminated Langerhans cell histiocytosis, unifocal eosinophilic granuloma, or multifocal eosinophilic granuloma.

Acute disseminated Langerhans cell histiocytosis (Letterer-Siwe disease) usually occurs before 2 years of age but occasionally may involve adults. The dominant clinical feature is the development of cutaneous lesions that resemble seborrheic skin eruptions, secondary to infiltrations of Langerhans histiocytes. Most of those affected have concurrent hepatosplenomegaly, lymphadenopathy, pulmonary lesions, and eventually, destructive osteolytic bone lesions. Extensive infiltration of the marrow often leads to anemia, thrombocytopenia, and predisposition to recurrent infections such as otitis media and mastoiditis. Thus, the clinical picture may resemble that of an acute leukemia. The course of untreated disease is rapidly fatal. With intensive chemotherapy, 50% of patients survive 5 years.

Both unifocal and multifocal Langerhans cell histiocytosis (unifocal and multifocal eosinophilic granuloma) are characterized by expanding, erosive accumulations of Langerhans cells, usually within the medullary cavities of bones. Histiocytes are variably admixed with eosinophils, lymphocytes, plasma cells, and neutrophils. The eosinophilic component ranges from scattered mature cells to sheetlike masses of cells. Virtually any bone in the skeletal system may be involved, most commonly the calvarium, ribs, and femur. Similar lesions may be found in the skin, lungs, or stomach, either as unifocal lesions or as components of the multifocal disease.

Unifocal lesions usually affect the skeletal system. They may be asymptomatic or may cause pain and tenderness and, in some instances, pathologic fractures. This is an indolent disorder that may heal spontaneously or may be cured by local excision or irradiation.

Multifocal Langerhans cell histiocytosis usually affects children, who present with fever; diffuse eruptions, particularly on the scalp and in the ear canals; and frequent bouts of otitis media, mastoiditis, and upper respiratory tract infections. An infiltrate of Langerhans cells may lead to mild lymphadenopathy, hepatomegaly, and splenomegaly. In about 50% of patients, involvement of the posterior pituitary stalk of the hypothalamus leads to diabetes insipidus.

The combination of calvarial bone defects, diabetes insipidus, and exophthalmos is referred to as the *Hand-Schüller-Christian triad*. Many patients experience spontaneous regression; others can be treated with chemotherapy.

Etiologic and Pathogenetic Factors in White Cell Neoplasia: Summary and Perspectives

Having described the many types of white cell neoplasms, it is worth reviewing common themes pertaining to their etiology and pathogenetic mechanisms.

CHROMOSOMAL TRANSLOCATIONS AND ONCOGENES

As we have seen, nonrandom karyotypic abnormalities, most commonly translocations, are present in the majority of white cell neoplasms; the most common of these are listed in Table 12–13. At a molecular level, translocations typically result in the fusion of elements from two genes. In some translocations, the DNA breaks fall within the coding sequence of both involved genes, leading to formation of a fusion gene encoding a novel chimeric protein. In other translocations, the coding sequence of one gene is juxtaposed to the noncoding regulatory elements of the second gene (often an immunoglobulin or T-cell receptor locus), resulting in inappropriate expression.

In the case of lymphoid neoplasms, many of the chromosomal translocations appear to occur during attempted normal immunoglobulin or T-cell receptor gene rearrangement. In other words, the genomic rearrangements that create the diversity of antigen receptor genes also carry an inherent risk of aberrant recombination and chromosome translocation. Indirect but compelling evidence of the importance of lymphoid recombinases can be seen in the karyotypic differences between B- and T-cell neoplasms. In the case of T cells, rearrangement of

■

Table 12–13. SUMMARY OF CHARACTERISTIC CHROMOSOMAL ABERRATIONS IN MYELOID AND LYMPHOID NEOPLASMS

Entity	Chromosomal Aberration(s)	Proposed Contribution to Transformation
B-Cell Neoplasms		
Precursor B-cell leukemia/lymphoma	Hyperdiploidy; t(12;21); t(1;19); 11q23 rearrangements; t(9;22) (Ph chromosome); many others	Creation of fusion genes encoding chimeric transcription factors that block differentiation. Increased proliferation in the case of BCR-ABL (created by the Ph chromosome) elevated tyrosine kinase activity
Lymphoplasmacytic lymphoma	t(9;14); dysregulates PAX5	Unknown. The PAX transcription factor is required for normal B-cell differentiation
Mantle cell lymphoma	t(11;14); dysregulates Cyclin D1	Increased proliferation caused by abnormal cell cycle progression
Follicular lymphoma	t(14;18); dysregulates BCL2	Resistance to cell death
Extranodal marginal zone lymphoma (MALT lymphoma)	t(1;14); t(11;18); dysregulate BCL10 and MALT1, respectively	Unknown. Normal BCL10 and MALT1 proteins form a complex that may regulate cell death
Plasmacytoma/plasma cell myeloma	t(4;14), involving FGFR3; many other rearrangements involving the IgH locus on 14q32	FGFR3 encodes a tyrosine kinase; may increase the proliferation of plasma cells
Diffuse large B-cell lymphoma	t(14;18), involving BCL2; rearrangements involving 3q27 which dysregulate BCL6	BCL2; resistance to cell death. BCL6; encodes a transcription factor necessary for formation of germinal centers; role in lymphomagenesis unknown
Burkitt lymphoma	t(8;14), t(2;8), t(8;22); all dysregulate C-MYC	Increased proliferation; immortalization
T-Cell Neoplasms		
Precursor T-cell leukemia/lymphoma	t(1;14); interstitial deletions of chromosome 1; diverse uncommon rearrangements involving 14q11 or 7q35	Overexpression of transcription factors that block T-cell differentiation (most commonly TAL1)
T-cell prolymphocytic leukemia	inv(14); dysregulation of TCL1	Inhibition of cell death
Anaplastic large cell lymphoma, primary systemic type	t(2;5) (present in a subset); involves ALK	Formation of chimeric ALK fusion protein with increased tyrosine kinase activity; probably leads to increased proliferation
Myeloid Neoplasms		
Acute myeloblastic leukemia	t(8;21); inv(16); t(15;17); rearrangements of 11q23; many others	Formation of fusion genes encoding chimeric transcription factors that block differentiation
Chronic myelogenous leukemia	t(9;22) (Ph chromosome); creates activated tyrosine kinase (BCR-ABL)	Increased proliferation
Myelodysplastic syndromes	del(5); del(7)	Unknown

inv, inversion; del, deletion.

T-cell receptor genes is normally confined to thymic lymphoblasts, and among T-cell tumors, only T-lymphoblastic tumors commonly have translocations involving antigen receptor genes. In contrast, *Ig* breakage and rearrangement normally occurs in both B lymphoblasts and germinal center B cells, and translocations involving antigen receptor genes are common in diverse B-cell neoplasms, ranging from B-lymphoblastic tumors to multiple myeloma. The prolonged exposure of B cells to cellular recombinases may also underlie the relative frequency of B-cell tumors as compared to T-cell tumors. The basis for the DNA breaks that lead to the chromosomal translocations characteristic of myeloid tumors is unknown.

INHERITED GENETIC FACTORS

As was discussed in Chapter 6, individuals with genetic diseases that promote genomic instability, such as Bloom syndrome, Fanconi anemia, and ataxia-telangiectasia, are at increased risk for the development of acute leukemia. In addition, Down syndrome (trisomy 21) and neurofibromatosis type I are both associated with an increased incidence of childhood leukemia.

VIRUSES AND ENVIRONMENTAL AGENTS

Three viruses, HTLV-1, EBV, and HHV-8, have been implicated as causative agents of lymphohematopoietic neoplasms. The possible mechanisms of transformation by viral agents were discussed earlier (Chapter 6). HTLV-1 has been clearly associated only with adult T-cell leukemia/lymphoma. In contrast, clonal episomal EBV genomes are found in the tumor cells of African Burkitt lymphoma, 30% to 40% of cases of Hodgkin lymphoma, many diffuse large B-cell lymphomas occurring in the setting of immunodeficiency, and certain NK-cell tumors. HHV-8 is uniquely associated with an unusual subset of large B-cell lymphomas presenting as lymphomatous effusions.

Several environmental agents that lead to chronic immune stimulation predispose to lymphoid neoplasia. The most clear-cut associations are *H. pylori* infection and gastric marginal zone lymphoma and gluten-sensitive enteropathy and intestinal T-cell lymphoma. It remains to be seen if other lymphoid neoplasms are antigen driven, either directly or indirectly, at early stages of their development.

IATROGENIC FACTORS

Ironically, radiotherapy and certain forms of chemotherapy used to treat cancer increase the risk of subsequent hematolymphoid neoplasms, including myelodysplastic syndromes, AML, and NHL. This association is believed to stem from mutagenic effects of ionizing radiation and chemotherapeutic drugs on hematolymphoid progenitor cells.

Bleeding Disorders

These disorders are characterized clinically by abnormal bleeding, which may either be spontaneous or become evident after some inciting event (e.g., trauma or surgery). Abnormal bleeding may have as its cause (1) a defect in the vessel wall, (2) platelet deficiency or dysfunction, or (3) a derangement of coagulation factors. As will become evident, the pathogenesis of some disorders that cause increased bleeding involves the systemic activation and consumption of platelets and/or coagulation factors. In these consumptive coagulopathies, abnormal bleeding may be accompanied by abnormal clotting.

Before embarking on a discussion of disorders of coagulation, it would be profitable to review normal hemostasis and the common laboratory tests used in the evaluation of a bleeding diathesis. It should be recalled from the discussion in Chapter 4 that the normal hemostatic response involves the blood vessel wall, the platelets, and the clotting cascade. The various tests used in the initial evaluation of patients with bleeding disorders are as follows:

- *Bleeding time.* This represents the time taken for a standardized skin puncture to stop bleeding. Measured in minutes, this procedure provides an in vivo assessment of platelet response to limited vascular injury. The reference range depends on the actual method employed and varies from 2 to 9 minutes. It is abnormal when there is a defect in platelet numbers or function.
- *Platelet counts.* These are obtained on anticoagulated blood by using an electronic particle counter. The reference range is 150 to 450 × 10^3/mm^3. Counts outside

this range must be confirmed by a visual inspection of a peripheral blood smear.

■ *Prothrombin time (PT).* Measured in seconds, this procedure tests the adequacy of the extrinsic and common coagulation pathways. It represents the time needed for plasma to clot in the presence of an exogenously added source of tissue thromboplastin (e.g., brain extract) and Ca^{++} ions. A prolonged PT may result from a deficiency of factors V, VII, or X; prothrombin; or fibrinogen.

■ *Partial thromboplastin time (PTT).* This test is designed to assess the integrity of the intrinsic and common clotting pathways. In this test, the time (in seconds) needed for the plasma to clot in the presence of kaolin, cephalin, and calcium is measured. Kaolin serves to activate the contact-dependent factor XII, and cephalin substitutes for platelet phospholipids. Prolongation of PTT may occur because of a deficiency of factors V, VIII, IX, X, XI, or XII or prothrombin or fibrinogen or an acquired inhibitor (typically an antibody) that interferes with the intrinsic pathway.

In addition to these, more specialized tests include measurement of the levels of specific clotting factors, fibrinogen, and fibrin split products; determination of the presence of circulating anticoagulants; and platelet function tests. With this overview, we can return to the three important categories of bleeding disorders.

Abnormalities of vessels can contribute to bleeding in several ways. *Increased fragility* of the vessels is associated with severe vitamin C deficiency (scurvy) (Chapter 8), systemic amyloidosis (Chapter 5), chronic glucocorticoid use, rare inherited conditions affecting the connective tissues, and a large number of infectious and hypersensitivity vasculitides. The latter include meningococcemia, infective endocarditis, the rickettsial diseases, typhoid, and Henoch-Schönlein purpura. Some of these conditions are discussed in other chapters; others are beyond the scope of this book. A *hemorrhagic diathesis that is purely the result of vascular fragility is characterized by* (1) the apparently spontaneous appearance of petechiae and ecchymoses in the skin and mucous membranes (probably from minor trauma), (2) a normal platelet count and tests of coagulation (PT, PTT), and (3) a bleeding time that is usually normal. Alternatively, as will be seen, consumptive coagulopathies sometimes stem from systemic conditions that make endothelial cell surfaces prothrombotic.

Deficiencies of platelets (thrombocytopenia) are important causes of hemorrhage. They may occur in a variety of clinical settings that are discussed later. There are disorders in which platelet function is impaired despite a normal platelet count. Such qualitative defects may be acquired, as in uremia, after aspirin ingestion, and in certain myeloproliferative disorders, or inherited, as in von Willebrand disease and other rare congenital disorders. Thrombocytopenia and platelet dysfunction are similar to increased vascular fragility in that petechiae and ecchymoses are present, as well as easy bruising, nosebleeds, excessive bleeding from minor trauma, and menorrhagia. Similarly, the PT and PTT are normal, although *in contrast to the vascular disorders, the bleeding time is always prolonged.*

Bleeding diatheses based purely on a *derangement of blood clotting* differ in several respects from those resulting from defects in the vessel walls or in platelets. The PT, PTT, or both, are prolonged, whereas the bleeding time is normal. Petechiae and other evidence of bleeding from very minor surface trauma are usually absent. However, massive hemorrhage may follow operative or dental procedures or severe trauma. Moreover, hemorrhages into areas of the body subject to trauma, such as the joints of the lower extremities, are characteristic. In this category is a group of congenital coagulation disorders.

One of the most complex of the bleeding diatheses, disseminated intravascular coagulation (DIC), discussed later, involves consumption of both platelets and the clotting factors, so it presents laboratory and clinical features of both thrombocytopenia and a coagulation disorder. von Willebrand disease also involves derangements in both modalities.

In this section the following hemorrhagic disorders are discussed: DIC (consumption of fibrinogen and platelets), thrombocytopenia (deficiency of platelets), and coagulation disorders (deficiency in clotting factors).

DISSEMINATED INTRAVASCULAR COAGULATION

An acute, subacute, or chronic thrombohemorrhagic disorder, DIC occurs as a secondary complication in a variety of diseases. *It is characterized by activation of the coagulation sequence, leading to formation of thrombi throughout the microcirculation. As a consequence of the widespread thromboses, there is consumption of platelets and coagulation factors and, secondarily, activation of fibrinolysis.* Thus, DIC may give rise either to tissue hypoxia and microinfarcts caused by myriad microthrombi or to a bleeding disorder related to pathologic activation of fibrinolysis and/or depletion of the elements required for hemostasis (hence the term *consumption coagulopathy*). This entity is probably a more common cause of bleeding than all of the congenital coagulation disorders, which will be discussed later.

Etiology and Pathogenesis. Before presenting the specific disorders associated with DIC, we will discuss in a general way the pathogenetic mechanisms by which intravascular clotting can occur. Reference to earlier comments on normal blood coagulation (Chapter 4) may be helpful at this point. It suffices here to recall that clotting may be initiated by either of two pathways: the extrinsic pathway, which is triggered by the release of tissue factor (tissue thromboplastin), or the intrinsic pathway, which involves the activation within the blood of factor XII by surface contact, collagen, or other negatively charged substances. Both pathways lead to the generation of thrombin. Clot-inhibiting influences include the rapid clearance of activated clotting factors by the mononuclear phagocytic system or by the liver, activation of endogenous anticoagulants (e.g., protein C), and activation of fibrinolysis.

Two major mechanisms may trigger DIC: (1) release of tissue factor or thromboplastic substances into the circulation and (2) widespread injury to endothelial cells (Fig. 12–29).

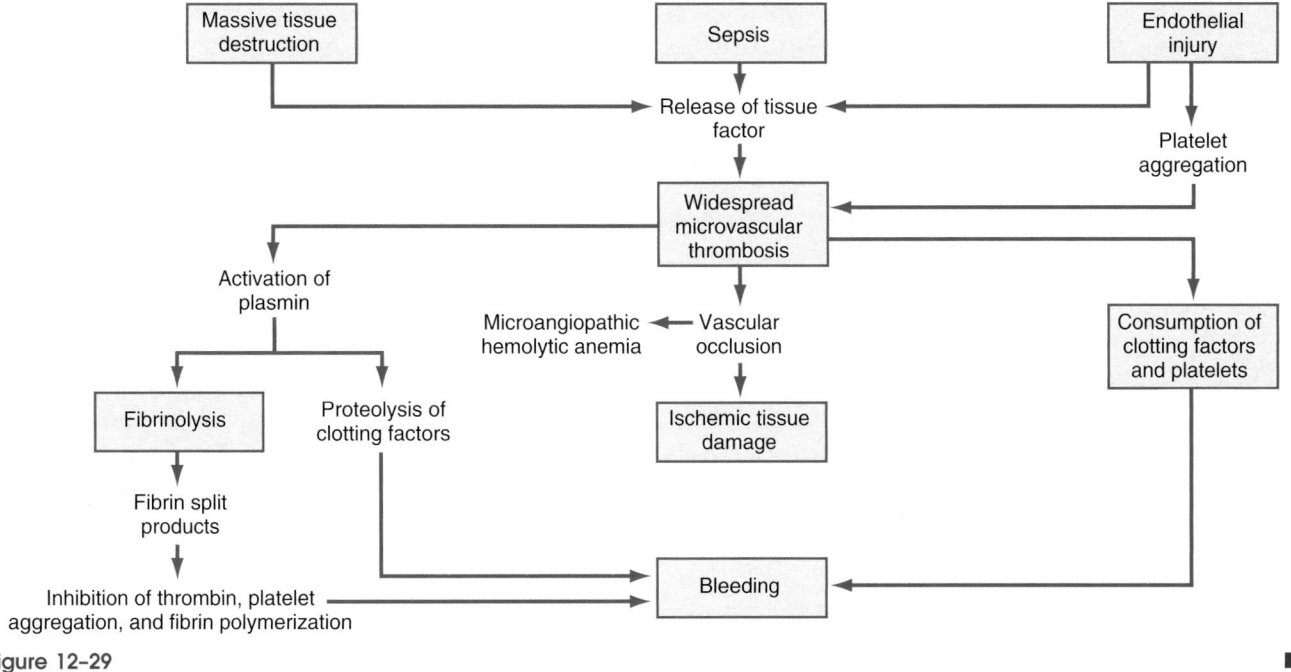

Figure 12-29

Pathophysiology of disseminated intravascular coagulation.

The tissue thromboplastic substances released into the circulation may be derived from a variety of sources—for example from the placenta in obstetric complications, from the cytoplasmic granules in the leukemic cells of acute promyelocytic leukemia, or from neoplastic cells in mucin-secreting adenocarcinomas. Carcinomas may also release other procoagulant substances, such as proteolytic enzymes, mucin, and other undefined tumor products. Some tumors express tissue factor on the cell membrane. In gram-negative and gram-positive sepsis (important causes of DIC), endotoxins or exotoxins cause increased synthesis, membrane exposure, and release of tissue factor from monocytes. Furthermore, activated monocytes release IL-1 and TNF, both of which increase the expression of tissue factor on endothelial cell membranes and simultaneously decrease the expression of thrombomodulin. The latter, you may recall, activates protein C, an anticoagulant (Chapter 4). The result is both activation of the extrinsic clotting system and inhibition of coagulation control.

Endothelial cell injury can initiate DIC by causing release of tissue factor and by promoting platelet aggregation and activation of the intrinsic coagulation cascade as a result of the exposure of subendothelial collagen. Even subtle damage to the endothelium can unleash procoagulant activity by enhancing membrane expression of tissue factor. Widespread endothelial injury may be produced by deposition of antigen-antibody complexes (e.g., in SLE), by temperature extremes (e.g., in heat stroke or burns), or by microorganisms (e.g., meningococci and rickettsiae). As discussed in Chapter 4, endothelial injury is an important consequence of endotoxemia, and, not surprisingly, DIC is a frequent complication of gram-negative sepsis.

Several additional disorders associated with DIC are listed in Table 12–14. Of these, *DIC is most likely to fol-*

low sepsis, obstetric complications, malignancy, and major trauma (especially trauma to the brain). The initiating factors in these conditions are multiple and often interrelated. For example, in obstetric conditions, tissue factor derived from the placenta, retained dead fetus, or amniotic fluid

■

Table 12-14. MAJOR DISORDERS ASSOCIATED WITH DISSEMINATED INTRAVASCULAR COAGULATION

Obstetric Complications

Abruptio placentae
Retained dead fetus
Septic abortion
Amniotic fluid embolism
Toxemia

Infections

Sepsis (gram-negative and gram-positive)
Meningococcemia
Rocky Mountain spotted fever
Histoplasmosis
Aspergillosis
Malaria

Neoplasms

Carcinomas of pancreas, prostate, lung, and stomach
Acute promyelocytic leukemia

Massive Tissue Injury

Trauma
Burns
Extensive surgery

Miscellaneous

Acute intravascular hemolysis, snake bite, giant hemangioma, shock, heat stroke, vasculitis, aortic aneurysm, liver disease may enter the circulation; however, shock, hypoxia, and acidosis often coexist and may cause widespread endothelial injury. Supervening infections may complicate the problem further. Trauma to the brain releases fat and phospholipids, and there is systemic activation of proinflammatory cytokines that affect endothelium.

Whatever the pathogenetic mechanism, DIC has two consequences. First, *there is widespread fibrin deposition within the microcirculation.* This leads to ischemia in the more severely affected or more vulnerable organs and to hemolysis as the RBCs are traumatized while passing through the fibrin strands *(microangiopathic hemolytic anemia).* Second, a *bleeding diathesis* ensues as the platelets and clotting factors are consumed and there is secondary release of plasminogen activators. Plasmin can not only cleave fibrin (fibrinolysis) but also digest factors V and VIII, thereby reducing their concentration further. In addition, fibrinolysis leads to the formation of fibrin degradation products, which have an inhibitory effect on platelet aggregation, have antithrombin activity, and impair fibrin polymerization, all of which contribute to the hemostatic failure (see Fig. 12–29).

MORPHOLOGY

Microthrombi are found principally in the arterioles and capillaries of the kidneys, adrenals, brain, and heart, but no organ is spared, and the lungs, liver, and gastrointestinal mucosa may also be prominently involved. The glomeruli contain small fibrin thrombi, which may evoke only a reactive swelling of the endothelial cells or may be surrounded by a florid focal glomerulitis. The resultant ischemia leads to microinfarcts in the renal cortex. In severe cases, the ischemia may even extend to destroy the entire cortex and cause bilateral renal cortical necrosis. Involvement of the adrenal glands reproduces the picture of the **Waterhouse-Friderichsen syndrome** (Chapter 20). Microinfarcts are also commonly encountered in the brain, surrounded by microscopic or gross foci of hemorrhage. These may give rise to bizarre neurologic signs. Similar changes are seen in the heart and often in the anterior pituitary. It has been suggested that DIC may contribute to **Sheehan postpartum pituitary necrosis** (Chapter 20).

When the underlying disorder is toxemia of pregnancy, the placenta is the site of capillary thromboses and, occasionally, florid degeneration of the vessel walls. Such changes are in all likelihood responsible for the premature loss of cytotrophoblasts and syncytiotrophoblasts that characterizes this condition.

The bleeding tendency associated with DIC is manifested not only by larger than expected hemorrhages near foci of infarction but also by diffuse petechiae and ecchymoses, which may be found on the skin, serosal linings of the body cavities, epicardium, endocardium, lungs, and mucosal lining of the urinary tract.

Clinical Course. The clinical picture is an apparent paradox, with a bleeding tendency in the presence of evidence of widespread coagulation. It is almost impossible to detail all the potential clinical manifestations. In general, *acute DIC (e.g., that associated with obstetric complications) is dominated by a bleeding diathesis, whereas chronic DIC (e.g., as may occur in a patient with cancer) tends to present as thrombotic complications.* Typically, the abnormal clotting occurs only in the microcirculation, although large vessels are involved occasionally. The manifestations may be minimal, or there may be shock, with acute renal failure, dyspnea, cyanosis, convulsions, and coma. Hypotension is characteristic. Most often, attention is called to the presence of a bleeding diathesis by prolonged and copious postpartum bleeding or by the presence of petechiae and ecchymoses on the skin. These may be the only manifestations, or there may be severe hemorrhage into the gut or urinary tract. Laboratory evaluation reveals *thrombocytopenia and prolongation of PT and PTT* (owing to consumption of platelets, clotting factors, and fibrinogen). *Fibrin split products* are increased in the plasma.

The prognosis for patients with DIC is highly variable and depends on the underlying disorder as well as on the degree of intravascular clotting, the activity of the mononuclear phagocyte system, and the amount of fibrinolysis. In some cases it can be life threatening; in others it can be treated with anticoagulants such as heparin or coagulants contained in fresh-frozen plasma. The underlying disorder must be treated simultaneously to prevent the progressive derangement of hemostasis.

THROMBOCYTOPENIA

Thrombocytopenia is characterized by spontaneous bleeding, a prolonged bleeding time, and normal PT and PTT. A platelet count of 100,000/μL or less is generally considered to constitute thrombocytopenia, although spontaneous bleeding does not become evident until the count falls below 20,000/μL. Platelet counts in the range of 20,000 to 50,000 may lead to post-traumatic bleeding. Thrombocytopenia is associated with bleeding from small blood vessels. Petechiae or large ecchymoses are commonly found in the skin and the mucous membranes of the gastrointestinal and urinary tracts, but no site is excluded. Bleeding into the central nervous system constitutes a major hazard in patients whose platelet count is markedly depressed. The etiologic groups of thrombocytopenia are listed in Table 12–15. Of these, reduced production and increased destruction are the most important categories.

■ A decrease in the production of platelets is associated with various forms of marrow failure or injury; these include idiopathic aplastic anemias, drug-induced marrow failure, and marrow infiltration by tumors. Thrombocytopenia is also an important hazard after bone marrow transplantation. Platelet recovery occurs much more slowly than recovery of other lineages. In all of these settings, the cytopenia is associated with a decrease in marrow megakaryocytes.

Table 12-15. CAUSES OF THROMBOCYTOPENIA

Decreased Production of Platelets

Generalized disease of bone marrow
    Aplastic anemia: congenital and acquired
    Marrow infiltration: leukemia, disseminated cancer
Selective impairment of platelet production
    Drug-induced: alcohol, thiazides, cytotoxic drugs
    Infections: measles, HIV infection
Ineffective megakaryopoiesis
    Megaloblastic anemia
    Paroxysmal nocturnal hemoglobinuria

Decreased Platelet Survival

Immunologic destruction
    Autoimmune: idiopathic thrombocytopenic purpura, systemic lupus erythematosus
    Isoimmune: post-transfusion and neonatal
    Drug-associated: quinidine, heparin, sulfa compounds
    Infections: infectious mononucleosis, HIV infection, cytomegalovirus infection
Nonimmunologic destruction
    Disseminated intravascular coagulation
    Thrombotic thrombocytopenic purpura
    Giant hemangiomas
    Microangiopathic hemolytic anemias

Sequestration

Hypersplenism

Dilutional

HIV, human immunodeficiency virus.

■ Accelerated destruction of platelets is often immunologically mediated, resulting from formation of antiplatelet antibodies or adsorption by platelets of immune complexes formed in the circulation. Antibody-mediated destruction of platelets may be associated with well-known autoimmune diseases such as SLE, or it may appear as an apparently isolated derangement (idiopathic thrombocytopenic purpura). Some of the drug-induced thrombocytopenias are also immunologically mediated.

■ Excessive destruction of platelets is mediated in some cases by nonimmunologic means. As mentioned earlier, excessive utilization of platelets occurs in DIC. Other nonimmunologic causes include prosthetic heart valves and the rare disorder called thrombotic thrombocytopenic purpura, described later. Whatever the cause of accelerated destruction, the bone marrow reveals a normal or a compensatory increase in megakaryocytes. Hence, bone marrow examination allows a ready distinction between the two major categories of thrombocytopenia.

Thrombocytopenia is one of the most common hematologic manifestations of the acquired immunodeficiency syndrome. It may occur early in the course of HIV infection and is believed to result from immune complex–mediated injury of platelets, autoantibodies, and HIV-mediated suppression of megakaryocytes.

Idiopathic Thrombocytopenic Purpura

A disorder of autoimmune origin, idiopathic thrombocytopenic purpura (ITP) most often occurs as an apparently isolated derangement but sometimes as a first manifestation of SLE. Although an acute, self-limited form that follows viral infections has been described in children, most patients are adult females between the ages of 20 and 40 years in whom the condition is designated "chronic ITP." It may occur in isolation or in association with an underlying condition such as lymphoma or collagen vascular disease (e.g., SLE).

Antiplatelet immunoglobulins directed against platelet membrane glycoproteins IIb/IIIa or Ib/IX complexes can be identified in many patients with ITP. In some patients, the autoantibodies may bind to megakaryocytes and impair platelet production as well. In most cases megakaryocyte injury is not significant enough to deplete their numbers. The spleen plays an important role in the pathogenesis of this disorder. It is the major site of production of the antiplatelet antibodies and destruction of the IgG-coated platelets. In more than two thirds of patients, splenectomy is followed by the return of normal platelet counts and complete remission of the disease. The spleen usually appears remarkably normal, with only minimal, if any, enlargement. The presence of splenomegaly or lymphadenopathy should lead one to consider other possible diagnoses. Histologically, the marrow may appear normal but usually reveals increased numbers of megakaryocytes, some of which have only a single nucleus and are thought to be young. A similar marrow picture is noted in most forms of thrombocytopenia that result from accelerated platelet destruction. Marrow examination may be used to rule out thrombocytopenia resulting from marrow failure.

The onset of chronic ITP is usually insidious. The patients manifest petechiae, easy bruisability, epistaxis, gum bleeding, and hemorrhages after minor trauma. More serious intracerebral or subarachnoid hemorrhages are much less common, especially in patients treated with steroids. The diagnosis is based on clinical features, the presence of thrombocytopenia, marrow examination, and exclusion of secondary causes of thrombocytopenia. Reliable tests for specific antiplatelet antibodies are not widely available.

Heparin-Induced Thrombocytopenia

This special type of drug-induced thrombocytopenia merits brief mention because of its clinical importance. Three percent to 5% of patients treated with unfractionated heparin become moderately to severely thrombocytopenic after 1 to 2 weeks of therapy. The thrombocytopenia is caused by acquired IgG antibodies that recognize platelet factor 4/heparin complexes on platelet surfaces. Through mechanisms that are still being elucidated, antibody binding results in platelet activation and aggregation, thus exacerbating the condition that heparin is used to treat: thrombosis. Both venous and arterial thromboses occur, even in the setting of severe thrombocytopenia, and may cause severe morbidity (e.g., loss of limbs because of vascular insufficiency) or death. Cessation of heparin therapy breaks the cycle of platelet activation and consumption.

Thrombotic Microangiopathies: Thrombotic Thrombocytopenic Purpura and Hemolytic-Uremic Syndrome

The term *thrombotic microangiopathies* encompasses a spectrum of clinical syndromes that includes thrombotic thrombocytopenic purpura (TTP) and hemolytic-uremic syndrome (HUS). Traditionally, *TTP has been characterized by its occurrence in adult females and the pentad of fever, thrombocytopenia, microangiopathic hemolytic anemia, transient neurologic deficits, and renal failure.* HUS, like TTP, is also associated with microangiopathic hemolytic anemia and thrombocytopenia but is distinguished from it by the absence of neurologic symptoms, the dominance of acute renal failure, and onset in childhood (Chapter 14). Recent studies have blurred these distinctions, because many adults with TTP lack one or more of the five criteria, and some patients with HUS have fever and neurologic dysfunction. *Fundamental to both of these conditions is widespread formation of hyaline thrombi in the microcirculation that are composed primarily of dense aggregates of platelets surrounded by fibrin.* Formation of myriads of platelet aggregates causes thrombocytopenia, and the narrowing of blood vessels by the thrombi results in microangiopathic hemolytic anemia.

For many years, the pathogenesis of TTP was enigmatic, although treatment with plasma exchange (initiated in the early 1970s) converted a disease that was almost uniformly fatal into one that is successfully treated in more than 80% of cases. Recently, the underlying cause of most, but not all, cases of TTP has been elucidated. In brief, *it has been found that symptomatic patients are deficient in an enzyme (designated "metalloprotease" but unrelated to better characterized "tissue metalloproteases") that normally degrades very-high-molecular-weight multimers of von Willebrand factor (vWF)* (see discussion of vWF later). In the absence of this enzyme, very-high-molecular-weight multimers of vWF accumulate in plasma and, under some circumstances, promote platelet microaggregate formation throughout the microcirculation, leading to the symptoms of the disease. Superimposition of endothelial cell injury (caused by some other condition) may further predispose the patient to microaggregate formation, thus initiating or exacerbating clinically evident TTP.

The deficiency of vWF-cleaving protease may be familial and genetic or more commonly may be acquired due to the formation of an autoantibody that inhibits the vWF metalloprotease. This protease has recently been cloned. TTP needs to be considered in any patient who presents with unexplained thrombocytopenia and microangiopathic hemolytic anemia, because failure to make an early diagnosis can be fatal.

Although clinically overlapping, HUS is pathogenetically distinct from TTP. HUS of childhood usually follows infectious gastroenteritis caused by *E. coli* strain O157:H7. This strain elaborates a *Shiga*-like toxin that damages endothelial cells, which then initiate platelet activation and aggregation. The affected children present with bloody diarrhea, and a few days later HUS makes its appearance. With supportive care and plasma exchange, affected children often recover completely, but irreversible renal damage and death may occur in more severe cases. HUS may also be seen in adults after

exposures (e.g., to certain drugs, radiation therapy) that damage endothelial cells. The prognosis of adults with HUS is more guarded, in part because it is most often seen in the setting of other chronic, life-threatenining conditions.

Although DIC and the thrombotic microangiopathies share features such as microvascular occlusion and microangiopathic hemolytic anemia, they are pathogenetically distinct. In TTP and HUS, unlike in DIC, activation of the coagulation cascade is not of primary importance, and thus results of laboratory tests of coagulation, such as PT and PTT, are usually normal.

COAGULATION DISORDERS

These disorders result from either congenital or acquired deficiencies of clotting factors. The latter, which are much more common and relatively straightforward, are considered first.

Acquired coagulation disorders are usually associated with deficiencies of multiple clotting factors. As discussed in Chapter 8, *vitamin K deficiency* may be associated with a severe coagulation defect, because this nutrient is essential for the synthesis of prothrombin and clotting factors VII, IX, and X. The liver is the site of synthesis of several coagulation factors; thus, *parenchymal diseases of the liver are common causes of hemorrhagic diatheses.* In addition, several liver diseases are associated with complex derangements of platelet function and fibrinogen metabolism, all of which contribute to the coagulopathy in liver disease.

Hereditary deficiencies have been identified for each of the coagulation factors. These deficiencies characteristically occur singly. Hemophilia A, resulting from deficiency of factor VIII, and hemophilia B (Christmas disease), resulting from deficiency of factor IX, are transmitted as X-linked recessive disorders, whereas most others are autosomal disorders. Most of these conditions are rare; only von Willebrand disease, hemophilia A, and hemophilia B are sufficiently common to warrant further consideration here.

Deficiencies of Factor VIII/von Willebrand Factor Complex

Hemophilia A and von Willebrand disease, two of the most common inherited disorders of bleeding, are caused by qualitative or quantitative defects involving factor VIII/vWF complex. Before we can discuss these disorders, it is essential to review the structure and function of these proteins.

Plasma factor VIII/vWF is a complex made up of two separate proteins that can be distinguished by functional, biochemical, and immunologic criteria. One component, which is required for the activation of factor X in the intrinsic coagulation pathway, is called *factor VIII procoagulant protein,* or *factor VIII* (Fig. 12–30). Deficiency of factor VIII gives rise to hemophilia A. Through noncovalent bonds, factor VIII is linked to a much larger protein, vWF, which forms approximately 99% of the vWF/factor VIII complex. vWF is not a discrete protein but exists in the form of a series of high-molecular-weight multimers. It is present normally in the cir-

Figure 12–30   ■

Structure and function of factor VIII/von Willebrand factor (vWF) complex. Factor VIII is synthesized by the liver and vWF in the endothelial cells. The two circulate as a complex in the circulation. vWF is also present in the subendothelial matrix of normal blood vessels. Factor VIII takes part in the coagulation cascade by activating factor X. vWF causes adhesion of platelets to subendothelial collagen, primarily via GpIb platelet receptor. Ristocetin activates GpIb receptors in vitro and causes platelet aggregation if vWF is present.

culation (in association with factor VIII) and in the subendothelium, where it binds to collagen.

When endothelial cells are stripped away by trauma or injury, subendothelial vWF becomes exposed and binds to platelets through the receptors glycoproteins Ib and IIb/IIIa (see Fig. 12–30). Indeed, *the most important function of vWF in vivo is to facilitate the adhesion of platelets to damaged blood vessel walls.* Thus, vWF is crucial to the normal process of hemostasis, and its absence in von Willebrand disease leads to a bleeding diathesis. In addition to its function in platelet adhesion, vWF also serves as a carrier for factor VIII. When factor VIII is activated by thrombin, it dissociates from vWF and serves its coagulant function.

The various forms of von Willebrand disease can be characterized by immunologic techniques and the so-called ristocetin agglutination test. Ristocetin (developed as an antibiotic) binds platelets and promotes the interaction between vWF and platelet membrane glycoprotein Ib. The binding of vWF creates interplatelet "bridges" that lead to the formation of platelet clumps (agglutination), an event that can be easily measured. Thus, the degree of ristocetin-dependent platelet agglutination caused by the addition of patient plasma serves as a bioassay for vWF.

The two components of the factor VIII/vWF complex are coded by separate genes and are synthesized by different cells. Although vWF is produced by both endothelial cells and megakaryocytes, the former cells are the major source of plasma vWF. Factor VIII can be synthesized by several tissues, but liver is the major source of this protein. *To summarize, the two components of factor VIII/vWF complex, synthesized separately, come together and circulate in the plasma as a unit that serves to promote clotting as well as the platelet–vessel wall interactions necessary to ensure hemostasis.* With this background we can turn to the discussion of diseases resulting from deficiencies of factor VIII/vWF complex.

vON WILLEBRAND DISEASE

von Willebrand disease is characterized clinically by spontaneous bleeding from mucous membranes, excessive bleeding from wounds, menorrhagia, and a prolonged bleeding time in the presence of a normal platelet count. In most cases it is transmitted as an autosomal dominant disorder, but several rare autosomal recessive variants have been identified. Its precise incidence is difficult to estimate, because in many instances the clinical manifestations are mild and the diagnosis requires sophisticated tests; it may well be the most common inherited bleeding disorder.

Without delving into great complexity, we can state that the classic and most common variant (type I) of von Willebrand disease is characterized by a reduced quantity of circulating vWF. Because vWF stabilizes factor VIII by binding to it, a deficiency of vWF is associated with a secondary decrease in the levels of factor VIII. The other less common varieties of von Willebrand disease tend to show qualitative and quantitative defects in vWF. Type II is divided into several subtypes that are all characterized by a selective loss of high molecular-weight multimers of vWF. Because these multimers are the most active form of vWF, there is a functional deficiency. In type IIA, the high-molecular-weight multimers are not synthesized, leading to a true deficiency. In type IIB, functionally abnormal high-molecular-weight multimers are synthesized that are rapidly removed from the circulation. These high-molecular-weight multimers may cause spontaneous platelet aggregation (reminiscent of the very-high-molecular-weight multimer aggregates seen in TTP), and indeed some patients with type IIB von Willebrand disease have chronic mild thrombocytopenia that is presumably caused by platelet consumption. To summarize, patients with von Willebrand disease have a compound defect involving platelet function and the coagulation pathway. However, except in severely affected patients (e.g., rare homozygous patients with type III von Willebrand disease), the effects of factor VIII deficiency that characterize hemophilia, such as bleeding into the joints, are uncommon.

FACTOR VIII DEFICIENCY (HEMOPHILIA A, CLASSIC HEMOPHILIA)

Hemophilia A is the most common hereditary disease associated with serious bleeding. It is caused by a reduced amount or reduced activity of factor VIII. As an X-linked recessive trait, it occurs in males or in homozygous females. However, excessive bleeding has been described in heterozygous females, presumably owing to extremely unfavorable lyonization (inactivation of the normal X chromosome in most of the cells). *Approximately 30% of cases are caused by new mutations and hence do not have a family history.* Overt clinical symptoms develop only in the presence of severe deficiency (less than 1% factor VIII activity). Mild (1% to 5% activity) or moderate (5% to 75% activity) degrees of deficiency are usually asymptomatic, although post-traumatic bleeding may be somewhat excessive. The variable degrees of deficiency in the level of factor VIII procoagulant are related to the type of mutation in the factor VIII gene. As with thalassemia, several genetic lesions (e.g., deletions, splice junction mutations, nonsense mutations) have been identified. To add to the complexities, in about 10% of patients levels of factor VIII appear normal by immunoassay, but the coagulant activity detected by bioassay is low. In these patients a mutation causes the synthesis of an antigenically normal but functionally abnormal protein. Approximately 15% of the most severely affected patients have antibodies against factor VIII. The basis of such autoantibody formation is not clear. Their presence complicates replacement therapy.

In all symptomatic cases there is a tendency toward easy bruising and massive hemorrhage after trauma or operative procedures. In addition, "spontaneous" hemorrhages are frequently encountered in regions of the body normally subject to trauma, particularly the joints, where they are known as *hemarthroses.* Recurrent bleeding into the joints leads to progressive deformities that may be crippling. *Petechiae are characteristically absent.* Typically, patients with hemophilia A have a normal bleeding time, normal platelet counts, and a normal PT, with a prolonged PTT that is corrected by mixing with normal plasma. If antibody against factor VIII is present in the patient's plasma, then mixing fails to correct the PTT. Factor VIII assays are required for diagnosis.

Treatment of hemophilia A involves infusion of factor VIII. Historically, replacement therapy involved infusion of factor VIII prepared from human plasma, carrying with it the risk of transmission of viral diseases. As discussed in Chapter 5, before 1985 thousands of hemophiliacs received factor VIII preparations contaminated with HIV. Subsequently, many became seropositive and developed the acquired immunodeficiency syndrome. With current blood banking practices, the risk of HIV transmission has been virtually eliminated, but the threat of other undetected infections remains. The availability and widespread use of recombinant factor VIII has now eliminated the infectious risk of factor VIII replacement therapy.

FACTOR IX DEFICIENCY (HEMOPHILIA B, CHRISTMAS DISEASE)

Severe factor IX deficiency is a disorder that is clinically indistinguishable from hemophilia A. Moreover, it is also inherited as an X-linked recessive trait and may occur asymptomatically or with associated hemorrhage. It is much less common than hemophilia A. The PTT is prolonged; bleeding time is normal. Identification of Christmas disease (named after the first patient with this condition) is possible only by assay of the factor levels. Treatment involves infusion of recombinant factor IX, now widely available.

■
■
■ | Disorders That Affect the Spleen and Thymus

● SPLENOMEGALY

The spleen is frequently involved in a wide variety of systemic diseases. In virtually all cases, the splenic changes are secondary to disease that is primary elsewhere, and in almost all instances the presentation of the splenic lesion is enlargement. Excessive destruction by the spleen of RBCs, leuko-cytes, and platelets may ensue. Evaluation of splenomegaly is a common clinical problem that is aided considerably by knowledge of the usual limits of splenic enlargement caused by the disorders being considered. Obviously, it would be erroneous to attribute enlargement of the spleen into the pelvis to vitamin B_{12} deficiency and equally erroneous to accept as classic a case of chronic myeloid leukemia unless there is significant splenomegaly. As an aid to diagnosis, then, we present the following list of disorders, classified according to the degree of splenomegaly characteristically produced:

A. Massive splenomegaly (weight more than 1000 g)

1. Chronic myeloproliferative disorders (chronic myeloid leukemia, myeloid metaplasia with myelofibrosis)
2. Chronic lymphocytic leukemia (less massive)
3. Hairy cell leukemia
4. Lymphomas
5. Malaria
6. Gaucher disease
7. Primary tumors of the spleen (rare)

B. Moderate splenomegaly (weight 500 to 1000 g)

1. Chronic congestive splenomegaly (portal hypertension or splenic vein obstruction)
2. Acute leukemias (inconstant)
3. Hereditary spherocytosis
4. Thalassemia major
5. Autoimmune hemolytic anemia
6. Amyloidosis
7. Niemann-Pick disease
8. Langerhans histiocytosis
9. Chronic splenitis (especially with infective endocarditis)
10. Tuberculosis, sarcoidosis, typhoid
11. Metastatic carcinoma or sarcoma

C. Mild splenomegaly (weight less than 500 g)

1. Acute splenitis
2. Acute splenic congestion
3. Infectious mononucleosis
4. Miscellaneous acute febrile disorders, including septicemia, systemic lupus erythematosus, and intra-abdominal infections

The microscopic changes associated with most of the previously mentioned diseases need not be described here, because they have been discussed in the relevant sections of this and other chapters.

An enlarged spleen may remove excessive amounts of one or more of the formed elements of blood, resulting in anemia, leukopenia, or thrombocytopenia. This is referred to as *hypersplenism* and may be associated with many of the diseases of the spleen listed previously. In some cases, however, hypersplenism is associated with an apparently normal spleen, without any known cause for splenic hyperfunction. These cases are labeled *primary hypersplenism.*

DISORDERS OF THE THYMUS

As is well known, the thymus is a central lymphoid organ that plays a critical role in T-cell differentiation. It is not surprising, therefore, that the thymus can be involved in lymphomas, particularly those of T-cell lineage. These were discussed earlier in this chapter. Here we will focus on the two most frequent (albeit uncommon) disorders of the thymus: thymic hyperplasias and thymomas.

Hyperplasia

The normal thymus is devoid of lymphoid follicles. *Hyperplasia of the thymus is characterized by the appearance of lymphoid follicles within the medulla.* Immunochemical staining techniques reveal that the follicles are rich in immunoglobulins. Thymic hyperplasia is present in most patients with myasthenia gravis and is also present in various other autoimmune diseases such as SLE and rheumatoid arthritis. The relationship between the thymus and myasthenia gravis is discussed in Chapter 21; for now, it suffices that T cells generated in the thymus and sensitized to its myoid cells cooperate with B cells in the lymphoid follicles to produce the autoantibodies that underlie the autoimmune reaction to acetylcholine receptors at the neuromuscular junction, a characteristic of this grave neuromuscular disorder. Significantly, removal of a hyperplastic thymus is beneficial early in the disease.

Thymoma

Although the normal thymus is a lymphoepithelial organ, the term *thymoma* is restricted to tumors in which epithelial cells constitute the neoplastic element. Scant or abundant thymic lymphocytes may also be present in these tumors, but they are normal, non-neoplastic thymocytes. Lymphomas arising in the lymphoid elements of the thymus gland are therefore not classified as thymomas. Numerous subtypes of thymoma have been established, based on cytologic and biologic criteria. A commonly used classification is as follows:

■ Benign thymoma: cytologically and biologically benign
■ Malignant thymoma

   Type I: cytologically benign but biologically aggressive and capable of local invasion and, rarely, distant spread
   Type II: also called *thymic carcinoma:* cytologically malignant with all of the features of cancer and comparable behavior

MORPHOLOGY

Macroscopically, thymomas are lobulated, firm, gray-white masses up to 15 to 20 cm in longest dimension. Most appear encapsulated, but in 20% to 25% there is apparent penetration of the capsule and infiltration of perithymic tissues and structures.

Microscopically, virtually all thymomas are made up of a mixture of epithelial cells and a variable infiltrate of non-neoplastic lymphocytes. The relative proportions of the epithelial and lymphocytic components are of little significance. In **benign thymomas,** the epithelial cells tend to resemble those of the medulla and are often elongated or spindle shaped, producing what is called a **medullary thymoma.** Frequently, there is an admixture of the plumper, rounder, cortical-type epithelial cells, and some are composed largely of such cells. This pattern of thymoma often has few lymphocytes. Some experts would call this pattern a **mixed thymoma.** The medullary and mixed patterns account for 60% to 70% of all thymomas.

The designation **malignant thymoma type I** implies a cytologically benign tumor that is locally invasive and sometimes has the capacity for widespread metastasis. These tumors account for 20% to 25% of all thymomas. They are composed of varying proportions of epithelial cells and lymphocytes; the epithelial cells, however, tend to be of the cortical variety, with abundant cytoplasm and rounded vesicular nuclei. Palisading of these cells about blood vessels is sometimes seen. Some spindled epithelial cells may be present as well. **The critical distinguishing feature of these neoplasms is penetration of the capsule with invasion into surrounding structures.**

Malignant thymoma type II is better designated **thymic carcinoma.** These represent about 5% of thymomas. In contrast to the type I malignant thymomas, these are cytologically malignant. Macroscopically, they are usually fleshy, obviously invasive masses sometimes accompanied by metastases to such sites as the lungs. Most are **squamous cell carcinomas, either well or poorly differentiated.** The next most common malignant pattern is the so-called **lymphoepithelioma,** composed of cytologically anaplastic cortical-type epithelial cells scattered against a dense background of benign-appearing lymphocytes. Some of these tumors contain the EBV genome and hence resemble nasopharyngeal carcinomas.

Clinical Features. All thymomas are rarities, the malignant more so than the benign. They may arise at any age but typically occur in middle adult life. In a large series, about 30% were asymptomatic; 30% to 40% produced local manifestations such as a mass demonstrable on computed tomography in the anterosuperior mediastinum associated with cough, dyspnea, and superior vena caval syndrome; and the remainder were associated with some systemic disease, principally myasthenia gravis. Fifteen to 20% of patients with this disorder have a thymoma. Removal of the tumor often leads to improvement in the neuromuscular disorder. Additional associations with thymomas include hypogammaglobulinemia, SLE, pure red cell aplasia, and nonthymic cancers.

BIBLIOGRAPHY

Red Cell Disorders

Andrews NC: Disorders of iron metabolism. N Engl J Med 341:1986, 1999. (An excellent review of all aspects of iron metabolism, including those relevant to iron deficiency and the anemia of chronic disease.)

Beutler E, Luzzatto L: Hemolytic anemia. Semin Hematol 36:38, 1999. (An excellent overview of the hemolytic anemias.)

Bunn HF: Pathogenesis and treatment of sickle cell disease. N Engl J Med 337:762, 1997. (Discussion of why sickle crises occur, and the role of hydroxyurea in their prevention.)

Luzzatto L, Bessler M: The dual pathogenesis of paroxysmal nocturnal hemoglobinuria. Curr Opin Hematol 3:101, 1996. (Discussion of the dual role of somatic mutation and autoimmunity in PNH.)

Pasloske BL, et al: Malaria, the red cell, and the endothelium. Annu Rev Med 45:283, 1994. (A review of the importance of endothelial cell:RBC interactions in cerebral malaria.)

Young NS: Hematopoietic cell destruction by immune mechanisms in acquired aplastic anemia. Semin Hematol 37:3, 2000. (An updated perspective on the causes and management of AA.)

White Cell Disorders

Bartolo C, Viswanatha DS: Molecular diagnosis in pediatric acute leukemias. Clin Lab Med 20:139, 2000. (A review of the molecular pathogenesis and diagnosis of ALL.)

Chaganti RS: Recurring chromosomal abnormalities in non-Hodgkin's lymphoma: histologic and clinical significance. Semin Hematol 37:396, 2000. (A summary of the chromosomal changes seen in the non-Hodgkin lymphomas.)

Daley GQ, et al: Induction of chronic myelogenous leukemia in mice by the Ph[1] bcr/abl gene of the Philadelphia chromosome. Science 247:824, 1990. (A classic paper demonstrating the role of the bcr-abl fusion protein in CML.)

Harris NL, et al: A revised European-American classification of lymphoid neoplasms: a proposal from the International Lymphoma Study Group. Blood 84:1361, 1994. (The widely accepted REAL classification for lymphoid neoplasms.)

Harris NL, et al: World Health Organization classification of neoplastic diseases of the hematopoietic and lymphoid tissues: report of the Clinical Advisory Committee meeting—Airlie House, Virginia, November 1997. J Clin Oncol 17:3835, 1999. (A progress report confirming the utility of the REAL classification for lymphoid neoplasms, and proposing new classification schemes for myeloid neoplasms.)

Kantargian H, et al: Hematologic and cytogenetic responses to imatinib mesylate in chronic myelogenous leukemia. N Engl J Med 346:645, 2002. (An elegant example of how understanding the molecular biology of CML has led to its treatment.)

Klein B, et al: Interleukin-6 in human multiple myeloma. Blood 85:863, 1995. (A summary of the role of IL-6 in the pathogenesis of multiple myeloma.)

Kuppers R, et al: Cellular origin of human B-cell lymphomas. N Engl J Med 341:1520, 1999. (A clear discussion of the origin of diverse B-cell malignancies.)

Kuppers R, Rajewsky K: The origin of Hodgkin and Reed/Sternberg cells in Hodgkin's disease. Annu Rev Immunol 16:471, 1998. (Discussion of the compelling data supporting a B-cell origin for RS cells and variants.)

Marcucci C, et al: Molecular and clinical advances in core binding factor primary acute myeloid leukemia: a paradigm for translational research in malignant hematology. Cancer Invest 18:768, 2000. (A review of the salient features of common forms of AML associated with the t[8;21] and inv[16].)

Schipp MA, et al: Diffuse B-cell lymphoma outcome prediction by gene expression profiling and supervised machine learning. Nat Med 8:68, 2002. (An example of how molecular profiling can predict clinical outcome in large B-cell lymphoma.)

Slack JL: Biology and treatment of acute progranulocytic leukemia. Curr Opin Hematol 6:236, 1999. (A discussion of the uncommon but important AML variant associated with the t[15;17].)

Young NS: Agranulocytosis. JAMA 271:935, 1994. (A practical approach to the etiology and management of agranulocytosis.)

Coagulation Disorders

Boyce TG, et al: *Escherichia coli* O157:H7 and the hemolytic-uremic syndrome. N Engl J Med 333:364, 1995. (An article on the etiology and pathogenesis of the hemolytic-uremic syndrome.)

Dahlback B: Blood coagulation. Lancet 355:1627, 2001. (A succinct review of coagulation and bleeding disorders.)

Kashansky K: The vWF-clearing protease: new opportunities in TTP. Blood 98:1643, 2001. (A brief editiorial on the cloning of vWF-clearing protease and pathogenesis of TTP.)

Keeney A, Cummings AM: The molecular biology of von Willebrand disease. Clin Lab Hematol 4:209, 2001. (An update on this disorder.)

Levi M, Cate HT: Disseminated intravascular coagulation. N Engl J Med 341:586, 1999. (A clinically oriented review of the causes, pathogenesis, and treatment of this disorder.)

Visentin CP: Heparin-induced thrombocytopenia: molecular pathogenesis. Thromb Haemost 82:448, 1999. (A discussion of the role of autoantibodies against platelet factor 4 and heparin in heparin-induced thrombocytopenia.)

The Lung and the Upper Respiratory Tract

ANIRBAN MAITRA, MD
VINAY KUMAR, MD

The major function of the lung is to excrete carbon dioxide from blood and replenish oxygen. The chest wall and diaphragm act as a bellows to move air in and out of the lungs, allowing gas exchange across the alveolocapillary membrane. Obviously, opportunities for disease in this important organ system are legion. A common approach in the study of lung pathology, and one that provides the framework for this chapter, is to organize lung diseases into those affecting (1) the airways, (2) the interstitium, and (3) the pulmonary vascular system. This division into discrete compartments is, of course, deceptively neat. In reality, disease in one compartment is generally accompanied by alterations of morphology and function in another.

The respiratory system includes, in addition to the lungs, (1) the diaphragm and muscles of the chest wall, (2) the regulatory neural circuits, (3) the pleural spaces, and (4) the upper respiratory tract (the nasopharynx and trachea, including the larynx). Diseases affecting the first two will not be discussed, but those affecting the pleura and upper respiratory tract will be considered after a discussion of diseases of the lung. We begin our discussion with atelectasis, because it can complicate many primary lung disorders.

ATELECTASIS (COLLAPSE)

Atelectasis, also known as collapse, is loss of lung volume caused by inadequate *expansion of airspaces*. It is associated with shunting of inadequately oxygenated blood from pulmonary arteries into veins, thus giving rise to a ventilation-perfusion imbalance and hypoxia. On the basis of the underlying mechanism or the distribution of alveolar collapse, atelectasis is divided into four categories (Fig. 13–1).

Resorption Atelectasis. Resorption atelectasis occurs when an obstruction prevents air from reaching distal airways. The air already present gradually becomes absorbed, and alveolar collapse follows. Depending on the level of airway obstruction, an entire lung, a complete lobe, or one or more segments may be involved. The most common cause of resorption collapse is obstruction of a bronchus by a mucous or mucopurulent plug. This frequently occurs postoperatively but may also complicate bronchial asthma, bronchiectasis, or chronic bronchitis. Sometimes obstruction is caused by the aspiration of foreign bodies, particularly in children, or blood clots during oral surgery or anesthesia. Airways may also be obstructed by tumors (especially bronchogenic carcinoma), by enlarged lymph nodes (as from tuberculosis), and (rarely) by vascular aneurysms.

Compression Atelectasis. Compression atelectasis (sometimes called *passive* or *relaxation atelectasis*) is usually associated with accumulations of fluid, blood, or air within the pleural cavity, which mechanically collapse the adjacent lung. This is a frequent occurrence with pleural effusions, caused most commonly by congestive heart failure. Leakage of air into the pleural cavity (pneumothorax) also leads to compression atelectasis. Basal at-

electasis resulting from the elevated position of the diaphragm commonly occurs in bedridden patients, in patients with ascites, and in patients during and after surgery.

Microatelectasis. Microatelectasis (or nonobstructive atelectasis) is a generalized loss of lung expansion caused by a complex set of events, the most important of which is loss of surfactant. Microatelectasis is present in both acute and neonatal respiratory distress syndromes and in several lung diseases associated with interstitial inflammation. Microatelectasis also occurs in the setting of postsurgical atelectasis.

Contraction Atelectasis. Contraction (or *cicatrization*) atelectasis occurs when either local or generalized fibrotic changes in the lung or pleura hamper expansion and increase elastic recoil during expiration.

Atelectasis (except that caused by contraction) is potentially reversible and should be treated promptly to prevent hypoxemia and superimposed infection of the collapsed lung.

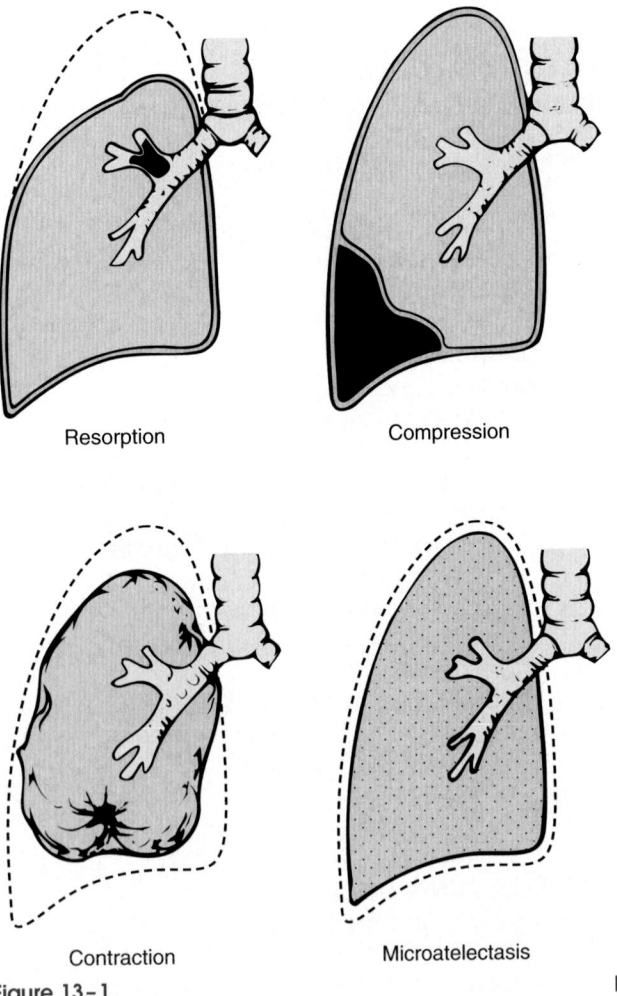

Resorption   Compression

Contraction   Microatelectasis

Figure 13–1   ■

Various forms of atelectasis.

OBSTRUCTIVE AND RESTRICTIVE LUNG DISEASES

Diffuse pulmonary diseases can be classified in two categories: (1) obstructive disease (airway disease), characterized by limitation of airflow usually resulting from an increase in resistance from partial or complete obstruction at any level; and (2) restrictive disease, characterized by reduced expansion of lung parenchyma accompanied by decreased total lung capacity.

The major obstructive disorders (excluding tumors or inhalation of a foreign body) are *asthma, emphysema, chronic bronchitis, bronchiectasis, cystic fibrosis*, and *bronchiolitis*. In patients with these diseases, total lung capacity and forced vital capacity (FVC) are either normal or increased, but the hallmark is a decreased expiratory flow rate, usually measured by forced expiratory volume at 1 second (FEV_1). Thus, *the ratio of FEV_1 and FVC is characteristically decreased.* Expiratory obstruction may result either from anatomic airway narrowing, classically observed in asthma, or from loss of elastic recoil, characteristic of emphysema.

In contrast, in *restrictive diseases*, FVC is reduced and the expiratory flow rate is normal or reduced proportionately. Hence, *the ratio of FEV_1 and FVC is near normal.* The restrictive defect occurs in two general conditions: (1) *extrapulmonary disorders* that affect the ability of the chest wall to act as a bellows (e.g., severe obesity, kyphoscoliosis, and neuromuscular disorders, such as the Guillain-Barré syndrome [Chapter 23], that affect the respiratory muscles) and (2) *acute or chronic interstitial lung diseases*. The classic acute restrictive disease is acute respiratory distress syndrome (ARDS). *Chronic* restrictive diseases include the pneumoconioses (Chapter 8), sarcoidosis, and idiopathic pulmonary fibrosis (IPF).

Obstructive Lung Diseases

ASTHMA

Asthma is characterized by episodic, reversible bronchospasm resulting from an exaggerated bronchoconstrictor response to various stimuli. The basis of bronchial hyperreactivity is not entirely clear, but it is widely believed to result from persistent bronchial inflammation. Hence, bronchial asthma is best considered a chronic inflammatory disorder of the airways. Clinically, asthma is manifested by episodic dyspnea, cough, and wheezing (a soft whistling sound during expiration). This common disease affects about 5% of adults and 7% to 10% of children.

Because asthma is a heterogeneous disease triggered by a variety of inciting agents, there is no universally accepted simple classification. Nevertheless, it is customary to classify asthma into two major categories based on the presence or absence of an underlying immune disorder:

1. *Extrinsic asthma*, in which the asthmatic episode is typically initiated by a type I hypersensitivity reaction induced by exposure to an extrinsic antigen(Chapter 5).

Three types of extrinsic asthma are recognized: *atopic asthma, occupational asthma* (many forms), and *allergic bronchopulmonary aspergillosis* (bronchial colonization with *Aspergillus* organisms followed by development of immunoglobulin E [IgE] antibodies). Atopic asthma is the most common type of asthma; its onset is usually in the first two decades of life, and it is commonly associated with other allergic manifestations in the patient as well as in other family members. Serum IgE levels are usually elevated, as is the blood eosinophil count. This form of asthma is believed to be driven by the T_H2 subset of CD4+ T cells.

2. *Intrinsic asthma*, in which the triggering mechanisms are nonimmune. In this form, a number of stimuli that have little or no effect in normal subjects can trigger bronchospasm. Such factors include aspirin; pulmonary infections, especially those caused by viruses; cold; psychological stress; exercise; and inhaled irritants such as ozone and sulfur dioxide. There is usually no personal or family history of allergic manifestations, and serum IgE levels are normal. These patients are said to have an *asthmatic diathesis*.

In general, asthma that develops early in life has a strong allergic (extrinsic) component, while asthma developing later in life is more often of the intrinsic subtype. It must be emphasized, however, that, because of inherent tracheobronchial hyperreactivity, a person who has extrinsic asthma is also susceptible to developing an asthmatic attack when exposed to factors implicated in intrinsic asthma. Moreover, as the cellular and molecular basis of asthma is becoming evident, the commonality of their pathways is making this rigid dichotomy increasingly redundant.

Pathogenesis. As emphasized at the outset, the common denominator underlying all forms of asthma is an exaggerated bronchoconstrictor response (also called airway *hyperresponsiveness*) to a variety of stimuli. Airway hyperresponsiveness can be readily demonstrated in the form of increased sensitivity to bronchoconstrictive agents such as histamine or methacholine (a cholinergic agonist).

Although the importance of increased airway reactivity is established, the basis of the abnormal bronchial response is not fully understood. Most current evidence suggests that *bronchial inflammation is the substrate for hyperresponsiveness.* Persistent inflammation of bronchi, manifested by the presence of inflammatory cells (particularly eosinophils, lymphocytes, and mast cells) and by damage to the bronchial epithelium, is a constant feature of bronchial asthma.

What causes the bronchial inflammation? In extrinsic (allergic) asthma, it is readily explained by type I hypersensitivity reactions, but the cause is much less clear in patients with intrinsic asthma. Because the basis of bronchial inflammation is better understood in extrinsic asthma, this will be considered first.

Extrinsic (Allergic) Asthma. The details of type I hypersensitivity were discussed in an earlier chapter (Chapter 5), so only mechanisms of particular importance in the pathogenesis of asthma are reviewed here

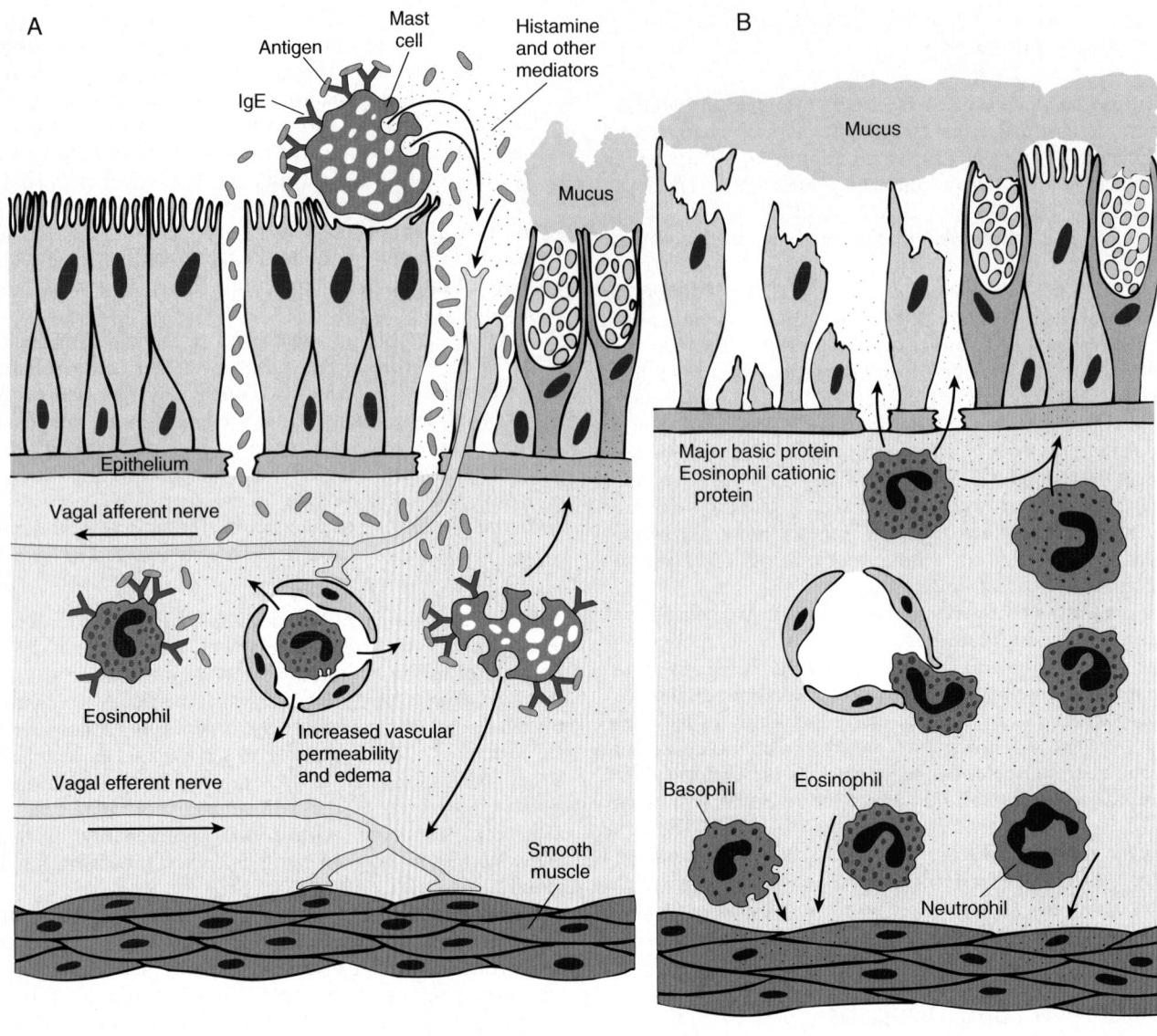

Figure 13-2 ■

A model for immediate and late stages of allergic asthma. *A,* The immediate reaction is triggered by antigen-induced cross-linking of IgE bound to IgE receptors (FcRε) on mast cells (and possibly FcRε-expressing eosinophils and macrophages) in the airways. These cells release preformed mediators that open tight junctions between epithelial cells. Antigen can then enter the mucosa to activate mucosal mast cells and eosinophils, which, in turn, release additional mediators. Collectively, the mediators, either directly or via neuronal reflexes, induce bronchospasm, increased vascular permeability, and mucus production and also recruit additional mediator-releasing cells from the blood. *B,* The arrival of recruited cells signals the initiation of the late stage of asthma, in which residual antigen binding to IgE (not shown) may trigger a fresh round of mediator release. Factors, particularly from eosinophils, may also stimulate release of mediators from other inflammatory cells and cause damage to the epithelium. (Reproduced with permission. Modified from Lichtenstein L: The nasal late phase response—an in vivo model. Hosp Pract 23(1):119, 1988. ©1988, The McGraw-Hill Companies. Illustration by Ilil Arbel.)

(Fig. 13–2). Like all type I hypersensitivity reactions, extrinsic asthma is driven by sensitization of CD4+ cells of the T$_H$2 type. It may be recalled that T$_H$2 cells release cytokines, specifically interleukins 4, 5, and 13 (IL-4, IL-5, and IL-13), which favor the synthesis of IgE, growth of mast cells, and growth and activation of eosinophils. *Induction of the T$_H$2 response is fundamental to the pathogenesis of allergic asthma, and IgE, mast cells, and eosinophils are key players in mediating it.* Attacks of atopic asthma often demonstrate two phases: an *early phase,* beginning 30 to 60 minutes after inhalation of antigen and then remitting, followed 4 to 8 hours later by a more protracted *late phase.* As might be expected, the initial triggering of mast cells occurs on the mucosal surface; the resultant mediator release opens mucosal intercellular junctions, allowing penetration of the antigen to more numerous mucosal mast cells. In addition, direct stimulation of subepithelial vagal (parasympathetic) receptors provokes reflex bronchoconstriction. As detailed in Chapter 5, mast cell activation leads to the release of a variety of primary and secondary mediators that function in both the early and late phases of asthma.

Early phase mediators include

- *Leukotrienes C_4, D_4, and E_4:* extremely potent mediators that cause prolonged bronchoconstriction, increase vascular permeability, and increase mucin secretion
- *Prostaglandins D_2, E_2 and $F_{2\alpha}$,* elicit bronchoconstriction and vasodilatation
- *Histamine:* causes bronchospasm and increases vascular permeability
- *Platelet-activating factor:* causes aggregation of platelets and release of histamine from their granules
- *Mast-cell tryptase:* inactivates normal bronchodilatory peptide (vasoactive intestinal peptide)

These initial reactions are followed by the late (or cellular) phase, which is dominated by additional recruitment of leukocytes: basophils, neutrophils, and eosinophils. *The mast cell mediators responsible for the recruitment of inflammatory cells include*

- Eosinophilic and neutrophilic chemotactic factors and leukotriene B_4: recruit and activate eosinophils and neutrophils
- IL-4 and IL-5: augment the T_H2 response of CD4+ T cells by increasing IgE synthesis and eosinophil chemotaxis and proliferation
- Platelet-activating factor: strongly chemotactic for eosinophils in the presence of IL-5
- Tumor necrosis factor: up-regulates adhesion molecules on vascular endothelium and also on inflammatory cells

The arrival of leukocytes at the site of mast cell degranulation leads to two effects: (1) these cells release additional waves of mediators that activate mast cells and intensify the initial response, and (2) they cause epithelial cell damage characteristic of asthmatic attacks. Epithelial cells themselves are sources of mediators, such as endothelin and nitric oxide, that can cause smooth muscle contraction and relaxation, respectively. Loss of epithelial integrity, by reducing available nitric oxide, may also contribute to airway hyperresponsiveness.

Eosinophils are particularly important in the late phase. As mentioned earlier, their accumulation at sites of allergic inflammation is favored by several mast cell–derived chemotactic factors. Studies have implicated other chemokines in eosinophil chemotaxis as well. The most potent of these appears to be *eotaxin,* produced by activated bronchial epithelial cells, macrophages, and airway smooth muscle. The accumulated eosinophils exert a variety of effects. Their armamentarium of mediators is as extensive as that of mast cells and includes *major basic protein (MBP)* and *eosinophil cationic protein (ECP),* which are directly toxic to the epithelial cells. *Eosinophil peroxidase* causes tissue damage through oxidative stress. Activated eosinophils are also a rich source of leukotrienes, especially leukotriene C_4, as well as of platelet-activating factor. *Thus, eosinophils can amplify and sustain the inflammatory response without additional exposure to the triggering antigen.*

Intrinsic Asthma. The mechanism of bronchial inflammation and hyperresponsiveness is much less clear in patients with intrinsic (nonatopic) asthma. Incriminated in such cases are *viral infections of the respiratory tract and inhaled air* pollutants such as sulfur dioxide, ozone, and nitrogen dioxide. These agents increase airway hyperreactivity in both normal and asthmatic subjects. In the latter, however, the bronchial response, manifested as spasm, is much more severe and sustained. *Recent experimental studies have demonstrated that the cellular and humoral effectors of intrinsic asthma show considerable overlap with those of extrinsic asthma.* For example, among the viral infections, respiratory syncytial virus infection has been implicated in inciting bronchospasm in susceptible individuals during early childhood. It is postulated that respiratory syncytial virus promotes secretion of a T_H2-dominant cytokine profile from antigen-specific T cells and therefore promotes eosinophilic infiltration. The bronchial epithelium itself is a rich source of proinflammatory cytokines during viral infections, and some of these are also involved in eosinophil maturation and chemotaxis. Thus, *the eosinophil has emerged as a key player in both subtypes of asthma.* Similarly, aspirin-induced asthma is presumed to be largely mediated by the effects of the leukotrienes, particularly leukotriene C_4; recall the important role played by leukotrienes in extrinsic asthma as well. Even as the "downstream" effectors of airway hyperresponsiveness continue to be unraveled, the basic mechanism of susceptibility remains largely unknown.

MORPHOLOGY

The morphologic changes in asthma have been described in patients who die of prolonged severe attacks (status asthmaticus) and in mucosal biopsy specimens of patients challenged with allergens. In fatal cases, grossly, the lungs are overdistended because of overinflation, and there may be small areas of atelectasis. **The most striking macroscopic finding is occlusion of bronchi and bronchioles by thick, tenacious mucus plugs.** Histologically, the mucus plugs contain whorls of shed epithelium (Curschmann spirals). Numerous eosinophils and Charcot-Leyden crystals (collections of crystalloids made up of eosinophil proteins) are also present. In addition, characteristic histologic findings in both nonfatal and fatal cases include the following:

- Edema, hyperemia, and an inflammatory infiltrate in the bronchial walls, with prominent eosinophils, which may constitute 5% to 50% of the cellular infiltrate. Also present are mast cells and basophils, macrophages, lymphocytes, plasma cells, and some neutrophils; many of the lymphocytes are CD4+ cells of the T_H2 type that secrete IL-4 and IL-5.
- An increase in size of the submucosal mucous glands (or increased numbers of goblet cells in bronchiolar epithelium).
- Patchy necrosis and shedding of epithelial cells.
- An increase in collagen immediately beneath the basement membrane, giving the appearance of a thickened basement membrane. This change is

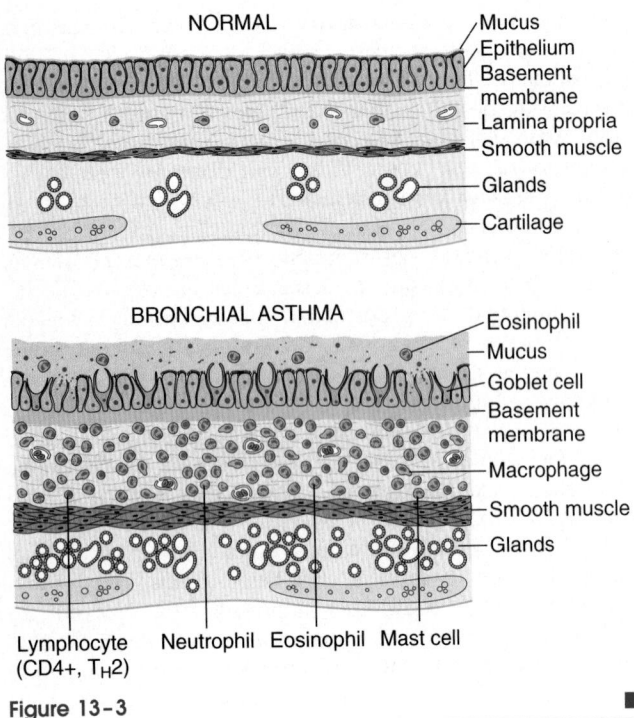

Figure 13–3 ■

Comparison of a normal bronchiole with that in a patient with asthma. Note the accumulation of mucus in the bronchial lumen resulting from an increase in the number of mucus-secreting goblet cells in the mucosa and hypertrophy of submucosal mucous glands. In addition, there is intense chronic inflammation caused by recruitment of eosinophils, macrophages, and other inflammatory cells. Basement membrane underlying the mucosal epithelium is thickened, and there is hypertrophy and hyperplasia of smooth muscle cells.

believed to result from cytokine-mediated activation of myofibroblasts that secrete collagen. Such remodeling of the basement membrane is not present in patients with chronic bronchitis (see later).

■ Hypertrophy and hyperplasia of the smooth muscle in the bronchial wall (Fig. 13–3). Unlike in chronic bronchiolitis (see later), the smooth muscle hyperplasia in asthma occurs at the level of large and medium airways.

Clinical Course. An attack of asthma is characterized by severe dyspnea with wheezing; the chief difficulty lies in expiration. The victim labors to get air into the lungs and then cannot get it out, so that there is progressive hyperinflation of the lungs with air trapped distal to the bronchi, which are constricted and filled with mucus and debris. In the usual case, attacks last from 1 to several hours and subside either spontaneously or with therapy, usually bronchodilators and corticosteroids. Intervals between attacks are characteristically free from respiratory difficulty, but persistent, subtle respiratory deficits can be detected by spirometric methods. Occasionally, a severe paroxysm occurs that does not respond to therapy and persists for days and even weeks (*status asthmaticus*). The associated hypercapnia, acidosis, and severe hypoxia may be fatal, although in most cases the disease is more disabling than lethal. In recent years, however, there has been an alarming increase in deaths from severe asthma. The basis of this trend is not clear.

CHRONIC OBSTRUCTIVE PULMONARY DISEASES

Chronic obstructive pulmonary disease (COPD) affects more than 10% of the US adult population and is the fourth leading cause of death in this country. Despite the wide use of the designation COPD, there is no general agreement on its precise definition. According to some, it is defined strictly on the basis of pulmonary function tests and is said to exist when there is objective evidence of persisting (and irreversible) airflow obstruction. Others use the term more broadly to include two common conditions—chronic bronchitis and emphysema—recognizing that in some cases either of these conditions can exist without significant airflow obstruction. Despite these uncertainties, one thing is clear: by the time patients with chronic bronchitis or emphysema develop sufficient dyspnea (breathlessness) to seek medical attention, airway obstruction can be readily demonstrated. Furthermore, as will be emphasized again, these two conditions often coexist, so on practical clinical grounds the grouping of chronic bronchitis and emphysema under the rubric of COPD is justified. The primarily *irreversible* airflow obstruction of COPD distinguishes it from asthma, which, as discussed previously, is characterized largely by *reversible* airflow obstruction.

Emphysema

Emphysema is characterized by *permanent enlargement* of the airspaces distal to the terminal bronchioles accompanied by *destruction of their walls*. There are several conditions in which enlargement of airspaces is not accompanied by destruction; this is more correctly called *overinflation*. For example, the distention of airspaces in the opposite lung after unilateral pneumonectomy is compensatory overinflation rather than emphysema.

The relationship between chronic bronchitis and emphysema is complicated, but the use of precise definitions has helped bring some order to what was once chaos. At the outset, it should be emphasized that the definition of emphysema is a morphologic one, whereas chronic bronchitis (see later) is defined on the basis of clinical features such as the presence of chronic and recurrent cough with excess mucus secretion. Second, the anatomic pattern of distribution is also different—chronic bronchitis affects both the large and small airways (the latter component has been called chronic bronchiolitis to indicate the level of involvement); by contrast, emphysema is restricted to the *acinus*, the structure distal to the terminal bronchioles (Fig. 13–4). Although chronic bronchitis may exist without demonstrable emphysema, and almost pure emphysema may occur (particularly in patients with inherited α_1-antitrypsin deficiency), the two diseases usually coexist because the major pathogenic mechanism, cigarette smoking, is common to both. Predictably, when the two entities coexist, the clinical and physiologic features overlap.

Types of Emphysema. Emphysema is defined not only in terms of the anatomic nature of the lesion but also according to its distribution in the lobule and acinus. The

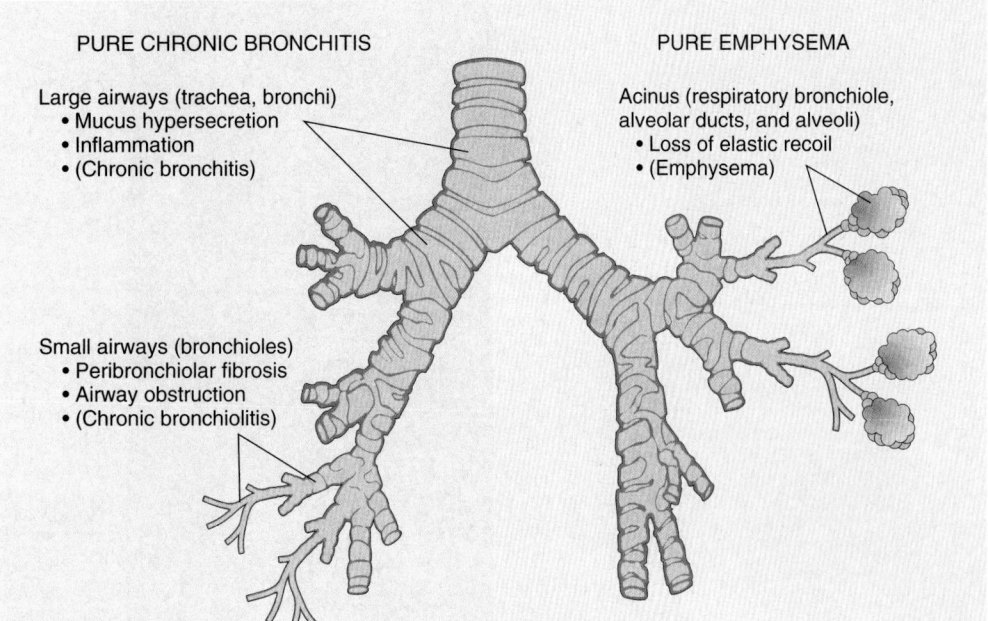

Figure 13-4 ■

Anatomic distribution of pure chronic bronchitis and pure emphysema. In chronic bronchitis, the small airway disease (chronic bronchiolitis) results in airflow obstruction, while the large airway disease is primarily responsible for the mucus hypersecretion.

acinus is the part of the lung distal to the terminal bronchiole and includes the respiratory bronchiole, alveolar ducts, and alveoli; a cluster of three to five acini is referred to as a lobule. There are three types of emphysema: (1) centriacinar, (2) panacinar, and (3) distal acinar. The first two are more important, but their differentiation is often difficult in advanced disease, and so they are diagrammed in Figure 13–5 and briefly described here.

Centriacinar (Centrilobular) Emphysema. The distinctive feature of this type of emphysema is the pattern of involvement of the lobules: the central or proximal parts of the acini, formed by respiratory bronchioles, are affected, while

Figure 13-5 ■

A, Diagram of normal structures within the acinus, the fundamental unit of the lung. A terminal bronchiole (not shown) is immediately proximal to the respiratory bronchiole. *B,* Centrilobular emphysema with dilation that initially affects the respiratory bronchioles. *C,* Panacinar emphysema with initial distention of the peripheral structures (i.e., the alveolus and alveolar duct); the disease later extends to affect the respiratory bronchioles.

Figure 13-6 ■

A, Centrilobular emphysema (magnification ×5). The pulmonary arteries contain injected barium. The emphysematous foci (E) abut the arteries, but normal alveolar spaces are adjacent to the septa (S). *B,* Panacinar emphysema (magnification ×5) demonstrates a more generalized distribution of the permanently enlarged emphysematous foci. Compare with *A.* (From Bates DV, et al: Respiratory Function in Disease, 2nd ed. Philadelphia, WB Saunders, 1971.)

distal alveoli are spared. Thus, both emphysematous and normal airspaces exist within the same acinus and lobule (Fig. 13–6*A*). The lesions are more common and severe in the upper lobes, particularly in the apical segments. In severe centriacinar emphysema the distal acinus also becomes involved, and so, as noted, the differentiation from panacinar emphysema becomes difficult. This type of emphysema is most commonly seen as a consequence of cigarette smoking in people who do not have congenital deficiency of α_1-antitrypsin.

Panacinar (Panlobular) Emphysema. In this type of emphysema, the acini are uniformly enlarged from the level of the respiratory bronchiole to the terminal blind alveoli (Fig. 13–6*B*). In contrast to centriacinar emphysema, panacinar

emphysema tends to occur more commonly in the lower lung zones and is the type of emphysema that occurs in α_1-antitrypsin deficiency.

Distal Acinar (Paraseptal) Emphysema. In this form, the proximal portion of the acinus is normal but the distal part is dominantly involved. The emphysema is more striking adjacent to the pleura, along the lobular connective tissue septa, and at the margins of the lobules. It occurs adjacent to areas of fibrosis, scarring, or atelectasis and is usually more severe in the upper half of the lungs. The characteristic findings are the presence of multiple, contiguous, enlarged airspaces that range in diameter from less than 0.5 mm to more than 2.0 cm, sometimes forming cystlike structures that with progressive enlargement are referred to as bullae. This type of emphysema probably underlies many of the cases of spontaneous pneumothorax in young adults.

Incidence. Emphysema is a common disease, but its precise incidence is difficult to estimate because a definite diagnosis, which is based on morphology, can be made only by examination of the lungs at autopsy. It is generally agreed that emphysema is present in approximately 50% of adults who come to autopsy. Most of those found to have emphysema at autopsy are asymptomatic. Emphysema, especially centriacinar, is much more common and more severe in men than in women. *There is a clear association between heavy cigarette smoking and emphysema*, and the most severe type occurs in those who smoke heavily. Although emphysema does not become disabling until the fifth to eighth decades of life, ventilatory deficits may become clinically evident decades earlier.

Pathogenesis. The genesis of the two common forms of emphysema, centriacinar and panacinar, is not completely understood. The current opinion favors emphysema arising as a consequence of *two critical imbalances—the protease-antiprotease imbalance and oxidant-antioxidant imbalance* (Fig. 13–7). Such imbalances almost always coexist, and in fact, their effects are additive in producing the end result of tissue damage.

The *protease-antiprotease imbalance* hypothesis is based on the observation that patients with a genetic deficiency of the antiprotease α_1-antitrypsin have a markedly enhanced tendency to develop pulmonary emphysema, which is compounded by smoking. About 1% of all patients with emphysema have this defect. α_1-Antitrypsin, normally present in serum, tissue fluids, and macrophages, is a major inhibitor of proteases (particularly elastase) secreted by neutrophils during inflammation. This enzyme is encoded by codominantly expressed genes on the proteinase inhibitor *(Pi)* locus on chromosome 14. The *Pi* locus is extremely polymorphic, with many different alleles. Most common is the normal *(M)* allele and the corresponding *PiMM* phenotype. Approximately 0.012% of the US population is homozygous for the *Z* allele *(PiZZ)*, associated with markedly decreased serum levels of α_1-antitrypsin. *Many of these persons develop symptomatic emphysema.*

The following sequence is postulated:

1. Neutrophils (the principal source of cellular proteases) are normally sequestered in peripheral capillaries, including those in the lung, and a few gain access to the alveolar spaces.
2. Any stimulus that increases either the number of leukocytes (neutrophils and macrophages) in the lung or the release of their protease-containing granules increases proteolytic activity.
3. With low levels of serum α_1-antitrypsin, elastic tissue destruction is unchecked and emphysema results.

Thus, *emphysema is seen to result from the destructive effect of high protease activity in subjects with low antiprotease activity.* This hypothesis is strongly supported by studies in experimental animals in which intratracheal instillation of the proteolytic enzymes papain and, more importantly, human neutrophil elastase results in the degradation of elastin accompanied by the development of emphysema.

The protease-antiprotease imbalance hypothesis also helps explain the effect of cigarette smoking in the development of emphysema, particularly the centriacinar form in subjects with normal α_1-antitrypsin levels (see Fig. 13–7):

■ *In smokers, neutrophils and macrophages accumulate in alveoli.* The mechanism of inflammation is not entirely clear but possibly involves the direct chemoattractant effects of nicotine as well as the effects of reactive oxygen species contained in smoke. These activate the transcription of nuclear factor κB (NF-κB), which switches on genes for tumor necrosis factor (TNF) and interleukin 8 (IL-8). These, in turn, attract and activate neutrophils.

■ Accumulated neutrophils are activated and release their granules, rich in a variety of cellular proteases (neutrophil elastase, proteinase 3, and cathepsin G), resulting in tissue damage.

■ Smoking also enhances elastase activity in macrophages; macrophage elastase is not inhibited by α_1-antitrypsin and, indeed, can proteolytically digest this antiprotease. There is now increasing evidence that in addition to elastase, matrix

Figure 13–7 ■

Pathogenesis of emphysema. The protease-antiprotease imbalance and oxidant-antioxidant imbalance are additive in their effects and contribute to tissue damage. α_1-Antitrypsin (α_1AT) deficiency can be either congenital or "functional" as a result of oxidative inactivation. See text for details. IL-8, interleukin 8; LTB$_4$, leukotriene B$_4$; TNF, tumor necrosis factor.

metalloproteinases derived from macrophages and neutrophils have a role in tissue destruction.

■ Smoking also plays a seminal role in perpetuating the *oxidant-antioxidant imbalance* in the pathogenesis of emphysema. Normally, the lung contains a healthy complement of antioxidants (superoxide dismutase, glutathione) that keep oxidative damage to a minimum. Tobacco smoke contains abundant reactive oxygen species (free radicals), which deplete these antioxidant mechanisms, thereby inciting tissue damage (Chapter 1). Activated neutrophils also add to the pool of reactive oxygen species in the alveoli. A secondary consequence of oxidative injury is inactivation of native antiproteases, resulting in "functional" α_1-antitrypsin deficiency even in patients without enzyme deficiency.

In summary, it is likely that the impaction of smoke particles, predominantly at the bifurcation of respiratory bronchioles, results in the influx of neutrophils and macrophages, both of which secrete proteases. An increase in protease activity localized in the centriacinar region, together with the smoke-induced oxidative damage, causes the centriacinar pattern of emphysema seen in smokers. Tissue breakdown is enhanced as a consequence of inactivation of protective antiproteases by reactive oxygen species in cigarette smoke. This schema also explains the additive influence of smoking and α_1-antitrypsin deficiency in inducing serious obstructive airway disease.

Figure 13-8 ■

Bullous emphysema with large apical and subpleural bullae. (From the teaching collection of the Department of Pathology, University of Texas Southwestern Medical School, Dallas.)

MORPHOLOGY

The diagnosis and classification of emphysema depend largely on the macroscopic appearance of the lung. Panacinar emphysema, when well developed, produces pale, voluminous lungs that often obscure the heart when the anterior chest wall is removed at autopsy. The macroscopic features of centriacinar emphysema are less impressive. The lungs are a deeper pink than in panacinar emphysema and less voluminous, unless the disease is well advanced. Generally, in centriacinar emphysema the upper two thirds of the lungs is more severely affected than the lower lungs, and in extreme cases emphysematous bullae may be grossly visible (Fig. 13-8).

Histologically, there is thinning and destruction of alveolar walls. With advanced disease, adjacent alveoli become confluent, creating large airspaces (Fig. 13-9). Terminal and respiratory bronchioles may be deformed because of the loss of septa that help tether these structures in the parenchyma. With the loss of elastic tissue in the surrounding alveolar septa, there is reduced radial traction on the small airways. As a result, they tend to collapse during expiration—an important cause of chronic airflow obstruction in severe emphysema. In addition to alveolar loss, the number of alveolar capillaries is diminished. There is fibrosis of respiratory bronchioles, and there may also be evidence of accompanying bronchitis and bronchiolitis.

Clinical Course. Dyspnea is usually the first symptom; it begins insidiously but is steadily progressive. In patients with underlying chronic bronchitis or chronic asthmatic bronchitis, cough and wheezing may be initial complaints. Weight loss is common and may be so severe as to suggest a hidden malignant tumor. Pulmonary function tests reveal reduced FEV_1 with normal or near-normal FVC. Hence, the ratio of FEV_1 to FVC is reduced.

The classic presentation in individuals who have no "bronchitic" component is one in which the patient is barrel-chested and dyspneic, with obviously prolonged expiration, sitting forward in a hunched-over position, attempting to squeeze the air out of the lungs with each expiratory effort. In these patients, airspace enlargement is severe and diffusing capacity is low. Dyspnea and hyperventilation are prominent, so that until very late in the disease gas exchange is adequate and blood gas values are relatively

Figure 13-9 ■

Pulmonary emphysema. There is marked enlargement of airspaces, with thinning and destruction of alveolar septa. (From the teaching collection of the Department of Pathology, University of Texas Southwestern Medical School, Dallas.)

normal. Because of prominent dyspnea and adequate oxygenation of hemoglobin, these patients are sometimes called "pink puffers."

On the other extreme are patients with emphysema who also have pronounced chronic bronchitis and a history of recurrent infections with purulent sputum. They usually have less prominent dyspnea and respiratory drive, so they retain carbon dioxide, become hypoxic, and are often cyanotic. For reasons not entirely clear, they tend to be obese. Often they seek medical help after the onset of congestive heart failure (cor pulmonale; Chapter 11) and associated edema. Patients with this clinical picture are sometimes called "blue bloaters."

Most patients with emphysema and COPD fall somewhere between these two classic extremes. In all patients, *secondary pulmonary hypertension develops gradually*, arising from (1) hypoxia-induced pulmonary vascular spasm and (2) loss of pulmonary capillary surface area from alveolar destruction. Death from emphysema is related to (1) pulmonary failure with respiratory acidosis, hypoxia, and coma or (2) right-sided heart failure (cor pulmonale).

Conditions Related to Emphysema. Several conditions resemble emphysema only superficially and are inappropriately referred to as such.

Compensatory emphysema is a term used to designate the compensatory dilation of alveoli in response to loss of lung substance elsewhere, such as occurs in residual lung parenchyma after surgical removal of a diseased lung or lobe.

Senile emphysema refers to the overdistended lungs of elders, resulting from age-related alterations of the internal geometry of the lung (e.g., larger alveolar ducts and smaller alveoli). There is no significant tissue destruction, and a better designation for such aging lungs would be *senile hyperinflation.*

Obstructive overinflation refers to the condition in which the lung expands because air is trapped within it. A common cause is subtotal obstruction by a tumor or foreign object. Obstructive overinflation can be a life-threatening emergency if the affected portion extends sufficiently to compress the remaining normal lung.

Mediastinal (interstitial) emphysema designates the entrance of air into the connective tissue stroma of the lung, mediastinum, and subcutaneous tissue. This may occur spontaneously with a sudden increase in intra-alveolar pressure (as with vomiting or violent coughing) that causes a tear, with dissection of air into the interstitium. Sometimes it occurs in children with whooping cough. It is particularly likely to occur in patients on respirators who have partial bronchiolar obstruction or in persons who suffer a perforating injury (e.g., a fractured rib). When the interstitial air enters the subcutaneous tissue, the patient may literally blow up like a balloon, with marked swelling of the head and neck and crackling crepitation all over the chest. In most instances the air is resorbed spontaneously when the site of entry is sealed.

Chronic Bronchitis

Chronic bronchitis is common among cigarette smokers and urban dwellers in smog-ridden cities; some studies of men in the 40- to 65-year age group indicate that 20% to 25% have the disease. The diagnosis of chronic bronchitis is made on clinical grounds: it is defined as *a persistent productive cough for at least 3 consecutive months in at least 2 consecutive years.* It can occur in several forms:

■ Most patients have *simple chronic bronchitis*: the productive cough raises mucoid sputum, but airflow is not obstructed.

■ If the sputum contains pus, presumably because of secondary infections, the patient is said to have *chronic mucopurulent bronchitis.*

■ Some patients with chronic bronchitis may demonstrate hyperresponsive airways and intermittent episodes of asthma. This condition, termed *chronic asthmatic bronchitis*, is often difficult to distinguish from atopic asthma.

■ A subpopulation of bronchitic patients develops chronic outflow obstruction as measured by pulmonary function tests. They are said to have *chronic obstructive bronchitis.*

Whereas the defining feature of chronic bronchitis (mucus hypersecretion) is primarily a reflection of large bronchial involvement, the morphologic basis of airflow obstruction in chronic bronchitis is more peripheral and results from (1) inflammation, fibrosis, and resultant narrowing of bronchioles ("small airway disease") and (2) coexistent emphysema. It is generally believed that while small airway disease (chronic bronchiolitis) does contribute to airflow obstruction, chronic bronchitis with significant airflow obstruction is almost always complicated by emphysema. Between 5% and 15% of smokers develop physiologic evidence of COPD, and many of these present initially with chronic bronchitis. At present, it is not possible to determine which cigarette smokers, including those with chronic bronchitis, will develop clinically significant COPD, with its potentially dire consequences. Clearly, some genetic factors are involved. Much effort is focused on defining polymorphisms of several genes that may be associated with COPD.

Pathogenesis. The distinctive feature of chronic bronchitis is hypersecretion of mucus, beginning in the large airways. Although the single most important causative factor is cigarette smoking, other air pollutants, such as sulfur dioxide and nitrogen dioxide, may contribute. These irritants *induce hypersecretion of the bronchial mucous glands, cause hypertrophy of mucous glands, and lead to metaplastic formation of mucin-secreting goblet cells in the surface epithelium of bronchi.* In addition, they cause inflammation with infiltration of CD8+ T cells, macrophages, and neutrophils. In contrast to asthma, in chronic bronchitis eosinphils are lacking unless the patient has asthmatic bronchitis. It is postulated that many of the respiratory epithelial effects of environmental irritants are mediated through the epidermal growth factor receptor. For example, transcription of the mucin gene *MUC5AC*, which is increased as a consequence of exposure to tobacco smoke in both in vitro and in vivo experimental models, is in part mediated by epithelial growth factor receptor pathways. Microbial

Figure 13-10 ■

Chronic bronchitis. The lumen of the bronchus is above. Note the marked thickening of the mucous gland layer (approximately twice normal) and squamous metaplasia of lung epithelium. (From the teaching collection of the Department of Pathology, University of Texas Southwestern Medical School, Dallas.)

infection is often present but plays a secondary role, chiefly by maintaining the inflammation and exacerbating symptoms.

MORPHOLOGY

Grossly, the mucosal lining of the larger airways is usually hyperemic and swollen by edema fluid. It is often covered by a layer of mucinous or mucopurulent secretions. The smaller bronchi and bronchioles may also be filled with similar secretions. Histologically, the diagnostic feature of chronic bronchitis in the trachea and larger bronchi is **enlargement of the mucus-secreting glands** (Fig. 13-10). The magnitude of the increase in size is assessed by the ratio of the thickness of the submucosal gland layer to that of the bronchial wall (Reid index). Often, an increased number of goblet cells is seen in the lining epithelium, with concomitant loss of ciliated epithelial cells. Squamous metaplasia frequently develops (see Fig. 13-10), followed by dysplastic changes in the lining epithelial cells, a sequence of events that may lead to the evolution of bronchogenic carcinoma. A variable density of inflammatory cells, largely mononuclear but sometimes admixed with neutrophils, is frequently present in the bronchial mucosa. The tissue neutrophilia increases dramatically during bronchitic exacerbations, and some studies have shown a relationship between the intensity of neutrophilic infiltrate and severity of disease. Unlike asthma, eosinophils do not constitute a prominent component of the inflammatory infiltrate, except in patients with hyperresponsive airways (asthmatic bronchitis). **Chronic bronchiolitis** (small airway disease), characterized by goblet cell metaplasia (normally the number of goblet cells is small in peripheral airways), inflammation, fibrosis in the walls, and smooth muscle hyperplasia, is also present. As previously stated, it is the peribronchiolar fibrosis and luminal narrowing that results in airway obstruction.

Clinical Course. In patients with chronic bronchitis, a prominent cough and the production of sputum may persist indefinitely without ventilatory dysfunction. However, as alluded to earlier, some patients develop significant COPD with outflow obstruction. This is accompanied by hypercapnia, hypoxemia, and (in severe cases) cyanosis. Differentiation of this form of COPD from that caused by emphysema can be made in the classic case, but, as mentioned, many patients have both conditions. With progression, chronic bronchitis is complicated by pulmonary hypertension and cardiac failure (Chapter 11). Recurrent infections and respiratory failure are constant threats.

BRONCHIECTASIS

Bronchiectasis is the permanent dilation of bronchi and bronchioles caused by destruction of the muscle and elastic supporting tissue, resulting from or associated with chronic necrotizing infections. It is not a primary disease but rather is secondary to persisting infection or obstruction caused by a variety of conditions. Once developed, it gives rise to a characteristic symptom complex dominated by cough and expectoration of copious amounts of purulent sputum. Diagnosis depends on an appropriate history along with radiographic demonstration of bronchial dilation. The conditions that most commonly predispose to bronchiectasis include the following:

1. *Bronchial obstruction.* Common causes are tumors, foreign bodies, and occasionally impaction of mucus. Under these conditions, the bronchiectasis is localized to the obstructed lung segment. Bronchiectasis can also complicate atopic asthma and chronic bronchitis.

2. *Congenital or hereditary conditions.* Only a few are cited:

   ■ In cystic fibrosis, widespread severe bronchiectasis results from obstruction and infection caused by the secretion of abnormally viscid mucus. This is an important and serious complication (Chapter 7).

   ■ In immunodeficiency states, particularly immunoglobulin deficiencies, bronchiectasis is prone to develop because of an increased susceptibility to repeated bacterial infections; localized or diffuse bronchiectasis can occur.

   ■ Kartagener syndrome, an autosomal recessive disorder, is frequently associated with bronchiectasis, and with sterility in males. Structural abnormalities of the cilia impair mucociliary clearance in the airways, leading to persistent infections, and reduce the mobility of spermatozoa.

3. *Necrotizing*, or *suppurative*, *pneumonia*, particularly with virulent organisms such as *Staphylococcus aureus* or *Klebsiella* spp., may predispose to bronchiectasis. In the past, postinfective bronchiectasis was sometimes a sequela to childhood pneumonias that complicated measles, whooping cough, and influenza, but this has substantially decreased with the advent of successful immunization. Post-tubercular bronchiectasis continues to be a significant cause of morbidity in endemic areas.

Pathogenesis. *Two processes are critical and intertwined in the pathogenesis of bronchiectasis: (1) obstruction and (2) chronic persistent infection.* Either of these two processes may come first. Normal clearance mechanisms are hampered by obstruction, so secondary infection soon follows; conversely, chronic infection in time causes damage to bronchial walls, leading to weakening and dilation. For example, obstruction caused by a bronchogenic carcinoma or a foreign body impairs clearance of secretions, providing a fertile soil for superimposed infection. The resultant inflammatory damage to the bronchial wall and the accumulating exudate further distend the airways, leading to irreversible dilation. Conversely, a persistent necrotizing inflammation in the bronchi or bronchioles may cause obstructive secretions, inflammation throughout the wall (with peribronchial fibrosis and scarring traction on the walls), and eventually the train of events already described.

In the usual case, a mixed flora can be cultured from the involved bronchi, including staphylococci, streptococci, pneumococci, enteric organisms, anaerobic and microaerophilic bacteria, and (particularly in children) *Haemophilus influenzae* and *Pseudomonas aeruginosa.*

Figure 13-11   ■

Bronchiectasis. Cross-section of lung demonstrating dilated bronchi extending almost to the pleura. (Courtesy of Dr. Linda Margraf, Department of Pathology, University of Texas Southwestern Medical School, Dallas.)

MORPHOLOGY

Bronchiectatic involvement of the lungs usually affects the lower lobes bilaterally, particularly those air passages that are most vertical. When tumors or aspiration of foreign bodies lead to bronchiectasis, involvement may be sharply localized to a single segment of the lungs. Usually, the most severe involvement is found in the more distal bronchi and bronchioles. The airways may be dilated to as much as four times their usual diameter and on gross examination of the lung can be followed almost to the pleural surfaces (Fig. 13-11). (By contrast, in normal lungs the bronchioles cannot be followed by ordinary gross examination beyond a point 2 to 3 cm from the pleural surfaces.)

The histologic findings vary with the activity and chronicity of the disease. In the full-blown active case, an intense acute and chronic inflammatory exudate within the walls of the bronchi and bronchioles and the desquamation of lining epithelium cause extensive areas of ulceration. Fibrosis of the bronchial and bronchiolar walls and peribronchiolar fibrosis develop in more chronic cases. When healing occurs, the lining epithelium may regenerate completely; however, usually so much injury has occurred that abnormal dilation and scarring persist. In some instances, **the necrosis destroys the bronchial or bronchiolar walls and forms a lung abscess.**

Clinical Course. The clinical manifestations consist of severe, persistent cough with expectoration of mucopurulent, sometimes fetid, sputum. The sputum may contain flecks of blood; frank hemoptysis can occur. Symptoms are often episodic and are precipitated by upper respiratory tract infections or the introduction of new pathogenic agents. Clubbing of the fingers may develop. In cases of severe, widespread bronchiectasis, significant obstructive ventilatory defects develop, with hypoxemia, hypercapnia, pulmonary hypertension, and (rarely) cor pulmonale. Metastatic brain abscesses and reactive amyloidosis (Chapter 5) are other, less frequent complications of bronchiectasis.

Restrictive Lung Diseases

Restrictive lung diseases are characterized by reduced compliance (i.e., more pressure is required to expand the lungs because they are stiff). Although chest wall abnormalities, some of which were mentioned earlier, can also cause restrictive disease, this discussion will concentrate on parenchymal causes.

Before we discuss the individual disorders, it is useful to consider two general features of restrictive pulmonary diseases, beginning with a brief review of the microanatomy of the septal wall.

■ As noted in Figure 13-12, only a thin basement membrane, scant pericapillary interstitial tissue, and the cytoplasm of two very flat cells, endothelium and alveolar epithelium, are interposed between air and blood. The initiating injury in these diseases usually affects either of these two cell types, although, with chronicity, changes in the interstitium tend to dominate the picture. Because of prominent changes in the interstitium, these disorders are often referred to as *interstitial lung disease*. It should be evident from Figure 13-12, however, that because of their intimate relationship, changes in the interstitium can affect both alveoli and capillaries.

■ The important signs and symptoms of restrictive lung disease can be inferred from the morphologic changes. Interstitial fluid or fibrosis produces a "stiff lung," which in turn reduces lung compliance and necessitates increased effort of breathing (dyspnea). Furthermore, damage to the alveolar epithelium and interstitial vasculature produces abnormalities in the ventilation-perfusion ratio, leading to hypoxia. For example, damaged or underventilated air units (alveoli) may still be perfused, and, conversely, with

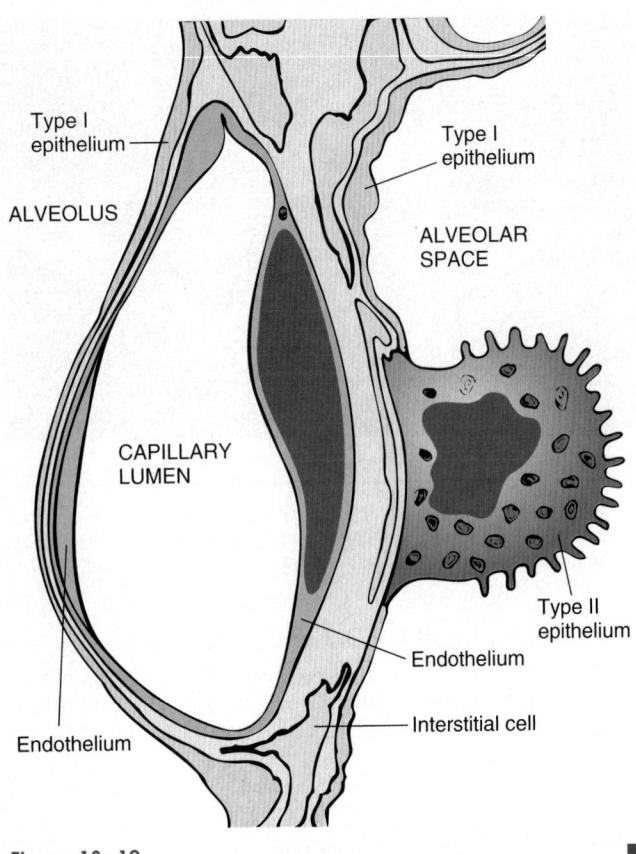

Figure 13-12 ■

Microscopic structure of the alveolar wall. Note that the basement membrane *(yellow)* is thin on one side and widened where it is continuous with the interstitial space. Portions of interstitial cells are shown.

damage to the capillaries, underperfusion of ventilated airspaces occurs. With progression, patients develop severe hypoxia and respiratory failure, often in association with pulmonary hypertension and cor pulmonale (Chapter 11).

Restrictive lung disease can be either (1) acute, associated with an abrupt decrement in respiratory function and demonstrable pulmonary edema, often with accompanying inflammation, or (2) chronic, associated with insidious development of respiratory dysfunction. Chronic restrictive lung disorders demonstrate variable amounts of chronic inflammation and fibrosis; in addition, some reveal unique features described later. In the discussion that follows, we first consider acute respiratory distress syndrome, the prototypic and most important acute restrictive lung disease, and then several examples of chronic interstitial disorders.

ACUTE RESTRICTIVE LUNG DISEASES

Acute Lung Injury and Acute Respiratory Distress Syndrome

Acute lung injury (ALI) and acute respiratory distress syndrome (ARDS) represent a continuum of progressive respiratory failure defined by (1) the acute onset of dyspnea, (2) decreased arterial oxygen pressure (hypoxemia), (3) development of bilateral pulmonary infiltrates on radiographs, and (4) absence of clinical evidence of primary left-sided heart failure. ALI is considered to be an early

stage of ARDS, with mild abnormalities of respiratory function that may subsequently evolve into the more typical, clinically severe syndrome of ARDS. Since the pulmonary infiltrates in ALI and ARDS are caused by damage to the alveolar capillary membrane, rather than left-sided heart failure, they represent the most common cause of *noncardiogenic pulmonary edema*. ALI and ARDS can occur in a multitude of clinical settings and are associated with either (1) direct injury to the lung or (2) indirect injury in the setting of a systemic process (Table 13-1).

Pathogenesis. The alveolar capillary membrane is formed by two separate barriers—the microvascular endothelium and the alveolar epithelium. In ALI and ARDS the integrity of this barrier is compromised by either endothelial or epithelial injury, or, more commonly, both. The acute consequences of damage to the alveolar capillary membrane include increased vascular permeability and alveolar flooding, loss of diffusion capacity, and widespread surfactant abnormalities caused by damage to type II pneumocytes (Fig. 13-13). Although the cellular and molecular basis of ALI and ARDS remains an area of active investigation, recent work suggests that *lung injury is caused by an imbalance of proinflammatory and anti-inflammatory cytokines.* The most proximate signals leading to uncontrolled activation of the acute inflammatory response are not yet understood. However, as early as 30 minutes after an acute insult (e.g., acid aspiration, trauma, or exposure to bacterial lipopolysaccharide) there is increased synthesis of IL-8, a potent neutrophil chemotactic and activating agent, by pulmonary macrophages. Release of this and similar compounds, such as interleukin 1 (IL-1) and TNF, leads to pulmonary microvascular sequestration and activation of neutrophils. *Neutrophils are thought to play an important role in the pathogenesis of ALI and ARDS.* Histologic examination of lungs early in the disease process has shown increased numbers of neutrophils within the vascular space, the interstitium, and the alveoli. Activated neutrophils release a variety of products (e.g., oxidants, proteases, platelet activating factor, and leukotrienes) that cause active tissue damage and maintain the inflammatory cascade. Macrophage inhibitory factor, a cytokine whose levels are increased in the milieu of lung injury,

■

Table 13-1. CLINICAL DISORDERS ASSOCIATED WITH THE DEVELOPMENT OF ACUTE LUNG INJURY AND THE ACUTE RESPIRATORY DISTRESS SYNDROME

Direct Lung Injury	Indirect Lung Injury
Common Causes	*Common Causes*
Pneumonia	Sepsis
Aspiration of gastric contents	Severe trauma with shock
Uncommon Causes	*Uncommon Causes*
Pulmonary contusion	Cardiopulmonary bypass
Fat embolism	Acute pancreatitis
Near-drowning	Drug overdose
Inhalational injury	Transfusion of blood products
Post–lung transplantation reperfusion injury	Uremia

Modified with permission from Ware LB, Matthay MA: The acute respiratory distress syndrome. N Engl J Med 342:1334, 2000.

Figure 13-13

The normal alveolus (left side) compared with the injured alveolus in the early phase of acute lung injury and the acute respiratory distress syndrome. Under the influence of proinflammatory cytokines such as interleukin 8 (IL-8), interleukin 1 (IL-1), and tumor necrosis factor (TNF) (released by macrophages), neutrophils initially undergo sequestration in the pulmonary microvasculature, followed by margination and egress into the alveolar space, where they undergo activation. Activated neutrophils release a variety of factors such as leukotrienes, oxidants, proteases, and platelet activating factor (PAF), which contribute to local tissue damage, accumulation of edema fluid in the airspaces, surfactant inactivation, and hyaline membrane formation. Macrophage inhibitory factor (MIF) released into the local milieu sustains the ongoing proinflammatory response. Subsequently, the release of macrophage-derived fibrogenic cytokines such as transforming growth factor β (TGF-β) and platelet-derived growth factor (PGDF) stimulate fibroblast growth and collagen deposition associated with the healing phase of injury. (Modified with permission from Ware LB, Matthay MA: The acute respiratory distress syndrome. N Engl J Med 342:1334, 2000.)

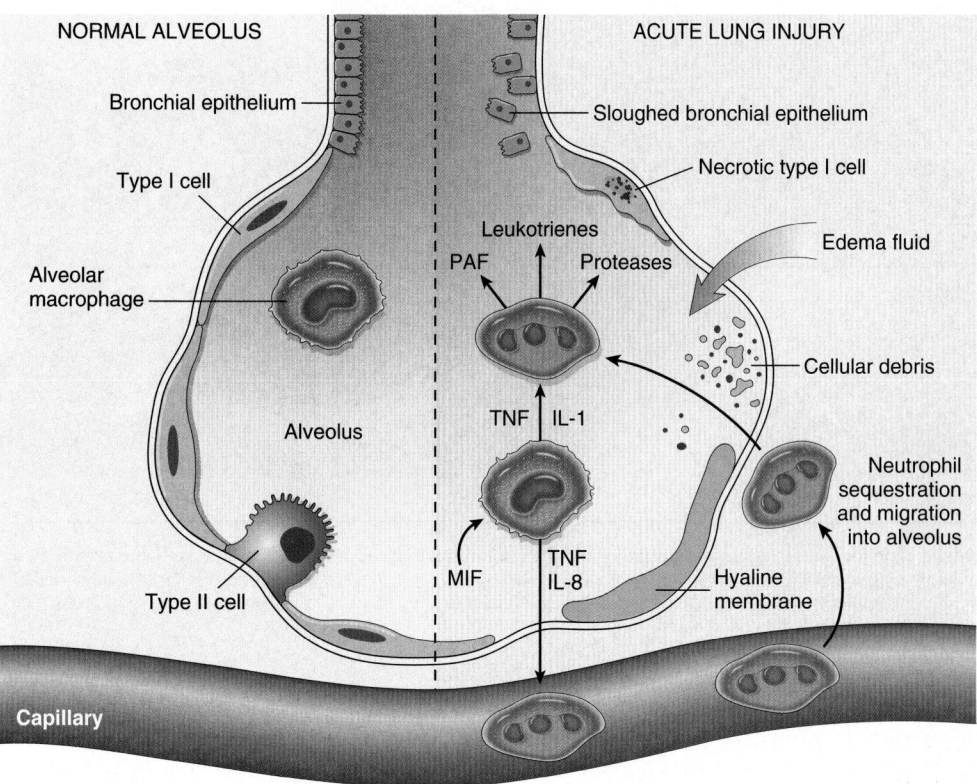

sustains inflammation in the alveolar spaces by promoting the release of proinflammatory mediators, such as IL-1 and TNF. Besides their role in the acute phase, cytokines such as transforming growth factor α (TGF-α) and platelet-derived growth factor (PDGF), which recruit fibroblasts and stimulate collagen production, contribute to the repair process after lung injury.

MORPHOLOGY

Diffuse alveolar damage is the morphologic counterpart of ALI and ARDS. The anatomic changes in diffuse alveolar damage are remarkably consistent, irrespective of the precipitating condition. The sequence of events in diffuse alveolar damage can be divided into exudative, proliferative, and fibrotic phases. On gross examination early in the disease, the lungs resemble the liver; they are dark red, firm, airless, and heavy. Microscopically, the exudative phase (0 to 7 days) demonstrates capillary congestion, necrosis of alveolar epithelial cells, interstitial and intra-alveolar edema and hemorrhage, and (particularly with sepsis) collections of neutrophils in capillaries. The alveolar ducts are dilated, and alveoli tend to collapse, in all likelihood owing to a secondary impairment of surfactant synthesis (see microatelectasis, p 454). Fibrin thrombi may be present in capillaries and large vessels. **The most** characteristic finding, however, is hyaline membranes, particularly lining the distended alveolar ducts (Fig. 13-14). Such membranes consist of protein-rich edema fluid admixed with remnants of necrotic epithelial cells. Overall, the picture is remarkably similar to that seen in respiratory distress syndrome in the newborn (Chapter 7). For that reason, acute respiratory distress syndrome was formerly called adult respiratory distress syndrome. The proliferative phase (1 to 3 weeks) is marked by proliferation of type II pneumocytes and by phagocytosis of remnant hyaline membranes by pulmonary macrophages. Type II pneumocyte hyperplasia is thought to be a **reparative phenomenon** in that these cells replace sloughed type I pneumocytes and then differentiate into type I cells once the initial insult has passed. There is also expansion of alveolar septa by proliferating interstitial fibroblasts and connective tissue. In patients who survive the acute episode, lung injury may either resolve with sparse histologic sequelae or cause progressive fibrosis involving the interstitium and alveolar spaces. The latter outcome results in marked distortion of lung parenchyma, usually leading to diffuse interstitial fibrosis interspersed with dilated and distorted airspaces (honeycomb lung).

Figure 13-14

Diffuse alveolar damage in acute lung injury and the acute respiratory distress syndrome *(left)*. Some alveoli are collapsed; others are distended. Many are lined by bright pink hyaline membranes *(arrow)*. In the healing stage *(right)*, there is resorption of hyaline membranes with thickened alveolar septa containing inflammatory cells, fibroblasts, and collagen. Numerous atypical type II pneumocytes are seen at this stage *(arrows)*, associated with regeneration and repair.

Clinical Course. Approximately 85% of patients develop the clinical syndrome of ALI or ARDS within 72 hours of the initiating insult. The prognosis of ALI and ARDS is grim, and in the past, mortality rates approached 100%. With improved methods of management, mortality is still between 30% to 40%; the toll exacted by sepsis-associated ALI/ARDS is significantly higher. Other predictors of poor prognosis include advanced age and the development of multisystemic (especially cardiac, renal, or hepatic) failure. High levels of the proinflammatory cytokine IL-1 and procollagen peptide III (a marker of collagen synthesis) in bronchoalveolar lavage fluid have also been associated with an increased risk of death. Should the patient survive the acute stage, diffuse interstitial fibrosis may occur and continue to compromise respiratory function. However, in most patients who survive the acute insult and are spared the chronic sequelae, normal respiratory function returns within 6 to 12 months.

CHRONIC RESTRICTIVE LUNG DISEASES

The chronic restrictive (interstitial) diseases of the lung parenchyma are a heterogeneous group with little uniformity regarding terminology and classification. Many entities are of unknown cause and pathogenesis; some have an intra-alveolar as well as an interstitial component, and there is frequent overlap in histologic features among the different conditions. Nevertheless, the presence of similar clinical signs, symptoms, radiographic alterations, and pathophysiologic changes justifies their consideration as a group. As stated earlier, *these patients have reduced FVC with proportionate reduction of FEV_1, and hence (unlike the situation in obstructive lung diseases) the FEV_1-to-FVC ratio is not reduced.*

Chronic restrictive lung disorders account for about 15% of noninfectious diseases seen by pulmonary physicians. A simplified etiologic classification is presented in Table 13-2.

While the end stage of most chronic restrictive lung diseases, irrespective of etiology, is diffuse interstitial pulmonary fibrosis with or without honeycombing, there are often sufficient histologic pointers in biopsy material (e.g., the existence of

Table 13-2. SELECTED CAUSES OF CHRONIC INTERSTITIAL LUNG DISEASE

Occupational and Environmental Exposure

Inorganic
   Asbestosis
   Silicosis
   Coal workers' pneumoconiosis
Organic
   Hypersensitivity pneumonitis*

Drug or Treatment Related

Chemotherapeutic agents
   Busulfan
   Bleomycin
   Methotrexate
Ionizing radiation
Oxygen

Immunologic Lung Disease

Sarcoidosis*
Wegener granulomatosis*
Collagen vascular diseases
   Systemic lupus erythematosus
   Rheumatoid arthritis
   Scleroderma
   Dermatomyositis-polymyositis
Goodpasture syndrome
Allograft rejection

Miscellaneous

Post acute respiratory distress syndrome
Idiopathic pulmonary fibrosis

*Associated with granulomas.

granulomas or telltale foreign material) to narrow, if not pin-point, the diagnosis. An accurate social and occupational history is indispensable for the surgical pathologist examining the histologic tissue. Although there are more than 150 causes of chronic interstitial lung disease, the etiopathogenesis of the most common subtype—idiopathic pulmonary fibrosis—is largely unknown.

Idiopathic Pulmonary Fibrosis

Idiopathic pulmonary fibrosis (IPF)—also known as cryptogenic fibrosing alveolitis—refers to a pulmonary disorder of unknown etiology characterized histologically by diffuse interstitial fibrosis, which in advanced cases results in severe hypoxemia and cyanosis. Males are affected more often than are females, and approximately two thirds of patients are older than 60 years of age at presentation. It should be stressed that similar clinical and pathologic findings may be noted with well-defined entities such as asbestosis, the connective tissue diseases, and a number of other conditions. Therefore, known causes must be ruled out before the appellation of "idiopathic" is used.

The proposed sequence of events in IPF begins with some form of alveolar wall injury, which results in interstitial edema and accumulation of inflammatory cells (alveolitis). If the injury is mild and self-limited, resolution with restoration of normal architecture follows. However, with persistence of the injurious agent, *cellular interactions involving lymphocytes, macrophages, neutrophils, and alveolar epithelial cells lead to proliferation of fibroblasts and progressive interstitial fibrosis.* It is suspected that immune mechanisms trigger this sequence of events (Fig. 13–15). In some patients, circulating immune complexes may bind to the Fc receptors of alveolar macrophages and stimulate them. In other instances, macrophages are activated by cytokines derived from T cells responding to unknown antigens. Regardless of whether the macrophages are driven by T cells or by immune complexes, they secrete factors (e.g., IL-8 and leukotrienes) that recruit and activate neutrophils. The soluble mediators released from macrophages and recruited neutrophils injure alveolar epithelial cells and degrade connective tissue. Alveolar macrophages from patients with IPF secrete a host of other factors, including fibroblast growth factor, transforming growth factor β (TGF-β), and PDGF, which can attract fibroblasts as well as stimulate their proliferation, thus setting in motion a repair response. It is now believed that alveolar epithelial cells are not merely passive

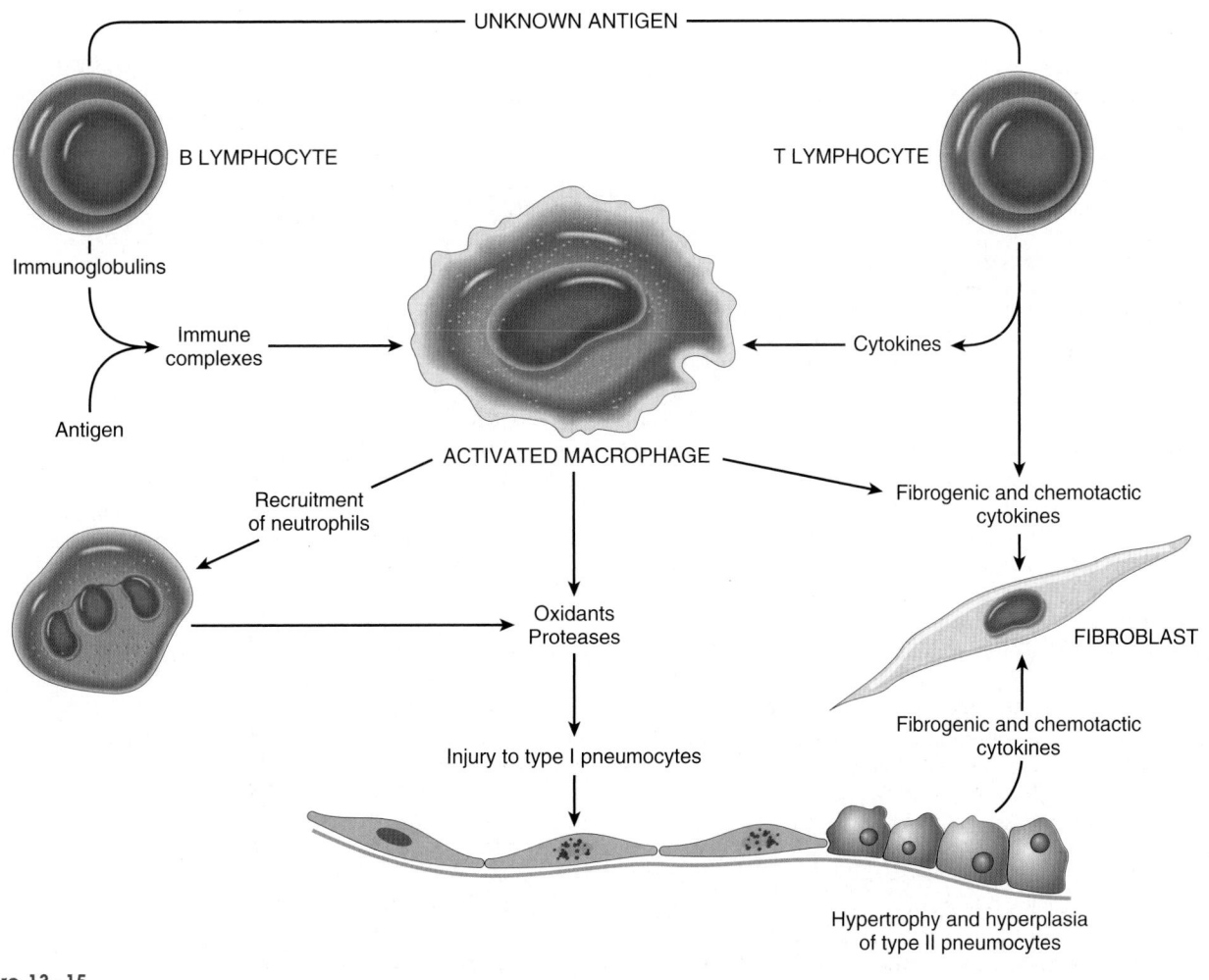

Figure 13-15

A possible schema of the pathogenesis of idiopathic pulmonary fibrosis. See text for details.

Figure 13-16

Idiopathic pulmonary fibrosis. *A*, The alveolar walls are thickened by fibrosis *(arrows)*. In addition, there is a sparse interstitial infiltrate of mononuclear cells. *B*, The interstitial fibrosis is better depicted with a Masson trichrome stain, which imparts a deep blue color to collagen.

targets in this process. Destruction of type I pneumocytes is often accompanied by proliferation of type II pneumocytes. These cells secrete chemotactic factors (e.g., macrophage chemotactic protein 1) that attract macrophages and T cells. In addition, they can contribute to fibrosis by secreting PDGF and other fibrogenic cytokines, such as TGF-β.

MORPHOLOGY

As stated in the preceding discussion, IPF is initiated as an inflammatory response to injury that subsequently heals by fibrosis. Hence, some degree of interstitial inflammation or pneumonitis is usually present in biopsy specimens from patients with IPF, especially in the early stages. The interstitial pneumonias can be divided into several distinct histologic subtypes, and there has been considerable confusion regarding which of these specifically accompanies IPF. This distinction is important, because any of the interstitial pneumonias may be associated with fibrosis, but the diagnosis of IPF-related interstitial pneumonia portends a worse prognosis and treatment refractoriness than the others. **By recent consensus, the term "IPF" is reserved for the clinical syndrome associated with the histologic subtype known as usual interstitial pneumonia.** The hallmark of usual interstitial pneumonia is a **heterogeneous appearance** at low magnification, with alternating areas of normal lung, interstitial inflammation, and fibrosis. The interstitial inflammation is usually patchy and consists of an alveolar septal infiltrate of lymphocytes and plasma cells, associated with type II pneumocyte hyperplasia. The fibrotic areas are composed primarily of dense

acellular collagen (Fig. 13-16). In the advanced stages, the lung shows airspaces lined by type II pneumocytes separated by inflammatory fibrous tissue. This so-called **honeycomb change** is not specific to usual interstitial pneumonia; it represents "end-stage" lung consequent to a variety of causes that result in lung injury and scarring.

Clinical Course. IPF usually presents insidiously, with the gradual onset of a nonproductive cough and progressive dyspnea. On physical examination, most patients have characteristic "dry" or "Velcro"-like crackles during inspiration. Cyanosis, cor pulmonale, and peripheral edema may be demonstrable in the later stages of the disease. Virtually all patients with IPF have an abnormal chest radiograph at the time of presentation. The availability of high-resolution computerized axial tomography has markedly improved the sensitivity of detecting IPF in its early stages. Surgical lung biopsy remains the gold standard for diagnosing IPF and for excluding other causes of pulmonary fibrosis. To date, most treatment strategies have focused on eliminating or suppressing the inflammatory component, such as with corticosteroids. Unfortunately, the progress of IPF is relentless despite therapy, and the mean survival in recent clinical series has ranged from 2 to 4 years.

Sarcoidosis

Although considered here as an example of a restrictive lung disease, it should be remembered that sarcoidosis is a *multisystemic disease of unknown etiology characterized by noncaseating granulomas in many tissues and organs.* Other diseases, including mycobacterial or fungal infections and berylliosis, sometimes also produce noncaseating granulomas; therefore, the histologic *diagnosis of sarcoidosis is one of exclusion.* Although the multisystemic involvement of sarcoidosis can present in many clinical guises, bilateral hilar lymphadenopathy or lung involvement (or both), visible on chest radiographs, is the major presenting manifestation in most cases. Eye and skin involvement each occur in about 25% of cases and may occasionally be the presenting feature of the disease.

Epidemiology. Sarcoidosis occurs throughout the world, affecting both sexes and all races and ages. There are, however, certain interesting epidemiologic trends, including the following:

- There is a consistent predilection for adults younger than 40 years of age.
- A high incidence has been noted in the Danish and Swedish population and among US blacks (in whom the frequency of involvement is 10 times greater than in US whites).
- Sarcoidosis is one of the few pulmonary diseases with a higher prevalence among *nonsmokers.*

Etiology and Pathogenesis. Although the etiology of sarcoidosis remains unknown, several lines of evidence suggest that it is a disease of disordered immune regulation in genetically predisposed individuals exposed to certain environmental agents. The role of each of these three contributory factors is summarized below.

Immunologic Factors. There are several *immunologic abnormalities* in the local milieu of sarcoid granulomas that suggest the development of a cell-mediated response to an unidentified antigen. The process is driven by CD4+ helper/inducer T cells. These include

- Intra-alveolar and interstitial accumulation of CD4+ T cells with helper-inducer activity, resulting in CD4:CD8 T-cell ratios greater than 3.5
- Oligoclonal expansion of T-cell subsets as determined by analysis of T-cell receptor rearrangement
- Increased levels of T cell–derived T_H1 cytokines such as IL-2 and interferon-γ (IFN-γ), resulting in T-cell expansion and macrophage activation, respectively
- Increased levels of several cytokines in the local environment (IL-8, TNF, macrophage inflammatory protein 1α [MIP-1α]) that favor recruitment of additional T cells and monocytes and contribute to the formation of granulomas

Additionally, there are *systemic immunologic abnormalities* in patients with sarcoidosis:

- Anergy to common skin test antigens such as *Candida* or purified protein derivative (PPD), thought to result from pulmonary recruitment of CD4+ T cells and consequent peripheral depletion
- Polyclonal hypergammaglobulinemia, another manifestation of helper T cell dysregulation

Genetic Factors. Evidence of genetic influences can be seen:

- Familial and racial clustering of cases
- Association with certain HLA genotypes (e.g., class I HLA-A1 and HLA-B8)

Environmental Factors. This is possibly the most tenuous of all the associations in the pathogenesis of sarcoidosis:

- Several putative "antigens" have been proposed as the inciting agent for sarcoidosis (e.g., viruses, mycobacteria, *Borrelia*, pollen).
- To date, *there is no unequivocal evidence to suggest that sarcoidosis is caused by an infectious agent.*

MORPHOLOGY

The histopathologic sine qua non of sarcoidosis is the noncaseating epithelioid granuloma, irrespective of the organ involved (Fig. 13–17). This is a discrete, compact collection of epithelioid histiocytes—highly differentiated mononuclear phagocytes—rimmed by an outer zone of largely CD4+ helper T cells. The epithelioid histiocytes are characterized by abundant eosinophilic cytoplasm and vesicular nuclei. It is not uncommon to see intermixed multinucleated giant cells formed by fusion of macrophages. A thin layer of laminated fibroblasts is present peripheral to the granuloma; over time, these proliferate and lay down collagen that replaces the entire granuloma with a hyalinized scar. Two other microscopic features are sometimes seen in the granulomas: (1) Schaumann bodies, laminated concretions composed of calcium and proteins; and (2) asteroid bodies, stellate inclusions enclosed within giant cells. Their presence is not required for diagnosis of sarcoidosis; they may also occur in granulomas of other origins. Rarely, foci of central necrosis may be present in sarcoid granulomas, suggesting an infectious process. Caseation necrosis typical of tuberculosis is absent.

Intrathoracic hilar and paratracheal **lymph nodes** are enlarged in 75% to 90% of patients, while a third present with peripheral lymphadenopathy. The

Figure 13–17 ■

Characteristic sarcoid noncaseating granulomas in lung with many giant cells. (Courtesy of Dr. Ramon Bianco, Department of Pathology, Brigham and Women's Hospital, Boston.)

nodes are characteristically painless and have a firm, rubbery texture. Unlike in tuberculosis, lymph nodes in sarcoidosis are "nonmatted" (nonadherent) and do not ulcerate.

The lungs are involved at some stage of the disease in 90% of patients. The granulomas predominantly involve the interstitium rather than air spaces, with some tendency to localize in the connective tissue around bronchioles and pulmonary venules and in the pleura ("lymphangitic" distribution). In 5% to 15% of patients, the granulomas are eventually replaced by diffuse interstitial fibrosis resulting in a honeycomb lung, accompanied by pulmonary hypertensive arteriopathy and **cor pulmonale.**

Skin lesions are encountered in approximately 25% of patients. Erythema nodosum, the hallmark of acute sarcoidosis, consists of raised, red, tender nodules on the anterior aspects of the legs. Sarcoidal granulomas are uncommon in these lesions. In contrast, discrete painless subcutaneous nodules can also occur in sarcoidosis, and these usually reveal abundant noncaseating granulomas. Another characteristic skin lesion of sarcoidosis consists of indurated plaques associated with a violaceous discoloration in the region of the nose, cheeks, and lips **(lupus pernio).**

Involvement of the eye and lacrimal glands occurs in about one fifth to one half of patients. The ocular involvement takes the form of iritis or iridocyclitis and may be unilateral or bilateral. As a consequence, corneal opacities, glaucoma, and (less commonly) total loss of vision may develop. The posterior uveal tract is also affected, with resultant choroiditis, retinitis, and optic nerve involvement. These ocular lesions are frequently accompanied by inflammation in the lacrimal glands, with suppression of lacrimation (sicca syndrome). **Unilateral or bilateral parotitis with painful enlargement of the parotid glands** occurs in less than 10% of the patients; some go on to develop xerostomia (dry mouth).

The spleen may appear unaffected grossly, but in about three fourths of cases it contains granulomas. In approximately 10% it becomes clinically enlarged. **The liver** demonstrates microscopic granulomatous lesions, usually in the portal triads, about as often as the spleen, but only about one third of the patients demonstrate hepatomegaly or abnormal liver function. Sarcoid involvement of **bone marrow** is reported in up to 40% of patients, although it rarely causes severe manifestations.

Less frequently affected sites include kidneys, the musculoskeletal system, and cranial nerves, although virtually any organ may demonstrate sarcoidal granulomas histologically. Sometimes there is hypercalcemia and hypercalciuria. This is not related to bone destruction but rather is caused by increased calcium absorption secondary to production of active vitamin D by the mononuclear phagocytes in the granulomas.

Clinical Course. In many patients the disease is entirely asymptomatic, discovered on routine chest films as bilateral hilar adenopathy or as an incidental finding at autopsy. In others, peripheral lymphadenopathy, cutaneous lesions, eye involvement, splenomegaly, or hepatomegaly may be presenting manifestations. In about two thirds of symptomatic cases, there is a gradual appearance of respiratory symptoms (shortness of breath, dry cough, or vague substernal discomfort) or constitutional signs and symptoms (fever, fatigue, weight loss, anorexia, night sweats). Occasionally, the presentation takes the form of a systemic hypersensitivity reaction with fever, erythema nodosum, and polyarthritis associated with bilateral hilar adenopathy (acute sarcoidosis). Combined uveoparotid involvement is designated *Mikulicz syndrome.* Because of the variable and nondiagnostic clinical features, resort is frequently made to lung or lymph node biopsy. *The presence of noncaseating granulomas is suggestive of sarcoidosis, but other identifiable causes of granulomatous inflammation must be excluded.*

Sarcoidosis follows an unpredictable course characterized by either progressive chronicity or periods of activity interspersed with remissions. The remissions may be spontaneous or initiated by steroid therapy and are often permanent. Overall, 65% to 70% of affected patients recover with minimal or no residual manifestations. Twenty percent develop permanent lung dysfunction or visual impairment. Of the remaining 10% to 15%, most succumb to progressive pulmonary fibrosis and cor pulmonale.

Hypersensitivity Pneumonitis

Hypersensitivity pneumonitis is an immunologically mediated inflammatory lung disease that primarily affects the alveoli and is therefore often called *allergic alveolitis.* Most often it is an occupational disease that results from heightened sensitivity to inhaled antigens such as moldy hay (Table 13–3). Unlike bronchial asthma, in which *bronchi are the focus of immunologically mediated injury, the damage in hypersensitivity pneumonitis occurs at the level of alveoli.* Hence, it presents as a predominantly restrictive lung disease with decreased diffusion capacity, lung compliance, and total lung volume. The occupational exposures are diverse, but the syndromes share common clinical and pathologic findings and probably have very similar pathophysiology.

Hypersensitivity pneumonitis may present either as an *acute reaction* with fever, cough, dyspnea, and constitutional complaints 4 to 8 hours after exposure or as a *chronic disease* with insidious onset of cough, dyspnea, malaise, and weight loss. Several lines of evidence suggest that hypersensitivity pneumonitis is an immunologically mediated disease:

■ Bronchoalveolar lavage specimens obtained during the acute phase have shown increased levels of proinflammatory chemokines such as MIP-1α and IL-8.
■ Bronchoalveolar lavage specimens also consistently demonstrate increased numbers of T lymphocytes of both CD4+ and CD8+ phenotype.
■ Most patients have specific precipitating antibodies in their serum, a feature supportive of type III (immune complex) hypersensitivity.

Table 13-3. SELECTED CAUSES OF HYPERSENSITIVITY PNEUMONITIS

Syndrome	Exposure	Antigens
Fungal and Bacterial Antigens		
Farmer's lung	Moldy hay	*Micropolyspora faeni*
Bagassosis	Moldy pressed sugar cane (bagasse)	Thermophilic actinomycetes
Maple bark disease	Moldy maple bark	*Cryptostroma corticale*
Humidifier lung	Cool-mist humidifier	Thermophilic actinomycetes, *Aureobasidium pullulans*
Malt worker's lung	Moldy barley	*Aspergillus clavatus*
Cheese washer's lung	Moldy cheese	*Penicillium casei*
Insect Products		
Miller's lung	Dust-contaminated grain	*Sitophilus granarius* (wheat weevil)
Animal Products		
Pigeon breeder's lung	Pigeons	Pigeon serum proteins in droppings
Chemicals		
Chemical worker's lung	Chemical industry	Trimellitic anhydride, isocyanates

- Complement and immunoglobulins have been demonstrated within vessel walls by immunofluorescence, also indicating a type III hypersensitivity.
- Finally, the presence of noncaseating granulomas in two thirds of the patients suggests development of a type IV hypersensitivity against the implicated antigen(s).

In summary, hypersensitivity pneumonitis is an immunologically mediated response to an extrinsic antigen that involves both type III (immune complex) and type IV (delayed type) hypersensitivity reactions.

MORPHOLOGY

The histopathology of both acute and chronic forms of hypersensitivity pneumonitis demonstrates patchy mononuclear cell infiltrates in the pulmonary interstitium, with a characteristic peribronchiolar accentuation. Lymphocytes predominate, but plasma cells and epithelioid histiocytes are also present. In acute forms of the disease, variable numbers of neutrophils also may be seen. Interstitial noncaseating granulomas are present in more than two thirds of cases, usually in a peribronchiolar location. In advanced chronic cases, diffuse interstitial fibrosis occurs.

The diagnosis of the acute form of this disease is usually obvious because of the temporal relationship of symptoms to exposure to the incriminating antigen. The etiology of the chronic form of the disease is less obvious and may require tissue examination for diagnosis. The presence of specific precipitating antibodies in the serum or positive skin tests may be helpful. The clinical course is variable. If antigenic exposure is terminated after acute attacks of the disease, fever and cough usually last a few days, and constitutional complaints clear in several weeks.

The chronic form of the disease resolves more slowly, and most patients continue to experience mild to moderate symptoms. In a small number of cases (about 5%), respiratory failure and death may occur.

Diffuse Alveolar Hemorrhage Syndromes

While there may be several "secondary" causes of pulmonary hemorrhage (necrotizing bacterial pneumonia, passive venous congestion, bleeding diathesis), the diffuse alveolar hemorrhage syndromes are a group of "primary" immune-mediated diseases that present as the *triad of hemoptysis, anemia, and diffuse pulmonary infiltrates.*

Goodpasture syndrome, the prototype disorder of this group, is an uncommon but intriguing condition characterized by a crescentic, usually rapidly progressive, glomerulonephritis (Chapter 14) and hemorrhagic interstitial pneumonitis. Both the renal and the pulmonary lesions are caused by antibodies to antigens common to glomerular and pulmonary basement membranes (thus, it is an example of type II cytotoxic antibody-mediated hypersensitivity). These antibodies can be detected in the serum of over 90% of patients. The immunopathogenesis of Goodpasture syndrome and the changes in the glomeruli are discussed in Chapter 14. Suffice it to say here that the characteristic linear pattern of immunoglobulin deposition (usually IgG, sometimes IgA or IgM) that is the sine qua non of diagnosis in renal biopsy specimens is also seen along the alveolar septa.

MORPHOLOGY

Microscopic examination of the lungs demonstrates focal necrosis of alveolar walls associated with intra-alveolar hemorrhages, fibrous thickening of the septa, and hypertrophy of septal lining cells. The presence of hemosiderin, either within macrophages or extracellularly, is characteristically seen for a few days after an acute presentation

Figure 13–18

A, Lung biopsy specimen from a patient with a diffuse alveolar hemorrhage syndrome demonstrates large numbers of intra-alveolar hemosiderin-laden macrophages on a background of thickened fibrous septa. *B,* The tissue has been stained with Prussian blue, an iron stain that highlights the abundant intracellular hemosiderin. (From the teaching collection of the Department of Pathology, Children's Medical Center, Dallas.)

(Fig. 13–18). Plasmapheresis and immunosuppressive therapy have markedly improved the once dismal prognosis for this disease. Plasma exchange removes offending antibodies, and immunosuppressive drugs inhibit antibody production. With severe renal disease, renal transplantation is eventually required.

Idiopathic pulmonary hemosiderosis is a disease of uncertain etiology that has pulmonary manifestations and histology similar to those of Goodpasture syndrome, but there is no associated renal disease or circulating anti–basement membrane antibody. Clinically, the course is usually mild to moderate, with periods of activity followed by prolonged remissions, and often remission is spontaneous. Notably, other immunologic diseases such as Wegener granulomatosis and connective tissue disorders can also present as diffuse alveolar hemorrhage.

Pulmonary Angiitis and Granulomatosis (Wegener Granulomatosis)

Wegener granulomatosis (WG) is the prototype disorder of the group of vasculitides known as pulmonary angiitis and granulomatosis and has been discussed in Chapter 10. In this section we will focus on the manifestations of WG in the respiratory system. More than 80% of patients with WG develop upper respiratory or pulmonary manifestations at some time in the course of their disease. The lung lesions in WG are characterized by a combination of necrotizing vasculitis ("angiitis") and parenchymal necrotizing granulomatous inflammation. The pulmonary vessels may also show necrotizing granulomas, although most often acute and chronic inflammation are intermingled with fibrinoid necrosis. The manifestations of WG can include both upper respiratory

symptoms (chronic sinusitis, epistaxis, nasal perforation) and pulmonary symptoms (cough, hemoptysis, chest pain). Radiologically, multiple nodular densities, representing confluence of the necrotizing granulomas, are seen, some of which may undergo cavitation. Although WG is classically a multisystemic disease, it may be restricted to the lung without upper respiratory tract or renal involvement ("limited" WG).

The Lung in Collagen Vascular Disorders

Several of the collagen vascular disorders (e.g., systemic lupus erythematosus, rheumatoid arthritis, scleroderma, and dermatomyositis-polymyositis) are associated with pulmonary manifestations. *Interstitial pneumonitis, accompanied by or terminating in diffuse interstitial fibrosis, is the most common pathologic finding in the lung.* The histology resembles that seen in the course of IPF, culminating as end-stage honeycomb lung. The frequency of other pulmonary manifestations, which include pulmonary hypertension, pulmonary vasculitis and diffuse alveolar hemorrhage, and pleuritis, varies depending on the specific disease entity. The pathology of Caplan syndrome, a form of accelerated pneumoconiosis seen in patients with rheumatoid arthritis who are exposed to coal, silica, or asbestos, is discussed in Chapter 8.

Transplantation Pathology

With the advent of better immunosuppressive agents, both combined heart-lung transplantation and single or sequential lung transplantation have become more frequent therapies of choice in patients with end-stage lung disease from a variety of causes (irreversible pulmonary hypertension, severe emphysema, and cystic fibrosis among others). Similar to cardiac and renal transplants, lung allografts are susceptible to the ravages of immunologic rejection. For the purposes of grading and therapy, pulmonary rejection has been divided into two forms—*acute* and *chronic*—with further subcategorization within each. *The grading of pulmonary rejection by the pathologist requires the evaluation of both airways and vessels.* By convention, *acute rejection* is classified on the basis of the nature and extent of perivascular infiltrates. The four grades of acute rejection, representing a continuum of increasing severity, are as follows:

- Minimal—subtle perivascular infiltrates of "activated" lymphocytes and histiocytes
- Mild—more obvious perivascular cuffing by mononuclear cells, with or without subendothelial infiltration by lymphocytes (endothelialitis)
- Moderate—intense perivascular cuffing by mononuclear cells, endothelialitis, and a lymphocytic interstitial pneumonitis
- Severe—diffuse alveolar damage, with hyaline membrane formation and fibrinoid necrosis within vessels

Although not required for the diagnosis or grading of acute rejection, it is important that airways be evaluated for the presence of *lymphocytic bronchitis* or *bronchiolitis*, because this may herald the onset of chronic airway rejection.

Chronic rejection targets both airways *(chronic airway rejection)* and vessels *(chronic vascular rejection)* and is the most important determinant of long-term graft survival. The form of chronic rejection affecting the airways is known as *bronchiolitis obliterans* and, as the name suggests, represents progressive obliteration of the bronchiolar lumina by a fibrosing inflammatory process. The proposed sequence of events begins with a lymphocytic bronchiolitis that causes destruction and denudation of respiratory epithelium, followed by ingrowth of submucosal fibroblasts that lay down collagen over the ulcerated mucosa. This "healing by fibrosis" results in scarring and loss in bronchiolar luminal diameter that over time may be reduced to a slitlike space or become completely obliterated. Chronic vascular rejection affects both pulmonary arteries and veins and results in intimal hyperplasia and mononuclear cell infiltrates (the "cellular" phase) with subsequent intimal sclerosis and luminal obliteration (the "burnt-out" phase). Sometimes, lipid-laden macrophages are found within the fibrous plaques, and hence chronic vascular rejection also carries the name of "graft atherosclerosis."

The diagnosis of acute rejection should be suspected in any lung transplant recipient who develops fever, leukocytosis, and bilateral lung infiltrates. *It must be remembered, however, that transplant patients are almost always immunosuppressed and hence are susceptible to a variety of opportunistic infections that may clinically and histologically mimic rejection.* This can be a vexing issue, since the treatment of acute rejection requires higher doses of immunosuppressive agents, while an infectious process would warrant attenuation of immunosuppression. Microbiologic studies and special stains to exclude organisms in the biopsy material are critical in resolving this dilemma. Chronic rejection results in progressive decline of pulmonary function (manifested as decrease in FEV_1), with little or no improvement on prolonged immunosuppression and eventual graft failure.

VASCULAR LUNG DISEASES

Pulmonary Thromboembolism, Hemorrhage, and Infarction

The embolization of venous and right-sided cardiac thrombi to the lungs is an extremely important clinical problem. Indeed, pulmonary thromboembolism is the most common preventable cause of death in hospitalized patients. In total, thromboembolism causes approximately 50,000 deaths per year in the United States. Even when not directly fatal, it can complicate the course of other diseases. The true incidence of nonfatal pulmonary embolism is not known. Some emboli undoubtedly occur outside the hospital in ambulatory patients and are small and clinically silent. Even among hospitalized patients, not more than one third are diagnosed before death. Moreover, when the diagnosis of a fatal pulmonary embolism is made clinically, postmortem examination fails to document the presence of emboli in approximately 50% of cases. Unfortunately, autopsy data on the incidence of pulmonary emboli vary widely, ranging from less than 1% to the extreme of 64%. If only fatal pulmonary emboli are considered, they are detected at postmortem examination in about 0.3% of hospitalized patients who have medical diseases, 1% of patients who have undergone surgery, and 5% to 8% of patients with hip fractures.

More than 95% of all pulmonary emboli arise from thrombi within the large deep veins of the lower legs, typically originating in the popliteal vein and larger veins above it. Thromboemboli do not commonly arise from superficial or smaller leg veins. Even when a patient has a well-documented pulmonary embolus, deep vein thrombosis can be identified clinically in only 20% to 70% of instances; this variation reflects whether invasive procedures such as venography were used.

The influences that predispose to venous thrombosis in the legs were discussed in Chapter 4, but the following risk factors should be emphasized: (1) prolonged bed rest (particularly with immobilization of the legs), (2) surgery on the legs (as following knee surgery), (3) severe trauma (including burns or multiple fractures), (4) congestive heart failure, (5) women in the period around parturition or who take birth control pills with high estrogen content (those who are carriers of a mutation in factor V are particularly vulnerable) (Chapters 4 and 8), and (6) disseminated cancer.

The pathophysiologic consequences of thromboembolism in the lung depend largely on the size of the embolus, which in turn dictates the size of the occluded pulmonary artery, and on the cardiopulmonary status of the patient. There are two important consequences of embolic pulmonary arterial occlusion: (1) an increase in pulmonary artery pressure from blockage of flow and, possibly, vasospasm caused by neurogenic mechanisms and/or release of mediators (e.g., thromboxane A_2 and serotonin); and (2) ischemia of the down-stream pulmonary parenchyma. Thus, occlusion of a *major vessel* results in a sudden increase in pulmonary artery pressure, diminished cardiac output, right-sided heart failure (acute cor pulmonale), or even death. Usually hypoxemia develops, as a result of multiple mechanisms:

■ *Perfusion of lung zones that have become atelectatic.* The alveolar collapse occurs in the ischemic areas because of a reduction in surfactant production and because pain associated with embolism leads to reduced movement of the chest wall; in addition, some of the pulmonary blood flow is redirected through areas of the lung that are normally hypoventilated.

■ The decrease in cardiac output causes a *widening of the difference in arterial-venous oxygen saturation.*

■ *Right-to-left shunting* of blood may occur in some patients through a patent foramen ovale, present in 30% of normal persons.

If *smaller vessels* are occluded, the result is less catastrophic, and the event may even be clinically silent.

Recall that lung is oxygenated not only by the pulmonary arteries but also by bronchial arteries and directly from air in the alveoli. If the bronchial circulation is normal and adequate ventilation is maintained, the resultant decrease in blood flow does not cause tissue necrosis. Indeed, ischemic necrosis (infarction) resulting from pulmonary thromboembolism is the exception rather than the rule, occurring in as few as 10% of cases. It occurs only if there is compromise in cardiac function or bronchial circulation, or if the region of the lung at risk is underventilated, owing to underlying pulmonary disease.

Figure 13–19 ■

Large saddle embolus from the femoral vein lying astride the main left and right pulmonary arteries. (Courtesy of Dr. Linda Margraf, Department of Pathology, University of Texas Southwestern Medical School, Dallas.)

MORPHOLOGY

The morphologic consequences of pulmonary embolism, as noted, depend on the size of the embolic mass and the general state of the circulation. Large emboli impact in the main pulmonary artery or its major branches or lodge astride the bifurcation as a **saddle embolus** (Fig. 13–19). Death usually follows so suddenly from hypoxia or acute failure of the right side of the heart (acute cor pulmonale) that there is no time for morphologic alterations in the lung.

Smaller emboli become impacted in medium-sized and small pulmonary arteries. With adequate circulation and bronchial arterial flow, the vitality of the lung parenchyma is maintained, but the alveolar spaces may fill with blood to produce pulmonary hemorrhage as a result of ischemic damage to the endothelial cells.

With compromised cardiovascular status, as may occur with congestive heart failure, **infarction** results. The more peripheral the embolic occlusion, the more likely is infarction. About three fourths of all infarcts affect the lower lobes, and more than half are multiple. They vary in size from lesions that are barely visible to involvement of large parts of a lobe. Characteristically, they are wedge shaped, with their base at the pleural surface and the apex pointing toward the hilus of the lung. Pulmonary infarcts are typically hemorrhagic and appear as raised, red-blue areas in the early stages (Fig. 13–20). The adjacent pleural surface is often covered by a fibrinous exudate. If the occluded vessel

can be identified, it is usually found near the apex of the infarcted area. The red cells begin to lyse within 48 hours, and the infarct pales, eventually becoming red-brown as hemosiderin is produced. In time, fibrous replacement begins at the margins as a gray-white peripheral zone and eventually converts the infarct into a scar that is contracted below the level of the lung substance. Histologically, the hallmark of fresh infarcts is coagulative necrosis of the lung parenchyma in the area of hemorrhage.

Figure 13–20 ■

A recent small, roughly wedge-shaped hemorrhagic pulmonary infarct.

Clinical Course. The clinical consequences of pulmonary thromboembolism are summarized here:

■ Most pulmonary emboli (60% to 80%) are clinically silent because they are small; the embolic mass is rapidly removed by fibrinolytic activity, and the bronchial circulation sustains the viability of the affected lung parenchyma until this is accomplished.

■ In 5% of cases, sudden death, acute right-sided heart failure (acute cor pulmonale), or cardiovascular collapse (shock) may occur when more than 60% of the total pulmonary vasculature is obstructed by a large embolus or multiple, simultaneous, small emboli. Massive pulmonary embolism is one of the few causes of literally instantaneous death, even before the patient experiences chest pain or dyspnea.

■ Obstruction of relatively small to medium pulmonary branches (10% to 15% of cases) that behave as end-arteries causes pulmonary infarction when some element of circulatory insufficiency is present. Typically, patients who sustain an infarct manifest dyspnea, the basis of which is not fully understood.

■ In a small but significant subset of patients (less than 3%), recurrent multiple emboli lead to pulmonary hypertension, chronic right-sided heart strain (chronic cor pulmonale), and, in time, pulmonary vascular sclerosis with progressively worsening dyspnea.

Emboli usually resolve after the initial acute insult. They contract, and endogenous fibrinolytic activity may cause total lysis of the thrombus. However, in the presence of an underlying predisposing factor, a small innocuous embolus may presage a larger one, and *patients who have experienced one pulmonary embolus have a 30% chance of developing a second.* Thus, recognition and appropriate preventive treatment are essential. Prophylactic therapy includes early ambulation for postoperative and postpartum patients, elastic stockings, and isometric leg exercises for bedridden patients. Anticoagulation is warranted for persons at high risk. Patients with pulmonary embolism are given thrombolytic and anticoagulation therapy.

In passing, mention should be made of nonthrombotic forms of pulmonary embolism, which include several uncommon, but potentially lethal, forms, such as air embolism, fat embolism, and amniotic fluid embolism, that were discussed in Chapter 4. Intravenous drug abuse is often associated with foreign body embolism in the pulmonary microvasculature; the presence of magnesium trisilicate (talc) in the intravenous mixture elicits a granulomatous response within the interstitium or pulmonary arteries. Involvement of the interstitium may lead to fibrosis, while the latter leads to pulmonary hypertension. Residual talc crystals can be demonstrated within the granulomas using polarized light. Bone marrow embolism (presence of hematopoietic and fat elements within pulmonary circulation) can occur after massive trauma and in patients with bone infarction secondary to sickle cell anemia.

Pulmonary Hypertension and Vascular Sclerosis

Pulmonary hypertension is most often caused by a decrease in the cross-sectional area of the pulmonary vascular

Table 13-4. CAUSES OF PULMONARY HYPERTENSION AND VASCULAR SCLEROSIS

Secondary Pulmonary Hypertension

Cardiac disease: left-to-right shunts: septal defects; mechanical obstructions: atrial myxoma, mitral stenosis
Inflammatory vascular disease: scleroderma and other connective tissue diseases; other forms of vasculitis
Lung disease: chronic hypoxia: high-altitude hypoxia, extraparenchymal restrictive lung diseases (obesity); chronic hypoxia with destruction of vascular bed: chronic obstructive pulmonary disease, chronic interstitial fibrosing diseases, pneumoconiosis
Recurrent thromboembolism*

Primary Pulmonary Hypertension

Plexiform pulmonary arteriopathy (30%–70% of cases)
Thrombotic pulmonary arteriopathy (20%–50% of cases)*
Pulmonary venoocclusive disease (10% of cases)

*These two diseases are difficult to distinguish clinically or morphologically.

bed, but it may also result from increased pulmonary vascular blood flow. It is most frequently *secondary* to (1) chronic obstructive or interstitial lung disease, (2) recurrent pulmonary emboli, or (3) heart disease in which there is a left-to-right shunt. Rarely (less than 5% of cases), pulmonary hypertension exists even though all known causes of increased pulmonary pressure can be excluded; this is referred to as *primary*, or idiopathic, pulmonary hypertension. Distinction of primary hypertension from that caused by recurrent thromboembolism may be particularly difficult, but angiography and radioisotope scanning may be helpful. Table 13–4 provides an overview of causes of pulmonary hypertension.

Because many of the diseases that give rise to secondary pulmonary vascular hypertension have already been discussed, only primary pulmonary hypertension is considered here. It should be stated at the outset that the mechanism of primary pulmonary hypertension is not known. According to current thinking, chronic vasoconstriction resulting from vascular hyperreactivity gives rise to pulmonary hypertension and, in time, its morphologic counterpart, intimal and medial vascular hypertrophy. The importance of vascular hyperreactivity is supported by the fact that about 10% of patients with primary pulmonary hypertension suffer from vasospastic disorders such as Raynaud phenomenon (Chapter 10). In addition, pulmonary vascular resistance can sometimes be rapidly decreased with vasodilators. The hyperreactivity is believed to be secondary to endothelial dysfunction and injury, idiopathic in most cases but sometimes associated with autoimmune diseases such as scleroderma and systemic lupus erythematosus. Endothelial dysfunction manifests as reduced production of prostacyclin and nitric oxide and increased generation of endothelin, all of which promote vasoconstriction. Endothelial cells may also elaborate growth factors that induce migration and proliferation of smooth muscle cells, responsible for vascular thickening. Studies on the rare familial pulmonary hypertension point to defects in TGF-β receptor family as being responsible for the vascular thickening. Apparently, mutations in these receptors prevent TGF-β and related molecules from exerting inhibition of vascular smooth muscle and endothelial cell proliferation. These studies suggest that other acquired defects in TGF-β receptor signaling may be important in the pathogenesis of nonfamilial primary pulmonary hypertension.

MORPHOLOGY

Vascular alterations in all forms of pulmonary sclerosis (primary and secondary) involve the entire arterial tree and include (1) in the main elastic arteries, atheromas similar to those in systemic atherosclerosis; (2) in medium-sized muscular arteries (Fig. 13–21A), proliferation of myointimal cells and smooth muscle cells, causing thickening of the intima and media with narrowing of the lumina (Fig. 13–21B); and (3) in smaller arteries and arterioles, thickening, medial hypertrophy, and reduplication of the internal and external elastic membranes. In these vessels, the wall thickness may exceed the diameter of the lumen, which is sometimes narrowed to the point of near-obliteration. In patients with severe, long-standing primary pulmonary hypertension, additional changes take the form of plexiform lesions and necrotizing arteritis with fibrinoid necrosis and thrombosis. The plexiform lesions consist of a multichanneled outpouching of the pulmonary arterial wall (Fig. 13–21C). These may represent aneurysmal dilation of the vessel wall or reparative lesions in areas of previous fibrinoid necrosis.

Clinical Course. *Secondary pulmonary vascular sclerosis* may develop at any age. The clinical features reflect the underlying disease, usually pulmonary or cardiac, with accentuation of respiratory insufficiency and right-

sided heart strain. *Primary pulmonary vascular sclerosis,* on the other hand, is almost always encountered in young persons, more commonly women, and is marked by fatigue, syncope (particularly on exercise), dyspnea on exertion, and sometimes chest pain. These patients eventually develop severe respiratory insufficiency and sometimes cyanosis. In patients with primary pulmonary hypertension, death usually results from right-sided heart failure within a few years of the diagnosis. Some amelioration of the respiratory distress can be achieved by vasodilators, but without lung transplantation the prognosis is grim.

PULMONARY INFECTIONS

Pulmonary infections in the form of pneumonia are responsible for one sixth of all deaths in the United States. This is not surprising because (1) the epithelial surfaces of the lung are constantly exposed to liters of variously contaminated air; (2) nasopharyngeal flora are regularly aspirated during sleep, even by healthy persons; and (3) other common lung diseases render the lung parenchyma vulnerable to virulent organisms. It is therefore a small miracle that the normal lung parenchyma remains sterile. This attests to the efficiency of a series of pulmonary defense mechanisms. A plethora of immune and nonimmune defense mechanisms exists in the respiratory system, extending from the nasopharynx all the way into the alveolar airspaces. Summarized in Table 13–5 and illustrated in Figure 13–22, they pose an impressive barrier to an infectious onslaught.

Despite the multitude of defense mechanisms, "chinks in the armor" do exist, and they predispose the individual to infections. *Defects in innate immunity (including neutrophil and complement defects) and humoral immunodeficiency*

Figure 13–21

Panel illustrating the morphologic alterations seen in pulmonary hypertension. *A,* Normal pulmonary muscular artery, identified by the presence of a muscular media lined by internal elastic lamina (IEL) and external elastic lamina (EEL). Note that the intima is scarcely visible and consists of a layer of endothelium apposed to the IEL. The tissue has been stained with a Verhoeff–van Gieson stain, which highlights elastic fibers that comprise the IEL and EEL. *B,* Intimal hyperplasia *(arrow),* in addition to medial hypertrophy. This is the stage of mild to moderate pulmonary hypertension and is usually reversible. *C,* Advanced grade of pulmonary hypertension with the formation of so-called *plexiform lesion.* These structures are presumably formed by aneurysmal disruption of the wall of small muscular arteries *(arrow)* from the high pulmonary pressures, with secondary thrombosis and recanalization occurring within the disrupted segment. (Courtesy of Dr. Linda Margraf, Department of Pathology, University of Texas Southwestern Medical School, Dallas.)

Reproduced with permission from Mandell GL, et al (eds): Mandell, Douglas and Bennett's Principles and Practice of Infectious Diseases, 5th ed. Philadelphia, Churchill Livingstone, p 718.

Table 13-5. PULMONARY HOST DEFENSES

Location	Host Defense Mechanism
Upper Airways	
Nasopharynx	Nasal hair
	Turbinates
	Mucociliary apparatus
	IgA secretion
Oropharynx	Saliva
	Sloughing of epithelial cells
	Local complement production
	Interference from resident flora
Conducting Airways	
Trachea, bronchi	Cough, epiglottic reflexes
	Sharp-angled branching of airways
	Mucociliary apparatus
	Immunoglobulin production (IgG, IgM, IgA)
Lower Respiratory Tract	
Terminal airways, alveoli	Alveolar lining fluid (surfactant, immunoglobulin, complement, fibronectin)
	Cytokines (interleukin 1, tumor necrosis factor)
	Alveolar macrophages
	Polymorphonuclear leukocytes
	Cell-mediated immunity

typically lead to an increased incidence of infections with pyogenic bacteria. On the other hand, cell-mediated immune defects lead to increased infections with intracellular microbes such as mycobacteria and herpesviruses as well as with microorganisms of very low virulence such as Pneumocystis carinii. Several exogenous lifestyle factors interfere with host immune defense mechanisms and facilitate infections. For example, cigarette smoke compromises mucociliary clearance and pulmonary macrophage activity, while alcohol not only impairs cough and epiglottic reflexes, thereby increasing the risk of aspiration, but also interferes with neutrophil mobilization and chemotaxis.

Pneumonia can be very broadly defined as any infection in the lung. It may present as acute, fulminant clinical disease or as chronic disease with a more protracted course. The histologic spectrum of pneumonia may vary from a fibrinopurulent alveolar exudate seen in acute bacterial pneumonias, to mononuclear interstitial infiltrates in viral and other atypical pneumonias, to granulomas and cavitation seen in many of the chronic pneumonias. Acute bacterial pneumonias can present as one of two anatomic and radiographic patterns, referred to as bronchopneumonia and lobar pneumonia. Bronchopneumonia implies a patchy distribution of inflammation that generally involves more than one lobe (Fig. 13-23). This pattern results from an initial infection of the bronchi and bronchioles with extension into the adjacent alveoli. By contrast, in lobar pneumonia the contiguous airspaces of part or all of a lobe are homogeneously filled with an exudate that can be visualized on radiographs as a lobar or segmental consolidation (see Fig. 13-23). Streptococcus pneumoniae is responsible for more than 90% of lobar pneumonias. The anatomic distinction between lobar pneumonia and bronchopneumonia can often become blurry because (1) many organisms present with either of the two patterns of distribution and (2) confluent bronchopneumonia can be hard to distinguish radiologically from lobar pneumonia. Therefore, it is best to classify pneumonias either by the specific etiologic agent or, if no pathogen can be isolated, by the clinical setting in which infection occurs. Classifying pneumonias by the setting in which they arise considerably narrows the list of suspected pathogens for administering empirical antimicrobial therapy. As illustrated in Table 13-6, pneumonia can arise in seven distinct clinical settings ("pneumonia syndromes"), and the implicated pathogens are reasonably specific to each category.

Community-Acquired Acute Pneumonias

Community-acquired acute pneumonias are bacterial in origin. Not uncommonly, the infection follows a viral upper respiratory tract infection. The onset is usually abrupt, with high fever, shaking chills, pleuritic chest pain, and a productive mucopurulent cough; occasional patients may have hemoptysis. Streptococcus pneumoniae (or pneumococcus) is the most common cause of community-acquired acute pneumonia; hence, pneumococcal pneumonia will be discussed as the prototype for this subgroup. Pneumococcal infections occur with increased frequency in three groups of individuals: (1) those with underlying chronic diseases such as congestive heart failure, COPD, or diabetes; (2) those with either congenital or acquired immunoglobulin defects (e.g., the acquired immunodeficiency syndrome [AIDS]); and (3) those with decreased or absent splenic function (e.g., sickle cell disease or post splenectomy). The last occurs because the spleen is the major organ responsible for removing pneumococcus from the blood.

MORPHOLOGY

With pneumococcal lung infection, either pattern of pneumonia, lobar or bronchopneumonia, may occur; the latter is much more prevalent at the extremes of age. Regardless of the distribution of the pneumonia, because pneumococcal lung infections usually originate by aspiration of pharyngeal flora (20% of adults harbor S. pneumoniae in their throats), the lower lobes or the right middle lobe are most frequently involved.

In the preantibiotic era, pneumococcal pneumonia involved entire or almost entire lobes and evolved through four stages: **congestion, red hepatization, gray hepatization,** and **resolution.** Early antibiotic therapy alters or halts this typical progression, so if the patient dies, the anatomic changes seen at autopsy may not conform to the classic stages.

During the first stage, that of **congestion,** the affected lobe(s) is (are) heavy, red, and boggy;

Ciliated respiratory epithelial cell

Lymph node 5

Mucous blanket

Mucous gland

"Upper" respiratory tract

Lymphatic

Macrophage

1

2

"Lower" respiratory tract

4

3

Microorganism

Capillary

Complement

PMN

A. NONIMMUNE LUNG

Plasma cell

Lymph node

"Upper" respiratory tract

1

IgA

Microorganism

Macrophage

"Lower" respiratory tract

PMN

2

3

IgG

Immune T cells

B. IMMUNE LUNG

Figure 13-22 ■

Lung defense mechanisms. *A,* In the nonimmune lung, removal of microbial organisms depends on (1) entrapment in the mucous blanket and removal via the mucociliary elevator, (2) phagocytosis by alveolar macrophages that can kill and degrade organisms and remove them from the airspaces by migrating onto the mucociliary elevator, or (3) phagocytosis and killing by neutrophils recruited by macrophage factors. 4, Serum complement may enter the alveoli and be activated by the alternative pathway to provide the opsonin C3b that enhances phagocytosis. 5, Organisms, including those ingested by phagocytes, may reach the draining lymph nodes to initiate immune responses. *B,* Additional mechanisms operate in the immune lung. 1, Secreted IgA can block attachment of the microorganism to epithelium in the upper respiratory tract. 2, In the lower respiratory tract, serum antibodies (IgM, IgG) are present in the alveolar lining fluid. They activate complement more efficiently by the classic pathway, yielding C3b (not shown). In addition, IgG is opsonic. 3, The accumulation of immune T cells is important for controlling infections by viruses and other intracellular microorganisms.

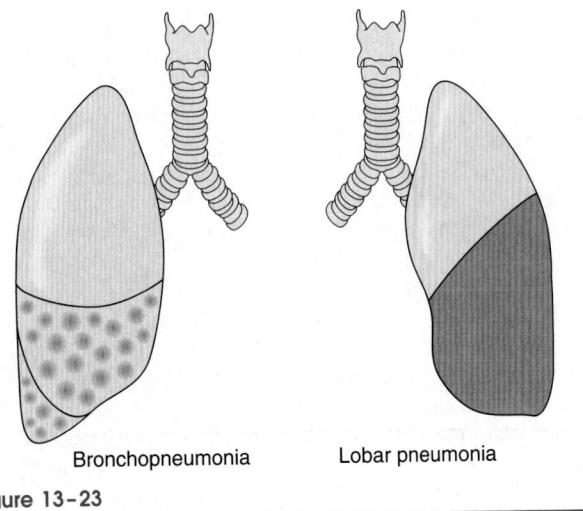

Bronchopneumonia

Lobar pneumonia

Figure 13-23 ■

The anatomic distribution of bronchopneumonia and lobar pneumonia.

histologically, vascular congestion can be seen, with proteinaceous fluid, scattered neutrophils, and many bacteria in the alveoli. Within a few days, the stage of **red hepatization** ensues, in which the lung lobe has a liver-like consistency; the alveolar spaces are packed with neutrophils, red cells, and fibrin (Fig. 13-24); and the pleura usually demonstrates a fibrinous or fibrinopurulent exudate. In the next stage, **gray hepatization,** the lung is dry, gray, and firm, because the red cells get lysed, while the fibrinous exudate persists within the alveoli (Fig. 13-25). **Resolution** follows in uncomplicated cases, as exudates within the alveoli are enzymatically digested and either resorbed or expectorated, leaving the basic architecture intact. The pleural reaction may similarly resolve or undergo organization, leaving fibrous thickening or permanent adhesions.

Table 13-6. THE PNEUMONIA SYNDROMES

Community-Acquired Acute Pneumonia

Streptococcus pneumoniae
Haemophilus influenzae
Moraxella catarrhalis
Staphylococcus aureus
Legionella pneumophila
Enterobacteriaceae (*Klebsiella pneumoniae*) and *Pseudomonas* spp.

Community-Acquired Atypical Pneumonia

Mycoplasma pneumoniae
Chlamydia spp. (*C. pneumoniae, C. psittaci, C. trachomatis*)
Coxiella burnetti (Q fever)
Viruses: respiratory syncytial virus, parainfluenza virus (children);
   influenza A and B (adults); adenovirus (military recruits)

Nosocomial Pneumonia

Gram-negative rods belonging to Enterobacteriaceae (*Klebsiella* spp.,
   Serratia marcescens, Escherichia coli) and *Pseudomonas* spp.
Staphylococcus aureus (usually penicillin-resistant)

Aspiration Pneumonia

Anaerobic oral flora (*Bacteroides, Prevotella, Fusobacterium,*
   Peptostreptococcus), admixed with aerobic bacteria (*Streptococcus*
   pneumoniae, Staphylococcus aureus, Haemophilas influenzae, and
   Pseudomonas aeruginosa)

Chronic Pneumonia

Nocardia
Actinomyces
Granulomatous: *Mycobacterium tuberculosis* and atypical mycobacteria,
   Histoplasma capsulatum, Coccidioides immitis, Blastomyces dermatitidis

Necrotizing Pneumonia and Lung Abscess

Anaerobic bacteria (extremely common), with or without mixed aerobic
   infection
Staphylococcus aureus, Klebsiella pneumoniae, Streptococcus pyogenes,
   and type 3 pneumococcus (uncommon)

Pneumonia in the Immunocompromised Host

Cytomegalovirus
Pneumocystis carinii
Mycobacterium avium-intracellulare
Invasive aspergillosis
Invasive candidiasis
"Usual" bacterial, viral, and fungal organisms (listed above)

Figure 13-24 ■

The histopathologic hallmark of acute pneumonia, irrespective of etiology and anatomic distribution, is the presence of *neutrophils* within the alveolar spaces. This is accompanied by septal capillary congestion and fibrinous exudates, resulting from increased capillary permeability. The term *fibrinopurulent* is applied to the combination of fibrin and neutrophils (pus) within the alveolar spaces.

material may accumulate in the pleural cavity, producing an **empyema;** (3) organization of the intra-alveolar exudate may convert areas of the lung into solid fibrous tissue; and (4) bacteremic dissemination may lead to **meningitis, arthritis,** or **infective endocarditis.** Complications are much more likely with serotype 3 pneumococci.

In the bronchopneumonic pattern, foci of inflammatory consolidation are distributed in patches throughout one or several lobes, most frequently bilateral and basal. Well-developed lesions up to 3 or 4 cm in diameter are slightly elevated and are gray-red to yellow; confluence of these foci may occur in severe cases, producing the appearance of a lobar consolidation. The lung substance immediately surrounding areas of consolidation is usually hyperemic and edematous, but the large intervening areas are generally normal. Pleural involvement is less common than in lobar pneumonia. Histologically, the reaction consists of focal suppurative exudate that fills the bronchi, bronchioles, and adjacent alveolar spaces.

With appropriate therapy, complete restitution of the lung is the rule for both forms of pneumococcal pneumonia, but in occasional cases complications may occur: (1) tissue destruction and necrosis may lead to **abscess** formation; (2) suppurative

Figure 13-25 ■

Gross view of lobar pneumonia with gray hepatization. The lower lobe is uniformly consolidated.

Examination of Gram-stained sputum is an important step in the diagnosis of acute pneumonia. The presence of numerous neutrophils containing the typical gram-positive, lancet-shaped diplococci is good evidence of pneumococcal pneumonia, but it must be remembered that *S. pneumoniae* is a part of the endogenous flora and therefore false-positive results may be obtained by this method. Isolation of pneumococci from blood cultures is more specific. During early phases of illness, blood cultures may be positive in 20% to 30% of patients.

Pneumococcal pneumonias respond readily to penicillin treatment, but there are increasing numbers of penicillin-resistant strains of pneumococci, so whenever possible antibiotic sensitivity should be determined. Commercial pneumococcal vaccines containing capsular polysaccharides from the common serotypes of pneumococcus are available, and their proven efficacy mandates their use in patients at risk for pneumococcal infections (see earlier).

Other organisms commonly implicated in community-acquired acute pneumonias include the following:

Haemophilus influenzae

- Both unencapsulated and encapsulated forms are important causes of community-acquired pneumonias.
- Individuals at risk for developing infections include those with chronic pulmonary diseases such as chronic bronchitis, cystic fibrosis, and bronchiectasis. *H. influenzae is the most common bacterial cause of acute exacerbation of COPD.*
- Encapsulated *H. influenzae* type b is also an important cause of epiglottitis in children.

Moraxella catarrhalis

- *M. catarrhalis* is being increasingly recognized as a cause of bacterial pneumonia, especially in the elderly.
- It is the second most common bacterial cause of acute exacerbation in adults who have underlying COPD.
- Along with *S. pneumoniae* and *H. influenzae*, *M. catarrhalis* constitutes one of the three most common causes of otitis media (infection of the middle ear) in children.

Staphylococcus aureus

- *S. aureus* is an important cause of secondary bacterial pneumonia in children and healthy adults following viral respiratory illnesses (e.g., measles in children and influenza in both children and adults).
- Staphylococcal pneumonia is associated with a high incidence of complications, such as lung abscess and empyema.
- Staphylococcal pneumonia occurring in association with right-sided staphylococcal endocarditis is a serious complication of *intravenous drug abuse*.
- Staphylococcal pneumonia is also an important cause of nosocomial pneumonia (see later).

Klebsiella pneumoniae

- *K. pneumoniae* is the most frequent cause of gram-negative bacterial pneumonia.
- It frequently afflicts debilitated and malnourished persons, particularly *chronic alcoholics*.
- Thick and gelatinous sputum is characteristic because the organism produces an abundant viscid capsular polysaccharide, which the patient may have difficulty coughing up.

Pseudomonas aeruginosa

- Although discussed here with community-acquired pathogens because of its association with infections in cystic fibrosis, *P. aeruginosa* is most commonly seen in nosocomial settings (see later).
- *Pseudomonas* pneumonia is also common in patients who are neutropenic, usually secondary to chemotherapy; in patients with extensive burns; and in those requiring mechanical ventilation.
- *P. aeruginosa* has a propensity to invade blood vessels at the site of infection with consequent extrapulmonary spread; *Pseudomonas* bacteremia is a fulminant disease, with death often occurring within a matter of days.
- Histologic examination reveals coagulation necrosis of the pulmonary parenchyma with organisms invading the walls of necrotic blood vessels (*Pseudomonas* vasculitis) (Fig. 13–26).

Legionella pneumophila

- *L. pneumophila* is the agent of legionnaire's disease, an eponym for the epidemic and sporadic forms of pneumonia caused by this organism. Pontiac fever is a related self-limited upper respiratory tract infection caused by *L. pneumophila*, without pneumonic symptoms.
- *L. pneumophila* flourishes in artificial aquatic environments, such as water-cooling towers and within the tubing system of domestic (potable) water supplies. The mode of transmission is thought to be either inhalation of aerosolized organisms or aspiration of contaminated drinking water.
- *Legionella* pneumonia is common in persons with some predisposing condition such as cardiac, renal, immunologic, or hematologic disease. *Organ transplant recipients are particularly susceptible.*
- *Legionella* pneumonia can be quite severe, frequently requiring hospitalization, and immunosuppressed individuals may have a fatality rate of 30% to 50%.
- Rapid diagnosis is facilitated by demonstration of *Legionella* antigens in the urine or by a positive fluorescent antibody test on sputum samples; culture remains the gold standard of diagnosis.

Community-Acquired Atypical Pneumonias

The concept of community-acquired atypical pneumonia was set forth in 1938 with the description of eight cases in which pharyngitis and systemic flulike symptoms evolved into laryngitis and finally tracheobronchitis and pneumonia. Unlike in "typical" acute pneumonias, sputum production was modest, there were no physical findings of consolidation, the white cell count was only moderately elevated, and bacteria and influenza A viruses could not be isolated. In retrospect, these cases were probably caused by *Mycoplasma pneumoniae*. This agent is the most common cause of atypical pneumonias, particularly at times when influenza A epidemics are not present in the community. A

Figure 13-26   ■

Lung sections from a patient who had nosocomial *Pseudomonas* pneumonia. *A,* There is extensive destruction of pulmonary parenchyma *(arrowhead),* with full-thickness fibrinoid necrosis of the arterial wall in the upper portion of the field *(arrow). B,* High-power photomicrograph demonstrates abundant bacteria *(deep blue)* invading the wall of the blood vessel; star indicates the vessel lumen (Steiner tissue stain).

similar syndrome may occur with a number of other agents, including viruses, chlamydiae, and rickettsiae (see Table 13-6). Among these, *Chlamydia pneumoniae* is being increasingly recognized as an important cause of community-acquired atypical pneumonias. Nearly all of these agents can also cause a primarily upper respiratory tract infection with coryza (inflammation with diffuse discharge from the nasal mucosa), pharyngitis, laryngitis, and tracheobronchitis. The common pathogenetic mechanism is attachment of the organisms to the respiratory epithelium followed by necrosis of the cells and an inflammatory response. When the process extends to alveoli, there is usually *interstitial* inflammation, but there may also be some outpouring of fluid into alveolar spaces so that on chest films the changes may mimic bacterial pneumonia. Damage to and denudation of the respiratory epithelium inhibits mucociliary clearance and predisposes to secondary bacterial infections. Viral infections of the respiratory tract are well known for this complication.

Mycoplasma infections are particularly common among children and young adults. They occur sporadically or as local epidemics in closed communities (schools, military camps, prisons). Viral lower respiratory tract infections may occur at any age, and in adults they are most often caused by influenza viruses A and B (see Table 13-6). Less common offenders are parainfluenza and respiratory syncytial viruses, the latter especially in infants and children. Adenovirus pneumonias are particularly common in young army recruits. A number of other viruses are sometimes implicated, including those that cause measles and chickenpox. Much depends on the resistance of the host, so atypical pneumonias range from mild to severe. More serious lower respiratory tract infection is favored by infancy, old age, malnourishment, alcoholism, and immunosuppression. Not surprisingly, viruses and mycoplasmas are frequently involved in outbreaks of infection in hospitals.

MORPHOLOGY

Regardless of cause, the morphologic patterns in atypical pneumonias are similar. The process may be patchy, or it may involve whole lobes bilaterally or unilaterally. Macroscopically, the affected areas are red-blue, congested, and subcrepitant. Histologically, the inflammatory reaction is largely confined within the walls of the alveoli (Fig. 13-27). The septa are widened and edematous; they usually contain a mononuclear inflammatory infiltrate of lymphocytes, histiocytes, and, occasionally, plasma cells. In contrast to bacterial pneumonias, alveolar spaces in atypical pneumonias are remarkably free of cellular exudate. In severe cases, however,

Figure 13-27   ■

Viral pneumonia. The thickened alveolar walls are heavily infiltrated with mononuclear leukocytes.

full-blown **diffuse alveolar damage with hyaline membranes may develop.** In less severe, uncomplicated cases, subsidence of the disease is followed by reconstitution of the native architecture. Superimposed bacterial infection, as expected, results in a mixed histologic picture.

Clinical Course. The clinical course of primary atypical pneumonia is extremely varied, even among cases caused by a single pathogen. It may masquerade as a severe upper respiratory tract infection or "chest cold" that goes undiagnosed, or it may present as a fulminant, life-threatening infection in immunocompromised patients. More typically, the onset is that of an acute, nonspecific febrile illness characterized by fever, headache, and malaise, and, later, cough with minimal sputum. Chest radiographs usually reveal transient, ill-defined patches, mainly in the lower lobes. Physical findings are characteristically minimal and indistinguishable from bronchopneumonia, although, particularly with *Mycoplasma*, lobar consolidations may occur. Because the edema and exudation are both in a strategic position to cause an alveolocapillary block, there may be respiratory distress seemingly out of proportion to the physical and radiographic findings.

Identifying the causative agent is difficult. Indeed, in most cases the pathogen remains undetermined. Culture of the organism is possible but is often difficult. Rising titers of specific antibodies point to the diagnosis, but these results are usually obtained after the patient has begun to recover. Elevations in the titers of cold agglutinins occur in mycoplasmal infection, but this is present in only 50% of cases. Because this test is not specific, it is of only historic interest. Tests for *Mycoplasma* antigens and polymerase chain reaction (PCR) testing for *Mycoplasma* DNA are available. As a practical matter, patients with community-acquired pneumonia for which a bacterial agent seems unlikely are treated with an antibiotic (erythromycin) effective against *Mycoplasma* and *Chlamydia pneumoniae*, because these are the most common treatable pathogens.

The prognosis for uncomplicated cases is good; generally, complete recovery is the rule. The most serious infections, caused by influenza viruses in infirm and elderly persons, are often complicated by bacterial superinfection.

Nosocomial Pneumonia

Nosocomial, or hospital-acquired, pneumonias are defined as pulmonary infections acquired in the course of a hospital stay. The specter of nosocomial pneumonia places an immense burden on the burgeoning costs of health care, besides the expected adverse impact on patient outcome. Nosocomial infections are common in patients with severe underlying disease, immunosuppression, prolonged antibiotic therapy, or invasive access devices such as intravascular catheters. Patients on mechanical ventilation represent a particularly high-risk group, and infections acquired in this setting are given the distinctive moniker *ventilator-associated pneumonia.* Gram-negative rods (Enterobacteriaceae and *Pseudomonas*

species) and *S. aureus* are the most common isolates; unlike community-acquired pneumonias, *S. pneumoniae* is not a major pathogen in nosocomial infections.

Aspiration Pneumonia

Aspiration pneumonia occurs in markedly debilitated patients or those who aspirate gastric contents either while unconscious (e.g., after a stroke) or during repeated vomiting. These patients have abnormal gag and swallowing reflexes that facilitate aspiration. The resultant pneumonia is partly chemical, owing to the extremely irritating effects of the gastric acid, and partly bacterial. Although it is commonly assumed that anaerobic bacteria predominate, recent studies implicate aerobes more commonly than anaerobes (see Table 13–6). This type of pneumonia is often necrotizing, pursues a fulminant clinical course, and is a frequent cause of death in patients predisposed to aspiration. In those who survive, abscess formation is a common complication.

Tuberculosis

Tuberculosis is a communicable chronic granulomatous disease caused by *Mycobacterium tuberculosis*. It usually involves the lungs but may affect any organ or tissue in the body. Typically, the centers of tubercular granulomas undergo caseous necrosis.

Epidemiology. Among medically and economically deprived persons throughout the world, tuberculosis remains a leading cause of death. It is estimated that 1.7 billion individuals are infected worldwide, with 8 to 10 million new cases and 3 million deaths per year. The World Health Organization estimates that tuberculosis causes 6% of all deaths worldwide, making it the most common cause of death resulting from a single infectious agent. In the Western world, deaths from tuberculosis peaked in 1800 and steadily declined throughout the 1800s and 1900s. However, in 1984 the decline in new cases stopped abruptly, a change that resulted from the increased incidence of tuberculosis in human immunodeficiency virus (HIV)-infected persons. Following intensive surveillance and tuberculosis prophylaxis among immunosuppressed individuals, the incidence of tuberculosis in US-born individuals has declined since 1992. Currently, it is estimated that about 25,000 new cases with active tuberculosis arise in the United States annually, and nearly 40% of these are in immigrants from countries where tuberculosis is highly prevalent.

Tuberculosis flourishes wherever there is poverty, crowding, and chronic debilitating illness. Similarly, elderly persons, with their weakened defenses, are vulnerable. In the United States, tuberculosis is a disease of the elderly, the urban poor, patients with acquired immunodeficiency syndrome (AIDS), and those belonging to minority communities. African Americans, Native Americans, the Inuit (from Alaska), Hispanics, and immigrants from Southeast Asia have higher attack rates than other segments of the population. *Certain disease states also increase the risk:* diabetes mellitus, Hodgkin disease, chronic lung disease (particularly silicosis), chronic renal failure, malnutrition, alcoholism, and immunosuppression. In areas of the world where HIV infection is prevalent, *it has become the single most important risk factor for the development of tuberculosis.* Most, perhaps all, of these predisposing conditions are related to a decrease in the capacity to develop and maintain T-cell–mediated immunity against the infectious agent.

It is important that *infection* be differentiated from *disease.* Infection implies seeding of a focus with organisms, which may or may not cause clinically significant tissue damage (i.e., disease). Although other routes may be involved, most infections are acquired by direct person-to-person transmission of airborne droplets of organisms from an active case to a susceptible host. In most persons, an asymptomatic focus of pulmonary infection appears that is self-limited, although, uncommonly, primary tuberculosis may result in the development of fever and pleural effusion. Generally, the only evidence of infection, if any remains, is a tiny, telltale fibrocalcific nodule at the site of the infection. Viable organisms may remain dormant in such loci for decades, and possibly for the life of the host. Such persons are infected but do not have active disease and so cannot transmit organisms to others. Yet when their defenses are lowered, the infection may reactivate to produce communicable and potentially life-threatening disease.

Infection with *M. tuberculosis* typically leads to the development of delayed hypersensitivity, which can be detected by the tuberculin (Mantoux) test. About 2 to 4 weeks after the infection has begun, intracutaneous injection of 0.1 mL of purified protein derivative (PPD) induces a visible and palpable induration (at least 5 mm in diameter) that peaks in 48 to 72 hours. Sometimes, more PPD is required to elicit the reaction, and unfortunately, in some responders, the standard dose may produce a large, necrotizing lesion. *A positive tuberculin test result* signifies cell-mediated hypersensitivity to tubercular antigens. It does not differentiate between infection and disease. It is well recognized that *false-negative reactions (or skin test anergy) may be produced by certain viral infections, sarcoidosis, malnutrition, Hodgkin disease, immunosuppression, and (notably) overwhelming active tuberculous disease.* False-positive reactions may also result from infection by atypical mycobacteria.

About 80% of the population in certain Asian and African countries are tuberculin positive. By contrast, in 1980, 5% to 10% of the US population reacted positively to tuberculin, indicating the marked difference in rates of exposure to the tubercle bacillus. In general, 3% to 4% of previously unexposed individuals acquire active tuberculosis during the first year after "tuberculin conversion," and no more than 15% do so thereafter. Thus, *only a small fraction of those who contract an infection develop active disease.*

Etiology. Mycobacteria are slender rods that are acid fast (i.e., they have a high content of complex lipids that readily bind the Ziehl-Neelsen [carbol fuchsin] stain and subsequently stubbornly resist decolorization). *M. tuberculosis hominis* is responsible for most cases of tuberculosis; the reservoir of infection is usually found in humans with active pulmonary disease. Transmission is usually direct, by inhalation of airborne organisms in aerosols generated by expectoration or by exposure to contaminated patient secretions. Oropharyngeal and intestinal tuberculosis contracted by drinking milk contaminated with *M. bovis* is now rare in

developed nations, but it is still seen in countries that have tuberculous dairy cows and unpasteurized milk. Both *M. hominis* and *M. bovis* species are obligate aerobes whose slow growth is retarded by a pH lower than 6.5 and by long-chain fatty acids, hence the difficulty of finding tubercle bacilli in the centers of large caseating lesions where anaerobiosis, low pH, and increased levels of fatty acids are present. Other mycobacteria, particularly *M. avium-intracellulare*, are much less virulent than *M. tuberculosis* and rarely cause disease in immunocompetent individuals. However, in patients with AIDS, these strains are frequently found, affecting 10% to 30% of patients.

Pathogenesis. The pathogenesis of tuberculosis in the previously *unexposed immunocompetent* individual is centered on the development of a targeted cell-mediated immunity that confers *resistance* to the organism and results in development of *tissue hypersensitivity* to tubercular antigens. The pathologic features of tuberculosis, such as caseating granulomas and cavitation, are the result of the destructive tissue hypersensitivity that is part and parcel of the host immune response. Because the effector cells for both processes are the same, the appearance of tissue hypersensitivity also signals the acquisition of immunity to the organism. The sequence of events from inhalation of the infectious inoculum to containment of the primary focus is illustrated in Figure 13–28A and B and outlined in the text below.

- Once virulent strains of mycobacteria gain entry into the macrophage endosomes (a process mediated by the macrophage mannose receptor that recognizes mannose-capped glycolipids on tubercular cell walls), the organisms are able to inhibit normal microbicidal responses by manipulation of endosomal pH and arrest of endosomal maturation. The end result of this "endosomal manipulation" is impairment of effective phagolysosome formation and unhindered mycobacterial proliferation.
- Recently, a gene called *NRAMP1* (or natural resistance–associated macrophage protein 1) has been implicated in early microbicidal activity, and it may play a role in the progression of human tuberculosis. Certain polymorphisms of the *NRAMP1* allele have been shown to be associated with an increased incidence of tuberculosis (especially among African Americans), and it is postulated that these genotypic variations of *NRAMP1* may result in decreased microbicidal function.
- Thus, the earliest phase of primary tuberculosis (<3 weeks) in the nonsensitized individual is characterized by unchecked bacillary proliferation within the pulmonary alveolar macrophages and airspaces, with resulting bacteremia and seeding of multiple sites.
- *Despite the bacteremia, most patients at this stage are asymptomatic or have a mild flulike illness.*
- The development of cell-mediated immunity occurs approximately 3 weeks after exposure. Processed mycobacterial antigens reach the draining lymph nodes and are presented in a major histocompatibility class II context by macrophages to uncommitted CD4+ T_H0 cells bearing the $\alpha\beta$ T-cell receptor.
- Under the influence of macrophage-secreted *IL-12*, these T_H0 cells "mature" into CD4+ T cells of T_H1 subtype, capable of secreting IFN-γ.

A. PRIMARY PULMONARY TUBERCULOSIS (0–3 weeks)

B. PRIMARY PULMONARY TUBERCULOSIS (>3 weeks)

Figure 13–28

The sequence of events in primary pulmonary tuberculosis, commencing with inhalation of virulent strains of *Mycobacterium* and culminating with the development of immunity and delayed hypersensitivity to the organism. *A,* Events occurring in the first 3 weeks after exposure; *B,* events thereafter. The development of resistance to the organism is accompanied by the appearance of a positive tuberculin test. Cells and bacteria not drawn to scale. iNOS, inducible nitric oxide synthase; MHC, major histocompatibility complex; MTB, *Mycobacterium tuberculosis*; NRAMP1, natural resistance–associated macrophage protein.

■ *IFN-γ released by the CD4+ T cells is critical in activating macrophages.* Activated macrophages release a variety of mediators with important downstream effects:

■ *TNF* is responsible for recruitment of monocytes, which in turn undergo activation and differentiation into the "epithelioid histiocytes" that characterize the granulomatous response.

■ IFN-γ in conjunction with TNF turns on the *inducible nitric oxide synthase (iNOS)* gene, which results in elevated *nitric oxide* levels at the site of infection. Nitric oxide is a powerful oxidizing agent and results in generation of reactive nitrogen intermediates and other free radicals capable of oxidative destruction of several mycobacterial constituents, from cell wall to DNA.

■ Besides activating macrophages, CD4+ T cells also facilitate the development of CD8+ cytotoxic T cells, which can kill tuberculosis-infected macrophages. While most of the T-cell mediated immune response is performed by cells bearing the αβ T-cell receptor, recent studies have focused on the complementary role of gamma-delta (γδ) T cells in host resistance to intracellular pathogens such as mycobacteria. γδ T cells not only secrete IFN-γ (thereby activating macrophages) but also can function as cytotoxic effector cells causing destruction of tuberculosis-infected macrophages.

■ Defects in any of the steps of a T$_H$1 response (including IL-12, IFN-γ, TNF, or nitric oxide production) result in poorly formed granulomas, absence of resistance, and disease progression.

In summary, immunity to a tubercular infection is primarily mediated by T cells and is characterized by the two-pronged development of hypersensitivity and the appearance of resistance to the organism. Hypersensitivity is accompanied by a destructive tissue response, such that reactivation or re-exposure to the bacilli in a previously sensitized host results in rapid mobilization of a defensive reaction but increased tissue necrosis. Just as hypersensitivity and resistance appear in parallel, so, too, the loss of hypersensitivity (such as tuberculin negativity in a previously tuberculin-positive individual) may be an ominous sign that resistance to the organism has faded as well.

PRIMARY TUBERCULOSIS

Primary tuberculosis is the form of disease that develops in a previously unexposed, and therefore unsensitized, person. Elderly persons and profoundly immunosuppressed persons may lose their sensitivity to the tubercle bacillus and so may develop primary tuberculosis more than once. With primary tuberculosis, the source of the organism is exogenous. About 5% of those newly infected develop significant disease.

Figure 13-29   ■

Primary pulmonary tuberculosis, Ghon complex. The gray-white parenchymal focus is under the pleura in the lower part of the upper lobe. Hilar lymph nodes with caseation are seen on the left.

MORPHOLOGY

In countries where bovine tuberculosis and infected milk have largely disappeared, primary tuberculosis almost always begins in the lungs. Typically, the inhaled bacilli implant in the distal airspaces of the lower part of the upper lobe or the upper part of the lower lobe, usually close to the pleura. As sensitization develops, a 1- to 1.5-cm area of gray-white inflammatory consolidation emerges, the **Ghon focus.** In most cases the center of this focus undergoes caseous necrosis. Tubercle bacilli, either free or within phagocytes, drain to the regional nodes, which also often caseate. **This combination of parenchymal lesion and nodal involvement is referred to as the Ghon complex** (Fig. 13-29). During the first few weeks, there is also lymphatic and hematogenous dissemination to other parts of the body. In approximately 95% of cases, development of cell-mediated immunity controls the infection. Hence, the Ghon complex undergoes progressive fibrosis, often followed by radiologically detectable calcification **(Ranke complex),** and, despite seeding of other organs, no lesions develop.

Histologically, sites of active involvement are marked by a characteristic granulomatous inflammatory reaction that forms both caseating and noncaseating tubercles (Fig. 13-30A–C). Individual tubercles are microscopic; it is only when multiple granulomas coalesce that they become macroscopically visible. The granulomas are usually enclosed within a fibroblastic rim punctuated by lymphocytes. Multinucleate giant cells are present in the granulomas.

The chief implications of primary tuberculosis are that (1) it induces hypersensitivity and increased resistance; (2) the foci of scarring may harbor viable bacilli for years, perhaps for life, and thus be the nidus for *reactivation* at a later time when host defenses are compromised; and (3) uncommonly, the disease may develop without interruption into so-called *progressive primary tuberculosis.* This occurs in individuals who are immunocompromised because of a well-defined illness such as AIDS or because of nonspecific impairment of host defenses, as may occur in malnourished children or in the elderly. Certain racial groups, such as Eskimos, are also more prone to develop progressive primary tuberculosis. The incidence of progressive primary tuberculosis is particularly high in HIV-positive patients with an advanced degree of immunosuppression (i.e., CD4+ counts less than 200 cells/mm^3). Immunosuppression results in an inability to mount a CD4+ T-cell–mediated immunologic reaction that would contain the primary focus; because hypersensitivity and resistance are most often concomitant, the lack of a tissue hypersensitivity reaction results in the absence of the characteristic caseating granulomas *(nonreactive tuberculosis)* (Fig. 13-30D).

The diagnosis of progressive primary tuberculosis in adults can be difficult. Contrary to the usual picture of "adult-type" (or reactivation) tuberculosis (apical disease with cavitation, see later), progressive primary tuberculosis more often resembles an acute bacterial pneumonia, with lower and middle lobe consolidation, hilar adenopathy, and pleural effusion; cavitation is rare, especially in patients with severe immunosuppression. Lymphohematogenous dissemination is a dreaded complication and may result in the development of *tuberculous meningitis* and *miliary tuberculosis.* Because similar lesions also occur after progression of secondary tuberculosis, these will be discussed later.

Figure 13-30

The morphologic spectrum of tuberculosis. A characteristic tubercle at low magnification *(A)* and in detail *(B)* illustrates central granular *caseation* surrounded by epithelioid and multinucleated giant cells. This is the usual response seen in patients who have developed cell-mediated immunity to the organism. Occasionally, even in immunocompetent individuals, tubercular granulomas may not show central caseation *(C)*; hence, irrespective of the presence or absence of caseous necrosis, special stains for acid-fast organisms need to be performed when granulomas are present in histologic sections. In *immunosuppressed* individuals, tuberculosis may not elicit a granulomatous response ("nonreactive tuberculosis"); instead, sheets of foamy histiocytes are seen, packed with mycobacteria that are demonstrable with acid-fast stains *(D)*. *(D,* Courtesy of Dr. Dominick Cavuoti, Department of Pathology, University of Texas Southwestern Medical School, Dallas.)

SECONDARY TUBERCULOSIS (REACTIVATION TUBERCULOSIS)

Secondary (or postprimary) tuberculosis is the pattern of disease that arises in a previously sensitized host. It may follow shortly after primary tuberculosis, but more commonly it arises from reactivation of dormant primary lesions many decades after initial infection, particularly when host resistance is weakened. It may also result from exogenous reinfection because of waning of the protection afforded by the primary disease or because of a large inoculum of virulent bacilli. Reactivation of endogenous tuberculosis is more common in low prevalence areas, whereas reinfection plays an important role in regions of high contagion. Whatever the source of the organism, only

a few patients (less than 5%) with primary disease subsequently develop secondary tuberculosis.

Secondary pulmonary tuberculosis is classically localized to the apex of one or both upper lobes. The reason is obscure but may relate to high oxygen tension in the apices. Because of the preexistence of hypersensitivity, the bacilli excite a prompt and marked tissue response that tends to wall off the focus. As a result of this localization, the regional lymph nodes are less prominently involved early in the developing disease than they are in primary tuberculosis. On the other hand, cavitation occurs readily in the secondary form, resulting in dissemination along the airways. Indeed, cavitation is almost inevitable in neglected secondary tuberculosis, and erosion into an airway becomes an important source of infectivity because the patient now raises sputum containing bacilli.

Secondary tuberculosis should always be an important consideration in HIV-positive patients who present with pulmonary disease. It is noteworthy that *while HIV infection is associated with an increased risk of tuberculosis at all stages of HIV disease, the manifestations differ depending on the degree of immunosuppression.* For example, patients with less severe immunosuppression (CD4+ counts greater than 300 cells/mm³) present with "usual" secondary tuberculosis (apical disease with cavitation). On the contrary, patients with more advanced immunosuppression (CD4+ counts less than 200 cells/mm³) present with a clinical picture that resembles progressive primary tuberculosis (lower and middle lobe consolidation, hilar lymphadenopathy, and noncavitary disease). The extent of immunosuppression also determines the frequency of extrapulmonary involvement, rising from 10% to 15% in mildly immunosuppressed patients to greater than 50% in those with severe immune deficiency. *Other atypical features* in HIV-positive patients that make the diagnosis of tuberculosis particularly challenging include an increased frequency of sputum-smear negativity for acid-fast bacilli compared with HIV-negative controls, false-negative PPD because of tuberculin anergy, and the lack of characteristic granulomas in tissues, particularly in the late stages of HIV infection.

Figure 13–31 ■

Secondary pulmonary tuberculosis. The upper parts of both lungs are riddled with gray-white areas of caseation and multiple areas of softening and cavitation.

MORPHOLOGY

The initial lesion is usually a small focus of consolidation, less than 2 cm in diameter, within 1 to 2 cm of the apical pleura. Such foci are sharply circumscribed, firm, gray-white to yellow areas that have a variable amount of central caseation and peripheral fibrosis. In favorable cases the initial parenchymal focus undergoes progressive fibrous encapsulation, leaving only fibrocalcific scars. Histologically, the active lesions show characteristic coalescent tubercles with central caseation. Although tubercle bacilli can be demonstrated by appropriate methods in early exudative and caseous phases of granuloma formation, it is usually impossible to find them in the late, fibrocalcific stages. Localized, apical, secondary pulmonary tuberculosis may heal with fibrosis either spontaneously or after therapy, or the disease may progress and extend along several different pathways:

■ **Progressive pulmonary tuberculosis** may ensue. The apical lesion enlarges with expansion of the area of caseation. Erosion into a bronchus evacuates the caseous center, creating a ragged, irregular cavity lined by caseous material that is poorly walled off by fibrous tissue (Fig. 13–31). Erosion of blood vessels results in hemoptysis. With adequate treatment, the process may be arrested, although healing by fibrosis often distorts the pulmonary architecture. Irregular cavities, now free of caseation

necrosis, may remain or collapse in the surrounding fibrosis. If the treatment is inadequate, or if host defenses are impaired, the infection may spread by direct expansion, via dissemination through airways, lymphatic channels, or the vascular system. **Miliary pulmonary disease** occurs when organisms drain through lymphatics into the lymphatic ducts, which empty into the venous return to the right side of the heart and thence into the pulmonary arteries. Individual lesions are either microscopic or small, visible (2-mm) foci of yellow-white consolidation scattered through the lung parenchyma (the word "miliary" is derived from the resemblance of these foci to millet seeds). Miliary lesions may expand and coalesce to yield almost total consolidation of large regions or even whole lobes of the lung. With progressive pulmonary tuberculosis, the pleural cavity is invariably involved and serous **pleural effusions, tuberculous empyema,** or **obliterative fibrous pleuritis** may develop.

■ **Endobronchial, endotracheal, and laryngeal tuberculosis** may develop when infective material is spread either through lymphatic channels or from expectorated infectious material. The mucosal lining may be studded with minute granulomatous lesions, sometimes apparent only on microscopic examination.

■ **Systemic miliary tuberculosis** ensues when infective foci in the lungs seed the pulmonary venous return to the heart; the organisms subsequently disseminate through the systemic arterial system. Almost every organ in the body may be seeded. Lesions resemble those in the lung. Miliary tuberculosis is most prominent in the liver, bone marrow, spleen, adrenals, meninges,

Figure 13–32 ■

Miliary tuberculosis of the spleen. The cut surface shows numerous gray-white granulomas.

kidneys, fallopian tubes, and epididymis (Fig. 13–32).

- ■ **Isolated-organ tuberculosis** may appear in any one of the organs or tissues seeded hematogenously and may be the presenting manifestation of tuberculosis. Organs typically involved include the meninges (tuberculous meningitis), kidneys (renal tuberculosis), adrenals (formerly an important cause of Addison disease), bones (osteomyelitis), and fallopian tubes (salpingitis). When the vertebrae are affected, the disease is referred to as Pott disease. Paraspinal "cold" abscesses in these patients may track along the tissue planes to present as an abdominal or pelvic mass.

- ■ **Lymphadenitis** is the most frequent form of extrapulmonary tuberculosis, usually occurring in the cervical region ("scrofula"). In HIV-negative individuals, lymphadenopathy tends to be unifocal, and most patients do not have evidence of ongoing extranodal disease. HIV-positive patients, on the other hand, almost always demonstrate multifocal disease, systemic symptoms, and either pulmonary or other organ involvement by active tuberculosis.

- ■ In years past, **intestinal tuberculosis** contracted by the drinking of contaminated milk was fairly common as a primary focus of tuberculosis. In developed countries today, intestinal tuberculosis is more often a complication of protracted advanced secondary tuberculosis, secondary to the swallowing of coughed-up infective material. Typically, the organisms are trapped in mucosal lymphoid aggregations of the small and large bowel, which then undergo inflammatory enlargement with ulceration of the overlying mucosa, particularly in the ileum.

The many patterns of tuberculosis are depicted in Figure 13–33.

Clinical Course. Localized secondary tuberculosis may be asymptomatic. When manifestations appear, they are usually *insidious* in onset; there is gradual development of both systemic and localizing symptoms. Systemic symptoms, probably related to cytokines released by activated macrophages (e.g., TNF and IL-1), often appear early in the course and include malaise, anorexia, weight loss, and fever. Commonly, the *fever is low grade* and remittent (appearing late each afternoon and then subsiding), and *night sweats* occur. With progressive pulmonary involvement, increasing amounts of sputum, at first mucoid and later purulent, appear. When cavitation is present, the sputum contains tubercle bacilli. Some degree of *hemoptysis* is present in about half of all cases of pulmonary tuberculosis. *Pleuritic pain* may result from extension of the infection to the pleural surfaces. Extrapulmonary manifestations of tuberculosis are legion and depend on the organ system involved (for example, tuberculous salpingitis may present as infertility, tuberculous meningitis with headache and neurologic deficits, Pott disease with paraplegia). The diagnosis of pulmonary disease is based in part on the history and on physical and radiographic findings of *consolidation or cavitation in the apices of the lungs*. Ultimately, however, *tubercle bacilli must be identified*. Acid-fast smears and cultures of the sputum of patients suspected of having tuberculosis should be performed. Conventional cultures required up to 10 weeks, but recent liquid media–based radiometric assays that detect mycobacterial metabolism are able to provide an answer within 2 weeks. PCR amplification of *M. tuberculosis* DNA allows for even greater rapidity of diagnosis, and two such assays are currently approved for use in the United States. PCR assays can detect as few as 10 organisms in clinical specimens, compared with greater than 10,000 organisms required for smear positivity. However, culture remains the gold standard because it also allows testing of drug susceptibility. Multidrug resistance is now seen more commonly, and hence currently all newly diagnosed cases in the United States are treated with multiple agents. The prognosis is generally good if infections are localized to the lungs, except when they are caused by drug-resistant strains or occur in aged, debilitated, or immunosuppressed persons, who are at high risk for developing miliary tuberculosis. Amyloidosis may appear in persistent cases.

Nontuberculous Mycobacterial Disease

Chronic pulmonary disease in *immunocompetent individuals* is the most common localized clinical disease caused by nontuberculous mycobacteria. In the United States, strains implicated most frequently include *M. avium-intracellulare* (also called *M. avium* complex), *M. kansasii*, and *M. abscessus*. It is not uncommon for nontuberculous mycobacteria to present as upper lobe cavitary disease, mimicking tuberculosis, especially in patients with a longstanding history of smoking or alcoholism. The presence of concomitant chronic pulmonary disease (chronic obstructive airway disease, cystic fibrosis, pneumoconiosis) is

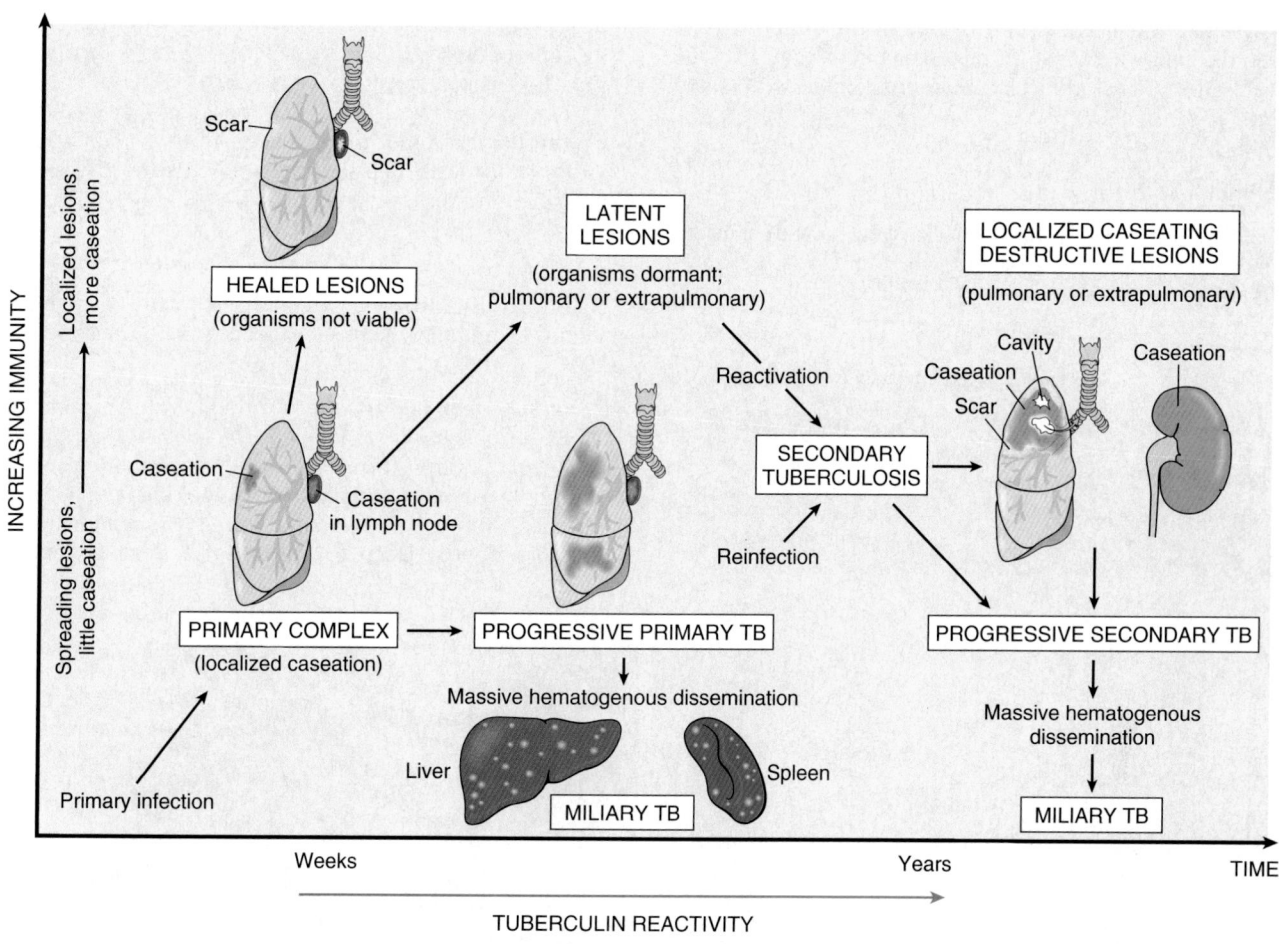

Figure 13-33   ■

The natural history and spectrum of tuberculosis. (Adapted from a sketch provided by Dr. R. K. Kumar, The University of New South Wales, School of Pathology, Sydney, Australia.)

an important risk factor associated with nontuberculous mycobacterial infection.

In *immunosuppressed individuals* (primarily, HIV-positive patients), *M. avium* complex presents as disseminated disease, associated with systemic symptoms (fever, night sweats, weight loss). Hepatosplenomegaly and lymphadenopathy, signifying involvement of the reticuloendothelial system by the opportunistic pathogen, is common, as are gastrointestinal symptoms such as diarrhea and malabsorption. Pulmonary involvement is often indistinguishable from tuberculosis in AIDS patients. Disseminated *M. avium* complex infection in AIDS patients tends to occur late in the course of the disease, when CD4 counts have fallen below 100 cells/mm^3; hence, tissue examination usually does not reveal granulomas and, instead, foamy histiocytes "plugged" with atypical mycobacteria are typically seen.

Fungal Infections

Fungi are classified into "yeasts" and "molds." The former are round or oval and divide by budding, while the latter form tubular structures called hyphae and grow by branching and longitudinal extension. This dichotomy has a

degree of overlap, because some fungi (e.g., *Histoplasma capsulatum*, *Coccidioides immitis*, and *Blastomyces dermatitidis*) are *dimorphic* (i.e., they grow as yeasts in tissues but grow in vitro at room temperature as molds). A simplified "clinical classification" of human mycoses has been used to divide them into *superficial*, *subcutaneous*, *deep-seated*, and *opportunistic* pathogenic fungi. As the names suggest, the superficial and subcutaneous fungi (e.g., the dermatophytes or the agents of chromoblastomycoses) almost always limit their activities to the skin and subcutaneous tissues. Deep-seated mycoses are caused by highly virulent organisms (classically, dimorphic fungi) with an ability to invade deeply into tissues and organs and thereby cause systemic disease. While ostensibly normal hosts can suffer from pulmonary disease after inhalation of the infective forms of the organism, deep-seated mycoses are more severe in immunosuppressed persons, as might be expected. By contrast, opportunistic fungi are organisms with a low virulence that can nevertheless cause localized or systemic infections in patients who are immunocompromised, are debilitated, or carry long-term intravascular access devices. Examples of opportunistic fungi include molds (*Aspergillus* species and the agents of mucormycosis) as well as yeast-like fungi (*Candida* species and *Cryptococcus neoformans*).

All systemic fungi, either deep-seated or opportunistic, can infect the lung, although extrapulmonary disease may be more frequent and clinically more important with some agents.

CANDIDIASIS

Candida albicans is the most frequent disease-causing fungus. It is a normal inhabitant of the oral cavity, gastrointestinal tract, and vagina in many individuals.

MORPHOLOGY

In tissue sections, *C. albicans* demonstrates yeast-like forms (blastoconidia), pseudohyphae, and true hyphae (Fig. 13–34A and B). Pseudohyphae are an important diagnostic clue for *C. albicans* and represent budding yeast cells joined end to end at

constrictions, thus simulating true fungal hyphae. The organisms may be visible with routine hematoxylin and eosin stains, but a variety of special "fungal" stains (Gomori methenamine-silver, periodic acid–Schiff) are commonly used to better highlight the pathogens.

Clinical Syndromes. Candidiasis can involve the mucous membranes, skin, and deep organs (invasive candidiasis).

■ *The most common pattern of candidiasis takes the form of a superficial infection on mucosal surfaces of the oral cavity (thrush).* Florid proliferation of the fungi creates gray-white, dirty-looking pseudomembranes composed of matted organisms and inflammatory debris. Deep to the surface, there is mucosal

Figure 13–34

The morphology of fungal infections. *A,* Invasive candidiasis in an immunocompromised patient, demonstrating the fungal organisms within the wall of a pulmonary vessel. *B,* The diagnosis of candidiasis is made by observing the characteristic pseudohyphae and blastoconidia (budding yeasts) in tissue sections or exudates. *C,* Invasive aspergillosis of the lung in a bone marrow transplant patient. *D,* Histologic sections from this case, stained with Gomori methenamine-silver (GMS) stain, show septate hyphae with acute-angle branching, features consistent with *Aspergillus.* Occasionally, *Aspergillus* may demonstrate so-called fruiting bodies *(inset)* when it grows in areas that are well-aerated (such as the upper respiratory tract).

Figure 13–34 Continued

E, Cryptococcosis of the lung in a patient with AIDS. The yeast forms are somewhat variable in size; unlike in *Candida,* pseudohyphae are not seen. In routine H & E stains, the capsule is not directly visible but often a clear "halo" can be seen surrounding the individual fungi representing the area occupied by the capsule. *F,* Disseminated histoplasmosis in a patient with AIDS. *Histoplasma capsulatum* is a dimorphic fungus and exists only in yeast form at body temperature. In GMS-stained tissue sections, the fungi are demonstrable within macrophages and are smaller and more uniform in size than *Cryptococcus. G,* Pulmonary coccidioidomycosis. *C. immitis* elicits a granulomatous response similar to tuberculosis in immunocompetent individuals (notice plump histiocytes lymphocytes and giant cell in photomicrograph). The fungi are present to the left side of the field. *Inset* illustrates the thick-walled nonbudding spherule of *C. immitis,* filled with endospores. *H,* Pulmonary blastomycosis. *Blastomyces dermatitidis* also elicits a granulomatous response in immunocompetent hosts. *Inset* illustrates the characteristic "broad-based" budding pattern seen in *Blastomyces.* (All figures courtesy of Dr. Dominick Cavuoti, Department of Pathology, University of Texas Southwestern Medical School, Dallas.)

hyperemia and inflammation. This form of candidiasis is seen in newborns, debilitated patients, children receiving oral corticosteroids for asthma, and after a course of broad-spectrum antibiotics that destroy competing normal bacterial flora. *The other major risk group includes HIV-positive patients;* patients with oral thrush for no obvious reason should be evaluated for HIV infection.

■ *Candida vaginitis* is an extremely common form of vaginal infection in women, especially those who are diabetic or pregnant or on oral contraceptive pills. It is usually associated with intense itching and a thick, curdlike discharge.

■ *Candida esophagitis* is common in AIDS patients and in those with hematolymphoid malignancies. These patients present with dysphagia (painful swallowing) and retrosternal pain; endoscopy demonstrates white plaques and pseudomembranes resembling oral thrush on the esophageal mucosa.

■ *Cutaneous candidiasis* can present in many different forms, including infection of the nail proper ("onychomycosis"), nail folds ("paronychia"), hair follicles ("folliculitis"), moist, intertriginous skin such as armpits or webs of the fingers and toes ("intertrigo"), and penile skin ("balanitis"). "Diaper rash" is a cutaneous candidial infection seen in the perineum of infants, in the region of contact of wet diapers.

■ *Chronic mucocutaneous candidiasis* is a chronic refractory disease afflicting the mucous membranes, skin, hair, and nails; it is associated with underlying T-cell defects. Associated conditions include endocrinopathies (most commonly hypoparathyroidism and Addison disease) and the presence of autoantibodies. Disseminated candidiasis is rare in this disease.

■ *Invasive candidiasis* implies bloodborne dissemination of organisms to various tissues or organs. Common patterns include (1) renal abscesses, (2) myocardial abscesses and endocarditis, (3) brain involvement (most commonly meningitis, but parenchymal microabscesses occur), (4) endophthalmitis (virtually any eye structure can be involved), (5) hepatic abscesses, and (6) *Candida* pneumonia, usually presenting as bilateral nodular infiltrates, resembling *Pneumocystis* pneumonia (see later). Patients with acute leukemias who are profoundly neutropenic post chemotherapy are particularly prone to developing systemic disease. *Candida* endocarditis is the most common fungal endocarditis, usually occurring in patients with prosthetic heart valves or in intravenous drug abusers.

CRYPTOCOCCOSIS

Cryptococcosis, caused by *C. neoformans*, rarely occurs in healthy persons. It almost exclusively presents as an opportunistic infection in immunocompromised hosts, particularly those with AIDS or hematolymphoid malignancies.

MORPHOLOGY

The fungus, a 5- to 10-μm yeast, has a thick, gelatinous capsule and reproduces by budding (Fig. 13–34E). Unlike in *Candida,* however, pseudohyphal or true hyphal forms are not seen. **The capsule is invaluable to diagnosis:** (1) It is stained by India ink or periodic acid–Schiff stains and effectively highlights the fungus; and (2) the capsular polysaccharide antigen is the substrate for the cryptococcal latex agglutination assay, which is positive in greater than 95% of patients infected with the organism.

Clinical Syndromes. Human cryptococcosis usually manifests as *pulmonary, central nervous system, or disseminated* disease. *Cryptococcus* is most likely acquired by inhalation from the soil or from bird droppings. *The fungus initially localizes in the lungs and then disseminates to other sites, particularly the meninges.* Sites of involvement are marked by a variable tissue response, which ranges from florid proliferation of gelatinous organisms with a minimal or absent inflammatory cell infiltrate (in immunodeficient hosts) to a granulomatous reaction (in the more reactive host). In immunosuppressed patients, fungi grow in gelatinous masses within the meninges or expand the perivascular Virchow-Robin spaces, producing the so-called soap-bubble lesions.

THE OPPORTUNISTIC MOLDS

Mucormycosis and *invasive aspergillosis* are uncommon infections almost always limited to immunocompromised hosts, particularly those with hematolymphoid malignancies, profound neutropenia, corticosteroid therapy, or post allogeneic bone marrow transplantation.

MORPHOLOGY

Mucormycosis is caused by the class of fungi known as Zygomycetes. Their hyphae are **nonseptate** and branch at right angles; in contrast, the hyphae of *Aspergillus* species are **septate** and branch at more acute angles (see Fig. 13–34D). *Rhizopus* and *Mucor* are the two fungi of medical importance within the Zygomycetes class. Both Zygomycetes and *Aspergillus* cause a nondistinctive, suppurative, sometimes granulomatous reaction with a **predilection for invading blood vessel walls, causing vascular necrosis and infarction.**

Clinical Syndromes

■ *Rhinocerebral* and *pulmonary mucormycosis:* Zygomycetes have a propensity to colonize the nasal cavity or sinuses and then spread by direct extension into the brain, orbit, and other head and neck structures. Patients with diabetic ketoacidosis are most likely to develop a fulminant invasive form of rhinocerebral mucormycosis. Pulmonary disease can be localized (e.g., cavitary lesions) or may present radiologically with diffuse "miliary" involvement.
■ *Invasive aspergillosis* occurs almost exclusively in patients who are immunosuppressed. The fungus preferentially localizes to the lungs, and it most often presents as a necrotizing pneumonia (see Fig. 13–34C and D). As mentioned previously, *Aspergillus* species have a propensity to invade blood vessels, and thus systemic dissemination, especially to the brain, is often a fatal complication.
■ *Allergic bronchopulmonary aspergillosis* occurs in patients with asthma who develop an exacerbation of symptoms caused by a type I hypersensitivity against the fungus growing in the bronchi. These patients often have circulating IgE antibodies against *Aspergillus* and peripheral eosinophilia.
■ *Aspergilloma* ("fungus ball") occurs by colonization of preexisting pulmonary cavities (e.g., ectatic bronchi or lung cysts, post-tuberculous cavitary lesions) by the fungus; these may act as ball valves, occluding the cavity and thus predisposing to infection and hemoptysis.

THE DIMORPHIC FUNGI

The dimorphic fungi, which include *Histoplasma capsulatum, Coccidioides immitis,* and *Blastomyces dermatitidis,* present as the so-called deep-seated mycoses. Isolated pulmonary involvement is commonly seen in infected immunocompetent individuals, whereas immunocompromised patients present with disseminated disease. In part owing to the overlap in clinical presentations, all three dimorphic fungi will be considered together in this section.

MORPHOLOGY

The yeast forms are fairly distinctive, which helps in the identification of individual fungi in tissue sections.

- **H. capsulatum:** round to oval and small yeast forms measuring 2 to 5 μm in diameter (Fig. 13–34F).
- **C. immitis:** thick-walled, **nonbudding spherules,** 20 to 60 μm in diameter, often filled with small endospores (Fig. 13–34G).
- **B. dermatitidis:** round to oval and larger than *Histoplasma* (5 to 25 μm in diameter); reproduce by characteristic "broad-based" budding (Fig. 13–34H).

Epidemiology. Each of the dimorphic fungi has a typical geographic distribution.

- **H. capsulatum:** endemic in the Ohio and central Mississippi River valleys and along the Appalachian mountains in the southeastern United States. Warm, moist soil, enriched by droppings from bats and birds, provides the ideal medium for the growth of the mycelial form, which produces infectious spores.
- **C. immitis:** endemic in the southwest and far west of the United States, particularly in the San Joaquin Valley, where it is known as "valley fever."
- **B. dermatitidis:** endemic area is confined in the United States to areas overlapping with those where histoplasmosis is found.

Clinical Syndromes. Clinical manifestations may take the form of (1) *acute (primary) pulmonary infection*, (2) *chronic (cavitary) pulmonary disease*, or (3) *disseminated miliary disease*. The primary pulmonary nodules, composed of aggregates of macrophages stuffed with organisms, are associated with similar lesions in the regional lymph nodes. These lesions develop into small granulomas complete with giant cells and may develop central necrosis and later fibrosis and calcification. *The similarity to primary tuberculosis is striking*, and differentiation requires identification of the yeast forms (best seen with periodic acid–Schiff or silver stains). The clinical manifestations resemble a "flulike" syndrome, most often self-limited. In the vulnerable host, chronic cavitary pulmonary disease develops, with a predilection for the upper lobe, resembling the secondary form of tuberculosis. It is not uncommon for these fungi to give rise to perihilar mass lesions that resemble bronchogenic carcinoma radiologically. At this stage, cough, hemoptysis, and even dyspnea and chest pain may appear.

In infants or immunocompromised adults, particularly those with HIV infection, disseminated disease (analogous to miliary tuberculosis) may develop. Under these circumstances, when T-cell–mediated immunity is markedly impaired, there is no granuloma formation. Instead, focal collections of phagocytes stuffed with yeast forms are seen within cells of the mononuclear phagocyte system, including in the liver, spleen, lymph nodes, lymphoid tissue of the gastrointestinal tract, and bone marrow. The adrenals and meninges may also be involved, and in a minority of cases ulcers form in the nose and mouth, on the tongue, or in the larynx. Disseminated disease is a hectic, febrile illness with hepatosplenomegaly, anemia, leukopenia, and thrombocytopenia. Cutaneous infections in disseminated *Blastomyces* frequently induce striking pseudoepitheliomatous hyperplasia, which may be mistaken for squamous cell carcinoma.

Skin tests (analogous to the tuberculin delayed hypersensitivity reaction) can be used to detect exposure to *Histoplasma* (histoplasmin) and *Coccidioides* (coccidioidin), respectively; a reliable skin test for *Blastomyces* does not exist. The diagnosis of active infection is best made by direct visualization of the organism in tissue sections and by culture of sputum, bone marrow, or liver biopsy. Serologic tests detecting antibodies against individual fungi are available but lack sensitivity and specificity. *A capsular antigen assay now available for detection of* Histoplasma *in urine or serum has become the mainstay of diagnosis for disseminated histoplasmosis.*

Lung Abscess

Lung abscess refers to a localized area of suppurative necrosis within the pulmonary parenchyma, resulting in the formation of one or more large cavities. The term *necrotizing pneumonia* has been used for a similar process resulting in multiple small cavitations; necrotizing pneumonia often coexists or evolves into lung abscess, making this distinction somewhat arbitrary. The causative organism may be introduced into the lung by any of the following mechanisms:

- *Aspiration of infective material* from carious teeth or infected sinuses or tonsils, particularly likely during oral surgery, anesthesia, coma, or alcoholic intoxication and in debilitated patients with depressed cough reflexes.
- *Aspiration of gastric contents*, usually accompanied by infectious organisms from the oropharynx.
- *As a complication of necrotizing bacterial pneumonias*, particularly those caused by *Staphylococcus aureus*, *Streptococcus pyogenes*, *K. pneumoniae*, *Pseudomonas* species, and, rarely, type 3 pneumococci. Mycotic infections and bronchiectasis may also lead to lung abscesses.
- *Bronchial obstruction*, particularly with bronchogenic carcinoma obstructing a bronchus or bronchiole. Impaired drainage, distal atelectasis, and aspiration of blood and tumor fragments all contribute to the development of abscesses. An abscess may also form within an excavated necrotic portion of a tumor.
- *Septic embolism*, from septic thrombophlebitis or from infective endocarditis of the right side of the heart.
- In addition, lung abscesses may result from *hematogenous spread of bacteria* in disseminated pyogenic infection. This occurs most characteristically in staphylococcal bacteremia and often results in multiple lung abscesses.

Anaerobic bacteria are present in almost all lung abscesses, sometimes in vast numbers, and they are the exclusive isolates in one third to two thirds of cases. The most frequently encountered anaerobes are commensals normally found in the oral cavity, principally species of *Prevotella*, *Fusobacterium*, *Bacteroides*, *Peptostreptococcus*, and microaerophilic streptococci. Often there is a mixed anaerobic-aerobic infection; the most commonly isolated aerobic organisms are *S. aureus*, β-hemolytic streptococci, *Nocardia*, and gram-negative organisms.

Abscesses vary in diameter from a few millimeters to large cavities of 5 to 6 cm. The localization and number of abscesses depend on their mode of development. Pulmonary abscesses resulting from aspiration of infective material are much more common on the right side (more vertical airways) than on the left, and most are single. On the right side, they tend to occur in the posterior segment of the upper lobe and in the apical segments of the lower lobe, because these locations reflect the likely course of aspirated material when the patient is recumbent. Abscesses that develop in the course of pneumonia or bronchiectasis are commonly multiple, basal, and diffusely scattered. Septic emboli and abscesses arising from hematogenous seeding are commonly multiple and may affect any region of the lungs.

As the focus of suppuration enlarges, it almost inevitably ruptures into airways. Thus, the contained exudate may be partially drained, producing an air-fluid level on radiographic examination. Occasionally, abscesses rupture into the pleural cavity and produce bronchopleural fistulas, the consequence of which is **pneumothorax** or **empyema**. Other complications arise from embolization of septic material to the brain, giving rise to meningitis or brain abscess. Histologically, as expected with any abscess, there is suppuration surrounded by variable amounts of fibrous scarring and mononuclear infiltration (lymphocytes, plasma cells, macrophages), depending on the chronicity of the lesion.

Clinical Course. The manifestations of a lung abscess are much like those of bronchiectasis and include a prominent cough that usually yields copious amounts of foul-smelling, purulent, or sanguineous sputum; occasionally, hemoptysis occurs. Spiking fever and malaise are common. Clubbing of the fingers, weight loss, and anemia may all occur. Infective abscesses occur in 10% to 15% of patients with bronchogenic carcinoma; thus, when a lung abscess is suspected in an older patient, underlying carcinoma must be considered. Secondary amyloidosis may develop in chronic cases. Treatment includes antibiotic therapy and, if needed, surgical drainage. Overall, the mortality rate is in the range of 10%.

Cytomegalovirus Infections

Cytomegalovirus (CMV), a member of the herpesvirus family, may produce a variety of disease manifestations, depending partly on the age of the infected host but even more on the host's immune status. Cells infected by the virus exhibit gigantism of both the entire cell and its nucleus. Within the nucleus is an enlarged inclusion surrounded by a clear halo ("owl's eye"), which gives the name to the classic form of symptomatic disease that occurs in neonates, cytomegalic inclusion disease. Although classic cytomegalic inclusion disease is a multisystemic disease, CMV infections are discussed here because in immunosuppressed adults, particularly AIDS patients and recipients of allogeneic bone marrow transplants, CMV pneumonitis is a serious problem.

Transmission of CMV can occur by several mechanisms, depending on the age group affected:

■ Transplacentally from a newly acquired or primary infection in the mother ("congenital CMV").
■ By transmission of the virus through cervical or vaginal secretions at birth, or, later, through breast milk from a mother who has active infection ("perinatal CMV").
■ During preschool years, especially in day care centers, through saliva. Toddlers so infected readily transmit the virus to their parents.
■ After 15 years of age, the venereal route is the dominant mode of transmission, but spread may also occur via respiratory secretions and the fecal-oral route.
■ Iatrogenic transmission can occur at any age through organ transplants or by blood transfusions.

Congenital Infections. Infection acquired in utero may take many forms. In approximately 95% of cases it is asymptomatic, but in some, mainly those who acquire the virus from a mother with primary infection (who does not have protective immunoglobulins), classic cytomegalic inclusion disease develops. Affected infants may suffer intrauterine growth retardation (Chapter 7), be profoundly ill, and manifest jaundice, hepatosplenomegaly, anemia, bleeding caused by thrombocytopenia, and encephalitis. In fatal cases the brain is often smaller than normal (microcephaly) and may show foci of calcification.

Histologically, the characteristic enlargement of cells can be appreciated. In the glandular organs, the parenchymal epithelial cells are affected; in the brain, the neurons; in the lungs, the alveolar macrophages and epithelial and endothelial cells; and in the kidneys, the tubular epithelial and glomerular endothelial cells. Affected cells are strikingly enlarged, often to a diameter of 40 μm, and they show cellular and nuclear polymorphism. Prominent intranuclear basophilic inclusions spanning half the nuclear diameter are usually set off from the nuclear membrane by a clear halo (Fig. 13–35). Within the cytoplasm of these cells, smaller basophilic inclusions may also be seen.

Those infants who survive usually bear permanent residual effects, including mental retardation, hearing loss, and other neurologic impairments. The congenital infection is not always devastating, however, and may take the form of interstitial pneumonitis, hepatitis, or a hematologic disorder. Most infants with this milder form of cytomegalic inclusion disease recover, although a few may develop mental retardation later. Uncommonly, a totally asymptomatic infection may be followed months to years

Figure 13-35

Cytomegalovirus infection of the lung. A typical distinct nuclear and ill-defined cytoplasmic inclusion is seen. (Courtesy of Dr. Arlene Sharpe, Brigham and Women's Hospital, Boston.)

later by neurologic sequelae, including delayed-onset mental retardation and hearing deficits.

Perinatal Infections. Infection acquired during passage through the birth canal or from breast milk is asymptomatic in the vast majority of cases, although uncommonly infants may develop an interstitial pneumonitis, failure to thrive, rash, or hepatitis. Despite the lack of symptoms, many of these patients continue to excrete CMV in their urine or saliva for months to years. Subtle effects on hearing and intelligence later in life have been reported in some studies.

Cytomegalovirus Mononucleosis. In healthy young children and adults, the disease is nearly always asymptomatic. In surveys around the world, 50% to 100% of adults demonstrate anti-CMV antibodies in the serum, indicating previous exposure. The most common *clinical manifestation of CMV* infection in immunocompetent hosts beyond the neonatal period is an infectious mononucleosis–like illness, with fever, atypical lymphocytosis, lymphadenopathy, and hepatomegaly accompanied by abnormal liver function test results, suggesting mild hepatitis. Most patients recover without any sequelae, although excretion of the virus may occur in body fluids for months to years.

Irrespective of the presence or absence of symptoms following infection, a person once infected becomes seropositive for life. The virus remains latent within leukocytes, which are the major reservoirs.

CMV in Immunosuppressed Individuals. This occurs most commonly in three groups of patients:

■ *Recipients of organ transplants* (heart, liver, kidney) from seropositive donors. These patients typically receive immunosuppressive therapy, and the CMV is usually derived from the donor organ, but reactivation of latent CMV infection in the host may also occur.
■ *Recipients of allogeneic bone marrow transplants.* These patients are immunosuppressed not only because of drug therapy but also because of graft-versus-host disease. In this setting, there is usually reactivation of latent CMV in the recipient.
■ *Patients with AIDS.* These immunosuppressed individuals have reactivation of latent infection and are also infected

by their sexual partners. *CMV is the most common opportunistic viral pathogen in AIDS.*

In all these settings, serious, life-threatening disseminated CMV infections primarily affect the lungs (pneumonitis), gastrointestinal tract (colitis), and retina (retinitis); the central nervous system is usually spared.

In the pulmonary infection, an interstitial mononuclear infiltrate with foci of necrosis develops, accompanied by the typical enlarged cells with inclusions. The pneumonitis can progress to full-blown acute respiratory distress syndrome. Intestinal necrosis and ulceration can develop and be extensive, leading to the formation of "pseudomembranes" (Chapter 15) and debilitating diarrhea. CMV retinitis, by far the most common form of opportunistic CMV disease, can occur either alone or in combination with involvement of the lungs and intestinal tract. Diagnosis of CMV infections is made by demonstration of characteristic morphologic alterations in tissue sections, successful viral culture, rising antiviral antibody titer, and qualitative or quantitative PCR-based detection of CMV DNA. The last approach has revolutionized the approach to monitoring patients post transplantation.

Pneumocystis Pneumonia

P. carinii, an opportunistic infectious agent long considered to be a protozoan, is now believed to be more closely related to fungi. Serologic evidence indicates that virtually all persons are exposed to *Pneumocystis* during the first few years of life, but in most the infection remains latent. Reactivation and clinical disease occurs almost exclusively in those who are immunocompromised. Indeed, *P. carinii* is an extremely common cause of infection in patients with AIDS, and it may also infect severely malnourished infants and immunosuppressed individuals (especially following organ transplantation or in patients receiving cytotoxic chemotherapy or corticosteroids). In AIDS patients, the risk of acquiring *P. carinii* infections increases in direct proportion to the fall in CD4 count, with counts less than 200 cells/mm³ having a strong predictive value. *Pneumocystis* infections are largely confined to the lung, where they produce an interstitial pneumonitis.

MORPHOLOGY

Microscopically, involved areas of the lung demonstrate a characteristic intra-alveolar foamy, pink-staining exudate with hematoxylin and eosin stains ("cotton candy" exudate) (Fig. 13-36A), and the septa are thickened by edema and a minimal mononuclear infiltrate. Special stains are required to visualize the organism in either the trophozoite or encysted form. Silver stains of tissue sections reveal cup-shaped cyst walls (5 to 8 μm in diameter) in the alveolar exudates (Fig. 13-36B). If sputum production can be successfully induced in the patient, Giemsa or methylene blue stains can demonstrate the trophozoite forms of the organism (about 4 μm in diameter with long filopodia) in about 50% of patients.

Figure 13-36 ■

Pneumocystis pneumonia. The alveoli are filled with a characteristic foamy "cotton candy" exudate *(left)*. GMS stain demonstrates cup-shaped cyst walls within the exudate *(right)*.

The diagnosis of Pneumocystis pneumonia should be considered in any immunocompromised patient with respiratory symptoms and an abnormal chest radiograph. Fever, dry cough, and dyspnea occur in 90% to 95% of patients, who typically demonstrate bilateral perihilar and basilar infiltrates. Hypoxia is frequent; pulmonary function studies show a restrictive lung defect. The most sensitive and effective method of diagnosis is to identify the organism in bronchoalveolar lavage fluids or in a transbronchial biopsy specimen. Besides the histologic stains mentioned previously, immunofluorescence antibody kits and PCR-based assays have also become available for use on clinical specimens. If treatment is initiated before widespread involvement, the outlook for recovery is good; however, because residual organisms are likely to remain, particularly in AIDS patients, relapses are common unless the underlying immunosuppression is reversed.

Pulmonary Disease in Human Immunodeficiency Virus Infection

Pulmonary disease continues to be the leading cause of morbidity and mortality in HIV-infected patients. Although the use of potent antiretroviral agents and effective chemoprophylaxis has dramatically altered the incidence and outcome of pulmonary disease in HIV-infected patients, the plethora of entities involved makes diagnosis and treatment a distinct challenge. Some of the individual microbial agents afflicting HIV-infected patients have already been discussed; this section will focus only on the general principles of HIV-associated pulmonary disease.

■ Despite the emphasis on "opportunistic" infections, it must be remembered that bacterial lower respiratory tract infection caused by the "usual" pathogens is one of the most serious pulmonary disorders in HIV infection. The implicated organisms include *S. pneumoniae*, *S. aureus*, *H. influenzae*, and gram-negative rods. Bacterial pneumonias in HIV-infected patients are more common, more severe, and more often associated with bacteremia than in those without HIV infection.
■ Not all pulmonary infiltrates in HIV-infected individuals are infectious in etiology. A host of noninfectious

diseases, including Kaposi sarcoma (Chapters 5 and 10), pulmonary non-Hodgkin lymphoma (Chapter 12), and primary lung cancer, occur with increased frequency and need to be excluded.
■ *The CD4+ count is often useful in narrowing the differential diagnosis.* As a rule of thumb, bacterial and tubercular infections are more likely at higher CD4+ counts (>200 cells/mm^3), Pneumocystis pneumonia usually strikes at CD4+ counts below 200 cells/mm^3, while cytomegalovirus and *Mycobacterium avium* complex infections are uncommon until the very late stages of immunosuppression (CD4+ counts <50 cells/mm^3).

Finally, it is useful to remember that pulmonary disease in HIV-infected patients may result from more than one cause, and even common pathogens may present with atypical manifestations. Therefore, the diagnostic work-up of these patients may be more extensive (and expensive) than would be mandated in an immunocompetent individual.

LUNG TUMORS

Although lungs are frequently the site of metastases from cancers in extrathoracic organs, primary lung cancer is also a common disease. Ninety-five percent of primary lung tumors arise from the bronchial epithelium (bronchogenic carcinomas); the remaining 5% are a miscellaneous group that includes bronchial carcinoids, bronchial gland tumors (adenoid cystic and mucoepidermoid carcinomas), mesenchymal malignancies (e.g., fibrosarcomas, leiomyomas), lymphomas, and a few benign lesions. The most common benign lesions are spherical, small (3 to 4 cm), discrete hamartomas that often show up as "coin" lesions on chest radiographs. They consist mainly of mature cartilage but are often admixed with fat, fibrous tissue, and blood vessels in varying proportions.

Bronchogenic Carcinoma

Bronchogenic carcinoma (bronchial carcinoma) is without doubt the number one cause of cancer-related deaths in industrialized countries. It has long held this position among males in the United States, accounting for about one third of cancer deaths in men, and has become the leading cause of cancer deaths in women as well. It is expected that during the year 2002, there will be about 169,400 new cases of lung cancer in the United States and about 154,900 people will die of this disease. The rate of increase among males is slowing down, but it continues to accelerate among females (Chapter 6). These statistics are undoubtedly related to the causal relationship of cigarette smoking and bronchogenic carcinoma. The peak incidence of lung cancer occurs between ages 55 and 65 years; currently, the male-to-female ratio is about 2:1. At diagnosis, greater than 50% of patients already have distant metastatic disease, while a fourth have disease in the regional lymph nodes. The prognosis of lung cancer is dismal: the 5-year survival rate for all stages of lung cancer combined is about 14%; even patients with disease localized to the lung have a 5-year survival of approximately 45%.

The four major histologic types of bronchogenic carcinoma are squamous cell carcinoma, adenocarcinoma, large cell undifferentiated carcinoma, and small cell carcinoma (Table 13–7). In some cases there is a combination of histologic patterns. For reasons not entirely understood, adenocarcinoma has replaced squamous cell carcinoma as the most common primary lung tumor in recent years. Adenocarcinomas are also by far the most common primary tumors arising in women, in lifetime nonsmokers, and in patients younger than 45 years. Before the individual histologic types are discussed, some general principles underlying classification of lung tumors are presented.

Table 13–7. HISTOLOGIC CLASSIFICATION OF BRONCHOGENIC CARCINOMA AND APPROXIMATE INCIDENCE

I. Non-Small Cell Lung Carcinoma (NSCLC) (70%–75%)
1. Squamous cell (epidermoid) carcinoma (25%–30%)
2. Adenocarcinoma, including bronchioloalveolar carcinoma (30%–35%)
3. Large cell carcinoma (10%–15%)

II. Small Cell Lung Carcinoma (SCLC) (20%–25%)

III. Combined Patterns (5%–10%)

Most frequently
Mixed squamous cell carcinoma and adenocarcinoma
Mixed squamous cell carcinoma and SCLC

■ For therapeutic purposes, bronchogenic carcinomas are classified into two broad groups: small cell lung cancer (SCLC) and non–small cell lung cancer (NSCLC). The latter category includes squamous cell, adenocarcinomas, and large cell undifferentiated carcinomas.

■ *The key reason for this distinction is that virtually all SCLCs have metastasized by the time of diagnosis and hence are not amenable to curative surgery. Therefore, they are best treated by chemotherapy, with or without radiation.* In contrast, NSCLCs usually respond poorly to chemotherapy and are better treated by surgery.

■ Besides the differences in morphology, immunophenotypic characteristics, and response to treatment (Table 13–8), there are also pertinent genetic differences be-

Table 13–8. COMPARISON OF SMALL CELL LUNG CARCINOMA (SCLC) AND NON–SMALL CELL LUNG CARCINOMA (NSCLC)

	SCLC	NSCLC
Histology	Scant cytoplasm; small, hyperchromatic nuclei with fine chromatin pattern; nucleoli indistinct; diffuse sheets of cells	Abudant cytoplasm; pleomorphic nuclei with coarse chromatin pattern; nucleoli often prominent; glandular or squamous architecture
Neuroendocrine markers (e.g., dense core granules on electron microscopy; expression of chromogranin, neuron-specific enolase and synaptophysin)	Usually present	Usually absent
Epithelial markers (epithelial membrane antigen, carcinoembryonic antigen, and cytokeratin intermediate filaments)	Present	Present
Mucin	Absent	Present in adenocarcinomas
Peptide hormone production	Adrenocorticotropic hormone, antidiuretic hormone, gastrin-releasing peptide, calcitonin	Parathyroid hormone–related peptide (PTH-rp)
Tumor suppressor gene abnormalities		
3p deletions	>90%	>80%
RB mutations	~90%	~20%
p16/CDKN2A mutations	~10%	>50%
TP53 mutations	>90%	>50%
Dominant oncogene abnormalities		
K-RAS mutations	<1%	~30% (adenocarcinomas)
MYC family overexpression	>50%	>50%
Response to chemotherapy and radiotherapy	Often complete response	Uncommonly complete response

Adapted with permission from Minna JD: Neoplasms of the lung. In Fauci A, et al (eds): In Harrison's Principles of Internal Medicine, 14th ed. New York, McGraw-Hill, 1998.

tween SCLCs and NSCLCs. For example, SCLCs are characterized by a high frequency of *TP53* and *RB* gene mutations, while *p16/CDKN2A* is commonly inactivated in NSCLCs. Similarly, activating *K-RAS* oncogene mutations are virtually restricted to adenocarcinomas within the NSCLC group and are rare in SCLCs.

Etiology and Pathogenesis. Bronchogenic carcinomas, similar to cancers at many other anatomic sites, arise by a stepwise accumulation of genetic abnormalities that result in transformation of benign bronchial epithelium into neoplastic tissue. The developmental sequence of molecular changes is not random but follows a predictable sequence that parallels the histologic progression toward cancer. For example, inactivation of the putative tumor suppressor genes located on 3p is a very early event, whereas *TP53* mutations or activation of the *K-RAS* oncogene occurs relatively late. More importantly, it appears that certain genetic changes such as loss of chromosome 3p material can be found even in benign bronchial epithelium of patients with lung cancer, as well as in the respiratory epithelium of smokers *without* lung cancers, suggesting that large areas of the respiratory mucosa are mutagenized after exposure to carcinogens ("field effect"). On this fertile soil, those cells that accumulate additional mutations ultimately develop into cancer.

With regard to carcinogenic influences, there is strong evidence that smoking and, to a much lesser extent, other environmental insults are the main culprits responsible for the genetic changes that give rise to lung cancers. First, the evidence relating to cigarette smoking will be given, followed by a few brief comments on the less important factors.

An impressive body of statistical, clinical, and experimental evidence incriminates cigarette smoking. Statistically, about 90% of lung cancers occur in active smokers or those who stopped recently. There is a nearly linear correlation between the frequency of lung cancer and pack-years of cigarette smoking. The increased risk becomes 60 times greater among habitual heavy smokers (two packs a day for 20 years) compared with nonsmokers. For reasons not entirely clear, women have a higher susceptibility to tobacco carcinogens than men. Although cessation of smoking decreases the risk of developing lung cancer over time, it may never return to baseline levels. In fact, genetic changes that predate lung cancer can persist for many years in the bronchial epithelium of former smokers. Passive smoking (proximity to cigarette smokers) increases the risk of developing lung cancer to approximately twice that of nonsmokers. The smoking of pipes and cigars also increases the risk, but only modestly.

The *clinical evidence* is largely composed of the documentation of progressive alterations in the lining epithelium of the respiratory tract in habitual cigarette smokers. These sequential changes have been best documented for squamous cell carcinomas, but they may also be present in other histologic subtypes. In essence, there is a linear correlation between the intensity of exposure to cigarette smoke and the appearance of ever more worrisome epithelial changes that begin with rather innocuous basal cell hyperplasia and squamous metaplasia and progress to squamous dysplasia and carcinoma in situ, before culminating in invasive cancer. *Among the major histologic subtypes of lung cancer, squamous and small cell carcinomas show the strongest association with tobacco exposure.*

The *experimental evidence*, although it mounts with each passing year, lacks one important link: it has not so far been possible to produce lung cancer in an experimental animal by exposing it to cigarette smoke. Nonetheless, cigarette smoke condensate is a witches' brew of tumorigenic delicacies such as polycyclic hydrocarbons and other potent mutagens and carcinogens. Despite the lack of an experimental model, the chain of evidence linking cigarette smoking to lung cancer grows ever stronger.

Other influences may act in concert with smoking or may by themselves be responsible for some lung cancers; witness the increased incidence of this form of neoplasia in miners of radioactive ores; asbestos workers; and workers exposed to dusts containing arsenic, chromium, uranium, nickel, vinyl chloride, and mustard gas. Exposure to asbestos increases the risk of lung cancer five-fold in nonsmokers. By contrast, *heavy smokers exposed to asbestos have an approximately 55 times greater risk of lung cancer than do nonsmokers not exposed to asbestos.*

Despite the fact that smoking and other environmental factors are paramount in the causation of lung cancer, it is well known that all persons exposed to tobacco smoke do not develop cancer. It is very likely that the mutagenic effect of carcinogens is conditioned by hereditary (genetic) factors. Recall that many chemicals (procarcinogens) require metabolic activation via the P-450 monooxygenase enzyme system for conversion into ultimate carcinogens (Chapter 6). There is evidence that persons with specific genetic polymorphisms involving the P-450 genes have an increased capacity to metabolize procarcinogens derived from cigarette smoke and, conceivably, incur the greatest risk of developing lung cancer. Similarly, individuals whose peripheral blood lymphocytes undergo chromosomal breakages following exposure to tobacco-related carcinogens (mutagen sensitivity genotype) have a greater than ten-fold risk of developing lung cancer compared with controls.

MORPHOLOGY

Bronchogenic carcinomas begin as small mucosal lesions that are usually firm and gray-white. They may form intraluminal masses, invade the bronchial mucosa, or form large bulky masses pushing into adjacent lung parenchyma. Some large masses undergo cavitation caused by central necrosis or develop focal areas of hemorrhage. Finally, these tumors may extend to the pleura, invade the pleural cavity and chest wall, and spread to adjacent intrathoracic structures. More distant spread can occur via the lymphatics or the hematogenous route.

Squamous cell carcinomas are more common in men than in women; they tend to arise centrally in major bronchi and eventually spread to local hilar nodes, but they disseminate outside the thorax later than other histologic types. Large lesions may undergo central necrosis, giving rise to cavitation. The preneoplastic lesions that antedate, and usually accompany, invasive squamous cell carcinoma are well characterized. Squamous cell carcinomas

Figure 13-37

The precursor lesions of squamous cell carcinomas may antedate the appearance of invasive tumor by years. Some of the earliest (and "mild") changes in smoking-damaged respiratory epithelium include goblet-cell hyperplasia *(A)*, basal cell (or reserve cell) hyperplasia *(B)*, and squamous metaplasia *(C)*. More ominous changes include the appearance of squamous dysplasia *(D)*, characterized by the presence of disordered squamous epithelium, with *loss of nuclear polarity, nuclear hyperchromasia, pleomorphism, and mitotic figures.* Squamous dysplasia may, in turn, progress through the stages of mild, moderate, and severe dysplasia. Carcinoma-in-situ (CIS) *(E)* is the stage that immediately precedes invasive squamous carcinoma *(F)*, and apart from the lack of basement membrane disruption in CIS, the cytologic features are similar to those in frank carcinoma. Unless treated, CIS will eventually progress to invasive cancer. *(A to E,* Courtesy of Dr. Adi Gazdar, Department of Pathology, University of Texas Southwestern Medical School, Dallas; *F,* reproduced with permission from Travis WD, et al [eds]: World Health Organization Histological Typing of Lung and Pleural Tumors. Heidelberg, Springer, 1999.)

are often preceded for years by squamous metaplasia or dysplasia in the bronchial epithelium, which then transforms to carcinoma in situ, a phase that may last for several years (Fig. 13-37). By this time, atypical cells may be identified in cytologic smears of sputum or in bronchial lavage fluids or brushings, although the lesion is asymptomatic and undetectable on radiographs. Eventually, the small neoplasm reaches a symptomatic stage, when a well-defined tumor mass begins to obstruct the lumen of a major bronchus, often producing distal atelectasis and infection. Simultaneously, the lesion invades surrounding pulmonary substance (Fig. 13-38).

Histologically, these tumors range from well-differentiated squamous cell neoplasms showing keratin pearls and intercellular bridges to poorly differentiated neoplasms having only minimal residual squamous cell features.

Figure 13-38

Squamous cell carcinomas usually begin as central (hilar) masses and grow contiguously into the peripheral parenchyma. It is not uncommon for squamous cell carcinomas to undergo cavitary necrosis during intrapulmonary spread.

Adenocarcinomas may occur as central lesions like the squamous cell variant but are usually more peripherally located, many arising in relation to peripheral lung scars ("scar carcinomas"). The basis of this association with lung scars is not clear, although the current thinking is that most often the scarring occurs secondary to the tumor (i.e., desmoplasia) rather than being a contributory factor. Adenocarcinomas have the weakest association with a previous history of smoking among the four major subtypes of bronchogenic carcinomas. In general, these tumors grow slowly and form smaller masses than do the other subtypes, but they tend to metastasize widely at an early stage. Histologically, they assume a variety of forms, including acinar (gland forming), papillary, and solid types. The last variant often requires demonstration of intracellular mucin production by special stains to establish its adenocarcinomatous lineage. Although foci of squamous metaplasia and dysplasia may be present in the epithelium proximal to resected adenocarcinomas, these are not the precursor lesions for this tumor. The putative precursor of peripheral adenocarcinomas has been described as **atypical adenomatous hyperplasia** (AAH) (Fig. 13-39A). Microscopically, AAH is recognized as a well-demarcated focus of epithelial proliferation composed of cuboidal to low-columnar cells resembling Clara cells or type 2 alveolar pneumocytes, which demonstrate various degrees of cytologic atypia (nuclear hyperchromasia, pleomorphism, prominent nucleoli), but not to the extent seen in frank adenocarcinomas. AAH can be multifocal and is found predominantly in lungs of patients with an existing adenocarcinoma or bronchioloalveolar carcinoma (see later). Genetic analyses have shown that lesions of AAH are mon-

oclonal, and they share many of the molecular aberrations associated with bronchogenic carcinomas in general (3p deletions) and with adenocarcinomas in particular (*K-RAS* mutations).

Bronchioloalveolar carcinomas (BAC) are included as a subtype of adenocarcinomas in the current World Health Organization classification of lung tumors. They involve peripheral parts of the lung, either as a single nodule or, more often, as multiple diffuse nodules that may coalesce to produce pneumonia-like consolidation. **The key feature of BAC is their growth along preexisting structures and preservation of alveolar architecture** (see Fig. 13-39B). The tumor cells grow in a mono layer on top of the alveolar septa, which serve as a scaffold (this has been termed a "lepidic" growth pattern, an allusion to the neoplastic cells resembling butterflies sitting on a fence). The neoplastic cells lining the alveoli resemble those in AAH but exhibit a qualitatively higher degree of nuclear pleomorphism and complex growth pattern, including occasional papillary formations. By definition, BAC do not demonstrate destruction of alveolar architecture or stromal invasion with desmoplasia, features that would merit their classification as frank adenocarcinomas.

Currently, the concept of sequential evolution of peripheral adenocarcinomas draws a parallel from the **adenoma-carcinoma sequence in the colon**, wherein AAH is thought to represent the earliest precursor lesion (the "adenoma"), and it may progress to bronchioloalveolar carcinoma ("in situ adenocarcinoma") and, finally, invasive adenocarcinoma, which is associated with disruption of the basement membrane and stromal invasion (see Fig. 13-39). It is not clear, as yet, whether all pulmonary adenocarcinomas arise by this pathway,

Figure 13-39 ■

The evolution of peripheral adenocarcinomas of the lung is thought to occur through a sequence that begins with a small, well-demarcated lesion known as atypical adenomatous hyperplasia, or AAH *(arrowheads) (A)*, that progresses to bronchioloalveolar carcinomas, or BAC (an in situ phase that grows along existing structures and does not demonstrate stromal invasion) *(B)*, and culminates in invasive adenocarcinoma, with stromal invasion and parenchymal destruction *(C)*. (*A* and *B* with permission from Travis WD, et al [eds]: World Health Organization Histological Typing of Lung and Pleural Tumors. Heidelberg, Springer, 1999; *C*, courtesy of Dr. Adi Gazdar, Department of Pathology, University of Texas Southwestern Medical School, Dallas.)

and the final picture may prove to be more complex than presently understood.

Large cell carcinomas constitute a group of neoplasms that lack cytologic differentiation and probably represent squamous cell or glandular neoplasms that are too undifferentiated to permit categorization. The cells are large, are usually anaplastic, and have large vesicular nuclei with prominent nucleoli. Occasional tumors have a prominent component of giant cells, many of which are multinucleated ("giant cell carcinoma"), while others are composed of spindle-shaped cells resembling a sarcoma ("spindle cell carcinoma"); some have a mixture of both ("spindle and giant cell carcinoma"). Large cell carcinomas have a poor prognosis because of their tendency to spread to distant sites early in their course.

Small cell lung carcinomas generally appear as pale gray, centrally located masses with extension into the lung parenchyma and early involvement of the hilar and mediastinal nodes. These cancers are composed of tumor cells with a round to fusiform shape, scant cytoplasm, and finely granular chromatin. Mitotic figures are frequently seen (Fig. 13–40A). Despite the appellation of "small," the neoplastic cells are usually twice the size of resting lymphocytes. Necrosis is invariably present and may be extensive. The tumor cells are markedly fragile and often show fragmentation and "crush artifact" in small biopsy specimens. Another feature of small cell carcinomas, best appreciated in cytologic specimens, is nuclear molding resulting from close apposition of tumor cells that have scant cytoplasm (Fig. 13–40B). These tumors are derived from neuroendocrine cells of the lung,

and hence they express a variety of neuroendocrine markers (see Table 13–8) in addition to a host of polypeptide hormones that may result in paraneoplastic syndromes (see later).

Combined patterns require no further comment, but it should be noted that a significant minority of bronchogenic carcinomas reveal more than one line of differentiation, sometimes several (see Table 13–7), suggesting that all are derived from a multipotential progenitor cell.

For all of these neoplasms, one can trace involvement of successive chains of nodes about the carina, in the mediastinum, and in the neck (scalene nodes) and clavicular regions and, sooner or later, distant metastases. Involvement of the supraclavicular node (Virchow node) is particularly characteristic and sometimes calls attention to an occult primary tumor. These cancers, when advanced, often extend into the pericardial or pleural spaces, leading to inflammation and effusions. They may compress or infiltrate the superior vena cava to cause either venous congestion or the full-blown vena caval syndrome (Chapter 10). Apical neoplasms may invade the brachial or cervical sympathetic plexus to cause severe pain in the distribution of the ulnar nerve or to produce Horner syndrome (ipsilateral enophthalmos, ptosis, meiosis, and anhidrosis). Such apical neoplasms are sometimes called Pancoast tumors, and the combination of clinical findings is known as Pancoast syndrome. Pancoast tumor is often accompanied by destruction of the first and second ribs and sometimes thoracic vertebrae. As with other cancers, tumor-node-metastasis (TNM) categories have been established to indicate the size and spread of the primary neoplasm.

Figure 13–40   ■

Small cell lung carcinoma. *A,* Nests and cords of round to polygonal cells with scant cytoplasm, granular chromatin, and inconspicuous nucleoli. Note mitotic figure in center. *B,* Cytologic preparation from a case of small cell carcinoma demonstrating "nuclear molding" of adjacent cells *(arrows).* This is a useful feature in bronchioloalveolar lavage samples or fine-needle aspiration specimens for diagnosing small cell carcinoma.

Clinical Course. Bronchogenic carcinomas are silent, insidious lesions that more often than not have spread so as to be unresectable before they produce symptoms. In some instances, chronic cough and expectoration call attention to still localized, resectable disease. When hoarseness, chest pain, superior vena caval syndrome, pericardial or pleural effusion, or persistent segmental atelectasis or pneumonitis makes its appearance, the prognosis is grim. Too often the tumor presents with symptoms emanating from metastatic spread to the brain (mental or neurologic changes), liver (hepatomegaly), or bones (pain). Although the adrenals may be nearly obliterated by metastatic disease, adrenal insufficiency (Addison disease) is uncommon because islands of cortical cells sufficient to maintain adrenal function usually persist.

Overall, NSCLCs have a better prognosis than SCLCs. When NSCLCs (squamous cell carcinomas or adenocarcinomas) are detected before metastasis or local spread, cure is possible by lobectomy or pneumonectomy. SCLCs, on the other hand, have invariably spread by the time they are first detected, even if the primary tumor appears small and localized. Thus, surgical resection is not a viable treatment. They are very sensitive to chemotherapy but invariably recur. Median survival even with treatment is 1 year.

It is variously estimated that 3% to 10% of all lung cancer patients develop clinically overt paraneoplastic syndromes. These include (1) hypercalcemia caused by secretion of a parathyroid hormone–related peptide (osteolytic lesions may also cause hypercalcemia, but this would not be a paraneoplastic syndrome [Chapter 6]); (2) Cushing syndrome (from increased production of adrenocorticotropic hormone); (3) syndrome of inappropriate secretion of antidiuretic hormone (SIADH); (4) neuromuscular syndromes, including a myasthenic syndrome, peripheral neuropathy, and polymyositis; (5) clubbing of the fingers and hypertrophic pulmonary osteoarthropathy; and (6) hematologic manifestations, including migratory thrombophlebitis, nonbacterial endocarditis, and disseminated intravascular coagulation. Secretion of calcitonin and other ectopic hormones has also been documented by assays, but these products usually do not provoke distinctive syndromes. Hypercalcemia is most often encountered with squamous cell neoplasms, the hematologic syndromes with adenocarcinomas. The remaining syndromes are much more common with small cell neoplasms, but exceptions abound.

Bronchial Carcinoid

Bronchial carcinoids are thought to arise from the Kulchitsky cells (neuroendocrine cells that line the bronchial mucosa) and resemble intestinal carcinoids (Chapter 15). The neoplastic cells contain dense core neurosecretory granules in their cytoplasm and, rarely, may secrete hormonally active polypeptides. They occasionally occur as part of multiple endocrine neoplasia (Chapter 20). Bronchial carcinoids appear at an early age (mean 40 years) and represent about 5% of all pulmonary neoplasms. In happy contrast to their more ominous neuroendocrine counterpart, small cell carcinomas, carcinoids are often resectable and curable.

MORPHOLOGY

Most bronchial carcinoids originate in mainstem bronchi and grow in one of two patterns: (1) an obstructing polypoid, spherical, intraluminal mass; or (2) a mucosal plaque penetrating the bronchial wall to fan out in the peribronchial tissue—the so-called collar-button lesion. Even these penetrating lesions push into the lung substance along a broad front and are therefore reasonably well demarcated. Five to 15 percent of these tumors have metastasized to the hilar nodes at presentation, although distant metastasis is rare. Histologically, these neoplasms, like their counterparts in the intestinal tract, are composed of nests of uniform cells that have regular round nuclei with "salt and pepper" chromatin, absent or rare mitoses, and little pleomorphism. Occasional tumors display a higher mitotic rate, increased cytologic variability, and focal necrosis—features that qualify for a designation of **atypical carcinoid.** The latter tumors have a higher incidence of lymph node and distant metastasis than "typical" carcinoids, and understandably patients fare worse in the long run. **Typical carcinoid, atypical carcinoid, and small cell carcinoma can be considered to represent a continuum of increasing histologic aggressiveness and malignant potential within the spectrum of pulmonary neuroendocrine neoplasms.**

Most bronchial carcinoids present with findings related to their intraluminal growth (i.e., they cause cough, hemoptysis, and recurrent bronchial and pulmonary infections). Some are asymptomatic and discovered by chance on chest radiographs. Only rarely do they induce the carcinoid syndrome. In any case, because they are slow-growing lesions that rarely spread beyond the local hilar nodes, these tumors are amenable to conservative resection. The reported 5- to 10-year survival rate ranges from 50% to 95%, but late recurrences sometimes develop.

PLEURAL LESIONS

Lesions of the pleura may be inflammatory or neoplastic. Although inflammatory processes are far more common, we will begin our discussion with the more ominous, but fortunately rare, malignant tumor of the pleura.

Malignant Mesothelioma

Malignant mesothelioma is a rare cancer of mesothelial cells, usually arising in the parietal or visceral pleura, although it also occurs, much less commonly, in the peritoneum and pericardium. It has assumed great importance because it is related to occupational exposure to asbestos in the air (Chapter 8). Approximately 50% of the patients have a history of exposure to asbestos. Those who work directly with asbestos (shipyard workers, miners, insulators) are at greatest risk, but malignant mesotheliomas have appeared in persons whose only exposure was living in proximity to an asbestos factory or being a relative of an asbestos worker. The latent period for developing malignant mesotheliomas is long, often 25 to 40 years after initial asbestos exposure, suggesting that multiple somatic genetic events are required for tumorigenic conversion of a mesothelial cell. As stated earlier, *the combination of cigarette smoking and asbestos exposure greatly increases the risk of bronchogenic carcinoma, but it does not increase the risk of developing malignant mesotheliomas.*

The basis for the carcinogenicity of asbestos is still a mystery. Clearly, the physical form of the asbestos is critical; very nearly all cases are related to exposure to amphibole asbestos, which has long, straight fibers, but not to serpentine chrysotile (Chapter 8). Asbestos is not removed or metabolized from the lung, and hence the fibers remain in the body for life. Thus, there is a lifetime risk after exposure that does not diminish with time (unlike smoking, in which the risk decreases after cessation). It has been hypothesized that asbestos fibers preferentially gather near the mesothelial cell layer, where they generate reactive oxygen species that cause DNA damage and potentially oncogenic mutations. Somatic mutations of two tumor suppressor genes—*p16/CDKN2A* on chromosome 9p21 and *neurofibromatosis 2 (NF2)* gene on chromosome 22q12—have been observed in malignant mesotheliomas. Recent work has demonstrated the presence of SV40 (simian virus 40) viral DNA sequences in 60% to 80% of pleural malignant mesotheliomas and in a smaller fraction of peritoneal cases. The SV40 T-antigen is a potent carcinogen that binds to and inactivates several critical regulators of growth, such as TP53 and RB. Currently, the interaction of asbestos and SV40 in mesothelioma pathogenesis is an area of active investigation.

Figure 13-41

Malignant mesothelioma. Note the thick, firm, white, pleural tumor that ensheathes this bisected lung.

sheets; and (3) biphasic, having both sarcomatoid and epithelioid areas.

Benign mesotheliomas (i.e., solitary fibrous tumors) can also arise from the pleura. These tumors have no relationship to asbestos exposure.

Pleural Effusion and Pleuritis

Pleural effusion, the presence of fluid in the pleural space, can be either a transudate or an exudate. A pleural effusion that is a transudate is termed *hydrothorax*. Hydrothorax from congestive heart failure is probably the most common cause of fluid in the pleural cavity. An exudate, characterized by a specific gravity greater than 1.020 and, often, inflammatory cells, suggests pleuritis. The four principal causes of pleural exudate are (1) microbial invasion via either direct extension of a pulmonary infection or bloodborne seeding; (2) cancer (bronchogenic carcinoma, metastatic neoplasms to the lung or pleural surface, mesothelioma); (3) pulmonary infarction; and (4) viral pleuritis. Other, less common causes of exudative pleural effusions are systemic lupus erythematosus, rheumatoid arthritis, or uremia and following thoracic surgery. Cancer should be suspected as the underlying cause of an exudative effusion in any patient older than the age of 40, particularly when there is no febrile illness, no pain, and a negative tuberculin test result. These effusions characteristically are large and frequently are serosanguineous. Cytologic examination may reveal malignant and inflammatory cells.

Whatever the cause, transudates and serous exudates are usually resorbed without residual effects if the inciting cause is controlled or remits. In contrast, fibrinous, hemorrhagic, and suppurative exudates may lead to fibrous organization, yielding adhesions or fibrous pleural thickening, and sometimes minimal to massive calcifications.

MORPHOLOGY

Malignant mesotheliomas are often preceded by extensive pleural fibrosis and plaque formation, readily seen in computed tomographic scans. These tumors begin in a localized area and in the course of time spread widely, either by contiguous growth or by diffusely seeding the pleural surfaces. At autopsy, the affected lung is typically ensheathed by a yellow-white, firm, sometimes gelatinous layer of tumor that obliterates the pleural space (Fig. 13-41). Distant metastases are rare. The neoplasm may directly invade the thoracic wall or the subpleural lung tissue. Normal mesothelial cells are biphasic, giving rise to pleural lining cells as well as the underlying fibrous tissue. Therefore, histologically, mesotheliomas conform to one of three patterns: (1) epithelial, in which cuboidal cells line tubular and microcystic spaces, into which small papillary buds project; this is the most common pattern and also the one most likely to be confused with a pulmonary adenocarcinoma; (2) sarcomatoid, in which spindled and sometimes fibroblastic-appearing cells grow in nondistinctive

Pneumothorax, Hemothorax, and Chylothorax

Pneumothorax refers to air or other gas in the pleural sac. It may occur in young, apparently healthy adults, usually men without any known pulmonary disease (simple or spontaneous pneumothorax), or as a result of some thoracic or lung disorder (secondary pneumothorax), such as emphysema or a fractured rib. Secondary pneumothorax occurs with rupture of any pulmonary lesion situated close to the pleural surface that allows inspired air to gain access to the pleural cavity. Such pulmonary lesions include emphysema, lung abscess, tuberculosis, carcinoma, and many other, less common, processes. Mechanical ventilatory support with high pressure may also trigger secondary pneumothorax.

There are several possible complications of pneumothorax. A ball-valve leak may create a tension pneumothorax that shifts the mediastinum. Compromise of the pulmonary circulation may follow and may even be fatal. If the leak seals and the lung is not re-expanded within a few weeks (either spontaneously or through medical or surgical intervention), so much scarring may occur that it can never be fully re-expanded. In these cases, serous fluid collects in the pleural cavity and creates hydropneumothorax. With prolonged collapse, the lung becomes vulnerable to infection, as does the pleural cavity when communication between it and the lung persists. Empyema is thus an important complication of pneumothorax (pyopneumothorax). Secondary pneumothorax tends to be recurrent if the predisposing condition remains. What is less well recognized is that simple pneumothorax is also recurrent.

Hemothorax, the collection of whole blood (in contrast to bloody effusion) in the pleural cavity, is a complication of a ruptured intrathoracic aortic aneurysm that is almost always fatal. With hemothorax, in contrast to bloody pleural effusions, the blood clots within the pleural cavity.

Chylothorax is a pleural collection of a milky lymphatic fluid containing microglobules of lipid. The total volume of fluid may not be large, but chylothorax is always significant because it implies obstruction of the major lymph ducts, usually by an intrathoracic cancer (e.g., a primary or secondary mediastinal neoplasm, such as a lymphoma).

LESIONS OF THE UPPER RESPIRATORY TRACT

Acute Infections

Acute infections of the upper respiratory tract are among the most common afflictions of humans, most frequently presenting as the "common cold." The clinical features are well known to all: nasal congestion accompanied by watery discharge; sneezing; scratchy, dry sore throat; and a slight increase in temperature that is more pronounced in young children. The most common pathogens are rhinoviruses, but coronaviruses, respiratory syncytial viruses, parainfluenza and influenza viruses, adenoviruses, enteroviruses, and even group A β-hemolytic streptococci have been implicated. In a significant number of cases (around 40%) the cause cannot

be determined; perhaps new viruses will be discovered. Most of these infections occur in the fall and winter and are self-limiting (usually lasting for a week or less). In a minority of cases, colds may be complicated by the development of bacterial otitis media or sinusitis.

In addition to the common cold, infections of the upper respiratory tract may present as signs and symptoms localized to the pharynx, epiglottis, or larynx. *Acute pharyngitis*, manifesting as a sore throat, may be caused by a host of agents. Mild pharyngitis with minimal physical findings frequently accompanies a cold and is the most common form of pharyngitis. More severe forms with tonsillitis, associated with marked hyperemia and exudates, occur with β-hemolytic streptococci and adenovirus infections. Streptococcal tonsillitis is important to recognize and treat early, because of its potential to develop peritonsillar abscesses ("quinsy") or result in post-streptococcal glomerulonephritis and acute rheumatic fever. Coxsackievirus A may produce pharyngeal vesicles and ulcers (herpangina). Infectious mononucleosis, caused by Epstein-Barr virus (EBV), is an important cause of pharyngitis and bears the moniker of "kissing disease," a reflection on the common mode of transmission in previously nonexposed individuals.

Acute *bacterial epiglottitis* is a syndrome predominantly of young children who have an infection of the epiglottis by *H. influenzae*, in which pain and airway obstruction are the major findings. The onset is abrupt. Failure to appreciate the need to maintain an open airway for a child with this condition can be fatal. The advent of vaccination against *H. influenzae* has greatly decreased the incidence of this disease.

Acute laryngitis can result from inhalation of irritants or may be caused by allergic reactions. It may also be caused by the agents that produce the common cold and usually involve the pharynx and nasal passages as well as the larynx. Brief mention should be made of two uncommon but important forms of laryngitis: *tuberculous* and *diphtheritic*. The former is almost always a consequence of protracted active tuberculosis, during which infected sputum is coughed up. Diphtheritic laryngitis has fortunately become uncommon because of the widespread immunization of young children against diphtheria toxin. After it is inhaled, *Corynebacterium diphtheriae* implants on the mucosa of the upper airways and elaborates a powerful exotoxin that causes necrosis of the mucosal epithelium accompanied by a dense fibrinopurulent exudate that creates the classic superficial, dirty-gray pseudomembrane of diphtheria. The major hazards of this infection are sloughing and aspiration of the pseudomembrane (causing obstruction of major airways) and absorption of bacterial exotoxins (producing myocarditis, peripheral neuropathy, or other tissue injury).

In children, parainfluenza virus is the most common cause of laryngotracheobronchitis, more commonly known as *croup*, but other agents such as respiratory syncytial virus may also precipitate this condition. Although self-limited, croup may cause frightening inspiratory stridor and harsh, persistent cough. In occasional cases the laryngeal inflammatory reaction may narrow the airway sufficiently to cause respiratory failure. Viral infections in the upper respiratory tract predispose the patient to secondary bacterial infection, particularly by staphylococci, streptococci, and *H. influenzae*.

Nasopharyngeal Carcinoma

This rare neoplasm merits comment because of (1) the strong epidemiologic links to EBV and (2) the high frequency of this form of cancer in the Chinese, which raises the possibility of viral oncogenesis on a background of genetic susceptibility. EBV infects the host by first replicating in the nasopharyngeal epithelium and then infecting nearby tonsillar B lymphocytes. In some persons this leads to transformation of the epithelial cells. Unlike the case with Burkitt lymphoma (Chapter 12), another EBV-associated tumor, the EBV genome is found in virtually all nasopharyngeal carcinomas, including those that occur outside the endemic areas in Asia.

The three histologic variants are keratinizing squamous cell carcinoma, nonkeratinizing squamous cell carcinoma, and undifferentiated carcinoma; the last-mentioned is the most common and the one most closely linked with EBV. The undifferentiated neoplasm is characterized by large epithelial cells having indistinct cell borders ("syncytial" growth) and prominent eosinophilic nucleoli. It should be recalled that in infectious mononucleosis, EBV directly infects B lymphocytes, after which a marked proliferation of reactive T lymphocytes causes atypical lymphocytosis, seen in the peripheral blood, and enlarged lymph nodes (Chapter 12). Similarly, in nasopharyngeal carcinomas a striking influx of mature lymphocytes can often be seen. These neoplasms are therefore referred to as "lymphoepitheliomas," a misnomer because the lymphocytes are not part of the neoplastic process, nor is the tumor benign. The presence of large neoplastic cells in a background of reactive lymphocytes may give rise to an appearance similar to non-Hodgkin lymphomas, and immunohistochemical stains may be required to prove the epithelial nature of the malignant cells. Nasopharyngeal carcinomas invade locally, spread to cervical lymph nodes, and then metastasize to distant sites. They tend to be radiosensitive, and 5-year survival rates of 50% are reported for even advanced cancers.

Laryngeal Tumors

A variety of non-neoplastic, benign, and malignant neoplasms of squamous epithelial and mesenchymal origin may arise in the larynx, but only vocal cord nodules, papillomas, and squamous cell carcinomas are sufficiently common to merit comment. In all these conditions, the most common presenting feature is hoarseness.

NONMALIGNANT LESIONS

Vocal cord nodules ("polyps") are smooth, hemispherical protrusions (usually less than 0.5 cm in diameter) located, most often, on the true vocal cords. The nodules are composed of fibrous tissue and covered by stratified squamous mucosa that is usually intact but can be ulcerated by contact trauma with the other vocal cord. These lesions occur chiefly in heavy smokers or singers (singer's nodes), suggesting that they are the result of chronic irritation or abuse.

Laryngeal papilloma or *squamous papilloma* of the larynx is a benign neoplasm, usually on the true vocal cords, that forms a soft, raspberry-like excrescence rarely more than 1 cm in diameter. Histologically, it consists of multiple, slender, finger-like projections supported by central fibrovascular cores and covered by an orderly, typical, stratified squamous epithelium. When the papilloma is on the free edge of the vocal cord, trauma may lead to ulceration that can be accompanied by hemoptysis.

Papillomas are usually single in adults but are often multiple in children, in whom they are referred to as *juvenile laryngeal papillomatosis*. These lesions are caused by human papillomavirus types 6 and 11, do not become malignant, and often spontaneously regress at puberty. In children, the papillomas tend to recur after excision. Cancerous transformation is rare.

CARCINOMA OF THE LARYNX

Carcinoma of the larynx represents only 2% of all cancers. It most commonly occurs after age 40 years and is more common in men (7:1) than in women. Environmental influences are very important in its causation; nearly all cases occur in smokers, and alcohol and asbestos exposure may also play roles.

About 95% of laryngeal carcinomas are typical squamous cell lesions. Rarely, adenocarcinomas are seen, presumably arising from mucous glands. The tumor usually develops directly on the vocal cords (glottic tumors) in 60% to 75% of cases, but it may arise above the cords (supraglottic; 25% to 40%) or below the cords (subglottic; less than 5%). The major etiologic factors associated with laryngeal squamous carcinomas include most importantly smoking, but also alcohol and previous radiation exposure. Human papillomavirus sequences have been detected in a minority of cases. Squamous cell carcinomas of the larynx follow the growth pattern of all squamous cell carcinomas. They begin as in situ lesions that later appear as pearly gray, wrinkled plaques on the mucosal surface, ultimately ulcerating and fungating (Fig. 13–42). The glottic tumors are usually keratinizing, well- to moderately differentiated squamous cell carcinomas, although nonkeratinizing, poorly differentiated carcinomas may also be seen. As expected with lesions aris-

Figure 13–42 ■

Laryngeal squamous cell carcinoma *(arrow)* arising in a supraglottic location (above the true vocal cord).

ing from recurrent exposure to environmental carcinogens, adjacent mucosa may demonstrate squamous cell hyperplasia with foci of dysplasia, or even carcinoma in situ.

Carcinoma of the larynx manifests itself clinically by persistent hoarseness. The location of the tumor within the larynx has a significant bearing on prognosis. For example, about 90% of glottic tumors are confined to the larynx at diagnosis. First, as a result of interference with vocal cord mobility, they develop symptoms early in the course of disease; second, the glottic region has a sparse lymphatic supply, and spread beyond the larynx is uncommon. By contrast, the supraglottic larynx is rich in lymphatic spaces, and nearly a third of these tumors metastasize to regional (cervical) lymph nodes. The subglottic tumors tend to remain clinically quiescent, usually presenting as advanced disease. With surgery, radiation, or combined therapeutic treatments many patients can be cured, but about one third die of the disease. The usual cause of death is infection of the distal respiratory passages or widespread metastases and cachexia.

BIBLIOGRAPHY

Ando M, et al: A new look at hypersensitivity pneumonitis. Curr Opin Pulm Med 5:299, 1999. (An update on the pathogenesis of hypersensitivity pneumonia, with emphasis on the immunologic aspects of this disease.)

Barnes PJ: Chronic obstructive pulmonary disease. N Engl J Med 343:269, 2000. (An excellent review of the pathogenesis of COPD.)

Bisno AL: Acute pharyngitis. N Engl J Med 344:205, 2001. (An excellent discussion of this common condition, typically ignored in the medical literature.)

Busse WW, Lemanske RF: Asthma. N Engl J Med 344:350, 2001. (An excellent review of the pathogenesis of allergic asthma.)

Fong K, et al: Molecular pathogenesis of lung cancer. J Thorac Cardiovasc Surg 118:1136, 1999. (A scholarly review of the molecular biol-ogy of lung carcinoma by one of the foremost research groups in the field.)

Idiopathic Pulmonary Fibrosis: Diagnosis and Treatment. International Consensus Statement of the American Thoracic Society and the European Respiratory Society. Am J Respir Crit Care Med 161:646, 2000. (The authoritative statement on what exactly constitutes IPF from the experts!)

Jeffery PK: Comparison of the structural and inflammatory features of COPD and asthma. Chest 117:S251, 2000. (A comparison of the histopathologic features in the two obstructive airway diseases, with a concurrent discussion of underlying pathogenetic mechanisms.)

Kitamura H, et al: Atypical adenomatous hyperplasia of the lung: implications for the pathogenesis of peripheral lung adenocarcinoma. Am J Clin Pathol 111:610, 1999. (Compelling histopathologic and molecular evidence is presented to link the putative precursor lesions to the development of subsequent adenocarcinomas.)

Marik PE: Aspiration pneumonitis and aspiration pneumonia. N Engl J Med 344:665, 2001. (A clinically oriented review of the subject.)

Mayaud C, et al: Tuberculosis in AIDS: past or new problems. Thorax 54:576, 1999. (A contemporary review of tuberculosis in patients with AIDS.)

Murthy SS, et al: Asbestos, chromosomal deletions, and tumor suppressor gene alterations in human malignant mesothelioma. J Cell Physiol 180:150, 1999. (An excellent review of the molecular biology of malignant mesotheliomas, all under one roof.)

Schwartz RS: The new element in the mechanism of asthma. N Engl J Med 346:857, 2002. (A succinct review of evidence supporting the primacy of T_H2 response in causation of asthma.)

Statement on Sarcoidosis: the Joint Statement of the American Thoracic Society, the European Respiratory Society and the World Association of Sarcoidosis and other Granulomatous Disorders. Am J Respir Crit Care Med 160:736; 1999. (A definitive review of sarcoidosis!)

Walter R, et al: Environmental and genetic risk factors and gene-environment interactions in the pathogenesis of chronic obstructive lung disease. Environ Health Perspect 108:733; 2000. (A review of various environmental and genetic factors and their interaction in the pathogenesis of COPD.)

Ware LB, Matthay MA: The acute respiratory distress syndrome. N Engl J Med 342:1334, 2000. (An overview of the current definitions, epidemiology, pathology, and clinical features of ARDS.)

The Kidney and Its Collecting System

RAMZI S. COTRAN, MD*
HELMUT RENNKE, MD
VINAY KUMAR, MD

CLINICAL MANIFESTATIONS OF RENAL DISEASES

GLOMERULAR DISEASES
Pathogenesis of Glomerular Diseases
Circulating Immune Complex Nephritis
Immune Complex Nephritis in Situ
Cell-Mediated Immune Glomerulonephritis
Mediators of Immune Injury
Other Mechanisms of Glomerular Injury
Glomerular Syndromes and Disorders
The Nephrotic Syndrome
Minimal Change Disease (Lipoid Nephrosis)
Membranous Glomerulonephritis (Membranous Nephropathy)
Focal Segmental Glomerulosclerosis
Membranoproliferative Glomerulonephritis
The Nephritic Syndrome
Acute Proliferative (Poststreptococcal, Postinfectious) Glomerulonephritis
Rapidly Progressive (Crescentic) Glomerulonephritis

IgA Nephropathy (Berger Disease)
Hereditary Nephritis
Chronic Glomerulonephritis

DISEASES AFFECTING TUBULES AND INTERSTITIUM
Tubulointerstitial Nephritis
Acute Pyelonephritis
Chronic Pyelonephritis and Reflux Nephropathy
Drug-Induced Interstitial Nephritis
Acute Drug-Induced Interstitial Nephritis
Analgesic Nephropathy
Acute Tubular Necrosis

DISEASES INVOLVING BLOOD VESSELS
Benign Nephrosclerosis
Malignant Hypertension and Malignant Nephrosclerosis
Thrombotic Microangiopathies

CYSTIC DISEASES OF THE KIDNEY
Simple Cysts
Autosomal Dominant (Adult) Polycystic Kidney Disease
Autosomal Recessive (Childhood) Polycystic Kidney Disease

*Deceased

509

URINARY OUTFLOW OBSTRUCTION
Renal Stones
Hydronephrosis
TUMORS
Renal Cell Carcinoma
Wilms Tumor

Tumors of the Urinary Bladder and Collecting System (Renal Calyces, Renal Pelvis, Ureter, and Urethra)

[handwritten margin notes:]

① Azotemia → ↑ NH₃ & Creatine markers to ↓ GFR)
- Prerenal → hypoperfusion of kidney in absence of parenchymal damage
- Postrenal → urine flow is obstructed below level of kidney

① ANS Synd → hematuria, proteinuria, azotemia
in... classic pres. of post strep. glomnephritis
② Neph Syn → heavy proteinuria, hypoalb, severe edema, hyperlipidemia

---

The kidney is a structurally complex organ that has evolved to subserve a number of important functions: excretion of the waste products of metabolism, regulation of body water and salt, maintenance of appropriate acid balance, and secretion of a variety of hormones and autocoids. Diseases of the kidney are as complex as its structure, but their study is facilitated by dividing them into those that affect the four basic morphologic components: glomeruli, tubules, interstitium, and blood vessels. This traditional approach is useful because the early manifestations of diseases that affect each of these components tend to be distinctive. Furthermore, some components appear to be more vulnerable to specific forms of renal injury; for example, glomerular diseases are often immunologically mediated, whereas tubular and interstitial disorders are more likely to be caused by toxic or infectious agents. Nevertheless, some disorders affect more than one structure. In addition, the anatomic interdependence of structures in the kidney implies that damage to one almost always secondarily affects the others. Thus, severe glomerular damage impairs the flow through the peritubular vascular system; conversely, tubular destruction, by increasing intraglomerular pressure, may induce glomerular atrophy. Thus, whatever the origin, there is a tendency for all forms of chronic renal disease ultimately to destroy all four components of the kidney, culminating in chronic renal failure and what has been called *end-stage contracted kidneys*. The functional reserve of the kidney is large, and much damage may occur before functional impairment is evident. For these reasons, the early signs and symptoms are particularly important to the clinician, and these are referred to in the discussion of individual diseases.

CLINICAL MANIFESTATIONS OF RENAL DISEASES

The clinical manifestations of renal disease can be grouped into reasonably well defined syndromes. Some are peculiar to glomerular diseases; others are present in diseases that affect any one of the components. Before we list the syndromes, a few terms must be clarified.

Azotemia is a biochemical abnormality that refers to an elevation of blood urea nitrogen and creatinine levels and is largely related to a decreased glomerular filtration rate (GFR). Azotemia is produced by many renal disorders, but it also arises from extrarenal disorders. *Prerenal azotemia* is encountered when there is hypoperfusion of the kidneys, which impairs renal function *in the absence of parenchymal*

damage. Similarly, *postrenal azotemia* is seen whenever urine flow is obstructed below the level of the kidney. Relief of the obstruction is followed by prompt correction of the azotemia.

When azotemia becomes associated with a constellation of clinical signs and symptoms and biochemical abnormalities, it is termed *uremia*. Uremia is characterized not only by failure of renal excretory function but also by a host of metabolic and endocrine alterations incident to renal damage. There is, in addition, secondary gastrointestinal (e.g., uremic gastroenteritis), neuromuscular (e.g., peripheral neuropathy), and cardiovascular (e.g., uremic fibrinous pericarditis) involvement.

We can now turn to a brief description of the major renal syndromes:

1. *Acute nephritic syndrome* is a glomerular syndrome dominated by the acute onset of usually grossly visible hematuria (red blood cells in urine), mild to moderate proteinuria, azotemia, edema, and hypertension; it is the classic presentation of acute poststreptococcal glomerulonephritis.
2. The *nephrotic syndrome* is characterized by heavy proteinuria (excretion of more than 3.5 g of protein/day), hypoalbuminemia, severe edema, hyperlipidemia, and lipiduria (lipid in the urine).
3. *Asymptomatic hematuria* or *proteinuria*, or a combination of these two, is usually a manifestation of subtle or mild glomerular abnormalities.
4. *Rapidly progressive glomerulonephritis* results in loss of renal function in a few days or weeks and is manifested by an active urine sediment (hematuria, dysmorphic red blood cells, red blood cell casts).
5. *Acute renal failure* is dominated by oliguria or anuria (no urine flow), with recent onset of azotemia. It can result from glomerular injury (such as crescentic glomerulonephritis), interstitial injury, or acute tubular necrosis.
6. *Chronic renal failure*, characterized by prolonged symptoms and signs of uremia, is the end result of all chronic renal diseases.
7. *Urinary tract infection* is characterized by bacteriuria and pyuria (bacteria and leukocytes in the urine). The infection may be symptomatic or asymptomatic, and it may affect the kidney (*pyelonephritis*) or the bladder (*cystitis*) only.
8. *Nephrolithiasis* (renal stones) is manifested by renal colic, hematuria, and recurrent stone formation.

In addition to these renal syndromes, *urinary tract obstruction* and *renal tumors*, discussed later, represent specific anatomic lesions that often have varied manifestations.

GLOMERULAR DISEASES

Glomerular diseases constitute some of the major problems encountered in nephrology; indeed, chronic glomerulonephritis (GN) is one of the most common causes of chronic renal failure in humans. Recall that the glomerulus consists of an anastomosing network of capillaries invested by two layers of epithelium. The visceral epithelium is incorporated into and becomes an intrinsic part of the capillary wall, whereas the parietal epithelium lines Bowman's space (urinary space), the cavity in which plasma ultrafiltrate first collects. The glomerular capillary wall is the filtering membrane and consists of the following structures (Figs. 14–1 and 14–2):

1. A thin layer of fenestrated *endothelial cells*, each fenestra being 70 to 100 nm in diameter.
2. A *glomerular basement membrane* (GBM) with a thick, electron-dense central layer, the *lamina densa*, and

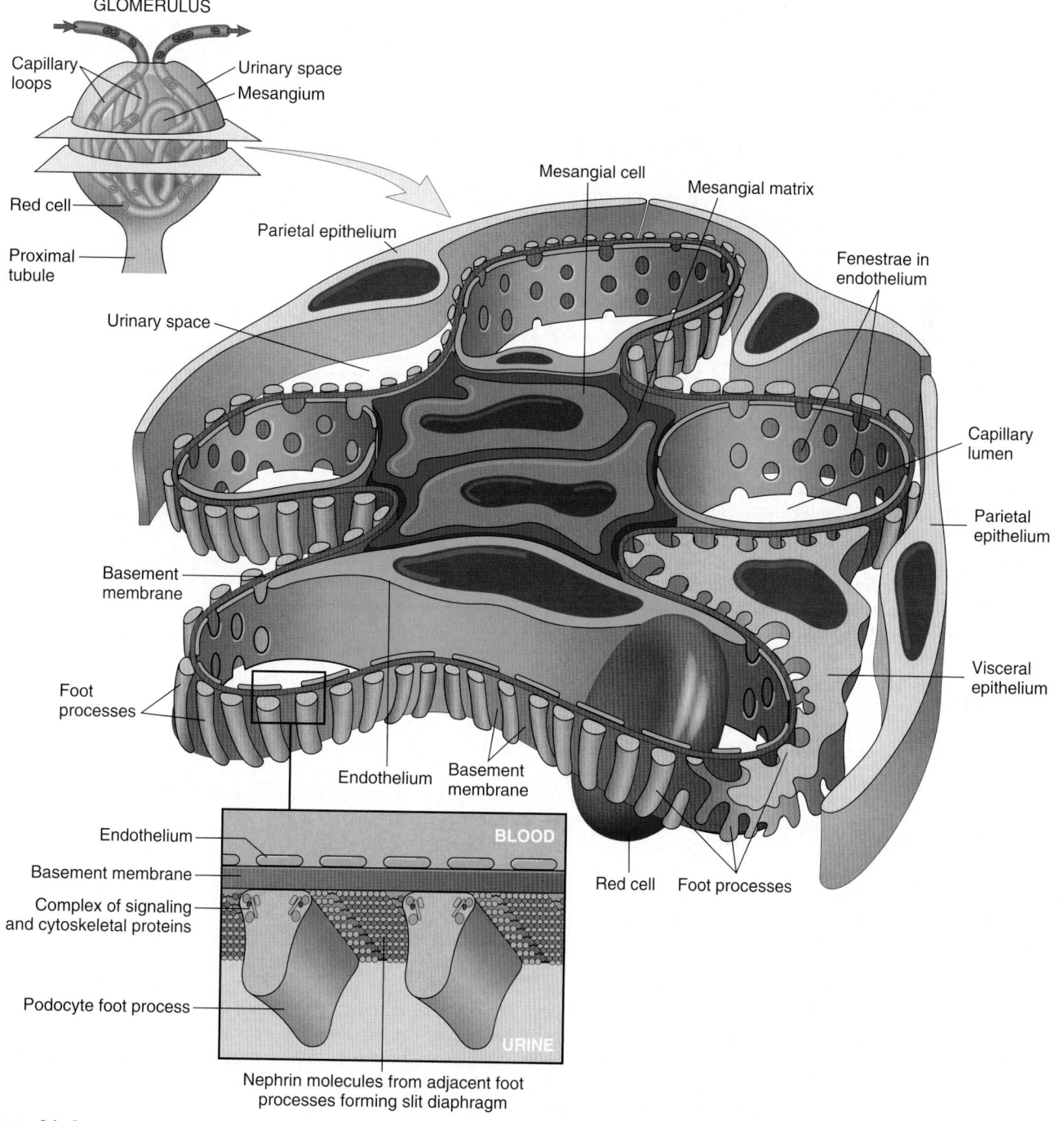

Figure 14-1

Schematic representation of a glomerular lobe.

Figure 14-2

Low-power electron micrograph of rat glomerulus. B, basement membrane; CL, capillary lumen; End, endothelium; Ep, visceral epithelial cells with foot processes; Mes, mesangium; US, urinary space.

thinner, electron-lucent peripheral layers, the *lamina rara interna* and *lamina rara externa.* The GBM consists of collagen (mostly type IV), laminin, polyanionic proteoglycans, fibronectin, and several other glycoproteins.

3. The *visceral epithelial cells* (podocytes), structurally complex cells that possess interdigitating processes embedded in and adherent to the lamina rara externa of the basement membrane. Adjacent *foot processes* (pedicels) are separated by 20- to 30-nm-wide *filtration slits,* which are bridged by a thin diaphragm composed of nephrin (see later).

4. The entire glomerular tuft is supported by *mesangial cells* lying between the capillaries. Basement membrane–like mesangial matrix forms a meshwork through which the mesangial cells are scattered. These cells, of mesenchymal origin, are contractile and are capable of proliferation, of laying down both matrix and collagen, and of secreting a number of biologically active mediators, as we shall see. The mesangium also contains a variable number of monocytes.

The major characteristics of glomerular filtration are an extraordinarily high permeability to water and small solutes and an almost complete impermeability to molecules of the size and molecular charge of albumin (±3.6 nm radius; 70,000 kD). The latter characteristic, called glomerular barrier function, discriminates among protein molecules depending on their size (the larger, the less permeable), their charge (the more cationic, the more permeable), and their configuration. This size-dependent and

charge-dependent barrier function is accounted for by the complex structure of the capillary wall, the integrity of the GBM, and the many anionic moieties present within the wall, including the acidic proteoglycans of the GBM and the sialoglycoproteins of epithelial and endothelial cell coats. The *visceral epithelial cell* is critical to the maintenance of glomerular barrier function: its filtration slit diaphragm presents a distal resistance to the flow of water and a diffusion barrier to the filtration of proteins, and it is the cell type that is largely responsible for synthesis of GBM components.

In the past few years much has been learned about the molecular architecture of the glomerular filtration barrier. Nephrin, a transmembrane glycoprotein, is the major component of the slit diaphragms between adjacent foot processes. Nephrin molecules from adjacent foot processes bind to each other through disulfide bridges at the center of the slit diaphragm. The intracellular part of nephrin molecules binds to and interacts with several cytoskeletal and signaling proteins (see Fig. 14–1). Nephrin and its associated proteins play a critical role in maintaining the selective permeability of the GBM. This is dramatically illustrated by rare hereditary diseases in which mutations of nephrin or its partner proteins are associated with abnormal leakage of plasma proteins, giving rise to the nephrotic syndrome (discussed later). This syndrome is one of the most common manifestations of glomerular disease, suggesting that acquired defects in the function or structure of slit diaphragms may constitute an important mechanism of renal disease.

Q Small , ⊖ molecules → pass through (G.F.B).

Table 14-1.   GLOMERULAR DISEASES

Primary Glomerulonephritis

Diffuse proliferative glomerulonephritis (GN)
Crescentic GN
Membranous GN
Lipoid nephrosis (minimal change disease)
Focal segmental glomerulosclerosis
Membranoproliferative GN
IgA nephropathy
Chronic GN

Secondary (Systemic) Diseases

Systemic lupus erythematosus
Diabetes mellitus
Amyloidosis
Goodpasture syndrome
Polyarteritis nodosa
Wegener granulomatosis
Henoch-Schönlein purpura
Bacterial endocarditis

Hereditary Disorders

Alport syndrome
Fabry disease

[handwritten marginal notes:]
Q Gr ↓ L Mp
- glomerulus is "innocent by stander"
- antigen not of glomerular origin... can be endogenous or exogenous
- complexes lie at 3 spots
1) mesangium
2) subendothelial
3) subepithelial
- seen as granular deposits

Glomeruli may be injured by a variety of factors and in the course of a number of systemic diseases. Immune diseases such as systemic lupus erythematosus (SLE), vascular disorders such as hypertension and polyarteritis nodosa, metabolic diseases such as diabetes mellitus, and some purely hereditary conditions such as Alport syndrome often affect the glomerulus. These are termed *secondary glomerular diseases* to differentiate them from those in which the kidney is the only or predominant organ involved. The latter constitute the various types of *primary GN* or *glomerulopathy*. Here we shall discuss the various types of primary GN. The glomerular alterations in systemic diseases are discussed in other parts of this book.

Table 14–1 lists the most common forms of GN that have reasonably well defined morphologic and clinical manifestations.

Pathogenesis of Glomerular Diseases

Although we know little of etiologic agents or triggering events, it is clear that immune mechanisms underlie most cases of primary GN and many of the secondary glomerular diseases. Experimentally, GN can be readily induced by antigen-antibody reactions, and glomerular deposits of immunoglobulins, often with various components of complement, are found in more than 70% of patients with GN. Cell-mediated immune mechanisms also play a role in certain glomerular diseases.

Two forms of antibody-associated injury have been established: (1) injury resulting from deposition of soluble circulating antigen-antibody complexes in the glomerulus and (2) injury by antibodies reacting in situ within the glomerulus, either with insoluble fixed (intrinsic) glomerular antigens or with molecules planted within the glomerulus (Fig. 14–3). In addition, cytotoxic antibodies directed

[handwritten note at bottom:]
Q Antibody ass. injury → 1) deposition of complexes
2) antibodies acting on fixed antigens

against glomerular cell components may cause glomerular injury. These pathways are not mutually exclusive, and in humans all may contribute to injury.

CIRCULATING IMMUNE COMPLEX NEPHRITIS

The pathogenesis of immune complex diseases (type III hypersensitivity reactions) was discussed in detail in Chapter 5. Here we shall briefly review the salient features that relate to glomerular injury. With circulating immune complex disease, the glomerulus may be considered an "innocent bystander" because it does not incite the reaction. The antigen is not of glomerular origin. It may be endogenous, as in the glomerulopathy associated with SLE, or it may be exogenous, as is likely in the GN that follows certain bacterial (streptococcal), viral (hepatitis B), parasitic (*Plasmodium falciparum* malaria), and spirochetal (*Treponema pallidum*) infections. Sometimes the inciting antigen is unknown.

Whatever the antigen may be, antigen-antibody complexes are formed in situ or in the circulation and are then trapped in the glomeruli, where they produce injury, in large part through the binding of complement, although complement-independent injury may also occur (see later). The glomerular lesions usually consist of leukocytic infiltration into glomeruli and proliferation of endothelial, mesangial, and parietal epithelial cells. Electron microscopy reveals the complexes as electron-dense deposits or clumps that lie at one of three sites: in the mesangium, between the endothelial cells and the GBM (subendothelial deposits), or between the outer surface of the GBM and the podocytes (subepithelial deposits). Deposits may be located at more than one site in a given case. The presence of immunoglobulins and complement in these deposits can be demonstrated by immunofluorescence microscopy. *When fluorescinated anti-immunoglobulin or anticomplement antibodies are used, the immune complexes are seen as granular deposits in the glomerulus* (Fig. 14–4A). Once deposited in the kidney, immune complexes may eventually be degraded, mostly by infiltrating monocytes and phagocytic mesangial cells, and the inflammatory changes may then subside. Such a course occurs when the exposure to the inciting antigen is short-lived and limited, as in most cases of poststreptococcal GN. However, if the shower of antigens is continuous, repeated cycles of immune complex formation, deposition, and injury may occur, leading to chronic GN. In some cases the source of chronic antigenic exposure is clear, such as in hepatitis B virus and human immunodeficiency virus (HIV) infection and in SLE. In SLE, autoimmune injury to the tissues constantly releases nuclear and cytoplasmic antigens. In other cases, however, the antigen is unknown.

IMMUNE COMPLEX NEPHRITIS IN SITU

As noted, antibodies in this form of injury react directly with fixed or planted antigens in the glomerulus.

Anti–Glomerular Basement Membrane Disease. The best-established model is so-called classic anti-GBM nephritis (see Fig. 14–3B). In this type of injury, antibodies are directed against fixed antigens in the GBM. It has its experimental counterpart in the nephritis of rabbits called

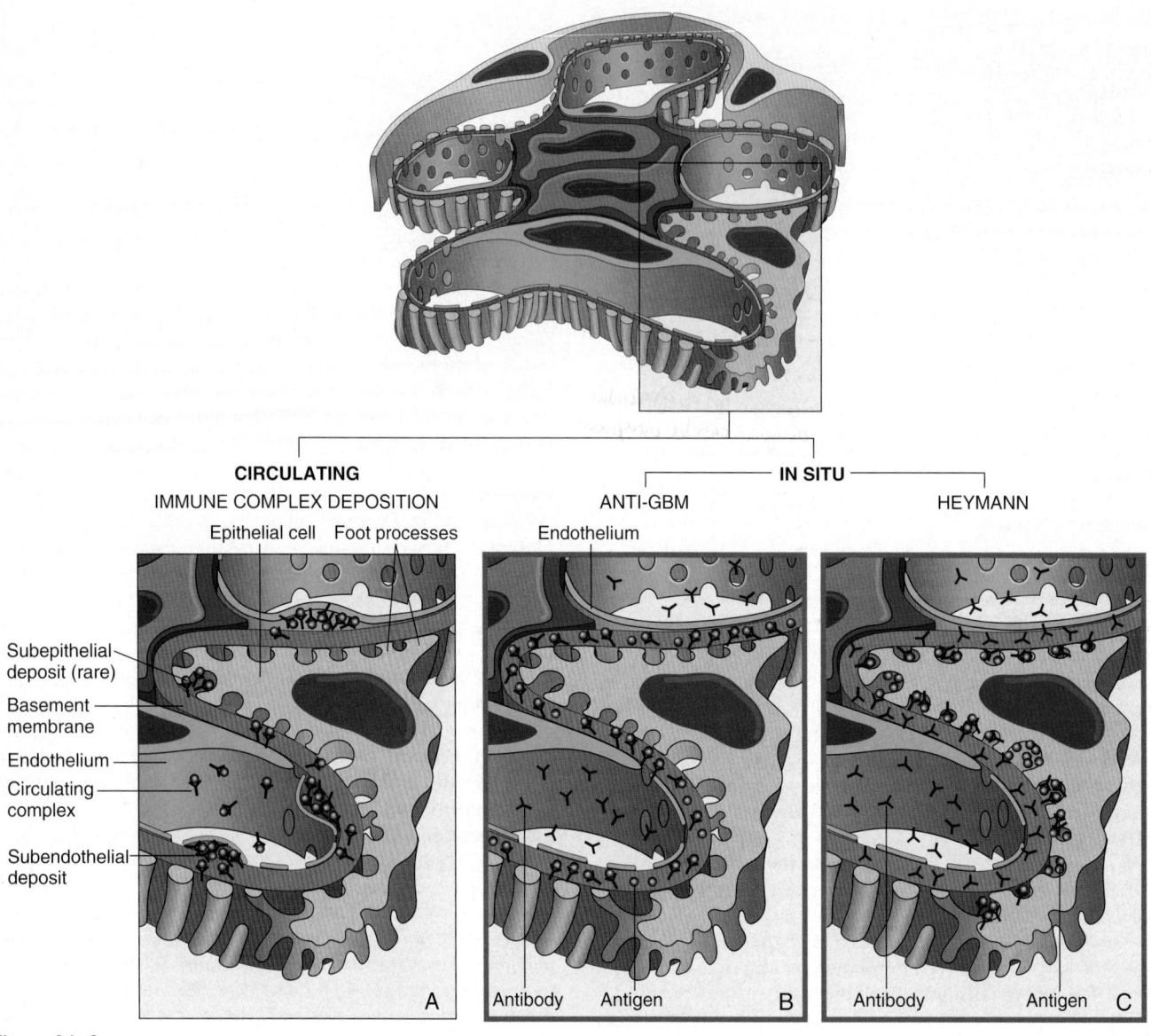

CIRCULATING

IMMUNE COMPLEX DEPOSITION

Epithelial cell   Foot processes

Subepithelial deposit (rare)

Basement membrane

Endothelium

Circulating complex

Subendothelial deposit

A

IN SITU

ANTI-GBM

Endothelium

Antibody   Antigen

B

HEYMANN

Antibody   Antigen

C

Figure 14–3 ■

Antibody-mediated glomerular injury can result either from the deposition of circulating immune complexes *(A)* or from formation in situ of complexes *(B* and *C).* Anti–glomerular basement membrane (GBM) disease *(B)* is characterized by linear immunofluorescence patterns, whereas lesions caused by immune complexes reveal granular patterns.

Masugi nephritis or *nephrotoxic serum nephritis.* This is produced by injecting rats with anti-GBM antibodies produced by immunization of rabbits with rat kidney. Although in the experimental model anti-GBM antibodies are produced by injecting "foreign" kidney antigens into an animal, *spontaneous anti-GBM nephritis in humans results from the formation of autoantibodies directed against GBM.* The antibodies directly bind along the GBM to cross-linked collagen molecules, creating a *linear pattern,* as is seen with immunofluorescence microscopy techniques, in contrast to the granular pattern described for other forms of immune complex–mediated nephritis (see Fig. 14–4*B*). Sometimes the anti-GBM antibodies cross-react with basement membranes of lung alveoli, resulting in simultaneous lung and kidney lesions *(Goodpasture syndrome).* It is

clear that this form of GN is an autoimmune disease, so any one of the several mechanisms discussed earlier (Chapter 5) in relation to autoimmunity may be involved in triggering the disease.

Anti-GBM nephritis accounts for less than 1% of human GN cases. It is established as the cause of injury in Goodpasture syndrome (Chapter 13). Many instances of anti-GBM nephritis are characterized by very severe glomerular damage and the development of rapidly progressive crescentic GN. The basement membrane antigen responsible for classic anti-GBM nephritis of Goodpasture syndrome is a component of the noncollagenous domain of the α3 chain of collagen type IV.

Heymann Nephritis. This is a model of human membranous GN. It was induced by immunizing rats with

Figure 14-4

Two patterns of deposition of immune complexes as seen by immunofluorescence microscopy. *A,* Granular, characteristic of circulating and in situ immune complex nephritis; *B,* linear, characteristic of classic anti–glomerular basement membrane disease. *Ig complexes deposited in proximal GBM = inflm. " " " distal " " = noninfl.*

preparations of proximal tubular brush border. The rats develop antibodies to brush border antigens and a membranous type of GN that closely resembles human membranous GN (discussed later). This is characterized on immunofluorescence microscopy by diffuse deposition of immunoglobulins and complement in a *granular* (rather than linear) pattern along the GBM. It is now clear that the GN results from the reaction of antibodies to an antigen complex located in the coated pits of visceral epithelial cells of the glomerulus in a discontinuous distribution and cross-reactive with a brush border antigen. The antigen consists of a large protein, ~330 kD, called *megalin,* that has homology to the low-density lipoprotein receptor and is complexed to a smaller 44-kD protein called *receptor-associated protein.* In human membranous GN, the epithelial cell antigen also appears to be a homologue of the megalin complex.

Antibodies may also react in situ with previously "planted" nonglomerular antigens, which may localize in the kidney by interacting with various intrinsic components of the glomerulus. Planted antigens include cationic molecules that bind to glomerular capillary anionic sites; DNA, which has an affinity for GBM components; bacterial products, such as endostreptosin, a protein of group A streptococci; large aggregated proteins (e.g., aggregated IgG), which deposit in the mesangium because of their size; and immune complexes themselves, because they continue to have reactive sites for further interactions with free antibody, free antigen, or complement. Most of these planted antigens induce a granular pattern of immunoglobulin deposition by immunofluorescence microscopy.

Several factors affect glomerular localization of antigen, antibody, or complexes. The molecular charge and size of these reactants are clearly important. The pattern of localization is also affected by changes in glomerular hemodynamics, mesangial function, and the integrity of the charge-selective barrier in the glomerulus. These influences may well explain the variable pattern of immune reactant

deposition and histologic change in GN. Studies in experimental models have shown that complexes deposited in the proximal zones of the GBM (endothelium or subendothelium) elicit an inflammatory reaction in the glomerulus with infiltration of leukocytes. In contrast, antibodies directed to distal zones of the GBM (epithelium and subepithelium) are largely noninflammatory and elicit lesions similar to those of Heymann or membranous GN.

To conclude the discussion of antibody-mediated injury, it must be stated that antigen-antibody deposition in the glomerulus is a major pathway of glomerular injury and that immune reactions in situ, trapping of circulating complexes, interactions between these two events, and local hemodynamic and structural determinants in the glomerulus all contribute to the morphologic and functional alterations in GN.

CELL-MEDIATED IMMUNE GLOMERULONEPHRITIS

There is increasing evidence that sensitized T cells, formed during the course of a cell-mediated immune reaction, can cause glomerular injury. In some forms of experimental GN in rodents, the disease can be induced by transfer of sensitized T cells. The idea is an attractive one, because it may account for the instances of GN in which either there are no immune deposits or the deposits do not correlate with the severity of damage. Even when antibodies are present, T-cell–mediated injury cannot be excluded. Recent evidence suggests that this may be the case in some forms of rapidly progressive GN (discussed later).

MEDIATORS OF IMMUNE INJURY

Once immune reactants are localized in the glomerulus, how does glomerular damage ensue? *Glomerular damage, reflected physiologically by loss of glomerular barrier function, is manifested by proteinuria and, in some instances,*

Ab deposition → Imm. Complexes → C5b-C9 → lysis & E&M
complement → C5a → neutrophils → damage

Q Other mediators 1) MACs 2) Platelets 3) resident glomerular cells 4) Fibrin related products

Figure 14-5 ■

A, Mediators of immune glomerular injury (see text). *B,* Epithelial cell injury. The postulated sequence is a consequence of antibodies to epithelial cell antigens, or toxins, cytokines, or other factors causing injury and detachment of epithelial cells, and protein leakage through defective GBM and filtration slits. (Adapted from Couser WG: Mediation of immune glomerular injury. Am Soc Nephrol 1:13, 1990.)

by reductions in GFR. One well-established pathway is the *complement-leukocyte–mediated mechanism* (Fig. 14–5A). Activation of complement initiates the generation of chemotactic agents (mainly C5a) and the recruitment of neutrophils and monocytes. Neutrophils release proteases, which cause GBM degradation; oxygen-derived free radicals, which cause cell damage; and arachidonic acid metabolites, which contribute to the reductions in GFR. However, this mechanism applies only to some types of GN, because many types show few neutrophils in the damaged glomeruli. Some models suggest complement-dependent but not neutrophil-dependent injury, due to an effect of the *C5–C9 lytic component* (membrane attack complex) of complement, which causes epithelial cell detachment and stimulates mesangial and epithelial cells to secrete damaging chemical mediators. The membrane attack complex also up-regulates transforming growth factor receptors on

epithelial cells; this leads to excessive synthesis of extracellular matrix, thus giving rise to GBM thickening.

In addition to producing immune complexes, antibodies directed to glomerular cell antigens may cause direct cytotoxicity. Such cytotoxic antibodies may mediate damage in those disorders in which immune complexes are not found. Other mediators of glomerular damage include (1) *monocytes and macrophages,* which infiltrate the glomerulus in antibody- and cell-mediated reactions and, when activated, release a vast number of biologically active molecules; (2) *platelets,* which aggregate in the glomerulus during immune-mediated injury and release prostaglandins and growth factors; (3) *resident glomerular cells* (epithelial, mesangial, and endothelial), which can be stimulated to secrete mediators such as cytokines (interleukin 1), arachidonic acid metabolites, growth factors, nitric oxide, and endothelin; and (4) *fibrin-related products,* which cause leukocyte infiltration and glomerular cell proliferation. In essence, virtually all the mediators described in our discussion of inflammation in Chapter 2 may contribute to glomerular injury.

proteinuria

OTHER MECHANISMS OF GLOMERULAR INJURY

Epithelial → induced by Ab to Cell inj.   VSC. Cell antigens

Other mechanisms may contribute to glomerular damage in certain primary renal disorders. Two that deserve special mention are epithelial cell injury and renal ablation glomerulopathy.

Epithelial Cell Injury. This can be induced by antibodies to visceral epithelial cell antigens; by toxins, as in an experimental model of proteinuria induced by puromycin aminonucleoside; conceivably by certain cytokines; or by still poorly characterized factors, as is the case in focal glomerulosclerosis (see later). Such injury is reflected by morphologic changes in the visceral epithelial cells, which include loss of foot processes, vacuolization, and retraction and detachment of cells from the GBM, and functionally by proteinuria. It is hypothesized that the detachment of visceral epithelial cells is caused by alterations in nephrin and its associated cytoskeletal proteins, and that this detachment leads to protein leakage (Fig. 14–5B).

Renal Ablation Glomerulopathy. Once any renal disease, glomerular or otherwise, destroys sufficient functioning nephrons to reduce the GFR to 30% to 50% of normal, progression to end-stage renal failure often proceeds inexorably, although the rate varies. Such patients develop proteinuria, and their kidneys show widespread *glomerulosclerosis.* Such progressive sclerosis may be initiated, at least in part, by the adaptive changes that occur in the relatively unaffected glomeruli of diseased kidneys. The remaining glomeruli undergo hypertrophy to maintain renal function. This is associated with hemodynamic changes, including increases in single-nephron GFR, blood flow, and transcapillary pressure (capillary hypertension). The additional load on the intact glomeruli leads ultimately to endothelial and epithelial cell injury, increased glomerular permeability to proteins, accumulation of proteins and lipids in the mesangial matrix, and fibrin deposition. This is followed by capillary collapse and by obsolescence, hyaline entrapment, and proliferation of mesangial cells; by increased deposition of mesangial matrix; and by

RAG → ↓ GFR 30-50% → renal failure
— overwork intact glomeruli → glomerulosclerosis

— nephrotic syndrome
— massive proteinuria, hypoalbuminemia, edema, hyperlipidemia
— due to derangement of capillary walls → ↑ perm. to plasma proteins
— comp. secretion of Aldosterone → salt/water retention → exacerbates edema

Chapter 14   THE KIDNEY AND ITS COLLECTING SYSTEM   ■   517

sclerosis of glomeruli. The last results in further reductions in nephron mass and a vicious cycle of continuing glomerulosclerosis.

We now turn to a consideration of specific types of GN and the glomerular syndromes they produce.

Glomerular Syndromes and Disorders

THE NEPHROTIC SYNDROME

The nephrotic syndrome refers to a clinical complex that includes the following: (1) massive proteinuria, with the daily loss in the urine of 3.5 g or more of protein; (2) hypoalbuminemia, with plasma albumin levels less than 3 g/dL; (3) generalized edema, the most obvious clinical manifestation; and (4) hyperlipidemia and lipiduria. At the onset there is little or no azotemia, hematuria, or hypertension.

The components of the nephrotic syndrome bear a logical relationship to one another. The initial event is a derangement in the capillary walls of the glomeruli, resulting in increased permeability to the plasma proteins. It will be remembered from the previous discussion of the normal kidney that the glomerular capillary wall, with its endothelium, GBM, and visceral epithelial cells, acts as a barrier through which the glomerular filtrate must pass. Any increased permeability resulting from either structural or physicochemical alterations allows protein to escape from the plasma into the glomerular filtrate. Massive proteinuria may result. With long-standing or extremely heavy proteinuria, serum albumin tends to become depleted, resulting in hypoalbuminemia and a reversed albumin-globulin ratio. The generalized edema of the nephrotic syndrome is, in turn, a consequence of the drop in osmotic pressure produced by hypoalbuminemia and primary retention of salt and water by the kidney. As fluid escapes from the vascular tree into the tissues, there is a concomitant drop in plasma volume, with diminished glomerular filtration. Compensatory secretion of aldosterone, along with the reduced GFR and reduction of secretion of natriuretic peptides, promotes retention of salt and water by the kidneys, thus further aggravating the edema. By repetition of this chain of events, massive amounts of edematous fluid (termed *anasarca*) may accumulate. The genesis of the hyperlipidemia is more obscure. Presumably, hypoalbuminemia triggers increased synthesis of lipoproteins in the liver. There is also abnormal transport of circulating lipid particles and impairment of peripheral breakdown of lipoproteins. The lipiduria, in turn, reflects the increased GBM permeability to lipoproteins.

The relative frequencies of the several causes of the nephrotic syndrome vary according to age. *In children younger than 15 years of age, for example, the nephrotic syndrome is almost always caused by a lesion primary to the kidney, whereas among adults it may often be associated with a systemic disease.* Table 14–2 represents a composite derived from several studies of the causes of the nephrotic syndrome. As the table indicates, the most frequent *systemic* causes of the nephrotic syndrome are diabetes, amyloidosis, and SLE. The renal lesions produced by these disorders are described in Chapter 5. The most important of the *primary* glomerular lesions that characteristically lead to the nephrotic syndrome are *membranous GN* and *lipoid nephrosis (minimal change disease)*. The latter is more important in children; the former in adults. Two other primary lesions, *focal glomerulosclerosis* and *membranoproliferative GN*, also produce the nephrotic syndrome. These four lesions are discussed individually below. The fifth possible primary cause of this syndrome, *proliferative GN*, is not considered in this section because this lesion frequently presents as the nephritic syndrome.

Q – children → neph. syn. caused by 1° lesion
— adults → " " " by 2°

— most frequent 2° → diabetes, amyloidosis, SLE
— most imp. 1° → memb. GN & lipoid nephrosis

Table 14–2. CAUSES OF NEPHROTIC SYNDROME

	Prevalence (%)*	
	Children	Adults
Primary Glomerular Disease		
Membranous glomerulonephritis (GN)	5	40
Lipoid nephrosis	65	15
Focal segmental glomerulosclerosis	10	15
Membranoproliferative GN	10	7
Proliferative GN (focal, "pure mesangial," IgA nephropathy)	10	23
Systemic Disease		
Diabetes mellitus		
Amyloidosis		
Systemic lupus erythematosus		
Drugs (gold, penicillamine, "street heroin")	} Most common systemic causes	
Infections (malaria, syphilis, hepatitis B, AIDS)		
Malignancy (carcinoma, melanoma)		
Miscellaneous (bee-sting allergy, hereditary nephritis)		

*Approximate prevalence of primary disease is 95% of the cases in children, 60% in adults. Approximate prevalence of systemic disease is 5% of the cases in children, 40% in adults.

MINIMAL CHANGE DISEASE (LIPOID NEPHROSIS)

This relatively benign disorder is the most frequent cause of the nephrotic syndrome in children. *It is characterized by glomeruli that have a normal appearance under the light microscope but disclose diffuse loss of visceral epithelial foot processes when viewed with the electron microscope.* Although it may develop at any age, this condition is most common between ages 2 and 3 years.

Pathogenesis. The pathogenesis of proteinuria in lipid nephrosis remains to be fully elucidated. Current evidence suggests that minimal change disease results from a disorder of T cells. By mechanisms not entirely clear, T cells elaborate a cytokine or a circulating factor that causes loss of epithelial foot processes and proteinuria. A variety of T-cell derived candidate circulating factors that can induce a similar disease in rats have been implicated. These include interleukin 8, tumor necrosis factor, and other poorly defined permeability factors. None of these, however, can be reproducibly demonstrated to be active in most patients with minimal change disease. The recent discovery that mutations in the nephrin gene give rise to congenital nephrotic syndrome (Finnish type) with minimal change morphology has focused attention on nephrin as the target of injury in lipoid nephrosis. It is thus postulated that a primary defect in T cells causes elaboration of a factor that affects nephrin synthesis (see Fig. 14–1). In support of this postulate, reduced nephrin expression and abnormal distribution have been reported in a small group of patients with minimal change disease.

MORPHOLOGY

With the light microscope the glomeruli appear nearly normal (Fig. 14–6A). The cells of the proximal convoluted tubules are often heavily laden with lipids, but this is secondary to tubular reabsorption of the lipoproteins passing through the diseased glomeruli. This appearance of the proximal convoluted tubules is the basis for the older term for this disorder, **lipoid nephrosis.** Even with the electron microscope, the glomerular capillary wall appears normal. The only obvious glomerular abnormality is the uniform and diffuse loss of the foot processes of the podocytes (Fig. 14–6C). The cytoplasm of the podocytes thus appears smeared over the external aspect of the GBM, obliterating the network of arcades between the podocytes and the GBM. There are also epithelial cell vacuolization, microvillus formation, and occasional focal detachments. The changes in the podocytes are reversible after remission of the proteinuria.

Clinical Course. The disease manifests by the insidious development of the nephrotic syndrome in an otherwise healthy child. There is no hypertension, and renal function is preserved in most patients. The protein loss is usually confined to the smaller serum proteins, chiefly albumin (selective proteinuria). The prognosis in children with this disorder is good. More than 90% of cases respond to a short course of corticosteroid therapy; however, proteinuria recurs in more than two thirds of the initial responders, some of whom become steroid dependent. Less than 5% develop chronic renal failure after 25 years. Because of its responsiveness to therapy in children, minimal change disease must be differentiated from other causes of the nephrotic syndrome in nonresponders. Adults also respond to steroid therapy, but the response is slower and relapses are more common.

MEMBRANOUS GLOMERULONEPHRITIS (MEMBRANOUS NEPHROPATHY)

This slowly progressive disease, most common between ages 30 and 50 years, *is characterized morphologically by the presence of subepithelial immunoglobulin-containing deposits along the GBM.* Early in the disease, the glomeruli may appear normal by light microscopy, but well-developed cases show *diffuse thickening of the capillary wall.*

Membranous GN (MGN) may occur in association with known disorders or agents (secondary MGN): (1) infections (chronic hepatitis B, syphilis, schistosomiasis, malaria); (2) malignant tumors, particularly carcinoma of the lung and colon and melanoma; (3) SLE and other autoimmune conditions; (4) exposure to inorganic salts (gold, mercury); and (5) drugs (penicillamine, captopril, nonsteroidal anti-inflammatory agents). In about 85% of cases the condition is truly idiopathic (primary).

Pathogenesis. Membranous GN is a form of chronic immune complex nephritis. Although circulating complexes of known exogenous (e.g., hepatitis B virus) or endogenous (DNA in SLE) antigen can cause MGN, it is now thought that most idiopathic forms are induced by antibodies reacting in situ to endogenous or planted glomerular antigens.

The lesions bear a striking resemblance to those of experimental Heymann nephritis, which, as you may recall, is induced by antibodies to a megalin antigenic complex, and a similar antigen is present in humans. Susceptibility to Heymann nephritis in rats and to MGN in humans is linked to the HLA locus, which influences the ability to elaborate antibodies to the *nephritogenic* antigen. Thus, idiopathic MGN, like Heymann nephritis, is considered an autoimmune disease linked to susceptibility genes and caused by antibodies to a renal autoantigen.

Relevant to the role of the immune deposits, how does the glomerular capillary wall become leaky? In the absence of neutrophils, monocytes, or platelets and the virtually uniform presence of complement, current work points to a direct action of C5b–C9, the membrane attack complex of complement, on the glomerular epithelial cell. The membrane attack complex causes activation of glomerular mesangial and epithelial cells, inducing them to liberate proteases and oxidants that can damage capillary walls. The epithelial mediators also seem to reduce nephrin synthesis and distribution.

Figure 14-6

Lipoid nephrosis *(A and C)* and membranous glomerulonephritis (GN) *(B and D)*. Note that under the light microscope the periodic acid–Schiff (PAS)-stained glomerulus appears normal, with a thin basement membrane, in lipoid nephrosis *(A)*. Compare this with the diffuse thickening of the basement membrane in membranous glomerulonephritis *(B)*. Lipoid nephrosis exhibits diffuse loss of foot processes of visceral epithelial cells *(C)*, whereas membranous glomerulonephritis *(D)* is characterized by electron-dense subepithelial deposits as well as loss of foot processes.

MGN → slowly progressive; 30-50 y.o; subepithelial Ig deposits + thickend BM
→ idiopathic forms induced by endogenous or planted antigens in situ; Abs to renal auto-antigen

MORPHOLOGY

Seen by light microscopy, the basic change appears to be diffuse thickening of the GBM (Fig. 14-6B). By electron microscopy, the apparent thickening is caused in part by subepithelial deposits that nestle against the GBM and are separated from each other by small, spikelike protrusions of GBM matrix ("spike and dome" pattern) (Fig. 14-6D). As the disease progresses, these spikes close over the deposits, incorporating them into the GBM. In addition, the podocytes lose their foot processes. Later in the disease, the incorporated

- direct action of C5b-C9 MAC → activation of mesangial epithelial cells → damage walls
- Granular deposition... insidious onset of nephrotic syndrome - minority renal failure
- Proteinuria non-specific → NO RESPOND to corticosteroids

[handwritten notes at top of page:] FSG → sclerosis as only some segments of only some glomeruli. — in children → nonselective proteinuria, poor response to corticosteroids, ↑ hematuria ohta than lipoid nephrosis

deposits are catabolized and eventually disappear, leaving for a time cavities within the GBM. These are later filled in by deposition of GBM-like material. With further progression, the glomeruli become sclerosed and, finally, completely hyalinized. Immunofluorescence microscopy shows typical granular deposition of immunoglobulins and complement along the GBM (see Fig. 14-4A).

Clinical Course. The onset in idiopathic cases is characterized by the insidious development of the nephrotic syndrome, usually without antecedent illness; however, proteinuria may be present without the full-blown nephrotic syndrome. In contrast to minimal change disease, the proteinuria is nonselective and does not usually respond to corticosteroid therapy. Globulins are lost in the urine, as are the smaller albumin molecules. It is necessary in any patient to rule out the secondary causes first. MGN follows a notoriously variable and often indolent course. Overall, although proteinuria persists in over 60% of patients, only about 40% of patients suffer progressive disease terminating in renal failure after 2 to 20 years. An additional 10% to 30% have a more benign course with partial or complete remission of proteinuria.

FOCAL SEGMENTAL GLOMERULOSCLEROSIS

Focal segmental glomerulosclerosis (FSG) is characterized histologically by sclerosis affecting some but not all glomeruli and involving only segments of each glomerulus. This histologic picture is often associated with the nephrotic syndrome and can occur (1) in association with other known conditions, such as HIV infection heroin addiction (HIV nephropathy, heroin addiction nephropathy); (2) as a secondary event in other forms of GN (e.g., IgA nephropathy); (3) as a component of glomerular ablation nephropathy (described earlier); (4) in an inherited congenital form resulting from mutations in cytoskeletal genes expressed in podocytes; or (5) as a primary disease.

Primary (or idiopathic) FSG accounts for approximately 10% of all cases of the nephrotic syndrome. It is becoming an increasingly common cause of nephrotic syndrome in adults and remains a frequent cause in children. *In children it is important to distinguish this cause of the nephrotic syndrome from minimal change disease (lipoid nephrosis),* because the clinical courses are markedly different. Unlike the case with minimal change disease, patients with this lesion have a higher incidence of hematuria and hypertension, their proteinuria is nonselective, and in general their response to corticosteroid therapy is poor. At least 50% of patients develop end-stage renal failure within 10 years of diagnosis. Adults in general fare even less well than children.

Pathogenesis. The pathogenesis of primary FSG is unknown. Some investigators have suggested that FSG is a variant, albeit an aggressive one, of minimal change disease. Others believe it to be a distinct clinicopathologic entity. In any case, *injury to the visceral epithelial cells and the resultant disruption of visceral epithelial cells is*

thought to represent the hallmark of FSG. As with minimal change disease, circulating permeability-increasing factors are implicated. The hyalinosis and sclerosis represent the entrapment of plasma proteins and lipids in hyperpermeable foci and the mesangial cell reaction to such proteins and to fibrin deposits. IgM and complement proteins seen in the lesion are also believed to result from nonspecific insudation and entrapment in damaged glomeruli. The recurrence of proteinuria in patients with focal sclerosis who receive renal allografts, sometimes within 24 hours of transplantation, supports the idea that a circulating mediator is the cause of the epithelial damage.

MORPHOLOGY

The disease first affects only some of the glomeruli (hence the term "focal") and initially only the juxtamedullary glomeruli. With progression, eventually all levels of the cortex are affected. Histologically, FSG is characterized by lesions occurring in some tufts within a glomerulus and sparing of the others (hence the term "segmental"). Thus, the involvement is both focal and segmental (Fig. 14-7). The lesions exhibit increased mesangial matrix, collapsed basement membranes, and deposition of hyaline masses (hyalinosis) and lipid droplets. Occasionally, glomeruli are completely sclerosed (global sclerosis). In affected glomeruli, immunofluorescence microscopy reveals deposits of immunoglobulins, usually IgM, and complement in the areas of hyalinosis. On electron microscopy, the visceral epithelial cells exhibit loss of foot processes, as in lipoid nephrosis, but also a **greater degree of epithelial cell detachment** with denudation of the underlying GBM.

In time, progression of the disease leads to global sclerosis of the glomeruli with pronounced

Figure 14-7

High-power view of focal segmental glomerulosclerosis (PAS stain), seen as a hyaline mass that has replaced a portion of the glomerulus. (Courtesy of Dr. H. Rennke, Department of Pathology, Brigham and Women's Hospital, Boston.)

[handwritten notes at top of page]
- hyalinosis, sclerosis, lipid droplets
- poor prognosis... 50% renal failure

tubular atrophy and interstitial fibrosis. This advanced picture is difficult to differentiate from other forms of chronic GN, described later.

A morphologic variant called **collapsing FSG** is being increasingly reported. It is characterized by collapse and sclerosis of the entire glomerular tuft. This is a more severe disease that may be idiopathic or, more commonly, the form associated with HIV infection. It carries a particularly poor prognosis.

There is little tendency for spontaneous remission of idiopathic FSG, and responses to corticosteroid therapy are poor. Progression to renal failure occurs at varying rates, and about 50% of patients suffer renal failure after 10 years.

MEMBRANOPROLIFERATIVE GLOMERULONEPHRITIS

Membranoproliferative GN (MPGN) is manifested histologically by alterations in the basement membrane and mesangium and by proliferation of glomerular cells. It accounts for 5% to 10% of cases of idiopathic nephrotic syndrome in children and adults. Some patients present only

with hematuria or proteinuria in the non-nephrotic range; others have a combined nephrotic-nephritic picture. Two major types of MPGN (I and II) are recognized on the basis of distinct ultrastructural, immunofluorescence microscopic, and pathogenic findings.

MORPHOLOGY

By light microscopy, both types are similar. The glomeruli are large and show proliferation of mesangial cells as well as infiltrating leukocytes (Fig. 14–8A). They have a lobular appearance. The GBM is thickened, and the glomerular capillary wall often shows a double contour or "tram track" appearance, especially evident in silver or periodic acid–Schiff (PAS) stains. This is caused by "splitting" of the GBM due to the inclusion within it of processes of mesangial and inflammatory cells extending into the peripheral capillary loops (Fig. 14–8B).

Types I and II have different ultrastructural and immunofluorescence microscopy features (see Fig. 14–8B). **Type I MPGN** (two thirds of cases) is characterized by subendothelial electron-dense deposits. By immunofluorescence microscopy, C3 is deposited in a granular pattern and IgG and early

[handwritten notes]
- MPGN → BM thickening, mesangial cell prolif., leukocyte infilt.
- Type 1
  - subendothelial deposits
  - caused by circ. immune complexes
  - poor prog.
  - ideopathic ass. w/ Hep C
- Type 2
  - intramembranous dep.
  - C3 Nef → activates alt. pathway → leads to hypocomplementemia
  - worse than poor

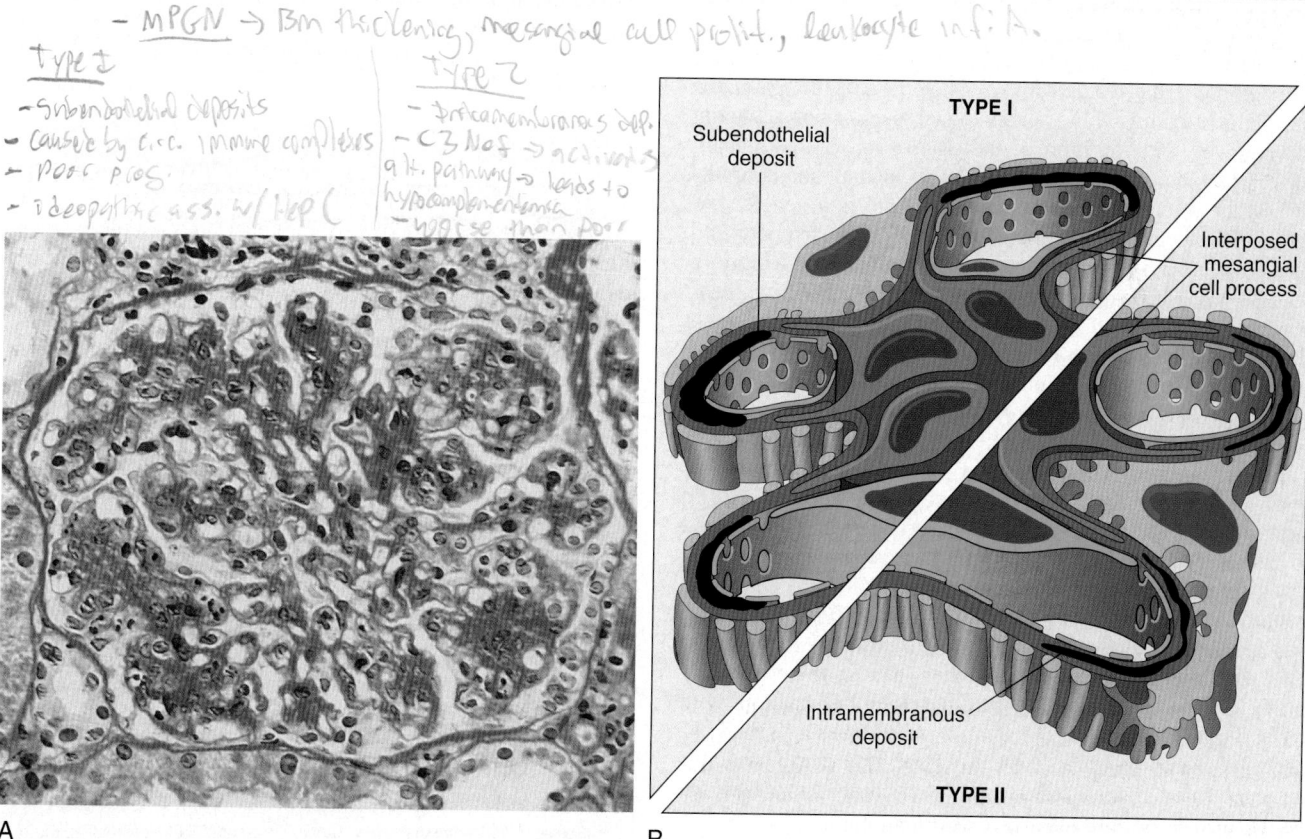

Figure 14–8

A, Membranoproliferative glomerulonephritis, showing mesangial cell proliferation, basement membrane thickening, leukocyte infiltration, and accentuation of lobular architecture. *B,* Schematic representation of patterns in the two types of membranoproliferative glomerulonephritis. In type I there are subendothelial deposits; type II is characterized by intramembranous dense deposits (dense deposit disease). In both, mesangial interposition gives the appearance of split basement membranes when viewed in the light microscope.

[handwritten notes at top of page: Nephritic Syndrome → hematuria, oliguria & azotemia & hta - lesions from prolif. of cells in glomeruli w/ leukocytic infiltrate → injures cap walls→ RBC escape to urine → also ↓GFR→ oliguria + az.]

complement components (C1q and C4) are often also present, suggesting an immune complex pathogenesis.

In **type II lesions,** the lamina densa and the subendothelial space of the GBM are transformed into an irregular, ribbon-like, extremely electron-dense structure, owing to the deposition of material of unknown composition, giving rise to the term **dense deposit disease.** C3 is present in irregular granular-linear foci in the basement membranes and mesangium in characteristic circular aggregates (mesangial rings). IgG is usually absent, as are the early-acting complement components (C1q and C4).

Pathogenesis. Although there is considerable overlap, different pathogenic mechanisms are involved in the development of type I and type II disease. Most cases of type I MPGN appear to be caused by circulating immune complexes, akin to chronic serum sickness, but the inciting antigen is not known. Type I MPGN also occurs in association with hepatitis B and C antigenemia, SLE, infected atrioventricular shunts, and secondary infections with persistent or episodic antigenemia. The pathogenesis of type II MPGN is less clear. The serum of patients with type II MPGN has a factor called *C3 nephritic factor* (C3NeF), which can activate the alternative complement pathway. This factor is an immunoglobulin that reacts with C3 convertase of the alternative complement pathway and serves to stabilize it, thus activating the pathway and resulting in the elaboration of biologically active complement fragments. C3NeF is thus an autoantibody, and, as in other autoimmune diseases, there is a genetic predisposition to the development of MPGN. The hypocomplementemia, more marked in type II, is produced in part by excessive consumption of C3 and in part by reduced synthesis of C3 by the liver. It is still not clear how the complement abnormality induces the glomerular changes.

Clinical Course. The principal mode of presentation (in ~50% of cases) is the nephrotic syndrome, although MPGN may begin as acute nephritis or more insidiously as mild proteinuria. The prognosis of MPGN is uniformly poor. In one study, none of 60 patients followed for 1 to 20 years showed complete remission. Forty percent progressed to end-stage renal failure, 30% had variable degrees of renal insufficiency, and the remaining 30% had persistent nephrotic syndrome without renal failure. Type II disease has a worse prognosis, and it tends to recur in renal transplant recipients. Like many other glomerulonephritides, MPGN, usually of type I, may occur in association with other known disorders *(secondary MPGN),* such as SLE, hepatitis B and C, chronic liver disease, and chronic bacterial infections. Indeed, many so-called idiopathic cases are believed to be associated with hepatitis C.

THE NEPHRITIC SYNDROME

The nephritic syndrome is a clinical complex, usually of acute onset, characterized by (1) *hematuria* with dysmorphic red cells and red blood cell casts in the urine, (2)

some degree of *oliguria* and azotemia, and (3) *hypertension.* Although there may also be some proteinuria and even edema, these are usually not sufficiently marked to cause the nephrotic syndrome. The lesions that cause the nephritic syndrome have in common proliferation of the cells within the glomeruli, accompanied by a leukocytic infiltrate. This inflammatory reaction injures the capillary walls, permitting escape of red cells into the urine, and induces hemodynamic changes that lead to a reduction in the GFR. The reduced GFR is manifested clinically by oliguria, reciprocal fluid retention, and azotemia. Hypertension is probably a result of both the fluid retention and some augmented renin release from the ischemic kidneys.

The acute nephritic syndrome may be produced by systemic disorders such as SLE, or it may be the result of primary glomerular disease. The latter is exemplified by acute diffuse proliferative GN.

Acute Proliferative (Poststreptococcal, Postinfectious) Glomerulonephritis

Diffuse proliferative GN (PGN), one of the more frequent of the glomerular disorders, is typically caused by immune complexes. The inciting antigen may be exogenous or endogenous. The prototype exogenous pattern is postinfectious GN, whereas that produced by an endogenous antigen is lupus nephritis, seen in SLE (Chapter 5). Infections by organisms other than the streptococci may also be associated with diffuse PGN. These include certain pneumococcal and staphylococcal infections as well as a number of common viral diseases such as mumps, measles, chickenpox, and hepatitis B and C.

The classic case of poststreptococcal GN develops in a child 1 to 4 weeks after the patient recovers from a group A streptococcal infection. Only certain "nephritogenic" strains of the β-hemolytic streptococci are capable of evoking glomerular disease. In most cases the initial infection is localized to the pharynx or skin.

Pathogenesis. It is generally agreed that immune complex formation is involved in the pathogenesis of acute poststreptococcal GN. *Typical features of immune complex disease, such as hypocomplementemia and granular deposits of IgG and complement on the GBM,* are seen. Nevertheless, the nature of the pathogenic antigen remains mysterious, and it is not clear whether circulating complexes or those formed in situ are the predominant forms. Studies indicate that C3 is deposited on the GBM before IgG deposition; hence, the primary injury might be by complement activation. Eventually, immune complexes are formed. The implicated antigens seem to be endostreptosin and nephritis–plasmin-binding protein.

MORPHOLOGY

Under the light microscope, the most characteristic change is a fairly uniformly increased cellularity of the glomerular tufts that affects nearly all glomeruli, hence the term "diffuse" (Fig. 14–9A). The increased cellularity is caused both by proliferation and swelling of endothelial and mesangial cells and by a neutrophilic and monocytic infiltrate. Sometimes

IO N

exogenous Ag → poststreptococcal (strep) → devlps weeks after step A inf.
endogenous Ag → lupus nephritis   immune complex formation → hypocomplementemia, granular dep of IgG & complement
→ ↑ cellularity b/c ↑ prolif. of glomeruli   Ags → endostreptosin &   nephritis - plasma binding protein
+ leuk. infil.

Chapter 14   THE KIDNEY AND ITS COLLECTING SYSTEM   ■   **523**

Figure 14–9

Poststreptococcal glomerulonephritis. *A,* Glomerular hypercellularity is caused by intracapillary leukocytes and proliferation of intrinsic glomerular cells. Note the red cell casts in the tubules. *B,* Typical electron-dense subepithelial "hump" and intramembranous deposits *(arrow).* BM, basement membrane; CL, capillary lumen; E, endothelial cell; Ep, epithelial cells.

RPGN → rapid & progressive loss of renal fxn
~ crescents present in glomeruli from
prolif. of parietal epithe

there are thrombi within the capillary lumina and necrosis of the capillary walls. In a few cases there may also be "crescents" (described next) inside Bowman's capsule. In general, these findings are ominous. When they involve most of the glomeruli, the pattern merges with that of rapidly progressive GN (see later). The electron microscope shows the immune complexes arrayed as subendothelial, intramembranous, or often subepithelial "humps" nestled against the GBM (Fig. 14–9B). Immunofluorescence studies reveal IgG and complement within the deposits. These deposits are usually cleared over a period of about 2 months.

Clinical Course. The onset of the kidney disease tends to be abrupt, heralded by malaise, a slight fever, nausea, and the nephritic syndrome. In the usual case, oliguria, azotemia, and hypertension are only mild to moderate. Characteristically, there is gross hematuria, the urine appearing smoky brown rather than bright red. Some proteinuria is a constant feature of the disease, and as mentioned earlier it may occasionally be severe enough to produce the nephrotic syndrome. Serum complement levels are low during the active phase of the disease, and serum antistreptolysin O titers are elevated in poststreptococcal cases.

Recovery occurs in most children in epidemic cases. Some children develop rapidly progressive GN or chronic renal disease. The prognosis in sporadic cases is less clear. In adults, 15% to 50% of patients develop end-stage renal disease over the ensuing few years or 1 to 2 decades, depending on the clinical and histologic severity. In contrast, the prevalence of chronicity after sporadic cases of acute GN in children is much lower.

Rapidly Progressive (Crescentic) Glomerulonephritis

Rapidly progressive glomerulonephritis (RPGN) is a clinical syndrome and not a specific etiologic form of GN. Clinically, it is characterized by rapid and progressive loss of renal function associated with severe oliguria and (if untreated) death from renal failure within weeks to months. *Regardless of the cause, the histologic picture is characterized by the presence of crescents in most of the glomeruli* (crescentic GN). These are produced in part by proliferation of the parietal epithelial cells of Bowman's capsule and in part by infiltration of monocytes and macrophages.

Pathogenesis. Crescentic glomerulonephritis (CrGN) may be caused by a number of different diseases, some restricted to the kidney and others systemic. Although no single mechanism can explain all cases, there is little doubt that in most cases the glomerular injury is immunologically mediated. Thus, a practical classification divides CrGN into three groups on the basis of immunologic findings (Table 14–3). In each group, the disease may be associated with a known disorder or it may be idiopathic.

Type I CrGN is best remembered as *anti-GBM disease* and hence is characterized by linear deposits of IgG and, in many cases, C3 on the GBM, as previously described. In some of these patients the anti-GBM antibodies also bind to pulmonary alveolar capillary basement membranes to produce the clinical picture of pulmonary hemorrhages associated with renal failure. These patients are said to have *Goodpasture syndrome,* to distinguish their condition from so-called idiopathic cases in which renal involvement occurs in the absence of pulmonary disease. Anti-GBM antibodies are present in the serum and are helpful in diagnosis. It is important to recognize type I CrGN, because these patients benefit from plasmapheresis, which removes pathogenic antibodies from the circulation.

→ ↓ prev chronicity   ~ constitutional symptoms &
in children   nephrotic syndrome

→ smoky brown urine from hematuria

Table 14-3. CRESCENTIC GLOMERULONEPHRITIS (CrGN)

Type I CrGN (Anti-GBM) *— linear dep. of IgE & C3*
Idiopathic *— helped by plasmaphorosis*
Goodpasture syndrome

Type II CrGN (Immune Complex) *— "lumpy bumpy" granular ptn*
Idiopathic *— not helped by plasmaphorosis*
Systemic lupus erythematosus
Postinfectious
Henoch-Schönlein purpura

Type III CrGN (Pauci-immune) ANCA-Associated
Idiopathic *— ANCA in serum → vasculitis*
Wegener granulomatosis
Microscopic polyarteritis

ANCA, antineutrophil cytoplasmic antibody.

Type II CrGN is an *immune complex–mediated disorder.* It can be a complication of any of the immune complex nephritides, including poststreptococcal GN, SLE, IgA nephropathy, and Henoch-Schönlein purpura. In some cases, immune complexes can be demonstrated but the underlying cause is undetermined. In all of these cases, immunofluorescence studies reveal the characteristic granular ("lumpy bumpy") pattern of staining. These patients cannot usually be helped by plasmapheresis, and they require treatment for the underlying disease.

Type III CrGN, also called *pauci-immune type CrGN*, is defined by the lack of anti-GBM antibodies or immune complexes by immunofluorescence and electron microscopy. Most of these patients have antineutrophil cytoplasm antibodies (ANCA) in the serum, which, as we have seen (Chapter 10), play a role in some vasculitides. Therefore, in some cases type III CrGN is a component of a systemic vasculitis such as microscopic polyarteritis nodosa or Wegener granulomatosis. In many cases, however, pauci-immune CrGN is limited to the kidney and is thus called idiopathic.

It should be obvious from this discussion that although all three types of CrGN may be associated with a well-defined renal or extrarenal disease, in some cases CrGN is idiopathic. When the cause can be identified, about 12% of patients have anti-GBM disease (type I CrGN) with or without lung involvement; 44% have type II CrGN; and the remaining 44% have pauci-immune type III CrGN. All have severe glomerular injury.

MORPHOLOGY

The kidneys are enlarged and pale, often with petechial hemorrhages on the cortical surfaces. Depending on the stage of the underlying disease, the glomeruli may show focal necrosis and thrombosis, diffuse or focal endothelial proliferation, and mesangial proliferation. However, the histologic picture is dominated by the formation of distinctive crescents (Fig. 14-10). Crescents are formed by proliferation of parietal cells and by migration of

Figure 14-10 ■

Crescentic glomerulonephritis. (PAS stain.) Note the collapsed glomerular tufts and the crescent-shaped mass of proliferating cells and leukocytes internal to Bowman's capsule. (Courtesy of Dr. M. A. Venkatachalam, Department of Pathology, University of Texas Health Sciences Center, San Antonio, TX.)

monocytes into Bowman's space, sometimes with multinucleated giant cells. T cells are also found in the crescents and Bowman's space. In the pauci-immune type they are believed to play a role in recruiting macrophages to the glomerulus. The crescents eventually obliterate Bowman's space and compress the glomeruli. Fibrin strands are prominent between the cellular layers in the crescents. Electron microscopy may disclose subepithelial deposits in some cases, as expected, but in all cases it shows distinct ruptures in the GBM. In time, crescents may undergo scarring.

— more pronounced
— prog. related to # of crescents

Clinical Course. The onset of RPGN is much like that of the nephritic syndrome except that the oliguria and azotemia are more pronounced. Proteinuria sometimes approaching nephrotic range may occur. Some of these patients become anuric and require long-term dialysis or transplantation. The prognosis can be roughly related to the number of crescents: patients with crescents in less than 80% of the glomeruli have a slightly better prognosis than those with higher percentages of crescents. Plasma exchange benefits some patients, particularly those with anti-GBM disease and Goodpasture syndrome.

IgA Nephropathy (Berger Disease)

This condition usually affects children and young adults and begins as an episode of gross hematuria that occurs within 1 or 2 days of a nonspecific upper respiratory tract infection. Typically, the hematuria lasts several days and then subsides, only to recur every few months. It is often associated with loin pain. *IgA nephropathy is one of the most common causes of recurrent microscopic or gross hematuria and is the most common glomerular disease worldwide.*

The pathogenic hallmark is the deposition of IgA in the mesangium. Some have considered Berger disease to be a

r.) Postoperatively, the infant is observed
of increased ICP, infection, bowel and blad-
nd movement of extremities. Prognosis is
ding on the location and severity of the

siderations

rotect the integrity of the sac until surgical
be completed. This is done by wearing
d using sterile linens to cover the defect.
ng the sac are kept moist with saline. The
ositioned so as not to exert pressure on the
gure 15-8C). A prone position is typically
must monitor carefully for symptoms of
fant should be kept warm. An isolette is
id placing heavy covers over the sac.
e and tactile stimulation are still vital for
rage parents to hold their baby's hand and
or her. For feeding, the baby may need to
arent's lap in a prone position with the
e side. Parents will need assistance from
plish feeding because the baby cannot be
ling positions.
the nurse will observe the child for signs
es in vital signs, and neurologic changes.
losely to prevent breakdown from bony
pelvis as the child lies in the prone posi-
hild's position to side-lying or hold the
ve range-of-motion exercises are impor-
tractures. The nurse should observe the
d bowel retention because this disorder
loss and loss of sphincter control. Older
ents with spina bifida will be taught to
ittent catheterization to maintain uri-
r defects are present.

alus

s from increased production, decreased
e of the flow of CSF. Blockage can be
pathologies, including infections, ven-
s, tumors, cysts, or malformations
rmations include:

n (downward displacement of the
m, and fourth ventricle, along with
he foramen magnum into the cervi-

uct of Sylvius, a recessive X-linked

me (a disruption of fetal brain devel-
fourth ventricle enlarges into a
e seen in Figure 15-12.

A

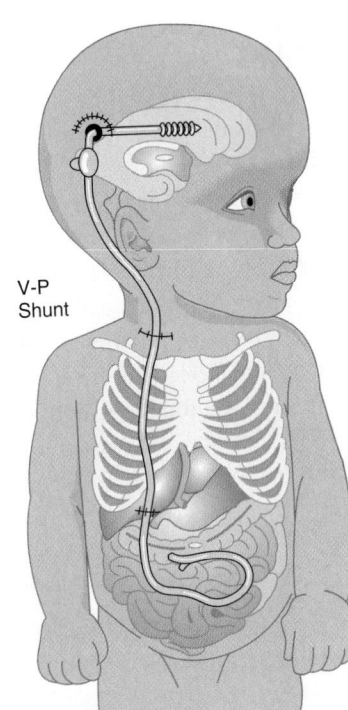

B

Figure 15-9. ■ (**A**) Infant with hydrocephalus. (**B**) A ventriculoperitoneal shunt, which allows fluid to leave the cranial cavity
and so reduces intracranial pressure, is usually placed at 3 to
4 months of age.

V-P
Shunt

Manifestations

Sometimes hydrocephalus is obvious at birth, but more
commonly it develops over time. The classic symptoms of
hydrocephalus include the child's head circumference
being greater than normal, with the forehead and top of

PHYSICAL

Infants

- Measure head circumference. Compare the measurements with the normal range for the age of the child.
- Palpate the spine for intactness.

- Observe the infant's posture.
- Test the infant's reflexes and reaction to stimuli.
  See Procedure 8-13, Eliciting Newborn
  Reflexes ⚌.
- Assess level of consciousness; the Glasgow Coma Scale
  can be used. See Procedure 15-1 ■.

PROCEDURE 15-1   Glasgow Coma Scale

Purpose

- To provide a score related to level of consciousness
- To allow health care providers a benchmark assessment that
  will allow them to document either improvement or
  deterioration of the child's neurologic condition

Equipment

- Glasgow Coma Scale (Table 15-1 ■)

Check order + Gather equipment + Introduce yourself + Identify client + Provide privacy + Explain procedure + Hand hygiene + Gloves as needed

Interventions and Rationales

1. Perform preparatory steps (see icon bar above).
2. Use the Glasgow Coma Scale to assess the child with a
   neurologic injury or disorder. Assign a score, based on
   the criteria outlined, for eye opening, verbal response,
   and motor response.
3. A total score of 15 indicates adequate neurologic
   function. A total score of 3 indicates neurologic
   unresponsiveness.
4. Document results and report scores below 15 to the
   charge nurse.
5. Repeat the Glasgow Coma Scale as necessary.

SAMPLE DOCUMENTATION

(date) 1500   4-year-old-male admitted to
               pediatric intensive care following
               closed head injury due to 6-foot
               fall from tree as reported by
               father. Glasgow Coma Scale
               score 5. Score reported to
               charge nurse. _____
               R. Roberts, LPN.

TABLE 15-1

Glasgow Coma Scale

FACULTY MEASURED	RESPONSE	SCORE
Eye opening	Spontaneous	4
	To verbal command	3
	To pain	2
	No response	1
Motor response	To verbal command	6
	To localized pain	5
	Flexes and withdraws	4
	Flexes abnormally	3
	Extends abnormally	2
	No response	1
Verbal response	Oriented, converses	5
	Disoriented, converses	4
	Uses inappropriate words	3
	Makes incomprehensible sounds	2
	No response	1

Note: 15 points = alert and oriented; 8 or less = comatose; totally
unresponsive = 3.

Toddlers, Preschoolers, School-Age Children, and Adolescents

- Note general behavior, such as responsiveness and activity level. (See more about behavior and thought process disorders in Chapter 16 ⚯.)
- Test balance, coordination, and accuracy related to motor skills.
- Assess sensations of touch, temperature, and pain.
- Assess deep tendon reflexes.
- Assess the child's short- and long-term memory.
- Observe for any signs of abuse. Suspected abuse should be reported to the charge nurse. (See legal information in Chapter 3 and discussion of abuse in Chapter 16 ⚯.)

Pain

PHYSIOLOGY

Pain in children can be a result of ischemia, tissue pressure, injury, or tension created by air or fluid filling a body cavity. A pain impulse stimulates the nociceptor, causing *transduction* of pain sensation. The **nociceptors** are sensory receptors that detect and differentiate pain sensation. Following transduction, the pain impulse is transmitted along peripheral sensory nerves to the spinal cord and brain.

PERCEPTION

Pain perception occurs as the pain impulse reaches the brain. Depending on which sensory receptor is stimulated, the child may perceive dull, burning, sharp, localized, cutaneous, somatic, visceral, or chronic pain. The child may express the pain verbally or nonverbally. Verbal expressions of pain include crying, moaning, groaning, or screaming. Nonverbal expressions of pain include facial grimacing, posturing, splinting, restlessness, and sleep disturbances. Box 15-3 ■ provides one mnemonic for assessing pain. See the Pain Assessment section of Chapter 8 ⚯ for more nursing information about assessing the child in pain.

PAIN THEORIES

The gate control theory (Figure 15-7 ■), developed by Melzack and Wall in 1965, is the most commonly used theory of pain and pain management. The gate control theory

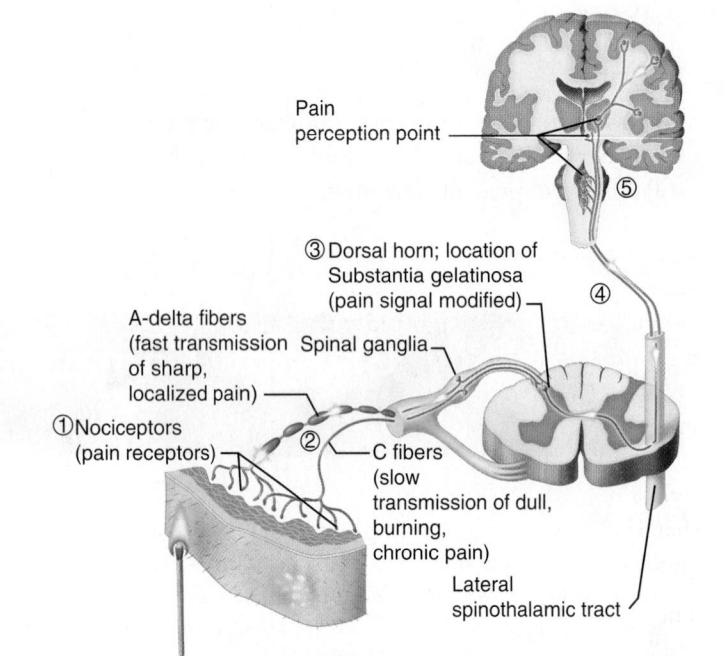

Figure 15-7. ■ In the gate control theory of pain, (1) nerve endings (*nociceptors*) transmit information about injury to the spinal cord via specialized nerve fibers. Biochemical mediators activate the nerve response or sensitize nerve endings. C fibers slowly transmit dull, burning, diffuse, or chronic pain. (2) A-delta fibers quickly transmit sharp, well-localized pain. (3) Depending on other stimuli, the pain signal may be modified at the dorsal horn of the spinal cord (*lower right*). (4) The pain signal is then transmitted to the brain, where perception occurs. (5) At the brain, emotional responses may increase or decrease the intensity of the pain perceived.

proposes that certain actions, if employed, can block pain transduction at the spinal cord before it reaches the brain. These behaviors include touch, distraction, and breathing and relaxation techniques. These are considered nonpharmacologic approaches to pain management.

PAIN MANAGEMENT

Treatment of Pain

The pharmacologic management of pain includes the use of narcotic and nonnarcotic medication. (Refer to Chapter 8 ⚯ for discussion of pain as the "fifth vital sign" and for pain assessment, Procedure 8-6 ⚯.) When possible, the oral route of administration is preferred for children. Careful dosage

---

BOX 15-3 **ASSESSMENT**

Pain in Children

Here is a quick way to remember how to assess for pain in children. Use the abbreviation PQRST:

- **P** Precipitating Factors—What caused the pain?
- **Q** Quality and Quantity—Describe the pain. Is it steady, or does it come and go?
- **R** Region, Radiation, and Related Symptoms—Describe the exact location of the pain. Does it radiate to other

parts of the body? What symptoms are associated with the pain?
- **S** Severity—Rate the pain as to its impact (e.g., Can you walk during the pain? Can you continue talking during the pain?).
- **T** Timing—What time of the day or night does the pain occur? Does it occur every day? Is it associated with other activities, such as breathing, lying down, or walking?

---

calculation is essential in preventing an overdose. If narcotics are used, monitoring the respiratory status is vital because narcotics can depress respiration. Narcotics are usually held if the respiratory is 12 or less. In cases of severe or prolonged pain, a PCA pump may be used (see Figure 7-11 ⚯).

Other nonpharmacologic nursing measures may be effective in the control of pain or enhance the use of pharmacologic methods. Distraction or involving the child in other activities and play can reduce anxiety and the awareness of pain. Massaging or rubbing the area of pain, or rocking and

CONGENITAL NEUROLOGIC DEF[...]

Congenital neurologic defects can have a profound impact on quality of life. Defects vary from spina bifida to Down syndrome (discussed later in this chapter under Mental Retardation).

Spina Bifida

Spina bifida is an incomplete closure of the vertebra and **neural tube** (the fetal tissue that develops into the CNS). The cause of spina bifida is a genetic predisposition with a deficiency of the essential nutrient folic acid. If spina bifida exists, there is a high probability of other congenital defects, including clubfoot, hip defects, and hydrocephalus. The defect can be found anywhere along the spinal column and results in a variety of pathologies. Most commonly, the defect is located in the lumbosacral region. Defects affecting only the vertebrae may not be obvious until the toddler tries to walk.

In larger defects, meningocele or meningomyelocele may result. **Meningocele** is the herniation of the meninges through the vertebral defect. **Myelomeningocele** is a

Figure 15-8. ■ (**A**) Meningocele. A saclike protrusion through the bony defe[ct] brospinal fluid. Sac may be transparent or membranous. (**B**) Myelomeningoc[ele] cerebrospinal fluid, and a portion of spinal cord or nerve root. Fluid leakage [...] defect is more common than the meningocele; 99% of children with this def[ect] placed prone or in a side-lying position, and the exposed sac is protected ca[...]

A Meningocele   B Myelomeningocele

---

in this chapte[...]
closely for sign[...]
der function, a[...]
variable, depe[...]
defect.

Nursing Co[...]

It is critical to p[...]
correction can [...]
sterile gloves ar[...]
The linens cover[...]
infant must be p[...]
meninges (see F[...]
used. The nurse[...]
infection. The in[...]
appropriate to av[...]
Emotional care[...]
this infant. Encou[...]
talk gently to him[...]
be placed on the [...]
head turned to or[...]
the nurse to accom[...]
held in typical fee[...]
Postoperatively[...]
of infection, chang[...]
Observe the skin [...]
prominences of the[...]
tion. Change the c[...]
child upright. Pass[...]
tant to prevent con[...]
infant for urinary a[...]
often causes sensory[...]
children and adolesc[...]
perform clean intern[...]
nary health if bladde[...]

herniation of [...]
meninges, th[...]
The outer cov[...]
parent, fragile[...]
are affected, [...]
der incontin[...]

Diagnosi[...]

During preg[...]
between 16 [...]
cate the pre[...]
confirmed [...]
After birth [...]
can determ[...]
other orga[...]

Treatm[...]

Surgical [...]
as possi[...]
placed a[...]

Hydroceph[...]

Hydrocephalus result[...]
absorption, or blocka[...]
caused by a variety of[...]
tricular hemorrhag[...]
(Figure 15-9 ■). Malf[...]

- *Chiari II malformati[...]* cerebellum, brainst[...] herniation through [...] cal spaces)
- Stenosis of the aquee[...] disorder
- *Dandy-Walker syndro[...]* opment in which the[...] cyst). Ventricles can [...]

the head being out of proportion to the face. The anterior fontanel bulges with the increasing ICP. The sclera of the eyes often can be seen above the iris, giving a "setting sun" appearance to the eyes. The child may be irritable or lethargic and experience nausea and vomiting because of increased ICP.

Diagnosis

Head circumference is monitored daily in the hospital setting. Increasing circumference may be indicative of hydrocephalus. In infants, prior to closure of the fontanels, an ultrasound can be used to diagnose the condition. In the older child, CT scans and MRIs are used.

Treatment

Surgical placement of a ventriculoperitoneal shunt can relieve the increasing ICP. As the child grows, a longer shunt may need to replace the initial shunt. If the blockage is caused by a tumor or cyst, surgical removal of the growth may correct the hydrocephalus.

Nursing Considerations

Nursing strategies for the child with hydrocephalus include measuring the child's head circumference regularly (see Procedure 8-10 ⬯). Before and after corrective surgery, the child must be monitored for symptoms of increased ICP. The nurse must carefully support the head when transferring the infant to avoid strain on the neck muscles.

Because the skin of the cranium is stretched and thin in hydrocephalus, the nurse should handle the infant gently and be careful to prevent skin breakdown on the cranium. Vomiting due to increased ICP is common with hydrocephalus, so feedings should be frequent and small in amount.

clinical ALERT

In the immediate postoperative period, the infant will need to lie flat to prevent rapid CSF drainage. The supine position is best with the head of the bed lowered. The head of the bed can be slowly raised in the absence of symptoms of increased ICP. Proper positioning should prevent tears in the cerebral arteries caused by rapid drainage of CSF. Assess for the return of bowel sounds, and avoid introducing fluids too quickly. This will prevent vomiting and the risk of increased ICP. ICP can also be increased while the child is straining for a bowel movement. Therefore, the nurse should assist with prevention of constipation by providing adequate fluids, administering stool softeners as ordered, and increasing activity in the absence of ICP.

Following shunt placement, there will be two surgical sites—most likely one behind the ear and one in the chest or abdomen. These sites need to be observed for integrity and signs of infection. Teach parents to avoid pressure on these incision sites and to prevent the child from "playing" with them.

Amyotrophic Lateral Sclerosis

Although rare in children, amyotrophic lateral sclerosis (ALS) may appear as a familial disorder linked to chromosome 21 defects. ALS (sometimes called *Lou Gehrig disease*) is a progressive, degenerative neurologic disease in which muscle weakness and wasting progress from the extremities to the core. In about 50% of cases, death results 2 to 5 years after the onset of symptoms, usually as a result of respiratory failure. In clients with such severe degenerative disorders, much special care is needed (see Health Promotion Issue on pages 392 and 393). Referrals are crucial for support for family and caregivers. Refer to a medical-surgical book for in-depth information on diagnosis and treatment.

NERVOUS SYSTEM DISORDERS

Seizures

Seizures are periods of sudden discharge of electrical activity in the brain that cause involuntary muscle activity, change in LOC, or altered behavior and sensory manifestation. Seizures may be the result of genetic factors; pathologic conditions such as tumors, trauma, infection, and toxins; or a rapid elevation in temperature above 102 °F (39 °C), called **febrile seizures**.

FEBRILE SEIZURES

A febrile seizure is a generalized seizure that usually occurs when a child's temperature rises rapidly to above 102 °F (39 °C). These seizures are most commonly associated with an illness. The seizures in children involve general **tonic-clonic movements** lasting less than 15 minutes (usually 1–2 minutes). Tonic-clonic movements are sustained contractions of skeletal muscles that occur involuntarily. These contractions are followed by the clonic phase where muscles contract and are followed by periods of relaxation. Respirations may be affected during tonic-clonic contractions. Rarely, the seizure may be complex, lasting longer than 15 minutes and recurring within 24 hours. In newborns, seizures may present as rhythmic repetitive movement of an extremity; repetitive blinking, lip smacking, sucking, tongue thrusting; or horizontal deviation of the eyes (Ball & Bindler, 2006).

Seizures are quite frightening to parents. Anticonvulsants may be prescribed to prevent recurrence of seizures

HEALTH PROMOTION ISSUE

AMYOTROPHIC LATERAL SCLEROSIS (ALS) IN A TEEN

Jamie, an 18-year-old Caucasian male, was diagnosed with amyotrophic lateral sclerosis (ALS) 3 years ago. His muscle weakness has progressively gotten worse until his speech, swallowing, chewing, and finally his breathing have all been affected. He has a feeding tube and is on continual oxygen. Jamie is in and out of the hospital frequently. His parents provide his care at home, although they have a home health nurse who provides a weekly assessment of his status. Jamie and his family developed a living will shortly after his initial diagnosis that includes Jamie's request not to be placed on a respirator should his breathing be compromised.

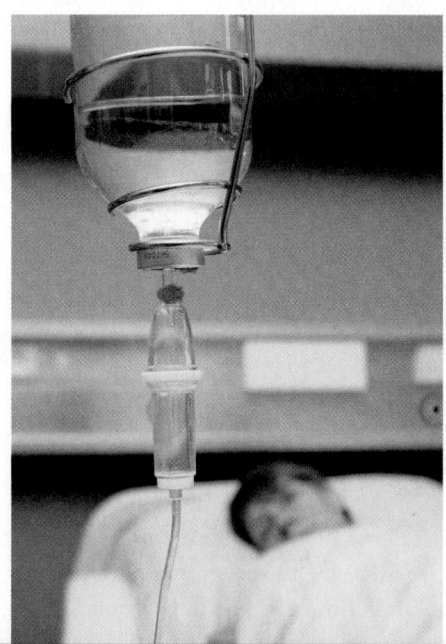

Jamie's physician discussed the rapid progression of his disease and encouraged the family to make some decisions about end-of-life care. The physician suggested contracting with a hospice agency to provide Jamie's care. After the physician leaves the exam room, Jamie's mother breaks down and sobs to the nurse. She states that she just cannot call hospice because that would mean she is giving up and will give Jamie the message that they have no hope. She also states that she does not know what hospice can do that she and her husband and the home health nurse are not already doing for Jamie.

DISCUSSION

Empowering the dying client by allowing a say in how and where death occurs can facilitate emotional acceptance of the eventual death. Because saying goodbye to a loved one is difficult, providing physical care to the dying client may become overwhelming to the caregivers. The answer for many clients and their families are health care agencies that focus on providing dignity in the last days by giving the client control and relieving stress on the family.

One agency that provides this type of care is the hospice agency. Hospice provides palliative nursing and medical care, including nutrition, comfort

measures, and pain management. The hospice caregiver also provides supportive social, emotional, and spiritual services. This care is most often given in the client's home. Care can be provided weekly, daily, or 24 hours/day. If the client has to be admitted to the hospital, the hospice caregiver is available to continue care during the time of hospitalization. In all states, it is required that the hospice agency be certified to provide health care services. Many state boards of health require that the agency also be licensed.

Hospice Services

A physician coordinates the care given to the client who has contracted the services of hospice. Registered nurses and licensed practical nurses provide hygiene, wound care, medication administration, nutritional support, pain management, and other services as necessary. A social worker may be assigned to assist the family in taking advantage of community resources. Aides or volunteers can assist the family with meal preparation, grooming, laundry services, running errands, car pooling, or babysitting. The agency may also offer physical, occupational, or speech therapies provided by a professional. Grief counseling is a standard of care for hospice agencies. The agencies assess the grief of the client and the family and continue this assessment

for the remainder of a febrile illness. However, the American Academy of Pediatrics (AAP, 1999; Millar, 2006) does not recommend long-term anticonvulsant therapy for febrile seizures. Instead, parents are taught methods of lowering fevers, such as administering nonaspirin antipyretic medication, dressing the child who

has fever in light clothing, and cooling the body with tepid compresses or baths. (*Note*: Alcohol compresses or baths are no longer recommended for use in children with high fevers.) Parents must also be taught safety measures to protect a child who is having a seizure (see Nursing Considerations section).

and care following the death of the client.

Costs

To be eligible for third-party reimbursement, a physician must provide documentation that the client may live less than 6 months. Medicare, Medicaid, and private health insurance policies can be used to pay for the services of hospice. Clients may also pay for the services, and hospice agencies frequently provide care free of charge when other resources are not available.

PLANNING AND IMPLEMENTATION

The nurse provides Jamie's mother with emotional comfort measures. She also uses therapeutic communication techniques to discover more about the feelings Jamie's mother has about his illness and probable death in the near future.

The nurse understands that in order for Jamie and his family to move to the acceptance phase of grief, they must acknowledge that Jamie's illness is incurable. The nurse also understands that Jamie's mom equates hospice care with Jamie's death. As long as Jamie

was receiving treatment, there was a shred of hope that a cure could be found.

The nurse also interviews Jamie's father and Jamie individually to ascertain their feelings regarding Jamie's illness, impending death, and hospice care. The nurse understands that in order for hospice care to be effective for the family, each member must believe that the care provided is necessary and can contribute to their well-being. The nurse asks Jamie and his parents for permission to tell them more about hospice. She also provides them with literature for further study. She has secured a list of clients within the practice who have benefited from hospice care. She encourages Jamie and his family to call these families to discuss their experiences with hospice.

The nurse schedules a home visit with Jamie and his family several days later to continue the discussion about hospice. During this visit, Jamie and his family tell the nurse they are ready to begin hospice care in their home. Jamie's mother thanks the nurse for helping them make the decision. She is especially grateful for the client referrals. She found them both helpful and encouraging.

The nurse and Jamie's family discuss the process for selecting a hospice agency. They call several agencies and set up in-home interviews.

In 1 week, the nurse telephones Jamie's family and learns that the hospice agency is already providing care, and that the family is quite satisfied with the care. In 1 month, Jamie dies at home in the presence of his family and the hospice nurse. Several weeks later, the nurse receives a thank-you note from the family expressing their gratefulness to the nurse for encouraging them to seek hospice care.

SELF-REFLECTION

Imagine that you have a terminal illness. What would be important to you related to your final days on earth? Where would you like to be? Who would you like to be around you? What type of care do you want to ensure that you have? What type of care do you want to avoid? Communicate these wishes and desires to a trusted individual or, better yet, record them officially in a living will.

SUGGESTED RESOURCES

For the Nurse

Acello, B. (2005). *The long-term care nursing desk reference.* Marblehead, MA: HCPro.

Addington-Hall, J., & Higginson, I. (Eds.). (2001). *Palliative care for non-cancer patient.* London: Oxford University Press.

For the Client

Marx, R., & Davidson, S. (2003). *Facing the ultimate loss: Coping with the death of a child.* Belgium, WI: Champion.

Rice, E. (Ed.). (2005). *If they could only hear me: A collection of personal stories about ALS and the families that have been affected.* Charleston, SC: BookSurge.

EPILEPSY

Epilepsy is a chronic disorder characterized by repeated seizure activity. **Status epilepticus** is a continuous seizure for more than 30 minutes accompanied by loss of consciousness. In status epilepticus, seizures can occur sequentially.

Manifestations

Partial or **focal seizures** are caused by abnormal electrical activity in a specific area of the brain, most commonly in the temporal, frontal, or parietal lobes of the cerebrum. Common symptoms include a momentary blank stare, facial movement, or report of hearing abnormal sounds. There is no loss of consciousness with focal seizures.

Generalized seizures result from diffuse electrical activity that begins in one area of the brain and spreads to involve the entire cerebral cortex and brainstem. General seizures begin with a tonic phase in which the child loses consciousness and has continuous muscle contractions. This is followed by a clonic phase characterized by alternating muscle contraction and relaxation. Some seizures are preceded by an **aura** (a recognizable sensation that signals a seizure is about to occur). A **postictal** period (period following a seizure) of confusion, sleepiness, slurred speech, poor coordination, or headache is common following a generalized seizure. Because of the limited communication ability of the infant, an aura may be impossible to detect. Older children, however, may be able to describe this activity in detail.

Diagnosis

Recognition of symptoms and a thorough health history assist in the diagnosis of epilepsy. Other tests may include complete blood counts, urine cultures and lumbar punctures if the seizure is accompanied by fever. CT scans and MRIs are not necessary for febrile seizures but may provide information about cerebral lesions in children with epilepsy. An electroencephalogram (EEG) is used to monitor brain wave activity and note changes.

Treatment

Anticonvulsants may be prescribed for the child to prevent further seizure activity (Table 15-2 ■). Depending on the cause and number of seizures, medication may be prescribed long term. It is important to administer medication on time to maintain therapeutic levels of medication. The child should be observed closely for repeated seizure activity until therapeutic levels of medications are established. Periodic or routine blood tests may be ordered to evaluate these therapeutic levels.

Nursing Considerations

Seizure precautions, including padding side rails and having suction equipment available, should be implemented for all children who have a history of seizures or who are at risk for seizures. These precautions will help prevent injury to the child during a seizure.

In the event of a seizure, the first priority is to establish a safe environment for the child. (Figure 15-10 ■). The child should not be restrained, but the head and extremities should be protected from hitting furniture, side rails, or the floor. Nothing should be put into the child's mouth during a seizure. Because the child does not breathe during the tonic phase of the seizure, circumoral cyanosis is common (LeMone & Burke, 2004). Where the seizure began, the specific movements or behavior, eye movements and pupil response as well as the length of the seizure should be documented.

TABLE 15-2				
Pharmacology: Drugs Used to Prevent Seizures				
DRUG (GENERIC AND COMMON BRAND NAME)	**USUAL ROUTE/DOSE**	**CLASSIFICATION AND PURPOSE**	**SELECTED SIDE EFFECTS**	**DON'T GIVE IF**
Phenytoin (Dilantin)	PO 15–20 mg/kg loading dose, then 5 mg/kg in two to three divided doses	Anticonvulsant for seizure prevention	Drowsiness, hypotension, gingival hyperplasia	Bradycardia
Carbamazepine (Tegretol)	Children less than 6 years: PO 10–35 mg/kg/day in three to four divided doses Children greater than 6–12 years: PO 100–800 mg/day in three to four divided doses	Anticonvulsant for seizure prevention	Leukopenia, vomiting, fatigue	Children less than 6 months
Phenobarbital (Barbital)	Neonate: PO or IV 3–4 mg/kg/day Child: PO or IV 3–8 mg/kg/day	Anticonvulsant for seizure prevention	Drowsiness, hypotension, vomiting	Serum concentration greater than 50 mcg/mL In liquid form, do not give without shaking bottle thoroughly. Shaking ensures accurate dosage

Figure 15-10. ■ A child who has a seizure when standing should be gently assisted to the floor and placed in a side-lying position. The area around the child should be cleared of any objects that might injure the child.

Immediately following the seizure, position the child on his or her side, remove mucus and drainage from the airway, and assess for airway patency. Oxygen may be needed if SpO_2 levels are less than 95%. The child may have been incontinent of urine and stool, so skin care may be needed. After the seizure, check neurologic function, including LOC, pupil response, equal bilateral movement and strength of extremities, and signs of injury if a fall occurred during the seizure. Remain with the child until consciousness returns and the airway is patent.

Seizure activity can be frightening for the parents and family. The nurse should remain calm during the child's seizure to inspire confidence and provide support to the family. Parents should be taught how to care for the child at home, during and after a seizure, as well as administration and side effects of medications. Parents, fearful for their child's safety, may become overprotective. With proper diagnosis and treatment, most children can have an active life. Parents should be encouraged to help their child reach developmental milestones.

Cerebral Palsy

Cerebral palsy (CP) is a motor disorder affecting motor function and posture. CP develops secondary to lesions or anomalies of the brain, hypoxic damage, or birth trauma to the motor center of the brain. The damage can occur during the prenatal, perinatal, or postnatal periods and up to 2 to 3 years of age. Neonatal infections (e.g., meningitis), as well as **kernicterus** (a toxic accumulation of bilirubin found in infants with hyperbilirubinemia), can result in CP. CP occurs more often in children born in the occipitoposterior position than in children born in the occipitoanterior position. CP occurs most frequently in very low-birth-weight and small-for-gestational-age infants. Some children may have a condition that mimics it (Box 15-4 ■).

Manifestations

Cerebral palsy is characterized by abnormal muscle tone and lack of coordination. Children with CP are frequently delayed in meeting growth and development milestones. Other neurologic problems may also be present, including hearing loss, visual defects such as nystagmus or strabismus, speech delay or impediment, seizures, or mental retardation.

Characteristic signs of CP, which may be present shortly after birth, include weak or absent sucking or swallowing, jitteriness, and slow or absent reflexes. Children with CP are at risk for notable delays in reaching developmental milestones. Infants may exhibit an abnormal or asymmetric crawl. Spastic movements may be noted. If the child learns to walk, a scissor gait and toe walking are common.

Diagnosis

Diagnosis of CP may require a longitudinal study of motor function and developmental delays. The physician may use electromyography and nerve conduction studies to document abnormal motor function. Intelligence testing may also be used to evaluate mental status. A number of diagnostic procedures and tests may be used to rule out other conditions that may cause symptoms similar to CP. These include ultrasound, MRI, CT scans, genetic testing, thyroid function studies, and ammonia levels.

Treatment

The focus of treatment for the child with CP is to improve motor function and communication skills. CP does not have a cure. Devices that assist with motor function, such as braces, walkers, and wheelchairs, enable the child to achieve a level of independence (Figure 15-11 ■). Physical, occupational, and speech therapists are used to assist the child.

Several surgical procedures may also be necessary to improve motor function in the child with CP. The Achilles tendon can be lengthened, the hamstring can be released, hip adduction can be improved, and the feet can be repositioned to improve the child's gait. Medications can also be administered to control muscle spasms and seizures (muscle relaxants and benzodiazepines) and to decrease gastrointestinal symptoms (H2 receptor antagonists). Box 15-5 ■ provides for more information on delivering baclofen (Lioresal) through an intrathecal pump.

Nursing Considerations

It is important for the nurse to teach the parents and family members how to care for the child with cerebral palsy. The child with CP will need long-term physical therapy to maintain joint mobility and prevent contractures. Parents should be referred to the appropriate resources to

Figure 15-11. ■ A child with cerebral palsy has abnormal muscle tone and lack of physical coordination. Muscles can be strengthened by periods of standing with support.

BOX 15-5 LIFE SPAN CONSIDERATIONS

Intrathecal Baclofen for Cerebral Palsy

Children with CP who weigh at least 30 pounds and are determined to be a low risk for surgical intervention may have an intrathecal baclofen pump inserted to reduce muscle hyperactivity. Baclofen blocks the neurotransmitters that cause the involuntary spasms and increased muscle tone associated with CP. Intrathecal baclofen is preferred to the oral route because direct administration to the spinal fluid decreases unwanted side effects of the medication.

Children who are deemed appropriate for this delivery method will have the medication injected into the spinal canal during a test dose to determine if this type of medication will assist them in reducing spastic movements. The child will be observed at least 8 to 10 hours. When effectiveness is determined, the child is scheduled for surgical implantation of the pump.

Younger children are most often given general anesthesia for the procedure. However, the older child and adolescent may only require local anesthesia. The pump is implanted into the abdomen with a catheter leading directly to the spinal canal. The pump is programmed to deliver a prescribed dosage of baclofen. The pump needs refilling and adjusting every 2 to 3 months. It will be replaced every 3 to 5 years at the end of the battery life (Stempien, 2000).

---

obtain adaptive appliances such as customized wheelchairs, braces, and eating utensils. Parents should be taught the importance of safety belts and helmets to prevent injury.

The child with CP may not be intellectually disabled. Use terminology for the developmental stage of the child. The nurse teaches the parents how to encourage and support the child in order to foster positive self-esteem. Because of the long-term nature of the disorder, the child and parents should be referred to appropriate counseling and support groups. Parents may need financial assistance to provide the needed care.

Fibromyalgia

Fibromyalgia is a disorder characterized by widespread musculoskeletal pain and fatigue. It may also be accompanied by irritable bowel syndrome, chronic headaches, temporomandibular joint dysfunction, PMS in the adolescent, skin sensitivities, and impaired coordination. The child with fibromyalgia will be treated for pain and fatigue. Exercise, such as water therapy, has been shown to be beneficial in assisting the child to manage clinical manifestations. The nurse can assist children and parents to modify the child's lifestyle to conserve energy and minimize pain.

NERVOUS SYSTEM INFECTIONS

Meningitis and Encephalitis

Meningitis illustrates an inflammation of the meninges by either a bacteria or a virus (Figure 15-12 ■). The majority of cases of meningitis in children occur before the age of 5 years. Bacterial meningitis is the more serious of the two types, causing neurologic damage and possible death. Causative agents of bacterial meningitis include *Haemophilus influenzae, Streptococcus pneumoniae* (causes pneumococcal meningitis), *Neisseria meningitidis* (causes meningococcal meningitis), and *Escherichia coli*. Viral meningitis can be caused by enterovirus, adenovirus, mumps, and arbovirus. See Chapter 10 ⃝⃝ for further discussion of communicable diseases.

Manifestations

Symptoms of bacterial or viral meningitis include fever, change in appetite, vomiting, and diarrhea. These may occur suddenly or progress over a week, depending on the causative organism. The child may be lethargic or extremely irritable. Rocking or cuddling, which usually calms the child, may make the child more irritable. The child may also have a headache, photophobia, nuchal rigidity, or a stiff neck. The child is comfortable only when lying on his or her side with the neck hyperextended and may have a positive Kernig's or Brudzinski's sign or both (Figure 15-13 ■). A hemorrhagic rash beginning as

A

B

Figure 15-12. ■ Central nervous system infections. Once bacteria reach the central nervous system, the pia mater, the arachnoid, and the cerebrospinal fluid–filled subarachnoid space all become infected. The cerebrospinal fluid (see *darkened arrows*) then circulates the pathogens throughout the brain and spinal cord.

C

Figure 15-13. ■ (**A**) The child with bacterial meningitis assumes an *opisthotonic* position (lying with the neck and head hyperextended) to relieve discomfort. (**B**) Kernig's and Brudzinski's signs are common findings in meningitis. To test for Kernig's sign, raise the child's leg with the knee flexed. Then extend the child's leg at the knee. If any resistance is noted or pain is felt, the result is a positive Kernig's sign. (**C**) To test Brudzinski's sign, flex the child's head while the child is supine. If this action makes the knees or hips flex involuntarily, a positive Brudzinski's sign is present.

TABLE 15-3	
Clinical Manifestations of Meningitis _Versus_ Encephalitis	
MENINGITIS	**ENCEPHALITIS**
Sudden onset	Sudden or gradual onset
Irritability or agitation	Malaise
Fever	Fever
Headache	Headache
Neck stiffness	Neck stiffness
Opisthotonos (back muscle spasms causing the back to arch)	Ataxia (uncoordinated movement)
Seizures (initial symptom)	Seizures (later symptom)
Joint pain seen in meningococcal and _H. influenzae_	
Fluid draining from ear seen in pneumococcal meningitis	
Petechial rash seen in meningococcal meningitis	

petechiae and progressing to larger lesions may be seen with meningococcal meningitis. Meningitis and encephalitis may sometimes be confused. Table 15-3 ■ compares and contrasts these two disorders.

Diagnosis

Meningitis is diagnosed primarily by evaluating CSF obtained from a lumbar puncture (see Procedure 8-20 ⬢). White blood cell counts will be elevated. Blood glucose can be decreased. Nose and throat cultures may also be obtained.

Treatment

Oral fluids are provided to the child with meningitis if the child is responsive and able to swallow. Otherwise, fluids may be given intravenously to prevent dehydration. Broad-spectrum antibiotics may also be administered intravenously until the bacterium is identified from the lumbar puncture.

To control the fever and alleviate pain, nonsteroidal anti-inflammatory drugs are administered. If the fever is extreme, tepid baths or a cooling blanket may be needed.

Parents should be encouraged to verbalize their feelings and concerns. Involving them in the care of their child can help relieve their fears. Because bacterial meningitis can damage the nervous system, long-term rehabilitation may be needed. Referral to social workers or clergy may be necessary for added support.

Nursing Considerations

The nurse will be responsible for frequent monitoring of vital signs and LOC. Measure and record head circumference daily because of the potential for increased ICP. The child with meningitis is at increased risk for seizures. See the previous section on the care of a child with seizures and epilepsy. Signs of sensory and/or movement deficiencies should be monitored. For example, the child may lose the ability to hold the bottle, drink, or manage oral secretions. The child could develop respiratory distress, including periods of apnea due to cerebral edema, electrolyte imbalances, or other neurologic changes.

The child with meningitis should be placed in a private room to prevent spread of the infection to others. Keep the room dark and quiet to prevent photophobia and to decrease the risk of seizures because increased activity can induce seizures. Until the causative agent is determined, the child should be placed in respiratory precautions. All individuals entering the room should wear gown, gloves, and mask.

Encephalitis is inflammation of the brain, most often caused by a viral infection. Common causative organisms include St. Louis encephalitis virus, West Nile virus, eastern and western equine virus transmitted by ticks and mosquitoes, herpes simplex virus, or rabies virus. It may also occur after vaccination with measles, mumps, or rubella vaccines.

Herpes simplex type I is the most common cause of encephalitis after the newborn period. It is associated with a high mortality rate. Surviving children often have significant neurologic deficits (cognitive, auditory, motor, or visual). The cardiovascular system, as well as the lungs or liver, may be affected.

clinical ALERT

Younger children generally have a more serious illness and greater residual effects from encephalitis.

Reye's Syndrome

Reye's syndrome is a complication of viral infection. It is an acute encephalitis characterized by an onset of symptoms 1 to 3 weeks following a viral infection. Because the syndrome seems to be associated with salicylate use during viral infections, parents should be taught to avoid giving the child products containing salicylate for pain or fever relief during a viral infection. (See Chapter 10 ⬢ for information on communicable diseases.)

clinical ALERT

Teach parents to avoid products containing _salicylate_ (aspirin). Inform them of the following over-the-counter products that contain salicylate: Pepto-Bismol, Triaminicin, Coricidin, and Alka-Seltzer.

Guillain-Barré Syndrome

Guillain-Barré syndrome (postinfectious polyneuritis) is a relatively rare disorder characterized by ascending paralysis (toe to head) and then descending (head to toe) remyelination. It can be an acute viral infection caused by *Campylobacter jejuni* (most common), cytomegalovirus, or Epstein-Barr virus. It has also been associated with administration of vaccines. Although Guillain-Barré syndrome can affect anyone at any age, it is most commonly seen in children between 4 and 9 years of age.

Manifestations

Typically, Guillain-Barré syndrome begins with pain and weakness in the lower extremities. The muscle weakness and paralysis can progress upward to involve the abdomen, chest, upper extremities, and possibly the entire body. The paralysis can stop at any point and recede. Respiratory efforts may be compromised. The child may have difficulty talking, chewing, and swallowing. Dysfunction of the autonomic nervous system may cause hypertension, postural hypotension, cardiac arrhythmias, diaphoresis, and urinary and bowel incontinence.

Diagnosis

The syndrome is diagnosed by the presence of symptoms, lumbar puncture (see Figure 8-20 ⬤◯ for positioning), and CSF evaluation and electroconduction tests.

Treatment

Medical and nursing care is supportive until the paralysis resolves in 2 to 4 weeks.

Nursing Considerations

The focus of nursing care for Guillain-Barré syndrome is maintaining respiratory function, preventing malnutrition, preventing complications associated with immobility, providing emotional support, and teaching the family to care for the child at home.

The child's respiratory function must be continuously monitored in the early phase of the disease. Signs of labored breathing, color changes, fatigue, and low oxygen saturation indicate the need for medical intervention. The child may be intubated and placed on mechanical ventilation until the paralysis subsides.

The child's ability to swallow should be evaluated frequently, especially before feeding. If the child drools instead of swallowing saliva, oral liquid or food should not be given because of the risk of aspiration. To meet nutritional requirements, the child will need IV supplements or enteral feedings.

Within a few days of onset of the disease, the child will become either partially or totally immobile. The child can develop complications of immobility, such as constipation and skin breakdown. The concepts of basic nursing care for the immobilized client should be followed and taught to the family. These include turning and maintaining proper alignment every 2 hours, active and passive range of motion, skin care, bowel care, and diversion activities.

The entire family will need support to deal with this sudden life-threatening disorder that may have long-term effects on the child. Referral should be made to a home care nurse, social worker, and rehabilitation specialist. With aggressive rehabilitation, children usually recover with few permanent deficits.

NEUROLOGIC TRAUMA

Neurologic trauma is defined as any injury to the head or spinal cord due to force, anoxia, or penetration. **Closed head injury** is a result of head trauma, either from an external force, such as a blow to the head, or an internal force, such as shaking the infant hard enough for the brain to strike the inside of the skull (called *shaken-baby syndrome*; see Chapter 16 ⬤◯). Head injuries are the most common serious injury in childhood. The younger the child, the greater the risk of head trauma because the head is proportionately larger and heavier than the rest of the body.

Hematoma

The impact of the head injury can cause several types of **hematomas,** or blood trapped within the brain tissue. These hematomas can be subdural, epidural, or intracerebral.

Subdural hematomas (Figure 15-14 ■), bleeding between the dura and the brain, are caused by falls, motor vehicle accidents, and shaken-baby syndrome. Epidural hematomas, bleeding between the dura and the skull, are caused by

Figure 15-14. ■ Intracranial hematomas (**A**) In subdural hematoma (*subdural* literally means under the dura), bleeding occurs between the dura and the brain. (**B**) In epidural hematoma, bleeding occurs between the dura and the skull.

blunt traumas such as an injury from a baseball. Bleeding within the cerebrum is called an intracerebral hematoma. This type of hematoma is caused by deep contusions or penetrating injuries to the skull.

Spinal cord injury can result from hyperflexion, lateral flexion, and extension or compression of the vertebrae. The specific trauma and area of injury determines the type of damage. The injury could range from a bruising to partial or complete laceration of the spinal cord. At the time of injury, the child becomes flaccid below the injury. Cervical injuries are the most common because of the weight of the head and flexibility of the neck, and they are the most serious because of respiratory complications.

Manifestations

The signs of head trauma depend on the severity of the injury. The child may lose consciousness, have amnesia, have a headache, or be nauseated and vomit. The child may have signs of increased ICP including decreasing LOC, fixed dilated pupils, decorticate or decerebrate posturing (Figure 15-15 ■), alteration in reflexes, and seizures. Hypoxic or anoxic neurologic trauma may result from drowning, carbon monoxide poisoning, or aspiration.

Diagnosis

Determining a diagnosis of head injury or spinal cord injury includes gathering data in the history and physical. The neurologic assessment is critical. To determine specific injuries, the health care provider will order x-rays,

computer tomography (CT) scan, and/or magnetic resonance imaging (MRI).

Treatment

Treatment of head injuries may be extensive and require intensive and long-term care. In some cases, oxygenation is facilitated by intubation. ICP must be controlled by the use of diuretics, sedation, and environmental control to decrease stimuli.

Nursing Considerations

It is important for the nurse to determine the exact time of the injury, the events surrounding the injury, the exact location of the injury, and whether the child lost consciousness. Nursing care begins with airway management. Evaluation of ICP is essential. Skin integrity becomes an issue if the child is immobilized for long periods of time.

Parents of a child with neurologic injury need to be able to vent their feelings. Care must be provided in a nonjudgmental manner. Parents may need assistance deciding whether to take a comatose child home or place the child in a long-term care facility. The nurse should assist the family as needed.

Prevention of neurologic trauma is an essential component of client and family teaching, including the use of car seats, bicycle (and other) helmets, and firearm safety. In order to prevent shaken-baby syndrome, a potentially lethal form of closed head injury, caregivers must be taught not to shake infants. (Shaken-baby syndrome is discussed in

A

B

Figure 15-15. ■ (A) Decorticate posturing, characterized by rigid flexion, is associated with lesions above the brainstem in the corticospinal tracts. **(B)** Decerebrate posturing, distinguished by rigid extension, is associated with lesions of the brainstem.

Chapter 16 ⬤.) The nurse needs to be aware of the possibility of parental abuse as a cause of trauma.

Concussion

A **concussion** is an injury that causes temporary neurologic impairment but no permanent damage to brain tissue. It may be caused by blunt injury to the head or by shaking an infant or child. A concussion is caused by stretching, compression, or tearing of the nerve fibers near the brain.

Manifestations

Clinical manifestations of a concussion include altered mental status or loss of consciousness, nausea, vomiting, headache, dizziness, and amnesia.

Diagnosis and Treatment

An x-ray will be ordered to rule out skull fracture. The child should also be observed closely for 24 hours following the injury for decreasing LOC and disorientation. The child with a concussion may have difficulty staying awake because of the trauma/swelling to the brain. The child can be allowed to sleep following a concussion but must be awakened frequently (every 1 to 2 hours) to check LOC. (Review the Glasgow Coma Scale, in Procedure 15-1.) The child should receive no analgesics or sedatives while under observation.

Drowning or Near-Drowning

Drowning, loss of life within 24 hours following submersion in water or other liquid, is the second leading cause of injury-related death for children ages 1 to 14. **Near-drowning** is defined as suffocation from submersion in liquid that is survived in the first 24 hours following the incident. Children lose consciousness within 3 to 5 minutes. Neurologic and circulatory impairment occurs within 5 to 10 minutes following submersion. Asphyxia and aspiration are the physical conditions most often associated with near-drowning.

Manifestations

Clinical manifestations of near-drowning include restlessness, loss of consciousness, vomiting, cyanosis, tachypnea, tachycardia, hypotension, and hypothermia. The child is at risk for pneumonia if bacteria and debris were ingested. Children who have had a near-drowning experience in saltwater are at risk of severe electrolyte imbalance that may cause death (Figure 15-16 ■). Box 15-6 ■ provides questions to ask when assessing a drowning victim.

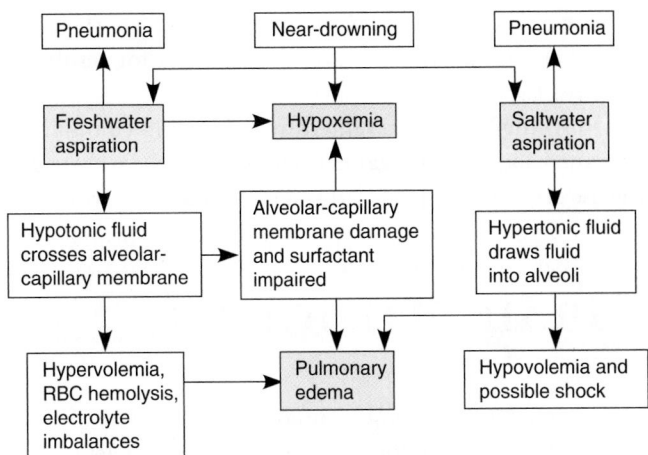

Figure 15-16. ■ Flowchart of near-drowning in fresh- or saltwater. Note the electrolyte imbalances that can occur.

Diagnosis

Lab tests required include blood gas evaluation, serum chemistries, and blood cultures. X-rays may also be done to observe for head or lung damage.

Treatment

Immediate treatment of the near-drowning victim includes cardiopulmonary resuscitation (CPR), correction of hypothermia, correction of electrolyte imbalance, and prevention of hyper- or hypovolemic shock. Neurologic dysfunctions such as increased ICP, cerebral edema, and seizures may need to be managed. Oxygen is given by nonrebreather face mask. Positive end-expiratory pressure (PEEP) can be used to keep the alveoli open. Administration of vasopressor medication may be necessary to maintain the child's blood pressure. Antibiotics are administered to children who develop pneumonia.

Nursing Considerations

Nursing care is focused on improving neurologic function, providing oxygenation, and decreasing the risk of infection. The child who has survived a drowning accident may

BOX 15-6	NURSING CARE CHECKLIST

Collecting Data on Drowning Victims

Adequate information about the near drowning incident must be obtained in order to treat the child appropriately.

☑ Ask how long the child was under water.

☑ Determine the type of water.

☑ What was the temperature of the water?

☑ What was the child's immediate response when pulled from the water?

☑ What rescue methods were employed?

develop a fear of water. The nurse can encourage the child to verbalize fears and to develop strategies for resolving these fears.

Drowning can be prevented by promoting community education and by encouraging environmental changes such as the use of fences and pool alarms. Pools should be surrounded with fences taller than 5 feet that are difficult for a child to climb. Buckets should be kept empty when not in use, and children should be supervised when near pools, at the beach, or in the bathtub. Families with pools should keep a phone near the pool and learn CPR techniques. See Figure 12-7 for photos of CPR equipment and techniques.

BRAIN TUMORS

Brain tumors are the most common solid tumor in children and the second most common malignancy after leukemia. Most brain tumors in children involve the cerebellum, midbrain, and brainstem (Figure 15-17 ■). The most common brain tumors in children are medulloblastoma, cerebellar astrocytoma, ependymoma, and brainstem glioma. Common tumors in children by age group are listed in Table 15-4 ■.

Manifestations

Symptoms of brain tumors differ depending on the type and location of the tumor. Table 15-5 ■ identifies the symptoms and medical treatment of the four common brain tumors in children. The nurse must be alert for atypical, nonspecific symptoms. These include slight behavior change, poor school performance, and change in coordination. Tumors in the area of the hypothalamus or pituitary gland can induce diabetes insipidus and growth abnormalities caused by excess excretion of hormones.

Diagnosis

Diagnosis of brain tumors is facilitated by parental information about the onset of symptoms. Tumor growth rate is related to how slowly or quickly symptoms occurred.

To determine type and location of the tumor, CT scans, MRIs, positron emission tomography scans, and single-photon emission computed tomography scans are used. Lumbar punctures are used to identify malignant cells in the CSF. Bone marrow aspiration and bone scans detect metastasis to other areas of the body (Ball & Bindler, 2006).

Treatment

Medical treatment of brain tumors includes surgery, radiation, chemotherapy, or a combination of these treatments. The goal of treatment is to destroy as much of the tumor as possible, with a minimum of complications. Laser surgery is used when tumors are located close to vital tissue or blood vessels. The use of radiation and improved chemotherapeutic agents have improved the prognosis of many types of brain cancer such as medulloblastoma and ependymoma. Complications of radiation and chemotherapy include infection, seizure activity, hydrocephalus, growth problems, and neurologic deficits.

TABLE 15-4				
Tumor Sites by Age Group				
	Up to 5 Years	5–9 Years	10–14 Years	15–19 Years
Leukemia	36%	31%	18%	12%
Brain	13%	25%	18%	10%
Lymphoma	10%	16%	25%	27%
Kidney	10%	5%	N/A	N/A
Eye	6%	2%	N/A	4%
Soft tissue	7%	5%	5%	5%
Bone	13%	3%	11%	7%
Ovary/testis	2%	N/A	3%	11%
Neuroblastoma	7%	3%	N/A	N/A
Thyroid	N/A	N/A	4%	8%
Skin	N/A	N/A	N/A	6%
Other	2%	10%	16%	10%

Source: Data from Crist, W. M. (2000). Neoplastic disease and tumors. In R. E. Behrman, R. M. Kliegman, & H. B. Jenson (Eds.), *Nelson textbook of pediatrics* (16th ed.). Philadelphia: Saunders; p.1531. Reprinted with permission from Elsevier.

Supratentorial tumors (**cerebral astrocytoma, ependymoma,** optic nerve gliomas)
Tentorial notch tumors (pineal region tumors, hypothalamic glioma)
Tentorial tumors
Infratentorial tumors (**brainstem gliomas, medulloblastoma,** cerebellar astrocytoma, ependymoma)
Foramen magnum tumors

Figure 15-17. ■ Sites of brain tumors in children. Approximately 1,500 children younger than 15 years are diagnosed annually as having tumors of the brain and central nervous system. The four most common brain tumors in children are medulloblastoma, cerebral astrocytoma, ependymoma, and brainstem glioma.

TABLE 15-5

Manifestations and Treatment of Brain Tumors

TUMOR	ETIOLOGY	CLINICAL MANIFESTATIONS	CLINICAL THERAPY
Medulloblastoma	External layer of cerebellum	Headache, vomiting, ataxia	Surgery; chemotherapy with lomustine, vincristine, prednisone, cisplatin; radiation
Astrocytomas	Glial cells, supratentorial or infratentorial	Seizures, visual disturbances, increased intracranial pressure, vomiting	Surgery; chemotherapy with vincristine, dactinomycin; radiation
Ependymoma	Fourth ventricle, posterior fossa	Hydrocephalus	Surgery, radiation
Brainstem gliomas	Pons	Cranial nerve (VI + VII) tract signs: nystagmus, ataxia, motor symptoms	Surgery, radiation

Nursing Considerations

Nursing care requires a multidisciplinary approach. The oncologist and neurosurgeon work closely with the pediatrician in providing medical treatment. The nurse coordinates with the dietitian, social worker, and physical and occupational therapist in managing complications of treatment. Parents can be taught to provide home care, including the administration of medication, and physical exercises. In addition, the parents must be taught the importance of follow-up examinations. The child and family members need support when the child has permanent deficits.

Sympathetic Nervous System Tumor

NEUROBLASTOMA

Neuroblastoma is a malignancy of the sympathetic nervous system. Solid tumors may be found in the abdomen, brain, adrenal medulla, thorax, or pelvis. It usually occurs in children between 2 and 5 years and rarely occurs after the age of 10.

Manifestations

The original tumor site may not produce symptoms until metastasis has occurred. Location of the tumor determines presenting symptoms. Abdominal or pelvic tumors may cause changes in bladder and bowel function, weight loss, and abdominal distention. Thorax tumors may produce dyspnea and chest pain. Brain tumors can cause changes in neurological status.

Diagnosis

Abdominal tumors are often palpable. Once the tumor is located, a biopsy is performed. CT scans, MRIs and X-rays assist in discovering metastases.

Treatment

Management of neuroblastoma includes surgery to excise the tumor, followed by chemotherapy and radiation. The actual course of treatment will depend on the severity of the child's condition at the time of diagnosis. The younger the child at diagnosis, the better the survival rate. The nursing care of children with neuroblastoma is similar to that of children with brain tumors.

MENTAL RETARDATION

Mental retardation (MR) is defined by the American Association of Mental Retardation (2002) as "a disability characterized by significant limitations both in intellectual functioning and in adaptive behavior as expressed in conceptual, social, and practical adaptive skills. This disability originates before age 18." Specific limitations include communication, social skills, activities of daily living, school work, and employment. Intelligence quotient (IQ) test scores of individuals with MR are typically less than 70 to 75. The child with mild MR has an IQ between 50 and 70.

For moderate MR, the IQ is between 35 and 50. For severe MR, the IQ is between 20 and 35. Profound retardation is characterized by an IQ of less than 20.

Mental retardation is associated with other conditions such as Down syndrome, fetal alcohol syndrome (discussed in Chapter 16 ⚭), and maternal infections passed on to the child prenatally, such as rubella and cytomegalovirus. Other causes of MR include hypoxia, infections such as meningitis or encephalitis, neurologic trauma, and ingestion of poisons such as lead.

Manifestations

Infants with MR appear unresponsive to contact. They do not maintain eye contact during feeding. They are often irritable and take longer periods of time to feed. As these children age, they will exhibit developmental delays in language, social skills, cognitive skills, and motor skills. Learning is difficult for the child with MR, and he or she often does not do well in school.

Diagnosis

A careful history and physical examination are important in determining both the cause and the extent of MR. Laboratory tests may help determine the cause of MR. These tests include chromosomal analyses, blood enzyme levels, toxicology screens, and cranial imaging. A standardized test used to screen for developmental delays is the Denver Developmental Screening Test II (see Appendix III 🔗). A test used to screen for the child's cognitive functioning is the Stanford-Binet Intelligence Scale. This can be found in a child development text. These tools used for screening are typically administered by mental health professionals.

Treatment

Because the degree of MR varies, each child will require a specific plan to assist the child to function at the highest level achievable. The child's family, physician, nurse, social worker, physical therapist, teachers, and school administrators all play a significant role in managing the care of the child with MR. Education programs must be adapted to accommodate the needs of the child with MR. The infant needs increased visual and physical stimulation. The preschooler needs a learning environment where the teacher can devote the necessary time to help the child learn. The school-age child can benefit from special education programs and perhaps progress to a regular classroom. The adolescent with an IQ in the higher range of MR can obtain job training. Families may need assistance finding alternative living options for the child with MR.

Nursing Considerations

Families with children who are diagnosed with MR often experience grief and have difficulty coping. The nurse can play an important role in helping the family work through these emotions. The Nursing Care Plan Chart below describes interventions for families with a child with mental retardation. Providing referrals to agencies that can assist the family in caring for the child with MR is a much-needed nursing strategy.

Children with MR do not have sound judgment. Because their safety may be compromised, they often require close supervision. The nurse can provide teaching to help the child avoid physical harm, and assist the parents in removing environmental hazards.

NURSING CARE PLAN CHART

Child with Mental Retardation

GOAL	INTERVENTION	RATIONALE	EXPECTED OUTCOME
1. Delayed Growth and Development related to neurologic deficits			
The child will achieve appropriate growth and development	Assess the child's developmental progress regularly	*Allows for a revision of the plan of care*	The child performs age-appropriate activities of daily living with minimal assistance.
	Encourage the child using positive reinforcement	*Positive reinforcement helps to motivate the child and increase his potential for learning*	
	Provide opportunities for the child to interact with other children at the same developmental level. Also provide appropriate toys and learning aids	*The child will learn from other children and mimic their behavior*	
The family will act positively to promote growth and development	Teach parents to recognize signs of readiness to learn	*Recognizing these signs will assist parents in providing educational opportunities*	The family is actively pursuing appropriate opportunities to assist the child's progress developmentally.
	Help parents to set appropriate goals for progress developmentally	*Realistic goals will promote self-esteem in the child and decrease frustration*	

GOAL	INTERVENTION	RATIONALE	EXPECTED OUTCOME
2. Interrupted Family Processes related to developmental crises of the child with mental retardation			
The family will obtain necessary support to manage the care of their child with mental retardation	Ensure that the family understands the child's condition and probable limitations	*Knowledge will allow the parents to form appropriate expectations*	The family is accepting of referrals and assistance.
	Discuss the child's strengths and abilities with the family	*Assists parents to understand their child's capabilities*	
	Assist the family to explore available options for caring for the child	*Families should understand home care and long-term care options in an effort to make decisions that will best suit their situation*	
	Discuss respite care options with the family	*Respite care can provide families time away to travel and rest while knowing their child is receiving proper care*	
	If the family decides on residential care for their child, provide them with suggestions for promoting meaningful relationships	*Relationships with the child in residential care can grow and thrive even though the parents are unable to be with the child day and night*	

Parents should be encouraged to allow the child to perform as many activities of daily living as possible. This will require patience and kindness. Children with MR benefit from being able to care for their own needs, including dressing themselves, brushing their own teeth, and feeding themselves.

The nurse should discuss issues of sexuality and living apart from their parents with the adolescent with mental retardation. These issues include safety, birth control, prevention of sexually transmitted infections, money management, and responsibility. The nurse can refer the family to community resources to assist in dealing with these issues.

Down Syndrome

Down syndrome is the most common chromosomal abnormality seen in infants causing moderate to severe MR. It occurs when there are three chromosomes at position 21 (Figure 15-18 ■) and is also called *trisomy 21*. The frequency of Down syndrome increases with maternal age.

Manifestations

The infant with Down syndrome presents with a short head (*bradycephaly*), flat forehead, short limbs, and a short, wide neck (Figure 15-18B). The tongue may be protruding because of a high-arched palate. **Epicanthal folds** (a fold of skin over the inner canthus of the eye) are common. Hands are short and wide with a **simian crease** (a horizontal crease extending across the entire palm). There is a wide space between the great and second toe. Moro reflex is absent, and the newborn exhibits sluggish reflexes (*hypotonia*). See Procedure 8-13, Eliciting Newborn Reflexes ⬤⬤ . The eyes may have **Brushfield spots** (white speckles on the edge of the iris).

The child with Down syndrome has an increased risk for congenital heart defects, diabetes, leukemia, and hearing loss. The degree of mental retardation varies among children with Down syndrome and is not able to be assessed at birth.

Down syndrome alone would not necessitate keeping the newborn in the neonatal intensive care unit (NICU). The newborn with Down syndrome may be hospitalized for some time after birth to allow time for the parents to adjust

MediaLink ⬤ Down Syndrome

A

B

Figure 15-18. ■ (**A**) Karyotype for a child with Down syndrome (trisomy 21). Note the extra chromosome at position 21. (**B**) This child with Down syndrome has typical characteristics, including Mongolian slant, short wide neck, and a protruding tongue.

to the diagnosis and to learn any special care that might be necessary.

Diagnosis

Prenatal tests to screen for Down syndrome include alpha-fetoprotein testing, chorionic villus sampling, amniocentesis, ultrasound, and nuchal translucency screening. Initial diagnosis is by clinical findings most often evident at birth. Cardiac defects may be diagnosed by x-ray or ultrasound. Definitive diagnosis is by chromosomal analysis.

Treatment

The need for medical treatment of a congenital heart disorder (discussed in Chapter 13 ⌘) will be a priority intervention. Surgery may be necessary to correct cardiac, gastrointestinal, or cranial deformities. A team approach will be instituted to assist the parents in coping with the child's physical and mental condition and in obtaining help through community resources.

Nursing Considerations

Parents of children with Down syndrome will need emotional support in coping with the new infant. There will be grief over the loss of their "perfect child." Nurses can model a loving and positive response to the neonate. They may need to repeat information that was provided because the parents may be overwhelmed at the thought of caring for a child with this disorder. Children with Down syndrome require lifelong assistance. With support, many children with Down syndrome are "mainstreamed" in schools and live in group homes as adults. Before discharge, the nurse must ensure that the parents are provided with information about the disorder and any necessary referrals.

SENSORY DISORDERS

Eye Disorders

ANATOMY AND PHYSIOLOGY

A child's eye is composed of external and internal structures. Figure 15-19 ■ reviews the eye's anatomy. Six muscles are responsible for the eye's movement. Vision occurs as light comes into the eye by way of the clear cornea. It then passes through the lens and is focused by the ciliary muscles onto the retina. The rods and cones relay the light impulses via the optic nerve to the occipital region of the brain.

BRIEF ASSESSMENT REVIEW

History

- Ask about loss of vision, eye pain, **diplopia** (double vision), excessive or deficient tearing, drainage, and blurred vision.
- In a young child, the nurse may have to phrase questions to explain what is meant. For example, to check for double vision, the nurse may hold up one finger and ask, "How many fingers do you see?"
- Inquire about corrective lenses or glasses.

Figure 15-19. ■ (**A**) Internal structure of the eye. (**B**) External structure of the eye.

■ Ask the parent for any behavior that would suggest the child is having difficulty seeing.

Physical

■ Observe for anatomic variations of the eye and the surrounding adnexa.
■ Inspect the conjunctivae, sclerae, iris, and pupils.
■ Use the pen light to determine **PERRLA** (pupils equally round and react to light and accommodation).
■ Assess visual acuity. Procedures 15-2 and 15-3 describe visual acuity testing with eye charts.

Eye Conditions

ACUTE CONJUNCTIVITIS

Acute conjunctivitis is commonly called *pinkeye* (Figure 15-20 ■). It is the inflammation of the conjunctiva caused by allergies, bacteria, or viruses. Bacterial and viral conjunctivitis are contagious and easily transmitted among children, to siblings, parents or caregivers.

Manifestations

Children with acute conjunctivitis can present with eye irritation, photophobia, redness, inflammation, and drainage, which may be purulent or watery. Conjunctivitis caused by an allergen will usually be accompanied by pruritus.

Diagnosis

Presentation of symptoms leads the practitioner to a diagnosis of acute conjunctivitis. Cultures of the drainage can assist in the differentiation between bacterial and viral conjunctivitis.

Treatment

Treatment for acute bacterial conjunctivitis includes ophthalmic antibiotics in the form of drops or ointment. Antiviral agents are available for viral conditions. Comfort measures for children with conjunctivitis caused by an allergen include cool compresses and antihistamines.

Nursing Considerations

The nurse should assist parents with the child's eye hygiene. To prevent transferring the harmful organism to others, the nurse can teach the child and parents to practice frequent hand washing, practice proper ophthalmic administration, change linens

Figure 15-20. ■ Acute conjunctivitis. The discharge from bacterial conjunctivitis is purulent discharge and may cause crusting. The discharge from viral conjunctivitis is *serous* (watery). Allergic conjunctivitis produces watery to thick drainage and is characterized by itching. (Phototake NYC.)

frequently, and avoid rubbing the eyes. The child should not go to school or day care while the infection is present.

STYE

A stye is an infection of a sebaceous gland or oil gland of the eyelid. *Staphylococcus* is the most common causative agent. The child with a stye may have pain, redness, and edema of the eyelid. The preauricular lymph nodes may also be enlarged. Styes are treated with ophthalmic antibiotic ointment and warm, moist compresses to relieve discomfort.

PERIORBITAL CELLULITIS

Periorbital cellulitis (Figure 15-21 ■) is an inflammation of the subcutaneous tissue of the eyelid. It may be caused by a preexisting infection, insect bites, or trauma.

Manifestations

The early symptoms of periorbital cellulitis often mimic those of acute conjunctivitis. The child may also have a fever, elevated white blood cells, malaise, and decreased visual acuity.

Figure 15-21. ■ Periorbital cellulitis is an infection of the eyelid and surrounding tissues, not of the eye itself. It is a serious bacterial infection that can spread to the optic nerve if not treated promptly with intravenous antibiotics. (Phototake NYC.)

Treatment

The child will be hospitalized to administer IV antibiotics. Prompt treatment prevents damage to the optic nerve.

RETINOBLASTOMA

Retinoblastoma is a congenital, malignant tumor of the retina. It may occur unilaterally or bilaterally. It is usually discovered in children under 5 years of age.

Manifestations

Parents usually note a white glow or reflection in the child's eye. This sign is called the cat's-eye reflex or **leukokoria.** The child may also have **strabismus** (a condition in which

---

TABLE 15-6

Communicating Across the Life Span: Child with Visual Impairment

	TODDLER	PRESCHOOLER	SCHOOL-AGE CHILD	ADOLESCENT
Client	Parent: I'm concerned about finding appropriate toys to stimulate my child who cannot see well.	Parent: I want my child to learn to read, but most of the preschool learning aids are not appropriate.	I'd love to play video games like my friends, but I can't even see the TV.	I'm graduating from high school next year and I really don't want my blindness to keep me from going to college.
Nurse	Look for toys that are lighted, produce sounds, musical instruments, puzzles that make noise and flash light when the pieces are placed correctly, textured balls, videos developed with high contrast images and verbal enhancements to promote auditory stimulation and language development.	Large magnifiers are available for books, newspapers, and computers. Be sure your child has a good source of lighting when attempting to read. Purchase audio books and have the child follow along in the printed version.	Several companies produce computers that are voice activated. Computer games are also available that verbally instruct the participant and describe the game scene.	Seeing eye dogs are available to assist you in all manner of living alone. If you and your parents are interested in exploring this option, we might want to pursue it now so that you could be comfortable with the dog before you leave for college.

the eyes do not track together; one eye is often fixed), orbital inflammation causing pain and redness, glaucoma, **heterochromia** (different colored eyes), and visual impairment leading to blindness. Table 15-6 ■ provides some ways of discussing blindness with children and their parents.

Diagnosis

Prenatal genetic screening is available for families with a history of retinoblastoma. An ophthalmic examination is necessary. For younger children, general anesthesia may be necessary to allow complete visualization.

Treatment

Retinal damage may require surgical removal of the eye and placement of a prosthesis. This surgical procedure is called **enucleation.** Laser surgery may be used to reduce circulation to the tumor. Chemotherapy is often used to further reduce tumor size and metastasis. The prognosis for children with retinoblastoma is favorable for more than 90% of children. These children are at risk for decreased visual acuity, osteogenic sarcoma, and melanoma.

Nursing Considerations

The care of the child with retinoblastoma depends on the treatment ordered. Chemotherapy requires care similar to other malignancies. See Nursing Care Plan Chart: Child Undergoing Chemotherapy, Chapter 14 ∞. The child who has had an enucleation requires sensitive nursing care. Parents and the child need detailed explanation about the child's expected appearance following surgery. The eye will be patched, but the face may be edematous and have bruising. The nurse can assist the child and parents to understand that prior to prosthesis placement (usually 3 weeks postoperative) a surgical sphere will be placed in the eye cavity and covered with conjunctiva. Parents can be taught to observe the surgical site for drainage and to keep the site dressed and changed daily to prevent infection. Special care should be given to the emotional adjustment of both parents and the child who has had an eye removed. The nurse can assist the discussion of feelings and refer to appropriate health care providers if necessary.

Eye Injuries

The cornea of the infant and young child is proportionally larger than that of an adult. The structures of the eye are not protected as well, especially from the side. Eye injuries cause the child intense pain, excessive tearing, light sensitivity, and changes in vision. Eye injuries are classified as

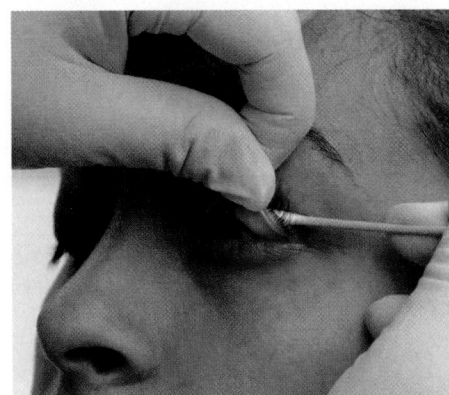

Figure 15-22. ■ Small pieces of debris or foreign objects can be visualized more readily by rolling the eyelid up over a cotton swab.

penetrating or nonpenetrating. Prompt treatment of any eye injury is of utmost importance.

PENETRATING INJURIES

Penetrating injuries to children's eyes are typically caused by toys, glass, pencils, and other sharp objects. The object, if it remains in the eye, should not be removed until the child is sedated and an ophthalmologist or eye surgeon is available. Ophthalmic antibiotics are administered, the affected eye patched, and a tetanus booster administered if necessary.

NONPENETRATING INJURIES

Nonpenetrating eye injuries include corneal abrasion; foreign object trauma that does not penetrate the eye such as air bags or baseball bats; hyphema; and chemical burns. To remove a superficial foreign object from the eye, grasp the eyelashes of the upper eyelid and stretch downward. Place a cotton-tipped applicator in the center of the eyelid, and pull the eyelid up and over the applicator (Figure 15-22 ■). Observe for the foreign object. If it is not embedded, it will be gently removed with another moist, cotton-tipped applicator. An ophthalmic antibiotic ointment will be prescribed. Water or saline eye irrigation in copious amounts is used for a chemical burn to the eye to flush out as much of the causative agent as possible.

HYPHEMA

Hyphema is a hemorrhage into the anterior chamber of the eye. Both of the child's eyes are patched. The child is placed on bed rest to prevent an increase in intraocular pressure and to allow for the reabsorption of the blood in the anterior chamber.

A Hyperopia

B Myopia

C Astigmatism

Figure 15-23. ■ (A) Hyperopia. In hyperopia, light rays focus behind the retina, making it difficult to focus on objects at close range. (B) Myopia. In myopia, light rays focus in front of the retina, making it difficult to focus on objects that are far away. (C) Astigmatism. In astigmatism, light rays do not uniformly focus on the eye because of abnormal curvature of cornea or lens.

Visual Impairment

Several conditions can occur that interfere with a child's vision. Visual impairment can cause learning difficulties. Visual acuity screenings are available to determine light refraction disorders such as **hyperopia** (farsightedness), **myopia** (nearsightedness), and **astigmatism** (an uneven focusing of light resulting in blurred images) (Figure 15-23 ■). See Procedures 15-2 and 15-3 ■. Lenses may be needed to correct the child's visual deficiencies.

PROCEDURE 15-2 Snellen Letter Chart

Purpose
■ To determine visual acuity for the child who can read the alphabet

Equipment
■ Snellen letter chart (Figure 15-24 ■)

Figure 15-24. ■ Snellen letter chart. The client stands 20 feet from the chart and reads letters one eye at a time, and then with both eyes together.

Interventions and Rationales

1. Perform preparatory steps (see icon bar on p. 410).
2. Position the child 20 feet from the chart. *At this distance, results are accurate.*
3. To test the right eye, cover the left eye completely, and ask the child to read the line on the chart indicated. *Testing eyes singly provides accurate results.*
4. To test the left eye, repeat as above, except cover the right eye completely.
5. Interpret the findings. *If the child can read the line marked 20 feet, his or her vision is considered to be 20/20. If, however, the child can only read lines labeled 40 to 200 feet, the vision is considered to be 20/40 to 20/200. Note: Charts are available using a distance of 10 feet. Appropriate visual acuity in children older than 3 years is 20/20.*
6. Report visual acuity findings to charge nurse.
7. Document findings.

SAMPLE DOCUMENTATION

(Date) 0800   Snellen letter chart used. Right eye 20/20. Left eye 20/20.
B. Darnell, LVN

PROCEDURE 15-3 ## Snellen E or Picture Chart

Purpose

■ To determine visual acuity for the child who cannot read the alphabet

Equipment

■ Snellen E chart (also called Tumbling E chart) or Snellen picture chart (Figure 15-25 ■)

Interventions and Rationales

1. Perform preparatory steps (see icon bar above).
2. Position the child 20 feet from the chart. *At this distance, results are accurate.*

3. Start with the right eye. *Testing eyes singly provides accurate results.*
4. Snellen E chart: Cover one eye and point to the direction the legs of the letter are pointing. The child can also be

given a card with a letter E on it. Ask the child to turn the card to match what he or she sees on the chart. Repeat with the other eye.

5. Snellen picture chart: Cover one eye, and identify the pictures on the chart in order. Repeat with other eye.

6. Record the findings. *If the child can read the line marked 20 feet, his or her vision is considered to be 20/20. If, however, only lines labeled 40 to 200 feet can be read, his or her vision is considered to be 20/40 to 20/200. Note: Charts are also available using a distance of 10 feet.*

7. Report visual acuity findings to charge nurse.

8. Document finding in the chart.

SAMPLE DOCUMENTATION

(Date) 1000 Visual acuity assessed with Snellen picture chart. Right eye 20/20. Left eye 20/20. _____
 V. Gates, LPN

A

B

Figure 15-25. ■ (A) Snellen E chart is often used for young school-age children. (B) Snellen picture chart is used for very young children who can talk.

STRABISMUS

Strabismus (Figure 15-26 ■), commonly known as *cross-eye* or *wall-eye*, occurs when eye muscles are uncoordinated and fail to maintain proper eye alignment. Strabismus is a common finding in infants younger than 2 months old because the child is trying to focus and muscles are immature. **Esotropia** is the turning of the eye inward. **Exotropia** is the turning of the eye outward. **Hypertropia,** also called *anoopsia*, is a vertical deviation of one eye.

The child with strabismus has difficulty seeing objects clearly and may be clumsy. The child may close one eye frequently in an effort to see more clearly. The cover test may be used to diagnose strabismus. In the cover test, the nurse gives the child an object with which to play. The nurse covers one of the child's eyes and observes the movement of the uncovered eye. Inward movement, outward movement, or vertical deviation of at least one eye indicates that the eye was not fixed on the toy and strabismus is present. Strabismus can be treated with corrective lenses, patching, **orthoptics** or eye exercises, or miotic medications to improve muscle function, or by surgery.

Esotropia

Exotropia

Figure 15-26. ■ Strabismus. In strabismus, the muscles of the eyes are not coordinated. (Pearson Education/PH College.)

Figure 15-27. ■ An eye patch is used with amblyopia ("lazy eye") to strengthen the weaker eye. (Photo Researchers Inc.)

AMBLYOPIA

Amblyopia, or *lazy eye*, is a reduction of vision in one eye. Without treatment, the child may lose vision in the eye. Strabismus may lead to amblyopia. However, the child may also not have any symptoms. The condition can be detected in routine visual screening. Referral to an ophthalmologist or optometrist is important. Amblyopia can be treated with corrective lenses, patching (Figure 15-27 ■), or orthoptics. Treatment should be initiated by ages 5 to 6 for the best chance of success. Some nursing interventions for children with amblyopia are provided in Box 15-7 ■. Nurses can teach parents these guidelines as well.

DYSLEXIA

Dyslexia is a specific, common learning disability that is neurologic in origin (International Dyslexia Association, 2002). Children with dyslexia often see mirror images of

BOX 15-7	NURSING CARE CHECKLIST

Guidelines for a Child with Amblyopia

☑ Male children in particular may enjoy pretending to be a pirate with an eye patch. This may also encourage them to be compliant with care.

☑ Secure patch with adhesive underneath the patch, tape over the patch, and/or a bandage or elastic band around the head.

☑ Use restraints only if necessary.

☑ Ensure that the child has the patch removed at least 2 hours daily.

☑ Assess for improvement of the eye's condition while the patch is removed.

☑ Document appropriately.

letters, numbers, and symbols. This condition makes speaking, writing, memorizing, working math problems, reading, and spelling difficult. Although the child may have other visual impairments, dyslexia is not treated by correcting the vision. Children with dyslexia (or other neurologically based learning disorders) need specialized assistance with learning. Learning techniques often involve stimulating several of the senses simultaneously, such as providing the material orally, in written form, and by three-dimensional model.

CATARACTS

Cataracts are opacities of the lens of one or both eyes (Figure 15-28 ■). Very dense cataracts may prevent light from reaching the retina. Cataracts can be acquired or congenital. Acquired cataracts are due to infections during pregnancy, trauma, or other disease processes. Congenital cataracts can be caused by an inherited autosomal dominant trait.

The nurse may be able to observe severe cataracts. The normal red reflex (the reflection of light off the retina when using an ophthalmoscope) may also be distorted or absent. An infant may not be able to focus on close objects or may demonstrate **nystagmus** (involuntary movement of the eyes). The older child may report blurred vision. Cataracts are removed surgically to restore the child's vision. Corrective lenses or artificial lens implants will be necessary to restore vision. Surgery is necessary before age 2 months in the infant with severe cataracts in an effort to prevent permanent visual impairment.

GLAUCOMA

Glaucoma is a condition caused by increased intraocular pressure (IOP) due to inadequate drainage of the aqueous humor (Figure 15-29 ■). Increased IOP from the anterior chamber of the eye has the potential to cause retinal damage, compression of the optic disc tissue, and eventually visual field defects or blindness.

Glaucoma in the pediatric client can be congenital or acquired. The child with congenital glaucoma may have increased tearing (called **epiphora**), eyelid spasms, enlargement of the eyeball (called **buphthalmos**), and

Figure 15-28. ■ Congenital cataract. The cataract reduces or prevents light from reaching the retina. (From Vaughan, D., Asbury, T., & Riordan-Eva, P. [1992]. *General ophthalmology*, [13th ed.]. New York: McGraw-Hill, p. 172.)

Figure 15-29. ■ Congenital glaucoma can be seen in this child's right eye as a cloudy film. (From Vaughan, D., Asbury, T., & Riordan-Eva, P. [1992]. *General ophthalmology* [13th ed.]. New York: McGraw-Hill, p. 172.)

sensitivity to light (called **photophobia**). The child with acquired glaucoma, if able to walk, may bump into objects because he or she has difficulty seeing objects in his or her peripheral vision as a result of visual field defects. The child may also report seeing halos around objects.

IOP is measured by a **tonometer.** In children, this procedure may require anesthesia because the device must be placed against the anterior eye globe. Normal IOP is 12 to 20 mm Hg. Increased IOP, above 30 mm Hg pressure, may require prompt surgical correction. One surgical technique is called a **goniotomy.** During a goniotomy, the flow of aqueous humor is increased from the anterior chamber. More than one surgery may be necessary to reduce the IOP to a level at which the risk of damage is reduced.

Ear Disorders

ANATOMY AND PHYSIOLOGY

The ear is composed of three sections: the external ear, the middle ear, and the inner ear (Figure 15-30 ■). The auricle, tympanic membrane, and external ear canal are parts of the *external ear*. The eustachian tube, malleus, incus, and stapes

Figure 15-31. ■ The correct placement of the external ears is found by drawing an imaginary line through the medial and lateral canthi of the eye toward the ear. This line normally passes through the upper portion of the pinna. The pinna is considered "low set" when the top lies completely below the imaginary line. Low-set ears are often associated with renal disorders.

are parts of the *middle ear*. The semicircular canals, cochlea, and cranial nerve VIII are parts of the inner ear.

The most important thing for the nurse to understand when assessing a child's hearing is the difference in the anatomic shape of the eustachian tube of young children (see Figure 15-30B). The eustachian tube of the young child is shorter, wider, more horizontal, and more flaccid. This shape increases the risk for otitis media because fluid and harmful bacteria more easily accumulate.

BRIEF ASSESSMENT REVIEW

History

■ Ask about hearing loss, vertigo, **tinnitus** (ringing or other sound in the ears), drainage, and ear pain.

Physical

■ Observe for placement of the ear on the head (Figure 15-31 ■). (Low-set ears are often associated with renal disorders.)

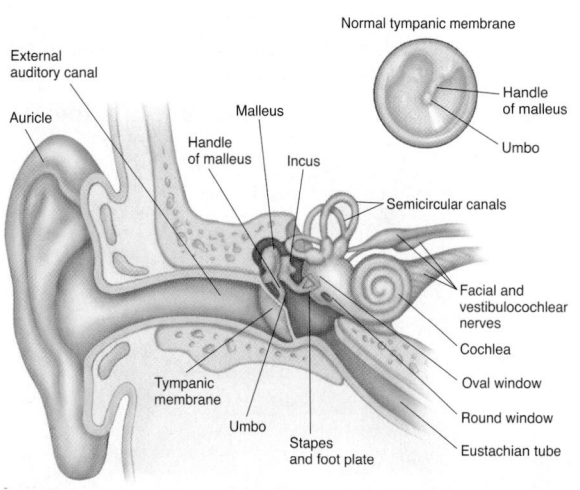

External
auditory canal

Auricle

Malleus

Handle
of malleus

Incus

Normal tympanic membrane

Handle
of malleus

Umbo

Semicircular canals

Facial and
vestibulocochlear
nerves

Cochlea

Oval window

Round window

Eustachian tube

Tympanic
membrane

Umbo

Stapes
and foot plate

A

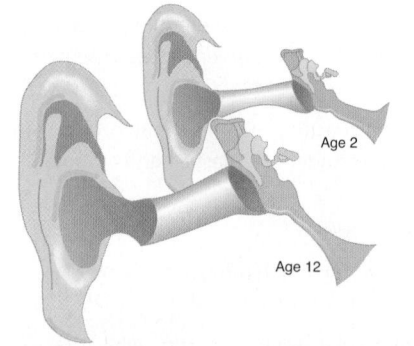

Position of eustachian tube
is at less of an angle (more
horizontal) in the young
child, resulting in decreased
drainage.

Age 2

End of eustachian tube in
nasal pharynx opens during
sucking.

Age 12

Eustachian tube equalizes
air pressure between the
middle ear and the outside
environment and allows for
drainage of secretions from
middle ear mucosa.

B

Figure 15-30. ■ **(A)** Ear anatomy. **(B)** Difference in the eustachian tube between an infant and an adult. In the infant and young child, it is more horizontal, resulting in decreased drainage. The end of the Eustachian tube (in the nasal pharynx) opens during sucking. It equalizes air pressure between the middle ear and the outside environment and allow drainage of secretions from middle ear mucosa.

- Inspect the external ear for symmetry, proportion, and color.
- Inspect the external ear canal for drainage, color, and the presence of wax (*cerumen*).
- Test for pain and tenderness by pulling on the auricle (down and back) and by palpating the mastoid process directly behind the ear.
- Assess for hearing acuity. (Hearing acuity testing is addressed later in this section.)

Ear Conditions

HEARING IMPAIRMENT

Sound is received through the external auditory canal and directed toward the tympanic membrane, causing it to vibrate (see Figure 15-30A). This vibration conducts the sound waves to the malleus, incus, and stapes, and then to the nerve endings in the cochlea. The cochlea transmits sound waves to the brain, where the child perceives the sound.

Hearing impairment can occur from birth or be acquired later in childhood. Hearing impairment can range from a slight hearing loss to total deafness. Three of every 1,000 babies are born with a hearing loss (Peck, 2005b). Causes of hearing loss include autosomal dominant inherited diseases; prenatal infections such as rubella and toxoplasmosis; perinatal asphyxia and anoxia caused by birth trauma; ototoxic drugs; radiation; childhood infections such as measles, mumps, and otitis media; head trauma; and excessive environmental noise (Figure 15-32 ■). Table 15-7 ■ provides information about degrees of hearing loss.

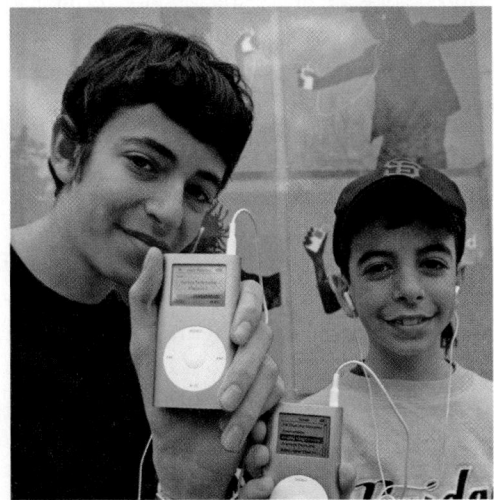

Figure 15-32. ■ Listening to loud music with headphones or at rock concerts is a frequent cause of hearing loss among teenagers and young adults. Children need guidelines about this activity. (AP Wide World Photos)

TABLE 15-7

Degree of Hearing Loss

TYPE OF LOSS	IMPAIRMENT	NURSING CONSIDERATIONS
Slight	Cannot hear whispers, no speech impairment, compensates by leaning forward and speaking loudly	Speak directly to the child so that the nurse's face is visible
Mild	Slight speech impairment, tries to face person to read lips	Assist the child with using alternate methods of communication, such as writing or typing requests
Moderate	Speech impairment present, difficulty with normal conversations, schoolwork is affected, may need a hearing aid	Consider referral for hearing aid. May need to learn sign language
Severe	Hearing aid is needed for all sounds, speech therapy required	Sign language training is necessary
Profound	Sounds are not heard, severe speech deficits	Referral to special schools for the deaf is necessary

Manifestations

Clinical manifestations of hearing impairment differ according to a child's age. The infant may not startle at loud noises or may fail to be soothed by his or her mother's voice. The older infant may not imitate sounds. Calling the name of a toddler may not elicit a response. The sound of a train approaching may go unnoticed. The toddler may also use nonverbal language instead of attempting to communicate verbally. The preschooler looks curious when given instructions or frequently asks for them to be repeated. The preschooler also may need to watch a person's lips in order to understand what is being said.

Diagnosis

See Hearing Acuity Screening section and Procedure 15-4.

Treatment

A child with hearing impairment may benefit from speech therapy or from learning to read lips or use sign language. (Some basic sign language is provided in Appendix VI ⚭.) A hearing aid may be necessary for the child to develop language skills. Infants younger than 6 months may be

A

B

Figure 15-33. ■ **(A)** Structure and positioning of cochlear implant. **(B)** Child with cochlear implant. Success with this surgery is greatest when the child is young. (AP Wide World Photos)

fitted for hearing aids. A hearing aid uses a microphone to convert sound waves into electrical impulses. These impulses are then broadcast across the tympanic membrane. The hearing aid is battery operated and fits into the child's ear. Parents will need assistance in changing the batteries. It requires a transmitter that fits behind the ear, on the child's glasses, or at the waist. Hearing aids can be costly, and it is likely that health insurance will not cover the expense.

COCHLEAR IMPLANTS. **Cochlear implants** are devices that can assist children who are deaf to hear (Figure 15-33 ■). In cochlear implant surgery, an electrode is implanted behind the ear with a wire leading to the cochlea. The child wears a headpiece behind the ear that contains a transmitter that transfers sound. The headpiece also contains a microphone to amplify sound. The speech processor is worn at the waist.

FOREIGN OBJECT IN EAR

Hearing may also be temporarily impaired by the presence of a foreign object in the ear. Curious children may take small objects and place them in the external ear canal. On otoscopic examination by the health care practitioner, the foreign object may be visualized. The nurse may assist in irrigation of the ear to remove the foreign object (see Procedure 8-33 🔗). The health care practitioner may use sterile forceps to remove the foreign object if irrigation is unsuccessful. Caution parents against attempting to remove the foreign object themselves. This may force the object further into the ear canal.

OTITIS MEDIA

Otitis media is inflammation of the middle ear that may be accompanied by fluid in the middle ear. Increased incidence of otitis media is seen in children with upper respiratory infections, cleft palate, and immunodeficiencies. Otitis media is also seen more commonly in children who are bottle fed, who use a pacifier, and who are exposed to cigarette smoke. Bottle-propping, which leads to formula pooling in the eustachian tube, provides a medium for bacterial growth. Pacifier use raises the soft palate and alters the direction of the eustachian tube. This provides an entry point for harmful bacteria from the nasopharynx (Ball & Bindler, 2006). Children exposed to second-hand smoke are at greater risk for respiratory infections that can lead to otitis media. During the winter and spring of the year when upper respiratory infections are common, more children will develop otitis media.

Manifestations

Clinical manifestations of otitis media include symptoms of an upper respiratory infection accompanied by fever and **otalgia** (ear pain). Although the older child can report pain, the infant and toddler may be observed pulling at the ear in an attempt to relieve the pain (Figure 15-34 ■). Irritability, vomiting, and diarrhea may also accompany otitis media because of accompanying illness, cold, or flu.

clinical ALERT

Because of the connection of the eustachian tube with the pharynx, the child with an ear infection may also have a throat infection.

A

B

Figure 15-34. ■ (**A**) This young child is pulling at an ear and act-ing fussy, two important signs of otitis media. (**B**) Acute otitis media is characterized by pain and a red, bulging nonmobile tym-panic membrane. (Phototake, NYC)

Diagnosis

Diagnosis of otitis media includes recognition of symptoms and ophthalmic examination of the tympanic membrane by the health care practitioner. The tympanic membrane is normally a pearl gray color with a light reflex. In otitis media, the tympanic membrane appears red and bulging, and the light reflex is diminished or absent (see Figure 15-34B).

Treatment

Otitis media is treated with broad-spectrum antibiotics, decongestants, analgesics, and antipyretics. Parents need to understand that hearing can be diminished for up to 6 months following treatment. Recurrent otitis media may require a surgical procedure called a **myringotomy.** During the myringotomy, a small plastic tube is inserted through the tympanic membrane to facilitate drainage of

fluid and ventilation of the middle ear. This procedure can be done on an outpatient basis with local anesthesia. The tubes are usually effective for 6 to 12 months and may fall out naturally or be removed by the health care practitioner.

Nursing Considerations

Hospitalization is rare for the child with otitis media. Most of the care provided to this child will be in an outpatient setting or in the home. The child with otitis media can experience a significant amount of pain. The nurse should provide information to parents on the proper administra-tion of analgesics, including topical anesthetic ear drops. Parents should be taught how to straighten the ear canal for proper administration of otic medication in infants or older children (see Figure 8-38 ⬭).

Prevention methods should be discussed with the child's family. Smoking cessation should be discussed with the parents because exposure to second-hand smoke challenges the respiratory system and is associated with an increased incidence of otitis media. Pacifier use should be discour-aged at bedtime in infants with prior infection because it may also increase incidence (Niemala, Pihakari, Pokka, & Uhari, 2000). Parents of children who are in day care and who have frequent episodes of otitis media should consider alternative forms of child care to avoid exposure to pathogens.

clinical ALERT

The nurse must teach the parents about care of the child with myringotomy tubes. Parents should be cautioned against allow-ing water to enter the child's ears. During bathing, showering, swimming, or other water activities, ear plugs should be used to prevent infection from outside microorganisms.

HEARING ACUITY SCREENING

Delayed speech and language development may be the result of poor hearing acuity. It is important to perform hearing acuity screening to identify hearing impairment from an early age. The American Academy of Pediatrics (AAP) has endorsed universal newborn hearing screening in birthing units as the standard of care (Johnson, 2002). Currently the goal is to screen all infants by 1 month of age and to provide early treatment interventions before 6 months to all affected children (AAP & American College of Obstetricians and Gynecologists [ACOG], 2002). Periodic screening is done at schools and in pediatrician's offices. Procedures 15-4 and 15-5 ■ describe hearing screening tests. These tests are usually performed in the clinic setting.

MediaLink   Otitis Media

PROCEDURE 15-4 Pure Tone Audiometry

Purpose

- To determine the auditory acuity of a child older than 3.

Equipment

- Private room, free of distractions
- Calibrated audiometer, including earphones
- Alcohol pads

Check order + Gather equipment + Introduce yourself + Identify client + Provide privacy + Explain procedure + Hand hygiene + Gloves as needed

Interventions and Rationales

1. Perform preparatory steps (see icon bar above).

2. Clean the earphones with alcohol pads. *Harmful bacteria could be transmitted via the earphones.*

3. Explain the procedure thoroughly to the child and parent.

4. Demonstrate the equipment, sounds, and method used to test hearing. *The usual method for testing hearing is to have the child raise a hand on the side where the sound is heard.*

5. Have the child return demonstration of hand signals. *Do not proceed until proper understanding is determined.*

6. Position the child with the back toward the machine. *This ensures that the child cannot see the machine or the examiner and thus cannot receive visual cues about sounds heard.*

7. Place the earphones on the child and deliver sounds randomly to both ears. Each ear should be tested with the following pitches: 500, 1,000, 2,000, and 4,000 Hz.

8. Interpret the findings. *Passing auditory acuity findings are 20 to 25 decibels (dB) for 500, 1,000 and 2,000 Hz and 25 dB for 4,000 Hz.*

9. Report findings to the charge nurse and document them in the chart.

10. Repeat the test in 2 weeks if the child does not pass the test. If the second test is also unsuccessful, further evaluation is necessary.

SAMPLE DOCUMENTATION

(date) 0900   Pure tone audiometry indicates
20 dB at 500 and 1,000 Hz;
25 dB at 2,000 and 4,000 Hz
in both ears. D. Bryant, LPN

PROCEDURE 15-5 Tympanometry

Purpose

- To determine an estimate of middle ear pressure and tympanic membrane movement in older infants and children

Equipment

- Calibrated tympanometer
- Disposable probe
- Graph paper

Check order + Gather equipment + Introduce yourself + Identify client + Provide privacy + Explain procedure + Hand hygiene + Gloves as needed

A

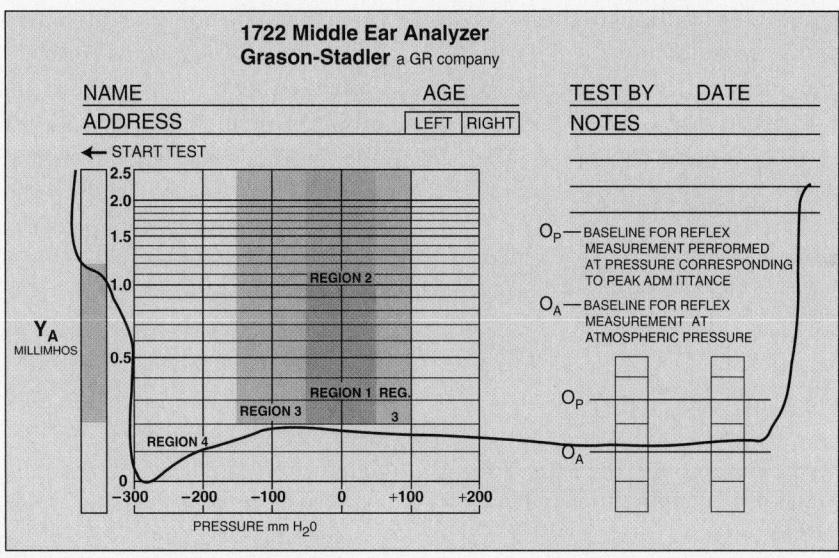

B

Figure 15-35. ■ (**A**) This tympanogram demonstrates normal hearing as evidenced by the curve showing the tympanic membrane's movement when a sound wave is emitted into the ear canal. Mobility is between 0.2 and 1.0 mL, the normal range. (**B**) In contrast, note the flat pattern in the second tympanogram, which shows restricted mobility of the tympanic membrane in response to sound.

Interventions and Rationales

1. Perform preparatory steps (see icon bar on p. 418).

2. Explain the procedure and the importance of remaining still to the child and his or her parents. *The risk of pain and injury to the auditory canal from the earpiece is reduced.*

3. Insert the earpiece covered with the disposable probe into the auditory canal. Ensure a seal. *The tight seal will provide an accurate measurement.*

4. Provide a tone from the tympanometer.

5. Repeat on the other ear.

6. Interpret findings plotted on graph paper (Figure 15-35 ■).

7. Report findings to charge nurse and document them in the chart.

SAMPLE DOCUMENTATION

(date) 1400   Tympanometry indicates fluid accumulation or pressure changes in the middle ear. Findings reported to charge nurse.
T. Edward, LVN

NURSING CARE

PRIORITIES IN NURSING CARE

The priorities in assessing a child with a neurologic impairment are determined by the type and degree of impairment. In general, the nurse ensures that the child has a patent airway and is well oxygenated. These children need protection from injury due to their altered mobility or their cognitive impairment. The nurse should perform a neurologic assessment every 2 hours to include level of consciousness, verbal responses, and motor responses.

ASSESSING

Children with nervous system disorders should be assessed for changes in LOC, reaction to stimuli, and ability to respond to stimuli. The nurse must monitor closely for signs of seizures, increased intracranial pressure (ICP), changes in LOC, and poor oxygenation.

clinical ALERT

Neurologic deterioration can occur rapidly in infants and young children. Changes in baseline vital signs and LOC must be recorded and reported immediately.

DIAGNOSING, PLANNING, AND IMPLEMENTING

The following nursing diagnoses may apply to the infant with a nervous system disorder:

- Ineffective Airway Clearance related to excessive mucus
- Risk for Deficient Fluid Volume related to imbalance of fluids and electrolytes
- Anticipatory Grieving (Parent) related to potential loss of neurologic function
- Risk for Injury related to impaired mobility due to neurologic deficit
- Impaired Communication: Verbal related to hearing impairment
- Self-Care Deficit: Hygiene, feeding, dressing, toileting related to neuromuscular impairment
- Disturbed Body Image related to head injury

Some outcomes for pediatric clients with neurologic disorders might include the following:

The client and/or parent will:

- Have a patent airway.
- Maintain fluid and electrolyte balance as evidenced by vital signs and lab values within normal limits.

- Demonstrate coping mechanisms.
- Provide a safe environment that prevents injury.
- Learn alternate methods to communicate effectively.
- Accept assistance in hygiene, feeding, dressing, and toileting.
- Demonstrate an understanding and acceptance of disfigurement.

The following nursing interventions are appropriate for children with neurologic impairment. (*Note:* Nursing interventions for some of these nursing diagnoses have been discussed previously in the context of particular disorders. They are not repeated here.)

- Adapt communication techniques for cognitive ability, not chronologic age. *Neurologic disorders can delay cognitive ability or the child may demonstrate regression of cognitive ability. Sometimes cognitive development stops and may never show normal progression.*
- Face the child and make eye contact when speaking. *This allows the child with a visual or moderate hearing defect to receive nonverbal cues.*
- Allow children to do as much for themselves as they are able. Provide assistance and encouragement toward self-care. Encourage family to allow the child as much independence as possible. Complete any care the child or family is unable to perform. *The amount of self-care depends on the degree of neurologic damage. Allowing the child to complete as much self-care as possible fosters independence and self-esteem.*
- Provide factual information to the child and family to assist in dealing with disturbed body image. Allow the young child expression of feeling through puppet play. Include other specialists such as physical therapist, occupational therapist, and speech therapist as needed. *Young children may not perceive disfigurement to the same extent as family members. Nursing care should focus on the family as the primary support for the child.*
- Reinforce teaching about the condition, and provide written materials and referrals as needed. *Parents may need information repeated so they can cope with the necessary adjustments at home, learn about the disorder, and follow up appropriately.*

EVALUATING

Evaluate airway patency by assessing the child's color, oxygen saturation, and respirations. The effectiveness of seizure medications is evaluated by recording the number, frequency, and type of seizures that occur. Evaluate for respiratory infection, malnutrition, constipation, and skin breakdown due to altered mobility. Watch family interaction with the child to determine the degree of their acceptance of the child's physical and mental limitations.

NURSING PROCESS CARE PLAN
Child with Cerebral Palsy

Daniel, a 9-year-old with CP, has moved to different city and will begin school in several weeks at a public elementary school. Daniel's parents, his pediatrician, and the school nurse meet to develop a plan to manage Daniel's health care while he is at school. The pediatrician tells the school nurse that Daniel is taking antiseizure medication but that the medication is not yet regulated. Daniel continues to have seizures approximately two times a week. Daniel's mom states that Daniel has fallen out of his wheelchair during seizures lately. However, he has not been injured during these falls.

Assessment

- Taking antiseizure medication
- Seizures twice weekly
- Falls during seizure activity
- Medical diagnosis—cerebral palsy

Nursing Diagnosis.
The following important nursing diagnosis (among others) is established for this client:

- Risk for **I**njury related to seizure activity

Expected Outcomes
- No sign of trauma following seizure activity

Planning and Implementation

- Teach school staff to recognize and manage seizures. *Daniel's safety will increase if all staff members have proper training in management of seizure activity.*
- Have oxygen and suction equipment available. *Seizures may cause hypoxia and/or airway obstruction.*
- Administer antiseizure medications as prescribed. *Proper administration of medication will assist in preventing seizure activity.*
- Teach Daniel to report aural warnings promptly. *Aural warnings may predict seizure activity and allow staff to better manage the seizure.*

- Consider protective headgear for Daniel. *The headgear may protect Daniel's head from injury.*
- Emphasize to the staff the importance of remaining with Daniel during the entire seizure. *Physical safety can be managed better, and documentation of events can be achieved.*
- Avoid restraining Daniel during the seizure. *Restraint may cause physical injury.*
- If necessary, use a chin-lift maneuver to open Daniel's airway during the seizure. *This maneuver maintains patent airway and prevents hypoxia.*
- Following the seizure, reassure Daniel and monitor neurologic status. *Return to expected neurologic status documents that the seizure is over.*
- Clearly document the seizure activity. *Management of the seizure activity is facilitated with correct documentation of aura, type and duration of movement, changes in level of consciousness, eye movement, pupil size, bowel and bladder incontinence, and teeth clenching.*

Evaluation.
In children with seizure activity, evaluate orientation and LOC regularly. Slight changes in these findings should be reported promptly. The nurse can evaluate the child's environment to determine the safety risk and make suggestions for improving the environment.

Critical Thinking Questions

1. What other physical challenges would the school nurse have in managing Daniel's case?
2. What social challenges will Daniel meet as he enters a new school with a disability?
3. What can the school nurse do to help Daniel overcome these social challenges?

Note: Discussion of Critical Thinking questions appears in Appendix I.

Note: The reference and resource listings for this and all chapters have been compiled at the back of the book.

Chapter Review

KEY TERMS by Topic

Use the audio glossary feature of either the CD-ROM or the Companion Website to hear the correct pronunciation of the following key terms.

Anatomy and Physiology
ganglia, neurons, axon, cell body, dendrite, myelination, myelin sheath, cephalocaudala, organogenesis, cranium, intracranial pressure, somatic reflexes, autonomic reflexes, sympathetic nervous system, parasympathetic nervous system

Pain
nociceptors

Congenital Neurologic Defects
spina bifida, neural tube, meningocele, myelomeningocele

Nervous System Disorders
seizures, febrile seizures, tonic-clonic movements, epilepsy, status epilepticus, focal seizures, generalized seizures, aura, postictal, kernicterus, fibromyalgia

Nervous System Infections
meningitis, encephalitis, Reye's syndrome, Guillain-Barré syndrome, postinfectious polyneuritis

Neurologic Trauma
neurologic trauma, closed head injury, hematomas, concussion, drowning, near-drowning

Mental Retardation
mental retardation, Down syndrome, epicanthal folds, simian crease, Brushfield spots

Eye Disorders
diplopia, PERRLA

Eye Conditions
acute conjunctivitis, leukokoria, strabismus, heterochromia, enucleation

Eye Injuries
hyphema

Visual Impairment
hyperopia, myopia, astigmatism, esotropia, exotropia, hypertropia, orthoptics, amblyopia, dyslexia, cataracts, nystagmus, glaucoma, epiphora, buphthalmos, photophobia, tonometer, goniotomy

Ear Disorders
tinnitus, cochlear implants, otitis media, otalgia, myringotomy

KEY Points

- The nurse needs to understand the anatomy and physiology of the child's nervous system in order to have an adequate understanding of the disorders of the neurologic system.

- Neurologic assessments include assessing for level of consciousness (LOC) and verbal and motor response to stimuli.

- Early signs of increased ICP are headache, vomiting, LOC changes, asymmetric pupils, and seizures. In the infant, a high-pitched cry, bulging fontanels, dilated scalp veins, and irritability may be noted. Later signs include significant changes in LOC, respiratory distress, bradycardia, increased systolic blood pressure, fixed and dilated pupils, and death.

- The Glasgow Coma Scale is used to evaluate a child's LOC.

- Pain in the child can be difficult to assess. Verbal expressions of pain include crying, moaning, groaning, or screaming. Nonverbal expressions of pain include facial grimacing, posturing, splinting, restlessness, and sleep disturbances.

- Management of pain in children includes pharmacologic and nonpharmacologic methods. Pharmacologic methods include narcotic and nonnarcotic analgesics. Nonpharmacologic methods include distraction, touch, and application of cold or heat.

- During a seizure, the first priority is to establish a safe environment for the child. Immediately after the seizure, position the child on the side, remove mucus and drainage from the airway, and assess for airway patency.

- The Snellen letter chart, picture chart, and E chart are available to screen for visual acuity.

EXPLORE MediaLink

Additional interactive resources for this chapter can be found on the Companion Website at www. prenhall. com/ adams.

Click on Chapter 15 and "Begin" to select the activities for this chapter.

For chapter-related NCLEX®-style questions and an audio glossary, access the accompanying CD-ROM in this book.

Animations:
Middle ear   Conjunctivitis   Down syndrome   Child's ear   Adolescent ear   Otitis media   The culture of deafness

FOR FURTHER Study

See Chapter 3 for legal information.

A PCA pump is illustrated in Figure 7-11.

See Chapter 8 for procedures for pain assessment, measuring head circumference, irrigating the eye and ear, and positioning the child for lumbar puncture. Table 8-3 explains Apgar scoring.

The Health Promotion Issue in Chapter 9 discusses organ donation in a dying child.

See Chapter 10 for further discussion of communicable diseases.

See Figure 12-7 for CPR techniques.

Congenital heart disorders are discussed in Chapter 13.

See Nursing Care Plan Chart: Child Undergoing Chemotherapy, Chapter 14.

Chapter 16 has discussion of thought process disorders, fetal alcohol syndrome, child abuse, and shaken-baby syndrome.

For the Denver Developmental Screening Test II, see Appendix III.

Some basic sign language is provided in Appendix VII.

Caring for a Client with Meningitis

NCLEX-PN® Focus Area: Safety

Case Study: Jessie is a 4-year-old female who developed a fever, anorexia, and vomiting, and complains of pain in her neck. Jessie attends day care Monday through Friday while her mother works at the bank. Several of the children in her class have been ill. Her big brother is in second grade. Jessie's mom calls the pediatrician's office to ask for advice on caring for her child.

Nursing Diagnosis: Risk for **I**njury, related to environmental exposure to pathogens

COLLECT DATA

Subjective	Objective
_____	_____
_____	_____
_____	_____
_____	_____
_____	_____
_____	_____

Would you report this? Yes/No

If yes, to: _____

Nursing Care

_____
_____
_____
_____
_____
_____
_____
_____
_____
_____
_____

How would you document this? _____

_____
_____
_____

Compare your documentation to the sample provided in Appendix I.

Data Collected:
(use only those that apply)

- Vital signs: T 101.4, P 70, R 12, BP 90/60
- Pain level: 8 using Oucher scale
- Jessie states, "My tummy hurts right here."
- Positive Brudzinski's sign
- Weight: 29 lb
- Mom states, "She is very irritable."
- 24-hour diet history: two crackers, 50 mL Pedialyte
- Emesis: 30 mL green vomitus x1
- Mom states, "Several children in her class at day care are sick with the same thing."
- Positive Kernig's sign

Nursing Interventions
(use only those that apply;

list in priority order)

- Teach mom signs and symptoms of infection and when to seek medical attention.
- Monitor vital signs for subtle changes.
- Record intake and output.
- Review immunization record.
- Assess for Kernig's and Brudzinski's sign.
- Monitor pain levels for changes.
- Identify comfort measures that decrease the child's pain level.
- Administer pain medications as ordered.
- Discuss ways to prevent transmission of bacteria, including hand washing techniques and isolating the child from other sick children.
- Monitor CBC values for signs of infection.

NCLEX-PN® Exam Preparation

TEST-TAKING TIP When a question has the key word *avoid*, it indicates a "false-response" question. You will need to pick the action that is <u>contraindicated</u>.

1 A 10-month-old is admitted to the hospital with possible meningitis. An IV has been started in her left forearm, and a restraint is being used to prevent interference with the IV infusion. Her aunt has come to stay with her for the afternoon and asks if the restraint can be removed. The nurse's best response is:

1. "It can only be removed with a doctor's order."
2. "It can be removed only if you are staying in the room."
3. "It needs to be kept on at all times."
4. "It can be removed only if the nurse is in the room."

2 A child has an order for acetaminophen (Tylenol) 240 mg PO. The label on the bottle reads 160 mg/5 mL. How many mL should be administered to the child?

3 Seeing his son, who was born with spina bifida, for the first time, a father exclaims, "What is that on his back!" An appropriate response would be:

1. Describing the condition fully, including long-term complications.
2. Defining the term *spina bifida* and providing a simple explanation of the anomaly.
3. Directing his attention away from the defect.
4. Saying, "I don't know. I'll have the doctor call you."

4 The nurse is assessing the infant for signs and symptoms of pain following circumcision. Choose all of the following symptoms that could be indicators of pain.

1. Facial grimacing, tachycardia
2. Bradypnea, flushing
3. Pupil dilation, restlessness
4. Tachypnea, anorexia
5. Sleepiness, bradycardia

5 The physician orders phenobarbital IV 20 mg/kg/day for the infant with status epilepticus. Available is phenobarbital 30 mg/mL. How many total mL will the nurse give for the infant who weighs 7 lb 5 oz?

6 The nurse is preparing to test the visual acuity of a 2-year-old female client using a Snellen chart. The nurse performs the test knowing that which of the following identifies the accurate procedure for this type of visual acuity testing for 2-year-olds?

1. The child is held by her mother at approximately 40 feet from the chart.
2. Both eyes are tested at the same time, and then the left eye is tested first followed by the right eye.
3. The child is held by her mother at approximately 30 feet from the chart and asked to identify the characters on the chart that can be read from 200 feet away.

4. The right eye is tested first, then the left eye, and then both eyes are tested together.

7 A nurse is caring for a client with Reye's syndrome. The nurse realizes the client's father understands the teaching about this syndrome when he makes the following comment:

1. "I am going to give my son Pepto-Bismol if he has an upset stomach."
2. "I realize I will have to check labels to make sure we don't give our son anything containing aspirin or aspirin-like products."
3. "I understand that Reye's syndrome was caused by bacteria."
4. "I will give my son Triaminicin for his next cold."

8 The nurse is helping with a lumbar puncture for a 6-year-old client with suspected Guillain-Barré syndrome. The nurse places the client in which of the following positions?

1. Prone knee-chest position
2. Supine
3. Lateral position, with the knees flexed up to the abdomen, back bowed at the edge of the bed and chin resting on the chest
4. Immobilized with the client on a spinal backboard to prevent movement during the procedure

9 The nurse is instituting seizure precautions for a 3-year-old client being admitted from the emergency department with a closed head injury and suspected concussion. Which of the following nursing interventions would the nurse avoid in planning for this client's safety?

1. Keeping airway, suction, and oxygen equipment at the bedside
2. Taping a padded tongue blade at the head of the bed
3. Padding the bed side rails of the bed
4. Having IV equipment ready for quick insertion of an IV line

10 The nurse is caring for a client newly diagnosed with cerebral palsy (CP). The parents are overwhelmed and ask the nurse about CP. The nurse responds to the parents based on the understanding that CP is:

1. An infection of the central nervous system
2. Caused by a virus that causes an inflammation of the brain
3. A congenital condition resulting in severe mental retardation
4. A chronic disability that is characterized by difficulty in controlling muscles

Answers for NCLEX-PN® Review and Critical Thinking questions appear in Appendix I.

Care of the Child with Psychosocial Disorders

BRIEF Outline

Brief Assessment Review

Psychological Disorders and Associated Manifestations

Nursing Care

Anorexia Nervosa and Bulimia

Nursing Care

Abuse and Family Violence

Nursing Care

Traumatic Events

Therapies Used to Assist the Child with Psychosocial Disorders

NURSING PROCESS CARE PLAN: Client with Anorexia Nervosa

HEALTH PROMOTION ISSUE: Preventing Infant Abduction

NURSING CARE PLAN CHART: Care of the Child Who Is Physically Abused

CRITICAL THINKING CARE MAP: Caring for a Client with Attention Deficit/Hyperactivity Disorder

LEARNING Outcomes

After completing this chapter, you will be able to:

1. Define key terms.
2. Describe an appropriate psychosocial assessment of the child.
3. Describe psychosocial disorders to include autism, Asperger's syndrome, attention deficit disorder, Gilles de la Tourette syndrome, anxiety, depression, anorexia nervosa and bulimia, child abuse (physical and emotional), and substance abuse.
4. Describe associated manifestations of psychological disorders to include overeating and obesity and suicide.
5. Discuss clinical manifestations, diagnostic procedures, medical management, and nursing interventions related to psychosocial disorders.
6. Explain appropriate nursing interventions for children with psychosocial disorders.
7. Discuss the impact to children of traumatic events and natural disasters.

Psychosocial health includes mental, emotional, social and spiritual stability. Usually by the age of 8 years, children have rational thinking and perceive situations realistically. The emotionally healthy child feels appropriately about life's circumstances. Stress is tolerated and coping skills are demonstrated. The socially healthy child has effective relationships, and their actions are appropriate in social situations. Spiritual health encompasses the child's belief system, their set of values, and how they make choices; it includes the meaning given to life's circumstances (D'Amico & Barbarito, 2007). Psychosocial health is affected by many factors such as genetics, physical health, family, culture, where people live, and their economic status, as well as their self-concept. Alterations in a child's psychosocial health will affect about one-fourth of all children (Ball & Bindler, 2006). Some of these alterations will be short term, whereas others will have lifelong effects.

Brief Assessment Review

To accurately assess the child, the nurse must review physical health, mental health, and spiritual health. **Holistic health** is a concept that approaches an individual's health as an integrated system rather than divided into physical, emotional, intellectual, and spiritual parts. Belief in this concept allows the nurse to understand that any alteration in the child's psychosocial health could have an effect on the child's physical health. At the same time, alterations in physical health could have psychosocial ramifications.

HISTORY

- Determine the child's past emotional or psychiatric problems.
- Determine the family history of emotional or psychiatric problems.
- Ask about the child's growth and development.
- Inquire about the child's performance in school and other organized activities.
- Inquire about their relationships with others.
- Determine the child's emotional response to illness and crises. Ask them to define their greatest source of comfort during these stressful times.
- Ask older children and teens to define their concept of hope and faith.
- Determine self-concept. Ask them how they would describe themselves to others.
- Ask specifically about their use of alcohol and street drugs.
- Ask about laxative use.
- Ask them about eating disorders such as anorexia nervosa or bulimia.
- See the sections below for child abuse and sexual abuse screening.

PHYSICAL

- Observe the child's general appearance. Describe dress, hygiene, and grooming.
- If bulimia is suspected, inspect dental enamel of the teeth. Worn enamel can occur from gastric acid produced during purging.
- Describe the child's facial expression and affect.
- Observe the child's body posture, gait, and body movement.
- Describe the child's speech patterns. Is the content of their speech appropriate? What is the tone, pace, and volume of their speech? Do they talk to themselves? Are they aphasic or incoherent?

Psychological Disorders and Associated Manifestations

The *Diagnostic and Statistical Manual of Mental Disorders—Fourth Edition Text Revision* (DSM-IV TR), which is published by the American Psychiatric Association, serves as the main diagnostic reference of mental health professionals in the United States. This resource includes diagnostic criteria for the most common mental disorders. It is also used for research purposes and by insurance companies to apply charges for services offered by mental health professionals. Appropriate use of the diagnostic criteria is said to require clinical training. Please refer to a psychiatric nursing text for more information about this resource.

Psychological disorders include a wide range of disorders that may begin at birth or early childhood and may continue throughout life. These include psychological disorders such as autism, attention deficit disorders (ADD), attention deficit hyperactive disorders (ADHD), anxiety, phobias, and depression. Also see Chapter 15 ⚭ for a further discussion of cognitive disorders such as mental retardation.

Psychological disorders involve abnormalities in behavior, communication, and social interactions. Depending on the cause of the specific disorder, the child's development might progress to a point and then stop, progress to a point and then regress, or fail to develop beyond the infantile state.

Children with some psychological disorders engage in repetitive behaviors, including self-stimulating or self-destructive behaviors. The repetitive behaviors might include, but are not limited to, twirling in circles, head banging, and biting themselves. Some of these children may have difficulty sitting quietly for any length of time and focusing on a productive activity. They run around the room and "get into everything." Other children with psychological disorders focus on only one activity and seem to "block out" everything that is going on around them.

Difficulty with speech (both with talking and understanding the spoken word) is common. Although some children may eventually learn to talk, abnormal patterns may develop. Cognitive abilities may correspond with intellectual deficits. Learning may be difficult and the child may struggle in school. Other children may learn, but have difficulty expressing what they know.

Children with psychological disorders demonstrate a wide range of social skills. They may have difficulty establishing relationships because of speech problems or lack of focus. Disrupted thought processes may cause the child to be anxious, develop phobias, overeat, or become depressed and even consider suicide. Some children and adults may be fearful of children with a thought process disorder and avoid interacting with them, causing further feelings of isolation.

AUTISM AND ASPERGER'S SYNDROME

According to the Autism Society of America, **autism** is "a complex developmental disability that typically appears during the first three years of life and is the result of a neurological disorder that affects the normal functioning of the brain, impacting development in the areas of social interaction and communication skills." Children with autism have difficulty with verbal and nonverbal communication, social interactions, and leisure or play activities (Figure 16-1 ■).

Autism is found to affect boys more often than girls. There is no known cause for autism. It is thought to be genetically inherited. Autism is associated with congenital rubella syndrome, *fragile X syndrome* (a congenital disorder causing mental retardation), phenylketonuria, Down syndrome, and tuberous sclerosis.

Another disorder that is similar to autism is **Asperger's syndrome.** In this disorder the child exhibits social isolation and communication difficulties (but no language delay), clumsiness, and a focused area of interest and attention. For instance, the child may be preoccupied with automobiles, knowing the names of all makes and models. Asperger's syndrome usually has a later onset than autism and does not have a delay in cognitive development.

Figure 16-1. ■ A Child with autistic disorder. (PhotoEdit, Inc.)

Manifestations

Prior to diagnosis of autism, the infant may show a lack of response to sounds, have difficulty sleeping or sleep longer than expected, have difficulty feeding, avoid eye contact, or show little to no response to human interaction. The toddler who is autistic may suddenly be unable to communicate verbally. Words may be repeated over and over again. This is called **echolalia.** The toddler, who is expected to have stranger anxiety, demonstrates no fear in unfamiliar surroundings or around unfamiliar people. Toilet training may also be very difficult in the toddler with autism.

Autism is marked in the child by the presence of excessive repetitive behaviors such as hand movements or rocking. These rigid and obsessive behaviors are also called **stereotypy.** The child may appear stiff, be unwilling to cuddle, and have an awkward gait. Repetitive sounds and loud responses to being touched are also noticed. The child is unable to interact with others socially and is often observed playing alone. Certain objects or toys have significance, and the child may not be able to eat, go to school, or go to sleep without them. They will also have either exaggerated responses to pain or a minimal response.

Diagnosis

The diagnosis of autism is made by the presence of symptoms. Other conditions that may mimic symptoms of autism are ruled out by CT scans, MRIs, testing for lead poisoning, tests for hearing, metabolic studies, and electroencephalograms. There are also several instruments available to use in screening for autism. For more information on these instruments, please see psychiatric nursing text.

Treatment

Although there is no cure for autism, many researchers in the field agree that early, intensive interventions prior to age 5 can lead to behavior modification. A highly structured environment, with one-on-one interaction, is necessary for some children and therefore the parents and each caregiver will need extensive training to promote success. Children may also be mainstreamed into public school systems. Eye contact, appropriate language, social skills, and proper methods of play are encouraged. Negative behaviors are discouraged by close supervision and consistency. Restraint may be necessary until the behavior is changed. Stimulants, selective serotonin reuptake inhibitors, and mood stabilizers may be prescribed to assist the interventions.

Nursing Considerations

It is important for the nurse caring for the child in either the outpatient or inpatient setting to carefully determine the child's rituals and communication patterns. The setting for health care should be altered to accommodate the needs of the child. For instance, if the child has a specific toy that brings him comfort, he should be allowed to keep it with him. Parents should be encouraged to stay with the child to provide familiarity.

Children with autism may pose a safety risk due to repetitive behaviors such as head banging and the lack of fear of dangerous situations. The nurse can provide devices such as helmets and hand mittens to protect the child from injury. The environment should be carefully scrutinized, modified, and supervised to promote safety. Parents should receive referrals to agencies and support groups or long-term care facilities to assist them managing care of the child with autism.

ATTENTION DEFICIT DISORDER (ADD) AND ATTENTION DEFICIT/HYPERACTIVITY DISORDER (ADHD)

ADD and ADHD are most commonly identified as the older child enters school. ADD is a central nervous system disorder characterized by inappropriate behaviors related to attention. ADHD involves inattention as well as hyperactivity and impulsiveness. Worldwide, 6% to 8% of school age children are diagnosed with ADHD (Faraone, 2002). In the United States, 3.8 million school-age children have the disorder (Vlam, 2006).

Manifestations

Children with ADD have difficulty finishing tasks. They are easily distracted and may move from topic to topic in their speech as well as activities. Some children with ADD are quietly distractible. They may have difficulty working with others.

Children with ADHD also have difficulty finishing tasks but (unlike children with ADD), they fidget, may become loud, and disrupt others. Some children with ADD and ADHD have difficulty maintaining social relationships. They may be teased or shunned by other children.

Diagnosis

The child who is suspected of having ADD or ADHD should be evaluated by a mental health specialist, primary care physician, or advanced practice registered nurse. The health care professional reviews the medical and social history of the child. There are several tools available to assist in the diagnosis of ADHD. These include parent scales, teacher scales, and those that close relatives or caregivers complete. These scales assess achievement and performance in the classroom, self-esteem, interactions with others, impulsive behaviors, hyperactivity, ability to pay attention, and level of anxiety. The *Diagnostic and Statistical Manual of Mental Disorders—Fourth Edition Text Revision* (DSM-IV TR) of the American Psychiatric Association's criteria for diagnosis include:

- At least 6 of 9 inattentive symptoms and/or 6 of 9 hyperactive or 1 impulsive symptom

- Duration of these symptoms longer than 6 months
- Symptoms evident in more than one setting (home, school, church, or community)

Treatment

If a diagnosis of ADD or ADHD is made, treatment may vary depending on the type and degree of disability. Treatment may include changing the environment, behavior modification, and medication.

Environmental changes include having the child use a separate desk in an area of the room where other students cannot distract them. However, ADD and ADHD children should also be made to feel important, valuable, and a part of the class. Stimuli should be decreased. This can be accomplished by turning off the radio or television. However, some children benefit from listening to their head sets while working, because it shuts out other external stimuli. Structure and routine need to be built into the child's day. Helping the child develop organizational skills is of great importance.

Professional counselors may be helpful in modifying the child's behavior and should be included in the care planning team. Establishing a system of rewards for appropriate behavior can help the child learn and foster a positive self-image. The expected behavior must be realistically achievable. If the child cannot receive frequent rewards, the behavior may not change. If consequences are necessary, they should follow quickly after the offense so the child can relate the consequence to the behavior.

The most commonly prescribed medications are stimulants. Common stimulants used in the treatment of ADD/ADHD are methylphenidate (Ritalin), dextroamphetamine sulfate (Dexedrine), and amphetamine sulfate (Adderal). Atomoxetine (Strattera), a specific noradrenergic reuptake inhibitor, is a more recent drug that is showing positive results. Other drugs such as antidepressants, antihypertensives, and arousal agents may also be used. The most recent medication approved by the FDA is methylphenidate transdermal system (Daytrana). The patch is applied once daily. It is designed to provide a sustained dosage and to stay on even active children. Table 16-1 ■ lists some common medications used to treat ADD/ADHD and usual side effects. Some medications may need to be taken at school. School personnel giving the medication should understand the safe administration of the drugs. "Drug holidays" may be implemented during vacation periods or the summer months when academic performance is not required.

Nursing Considerations

The nurse should make sure parents understand the prescribed medication, including side effects. Insomnia can be prevented or corrected by taking the medication early in the day and by avoiding caffeine later in the day. It is also

TABLE 16-1

Pharmacology: Medications Used to Treat ADD/ADHD

DRUG (GENERIC AND COMMON BRAND NAME)	USUAL ROUTE/DOSE	CLASSIFICATION AND PURPOSE	SELECTED SIDE EFFECTS	DON'T GIVE IF
Methylphenidate hydrochloride (Ritalin)	5–10 mg before breakfast and lunch, increasing 5–10 mg/wk prn, PO	Cerebral stimulant to provide mental focus	Dizziness, nervousness, insomnia, increased P & BP, blurred vision, dry mouth, loss of appetite if taken before meals (sometimes reported to slow growth)	After 6 p.m. to avoid insomnia
Amphetamine sulfate (Adderall)	Child: 2.5–5 mg PO 1–2 times/day, increasing by 2.5–5 mg weekly; Adolescent: 10 mg extended release once daily PO in morning; may increase by 5–10 mg at weekly intervals	Cerebral stimulant to provide alertness	Irritability, euphoria, palpitations, insomnia, restlessness	Within 6 hours of bedtime to avoid insomnia. Do not crush extended release capsules
Atomoxetine hydrochloride (Strattera)	0.5–1.2 mg/kg/d PO	Psychotherapeutic agent to improve attentiveness and ability to follow through on tasks; diminishes hyperactivity	Anorexia, upset stomach, dizziness, tiredness, mood swings, insomnia, hypersomnia	The child reports hypotension or urinary retention
Bupropion hydrochloride (Wellbutrin)	6 mg/kg/day PO	Antidepressant	Dizziness, agitation, insomnia, blurred vision, headache, tremor, nausea, vomiting, constipation, dry mouth	On an empty stomach
Modafinil (Provigil)	100 mg/day PO	Cerebral stimulant, arousal agent	Headache, nausea	Child is less than 16 years old

important to remove the computer, television, radio and cell phone from the bedroom to eliminate activities that would prolong the initiation of sleep. The stimulant class of medications has a high potential for abuse. Discuss with the child and parents the need to secure all medication at all times.

Families of children with ADD and ADHD require support. Parents may become frustrated with a child's behavior and inflict inappropriate punishments. A stable, routine environment will help the child to focus. The parent needs to set boundaries and limits and help the child learn to act within them. Support groups may be beneficial to the parents.

The child with ADD or ADHD should be evaluated on a regular basis. Medications usually have an effect within the first 10 to 14 days of treatment. Behavior modification programs may take weeks or months to be effective. Small positive steps in behavioral change should be recognized.

ANXIETY

Anxiety is an emotion that everyone feels at some time in life. However, in some people the feeling is not related to actual past or upcoming events. When it exists consistently and out of proportion to reality, a diagnosis of anxiety may be made.

Manifestations

Subjective feelings of worry, helplessness, insecurity, and apprehension are characteristics of anxiety. Objective or physical symptoms often accompany these symptoms. These objective symptoms include tachycardia, restlessness, diaphoresis, and trembling. Regressive behaviors may occur in some children. The child may experience enuresis and/or **encopresis** (a condition where the child delays defecation or experiences frequent soiling of feces). (For more information on enuresis, see Chapter 18 .) Children with anxiety frequently learn to cope with anxiety by withdrawing, avoiding situations, or becoming overly dependent on parents or other caregivers.

Generalized anxiety disorder (GAD) is also called overanxious disorder. The child is prone to excessive worry about the future. These worries are often imagined. Even if the worries never materialize, the child continues to demonstrate a pattern of worry. The child with **separation**

anxiety disorder (SAD), also called *anaclitic depression*, is fearful of separation from individuals or locations. Panic may set in as the child approaches the time and location of separation.

School phobia, also called school avoidance or school refusal, may be a type of SAD, although there may be other reasons the child refuses to go to school. Physical complaints usually accompany school phobia. These include stomachaches, headaches, and fever. School phobia may be associated with real stressors such as physical abuse or bullies. See the section on bullying below for more information. School performance, sleep habits, and family and peer relationships are affected by school phobia. If the symptoms continue, the child's future education and employment may be affected. Children with school phobia have an increased risk of psychiatric disorders. Antidepressants may be effective in assisting the child to overcome the phobia.

Obsessive-compulsive disorder (OCD) is characterized by ritualistic thoughts or actions that interfere with activities of daily living. Children may have obsessions about germs, sexual activity, fears of traumatic events, or religious rituals. OCD may be associated with ADHD, tics (sudden, rapid, involuntary movements of head, eyes, and upper body), or hoarding behaviors. (*Note:* Tics may also occur in children as a result of high doses of medication.) Behavioral therapy can help the child learn to overcome fears and obsessions.

Diagnosis

Parents may bring their child to the health care provider, unaware of the possibility that anxiety is causing the manifestation of symptoms. A physical examination, lab work, and other diagnostic tests can be done to rule out physical conditions. A careful health history, review of symptoms, and discussion with the parent and child regarding the clinical manifestations of anxiety aid in the diagnosis.

Treatment

All anxiety disorders should be recognized and dealt with promptly. Families and school personnel should be given proper information about the disorder and encouraged to assist in the relief measures. Real threats to the child's safety must be assessed and resolved if present. Children need to learn coping skills and relaxation techniques. Antidepressants and antianxiety medications may be used to assist the child with the initial relief of symptoms.

Nursing Considerations

The nurse can help the child develop coping methods. The child can be taught to replace negative thoughts with positive ones. For example: when the child feels anxious, he or she could repeat the phrase, "I am calm. I am in control."

Physical activity decreases stress behaviors. Simply going on a 30-minute walk can help a child deal with symptoms of anxiety. Avoiding caffeine, tobacco, and other stimulants is essential to decreasing anxiety. The nurse should assess whether these habits are part of the child's life, and if so, encourage the child to replace these habits with healthy behaviors.

GILLES DE LA TOURETTE SYNDROME

Gilles de la Tourette syndrome is characterized by **tics** (sudden, rapid motor movements of the head, eyes, and upper body) and a variety of verbal noises. In Tourette syndrome, children may utter obscenities, profanities, or racial slurs (**coprolalia**) and may involuntarily gesture obscenely (**copropraxia**).

Tourette syndrome is thought be genetically caused and occurs more commonly in boys than girls. It is most often treated in children with pimozide (Orap), a dopamine receptor antagonist. The nurse must provide parental support and assist in helping the child to achieve normal development. Because the tic behavior can occur more commonly during stressful periods, stress reduction techniques can be taught. If the child is unable to attend school while the tics are uncontrolled, the nurse can assist the parents in arranging for home tutoring.

DEPRESSION

Depression is a persistent feeling of sadness or hopelessness. It affects approximately 2% of children and 5% of adolescents, with increased numbers in the older adolescent. This risk increases in the adolescent because of the biological changes, social pressures, and search for autonomy common to most children of this age group. Depression is thought to be genetically passed on to children or to be the result of a biochemical imbalance.

Manifestations

Characteristics of depression include declining school performance, irritability, withdrawal from social activities, sleep disorders (either unable to sleep or sleeping all the time), appetite disturbance (either overeating or anorexia), headache, stomachache, difficulty concentrating, and difficulty making decisions. Box 16-1 ■ highlights manifestations of depression in children (Simpson & Ivey, 2005).

Depression can be a primary condition or secondary to learned behavior due to dysfunctional family traits. Depression can be seen with other psychiatric disorders including attention deficit/hyperactivity disorder, anxiety, bipolar disorder, or personality disorders. At times the depressed child maintains some degree of functioning until some crisis (such as a fight with parents, ending of a close relationship, or the loss of a friend) becomes the catalyst for

BOX 16-1   ASSESSMENT

Depression in Children
- Chronically depressed mood occurring for most of the day, and on more days than not
- Demonstrating sad behaviors or describing their mood as sad
- Irritability
- Poor appetite or overeating
- Insomnia or hypersomnia
- Headaches
- Stomachaches
- Loss of interest in usual activities
- Low energy or fatigue
- Low self-esteem
- Poor concentration or difficulty making decisions
- Feelings of hopelessness
- Low interest
- Self-criticism; describing oneself as being uninteresting, incapable, or ineffective
- Suicidal thoughts

extreme behavior. The depressed child may strike out at authority figures, as exhibited by violence at school, or direct the anger inward and hurt himself or herself. Depression in children is associated with substance abuse, increased physical illness, teenage pregnancy, decreased success in academics, and suicidal behavior. See the section on Suicide found later in this chapter.

Diagnosis
A comprehensive history of the child's symptoms must be obtained. A thorough psychiatric evaluation is often performed by a specially trained clinician. Data should be sought from the child, the parents, other family members, and teachers if appropriate. The child and parents may be asked to keep a mood diary to obtain a log of symptoms over a longer period of time.

Treatment
Treatment of children with depression will depend on the degree of depression and the specific needs of the child and family. The child may be hospitalized if there is a threat to his or her physical safety. A combination of therapy and medications is usually prescribed, whether the child is treated in an inpatient or outpatient setting. Therapy involves a combination of individual and family therapy and usually is necessary for 6 to 12 months. About half of children will relapse into depression following therapy, so treatment may be extended as a preventative measure (American Academy of Child and Adolescent Psychiatry, 1998). Individual psychotherapy uses either play or talk to attempt to assist the child to resolve negative feelings

related to life events that may have triggered depression. Cognitive behavior therapy is more likely to be used with adolescents and seeks to identify and correct negative thought patterns. Children may be given antidepressant medication called selective serotonin reuptake inhibitors (SSRIs). Some examples of these medications are fluoxetine hydrochloride (Prozac) and sertraline hydrochloride (Zoloft).

Nursing Considerations
The nurse must seek to help the child and the parents identify symptoms of depression and report them promptly. Parents should be assisted in developing methods of building the child's self-esteem. Parents can encourage the child in activities they enjoy and in which they demonstrate competence. Listening is an important activity for the nurse, to assist in building self-esteem and to provide encouragement to the child.

The nurse must also help the child and parent to understand medications prescribed for depression. Information should be given about side effects, the dosage schedule, and the danger of overdose. Side effects include impulsiveness, silliness, agitation, daring behavior, diaphoresis, headaches, bruising, and changes in appetite. Storage and administration of the medication should be a parental responsibility to minimize the risk of overdose. The nurse should explain that it often takes 4 to 6 weeks to realize an improvement of symptoms when the child is taking SSRIs. The family must be warned against abrupt discontinuation of SSRIs because withdrawal may occur.

clinical ALERT
Because of reports of increased suicidal thinking or aggressive behavior in children and adolescents taking antidepressant medications for psychiatric disorders, clear warnings now appear on FDA-approved antidepressant drugs. Parents must be cautioned to watch children carefully for these changes, especially during the first few weeks of treatment.

BIPOLAR DISORDER
Bipolar disorder is also called *manic depression*. In this disorder, children have mood swings that vary between mania and depression. Manic episodes are characterized by hyperactivity, irritability, aggression, and possibly hallucinations. Depressive episodes are marked by periods of sadness, sleep and eating disturbances, and social withdrawal. Ten to twenty percent of those diagnosed with bipolar disorder commit suicide. Treatment is focused on stabilizing the child's mood by administering lithium, valproate (Depakote), or carbamazepine (Tegretol). Lamotrigine (Lamictal) is also used as a mood stabilizer (Keck & McElroy, 2003).

SUICIDE

Suicide, the taking of one's own life, is the second leading cause of death for 15- to 19-year-olds. The rate of suicide has tripled in the past 50 years. For every suicide that is completed, it is estimated that 100 to 200 attempts are made. Although females attempt suicide 3 to 4 times more often than males, males complete the act 4 times more often. Many suicides are reported as accidents because of family embarrassment or social stigma. Suicide can be an associated manifestation of psychological disorders.

Instability in the American family has increased. This lack of parental support, coupled with increased exposure to stressors at school, within peer groups, and at home, has caused the adolescent to have difficulty coping. Tired of trying to handle the pressure alone, the teen becomes depressed and sees suicide as a way out. With easy access to firearms and drugs, it is not surprising that these become the usual method of suicide.

Early detection of depression (see Box 16-1) is the key to preventing the tragedy of suicide or violence against others. When adolescents begin to contemplate suicide, their behavior may signal their thought processes, and immediate help is needed. It is important to seek help if the teen:

- Has behavior changes that last for a few weeks or longer
- Is showing four or more symptoms of depression
- Is doing poorly in school
- Is seriously withdrawn or isolated
- Is overly impulsive
- Is uninterested in activities that were once enjoyed
- Cries frequently
- Gives away treasured items
- Verbalizes suicidal thoughts such as, "I don't want to live any longer"

If a child expresses suicidal thoughts, the nurse should not ignore the statement. The nurse should question the teen about depression and thoughts of suicide using therapeutic communication skills. If the teen admits suicidal thoughts (called *suicidal ideation*), the plan for suicide should be explored, including method and opportunity. The more lethal the method and the more realistic the opportunity, the higher the probability the teen will attempt suicide. The nurse should not leave teen unattended until medical treatment is initiated.

The teen who is depressed should be referred immediately to a qualified professional for evaluation and treatment. Frequently, antidepressants are prescribed in conjunction with individual and family counseling. For more information, see the section on treatment of depression.

In many cases, the risk for depression and suicide lessens with time and treatment. As the adolescent matures, he or she learns skills to cope with stress. In mild cases, an herbal

BOX 16-2 COMPLEMENTARY THERAPIES

St. John's Wort and Depression

A 2003 study at Case Western Reserve University of 33 children with a mean age of 10.5 years found that St. John's wort may be effective in treating children diagnosed with depressive disorders. St. John's Wort, also called *Hypericum perforatum* or Klamathweed, occurs naturally as a shrub with yellow flowers. The plant can be processed into capsules, tablets, tinctures, teas or lotions and has been associated with reduced symptoms of mild to moderate depression. Side effects are nausea, hives, fatigue, photosensitivity, restlessness, headache, dry mouth, dizziness and confusion. Children must take St. John's wort only under the supervision of a physician. The following drugs have been found to interact negatively with St. John's wort: antidepressants, digoxin, immunosuppressants, antiretrovirals, loperamide, oral contraceptives, reserpine, theophylline, and warfarin (Lawvere & Mohoney, 2005). Some cases of negative interaction have also occurred in clients taking selective serotonin reuptake inhibitors for bipolar disorder (Moses & Mallinger, 2000).

remedy may be of use but should always be checked with the care provider (Findling et al., 1999). Box 16-2 describes one such herbal remedy. For more details on working with the adolescent who has mental health conditions, refer to an adult mental health text.

OVEREATING AND OBESITY

Obesity may be an associated manifestation of psychological disorders. Obesity in children affects 11% to 16% of American children (*Healthy People 2010*) and is considered by some to have reached epidemic proportions. Hispanics and Mexican Americans have higher rates of obesity than other ethnic groups. **Obesity** is defined as excessive weight and accumulation of body fat. Obesity is considered a BMI greater than or equal to the 95th percentile. Many children have learned a pattern of overeating from their families and appear well adjusted. Although the intake of "junk food" makes them feel good, the increased weight contributes to a poor body image, depression, and low self-esteem. Many children use overeating to compensate for insecurities, low self-esteem, poor body image, lack of parental attention, or feelings of stress, anxiety, and depression. The sedentary lifestyle of many children increases the risk of obesity. Watching television and playing video games instead of exercising greatly increases a child's risk of obesity.

A referral to a nutritionist may be appropriate to teach the child to make healthy food choices. If obesity is not corrected during adolescence, diabetes, orthopedic problems, and cardiovascular complications could develop in later years.

An extreme option for the severely obese adolescent is **bariatric surgery** (surgery to reduce stomach size). Strict criteria are required to even consider this life-altering option. The teen must have tried weight management techniques for longer than 6 months and failed. They must be physiologically mature and agree to psychological evaluations both before and after surgery. Psychiatric issues must be resolved or successfully managed prior to surgery. Female clients considering bariatric surgery must agree to avoid pregnancy for more than 1 year postoperatively. A supportive family is also required.

Nurses may not see the obese child until conditions related to obesity cause them to seek health care. Accurate weight and height are necessary. The nurse must carefully measure the child's blood pressure. Obtaining serum cholesterol, triglycerides, glucose, and hemoglobin A1c will assist in determining the presence of complications related to obesity. The nurse should focus on helping the family to meet the child's nutritional needs, managing related health conditions, and promoting self-esteem. The nurse can encourage exercise and activity programs that will not embarrass the child.

NURSING CARE

PRIORITIES IN NURSING CARE

When caring for children with psychological disorders, the nurse must assist the child and family to develop appropriate coping skills in order to manage the disorder effectively. The nurse can assist the family in helping the child achieve developmental milestones. Children with autism, Asperger's syndrome, ADD, ADHD, anxiety, and depression will benefit from nursing interventions aimed at assisting them to focus and communicate effectively. Preventing injury and ensuring the child's safety are also priority nursing interventions. Finally, the nurse should assist the child and his or her family to seek healthy behaviors related to nutrition, rest, exercise, medication administration, and stress relief measures.

ASSESSING

When assessing the child suffering from psychological disorders, the nurse should take a thorough health history including a birth history. Ask parents or caregivers to specifically describe the child's behavior. The nurse must also observe the child's behavior closely to validate these behaviors. Be sure to ask about these behaviors in a variety of settings. Determine if the child is behaving in a particular manner at school, at home, and in the community. A physical examination is also important, particularly for the child with depression and suicidal thoughts.

DIAGNOSING, PLANNING, AND IMPLEMENTING

Nursing diagnoses for children suffering from psychological disorders might include:

- **H**opelessness related to negative self-perception
- Chronic Low **S**elf-Esteem related to disturbance of thoughts
- **C**aregiver Role Strain related to intensive care required to manage the child with a psychological disorder
- Impaired Verbal **C**ommunication related to altered perceptions

Some outcomes for children suffering from psychological disorders might include:

- The child will express hope for the future.
- The child will demonstrate behaviors associated with appropriate self-esteem.
- The caregiver will describe interventions for managing role strain.
- The child will verbalize thoughts and needs appropriately.

The nurse's role in providing support to these clients would include the following:

- Explore with the child factors contributing to hopelessness. *Verbalization of feelings allows the child to better understand and deal with their emotions.*
- Positively reinforce behaviors that are desirable, such as making eye contact (in a child with autism) or putting things away (in a child with attention deficit). *Positive reinforcement yields encouragement for these behaviors.*
- Restrict negative comments about self, while allowing the child some opportunity to verbalize thoughts and feelings. *Decreases the chance of positively reinforcing negative behaviors.*
- Avoid any teasing or joking with the child who has low self-esteem. *These children are highly sensitive to negative comments, and even ones given in jest may be taken to heart.*
- Encourage small positive steps that can improve self-image. For example, a parent can provide a variety of outdoor activities to help an overweight child get more exercise. *Small changes in behavior followed by praise or other positive reinforcement can build a new life pattern.*
- Develop a plan of care with the caregiver to obtain assistance with household chores, mental health care for the entire family, and support groups that might provide emotional care. *These steps can assist the family in identifying coping mechanisms and availability of support.*
- Discuss with the family the need to lower expectations and be flexible about future goals. *Often holding on to impossible goals and expectations can complicate coping with the reality of the situation.*

- Assist the family in the grief process once goals are adjusted. *Unrealized expectations often elicit feelings of grief.*
- Assist the child in finding alternative methods of communicating such as pen and pencil or flash cards. *Children with psychological disorders often need to find different ways of expressing thoughts and ideas.*
- Always speak slowly and clearly when addressing the child. *Role modeling is a way of teaching the child to communicate properly.*
- Refer to mental health professionals and speech therapists as needed. *Collaborative activities will facilitate improvement for the child with a psychological disorder.*

EVALUATING

In order to evaluate the outcomes for the child with psychological disorders, the nurse must develop and maintain a trusting relationship that encourages the child to verbalize thoughts and feelings in a safe environment. Evaluation must include questioning the caregivers about their level of strain and their coping mechanisms. It will be important to report immediately any thoughts of self-inflicted harm or suicide to the nursing supervisor.

Anorexia Nervosa and Bulimia

Anorexia nervosa is an eating disorder characterized by weight loss, emaciation, and an exaggerated fear of gaining weight. Clients lose weight either by excessive dieting and laxative abuse or by eating and then purging by inducing vomiting and diarrhea. A closely related condition is **bulimia**, which is characterized by binge eating and purging. Binge eating is repeated episodes of consuming large quantities of foods in brief periods of time without purging. The foods are usually forbidden and high in calories. **Purging** is self-induced vomiting, abusing laxatives or diuretics, or both. The typical client is a White female, between 13 and 18 years of age, in a middle- to upper-middle-class family; however, the condition can affect males as well.

Many authorities view anorexia nervosa as a family problem. Often the parents are overly controlling and perfectionists. The adolescent's eating disorder is an attempt to achieve independence and resolve psychological conflicts. Society's preoccupation with being thin may contribute to the adolescent's view of her body shape and the fear of becoming fat (Figure 16-2 ■). The teen may also have a history of abuse. Families of bulimics may live in chaos and lack emotional connections.

Manifestations

Anorexia nervosa is characterized by body weight less than 85% of the expected weight. For example, if the expected body weight is 120 pounds, a weight of 102 pounds could

Figure 16-2. ■ Body image is the sum of a person's conscious and unconscious attitudes about his or her body. This illustration shows a disturbance in body image.

indicate a problem. In order to lose weight, the adolescent may not only decrease the caloric intake, but also indulge in strenuous exercise programs. Other symptoms include preoccupation with food and preparing elaborate meals for others, but consuming very few calories. People with anorexia may cut food and push it around on the plate. They act like they are eating, but they are not. Teens may cry frequently, feel depressed and lonely, and consider suicide. Anxiety and OCD may accompany other symptoms. The fear of becoming fat does not disappear with weight loss. Over time the adolescent becomes very emaciated. Malnutrition accompanied by fluid and electrolyte imbalance results in life-threatening cardiac arrhythmias.

Physical symptoms of anorexia nervosa include cold intolerance, dizziness, constipation, bloating, and amenorrhea. Teens who suffer from anorexia may develop osteoporosis, decreased bone density, and frequent fractures. *Lanugo* (fine, downy body hair) and bradycardia are also seen. Death may occur as a result of a weakened immune system, renal failure, or cardiac arrest.

Symptoms of bulimia include tooth and gum decay due to the frequent presence of gastric acid in the mouth.

The back of the teen's hand may have abrasions from scraping the teeth during purging episodes. Abdominal distention may also be noted.

Diagnosis

Thorough physical and psychological examinations assist in the diagnosis of anorexia nervosa and bulimia. Serial weights and body fat analysis are important measurements. Laboratory data include complete blood count and metabolic profiles.

Treatment

Treatment begins by correcting the malnutrition and continues with psychological counseling for the adolescent and the family. At times lifesaving measures such as the administration of total parenteral nutrition (TPN), IV fluids, and electrolytes, as well as cardiac medications, are the priority interventions. Once the adolescent is physically stable, intense counseling is begun. Usually the plan of care includes a contract with the adolescent regarding eating habits. The goal is to reestablish a normal eating pattern with adequate nutritional intake. Family counseling is needed to help the family understand the cause of the adolescent's eating disorder and to take steps toward a higher level of family functioning.

Nursing Considerations

Hospitalization is required for teens who have lost significant weight, have severe electrolyte imbalances, or need constant psychological intervention. The teen with anorexia may resist treatment. The nurse must firmly enforce prescribed treatments. Because these teens have altered self-perceptions and are likely to have been concealing their condition, they are masters at deception. Manipulative behaviors are common and must be identified by the nurse.

It is also important that the nurse obtain accurate weight measurements on the schedule that is ordered. (Daily weights may be avoided because of the teen's preoccupation with weight.) Intake and output measurements will also be necessary. Lab values must be closely monitored to detect complications.

NURSING CARE

PRIORITIES IN NURSING CARE

When caring for adolescents with eating disorders, the nurse must implement nursing interventions to prevent nutritional and fluid and electrolyte deficits. Another priority nursing strategy is developing a trusting relationship with the client. This effective nurse-client relationship will assist the nurse to enforce prescribed treatments and open lines of communication to address the issues of disturbed body image.

ASSESSING

The nurse must obtain an accurate body weight of the child suffering from an eating disorder. Some physicians order the weights be done with the client's back to the scale to discourage focusing on weight. The nurse must also obtain a nutritional history of their daily intake including beverages and their meal patterns as a baseline. A 24-hour diet recall can be helpful in obtaining this information. Determine the child's exercise habits, including type of exercise and frequency. If the female child has gone through puberty, obtain a menstrual history.

DIAGNOSING, PLANNING, AND IMPLEMENTING

Nursing diagnoses for children with eating disorders might include:

- Imbalanced <u>N</u>utrition: More than Body Requirements related to overeating
- Imbalanced <u>N</u>utrition: Less than Body Requirements related to induced vomiting or inadequate intake and excessive exercise.
- Deficient <u>F</u>luid Volume related to abuse of laxatives
- Disturbed <u>B</u>ody Image related to distorted perception of appearance
- <u>A</u>ctivity Intolerance related to sedentary lifestyle (obesity) or fatigue (anorexia nervosa)

Some outcomes for children with eating disorders might include:

- Child will meet weight and body mass index goal (decreased for obesity and increased for anorexia nervosa and bulimia).
- Child will maintain expected fluid volume.
- Child will view body size realistically.
- Child will be able to complete activities of daily living without fatigue.

The nurse's role in providing support to these clients would include the following:

- Establish a trusting relationship with the child/teen. *This relationship is essential so that the child/teen will listen to instructions and comply.*
- Communicate clear and simple expectations for food intake and the amount of exercise prescribed. *Compliance with the medical regime is improved with clear instructions. The child/teen suffering from obesity needs obtainable goals that will allow them to see progress. The child/teen suffering from anorexia nervosa or bulimia is goal oriented as well as manipulative, so clear expectations are necessary.*
- The child/teen with an eating disorder needs to be monitored *to avoid overeating or self-induced vomiting.*

- Assist the child/teen in learning how to make appropriate food choices. *Appropriate food choices can allow the child to achieve optimal nutrition and not gain excessive weight.*
- Teach the child/teen and their family about the physical risks associated with obesity and anorexia nervosa and bulimia. *Knowledge of the risks will increase compliance with the medical regime.*
- Take weight measurements on the schedule ordered by the physician. Weight needs to be as accurate as possible. This can be accomplished by weighing the child/teen consistently at the same time, with the same amount of clothing. Document carefully. *Monitoring weight gain or weight loss needs to be consistent to make necessary changes in the plan of care.*
- Carefully monitor hydration status by performing skin turgor test, observing mucous membranes, palpating pulses bilaterally, calculating intake and output, and monitoring laboratory values. *Fluid imbalances can shift quickly and cause serious risks to the child's/teen's health. These imbalances need to be reported promptly.*
- Encourage the child/teen to talk about his or her body perceptions. If necessary, have the child/teen draw his or her body image. *The nurse must understand the child's/teen's true feelings in order to deal appropriately with them.*
- Provide respect and privacy when giving care to this child/teen. *This will give the child/teen a sense that his body is worth respecting.*
- Schedule rest periods throughout the day. *Rest will help the child/teen avoid fatigue and promote conservation of energy for important activities.*
- Assist the child/teen with activities of daily living. *Until proper nutritional status is restored, the child/teen may need assistance to conserve energy.*

EVALUATING

Outcomes will be evaluated based on the child's weight, daily intake and output, perception of their body size, and ability to perform activities of daily living without fatigue. Because variations in fluid balance and nutrition can cause serious risks, it is important for the LPN/LVN to report significant changes immediately to the supervising nurse.

NURSING PROCESS CARE PLAN
Client with Anorexia Nervosa

Meghan, a 14-year-old White female, is brought to the family physician's office by her mother. Meghan's mother reports that Meghan had been losing weight and has been tired and irritable for months. Meghan states that it is important to her to be thin and attractive. She states,

"I'd do anything to avoid being fat like I am now. I really do not like the way I look and want to change it." Her weight today is 92 pounds. She states her last menstrual period was 6 months ago. Her hair is dry and brittle and her skin is lacking moisture.

Assessment

- "I'd do anything to avoid being fat like I am now."
- States desire to be thin and attractive
- Recent weight loss
- "I really do not like the way I look and want to change it."

Nursing Diagnosis. The following important nursing diagnosis (among others) is established for this client:

- Disturbed **B**ody Image related to difficulty coping with maturation

Expected Outcomes. Expected outcomes for Meghan are that:

- She will express a positive body image.
- She will be able to manage her weight in an appropriate manner.

Planning and Implementation

- Assess client's self-concept and body image. *Knowing exactly what the client believes will assist the nurse in developing a specific plan.*
- Assess the family structure and stressors in the client's life. *It is important to identify aspects of the client's life that may have contributed to her condition.*
- Assist the client in differentiating between thin and healthy body size. *The client may have a distorted view of what is a normal body weight and may not understand the health hazards associated with extreme weight loss.*
- Assist the client to develop a realistic body image and nutritional intake. *Recovery is facilitated when the client is involved in planning her care.*
- Refer client to an adolescent support group. *Adolescents respond well to peer counseling.*

Evaluation. Consistent care and follow-up with the client and her family will restore a positive body image, and she will develop appropriate skills to cope with her stressors.

Critical Thinking in the Nursing Process

1. What societal aspects may contribute to an unrealistic body image in the adolescent?
2. What type of family support will most likely help Meghan?
3. How could Meghan's friends assist with her recovery?

Note: Discussion of Critical Thinking questions appears in Appendix I.

Abuse and Family Violence

Child abuse is a crime punishable in all states. It can occur as physical abuse, emotional abuse or neglect, and sexual abuse. Unfortunately child abuse can occur in any household, with any race or religion, with males or females, and in children of any age (Box 16-3 ■). Caring for children is a difficult task even in the best of situations. There will be many times in the rearing of children when parental frustration and anger occur. Parents who are not equipped to channel this frustration and anger properly are at risk for abusing their children.

Many parents who abuse their children were also abused as children. They learned a pattern of discipline and child rearing from their parents and tend to implement the same forms of punishment. They may have never been shown love and nurturing. Because they did not develop a healthy sense of trust, it is difficult, without intervention, for them to pass on to their children a sense of security and love.

Lack of knowledge about normal growth and development of the child may create unrealistic expectations of the child. When these expectations are not met, frustration develops. Parents may be socially isolated and not have a support system that could teach them proper parenting techniques. Child abusers often abuse alcohol and other substances. These substances impair judgment and are associated with poor decision making.

Parents who choose to abuse their children may view them as different. There is a higher incidence of abuse among children born with birth defects or who were born prematurely. These situations may keep infants and parents separated for periods of time following birth and complicate efforts to bond. These situations are also stressful to the parents physically, emotionally, and financially. Child abuse is more likely to occur during periods of stress. The Health Promotion Issue on pages 438 and 439 cites one type of situation in which abuse may occur.

BOX 16-3   **CULTURAL PULSE POINTS**

Discipline in Appalachian Culture

The Appalachian mountain range spans 13 states—Alabama, Mississippi, Georgia, Virginia, West Virginia, North and South Carolina, Kentucky, Tennessee, Ohio, Maryland, New York, and Pennsylvania.

Especially in rural areas of these states, families usually are large, and they enforce a strict work ethic. Corporal and physical punishment is frequently used to discipline children.

If child abuse is suspected in a family from this region, consider that the parents *may* not perceive their forms of discipline as abusive and may not accept counsel from health care professionals.

REPORTING ABUSE

The nurse must report to agency supervisors, local or state child protective services, or law enforcement authorities any suspicion of child abuse. Agency policy will dictate the method of reporting but requires notification of the nursing supervisor in all situations. The report must also be made immediately when symptoms are recognized to prevent further danger to the child and to be able to document current abuse. Most child protective services have the authority to hold the child in their custody until a proper investigation can be implemented.

Documentation is a vital part of the report of child abuse. The nurse must be careful to clearly chart physical symptoms as well as subjective data gathered from the child and the parent. When charting physical findings, the nurse needs to be specific as to the location and size of the injury. Obtaining color pictures of the injury may be essential to proving abuse in a court of law.

State laws provide protection for the nurse from prosecution for reporting abuse. Although not required, it is advisable to notify the parents that a report of child abuse has been submitted. This can evoke anger on the part of the parent, yet it allows the health care personnel to communicate a rationale for holding the child in custody. If, however, the nurse fails to report suspected child abuse, a fine can be levied or the nursing license could be revoked. See Chapter 3 ∞ to obtain more information on the legal aspects of nursing.

PHYSICAL ABUSE

Physical abuse of a child is inflicting pain and injury in a deliberate manner. Injury may be inflicted on a child by hitting, burning, biting, choking, shaking, or throwing a child. The perpetrator may use his or her hands, fists, head, teeth, knees, or feet and legs to inflict punishment on the child. Weapons may also be used, such as electrical cords, ropes, sticks, baseball bats, or cigarette lighters. Physical abuse also includes administering excessive doses of medication or withholding needed medications.

Manifestations

Clinical manifestation of physical child abuse include bruises, burns (see Figure 21-14 ∞), rope or cord marks (usually on the back of the body), multiple fractures, shortness of breath, sedation from medication, or exacerbation of a chronic illness from withholding medications.

The nurse must be able to chart the color of the bruise objectively. Findings should be discussed with the physician and supervising nurse. A bruise that is less than 1 day old is red, blue, or bright purple with distinct margins (Figure 16-3 ■). The bruise that is 1 to 2 days old is bluish brown to dark purple. A 3- to 5-day old bruise is yellow-green

(*Text continues on p. 440.*)

MediaLink ● Identifying Child Abuse

Newborn Safety

MediaLink

HEALTH PROMOTION ISSUE

PREVENTING INFANT ABDUCTION

Janice Pope, a 29-year-old G2 P1, is touring the birthing facility prior to the birth of her second child. She is accompanied by her mother and her 5-year-old son, Cody. She discusses with the nurse conducting the tour that she is concerned about the safety of her newborn while he is hospitalized. Ms. Pope and her husband are in the midst of a divorce and custody battle. Her husband has threatened to steal the baby if she doesn't agree to give him custody of Cody. He also made the statement that he is not interested in having custody of the baby but he doesn't want her to have it either. Ms. Pope has reason to believe her husband because he has a history of violent behavior. Ms. Pope is visibly shaken by these threats to her newborn's safety. The nurse desires to respond appropriately to her concerns.

DISCUSSION

The Joint Commission on Accreditation of Healthcare Organizations (JCAHO) calls infant abduction a sentinel event

or critical incident. A *sentinel event* is an occurrence where death or serious physical or psychological injury could occur. Infant abductions could occur in the hospital or from a family's home.

The abductor could be a family member or a stranger. The typical abductor is a female with emotional difficulties related to her marriage or relationships or her reproductive life. She may have low self-esteem and exhibit compulsive behaviors. The National Center for Missing and Exploited Children list the following as typical characteristics of abductions: The abductor acts alone, dresses as medical personnel, tells the mother that the baby needs medical attention, seeks to befriend the mother, usually calls her by name, creates a distraction just prior to the abduction such as spilling a drink in the hallway, and thinks of the baby as her own immediately following the abduction.

JCAHO requires health care facilities to seriously address possible infant abductions. The Commission requires

these plans to be developed by health care personnel from many different disciplines such as medicine, nursing, security, social services, and public relations. The plan must include proper newborn identification, staff and parent education, and a physical environment that ensures newborn safety. Below is an example of a plan for prompt response to an infant abduction:

1. Prompt notification of assistive personnel to include unit and nursing supervisors, security, and hospital administration. Also, an overhead page is used to alert all hospital personnel.
2. Secure the area, especially the exits and elevators. Observe for suspicious behavior.
3. Attend to the needs of the family both during the event and afterward. Whether the infant is found or not, the family will experience stress.
4. Following the event, the staff must review the scenario. They will also need an opportunity to debrief.

PLANNING AND IMPLEMENTATION

The nurse discusses with Ms. Pope the specific plan her hospital uses to keep newborns safe. Newborns are identified in several ways. Immediately after birth, hospital identification bands are placed on the infant's wrist and opposite ankle. These bands have a five-digit number that matches the mother's and also has her name on it. The mother can choose one other family member to give a matching identification band to. Only the mother and this other individual may transport the baby to the nursery or receive the baby from the nursery. The infant will also have a security device placed on the ankle. Also, in the delivery room, the baby will be footprinted. These footprints will be on the same page as a fingerprint from the mother's index finger. Shortly after birth, the baby is transported by nursing personnel to the nursery. If the baby's temperature is stable, the baby will receive his first bath. After the bath, the baby's picture is taken with a digital camera before he leaves the nursery. The pictures are printed for the mother and stored digitally for retrieval at a later date if necessary. These pictures can be placed on the hospital's website, but no last names are given. Ms. Pope may decide not to place her baby's picture on the website.

The entire staff of the hospital is familiar with methods to avoid newborn abductions and safeguard the newborn while they are admitted to the hospital. The staff wears a unique style and color of scrubs that change weekly. All approved personnel have a picture identification badge. Babies are transported in their cribs, never in a nurse's arms. There will also be a daily security code that nurses are required to say when removing a baby from the mother's room. This security code word will be communicated to postpartum mothers at 0730 each morning.

The nurse tells Ms. Pope that all client identification is kept confidential and cannot be accessed by the public.

She also tells Ms. Pope about the policy for a confidential admission where her chart will be flagged to help staff be especially careful about her personal information. The infant may also be given a false name to further conceal his identity. Security can also be alerted to the potential for danger and extra surveillance can be arranged.

The nurse teaches Ms. Pope to carefully study each nurse's identification badge when they remove the newborn from her room. She has the right to question anybody who seems suspicious and to accompany the newborn to any tests or examinations. The newborn should never be left unattended in the hospital room, even when Ms. Pope needs to toilet or shower. The crib should not be placed next to the door.

Ms. Pope should also understand that the women's unit is equipped with safety measures designed to prevent infant abductions. All personnel wear an additional badge that allows them passage into the nursery and into the postpartum unit. These badges are signed out to each nurse and inventoried on a regular basis. The unit is also monitored by video cameras that are surveyed by security personnel. Signs are posted in the unit to alert the public that they are being monitored by video cameras. Finally, sensors would detect when an infant is removed from the nursery or postpartum areas, and alarms would sound.

When preparing for discharge, Ms. Pope should consider the following

safeguards. She should avoid any signs or decorations that alert the public that there is a newborn in the home. The nurse must communicate to Ms. Pope that the hospital does not have a postpartum home visit program and there should be no reason for health care personnel to appear unannounced at her home. The nurse can also encourage Ms. Pope to collect identification data about her infant. This data should include a color photograph, footprints, hair color, eye color, current length, current weight, date of birth, and a detailed description of any physical characteristics that might assist in identification.

SELF-REFLECTION

What safety measures have you observed in different health care facilities to prevent infant abductions? Which of these are most effective? Least effective? Think about your own practice of transporting infants within the health care facility. How could you improve this practice to ensure infant safety?

The fear of infant abduction creates fear and stress in hospital personnel as well as in new mothers. Describe these fears. What nursing interventions contribute to this fear? What nursing interventions help to dispel this fear? Look at your practice. Are you contributing to fear or dispelling it?

SUGGESTED RESOURCES

For the Nurse

Mertens, S. (2005). Neonatal security: It takes a community. *Nursing Management, 36*(8), 41–44.

Rabun, J., Jr. (2005). *For healthcare professionals: Guidelines on prevention of and response to infant abductions (8th ed.).* National Center for Missing and Exploited Children. Alexandria, VA: U.S. Department of Justice.

Shogan, M. G. (2002). Emergency management plan for newborn abductions. *JOGNN, 31*(3), 340–346.

Figure 16-3. ■ The timing of physical abuse can be assessed by the color of bruises in soft tissue. (PhotoEdit, Inc.)

Signs of Abuse

Child's Behavior

- Shows sudden changes in behavior or school performance.
- Has not received help for physical or medical problems brought to the parents' attention.
- Has learning problems (or difficulty concentrating) that cannot be attributed to specific physical or psychological causes.
- Is always watchful, as though preparing for something bad to happen.
- Lacks adult supervision.
- Is overly compliant, passive, or withdrawn.
- Comes to school or other activities early, stays late, and does not want to go home.

Parent's Behavior

- Shows little concern for the child.
- Denies the existence of—or blames the child for—the child's problems in school or at home.
- Asks teachers or other caretakers to use harsh physical discipline if the child misbehaves.
- Sees the child as entirely bad, worthless, or burdensome.
- Demands a level of physical or academic performance the child cannot achieve.
- Looks primarily to the child for care, attention, and satisfaction of emotional needs.

Parent and Child's Behavior

- Rarely touch or look at each other.
- Consider their relationship entirely negative.
- State that they do not like each other.

to brown, whereas one that is 5 to 7 days old is fading to yellow without distinct borders. Finally, a bruise that is older than 1 week has only slight yellow-brown discolorations. The nurse must carefully chart the subjective statements given by the parents regarding how the child became bruised. Box 16-4 ■ highlights some manifestations of abuse.

The nurse must be careful not to accuse a parent of abuse rashly. Some cultural healing methods such as cupping and coining (see Figure 10-5 ⊙⊙) may look, at first glance, like signs of abuse.

Treatment

Caring for a child who has been physically abused requires teamwork. The team will consist of physicians, nurses, social workers, school counselors and teachers, mental health professionals, and the family. These team members will work to ensure the child's physical safety and recovery from the inflicted injuries. Once abuse is reported, the child is removed from the situation in which the abuse occurred. (Table 16-2 ■ provides some ways of communicating with the child who is being removed from an abusive situation.) Mental health professionals will assist the child with emotional recovery

from this abuse. They can use a variety of therapies. See the section below for a further description. The social worker develops a plan to provide the child a home environment free of abuse.

SHAKEN BABY SYNDROME

A serious form of physical abuse against the infant is **shaken baby syndrome.** Infants are particularly susceptible to head injuries because their heads are large and their neck muscles are weak. If the caretaker shakes an infant, the jarring motion causes tearing of the nerve fibers in the brain, subdural hematoma, cerebral edema, and retinal hemorrhages.

The infant who has this type of head injury may have seizures, vomiting, lethargy, and respiratory difficulties. They also may present with failure to thrive. One-third of infants die from this injury, whereas another third have permanent damage. Permanent damage may include mental retardation, vision or hearing impairment, seizures, paralysis, or developmental delays.

TABLE 16-2

Communicating Across the Life Span: Talking to a Child Removed from an Abusive Home

	TODDLER	PRESCHOOLER	SCHOOL-AGE CHILD	ADOLESCENT
Client	"I want my mommy."	"Why can't I go home? That's where my sister is."	"You can make me go, but I won't ever be happy unless I get to go home."	"Being in another home is not going to change my father—he's going to always hit me when he's mad."
Nurse	"I know you want your mommy. What is your favorite toy? You can bring that with you on this adventure. For several days and nights you'll be staying at a special place with wonderful people who are going to take good care of you." Describe specifics about the home and family.	"It's important that you not get hurt again. You and your sister are going to go home with Lisa and John" (have them there when discussing this with the child). "Lisa and John have a turtle named Pokey. You and your sister can help feed him and give him water."	"Please tell me more about why you are so unhappy." (Allow the child to express all emotions.) "I want you to meet the family who will care for you over the next few days. This family is going to give you a safe place to live, cook you delicious meals, take you to school, and help you with your homework. They also have a membership to the community pool and would like to take you swimming, too."	"Going to another home is for you, to protect you. Your father is going to counseling to help him, too. The social worker will determine if the counseling has helped him with his anger. It's going to be very important for you to honestly communicate your feelings to the social worker."

BULLYING

Bullying is a type of physical and emotional abuse. A recent survey (Glewe, 2005) says that 22% of school-age children experience this form of abuse. The child may be teased, threatened, hit, shoved, kicked, or pushed. Bullying most commonly occurs during school hours, but can also occur at community activities, on a school bus, in the neighborhood, at religious activities, or via the Internet.

Children who are bullied feel anxious, isolated, depressed, and possibly suicidal. They often complain of headaches, stomachaches, and other vague complaints in an effort to avoid situations where they may be bullied. They may also express their anger toward the bully in the form of aggression to siblings, parents, or friends. The victim's grades begin to suffer, and they no longer feel safe at school.

Teachers and parents must recognize the signs of physical and emotional threats to the child's safety. The primary action is to remove the child from physical danger and to seek to restore their emotional health.

EMOTIONAL ABUSE AND NEGLECT

Emotional abuse of a child includes attacks on a child's self-esteem. The perpetrator uses words to control and frighten the child. The child may be shamed, ridiculed, or embarrassed by the abuser (often an adult). Emotional abuse can also include acts of violence against someone or something that the child loves, such as a pet or favorite toy.

A child may also be neglected either physically or emotionally. Physical neglect of a child is the deliberate withholding of physical care or resources to the child. The perpetrator may withhold food, water, hygiene, shelter, or health care. Children who are emotionally abused do not have nurturing care. The perpetrator is cold and insensitive to the child's needs.

Clinical manifestations of emotional abuse or neglect include poor self-esteem, lack of friends, lack of trust in adults, and impaired communication. The child may be sick frequently and may present with failure to thrive (see later discussion). They often do not do well academically and present with behavior problems at school. They may be depressed and think about suicide.

NONORGANIC FAILURE TO THRIVE

Nonorganic failure to thrive (NOFTT) is a disorder characterized by inadequate growth in height and weight. It usually occurs in infancy and early childhood. It occurs most commonly in children whose parents are depressed, abuse a variety of substances, are mentally retarded, or are psychotic. These parents are more likely to be poor, socially isolated, and have lower educational levels. Even if the parent has an education, they may not know the proper way to feed the child, such as formula preparation, methods of breastfeeding, or introducing solid foods.

Children with NOFTT will be below the 3rd to 5th percentile on the growth charts for height and weight. They may have little if any subcutaneous fat and reduced muscle mass. They appear lifeless and apathetic. They avoid eye contact with the caregiver and have no expression in their faces.

They will also be irritable and difficult to soothe and with poor sleeping habits. When they are held, children with NOFTT will not mold to the caregiver's body and quite frequently will arch the back in an effort not to be held. They have signs of neglect such as diaper rash; long, dirty fingernails; dirty clothes; and an unwashed body. They may have a foul odor. They also experience developmental delays.

Adequate nutritional support is the primary goal of treatment. Second, the care of this child must include promotion of bonding behaviors to help the parent and child attach. Parents who lack education must be taught about proper feeding methods and the need for physical interaction with the child. A thorough evaluation of the home environment must be performed, and monitoring of this environment must be ongoing.

SEXUAL ABUSE

Sexual abuse can be defined as sexual acts that are imposed on children who cannot protect themselves because of their lack of emotional or cognitive development. Sexual abuse can happen in a variety of ways. Box 16-5 ■ provides definitions related to sexual abuse. Between 100,000 and 500,000 children in the United States are sexually abused every year (Ball & Bindler, 2006).

Most perpetrators are males. The victim may be male or female; however, more females than males are victims. Several risk factors have been identified for sexual abuse. These include a stepfather living in the home instead of the biological father; poor parental relationships; a parent or caregiver who never finished high school; a parent or caregiver who has an annual income less than $10,000; a mother employed outside of the home; parental substance abuse; and a child with two or fewer friends.

Manifestations

Sexual abuse in children can be characterized by physical symptoms, mood changes, cognitive impairment, sexual symptoms, and lack of coping skills. Physical symptoms include a vaginal discharge, possibly with a strong odor; vaginal or anal bleeding or bruising (underpants or diaper may be blood-stained); genital irritation such as redness, pain, itching, or burning; recurrent urinary tract infections; sexually transmitted infections; a positive pregnancy test, particularly at a young age; enuresis; and encopresis. The child may also complain frequently of a headache or stomachache when there is no physical indication for these symptoms. Mood changes associated with sexual abuse includes depression, anxiety, withdrawal, hostility, irritability, fear of strangers and other phobias, and aggressive behaviors. The child who has been sexually abused will appear very afraid of a physical examination and may become combative during the exam. Symptoms of cognitive impairment related to sexual abuse include sudden changes in school performance and school attendance; low self-esteem; frequent daydreaming; and nightmares or night terrors.

Children who have been sexually abused may demonstrate sexual symptoms such as promiscuous behavior. They may express confusion about their sexual identity and begin to masturbate frequently. Many children who have been sexually abused pursue prostitution as a form of income. It seems the dissociation they developed to cope with the abuse also allows them to participate in prostitution.

These children may also demonstrate a lack of coping skills. They frequently abuse tobacco, alcohol, and drugs. They may run away from home. They may inflict pain on themselves and others. Sleeping and eating habits may change. The female victim of sexual abuse tends to act like a wife or mother.

Diagnosis and Treatment

History and physical evidence lead to the diagnosis of sexual abuse. However, the collection of forensic evidence is important to trace the perpetrator. Collection of body fluids and tissues needs to be done by a trained expert so that valuable evidence is not destroyed. These experts are also trained to address the emotional issues of the child related to the examination. The child will be treated for physical injuries and for sexually transmitted infections. A pregnancy test is also necessary. Referral to a mental health professional is necessary for the child who has been sexually abused. The child's physical safety must also be ensured.

BOX 16-5

Definitions Related to Sexual Abuse

- **Incest**—sexual activity between family members.
- **Assault**—a sudden, violent physical attack on someone. Assault is an unlawful act.
- **Rape**—sexual intercourse without consent that occurs as a result of threat or physical force.
- **Statutory rape**—sexual intercourse that occurs between a minor and an adult. There is consent given by the minor.
- **Date rape**—sexual intercourse during a social outing without consent, which occurs as a result of threat or physical force. The perpetrator is known socially by the victim.
- **Child molestation**—sexual involvement other than intercourse between a child and an older child, adolescent, or adult. Child molestation includes oral-genital contact, genital fondling, and masturbation in the presence of children.
- **Child exploitation**—the unethical use of child for one's own profit. Child exploitation may be in the form of prostitution or child pornography.
- **Child pornography**—the photography or visual representation of children nude and/or in sexual acts. These materials may be distributed in print media, in videos, or over the Internet.
- **Exhibitionism**—exposing the genitals to strangers.
- **Pedophile**—a person who has sexual interest in children.

Nursing Considerations

Because of the number of children who have been sexually abused, the nurse must explore the possibility of this type of abuse with all children. The following are questions that will assist the nurse in screening for sexual abuse.

- What sleeping arrangements do you have in your home?
- Tell me about bath time in your home.
- Do you keep secrets from anyone in your home? Who asked you to keep these secrets?

- Has anyone ever touched you when you didn't want them to? Tell me where.
- Has anyone ever asked you to touch them when you didn't want to? Tell me where.
- Would you tell me who has asked you to do these things? How often has it happened? Have you ever told anyone else about this? Who?

The Nursing Care Plan Chart below describes aspects of nursing care for a child who is being abused.

NURSING CARE PLAN CHART

Care of the Child Who Is Physically Abused

GOAL	INTERVENTION	RATIONALE	EXPECTED OUTCOME
1. Risk for Trauma related to inappropriate parental interactions			
The child will avoid physical injury	Document physical abuse thoroughly	*Correct documentation allows authorities to successfully keep the child from the environment where the abuse occurs*	There will be no evidence or report of bruising, fractures, contusions, burns, or other signs of physical injury.
	Assist social agencies in providing a safe environment for the child	*The child will need housing, food, clothing, health care, and financial assistance when removed from the unsafe environment*	
	Provide follow-up contact with the child in the new environment	*To ensure that the proper type of care is being administered and that the child is adjusting emotionally*	
The family will cease inappropriate parent-child interactions that cause physical and emotional harm	Refer family to counseling services	*Counseling services can assist the family in identifying anger, stress, and other causes of physical and emotional abuse*	The family will be able to identify dangerous parenting interactions and accept assistance in learning alternate parenting methods.
	Provide follow-up contact with the family and counselor	*Before the child can return to the home environment, the social worker must document that the family has learned alternative parenting methods that will ensure the child's safety*	
2. Powerlessness related to negative interpersonal reactions with parents			
The child will demonstrate increased power or control over his or her life	Encourage the child to be involved in choices related to his new environment such as personal items to bring from his old home or what breakfast foods to eat	*Allowing the child to be involved in making choices related to his care improves his self-esteem and self-responsibility*	The child is able to express feelings and demonstrates the ability to make decisions about life events
	Discuss past successes in the child's life. Emphasize these strengths. Explore ways to repeat these successes	*Past successes allow the child to have enhanced confidence in his or her abilities and strengths*	
	Allow the child the opportunity to express feelings, perceptions, fears, and anxieties	*Listening to the child in a non-judgmental manner provides the child with acceptance of these feelings and allows him to be able to develop coping mechanisms related to these feelings*	

MediaLink Child Abuse

SUBSTANCE ABUSE

Crossing all socioeconomic boundaries, substance abuse affects children of all ages. Children are particularly vulnerable to the hazards of substance abuse because of their incomplete physical development. The adolescent, struggling for identity and independence, may experience periods of confusion and sadness. At these times the teen is more vulnerable to substance abuse. Whereas some adolescents are exposed to addictive substances through peer contact, others witness their parents abusing substances and so believe using chemicals is the "adult" thing to do (Figure 16-4 ■). Flora (2006) found that 25% of children 18 and under live with alcoholic parents. Adolescents may experiment with only a few substances, and then stop using them altogether, whereas others move from substance to substance until they become dependent on chemicals to "feel good." Table 16-3 ■ identifies the stages of substance abuse.

Substance abuse includes tobacco, alcohol, illegal drugs, and some over-the-counter chemicals as well. The younger adolescent with limited financial resources may experiment with household chemicals such as glue, cold medicine, or herbs. Common household chemicals that are inhaled include paint thinner, spray paint, nail polish remover, gasoline, moth balls, and helium. Methamphetamine is an extremely dangerous drug that can be manufactured with common household substances. Children who live in households where this drug is manufactured and smoked are at risk for the effects of methamphetamine and injuries such as burns due to explosions of the chemicals. Methamphetamine causes hyperactivity, decreased appetite, a general sense of well-being, and possible agitation and violence. Long-term effects include a pattern of violent behavior, paranoia, auditory hallucinations, delusions, tooth decay, weight loss, and stroke.

Beer, wine, and other alcohol may also be available in the home. In order to purchase illegal drugs, the adolescent

Figure 16-4. ■ Alcoholism runs in families because of a combination of genetic and environmental factors. (*Source:* Tom & Dee Ann McCarthy/Corbis/Stock Market.)

may work, steal, or indulge in prostitution. The commonly abused drugs are identified in Table 16-4 ■.

Forms of tobacco abuse include cigarettes, cigars and smokeless tobacco including snuff and chewing tobacco. Imported cigarettes may appeal to children because they are typically less expensive; however, these forms of tobacco carry the same health risks. Examples of these imported cigarettes are *bidis* (fruit- or candy-flavored cigarettes) and *kretek* (clove cigarettes). Risks of tobacco abuse include oral or lung cancer, cardiovascular disease, chronic pulmonary obstructive disease, emphysema, and low-birth-weight babies. Even if the child does not smoke, living with family members who smoke puts him or her into the same risk category.

TABLE 16-3

Stages of Substance Abuse

STAGE		DESCRIPTION
0	Curiosity in a Do-Drugs World	Occasional experimentation with alcohol or other drugs. Initial use may be unpleasant.
1	Learning the Mood Swing	With continued use, learn to "get high." Learn that some drugs work faster or better than others.
2	Seeking the Mood Swing	Wanting the "high" more frequently, actively seeks alcohol or drugs.
3	Preoccupation with Mood Swing	Tolerance to substance builds with continued use. The majority of time is spent obtaining and using the drug.
4	Using Drugs to Feel Normal	Physical and psychological dependence ensues. Signs of withdrawal occur without drug.

TABLE 16-4

Commonly Abused Drugs and Their Effects

DRUG	EFFECTS	SIGNS OF WITHDRAWAL	TREATMENT
Nicotine	Vasoconstriction, tachycardia, increased adrenalin, elevated blood pressure	Anxiety, mood swings, cravings, dizziness, insomnia, headache, difficulty concentrating, increased appetite	Smoking cessation programs
Narcotics Heroin Morphine Meperidine (Demerol)	Euphoria, drowsiness, pinpoint pupils, respiratory depression	Yawning, tearing eyes, gooseflesh, abdominal cramps	Narcotic antagonist naloxone (Narcan); methadone (Dolophine)
Cocaine Amphetamines	CNS stimulation with marked euphoria and excitement	Depression, lethargy, psychosis, intense craving for drug	Frequent monitoring due to depression and fatigue. Manipulate to get drug
Depressants Barbiturates (phenobarbital, secobarbital)	Sleepy, dizzy	Abdominal cramps, weakness, tremors	Withdrawal dangerous, must be done slowly, seizures could ensue
Hallucinogens LSD PCP Marijuana	Visual illusions, hallucinations, altered perceptions	No physical symptoms, Psychotic episode, flashbacks	Monitor for psychosis
Alcohol	Euphoria, delayed reactions, unsteady gait	Hallucinations, tremors (delirium tremens), seizures	Monitor during withdrawal. Antianxiety drugs to prevent DTs

Manifestations

Symptoms of substance abuse vary depending on the specific substance(s) being abused. Physical symptoms might include:

- Dilated or pinpoint pupils, blood shot eyes
- Bruising or needle marks
- Runny nose
- Shaking hands
- Halitosis

Psychological or cognitive symptoms might include:

- Inconsistent behavior
- Drowsiness
- Restlessness or increased energy depending on whether stimulant or depressant
- Lack of concentration
- Agitation
- Decreased interest in school, decreased grades

Diagnosis

Toxicology studies can be done to determine if there are levels of harmful substances in the child's urine. Many schools are developing voluntary drug testing programs for students in an effort to promote positive peer pressure to avoid substance abuse.

Treatment

Treatment begins with removal of the abused substance. In many cases sedative-hypnotics or major tranquilizers may be needed to ease the withdrawal symptoms. Withdrawal from some drugs is dangerous and requires hospitalization and frequent monitoring. Once the adolescent is stabilized, psychological therapy to understand and treat the underlying cause is necessary.

Nursing Considerations

The nurse caring for children and adolescents must give priority to assessing risk factors related to substance abuse. The child's social history and self-concept are a critical piece of this assessment. The nurse should also determine the child's knowledge about the hazards of substance abuse, including chronic illnesses. These hazards can be communicated to the pediatric client by a number of methods such as peer counseling, posters, brochures, buttons, and formal presentations.

The nurse can encourage children to participate in activities that will increase their self-esteem such as sports or

Scouting. Children should be encouraged to be future minded and goal oriented. They should be helped to understand the negative impact that substance abuse may have on their future career and family life.

Family counseling is needed to assist the parents and siblings to understand and help the addicted adolescent. Support groups such as Ala-teen, Narc-Anon, and Al-Anon are available in most communities.

FETAL ALCOHOL SYNDROME

Fetal alcohol syndrome (FAS) can occur if a pregnant woman consumes alcohol during pregnancy. No amount of alcohol intake during pregnancy has been determined safe. Obviously, the greater the consumption of alcohol, the greater the risks. Newborns with FAS have three types of characteristics: growth retardation, CNS abnormalities and craniofacial abnormalities. Physically they demonstrate growth retardation (Figure 16-5 ■). Most notably, this growth retardation is marked by decreased weight, height, and head circumference, and decreased adipose tissue. CNS abnormalities include developmental and cognitive delays and behavioral problems such as irritability and hyperactivity. Craniofacial abnormalities include microcephaly, small eyes, short palpebral fissures, thin upper lip, and a flattened maxillary area.

Immediate care of these newborns will focus on nutritional support. They are often fussy and poor eaters. The nurse will closely monitor their intake and output. For this child to thrive, the mother must be referred to an alcohol rehabilitation program and her care of the baby must be closely monitored. The nurse should also help pregnant women understand the detrimental effects of alcohol consumption during pregnancy.

NURSING CARE

PRIORITIES IN NURSING CARE

Implementing nursing strategies to prevent abuse in all forms is a priority for the pediatric nurse. The nurse can provide parents and potential parents with teaching about the expected growth and development of children. Parents also need to be taught parenting techniques to promote nurturing and proper discipline. The pediatric nurse must closely assess each client for signs and symptoms of abuse. If abuse is noted, prompt reporting and clear, objective documentation are essential. The nurse must ensure that the victim of abuse is provided a safe environment where the child will be free from harm.

ASSESSING

Assessment for the children suffering from abuse and family violence includes a complete medical, family and social history. The use of subjective data will avoid bias. The nurse must assist with a thorough physical examination, being sensitive to the child who has not been touched properly. For the child suspected of substance abuse, the nurse should ask direct but nonjudgmental questions to determine the types of substances abused and how frequently they are used.

DIAGNOSING, PLANNING, AND IMPLEMENTING

Nursing diagnoses for children suffering from abuse and family violence might include:

- Deficient **K**nowledge related to dangers of hazardous substances such as tobacco, alcohol and illegal drugs
- Risk for **I**njury related to forms of abuse including substance, physical, emotional, and sexual
- Delayed **G**rowth and Development related to poor parenting
- **F**ear related to past experience with abuse
- **A**nxiety related to past experience with abuse or the unknown should the child be removed from the home environment

Some outcomes for children suffering from abuse and family violence might include that the child will:

- Understand the risks associated with substance abuse.
- Be free from evidence of injury from any form of abuse.

Figure 16-5. ■ Fetal alcohol syndrome is the result of a woman consuming alcohol during pregnancy, and it can have many severe effects on children. Among them are physical malformations, such as those shown here. (*Source:* George Steinmetz/San Francisco AIDS Foundation.)

- Demonstrate age-appropriate growth and developmental level.
- Develop skills to overcome fear.
- Be free of anxiety symptoms.

The nurse's role in providing support to these children would include the following:

- Provide teaching at the child's cognitive level about the hazards of substance abuse. *Factual information can change the child's behavior patterns.*
- Reinforce teaching with written materials and asking the child questions to validate understanding. *Evaluation of learning is important following teaching.*
- Parents and children should be taught how to recognize the symptoms of overdose. *Prompt action is necessary to restore health when the child has overdosed.*
- Report abuse promptly so that the child who has been physically, emotionally, or sexually abused can be removed from the home where the abuse occurred. *Child abuse is a repetitive behavior, and the child will not be safe with the perpetrator.*
- Provide the child with delayed growth and development opportunities to interact with child of appropriate growth and development. *The child may learn behaviors by watching other children role model.*
- Ensure that the child has age-appropriate toys and games. *This will promote appropriate growth and developmental levels.*
- For children with fear and anxiety as a result of abuse, the nurse must use a calm, soothing, nonjudgmental manner. *This approach will be reassuring and comforting to the child and assist the nurse in developing a trusting relationship.*
- Encourage the child to express his or her feelings of fear and anxiety. *The nurse will be able to assist the child in addressing these concerns and to assist in correcting those that are not based in reality.*
- Provide consistency for the child as well as comforting items such as a nightlight, favorite toy, or blanket. *Familiarity will help to decrease fear and anxiety.*
- Provide positive reinforcement when the child is able to demonstrate coping behaviors and continue with activities of daily living despite expressed fears and anxiety. *Positive reinforcement will assist the child in replacing negative emotions with positive ones.*
- Teach the child self-calming behaviors such as breathing techniques, relaxation methods, and self-talk. *Helping the fearful, anxious child develop coping mechanisms will assist him or her in overcoming these negative emotions.*

EVALUATING

To evaluate outcomes, the nurse must interview the child to determine knowledge of the risks of substance abuse. Frequent follow-up visits may be necessary to evaluate

future injury related to abuse, progress related to growth and developmental level, and symptoms of fear and anxiety. Ongoing accurate documentation will assist in the clinical treatment of these forms of abuse.

Traumatic Events

Children may experience trauma in their lives and be greatly affected. Children are exposed to violent crimes, sometimes in their neighborhood, on television, or in the movies. They may live through a natural disaster such as a flood, tornado, forest fire, mudslide, hurricane, or earthquake. Many will be involved in a motor vehicle crash. Abuse of any kind is also considered a traumatic event. Children can have negative effects from a traumatic event whether they experience it personally or witness it.

Children may be affected mentally, emotionally, physically, or morally. As children try to understand the traumatic event, they feel frightened, confused, and insecure. They may feel anger, isolation, and anxiety. Box 16-6 ■ outlines the effects of disasters on children depending on their age.

The nurse can play an instrumental role in assisting children who have experienced a traumatic event to deal with

BOX 16-6   LIFE SPAN CONSIDERATIONS

Effects of Disasters on Children

Infant
The infant experiences little to no effect.

Preschooler or Toddler
The preschooler or toddler may exhibit regressive behavior; cling to trusted adults; have difficulty sleeping; have changes in eating habits; complain of aches and pains without obvious cause; exhibit disobedient behavior; exhibit hyperactivity or aggressive behavior; withdraw; or tell exaggerated stories, particularly about the event.

School-Age Child
The school-age child often withdraws from friends; seeks to gain attention from parents; develops school phobia; has a sudden onset of poor school performance; exhibits aggressive behavior; has difficulty concentrating; or may begin acting in a childlike manner.

Adolescent
The adolescent has vague physical complaints; shirks responsibility of chores, school work, and extracurricular activities; competes for the attention of parents and other trusted adults; withdraws from friends; becomes resistant to authority; becomes disruptive in group settings, such as in class; begins to experiment with risky situations such as use of alcohol, drugs, and sex; feels helpless; feels guilty; or may try to deny any emotions related to the traumatic event.

their emotions. Openly and honestly discuss the particulars of the event in a manner appropriate to the child's developmental level. Help the parents of this child understand that the child needs to be protected from too much information about the event. Particularly if this is a national event, the child needs to be protected from too much media exposure. Graphic images, viewed over and over again, become difficult for children to rid from their minds.

The child needs reassurance, love, and physical contact in the form of cuddling, as well as verbal support. The child needs to feel safe asking any question and deserves to trust they will get a valid, honest answer. The child may be encouraged to express emotions through drawing and painting.

Encourage parents to maintain a normal routine as much as possible. Exercise will assist the child in dealing with feelings of aggression and anger. Parents also need to relax their expectations for the child's behavior until the initial trauma has passed and the child has time to assimilate the event. The nurse should be aware of symptoms of anxiety, depression, suicidal behavior, or deviant behavior and be quick to seek professional counseling for the child.

Therapies Used to Assist the Child with Psychosocial Disorders

The child with a psychosocial disorder will most likely be cared for in an outpatient setting. Therapies involve the child and his or her caregivers. The nurse can assist physicians and mental health professionals to administer these therapies. If the psychosocial disorder is in an acute phase, hospitalization may be necessary. In the hospital, a psychiatric unit can provide the necessary treatment. There are also free-standing facilities that provide care to the child with substance abuse or psychosocial disorders.

PLAY THERAPY

Most children are comfortable playing at some level. Play allows the child to express emotions through a nonthreatening medium (Figure 16-6 ■). The mental health professional may encourage the child to play with dolls, toys, or clay to express anxiety, stress, and fears. The play is used to determine the child's feelings and to teach them appropriate methods of dealing with these negative emotions.

GROUP THERAPY

The teenager is especially receptive to group therapy. Because the teen is more responsive to his or her peers and not an authority figure, this type of therapy can assist teens in verbalizing their feelings. Appropriate suggestions from their peer group can be accepted more readily than from a therapist or parent. One hazard of this type of therapy is the lack of control the therapist has on the direction of the conversation and suggested resolutions.

Figure 16-6. ■ The psychologist uses play therapy to help this girl reenact her car crash. This helps her gain control over the event so that it is not so frightening.

FAMILY THERAPY

Rarely is a problem within a family caused by only one member. Difficulties and their manifestations are typically due to the strength or weaknesses of the family unit. Family therapy seeks to build strong relationships that will promote healing of the child and future healthy relationships.

ART THERAPY

In art therapy children are given paper, colored pens, paint, glue, and scissors (if they are not at risk for inflicting injury on themselves or others). They asked to create something that depicts what they feel inside. The therapist is then able to use their drawings to discuss the children's feelings and help them develop methods of managing negative emotions. Art may also be used to discover hidden events of abuse or violence that children are not able to verbalize.

BEHAVIOR THERAPY

Behavior therapy is a technique used to encourage the child to replace negative, unwanted behaviors with more positive, desirable behaviors. Rewards are used to reinforce the positive behaviors. This type of therapy works best when the therapist and family members use it consistently.

COGNITIVE THERAPY

In cognitive therapy, the child is taught how to recognize negative emotions such as anxiety quickly. The child is also taught why it is detrimental to continue in these negative emotions and the benefits of avoiding them. In cognitive therapy, the mental health professional teaches the child mental activities such as breathing and relaxation techniques to counteract negative emotions.

Note: The reference and resource listings for this and all chapters have been compiled at the back of the book.

Chapter Review

 KEY TERMS by Topic

Use the audio glossary feature of either the CD-ROM or the Companion Website to hear the correct pronunciation of the following key terms.

Introduction
psychosocial health

Brief Assessment Review
holistic health

Psychological Disorders and Associated Manifestations
autism, Asperger's syndrome, echolalia, stereotypy, encopresis, generalized anxiety disorder, separation anxiety disorder, obsessive-compulsive disorder, tics, coprolalia, copropraxia, depression, bipolar disorder, suicide, obesity, bariatric surgery

Anorexia Nervosa and Bulimia
anorexia nervosa, bulimia, purging

Abuse and Family Violence
shaken baby syndrome, nonorganic failure to thrive, sexual abuse, incest, assault, rape, statutory rape, date rape, child molestation, child exploitation, child pornography, exhibitionism, pedophile

KEY Points

- Psychosocial health includes mental, emotional, social, and spiritual stability. Alterations in psychosocial health affect the child as well as the entire family.

- The *Diagnostic and Statistical Manual of Mental Disorders—Fourth Edition Text Revision* (DSM-IV TR) serves as the main diagnostic reference of mental health professionals in the United States.

- Children with autism have difficulty with verbal and nonverbal communication, social interactions, and leisure or play activities. Ensuring safety is a priority because of the child's repetitive behaviors such as head banging.

- The child with ADD has difficulty finishing tasks, is easily distracted, and may move from topic to topic. The child with ADHD also fidgets, may become loud, and disrupts others. Both ADD and ADHD children have difficulty maintaining social relationships.

- Anxiety is subjective feelings of worry, helplessness, insecurity, and apprehension. The nurse can teach the child coping skills and relaxation techniques.

- Characteristics of depression vary from child to child and include declining school performance, irritability, withdrawal from social activities, sleep disorders (either unable to sleep or sleeping all the time), appetite disturbance (either overeating or anorexia), headache, stomachache, difficulty concentrating, and difficulty making decisions.

- Anorexia nervosa is a serious disorder and may require hospitalization.

- The nurse is legally obligated to report to local or state child protective services or law enforcement authorities any suspicion of child abuse.

- Physical abuse of a child is inflicting pain and injury in a deliberate manner. Emotional abuse of a child includes attacks on a child's self-esteem and efforts to control and frighten and embarrass the child.

- Sexual abuse can be defined as sexual acts that are imposed on children who cannot protect themselves because of their lack of emotional or cognitive development.

- Children and teens are vulnerable to the hazards of substance abuse because of their developmental levels. The nurse must recognize the physical, psychological, or cognitive symptoms of substance abuse.

 EXPLORE Media Link

Additional interactive resources for this chapter can be found on the Companion Website at www.prenhall.com/adams.

Click on Chapter 16 and "Begin" to select the activities for this chapter.

For chapter-related NCLEX®-style questions and an audio glossary, access the accompanying CD-ROM in this book.

Animations:
What is autism?
Anorexia
Identifying child abuse
Children and obesity
ADD and ADHD

FOR FURTHER Study

For additional information on assessing fines and the revoking of the nursing license, see Chapter 3.

See Chapter 15 for a further discussion of cognitive disorders.

For more information on enuresis, see Chapter 18.

For additional physical signs of child abuse, see Figure 21-14.

Critical Thinking Care Map

Caring for a Client with Attention Deficit/Hyperactivity Disorder
NCLEX-PN® Focus Area: Psychosocial Integrity

Case Study: Jackson, age 6, is in first grade. Since the beginning of school he has not been able to complete his coursework in the expected time frame and is frequently isolated from his peers during lunch and recess in an effort to get his work done. Jackson is diagnosed with ADHD and has begun daily treatment with Adderall. Jackson's mother is concerned, among other things, that Jackson does not have any friends because of his hyperactive behavior. She is seeking assistance for this concern.

Nursing Diagnosis: Impaired **S**ocial Interaction related to altered thought processes, that is, hyperactivity

COLLECT DATA

Subjective	Objective
_____	_____
_____	_____
_____	_____
_____	_____
_____	_____

Would you report this? Yes/No

If yes, to: _____

Nursing Care

_____
_____
_____
_____
_____
_____
_____
_____
_____

How would you document this? _____
_____
_____
_____

Compare your documentation to the sample provided in Appendix I.

Data Collected
(use only those that apply)

- "I couldn't sleep last night."
- Teacher states that Jackson is better able to do his course work since he has been on Adderall.
- Jackson is observed attempting to talk to a group of boys in the lunchroom without success.
- Teacher's report of lack of peer interaction.
- "I'm not hungry for lunch right now."
- In P.E. class, Jackson is observed completing the obstacle course in the shortest amount of time.
- Jackson plays on the playground alone on the monkey bars.
- Jackson completes his English assignment during the allotted time.
- Mother's report of lack of peer interaction.
- Jackson brings his teacher a basket of apples.
- Jackson states that he has no friends.
- When buddies are picked for a class activity, Jackson is not picked.

Nursing Interventions
(use only those that apply; list in priority order)

- Develop a plan for self-administration of Adderall during the school day.
- Involve Jackson's parents and his teacher in developing a plan to improve social interactions between Jackson and his peers.
- Teach Jackson and his mother about the side effects of Adderall.
- Use role play to observe the social interaction between Jackson and his peers.
- Assist Jackson in developing social skills such as respect for others' privacy, and interpreting reactions from peers honestly.
- Plan an opportunity to observe Jackson in a social interaction during school hours.
- Refer Jackson to a tutoring program to enhance his school work.
- Help develop a plan for additional ways for Jackson to interact socially with other children.
- Develop a plan to reward Jackson for appropriate social interaction.

1 The nurse is assigned to care for a 4-year-old autistic child with an upper respiratory infection. The nurse observes the following behavior and knows this is a clinical manifestation of autism.

1. Conversing with others without shyness
2. Displaying repetitive behaviors such as rocking back and forth
3. Being able to work difficult math problems without assistance
4. Playing with other children but not being able to share

2 The parents of a newly diagnosed 2-year-old with autism are having difficulty with the child's diagnosis. The nurse has just finished talking with the parents and answering their questions and realizes additional information is needed when the mother states:

1. "I realize that with the proper care and medication our child will be cured."
2. "We understand we have to work with our child on behavior modification."
3. "I realize that we have to supervise our child constantly."
4. "We realize that when we talk with our son, we must maintain eye contact and be consistent."

3 The nurse is caring for an infant born with fetal alcohol syndrome (FAS). The nurse knows that there are some characteristics displayed in infants with FAS, and they are:

1. Hepatosplenomegaly, intussuception, and dysphagia
2. Hepatotoxemia, portal hypertension, and jejunoileitis
3. Growth retardation, CNS abnormalities, and craniofacial abnormalities
4. Club foot, hemophilia, and hepatitis

4 A nursing student is asked to identify the characteristics of drug abuse. The nursing instructor steps in to correct the student when the student identifies which incorrect characteristic of drug abuse?

1. Dilated or pinpoint pupils, bloodshot eyes
2. Bruising or needle marks
3. Runny nose
4. Psoriasis

5 The nurse is observing a child with ADD. The child has been taking amphetamine sulfate (Adderall) and is exhibiting irritability and restlessness. Based on these observations, the nurse's initial response would be:

1. Call the physician as these are abnormal side effects of the drug.
2. Prepare for a code situation as the child is in a serious situation.
3. Do nothing as these are common side effects of the drug.
4. Call the drug manufacturer and report these abnormal side effects of the drug.

6 An emergency department nurse is collecting data on a child with suspected sexual abuse. What findings are suspicious related to sexual abuse and indicate the need for further investigation?

1. Anorexia nervosa
2. Vaginal redness, pain, and bloody discharge
3. Fear of authority figures
4. Severe diarrhea

7 A nursing student is caring for a client with anorexia nervosa and developing a plan of care. The nursing instructor speaks with the nursing student about which of the following entries as an incorrect nursing intervention for this disorder?

1. Observe strenuous exercise activities.
2. Monitor food intake.
3. Monitor fluid and electrolyte levels.
4. Observe for binge eating and purging.

8 The nurse answers the phone in the Crisis Center. The call is from the mother of a 16-year-old female who has told her mother that she "doesn't want to live any longer." The nurse's most appropriate response to the mother would be:

1. "Don't worry, all teens go through this stage."
2. "Please stay with your daughter and bring her in for a consult with our psychologist."
3. "Have your daughter lie down and check on her in the morning."
4. "Why would she say such a thing!?"

9 The nurse is collecting data on a severely obese 16-year-old female in the physician's office who states she wants bariatric surgery to correct her obesity. Select all criteria required before an adolescent can be considered for this surgery.

1. Must have tried weight management techniques for longer than 6 months and failed
2. Must be physiologically mature
3. Must weigh over 150 pounds
4. Must agree to a psychological evaluation before surgery
5. Must agree to a psychological evaluation after surgery
6. Must avoid pregnancy for more than 1 year postoperatively

10 A nurse is preparing to admit an infant to the hospital with a diagnosis of shaken baby syndrome. Choose the correct statements about this syndrome.

1. Infants are susceptible to this injury because their neck muscles are weak
2. Jarring motion causes tearing of the nerve fibers in the brain
3. This type of injury always leads to death within 1 month
4. After this injury infants may have seizures, lethargy, and respiratory difficulties
5. Vision impairment or loss of hearing may result from this injury

Answers for NCLEX-PN® Review and Critical Thinking questions appear in Appendix I.

Chapter 17

Care of the Child with Gastrointestinal Disorders

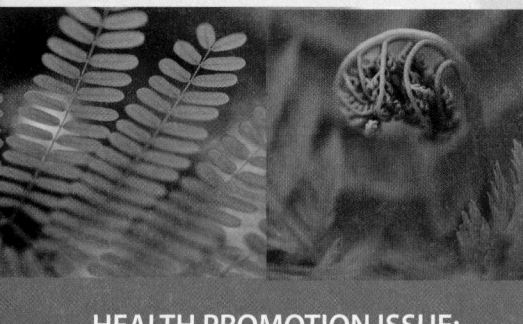

HEALTH PROMOTION ISSUE:
Childhood Obesity and Fast Foods

NURSING CARE PLAN CHART:
Infant with Colic

NURSING PROCESS CARE PLAN:
Care of a Child with Bilateral Cleft Lip

CRITICAL THINKING CARE MAP:
Caring for a Client with Gastroenteritis

BRIEF Outline

Anatomy and Physiology

Brief Assessment Review

Anatomic and Congenital Gastrointestinal Defects

Gastrointestinal Inflammation

Motility Disorders

Malabsorption and Inborn Metabolic Disorders

Nutrition Disorders

Intestinal Parasites

Poisonings

Hepatic Disorders

Nursing Care

LEARNING Outcomes

After completing this chapter, you will be able to:
1. Define key terms.
2. Describe the basic structures and functioning of the gastrointestinal tract and accessory structures.
3. Describe major gastrointestinal disorders in clear, simple terms.
4. Discuss clinical manifestations, diagnostic procedures, and medical management related to gastrointestinal disorders.
5. Explain appropriate nursing interventions for children with gastrointestinal disorders.

Gastrointestinal disorders in children include congenital malformation, malabsorption conditions, and problems with motility. The role of the LPN/LVN in caring for these children is one of assisting with data collection and monitoring the effectiveness of treatments. Most therapeutic interventions ordered for gastrointestinal disorders can be administered by the LPN/LVN.

Anatomy and Physiology

PRIMARY ORGANS

The primary organs of the gastrointestinal system consist of a series of hollow tubelike structures through which food is digested and solid waste is eliminated (Figure 17-1 ■). The entire system is lined with a mucous membrane. Food is propelled through the system by **peristalsis** (wavelike contractions of the smooth muscle that lies underneath the mucous membrane).

The oral cavity is formed by the hard and soft palate, the cheeks, and the tongue. Extending from the center of the soft palate is a cone-shaped process, the uvula. The soft palate and uvula prevent food and fluid from entering the nasal cavity during swallowing. The tongue is made of skeletal muscle attached to the mandible and hyoid bone in

the neck. A thin membrane or **lingual frenulum** attaches the tongue to the floor of the mouth. The tongue is covered with small raised bumps called **papillae.** The sensory receptors for salt, sour, sweet, and bitter are located on the sides of the papillae. The mucous membrane covering the front of the mouth and the inside of the lips is called the **gingiva.** The teeth formed in the mandible and maxilla erupt through the gingiva beginning at around 6 months of age and continue until all 20 deciduous teeth are in place by 2 years of age. Around 6 years of age, the deciduous teeth are replaced by permanent teeth. The 32 permanent teeth, including wisdom teeth, are generally in place between 17 and 24 years of age. Three pairs of salivary glands empty their secretions into the oral cavity. The largest of the salivary glands, the **parotid gland,** is located below and in front of the ears at the angle of the jaw. The parotid ducts open into the **buccal space** (area inside the cheek by the second molars). The **submandibular glands** lie behind the mandible and secrete saliva into the submandibular (Wharton's) ducts opening on each side of the lingual frenulum. The **sublingual glands** (glands under the tongue) open into the floor of the mouth. These structures are illustrated in Figure 17-2 ■.

The esophagus attaches the oral pharynx to the stomach. At the lower end of the esophagus, the **cardiac sphincter** acts to prevent food and gastric acid from being pushed from the stomach into the esophagus.

The stomach is a muscular backward "C"-shaped pouch located just under the diaphragm. The rounded top of the stomach is the **fundus.** The area around the cardiac sphincter is the **cardiac region.** The inner curved area of the stomach is the **lesser curvature,** and the outer area is the **greater curvature.** At the bottom of the stomach, surrounding the pyloric sphincter, is the **pylorus** (the

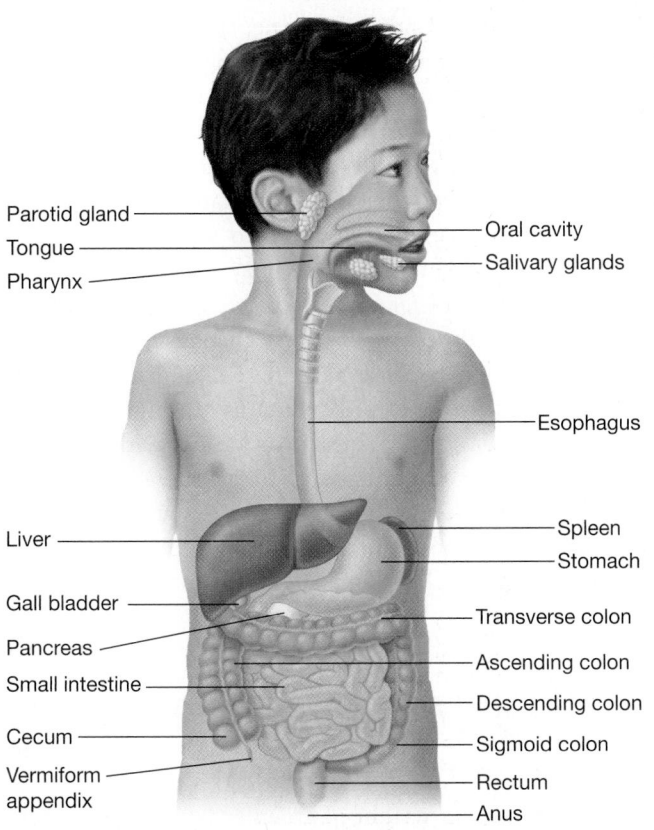

Figure 17-1. ■ Organs of the alimentary canal and related accessory organs.

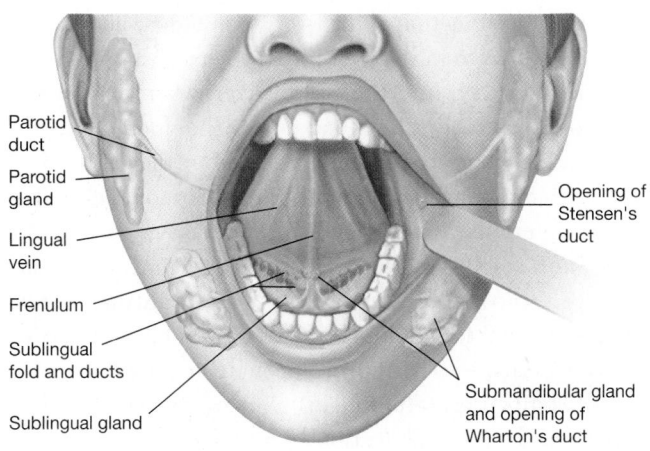

Figure 17-2. ■ Salivary glands and structures of the mouth.

muscular tissue surrounding and controlling the stomach outlet). When the stomach is empty, its lining lies in folds called **rugae.** When food enters the stomach, hydrochloric acid and digestive enzymes are released from the gastric glands inside the mucous membrane. Mucus is also produced to prevent damage to the mucous membrane from the potent gastric juices. Three layers of muscles contract to mix food with digestive acid and enzymes and form a semi-liquid substance called **chyme.** The chyme stays in the stomach several hours before it is propelled through the pyloric sphincter into the small intestine.

The small intestine is divided into three sections: the duodenum, small intestine, and ileum. The main processes of chemical digestion take place in the duodenum. Absorption of nutrients occurs mainly in the jejunum and ileum. The inner lining of the small intestine lies in folds called **plicae.** Covering each plica are small, fingerlike structures called **villi** (singular, *villus*). Inside each villus is a capillary network and lymph vessel into which nutrients are absorbed.

The large intestine or colon is divided into several sections. First, the *cecum* is located in the lower right quadrant of the abdomen. Hanging from the lower end of the cecum is the appendix. Chyme, entering the cecum, is propelled by peristalsis upward through the *ascending colon*, through the *transverse colon* and the *descending colon*, and into the *sigmoid colon*. As the chyme moves through the large intestine, water is removed, leaving the solid waste or feces in a compacted mass. Feces remains in the rectum and sigmoid colon until it is expelled through the anus.

ACCESSORY ORGANS

The two accessory organs of the digestive system are the liver and pancreas (see Figure 17-1).

Liver

The liver, located in the upper right quadrant of the abdomen, just below the diaphragm, is the largest gland in the body. One function of the liver is to produce and excrete bile. Bile flows from the liver into the hepatic duct and cystic duct and then into the gall bladder, where it is stored and concentrated. When food enters the duodenum, the gall bladder contracts, forcing the bile out the cystic duct, and the common bile duct and into the duodenum. Bile acts as an **emulsifier.** An emulsifier breaks large molecules of fat into smaller molecules of fat. All chemicals that are absorbed into the blood from the gastrointestinal system are transported to the liver for processing. The liver detoxifies chemicals, breaks down compounds (**catabolism**), and builds compounds (**anabolism**) of many substances necessary for normal body function. Some functions of the liver include production of blood clotting factors and plasma

proteins, breaking down of dead red blood cells, recycling of needed chemicals, and assisting in the regulation of blood glucose.

Pancreas

The pancreas is both an endocrine and an exocrine gland. As an exocrine gland, the pancreas releases pancreatic fluid into the pancreatic duct. The pancreatic duct joins the common bile duct at the entrance into the duodenum. Pancreatic fluid contains strong enzymes necessary for the chemical digestion of all food groups. As an endocrine gland, the pancreas produces both glycogen and insulin, which are necessary in the regulation of blood sugar.

CHEMICAL DIGESTION

Chemical digestion is the breakdown of food into small molecules that can be absorbed into the blood. To break many chemical bonds, a high temperature over a long period of time is necessary. This temperature would not be conducive to life. However, enzymes found in digestive fluid speed up chemical reactions and allow them to occur within the normal body temperature.

Chemical digestion begins in the mouth. *Amylase* found in saliva changes starch (a polysaccharide) into maltose (a disaccharide). If swallowing occurs too rapidly, this reaction will not take place. When food enters the stomach, hydrochloric acid and *protease* (pepsin) found in gastric fluid break large molecules of protein into smaller molecules. Many chemical reactions occur in the duodenum. Chyme leaving the stomach is highly acidic. The fluids in the duodenum are alkaline, changing the pH of the chyme. Bile is excreted over the chyme. As stated previously, bile breaks large molecules of fat into smaller molecules. Pancreatic fluid contains three enzymes. Lipase changes small molecules of fat into fatty acids, monoglycerides, and glycerol. Protease (trypsin) changes proteins into amino acids and peptides. Amylase changes starch into maltose. Intestinal fluid contains several enzymes. Peptidase changes peptides into amino acids. Maltase changes maltose into glucose. Lactase changes lactose into galactose and glucose. Sucrase changes sucrose into glucose. At the end of chemical digestion, glucose, galactose, amino acids, fatty acids, and glycerol are absorbed into the blood.

Brief Assessment Review

HISTORY

- Compare current weight to growth charts. Inquire about weight changes.
- Ask whether the child has any difficulty swallowing.

- Question the family about the child's symptoms, including appetite, vomiting, diarrhea, constipation, and abdominal pain.
- Inquire about specific foods the child has eaten in the past 24 hours. For the infant, ask about breast or formula feeding. This may be important when allergies or food-borne infections are being considered.
- Ask whether anyone else in the family has similar symptoms.
- Inquire about the child's bowel habits. Is the child toilet trained? Determine frequency, color, consistency and any changes in these habits.
- If constipation is reported, ask about fluid in the diet. Is the constipation associated with pain?

PHYSICAL

A child who appears far above average in weight may be one of the growing number of children for whom obesity will be a lifelong issue. The nurse can plan to provide client information about healthful diets and the importance of proper nutrition. The Health Promotion Issue on pages 456 and 457 discusses one aspect of this concern.

- Inspect the color and consistency of the child's bowel movements. Bowel movements usually begin within the first few hours after birth. In an infant, the stool, or *meconium*, is blackish green and sticky. It is made up of salts, amniotic fluid, mucus, bile, and epithelial cells. Meconium stools may persist for 2 to 3 days until the newborn begins to digest formula or breast milk.

clinical ALERT

If the newborn has not passed meconium stool within the first 24 hours, the primary care provider should be informed. Failure to pass stool could indicate congenital anomalies or other conditions of the gastrointestinal system.

- Observe the shape of the abdomen. The abdomen should be soft, rounded, and without palpable masses. In the infant, the umbilical cord should be clamped, and three blood vessels should be identifiable. In infants and children, there should be no distention or bulging of the abdominal muscles at the midline or around the umbilicus. Bulging could indicate the presence of hernias or other masses. If distention is present, the skin becomes tight and blood vessels appear.

clinical ALERT

Abdominal distention is a sign of many abnormalities of the gastrointestinal tract and should be reported to the primary care provider.

- Auscultate the abdomen using the diaphragm of the stethoscope. Auscultation is done prior to palpation because palpation can alter the frequency and quality of bowel sounds. Bowel sounds are present in four quadrants within an hour after birth and should occur every 10 to 30 seconds and have a high-pitched quality thereafter. Auscultate for at least 5 minutes before reporting that bowel sounds are absent. Absent bowel sounds may indicate peritonitis or paralytic ileus. Hyperactive bowel sounds indicate gastroenteritis or a partial obstruction.
- Palpate the abdomen using light palpation to assess the softness or firmness of the abdominal muscles and the presence of any tenderness. Deep palpation is used to assess the size and consistency of the liver and other organs, except in certain instances such as Wilms' tumor (discussed in Chapter 18 ⬛). Deep palpation is not a responsibility of the LPN, although it is important to understand. Palpation is best accomplished when the child is supine, with the knees bent. To help the small child relax, ask the child, "How soft can you make your tummy?" If the child is ticklish, firm pressure should be used. Do not pretend to tickle because the child will tighten the abdominal muscles, making it difficult to feel the underlying tissue.
- Inspect the anus if necessary. Observe for redness, swelling, fissures, and drainage. A rectal examination should only be performed by an advanced practice nurse or physician.

Gastrointestinal system disorders include congenital anomalies, as well as inflammation, malabsorption, and motility problems. The liver is an accessory organ to the gastrointestinal system, so hepatic disorders are also covered in this chapter. The focus of nursing care is to maintain nutrition and fluid balance and to promote elimination of solid waste.

Anatomic and Congenital Gastrointestinal Defects

Congenital defects of the gastrointestinal system, the most common of the congenital defects, require surgical correction but are not usually immediately life threatening. Without correction, however, aspiration, malnutrition, and obstruction could result if detection and correction are not made in a timely manner.

CLEFT LIP AND CLEFT PALATE

Cleft lip and cleft palate commonly occur together but can be found separately (Figure 17-3 ⬛). When the medial nasal and maxillary processes fail to join, the result is a **cleft**

(Text continues on page 458.)

HEALTH PROMOTION ISSUE

CHILDHOOD OBESITY AND FAST FOODS

An overweight single mother brings her two young children in for wellness checks. The 2-year-old is at the 50th percentile for height, the 98th for weight. The 5-year-old is at the 65th percentile for height, the 96th for weight. The mother insists that she does not have a lot of snack food around the house. "We usually just eat out when I pick them up on the way home from work."

DISCUSSION

Childhood obesity has increased since the mid-1980s and may be approaching epidemic status (Yuan et al., 2001). The National Health and Nutrition Examination Survey data indicate that 15% of children and teens between 6 and 19 years are overweight (Binns & Ariza, 2004). It is estimated that 25% to 30% are obese (Moran, 1999). What are some implications of obesity? What is causing this increase in childhood obesity?

Few problems in childhood have such an impact on the life of the individual as obesity. Obesity is associated with many physical complications, including type II diabetes mellitus, coronary artery disease, pulmonary dysfunction, stroke, and arthritis. Obesity can also disable the individual emotionally, including poor body image, low self-esteem, social isolation, and feelings of depression and rejection.

Obesity is not only an individual's problem, but also causes social concern. For example, the cost of treatment of the complications of obesity will put additional strain on the national health care budget. The obese individual may need to take more sick days off work and therefore be less productive.

What is the difference between being overweight and obesity? Being overweight and obese are both an unhealthy accumulation of body fat. The body mass index (BMI) is the standard for determining if an individual is overweight or obese. The BMI is determined by dividing the individual's weight in kilograms by their height in meters squared. For example, a child weighs 45 lb (20.45 kg) and is 42 inches tall. The height in meters squared would be 1.1 m² (42 inches = 105 cm = 1.05 m). The BMI would be 18%. Children with a BMI between the 85th and 95th percentile are considered to be overweight. Children over the 95th percentile are considered to be obese. (*Note:* See Appendix II 🔗 for growth charts to determine percentile.)

PLANNING AND IMPLEMENTATION

There are many causes of the increase in obesity in children. Heredity is one factor that cannot be changed. Other factors can be changed with positive results. In many households, children spend most of their personal time sitting in front of a computer or television. With little activity, children do not burn the calories they consume. By limiting a child's sedentary activities and encouraging participation in

physical, motion-oriented activities, parents can help children slow or prevent the deposition of body fat.

Diet is the second factor that can be adjusted. Fast food has become a prominent feature in the diet of families. Consumption of fast food by children increased fivefold between 1970 and 1995, while the number of fast-food restaurants doubled. Several dietary factors may cause excessive weight gain from fast food consumption. They include massive portion size; high energy-density foods; an appeal to taste preference for fats, sugar, and salt; high content of saturated and trans fat; high glycemic load; and low fiber.

Little research has been conducted on the effects of fast food on body weight. Without sufficient data, many support the claim that fast food can be part of a healthy diet. One study by Bowman, Gortmaker, Ebbeling, and colleagues (2002) included 6,212 children and adolescents from 4 to 19 years. On a typical day, more than 30% of the children ate fast food. These children consumed more total calories; more fat; more carbohydrates, including sugar and sweetened beverages; less fiber; less milk; and fewer fruits and vegetables. These same children made poorer food choices on days when they did not consume fast food. The study concluded that fast-food consumption has an adverse effect on dietary quality that could increase risk for obesity.

In response to political pressure, many fast-food restaurants are providing information about the nutrition content of their menu items. Some fast-food restaurants are offering nutritious choices, including salads, fruit, and milk. Advertisements for meat sandwiches complemented with vegetables are becoming more common. It will be up to parents to ensure that children select the healthier foods.

Nursing Concerns

When assessing a child's nutritional status, the nurse should ask about the frequency and content of fast-food meals. The child should be weighed and measured, and the BMI calculated.

Children over the 85th percentile should be evaluated for complications such as hypertension, diabetes, and hyperlipidemia. The child's activities should be assessed in relation to calories burned. It is important to assess the child's emotional status and the impact the child's weight has on quality of life.

Parents and children should be taught the impact that being overweight or obese has on their general health. Although it is necessary to discuss complications of being overweight, it is important to stress how well the child will feel when he or she has more energy following weight loss. Point out the benefits of weight loss, instead of dwelling on the risks and complications.

The family may need a referral to a nutritionist. It should be suggested that meals at a fast-food restaurant be reserved for a special occasion instead of being a daily event. Suggest that when fast food must be consumed, the restaurant selected should offer nutritious meals, and the food choices should reflect a balanced meal, with as low a fat content as possible.

Parents should encourage their children to become physically active. Limiting computer or television time may be necessary. Scheduling activities daily that require active participation will help burn calories and establish lifelong habits of physical exercise.

Obesity in children is becoming a major health concern. The problem results, in part, from the rapid pace at which parents live. The rush-rush of today's lifestyle necessitates rapid meal production and encourages parents to purchase fast foods for their families. These high-calorie, high-fat meals, coupled with sedentary activities of children, result in obesity. The nurse should provide teaching and support as families try to break the cycle and improve their health.

SELF-REFLECTION

Do I find time each day to take a break for some enjoyable physical activity? Do I give myself several portions of fruits and vegetables daily? If I am in a hurry, do I seek out healthful food options?

SUGGESTED RESOURCES

For the Nurse

Bowman, S., Gortmaker, S., Ebbeling, C., Pereira, M., & Ludwig, D. (2004). Effects of fast-food consumption on energy intake and diet quality among children in a national household survey. *Pediatrics, 113*(1), 112–118.

Freeland-Graves, J., & Nitzke, S. (2002). Position of the American Dietetic Association: Total diet approach to communicating food and nutrition information. *Journal of the American Dietetic Association, 102*, 100–108.

Nestle, M. (2002). *Food politics: How the food in industry influences nutrition and health.* Berkeley: University of California Press.

Taveras, E., Berkey, C., Rifas-Shiman, S., Ludwig, D., Rockett, H., Field, A., Colditz, G., & Gillman, M. (2005). Association of consumption of fried food away from home with body mass index and diet quality in older children and adolescents. *Pediatrics, 116*(4), e518–e524.

For the Client/Parent

Hassink, S. (Ed.). (2006). *A parent's guide to childhood obesity: A roadmap to health.* Washington, DC: American Academy of Pediatrics.

Okie, S. (2006). *Fed up: Winning the war against childhood obesity.* Washington, DC: National Academies Press.

A

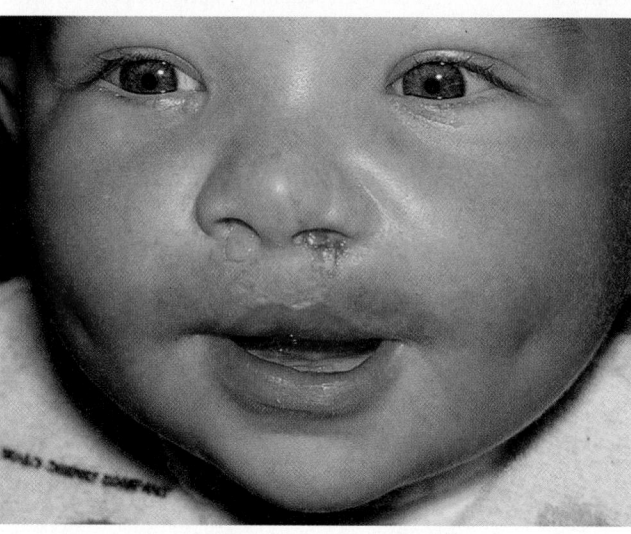

B

Figure 17-3. ■ **(A)** Bilateral cleft lip. **(B)** Repaired bilateral cleft lip. (Courtesy of Dr. Elizabeth Peterson, Spokane, WA.)

palate. There is an opening between the roof of the mouth and the floor of the nasal passage. If the upper lip fails to join medially, a **cleft lip** is the result. Cleft lip can be unilateral or bilateral. Cleft palate could be complete (through bone and tissue) or partial (involving the bone structure but not the overlying mucous membrane). So, when assessing every newborn, it is important not only to visualize the palate, but also to feel the palate with the little finger to be sure the bones are intact.

The cause of clefts is a combination of genetic and environmental influences. There is an increased incidence in families with a history of clefts. In the United States, cleft lip and cleft palate are more common in Native Americans

and Asians than in Whites and Blacks. Since 1996, when cereal was fortified with folate in an attempt to decrease neural tube defects, the incidence of cleft lip and palate has decreased. The data suggest a correlation between folate and facial formation (Wong et al., 1999).

Preoperative Nursing Considerations

The most immediate concern when a baby is born with a cleft lip or cleft palate is providing nutrition. The newborn with a cleft lip cannot make a seal around the nipple. Air leaking between the cleft in the lip and the nipple prevents adequate suction to draw the milk into the mouth. The small amounts of milk that do enter the mouth may leak out instead of being swallowed.

The newborn with a cleft palate will be unable to compress the nipple between the tongue and the palate. Milk that enters the mouth can enter the nasal cavity, and then drain from the nose or down the back of the throat. When milk drains down the throat without coordinated swallowing, the child is at risk for choking. Milk that pools in the nasal passages increases the risk for sinus and middle ear infections. Repeated middle ear infections can damage the tympanic membrane, resulting in hearing loss.

Prior to surgical repair, the infant must be fed. Special feeding equipment such as a long nipple with enlarged holes or a *Breck feeder* (syringe with a rubber tube) may be used. Parents will need instruction on the use of special equipment. The infant should be positioned in an upright position. The use of an angle-necked bottle will facilitate feeding. The nipple of the bottle should be positioned to the back and along the side of the mouth. Instruct the parent to squeeze the cheeks gently around the nipple to improve suction. Parents will also need encouragement and emotional support to handle this additional responsibility in the care of their child.

Sucking increases the strength of the muscles of the mouth that are needed for speech. When the lip and palate are not formed correctly, teeth may not erupt or may erupt out of alignment. A space may be present between the front teeth. The teeth, lips, and palate are used in forming sounds. When these structures are not formed properly, speech therapy is often required.

Surgical Correction of Cleft Lip

The surgical correction of cleft lip is usually accomplished in the first 3 months of life. To achieve the best cosmetic effect, the priority of care is to protect the suture line from trauma and infection. A **Logan clamp** (a metal bow taped to both sides of the suture line) or a butterfly bandage is frequently used to decrease tension on the suture line. Depending on the extent of the defect, the absence of infection, and the lack of suture line trauma, complete closure may be accomplished in one surgery. Cosmetic revision may need to be done at a later date.

Surgical Correction of Cleft Palate

Surgical closure of a cleft palate may need to be accomplished in stages, depending on the extent of the cleft. Closure of a cleft palate is usually begun at 4 to 6 months of age, with complete closure accomplished by age 2. As with cleft lip repair, preventing trauma and infection of the suture line is important. To prevent trauma, the nurse should teach the family to avoid putting hard or sharp objects into the child's mouth, including suction catheters, tongue blades, straws, forks, and toothbrushes. Once healing is complete, the child will need to be referred to a speech therapist.

Postoperative Nursing Considerations

Postoperatively, fluids are given through a dropper or syringe. No hard object is inserted into the infant's mouth. The infant cannot suck until the suture line has healed. The infant should be placed supine or in a side-lying position to avoid friction on the suture line from the bed. Soft restraints over the elbows may be used to keep the child from touching the suture line or sucking on the thumb or fingers. Antibiotic ointment is generally placed on the suture line to prevent infection. The infant should be medicated for pain as necessary to prevent crying and stress on the suture line.

Parents anticipate the birth of their "pretty" baby. When the child is born with an obvious facial defect, the family experiences the loss of their "perfect" child. Although in most cases corrective surgery can provide closure of the defect, a permanent scar remains. Nursing care is needed to allow families to express their grief or disappointment and to model a positive response to the newborn.

ESOPHAGEAL ATRESIA AND TRACHEOESOPHAGEAL FISTULA

Esophageal atresia and tracheoesophageal fistula may be found separately but are most commonly found together. When the esophagus ends in a blind pouch before entering the stomach, the anomaly is called **esophageal atresia.** The proximal end of the lower segment of the esophagus is also a closed pouch. **Tracheoesophageal fistula** is a connection between the trachea and the esophagus. The most common type of anomaly, illustrated in Figure 17-4 ■, occurs when the upper segment of the esophagus ends in a blind pouch connected to the trachea. The lower segment of the esophagus is connected to the trachea by a fistula. This formation is described as an esophageal atresia with proximal and distal tracheoesophageal fistula. Oral intake will be unable to enter the stomach (resulting in vomiting);

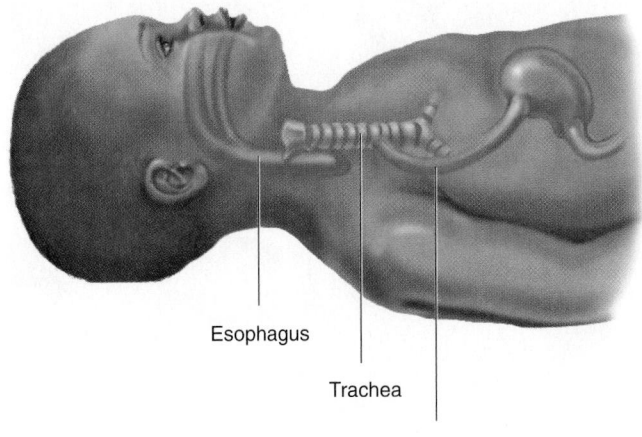

Figure 17-4. ■ Esophageal atresia and tracheoesophageal fistula. Most commonly, the upper segment of the esophagus ends in a blind pouch connected to the trachea; a fistula connects the lower segment to the trachea.

instead, it will enter the trachea through the fistula, causing aspiration. Esophageal atresia and tracheoesophageal fistula are potentially life threatening.

Manifestations

The infant with esophageal atresia and tracheoesophageal fistula presents with copious amounts of thin mucus shortly after birth. The secretions clear with suctioning, but they soon reappear. If a tracheoesophageal fistula is present, the stomach may become distended with trapped air. If the defects are not identified prior to feeding, the infant will regurgitate the feeding, or the feeding will be aspirated into the lungs. Severe respiratory distress will occur, and aspiration pneumonia may develop.

Diagnosis

To diagnose this disorder, an attempt is made to pass a 5 or 8 French nasogastric tube into the stomach. The tube meets resistance and can be advanced only a short distance. X-ray, ultrasound, and echocardiogram are performed to confirm diagnosis.

Treatment

Treatment is aimed at preventing respiratory complications until the defect can be surgically repaired. In the absence of other anomalies, surgical repair is usually completed in the first few days of life to separate the trachea from the esophagus and join the esophageal segments. If other anomalies are present, gastrostomy feedings may be necessary until the infant is stabilized (Figure 17-5 ■). See also Procedure 8-22 ⬭.

Figure 17-5. ■ Gastrostomy tube feeding into stomach. This type of feeding may be given to a child with tracheoesophageal fistula prior to surgery.

Figure 17-6. ■ Imperforate anus.

Postoperatively, the infant should not be fed orally for 7 to 14 days to allow for healing. Once oral feedings begin, they are usually tolerated.

IMPERFORATE ANUS

Imperforate anus occurs when the membrane between the anal pit and the colon fails to break down.

Manifestations

On inspection of the perineum, a thin membrane may be seen covering the anus or an obvious malformation can be seen, including a flat anus or deep dimple. Anomalies of the urinary and reproductive systems should be suspected, especially if meconium is present in the urine. Figure 17-6 ■ illustrates this anorectal anomaly.

Diagnosis

If meconium is not passed within 24 hours of birth, an imperforate anus should be suspected. The diagnosis can be confirmed with x-rays.

Treatment

Surgical correction, occurring shortly after birth, is a relatively simple procedure if no other anomaly is present. The baby should not receive oral intake until the anus is opened surgically. Feeding the infant would stimulate peristalsis and could cause rupture of the colon. If surgery is delayed, IV fluid and nutrition will be necessary.

OMPHALOCELE

Omphalocele is a congenital malformation of the abdominal wall allowing the abdominal contents to herniate into

the umbilical cord (Figure 17-7 ■). There is generally a thin translucent sac (peritoneum) covering the abdominal organs. The size of the sac varies depending on the degree of defect. Small defects may be repaired with good prognosis. Large defects may result in long-term gastrointestinal disorders.

HERNIAS

A **hernia** is a protrusion of the stomach or intestine through a malformation or enlarged opening in the normal musculature. In the infant, three locations are common:

■ Diaphragmatic hernia, the most life threatening
■ Umbilical hernia
■ Inguinal hernia.

Figure 17-7. ■ In omphalocele, the size of the sac depends on the extent of the protrusion of abdominal contents through the umbilical cord. (Reprinted, with permission, from McGraw-Hill Companies, Inc. Rudolph, A. M., Hoffman, J. L. E., & Rudolph, C. D. [Eds.]. [1991]. *Rudolph's pediatrics* [19th ed.]. Stamford, CT: Appleton & Lange, p. 1040.)

Diaphragmatic hernia is the result of a birth defect of the diaphragm that allows the organs of the abdomen to protrude into the thoracic cavity. It can appear in different degrees and is often visible on prenatal ultrasound. Intrauterine fetal surgery to repair the defect is available in larger hospitals. Infants born with diaphragmatic hernia often have severe respiratory distress due to the infant's inability to expand the lungs fully. Surgery is done as soon as the infant can be stabilized.

Umbilical hernia results from protrusion of abdominal contents through a weakened umbilical ring and is most common in African American girls. This hernia can be noted on inspection and palpation of the infant's abdomen. The defect may close spontaneously by age 1 to 2. If not, surgical repair may be necessary.

Inguinal hernia, a protrusion of abdominal contents through a weakened inguinal ring, is more common in boys. The hernia appears as a soft swelling below the umbilicus or in the groin or scrotum. The hernia grows larger with coughing, crying, or straining. Surgery is most often necessary but can be delayed until the infant is at least 3 months old.

Strangulation of the bowel may occur when the intestines become trapped in the hernia. Ischemia occurs in the affected intestine and an obstruction develops. Infants who develop strangulation will have intense pain, redness in the groin, vomiting, and abdominal distention. Strangulation is an emergency situation, and attempts may be made to reduce the hernia by applying pressure to the mass. If this is unsuccessful, surgical intervention is required.

clinical ALERT

Parents should be instructed not to push on the hernia or apply tape, straps, or coins. These actions can cause the intestine to strangulate (see Figure 17-12B).

Gastrointestinal Inflammation

GASTROENTERITIS

Gastroenteritis, or inflammation of the stomach, may be caused by bacteria (e.g., *Escherichia coli* or salmonella), virus (e.g., rotavirus), toxins, and allergies. The illness may resolve without complications or cause mild to severe dehydration.

Manifestations

Symptoms include nausea, vomiting, diarrhea, and fever. The child should be offered small amounts of clear fluid to help prevent dehydration. If symptoms do not resolve in 24 to 48 hours, or bleeding is present, the parents should consult a physician immediately. See Chapter 11 ⟳ for more information on fluid and electrolyte imbalances.

BOX 17-1 | COMPLEMENTARY THERAPIES

Probiotics

When children are given a long course of broad-spectrum antibiotics, the normal intestinal flora can be destroyed. In such situations, the use of **probiotics** (foods or supplements containing live beneficial organisms) may be helpful to restore the normal flora. Many dairy manufacturers are enhancing foods with probiotics. Fermented foods such as miso, tempeh, soy sauce, and yogurt contain active probiotic cultures.

Individuals who have been on long-term antibiotic therapy may need large quantities of these foods to reestablish the normal flora in the gastrointestinal tract. In these cases, probiotic supplements in the form of powder or capsules may be better. These supplements, which contain *Lactobacillus, Acidophilus*, and bifidobacteria, should be kept refrigerated. Symptoms of diarrhea, bloating, and flatus should resolve within a few weeks.

Some practitioners believe that the Western diet, which is high in sugar and animal fat, prevents the normal flora from flourishing. They recommend a diet high in fiber and probiotic supplements for everyone (Pick, 2006).

Probiotics may have helpful effects beyond the gastrointestinal tract. They have also been studied in relation to prevention of atopic dermatitis in children (Kalliomäki, Salminen, Poussa, Arvilommi, & Isolauri, 2003).

MediaLink Importance of Probiotics

Diagnosis

Diagnosis is based on history and clinical findings. Lab tests include CBC and urinalysis. Stool cultures may be done to determine the causative agent.

Treatment

If the child is hospitalized, the treatment would include IV fluids, administration of electrolytes, and antibiotics. The child would be placed on enteric precautions, and a gown and gloves would be required when caring for the child.

Once vomiting and diarrhea subside, the child's diet should be progressed to full liquids and soft foods for a few days. Box 17-1 ■ provides information that might assist digestion.

APPENDICITIS

Appendicitis is inflammation of the vermiform appendix, a small sac at the end of the cecum. Appendicitis is most common in boys between 10 and 16 and rarely occurs before 2 years of age. Initially, there is a blockage of the lumen of the appendix followed by infection and inflammation. If the infection is not relieved or the appendix removed, the risk of rupture and subsequent peritonitis is great (Figure 17-8 ■).

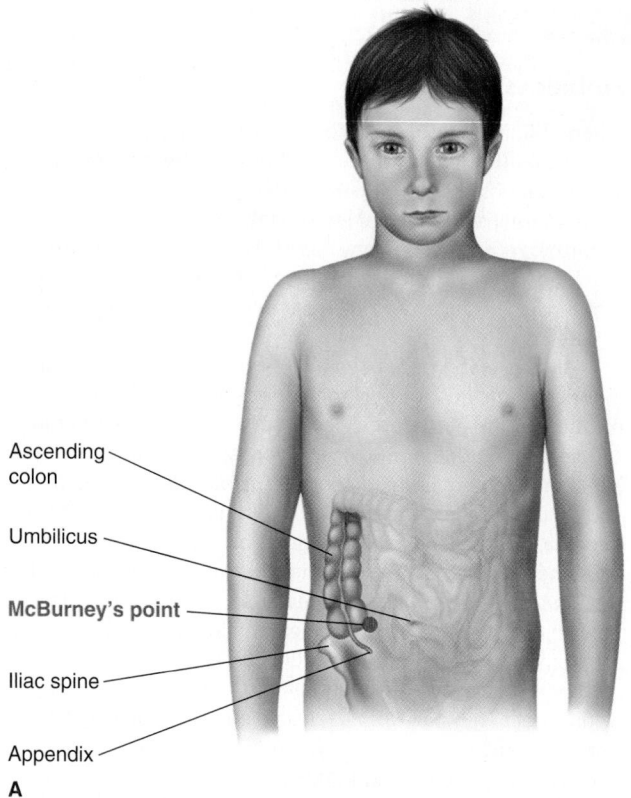

Ascending colon

Umbilicus

McBurney's point

Iliac spine

Appendix

A

B

Figure 17-8. ■ **(A)** McBurney's point is the common location of pain in children and adolescents with appendicitis. **(B)** Appendectomy. The appendix and cecum are brought through the incision to the surface of the abdomen. The base of the appendix is clamped and ligated. The appendix is then removed.

Manifestations

The child presents with constant right lower quadrant pain. There is usually **rebound tenderness** following palpation (increase in discomfort when abdominal pressure is released). The child usually exhibits a fever, nausea, and an elevated white blood cell count. The child may prefer a side-lying position with the knees flexed (fetal position). A sudden relief of pain may indicate that the appendix has ruptured.

Diagnosis

Diagnosis may be more difficult in a child than in an adult because a child's symptoms and pain perception may be more generalized. Computed tomography (CT) with contrast is increasingly used. X-rays may or may not show a **fecalith** (a hard mass of feces) in the right lower quadrant. Lab tests may be performed to rule out a variety of possible disorders, such as urinary tract infection, inguinal hernia, sickle cell crisis, testicular torsion, pelvic inflammatory disease, and gastroenteritis.

Treatment

The medical treatment of appendicitis is surgical intervention as soon as possible (see Figure 17-8B). Routine preoperative care should be provided, including surgical consent, an IV infusion, and sedation. With an uneventful surgical procedure, the child may be discharged within 12 to 24 hours. Routine discharge teaching should be given to the child and parents.

If the appendix ruptures prior to surgery, peritonitis spreads rapidly. If untreated, small-bowel obstruction, electrolyte imbalance, and septic shock result. In this case, the nurse should anticipate a longer, more complex course of nursing care.

Nursing Considerations

Following surgery, the child should be monitored frequently for signs of infection and small-bowel obstruction. Intravenous antibiotics will be administered, and IV fluids will be given until bowel function returns. Once bowel sounds are heard, small amounts of clear fluid are offered, and the diet is gradually progressed as tolerated. A small-bowel obstruction would be treated with nasogastric decompression.

The child will be hospitalized approximately 3 to 5 days postoperatively. Prior to discharge, the child and parents should be instructed in use of pain medication, antibiotic administration, incision care, and the need for follow-up visits to the surgeon.

Evaluation of well-being is based on a return of bowel function, a return of white blood cell count to normal, and a decrease in discomfort. The child and parents should verbalize an understanding of discharge instructions. The child should be able to return to normal activities within a few days. Vigorous activities such as contact sports should be avoided until approved by the physician.

INFLAMMATORY BOWEL DISEASE

Inflammatory bowel disease includes two separate chronic disorders of the intestine:

■ **Crohn's disease** (random inflammation of the entire gastrointestinal tract that involves all layers of the bowel wall)

■ **Ulcerative colitis** (inflammation with sloughing of the mucosa of the large intestine)

It was once believed that these were diseases of young adults. However, the incidence of both disorders has increased in adolescence. The etiology is uncertain, but there is a strong support for a genetic association (Box 17-2 ■).

BOX 17-2   CULTURAL PULSE POINTS

Prevalence of Inflammatory Bowel Disorders

Both Crohn's and ulcerative colitis are three to six times more prevalent in individuals of Jewish descent. When a Jewish child presents with recurrent abdominal pain and diarrhea, testing for inflammatory bowel disease is recommended.

Manifestations

Crohn's disease begins as a small, localized mucosal ulcer of the ileum, colon, or rectum, which grows in size and depth. The onset of symptoms is gradual, with abdominal cramps followed by diarrhea. These symptoms subside in a few days and then recur, becoming more severe each time. Over time, the child develops anorexia, weight loss, and general malaise.

Ulcerative colitis also begins with abdominal cramps and diarrhea. Lower abdominal pain occurs before and during a bowel movement and stops with the passage of stool and flatus. The stool is mixed with mucus and blood. Weight loss and delayed growth occur over time.

Diagnosis

Diagnosis is based on determining the location and extent of involvement. Stool specimens are used to rule out an infectious process. Biopsy can be taken during a colonoscopy.

Laboratory studies are useful in identifying secondary conditions such as anemia, electrolyte imbalance, and malnutrition.

Treatment

Medical treatment for both disorders (Table 17-1 ■) involves the administration of corticosteroids, antibiotics, and antidiarrheal medication (Ball & Bindler, 2006). For moderate to severe Crohn's disease, including fistula-forming disease, immunosuppresants such as infliximab (Remicade) are administered. The goal of nutritional therapy is to provide adequate calories and nutrients for growth without aggravating the inflammation and diarrhea. Total parenteral nutrition (TPN) is often given during an acute episode when the bowel must be rested. TPN can be used to improve nutrition by increasing the amount of protein, carbohydrates, vitamins, and minerals to aid in healing. At times, surgery is needed. A temporary colostomy or ileostomy is performed to allow the lower small intestine or colon to rest and heal. In ulcerative colitis, the removal of the affected tissue usually provides a cure. In Crohn's disease, ulceration tends to recur elsewhere.

Nursing Considerations

Nursing care focuses on the emotional impact of these chronic disorders, teaching the administration of prescribed medication, monitoring nutritional status, and providing referrals. Nursing management most commonly occurs in the home and school, and parents may need to arrange home tutoring during acute episodes of the disease. Table 17-2 ■ provides tips on communicating about ostomies with children of different ages.

Adolescence is an emotionally difficult time, given the normal changes in body image. Abdominal pain, diarrhea, fluid and electrolyte loss, blood loss, and side effects of medication all place additional stress on the adolescent's self-image. The need for a temporary or permanent ileostomy or

---

TABLE 17-1

Pharmacology: Drugs Used for Inflammatory Bowel Disease

DRUG (GENERIC AND COMMON BRAND NAMES)	USUAL ROUTE/DOSE	CLASSIFICATION	SELECTED SIDE EFFECTS	DON'T GIVE IF
Loperamide (Kaopectate, Imodium)	1–2 mg bid–tid; follow with 0.1 mg/kg/dose after each loose stool	Antidiarrheal	Constipation, toxic megacolon in patients with ulcerative colitis	Child has severe diarrhea. Consult care provider.
Infliximab (Remicade)	Child over 6 years: 5 mg/kg IV over 2 hours; may repeat 2 times at 4-week intervals	Immunosuppressant	Fatigue, fever, pain, headache, dizziness, infections	Suspected or identified infection is present.

TABLE 17-2				
Communicating Across the Life Span: Child with an Ostomy				
	TODDLER	**PRESCHOOLER**	**SCHOOL-AGE CHILD**	**ADOLESCENT**
Client	"What's this?"	"I don't like this bag here."	"Am I going to be able to play baseball with this attached to me?"	"I can't go to school with this thing. What if it stinks? Everyone will know it's me."
Nurse	"This is a plastic bag that will be taped to your belly. Your mommy and I will be changing it to keep it clean."	"The bag is helping your body to get rid of your poop while your body gets better."	"The bag is only temporary. While it's attached, you and your parents may decide it's safer to not play baseball."	"I'll show you how to take care of the ostomy and even add a deodorant if you like. If you still feel uncomfortable, we can talk about getting your assignments and completing them from home. Let's see what your parents think about that idea."

colostomy will compound the issue (Figure 17-9 ■). During an acute episode, the client may not be able to attend school, which may limit support from friends. Encourage the adolescent to maintain contact with friends by telephone, e-mail, cards, and visits. Referral to visiting nurses and support groups for children with ostomies and the Crohn's Colitis Foundation may be useful.

Because adolescents can provide a lot of their own care, instructions should be given to both the client and the parents. Demonstration and return demonstration in care of

central venous catheters and administration of TPN, including maintaining sterile technique, operating infusion pumps, and obtaining blood glucose levels, are important aspects of teaching. Teaching should also include the importance of adhering to the prescribed medication regimen, with an emphasis on continuing the medications even when the client is asymptomatic. If an ostomy is required, teaching must include the care of the site, bag change, and odor management. Procedure 17-1 ■ describes the steps in ostomy care.

Motility Disorders

Motility disorders prevent gastrointestinal contents from moving through the system in a normal manner.

GASTROESOPHAGEAL REFLUX

Gastroesophageal reflux disease (GERD) is a condition caused by a relaxation of the cardiac sphincter. The relaxation of the cardiac sphincter allows gastric contents to return to the esophagus. GERD is more common in premature infants and children with neurologic impairment.

Manifestations

Some "spitting up" is considered normal in infants, but continued regurgitation can lead to aspiration, pneumonia, or apnea. The child may complain of hunger or be irritable and may have a history of vomiting. He or she will eat but still lose weight. The adolescent may complain of heartburn, chest pain, or abdominal pain. If they vomit, it may contain food, stomach acid, blood, or bile. Breathing may become difficult, and they may develop a cough that is

Figure 17-9. ■ Nursing strategies to address altered perception of body image and to increase feelings of independence are important when working with an adolescent who has an ostomy. Support groups or a visit from another teenager who has had an ostomy can facilitate positive coping, as demonstrated by this teenage girl.

PROCEDURE 17-1   Ostomy Care

Purpose

- To assess and care for the skin around the stoma
- To collect stool
- To contain odors for client comfort and self-esteem

Equipment

- Disposable gloves
- Bedpan
- Solvent (presaturated sponges or liquid)
- Moisture-proof bag for disposal of pouches
- Cleaning materials, including toilet tissue, warm water, mild soap, washcloths, towel
- Skin barrier (paste, powder, water, or liquid skin sealant)
- Stoma measuring guide
- Pen or pencil, scissors
- Clean ostomy appliance (pouch) with belt (optional)
- Tail closure clamp
- Deodorant (liquid or tablet)

Check order + Gather equipment + Introduce yourself + Identify client + Provide privacy + Explain procedure + Hand hygiene + Gloves as needed

Interventions and Rationales

1. Perform prepatory steps (see icon bar above).

2. Determine the need for appliance change.
   - Assess the used appliance for fluid leakage. *Fluid leakage can irritate and damage skin*
   - Ask client about discomfort at or around the stoma. *Discomfort around stoma could indicate skin irritation and breakdown*
   - Assess fullness of pouch. *Pouch should be emptied or changed when one-third to one-half full. The weight of an overfilled pouch can cause it to detach from the skin, causing spillage and skin irritation*

3. Select appropriate time.
   - Avoid changing pouch close to meals or visiting hours. *Odor may reduce the appetite, offend visitors, or embarrass the client.*
   - Avoid times when increased peristalsis would increase drainage. *Food intake and certain medications will increase peristalsis. It is better to avoid these times so stool does not leak out of the stoma and onto the skin or linen.*

4. Prepare the client.
   - Position the client in a supine position, or sitting in the bathroom. *If the client is unable to get out of bed, the supine position is used. Sitting or standing in the bathroom may be the position used in the home and should also be used in the hospital.*

5. Empty the pouch.
   - Empty the pouch through the bottom tail by opening the clamp and squeezing the stool into the bedpan or toilet. *Emptying the pouch before removal prevents spillage onto the client's skin.*
   - Assess the amount, color, and consistency of stool. *Assessment is necessary to determine if bowel is functioning properly.*
   - If the pouch is attached to the skin and no leaks are apparent, the bag can be rinsed with warm water, drained into the bedpan or toilet, and the clamp reapplied. *As long as the appliance is attached to the skin and no skin irritation is apparent, the appliance can be reused. It should be changed every 48 to 72 hours.*

6. Remove the appliance.
   - Peel the pouch off slowly while supporting the client's skin. *Keeping the skin taut lessens discomfort and prevents skin abrasions.*
   - Dispose of the pouch in a moisture-proof bag.

7. Clean the stoma and surrounding skin.
   - Gently wipe any excess stool from the stoma with toilet tissue and dispose of it in moisture-proof bag or toilet.
   - Wash stoma and surrounding skin with warm water (and soap) using washcloth. Rinse and dry the skin with towel. *Soap may dry the skin and so may not be used. The stoma has no sensory neurons, so cleaning will not cause discomfort but may stimulate peristalsis.*
   - Use special cleanser to remove hard, dry stool, or remnants of old stoma adhesive. *Special cleansers emulsify to prevent damage to the skin.*
   - Rinse and pat dry. *Skin must be dry before new pouch is applied.*

Figure 17-10. ■ Healthy-appearing stoma. (Courtesy of Carol Williams, RN, BS, UC Davis Medical Center.)

8. Assess the stoma (Figure 17-10 ■).
   - Inspect stoma for redness, swelling, size, and bleeding.
   - Inspect skin for redness, ulceration, and irritation. *Slight redness after appliance removal is normal.*
9. Apply a new appliance.
   - Use the guide to measure the size of the stoma. *Stoma size varies and may change as the child grows.*
   - Be sure opening in the pouch adhesive is the correct size. Cut to fit if needed. *Some pouches come with standard size openings, whereas others need to be cut to fit. The entire stoma should fit through the opening.*

- Apply skin barrier (powder, paste, or liquid). Follow manufacturer's directions. *A variety of products are available. Parents should be taught to use the product(s) they will be using at home. Skin barrier protects the tissue from stool and moisture.*
- Center the pouch over the stoma. *The adhesive from the pouch should not touch the stoma. Adhesive can irritate and damage the stomal tissue.*
- Gently press against the skin.
- Place deodorant in the pouch. Close the tail of the pouch with the clamp. *Deodorant is optional.*
- Dispose of supplies. Air freshener may be needed.

SAMPLE DOCUMENTATION

(date/time) Ostomy appliance removed, skin and stoma cleansed with warm water. Fresh pouch applied with skin prep. Stoma moist, dark red, without bleeding. Peristomal skin without irritation or ulceration. Client denies discomfort. J. House, LPN

particularly worse at night or wheezing. Other symptoms include bad breath, dental erosions, sore throat, hoarseness, weight loss, or difficulty sleeping.

Diagnosis

Historical data should be gathered related to feeding patterns, patterns of gastric distress and vomiting, growth patterns, respiratory symptoms, and stress levels. An upper GI series may be used to rule out other conditions such as pyloric stenosis and hiatal hernia. Esophageal pH monitoring may be used to measure acid reflux.

Treatment

Treatment of gastroesophageal reflex depends on the severity of the disorder. Mild cases may be treated by changing an infant's formula to a hypoallergenic version, adding rice cereal to thicken the feedings, positioning the child upright 30 degrees after feeding, and avoiding acidic juices. The older child should be positioned on the left side for sleep.

Diet changes in the child and adolescent can assist in diminishing symptoms. Spicy foods, high-fat foods, foods containing acid, carbonated drinks, caffeine, and chocolate should be avoided. The teenager should understand that cigarette smoking and alcohol intake can complicate the

course of GERD. Meal size should be reduced and eating and drinking should be avoided 2 to 3 hours prior to bedtime. Drinking water has been proven effective in reducing symptoms as well.

Medications may also be prescribed to reduce stomach acid. Histamine-2 receptor antagonists such as cimetidine (Tagamet) or famotidine (Pepcid) produce relief of symptoms and promote mucosal healing. Proton pump inhibitors such as esomeprazole (Nexium) or omeprazole (Prilosec) suppress acid production. (NASPGHAN, 2001)

Severe cases of gastroesophageal reflux may require surgery such as a *Nissen fundoplication* (which anchors the lower esophageal sphincter below the diaphragm and reinforces the high-pressure area). A gastrostomy tube will be left in place for approximately 6 weeks. Parents will need to be taught to administer gastrostomy feedings and to care for the insertion site.

PYLORIC STENOSIS

Pyloric stenosis is an obstruction of the pyloric canal caused by a thickening of the pyloric sphincter and narrowing of the passageway between the stomach and the duodenum (Figure 17-11 ■). As the stomach tries to push food

Figure 17-11. ■ Pyloric stenosis results in symptoms of projectile vomiting and visible peristalsis.

through the narrowed lumen, the mucous membrane becomes inflamed and swollen, narrowing the lumen further and eventually causing total obstruction.

Manifestations

The disorder occurs most commonly in 5-week-old first-born boys. The infant with pyloric stenosis is usually asymptomatic until 2 to 4 weeks after birth, appearing healthy but possibly regurgitating a small amount of milk after feeding. Parents report the child to be a "good eater." As the pylorus narrows, the infant begins to vomit after every feeding. Within a few weeks, the vomiting becomes projectile, and the emesis may be ejected up to 3 feet from the infant. The infant becomes dehydrated, loses weight, and passes fewer and smaller stools.

A small round mass may be felt in the right upper quadrant, and peristaltic waves may be seen across the abdomen. The infant may appear irritable and uncomfortable, or, if severe dehydration is present, he or she may be lethargic. The infant with pyloric stenosis becomes very ill with dehydration in just a few days. It is important for the parents to obtain medical attention immediately.

Diagnosis

A thorough history assists in the diagnosis of pyloric stenosis. An abdominal ultrasound is most commonly used to diagnose this disorder; x-ray may also be performed. Laboratory data will also reveal dehydration.

Treatment

As soon as the diagnosis is made, plans for urgent surgery are developed. Surgical correction by **pyloroplasty** (procedure in which the pyloric canal is widened) is the treatment of choice. The infant usually recovers rapidly after surgery, with a very positive prognosis, and is usually discharged in a few days.

Nursing Considerations

Nursing care focuses on meeting the infant's needs for fluids and nutrition, promoting comfort, preventing infection, and supporting the parents. Because projectile vomiting will continue until surgery, the infant should be kept NPO. IV therapy will be used to establish fluid and electrolyte balance. By monitoring the infant's intake and output, including emesis and urine specific gravity, the nurse can evaluate the effectiveness of therapy.

Postoperatively, the infant is given small amounts of clear liquid. If clear liquids are tolerated, the infant will be advanced to formula or breastfeeding. To provide for the infant's comfort, acetaminophen or other analgesics are given as prescribed. Parents should be instructed to avoid pressure on the incision. When diapering the infant, slide the diaper under the buttocks instead of lifting the legs. Parents should be encouraged to swaddle, hold, and rock the infant.

In planning for discharge, parents should be taught the signs of incisional infection, including redness, swelling, discharge, and a fever higher than 101 °F (38.5 °C). The infant should not be submerged in bathwater until approved by the physician.

COLIC

Colic, also called paroxysmal abdominal pain, refers to acute abdominal pain caused by spasmodic contractions of the intestines. Colic occurs most commonly during the first 3 months of life. Infants cry loudly, pull their arms and legs up, and become red in the face. They may expel flatus or belch frequently, spitting up mucus and undigested milk or formula. The exact cause of colic is unknown, but contributing factors include swallowing air during feeding, eating too rapidly, overeating, overexcitement, and an anxious mother.

Colic may be relieved by picking the infant up and walking with the infant face down, the body across the parent's arm (this position applies gentle pressure to the stomach), burping (bubbling) gently, and giving some warm water to drink. Rocking and soothing the infant in a calm manner provides reassurance. A change in formula may also be necessary to rule out an allergic reaction. Colic is not serious, and most infants are healthy and continue to gain weight. If pharmacologic intervention becomes necessary, the physician may prescribe sedatives such as phenobarbital; antiflatulents such as simethicone (Mylicon); or antihistamines such as hydroxyzine hydrochloride (Atarax).

Nursing care of the infant with colic is described in the Nursing Care Plan Chart on page 468.

NURSING CARE PLAN CHART

Infant with Colic

GOAL	INTERVENTION	RATIONALE	EXPECTED OUTCOME
1. Acute Pain related to intestinal spasms			
The infant will have relieved pain	Assess the infant's feeding pattern	*Allows the nurse to determine frequency and volume of feeding as well as how often the parents are burping the infant*	The infant will have decreased crying, reduced abdominal distention, and a relaxed body position.
	Assess the infant's symptoms of colic and their duration	*Allows the nurse to determine onset, duration, and characteristics of the infant's cries*	
	Assess what methods the parents are using to comfort their infant	*Allows the nurse to determine effectiveness and ineffectiveness of the parental soothing methods*	
The family will develop methods of effectively dealing with colic	Teach parents to provide rhythmic movement and a variety of positions	*Rhythmic movement such as rocking, infant swings, and car rides soothes the infant's stomach. Positions include swaddling and other positions that apply gentle pressure to the infant's abdomen*	The family provides a variety of techniques that are effective in helping the infant deal with colic.
	Teach parents to reduce environmental stimuli and provide tactile stimuli	*Environmental stimuli can distract the infant as well as soothe him. Environmental stimuli include music, dim lights, warm temperatures. Tactile stimuli elicit the gate-control method of pain management and include sucking on a pacifier, a warm bath, and a gentle abdominal massage*	
2. Risk for Impaired Parent/Infant Attachment related to frequent fussy periods and resulting parental fatigue			
The family will demonstrate confidence in their soothing abilities	Assess the parents' feelings regarding the infant's colic	*Allows the nurse to plan care properly to help parents deal with negative feelings*	The family demonstrates confidence when using a variety of soothing methods.
	Assess the parents' level of fatigue	*Allows the nurse to determine number of hours of sleep parents are receiving*	
	Assess the parents' level of support	*Allows the nurse to determine whether the family has enough support to obtain adequate rest and properly care for the infant*	
The family will demonstrate attachment behaviors	Help the parents understand the pathophysiology of colic	*This helps parents understand that they are not responsible for the infant's colic*	The family and infant gaze at one another and the family responds appropriately to the infant's needs.
	Teach the parents how to interact positively with their infant when the infant is not exhibiting colic behaviors	*Between periods of colic behaviors is an important time for parent and infant to bond*	

INTUSSUSCEPTION

Intussusception is one of several causes of mechanical obstruction of the small bowel (Figure 17-12 ■) seen in children. It occurs when one portion of the intestine telescopes into another portion. The most common site for intussusception is the ileocecal valve. As telescoping occurs, the walls of the intestine rub together, producing inflammation, swelling, and obstruction. Swelling causes a decrease in

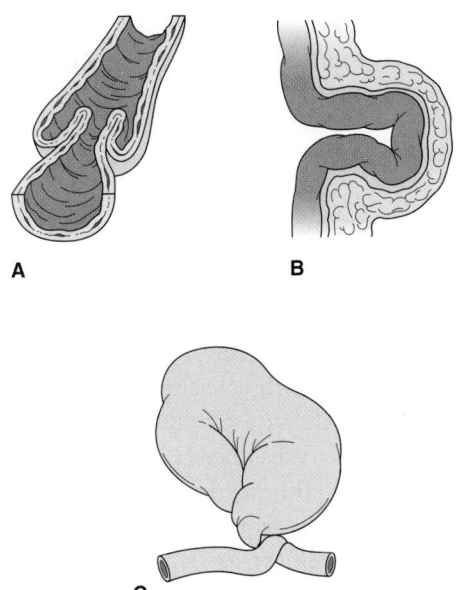

Figure 17-12. ■ Selective causes of mechanical obstruction.
(A) Intussusception. **(B)** Incarcerated hernia. **(C)** Volvulus.

blood flow to the intestine, resulting in ischemia, necrosis, perforation, and hemorrhage. Intussusception is one of the most common causes of intestinal obstruction in children. It occurs more frequently in boys between the ages of 2 months and 5 years than in other groups.

Manifestations

The child with intussusception presents with sudden severe abdominal pain, vomiting, and passage of brown stool. Periods of comfort may be followed by a recurrence of pain. As the condition worsens, the stool resembles currant jelly. A palpable abdominal mass may be felt.

Diagnosis and Treatment

Diagnosis is made from the history and barium enema studies. In some cases the installation of barium moves the intestine back into place. If this does not occur, surgery will be required to reduce the telescoping bowel and remove damaged tissue.

Nursing Considerations

Nursing care focuses on pain management, maintaining fluid balance and nutrition, and supporting parents. The child will be kept NPO and may have a nasogastric tube to suction until the bowel is returned to its normal location. Postoperative care is routine, including administration of IV fluids, analgesics, and assessments. After normal bowel function returns, the child is offered clear liquids and is advanced to full feedings as tolerated.

Parents should be taught to care for the child at home, including watching for infection and administering prescribed medication. Surgery is usually successful in cor-

recting the problem, but parents should be encouraged to seek medical attention if symptoms recur, if the child develops a fever, or if appetite decreases.

MECKEL'S DIVERTICULUM

Meckel's diverticulum occurs when the connection between the yolk sac and the intestine in the embryo fails to atrophy. The result is a **diverticulum** (an outpouching) in the ileum, usually near the ileocecal valve. The pouch contains gastric or pancreatic tissue that secretes acid and enzymes, causing irritation and ulceration.

Manifestations

Symptoms appear by 2 years of age. Painless bleeding, manifesting as either dark stools or bright red bleeding, occurs as a result of ulceration and obstruction. Abdominal pain is unusual, but when it occurs, it has a sudden onset and may resemble appendicitis, **volvulus** (twisted bowel; see Figure 17-12C), or intussusception.

Diagnosis and Treatment

Diagnosis is usually based on history because the diverticulum is small and does not fill with contrast medium. If untreated, perforation and peritonitis could result. Treatment involves surgical removal of the diverticulum and any damaged tissue. Once healing occurs, prognosis is good.

HIRSCHSPRUNG'S DISEASE

Hirschsprung's disease (also called **megacolon**) is a condition in which the autonomic parasympathetic ganglia that normally cause peristalsis in the intestine are absent. The resulting inadequate motility causes mechanical bowel obstruction of the large intestine. Hirschsprung's disease is more common in boys and often occurs with congenital heart defects, Down syndrome, and other neurologic syndromes.

Manifestations

Symptoms vary depending on the extent of the defect and the age of the child. In newborns, the first symptom may be failure to pass meconium, refusal to suck, abdominal distention, and meconium emesis. Older children may have a history of abdominal distention and constipation alternating with diarrhea.

clinical ALERT

Because newborns are frequently discharged from the hospital within 24 hours of birth, parents must be instructed to observe for meconium passage, abdominal distention, and vomiting. If the newborn fails to pass stool or the abdomen becomes distended, parents should contact the primary care provider.

Diagnosis and Treatment

Diagnosis is made by history, radiographic contrast studies, and biopsy. In mild cases, treatment includes high-fiber diet, adequate fluids, stool softeners, and isotonic enemas. More severe cases require surgery to remove the affected bowel. At times, a colostomy is performed. If a small portion of the bowel is affected, the colostomy may be reversed, and **reanastomosis** (reconnection) may be performed at a later date. If large areas of the bowel are affected, the colostomy may be permanent.

Nursing Considerations

Nursing care includes careful observation of the newborn for the passage of meconium. When the diagnosis is made later in infancy or childhood, a careful history of growth patterns, nutritional intake, and bowel habits must be obtained. Parents will need instruction on administering medication, giving saline enemas, and managing a colostomy, including proper drainage, skin care, and changing bags. Parents must be taught to watch for malabsorption of nutrients, including poor growth and malnutrition. Referral to an enterostomal nurse specialist and ostomy support groups may be helpful.

Malabsorption and Inborn Metabolic Disorders

Malabsorption disorders result from lack of nutrients in the diet, an inability of the small intestine to absorb nutrients, or liver disorders that result in lack of bile for digestion and alter metabolism of nutrients. Metabolic disorders are disorders in which the normal metabolic process is disrupted.

CELIAC DISEASE

Celiac disease (*gluten-sensitive enteropathy* or *sprue*) is a chronic malabsorption syndrome in which the child is unable to digest gluten, a protein found in wheat, barley, rye, and oats. The inability to digest gluten results in an increase in the amino acid glutamine, which is toxic to the mucous membrane in the small intestine. Over time, the intestinal villi are damaged. Initially, fat absorption is affected, resulting in **steatorrhea** (fat in the stool). Absorption of protein, carbohydrates, calcium, iron, and fat-soluble vitamins is affected. Research is being conducted to determine the existence of a genetic influence in the child developing celiac disease.

Manifestations

Symptoms do not begin until the child has ingested solid foods containing gluten, usually in the first 2 years of life. When gluten is introduced into the diet, the child experiences chronic diarrhea, vomiting, and failure to grow. The stools are large, foul-smelling, greasy, and frothy.

Diagnosis

Diagnosis is based on symptoms, fat content in the stool, and intestinal biopsy.

Treatment

The child improves rapidly when gluten is eliminated from the diet. Vitamin supplements may be prescribed if the child is malnourished. Growth patterns usually return to normal within a year.

Nursing Considerations

The family of a child with celiac disease must establish a plan for lifelong avoidance of gluten-containing foods. When any such serious disorder is identified, parents will need time to adjust to the diagnosis and to incorporate new information and lifestyle requirements. The nurse provides emotional support for this transition, as well as information and referrals. A nutritionist or celiac support group can assist the family in developing a variety of recipes focusing on viable foods (e.g., fruits, vegetables, meat, rice).

Teach parents that the child with celiac disease will need to avoid gluten (wheat, rye, barley) completely and for life. Parents must not reintroduce these foods once symptoms disappear. Reintroduction of gluten puts the child at risk for growth retardation and development of gastrointestinal cancer as an adult. Also, teach parents to read labels carefully for "hidden" sources of gluten. Some examples of unexpected gluten-containing foods are:

- Mayonnaise
- Many types of vinegar
- Catsup
- Canned soup

Diet will need to be reviewed and reinforced as the child grows (Box 17-3 ■). This is especially true for adolescence, when peer group pressure may cause the child to want to abandon the required diet in order to "fit in."

| BOX 17-3 | LIFE SPAN CONSIDERATIONS |

Children with Malabsorption or Inborn Metabolic Disorders

Children with malabsorption or inborn metabolic disorders must learn to avoid certain foods in order to live a healthy life. For the infant and toddler, parents are able to make these food choices and monitor their child's intake. The school-age child and adolescent must be involved in these food choices because they will be in many situations where parents are not present. The nurse can play an important role in helping these older children to understand the risks associated with ingesting the wrong nutrients. A dietitian may be effective in assisting the child in understanding which foods contain which nutrients.

LACTOSE INTOLERANCE

Lactose intolerance is a congenital or acquired disorder in which the child fails to produce lactase, an enzyme needed in the digestion of lactose. Lactose or milk sugar is found in milk and milk products. The child rapidly develops gastric distress including diarrhea as soon as milk is consumed.

Implementing a lactose-free diet relieves the symptoms. In the newborn, soy formulas are used instead of breastfeeding or milk-based formula. In the older child, eliminating milk and milk products from the diet is necessary. Soy substitutes may be used in place of milk, cheese, and yogurt. In some children, adding enzyme tablets such as LactAid to the milk or sprinkling powdered enzyme on food corrects the problem.

KWASHIORKOR

Kwashiorkor is a deficiency in protein in the diet that results in muscle wasting. It is most common in underdeveloped countries, where malnutrition is common. Frequently, the protein deficiency occurs even when the diet is nearly adequate in calories.

Manifestations

Symptoms may develop after the child has been weaned from breast milk. Because of the lack of protein in the diet, the child fails to grow, muscles waste, and the abdomen is protuberant. Anorexia, diarrhea, and vomiting may occur. The hair becomes thin, brittle, and lightens in color because of the lack of melanin. Skin breaks down and becomes infected. The child is irritable at first and then becomes mentally dull. Figure 17-13 ■ shows the multisystem effects of malnutrition.

Diagnosis

Physical examination of the child with kwashiorkor reveals hepatomegaly and generalized edema. Decreased renal function is evidenced by urinalysis and chemistry profile.

Treatment

Treatment is mainly preventive. Although kwashiorkor may never be totally eradicated worldwide, many organizations are working to supply sufficient quantities of protein in the diet to prevent starvation. Powdered protein, sprinkled on the culturally prepared food, can relieve the problem. In established cases of kwashiorkor, the addition of protein to the diet may prevent more serious growth retardation but may not correct the existing damage.

PHENYLKETONURIA

Phenylketonuria (PKU) is an autosomal recessive inherited disorder that affects the body's ability to use protein.

Normally, a liver enzyme, phenylalanine hydroxylase, breaks down the amino acid phenylalanine into tyrosine. Children with PKU have a deficiency in this enzyme.

Manifestations

As phenylalanine builds up in the blood, it causes a musty odor of the body and urine, as well as vomiting, irritability, seizures, hyperactivity, and rash. Over time, elevated levels of phenylalanine result in mental retardation.

Diagnosis

A screening test, required by law in all 50 states, determines the presence of an autosomal recessive disorder of amino acid metabolism in which the individual is unable to breakdown phenylalanine (Box 17-4 ■). In order to meet the legal requirements, facilities obtain the blood sample prior to discharge. For the results of the screening to be most accurate, the test must be done after the baby has received milk (either breast milk or formula). It may take 48 to 72 hours (or more) for the newborn to have an adequate consumption of milk. For this reason, the PKU test may need to be repeated in 1 to 2 weeks. The blood sample is obtained by heel stick. The blood is placed on a PKU specimen card and sent to the laboratory for analysis.

Treatment

Special formulas, such as albuamid XP, lofenalac, and minafen, are used in treatment until the child is ready for solid food. Then a diet low in phenylalanine is maintained for life. The diet must also meet the child's requirements for growth. The phenylalanine diet would be low in meat, milk products, and aspartame. Modified protein in which phenylalanine has been removed can be used. If diet modifications are not followed for at least the first 6 years, there will be a significant impact on the child's IQ. The modified diet must be followed for life. If adults fail to follow the diet, their IQ will remain the same, but they will have difficulty focusing on tasks and processing thoughts rapidly. Because this is a disorder that requires lifelong changes in diet, nursing considerations are similar to those for celiac disease.

BOX 17-4	CULTURAL PULSE POINTS

Phenylketonuria

PKU is more common in communities with numerous inter-marriages over several generations. It is rare in African, Jewish, and Japanese populations.

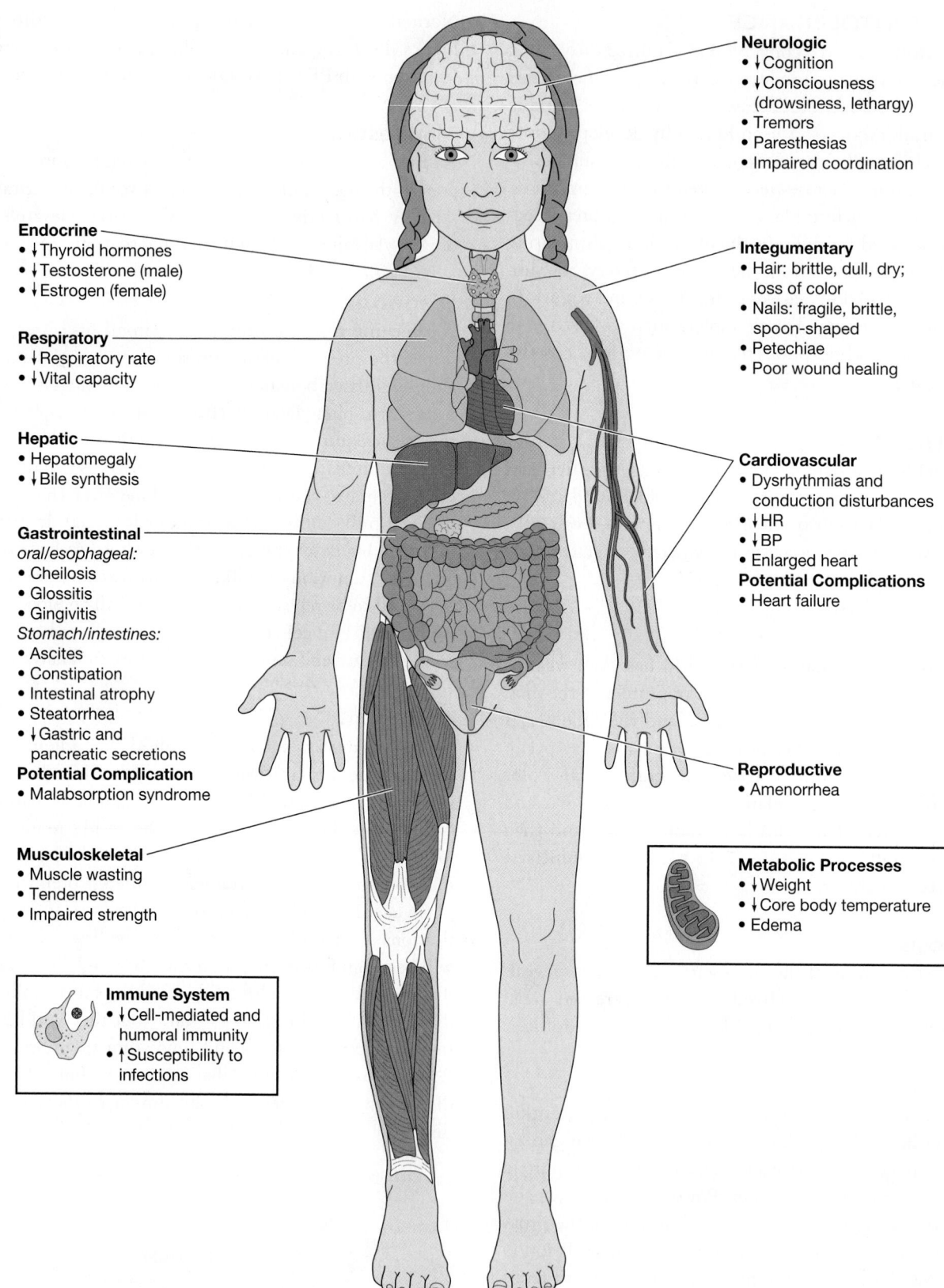

Neurologic
- ↓Cognition
- ↓Consciousness
  (drowsiness, lethargy)
- Tremors
- Paresthesias
- Impaired coordination

Endocrine
- ↓Thyroid hormones
- ↓Testosterone (male)
- ↓Estrogen (female)

Respiratory
- ↓Respiratory rate
- ↓Vital capacity

Hepatic
- Hepatomegaly
- ↓Bile synthesis

Gastrointestinal
oral/esophageal:
- Cheilosis
- Glossitis
- Gingivitis
Stomach/intestines:
- Ascites
- Constipation
- Intestinal atrophy
- Steatorrhea
- ↓Gastric and
  pancreatic secretions
Potential Complication
- Malabsorption syndrome

Musculoskeletal
- Muscle wasting
- Tenderness
- Impaired strength

Integumentary
- Hair: brittle, dull, dry;
  loss of color
- Nails: fragile, brittle,
  spoon-shaped
- Petechiae
- Poor wound healing

Cardiovascular
- Dysrhythmias and
  conduction disturbances
- ↓HR
- ↓BP
- Enlarged heart
Potential Complications
- Heart failure

Reproductive
- Amenorrhea

Metabolic Processes
- ↓Weight
- ↓Core body temperature
- Edema

Immune System
- ↓Cell-mediated and
  humoral immunity
- ↑Susceptibility to
  infections

Figure 17-13. ■ Multisystem effects of malnutrition.

Nutrition Disorders

RICKETS

Rickets is a condition caused by a vitamin D deficiency. Vitamin D is necessary for the proper absorption and utilization of calcium and phosphorus. When deficiency exists, the result is failure of the bones to develop. The child may manifest bow legs, knock-knees, beading along the ribs (*rachitic rosary*), and improper formation of teeth.

The widespread use of vitamins and fortified foods has nearly eliminated rickets in North America. However, parents should be encouraged to provide well-balanced meals and exercise in the sunlight (because the skin synthesizes vitamin D when exposed to the sun).

SCURVY

Scurvy is caused by a lack of vitamin C in the diet. Vitamin C is a water-soluble vitamin that is destroyed by heat. Because vitamin C is not stored in the body, daily intake is required. The main sources of vitamin C in the diet are citrus fruits and raw leafy vegetables. Vegetables should be cooked in small amounts of water at low heat to prevent destruction of vitamin C. Vitamin C tablets may be used to supplement the diet.

FAILURE TO THRIVE

Failure to thrive (FTT) is a general term used to describe the child who fails to gain weight or loses weight for unknown reasons. Causes can be physical (e.g., malabsorption, heart or liver disorders) or environmental (e.g., failure to bond with parents or neglect by caregivers). Nonorganic failure to thrive (NOFTT) is also discussed in Chapter 16 ⚭.

The FTT child may be irritable and weak. He or she may have vomiting, diarrhea, anorexia, or **pica** (ingestion of nonfood material). The child may appear apathetic, listless, and exhibit "rag doll" limpness.

The child may be admitted to the hospital for evaluation. Malabsorption and heart and liver disorders can be identified and treated with good success. When FTT is the result of environmental factors, the nurse must be alert in observing child-parent interaction to identify any areas of concern in the relationship. These situations are complex and may take time to identify the cause. If there are concerns about the child-parent relationship, a multidisciplinary approach involving the physician, nurses, social workers, counselors, and family agencies may be needed. If improvement cannot be demonstrated, the child may be placed in foster care. In the hospital environment, one nurse is selected to provide the nurturing and interaction that may be lacking at home.

The prognosis is questionable. It has been documented that children who have been starved emotionally can have lifelong problems involving language, social interactions, and intelligence. The importance of bonding is discussed in Box 15-1 ⚭.

OVEREATING AND OBESITY

Obesity may be an associated manifestation of psychological disorders. Obesity in children affects 11% to 16% of American children (*Healthy People 2010*) and is considered by some to have reached epidemic proportions. Hispanics and Mexican Americans have higher rates of obesity than other ethnic groups. **Obesity** is defined as excessive weight and accumulation of body fat. Obesity is considered a BMI greater than or equal to the 95th percentile. Many children have learned a pattern of overeating from their families and appear well adjusted. Although the intake of "junk food" makes them feel good, the increased weight contributes to a poor body image, depression, and low self-esteem. Many children use overeating to compensate for insecurities, low self-esteem, poor body image, lack of parental attention, or feelings of stress, anxiety, and depression. The sedentary lifestyle of many children increases the risk of obesity. Watching television and playing video games instead of exercising greatly increases a child's risk of obesity.

A referral to a nutritionist may be appropriate to teach the child to make healthy food choices. If obesity is not corrected during adolescence, diabetes, orthopedic problems, and cardiovascular complications could develop in later years.

An extreme option for the severely obese adolescent is **bariatric surgery** (surgery to reduce stomach size). Strict criteria are required to even consider this life-altering option. The teen must have tried weight management techniques for longer than 6 months and failed. Clients must be physiologically mature and agree to psychological evaluations both before and after surgery. Psychiatric issues must be resolved or successfully managed prior to surgery. Female clients considering bariatric surgery must agree to avoid pregnancy for more than 1 year postoperatively. A supportive family is also required.

Nurses may not see the obese child until conditions related to obesity cause them to seek health care. Accurate weight and height are necessary. The nurse must carefully measure the child's blood pressure. Obtaining serum cholesterol, triglycerides, glucose, and hemoglobin A1c will assist in determining the presence of complications related to obesity. The nurse should focus on helping the family to meet the child's nutritional needs, managing related health conditions, and promoting self-esteem. The nurse can encourage exercise and activity programs that will not embarrass the child.

Intestinal Parasites

Intestinal parasites occur most frequently in tropical regions but can occur in any area of the United States. Typically, outbreaks occur in areas where water is not treated, poor sanitation exists, or food is not properly cooked. However, children are also exposed to larvae or eggs from playing in contaminated dirt at playgrounds and in sandboxes. Infected children playing in wet or dirty diapers can transfer eggs or larvae to the soil, where others can become infected. The most common intestinal parasites are included in Table 17-3 ■.

Manifestations

Symptoms of intestinal parasites include abdominal cramps, diarrhea, and weight loss. Some parasites lay eggs at the anal opening, resulting in anal irritation and itching. Severe infections may result in intestinal obstruction and liver and lung involvement.

Diagnosis and Treatment

The organism is identified by laboratory examination of stool specimen. Treatment involves administration of prescribed medication. See Table 17-3 for medications commonly prescribed for specific parasites. Generally, all family members and others in direct contact with the infected child should be treated. Follow-up stool examination is necessary to ensure cure. Repeat medication regimen may be required. Prevention includes frequent hand washing, covering sandboxes when not in use, and frequent diaper changes with perineal care for infected children.

TABLE 17-3

Common Intestinal Parasites

PARASITE	TRANSMISSION	SYMPTOMS	TREATMENT
Giardiasis Organism: protozoan *Giardia lamblia*	Person to person, unfiltered water, infected food, animals. Organisms enter through mouth, feed in the duodenum and jejunum, and are excreted in stool.	Abdominal cramps; foul-smelling, loose, or watery stool containing gelatinous material.	Medication: furazolidone (has fewer side effects but is more expensive), quinacrine.
Pinworms Organism: nematode *Enterobius vermicularis*	Discharged eggs inhaled or hand to mouth. Eggs hatch in intestine in 15–28 days; larvae migrate to cecum. After mating, mature female leaves out the anus. Can move to vagina and urethra.	Worm movement causes intense itching, especially at night when female leaves anus.	Medication: mebendazole, pyrantel, pamoate, piperazine citrate. Repeat treatment in 2–3 weeks. All family members should be treated.
Roundworms (Ascariasis) Organism: nematode *Ascaris lumbricoides*	Eggs carried hand to mouth. Eggs hatch in small intestine. Larvae can penetrate intestinal villi, enter portal circulation and liver. Some ascend to upper respiratory tract, are swallowed, move to small intestine, and cycle repeats. Some eggs are excreted in stool.	Severe infection results in intestinal obstruction, peritonitis, jaundice, and lung involvement.	Medication: mebendazole, pyrantel, pamoate, piperazine citrate. Check stools in 2 weeks and monthly for 3 months. Intestinal obstruction may require surgery. All family members should be treated.
Hookworms Organism: nematode *Necator americanus*	Direct contact with infected soil. Larvae attach to and penetrate skin. Travel in blood to lungs, move in sputum to throat and are swallowed. Worms live in small intestine, feed on villi, causing bleeding. Eggs excreted in stool, hatch in damp shaded soil.	Severe infection results in anemia and malnutrition. Larvae on skin may cause irritation, burning, and itching.	Medication: mebendazole, pyrantel pamoate. Examine stool in 2 weeks and monthly for 3 months. All family members should be treated.
Visceral larva migrans (Toxocariasis) Organism: nematode *Toxocara canis* or *Toxocara catis* (commonly found in dogs and cats)	Ingestion of eggs from soil. Hatch in intestine. Mobile larva migrate to liver and eventually all organs, including brain. They encapsulate in dense fibrous tissue.	Low-grade fever, recurrent upper airway disease, hepatomegaly, pulmonary infiltration, neurologic problems. Hypereosinophili in blood.	None specific. Infection usually resolves spontaneously. Deworm household pets. Keep away from animal droppings.

Poisonings

Poisoning, the ingestion of a toxic substance, is a common cause of injury or death in children between 1 and 4 years of age. Recall from Chapter 5 ⚭ that the developmental task of children in this age group is to explore their environment. Young children frequently put objects and fluid into their mouths, potentially resulting in poisoning (Table 17-4 ■). The Poison Prevention Packaging Act of 1970 mandates child-protective devices for all potentially toxic substances such as household cleansers and medication. However, some adults find these protective lids difficult to remove and will not tighten them or will leave the lid off. Other substances found in the home are potentially hazardous and are not regulated by law. For example, many household plants, including Boston ivy, poinsettia, philodendron, lily-of-the-valley, daffodil, azalea, and rhododendron, are toxic if ingested. Cosmetics; nail care products; weed, bug, and rodent killers; paints; and furniture polish are also highly toxic.

Most poisonings occur in the home. Parents who suspect a child has ingested a poisonous substance should call the local poison control center (PCC) immediately. The PCC can ask the parents questions about the substance, advise the parents about treatment to begin at home, and direct the parents on the need for emergency treatment. The possibility of intentional ingestion should be considered with older children. If the child vomits, the emesis should be brought to the emergency department.

Emergency treatment for poisoning is based on the goal of preventing further absorption of the poison and reversing its effects.

clinical ALERT

The priorities of treatment for a child with poisoning can be recalled with the mnemonic SIRES:

- **S**tabilize the child's condition.
- **I**dentify the toxic substance.
- **R**everse its effects.
- **E**liminate the substance from the child's body.
- **S**upport the child (and parents) physically and psychologically.

When the child arrives in the emergency department, the airway, breathing, and circulation must be monitored continuously and cardiopulmonary resuscitation (CPR) performed if needed. An IV line should be established and blood drawn for toxicology. Parents, family, and child (if applicable) should be questioned about the events leading up to the poisoning. The type of poison, the amount of

TABLE 17-4

Poisons

TYPE OF POISON	SOURCES	CLINICAL MANIFESTATION	TREATMENT	PREVENTION
Corrosives: acids and alkaline	Cleansers: toilet cleaner, drain cleaners, bleach Batteries	Burns around mouth, throat, and stomach; respiratory obstruction; drooling; pain	Do NOT induce vomiting, dilute with water, give activated charcoal	Keep cleansers and batteries out of reach of children. Keep lids tightly closed.
Hydrocarbons: distillates of petroleum	Gasoline, kerosene, furniture polish, paint thinners, oils	Coughing, vomiting, respiratory distress, lethargy	Do NOT induce vomiting, provide gastric lavage, supportive care, decontaminate skin	Keep gasoline products out of reach of children. Do NOT store in other containers. Keep lids tightly closed.
Salicylates: aspirin	Products containing aspirin	Nausea/vomiting, tinnitus, bleeding, convulsions, death	If alert, induce vomiting, IV sodium bicarbonate, vitamin K	Keep in locked medicine cabinet. Keep lid tightly closed.
Acetaminophen	Many over-the-counter products, in combination with narcotics	Nausea/vomiting, pallor, hepatic involvement	Induce vomiting/gastric lavage; give charcoal, or Mucomyst	Keep in locked medicine cabinet; tell children drug is NOT candy.
Heavy metals: mercury, lead	Paints, pesticides, water from lead pipes, broken thermometers	Tremors, memory loss, cognitive defects	Remove causative agent, provide chelation therapy (see text)	Remove potential causes from environment. Use digital thermometers.

chemical, the amount of time the child was unsupervised, allergies, and preexisting disorders should be determined.

The process of reversal or elimination of the substance from the child's body depends on the specific agent ingested. See Table 17-5 ■ for methods commonly used to reverse the effect of poisons. Syrup of ipecac is no longer recommended because it can be harmful in some situations and may not remove all poison. Activated charcoal binds with poisonous chemicals to slow or prevent absorption.

Once the emergency phase of treatment is over, the child and parents will need continued physical and emotional support. Depending on the degree of damage from the toxic agent, the child may recover without deficit, or he or she may have life-changing deficits of gastrointestinal, neurologic, cardiovascular, hepatic, and renal functions. The age and development of the child will guide the amount of emotional support that will be needed. Parents, however,

will need emotional support to deal with feelings of guilt, blame, and shame. Conflict between parents might occur. If a babysitter or other care provider is involved, additional emotional stress will be placed on the family. In some instances, child protective services may be called and the child placed in protective custody while the situation is under investigation.

LEAD POISONING

Lead poisoning (toxic levels of lead in the blood) is decreasing in the United States but remains a concern in many poor families living in older housing in inner cities or rural areas. The main sources are from lead-based paint; drinking water flowing through lead pipes, lead holding tanks, or pipes and tanks soldered with lead; food grown in lead-contaminated dirt; and airborne lead from smelters and battery manufacturing plants.

Children are at greater risk for toxic levels because they absorb and retain more lead in proportion to body weight than adults. Children younger than 7 years are particularly at risk. Young children often chew on crib rails, pencils, or other painted surfaces when teething. They ingest small quantities of paint that over time can build to toxic levels. Lead interferes with normal cell function, particularly nervous system, blood cells, kidneys, and vitamin D and calcium metabolism. Once in the body, lead is deposited in bones and teeth. It is slowly released from the bones. Even when the source is removed, toxic levels can take time to be resolved.

Manifestations

Symptoms include cognitive deficit, learning disabilities, hearing impairment, and growth delays. Lead ingestion by pregnant women can cause fetal malformation, low birth weight, and premature birth.

Diagnosis and Treatment

A blood test (Pb-B) is the most useful tool in the screening, diagnosis, and monitoring of lead poisoning. Treatment is with **chelation therapy,** the administration of a chemical that will bind to the lead and increase the rate of excretion. Calcium disodium ethylenediamine tetraacetate (CaNa$_2$EDTA), dimercaprol (BAL), *d*-penicillamine, or succimer (DMSA) may be used alone or in combination for several days followed by a rest period and then repeated. Before the child is discharged, a lead-free environment must be ensured.

Nursing Considerations

Nursing implications include community teaching regarding lead poison risks, environmental assessment, and screening individuals at risk. The school nurse should suspect lead poisoning in children with learning

TABLE 17-5

Methods to Treat Poisoning

TYPE OF TREATMENT	PROCESS OR AGENT
Gastric lavage	■ Insert largest gastric tube possible through mouth. ■ Instill and aspirate normal saline until returns clear. ■ Less effective than vomiting, used for neurologically depressed, diminished gag reflex, or uncooperative children. ■ Use in acid ingestion to prevent continued damage. ■ Contraindicated in alkaline ingestion because of possible damage to esophagus.
Activated charcoal	■ Assess level of consciousness before giving orally. ■ Can be given by gastric tube. ■ Give in opaque cup with a lid and straw so child cannot see black liquid. ■ Give after vomiting stops; aspiration of charcoal can damage lung.
Cathartics	■ Increases elimination of toxic substance and minimize absorption.
Antidote and antagonist	■ There are only a few agents. ■ Narcan is common for opiate ingestion.
Other (depending on child's condition)	■ Diuretics ■ Fluids ■ Anticonvulsants ■ Hemodialysis ■ Antiarrhythmics ■ Exchange transfusion

BOX 17-5   CULTURAL PULSE POINTS

Use of Lead in Traditional Medicines or Cosmetics

Some traditional medicines and cosmetics contain large amounts of lead. Mexican Americans use azarcon and greta to treat empacho (a colic-like illness). Asian communities use chifong, tokuwan, pay-loo-ah, ghasard, bali goli, and kandu. Middle Eastern communities use alkohl, kohl, surma, saoot, and cebagin.

disabilities and children with growth delays. Nurses must teach the parents about individual risk, administration of chelation therapy, and the need to avoid all sources of lead. This teaching may find resistance in some cultures (Box 17-5 ■).

Hepatic Disorders

The liver is one of the most vital organs (see Figure 17-1). It is important to remember that the liver stores blood; produces blood clotting factors; stores proteins, fats, glucose, iron, and vitamins; and detoxifies drugs, hormones, and other substances. Two common liver disorders, biliary atresia and hepatits, are addressed in this chapter.

BILIARY ATRESIA

Biliary atresia occurs when the bile ducts outside the liver fail to form properly or become closed. As a result, bile backs up, destroying the liver and often requiring a liver transplant.

Manifestations

Initially, the baby appears healthy until jaundice develops in the 2nd or 3rd week of life. Elevated bilirubin levels are accompanied by abdominal distention and **hepatomegaly** (enlarged liver). The infant is easily bruised, has prolonged bleeding time, and experiences **pruritis** (itching). Within a short time, **splenomegaly** (enlarged spleen) develops. Because of the absence of bile, the stools become off-white or clay colored and are the consistency of putty. Bilirubin is excreted by the kidneys and turns the urine tea colored. Without bile, the infant is unable to digest fat and absorb the fat-soluble vitamins A, D, E, and K. The infant becomes malnourished and weak. Without a liver transplant, the infant dies.

Diagnosis

Early diagnosis is critical in the medical treatment of biliary atresia. Laboratory tests show elevated bilirubin, serum aminotransferase, and alkaline phosphatase and ammonia levels. Prothrombin time will be prolonged. Ultrasound will rule out other causes of illness.

Treatment

Surgery (*hepatoportoenterostomy* or *Kasai procedure*) may be done to connect the duodenum to the hepatic portal segment of bile duct inside the liver. This surgical procedure is done as a palliative measure to delay liver transplant. Advances in transplant procedures make it possible to perform partial liver transplantation. Because live donors can be used, transplant can be done when the baby is in optimum health instead of waiting for an appropriate-size cadaver liver. Close family members are often good tissue matches.

Nursing Considerations

When the serious nature of the disease becomes evident, parents will need increased emotional support and teaching. As the disease progresses, the baby will become irritable because of the intense itching and accumulation of toxins. Tepid baths may help relieve itching temporarily. Drying the skin by rubbing stimulates vasodilatation, which intensifies itching. Therefore, the skin should be patted dry.

Care following surgery for either hepatoportoenterostomy or transplant is the same as any other abdominal surgery. Parents must be taught to care for the incision and administer pain medication during the healing process. When liver transplant has been performed, parents must be taught to administer immunosuppressant medication and to recognize the actions and side effects of specific medication. Parents will need to be observant for signs of tissue rejection (nausea, vomiting, fever, and jaundice) and report them immediately to the primary care provider. See Chapter 22 ⬡ for more information about organ transplantation.

HEPATITIS

Hepatitis is inflammation of the liver caused by a viral infection. The most common infections in the United States are from hepatitis A virus (HAV), hepatitis B virus (HBV), hepatitis C virus (HCV), and hepatitis D virus (HDV). Hepatitis E virus (HEV) is more common in unclean water in developing countries. Table 17-6 ■ compares the common causes of hepatitis.

clinical ALERT

Nurses and other health care workers could come in contact with blood or body fluids containing hepatitis virus. Standard precautions should be used at all times. It is recommended that health care workers receive three doses of hepatitis B immunization.

TABLE 17-6

Common Causes of Hepatitis

ORGANISM	MODE OF TRANSMISSION	INCUBATION	CLINICAL MANIFESTATION	IMMUNIZATION AVAILABLE
Hepatitis A virus	Fecal-oral route, person to person, contaminated water or food (shellfish)	4 weeks (10–50 days)	Acute onset (may be less acute in young children). Children usually do not become jaundiced. Flulike symptoms.	Immune serum globulin Hepatitis A vaccine
Hepatitis B virus (HBV)	Blood and body fluids	1–6 months	Nausea, vomiting, anorexia, fatigue, upper right quadrant pain, hepatomegaly.	Hepatitis B immune globulin Hepatitis B vaccine
Hepatitis C virus	Blood and blood products	6–7 weeks	Frequent episodes of flulike symptoms without jaundice. Risk of liver cancer.	None
Hepatitis D virus	Blood and blood products Found with HBV infection	2–8 weeks	Same as HBV. Causes fulminating hepatitis.	Hepatitis B vaccine
Hepatitis E virus	Fecal-oral route from water in developing countries	2–9 weeks	Severe flulike symptoms. High mortality in pregnancy and fetal loss.	None

Hepatitis A, commonly called *infectious hepatitis*, is highly contagious. Because it is transmitted primarily by the fecal-oral route during the early stages of the illness, large numbers of people can become exposed. The HAV lives on surfaces for up to 1 month, so diaper changing tables should be cleansed frequently. Children often become infected from day care workers who change diapers and then prepare food. Although HAV is mild in most people, in those individuals with preexisting liver disease, HAV infection could cause liver failure and death.

Hepatitis B, commonly called *serum hepatitis*, is a serious illness. Transmission of HBV occurs through blood and body fluids exchange, including sexual contact, sharing IV needles, and from mother to fetus. Those individuals testing positive for HBV should also be tested for HDV.

Hepatitis C is transmitted through blood and blood products. Children requiring repeat blood transfusions such as for treatment of sickle cell disease or hemophilia are at risk for developing HVC. IV drug use, body piercing, and multiple sexual partners also increase the risk.

Hepatitis D is found in conjunction with HBV. When signs of liver failure are more acute than would be expected in an individual with HBV, HDV infection should be suspected. Children with HBV coupled with HDV are at extreme risk for developing **fulminating hepatitis** (progressive, total destruction of the liver). These children die within 2 weeks unless a liver transplant is completed.

Hepatitis E is transmitted in contaminated water in developing countries. Most commonly, outbreaks of HEV occur shortly after a heavy rain when groundwater becomes contaminated with runoff from outdoor septic systems.

The body's response to the hepatitis virus is the same. At first, the virus attacks the **parenchymal** cells (functional part of an organ), resulting in local degeneration and necrosis of the tissue (Figure 17-14 ■). This stimulates the inflammatory process. Swelling and an accumulation of white blood cells block the drainage of bile. The backup of bile further damages the liver tissue, resulting in an elevation in bilirubin, and ALT and alkaline phosphatase in the blood. The liver fails to produce enough albumins, resulting in generalized edema. In most cases, the body's immune system is able to destroy the hepatitis virus, stopping the liver destruction. Regeneration of liver tissue occurs in approximately 3 months. Serology studies would show positive for antibodies to one or more of the hepatitis viruses. For children with a preexisting liver disorder or an impaired immune system, continued liver destruction could result in death.

clinical ALERT

When hepatitis is present, the liver is unable to detoxify and metabolize drugs at the usual rate. Medications should be administered carefully and the child monitored closely for both side effects and toxic effects.

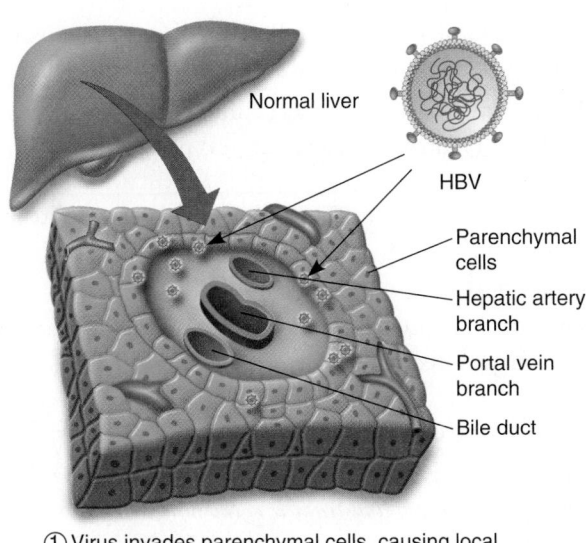

① Virus invades parenchymal cells, causing local degeneration and necrosis

Normal liver

HBV

Parenchymal cells

Hepatic artery branch

Portal vein branch

Bile duct

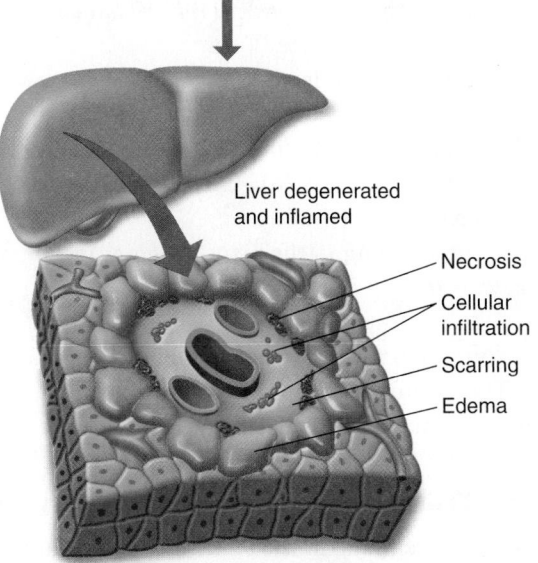

Liver degenerated and inflamed

Necrosis

Cellular infiltration

Scarring

Edema

② Infiltration by lymphocytes, macrophages, and other white blood cells causes inflammation that blocks drainage

③ Structural changes occur in parenchymal cells, resulting in altered liver function:

Impaired bile excretion

Elevated ALT and alkaline phosphatase levels

Decreased albumin synthesis

Figure 17-14. ■ Pathophysiology of hepatitis. The hepatitis virus causes degeneration and necrosis of the liver, which results in abnormal liver function and illness.

For more information about the transmission, clinical manifestations, diagnostic tests, medical treatment and nursing considerations related to hepatitis A and B, see Table 10-6 ∞.

NURSING CARE

PRIORITIES IN NURSING CARE

Priorities for the nurse in caring for children with gastrointestinal disorders include the following:

- Early detection and treatment of gastrointestinal conditions
- Prevention of fluid and electrolyte imbalance due to vomiting and diarrhea
- Maintaining adequate nutrition for growth requirements
- Promoting elimination of solid waste

ASSESSING

Children with gastrointestinal disorders should be assessed for the presence of active bowel sounds, abdominal tenderness, vomiting, diarrhea, and constipation. Parents of young children or the older client should be questioned about the frequency, color, amount, and odor of the stool. Questions should be asked about usual feeding habits and recent changes in those habits. When a child presents with flulike symptoms, it is important to ask whether the child has been around anyone testing positive for hepatitis, or whether there has been possible exposure from contaminated blood, blood products, or contaminated water.

DIAGNOSING, PLANNING, AND IMPLEMENTING

The following nursing diagnoses may be pertinent to the care of young children with gastrointestinal disorders:

- Deficient **F**luid Volume related to vomiting
- Imbalanced **N**utrition: Less Than Body Requirement related to inability to absorb nutrients
- Risk for **I**nfection related to postoperative condition
- Disturbed **B**ody Image related to jaundice (older child or teen)
- **P**ain related to disorder or surgery.

Expected outcomes for children with gastrointestinal disorders would include the following, among others:

- Maintain adequate hydration.
- Obtain necessary nutrients to provide for healing and growth.
- Remain free of infection.
- Express an understanding of the condition and how it is expected to resolve.
- State that pain is within acceptable limits.

Nursing interventions might include the following:

- Administer fluids (either intravenously or orally) as ordered. *Maintaining fluid balance is a high priority when the gastrointestinal system is not functioning properly. Refer to Chapter 11 ⚭ for more information.*

■ Advance diet from clear liquid to full liquid to soft as ordered and tolerated. *Often, the child will be NPO for diagnostic tests, surgery, or to rest the gastrointestinal system and allow for healing. Once a diet can be resumed, it is best to advance the diet slowly.*

■ Administer medication, including antiemetics, antibiotics, antidiarrheals, and laxatives, as ordered. *Medications are frequently ordered to stop vomiting and diarrhea and stimulate defecation if the child is constipated. Antibiotics may be ordered to treat gastrointestinal infections or prior to bowel surgery.*

■ Teach parents and child (if appropriate) the care of medical appliances in use at home. *Medical appliances such as intestinal tubes, tube feeding pumps, and colostomy drainage bags may be used in the treatment of gastrointestinal disorders. Parents (and older children) must be taught to care for insertion sites, skin around appliances, and any other equipment.*

■ Teach parents regarding follow-up care. *Many gastrointestinal disorders are chronic in nature and require continued medical supervision.*

EVALUATING

Signs of dehydration will subside, a normal elimination pattern will return, vomiting will stop, and the child will gain weight. Postoperatively, the child will be evaluated for return of normal gastrointestinal function. Parents should be able to verbalize understanding of home care.

NURSING PROCESS CARE PLAN
Care of a Child with Bilateral Cleft Lip

John was born with a bilateral cleft lip. He has been cared for at home and is strong enough for surgical correction. John has been admitted to the pediatric unit from surgery.

Assessment.   VS: T 99.2 (R), P 90, R 36, Wt 12.5 lb (5.7 kg). John is awake and crying. An IV of lactated Ringer's solution is infusing in his left hand. Logan clamp is present across the surgical site. His diaper is wet.

Nursing Diagnosis.   The following important nursing diagnoses (among others) are established for this client:

■ **P**ain related to surgical procedure
■ Risk for **T**rauma related to surgical procedure

Expected Outcomes.   The following expected outcomes have been identified:

■ Infant does not exhibit any signs of pain.
■ Operative site is without erythema, edema, tenderness, or signs of infection.

Planning and Implementation

■ Medicate for pain as ordered. *Keeping the infant comfortable will decrease crying and trauma to the suture line.*
■ Apply elbow restraints. Restrain on back. *Jacket restraint prevents bending the elbows and rubbing the face or sucking the thumb. Restraining on back prevents rubbing face on the bed. Restraint will also protect the IV site.*
■ Clean suture line as ordered. *Cleaning the suture line prevents infection and aids in healing.*
■ Teach parents use of restraints and suture line care at home. *Continued care will be needed after discharge until healing is complete in several weeks.*
■ Do not put anything in the mouth. *This prevents trauma to the suture line.*

Evaluation.   John will rest comfortably with minimal crying. The suture line will remain intact without signs of infection. Parents can verbalize home care.

Critical Thinking in the Nursing Process

1. How should pain medication and feeding schedules be managed?
2. If John cannot have anything put in his mouth, how will he be fed?
3. How will the nurse know that John is getting enough nutrition?

Note: Discussion of Critical Thinking questions appears in Appendix I.

Note: The reference and resource listings for this and all chapters have been compiled at the back of the book.

Chapter Review

 KEY TERMS by Topic

Use the audio glossary feature of either the CD-ROM or the Companion Website to hear the correct pronunciation of the following key terms.

Anatomy and Physiology

peristalsis, lingual frenulum, papillae, gingiva, parotid gland, buccal space, submandibular glands, sublingual glands, cardiac sphincter, fundus, cardiac region, lesser curvature, greater curvature, pylorus, rugae, chyme, plicae, villi, emulsifier, catabolism, anabolism

Anatomic and Congenital Gastrointestinal Defects

cleft palate, cleft lip, Logan clamp, esophageal atresia, tracheoesophageal fistula, omphalocele, hernia

Gastrointestinal Inflammation

gastroenteritis, probiotics, appendicitis, rebound tenderness, fecalith, Crohn's disease, ulcerative colitis

Motility Disorders

motility disorders, gastroesophageal reflux disease, pyloric stenosis, pyloroplasty, colic, intussusception, diverticulum, volvulus, Hirschsprung's disease, megacolon, reanastomosis

Malabsorption and Inborn Metabolic Disorders

celiac disease, steatorrhea, lactose intolerance, kwashiorkor, phenylketonuria

Nutrition Disorders

rickets, scurvy, failure to thrive, pica, obesity, bariatric surgery

Poisonings

poisoning, chelation therapy

Hepatic Disorders

biliary atresia, hepatomegaly, pruritis, splenomegaly, hepatitis, fulminating hepatitis, parenchymal

KEY Points

- Gastrointestinal disorders are potentially life threatening due to fluid and electrolyte imbalance and malnutrition.
- Vomiting and diarrhea must be treated rapidly in children to prevent dehydration.
- Congenital malformation of the gastrointestinal system may require multiple surgeries to correct; therefore, nutrition is provided by IV administration of TPN.
- Most metabolic disorders require lifelong treatment.
- Families may need to be taught to administer nutrition by tube feeding or IV when long-term treatment is required.
- Health promotion activities include a low-fat, high-fiber diet and exercise to prevent or treat obesity.

FOR FURTHER Study

For more information about transmission, clinical manifestations, diagnostic tests, medical treatment and nursing considerations of hepatitis A and B, see Table 10-6.

Children who have been starved emotionally can have lifelong problems involving language, social interactions, and intelligence (see Box 15-1).

Failure to thrive and obesity are also discussed in Chapter 17.

Wilms' tumor is discussed in Chapter 18.

See Chapter 22 for information about organ transplantation.

See Appendix II for growth charts to determine percentile.

EXPLORE MediaLink

Additional interactive resources for this chapter can be found on the Companion Website at www.prenhall.com/adams.

Click on Chapter 17 and "Begin" to select the activities for this chapter.

For chapter-related NCLEX®-style questions and an audio glossary, access the accompanying CD-ROM in this book.

Animations:

Digestive system

Gavage tube

Critical Thinking Care Map

Caring for a Client with Gastroenteritis

NCLEX-PN® Focus Area: Physiologic Integrity: Basic Care and Comfort

Case Study: Jonathan's mother calls the pediatrician's office and reports that Jonathan has been vomiting and having diarrhea for the past 2 days. He is lethargic and not drinking his bottle. The infant is 7 months old.

Nursing Diagnosis: Imbalanced **N**utrition: Less Than Body Requirements related to excessive vomiting and diarrhea

COLLECT DATA

Subjective	Objective
_____	_____
_____	_____
_____	_____
_____	_____
_____	_____
_____	

Would you report this? Yes/No

If yes, to: _____

Nursing Care

_____
_____
_____
_____
_____
_____
_____
_____
_____

How would you document this? _____
_____
_____
_____
_____

Compare your documentation to the sample provided in Appendix I.

Data Collected
(use only those that apply)

- Previous weight: 16 lb
- Diffuse red area across buttocks
- Mother reports no fluid or solid intake in the past 48 hours
- Mother states infant enjoys playing with trucks
- Mucous membranes pale
- Current weight: 12 lb
- Vomiting ×6/day
- Diarrhea ×10/day
- Immunizations up to date
- Hyperactive bowels sounds in all four quandrants
- Mother reports infant is lethargic

Nursing Interventions
(use only those that apply; list in priority order)

- Apply topical agents as ordered for rash.
- Monitor lab values carefully.
- Administer next series of immunizations.
- Assess for possible causes of vomiting and diarrhea.
- Develop a plan with the parents for nutritional and fluid replacement.
- Obtain a thorough nutrition history.
- Assess for signs and symptoms of dehydration.
- Administer antiemetics as ordered.
- Provide age-appropriate toys for play.
- Weigh daily.

NCLEX-PN® Exam Preparation

TEST-TAKING TIP   It is often possible to eliminate words that are meant to distract, such as "always" and "never," especially when discussing client outcomes.

1 A 2-week-old infant is recovering from surgery for pyloric stenosis. The mother comments, "Now that the surgery is over, Timmy should not have intestinal obstruction ever again." An appropriate nursing response would be:

1. "You need to talk with the doctor about your son's future."
2. "You are correct. Timmy will never again experience intestinal obstruction."
3. "Recurrence of obstruction is unlikely, but we will review symptoms you should watch for."
4. "Timmy will not have obstruction as a child but will have digestive problems as an adult."

2 A pediatric client has been diagnosed with rickets. The nurse knows that the child's mother understands the treatment when she states that she will give the child additional amounts of which of the following? Select all that apply.

1. Milk, cheese, and yogurt
2. Jell-O or rice pudding
3. Raisin bread and brown bread
4. Oranges, lemons, and grapefruit
5. Salmon and sardines

3 The symptom that the nurse must monitor most closely when pyloric stenosis is suspected is:

1. Anorexia.
2. Infrequent bowel movements.
3. Projectile vomiting.
4. Colicky abdominal cramps.

4 To prevent trauma to the surgical site after a cleft palate repair, the nurse should avoid the use of which of the following? Choose all that apply.

1. Oral thermometer
2. Spoon
3. Cup
4. Dropper
5. Syringe

5 The nurse is providing teaching to parents of an infant with Hirschsprung's disease. Which of the following statements best describes Hirschsprung's disease?

1. It results in frequent evacuation of solids, liquids, and gas.
2. There is passage of excessive amounts of meconium.
3. It results in excessive peristaltic movement within the gastrointestinal tract.
4. The colon has a segment with limited nerve supply that prevents normal movement.

6 A 4-month-old has gastroesophageal reflux but is thriving without other complications. Which of the following should the nurse suggest to minimize reflux?

1. Discontinue breastfeeding.
2. Position the baby with the head up after feeding.
3. Give continuous nasogastric tube feeding.
4. Decrease frequency of feedings as much as possible.

7 The nurse is caring for a baby with probable intussusception. The baby had diarrhea before admission but, while waiting for a barium enema, passed a normal brown stool. Which of the following is the most appropriate nursing action?

1. Notify the physician.
2. Measure abdominal girth.
3. Continue with preparation for barium enema.
4. Take vital signs, including blood pressure.

8 The nurse would consider which of the following as a positive outcome in evaluating an infant with failure to thrive?

1. The family depends on nursing staff for care.
2. The family demonstrates nurturing behaviors toward the infant.
3. The infant maintains admission weight.
4. The infant makes slow progress on developmental milestones.

9 Which of the following is most important when assessing a child with poisoning?

1. Determine what was taken and the treatment provided by parents.
2. Determine medication allergies.
3. Give ipecac before activated charcoal.
4. Induce vomiting.

10 A 12-year-old client has a fever and complains of abdominal pain. The school nurse:

1. Calls the physician.
2. Checks for rebound tenderness.
3. Recommends a laxative.
4. Applies a heating pad.

Answers for NCLEX-PN® Review and Critical Thinking Questions appear in Appendix I.

Chapter 18

Care of the Child with Genitourinary Disorders

NURSING PROCESS CARE PLAN:
Child with Nephrotic
Syndrome

HEALTH PROMOTION ISSUE:
Assisting the Young Teen with
Her First Pap Smear

NURSING CARE PLAN CHART:
Child with Recurrent Urinary
Tract Infection

CRITICAL THINKING CARE MAP:
Caring for a Client with
Vaginitis

BRIEF Outline

URINARY (RENAL) SYSTEM
Anatomy and Physiology
Brief Assessment Review
Congenital Urinary Defects
Urinary Tract Infections
Acute Postinfectious
Glomerulonephritis
Nephrotic Syndrome
Acute and Chronic Renal
Failure
Wilms' Tumor or
Nephroblastoma
Enuresis
Nursing Care

REPRODUCTIVE SYSTEM
Anatomy and Physiology
Brief Assessment Review
Ambiguous Genitalia
Male Disorders
Sexually Transmitted Infections
Female Disorders
Breast Disorders
Uterine Disorders
Ovarian Disorders
Nursing Care

LEARNING Outcomes

After completing this chapter, you will be able to:
1. Define key terms.
2. Discuss the anatomy and physiology of the pediatric urinary and reproductive systems.
3. Describe urinary and reproductive disorders to include male and female disorders.
4. Discuss clinical manifestations, diagnostic procedures, medical management, and nursing interventions related to urinary and reproductive disorders.
5. Explain appropriate nursing interventions for children with urinary and reproductive disorders.

The **genitourinary system** consists of structures of the urinary system and the reproductive system. In this chapter, the anatomy and physiology of both systems will be reviewed. Disorders of the urinary system and the reproductive system will also be discussed.

URINARY (RENAL) SYSTEM

Anatomy and Physiology

The structures of the urinary system include the kidneys, ureters, bladder, urethra, and renal arteries and veins (Figure 18-1 ■). The primary functions of the urinary system include waste excretion; homeostasis, fluid, electrolyte, and acid-base balance; regulation of blood pressure; regulation of calcium metabolism; and stimulation of erythrocyte development.

Early in pregnancy, the kidneys develop and begin to assist in the maintenance of amniotic fluid levels. Urine production begins during the 3rd month of pregnancy. The placenta filters the fetus's blood and maintains homeostasis. At birth the newborn's kidneys take over these functions.

Growth of the kidney continues until adolescence. The process of filtration becomes refined by age 2. Urine output also increases as the child ages. Urinary output is as follows:

- For an infant, 2 mL/kg/hr
- For a child, 0.5–1 mL/kg/hr
- For an adolescent, 40–80 mL/hr

An estimate of a child's bladder capacity can be made by adding 2 to the child's age in years. This approximates the ounces of bladder capacity in the child. For example, the normal amount of urine a 1-year-old child can hold is 3 ounces (90 mL).

Brief Assessment Review

HISTORY

- Ask about patterns of urination. Include amount, color, and number of times per day (for an infant, number of diapers per day).
- Ask if the child complains of pain, burning, frequency, or urgency when voiding. Any of these symptoms could indicate the presence of a urinary tract infection.
- Ask about toilet training.
- Ask about involuntary urination. Ask when and how often it occurs. In an older child (school-age), ask if there are situations that are associated with involuntary urination (such as sleeping in a strange place overnight).
- Inquire about recent weight gain. It is especially important to note sudden increases in weight that seem unusual to the parents, because this may indicate kidney malfunction.
- Inquire about past urinary disorders. Some people are prone to UTIs.
- Require family history as it relates to urinary disorders.

PHYSICAL

- Weigh the child.
- Inspect for adequate hydration. Perform test for skin turgor.
- Inspect extremities for edema.
- Observe for bladder distention. Improper functioning of the urinary system may result in bladder distention.

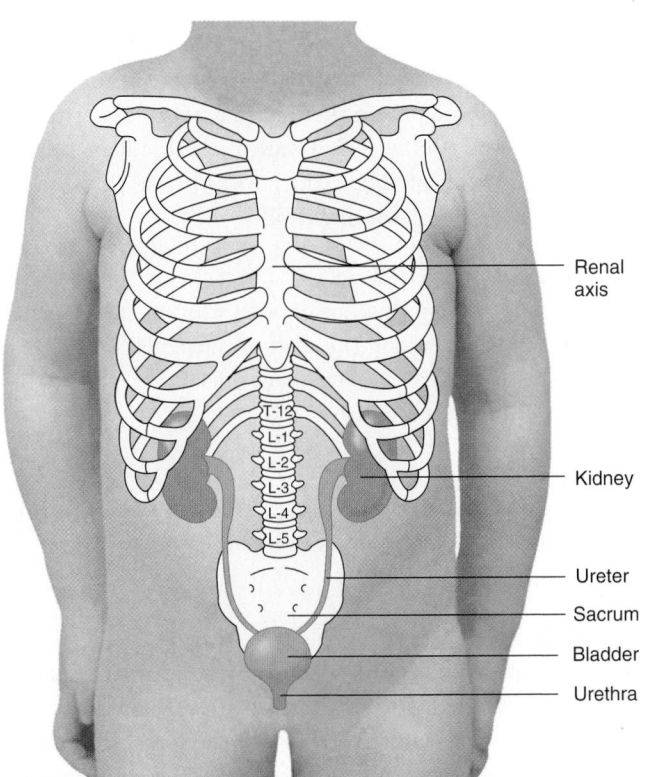

Figure 18-1. ■ ■ The kidneys are located between the twelfth thoracic (T12) and the third lumbar (L3) vertebrae.

Disorders of the urinary system that affect the child include congenital anomalies, infections, and tumors. Because one of the functions of the urinary system is to eliminate waste, disorders affecting the urinary system pose a significant risk to the health of the child.

Congenital Urinary Defects

Defects of the urinary system are commonly found with defects of the lower gastrointestinal tract and reproductive system. The first concern is to determine that the infant is able to urinate. Most commonly, the newborn voids in the first 24 hours of birth. If this does not occur, intervention must be more immediate. The newborn who does not void within 24 hours may be assessed for urethral stenosis or absent kidneys or ureters. Only common disorders of the urinary tract will be discussed here.

URETHRAL MALPOSITION

Typically in the male child, the urethra opens at the tip of the penis. **Hypospadias** occurs when the urethra opens on the *ventral* (lower) surface of the penis. **Epispadias** occurs when the urethra opens on the *dorsal* (upper) surface of the penis (Figure 18-2 ■). Epispadias may occur in females, but it is quite rare. In females, the urethra opens by a separation of the labia minora and a fissure of the clitoris.

Both hypospadias and epispadias are congenital anomalies that occur when the urethral folds fail to fuse over the urethral groove during fetal development. Hypospadias commonly occurs in combination with congenital inguinal hernias, undescended testes, and **chordee** (a congenital anomaly that causes a ventral curvature of the penis, which is caused by fibrous tissues along the corpus spongiosum).

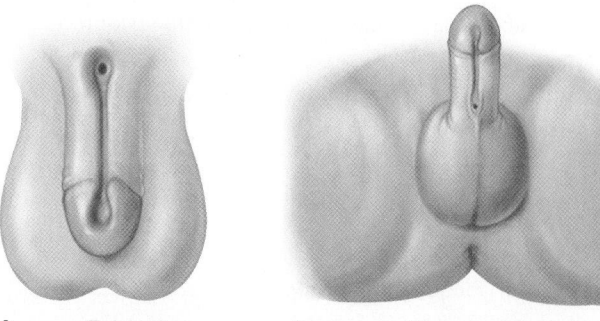

A Epispadias   **B** Hypospadias

Figure 18-2. ■ (A) In *epispadias* the urethra is on the dorsal surface of the penis. **(B)** In *hypospadias*, the urethra is on the ventral surface of the penis.

Figure 18-3. ■ This child has bladder exstrophy, noted by extrusion of the posterior bladder wall through the lower abdominal wall. Until surgery can be performed, the bladder mucosa must be protected from trauma and irritation. A sterile, saline-soaked dressing maintains moisture; it is covered with a sterile plastic wrap. The surrounding area must be cleaned daily. Skin sealant is applied to protect surrounding skin from leaking urine.

Epispadias can be associated with **bladder exstrophy** (Figure 18-3 ■), a defect usually corrected in the first 48 hours of life, in which there is an absence of part of the abdominal wall and anterior wall of the bladder, causing the posterior wall of the bladder to protrude through the defect, outside the abdominal wall.

Manifestations

The opening, in hypospadius or epispadius of the male, can be found anywhere along the shaft of the penis. A dimple or pit may be seen along the ventral or dorsal side of the penile shaft (see Figure 18-2).

Diagnosis

Diagnosis is made by documenting physical findings. Prenatally, the defect may be seen on ultrasound. Genetic testing may also be done.

Treatment

Surgical correction is needed for hypospadias and epispadias, usually during the first year of life. Infants are not circumcised in an effort to preserve the foreskin to use it in the cosmetic repair. The surgery moves the position of the urethra to correct urinary function. Following surgery, the infant will have a urethral stent to keep the urethra open.

Nursing Considerations

The nurse observes the infant postoperatively for edema, dysuria, bleeding, infection, and pain. Because of the urinary stent, the infant needs to be double diapered (Figure 18-4 ■). Maintaining hydration will assist adequate urinary output. The nurse needs to document the child's intake and output carefully, noting any lack of urinary drainage for one hour. (See intake and output, Procedure 11-1 ⬭ .) Be aware that the urine will be blood tinged for a few days.

Following surgery the infant may have bladder spasms. Anticholinergics and analgesics are administered by the nurse. Antibiotics are administered prophylactically to prevent infection. Box 18-1 ■ provides steps for the nurse to take to prevent and/or recognize symptoms of postoperative infection.

OBSTRUCTIVE UROPATHY

Obstructive uropathy is a condition in which the structure or function of the urinary system is altered, resulting in obstruction of urine flow (Figure 18-5 ■). Obstructions can be congenital or acquired. A congenital cause for urinary obstruction is **polycystic kidney.** In this condition, one or both kidneys are enlarged and contain fluid-filled cysts. Acquired causes include tumors, kidney stones (**nephrolithiasis**), and crystal formations caused by medications.

Manifestations

As urine flow from the kidney to the bladder is blocked, urine will back up, causing **stasis** (pooling of urine or other body fluids). Stasis can lead to UTIs, loss of renal function, and hydronephrosis. **Hydronephrosis** is the distension of the renal pelvis caused by increased pressure due to urine back up.

Figure 18-4. ■ The double diapering technique protects the urinary stent after surgery for hypospadias or epispadias repair. The inner diaper collects stool; the outer diaper, urine.

BOX 18-1	NURSING CARE CHECKLIST

Preventing Postoperative Infection

☑ Change all dressings with sterile technique.

☑ Keep drains and stents free of obstruction.

☑ Observe closely for signs of infection including:

- Change in vital signs: increased temperature, increased pulse
- White, puslike drainage from the wound
- Foul odor from the wound
- Edema and redness around the wound
- Increasing report of pain
- Increasing irritability
- Decreasing appetite

☑ Report symptoms of infection promptly to physician.

☑ Administer antibiotics properly.

☑ Teach caregiver, on discharge, to administer the entire course of prescribed antibiotics and to report symptoms of infection promptly.

Diagnosis

Obstructive uropathy is suspected when the child's urinary output is altered. The obstruction may be visualized by ultrasound or cystoscopy.

Kidney

Stenosis of the ureteropelvic valve

Ureter

Stenosis of the ureterovesicular junction

Bladder

Urethra

Stenosis of the posterior urethral valve

Figure 18-5. ■ The common sites of obstruction in the upper and lower urinary tract. Upper urinary tract infections are often unilateral. Renal failure is most likely to occur when both kidneys are affected by hydronephrosis.

Treatment

Once the obstruction is diagnosed, placement of a urethral or suprapubic catheter is necessary until surgical intervention can occur. Surgical corrections include **pyeloplasty** (removal of the obstructed ureter segment and replacement into the renal pelvis) and **valve ablation** (removal of a faulty valve).

Nursing Considerations

Preoperatively the nurse assists in the diagnostic process and ensures that the child and family understand the condition and the prescribed treatment. Postoperatively, the nurse observes for urinary retention and fluid and electrolyte imbalances.

On discharge, many children will have a stent, catheter, or urinary diversion device. Parents need specific instructions on how to care for these devices, how to maintain hygiene (see Figure 18-4), and when to report complications.

Urinary Tract Infections

Urinary tract infections (UTIs) are a group of bacterial infections that include **cystitis** (bladder infection) and **pyelonephritis** (kidney infection). Urinary tract infections can be a single acute episode or a chronic recurrent or persistent infection. In the infant, UTIs are more common in males primarily because of structural defects. In the young child, UTIs are more common in females, usually caused by

Escherichia coli entering the urethra and progressing to the bladder. Younger children also have shorter bladders, which increases their risk for UTIs.

UTIs can also be caused by **vesicoureteral reflux,** a defect of the vesicoureteral valve. Normally, when urine enters the bladder, pressure builds and closes the vesicoureteral valve. If there is a defect in this valve, closure does not occur and urine refluxes into the ureter. Urinary stasis leads to UTIs. Vesicoureteral reflux may resolve spontaneously. If dilation of the kidneys occurs, surgical intervention may be necessary.

Manifestations

Signs of UTI in the infant are less specific than in older children. Anytime an infant presents with unexplained illness, the possibility of UTI should suspected. Symptoms of UTI include fever, nausea and vomiting, anorexia, strong-smelling urine, abdominal pain, **dysuria** (painful urination), and **hematuria** (blood in the urine). In the infant and young child who is nonverbal, dysuria may be displayed as crying during urination. The continent child may suddenly develop incontinence or hesitancy, due to fear of pain.

Diagnosis

Urinalysis can detect hematuria and the presence of white blood cells and nitrites (Table 18-1 ■). However, to determine

TABLE 18-1		
Lab Values for Urinalysis		
CHARACTERISTIC	NORMAL VALUE	NURSING CONSIDERATIONS
Bacteria	None to few organisms present	Normally residing bacteria from the perineum may contaminate the specimen
pH	4.50–8.0	Normal urine is slightly acidic. Urinary tract infections may cause the urine to become alkaline
Color	Clear, straw colored, amber	Bacteria or vaginal discharge may cause cloudy urine. Concentrated urine is dark. Urine with blood is red.
Odor	Slight, nonoffensive odor	Urine containing bacteria may smell foul
Glucose	Negative	Presence of glucose in the urine may indicate high blood glucose levels
Protein	Negative	Presence of protein in the urine may indicate glomerular kidney disease
Red blood cells	Negative on gross examination; 0–5 per high powered field	Blood in the urine may indicate UTI or other kidney diseases
White blood cells	Negative; less than 2 per high-powered field	Presence may indicate UTI
Specific gravity	Newborn: 1.001–1.020; child: 1.005–1.030	Increased values may indicate renal disease
Ketones	Negative	Present in diabetes mellitus, in starvation, or in children who have ingested an excessive amount of aspirin

the exact causative agent, a urine culture is necessary. A sterile urine specimen is collected by the nurse (see description of this in Procedure 8-14 ⬭). Proper collection of the sample is essential to the accuracy of the findings. A clean-catch specimen may be obtained if the child is cooperative. A sterile single-use, self-adhering urinary bag or catheterization may be used to collect a sample in the incontinent child. (Urinary catheterization in a child is described in Procedure 8-24 ⬭.)

Treatment

The primary treatment for UTI is administration of antibiotics. Parenteral antibiotics are required for children with pyelonephritis. Oral or intravenous fluids can assist in maintaining urinary function.

Prophylactic antibiotic administration is indicated for children with structural defects such as vesicoureteral reflux.

Nursing Considerations

In most circumstances, a UTI can be prevented. The parents should be taught to clean the perineum thoroughly with each diaper change. The young child who is being toilet trained should be taught to wipe from front to back. The perineum should be washed daily. Discourage the use of bubble baths and hot tubs that can irritate the urethra and increase the chance of infection. Box 18-2 ■ provides information about preventing UTI. The Nursing Care Plan Chart on page 490 describes care of a child with recurrent UTI.

Acute Postinfectious Glomerulonephritis

Acute postinfectious **glomerulonephritis** (inflammation of the glomeruli), or APIGN, usually results from the body's immune response following an infection (Figure 18-6 ■). This condition is also called *acute poststreptococcal glumerulonephritis* if caused by *Streptococcus*. Infecting organisms related to glomerulonephritis are group A beta-hemolytic *Streptococcus*, *Staphylococcus*, *Pneumococcus*, and coxsackievirus. It is the most common type of kidney inflammation. It is most often seen in children between the ages of 2 and 12 years, and it is twice as common in boys as in girls. Antibiotic therapy to kill the infecting agent does not prevent this disorder from occurring. APIGN results when immune complexes, deposited in glomeruli, obstruct capillary blood flow. The condition can lead to acute or chronic renal failure.

Manifestations

Children with glomerulonephritis may be asymptomatic. Others have a sudden onset of flank pain, irritability, malaise, and fever. Other symptoms include gross or microscopic hematuria, dysuria, edema, hypertension, and oliguria.

BOX 18-2	COMPLEMENTARY THERAPIES

Preventing Urinary Tract Infections

There are several nonpharmacologic measures parents can use to help prevent UTI in their children.

Risk of bacterial contamination can be reduced by:

- In female children, wiping the perineum from front to back after urination, defecation, and during regular hygiene to keep harmful bacteria found in the stool away from the urethra.
- Avoiding the use of bubble baths, which are a skin irritant and which provide a medium for growth of harmful bacteria.
- Decreasing the use of harsh soaps, shampoos, and detergents, which can be skin irritants.
- Limiting bath times to 15 minutes. Children should urinate immediately following the bath to remove harmful bacteria.
- In the infant, changing diapers frequently.
- Supplying children with white cotton underwear. Synthetic fibers and fabric dyes can be skin irritants.
- Providing loose-fitting pants, shorts, tights, and underwear to avoid skin irritation.
- Quickly removing wet clothing such as dance or exercise wear and bathing suits to avoid skin irritation.
- Providing a diet with plenty of fiber helps to prevent constipation. Constipation distends the rectum and distorts the bladder, which hinders complete emptying of the bladder.
- Providing plenty of clear liquids routinely to flush harmful bacteria from the urinary tract. Cranberry juice may change the acidity of the urine and cause it to be less likely to become infected.
- Having the child empty the bladder every 4 hours during the day and once before bedtime to help remove harmful bacteria regularly.
- For males, retracting the foreskin and cleaning the head of the penis daily keeps an uncircumcised child clean.

Source: Data from National Women's Health Information Center. (2003). *A lifetime of good health: Your guide to staying healthy.* Washington, DC: U.S. Department of Health and Human Services; National Kidney and Urologic Diseases Clearinghouse. (2005). Urinary tract infections in children. NIH Publication no. 06-4246. Bethesda, MD: Author.

Diagnosis

Urinalysis and serum studies are performed. An electrocardiogram may also be done, to look for changes caused by circulatory overload.

Treatment

Treatment for children with glomerulonephritis is supportive, including bed rest in some cases, antihypertensive medication, and fluid restriction. The nurse should monitor the child's fluid status by planning fluid restriction and documenting intake and output. See Procedures 11-1 and

NURSING CARE PLAN CHART

The Child with Recurrent Urinary Tract Infection

GOAL	INTERVENTION	RATIONALE	EXPECTED OUTCOME
1. Impaired **U**rinary Elimination related to infectious process			
The child will have return of expected urinary elimination patterns related to age of child.	Monitor urinary output and characteristics of urine	*These assessments will assist the nurse in determining effectiveness of treatment*	The child's urine will be free of odor, blood, and particulate matter. Lab values will be within normal limits. The child reports no dysuria, frequency, or urgency.
	Encourage the child to drink water with meals and between meals	*Adequate fluid intake, especially water, will assist in the resolution of the infectious process. Other beverages may contribute to symptoms of urgency and dysuria*	
	Encourage the child to respond immediately to urge to void	*Prompt response to urgency will assist the child in avoiding accidents*	
The family will be able to recognize signs and symptoms of UTI.	Teach parents how to recognize a UTI.	*Prompt recognition of symptoms yields prompt reporting and therefore more effective treatment*	The family will report promptly signs and symptoms of UTI.
2. Ineffective **H**ealth Maintenance related to lack of child's ability to make deliberate judgments			
The child will demonstrate an awareness of healthy behaviors that will prevent UTIs.	Determine the child's level of understanding related to actions that increase risk of UTI	*This knowledge base will give the nurse the data needed to develop an appropriate teaching plan*	The child verbalizes at least three prevention measures related to UTIs and describes the manner in which they will incorporate them into their daily lives.
	Determine the child's ability to execute changes necessary in their life as well as their readiness to change	*The nurse must determine that the child has the skills necessary to implement preventative measures and desires to implement these*	
	Discuss preventative health measures related to UTIs such as perineal cleansing, use of appropriate cleansers, clothing, diet, fluids, urinary habits. Request verbalization of understanding	*Specific teaching will assist the child in changing harmful habits. Verbalization of understanding will allow the nurse to determine if teaching was effective*	
The family will participate in assisting the child to prevent UTIs.	Encourage parents to develop a motivational strategy to assist the child in maintaining healthy behaviors	*Motivation and encouragement reinforce positive behaviors and assist in making them lifelong habits*	The family will provide motivation, monitoring, and follow-up related to prevention methods.
	Encourage parents to review prevention strategies with the child on a regular basis	*Reviewing strategies will assist to reinforce behaviors and correct inappropriate behaviors and information*	

11-3 ⚭ . If tests are positive for streptococcal infection, antibiotics are administered and the family may be tested and treated for strep as well (Ball & Bindler, 2006). Further infection should be prevented by reducing exposure to pathogens.

Nursing Considerations

The child's skin integrity is compromised by bed rest. The nurse can reposition the child frequently and keep linens wrinkle free. Maintaining adequate nutritional intake may be a challenge for the nurse. The child with

Figure 18-6. ■ Pathophysiology of acute postinfectious glomerulonephritis.

glomerulonephritis has a decreased appetite, so the nurse will have to encourage the child to eat.

Most cases of APIGN resolve completely. Gross signs generally resolve in a few weeks. Lab values for microscopic hematuria may take up to 2 years to return to normal, whereas lab values for proteinuria may be abnormal for up to 12 months. Parents should be forewarned about these findings.

Nephrotic Syndrome

Nephrotic syndrome is a clinical state characterized by edema, **proteinuria** (protein in the urine), **hypoalbuminemia** (low blood albumin levels), **hyperlipidemia** (high blood lipids), and altered immunity. *Primary nephrotic syndrome*, also called minimal-change nephrotic syndrome (MCNS), affects only the kidneys and frequently follows an infection such as **pyelonephritis** (inflammation of the kidney pelvis). Primary nephrotic syndrome is seen most often in children. *Secondary nephrotic syndrome* results from a multi-system disorder such as diabetes, systemic lupus, or sickle

cell anemia. Nephrotic syndrome affects more male children between the ages of 2 and 7 than any other group.

In nephrotic syndrome, the glomerular permeability is altered, allowing albumin to move from the blood to the urine. This results in hypoalbuminemia and proteinuria. The shift in albumin changes the osmotic pressure of the blood. The kidney reabsorbs sodium and water, resulting in edema. A low osmotic pressure stimulates the liver to make lipoproteins (*cholesterol*), leading to hyperlipidemia. As immunoglobulins are excreted, the child's immunity is decreased.

Manifestations

Edema in the child with nephrotic syndrome develops rapidly over a few days to 2 weeks, resulting in a dramatic weight gain (Figure 18-7 ■). Notable edema can be seen in the face, especially **periorbital edema** (edema around the eyes). Edema is also seen in the abdomen (**ascites**), scrotum, and extremities. The blood pressure will increase. The child may become irritable, which might indicate increased intracranial pressure or discomfort. Albuminuria causes the

Figure 18-7. ■ Young boy exhibits edema characteristic of nephrotic syndrome.

urine to be foamy. The child will begin to appear malnourished with dull eyes; dull, brittle hair; and skin lesions.

Diagnosis

When nephrotic syndrome is suspected, a urinalysis is done to determine the presence of protein in the urine. Typical findings are 3+ to 4+ protein. A 24-hour urine specimen may reveal as much as 15 grams of protein. Hematuria may also be detected.

Treatment

Treatment of nephrotic syndrome is focused on reducing proteinuria and edema and preventing infection while the child is immunocompromised. Oral corticosteroids are given initially to reduce proteinuria and edema. Diuretic therapy may be necessary to further reduce the edema. Potassium supplementation may be necessary if hypokalemia develops in children taking diuretics. Cyclophosphamide (Cytoxan) can be given to improve symptoms, but this further compromises the child's immunological status.

Nursing Considerations

The child with nephrotic syndrome should be weighed daily to determine resolution of edema. The blood pressure should be monitored and hypertension reported to the supervising registered nurse and physician. Intravenous infusions will be established to administer albumin, and diuretics are given to decrease edema. Steroids may be given daily for several weeks to decrease inflammation of the glomeruli. The child will probably remain on steroids for 4 to 6 months.

In order to improve the nutritional status of the child, a regular diet is recommended that is low in sodium to prevent further protein loss by the kidneys and to allow return of normal blood protein levels. Methods of infection prevention should be implemented by the nurse. These include screening visitors for signs of infection, proper hand-washing techniques, and close observation for symptoms of infection in the child.

Children and parents are often fearful and anxious about the child's life-threatening illness. Parents may feel guilty they did not seek medical attention earlier. If nephrotic syndrome becomes a chronic condition, the child and parents may be frustrated and depressed.

Prior to discharge, the child and family should be provided with an explanation of the disease process and treatment plan. Parents should understand the administration and side effects of medications. Parents should monitor and record the urine protein and the child's weight daily and verbalize the need for routine medical follow-up care.

Acute and Chronic Renal Failure

Renal failure is the inability of the kidneys to remove liquid waste from the blood. Renal failure can result from lack of circulation to the kidney, damage to the glomerulus, or blockage that prevents any part of the kidney from draining. Factors that increase the risk of developing renal failure include severe dehydration, hypotension, accidental poisoning, repeated infection, and trauma.

Acute renal failure (ARF) is the sudden onset of diminished kidney function resulting in the imbalance of fluids and electrolytes. **Chronic renal failure** (CRF) is a progressive, irreversible loss of kidney function. CRF can progress to **end-stage renal disease** (ESRD), a condition in which kidney function is less than 10% and the child requires dialysis or kidney transplantation to survive.

Manifestations

Specific symptoms of ARF may not appear in the child until the disease is advanced. However, oliguria is usually one of the first symptoms noticed. Nonspecific symptoms include pale skin, headache, nausea, and fatigue. The child may have difficulty concentrating. As the disease progresses, edema (see Figure 18-7), tachycardia, and hypertension become evident. In addition to the symptoms just listed, children with CRF have decreased mental alertness, anemia, and growth retardation caused by demineralization of bone. In ESRD, all body systems become affected when waste is not eliminated. **Uremic syndrome** develops in ESRD (Figure 18-8 ■). Uremic syndrome is characterized by nausea, vomiting, anorexia, uremic breath odor, anemia, **uremic frost** (urea crystals deposited on the skin), pruritis,

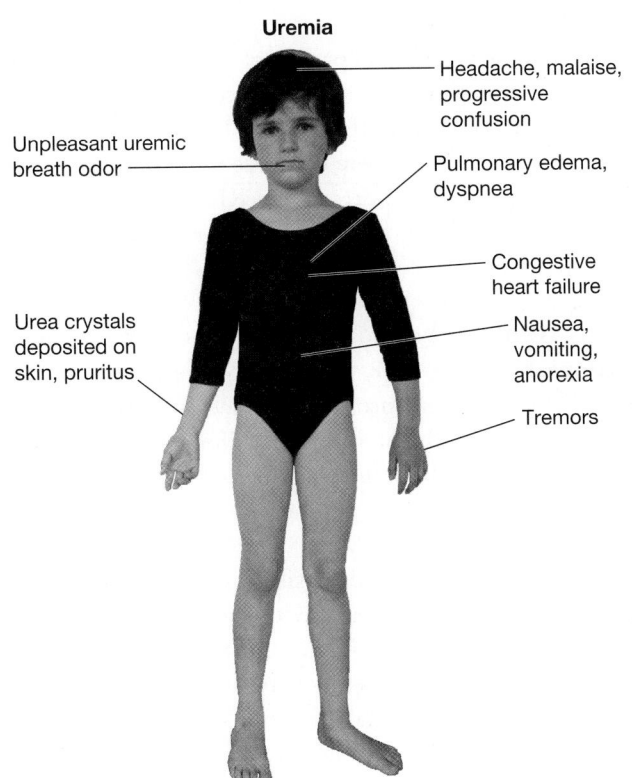

Uremia

- Headache, malaise, progressive confusion
- Pulmonary edema, dyspnea
- Congestive heart failure
- Nausea, vomiting, anorexia
- Tremors
- Unpleasant uremic breath odor
- Urea crystals deposited on skin, pruritus

Figure 18-8. ■ Multisystem effects of uremia.

TABLE 18-2		
Lab Values for Children with Renal Failure		
LAB	NORMAL	FINDING
Blood Urea Nitrogen (BUN)	Infant: 5–15 mg/dL	Increased
	Child: 5–20 mg/dL	Increased
Serum creatinine	Newborn: 0.8–1.4 mg/dL	Increased
	Infant: 0.7–1.7 mg/dL	Increased
	2- to 6-yr-old: 0.3–0.6 mg/dL	Increased
	More than 6 yr old: 0.4–1.2 mg/dL	Increased
Serum potassium	Infant: 3.6–5.8 mEq/L	Increased
	Child: 3.5–5.5 mEq/L	Increased
Serum sodium	Infant: 134–150 mEq/L	Increased or decreased
	Child: 135–145 mEq/L	Increased or decreased
Bicarbonate (HCO_3)	24–28 mEq/L	Decreased

malaise, headache, confusion, tremors, pulmonary edema, dyspnea, and congestive heart failure.

Diagnosis

Urinary output is measured carefully, usually by indwelling catheter (see Procedure 8-26 ⬤⬤). Oliguria in renal failure in children is defined as urine output less than 1 mL/kg/hr. For example: A child weighing 8 kg would have a urine output of less than 8 mL/hour. Increased laboratory values include serum creatinine, BUN, and serum potassium. Arterial bicarbonate may be decreased. Serum sodium may be increased or decreased depending on the child's fluid status. Table 18-2 ■ shows lab values in children with renal failure. Kidney function tests such as an intravenous pyelography (IVP) may be ordered to determine size, structure, and function of the kidneys, ureters, and bladder.

Glomerular filtration rate is used to determine the extent of CRF in children. The glomerular filtration rate depicts the kidney's ability to filter plasma properly. In CRF, this rate is decreased. Table 18-3 ■ reviews normal glomerular filtration rates for the pediatric client.

Treatment

Children in ARF who have fluid volume deficit are typically admitted to pediatric intensive care units for intravenous fluid replacement. Solutions used are normal saline or lactated Ringer's. If blood loss is the cause of fluid volume deficit, albumin is given.

Children in ARF with fluid overload require diuretic therapy and oral fluid restriction. Hyperkalemia is treated with Kayexalate. This medication can be given orally or by enema.

CRF requires strict dietary management in order to provide the child with adequate calories for growth needs while restricting foods that might complicate fluid and electrolyte imbalances. Pharmacologic agents for children with CRF include vitamin and mineral supplementation, phosphate-binding agents to prevent bone demineralization, growth

TABLE 18-3	
Normal Glomerular Filtration Rates (GFRs)	
AGE OF CHILD	NORMAL GFR
Infants, 1 week	40.6 ± 14.8 mean GFR
Infants, 2–8 weeks	65.8 ± 24.8 mean GFR
Infants, 8 weeks to 2 years	95.7 ± 21.7 mean GFR
Children, 2–12 years	133.0 ± 27.0 mean GFR
Males, 13–21 years	140.0 ± 30.0 mean GFR
Females, 13–21 years	126.0 ± 22.0 mean GFR

hormones to stimulate growth, hematopoietic growth factors and iron supplementation to treat anemia, and antihypertensive agents to treat hypertension.

Some children can be managed with a combination of medication and diet therapy, whereas other children progress rapidly to ESRD that requires dialysis or kidney transplant. See the following section for more information on dialysis. For more information about organ transplantation, see Chapter 22 ⊙⊙.

Nursing Considerations

The child with renal failure should be assessed for signs of fluid overload including weight gain, pitting edema, pulmonary edema, and ascites. A priority nursing task is strictly monitoring intake and output. See Chapter 11 ⊙⊙ for more information on this procedure. Urinary output should be monitored, including the color and odor of the urine. Blood values (including serum electrolytes, blood urea nitrogen [BUN], creatinine, and bicarbonate levels) should be monitored closely. Abnormal levels should be reported to the supervising RN and physician.

Medications must be administered as directed in order to achieve the desired effect. The child must be monitored for side effects of medication, signs of electrolyte imbalance, and alterations in blood pressure. The child will need small, frequent feedings in order to meet additional nutrition demands.

In a child with renal failure, infection places additional burden on the kidneys and can speed the progression of the disease. Sites for infection include respiratory, urinary, and gastrointestinal tracts and dialysis sites. The nurse must be an effective role model for the child and family in preventing infection.

The child and family should be assessed for signs of undue stress brought on by life-threatening chronic illness. The need for ongoing dialysis is expensive, and the limited number of dialysis facilities dictates the family's place of residence. The child and family need emotional support in dealing with a chronic life-threatening illness. The National Kidney Foundation and local support groups can be valuable resources for the nurse and the family.

In planning home care, the needs of the child and family should be identified well before discharge. Help the family to plan medication administration times that work around dialysis and that fit their routine. Stress the importance of consistency in diet, activity, and medication administration. If the child will be receiving peritoneal dialysis or hemodialysis at home, the family will need to be taught how to administer these treatments. Strict sterile technique must be used to prevent infection.

DIALYSIS

Dialysis is the mechanical process of removing wastes from blood or lymph through the processes of diffusion, osmosis, and ultrafiltration. Once the blood or lymph is filtered, it is returned to the body. There are three types of dialysis that may be used to treat children with CRF and/or ESRD: peritoneal, hemodialysis, and continuous renal replacement therapy.

Peritoneal Dialysis

Peritoneal dialysis involves placing a catheter through the child's abdomen into the peritoneal cavity to infuse *dialysate*, the dialysis solution. The dialysate draws wastes and extra fluids into the peritoneal cavity, where they are drained through the catheter. Two types of peritoneal dialysis are available. The first is continuous ambulatory peritoneal dialysis (CAPD). Dialysate is infused into the peritoneal cavity four or five times per day. Drainage of the fluid occurs when the collection chamber is lowered below the pelvis. The second method of peritoneal dialysis is called automated peritoneal dialysis. The process of infusing dialysate and removing it is automated and occurs approximately five times over a 10-hour period.

clinical ALERT

The nurse must carefully assess the child undergoing peritoneal dialysis for peritonitis and abdominal hernia. The child with peritonitis may have cloudy dialysate following dialysis, as well as fever, vomiting, diarrhea, and abdominal tenderness or pain.

Hemodialysis

In hemodialysis the child's blood is removed from the body, flows through a *dialyzer* (a machine that removes wastes and extra fluid), and then is returned to the body (Figure 18-9 ■). The child will have an external shunt or an arteriovenous fistula. Children with CRF and/or ESRD need hemodialysis three times weekly. Each dialysis session last 3 to 4 hours.

clinical ALERT

The nurse must be vigilant to observe for complications related to hemodialysis. These complications include hypotension, thrombosis, infection, fluid and electrolyte imbalances, and shock. **Disequilibrium syndrome** is a complication caused by cerebral edema. Symptoms of disequilibrium syndrome include fatigue, nausea, vomiting, and tremors that can progress to delirium, seizures, and coma.

A

B

Figure 18-9. ■ This child is undergoing hemodialysis. (**A**) A surgically implanted vascular graft is being used here. One needle is placed in the arterialized end of the graft (red tubing), and one needle is placed in the venous end (blue tubing) for blood return. (**B**) The child is able to draw or perform other quiet activities during dialysis treatment. Note that the child's blood pressure is monitored carefully throughout treatment.

Continuous Renal Replacement Therapy

Continuous renal replacement therapy (CRRT) provides the child with continuous hemodialysis, 24 hours per day. CRRT is an inpatient procedure, often requiring that the child be admitted to pediatric intensive care.

Wilms' Tumor or Nephroblastoma

Wilms' tumor or **nephroblastoma** is a highly metastatic, cancerous tumor of the kidney. It is most common in children between 2 and 5 years of age. Even in the absence of other anomalies, a genetic link is suggested. A gene that promotes normal kidney function is missing in a child with Wilms' tumor.

Manifestations

A child with Wilms' tumor may be asymptomatic. Commonly parents palpate an abdominal mass while bathing the child. The mass may be unilateral or bilateral; it is usually firm and contains several lobes. Hematuria, hypertension, and abdominal pain may be present.

Diagnosis

Diagnosis is made on the basis of ultrasound. MRI of the lungs, liver, spleen, and brain are necessary to determine metastasis. These procedures are frightening to the child and parents, and thorough explanation is important. Parents are usually allowed to stay with the child during diagnostic tests. The diagnosis will provide the staging of the tumor (Table 18-4 ■).

Treatment

Surgery to remove the kidney and affected lymph nodes is usually scheduled as soon as possible. Follow-up chemotherapy and/or radiation may be necessary to ensure destruction of the tumor. If the tumor has metastasized to the other kidney or to other organs, prognosis is poor.

TABLE 18-4	
Staging of Wilms' Tumor	
STAGE OF WILMS' TUMOR	**CANCER LOCATION**
Stage I	Cancer is found only in the kidney and can be completely removed by surgery.
Stage II	Cancer has spread beyond the kidney, to fat or soft tissue or blood vessels. The cancer can be completely removed by surgery.
Stage III	Cancer has spread within the abdomen and cannot be completely removed by surgery. The cancer may have spread to the lymph nodes (small bean-shaped structures found throughout the body that produce and store infection-fighting cells) near the kidney, blood vessels, or the peritoneum (tissue that lines the abdomen and covers most organs in the abdomen).
Stage IV	Cancer has spread to the lungs, liver, bone, or brain, or to lymph nodes outside of the abdomen and pelvis.
Stage V	Cancer cells are found in both kidneys when the disease is first diagnosed.

Nursing Considerations

Because of the highly metastatic nature of Wilms' tumor, signs should be placed on the chart and head of the bed warning all health care providers to avoid palpating the child's abdomen. Preoperative and postoperative care follows routine protocols.

> ### clinical ALERT
>
> **Do not** palpate the abdomen of a child with potential Wilms' tumor. These tumors are fragile. Palpation could cause the tumor to rupture, dispersing cancerous cells throughout the abdomen.

The postoperative nursing care focuses on pain management and fluid balance. A large incision is needed to remove the kidney, and the shift in the internal organs can cause discomfort for the child. Gentle handling is important, but the child will need encouragement to turn, cough, and deep breathe to prevent complications.

Fluid balance should be monitored by daily weight, intake and output, and urine specific gravity. The blood pressure should be monitored to assess shock and the function of the remaining kidney.

During chemotherapy, the child should be monitored for side effects, infection, and function of the remaining kidney. Parents should be taught home care and the need for continued follow-up visits prior the discharge. The remaining kidney needs to be protected from infection and injury. Parents may want to overprotect the child, but it will help the positive development of the child to maintain as normal lifestyle as possible.

Enuresis

Enuresis is urinary incontinence occurring in a child who is capable of obtaining bladder control. (Box 18-3 ■ describes physiologic factors that relate to toilet training.) *Nocturnal enuresis* occurs during the night, and *diurnal enuresis* occurs during the day. Enuresis can be a result of familial tendencies, difficulty in arousing, decreased bladder

---

BOX 18-3

Physiology of Toilet Training

At birth a child's bladder capacity is 20–50 mL. This capacity increases gradually until reaching 700 mL in adulthood. When "stretch receptors" found in the bladder wall are stimulated, urination is initiated. Children less than 2 years of age are incapable of maintaining bladder control because they do not have sufficient nerve development to be able to detect the stimulation of these stretch receptors. Complete bladder control may not be possible until age 4 or 5 years.

---

capacity, abnormal circadian rhythms, abnormalities of the urethra, developmental delays, or sleep apnea.

Diagnosis

To diagnose enuresis in children, historical data must be gathered. It is important to determine a family history of enuresis. There should be a discussion of how the family is currently managing the problem. It should be determined how the child was toilet trained, if applicable. It is also important to determine if there are any stressors in the child's life that may contribute to enuresis.

Other laboratory tests that can assist in the diagnosis are urinalysis and urine culture. Diagnostic studies done may include bladder capacity, uroflow measurement, and ultrasound scans of the bladder to measure residual urine.

Treatment

Treatment for enuresis can be a combination of medication and behavioral modifications. Medications used are antidiuretics, anticholinergics, or tricyclic antidepressants (Table 18-5 ■). The child's behavior related to fluid intake and voiding is modified in an effort to develop new habits that will assist the child in controlling the bladder at night. Total fluid intake for the day is divided portions administered as follows: 40% between 7 a.m. and noon; 40% between noon and 5 p.m.; and 20% after 5 p.m. For children over 7 years of age, an alarm that sounds when the child begins to void at night can assist the child in waking and voiding in the bathroom (Box 18-4 ■). Positive reinforcement and rewards can be implemented when the child is able to remain dry. These reinforcements should be specifically motivating for the child. If the child has diurnal enuresis, a 2-hour voiding schedule can be used to teach the child to empty the bladder completely.

NURSING CARE

PRIORITIES IN NURSING CARE

When caring for children with urinary disorders other than renal failure, the nurse should seek to maintain renal function and fluid balance. Children with infections should be monitored for changes in body temperature, elevated WBCs, and poor urine output. Monitor closely for signs and symptoms of fluid deficit or fluid overload. See Chapter 15 🔗 for more information on fluid and electrolyte imbalances. Oral and intravenous intake must be carefully assessed to avoid excess intake. The nurse carefully collects data and records daily intake and output.

TABLE 18-5

Pharmacology: Medications Used for Treatment of Enuresis

DRUG (GENERIC AND COMMON BRAND NAME)	USUAL ROUTE/DOSE	CLASSIFICATION AND PURPOSE	SELECTED SIDE EFFECTS	DON'T GIVE IF
Imipramine hydrochloride (Tofranil)	25–50 mg PO 1 hour before bedtime	Tricyclic antidepressant for nocturnal enuresis	Sedation, drowsiness, orthostatic hypotension, arrhythmias, blurred vision, dry mouth, urinary retention	Child has respiratory disorder, cardiovascular disorder, blood disorder, or hepatic disorder.
Hyoscyamine sulfate (Levsin or Levsinex Timecaps)	0.0625–0.125 mg PO prn, maximum dosage for child 2–12 is 0.75 mg/d	Anticholinergic (parasympatholytic) relaxes smooth muscle of the bladder, increasing bladder capacity	Drowsiness, blurred vision, dry mouth, constipation, urinary retention	Child has diabetes mellitus or cardiac disease.
Desmopressin acetate (DDAVP or Stimate)	5–40 mcg Intranasal spray at bedtime or 0.2–0.6 mg PO at bedtime for children 6 years or older	Vasopressin to relieve polyuria	Transient headache, nasal congestion, heartburn, shortness of breath	Child has cardiac disease, marked edema.
Oxybutynin chloride (Ditropan)	0.2 mg/kg PO 2–4 times/d for child 1–5 years; 5 mg PO 2 times/d for child over 5 years	Anticholinergic (parasympatholytic) relaxes smooth muscle of the bladder, increasing bladder capacity	Drowsiness, blurred vision, dry mouth, constipation	Child has GI obstruction, myasthenia gravis, glaucoma, severe colitis, urinary retention, severe cardiac disease.

BOX 18-4   CLIENT TEACHING

Use of Enuresis Alarm

Parents and children must understand how the enuresis alarm functions and how it is to be used (Mercer, 2003). Teach parents the following:

■ The average child will need to use the enuresis alarm for 10 to 12 weeks to achieve success in staying dry.

■ Attach the alarm to close-fitting cloth underwear. Do not attach it to loose clothing such as boxer shorts or pajamas. Do not attach it to disposable diapers.

■ When the alarm sounds, go to the child's room and observe the child's response. Tell the child to put feet on the floor and walk to the bathroom. Help the child if necessary. Turn off the alarm only after the child puts his or her feet on the floor.

■ Recognize that in the beginning, the child will have voided by the time he or she wakes up or the parents arrive. The measures of progress include:

• Reduced number of episodes of wetting per night

• Increased length of sleep time before wetting

• Decreased amount of urination (spotting) before the child puts feet on the floor

■ After a wetting episode, reattach the alarm to clean dry underpants.

■ Keep a chart to track events, and praise the child for progress.

■ Consider giving prizes for cooperation and improved performance. Prizes may include stickers for each time the child goes without assistance to the bathroom or a larger prize, such as a meal out or some form of entertainment, for the first completely dry night.

■ Remind parents that the greatest reward for the child is their praise.

■ Once the child is able to stay dry through the night, continue use of the alarm until there have been 2 continuous weeks without an episode of enuresis. Then use the alarm every other night for 2 or more weeks of consecutive dryness.

■ If the child has a wetting episode during this time, begin the 2-week "weaning period" again. Do not be hasty about this phase of the training. Relapse is common when training is cut off prematurely.

ASSESSING

Children with urinary disorders should be assessed for intake and output. Urine should be monitored for amount, color, clarity, odor, and specific gravity. (Normal specific gravity of urine is 1.010 to 1.025.) Assess the abdomen using light palpation to prevent damage to internal organs. Assess the child for signs of dehydration or fluid excess including the presence of edema and monitoring daily weights.

DIAGNOSING, PLANNING, AND IMPLEMENTING

Numerous nursing diagnoses could apply to children with urinary disorders and their families. Nursing diagnoses might include:

- Risk for **I**nfection related to urinary stasis
- Excess **F**luid Volume related to impaired kidney function
- Risk for Deficient **F**luid Volume related to impaired kidney function
- Impaired **U**rinary Elimination related to structural or function impairment of the urinary system

Some outcomes for pediatric clients with urinary disorders might include the following. The client and/or parent will:

- Demonstrate decreased risk factors for infection and will demonstrate appropriate infection prevention measures.
- Verbalize understanding of fluid and dietary restrictions.
- Achieve electrolyte and acid-base balance.
- Have no compromise of urinary elimination.

Nursing interventions follow the general health guidelines presented in previous chapters of this book. Adaptation of interventions with the child is addressed here.

- Encourage children to drink water and a variety of juices daily. Frozen pops and juice can be used to increase fluid intake. *Adequate fluid intake is essential to proper kidney function. Additional fluids may be needed during times of illness, infection, and fever.*
- Follow doctor's orders for fluid restriction in children with urinary disorders. See Procedure 11-3 ⚭ for more information on managing fluid restrictions. *When sodium and water retention are present, fluids should be limited.*
- Administer medications as ordered, such as analgesics and steroids. *Dysuria may make the child reluctant to void. If surgery is needed, the child must be medicated for comfort. Steroids reduce the immune response.*
- Provide instruction to the child and parents about care. Be aware of family strain and refer to RN and social worker as necessary. *The life-threatening nature of urinary disorders contributes to family strain. The long-term effects and treatment contribute to caregiver strain.*
- Provide client teaching concerning signs of infection after surgery (Box 18-5 ■).

BOX 18-5	CLIENT TEACHING

Signs of Infection After Surgery

Teach parents to understand the following signs and symptoms of infection and to report them promptly to the primary care provider. Signs of infection include:

- Increased temperature
- Cloudy urine
- Foul odor from the surgical site
- Purulent drainage
- Decreased feeding
- Increased fussiness

EVALUATING

The child's condition is evaluated by blood and urine analysis, weight loss, and a return of general health. Monitor closely for side effects of medications. The function of the kidneys (or a remaining kidney) must be evaluated frequently. Report any signs of urinary infection or renal failure to the physician immediately. Repeat urine samples may be done after treatment with antibiotics to determine complete eradication of the causative organism.

Because of the strain of acute life-threatening illness on the child and family, frequent evaluation of family functioning is important. Referral to support groups and agencies may be necessary.

NURSING PROCESS CARE PLAN: Child with Nephrotic Syndrome

James, a 22-month-old child, has been admitted to the pediatric unit with a diagnosis of possible nephrotic syndrome. James has gained 2 pounds in the last week and a half. His mother states, "His face is so swollen, I can hardly recognize my own child." Laboratory reports indicate a low blood albumin, and high proteinuria. James is irritable and whines most of the time.

Assessment

- 2+ edema
- Crackling lung sounds
- Pulse 150, Respirations 48

Nursing Diagnosis. The following important nursing diagnosis (among others) is established for this client:

- Excess **F**luid Volume related to altered urinary function

Expected Outcomes

■ Intake and output will be within 100 mL by 3rd hospital day.

Planning and Implementation

■ Measure and record I & O every 8 hours. *Accurate recording of I & O allows for close monitoring of the child's fluid status.*

■ Check output hourly. If no urinary catheter, weigh diapers. *Weighing diapers is a method of monitoring urinary output.*

■ Monitor specific gravity. *Urine specific gravity is a measure of fluid status.*

■ Take daily weights. *Daily weight is a measure of fluid status.*

■ Reposition every ¹/₂ hour. *The child's skin integrity is compromised when fluid status is overloaded.*

■ Anticipate respiratory distress by monitoring breath sounds, respiratory effort, and level of consciousness. *Respiratory distress is associated with fluid overload. The LPN should monitor closely so that appropriate actions can be taken to prevent oxygen deprivation.*

■ Administer IV fluids via appropriate equipment. *Intravenous fluid overload can compromise fluid status and must be monitored closely.*

■ Administer medications with attention to dosage and potential effect on electrolytes and blood protein levels. *The therapeutic effect of medications may be altered in fluid overload.*

Evaluation

■ Review intake and output record, to determine balance.

■ Edema in body will be less than on admission.

■ Lung sounds will be clear.

■ Weight will be same as 2 weeks ago.

Critical Thinking in the Nursing Process

1. Explain the importance of repositioning James every half hour.
2. What information would you obtain from weighing diapers and why is it important?
3. What actions might you take to support James's family during his hospitalization?

Note: Discussion of Critical Thinking questions appears in Appendix I.

REPRODUCTIVE SYSTEM

Anatomy and Physiology

The reproductive system consists of internal and external organs that will, when mature, assist the individual in achieving conception and assist the female in maintaining pregnancy and achieving childbirth. The organs of the male are the penis, scrotum, testes, prostate, and epididymis. These organs function to produce, protect, and transport sperm; regulate hormone production, and provide sexual pleasure later in life.

Female reproductive organs include the ovaries, fallopian tubes, uterus, cervix, vagina, and vulva. These organs function to produce, protect and transport ova, regulate hormone production, and provide sexual pleasure later in life (Figure 18-10 ■). The phases of sexual maturation (called *Tanner's stages*) are described in Table 5-12 ⦾.

Puberty is the maturation process of the reproductive system. At the end of this process, the individual is capable of

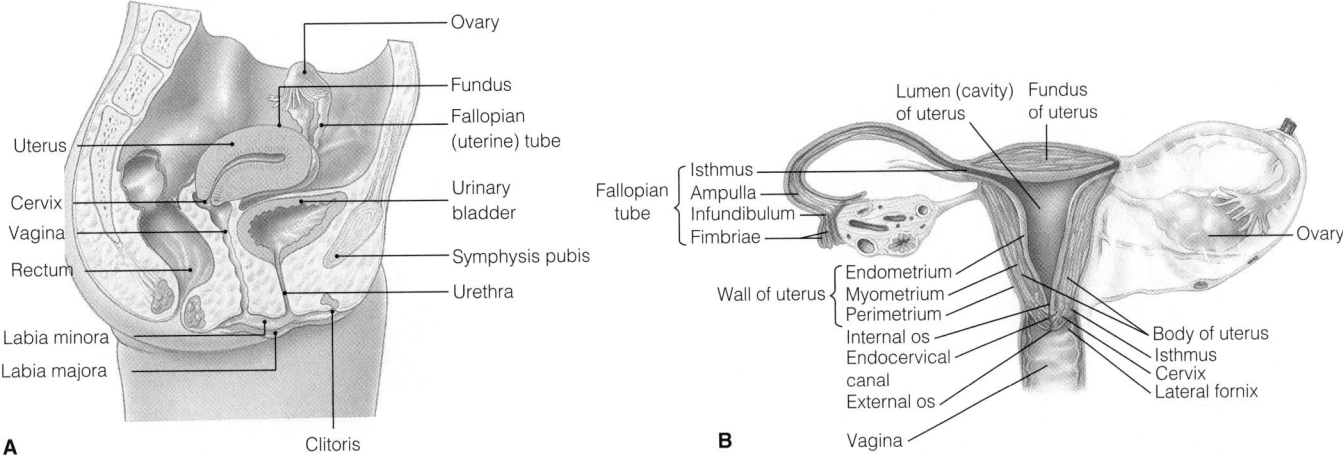

A

B

Figure 18-10. ■ Internal female reproductive structures. (**A**) Cross-section of the female reproductive system. (**B**) Internal organs of the female reproductive system.

reproduction. In males, the onset of puberty occurs between ages 10 and 15. During puberty, the penis, testes, and scrotum enlarge. New hair develops on the face, in the pubic area, and in the axillae. Mature sperm are able to be produced.

In females, the onset of puberty occurs between ages 8 and 13. During puberty, breasts enlarge, menstruation begins, and new hair develops in the pubic area and in the axillae.

Brief Assessment Review

HISTORY

- Ask about family history of reproductive disorders.
- Inquire about redness, swelling, or discharge from the genitalia.
- Ask about burning or itching of the genitalia.
- Inquire about lumps or masses on the child's genitalia.
- For the older child and adolescent, ask about sexual abuse. See Chapter 16 ⟨∞⟩ for a more detailed description of this assessment.

PHYSICAL

- Inspect external genitalia for color, size, hair distribution, lumps or masses, drainage, and symmetry of the organs.
- In males, note placement of the urinary meatus and determine whether the child is circumcised.

Although the reproductive system is immature until puberty, many congenital anomalies of the urinary system also affect the reproductive system as well.

Ambiguous Genitalia

Ambiguous genitalia (**pseudohermaphroditism**) is a rare condition in which it is difficult to determine the sex of the child (Figure 18-11 ■). In this circumstance, chromosomal analysis may be necessary to assist in the determination. Not only is the reproductive system affected, but in many cases, the urinary and intestinal systems are affected as well. Surgical reconstruction is usually done in stages, with the primary goal being normal functioning of the urinary and intestinal systems. Depending on the degree of defect, reproductive function may be lost.

Male Disorders

HYDROCELE

Hydrocele (Figure 18-12 ■) is the accumulation of fluid in the scrotum. During fetal development, fluid becomes trapped in the tunica vaginalis. When the scrotum is

Figure 18-11. ■ Newborn girl with ambiguous genitalia. (Courtesy of Patrick C. Walsh, MD.)

palpated, a round, smooth, and nontender mass is noted. The scrotal sac can also be *transilluminated* (have a light shone through it) to detect the presence of fluid. Most hydroceles resolve spontaneously in the first 2 years of life. The nurse should assist the family in understanding this disorder. Parents may also be concerned that the enlargement of the scrotum is permanent. The nurse should provide teaching about the probable spontaneous resolution of the condition.

PHIMOSIS

Phimosis is the inability to retract the foreskin of the penis due to a tightened prepuce. At birth, the infant's foreskin is not retractable because of adhesions. As the child grows, retraction of the foreskin should occur. Complications of phimosis include difficulty with urination, **balanoposthitis** (inflammation or infection of the glans penis), and **paraphimosis** (the inability to return the foreskin over the glans, causing constriction of the penis).

Figure 18-12. ■ Hydrocele is a nontender, fluid-filled mass within the tunica vaginalis.

Phimosis is treated surgically by *circumcision* (the removal of the foreskin). Circumcision in the older child can be traumatic and painful. The nurse can assist with anxiety-reducing techniques in the preoperative period.

Circumcision

Circumcision is the surgical removal of the foreskin (*prepuce*) of the penis. Table 18-6 ■ identifies the advantages and disadvantages of circumcision. Parents should make an informed decision prior to signing the consent form. Only full-term infants should be circumcised.

Before the procedure begins, an informed consent must be signed. The infant is kept NPO for several hours. The infant is restrained on a circumcision board and a blanket should be placed over the infant's chest to prevent heat loss. At this point, the infant frequently begins to cry because he is being held in extension. The physician may administer a local anesthetic in the form of an injection or cream. The physician then makes a slit in the prepuce and uses a Yellen (Gomco) clamp or Plastibell (Figure 18-13 ■) to control bleeding. The prepuce is then cut off. The Gomco clamp will be left in place for 5 minutes to ensure bleeding has stopped; it is then removed. When the Gomco clamp is used, vitamin A and D ointment or petroleum jelly may be applied to the penis to prevent the glans from sticking to the diaper. Ointment is not applied when the Plastibell is used. The Plastibell will fall off in 5 to 8 days.

After circumcision, the penis should be checked for bleeding at least every hour for 12 hours. If bleeding occurs, pressure should be applied with sterile 4 × 4 cotton gauze until bleeding stops. If bleeding cannot be controlled, the charge nurse and physician should be notified. The penis should be washed with warm water with each diaper change. Parents should be instructed to be alert for signs of infection until the circumcision has healed in 7 to 9 days.

TESTICULAR TORSION

If the spermatic cord becomes twisted, a condition called testicular torsion occurs (Figure 18-14 ■). This condition may occur in newborns, but more commonly occurs in early

Figure 18-13. ■ Circumcision using the *Plastibell*. The bell is fitted over the glans. A suture is tied around the bell's rim, and the excess prepuce is cut away. The plastic rim remains in place for 3 to 4 days until healing occurs. The bell may be allowed to fall off. It is removed if it is still in place after 8 days.

adolescence. The young male experiences intense scrotal pain accompanied by nausea and vomiting. Because ischemia develops quickly, surgical correction is necessary within 4 hours of the onset of symptoms.

CRYPTORCHIDISM

Cryptorchidism (undescended testicle) is a condition in which one or both of the testicles fail to descend into the scrotum. Descent of the testes may occur in utero or may take place by the time the infant is 3 months old. Cryptorchidism can occur as a result of lower testosterone levels or structural defect, such as a shortened spermatic cord.

Diagnosis

Diagnosis of cryptorchidism is made by physical examination and confirmed by ultrasound, CT scan, or MRI. At birth, the infant is screened for cryptorchidism by using the Ballard Gestational Assessment Scale. See Appendix II ⬳ to review

TABLE 18-6	
Advantages and Disadvantages of Circumcision	
ADVANTAGES	**DISADVANTAGES**
Religious conviction	Varied evidence of medical benefit
Culture	Painful procedure
Social norm	Risk of bleeding
Hygiene	Risk of infection

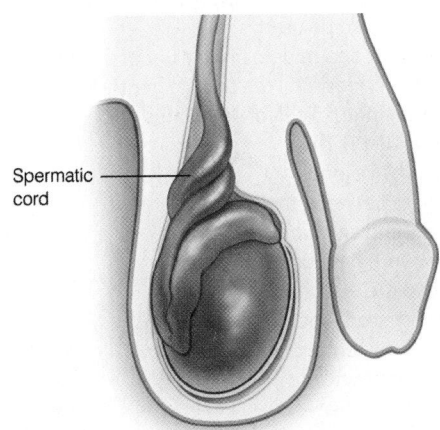

Spermatic cord

Figure 18-14. ■ Testicular torsion occurs most frequently in adolescents. It requires immediate surgical intervention.

this assessment tool. Findings of undescended testicles at birth require follow-up examinations.

Treatment

Medical treatment of cryptorchidism includes administration of human chorionic gonadotrophin, although this treatment is not widely accepted in America. Prior to age 2, a surgical procedure called an *orchiopexy* may be performed to reposition the testicle into the scrotal sac. Children with cyrptorchidism have a 35 to 50 times greater risk of testicular cancer. These children should be taught the technique of testicular self-examination (Box 18-6 ■ and Figure 18-15 ■).

TESTICULAR CANCER

Testicular cancer is the most common cancer of men between 15 and 35 years of age. Fortunately, testicular cancer has a greater than 90% cure rate. Most men with testicular cancer have no risk factors. Therefore, beginning at 15 years of age, all men should perform testicular self-exam.

Testicular cancer grows within the testicle, eventually replacing all normal tissue. Normal tissue will feel soft, whereas the tumor will be a hard, painless mass. Most commonly, only one testicle is affected. Testicular cancer spreads rapidly through the lymph vessels into the retroperitoneal lymph nodes (located behind the peritoneum but outside the abdominal/pelvic cavity). Enlarged

lymph nodes may be palpated in the groin. If the cancer cells reach the vascular system, they commonly metastasize to the lungs, liver, and bone.

Treatment usually involves a radical **orchiectomy** (removal of one testis and spermatic cord) with removal of the retroperitoneal lymph nodes. The surgery is accomplished through an inguinal incision, taking care not to damage the nerves needed for ejaculation. Following surgery, radiation and chemotherapy are used to destroy any remaining cancer cells. If only one testicle is removed, reproduction may still be possible. However, the banking of sperm prior to surgery, radiation, and chemotherapy should be discussed with the client and his partner, if appropriate. If the client is a minor, teaching and support must also be provided to the parents.

EPIDIDYMITIS AND ORCHITIS

An infection of the male reproductive system may result in epididymitis (inflammation of the epididymis) and orchitis (inflammation of the testes). In young men, the infection is most commonly caused by sexually transmitted infections (STIs) such as chlamydia or gonorrhea.

Manifestations of epididymitis include pain and swelling of the scrotum, at times interfering with ambulation. Medical treatment includes antibiotics and analgesics. Nursing care focuses on relieving symptoms with ice packs and scrotal support. Epididymitis can cause infertility and should be evaluated after the infection is resolved.

Orchitis may be caused by the same organisms as epididymitis, as well as by a mumps virus that is excreted in the urine, or by trauma. Manifestations include severe testicular pain and swelling. Complications include hydrocele and testicular abscess. These complications can result in infertility and erectile dysfunction.

Sexually Transmitted Infections

Sexually transmitted infections (STIs; also called sexually transmitted diseases or STDs) result from sexual contact with an infected person. Many people believe that sexual intercourse is necessary for an STI to develop. The reality is that infection can occur not only through sexual intercourse, but also through genital-genital, oral-genital, or rectal-genital contact. The most common STIs are chlamydia, genital herpes, gonorrhea, genital warts, trichomoniasis, and syphilis. Table 18-7 ■ lists these common infections, their manifestations, and their medical treatment.

CHLAMYDIA

Chlamydia is an infectious disease caused by *Chlamydia trachomatis*. In males, chlamydia is the major cause of nongonorrhea urethritis. In females, it infects the vagina, cervix, uterus, fallopian tubes, and urethra. The infection

---

BOX 18-6

Testicular Self Examination

Testicular self-examination is important for all males age 15 to 35, but especially for the young man with a history of cryptorchidism. Young men should choose a day of the week, perhaps their birthday, and examine the testicles in the following manner every month.

■ Examination can be done in front of a mirror or in the shower.

■ Lubrication makes the skin around the testicle move more easily. In the shower, soap is appropriate. Outside of the shower, lotion can be used.

■ Place the index and middle fingers under the testicle with thumbs on top. Roll the testicle gently between the thumbs and fingers. Feel for any lumps or masses (see Figure 18-15). This should not be painful.

■ Differentiate between the epididymis and any lumps. The epididymis lies above and behind the testicle. It is soft and smooth and may be slightly tender.

■ Contact your physician promptly if any masses, lumps, or unexpected pain or tenderness are noted.

Figure 18-15.

TABLE 18-7

Summary of Sexually Transmitted Infections

DISEASE	ORGANISM	MANIFESTATIONS	MEDICAL TREATMENT
Chlamydia	*Chlamydia trachomatis*	Males: urethritis Females: permanent scarring	Erythromycin Amoxicillin
Genital herpes	Herpes simplex virus (HSV-2)	Burning, itching sensation prior to blister formation; blisters break, resulting in painful open lesions	Acyclovir
Gonorrhea	*Neisseria gonorrhoeae*	Females: asymptomatic, permanent scarring Males: urethritis, purulent urethral drainage, burning on urination	Ceftriaxone Cefixime with erythromycin or amoxicillin
Genital warts (condylomata acuminata)	Human papillomavirus (HPV)	Grayish-pink cauliflowerlike lesions appear on the vulva or penis approximately 3 weeks after exposure	Cryotherapy Trichloroacetic acid
Trichomoniasis	*Trichomonas vaginalis*	Inflammation of the vagina and cervix, yellow-green, frothy, odorous discharge	Metronidazole *Note for pregnant adolescent:* Metronidazole (Flagyl) is contraindicated in the first trimester of pregnancy because of the teratogenic effects on the fetus.
Syphilis	*Treponema pallidum*	Stage 1: painless open sore, chancre, slight fever, and malaise Stage 2: fine red rash over the body, palms, and soles Stage 3: damage to heart, nervous system, bone, and skin Aneurysm, gait disturbances, blindness, dementia	Benzathine Penicillin G

can be passed to the newborn during the birth process, resulting in eye infection and pneumonia. Complications include pelvic inflammatory disease, scarring of the fallopian tubes, and ectopic pregnancy. The newborn of an infected untreated woman is at risk for developing ophthalmia neonatorum. In men, chlamydia can cause scarring of the urethral mucosa.

GONORRHEA

Gonorrhea is caused by *Neisseria gonorrhoeae*. In males, gonorrhea is associated with urethritis, purulent urethral drainage, and burning on urination. Females are usually asymptomatic. Prior to pregnancy, gonorrhea can ascend through the cervix and infect the uterus, the fallopian tubes, and the pelvis. After the 3rd month of pregnancy, the cervical mucous plug prevents gonorrhea from ascending into these organs. When the fetal membranes rupture during the birth process, gonorrhea can infect the infant's eyes and respiratory tract.

As with chlamydia, gonorrheal infection of the reproductive organs can lead to permanent scarring of the fallopian tubes and seminiferous tubules. The scarring may result in infertility.

Chlamydia and gonorrhea are commonly found together. Adequate treatment of both partners is essential to cure the infections. Abstinence or condom use is needed to prevent reinfection until cure is achieved. Further cultures must be taken to verify that treatment was successful.

SYPHILIS

Syphilis is an infection by the bacteria *Treponema pallidum*. Syphilis is divided into three stages with very different symptoms at each stage.

- Primary syphilis: Initially, a **chancre** (painless open sore) forms at the entry site (Figure 18-16A ■). General signs of infection, including slight fever and malaise, may occur. If left untreated, the chancre disappears in 3 to 4 weeks.

Figure 18-16. ■ Some sexually transmitted infections. (**A**) Primary syphilis. The entry point of syphilis develops a chancre. (**B**) Genital herpes blisters on the penile shaft signal the infectious phase. (**C**) Condylomata acuminata (*genital warts*) on the labia. (**A**: Custom Medical Stock Photo. **B**: Camera MD Studios, Carroll Weiss, Director, 8290 NW 26th Place, Sunrise, FL 33322. **C**: Ken Greer Visuals Unlimited.)

■ Secondary syphilis: Several months later, the symptoms of secondary syphilis appear. These include a fine red rash over the body, palms, and soles of the feet. Highly infectious moist papules may appear on the perineum. If untreated, these symptoms will also disappear in a few weeks. Symptoms of infection may not recur for many years.

■ Tertiary syphilis: In the tertiary stage, damage to the heart, nervous system, bone, and skin become apparent. Aneurysm, gait disturbances, blindness, and dementia are a few disorders that can result from untreated syphilis.

GENITAL HERPES

Herpes is caused by one of two types of herpes simplex virus (HSV). HSV-1 causes cold sores and typically occurs above the waist. HSV-1 is not sexually transmitted. HSV-2 is associated with sexual contact. The symptoms include a burning, itching sensation prior to blister formation (Figure 18-16B). The blisters break and result in painful open lesions. Many viruses are shed at this time, and an infection is highly contagious. Lesions heal spontaneously in several weeks.

Genital herpes results in lifelong health problems that will affect future partners as well. For example, during an acute outbreak, the couple should abstain from sexual intercourse. If a pregnant woman has an acute outbreak and goes into labor, a cesarean section delivery should be performed to prevent infection of the infant.

GENITAL WARTS

Genital warts (or *condylomata acuminata*) are caused by the human papillomavirus (HPV). There are more than 100 varieties of the virus with five of them being sexually transmitted. The grayish-pink cauliflowerlike lesions appear on the vulva (Figure 18-16C) or penis approximately 3 weeks

to 9 months after exposure. Because genital warts resemble other lesions and can undergo malignant transformation, they should be biopsied and treated. Some strains of HPV are associated with cancer of the cervix. A new vaccine has been recently approved to prevent cervical cancer related to HPV. Box 18-7 ■ describes the vaccine approved for prevention of some strains of HPV.

TRICHOMONIASIS

Trichomoniasis, caused by the protozoan *Trichomonas vaginalis*, is most commonly transmitted through sexual contact. It can also be transmitted through shared bath

---

BOX 18-7

Vaccine for Prevention of Cervical Cancer

In 2006 the Center for Disease Control and the Food and Drug Administration announced a recommendation that the vaccine Gardasil can prevent transmission of HPV and therefore serve as a preventative measure against cervical cancer. Gardasil protects against four types of HPV: two causing cervical cancer and two causing genital warts. Studies show that this vaccine is most effective when used in females prior to initiation of sexual activity. The CDC's Advisory Committee for Immunization Practices recommends the routine vaccination of 11- to 12-year-old girls.

The three series inactivated, recombinant vaccine is given intramuscularly initially and then repeated 2 months and 6 months later. The dosage of Gardasil is 0.5 mL. Current cost of the vaccine is $120 per dose.

Source: Data from Schmidt, J. (2007). HPV vaccine: Implications for nurse and patients. *Nursing for Women's Health, 11*(1), 83–87. CDC. (2006). *Human papillomavirus (HPV), cervical cancer, and HPV vaccine and recommendations: A Current Issues in Immunization NetConference* (Course number EV0378). Retrieved April 27, 2007; Frazer, I., Cox, J., Mayeaux, E., France, E., Moscicki, A., Palefsky, J., et al. (2006). Advances in prevention of cervical cancer and other human papillomavirus–related diseases. *Pediatric Infectious Disease Journal, 25*(2), S65–81.

facilities, wet towels, and wet swimwear. Symptoms in women include inflammation of the vagina and cervix as well as a yellow-green, frothy, odorous discharge. In men, trichomoniasis causes burning on urination due to urethral irritation. The treatment consists of administration of metronidazole (Flagyl) to all partners. Flagyl is contraindicated in the first trimester of pregnancy, because it acts as a **teratogen** (a chemical that can cause abnormal fetal development). Clotrimazole vaginal suppositories are used to provide symptomatic relief during the first 12 weeks of pregnancy, and then Flagyl can be given.

HUMAN IMMUNODEFICIENCY VIRUS AND ACQUIRED IMMUNODEFICIENCY SYNDROME (HIV/AIDS)

Human immunodeficiency virus (HIV) is a retrovirus that attacks and destroys the body's immune system. The method of transmission is by direct contact with body fluids. **Acquired immunodeficiency syndrome** (AIDS) is life-threatening, end-stage infection with HIV. Although HIV is being treated with increased success, HIV infection is still considered fatal. The main HIV/AIDS discussion is in Chapter 22 in this book. Refer to an adult medical-surgical textbook for further information.

CANDIDIASIS

Candidiasis (**monilia** or **yeast infection**) is a common organism causing vaginitis. Characteristics of a yeast infection are thick white areas of discharge resembling cottage cheese that adhere to the cervix, vaginal wall, and labia. There is intense itching of the vulva and vagina. The mucous membrane is red and inflamed. When a specimen is viewed under the microscope, *hyphae* (threadlike filaments) and spores may be seen.

Treatment includes medicated creams, vaginal tablets, or suppositories. The sexual partner should be treated as well, because *Candida* can grow under the foreskin and on the glans and outer skin of the penis.

Female Disorders

Routine care of female clients related to the reproductive system begins in the pediatrician or family practice office setting. Adolescent girls may decide to seek the care of a gynecologist, nurse practitioner, or certified nurse midwife. Regular gynecologic examinations often start during late adolescence or when the girl becomes sexually active. Nursing care involves sensitivity to the embarrassment or fear the client might feel when approaching a gynecologic exam. The Health Promotion Issue on pages 506 and 507 addresses this topic.

IMPERFORATE HYMEN

The **hymen** is the mucous membrane, skin, and fibrous tissue that covers the introitus of the vagina at birth. An *imperforate hymen* is a hymen that does not allow passage of vaginal secretions or menses. The female child may have no symptoms until the onset of puberty. Obstruction of menses increases uterine pressure and results in abdominal discomfort and distension.

The hymen may be removed surgically. Young girls will need information related to their anatomy. They will also need reassurance that this condition will not affect their future sexuality or childbearing.

FEMALE CIRCUMCISION

Female circumcision is a surgical procedure performed on young girls for cultural purposes rather than medical ones. In some cultures, this procedure may be performed on infants as young as 1 day old, whereas in other settings, it may be performed on the adolescent or young adult woman. Three types of female circumcision are typically seen:

- *Sunna* is the excision of part or all of the clitoris.
- The second type is the excision of the entire clitoris and the labia minora. Following this type of circumcision, the edges of the labia minora are sewn together.
- *Infibulation* is the third type of female circumcision. In this procedure the entire clitoris and labia minora are excised and the labia majora is scraped. The edges are then sewn together leaving only a small opening for urination and menstruation.

This cultural norm in some African, Asian, and Middle Eastern societies is said to be done to control a woman's sexuality, ensure her virginity until marriage, ensure expected cultural role is maintained, protect her from rape, enhance feminine hygiene, and as a religious ritual (Reichert, 1998).

Girls who have this surgical procedure are at risk for hemorrhage, pain, and infection. Psychological complications include anxiety, depression, and frigidity. Intercourse is painful if possible at all. Vaginal childbirth may not be possible either.

Nurses should learn about the practice of female circumcision, especially among the population they serve. Children who present with symptoms of complications from female circumcision should be treated with dignity and respect. For the child to be able to talk about her feelings related to her body, she must to be able to trust the nurse. The child and her family need to be educated about the possible complications of this practice.

MENSTRUAL DISORDERS

As puberty begins, adolescent girls may develop menstrual disorders. It can be helpful for the girl who is just beginning to menstruate to discuss what menstruation is and

(Text continues on p. 508.)

HEALTH PROMOTION ISSUE

ASSISTING THE YOUNG TEEN WITH HER FIRST PAP SMEAR

Seventeen-year-old Dana presents to the family planning clinic requesting birth control pills. She had a baby 18 months ago and states that she does not want to be pregnant again. She is accompanied by her mother and her toddler son, Gray.

The LPN takes Dana's history. Dana has been sexually active since she was 14 years old. She has never used any form of birth control, including condoms, and has had at least five sexual partners. Dana states that she has never had a Pap smear and confesses that she does not really know what one is. She says that her friend told her that it was painful and that she should never have one.

Dana says that she is afraid of having a Pap smear. She just wants the nurse practitioner to give her a prescription for birth control pills because she needs to go to work.

The LPN and nurse practitioner review Dana's history and discuss her situation. It is determined that a Pap smear is indicated based on her past medical history. Together, they devise a teaching plan to help Dana understand the importance of this procedure.

DISCUSSION

The Papanicolaou test, commonly called the Pap smear, is a screen for cervical cancer. A physician, nurse practitioner, nurse midwife, or physician's assistant will take a small sample of cervical cells, which are sent to the laboratory for examination. Prior to becoming cancer, cervical cells go through cellular changes. The Pap smear is designed to detect these cervical cellular changes prior to their becoming cancerous.

According to the American Cancer Society and the American College of Obstetricians and Gynecologists, a woman should have her first Pap smear at age 21 or within 3 years of becoming sexually active, whichever comes first. These recommendations were made based on the risk of cervical cancer to this age group. The most common cause of cervical cancer is infection with the human papillomavirus (HPV). This virus is most often transmitted sexually. The Pap smear can detect infection with HPV. Other risk factors for developing cervical cancer include smoking, having multiple partners (more than two), having sexual intercourse before age 18, having sexual intercourse with males who have multiple partners, and infection with sexually transmitted infections, including HIV.

The Pap smear is part of a complete gynecologic examination. The comprehensive examination can include, but is not limited to, personal and family medical history, weight measurement, urinalysis, hematocrit and hemoglobin check, blood pressure check, auscultation of heart and lungs, an abdominal exam, a breast exam, teaching about breast self-exam, a pelvic exam, and evaluation for contraception or conception readiness.

Prior to the Pap smear, the client must completely disrobe below the waist. The LPN will supply a disposable gown and drape. The client is placed in a private room and a chaperone, usually the nurse, is provided for the client's comfort and to assist the practitioner.

Most examination tables are covered with disposable paper. Tables are padded and have stirrups to support the woman's feet. Stirrups are metal and can be cold. The woman can wear socks to be more comfortable.

The practitioner uses a vaginal speculum to separate the vaginal walls and visualize the cervix. The nurse can position an examination light toward the perineum and apply water-soluble lubricant to ease insertion of the speculum. The speculum can be made of plastic or metal. Both the speculum and the lubricant can be prewarmed to promote comfort.

A small wooden spatula, plastic scraper, cotton swab, or brush is used by the practitioner to obtain cervical cells. The cells are then placed on a glass slide and may be sprayed or mixed with a fixative agent. The nurse is usually responsible for properly preparing, labeling, and processing the specimen and then sending it to the lab.

Most results from the Pap smear are available within 1 to 2 weeks. The clinic may send postcards through the mail for negative results. Clients are usually called when positive results are determined, meaning that abnormal cervical cells were identified. This positive result is classified as cervical inflammation or irritation. It may be caused by an infection; dysplasia; or early signs of cancers, carcinoma *in situ* (cancer cells detected only in the top layer of the cervix), or advanced cervical cancer.

PLANNING AND IMPLEMENTATION

The LPN and nurse practitioner understand that a woman's first experience with a Pap smear will affect her approach to this vital health screening for the rest of her life. Dana has expressed fear of the procedure and a lack of knowledge about its importance. Typical emotions that accompany the first Pap smear are anxiety, fear of finding cancer or other health issues, fear of pain, and embarrassment.

The LPN decides to discuss Dana's concerns with her first. She asks Dana to tell her about her fears regarding the Pap smear. Dana states that she is embarrassed and afraid that the nurse practitioner will think she has not kept herself clean enough. Dana asks if she can come back when she has recently used a vaginal douche. The LPN tells Dana that using douches or other feminine hygiene products can actually make the test invalid.

The nurse asks Dana the date of her last menstrual period. Dana does not understand why that matters. The nurse explains that having her period during the Pap smear also interferes with the test results. Dana states that her last menstrual period was 2 weeks ago.

Dana is still concerned about the discomfort she may experience during the Pap smear. The nurse explains the procedure step by step and answers Dana's questions carefully and patiently. The nurse is careful not to tell Dana that there will be no discomfort, but she does give her some suggestions for making the procedure less uncomfortable. She teaches Dana simple deep abdominal breathing. She also shows Dana which muscles are most likely to become tense and gives her some suggestions for releasing the tension in these muscles.

Dana is also concerned about bleeding after the procedure. Her friend reported that she bled heavily for several days. The nurse explains to Dana that a small amount of vaginal spotting is common for several hours after the Pap smear. There may be a need to wear a panty liner to protect her clothes, but the spotting should go away by the next morning. The nurse tells Dana that if she is still spotting the next morning or if there is bleeding heavier than spotting, she should call the clinic and report these symptoms.

The nurse has also assessed that Dana needs some further teaching. After the nurse validates that Dana has an understanding of the indications and results, she discusses with Dana the risks of her unprotected sexual activity.

Because the LPN and the nurse practitioner accurately assessed Dana's emotional and physical needs, Dana consented to the Pap smear. The procedure was performed easily by the nurse practitioner with the assistance of the LPN. Dana's need for birth control and protection from sexually transmitted infections was discussed, and she left the clinic after receiving an injection of Depo and several samples of condoms. The LPN made a follow-up appointment for Dana in 1 month.

SELF-REFLECTION

At what age did you have your first Pap smear? What was the indication for this procedure? Try to remember your feelings before, during, and after the Pap smear. Do you remember the nurse assisting with this procedure? Did he or she assess your emotional response to the procedure?

SUGGESTED RESOURCES

For the Nurse

Condon, M. (2004). *Women's health: Body, mind, spirit: An integrated approach to wellness and illness.* Upper Saddle River, NJ: Prentice Hall.

Lichtman, R. (2005). *Gynecology: Well-woman care* (2nd ed.). Upper Saddle River, NJ: Prentice Hall.

Varney Burst, H. (2004). *Varney's midwifery* (4th ed.). Sudbury, MA: Jones and Bartlett.

Youngkin, E., & Davis, M. (2004). *Women's health: A primary care clinical guide* (3rd ed.). Upper Saddle River, NJ: Prentice Hall.

For the Client

Greydanus, D. (2003). *American Academy of Pediatrics: Caring for your teenager.* New York: Bantam.

Lopez, R. I. (2003). *The teen health book: A parent's guide to adolescent health and well-being.* New York: W. W. Norton & Company.

Reisser, P. (2002). *Teen health guide.* Colorado Springs, CO: Focus on the Family.

TABLE 18-8

Communicating Across the Life Span: Preparing the Female Child for Menstruation

	TODDLER	PRESCHOOLER	SCHOOL-AGE CHILD	ADOLESCENT
Nurse	To the parent: "So that menses are not such a shock to your daughter, you can begin now to use the correct anatomical terms for the female body. For example, your child should be told that mommies have babies in their uterus, not in their tummies."	To the parent: "When you shop with your child, give a brief explanation of the use of the feminine products you are purchasing."	To the child: "Have you noticed any changes in your body? Pretty soon there will be changes that mean you are changing from a child into a young woman. There is a fun class at the hospital next Saturday that will help you learn more."	To the teen: "Now that your menstrual cycle has begun, it is important to keep a good record of when your period begins, how long it lasts, and how you feel during it. This information will help you and your primary care provider make decisions regarding your future health."
Parent/Client	"So I should use terms like vagina, uterus, and cervix?"	"Should I say something like, 'Mommy uses these pads once a month when she has her period or bleeds from her vagina. Every Mommy has a period. It doesn't mean I'm sick. It means my body is healthy.'"	"I don't feel as pudgy any more and sometimes my stomach hurts right here. Can my mom come to the class with me?"	"I don't want anybody else to see on my calendar that I've started my period. Maybe I could use symbols on my calendar to indicate when my period starts and when it stops."

what symptoms may be associated with it. Table 18-8 ■ provides some ways of communicating with girls who are at *menarche*. Menstruation may be painful (*dysmenorrhea*), or menstrual cycles may be irregular. Dysmenorrhea is due to the release of prostaglandins during the menstrual cycle, and it accompanies ovulatory cycles. Prostaglandin inhibitors such as ibuprofen are an effective treatment for dysmenorrhea. Nonpharmacologic pain relief methods for dysmenorrhea include a low-sodium diet to reduce bloating, heat application to the lower abdomen and back, rest, and exercise.

Adolescents can experience *metrorrhagia* or bleeding between menstrual cycles. Some young girls may spot during ovulation or experience breakthrough bleeding if they are on oral contraceptives. Vaginal irritation such as vaginitis may also cause bleeding. Any bleeding between periods that is not associated with these explanations should be reported to the physician, because it may be a sign of uterine cancer or ovarian cysts.

Amenorrhea (the absence of menses) can occur in the adolescent who is under severe stress, has a chronic illness, is dieting extremely, or is exercising strenuously. Amenorrhea is also a sign of pregnancy.

Premenstrual syndrome (PMS) is also a menstrual disorder that often affects teens. PMS is caused by estrogen and progesterone imbalance and increased prolactin and aldosterone levels. Rising aldosterone causes sodium and water retention. Manifestations include irritability, depression, edema, and breast tenderness that occurs prior to the start of the menstrual cycle each month. The manifestations of multisystem effects of PMS (Figure 18-17 ■) vary for each client.

Management of PMS focuses on diet, exercise, and relaxation techniques to reduce stress. A diet high in complex carbohydrates with limited simple sugars and alcohol is recommended. Restricting caffeine may reduce irritability. Limiting salt intake is useful in reducing fluid retention. An increased intake of calcium, magnesium, and vitamin B_6 may be helpful. A balance between exercise and rest can also help reduce irritability. Relaxation techniques and stress management include muscle relaxation, deep abdominal breathing, guided imagery, and meditation.

VAGINITIS

Vaginitis is inflammation of the vagina. Vaginal irritation may be caused by the insertion of foreign objects, infection with *Streptococcus* or *Escherichia coli*, infestation of pinworms, or chemical irritation from hygiene products such as douches, soaps, and perfumes. It may also be caused by *Candida albicans* (often appearing when a girl becomes sexually active) or trichomoniasis (the most frequently diagnosed STI). Sexual abuse must also be ruled out when a child or adolescent presents with vaginitis. For more

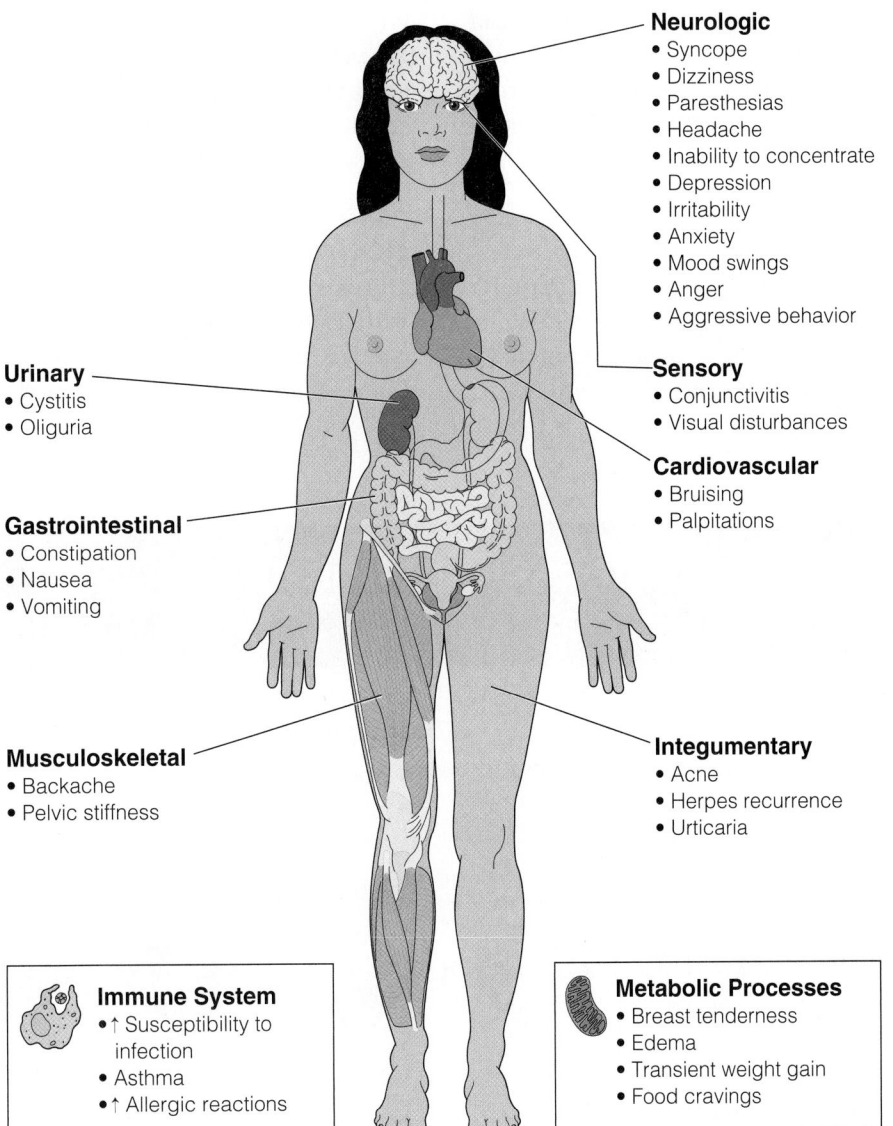

Neurologic
- Syncope
- Dizziness
- Paresthesias
- Headache
- Inability to concentrate
- Depression
- Irritability
- Anxiety
- Mood swings
- Anger
- Aggressive behavior

Sensory
- Conjunctivitis
- Visual disturbances

Cardiovascular
- Bruising
- Palpitations

Urinary
- Cystitis
- Oliguria

Gastrointestinal
- Constipation
- Nausea
- Vomiting

Musculoskeletal
- Backache
- Pelvic stiffness

Integumentary
- Acne
- Herpes recurrence
- Urticaria

Immune System
- ↑ Susceptibility to infection
- Asthma
- ↑ Allergic reactions

Metabolic Processes
- Breast tenderness
- Edema
- Transient weight gain
- Food cravings

Figure 18-17. ■ Multisystem effect of premenstrual syndrome (PMS).

information on caring for the child who has experienced sexual abuse, see Chapter 16 ⬭.

Manifestations

The client with vaginitis may complain of pruritus, pain, and vaginal discharge or bleeding. Discharge may have a foul odor.

Diagnosis

An examination of the child's external genitalia and collection of a specimen of the vaginal discharge is necessary. These specimens are collected by an advanced practice nurse or the physician. The LPN may be responsible for preparing the specimen for observation under the microscope.

Treatment

The drug of choice for *Candida albicans* is Nystatin ointment. Miconazole (Monistat) may also be ordered and administered as a vaginal suppository. For trichomoniasis, metronidazole (Flagyl) is often ordered.

Nursing Considerations

The nurse can help the young girl avoid contact vaginitis by teaching her to wipe her perineum from front to back, therefore avoiding infestation of the vagina with harmful bacteria from the rectum. The nurse can also discourage the use of bubble baths and feminine hygiene products such as douches or sprays. The nurse can encourage daily cleansing of the perineum with warm water and mild soap, as well as frequent changes of tampons and sanitary pads during

MediaLink   Premenstrual Syndrome

menstruation. Caution young girls that wet clothes can cause vaginal irritation. Wet swimsuits and exercise clothing should be removed promptly. Teach girls that cotton underwear absorbs moisture more effectively than synthetic materials.

Breast Disorders

Breast disorders may be detected by the woman during a monthly breast self-exam (BSE), during a physical examination by the primary care provider, or by **mammography** (diagnostic x-ray of the breast). Because early detection is

critical to the treatment of malignancy, adolescents should be taught the BSE technique (Procedure 18-1 ■) and encouraged to seek annual physical examination. Adolescents should also be taught the importance of the mammogram as a screening tool later in life.

NONMALIGNANT BREAST DISORDERS

Fibrosis is the replacement of inflamed or damaged tissue with connective or scar tissue. In the breast the result is a painless encapsulated tumor or fibroid. Frequently the fibroid degenerates, accumulating fluid in the process. This

---

PROCEDURE 18-1 Breast Self-Examination

Purpose

- To provide instruction in monthly self-examination of the breasts
- To identify abnormalities in the breast tissue

Equipment

- Mirror
- Small pillow or folded towel

Check order + Gather equipment + Introduce yourself + Identify client + Provide privacy + Explain procedure + Hand hygiene + Gloves as needed

Interventions and Rationales

1. Perform preparatory steps (see icon bar above).

2. Instruction is provided by demonstration, return demonstration, and written material. *Showing the client what to do and then watching her return the demonstration ensures proper technique. Written material is a useful reference when at home.*

3. Stand in front of a mirror in good light with both breasts exposed. *Standing in front of a mirror with good light provides the opportunity to visually inspect all areas of the breast.*

4. Observe the breasts individually for lumps, dimpling, deviation, recent nipple retraction, irregular shape, edema, or discharge. Compare the right and left breast for symmetry. *Tissue should be consistent throughout the breast. Inconsistent tissue could indicate abnormalities.*

5. Observe the breasts in these positions. *Changing position allows for adequate inspection.*
   - With her arms relaxed at her sides
   - With her arms lifted over her head

- With her hands pressed against her hips
- With her hands pressed together at her waist and leaning forward

6. While sitting or standing in the shower, place one hand behind the head. Use the finger pads of the other hand to palpate the breast, moving in small, dime-sized circles. *Soap and water make the skin slick and decrease discomfort.*

7. Palpate the area from the collarbone to below the breasts, and from the middle of the armpit to the breastbone (Figure 18-18 ■). Gently press the breast tissue against the chest wall, feeling for lumps or thickening of the tissue. *This pattern ensures that areas of the breast are examined.*

8. Repeat on the other side.

9. Position the body supine with a small pillow or folded towel under one shoulder. Place the arm on that side under the head. *In this position, gravity pulls the breast into a different position, allowing for more complete examination.*

Move the hand vertically down and up across the breasts, starting at the axilla and working toward the center of the body. Press with the finger-pads in small, dime-sized circles to feel the chest wall.

Repeat the same procedure sitting up with your hand still behind your head.

Figure 18-18. ■ **(A)** Check each breast using the pads of the fingers, feeling all parts of the breast. **(B)** While holding one hand behind the head, palpate the breast.

10. Using the pads of the fingers, palpate the breast again as in steps 6 and 7. Move down and up across the breast, starting at the axilla (see Figure 18-18A).

11. Repeat on the other side.

12. Palpate the areola and the nipple. Compress the nipple between the thumb and finger to check for discharge. *Gently compressing the nipple forces any drainage from the lactiferous duct.*

13. Use a calendar to record when BSE was performed. BSE should be performed once a month, usually on the fifth day after onset of menses. *Recording when BSE was performed is a useful reminder of when to do the next BSE as well as providing documentation should abnormalities occur. On the fifth day after menses begins, the breast tissue has the least hormonal influence.*

14. Report any lumps, dimpling, asymmetry, or discharge to the primary health care provider.

SAMPLE DOCUMENTATION

(date/time)   Instruction in BSE provided. Return demonstration indicates appropriate technique. Written material provided. _____
C. Downey, LPN

fluid-filled mass or **fibrocyst** puts pressure on surrounding tissue and becomes painful. Commonly, more than one fibrocyst forms in each breast, resulting in breast irregularities or "lumpiness." Occasionally the cyst will drain onto the nipple.

Fibrocystic breast disease is most common in women between 30 and 50 years of age; however, teaching the adolescent girl about the disease may aid detection later in life. Fibrocystic changes in the breast are an excessive response to cyclic hormonal changes. After menopause, these breast changes usually decrease. If cell growth occurs in conjunction with cyst formation, the woman is at a greater risk for breast cancer. Oral intake of caffeine found in coffee, tea, cola, and chocolate may contribute to fibrocystic breast disease. Medical management of fibrocystic breast disease focuses on diagnosis, screening for malignancy, and suppressing estrogen while stimulating progesterone. Aspirating fluid from the cysts is used for diagnosis as well as for relieving pressure and discomfort. There is no evidence that fibrocystic breast disease prevents breastfeeding.

Fibroadenoma is a freely movable rounded mass with well-defined borders and a solid rubbery texture. These nontender masses are most common in women in their teens and early twenties. Diagnosis is by history and fine-needle biopsy. Excision may be indicated, but caution is exercised to prevent damage to the developing breast structure. Fibroadenomas are not associated with breast cancer.

Intraductal papillomas are tumors growing in a mammary duct. They most commonly occur in women between 35 and 55. Although they are not malignant, they have the potential of becoming cancerous. These small ball-like tumors are often not palpable, but are found on mammography. If they occur near the nipple, a serosanguineous or brownish green discharge may be present. Because of the risk for malignancy, papillomas are usually removed surgically.

BREAST CANCER

Breast cancer is the second leading cause of cancer-related deaths among women. The most significant risk factor is the woman's age, with most breast cancer occurring after 50. Box 18-8 ■ describes breast cancer risk factors.

Breast cancer is an uncontrolled growth of abnormal cells in the breast. Women who have never had functioning ovaries and who have never had estrogen replacement do

BOX 18-8 **ASSESSMENT**

Breast Cancer Risk Factors

Personal Data: Female, over 50

Race: White

Family History: Mother or sister with breast cancer

Genetic History: Defective genes BRCA1 and BRCA2

Medical History: Cancer of breast, endometrial cancer, proliferative fibrocystic breast changes

Menstrual/Reproductive History: Early menarche (before age 12), late menopause (after age 50), use of estrogen replacement therapy more than 5 years

Radiation Exposure: Multiple chest x-rays or fluoroscopic exams, particularly before age 30

Lifestyle: More than two alcoholic drinks daily, obesity, smoking, high economic status, breast trauma

not develop breast cancer. Most cancerous tumors occur in the ductal areas of the breast.

Noninvasive (also called *in situ*) malignancies develop within the ducts or lobes of the breast without invading the surrounding tissue. Diagnosis of these tumors, which often lie under the areola and nipple, is usually made by mammography rather than palpation.

Invasive tumors grow from the intermediate ducts of the breast. Tumors are classified by cell type. However, prognosis and treatment depend on the progression of the disease (stage of development). Symptoms of breast cancer include small, hard painless lump, change in the size or shape of the breast, nipple discharge, dimpling, or pulling or retraction of the skin of the breast resembling an orange peel.

Breast cancer can metastasize to the ribs, sternum, or lungs. In this case the woman may also exhibit pain, spontaneous bone fractures, and respiratory symptoms including labored breathing, cough, and **hemoptysis** (bloody sputum).

Treatment of breast cancer is dependent on the stage of cancer progression. Surgical intervention may include a **lumpectomy** (removal of the lump), breast-conserving surgery (removal of the tumor, a disease-free margin surrounding the tumor, and adjacent lymph nodes), simple **mastectomy** (removal of the breast), or radical mastectomy with removal of the breast, surrounding lymph nodes, and underlying muscle structure. Radiation and chemotherapy may also be used to shrink and destroy the cancer cells. Long-term treatment with tamoxifen (Nolvadex) is usually recommended. See pharmacology Table 18-9 ■ for information on medications.

BREAST SURGERY

Surgery on the breast can be done for several reasons. As mentioned, surgery can be performed to remove a tumor or the entire breast and surrounding tissue due to a malignancy. Breast reconstruction (**mammoplasty**) may be performed at the time of the mastectomy or at a later date if extensive therapy is required. (This information is covered in depth in medical-surgical courses.)

Some women have breasts that are very large and heavy, putting strain on the shoulders and upper back. Some of these women request that a **reduction mammoplasty** be performed. If the woman is of childbearing age, the size of the breast will be reduced by removing fat tissue with an attempt to leave the mammary glands intact. This would allow the woman to breastfeed if she desires.

Some women have smaller breasts than they desire. Because the ability to breastfeed is not related to the size of the breast, breast augmentation (a surgical procedure using implants to increase the size of the breast) may help the woman improve her self-image. Implants contain either saline or silicone. In recent years there has been controversy over the safety of silicone implants. Continued research should resolve the controversy in the future. Parents and teens need to make this important decision together with the assistance of medical personnel.

Postoperatively, the woman may have drains coming from the surgical site. The dressings are usually large and may be cumbersome. It will take a week or more for the swelling and bruising to subside. Before discharge, she should be taught to care for the incision, apply dressings, and empty the drainage container. During this time the woman should be encouraged to look at the breast with a mirror, and to begin to adjust to her new image.

TABLE 18-9

Pharmacology: Common Drugs for Clients with Breast Cancer

DRUG (GENERIC AND COMMON BRAND NAMES)	USUAL ROUTE/DOSE	CLASSIFICATION	SELECTED SIDE EFFECTS	DON'T GIVE IF
Tamoxifen (Tamofen, Tamone)	10–20 mg once or twice a day for 5 years	Antiestrogen, antineoplastic	Bone pain, blood clot formation, alteration in CBC, GI upset	Call health care provider if there is suspicion of blood clots, signs of thrombophlebitis, or pulmonary embolism.

Uterine Disorders

Common uterine tumors include nonmalignant fibroids, endometrial cancer, and cervical cancer. Fibroid tumors of the uterus, common among women of all ages, are classified by their location within the uterus (Figure 18-19 ■) Although the exact cause of fibroid uterine tumor is unclear, they are probably related to estrogen secretion. Small tumors may go unnoticed for some time. Large tumors can enlarge the uterus, cause menorrhagia, put pressure on surrounding tissues, and cause lower abdominal and pelvic pain. In asymptomatic women who wish to bear children, the fibroid tumors are monitored. In some cases a laparoscopic **myomectomy** (removal of tumor and surrounding myometrium) may be performed. If tumors are large, a **hysterectomy** (removal of the uterus) may be necessary.

Endometriosis occurs when endometrial tissue grows outside of the uterine cavity (Figure 18-20 ■). Although the exact cause is unknown, it is theorized that endometrial cells migrate to deeper uterine tissue (myometrium) during fetal development or are washed through the fallopian tubes during menstruation. Endometrial cells can also be picked up in the lymph vessels and transported throughout the body. Endometrial cells that are **ectopic** (outside the uterus) respond to cyclic hormone influence just as uterine endometrium does. The cyclic bleeding results in inflammation, scar tissue formation, adhesions, and occlusions. Endometriosis may lead to infertility.

No single symptom is diagnostic of endometriosis. Often the teenager or young woman will complain of dysmenorrhea

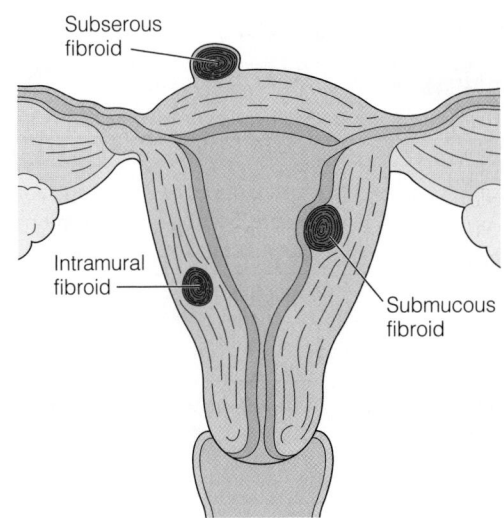

Figure 18-19. ■ Sites of uterine fibroid tumors.

with pelvic pain, or premenstrual **dyspareunia** (painful intercourse). Dysuria may indicate involvement of the urinary bladder. Premenstrual **tenesmus** (painful straining to defecate) and diarrhea may indicate colon involvement. Diagnosis is made by laparoscopic examination and biopsy of suspected tissue.

The goal of treatment is to preserve fertility for as long as possible. The woman who wishes to have children is encouraged to become pregnant as soon as possible. Hormones may be prescribed to cause endometrial atrophy. Table 18-10 ■ identifies common medications used to treat endometriosis.

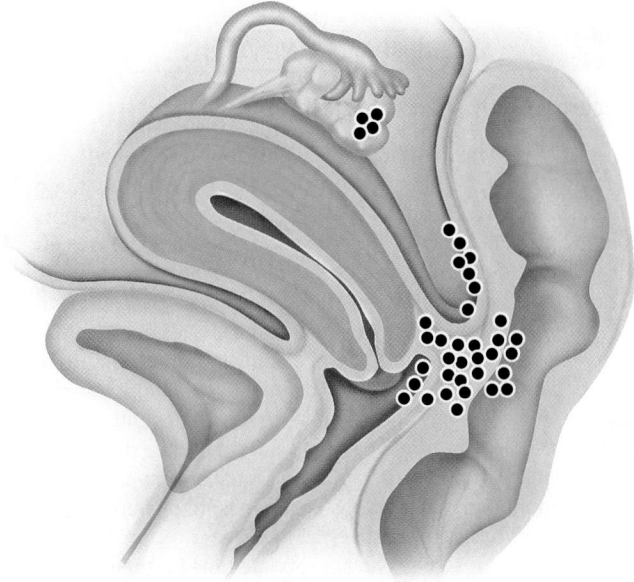

Figure 18-20. ■ Common sites for endometriosis. (Reproduced, with permission, from McGraw-Hill Companies, Inc. Way, L. W. [Ed.]. [1994]. *Current surgical diagnosis and treatment* [10th ed.]. Norwalk, CT: Appleton & Lange, p. 985.)

TABLE 18-10

Pharmacology: Drugs Used to Treat Endometriosis

DRUG (GENERIC AND COMMON BRAND NAMES)	USUAL ROUTE/DOSE	CLASSIFICATION	SELECTED SIDE EFFECTS	DON'T GIVE IF
Oral contraceptives	mg/tab depends on specific drug, one tablet daily	Contraceptive hormone	GI upset, depression, increased blood clotting, weight change	Call health care provider if there is a history of blood clotting disorders or if client is pregnant
Progesterone	Individual	Hormone	GI upset, depression, increase blood clotting, weight change	History of blood clotting disorders Pregnancy
Androgen hormone (Danozol)	100–400 mg twice daily	Androgen hormone	Decreased breast size, decreased libido, emotional lability	Pregnancy

Surgical treatment may include endometrial obliteration with a laser, or electrocautery via a laparoscope. If adequate symptom relief is not achieved, a hysterectomy with bilateral salpingo-oophorectomy may be required.

CERVICAL CANCER

Most cervical cancers result from an infection by the human papillomavirus (HPV). Please see the section on HPV in this chapter. Other risk factors also include early sexual intercourse, unprotected sex, multiple sex partners, HIV infection, smoking, and poor diet. Early detection and intervention have reduced the incidence of invasive cervical carcinoma. Box 18-9 ■ discusses lifespan considerations with the new vaccine against cervical cancer.

BOX 18-9   LIFE SPAN CONSIDERATIONS

Vaccine Against Human Papillomavirus

Parents have a new immunization decision to make with the recent recommendation from the FDA and the CDC regarding Gardasil, the vaccine against HPV. The nurse can assist parents in understanding how HPV is transmitted, how it relates to cervical cancer, and how it can be prevented. Parents should be taught that the vaccine is most effective when given prior to the initiation of sexual activity. Parents may have concerns that vaccinating their daughters is an acknowledgment that they will become sexually active. The nurse can help parents explore these feelings and compare risks and benefits related to the vaccine. The nurse can help parents understand that even if their daughters abstain from sexual activity until they are in a monogamous relationship, there is no guarantee that their partner has been abstinent. Therefore it is possible that he carries the virus. This is an appropriate time for the nurse to assist parents in health promotion teaching regarding sexual activity.

Most cervical cancers begin as **cervical dysplasia** (abnormal changes in the tissue of the cervix) or cervical intraepithelial neoplasia (CIN), including changes in the squamous cells of the cervix. Over time these cellular changes develop into carcinoma in situ, a localized cancer that becomes invasive if not treated. Cervical cancer invades the surrounding tissue including the vagina, urethra, bladder, and rectum.

In the early stages cervical cancer is asymptomatic. Once invasion occurs, bleeding, back and thigh pain, hematuria, bloody stools, and anemia are common. Diagnosis is made by a Papanicolaou (Pap) smear (see Health Promotion Issue). Cells and secretions from the cervix are collected on a glass slide, sprayed with a fixative, labeled, and sent to the laboratory for examination. If cancerous cells are identified, an MRI or CT of the pelvis, abdomen, and bones may be ordered to determine the extent of invasion.

When the tumor is localized within the cervix, it may be removed by laser, heated or cooled probes, or cauterization. A **conization** (removal of a cone-shaped wedge of cervical tissue) may be done if lesions extend into the endocervical canal (Figure 18-21 ■). If the client becomes pregnant, it is important for her to discuss the cervical conization with her health care provider. As the pregnancy progresses, the cervix may dilate under pressure, and premature delivery may result. If the cancer has spread to surrounding organs, radical surgery, radiation, and chemotherapy may be needed.

Ovarian Disorders

Cysts (fluid-filled sacs) commonly form in the ovary, whether from the graafian follicle or from the corpus luteum. Most cysts regress spontaneously in two or three

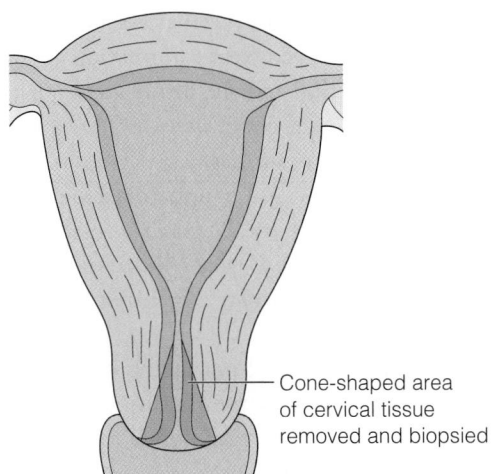

Cone-shaped area
of cervical tissue
removed and biopsied

Figure 18-21. ■ *Conization:* removal of a cone-shaped section of the cervix.

menstrual cycles. Some cysts can enlarge, rupture, and drain into the pelvis. Bleeding and a surgical emergency could occur.

Polycystic ovary syndrome (PCOS) results from numerous follicular cysts. This endocrine disorder is characterized by higher than normal LH, estrogen, and androgen levels and low FSH levels. This hormone imbalance results in irregular menstrual cycles, **hirsutism** (excessive hair growth), acne, obesity, and infertility. The woman may develop type II diabetes mellitus and has an increased risk for endometrial cancer, hypertension, and high cholesterol.

Diagnosis of ovarian cysts is made by pelvic ultrasound. Hormone levels are evaluated to diagnose PCOS. Laparoscopic surgery may be necessary to drain large cysts or control bleeding. Hormone therapy may be useful to prevent cyst formation.

Ovarian cancer is the most lethal of female reproductive cancers. Ovarian cancer is most commonly found in women over age 50, but it also may occur in much younger women. Ovarian cancer is asymptomatic until the cancer has spread to surrounding tissue or has been transported by the lymphatic system to other parts of the body. Risk factors for ovarian cancer include older age, early menarche, late menopause, history of infertility, treatment of infertility with Clomid (clomiphene), and a history of breast or ovarian cancer.

Diagnosis of ovarian cancer is made by pelvic ultrasound and laparoscopic biopsy. The treatment of choice is abdominal hysterectomy with bilateral salpingo-oophorectomy. The pelvic organs are examined for metastasis. Radiation and chemotherapy are used to destroy remaining malignant cells.

NURSING CARE

PRIORITIES IN NURSING CARE

Disorders related to the reproductive system can cause anxiety and embarrassment for children and their families. The nurse must be very sensitive to these emotions and take care to communicate (verbally and nonverbally) in a professional manner. The use of humor is <u>not</u> appropriate in these situations. Listen carefully to expressed concerns and assess carefully and respectfully for any unexpressed concerns. It is also important for the nurse not to assume that all families share Western values and viewpoints about sex and sexuality (Box 18-10 ■).

ASSESSING

Nursing assessments for children with reproductive disorders includes monitoring for signs and symptoms of infection. The nurse should carefully assess lab values, personal hygiene practices, and other factors that might increase the child's risk for infection. Assess for the child's verbal and nonverbal reactions to his or her physical characteristics. Pay close attention to statements that reflect self-criticism.

Acute pain is often associated with disorders of the reproductive system. The nurse should assess for verbal and nonverbal symptoms of pain using age-appropriate pain scales. Myths are prevalent related to disorders of the reproductive system. The nurse must be careful to determine the child's and the family's level of knowledge related to the condition and the prescribed treatment.

DIAGNOSING, PLANNING, AND IMPLEMENTING

Nursing diagnoses for children with reproductive disorders include

- Risk for **I**nfection related to surgical procedure
- Risk for Disturbed **B**ody Image related to anatomical alterations
- Acute **P**ain related to menstrual irregularities
- Deficient **K**nowledge related to changes of puberty

Some outcomes for children with reproductive disorders might include:

- Child will remain free of signs and symptoms of infection.
- Child and family will accept current body structure and function.
- Child will remain free of pain.
- Child and family will accurately state information regarding the condition and prescribed treatment.

BOX 18-10 CULTURAL PULSE POINTS

Conflict with "Western" Values

Young women of Egyptian heritage face many conflicts related to their sexuality. Egyptians and others from Middle Eastern or Eastern cultures have traditional religious beliefs that forbid sexual activity outside of marriage. It is expected that women will be virgins when they get married. Parents may be hesitant to discuss issues of birth control, sexually transmitted diseases, and teenage pregnancy with their daughters, because they fear it would promote premarital sexual activity. Parents may impose strict policies on their daughter's activities away from home. Some parents may consider returning to their native country with their daughter, rather than risk having her influenced by American values.

The nurse's role in providing support to these clients would include the following:

- Teach the child and family the importance of preventing infections of the reproductive system, especially in the postoperative period. *Knowledge of the risks of infection will motivate the child and family to use preventive measures.*
- Use hand washing between contacts with other clients and procedures with this child. *Harmful bacteria can be effectively removed by friction and running water.*
- Teach parents the importance of their responses to the child's physical characteristics. *Children often take their cues about their body image from their parents.*

- Parents of children with physical alterations in the reproductive system need clear information about the nature of the alteration and the future consequences. *Accurate information allows the family to form an accurate mindset about the child's condition.*
- Provide pharmacologic and nonpharmacologic pain relief measures as necessary. *Pharmacologic pain relief measures provide physiological relief of pain while nonpharmacologic pain relief measures reduce tension and therefore relieve psychological aspects of pain.*
- Select age-appropriate teaching methods to instruct the child and the family about the condition and prescribed treatment. *Cognitive development must be considered in order to convey information accurately.*

EVALUATING

The nurse reviews stated outcomes to determine if goals were met. Follow-up pain assessments are important when administering pharmacological pain medications. Signs and symptoms of infection should be reported promptly. The nurse confirms the child and the family's understanding of the condition and the prescribed treatment by having them verbalize information.

Note: The reference and resource listings for this and all chapters have been compiled at the back of the book.

Chapter Review

 KEY TERMS by Topic

Use the audio glossary feature of either the CD-ROM or the Companion Website to hear the correct pronunciation of the following key terms.

Introduction
genitourinary system

Congenital Urinary Defects
hypospadias, epispadias, chordee, bladder exstrophy, obstructive uropathy, polycystic kidney, nephrolithiasis, stasis, hydronephrosis, pyeloplasty, valve ablation

Urinary Tract Infections
cystitis, pyelonephritis, vesicoureteral reflux, dysuria, hematuria

Acute Postinfectious Glomerulonephritis
glomerulonephritis

Nephrotic Syndrome
nephrotic syndrome, proteinuria, hypoalbuminemia, hyperlipidemia, pyelonephritis, periorbital edema, ascites

Acute and Chronic Renal Failure
renal failure, acute renal failure, chronic renal failure, end-stage renal disease, uremic syndrome, uremic frost, dialysis, disequilibrium syndrome

Wilms' Tumor or Nephroblastoma
Wilms' tumor, nephroblastoma

Enuresis
enuresis

Ambiguous Genitalia
pseudohermaphroditism

Male Disorders
phimosis, balanoposthitis, paraphimosis, circumcision, cryptorchidism, orchiectomy

Sexually Transmitted Infections
chlamydia, gonorrhea, syphilis, chancre, genital warts, trichomoniasis, teratogen, human immunodeficiency virus, acquired immunodeficiency syndrome, candidiasis, monilia, yeast infection

Female Disorders
hymen, vaginitis

Breast Disorders
mammography, fibrosis, fibrocyst, fibroadenoma, intraductal papillomas, hemoptysis, lumpectomy, mastectomy, mammoplasty, reduction mammoplasty

Uterine Disorders
myomectomy, hysterectomy, endometriosis, ectopic, dyspareunia, tenesmus, cervical dysplasia, conization

Ovarian Disorders
cysts, polycystic ovary syndrome, hirsutism, ovarian cancer

KEY Points

- The primary functions of the urinary system include waste excretion; homeostasis, fluid, electrolyte, and acid-base balance; regulation of blood pressure; regulation of calcium metabolism; and stimulation of erythrocyte development.

- It is important for the nurse to know the normal bladder capacity for the child according to age group. Urinary output needs to be measured carefully.

- Most commonly, the newborn voids in the first 24 hours of birth. The newborn who does not void within 24 hours may be assessed for urethral stenosis or absent kidneys or ureters.

- In the infant, UTIs are more common in males primarily because of structural defects. In the young child, UTIs are more common in females, usually caused by *Escherichia coli* entering the urethra and progressing to the bladder. Younger children also have shorter ureters, which increases their risk for UTIs.

- The nurse should be able to recognize symptoms of UTI, which include fever, nausea and vomiting, anorexia, strong-smelling urine, abdominal pain, dysuria, and hematuria. In the infant and young child who is nonverbal, dysuria may be displayed as crying during urination. The continent child may suddenly develop incontinence or hesitancy, due to fear of pain.

- Renal failure is the inability of the kidneys to remove liquid waste from the blood. Renal failure can be acute or chronic.

- The child with renal failure should be assessed for signs of fluid overload including weight gain, pitting edema, pulmonary edema, and ascites.

- The nurse can help the young girl avoid contact vaginitis by teaching her to wipe her perineum from front to back, therefore avoiding infestation of the vagina with harmful bacteria from the rectum.

- Disorders related to the reproductive system can cause anxiety and embarrassment for children and their families. The nurse must be very sensitive to these emotions and take care to communicate (verbally and nonverbally) in a professional manner.

EXPLORE MediaLink

Additional interactive resources for this chapter can be found on the Companion Website at www.prenhall.com/adams.

Click on Chapter 18 and "Begin" to select the activities for this chapter.

For chapter-related NCLEX®-style questions and an audio glossary, access the accompanying CD-ROM in this book.

(continued)

Chapter Review

Animations:

Renal corpuscle

Erectile dysfunction

Conception

Oogenesis

H.I.V.

Spermatogenesis

Ovulation

Breast cancer

Circumcision

Gonorrhea

Premenstrual syndrome

∞ FOR FURTHER Study

The phases of sexual maturation (called *Tanner's stages*) are described in Table 5-12.

Collection of urine specimens is described in Procedure 8-14. Urinary catheterization in a child is described in Procedure 8-26.

For more information about transmission, clinical manifestations, diagnostic tests, medical treatment, and nursing considerations of hepatitis A and B, see Table 10-6.

For additional information on fluid and electrolyte imbalances, monitoring intake and output, and other fluid-related topics, see Chapter 11.

See Chapter 16 for a more detailed description of sexual abuse assessment.

For more information about organ transplantation and immune disorders, see Chapter 22.

Critical Thinking Care Map

Caring for a Client with Vaginitis
NCLEX-PN® Focus Area: Physiological Integrity

Case Study: Mrs. Friedman has made an appointment with the pediatrician for her 14-year-old daughter, Casey. Casey reported to her mother yesterday that her vulva was swollen and painful and that she was experiencing intense itching. Mrs. Friedman has accused Casey of having sexual intercourse because she understands that is the only way a woman can have the symptoms Casey is describing. Casey denies having sexual intercourse.

Nursing Diagnosis: Deficient **K**nowledge (Parent) related to causes of vaginitis

COLLECT DATA

Subjective
_____
_____
_____
_____
_____

Objective
_____
_____
_____
_____
_____

Would you report this? Yes/No

If yes, to: _____

Nursing Care
_____
_____
_____
_____
_____
_____
_____
_____
_____

How would you document this? _____
_____
_____
_____
_____

Data Collected
(use only those that apply)

- Report of swollen vulva
- Intact hymen
- Report of vulvar pain
- Vulva edematous
- Temp 98.6 °F, P 60, R 12, B/P 110/70
- Report of vulvar itching
- Mrs. Friedman is waving arms and pacing in examination room
- "Casey has had sex and that's why she has these symptoms."
- "I have not ever had sex with anyone."
- Vulva red
- Small amount of white vaginal discharge noted.

Nursing Interventions
(use only those that apply; list in priority order)

- Assist physician to obtain vaginal specimen.
- Describe methods of preventing vaginitis.
- Explain the physiology and causes of vaginitis.
- Obtain urine specimen for pregnancy test.
- Describe the signs and symptoms of vaginitis.
- Assess Mrs. Friedman's knowledge level regarding vaginitis.
- Explain medical treatment of vaginitis.
- Counsel Casey on the hazards of sexual activity.
- Present teaching in a nonjudgmental manner.

Compare your documentation to the sample provided in Appendix I.

NCLEX-PN® Exam Preparation

TEST-TAKING TIP Be sure to picture the different congenital defects as clearly as possible in your mind when studying. At times you will be able to use this knowledge and the process of elimination to determine the correct answer.

1 A nurse is caring for a child who has just returned from surgery where he underwent repair for epispadias. The parents are concerned when they see a slight amount of blood in the urinary collection bag. The nurse tells the parents:

1. "I will call the surgeon right away."
2. "Your child will probably need a blood transfusion."
3. "A slight amount of blood in the urine is normal following this surgery."
4. "The catheter will be taken out soon."

2 The nurse is discussing the discharge plans for a newborn with hypospadias. What statement by the parents indicates their understanding of the plan?

1. "Our child will have to have frequent blood tests."
2. "Our child will have to be catheterized frequently."
3. "A special support will have to be worn by our child until surgery."
4. "Our child won't be circumcised right away in order to save tissue for repair."

3 In a child with a diagnosis of urinary tract infection (UTI), the nurse knows the child may experience the following symptoms:

1. Hematuria, dysuria, nausea, and vomiting
2. Oliguria, hematuria, and seizures
3. Proteinuria, oliguria, and hypoalbuminemia
4. Hyperlipidemia, hypoalbuminemia, and hyperproteinuria

4 The nurse reviews the laboratory report of a child with possible glomerulonephritis. The nurse knows which finding is associated with a diagnosis of glomerulonephritis?

1. Hematuria
2. Decreased pH
3. Streptococcal infection
4. Glucosuria

5 A nurse is caring for a child with symptoms of uremic frost, nausea, vomiting, anorexia, uremic breath odor, anemia, pruritis, and pulmonary edema. The nurse knows these symptoms are most likely caused by:

1. Hypospadias
2. Bladder exstrophy
3. Epispadias
4. Uremic syndrome

6 The nurse is conducting an assessment of a child with a potential Wilms' tumor. In the course of the assessment, the nurse avoids which method of gathering data?

1. Obtaining a urine sample
2. Taking the child's temperature
3. Obtaining a radial pulse
4. Palpating the abdomen

7 The nurse is reviewing the plan of care for an infant with the diagnosis of bladder exstrophy and targets which of the following priority diagnoses?

1. Potential for infection
2. Alteration in comfort
3. Impaired tissue integrity
4. Deficient knowledge of parents

8 The parents of an infant with bladder exstrophy ask the nurse about the condition. The nurse explains this condition is caused by:

1. A congenital disorder inherited from the father
2. An intrusion of the bladder, which is abnormally located in the renal pelvis
3. An extrusion of the bladder through a lower abdominal wall defect
4. A condition due to low folic acid intake by the mother during pregnancy

9 The nurse is caring for a child admitted to the medical center with a diagnosis of nephrotic syndrome and selects the following data that can be found on assessment (choose all that apply):

1. Hypoalbuminemia
2. Protein in the urine
3. Edema
4. Uremic frost
5. Hyperlipidemia
6. Decreased immunity

10 The nurse selects the following teaching items for the parents of a 2-year-old, partially toilet-trained female child with a diagnosis of urinary tract infection (choose all that apply):

1. Clean the perineum after each diaper change
2. Wipe the child from front to back
3. Avoid bubble baths
4. Avoid putting the child in a commercial hot tub
5. Do not use disposable diapers

Answers for NCLEX-PN® Review and Critical Thinking questions appear in Appendix I.

Care of the Child with Endocrine Disorders

BRIEF Outline

Anatomy and Physiology
Brief Assessment Review
Inborn Errors of Metabolism
Pituitary Disorders

Thyroid Disorders
Adrenal Disorders
Pancreatic Islet Disorder
Nursing Care

LEARNING Outcomes

After completing this chapter, you will be able to:

1. Define key terms.
2. Identify the location of each endocrine gland, the hormones produced, and the function of each.
3. Discuss the interrelationship of the normally functioning endocrine system.
4. Discuss disorders of each endocrine gland including pathology, diagnostic procedures, and medical treatment.
5. Explain appropriate nursing interventions for children with endocrine disorders.
6. Discuss teaching topics for children with diabetes and their parents.

NURSING CARE PLAN CHART:
Child with Diabetes Mellitus

HEALTH PROMOTION ISSUE:
Metabolic Syndrome
(Metabolic X Syndrome)

NURSING PROCESS CARE PLAN:
Care of a Client with Growth
Hormone Deficiency

CRITICAL THINKING CARE MAP:
Caring for a Client with Type I
Diabetes Mellitus

Endocrine disorders are some of the most difficult disorders to diagnose, but they can have some of the farthest-reaching effects. Many endocrine disorders are identified only over time as other diagnoses are ruled out. Furthermore, once a disorder is identified, it can still take a great deal of time and effort before treatment is adjusted to an appropriate level. By recognizing and reporting symptoms, the LPN/LVN may assist in identification of an endocrine disorder.

Endocrine system disorders result from an overproduction or an underproduction of hormones or from not enough target cells responding to hormones. Because the endocrine system regulates metabolism, some metabolic disorders affecting children will be discussed here, even though they may not be directly related to a specific hormone.

Anatomy and Physiology

The endocrine system performs the function of communication and slow, long-lasting control of various other body systems (Figure 19-1 ▪). **Hormones,** proteins produced by endocrine glands, are secreted into the blood, where they

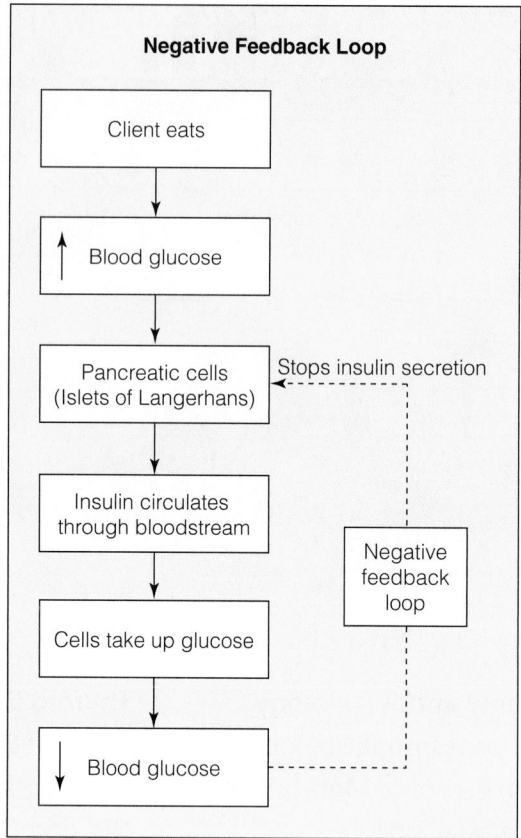

Figure 19-2. ▪ Negative feedback mechanism with blood glucose and insulin.

are transported to the target organs. Hormones are the main regulators of growth and development, metabolism, and reproduction.

The blood level of most hormones is regulated by a negative feedback mechanism. Negative feedback involves two or more substances working in opposition to each other. An increase in one causes a decrease in the other. In **negative feedback** mechanisms, high levels of a hormone in the blood inhibit (switch off) hormone production. Low levels trigger (switch on) hormone production, much as a thermostat would turn heat off or on in a house. Negative feedback can be illustrated using the regulation of blood glucose as an example (Figure 19-2 ▪). Following a meal, the blood glucose level increases. The islet cells in the pancreas register the high glucose level and cause the pancreas to secrete the hormone insulin. Insulin aids transport of glucose out of the blood and into body cells. When glucose moves out of the blood into cells, the blood glucose levels decrease, and the cells in the pancreas register reduced levels of glucose and "switch off" insulin production. This is a *negative feedback* mechanism, because production of a chemical (in this case, insulin) slows or stops when glandular tissue receives feedback that no more of the chemical is needed.

In **positive feedback** an increase in one substance causes an increased response until some major event occurs that causes

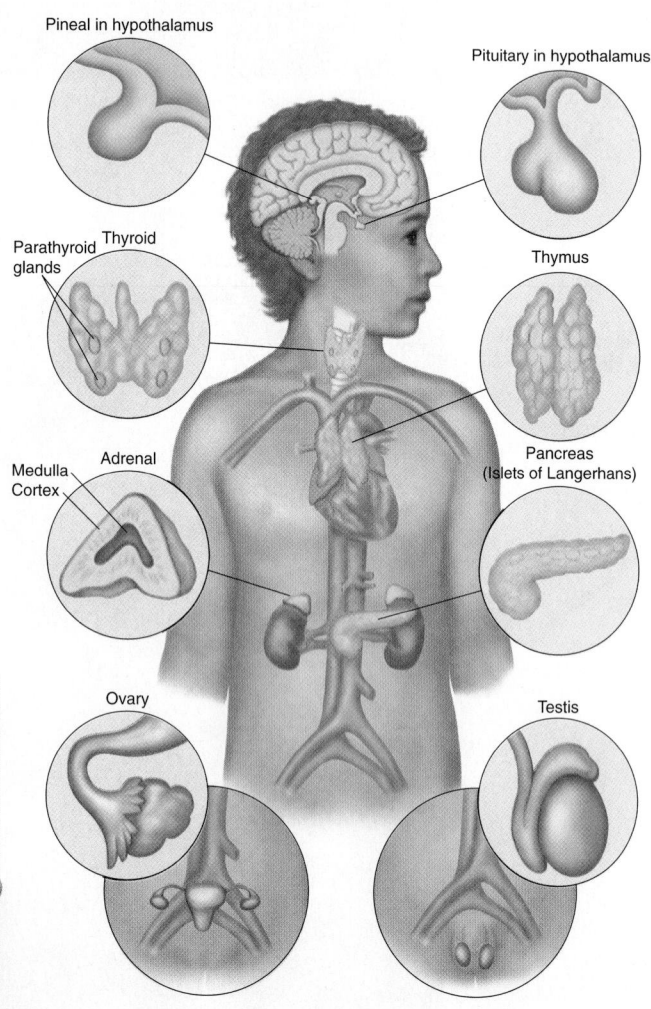

Figure 19-1. ▪ Major organs and glands of the endocrine system.

a decrease in the substance. The hormone oxytocin is regulated by a positive feedback mechanism. Oxytocin is responsible for stimulating contractions of the uterus during labor. Once started, secretion of oxytocin continues until delivery (the major event) has occurred. Then oxytocin secretion slows.

Whereas most hormones are produced and excreted by endocrine glands, one group, **prostaglandins,** is produced by various tissues in the body. Researchers are discovering that prostaglandins have an effect on respiration, blood pressure, gastrointestinal secretions, and reproduction. Through continued study of these complex hormones, causes of diseases and new treatments may be found.

Before studying specific pediatric endocrine disorders, a review of each endocrine gland and its specific hormones is warranted. Table 19-1 ■ provides an overview for review of the endocrine system.

TABLE 19-1

Review of Endocrine Glands and Effects

GLANDS	LOCATION	SECRETIONS	TARGET TISSUE	EFFECTS
Pineal	Located in third ventricle of the brain	Melatonin	Gonads, pigment cells	Regulates sleep/wake cycles and inhibits **gonadotropic** (sex-organ) hormones
Pituitary **Anterior** (adenohypophysis)	Located at the base of the skull behind the base of the nose in the sella turcica A strip of tissue (pars intermedia) seperates the anterior and posterior	Growth hormone (GH)	Many organs	Stimulates growth and is essential for proper metabolic regulation of fat and glucose
		Thyroid-stimulating hormone (TSH)	Thyroid gland	Stimulates thyroid secretions
		Adrenocorticotropic hormone (ACTH)	Adrenal cortex	Stimulates the adrenal cortex to release cortisol and aldosterone; regulates glucose homeostasis
		Follicle-stimulating hormone (FSH)	Gonads	Stimulates spermatogenesis in males. Stimulates ovarian follicles in females
		Luteinizing hormone (LH)	Gonads	Stimulates ovulation and corpus luteum formation; stimulates secretion of testosterone in males
		Prolactin (PRL)	Mammary gland	Stimulates breast milk production during pregnancy
Posterior (neurohypophysis)		Antidiuretic hormone (ADH)	Kidneys	Stimulates reabsorption of water by the kidneys. Important in preventing dehydration
		Oxytocin	Uterus Mammary gland	Stimulates contractions Stimulates milk ejection in pregnancy
Thyroid Gland	Located over the trachea	Thyroxine (T_4), Triiodothyronine (T_3)	Most cells	Regulates the rate of metabolism. Iodine in the diet is needed for production of these hormones
		Calcitonin	Bone	Decreases concentration of blood calcium by inhibiting the release of calcium from the bone
Parathyroid Glands	Beanlike structures embedded in the posterior surface of the thyroid gland	Parathormone (PTH).	Bone, kidneys, digestive tract	Maintain calcium and phosphate balance in the body, activates vitamin D
Thymus Gland	Consists of two lobes located in the mediastinum beneath the sternum	Thymosin		Development of the immune system

(continued)

TABLE 19-1

Review of Endocrine Glands and Effects (continued)

GLANDS	LOCATION	SECRETIONS	TARGET TISSUE	EFFECTS
Adrenal Glands (suprarenals)	Located on top of the kidneys Outer portion is the *adrenal cortex*, and the inner core is the *adrenal medulla*	**Cortex** Glucocorticoids (cortisol)	Kidney tubules, many organs	Maintain blood glucose levels, maintain blood pressure, work as an antiinflammatory, and are a first response to stress
		Mineralocorticoids (mainly aldosterone)		Regulate electrolyte (mainly sodium and potassium) and water balance
		Gonadocorticoids		Secrete sex hormones in small amounts
		Medulla Epinephrine (adrenalin)	Smooth muscle, cardiac muscle, blood vessels	Increase body metabolism, released during the "fight or flight" reaction
		Norepinephrine (noradrenalin)		Contract the blood vessels, increase the blood pressure, slow the GI tract, and dilate the pupils
		Dopamine		Dilate systemic arteries, increase cardiac and urinary output. Affect blood pressure.
Pancreas (islets of Langerhans)	Located in the left quadrant of the abdomen just below the stomach and is connected to the duodenum of the small intestines by the pancreatic duct	Glucagon	Liver, adipose tissue	Targets the liver to release glycogen, causing an increase in blood sugar
		Insulin	Liver, skeletal muscles, adipose tissue	Moves glucose out of the blood and into the cells, thereby decreasing blood sugar
		Somatostatin		Interferes with release of the growth hormone and glucagons
Ovaries		Estrogens	General female reproductive structures	Promote the growth and development of the female characteristics
		Progesterone	Uterus	Responsible for the secretion of the corpus luteum, maintenance of the lining of the uterus in pregnancy
			Mammary glands	Stimulate development
Testes		Testosterone	Many organs	Stimulate development of the male characteristics and growth spurt at puberty
			Male reproductive systems	Stimulate development of sex organs, and spermatogenesis

Brief Assessment Review

HISTORY

- Inquire about a family history of diabetes or thyroid disease.
- Ask the child or parent about excessive hunger, thirst, sweating, or urination.
- Inquire about abnormal hair distribution, or salty taste to the skin.
- Inquire about symptoms of precocious or delayed puberty.
- Inquire about activity level, especially energy level.
- Ask if the child is exhibiting symptoms of mental decline.
- Ask if the child is intolerant to cold or heat.
- Ask if the child has frequent headaches or is irritable.

PHYSICAL

To perform a brief focused assessment of the endocrine system, the nurse would:

- Observe the skin for moisture, hair distribution and moisture, and edema.
- Observe for sexual development.
- Assess and record height and weight. Compare to growth charts.
- Monitor body temperature, respiratory rate, and blood pressure (see Procedures 8-1, 8-3, and 8-4 ⬭).
- Test for muscle strength and tone.

Inborn Errors of Metabolism

Phenylketonuria was discussed in Chapter 17 ⬭.

GALACTOSEMIA

Galactosemia is an autosomal recessive disorder of carbohydrate metabolism. Galactosemia results from a deficiency in galactose-1-phosphate uridyltransferase (GALT), one of the three enzymes necessary for the conversion of sugar galatose into glucose. High levels of galactose in the blood result in damage to the kidneys, liver, brain, and eyes. Many children develop gram-negative infections.

Manifestations

Within a few days after birth, the baby develops vomiting and diarrhea, does not eat well, becomes hypoglycemic, and develops an enlarged liver. If not diagnosed and treated, the child will become mentally retarded and develop jaundice, ascites, cataracts, seizures, lethargy, and coma. Death usually occurs within a month.

Diagnosis

Routine screening of the newborn is done in all but six states. In these six states, diagnosis is made in symptomatic babies from history and laboratory tests.

Treatment

Infants with galactosemia are placed on lactose-free or galactose-free formulas. The child will be on a galactose-free diet (no milk or milk products) for life. Many children who follow a strict diet still develop complications of galactosemia including learning disabilities, speech defects, visual disturbances, and ovarian failure.

Nursing Considerations

Nursing responsibilities focus on teaching the parents and child about the prescribed diet and referring the family to a nutritionist for counseling. Parents must learn to screen foods and medication for hidden lactose that has been used as filler. The parents should be referred for genetic counseling.

Genetic Factors in Maple Syrup Urine Disease

Maple syrup urine disease (MSUD) is rare in the general population. However, there is a very high rate (1 in 380 live births) among the Pennsylvania Mennonites (a religious group) and in an intermarrying subgroup called the Amish. All newborns in this population should be tested for MSUD (Robinson & Drumm, 2001). Prompt recognition of the condition can allow preventive treatment that vastly increases quality of life.

MAPLE SYRUP URINE DISEASE

Maple syrup urine disease (MSUD) is an autosomal recessive disease that affects amino acid metabolism. A missing or defective enzyme prevents the breakdown of three essential amino acids, leucine, isoleucine, and valine (Box 19-1 ■). The result is alpha ketoacidosis. All three amino acids are necessary for normal hair, skin, and muscle formation. Leucine accumulates in the brain, causing cerebral edema, neurologic damage, and death.

Manifestations

Within days of birth, the infant becomes lethargic, has variable muscle tone, and becomes irritable with a high-pitched cry; the skin has a sweet smell.

Diagnosis

Diagnosis is made by documentation of manifestations and laboratory findings.

Treatment

Specially designed formulas with the three amino acids removed are prescribed. The diet should be rich in other amino acids, vitamins, minerals, and calories. The child needs special low-protein foods that are adequate for growth without causing a catabolic state (tissue breakdown). Daily urine testing for ketones is required to monitor the metabolic state.

Nursing Considerations

Nursing care includes teaching parents to maintain the prescribed diet. This includes mixing the special formula and developing a plan to prevent ketoacidosis on sick days. Referral to a nutritionist is helpful. Support groups can also help families by sharing tips for managing the child's condition.

TAY-SACHS DISEASE

Tay-Sachs disease is caused by an inherited abnormal gene. Because of this abnormal gene, the child does not have hexosaminidase A (HEXA), an enzyme that breaks down a fatty material called ganglioside GM2. Because the child lacks HEXA, the fatty material builds up in the brain, eventually causing nerve damage. Tay-Sachs is an autosomal recessive condition, which means both parents must carry the abnormal gene for them to pass it on to the baby (Box 19-2 ■).

Manifestations

Infants with Tay-Sachs disease usually show symptoms between 3 and 6 months. Symptoms include muscle weakness that progresses to paralysis. The child may become deaf and blind. Neurological damage continues until death occurs around age 5. Three related conditions have similar symptoms because they affect the same gene:

- A juvenile form appears between 2 and 5 years and progresses to death by age 15.
- A chronic form appears by age 5, with muscle weakness, slurred speech, tremors, and, sometimes, mental impairment.
- An adult form resembles the chronic form but appears between the teens and the 30s.

Diagnosis and Treatment

Diagnosis is through genetic testing. There is no effective treatment for Tay-Sachs disease. Medical management and nursing care is aimed at relieving symptoms, making the child comfortable, and preparing the child and family for death.

Those adults from high-risk groups should be encouraged to seek genetic counseling before becoming pregnant. If a woman is pregnant and both parents are carriers for Tay-Sachs disease, chorionic villus sampling can determine whether the fetus has the disease. Decisions can then be made about the status of the pregnancy.

Pituitary Disorders

Pituitary disorders in children may be caused by brain infections, infarction of the pituitary gland (associated with sickle-cell disease), cranial injury, hypothalmic or pituitary tumors, or psychosocial deprivation. The discussion below concerns the most common pituitary disorders in children.

GROWTH HORMONE DEFICIENCY

Growth hormone deficiency is a decrease in growth hormone that results from injury or disease of the hypothalamus or pituitary gland, inheritance, or genetic mutation. Because decreased function of the pituitary gland results in GHD, this disorder is often referred to as **hypopituitarism.**

Manifestations

Children with GHD have normal birth weights and lengths. Growing less than 2 inches (5 cm) a year, these children fall below the 3rd percentile in growth by 1 year of age. Children with GHD tend to be overweight. Because growth hormone affects all cells, these children also develop hypoglycemic seizures, hyponatremia, jaundice, pale optic disc, and male genital problems (micropenis and undescended testicles). They maintain youthful facial features, higher-pitched voices, and delayed skeletal and sexual maturity.

Diagnosis

Children below the 3rd percentile for height should be referred to a pediatric endocrinologist. It is recommended that blood testing for growth hormone levels be done every 3 to 4 months.

Treatment

Treatment depends on the cause of the deficiency. Many children will receive subcutaneous injections of growth hormone three to seven times a week for at least a year or until normal height is achieved. Frequent monitoring will continue every 3 to 4 months, and injections will resume as needed. In some cases, the onset of puberty is delayed with medication to allow more time to achieve adult height.

Nursing Considerations

Nursing care consists of monitoring growth, teaching the family about the disorder and the treatment, and providing emotional support. Parents need to be taught to administer the injections. Growth hormone injections are expensive and may not be covered by insurance. Parents may need financial assistance and resources.

If hormone injections are not initiated at an early age, normal growth may not be achieved. People often treat short individuals differently based on their height, not their age. It is not uncommon for these social prejudices to affect the child's self-esteem, as discussed in Box 19-3 ■. The emotional stress may be most notable during adolescence when the child is preoccupied by body image. Suggesting the child take part in sports that do not require a large physical stature (swimming, gymnastics, ice skating, etc.) and identifying positive role models who are successful despite their short stature may be helpful.

Children with Growth Hormone Deficiency

Children with growth hormone deficiency must manage body image disturbance issues related to their short stature. As the child ages, the difference in height is more recognizable and more of a concern to the child. Encouraging a healthy self-esteem is very important. This focus should begin early in life. The nurse can assist parents in promoting internal sources of strength, encouraging creativity, and accentuating academic success.

GROWTH HORMONE EXCESS

Growth hormone excess is rare in children. Most commonly it results from a pituitary tumor. If growth hormone excess is coupled with precocious puberty, a hypothalamic tumor should be suspected. Because tall stature is valued in our society, a tall or rapidly growing child (especially a boy) may not be evaluated in a timely manner. Any child whose height is greater than predicted by parental height should be evaluated.

Diagnosis

Diagnosis is made from history, laboratory findings, and radiological studies.

Treatment

Treatment depends on the cause. If the epiphyseal plates remain open, high doses of sex hormones may be given to close the epiphyseal plates and stop growth.

Nursing Considerations

Nursing care involves teaching and emotional support. Like short stature, tall stature may be emotionally stressful for the child. Tall children may be treated as though they are older than their chronological age.

PRECOCIOUS PUBERTY

Puberty normally begins between the age of 8 and 13 years in girls and 9 and 14 years in boys. **Precocious puberty** is the presence of any secondary sex characteristics before the age of 8 in girls and before the age of 9 in boys.

Manifestations

Children with precocious puberty have advanced bone age as well as reproductive changes. These children have a period of rapid growth followed by rapid closure of the epiphyseal plates. The end result is a short stature. Mood swings and emotional *lability* (changeability) may also be noted.

Diagnosis

Diagnosis is made by monitoring the sex steroids, FSH, and LH, as well as determining whether other pituitary dysfunction exists.

Treatment

Occasionally hormone treatment is necessary to suppress FSH and LH, but most commonly no medical treatment is required.

Nursing Considerations

The nurse should support parents and help them to explain to the child that the changes in his or her body are normal, but earlier than expected. It is important to remember that the child's emotional development will not match his or her physical development. The child may need support to deal with teasing by peers. Children with precocious puberty should be dressed for their chronological age, not their physical development. Parents can encourage loose-fitting clothing to hide the body changes that are occurring. Parents need to be advised to talk with their child about sexuality and reproduction at an earlier age. The child and parents may need referral for counseling.

DIABETES INSIPIDUS

Diabetes insipidus is a rare disorder of the posterior pituitary gland. There are two types of diabetes insipidus that affect children:

1. Inadequate pituitary production of ADH. The first type of diabetes insipidus is failure of the pituitary gland to produce an adequate amount of ADH. Any trauma, inflammation, or pressure on the pituitary gland can cause the gland to slow or stop production of ADH.
2. Lack of response to ADH. The second, called *nephrogenic* (kidney-induced) diabetes insipidus, results from failure of the renal tubules to respond to ADH. Recall that ADH normally causes reabsorption of water from the renal tubules. Without adequate ADH, or when the renal tubules fail to respond to ADH, water is not reabsorbed.

Manifestations

The end result of this disorder is excessive urine output (**polyuria**). When a large amount of water is lost, the child experiences **polydipsia** (excessive thirst). No matter how dehydrated the child becomes, the kidneys are unable to concentrate urine, as evidenced by a urine specific gravity of less than 1.010. Hypernatremia, increased serum sodium, is common. (See more on hypernatremia in Chapter 11 ⬤⬤.)

Diagnosis

Diagnostic tests include serum electrolytes, as well as serum and urine osmolality. Plasma arginine vasopressin (AVP) level before and during a fluid deprivation test confirms the diagnosis. During a fluid deprivation test, fluid is withheld from the child for up to 7 hours.

clinical ALERT

It is important to tell the parents that the child will become thirsty and irritable during the test. The test is stopped if the child loses 3% of body weight and develops a fever and hypotension.

Treatment

There are separate treatments for the two causes of diabetes insipidus. The treatment of ADH insufficiency is administration of desmopressin acetate (DDAVP). DDAVP is titrated so the urinary output is lowered, and the child retains adequate caloric intake. DDAVP is not effective in controlling nephrogenic diabetes insipidus.

For nephrogenic diabetes insipidus, children are treated with diuretics, increased fluid intake, and salt- and protein-restricted diet. Box 19-4 ■ provides information about salt- and protein-restricted diets.

Nursing Considerations

Nursing responsibilities are to teach the parents how to manage their child's disease, to administer medication, and to recognize signs of complications such as dehydration and

BOX 19-4   NUTRITION THERAPY

Foods for a Low-Salt, Low-Protein Diet

Low-Salt Diet

■ The health care professional will order the amount of restriction (such as a 2-g Na diet). Most foods do contain some sodium, so foods that are lowest in sodium should be selected.

■ The nurse reinforces the following guidelines to help the client (or parents) maintain a low-salt diet:
  • Check labels for Na (sodium)
  • Add no salt to foods
  • Avoid salty snacks (chips, salty popcorn, pretzels with salt)
  • Avoid processed, prepared foods because they tend to contain higher levels of sodium

Low-Protein Diet

■ The health care professional will order the amount of restriction (for example, a 40-g protein diet)

■ The nurse reinforces the following guidelines to help the client (or parents) maintain a low-protein diet:
  • All meats and milk are high in protein (about 3 oz meat = 8 g protein)
  • Cereal/bread and vegetables are moderate to low in protein:
    • $1/2$ cup cereal or 1 slice bread = 2 g protein
    • $1/2$ cup vegetables = 1 g protein
  • Avoid seafood
  • Limit meat to $1/2$ serving
  • Use bread and vegetables for food volume

BOX 19-5   CLIENT TEACHING

Child with Diabetes Insipidus

Teach parents that assisting the child with diabetes insipidus requires learning everyday maintenance, medicine administration, and warning signs of complications.

Medication Administration

■ Desmopressin acetate (DDAVP) is administered by intranasal drops or spray.
  • Put $1/2$ dose in each nostril. (Review Procedure 8-34 ⚭ for steps to teach parents about administering nasal medication)
  • Solution should be kept in refrigerator

Fluid Administration

■ Provide written signs of dehydration and discuss warning signs with parents.

■ Instruct parents to measure intake and output. Fluid intake must equal fluid output.

■ Forewarn parents that the child who has compensated for high urine output may have difficulty decreasing intake when output has slowed with treatment. They should expect the child will adjust in time.

■ Give fluids during the night as needed.

■ Acute illness increases metabolism and increases risk of dehydration and electrolyte imbalance. Parents need to notify the physician right away. They will also need to monitor I & O more closely during times of acute illness.

Follow-up Care

■ Remind parents to schedule an appointment for blood work to monitor electrolytes.

■ Instruct parents that follow-up medical care is important to monitor the diagnosis.

■ Instruct parents to seek medical attention during times of illness.

■ Provide referral resources for home health nurse and respite care.

electrolyte imbalance. When the child becomes ill, it is important for the parents to seek medical attention right away and to communicate to health care providers the child's diagnosis of diabetes insipidus. Box 19-5 ■ provides client teaching about care of a child with diabetes insipidus.

Thyroid Disorders

Thyroid disorders are rare in children. However, when they do occur, they must be diagnosed and treated in a timely manner, because thyroid hormones are necessary for cellular metabolism, mental functioning, and growth.

HYPOTHYROIDISM

Hypothyroidism is a disorder in which thyroid hormones are decreased. The cause can be congenital. It may also result from an autosomal recessive gene mutation, a deficiency in TSH, or inflammation of the thyroid gland.

Manifestations

Symptoms generally do not appear for a few months after birth (Figure 19-3 ■). The tongue and lips thicken, and the child has a dull expression. The child can also develop jaundice, hypotonia, bradycardia, lethargy, feeding problems, and cool extremities. Older children may develop precocious puberty, irregular menses, hair loss, slowing of growth, increased weight, and **goiter** (painless enlargement of thyroid gland).

Diagnosis

In the newborn, diagnosis is made by mandatory screening of TSH and T_4. If TSH is elevated, the hypothyroidism is caused by the thyroid gland, not the pituitary gland.

clinical ALERT

It is important to diagnose and treat hypothyroidism rapidly to prevent permanent mental retardation.

Treatment

Levothyroxin (Synthroid) is often prescribed to treat hypothyroidism. As the child grows, the dose will need to be adjusted to maintain a normal hormone level. It is important for the child to be followed by a pediatric endocrinologist.

Nursing Considerations

As with other endocrine disorders, the nursing management involves parent teaching about the condition, the administration of medication, and the signs of inadequate hormone replacement. It is important to stress to parents the need for lifelong thyroid replacement therapy. Table 19-2 ■ shows ways of discussing side effects related to thyroid replacement.

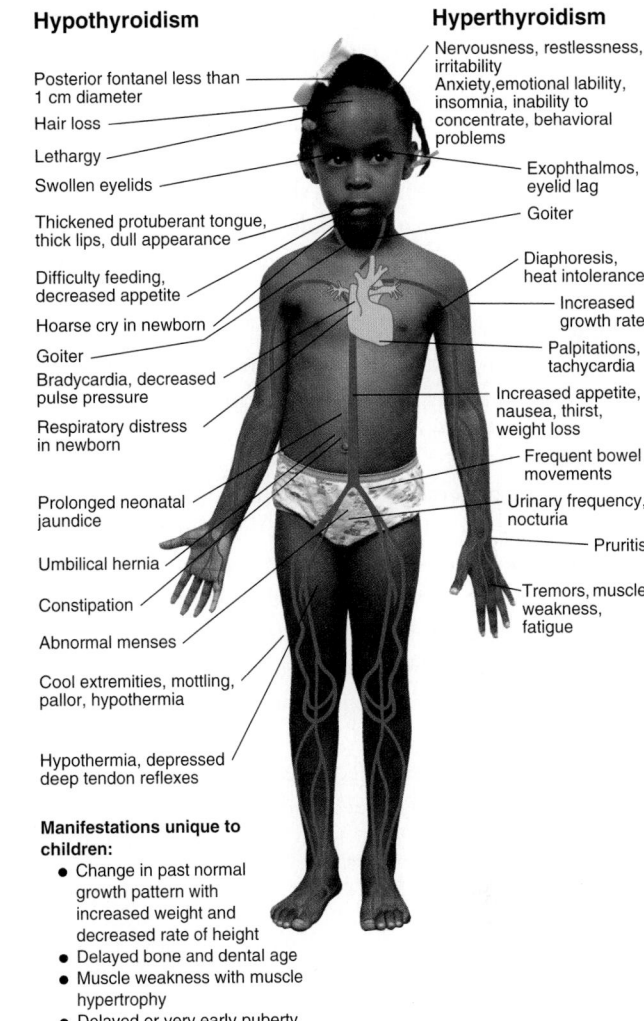

Hypothyroidism

Posterior fontanel less than 1 cm diameter
Hair loss
Lethargy
Swollen eyelids
Thickened protuberant tongue, thick lips, dull appearance
Difficulty feeding, decreased appetite
Hoarse cry in newborn
Goiter
Bradycardia, decreased pulse pressure
Respiratory distress in newborn
Prolonged neonatal jaundice
Umbilical hernia
Constipation
Abnormal menses
Cool extremities, mottling, pallor, hypothermia
Hypothermia, depressed deep tendon reflexes

Manifestations unique to children:
- Change in past normal growth pattern with increased weight and decreased rate of height
- Delayed bone and dental age
- Muscle weakness with muscle hypertrophy
- Delayed or very early puberty

Hyperthyroidism

Nervousness, restlessness, irritability
Anxiety, emotional lability, insomnia, inability to concentrate, behavioral problems
Exophthalmos, eyelid lag
Goiter
Diaphoresis, heat intolerance
Increased growth rate
Palpitations, tachycardia
Increased appetite, nausea, thirst, weight loss
Frequent bowel movements
Urinary frequency, nocturia
Pruritis
Tremors, muscle weakness, fatigue

Figure 19-3. ■ Multisystem effects of hypothyroidism and hyperthyroidism.

TABLE 19-2				
Communicating Across the Life Span: Discussing Side Effects Related to Thyroid Replacement				
	TODDLER	**PRESCHOOLER**	**SCHOOL-AGE CHILD**	**ADOLESCENT**
Parent/Child	Parent: Since beginning the medication, my child is not sleeping well at night.	Parent: I think my child's heart is racing since she's taking Synthroid.	Child: I seem to have more and more headaches and it's hard to concentrate at school.	Child: Every time I brush my hair, I think it's falling out! If it's the medicine, I'd rather not take it than be bald!
Nurse	To the parent: Give the medication 1 hour before breakfast to prevent insomnia.	To the parent: I'll show you how to count the pulse rate. If her heart rate gets above 100, please let the physician know.	To the child: This is sometimes a side effect of the medication. We'll talk to the doctor about it. Why don't you start recording how often you have the headaches and how much they bother you? In the meantime, let's talk about how you can manage the pain.	To the adolescent: Synthroid can cause temporary hair loss. Usually once your body is used to the medication, that side effect should go away. It is very important that you continue to take your medication daily as it is assisting your body to function properly. Can I give you a call next week to see how you are doing?

HYPERTHYROIDISM

Hyperthyroidism is extremely rare in children and adolescents. When it does occur, it is almost always associated with Graves' disease. **Graves' disease** is an autoimmune disorder in which antibodies attack the thyroid gland. When immunoglobulins attack the thyroid cells, the result is an overproduction of thyroid hormones. Congenital hyperthyroidism can occur in infants of mothers with Graves' disease when the immunoglobulins are transferred through the placenta. Other causes of hyperthyroidism are thyroid-secreting tumors of the thyroid, thyroiditis, and pituitary tumors that increase the production of TSH.

Manifestations

Symptoms of hyperthyroidism include an enlarged non-tender thyroid gland (*goiter*), prominent or bulging eyes (**exophthalmos**), nervousness, restlessness, and irritability. Increased weight loss with increased appetite, heat intolerance, and muscle weakness occur when the condition remains untreated. Symptoms generally begin in the school-age child and may be present for several years before they are recognized and treated. The child's performance in school declines because of decreased ability to concentrate. They rapidly become fatigued and overheated in physical education class. They may have difficulty relaxing and sleeping.

Diagnosis

Diagnosis is usually made with serum TSH, T_3, and T_4 autoantibodies specific for thyroid disorders, and thyroid scan.

Treatment

Antithyroid medications are usually the first choice of treatment. This treatment continues for approximately 2 years or until the thyroid decreases in size. Hyperthyroidism generally recurs every few years and requires repeated treatment.

The second choice of treatment is radiation with radioactive iodine to destroy the thyroid tissue. There is no evidence that this type of radiation increases the risk for cancer or birth defects in future children.

Thyroidectomy is the third option of treatment. Destruction or removal of the thyroid causes permanent hypothyroidism. After thyroidectomy, the client will require lifelong thyroid replacement therapy.

Nursing Considerations

Nursing care involves teaching the child and parents about the disorder and the chosen treatment. Because treatment is long-term and relapse can occur, the child and family need emotional support and encouragement. The child with hyperthyroidism is easily fatigued and may need periods of rest, even at school. Children receiving radiation and their families need reassurance about the safety of radioactive iodine treatment.

Families anticipating thyroid surgery in their child will need routine preoperative teaching as well as specific information about surgically induced hypothyroidism. Children may be very fearful of having their "throat cut" for thyroid surgery. They will need additional emotional support.

The priority for postoperative care is to maintain the airway and prevent blood loss. Swelling at the surgical site could obstruct the airway and the physician would need to insert a tracheostomy tube to maintain respirations. Anticipating the child's return from the operating room, the nurse should have a tracheostomy tray at the bedside in preparation for emergency treatment should it be required.

Postoperatively the nurse should observe closely for bleeding. The thyroid is a very vascular organ and bleeding could be excessive. When the child is lying flat, blood would drain onto the bed and pool under the child's head. The nurse should feel for wetness under the child's neck with each assessment until the risk for bleeding has passed.

clinical ALERT

Swelling of the surgical site can cause airway obstruction. The child should be assessed closely for swelling, bleeding, hoarseness, and difficulty breathing. If the parathyroid glands were accidentally removed, the blood calcium level can drop to life-threateningly low levels. Signs of hypocalcemia include tingling and tetany. A syringe containing calcium should be kept at the bedside.

All cases of hyperthyroidism require regular follow-up appointments with a pediatric endocrinologist. Serum thyroid levels should be drawn on a regular basis. The child should also wear a medical alert bracelet identifying hyperthyroidism, or surgically induced hypothyroidism, and the specific medications.

THYROID CANCER

In the United States, thyroid cancer is the most common pediatric endocrine cancer. Between 1997 and 2004, 6.2% of childhood cancers were thyroid cancers (Ries et al., 2007). In children younger than 15, thyroid cancer affects males and females equally. After 15, however, females are affected at higher rates.

Thyroid cancer is associated with exposure to radiation and chemotherapy. In fact, in 1986, following the explosion and radioactive contamination at the Chernobyl Nuclear Power Plant in Pripyat, Ukraine, there was a marked increase of cases in that area. Congenital hypothyroidism also increases the risk of thyroid cancer.

The typical presentation of thyroid cancer in children is a neck mass unaccompanied by additional symptoms. The diagnosis of thyroid cancer is assisted by the measure of calcitonin levels, antithyroid anitbodies, and serum carcinoembryonic antigen. Ultrasound, radionucleotide scans, fine needle biopsy, and CT scans assist in the diagnosis.

Treatment includes radioactive therapy with iodine-131, but most commonly surgery is indicated to remove the mass and affected tissue. Thyroid hormone replacement will be necessary. The 20-year survival rate for children is 92–100%.

Adrenal Disorders

Like other endocrine disorders, adrenal disorders are rare in children. However, when they do occur, prompt attention is needed.

CUSHING'S SYNDROME

Hyperfunction of the adrenal cortex is called **Cushing's syndrome.** Symptoms result from increased levels of glucocorticoids (especially cortisol). Cushing's syndrome can be caused by tumor of the adrenal cortex, by an increased secretion of ACTH by the pituitary gland, or by hyperplasia of the adrenal glands. In children the most common cause of Cushing's symptoms (*cushingoid* or Cushing's-like features) is administration of corticosteroids for the treatment of other disorders. These children do not have actual Cushing's syndrome, only the symptoms.

Manifestations

Symptoms of Cushing's syndrome include a gradual, excessive weight gain and slow growth. It generally takes 5 years for the characteristics of "**moon face**" (round cheeks and double chin) and "**buffalo hump**" (fat deposits on the back between the shoulders) to develop. Other changes include delayed puberty and mental changes.

Diagnosis

Diagnosis is based on clinical symptoms and abnormal laboratory findings of sodium, potassium, calcium, phosphorus, and glucose. Adrenal suppression tests reveal that adrenal cortisol output is not suppressed after administration of dexamethasone.

Treatment

If cushingoid features are the result of hydrocortisone administration, treatment would be geared to the symptoms, to obtain and maintain normal electrolyte and glucose levels. If Cushing's syndrome is the result of tumor, surgical intervention is warranted. The prognosis for malignant tumors of the adrenal gland is poor.

Nursing Considerations

Nursing care includes monitoring of lab values, as well as client teaching about the pathology of the disorder and prescribed treatment.

> ### clinical ALERT
> Children receiving hydrocortisone must not be withdrawn from the medication rapidly. Rapid withdrawal could result in a life-threatening condition called *adrenal crisis.*

A child with Cushing's syndrome or drug-induced cushingoid features should wear a medical alert bracelet at all times. In an emergency, the primary care providers may look at lab values and misdiagnose the child's condition. They may administer too high a dose of corticosteroids if they do not know the child is already taking these medications.

CONGENITAL ADRENAL HYPERPLASIA

Congenital adrenal hyperplasia (also called *adrenocortical hyperplasia*) is an autosomal recessive disorder that causes a deficiency in one of the enzymes needed for cortisol and aldosterone production. Congenital adrenal hyperplasia occurs more commonly in Native Alaskans (American Academy of Pediatrics Section on Endocrinology and Committee on Genetics, 2000). The most common form of congenital adrenal hyperplasia blocks the production of aldosterone, causing a loss of salt in the urine. A decrease in cortisol stimulates an increase in ACTH by the pituitary gland.

Manifestations

During fetal development, an increase in ACTH triggers an overproduction of androgens, resulting in ambiguous genitalia (**pseudohermaphroditism**). In older children, precocious genitalia (transition to adult genitalia) may occur by 6 to 8 years of age. Epiphyseal plates close early, resulting in small stature.

Diagnosis

Diagnosis is confirmed by elevated levels of serum 17-hydroxyprogesterone. Chromosome studies may be necessary to confirm the gender of the infant. These children may have life-threatening electrolyte imbalances. Because of this, lab tests must be performed often.

Treatment

Treatment involves administration of glucocorticoid medication to suppress production of ACTH and androgens. Mineralocorticoids or additional salt intake may be necessary. Reconstructive surgery of the genitals may be necessary.

Nursing Considerations

Nursing care includes teaching and emotional support. Siblings, grandparents, other family members, and day care workers will also need instructions about the condition, as well as teaching about symptoms of electrolyte imbalance.

Until gender is confirmed, the newborn should be referred to as "your infant" instead of "your son" or "your daughter." Genetic counseling and referral for counseling may be needed.

ADRENAL INSUFFICIENCY (ADDISON'S DISEASE)

Adrenal insufficiency (Addison's disease) is extremely rare in children. When it does occur, the child experiences a decrease in glucocorticoids and mineralocorticoids. The condition can be caused by trauma to the adrenal glands.

Symptoms progress slowly as the adrenal glands deteriorate. The child may present with weakness, fever, abdominal pain, hypoglycemia, dehydration, and shock. Client with Addison's disease may crave salt; the nurse can be aware of this while collecting data.

Addison's disease is diagnosed by low levels of serum cortisol and urinary 17-hydroxycorticoid. Serum values for sodium and glucose are low and potassium is high. Treatment includes the administration of deficient hormones. Nursing care includes teaching and emotional support.

PHEOCHROMOCYTOMA

Pheochromocytoma is an adrenal tumor, most commonly benign and curable. The tumor occurs between the ages of 6 and 14 years. The adrenal tumor releases the catecholamines epinephrine and norepinephrine.

Manifestations

Symptoms include severe hypertension with a systolic blood pressure that may reach 190 mm Hg. The child may also experience blurred vision, headache, palpitations, weakness, polyuria, and polydipsia. Because the release of epinephrine and norepinephrine is intermittent, symptoms come and go. Attacks may occur weekly, monthly, or in some cases only during periods of stress.

Diagnosis

Diagnosis is based on 24-hour urine studies to detect urinary catecholamines, vanillylmandelic acid (VMA) levels, and MRI to localize the tumor.

Treatment

Beta- and alpha-adrenergic blocking agents are given to control hypertension and catecholamine release. Surgical removal of the affected adrenal gland occurs approximately 14 days after medication has started. Following surgery, 24-hour urine studies are performed for several days to determine whether all of the tumor has been removed.

Nursing Considerations

Nursing care is mainly emotional support and preoperative and postoperative teaching. Families should be taught how to monitor the child's blood pressure. Follow-up urine screening is done on a regular basis for the rest of the child's life.

Pancreatic Islet Disorders

DIABETES MELLITUS

The most common metabolic disorder in children is **diabetes mellitus,** a disorder of carbohydrate, protein, and fat metabolism. There are two types of diabetes mellitus. The majority of children have type I or insulin-dependent diabetes mellitus (IDDM). Non-insulin-dependent diabetes mellitus (NIDDM) or type II is usually contracted as an adult. However, the incidence of children and adolescents acquiring type II diabetes mellitus is increasing. Therefore, both types will be discussed.

TYPE I DIABETES MELLITUS

The average age of onset of type I (insulin-dependent) diabetes mellitus (IDDM) is 10 to 14 years. Although there is a strong familial tendency to type I diabetes mellitus, there is no specific inheritance (American Diabetes Association). Current research has identified a genetic marker that increases the child's susceptibility to the disease. Other environmental factors, such as viruses or chemicals in the diet, stimulate an autoimmune response that damages the islets of Langerhans (where insulin is produced). Antigens generate the production of antibodies that indicate the continued destruction of the islet cells.

As you recall, insulin is necessary for the transport of glucose into all body cells. When the beta cells are destroyed, the level of insulin falls and the level of blood glucose increases. Because cells need glucose for energy, there is a steep decrease in cell metabolism and cells must convert protein and fat into glucose. When the level of blood glucose exceeds the renal threshold of 160 mg/dL, glucose is excreted in the urine (**glucosuria**). Glucose in the urine causes an increase in osmotic pressure that pulls additional water into the urine, resulting in increased urinary output (*polyuria*). With an excessive urinary output, the child will become thirsty (*polydipsia*). The cells become starved for glucose, triggering the appetite and resulting in **polyphagia** (excessive hunger).

To provide cells with needed energy, the liver metabolizes free fatty acids at an increased rate. Although this use of fatty acids increases the energy available to cells, it also results in an accumulation of acetyl coenzyme A (CoA) or *ketone bodies*. An increase in ketone bodies results in metabolic acidosis or **diabetic ketoacidosis** (DKA; discussed further later).

Manifestations

The classic signs of type I diabetes mellitus include:

- The three Ps (Figure 19-4 ■):
  - Polyuria
  - Polydipsia
  - Polyphagia
- Hyperglycemia
- Weight loss

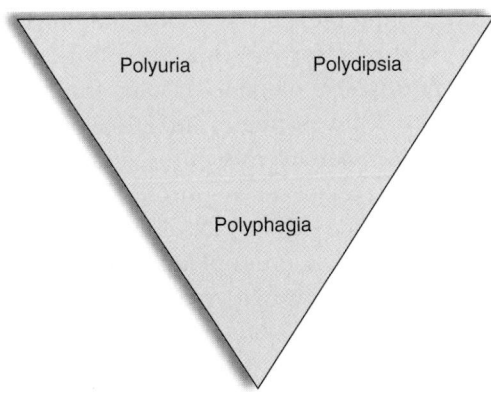

Figure 19-4. ■ Classic symptoms of diabetes mellitus.

Other symptoms include fatigue, headache, poor wound healing, and infection. Adolescent girls may have recurrent episodes of vaginitis caused by *Candida*, which thrives in a high-glucose environment. Symptoms generally develop

over time, but most have been present for less than a month. The parents may bring their child to the health care provider with recognizable symptoms, or the child may present in the emergency room with DKA.

Figure 19-5 ■ shows early and late symptoms of type I and type II diabetes. It also illustrates the progressive and long-term complications of this complex disorder. Diabetic ketoacidosis is discussed later.

Diagnosis

Type I diabetes mellitus is diagnosed by nonfasting blood glucose (random glucose) levels over 200 mg/dL. A follow-up fasting blood glucose level would also be elevated over 126 mg/dL. The primary care provider may monitor an insulin test to detect the blood level of insulin. A test for C-peptide, a by-product of insulin production, may also be used in diagnosis.

EARLY MANIFESTATIONS
- **Type 1 DM**
  - Polyuria (sometimes enuresis)
  - Polydipsia
  - Polyphagia
  - Weight loss
  - Glycosuria
  - Hyperglycemia
  - Fatigue
  - Vaginitis
- **Type 2 DM**
  - Obesity
  - Acanthosis nigricans
  - Polyuria
  - Polydipsia
  - Blurred vision
  - Glycosuria
  - Hyperglycemia

PROGRESSIVE COMPLICATIONS
- **Cardiovascular**
  - Lipid disorders
  - Hypertension
- **Metabolic**
  - Diabetic ketoacidosis
  - Hyperglycemic hyperosmolar nonketotic coma
  - Hypoglycemia
  - Androgen-mediated hirsutism, polycystic ovary syndrome, menstrual irregularities
- **Renal**
  - Albuminuria
- **Integumentary**
  - Impaired healing
  - Acne

LONG-TERM COMPLICATIONS
- **Eyes**
  - Diabetic retinopathy
  - Blurred vision
- **Cardiovascular**
  - Atherosclerotic heart disease
  - Peripheral vascular disease
- **Renal**
  - Proteinuria
  - Chronic renal failure
- **Neurologic**
  - Peripheral neuropathy
  - Paresthesias
  - Impotence in males
- **Impaired Immune System**
  - Recurrent infections

Immune System
- Impaired healing
- Chronic skin infections
- Periodontal disease
- Urinary tract infections
- Lung infections
- Vaginitis

Figure 19-5. ■ Multisystem effects of diabetes mellitus.

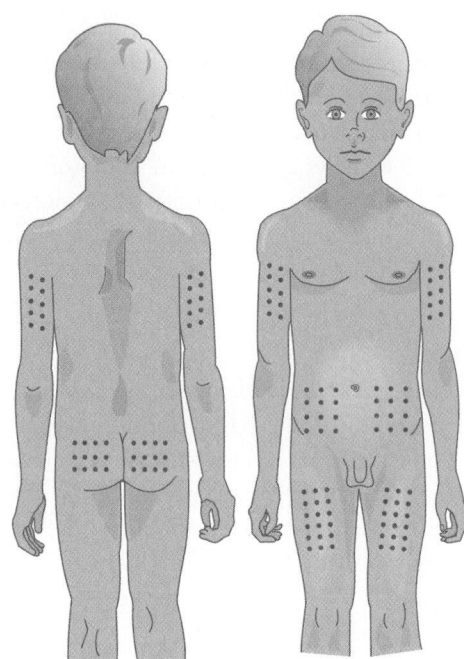

Figure 19-6. ■ Locations for rotating administering of insulin.

Treatment

The medical goal for type I diabetes mellitus is to regain a normal blood glucose level with the administration of insulin. Insulin administration may be either by repeated subcutaneous injections (Figure 19-6 ■) or by continuous subcutaneous insulin pump. The health care provider will prescribe a meal plan for the child to follow, in which approximately 50–60% of calories come from carbohydrates, 10–20% from protein, and 20–30% from fat. Exercise plays an important role in diabetes management by increasing the metabolism of glucose. Individuals who have high levels of activity may be able to have a higher caloric intake and lower doses of insulin. Exercise may result in decreased body weight, which decreases the need for insulin.

clinical ALERT

Blood glucose levels must be monitored during periods of exercise to prevent hypoglycemia. High-carbohydrate juice or snacks should be available to treat hypoglycemia should it occur.

More information about caring for the client with diabetes mellitus in provided in the Nursing Care Plan Chart below.

DIABETIC KETOACIDOSIS

Diabetic ketoacidosis is the most common cause of death in diabetic children. The child may be seen initially in the emergency department and then transferred to a pediatric intensive care unit for continuous monitoring and treatment. The only

NURSING CARE PLAN CHART

Child with Diabetes Mellitus

GOAL	INTERVENTION	RATIONALE	EXPECTED OUTCOME
1. Risk for Imbalanced Nutrition: Less than Body Requirements related to hyperglycemia			
The child will demonstrate a balanced diet and normal blood glucose levels.	Carefully review the child's pre-diagnosis diet	*These data will provide the nurse an opportunity to make a client-specific diet plan*	Child's weight is stable, stable HbA1c, and avoids complications related to imbalanced blood glucose.
	Determine the child's readiness to learn	*Behaviors change when there is a readiness to learn*	
	Discuss the dietary requirements related to diabetes mellitus. Present information in an age-appropriate manner	*Discussing the dietary requirements with the client and their family requires a presentation method that will be received in order for adequate utilization*	
The family will demonstrate understanding of dietary requirements and necessary changes in family meal planning.	Present the family with sample menus and shopping lists outlining dietary requirements	*Teaching should include handouts for the family to take home as a reference. This will reinforce the information given*	The family presents a sample menu plan incorporating necessary dietary requirements.
	Refer the child and family to a nutritionist for follow-up care	*Diabetes management is a lifelong issue that will require ongoing assistance from many health care providers.*	

GOAL	INTERVENTION	RATIONALE	EXPECTED OUTCOME
2. Deficient **K**nowledge related to medical condition requiring intense therapeutic regimen			
The child will demonstrate ability to monitor blood glucose and administer insulin correctly.	Demonstrate use of the glucometer, including correct interpretation of results. Require return demonstration	*Using demonstration and requiring return demonstration allows the nurse to assess comprehension of information*	The child demonstrates correct use of the glucometer and demonstrates correct subcutaneous injection technique.
	Assess child's anxiety level related to invasive procedures	*Anxiety may prevent appropriate learning of skills*	
	Demonstrate insulin administration. Require return demonstration	*Using demonstration and requiring return demonstration allows the nurse to assess comprehension of information*	
The family will assist the child in learning techniques of blood sugar analysis and insulin administration.	Provide printed handouts related to diabetic teaching	*Teaching should include handouts for the family to take home as a reference. This will reinforce the information given*	The family verbalizes necessary steps related to blood sugar analysis and insulin administration and demonstrates assistance to the child when appropriate.
	Refer parents to a diabetic educator for follow-up care	*Diabetes management is a lifelong issue that will require ongoing assistance from many health care providers*	

cause of DKA is insufficient amount of insulin. Precipitating factors can be infection, other illnesses, or omission of insulin.

Manifestations

The classic signs of diabetic ketoacidosis include those of type I diabetes mellitus plus fruity or **acetone breath** (breath with odor of nail polish remover or rotting apples), deep labored breathing (**Kussmaul respiration**), dehydration, decreased level of consciousness, and flushed dry skin. In late stages, DKA may present with electrolyte imbalances,

arrhythmias, shock, and death. Manifestations of DKA are listed in Box 19-6 ■.

Diagnosis and Treatment

Values shown in Box 19-6 establish the diagnosis of diabetic ketoacidosis. (London et al., 2007). DKA is a life-threatening emergency, and treatment must begin immediately to prevent further cell damage and death. If the child presents with DKA, immediate treatment involves intravenous infusion of isotonic fluids, most

BOX 19-6   ASSESSMENT

Diabetic Ketoacidosis

Lab Values
  Blood glucose greater than 300 mg/dL
  Serum ketones
  pH less than or equal to 7.3
  Bicarbonate less than 15 mEq/L
  Glycosuria
  Ketonuria
  Elevated blood urea nitrogen (BUN) and creatinine
  Possible electrolyte imbalances

Manifestations
  Weight loss
  Dehydration
  Flushed cheeks and ears
  Tachycardia
  Kussmaul respiration

Acetone breath
Altered level of consciousness
Hypotension
Abdominal or chest pain
Nausea and vomiting

Late-Stage Manifestations
  Electrolyte imbalances
  Arrhythmias
  Altered consciousness
  Shock
  Death

Complication of DKA
  Cerebral edema (potentially life-threatening; evidenced by headache, lethargy, very fast or very slow heartbeat, widening pulse pressure)

commonly normal saline. The rate of infusion is geared to replace the deficit in 24 to 48 hours.

Blood glucose levels are decreased with the intravenous infusion of regular insulin. Insulin must be given IV, because insulin cannot be absorbed from subcutaneous tissue when dehydration or acidosis is present. Because hypoglycemia could result if blood glucose levels are decreased rapidly, IV infusion of insulin is administered at a rate to decrease the blood glucose 100 to 150 mg/dL/hour. When the blood glucose level reaches 200 to 300 mg/dL, dextrose may be added to the intravenous fluids in order to prevent hypoglycemia.

clinical ALERT

Insulin will stick to plastic and glass tubing. Many hospitals are recommending that the pharmacy add albumin to the IV fluid to decrease this tendency. The tubing should be flushed to saturate the binding sites before the insulin is added to the solution.

DKA causes hydrogen ions to replace intracellular potassium. This initially causes serum potassium readings to be falsely elevated. In reality, the *total* body potassium is being depleted. Once urine output is established, intravenous potassium is administered. Other electrolytes must be closely monitored, and replacement may be necessary.

Nursing Considerations

The goals of nursing care are to stabilize the child's condition, to teach the child and family to manage the condition at home, and to prevent long-term complications. The first priority is to stabilize the child's condition. There is no protocol for the management of diabetes. Application of the entire nursing process on an ongoing basis is important. The nurse must be skilled in assessment, must understand the goals of treatment, and must be able to make rapid adjustments in the plan of care.

Nursing responsibilities in caring for the child with diabetic ketoacidosis are to administer isotonic IV fluids; to monitor electrolytes, blood glucose, and acid-base balance;

and to administer replacements as ordered. Once the child has stabilized, balanced nutrition will be given orally. Blood glucose will be monitored. Insulin will be administered subcutaneously to prevent further episodes of hyperglycemia.

Teaching the parents and the child is important for the long-term management of diabetes and the prevention of complications. Although the complete teaching plan is the responsibility of the registered nurse, the LPN/LVN may be asked to provide instruction on the following topics:

- Blood glucose testing (see Chapter 8 ⚭)
- Balanced nutrition with regular meals and snacks (the American Diabetes Association offers help in adapting food needs, including an adapted food pyramid)
- Regular daily activity
- Insulin administration (see Chapter 8 ⚭)
- Prescribed insulin including onset, peak, duration (Table 19-3 ■)
- Signs of hyperglycemia and hypoglycemia (Table 19-4 ■)
- Complications (see Figure 19-5)
- Health promotion activities to prevent injury to the feet:
  - Wearing shoes that fit the foot well
  - Filing nails straight across
  - Inspecting the feet daily for redness, swelling, or sores
- Health promotion activities to prevent infection:
  - Bathing daily
  - Avoiding contact with infected individuals
  - Cleaning wounds, applying antibiotic ointment, and keeping wounds covered
- Management of type I diabetes mellitus during times of minor illness, such as cold and flu. Client teaching about this is discussed further under Nursing Care. Box 19-7 ■ provides guidelines for client teaching about care of a client with type I diabetes mellitus during illness.

Children should be encouraged to learn to manage their health needs. The young child can help assemble the equipment, can make choices about which finger to use for blood glucose testing, and can help in the selection of nutritious

TABLE 19-3

Types of Insulin

TYPE OF INSULIN	ONSET (BEGIN EFFECT)	PEAK (MAXIMUM EFFECT)	DURATION (LENGTH OF EFFECT)
Lispro	15–25 minutes	30–90 minutes	3–5 hours
Regular	30–60 minutes	2–3 hours	4–6 hours
NPH	2–4 hours	4–10 hours	14–18 hours
Lente	3–4 hours	4–12 hours	16–20 hours

TABLE 19-4

Symptoms of Hyperglycemia and Hypoglycemia

HYPERGLYCEMIA (BG MORE THAN 120 mg/dl)	HYPOGLYCEMIA (BG LESS THAN 60 mg/dl)
Polyuria (excess urine)	Dizziness
Polydipsia (excess thirst)	Shakiness
Polyphagia (excess hunger)	Headache
Dry skin	Pallor
Flushed face	Visual disturbance
Blurred vision	Hunger
Muscle weakness	Fatigue
Weak, slow pulse	Tachycardia
Fruity or acetone breath	Disorientation (slow thought process)
Rapid respirations	Confusion
Confusion	Seizure
Coma	Coma
Death	Death

snacks. Older children can be taught to perform their own glucose testing, administer their insulin, and complete daily records.

The emotional support needed for the child depends on the age and stage of emotional development. Efforts should

BOX 19-7   CLIENT TEACHING

Managing Diabetes During Sick Days

Maintain Normal Blood Glucose
- Monitor blood glucose every 2 hours.
- Take insulin as prescribed.
- Increase caloric intake with simple sugars in small amounts (sweetened gelatin, juice).

Prevent Dehydration
- Maintain fluid intake with small amounts of liquids frequently.
- Take antiemetics or antidiarrhea medication as recommended.

Decrease Activity
- Provide adequate rest periods.

Know Resources
- Contact primary care provider if normal blood glucose cannot be maintained.
- Contact primary care provider if unable to maintain fluid balance.

be made to enhance the child's feeling of autonomy and independence. The fewer changes the family has to make, the more supportive family members can be. Printed material should be provided to help the family learn and adjust to the changes. The child may need additional emotional support to handle the pressures of adolescence (such as what to do if friends want to go get ice cream sundaes together). The family should be referred to home health or diabetes centers for continued in-depth teaching and support. The American Diabetes Association is also an excellent source of information. Most schools do not allow children to have medication in their possession at school. Therefore, a plan for blood testing and insulin administration needs to be established. The school nurse should be informed of the child's diagnosis and plan of care. The school nurse may need to help the young child with blood testing or insulin administration at school. If other school personnel are to help the child, they must receive adequate instruction and supervision.

The child with newly diagnosed type I diabetes mellitus should be evaluated by the nurse and health care provider every few weeks until the condition has stabilized. The child and family should be able to verbalize an understanding of all teaching. The daily record of diet, blood glucose values, and amount of insulin administered should be reviewed and used as a basis for changes in insulin dosage.

TYPE II DIABETES MELLITUS

Type II diabetes mellitus occurs most commonly in adults over age 40. However, the incidence of type II diabetes mellitus in individuals under 25 has increased in the past 10 years. Type II diabetes accounts for 16% of childhood/adolescent diabetes. Many of these children have relatives with type II diabetes, are overweight, and are of African American, Hispanic, Asian, or Native American descent.

In type II diabetes, the body produces enough insulin, but for some reason the body is unable to use the insulin effectively. This condition is called **insulin resistance** and is a precursor to type II diabetes mellitus. Over several years, the production of insulin decreases, resulting in hyperglycemia.

Manifestations

Symptoms of type II diabetes develop slowly. Children may have polydipsia, polyuria, and polyphagia. They may be tired and develop frequent infections, but they do not have ketoacidosis.

Diagnosis and Treatment

Diagnose by fasting blood glucose test. Medical treatment of type II diabetes mellitus includes diet, exercise, blood glucose monitoring, and in many cases oral hypoglycemic

TABLE 19-5

Pharmacology: Oral Hypoglycemics

DRUG (GENERIC AND COMMON BRAND NAME)	USUAL ROUTE/DOSE	CLASSIFICATION	SELECTED SIDE EFFECTS	DON'T GIVE IF
Metformin (Glucophage)	1 tablet 2–3 times a day	Oral antidiabetic drug	Dizziness, weakness, tired, shortness of breath, irregular pulse	Clients have abnormal renal function or congestive heart failure.
Glyburide (sulfonylurea)	2.5–5 mg every day	Oral antidiabetic drug	GI upset, weakness, tired	Client has low blood glucose levels.

agents or, less commonly, insulin (Table 19-5 ■). The diet should meet the nutritional needs of the growing child or adolescent, but be low enough in calories to allow for weight loss. Exercise is intended not only to decrease the need for insulin, but also to burn calories for additional weight loss.

Oral hypoglycemic agents are not insulin. They stimulate the pancreas to produce insulin, and they make cell receptor sites more sensitive to insulin. Because type II diabetes mellitus has been unusual in children and adolescents, research is currently being conducted about the use of oral hypoglycemic agents in children and adolescents (Jacobson-Dickman & Levitsky, 2005).

Nursing Considerations

Nursing responsibilities are similar to those for type I diabetes mellitus. Client and family teaching about the signs of hypoglycemia and hyperglycemia, the complications of diabetes, and treatment is consistent with all types of diabetes. Because oral hypoglycemic agents have not been used extensively in children and adolescents, it is important for the nurse to teach the family to monitor for side effects and report them to the health care provider in a timely manner.

METABOLIC SYNDROME (METABOLIC X SYNDROME)

In recent years a set of conditions related to glucose metabolism has been identified and named metabolic (or metabolic X) syndrome. The Health Promotion Issue on pages 540 and 541 discusses this increasingly prevalent disorder.

NURSING CARE

PRIORITIES IN NURSING CARE

- Monitor ordered lab values.
- Teach child/family to manage the condition at home.
- Provide information about specialists, support groups, and financial resources.

ASSESSING

The symptoms of many endocrine disorders are similar to symptoms of other disorders. Many affect the child's growth and development over time. The nurse should be *alert to compare* the client's data to the established standards of growth and development for the child's age.

DIAGNOSING, PLANNING, AND IMPLEMENTING

The specific endocrine disorder will determine the particular interventions needed. Diagnosis of disorders is usually made from serum levels of specific chemicals, as well as symptoms and eliminating other diagnoses.

Expected nursing diagnoses for children (and families) with endocrine disorders would include (but not be limited to) the following:

- Deficient **K**nowledge related to the particular disorder
- Risk for Imbalanced **F**luid Volume related to endocrine imbalance
- **C**aregiver Role Strain related to care demands of endocrine disorder

Outcomes for such nursing diagnoses would include:

- Expresses understanding of disorder, treatment, and ongoing management.
- Maintains adequate hydration.
- States plan to use personal network, support services, and referrals in long-term care of the child with an endocrine disorder.

Nursing interventions must be tailored to the specific needs of the client and family. Appropriate nursing actions include (but are not limited to) the following:

- Teach the child and family about the disorder and how to manage the day-to-day treatment. *Learning about a serious medical problem may be overwhelming. The family may need to hear information several times in order to retain learning.*

- Help the family plan alterations in diet, activity, and medication administration. Provide written materials for the parents' use later. *The parents can use the process of planning as a model. They may refer back to a sample plan when they are tired or overwhelmed.*
- Provide specific instructions and contact information concerning what to do when illness occurs in the child with an endocrine disorder. Stress the importance of Medic-Alert bracelets. *Acute illness may affect the endocrine disorder, and parents must keep the primary care provider informed of changes in the child's condition. Failure to notify medical personnel about the child's disorder may result in improper treatment and death.*
- Provide referrals to home health nurses and school nurses if possible. *They may be beneficial resources in planning and implementing care.*

EVALUATING

Endocrine disorders in children affect their health for the rest of their lives. Periodic monitoring of serum levels is necessary to ensure stability of a child's condition. Dietary requirements change as a child grows. Diet restrictions should be reviewed and changes made to meet changing needs. Family dynamics and individual coping should be evaluated to ensure all needs are met.

NURSING PROCESS CARE PLAN
Care of a Client with Growth Hormone Deficiency

Juanita received a concussion at 9 months of age from a fall. At the time, she seemed to recover without incident. She is now 2 years old and is being seen in the pediatric endocrinologist office for failure to grow. She is in the 2nd percentile for growth for her age, but in the 20th percentile for weight. Except for failure to grow, Juanita's development is consistent with her age.

Assessment.   Vital signs: T 97.2 (A) P 90, R 36. Wt 24.5 lbs (11 kg), Ht 30.5 in (77 cm). Juanita is alert and talkative. She is walking around the room holding a doll. Her speech is understandable, and she uses four- to five-word sentences. She has been referred from a health clinic because of slow growth.

Nursing Diagnosis.   The following important nursing diagnosis (among others) is established for this condition:

- Risk for Disproportionate **G**rowth related to hormone imbalance

Expected Outcomes.   The following expected outcome was identified:

- Juanita will grow 2 inches in the next year.

Planning and Implementation

- Obtain serum growth hormone level as ordered by the primary care provider. *Serum growth hormone is needed for diagnosis and a baseline for evaluation of treatment.*
- Discuss with parents the resources available to provide financial assistance to purchase prescribed growth hormone. *Growth hormone is expensive. Most parents will need financial assistance.*
- Teach parents the manifestations of growth hormone deficiency and the need for long-term follow-up assessments. *Parents need information in order to make informed choices. GHD requires treatment and follow-up assessment until the child reaches adult height.*
- Teach parents to administer the growth hormone injections as ordered. *Injections will be given 3 to 7 times a week. It is less expensive and more convenient for parents to administer the medication.*
- Provide emotional support for parents and child. *The long-term effects of GHD can be frightening for parents. Children also need support because of the frequent injections. When the child gets older, support may be needed because of social pressure from peers.*
- Schedule follow-up appointments to monitor Juanita's growth, obtain serum growth hormone level, and assess side effects of medication.

Evaluation.   Juanita will grow 0.5 inches in 3 months. Growth hormone level will be within normal range. No side effects of growth hormone replacement will be apparent.

Critical Thinking in the Nursing Process

1. What else can the nurse teach the parents that will help in Juanita's growth?
2. If Juanita does not receive growth hormone injections, will she grow any more?
3. What suggestions may be offered to help Juanita accept a shot every day?

Note: Discussion of Critical Thinking questions appears in Appendix I.

Note: The reference and resource listings for this and all chapters have been compiled at the back of the book.

HEALTH PROMOTION ISSUE

METABOLIC SYNDROME (METABOLIC X SYNDROME)

A young woman, unable to lose weight for over a year, seeks assistance from her primary care provider. She states she began putting on weight when she was 16 years old. She admits to a sedentary lifestyle, but states she does not have the energy to exercise. She is 62 pounds over the expected weight for her height. The majority of the weight is around her abdomen. Her blood pressure is 142/88. Her laboratory tests determine that blood glucose level is high, triglycerides are elevated, and HDL cholesterol is low. The primary care provides suspects she has a relatively newly identified disorder called metabolic syndrome.

DISCUSSION

Metabolic syndrome, also called metabolic X syndrome, is a group of related metabolic disorders, including obesity, insulin resistance, and complications of type II diabetes. Although these disorders

have been known for years, the relationship and linking of these and other disorders together is relatively new. Research is still underway to discover the cause of this life-altering syndrome and other disorders that may be linked to metabolic syndrome in the future.

One point is clear: central obesity is a key factor in this syndrome. As noted in Chapter 17 ⚭, obesity is rapidly increasing in children. Many individuals, when seeking medical help to lose weight, state that their weight problem began during their teenage years. They admit to a high-calorie intake and a sedentary lifestyle. As overweight children grow, many may develop metabolic syndrome. However, not everyone who is overweight and inactive will develop this disorder. Researchers believe a genetic factor plays an important role as well. Further research is needed in this area. (See the Health Promotion Issue in Chapter 17 ⚭ for information on high-calorie diets and obesity in children.)

Metabolic syndrome places the individual at risk for other potentially life-threatening disorders. A buildup of plaque inside blood vessels, resulting from low HDL cholesterol levels, leads to coronary artery disease (CAD), cerebral vascular disease leading to stroke, and peripheral vascular disease. Insulin resistance or glucose intolerance is a precursor to type II diabetes. Metabolic syndrome is also being linked to fatty deposits in the liver resulting in liver failure, renal failure, and cancer. Researchers in Australia have identified altered endocrine function related to metabolic syndrome. These include high estrogen levels in women, low testosterone levels in men, high cortisol levels, and low thyroid levels.

It is generally accepted that if clients exhibit three of the following criteria,

they can be diagnosed with metabolic syndrome:

- **Central obesity:** fat deposits in and around the abdomen
- **Atherogenic dyslipidemia:** blood fat disorders (especially high triglycerides and low HDL cholesterol) leading to plaque buildup in blood vessels
- Insulin resistance or glucose intolerance
- **Prothrombotic state:** increased fibrinogen or plasminogen activator inhibitor [−1] in the blood leading to increased chance of thrombosis.
- Elevated blood pressure of 130/85 mm Hg or higher
- **Preinflammatory state:** increased C-reactive protein in the blood indicating an inflammatory process is in the early stage.

Diagnosis is based on clinical findings and abnormal laboratory values. Most of the tests must be repeated over time. Many individuals do not exhibit all the symptoms for years, so diagnosis takes time. However, when the individual has central edema and states they have difficulty losing weight, the nurse should recommend laboratory testing be done to establish a baseline for future evaluation.

The waist measurement indicates central obesity. The waist measurement in women with central obesity is greater than 102 cm (40 inches); in men, it is greater than 88 cm (35 inches). The blood pressure may be elevated initially or gradually increase over time. The individual may have a history of polycystic ovarian disease. Depression, irritable bowel syndrome, chronic infections, and fatigue are all common complications seen with metabolic syndrome.

Laboratory findings show high blood glucose, low thyroid, and low HDL cholesterol. Estrogen levels will be elevated in women; testosterone levels will be lower in men. Estrogen results in calories being converted to fat. Liver function tests indicate a gradual decrease in liver function. Cortisol levels will be elevated.

PLANNING AND IMPLEMENTATION

There is no specific treatment for metabolic syndrome, nor is there a quick fix. Treatment is centered on weight loss, maintaining blood glucose in normal ranges, and increasing activity. Diets must be altered to decrease calories while increasing protein and fiber. Activity should be increased to improve the efficiency of cell metabolism. Insulin resistance and increased blood glucose are often treated with oral hypoglycemics. Hypothyroidism is treated with synthetic hormone replacement. By increasing metabolism with increased thyroid, cell metabolism is increased and more calories are burned. Anticholesterol and antitriglyceride medications may be given. Some herbal drugs such as pantethine, fish oil, and garlic can lower both cholesterol and triglycerides. Often these are enough to reduce weight, stabilize blood glucose, and increase the HDL cholesterol. Evaluation of these treatments is usually done at 3-month intervals.

Typically, the treatment for ovarian cysts is birth control pills that increase the estrogen and progesterone levels. Because of the high estrogen levels seen with metabolic syndrome, only low-level birth control pills can be used. An intrauterine device containing progesterone may be helpful in women who are unable to have additional estrogen.

Because of the multisystem effects of metabolic syndrome, it is important to prevent and treat central obesity in order to prevent the client from developing cardiac disease. Prevention begins in childhood by providing a diet that is adequate in fruits and vegetables, whole grain breads and cereals, meat, and milk products. The diet should be low in saturated fats. The nurse should teach children and parents to make healthy choices in their diet and to limit fast foods that are typically high in fats and calories.

Exercise is another key component in preventing obesity. Children should run, climb, or swim daily. Being involved in sports not only burns calories but also improves social skills such as teamwork and fair play. Some children, however, do not enjoy sports, and it is hard to get them involved in physical activity. Encouraging them to walk or ride their bicycle to school, or to park away from the building so they will have to walk farther, will help them increase their activity. The nurse should help the family problem find other ways to increase activity in the child.

When assessing every child, the nurse should pay attention to the child's weight and fat distribution. If the child's weight is increasing faster than is expected, the nurse should discuss the child's diet and activity with the parents. By teaching parents about the potential for metabolic syndrome and the effect of obesity on the endocrine and other body systems, these disorders may be prevented.

When metabolic syndrome occurs, the nurse is responsible for teaching the individual about the syndrome, the prescribed treatment, and how to monitor the blood glucose level. The nurse assists in monitoring the effects and side effects of medication, the laboratory values, and the client's weight. Decreasing stress can help to decrease the cortisol level, and therefore, decrease the effects on cell metabolism.

SELF-REFLECTION

Take notes for a day on your thoughts related to food and exercise. Do thoughts of food as a reward or a comfort pop into your mind? If you are planning to exercise, what are the thoughts that go through your mind? Do you recognize some thoughts that are self-defeating? Think of positive phrases that you can use as substitutes. For example, if you think, "I can't jog four blocks," you could substitute, "It doesn't matter if I jog or walk. What matters is that I am getting fresh air and exercise."

SUGGESTED RESOURCES

For the Nurse

Kidson, W. (1998). Polycystic ovary syndrome: A new direction in treatment. *Medical Journal of Australia, 169*, 537–540.

Largo, R. S., Gnatuk, C. L., Kunselman, A. R., & Dunaif, A. (2005). Change in glucose tolerance over time in women with polycystic ovarian syndrome: A controlled study. *Journal of Clinical Endocrinology and Metabolism, 90*(6), 3236–3242.

Chapter Review

 KEY TERMS by Topic

Use the audio glossary feature of either the CD-ROM or the Companion Website to hear the correct pronunciation of the following key terms.

Anatomy and Physiology
hormones, negative feedback, positive feedback, prostaglandins, gonadotropic

Pituitary Disorders
growth hormone deficiency, hypopituitarism, precocious puberty, polyuria, polydipsia

Thyroid Disorders
goiter, Graves' disease, exophthalmos

Adrenal Disorders
Cushing's syndrome, "moon face," "buffalo hump," pseudohermaphroditism, pheochromocytoma

Pancreatic Islet Disorders
diabetes mellitus, glucosuria, polyphagia, diabetic ketoacidosis, acetone breath, Kussmaul respiration, insulin resistance, atherogenic dyslipidemia, prothrombotic state, preinflammatory state

KEY Points

- Endocrine disorders are potentially life threatening because of lack of regulation of other body systems.
- Endocrine disorders display symptoms similar to those of other body systems, making diagnosis difficult at times.
- Endocrine disorders require long-term treatment.
- Some endocrine disorders are fatal.
- Diabetes mellitus is the most common endocrine disorder in children. The LPN must seek to implement nursing care that will stabilize the child's condition, to teach the child and family to manage the condition at home, and to prevent long-term complications.
- Diabetic ketoacidosis is the most common cause of death in diabetic children. The LPN must be able to recognize these symptoms and act promptly.
- Families may need to be taught to monitor the child's condition and administer treatments including medication
- Many treatments of endocrine disorders are expensive and may not be covered by insurance. The nurse may need to provide resource information
- Metabolic syndrome is an example of the complex nature of endocrine disorders.

 EXPLORE Media Link

Additional interactive resources for this chapter can be found on the Companion Website at www.prenhall.com/adams.

Click on Chapter 19 and "Begin" to select the activities for this chapter.

For chapter-related NCLEX®-style questions and an audio glossary, access the accompanying CD-ROM in this book.

Animations:
Diabetes
Endocrine system

FOR FURTHER Study

See Procedures in Chapter 8 for temperature, respiratory rate, and blood pressure, as well as blood glucose testing and insulin administration.

See more on hypernatremia in Chapter 11.

Sympathetic and parasympathetic responses are discussed in Chapter 15.

See Chapter 17 for a complete discussion on phenylketonuria and for additional information on the pancreas as an exocrine gland, high-calorie diets, and obesity.

Caring for a Client with Type I Diabetes Mellitus
NCLEX-PN® Focus Area: Physiological Integrity

Case Study: Grey Wolf, an 11-year-old American Indian boy, is admitted to the tribal clinic with a blood glucose of 48 mm/dL. He was diagnosed with type I diabetes mellitus 3 months ago. He has been having difficulty remembering to eat a snack before soccer practice.

Nursing Diagnosis: Risk for Injury related to hypoglycemia

COLLECT DATA

Subjective	Objective
_____	_____
_____	_____
_____	_____
_____	_____
_____	_____
_____	_____

Would you report this? Yes/No

If yes, to: _____

Nursing Care

_____

_____

_____

_____

_____

_____

_____

_____

How would you document these findings? _____

_____

_____

_____

_____

_____

Compare your documentation to the samples provided in Appendix I.

Data Collected
(use only those that apply)

- Irritable
- Thirsty
- Sweating
- Flushed
- Fruity/acetone breath
- Hungry
- Tremors
- Pulse 102
- Resp. 38

Nursing Interventions
(use only those that apply; list in priority order)

- Obtain a thorough nutrition history.
- Review causes and signs of hypoglycemia.
- Administer regular insulin as ordered.
- Give orange juice with 1 packet sugar added.
- Start an IV of normal saline as ordered or as per facility policy.
- Give 1 ampule of sodium bicarbonate as ordered.
- Monitor blood glucose every 30–60 minutes.
- Review insulin administration techniques.

NCLEX-PN® Exam Preparation

TEST-TAKING TIP When reading a question, be sure to note whether it is a regular multiple-choice question or not. If it is an alternate-style multiple choice, there will be more than one correct answer. You could get the answer wrong by not noting all the correct options.

1 Children are generally more physically active during the summer months. In caring for the child with type I diabetes mellitus, what changes in the plan of care should be expected?

1. Decrease food intake
2. Increase food intake
3. Increase insulin dose
4. Decrease insulin dose

2 The nurse is teaching an adolescent who has recently been diagnosed with type I diabetes mellitus. The nurse bases the teaching on the adolescent's:

1. Need to be unique, allowing them to select their diet without restriction.
2. Preoccupation with the future, allowing them to decline physical activity in favor of computer skills.
3. Need to feel in control, allowing them a larger share in decision making regarding their treatment plan.
4. Awareness of the severity of the disorder, motivating them to maintain a strict routine.

3 When a child develops diabetic ketoacidosis, the child's condition is:

1. An expected outcome of diabetes.
2. Best treated at home.
3. Extremely rare in children.
4. A life-threatening situation.

4 An adolescent with a new diagnosis of diabetes is learning to give her own insulin injection. She correctly prepares the injection, but cannot give herself the shot. The nurse should:

1. Give the shot and allow her to practice more.
2. Take her hand and make her give the shot.
3. Refer her to the doctor.
4. Tell her she can give the shot later.

5 A child with lupus has been placed on corticosteroids for an indefinite period of time. Which of the following are cushingoid symptoms associated with corticosteroid administration to children?

1. Weight gain and delayed puberty
2. Delayed growth and weight loss
3. Fat deposits and rapid growth
4. Moon face and precocious puberty

6 A diabetic adolescent has been admitted following an automobile crash. He is on bed rest and his condition is stable. At 11:30 a.m. he develops a flushed face, increased urinary output, and fruity breath. Place the following interventions in priority order.

1. Call the primary care provider.
2. Administer regular insulin on sliding scale.
3. Obtain a blood glucose level.
4. Increase oral intake of water.
5. Review the intake and output record.

7 The mother of an 8-year-old girl is concerned because her daughter is developing pubic hair and enlarged breast tissue. The nurse's best response would be:

1. "Don't worry, girls won't get their period until age 12."
2. "She is probably going to start her period soon, so you must get used to it."
3. "At what age did you begin puberty?"
4. "You had better tell her about menstruation soon."

8 After a thyroidectomy, a teenager is experiencing tingling and spasms of the hands. The nurse identifies this electrolyte imbalance as_____.

9 The nurse caring for a child with head trauma is ordered to monitor the urine specific gravity. The doctor is concerned the child will develop diabetes insipidus. Which of the following urine specific gravity values should be reported immediately?

1. 1.004
2. 1.015
3. 1.020
4. 1.025

10 The nurse realizes that her client, an overweight teenage male with type II diabetes, needs further instruction when he states:

1. "I have to walk at least 3 miles a day."
2. "I should eat fruit for dessert instead of cake."
3. "I can drink diet soda once a day."
4. "If I take these pills, I will never need to take insulin shots."

Answers for NCLEX-PN® Review and Critical Thinking questions appear in Appendix I.

Care of the Child with Musculoskeletal Disorders

BRIEF Outline

Anatomy and Physiology
Brief Assessment Review
Congenital Skeletal Defects
Musculoskeletal Disorders

Musculoskeletal Trauma
Musculoskeletal Infection
Musculoskeletal Tumors
Nursing Care

LEARNING Outcomes

After completing this chapter, you will be able to:

1. Define key terms.
2. Discuss the anatomy and physiology of the pediatric musculoskeletal system.
3. Describe musculoskeletal disorders to include developmental hip dysplasia, scoliosis, muscular dystrophy, osteomyelitis, osteosarcoma, and musculoskeletal injuries.
4. Discuss clinical manifestations, diagnostic procedures, and medical management related to musculoskeletal disorders.
5. Explain appropriate nursing interventions for children with musculoskeletal disorders.

HEALTH PROMOTION ISSUE:
Children and Body Building

NURSING CARE PLAN CHART:
Child with Scoliosis

NURSING PROCESS CARE PLAN:
Child with an Amputation

CRITICAL THINKING CARE MAP:
Caring for a Child with a Fracture

The muscular system at birth is essentially complete, except for the growth in length and circumference of muscle that occurs as the child ages. Skeletal growth, however, is extensive during the period of childhood and adolescence. For example, Figure 20-1 ■ illustrates changes in the hand from infant to adult.

Anatomy and Physiology

MUSCLES

There are three types of muscles in the body: cardiac, smooth, and skeletal. Skeletal muscles are typically voluntary striated. These striated muscles assist in movement and maintaining posture. Tendons attach bones to muscles and also continue to grow in length as the child ages.

SKELETON

Ossification or bone formation is almost complete at birth. Fontanels connect the cranial bones *in utero* and at birth to allow for molding of the head during the birth process. The anterior and posterior fontanels (see Figure 15-4 ⬤⬤) should be firm and flat in the newborn period. The long bones of a child's body continue to grow until he or she reaches adulthood at age 20 or 21.

The three sections of the long bone (Figure 20-2 ■) are the epiphysis, metaphysis, and diaphysis. The **epiphysis** is the attachment site for muscles and the site for ossification. The **epiphyseal plate** or *growth plate* remains open until late adolescence. Injuries to this area during childhood may affect the growth of the bone. This tissue can also be affected by nutrition and hormone levels, particularly growth hormone. There are some variations in bone mass and density related to race (Box 20-1 ■).

The **metaphysis** is responsible for converting new cartilage into bone. The **diaphysis** contains the medullary cavity, where **hematopoiesis** (production of blood cells) occurs. Fat is also stored in the medullary.

Figure 20-1. ■ These images show the remarkable development of bone as children grow. (Photo Researchers, Inc.)

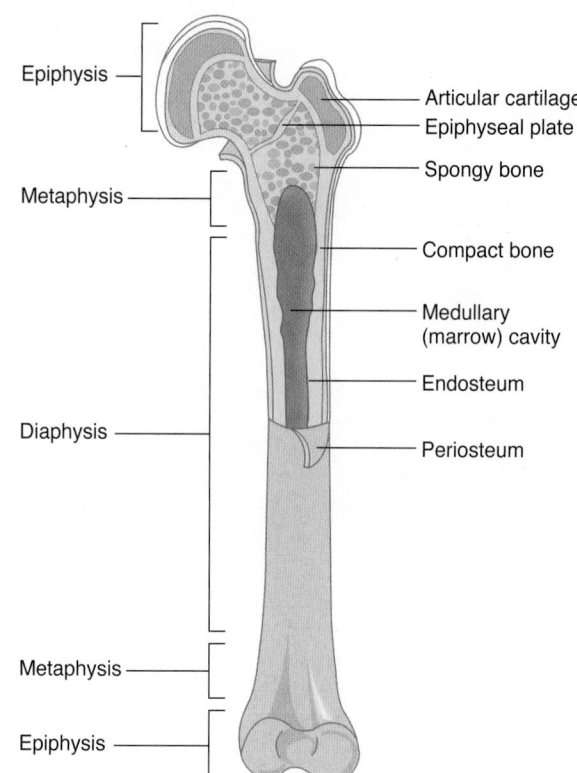

Figure 20-2. ■ The three sections of the long bone are the epiphysis, metaphysis, and diaphysis. Note the *growth plate* or *epiphyseal plate* near the top of the illustration.

Long bones in children are porous and less dense than in adults. Injuries to the long bone can therefore result in a bend or buckle in addition to a break. The bending or buckling of a long bone is called a **greenstick fracture** (discussed later in this chapter). During periods of rapid growth of long bones, the child may complain of aching or pain in the bones. Commonly called *growing pains*, this discomfort is the result of the stretching of muscles as the bone is growing.

BOX 20-1	CULTURAL PULSE POINTS

Variations in Musculoskeletal System by Ethnicity or Race

Children of Hindu heritage are at risk for osteomalacia. This disease is typically the result of calcium and vitamin D deficiency. In contrast, children of African heritage tend to have greater bone density.

Indians, as well as Ethiopians and Algerians, are at risk for a disease called lathyrism. *Lathyrism* (Stedman's, 1997) is a disorder associated with a diet high in certain plants (vetches, khasari, and allied species). Its manifestations include paralysis of the leg muscles, rendering the child crippled.

Localized and inbred populations of Amish (a religious community) are at risk for *dwarfism* (the condition of being abnormally undersized).

Sidebar (left margin): MediaLink • Skeleton

Figure 20-3. ■ Posture. (**A**) The infant's posture changes from a straight spine at about 10 to 15 months to the protruding abdomen and lumbar lordosis shown here in a toddler. (**B**) The school-age child has two curves in the spine that balance each other: thoracic (convex) and lumbar (concave) curves.

Figure 20-4. ■ (**A**) Genu valgum, or knock-knees. Note that the ankles are far apart while the knees are together. (**B**) Genu varum, or bowlegs. The legs are bowed so the knees are far apart as the child stands. This second condition is often associated with vitamin D deficiency (rickets) or Blount's disease if the genu varum persists beyond 2 years of age.

Postural changes occur as the child ages (Figure 20-3 ■). Prior to birth, the thoracic and sacral areas of the spine are convex curves. When the infant can hold his or her head up, the cervical area becomes concave. Then as the child learns to stand, the lumbar area also becomes concave.

The arch of a newborn's foot is absent. It normally develops gradually during the preschool years. The child may appear to have knock-knees (**genu valgum**) (Figure 20-4A ■). This condition usually resolves by late childhood or early adolescence. Infants may appear to have bowlegs (**genu varum**) (Figure 20-4B). Yet, this usually resolves as the child begins to walk. Further evaluation would be needed if these conditions do not resolve by the expected time frame.

Brief Assessment Review

HISTORY

■ With infants, review the history of birth. A child who experienced trauma or hypoxia during the birthing process may develop musculoskeletal trauma.
■ Obtain information on injuries to bones and muscles, such as the nature of the injury and treatment.
■ Inquire about deformities of limbs, spine, and fingers or toes.
■ Determine the child's activity level, including participation in sports activities.
■ Inquire about developmental delays.

PHYSICAL

■ Inspect posture and gait.
■ Note symmetry of shoulders and hips and any unusual curvature of the spine.
■ Assess for full range of motion (ROM) of joints.
■ Assess muscle strength.

Congenital Skeletal Defects

Skeletal defects can be minor and easy to correct, or they can be major malformations requiring long-term therapy. These defects are rarely life threatening. However, they require correction, if possible, in order for normal support and movement to occur. Two common defects are discussed here: developmental dysplasia of the hip and clubfoot.

DEVELOPMENTAL DYSPLASIA OF THE HIP

Developmental dyplasia of the hip (also called DDH) is a developmental abnormality of the femoral head (ball), **acetabulum** (socket), or both.

Manifestations

DDH is displayed by partial or complete dislocation of the hip joint. This results in shortening of the femur, uneven thigh and gluteal folds, and limited abduction on the affected side.

Diagnosis

DDH is usually diagnosed by physical exam during the newborn assessment, but at times it may be identified later. These assessments include Allis's sign and the Ortolani-Barlow maneuver.

ALLIS' SIGN. To evaluate for Allis' sign, the infant's hips and knees are flexed, with the heels placed close to the buttocks. Feet should be placed flat on the examination table. Dislocation of the hip is demonstrated by a lower position of the knee on the affected side.

ORTOLANI-BARLOW MANEUVER. To perform the Ortolani-Barlow maneuver, the practitioner places the infant on his or her back, flexing the hips and knees at 90-degree angles (Figure 20-5 ■) The practitioner holds the knees with the thumb over the inner thigh and the first two fingers over the upper femurs. The infant's knees are positioned together, and downward pressure is exerted on the femurs one at a time to determine dislocation. Next the hips are slowly abducted while maintaining pressure on the hip joints. The normal finding is equal hip abduction without resistance. Resistance or a clunking sound or movement indicates hip dislocation. LPNs/LVNs may be trained in this maneuver. If the LPN/LVN notices a hip click, the practitioner should be informed.

If the child is ambulatory, a notable limp is present. Box 20-2 ■ identifies signs of DDH. Symptoms and prognosis worsen when left untreated.

Treatment

Treatment of DDH should begin as soon as possible. If only a small amount of abnormality is present, triple diapering is used to support the hip in abduction, allowing the femoral head to remain in the acetabulum until ligaments are strong enough to maintain hip alignment permanently. If more support is needed, a Pavlik harness (Figure 20-6 ■) is commonly used for 3 to 4 months. Skin traction is used for older children. If the harness is unsuccessful, surgery followed by a **hip spica cast** (a cast covering the upper thighs and lower torso) may be necessary.

Nursing Considerations

The nursing care of children with DDH includes maintaining traction through triple diapering, the Pavlik harness, or skin traction, and providing cast care. Procedures for these nursing actions appear later in this chapter in the Musculoskeletal Trauma section.

BOX 20-2	ASSESSMENT

Developmental Dysplasia of the Hip

The following are signs of developmental dysplasia of the hip:
- Hip click with abduction (Ortolani-Barlow sign)
- Asymmetric thigh folds
- Uneven knee level (Allis' sign)
- Limited hip abduction

A

B

C

Figure 20-5. ■ (**A**) Hip integrity is assessed in a newborn by observing and feeling the smoothness of movement in the joint. (**B**) A "click" on return is an indication of possible hip dysplasia. (**C**) Skin folds can be noted with hip dysplasia.

Immobility and the resulting complications are a hazard to children with DDH. The nurse should frequently assess lung sounds, neurovascular symptoms, and skin. Children with a cast should change positions at least every 2 hours. Pillows

Figure 20-6. ■ Steps for Pavlik harness application: (1) Position the chest halter at nipple line and fasten with Velcro. (2) Position the legs and feet in the stirrups, being sure the hips are flexed and abducted. Fasten with Velcro. (3) Connect the chest halter and leg straps in front. (4) Connect the chest halter and leg straps in back. All straps are marked at the first fitting with indelible ink so they can be reattached easily after the harness is rinsed and dried.

can assist in positioning the child comfortably. Covering rough edges of the cast with moleskin or tape (called *petaling*) can protect the child's skin from injury. To enhance the child's bladder and bowel function, the nurse should encourage a diet high in fiber with adequate intake of fluids.

TALIPES (CLUBFOOT)

Talipes or clubfoot is a congenital, unilateral or bilateral twisting of the foot, usually inward (Figure 20-7 ■).

Manifestations

The foot cannot easily be moved into alignment because of deformity in three areas of the foot:

■ The **equines** or midfoot is directed downward.
■ The **varus** or hindfoot turns inward.
■ The forefoot curls toward the heel and upward.

Figure 20-7. ■ Clubfoot, with the midfoot (*equines*) directed downward, the hindfoot (*varus*) turned inward, and the forefoot curled toward the heel and upward. This condition is corrected surgically. (Custom Medical Stock Photo, Inc.)

The clubfoot is usually smaller than the other foot, and the child has a shortened Achilles tendon. The muscles of the lower leg are atrophied.

Diagnosis

Talipes is diagnosed by observation of the deformity as the child ambulates and is at rest. Prenatal ultrasound may detect the possibility of the deformity. After birth it can be confirmed by x-ray or CT scan.

Treatment

Nonsurgical treatment involves moving the foot into correct alignment and applying a cast to hold the foot in the corrected position. The cast is changed every 1 to 2 weeks for about 3 months until alignment is achieved. After the proper alignment is achieved, the child may need to wear orthopedic shoes and nighttime braces in order to maintain the alignment. Failure to achieve alignment could result in the need for surgical correction.

clinical ALERT

Infants can be frightened by the noise of a cast cutter. The cast can be removed easily by soaking skin in a warm bath until it disintegrates. This could be done in the health care facility with assistance from the LPN, if approved by the physician. Manual cast cutters may also be less frightening to the child.

A bottle, pacifier, or familiar toy can provide distraction during cast application. Depending on the age of the child, earphones to a battery-operated CD or MP3 player may be provided to listen to music while the cast is being removed. (Regular radios should never be used in proximity to water because of the risk of electrocution.)

Nursing Considerations

The LVN/LPN is responsible for assisting with cast application (see description in the Musculoskeletal Trauma section of this chapter). Proper cast care is taught to the parents. If the child has surgery, the nurse is responsible for pain management. Observation for drainage and bleeding from the surgical site is also essential.

Musculoskeletal Disorders

Musculoskeletal disorders are some of the most common disorders affecting the older child. Their frequency is partially due to changes in bone structure during periods of rapid growth and partially due to accidents as the child interacts with the environment.

MUSCULAR DYSTROPHY

Muscular dystrophy (MD) is a group of inherited diseases that cause muscle degeneration and wasting. There are several kinds of MD, but the most common form affecting children is Duchenne dystrophy. This sex-linked recessive disorder is carried by mothers and passed to their sons.

Manifestations

The onset of symptoms occurs in the first 3 to 4 years of life. The child with MD generally appears normal for the first year, but walking may be delayed. The child gradually gains enough muscle strength to walk but tires easily, especially when running or climbing. As muscles degenerate over time, the child trips and falls frequently, develops a waddling gait, and may walk on the toes. A classic symptom is a positive **Gower's maneuver,** in which the child uses the upper extremities to lift up from the floor. Figure 20-8 ■ illustrates a positive Gower's maneuver. Most children are wheelchair bound by age 12, and death from respiratory paralysis can occur during adolescence.

In examining the child with MD, the calf muscles appear to hypertrophy, but they are actually enlarged due to increased fatty tissue. As the chest muscles waste, the child will develop scoliosis, respiratory difficulty, and the inability to sit upright. Swallowing may be affected, leading to respiratory infection and malnutrition.

Diagnosis

Diagnosis of MD is made by observation of clinical manifestations. Serum creatine kinase will be elevated. A muscle biopsy is used to measure levels of dystrophin, which will be low. Electromyography, which measures electrical activity of skeletal muscles at rest and during voluntary muscle contractions, will show activity at rest and increased voluntary muscle contractions.

Treatment

There is no cure for muscular dystrophy. Deformities of the chest, including scoliosis, may need to be corrected surgically to promote adequate respiration. Respiratory infections must also be treated promptly. Physical therapy is implemented to maintain range of motion. However, the use of braces and wheelchairs may be necessary.

A

B

C

D

E

Figure 20-8. ■ Gower's maneuver in child with muscular dystrophy. (**A** and **B**) The child first maneuvers to a position supported by arms and legs. (**C**) The child pushes off the floor and rests one hand on the knee. (**D** and **E**) The child pushes the body up straight.

Nursing Considerations

The goals of nursing care are to prevent complications, promote independence for as long as possible, and support the family in dealing with this progressive, incapacitating, and ultimately fatal disease. Nursing interventions may include oxygen administration, respiratory therapy, administration of medications, tube feeding, monitoring for signs of infection, and preventing skin breakdown. Parents will need a lot of support and will need to be taught how to offer support to their child. The nurse can help the child and family design a plan of active and passive ROM exercise. They can be taught the advantages of controlling weight gain within the normal limits with a low-calorie, high-protein, and high-fiber diet, and they can be taught to drink plenty of fluids to prevent constipation. It also is important to refer the family to appropriate resources and support groups.

The child's development should be assessed periodically. Parents, teachers, therapists, and nurses should meet to devise plans to meet the child's learning and developmental needs. The focus should be on what the child *can do* instead of what the child *cannot do*.

LEGG-CALVÉ-PERTHES DISEASE

Legg-Calvé-Perthes disease is a self-limiting condition in which the circulation to the femoral head is interrupted. The femoral head dies from lack of blood supply, which gradually returns as healing occurs. The necrotic bone is reabsorbed and replaced with vascularized granulation tissue. In approximately 3 years, ossification occurs, forming a new femoral head.

The cause of Legg-Calvé-Perthes disease is unknown, but it is believed to occur following mild trauma. The disorder could be unilateral or bilateral. Boys between the ages of 4 and 8 are most commonly affected (Figure 20-9 ■). People of African and Chinese descent have a lower incidence of the disease.

Manifestations

Symptoms may be present for several months before the parents seek medical assistance. Early symptoms include mild hip and anterior thigh pain and a limp. The symptoms are worse with activity and relieved by rest. The child favors the leg and limits movement to decrease the pain. As the disease progresses, muscle wasting and decreased mobility occur. The affected thigh will be about 1 inch (2 to 3 cm) smaller in diameter than the unaffected thigh.

Diagnosis

Diagnosis is made by reviewing symptoms, x-rays, bone scans, and magnetic resonance imaging (MRI) scans.

Treatment

The medical treatment is directed at relieving pain and holding the femoral head in place while healing occurs. The femoral

Figure 20-9. ■ Toronto brace used for Legg-Calvé-Perthes disease. This young boy needs to use crutches to be able to walk in the Toronto brace for treatment of Perthes disease.

head is held abducted with internal rotation by use of a Toronto (see Figure 20-9) or a Scottish-Rite brace. These braces hold the hip in place and support the weight of the child on the ischium. The child should wear the braces for 23 hours a day.

Nursing Considerations

Nurses are involved in teaching parents how to apply the braces, monitoring for signs of skin breakdown under the braces, and providing skin care to prevent skin breakdown. The child will learn to ambulate with the braces but may need crutches to help with balance.

Helping the child and family deal with the long-term nature of the treatment may be a challenge for the nurse. Because the disease occurs at an age when the child is very active, the limitations of the brace cause stress to the child and family. Parents should be given suggestions to help direct the child's energy within the limitations of the brace (Box 20-3 ■). The child should return to school as soon as possible.

Follow-up visits are arranged at regular intervals to evaluate the healing process and make adjustments to the brace as the child grows. Toward the end of treatment, the child may be allowed periods of limited exercise without the brace. Activities such as swimming can increase muscle strength without stressing the growing bone. Prognosis is good as long as the femoral head is contained. If treatment is delayed or the child and family are noncompliant with the treatment plan, there is a high probability of permanent deformity and arthritis later in life.

BOX 20-3 CLIENT TEACHING

School-Age Children with Braces

School-age children are energetic and industrious. It is important to promote these developmental characteristics in children who must wear a brace. The nurse must ensure that the child is able to move and ambulate before discharge from the health care facility. Use the following suggestions when teaching children and their parents how to redirect the child's energy.

Fine motor skills:
- Encourage journaling about the experience of this disease.
- Teach the child a new craft, such as beaded jewelry.
- Supply the child with art supplies and encourage drawing or painting.

Gross motor skills:
- Teach the child to ride a horse.
- Join the YMCA and go swimming several times a week.
- Encourage the child to learn to play Ping-Pong or pool.

Cognitive activities:
- Supply the child with educational computer activities.
- Encourage reading or listening to books on tape.
- Challenge the child to competitions such as learning the capitals of the 50 states, memorizing the presidents in order, or memorizing Bible verses.

SCOLIOSIS

Scoliosis is a lateral S- or C-shaped curve of the spine, with rotation of the spine and ribs. Scoliosis is more common in girls between 10 and 13 years of age than in other groups. It is also associated with other musculoskeletal and nervous system deformities. Most commonly, there is a right-sided thoracic curve and a left-sided lumbar curve.

Manifestations

Symptoms of scoliosis develop slowly and without pain. In assessing the back, the shoulders and hips are different heights (Figure 20-10 ■), causing the clothing to hang unevenly. Rotation of the vertebrae and ribs cause a one-sided rib hump and a prominent scapula. The assessment includes comparing the level of the right and left hip and shoulders. The child is also asked to bend forward, and the posterior chest is inspected for symmetry. The school nurse routinely assesses many children for scoliosis.

Diagnosis

Moiré photography is projection of wavelike patterns onto the client's back to highlight asymmetry of bony landmarks. It can be used to document the degree of asymmetry in the spine. If scoliosis is suspected, the child is referred for spinal x-ray and follow-up care.

Treatment

The goal of treatment is to limit or stop the progression of spinal deformity. The method of treatment depends on the degree of curvature. Mild scoliosis can be treated with exercise to increase muscle tone and flexibility and to improve

Figure 20-10. ■ Scoliosis, showing deviation of the spine to the right. (Phototake NYC)

posture. See Health Promotion Issue on pages 554 and 555. Chiropractic adjustments may be used to realign vertebrae if there is a mild degree of curvature (Box 20-4 ■). A Boston or Milwaukee brace is used to treat moderate scoliosis. These braces are custom fitted for the child and should be worn 23 hours a day. During the hour without the brace, the child may bathe, shower, or take part in activities that the brace would restrict. Unless otherwise instructed by the physician, the

BOX 20-4 COMPLEMENTARY THERAPIES

Chiropractor

A chiropractor can check a child's spine for misalignments. These misalignments or subluxations (also called pinched nerves) are said to impair nervous system function affecting overall body function. Nervous system impairment results from bones or tissues irritating, stretching, or impinging on nerve fibers and therefore causing pain and discomfort. The chiropractor uses his hands or specialized instruments to realign the spine, relieving pressure on these nerve fibers.

The International Chiropractic Pediatric Association promotes regular adjustments for children beginning shortly after birth, with adaptations for the child's size and physical maturity. Several research studies have found that children who receive regular chiropractic adjustments have fewer ear infections, fewer allergies, lower incidence of tonsillitis, and less need for antibiotic therapy.

Source: Data from Lee, A. C., Li, D. H., & Kemper, K. J. (2000). Chiropractic care for children. *Archives of Pediatric and Adolescent Medicine, 154,* 401–407; Anrig, C. (2004). Relief versus wellness care in the family practice. *Dynamic Chiropractic 22(7);* and Fallon, J. M. (1997). The role of the chiropractic adjustment in the care and treatment of 332 children with otitis media. *Journal of Clinical Chiropractic Pediatrics, 2;* 167–183.

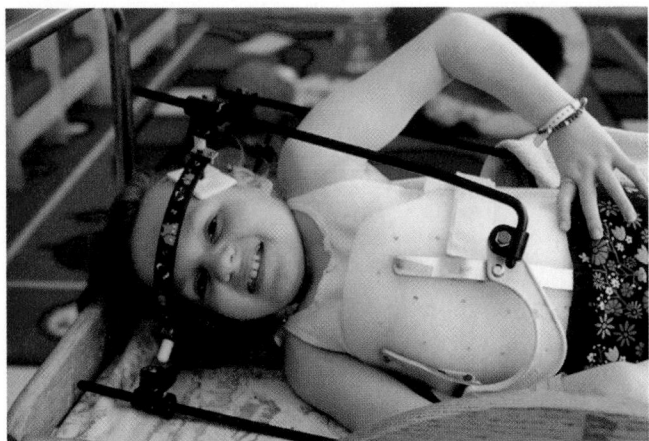

Figure 20-11. ■ In severe scoliosis, the child may wear a halo brace, shown here, to hold the body in position after surgery.

child is not prohibited from participating in sports activities (Hart, 2003).

Severe scoliosis requires surgery to fuse the spine, remove rib sections and/or insert screws and rods or wires to straighten the spine. A halo brace (Figure 20-11 ■) may be used after surgery to hold the body in alignment. The surgery consists of spinal fusion, possible bone grafting, and insertion of permanent wires to stabilize the spine. Some surgeons may perform the surgery laparoscopically.

Postoperatively, the child will remain on bed rest during recovery. Once the child is able to get up, a plastic anterior and posterior shell is used to stabilize the back until healing is complete. The rod may cause some limited range of motion, such as bending and twisting.

Scoliosis screening is routinely completed when the child is in the fifth and seventh grades. Any indication of scoliosis is discussed with the parents. If scoliosis is detected, treatment should begin immediately to slow or stop the progression. Follow-up evaluations would be made at regular intervals. Nursing care for a child with scoliosis is discussed in the Nursing Care Plan Chart about scoliosis on page 556.

OTHER SPINAL CURVATURES

Three other spinal curvatures warrant mention. **Kyphosis,** excessive convex curvature of the thoracic spine, is also know as *hunchback*. **Lordosis,** or *sway back*, is an excessive concave curvature of the lumbar spine. Frequently, these abnormal curvatures are found together. **Torticollis,** or wry neck, is a tilt of the head caused by rotation of the cervical spine. Injury to the sternocleidomastoid muscle is typically the cause. This injury occurs most commonly at birth. Table 20-1 ■ identifies the type and degree of curvature, the recommended treatment, and nursing interventions.

(*Text continues on p. 556.*)

TABLE 20-1

Spinal Curvatures

CONDITION	DIAGNOSIS AND TREATMENT	NURSING INTERVENTIONS
Lordosis: Excessive concave curvature of the lumbar spine	Diagnosis: Look at child from side. Observe lumbar curve. Confirm with spinal x-ray. Treatment: Exercises and postural awareness. Chiropractic therapy.	Encourage physical conditioning exercises. Reassure family that condition may be outgrown as child matures.
Kyphosis: Excessive convex curvature of thoracic spine	Diagnosis: Have child bend forward at waist. Look at thoracic spine at level of scapula. Confirmed with x-ray. Treatment: Mild condition requires exercise, moderate condition requires bracing, severe condition requires surgery. Chiropractic therapy.	Encourage strengthening exercises and posture awareness. Teach brace application and postoperative care. Help deal with altered body image.
Scoliosis: "S" curve of the spine, often with rotation of spine and hips	Diagnosis: Observe back for deformity, uneven scapula and hips, uneven ribcage. Confirmed with x-ray. Treatment: mild condition (10–20 degrees) requires exercise, chiropractic therapy. Moderate condition (20–40 degrees) requires bracing in addition to exercise. Severe condition (40 degrees or more) requires surgery with spinal fusion.	Promote compliance with treatment plan. Encourage diligence with exercise plan. Provide emotional support for child and family. Teach brace application and care. Teach postoperative care.
Torticollis: Tilt of the head caused by rotation of the cervical spine	Diagnosis: Observe position of head and rotation of cervical spine. Treatment: Surgery, heat application, immobilization of the neck in the correct position.	Encourage physical conditioning exercises. Provide emotional support for child and family. Instruct in proper use of the immobilization device.

HEALTH PROMOTION ISSUE

CHILDREN AND BODY BUILDING

Ten-year-old Michael has been playing baseball since he was 3 years old. He pitches for his community team, and the coach has placed him as lead-off batter. He enjoys playing baseball and talks often about playing professionally. Michael's father played professional baseball until a shoulder injury ended his career. Because Michael's father wants Michael to avoid such injuries, he has hired a trainer and pitching coach to work with Michael several times a week. Recently, the trainer has suggested that Michael begin a weight training regimen to strengthen his muscles. This concerns his mother, who is worried about the injuries Michael could sustain lifting heavy weights. She calls the pediatrician's office for information about the safety of weight training in children.

DISCUSSION

A study done in 1978 measured the muscle strength of preadolescent and adolescent boys following an 8-week resistance training program. The adolescent boys gained muscle strength while the preadolescent boys did not. Then, in 1988, another study reported that 12-year-old boys could not benefit from strength training that occurred three times a week for 4 to 6 weeks. Unfortunately, these studies were based on low resistance and only one or two sets of exercises per session. In 1983, the American Academy of Pediatrics (AAP) even published a statement that said preadolescent boys could not signifi-

cantly improve strength or muscle mass following weight training.

More recent studies with better methods of testing muscle strength have found different results. Muscle strength has been demonstrated to improve with resistance training in preadolescent boys. Other studies have found improvement in muscle coordination and greater flexibility. One study even reported that parents found children who participated in strength training to be more willing to do household chores and homework. There have, however, been no studies that can link weight training with improved sports performance.

Many of the studies that do link injuries with weight lifting are actually associated with weight lifting as a sport and not strength training or weight training. *Strength training* is defined as muscle conditioning using resistance in the form of free weights, weight machines, or resistance bands. *Weight lifting* and power lifting are competitive sports using a weighted barbell that is lifted from the ground to overhead.

In 2001, the AAP published a revised statement related to children and weight training. It reads, "Studies have shown that strength training, when properly structured with regard to frequency, mode (type of lifting), intensity, and duration of program, can increase strength in preadolescents and adolescents (p.1472)." The American College of Sports Medicine (ACSM) has also stated that strength training programs that are properly designed and supervised can enhance motor fitness skills and sports performance. The ACSM also states that strength training encourages healthy lifestyles, builds confidence, increases lean body mass, improves cholesterol levels, improves cardiac fitness and respiratory fitness, and improves bone fitness, self-image, and self-esteem.

PLANNING AND IMPLEMENTATION

The pediatric nurse should help Michael's mother understand the previous information. Michael should benefit from weight training if his regimen includes supervision, a well-planned program, and proper technique.

Supervision of the weight training program is a must. The nurse should suggest that the adult supervisor be trained and certified as a fitness expert. The supervisor should have experience working with children. He or she should also remain with Michael during the entire training session and provide proper spotting of the weights during lifts. Suggest to Michael's parents that the trainer have no more than 10 students to supervise at any given time.

Michael's parents should be encouraged to find a gym that is clean, safe, and spacious. The equipment should be child sized and have weight increments of 1 to 5 lb. Another important aspect is appropriate clothing and appropriate shoes. Clothing should not be large and baggy. Ill-fitting clothes can prove hazardous if they get caught on the weight machines. Shoes should provide foot and ankle stability and have adequate traction. The nurse should also suggest proper nutrition and hydration during the training period.

For Michael to achieve maximum benefit from weight training, proper technique must be implemented. Training should occur two to three times per week with 1 day off between training sessions. Experts suggest that every weight training session begin with time for stretching and aerobic activity. Each session should also end with a time for stretching. Weight can be increased when 15 repetitions become too easy, but should not be increased until Michael can do three sets of 15 repetitions of an exercise on three consecutive sessions.

Although the nurse may not be qualified to develop a specific workout plan for Michael, showing Michael's parents a sample weight training plan will assist them in approving an appropriate plan for Michael. Following is a sample plan for a preadolescent:

- 10 minutes stretching and brisk walk on the treadmill
- Shoulder exercises: 10–15 repetitions on deltoids, internal rotators, and external rotators
- Upper back exercises: 10–15 repetitions of bent-over lateral raises, bench rows, and latissumus pull-downs
- Lower back and abdomen exercises: 10–15 repetitions of crunches and reverse sit-ups
- 15 minutes of stretching and two laps around the track to cool down

SELF-REFLECTION

Motivation for activities may arise from the child or from the parent. What are your feelings regarding parents encouraging or coercing a child to participate in a physical activity? Where should the line be drawn between helping the child develop discipline and requiring participation in physical activities?

SUGGESTED RESOURCES

For the Nurse

American Academy of Pediatrics Committee on Sports Medicine and Fitness. Strength training by children and adolescents. (2001). *Pediatrics, 107,* 1470–1472.

Benjamin, H, & Glow, K. (2003). Strength training for children and adolescents: What can physicians recommend? *The Physician and Sportsmedicine, 31*(9).

Strength training in children and adolescents (2002, September). The American College of Sports Medicine.

For the Client

Antonio, J., & Stout, J. (2004). *Fit kids for life: A parent's guide to optimal nutrition and training for young athletes.* Laguna Beach, CA: Basic Health.

Metzl, J. (2003). Overtraining in children and adolescents. *Fit Society Page,* Spring, B1.

NURSING CARE PLAN CHART

Child with Scoliosis

GOAL	INTERVENTION	RATIONALE	EXPECTED OUTCOME
1. Impaired Physical Mobility related to spinal surgery and assistive devices/appliances			
The child will maintain mobility.	Demonstrate proper body mechanics and request return demonstration	*This prevents injury to muscles and joints*	The child adapts mobility needs and performs ADLs without assistance.
	Assess client's pain level	*Unmanaged pain can prevent mobilization*	
	Provide pain management as ordered	*Unmanaged pain can prevent mobilization*	
	Provide positive reinforcement when client ambulates correctly and accomplishes ADLs independently	*Positive reinforcement will provide encouragement for the client to continue these proper behaviors and contribute to their wellness*	
	Encourage a realistic view of physical limitations	*This promotes acceptance of limitations and decreases negative thinking*	
	Seek referral to physical therapist as needed	*A physical therapist can provide additional assistance in maintaining mobility*	
2. Risk for Impaired Skin Integrity related to spinal surgery, immobility, and assistive devices/appliances			
The child will not experience impaired skin integrity.	Teach the child methods of minimizing skin exposure to moisture, such as applying antiperspirant, bathing, and drying thoroughly at least daily and more often if perspiring	*Moisture increases the risk of skin irritation. Good hygiene practices can also minimize skin irritation*	Skin color, temperature, and sensation are WNL. Capillary refill is rapid and pulses are strong and equal bilaterally.
	Encourage the child to wear a cotton undershirt under the assistive devices/appliances	*Cotton is less apt to irritate the skin and provides a protective barrier to the skin*	
	Teach child and parents to daily inspect the skin that is in constant contact with the assistive devices/appliances.	*Prompt treatment can be implemented when signs of impaired skin integrity are recognized*	
	Encourage prompt reporting of skin irritation		
	Apply protective barriers if indicated	*Creams or lotions can provide a moisture barrier and prevent skin irritation*	

JUVENILE RHEUMATOID ARTHRITIS

Juvenile rheumatoid arthritis (JRA or Still's disease) is an autoimmune inflammatory disease that affects children 2 to 5 years of age and 9 to 12 years of age. The cause of JRA is unknown. The diagnosis is made on the basis of history and clinical symptoms. Discussion of this condition appears in Chapter 22 ⬤⬤.

Musculoskeletal Trauma

Musculoskeletal trauma can occur in the form of muscle strains and sprains or fractures of the bones. A **sprain**

occurs when the ligament associated with a joint is torn following trauma to the joint. Sprains are immobilized for the first 24 to 36 hours. Parents can be taught the RICE acronym for treatment of a sprain – rest, ice, compression, and elevation. Nonsteroidal antiinflammatory agents (NSAIAs) may be prescribed to help reduce inflammation and pain (Table 20-2 ■). After 36 hours, the child should gradually begin weight-bearing activities.

A **strain** is a more minor injury to the muscle or tendon. It can be caused by everyday activity (Box 20-5 ■), sports (Box 20-6 ■), or unusually strenuous exercise. A

TABLE 20-2

Pharmacology: Drugs Used to Reduce Inflammation (Nonsteroidal Antiinflammatory Agents or NSAIAs)

DRUG (GENERIC AND COMMON BRAND NAME)	USUAL ROUTE/DOSE	CLASSIFICATION AND PURPOSE	SELECTED SIDE EFFECTS	DON'T GIVE IF
Naproxen (Naprosyn)	For inflammation: 10–15 mg/kg/day PO, children greater than 2 years For pain: 5–7 mg/kg every 8–12 hours PO, children greater than 2 years	NSAIA for inflammation and pain	Headache, drowsiness, dizziness, anorexia, heartburn, nausea	Child has GI irritation such as peptic ulcer
Indomethacin (Indocin)	1–2 mg/kg/day or 150–200 mg/day PO	NSAIA for juvenile rheumatoid arthritis	Dizziness, nausea, vomiting, headache	Child has an allergy to other NSAIAs or aspirin

BOX 20-5   CLIENT TEACHING

Heavy Backpacks Cause Back Pain

Every day many children and teens strap on backpacks filled with lunch, textbooks, gym shoes and clothes, and numerous electronic devices. Many must walk to school, wait for the bus, or catch the subway with this weight straining their backs. The backpacks can be 10% to 20% of the child's body weight. It is generally acknowledged that a child carrying more than 15% of his or her body weight can suffer from severe back, neck, and shoulder pain, headaches, and other spinal discomfort.

One researcher at the University of California at San Diego developed a research project to measure the pressure exerted on a child's back when carrying a heavy backpack and to rate the pain this load causes (Macias, Murthy, Chambers & Hargens, 2005). He found that pressure exerted by the loaded backpacks was significantly greater than the pressure needed to occlude skin and muscle blood flow. Right shoulder pressures were also higher than left shoulder pressure. Back pain increased as the pressure that was exerted increased.

Parents and health care professionals need to develop methods of assisting children and teens to avoid added back strain from heavy backpacks. Health education programs can alert children and parents to the risks associated with carrying heavy backpacks and instruct children in proper body mechanics. Makers of backpacks have developed backpacks with wheels. Manufacturers should develop products that are appealing to the style-conscious child and yet are ergonomically correct.

Source: Data from Macias, B. R., Murthy, G., Chambers, H., & Hargens, A. (2005). High contact pressure beneath backpack straps of children contributes to pain. *Archives of Pediatrics and Adolescent Medicine, 159* (12), 1186–1187; Anrig, C. (2005). The backpack dilemma: Function vs. fashion. *Dynamic Chiropractic, 23* (18);. and Sheir-Neiss, G. I., Kruse, R. W., Rahman, T., Jacobsen, L. P., & Pelli, J. A. (2003). The association of backpack use and back pain in adolescents. *Spine, 28*(9), 922–930.

BOX 20-6

Cheerleading: A Source of Musculoskeletal Injury

Cheerleading is often not recognized by school officials as a sport. Therefore, training and certification for coaches may not be required. Without this training, students may not be taught safety measures to prevent injury.

Cheerleading activities include acrobatics, pyramid building, and tosses. The flyer, or person being tossed or placed on top of the pyramid, is at greatest risk for a fall-related injury. The base, or person on the bottom of the pyramid, is at greatest risk for muscle strain and sprain or back injuries.

A recent study found that between 1990 and 2002 more than 200,000 children ages 5 to 18 were treated in the emergency room for injuries related to cheerleading. The U.S. Consumer Product Safety Commission reported nearly 25,000 cheerleading-related injuries requiring emergency care in 2001 alone. Overall, cheerleading injuries have increased fivefold during the past 20 years. These injuries include strains, sprains, soft tissue injuries, fractures, dislocations, lacerations, concussions, and closed head injuries.

Source: Data from Shields, B., & Smith, G. (2006). Cheerleading related injuries to children 5 to 18 years of age: United States 1990–2002. *Pediatrics, 117*, 122–129; American Association of Cheerleading Coaches and Advisors. (2000); National Center for Health Statistics. (2001). *Sports-related injuries cause 2.6 million visits annually by children and young adults to emergency rooms.* Hyattsville, MD: Author.

OSGOOD-SCHLATTER DISEASE

Osgood-Schlatter disease (Figure 20-12 ▪) is an overgrowth of the tibial epiphysis due primarily to recurring inflammatory episodes. The repeated pull of the quadriceps femoris as seen in athletic children is believed to cause inflammation, new bone formation, and a bony prominence at the knee. The disease is most common in boys between 13 and 14 years and girls between 10 and 11 years. Treatment is aimed at resting the joint until healing occurs. Casting the knee may be necessary to relieve pain and swelling. Exercise

period of rest and support is needed for the muscle or tendon to heal before returning to weight-bearing activities.

A **fracture** results from an injury and causes the continuity of the bone to be altered. Osgood-Schlatter disease is also a cause of musculoskeletal trauma.

Figure 20-12. ■ Osgood-Schlatter disease often occurs in school-age children involved in running sports such as soccer. (Phototake NYC)

to strengthen the muscles above and below the knee is sometimes helpful. Surgery is rarely needed.

FRACTURES

Fractures are a common occurrence in childhood because of children's active nature. Injuries such as fractures, sprains, strains, and dislocations may result from sporting activities, play, or because the child is taking risks and not being careful.

Manifestations

Signs of fracture vary, depending on the type of fracture and the location. Generally, pain, abnormal positioning, edema, discoloration, and abnormal movement characterize fractures. The common locations of fractures are clavicle, tibia, femur, radius, and ulna. X-ray is used to determine the exact location and type of fracture (Figure 20-13 ■). When

assessing bruising and fracture, nurses must be alert to the possibility of child abuse (Box 20-7 ■).

When assessing the injured child, be alert for the possibility of fracture. The area should be immobilized prior to movement in order to prevent further injury. The child, parents, and family should be questioned to determine the cause of the injury.

BOX 20-7	ASSESSMENT

Possible Child Abuse

The nurse must consider physical child abuse when the following signs are noticed:

- Unexplained burns, bites, bruises, broken bones, or black eyes
- Fading bruises or other marks
- A child who is frightened of the parents and protests or cries when it is time to go home
- A child who shrinks at the approach of adults
- A child who reports injury by a parent or another adult caregiver.

Also consider the possibility of physical child abuse when the **parent or other adult caregiver:**

- Offers conflicting, unconvincing, or no explanation for the child's injury
- Describes the child as "evil," or in some other negative way
- Uses harsh physical discipline with the child
- Has a history of abuse as a child

For more information about child abuse, see Chapter 3 for legal aspects and Chapter 16 ⚭ for a detailed discussion of child abuse.

Source: Adapted from National Clearinghouse on Child Abuse and Neglect Information (DHHS). (2003). *Recognizing child abuse and neglect: Signs and symptoms.* Washington, DC: Department of Health and Human Services.

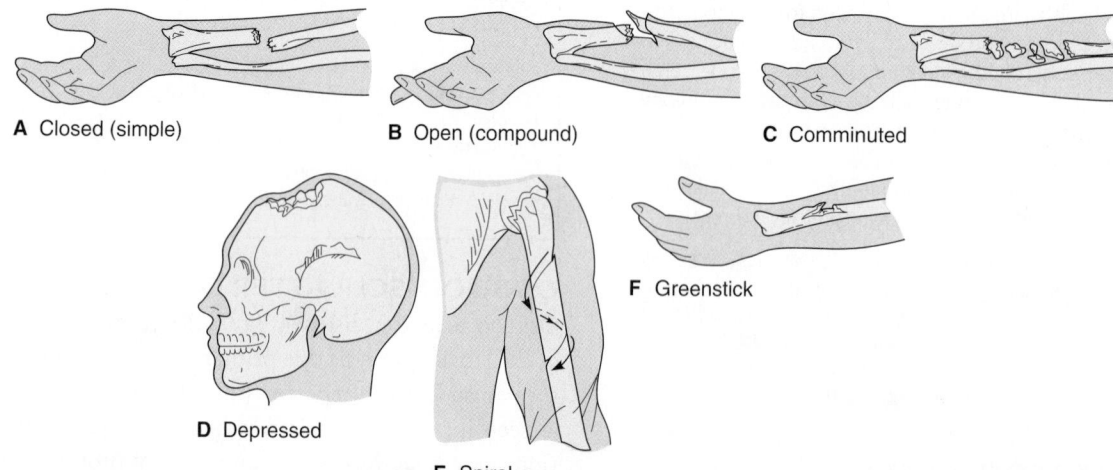

A Closed (simple) **B** Open (compound) **C** Comminuted

D Depressed **E** Spiral **F** Greenstick

Figure 20-13. ■ Fracture of the bone is defined as any disruption in the bone itself. It is classified as open or closed. (**A**) Closed (simple)—skin over the fracture remains intact. (**B**) Open (compound)—broken bone protrudes through the skin. (**C**) Comminuted—bone fragments into many pieces. (**D**) Depressed—broken bone is pressed inward (e.g., the skull). (**E**) Spiral—jagged break due to twisting force—often found in association with abuse. (**F**) Greenstick—incomplete break along the length of the bone (often found in young children).

The area of injury should be inspected for broken skin; circulation including pulse and bleeding; and normal sensation. If the skin has been broken, bleeding should be controlled and sterile dressings applied.

When fractures involve the epiphysis, they can disrupt the growth process. Figure 20-14 ■ illustrates the Salter-Harris classification of fractures and shows which types of fracture can cause the greatest threat to normal growth.

Diagnosis

Diagnosis of fractures is made by viewing x-rays of the affected injury.

Treatment

The goal of medical treatment is to reduce or realign the fracture, immobilize the bones until healing has occurred, and manage pain. The fractured bones can be realigned by **closed reduction** (manually moving the bones into alignment such as casting or bracing) or **open reduction** (surgically aligning the bone and stabilizing the ends with nails, plates, or screws). Sometimes traction is applied to immobilize the unstable bone ends. Figure 20-15 ■ illustrates the common types of traction used for children. At other times, external fixators or stabilizers (Figures 20-15E and F) are used to immobilize the fracture while allowing the child more freedom of activity.

Type I
Common
Growth plate undisturbed
Growth disturbances rare

Type II
Most common
Growth disturbances rare

Type III
Less common
Serious threat to growth and joint

 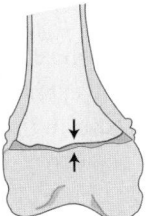

Type IV
Serious threat to growth

Type V
Rare
Crush injury causes cell death in growth plate, resulting in arrested growth and limited bone length
If growth plate is partially destroyed, angular deformities may result

Figure 20-14. ■ Salter-Harris classification system for fractures involving the epiphyses (growth plates).

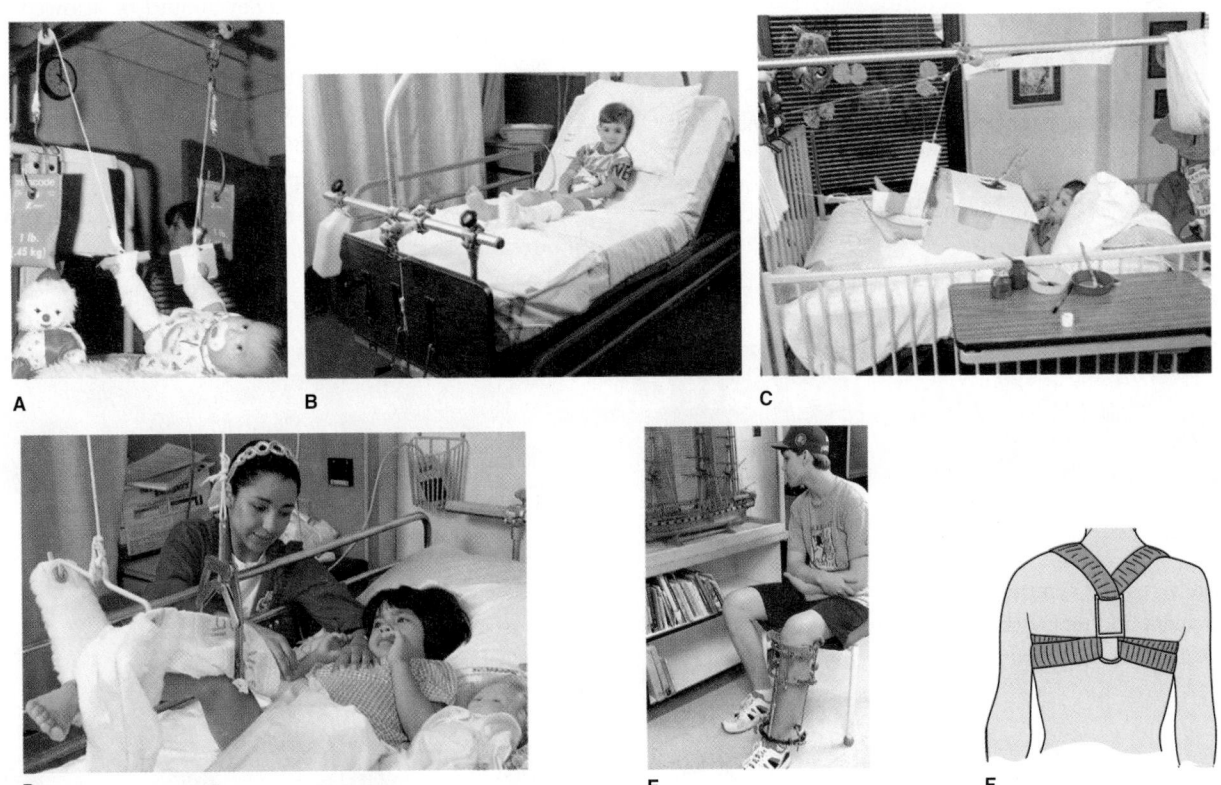

Figure 20-15. ■ Types of traction used for children. (**A**) Bryant traction. (**B**) Buck traction. (**C**) Russell traction. (**D**) 90-90 traction. (**E**) External traction (external fixator device). (**F**) Clavicle strap for stabilizing clavicle fracture.

A plaster or plastic cast may be used to immobilize the fractured bone. Removable casts may be used for children because they are light and easy to apply and remove.

Nursing Considerations

The care of the child in traction and external fixators is similar to that of an adult. The area should be assessed for circulation, movement, and sensation. Skin care must be given routinely to prevent breakdown. The weights used in traction should hang freely and the child must be kept in proper alignment. This is a challenge with the young or uncooperative child who moves around in the bed. The skin around the pins of external fixative devices should be cleaned and dressed using sterile technique. However, pin care should only be done if it is specifically ordered.

The nurse must be alert for the development of compartment syndrome in the child with a cast. **Compartment syndrome** occurs when increased pressure in a limited space compromises circulation and nerve innervation, leading to possible necrosis.

clinical ALERT

Symptoms of compartment syndrome include:

Paresthesia
Pain/Pressure
Pallor
Paralysis
Pulselessness

Deep pain unrelieved by analgesia, lack of sensation, and edema suggest compartment syndrome and should be reported immediately. The cast should be altered or removed promptly to prevent permanent damage to underlying tissue.

BOX 20-8 | LIFE SPAN CONSIDERATIONS

Teens with Fractures

The use of braces, crutches, and casts is probably most difficult for the adolescent client to accept. Because of the adolescent's developmental stage, adolescents are very conscious of their body image. These devices alter their body image, even if it is temporary in some cases. The nurse can play an important role in assisting the teen to accept the necessity of wearing these devices. Acceptance of the device will increase compliance. Be sure that the teen knows the extent of the injury or condition. They also need to know how the device will improve their condition and what the consequences of not wearing the device are. Be specific with how this teen's life can be altered. For example, the teen with a broken finger who is also a pianist will need to understand that a finger that is not straight or pliable may affect his or her ability to play the piano. Teens can also understand the relationship between joint injury and the onset of osteoarthritis.

Help the teen explore how the musculoskeletal device might be disguised. For example: choosing clothes that fit easily over the cast or brace such as a lightweight jacket that can be worn most of the day. Many teens enjoy allowing their friends to decorate their cast. Encourage the teen to keep a supply of different colored permanent markers available.

Children need special attention to deal with the anxiety related to orthopedic casts. They should be allowed to participate as much as possible in their care. Allowing children to choose a cast color or to "decorate" their casts is acceptable as long as decoration will not interfere with the function of the casts. Teens may need some special considerations when dealing with appliances (Box 20-8 ■).

Procedures 20-1 to 20-3 ■ review essential information about care for the client with fracture.

PROCEDURE 20-1 | Providing Cast Care

Purpose

■ To note signs and symptoms of neurovascular impairment and report them promptly
■ To maintain cast integrity, thus promoting healing

Equipment

■ Pillows with waterproof covering
■ Absorbent pads and protectors
■ Plastic bag
■ Permanent marker

Check order + Gather equipment + Introduce yourself + Identify client + Provide privacy + Explain procedure + Hand hygiene + Gloves as needed

Interventions and Rationales

1. Perform preparatory steps (see icon bar).

2. Elevate recently casted limb. *Elevating the limb reduces edema.*

3. Inspect the damp cast for indentations and handle only with the palms of the hand until the cast is completely dry. *Damp casts move under pressure. Indentations indicate potential pressure areas where skin breakdown could occur.*

4. Observe for drainage, noting amount by marking the outline of the drainage area, date, and time on the cast with permanent marker. *Water-based marker could be removed by drainage or cleaning.*

5. Observe for symptoms of neurovascular impairment every 15 minutes following cast placement progressing to every 2 hours. Report abnormal findings such as decreased or absent pulses, change in color of skin above or below the cast, warmth of the extremity, decreased sensation, decreased capillary refill, increased edema, limited movement of extremity, or pain, burning, or tingling. *These measures allow the nurse to recognize and prevent complications.*

6. Instruct children and parents to observe for the previous findings as well and report accordingly. *Much of the healing time will be at home. The child and parents must be taught to recognize and report symptoms.*

7. Cover cast with a plastic bag during bathing or toileting to keep it dry and clean (Figure 20-16 ■). *The cast will disintegrate if it gets wet. It must remain dry in order to support proper healing.*

8. Cover the edges of the cast by "petaling" them with adhesive tape or moleskin. *The edges of the cast can be rough and abrasive if they come in direct contact with skin.*

9. Avoid the use of lotions and powders under the cast. *These may cause skin irritation.*

10. Keep shirts or other clothing over the top edges of the cast on young children. *This helps keep the child from picking at the cast or putting small objects into the cast.*

11. Instruct children and their families about care of the cast at home, including:
    - The area under the cast and toes and fingers can be cleaned with alcohol and a cotton swab. Water should be avoided.
    - Use a cast shoe, sock, or sling to protect the cast.
    - Report unusual odor, damage to the cast, or unexplained fever. *This may be a sign of infection.*

SAMPLE DOCUMENTATION

(date/time)   Right forearm cast intact. No drainage noted. Fingers warm with adequate capillary refill. No edema noted. ROM without limitation. Cast covered with plastic and edges taped. Assisted to shower.

_____ L. Erskine, LPN

A   **B**

Figure 20-16. ■ Cast care. Plastic can be placed over the cast during bathing or toileting to keep materials dry and clean. (**A**) Nurses can protect children's skin from the rough edges of the cast by "petaling" it. (**B**) This is done by securing adhesive tape to the inside of the cast and pulling it over the edge, covering the jagged or broken pieces of plaster, and securing it to the outer surface of the cast. Moleskin may also be used on the cast.

PROCEDURE 20-2   Setting Crutch Height

Purpose
- To ensure proper fit of crutches and facilitate ambulation

Equipment
- Crutches
- Measuring tape, if desired

Check order + Gather equipment + Introduce yourself + Identify client + Provide privacy + Explain procedure + Hand hygiene + Gloves as needed

Interventions and Rationales

1. Perform preparatory steps (see icon bar above).

Figure 20-17. ■ Crutches should fit comfortably under the axillae so they do not rub against the skin. The child should not have to stoop to use the crutches.

2. Have the child stand with elbows slightly and comfortably flexed.
3. Place the tip of the crutches 3 to 6 inches from the upper, outer border of the toes of each foot. *This provides a wider base of support for improved balance.*
4. Adjust the crutches to proper height, ensuring that the upper pads on the crutches are placed lightly under the child's axillae (Figure 20-17 ■). *The crutches should not put pressure on the axillae.*
5. Check the child's posture. The back or neck should not be flexed. *This would indicate that the crutches are too short.*

SAMPLE DOCUMENTATION

(date/time)   Crutches placed in axillae. Height adjusted. Correct posture and pad placement noted. Instructions on proper crutch-walking given. Client verbalized understanding. J. Ness, LPN

PROCEDURE 20-3   Applying Traction

Purpose
- To ensure appropriate traction is applied
- To ensure proper body alignment is maintained
- To maintain safety and prevent further injury

Equipment
- Poles, pulleys, rope, weight, pads as ordered
- Elastic wrap for external traction

Check order + Gather equipment + Introduce yourself + Identify client + Provide privacy + Explain procedure + Hand hygiene + Gloves as needed

Interventions and Rationales

1. Perform preparatory steps (see icon bar).

2. Place weights as ordered.

3. Apply traction as ordered to affected extremity. *Proper weights and placement will ensure correct treatment.*

4. Make the following assessments every 30 minutes initially, and then every 1 to 2 hours when stable:
   - Proper position of traction.
   - Proper body alignment.
   - Neurovascular status of extremity (Figure 20-18 ■). Report any of the following: decreased or absent pulses, change in color of skin above or below site of traction, warmth of the extremity, decreased sensation, decreased capillary refill, increase edema, limited movement of extremity, or pain, burning, or tingling.

clinical ALERT

When assessing neurovascular status in a pediatric client with musculoskeletal injury, the nurse looks for **c**irculation, **m**ovement, and **s**ensation (CMS). Also, observe and document the five Ps: **P**aresthesia, **P**ain/pressure, **P**allor, **P**aralysis, **P**ulselessness.

   - Condition of skin under and around traction application.
   - Skin over bony prominences.
   - Vital signs
   - Pain.
   - Emotional state. *These assessments will ensure quality of care.*

5. Perform sterile pin care according to agency policy for internal traction or as ordered by physician. *Sterile cleansing is necessary to prevent introduction of microorganisms to compromised skin.*

6. Provide teaching and evaluation of technique if the family will maintain traction at home.

Figure 20-18. ■ The skin of the extremities should be warm. It should blanch when slight pressure is applied and then return to its normal color within 3 seconds.

Client teaching and return demonstration will provide the family with the knowledge and skills they need to support the healing process.

SAMPLE DOCUMENTATION

(date/time)   Traction to left lower extremity applied per order. Toes warm, pink, with appropriate ROM. Client is without complaint at present. Verbalized understanding of plan of care. Video provided for distraction. Call bell within reach. L. Atchley, LPN

CLIENT TEACHING

Most fractures can be managed at home. The child and family should be taught to care for any orthopedic appliance, to administer medication, and to recognize complications. Follow-up visits to the health care provider are essential to evaluate bone healing. Table 20-3 ■ provides information on ways communicate about cast care with parents and children.

Evaluation of the effectiveness of treatment includes skin integrity, body alignment, neurovascular status, and bone healing. Because children's fractures heal faster than adults, follow-up evaluation should occur every few weeks. Parents should be able to verbalize any modification that may be needed at home or school. The nurse should refer parents to home health nurses if indicated.

Musculoskeletal Infection

OSTEOMYELITIS

Osteomyelitis (Figure 20-19 ■) is an infection of the bone that may spread to surrounding tissues.

The infection typically follows an injury or surgery and is the result of bacteria, virus, or fungi. The most common causative agent is *Staphylococcus aureus*. Children ages 1 to

TABLE 20-3

Communicating Across the Life Span: Providing Cast Care Instructions

COMMUNICATOR	TODDLER	PRESCHOOLER	SCHOOL-AGE CHILD	ADOLESCENT
Client/Parent	How can I help my child get exercise while they have this cast on their leg?	My child usually takes showers. How can we do that with this arm cast?	I caught my child using his cast as a hammer. Now we have to get the cast replaced. How can I get him to understand how to take better care of the cast?	I'm going to summer camp. I know there will be fishing, boating, and swimming. I guess I'll just sit on the riverbank and watch.
Nurse (to the parents)	Determine what activities the child usually participates in. Try to modify something they enjoy doing. For example: If the child enjoys climbing on the jungle gym in the backyard, suggest that the child swing instead. Encourage the parents to supervise this activity and to teach the child not to jump from the swing.	Showers will cause the cast to get wet. During the time your child has the cast, baths will be more appropriate. It will still be important to wrap the cast in a plastic trash bag for each bath and to monitor the entire bath time.	It's important that your child understand the reason for the cast, how the cast will protect his arm, and what can happen if the bone doesn't heal properly. When you come in to the office, we'll get the x-rays out and show him the break. We'll also review the teaching about cast care. Doesn't your child play baseball? Maybe he'll understand how a bone that is not healed properly will affect his performance in this sport.	Let's think about how you can participate in these activities. What could you use to cover your cast to keep it from getting wet? How about a raincoat, trash bag, plastic wrap? You should be able to go fishing and boating as long as you do not get into the water. Swimming is going to be something you'll have to do after your cast comes off. Maybe you could talk to the camp lifeguards and get them to let you assist them.

12 years are most likely to have osteomyelitis, and boys are more likely to have it than girls.

Manifestations

The child may present with symptoms of constant pain in the affected area and surrounding tissues. The affected surrounding tissues may be edematous, and there may be decreased mobility of the joint. The child may refuse to use the affected limb or may limp. There may also be redness over the site of injury, and the child may have a fever.

Diagnosis

Diagnosis is made by a careful review of the child's history, including incidents of trauma. Laboratory results may indicate an increase white blood cell count and erythrocyte sedimentation rate. X-rays and bone scans are used to view the site of injury. Needle aspiration of fluid from the site allows the health care provider to culture the specimen for the causative agent.

Treatment

The child with osteomyelitis is hospitalized and administered IV antibiotics. Some form of antibiotic treatment is usually administered for 3 to 6 weeks. If the child is discharged from the hospital, antibiotic treatment will be continued at home either orally or intravenously. For the child who is discharged on IV antibiotics, a home health care nurse can assist in the administration and care of the IV site.

Figure 20-19. ■ Osteomyelitis. (**A**) Bacteria enter and multiply in the bone. (**B**) The infection spreads to other parts of the bone, and the periosteum separates from the surface of the bone.

A Initial infection

Initial infection

Periosteum

B Acute phase

Blood supply blocked

Pus-filled abscess

Musculoskeletal Tumors

OSTEOSARCOMA
Bone tumors are rare, but periods of rapid growth are the most common times for occurrence in adolescent boys. Bone tumors are usually found in the distal femur, proximal tibia, or proximal humerus.

Manifestations
Clinical manifestations include pain, swelling, and mobility or gait problems. Fever, elevated white blood cell count, and elevated erythrocyte sedimentation rate may be seen.

Diagnosis
X-ray, computed tomography (CT) or MRI scan, and tissue biopsy are used to reach a diagnosis of osteosarcoma.

Treatment
Treatment involves surgery and the use of chemotherapy and radiation. Depending on the extent of the tumor, limb-sparing surgery may be used to remove the tumor and surrounding bone. An internal prosthesis is then inserted. Amputation must be performed if the tumor is large or involves surrounding soft tissue, including nerves. Chemotherapy and radiation are given to treat nondetectable metastasis.

Nursing Considerations
Nursing management includes standard preoperative and postoperative care. Psychological assessment of the adolescent and the family is necessary. Body image disturbances occur when a limb is lost. Signs of disturbed body image include:

- Refusal to look at or touch the altered body part
- Hiding the affected body part
- Preoccupation with the loss or change
- Overexposure of the body part
- Feelings of guilt, shame, or embarrassment

Client and family support systems should be identified and contacted as soon as possible. The older child or adolescent will need to learn to care for the stump (Figure 20-20 ■ and Box 20-9 ■). Rehabilitation will be needed to help the child learn to use the prosthesis and adapt to the amputation (Figure 20-21 ■). With practice and at times with special devices, many children continue their involvement with sports.

Prosthetics can be expensive, and parents may need financial support beyond insurance. Referral to special hospitals such as the Shriner's Hospitals may be an option. The school should be contacted and plans made for the

Figure 20-20. ■ With an above-the-knee amputation, a figure-eight bandage is wrapped around the waist, then brought down over the stump and back up around the hip.

adolescent's return. Some adaptation may be needed to accommodate wheelchair, crutches, or other appliances and to plan for emergency evacuation.

EWING'S SARCOMA
Ewing's sarcoma is a malignant tumor found most commonly on the femur, pelvis, tibia, fibula, ribs, humerus, scapula, and clavicle. Whites and Hispanics are most commonly affected. Children ages 10 to 20 years have the highest incidence of Ewing's sarcoma.

BOX 20-9   NURSING CARE CHECKLIST

Care of the Stump Following Amputation

- ☑ Carefully monitor vital signs and drainage from dressing.
- ☑ Keep a surgical tourniquet available to control bleeding if necessary.
- ☑ Observe strict sterile technique for dressing changes to prevent infection.
- ☑ Apply compression bandage as ordered (see Figure 20-20).
- ☑ Change bandages twice daily to observe for wound healing.
- ☑ Avoid hip flexion contractures by limiting sitting in chair to less than 1 hour. Also avoid pillows under the limb.
- ☑ Explain phantom limb pain to the child and parents. Symptoms include coolness, heaviness, and pain.
- ☑ Administer pain medications as ordered to control the child's comfort.
- ☑ Assist with temporary prosthesis fitting.
- ☑ Assist with ROM exercises as ordered.
- ☑ Teach crutch walking with lower limb amputation as ordered.

Figure 20-21. ■ A role model can provide support and encouragement to a child learning to adapt to life with a prosthetic limb. (Photo Researchers, Inc.)

Manifestations

Clinical manifestations are similar to those of osteosarcoma. Fractures of the affected bone may occur.

Diagnosis

Diagnosis is made by biopsy of the tumor.

Treatment

Treatment includes chemotherapy to reduce the tumor size, followed by surgery to remove the bone. High-dose radiation may also be implemented. Chemotherapy typically follows surgery. Nursing care for children with Ewing's sarcoma is the same as outlined above for osteosarcoma.

NURSING CARE

PRIORITIES IN NURSING CARE

When caring for children with musculoskeletal disorders, the LVN/LPN must promote independence of the child. Nursing care will also focus on the child's mobility and maintaining safety. The nurse must use available resources to assist the child and the family in getting support and establishing proper home care.

ASSESSING

Monitor cardiac, respiratory, urinary, and bowel function. Assess range of motion, mobility, posture, and muscle strength. Note any swelling or redness that may be associated with muscle sprain. If the child uses assistive devices, the nurse must assess the correct use of the devices and the effectiveness of the devices in aiding the child's mobility.

For chronic disorders such as muscular dystrophy, the nurse collects data about the family's ability to care for the child long term in the home both physically and emotionally.

DIAGNOSING, PLANNING, AND IMPLEMENTING

The following nursing diagnoses may be used in planning nursing care for the child with a musculoskeletal disorder:

- Impaired Physical **M**obility related to musculoskeletal impairment
- **A**ctivity Intolerance related to weakness
- Risk for **I**njury related to altered mobility
- Compromised **C**oping: Family related to caring for a child with a chronic condition

Typical outcomes for the child or family with a musculoskeletal disorder might include these as well as others:

- Mobility will be restored through the use of assistive devices.
- Tolerance for activity will be demonstrated as evidenced by vital signs within normal limits.
- Family will create a safe environment.
- Family will participate effectively in developing a plan to care for the child.

Nursing interventions related to children with musculoskeletal disorders include:

- Teach client to use assistive devices. *Crutches, canes, braces, walkers, and wheelchairs require specific instruction to operate properly. Demonstration and return demonstration of the use of these devices will promote mobility.*
- Provide positive encouragement before, during, and after use of assistive devices. *Encouragement will promote well-being and the desire to continue working on using the devices properly.*
- Assist the family in planning daily activities to include periods of rest. *Adequate rest is essential for energy conservation.*
- Keep frequently used objects within easy reach. *Reducing the number of steps required to complete activities of daily living will assist in energy conservation.*
- Assist the parents in assessing their home environment for safety hazards. *Safety hazards must be identified in order to correct them.*
- Provide information about correcting identified hazards. *Instructing families in how to correct hazards will help them manage their environment correctly and prevent injury.*
- Discuss with the family the common responses to caring for a child with a musculoskeletal disorder. *The nurse can assist the family in identifying anxiety, fear, and depression as normal responses of families in their situation.*

- Provide the family with specific information on caring for their child with a musculoskeletal disorder. *Families can develop coping mechanisms when they are able to view the task before them and understand how it can be managed effectively.*

EVALUATING

The child is evaluated for mobility, tolerance to activity, and safety. The family can be evaluated for coping with the care of the child. These evaluations should be made on a regular basis because these criteria can change throughout the child's care.

NURSING PROCESS CARE PLAN
Child with an Amputation

Jake is a 14-year-old who was admitted 1 week ago with a diagnosis of osteosarcoma and is scheduled for surgery tomorrow. Jake's physician has informed Jake and his parents that Jake's leg may have to be amputated to ensure complete removal of the tumor. Jake has spent the last 5 years playing baseball and is "depressed" that he will no longer be able to play sports.

Assessment.   The following data should be collected as soon as possible:

- Vital signs
- Condition of surgical site, preoperatively
- Client's and family's understanding of the disease process
- Client's and family's understanding of the treatment regimen
- Feelings and concerns about the possible amputation
- Client's understanding of the use of a prosthesis
- Level of familial support.

Nursing Diagnosis.   The following important nursing diagnosis (among others) is established for this client:

- Disturbed **B**ody Image related to surgical alteration of limb

Expected Outcomes

- Will demonstrate a positive body image
- Will express the desire to learn how to use a prosthesis

Planning and Implementation

- Listen attentively to Jake's concerns in a nonjudgmental manner. *Therapeutic listening will provide a safe environment.*
- Encourage grief behaviors. *Dealing with emotions is part of healing.*
- Assist Jake and his family in developing coping mechanisms, using personal strengths.
- Encourage Jake to begin regular activities of daily living as soon as possible after surgery. *Independent self-care increases self-esteem.*
- Teach Jake's parents the importance of their responses related to his body changes. *Their modeling of acceptance and a positive attitude toward Jake's changed physical appearance will encourage similar changes in Jake.*
- Refer the family to social services for home care and follow-up. *Support services are essential in making this transition. Both parents and child may benefit from participation in a support group.*

Evaluation.   Jake begins to care for his amputation shortly after surgery and readily accepts the duties related to stump and prosthesis care. He discusses life after amputation with a young girl who had an amputation 1 year ago. On discharge, he tells the nurse that he would love to learn more about playing sports with a prosthesis.

Critical Thinking in the Nursing Process

1. What competitive sporting activities could the nurse suggest for Jake to try?
2. Managing a prosthesis requires additional energy. What suggestions should the nurse make to assist Jake in having adequate energy?
3. List two caring responses to the following concern expressed by Jake: "I'm afraid people will stare at me when I walk by."

Note: Discussion of Critical Thinking questions appears in Appendix I.

Note: The reference and resource listings for this and all chapters have been compiled at the back of the book.

Chapter Review

 KEY TERMS by Topic

Use the audio glossary feature of either the CD-ROM or the Companion Website to hear the correct pronunciation of the following key terms.

Anatomy and Physiology
ossification, epiphysis, epiphyseal plate, metaphysis, diaphysis, hematopoiesis,

greenstick fracture, genu valgum, genu varum

Congenital Skeletal Defects
acetabulum, hip spica cast, talipes, equines, varus

Musculoskeletal Disorders
muscular dystrophy, Gower's maneuver, kyphosis, lordosis, torticollis

Musculoskeletal Trauma
sprain, strain, fracture, closed reduction, open reduction, compartment syndrome

KEY Points

- Injuries to a child's bones may be due to the fact that the growth plate is still open and the child's long bones are less dense than an adult's. Children are also naturally curious and adventurous.

- A priority nursing role when caring for children with musculoskeletal disorders is to promote independence.

- An essential assessment for the nurse to make when caring for a child with a cast is observing for compartment syndrome, which occurs when increased pressure in a limited space compromises circulation and nerve innervation, leading to possible necrosis. Symptoms of compartment syndrome include paresthesia, pain/pressure, pallor, paralysis, and pulselessness.

- The nurse should teach the child and parents to prevent complications with a cast by teaching them to keep the cast dry and clean, avoid using powders or lotions, avoid sticking objects into the cast, and cover the cast to protect it from injury.

- When providing instruction to a child who is learning to walk with crutches, the nurse should ensure that the crutches are not pressing on the axillae and that the child is able to maintain a straight spine when walking.

- Besides physical care, children in traction need their emotional needs to be addressed.

- The nurse should observe the child with a musculoskeletal disorder for body image disturbance by recognizing the following signs: refusal to look at or touch the altered body part, hiding the affected body part, preoccupation with the loss or change, overexposure of the body part, and/or feelings of guilt, shame, or embarrassment.

 EXPLORE MediaLink

Additional interactive resources for this chapter can be found on the Companion Website at www.prenhall.com/adams.

Click on Chapter 20 and "Begin" to select the activities for this chapter.

For chapter-related NCLEX®-style questions and an audio glossary, access the accompanying CD-ROM in this book.

Animations:

Skeleton

FOR FURTHER Study

For more information about legal aspects of child abuse, see Chapter 3.

See Figure 15-4 for anterior and posterior fotanels.

For psychosocial aspects of child abuse, see Chapter 16.

For more information on juvenile rheumatoid arthritis, see Chapter 22.

Caring for a Child with a Fracture

NCLEX-PN® Focus Area: Physiologic Integrity

Case Study: Billy, an 8-year-old, is brought to the urgent care clinic for a possible fractured left lower leg. Billy had been rollerblading when he fell, twisting his left ankle. He is hopping on his right leg. He has been crying and states, "It hurts real bad."

Nursing Diagnosis: Impaired Physical **M**obility related to fractured leg

COLLECT DATA

Subjective	Objective
_____	_____
_____	_____
_____	_____
_____	_____
_____	_____

Would you report this? Yes/No

If yes, to: _____

Nursing Care

_____

How would you document this? _____

Compare your documentation to the sample provided in Appendix I.

Data Collected
(use only those that apply)

- Pedal pulses present
- Crying
- States, "It hurts real bad."
- Ankle swollen, bruised
- Mother states child has history of asthma
- Non-weight-bearing

Nursing Interventions
(use only those that apply; list in priority order)

- Apply ice pack to ankle.
- Instruct not to put anything inside cast.
- Offer milk three times a day.
- Apply heat lamp to ankle.
- Instruct to support cast on pillows until dry.
- Teach crutch walking.
- Instruct regarding signs of impaired circulation.

NCLEX-PN® Exam Preparation

TEST-TAKING TIP   Notice any question with the key word *avoids*. This word indicates a "false-response" question (it asks you to select the *wrong* intervention). Use the process of elimination and your knowledge about caring for children to arrive at the correct response.

1 A 12-year-old asks, "Do I really have to wear this Milwaukee brace when I go school? I look like a freak!" The nurse's best response would be:

   1. "It is important that you wear the brace 23 hours a day."
   2. "I know the brace does not look very stylish; let's see if we can find some pictures of cute shirts that may help."
   3. "I will ask the doctor if you can wear another type of brace."
   4. "I guess it will be alright for you to leave the brace off while you are at school."

2 The nurse is caring for a client with osteosarcoma. Which of the following symptoms would the nurse expect?

   1. Swelling in the area of the clavicle
   2. Difficulty using either hand
   3. Pain in the femur
   4. Frequently stiff back

3 A 17-year-old is 3 days postop below-the-knee amputation for osteosarcoma. The LPN is gathering data in a psychological assessment. Which of the following findings should be reported to the RN?

   1. Client removed the bandage and looked at the wound.
   2. Client discusses what it will be like without a leg.
   3. Client keeps leg under the covers.
   4. Client discusses the surgery with his best friend.

4 An infant was born with developmental dysplasia of the hip. His father states, "I am glad we will only have to triple his diaper for a few days. They look so uncomfortable." The nurse should reply:

   1. "Tell me what you understand about the infant's hip problem."
   2. "You are wrong, he will have to wear triple diapers for 3 to 4 months."
   3. "You are right, he will only need triple diapers for a few days."
   4. "Triple diapers are uncomfortable, so you will need to medicate your infant every 4 hours."

5 The nurse is providing instruction to parents about a synthetic cast applied to the child for treatment of clubfoot. Which of the following statements is true about synthetic casting?

   1. "Make sure the cast is allowed to dry for 24 hours."
   2. "Synthetic casts are best because they are stronger than plaster casts."
   3. "This cast is heavier than a plaster cast."
   4. "Synthetic casts allow for greater mobility."

6 The nurse is assisting the physician during an examination of an infant with a diagnosis of hip dysplasia. The physician is planning on performing an Ortolani-Barlow maneuver. The nurse understands that the physician is assessing the infant's hips for _____.

7 A nurse is taking care of a child in skeletal traction and avoids which action when caring for this child?

   1. Ensuring the weights are hanging freely
   2. Putting the bed linens on the traction ropes
   3. Making sure the weights are out of the child's reach
   4. Checking to ensure the weights are in the pulleys

8 The nurse is caring for a child with a right leg cast and is checking the capillary refill of the extremity. The nurse presses the nail bed of the great toe and it returns to the original color in 2 seconds. The nurse's next action is to:

   1. Document the findings.
   2. Prepare the child for immediate cast removal.
   3. Elevate the extremity on two pillows and recheck the capillary refill.
   4. Notify the physician.

9 A nurse is checking off instructions for the parents for care of a child with a newly applied cast to the right lower leg. Select all instructions that would be included on this list.

   1. Observe the cast for drainage.
   2. Contact the physician if the child complains of numbness or tingling in the leg.
   3. Elevate the leg on pillows for the first 24 to 48 hours after the cast application.
   4. Observe the toes for changes in color (blue color, pallor).
   5. Cover cast with plastic bag during bathing.
   6. Sprinkle powder inside the cast to keep the leg dry.

10 The nurse is providing instruction for the mother of an adolescent girl with scoliosis who has just been fitted for a Milwaukee brace. The nurse realizes additional instruction is needed when the mother states:

   1. "I understand that the brace must be worn for 2 hours on and 2 hours off."
   2. "I know I have to check around the brace for skin breakdown."
   3. "I will provide skin care to prevent breakdown."
   4. "I will work with my daughter so she can learn how to sit, stand, and walk with the brace."

Answers for NCLEX-PN® Review and Critical Thinking questions appear in Appendix I.

Care of the Child with Integumentary Disorders

BRIEF Outline

Anatomy and Physiology

Brief Assessment Review

Congenital Lesions

Skin Disorders

Inflammatory Disorders

Nursing Care

Parasitic Infestations

Skin Infections

Fungal Infections

Nursing Care

Burns

Nursing Care

Trauma to the Skin from the Environment

Nursing Care

NURSING PROCESS CARE PLAN:
Client with Cellulitis

NURSING CARE PLAN CHART:
Child with a Burn

HEALTH PROMOTION ISSUE:
Teens and Tanning

CRITICAL THINKING CARE MAP:
Caring for a Child with Eczema

LEARNING Outcomes

After completing this chapter, you will be able to:

1. Define key terms.
2. Review the basic structure and function of skin and describe differences between the skin of a child and an adult.
3. Discuss common congenital disorders of skin, their treatment, and nursing care.
4. Discuss common infections and infestations of skin in children, as well as treatment and nursing care.
5. Discuss various types of skin trauma in children, as well as treatment and nursing care.

Many changes occur in the skin from the time of birth through adolescence. Skin disorders are common among pediatric clients. The LPN/LVN plays an important role in assisting the client and the family as they cope with common skin disorders. Important priorities for the LPN/LVN are promoting healthy skin care to the pediatric client and providing methods to prevent skin infections while decreasing pain and discomfort. Psychological and social development may be altered if skin disorders lead to disfigurement.

Skin serves several functions. The main function of the skin is to protect the body from pathogens that may cause infections. Temperature is regulated by the skin when the blood vessels dilate (allowing heat to dissipate from the body), and through perspiration (allowing evaporation of fluids). Production of serum creates an oily barrier that prevents fluid loss. Sensory receptors provide information about pain, touch, pressure, and temperature. The outer layer of the skin participates in the production of vitamin D.

Anatomy and Physiology

The integumentary system is the largest organ system in the body. The integumentary system includes the skin and its associated structures: hair, nails, sebaceous and sweat glands, blood vessels, nerve endings, and sensory organs (Figure 21-1 ■). The skin is the first line of defense against infection.

The **epidermis** is the outer thin layer of the skin. It consists of two layers:

■ *Stratum corneum* (horny cell layer), which consists of flattened dead, keratinized cells.

Figure 21-1. ■ Anatomic view of skin and accessory structures.

■ *Stratum germinativum* (basal cell layer), where cells multiply, grow, and move toward the skin's surface, causing the surface layer to be replaced about every 4 weeks. The stratum germinativum also contains melanocytes, which secrete **melanin,** a pigment that adds color to the skin.

The **dermis** is the inner, thicker layer of the skin, which contains most of the associated structures (such as hair, nails, sebaceous and sweat glands, blood vessels, nerve endings, and sensory organs). The dermal layer is highly vascular and provides nourishment to the epidermis. Fibrous connective and collagen tissue within the dermis provides strength and allows the skin to stretch with body movements. Collagen is produced by *fibroblast cells* (the primary cell type in the dermis). Nerve endings within the dermis provide sensations of pain, pressure, temperature and touch.

ASSOCIATED STRUCTURES

Hair

Hair covers the majority of the body except the lips, palms of the hands, and the soles of the feet. Hair consists of the shaft (the visible part of the hair) located in the epidermis and the root located deep within the dermal layer of the skin, all of which make up the hair follicle. The **arrector pili,** an involuntary muscle, surrounds the hair follicle and pulls the hair upright when it contracts when the child is exposed to cold external temperatures or fear. Hair located on the scalp, eyelids, eyebrows, and ear canals aids in keeping dust and insects from entering the body. Hair that is shiny, lustrous, and not easily plucked reflects good nutritional status in the client. Hair that is dry, brittle, thinning, and easily plucked indicates poor nutritional status. The color of the hair is provided by melanocytes (found in the hair shaft).

Nails

Nails consist of keratinized epidermal cells. The body of the nail is visible and pink in color because of the vascular nail bed underneath. Nail growth takes place at the nail root, which lies under the cuticle. Healthy nails are firm and transparent but may appear pink over the body of the nail. Nails that are brittle may often indicate poor nutritional status.

Sebaceous Glands

Sebaceous glands are located in the dermis and secrete sebum. Sebum has a lubricating effect on the skin, keeping the skin soft and the hair supple, and aids in preventing the growth of bacteria. Secretion of sebum from the sebaceous glands is stimulated by sex hormones, which increase during puberty. Sebaceous glands are located over the entire body except the palms of the hand and soles of the feet. The face, scalp, upper chest, and back contain more sebaceous glands than other parts of the body.

Sweat Glands (Sudoriferous Glands)

Sweat glands (sudoriferous glands) are *exocrine* glands (i.e., they have ducts). Eccrine glands and apocrine glands are two types of sweat glands that secrete fluids to the surface of the skin.

- *Eccrine glands* are small but distributed throughout the body. They play a role in maintaining body temperature by allowing body heat to dissipate as sweat when it is brought to the top of the skin for evaporation.
- *Apocrine glands* are deeper in the dermis and open into the hair follicles. These sweat glands are larger, are found in the axillae and genital areas, and begin functioning at the onset of puberty. Once the sweat produced by the apocrine glands comes in contact with bacteria on the skin, it produces a distinct body odor.

SUBCUTANEOUS LAYER

The subcutaneous layer, also referred to as the *superficial fascia*, is directly under the dermis. (The word *subcutaneous* means "under the skin.") The subcutaneous layer includes elastic, fibrous, and adipose tissue. The main functions of this layer are to cushion internal organs, store fat for energy, insulate the body, and connect the skin to the surface of the muscles.

GROWTH AND DEVELOPMENT

The skin of the newborn is high in water content and very thin (Figure 21-2 ■). It can absorb harmful chemicals more readily than older skin. Because the epidermis is not strongly attached to the underlying dermis, friction may cause blistering. Care must be taken to handle the newborn's skin gently.

Newborns have little subcutaneous fat, so heat loss is rapid. The newborn's body regulates temperature through the eccrine sweat glands; the apocrine sweat glands do not yet function. Skin contains little melanin at birth, so skin tones are lighter.

As children grow, the skin thickens and the epidermis and dermis become more tightly bound. Eccrine glands increase their function, and apocrine glands begin functioning at puberty. Increased melanin creates a full skin tone and protects the body against harmful rays of the sun.

Pediatric clients are more prone to skin infections than adults. If a skin infection develops, it is more likely to produce systemic symptoms in children. Subcutaneous fat is decreased in preterm and term newborns, making them more sensitive to environmental changes. The epidermis of the newborn is thinner, which makes it more susceptible to blisters from friction if careful handing is not practiced. The pH level of the newborn's skin is more alkaline than that of the older child; because of this, it is more prone to infections. The eccrine glands mature around 2 to 3 years of age, allowing the child to regulate body temperature more easily. The skin of the young child is drier and chaps easily, because sebum is not excreted by the sebaceous glands until 8 to 10 years of age. The hormonal surge during adolescence increases sebum production, leading to increased incidence of acne vulgaris (discussed later in the chapter).

Brief Assessment Review

Assessment of the skin can be a window into systemic problems involving oxygenation, circulation, nutrition, and hydration.

HISTORY

- Review past health history and family history for any skin health issues such as eczema, pruritus, lesions, lice, scabies, change in hair or hair loss, changes in nails, or any other infections or infestations.
- Inquire about allergies (food, medication, fabrics, metals, or pollens).
- Inquire about current medications (topical or systemic).
- Ask the parent and/or child about skin care habits (bathing, use of skin care products, and use of sunscreen).

PHYSICAL

- Inspect the skin for color pigment changes (pallor, jaundice, cyanosis, or erythema). Use a penlight if focused lighting is necessary.

Body surface area of adult much greater in relation to internal organs

Sebaceous glands increase production in adolescence

Sweat glands have greater production in adolescents and young adults

Epidermis thicker in adult with more fat and subcutaneous tissue

Figure 21-2. ■ Adult versus child integumentary system.

- Inspect for location of birthmarks such as port-wine stains or strawberry hemangiomas (discussed later).
- Palpate the skin to assess moisture, texture, turgor, and temperature. The dorsal side of the examiner's hand is used, because it is more sensitive to temperature changes.
- Use a clear, flexible metric ruler to measure the size of lesions, patches of skin discolorations, and wound size. A marking pen may be used to define borders so the primary health care provider can inspect for increasing or decreasing size of lesions, skin discolorations, and wounds.

- Identify the major types of lesions (including tattoos and piercings) and note location, shape, and size. It is important to differentiate between primary lesions and secondary lesions. (Box 21-1 ■ and Figure 21-3 ■ provide descriptions and pictures.)

clinical ALERT

Inspect suspicious or possible malignant lesions by using the acronym ABCDE: **A**, asymmetry of shape; **B**, border irregularity; **C**, color variation; **D**, diameter larger than 6 mm; **E**, elevation of lesion.

BOX 21-1

Common Skin Lesions

Primary Lesions (see Figure 21-3)
Cyst—a fluid-filled or semisolid sac originating in the subcutaneous tissue or dermis.
Examples: epidermoid (skin) cyst or sebaceous cyst seen in acne
Macule, patch—a discolored spot that is even with the skin's surface; macules are less than 1 cm, patches are greater than 1 cm
Examples: (of macule) freckles, petechiae; (of patch) port wine stains, mongolian spots
Papule, plaque—a circumscribed, solid elevation of the skin
Examples: (of papule) elevated mole, warts; (of plaques) psoriasis, actinic keratosis
Nodule, tumor—a circumscribed, elevated mass of tissue extending deeper into the dermis than a papule; nodules are 0.5–2 cm; tumors are greater than 2 cm and may have irregular borders
Examples: (of nodule) squamous cell carcinoma or small lipoma (fatty growth); (of tumor) hemangioma, carcinoma
Pustule—a small, circumscribed elevation of the skin containing purulent matter
Examples: infected pimple
Vesicle, Bulla—a small, circumscribed elevation of the skin containing fluid; vesicles are less than 0.5 cm; bullae are greater than 0.5 cm
Examples: (of vesicle) herpes simplex or cold sore; (of bulla) contact dermatitis or large burn blisters
Wheal—a circumscribed, slightly reddened, papule or irregular plaque of edema of the skin, usually accompanied by intense itching
Examples: insect bites, hives

Secondary Lesions (see Figure 21-3)
Atrophy—a semitransparent, paperlike, sometimes wrinkled skin surface; a wasting of the skin
Examples: aged or sun-damaged skin, striae ("stretch marks")
Crust—blood, pus, or serum that has dried on the surface of the skin after injury
Examples: scab (after abrasion injury), eczema

Erosion—a wearing away of the superficial epidermis by friction or pressure
Examples: scratches, ruptured vesicles
Fissure—a deep furrow or slit extending into the dermis
Examples: athlete's foot lesions, cracks at the sides of the mouth with dehydration
Keloid—excess scar tissue; hyperplastic scar tissue with irregular bands of collagen, usually formed after trauma, surgery, burn of severe skin disease
Examples: enlarged scars from ear piercing
Lichenification—leathery hardening and thickening of the skin, caused by scratching or rubbing
Examples: chronic dermatitis
Scales—a small thin plate of epidermis that is shed from skin tissue
Examples: dandruff, eczema, dry skin
Scar—fibrous tissue that replaces normal tissue after injury
Examples: healed surgical wound, healed acne
Ulcer—superficial loss of tissue, usually with inflammation, on the surface of the skin or mucous membrane
Examples: decubitus ulcers (pressure sores), chancres

Vascular Lesions
Ecchymosis—purplish patch caused by extravasation (leaking) of blood into the skin; like petechiae but greater than 3 mm diameter
Hematoma—localized mass of extravasated blood that is confined within an organ or tissue
Petechiae—tiny hemorrhagic spots, from pinpoint to pinhead size
Port-wine stain—a large, congenital vascular nevus with a purplish color; usually found on the head and neck (see Figure 21-3)
Purpura—condition characterized by hemorrhaging into the skin
Spider angioma—dilated arteriole in the skin with radiating capillary branches that look like the legs of a spider
Strawberry mark—a small capillary hemangioma that resembles a strawberry in size, shape, and color; usually disappears in early childhood

Source: Ramont, R., & Niedringhaus, D. (2006). *Comprehensive nursing care.* Upper Saddle River, NJ: Prentice Hall, Box 22-2, p. 529.

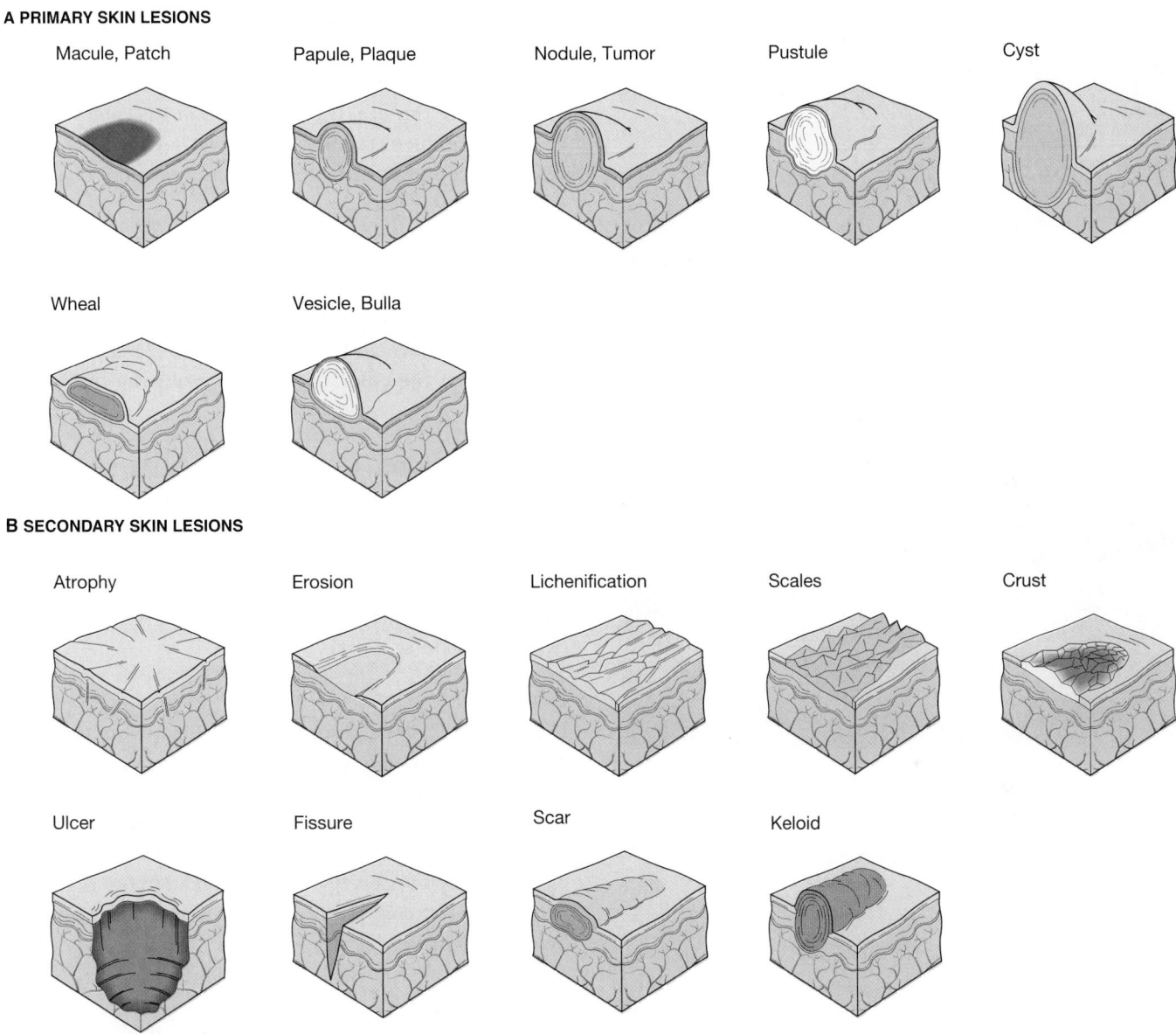

A PRIMARY SKIN LESIONS

Macule, Patch Papule, Plaque Nodule, Tumor Pustule Cyst

Wheal Vesicle, Bulla

B SECONDARY SKIN LESIONS

Atrophy Erosion Lichenification Scales Crust

Ulcer Fissure Scar Keloid

Figure 21-3. ■ Vascular skin lesions. (**A**) Primary skin lesions. (**B**) Secondary skin lesions.

Congenital Lesions

Birthmarks are discolorations of the skin. They can be a common finding among newborns. All birthmarks should be examined for color, size, location, texture, and elevation. Some birthmarks may be an indicator of disease and may require further investigation. Appearance of birthmarks may be upsetting to parents. The LPN/LVN provides support and education to the family about birthmarks.

Several discolored areas are commonly found on newborn's skin. A **mongolian spot** is a dark discolored area found over the lower back and sacrum of infants of Black, Hispanic, South Asian, or East Asian descent. Over time, the infant's skin tones darken to become the same color as the mongolian spot. Some infants are born with dark red spots on the eyelids, forehead, or nape of the neck. These red areas, called **telangiectactic nevi** or **stork bites,** usually fade in time. Parental concern for these and other birthmarks should be discussed with the pediatrician. Consultation with a plastic surgeon may be needed. The sebaceous glands on the face become distended a few days after birth, resulting in **milia** or white pinpoint spots resembling whiteheads. A few weeks of bathing opens the sebaceous glands, and the milia disappear.

CAPILLARY (STRAWBERRY) HEMANGIOMA

Strawberry (or capillary) hemangioma is a benign cutaneous tumor that involves the capillaries in the dermis. Strawberry hemangiomas (Figure 21-4 ■) may appear a few weeks after birth and are more common in girls and in

A

B

Figure 21-4. ■ (**A**) Capillary (strawberry) hemangioma.
(**B**) Port-wine stain. (**A**. H. C. Robinson/Science Photo Library/Photo
Researchers, Inc. **B**. Custom Medical Stock Photo, Inc.)

premature infants. During the first year, capillary hemangiomas may enlarge. By 2 to 3 years of age, the hemangiomas will begin to decrease.

Manifestations

Clinical manifestations include a bright red area of skin
that is flat in the beginning but will elevate with growth.
The surface is rough and has a rubbery feel to it. The margins are well defined. Most hemangiomas are found on the
face and head.

Diagnosis

Diagnosis is made by inspection and palpation of the
hemangioma, documenting location, color, and size.
Monitoring the growth of the vascular tumor is also helpful
for diagnostic purposes.

Treatment

Medical treatment may not be indicated once the hemangioma begins to resolve spontaneously. Oral prednisone
may be given once a day for 7 to 10 days then tapered to the
lowest most effective dose for 4 to 6 weeks to help slow the

growth of the hemangioma. A rest period of 2 to 4 weeks
may be needed between prednisone treatments. For some
children, hemangiomas treatment may include laser therapy to reduce the size. If the hemangioma is extensive and
causing a problem to the airway, eyes, or ear canal, or if
feeding is compromised, subcutaneous injections of alfa-2a
or alfa-2b interferon may be needed.

PORT-WINE STAINS

Port-wine stains are permanent vascular stains that involve
the vascular bed in the dermis. They are most commonly
found on the face and head (see Figure 21-4B). As the
child grows, the color may darken, and the birthmark
thickens.

Manifestations

Clinical manifestations include a pink to reddish purple
stain on the face or head. The color may depend on the
depth of dermal tissue involved. When deeper vessels of the
dermis are involved, the port-wine stain darkens. If located
on the face, the birthmark becomes thick with a *verrucose*
(wartlike) nodular surface.

Diagnosis

Diagnosis is made by inspection and palpation of the port-
wine stain in relation to the location, color, and size. Port-
wine stains do not blanch. Examination should rule out any
structural malformations which are sometimes associated
with port-wine stains, such as glaucoma or tumors of the
blood or lymph vessels in the piaarachnoid (refers to the pia
mater and arachnoid layers of the meninges protecting the
brain and spinal cord).

Treatment

Medical treatment may depend on the location and size of
the port-wine stain. If the birthmark is small, cosmetics
may be used to cover the stain. If large, a series of laser
treatments may be necessary.

Nursing Considerations

Support and encouragement are vital to families of
infants with congenital lesions. For children with strawberry hemangiomas, a series of photographs may be taken
over time. This visual record of progressive involution of
the hemangioma will offer encouragement. If laser treatments are used to correct strawberry hemangiomas or
port-wine stains, care should be given to prevent any
trauma such as picking at the scab. Only water is used to
clean these areas and to blot them dry. Sometimes a topical antibiotic ointment is applied to the area. Sunlight
should be avoided for a few weeks; then sunscreen (at
least SPF 15 or higher) should be applied for continual
protection.

Skin Disorders

MILIARIA

Miliaria is also known as *prickly heat* or *heat rash*. Eccrine (sweat) glands become blocked when the child is exposed to high environmental temperatures and increased humidity. This reaction may cause backup pressure of sweat, which escapes to surrounding tissue and causes the skin to itch and feel prickly.

Manifestations

Clinical manifestations include minute vesicles with papules. Erythema surrounds the vesicles and papules (see Figure 21-3). Itching is present.

Diagnosis

Diagnosis is made by inspection and palpation of the skin.

Treatment

Medical management involves providing a cool environment and allowing for good ventilation. Cool baths and dusting powders may decrease itching.

Nursing Considerations

Nursing care includes advising parents to monitor the room temperature and to avoid being outside if the temperature is too humid.

INTERTRIGO

Intertrigo is skin irritation caused when opposing skin creates friction. Excessive heat and moisture may cause sweat to be retained between skin folds or in areas where skin rubs together. Areas commonly irritated include the neck, axillae, groin, and intergluteal folds. Obese children are more prone to intertrigo.

Manifestations

Clinical manifestations include inflammation and erythema of the skin, especially in areas where skin has rubbed together. Skin may appear warm and moist. *Candida* infection (discussed later) may also be present.

Diagnosis

Diagnosis is made by inspection and palpation of the skin and skin folds for inflammation, moisture, and redness.

Treatment

Medical treatment involves applying nonmedicated powder to affected areas. Treatment using 1% hydrocortisone cream and antifungal medication may also be needed if a candidal infection is present. Weight loss may help prevent rubbing of skin folds.

Nursing Considerations

Nursing care is directed by keeping the affected area clean and dry. Encourage parents to expose the child's skin to air and light for short periods of time to help dry the skin. Instruct parents that clothing should be appropriate for environmental temperature and should not be tight or binding.

Inflammatory Disorders

ERYTHEMA TOXICUM NEONATORUM

Erythema toxicum neonatorum is a raised pink papule with a light-colored center resembling a mosquito bite on the newborn. These lesions appear suddenly on the chest, abdomen, and back 24 to 48 hours after birth. They are benign and will disappear without treatment.

DERMATITIS

Dermatitis is a general term meaning inflammation of the dermis or skin. When a foreign substance, known as an **irritant,** irritates the skin, the cells release histamine. Histamine causes blood vessels to dilate, resulting in redness, heat, and swelling. Itching and pain are also common. At times vesicles or blisters form, open, drain, and develop a crust. Dermatitis is classified by the location and cause of the irritation, which may stem from an allergen or an irritant. Contact dermatitis, diaper dermatitis, and seborrheic dermatitis are common inflammatory conditions of the skin and are prevalent in infants and children.

CONTACT DERMATITIS

Contact dermatitis can stem from allergens (poison ivy, poison oak, latex, or nickel) or from repeated exposure to irritants (detergents, bleaches, soaps, lotions, urine, and stool). Inflammation is usually limited to the area of contact. Latex may cause both an allergic and an irritant reaction in some infants and children.

Manifestations

Clinical manifestations of allergic contact dermatitis include reddened papules that ooze, crust, itch, and are edematous (see Figure 22-6). Reactions to allergens may develop within 12 to 72 hours after exposure and last up to 3 to 4 weeks. Contact dermatitis caused by irritants manifests itself by localized redness, edema, and scaling of the skin. Reactions appear shortly after exposure to the irritant. They disappear quickly once the irritant is removed.

Diagnosis

Diagnosis is made by obtaining a thorough history of any repeated or prolonged use of common substances known to cause contact dermatitis. Physical examination is done by inspection and palpation of the lesions. Skin testing may be ordered to identify specific allergens and/or irritants that affect the skin.

Treatment

Medical treatment includes proper cleansing of the affected area with mild soap and thorough rinsing of the skin. Hydrocortisone topical ointment may be prescribed to relieve the inflammation. Topical antihistamines may be prescribed to relieve pruritis. Advise the family to avoid irritants known to affect the skin.

Nursing Considerations

Nursing care begins by collecting data to identify any irritants that have come in contact with the skin. The nurse educates the family on methods to avoid common household products known to cause contact dermatitis.

If the contact dermatitis covers a large area of the body, fails to resolve, or gets worse in a short time, or if signs of infection are present, the infant should be seen by a physician or health care provider. Instruct the family on how to recognize signs of infections.

DIAPER DERMATITIS

Diaper dermatitis (Figure 21-5 ■) is caused by irritation from urine and/or stool and is more common in infants. Breastfed infants have a lower pH and therefore are not as prone to diaper dermatitis as are bottle-fed infants. Introduction of formula or solid foods changes the pH level,

Figure 21-5. ■ Diaper dermatitis. (Courtesy of the Centers for Disease Control and Prevention, Atlanta, GA.)

leaving the infant more prone to diaper dermatitis. At times the diaper area can become infected with *Candida albicans*.

Manifestations

Clinical manifestation includes red, edematous, and blistered skin in the diaper region. Skin folds may be free of irritation because they do not come in contact with the soiled diaper.

Diagnosis

Diagnosis is made by inspection and palpation of the lesions located in the diaper area.

Treatment

Medical management may include treating the area with a 0.25% to 1% hydrocortisone cream with each diaper change and then applying a sealant to help protect against moisture. The area should be cleansed with mild soap and water at each diaper change, and the diaper area should be allowed to air dry. Application of 1% hydrocortisone cream and antifungal creams may be used to treat *Candida albicans*.

Nursing Considerations

Nursing care begins by educating the parents on prevention methods that decrease the risk of diaper dermatitis. Encourage parents to use super-absorbent diapers. Instruct parents to change soiled diapers immediately and thoroughly cleanse the area with mild soap and water. Tell parents to avoid using diaper wipes because the solution may further irritate the skin. Barrier creams or sealants (Balmex, Desitin, or zinc oxide) may be used to protect the skin from moisture. With a doctor's order, a 0.25% to 1% hydrocortisone ointment may be applied before any ointment to seal out moisture.

SEBORRHEIC DERMATITIS

Seborrheic dermatitis, known as *cradle cap* in babies, may be a result of changes in sebaceous glands. Adolescents may also present with seborrheic dermatitis commonly known as *dandruff*, which may begin with the onset of puberty.

Manifestations

Clinical manifestations include oily yellow scaly patches on the scalp and forehead with mildly erythematous skin underneath.

Diagnosis

Diagnosis is made by inspection and palpation of lesions on the scalp and forehead.

Treatment

Medical treatment for infants includes daily shampooing with a mild nonmedicated shampoo. Emollients can be left in place for a few minutes to loosen and lift the crusts, then be removed with a soft-bristle hairbrush or fingertips. Adolescents may use a medicated dandruff shampoo.

Nursing Considerations

Nursing care includes educating parents on proper cleansing of scalp and forehead. Demonstrate proper holding during the shampoo to avoid getting it in the child's eyes. The cheeks and eyelids can be washed with baby shampoo. Encourage parents to apply an emollient on the scalp for 20 minutes prior to cleansing. Vigorous brushing with a soft baby hair brush is helpful in removing the scales. Instruct adolescents to adapt a regular hygiene regime for shampooing and to switch to a medicated shampoo product. Encourage adolescents to seek treatment as soon as symptoms begin.

ECZEMA

Eczema (Figure 21-6 ■) is a chronic inflammatory skin disorder. The cause of eczema is unknown but has been associated with an immune dysfunction of the skin. A combination of external factors (allergens/irritants) and a family history of allergies, asthma, or hay fever have been linked to eczema. If the eczema is severe in the infant or appears before age 2 years, the cause is likely to be related to food allergies. Common food allergies include eggs, milk, peanuts, wheat, soy, and fish. Common irritants include wool, soaps and detergents, some perfumes and cosmetics, chlorine, dust, sand, and even cigarette smoke. If eczema persists during childhood and into adolescence, it is less acute. Self-esteem is an issue with children and adolescents because of changes in appearance of skin during flare-ups. Eczema flare-ups are more common during the winter months when the air is dry.

Figure 21-6. ■ Chronic eczema.

Manifestations

INFANTS.   Clinical manifestations for infants with eczema include erythematous areas of skin with papulovesicular lesions that rupture and crust. Areas that are affected in infants include cheeks, scalp, forehead, neck, trunk, and extensor surfaces of extremities. The infant is irritable and restless because of intense pruritis (Box 21-2 ■).

CHILDREN.   For children over age 2 years to puberty, the skin appears erythematous, dry and scaly, and may include papules that rupture and *weep* (drip serous fluid). Pruritis is also present. Skin behind the knees, around the wrist, sides of the neck, and around the mouth is most commonly affected. Adolescents may also develop lesions on the eyelids, earlobes, fingertips, toes, and nipple area

Diagnosis

Diagnosis begins by collecting a comprehensive health history. Data relating to age of onset, presence of asthma or hay fever in parents, location of flare-ups on the body, flare-ups occurring prior to age 4, skin rash prior to age 2, and episodes of dry skin in the past year are helpful for diagnosis. Physical exam includes inspection and palpation of papules and vesicles that have ruptured and formed a yellow crusty exudate. Skin testing may be done to isolate food allergies.

Treatment

Medical treatment involves hydrating and lubricating the skin to minimize pruritis, while determining triggers that lead to flare-ups. Emollients (Eucerin), oral antihistamines (Benadryl), and topical (1% to 2.5% hydrocortisone) and oral corticosteroids are used to treat eczema. If lesions become infected, topical or oral antibiotics may be prescribed.

BOX 21-2   LIFE SPAN CONSIDERATIONS

Infant with Eczema

The distribution and appearance of the lesions associated with eczema vary according to the age of the child. The infant with eczema can have the lesions all over the body and appear as vesicles or papules and may ooze or be scaly or crusty. The infant will experience itching, which may be manifested as irritability. Parents should be encouraged to provide prompt attention to irritability. Children will have lesions mainly in the crevices of the body. These areas will be dry and hyperpigmented, and the skin can be thickened. Children can be taught to assist in controlling itching by applying topical medications and employing distraction techniques. Adolescents may have eczema lesions on the face and arms that appear much like the childhood lesions. Adolescents will need assistance dealing with body image issues. They can be encouraged to appropriately use their medications and wear clothing that covers their lesions.

Nursing Considerations

The LPN/LVN works closely with children and their families to identify and remove allergens or irritants that cause flare-ups. Encourage regular use of moisturizing lotions and creams to keep skin lubricated to prevent drying and cracking of skin. Apply wet compresses soaked in aluminum acetate solution to help remove crusts and decrease inflammation. Encourage children and adolescents to shower after swimming in pools with chlorine water and after excessive sweating. Encourage children to apply a lubricant after bathing to help seal in moisture. Loose-fitting clothing and soft fabrics help to minimize skin irritation. Wash clothes in mild detergents and rinse well. During winter months, keep the environment cool with constant humidity levels. Fingernails should be cut short in infants and children to prevent excessive skin irritation from scratching. Antihistamines may be used at night to decrease itching so the child can rest well. Educate parents to recognize signs of infections and to report them immediately. Encourage children and adolescents to express feelings about their appearance. Low self-esteem is common in children with eczema.

ACNE VULGARIS

Acne vulgaris (acne) is a very common skin condition that mostly affects adolescents (Figure 21-7 ■). During puberty sebum (oil) production from the sebaceous glands increases (under the influence of androgens), and epithelial cells shed at a faster rate. Hair follicles in the skin become blocked, trapping sebum under the skin and causing **comedones** (whiteheads and blackheads) to develop. These blocked follicles provide a rich environment for *Propionibacterium* acnes

to grow, causing inflammation. Papules, pustules, and nodules develop in the skin. Acne lesions are commonly found on the face, chest, shoulders, and back.

Manifestations

Clinical manifestations include formation of comedones (whiteheads and blackheads), pustules, and papules over the surface of the skin.

Diagnosis

Identification of comedones, pustules, and papules is used to diagnosis acne vulgaris. Physical exam includes inspection and palpation of the lesion.

Treatment

Topical medications such as tretinoin (Retin-A) or adapalene (Differin) are used to treat mild acne. Medical treatment also includes the use of systemic antibiotics such as doxycycline, erythromycin, or tetracycline for 3 months. For more severe acne, isotretinoin (Accutane) may be prescribed.

Nursing Considerations

Nursing management includes supporting and educating the adolescent on proper care of acne lesions. Educate the adolescent to care for skin properly and avoid oil-based cosmetics or lotions. Encourage the client to maintain prescribed medical treatments and explain that improvement of skin lesions may take up to 3 months. Some acne medications make the skin more sensitive to sunlight, so use of sunscreen should be encouraged. Advise the client to avoid picking or squeezing the lesions, which may push the infected material deeper into the follicle, prolonging inflammation and infection.

> **clinical ALERT**
>
> If Accutane is prescribed, explain that pregnancy should be avoided. Accutane has a teratogenic effect on the developing fetus. Girls who are sexually active should be informed about alternative methods of birth control.

NURSING CARE

PRIORITIES IN NURSING CARE

The priority for nursing care of children with inflammatory skin conditions focuses on identification of the lesions so appropriate medical treatments may begin as soon as possible. The LPN/LVN assists the family and child in identifying any irritants that may have come in contact with the skin. It is important to assist the adolescent with acne vulgaris to identify any triggers that may have precipitated

Figure 21-7. ■ Acne lesions. (Medical-On-Line Ltd.)

the outbreak. The LPN/LVN educates families on proper hygiene methods for bathing and shampooing.

ASSESSING

Children with inflammatory skin conditions should be assessed for any change in color, texture, temperature, and moisture of the skin. Document the location of the lesions and assess whether the lesions are spreading to other areas of the body. Collect data concerning any irritants that may have been in contact with the skin. Assess for the presence of pruritis, which may lead to secondary infections if the child scratches the lesions. Assess effectiveness of treatments for the lesions with lotions and ointments. Collect data about the child's ability to cope with changes in body image, especially in clients with eczema and acne vulgaris.

DIAGNOSING, PLANNING, AND IMPLEMENTING

The following nursing diagnoses may be used in planning nursing care for the child with an inflammatory disorder:

- Impaired **S**kin Integrity related to allergies or irritants
- Acute **P**ain related to itching and scratching
- Risk for **I**nfection for related to open lesions
- Disturbed **B**ody Image related to prolonged treatments for healing.

Typical outcomes for a child with an inflammatory skin disorder might include:

- Skin lesions identified and healed.
- Irritants removed.
- Pain level is decreased.
- No signs of secondary infections.
- Verbalizes understanding of the healing process.
- Nursing interventions related to children with inflammatory disorders include:

For Diaper Rash and Infants' Skin

- Encourage frequent diaper changes. *Removes irritants (urine and stool) away from skin to promote healing.*
- Expose diaper area to open air. *Moisture increases skin irritation. Exposing skin to open air allows skin to dry.*
- Assist families to identify irritants that cause skin to become inflamed. *Eliminating exposure to common irritants will decrease flare-ups and allow skin to heal.*

For Infections, Infestations, Bites, and Contact Dermatitis

- Encourage child to avoid picking and scratching lesions. *Scratching skin lesions increases the chance of infection entering the skin tissue.*
- Educate parents to recognize signs of infection. *Secondary infections may occur if the lesions are exposed to bacteria.*

- Instruct parents how to cleanse the affected area. *Proper cleansing and drying are vital to reducing risk for infection and promoting the healing process.*
- Administer medicated creams and lotions as scheduled. *Adhering to the prescribed medication schedule will promote healing.*

For Acne and Other Conditions of Adolescents

- Encourage the adolescent to express concerns about appearance of skin associated with acne. *This allows the adolescent to convey feelings about altered skin condition. The nurse is able to dispel any misconceptions about causes and treatments with acne.*

EVALUATING

The LPN/LVN documents whether redness or swelling have increased or decreased over a period of time and whether the client perceives that the itching has increased or decreased. Improvement of skin texture is also documented. Medicated lotions and creams are evaluated for effectiveness. Evaluate the family's ability to adopt good hygiene practices. Determine whether the child understands the healing process and the time involved. The family and child verbalize common allergens and irritants that affect outbreaks of eczema or contact dermatitis.

Parasitic Infestations

Parasites are living organisms that get their food source from another living host. *Pediculosis* and *scabies* are infestations by lice and *Sarcoptes* mites, respectively. Lice and mites are arthropods that get their food supply by sucking blood from a human host. These infestations are transmitted by direct skin-to-skin contact or by sharing of personal items that have come into contact with the infestation.

PEDICULOSIS

Pediculosis is an infestation with parasites (lice) that live on the outside of a human host. *Pediculus capitis* (head lice) is found most commonly in children from 3 to 10 years of age (Figure 21-8 ■). Preschools and elementary schools have occasional outbreaks of head lice among children in the same classroom. Lice are often found behind the ears on the back of the scalp where the female louse lays eggs (viable **nits**) that hatch within 8 to 10 days. *Pediculus corporis* (body lice) and *Phthirus pubis* (pubic lice or **crabs**) are two other forms of lice infestations.

Manifestations

Clinical manifestations include intense itching over the scalp area and viable nits (eggs) located on one side of the hair shaft.

Nit

Figure 21-8. ■ Head lice nits in the hair.

Diagnosis

Diagnosis is made by inspection, using a bright light and magnifying glass over the affected area. Detection of head lice is aided by inspecting sections of hair and the back of the scalp (over the occipital area and behind the ears) for tiny viable nits attached to the base of hair shafts. In severe cases, lice are visible to the naked eye.

Treatment

Medical treatment involves using a *pediculicide* (lice-killing) shampoo, such as permethrin (Nix). The hair is combed with a fine-tooth comb dipped in vinegar or hair conditioner to help remove stubborn nits and nit shells. A second treatment is applied in 7 days to ensure that all nits are killed.

Nursing Considerations

Nursing care focuses on teaching parents and/or children how to kill the parasite and alleviate itching. Demonstrate how to inspect for lice by checking the scalp over the occipital area of the head and by separating small amounts of hair to look for any nits. Instruct parents to remove any nits before they hatch. All family members should be examined for the presence of lice so treatment may be initiated immediately. Instruct parents to inform the child's school so precautions may be taken in the classroom to prevent spread of the infestation. Advise parents to follow directions carefully on the prescribed shampoo. Some providers then suggest drying the hair and combing it with a fine-toothed comb dipped in vinegar to remove stubborn nits. This process may need to be repeated again in 7 days to kill any eggs that may have hatched after shampooing.

It must be stressed that parents will need to wash all bedding, towels, and hair accessories in hot water and dry

them in a hot dryer. Upholstered furniture should be vacuumed and the vacuum bag should be discarded. Personal items that cannot be washed, such as pillows, toys, and stuffed animals, should be sealed in a plastic bag for 2 weeks. This breaks the cycle of infestation by preventing any lice that hatch from finding a new host.

SCABIES

Scabies is an infestation caused by the mite *Sarcoptes scabiei*. The lesions are mainly found on the hands and feet and in the folds of the skin. Once the scabies mite finds a human host, it burrows into the epidermis and lays eggs. In 2 to 4 days the eggs hatch and the immature mites travel toward the surface of the skin, where they mature and grow. If left untreated, scabies mites continue this cycle every 14 to 17 days. Ova and feces from the scabies mites come in contact with the skin and cause irritation and pruritus (Figure 21-9 ■). This usually appears about 1 month after infestation.

Manifestations

Clinical manifestations include erythematous papules, vesicles, and even pustules. Pruritus is present and is more severe at night. Lesions may appear on the face, head, neck, chest, abdomen, waist, axillae, webs of fingers, buttocks, intergluteal folds, palms of the hands, and soles of the feet, Lesions may appear as a thin gray burrow that ends with a *vesicle* (blister).

Figure 21-9. ■ Diffuse scabies in an infant. The lesions are most numerous around the axillae, chest, and abdomen. (From Habif, T. P. [1990]. *Clinical dermatology: A color guide to diagnosis and therapy* [2nd ed.]. St. Louis, MO: Mosby-Year Book, p. 298. With permission from Elsevier.)

Diagnosis

Diagnosis is made by obtaining a complete history and general physical examination. Skin scrapings are inspected under the microscope for the presence of mites, eggs, or feces.

Treatment

Medical treatment may include treatment with permethrin cream (Elimite) and good hygiene practices to prevent recurrent infestations. Recommend washing all clothing, linens, and towels in hot (140 °F) water and drying them at high heat to kill any remaining mites.

Nursing Considerations

Once diagnosis is made, the child needs to shower, dry thoroughly, and apply 5% permethrin lotion. All household members should be treated at the same time, whether they have symptoms or not. Instruct the child to leave the cream or lotion on for 8 to 12 hours before showering again. Much of the care for scabies resembles the care for pediculosis. The nurse teaches good hygiene practices and instructs parents to wash clothes, bed linens, and towels on a regular basis. Items that cannot be washed or dry cleaned should be sealed in a plastic bag for 5 days. Nonjudgmental nursing care will increase the family's compliance with treatment regimens and will lessen embarrassment about the situation.

Skin Infections

Any break in skin integrity provides an opportunity for infection to take hold (see chain of infection, Figure 10-1 ⚭). Introduced lesions, such as piercings and tattoos, increase the risk of infection. Box 21-3 ■ discusses some of the issues involved in these forms of ornamentation.

WARTS (PAPILLOMAVIRUS)

Warts are benign tumors in the epithelial cells of the skin that are caused by the human papillomavirus. Common warts are found on the skin surface, and plantar warts are found on the feet. Warts can be transmitted from person to person, or the infection may transfer from one site to another on the same person (referred to as *autoinoculation*). Plantar warts may develop from contact on surfaces such as locker room floors. A compromised immune system in children may increase the risk for developing HPV, therefore leaving children more susceptible to warts.

BOX 21-3   **CULTURAL PULSE POINTS**

Tattoos and Piercings

Among some cultures and subcultures, tattoos and body piercings are considered important adornments. Parents may have piercings performed on their children while they are still infants, or tattoos and piercings may be a way of celebrating the onset of puberty or the approach of adulthood. Nurses should be informed about the care involved when having these procedures, so that they can provide teaching.

Youth who want tattoos or piercings must follow state regulations. Parental consent may be required. Because piercings and tattoos both compromise skin integrity, these procedures carry certain risks of infection. In all cases, proper care of the skin as it heals is essential to prevent local infection. More importantly, safety guidelines need to be followed by those performing the piercings or tattooing to prevent systemic infections, including life-threatening ones such as hepatitis, tetanus, or HIV.

According to La Leche League (2005), proper tattooing procedures include:

■ Sterilization of equipment with an autoclave
■ Bagging of equipment after use
■ Single-use needles, gloves, ink, cups, posts
■ Thorough hand washing with disinfectant soap

Likewise, piercings should only be done with new needles, and universal precautions should be followed during the procedure.

Care of the skin while it heals after tattooing includes:

■ Daily washing with a mild soap and water
■ No picking of scabs
■ No sun exposure

Care of the skin after piercing is done one to five times per day until healing is complete (Children's Hospital Boston, 2006). Healing time ranges from about 4 weeks (for the tongue) to a year (for ear cartilage or the navel). Care includes:

■ Washing the hands before touching the pierced area.
■ Removing crusty skin from the site and jewelry with warm water.
■ Washing the skin and jewelry with antibacterial soap, rinsing well, and patting the area dry with a paper towel. (Note: Cloth towels are not used because they may harbor bacteria.)
■ Allowing air to the site to promote healing. (Antibacterial ointment is not used.)
■ Preventing sweat, dirt, body fluids, alcohol or hydrogen peroxide, or tight clothing from coming into contact with the site until healing is complete. These may cause irritation or infection.
■ Avoiding hot tubs and swimming pools until skin has completely healed.

There is no evidence to suggest that tattooing, or tattoo removal, affects breastfeeding (La Leche League, 2005). However, most professionals will not tattoo a woman who is pregnant, and it is recommended that a woman wait a year after childbirth before getting a new tattoo.

Manifestations

Warts (Figure 21-10 ■) appear on the surface of the skin as rough, scaly papules and nodules that are the same color as the skin. They are painless and are most commonly found on the dorsal surface of the hand and around the nails of the fingertips. Plantar warts are more common in adolescents; they appear as papules and plaques on the bottom of the feet. Because of the pressure and irritation of walking, they can be very painful.

Diagnosis

Diagnosis is made by inspection of papules and nodules that appear rough and scaly.

Treatment

Medical treatment is individualized, ranging from no treatment to destroying the wart by physical or chemical methods. Removal of the wart may require the use of chemical substances or peeling agents, **cryotherapy** (freezing with liquid nitrogen), laser therapy, or applying duct tape over the wart.

Nursing Considerations

The nurse explains that treatments involving the applications of peeling agents may take up to several months to see improvement. If pain is associated with treatment, encourage parents to reduce the frequency. Once the pain decreases, instruct them to continue therapy as directed. Encourage the child to avoid picking the wart. This will reduce the risk of autoinoculation.

IMPETIGO

Impetigo is a superficial skin infection that appears on the face, hands, neck, or extremities and is caused by streptococci or staphylococci. Insect bites, burns, scratches and lacerations provide a portal of entry for the bacteria. It is highly contagious and can be transferred between children and adults, especially if towels, linens, and clothing are shared with the infected person. Poor sanitation and close living conditions place children at risk for contracting impetigo. This infection is primarily seen in children during the summer months when the temperature is hot and humid and children are more prone to insect bites, scratches, and lacerations.

Manifestations

Clinical manifestations include vesicles or pustules, edema, and redness surrounding the lesion (Figure 21-11 ■). Once the vesicle ruptures, the lesion is covered with a loosely adherent, honey-yellow crust. If the crust is removed, a new honey-yellow crust will form.

Diagnosis

Diagnosis is made by inspecting and palpating the lesions for a honey-yellow colored crust and exudate. Disposable gloves should be worn by the LPN/LVN during assessment. Bacterial cultures may be obtained for diagnosis.

Treatment

Medical treatment involves soaking the crusted lesion in warm water, scrubbing with medicated soap to remove the crust, and applying a topical bactericidal ointment (such as mupirocin or bacitracin) to the lesion for 1 week. A systemic antibiotic may be used if no improvement is seen with topical ointments.

Nursing Considerations

The nurse educates the family that even minor cuts and scratches to the skin pose a threat for invasion of bacteria. Remind the family that impetigo is highly contagious and

Figure 21-10. ■ Warts on a child's hand. (Phototake NYC)

Figure 21-11. ■ Bullous impetigo. (Courtesy of Dr. William H. Sorey, University of Mississippi Medical Center.)

that towels, bed linens, and clothes must not be shared with a family member who is infected with impetigo. Instruct parents to wash and remove the crust several times a day and to follow orders for applying topical bactericidal ointment. Tell them to return to the clinic if the lesions do not improve, because a systemic antibiotic may be necessary.

CELLULITIS

Cellulitis is a bacterial infection of the dermis and subcutaneous tissue. Recent upper respiratory infections, sinusitis, otitis media, or an abscessed tooth may result in cellulitis affecting the face and neck region. Injury that compromises the skin barrier such as trauma, scratches, or bug bites may cause cellulitis in the extremities. Cellulitis may also occur at an intravenous insertion site if standard precautions are not followed by the LPN/LVN. *Staphylococcus aureus, Streptococcus pneumoniae, Haemophilus influenzae,* and beta-hemolyytic and group A *Streptococcus* are common causative organisms. Onset is usually rapid.

> ### clinical ALERT
>
> If cellulitis is not treated, the infection may become widespread and may result in septicemia, septic arthritis or meningitis. These conditions constitute a medical emergency and the pediatrician should be notified immediately.

Manifestations

Clinical manifestations of local symptoms around the infected site include edematous skin that is red, tender, and warm to touch (Figure 21-12 ■). There may be red streaks

Figure 21-12. ■ Cellulitis. Markings on leg show fullest extent of infection. (Medical-On-Line Ltd.)

extending out from the infected area. Systemic symptoms indicating septicemia include fever, headache, pain, chills, malaise, and lymphangitis.

Diagnosis

Diagnosis is made by evaluating lab results for a complete blood cell count (including a differential) and by analyzing results from cultures drawn from the infected site. Blood cultures may be taken if child appears toxic.

Treatment

Children with cellulitis of the trunk, extremities, or perianal area may be treated with oral antibiotics on an outpatient basis. When the case is severe or the face and larger areas of the body are affected, the child may be hospitalized and treated with IV antibiotics.

Nursing Considerations

Nursing considerations include strict adherence to antibiotics administration to achieve therapeutic blood levels and prevent sepsis. The nurse ensures that the child has an opportunity to rest and elevate the affected area. Warm compresses are applied to improve circulation and promote healing of the skin tissues. To avoid spread of infection, parents and child are taught to wash hands frequently, especially when caring for the infected area. Instruct the parents to return to the pediatrician's office immediately if they notice any signs of sepsis or spread of infection.

HERPES SIMPLEX TYPE I

Herpes simplex type I ("fever blister," "cold sore," or "canker sore") is a viral infection caused by herpes simplex virus type I (HSV-I). The virus is passed from the infected person to another by direct contact. The virus remains latent, possibly from childhood, until individual triggers activate a response. Fever, emotional upset, menses, cold, or sun exposure are triggers that initiate an outbreak of the virus. HSV-I poses a serious threat to newborns. (See Chapter 18 ⬭ for more information about herpes simplex type II.)

Manifestations

Clinical manifestations include a tingling or burning sensation at the affected site. A single vesicle or a cluster of vesicles appears over red inflamed skin. Lesions are found near the mouth, and some are found on the buccal mucosa. Usually the vesicles dry and heal in 8 to 10 days.

Diagnosis

Medical diagnosis is made by inspection of the lesion with attention to the presence of vesicles that appear reddened and crusted. A culture may be obtained for analysis.

Treatment

Topical treatment of the lesion can shorten the duration of the cold sore. The child should be instructed to avoid picking at the lesion to avoid secondary infection. Keeping the child's nails trimmed or applying mittens in the small child may be necessary.

Nursing Considerations

The nurse encourages the child to report symptoms of a herpes outbreak early so medication can begin as soon as possible to decrease the length of the outbreak. Instruct the child on methods to prevent spreading of the lesions by using good hand washing techniques. Help the child identify what triggers the outbreak of the lesions and develop a plan to minimize the triggers (Table 21-1 ■).

Fungal Infections

DERMATOPHYTES (RINGWORM)

Dermatophytes are fungi that mainly affect the surface of the skin, hair, and nails. Tinea (sometimes called **ringworm**) is a term used to describe a group of fungal infections of the skin that are transmitted from human to human or from animals to human. The different types of fungal (tinea) infections are named after the location of the fungal infection on the body: tinea capitis (of the head), tinea corporis (of the body), tinea pedis (of the foot), and tinea cruris (of the groin).

Manifestations

- **Tinea capitis** is a scalp fungus. It most commonly affects children between the ages of 3 and 10 years. When the fungus invades the scalp, the hair becomes brittle and breaks off, leaving circular patches of scalp showing the hair loss. Papules form around the edges of the ring and become scaly and red in color (Figure 21-13 ■).

- **Tinea corporis** has a circular reddened patch on the skin with raised borders. The lesions can become scaly (see Figure 21-13B).
- **Tinea pedis** is referred to as *athlete's foot*. The skin between the toes and on the soles of the feet becomes red, with deep scaly fissures that are painful and itchy.
- **Tinea cruris,** referred to as *jock itch*, causes the skin in the groin area to become red and scaly, with raised papules or vesicles forming a circular rash.

Diagnosis

Diagnosis is made by obtaining a skin scraping of the lesion and viewing it under a microscope to detect fungal growth. A Wood's lamp may be used to diagnose tinea capitis.

Treatment

Medical treatment involves the use of antifungal topical ointments, powders, or sprays. Superficial fungal infections may be treated with over-the-counter medications such as Tinactin, Micatin, Lotrimin, and Lamisil. If the fungal infection is deep into the skin, Diflucan or Sporonax may be prescribed. Griseofulvin is treatment of choice for tinea capitis.

Nursing Considerations

Nursing care focuses on preventing the spread of infection, encouraging good hygiene practices, and promoting comfort. To prevent spread of tinea capitis and tinea corporis, instruct children to not share hair brushes, combs, pillows, towels, clothes, or hats. Advise children with tinea cruris and tinea pedis to keep the infected area clean and dry. Recommend loose-fitting clothing that will keep moisture out and decrease friction from fabric that can cause skin irritation. Teach children that, to prevent tinea pedis, they must wear shoes at all times in public locker rooms and showers. Encourage parents to administer medication for

---

TABLE 21-1

Communicating Across the Life Span: Skin Care Related to Herpes Lesions

	TODDLER	PRESCHOOLER	SCHOOL-AGE CHILD	ADOLESCENT
Nurse	To the toddler's parent: Scratching or picking at the lesion could cause scarring. I think you should put mittens on your child during the night.	To the preschooler's parent: Try to keep the child's mouth as dry as possible to allow the lesion to heal more quickly.	To the child: We want the lesion to dry and heal. You should avoid lip balm and only use the ointment prescribed by the physician.	To the adolescent: Applying makeup and lip gloss will only keep the lesion moist and delay healing.
Parent/Client	I think I'll put these mittens on him after he goes to sleep because he would probably protest otherwise.	Maybe I should get my child to drink from a straw to avoid additional moisture on his mouth when he is drinking.	I guess I can lay off the lip balm for a while. It's a habit though, so it'll be tough.	Do you mean all the cover stick I've been putting on it could make it worse? I never thought about that!

A Tinea capitis

B Tinea corporis

Figure 21-13. ■ (**A**) Tinea capitis. (**B**) Tinea corporis. (Courtesy of the Centers for Disease Control and Prevention, Atlanta, GA.)

the entire prescribed period, even up to 7 days after the infection has resided. Fungal infections may need to be treated for 6 months to a year.

ORAL CANDIDIASIS (THRUSH)

Oral candidiasis (**thrush**) is a yeast-like fungal infection that is caused by *Candida albicans* (see Figure 22-3 ⬯). It generally affects newborns born vaginally from an infected mother. It may also be a chronic condition in young children receiving antibiotics or corticosteroids, or those who have an immune disorder.

Manifestations

Oral candidiasis (thrush) appears as white plaques on the tongue, palate, or buccal mucosa that bleed easily. Nutritional intake may be decreased because of pain and discomfort with breastfeeding or feeding. Candida lesions may also be present in the diaper area of an infant who has diaper dermatitis.

Diagnosis

Oral candidiasis is diagnosed by inspection of the oral mucosa or by fungal culture. Microscopic examination from skin scrapings of the lesion is also used for diagnosis.

Treatment

Medical treatment for thrush includes the use of oral and topical antifungal medications such as nystatin oral suspension or clotrimazole. Fluconazole or itraconazole may be prescribed if the infection is severe or if immunocompromised children have oropharyngeal candidiasis. Systemic *Candida* infections are treated with intravenous amphotericin B.

Nursing Considerations

Nursing care involves teaching the parents to use a swab when applying nystatin oral suspension to the tongue surface and buccal mucosa, then allowing the infant to swallow the remaining suspension. This procedure is done following feedings. Older children can be taught to swish the suspension in the mouth before swallowing. Nursing care also focuses on decreasing the risk of reinfection by instructing the parents to sterilize bottle nipples and pacifiers for 20 minutes in boiling water. Instruct parents to follow directions on antiseptic sprays when disinfecting toys that cannot be autoclaved. The child who uses a corticosteroid inhaler should be taught to rinse the mouth well with water after use. Spacers should also be rinsed in water after use. Instruct breastfeeding mothers to apply nystatin oral suspension to the nipple area to prevent reinfection.

NURSING CARE

PRIORITIES IN NURSING CARE

When caring for children with skin infections or infestations, the priority of care revolves around diagnosing the organism. Focus care on preventing the spread of infection and eradicating the infestation (head lice or mites). Explain to families how skin infections such as impetigo and herpes simplex I are spread from person to person. Instruct families how to eliminate parasites by educating families on establishing good hygiene practices and protecting the home environment. Provide nursing care in a nonjudgmental way to decrease embarrassment about fungal and parasitic infections. Promote compliance with prescribed medication procedures.

ASSESSING

Children with skin infections should be assessed for signs of erythema, vesicles or pustules, edema, fever, malaise, and texture of skin lesions. Collect data on drainage from lesions, documenting color, order, and crusting. Assess oral mucosa for white plaques. Assess presence of pruritis. Inspect hair shafts at base of head for presence of female louse eggs (viable nits). Assess the family's compliance with medication routines.

DIAGNOSING, PLANNING, AND IMPLEMENTING

The following nursing diagnoses may be used in planning nursing care for the child with skin infections and infestations:

- Ineffective **H**ealth Maintenance related to poor hygiene practices
- Impaired **S**kin Integrity related to ruptured vesicles and crusting of lesions
- Disturbed **B**ody Image related to visible parasites on hair and skin
- Interrupted **B**reastfeeding related to pain and discomfort from infected oral mucosa
- Risk for **I**nfection related to spread of organisms from person to person
- **S**elf-Care Deficit: Bathing/Hygiene related to lack of knowledge on bathing and shampooing

Typical outcomes for a child with a skin infection or infestation might include:

- Regular hygiene practices are followed.
- Skin remains intact and free of drainage from lesions.
- Body image improved.
- Breastfeeding resumed.
- No signs of infection are noted among family members.
- Verbalizes the importance of good hygiene practices.

Nursing interventions for some of the nursing diagnoses have been discussed previously in this chapter and will not be repeated.

- Instruct parents how to soak and remove crusts from impetigo lesions several times a day. *Promotes healing.*
- Educate parents to recognize signs of infection. *Prompt medical attention is needed to prevent spread of infection.*
- Apply warm compresses over skin infected with cellulitis. *Improves circulation and promotes healing.*
- Monitor antibiotic therapy. *Helps to achieve a therapeutic blood level to decrease infection.*

- Encourage frequent hand washing. *To prevent spread of infection.*
- Educate parents how to apply medicated lotions or creams to lesions. *Protects skin and improves healing.*
- Inform parents to wash all towels, bed linens, and clothes when lice and scabies are detected. *Prevents spread of lice to other members of the family. Washing in hot water and heated drying will eradicate lice and scabies.*
- Demonstrate proper application of antifungal medication to the oral mucosa in infants. *Swabbing nystatin oral suspension to the tongue and oral mucosa to infants following feedings will help promote healing of thrush and continued breastfeeding. Older children should be taught how to swish and swallow.*

EVALUATING

The LPN/LVN documents no signs of infection. Infections are not spread to other members of the family. The LPN/LVN verifies that the parents are following recommendations for washing towels, linens, and clothing to eradicate parasites. The LPN/LVN observes the parent as she/he applies medicated lotion and creams to infected skin tissue. Listen to determine if parents can recall signs of infections and verbalize when to return to the pediatrician's office.

NURSING PROCESS CARE PLAN
Client with Cellulitis

Mrs. B calls the pediatrician's office to report that her daughter Lucy, age 12, woke up this morning complaining of headache, chills, and pain in her right calf. Last week at camp Lucy injured her leg on a piece of old wood in the lake while canoeing. The camp nurse accompanied Lucy to the emergency room where she received stitches in her right calf. The mother states the leg is swollen with red streaks spreading out from the wound.

Assessment. The LPN/LVN should gather the following information over the telephone:

- Onset of symptoms
- Complaints of chills, fever, or malaise
- Color of skin around the wound
- Swelling in the leg
- Drainage from the wound
- Pain associated with walking
- Pain level

When the child is seen in the pediatrician's office, gather the following data:

- Vital signs
- Condition of skin around the wound
- Lab work
- Inspect stitches and approximation of wound
- Assess for lymphangitis

Nursing Diagnosis.   The following important nursing diagnosis (among others) is established for this client:

- Risk for **I**nfection related to tissue trauma from a foreign object.

Expected Outcomes

- Will be free of infection.
- Will remain pain free with weight bearing.

Planning and Implementation

- Review lab work and report abnormalities immediately. *To identify infection and type of bacteria.*
- Instruct child to rest and elevate leg. *To reduce swelling and promote comfort.*
- Explain the importance of following the advised medical regimen for antibiotic therapy. *To prevent complications associated with systemic infections and to achieve therapeutic blood levels of antibiotics.*
- Explain the importance of hand washing while caring for the wound. *To prevent spread of infection.*
- Demonstrate proper technique for dressing changes. *To ensure proper care of wound.*
- Apply warm compresses over the infected area. *To enhance circulation to the area and promote healing.*
- Instruct parents to recognize signs of infection. *Cellulitis may lead to septicemia.*
- Explain to parents the need to return to the pediatrician's office if infection worsens. *Spread of infection could cause the child to become seriously ill and require hospitalization.*

Evaluation.   Inflammation of the skin tissue should begin to subside within 48 hours after initiating antibiotic therapy. Temperature will return to normal range. The child should be able to bear weight on the leg once inflammation and pain decrease. Skin tissue will be free of redness, drainage, and edema. Complications leading to septicemia are prevented.

Critical Thinking in the Nursing Process

1. Lucy notices that the redness in her right calf has traveled above her knee and appears to have red streaks that lead to the wound. What is causing changes in the skin tissue?

2. Lucy has been admitted to the hospital and is placed on IV antibiotics. How do you explain to Lucy why she now has IV medication?

3. Mrs. B. asks what she can do to help Lucy be more comfortable at home. How do you respond?

Note: Discussion of Critical Thinking questions appears in Appendix I.

Burns

Burns can happen at any age; however, in the young child burns are more common in boys between 1 and 4 years of age. At this age, children are exploring their environment. They can reach hot pans on the stove, pull and chew on electrical cords, ingest cleaning agents and chemicals, grab a hot curling iron, and explore the fire in the fireplace. School-aged children and adolescents venture outside to explore. They may come in contact with matches, fireworks, and electrical wires (when climbing trees and voltage towers). They may experiment with mixing chemicals. Most burns can be prevented, and parents must be alert to hazards in and around the child's environment. There are four types of burns (Figure 21-14 ■):

- **Thermal burns** are caused by flame, or by hot objects such as coffee, grease, or stoves (Figure 21-14A and B).
- **Chemical burns** are caused by strong acids or alkalis, such as the chemical found in cleansers containing lye, toilet cleaners, or preparations used to open clogged drains.
- **Electrical burns** (see Figure 21-14C) are caused by contact with exposed electric wires. As the electricity travels through the body, it burns the tissue at point of entrance and at point of exit.
- **Radiation burns** are caused by exposure to radiation, the most common type being sunburn.

Burns may also be evidence of child abuse. Any unusual burn occurring in a pattern could suggest deliberately induced burns. Examples are the circles of cigarette burns or a burn that covers the area like a glove or a stocking. For more on child abuse, see Chapter 16 ⊂⊃.

Manifestations

Burns are assessed for burn depth (thickness) and burn area (percentage of body surface area, BSA). Burn depth is described as partial thickness or full thickness. Partial-thickness burns (sometimes called first- and second-degree burns) may be superficial or deep. Skin appears red, may blister, blanches with pressure, and is painful and sensitive to cold air. The skin may regenerate, but some scarring may result. Full-thickness burns include third-degree burns. Skin will appear brown, may form **eschar** (dead matter that is sloughed off the skin), and may appear white to gray in

Figure 21-14. ■ (**A**) Thermal (scald) burns are the most common burn injury in infancy. (**B**) Burns of the hands or feet that are distributed like gloves or stockings are associated with child abuse. (**C**) Electrical burn caused by biting an electric cord. (**B**: Robert A. Felter, MD. **C**: Courtesy of Dr. Lezley McIlveen, Department of Dentistry, Children's National Medical Center, Washington, DC.)

color. Decreased sensation to pain is associated with full-thickness burns. These burns require skin grafting because the skin cannot regenerate.

Burn area, a percentage of body surface area, is an estimate of the amount of body surface damaged (Figure 21-15 ■). The process for estimating the amount of body surface damage is the same as for an adult. However, the percent of body surface is different for a child than for an adult because of the different body proportions. For example, if a 1-year-old were burned on the back of the head (8.5%) and upper back (6.5%), the burn area would be 15%. For an adult, it would be 13.5%.

Diagnosis

Diagnosis for burns is based on assessment of the thickness of the burn and use of the Lund and Browder chart (see Figure 21-15) to determine the percentage of body surface area burned.

Treatment

The initial treatment of a burn is to stop the burning process by removing the cause. Because the child's status may change rapidly as a result of smoke inhalation and swelling of the airway, monitoring of airway, breathing, and circulation (the ABCs) is essential. Medical treatment also focuses on replacing fluid loss, managing pain control, preventing infection, promoting nutrition to improve tissue healing, and salvaging viable burned tissue. Box 21-4 ■ describes a common remedy for mild superficial burns.

Nursing Considerations

A serious burn is an emergency. Continued monitoring of the ABCs is a priority. Shortly after a burn, fluid shifts from the blood vessels to the interstitial space (see Figure 11-3 ∞), resulting in low blood volume. With severe burn injuries, fluid volume must be replaced to prevent hypovolemic shock. Intravenous hydration should be initiated with lactated Ringer's or normal saline. Nutritional requirements for

---

BOX 21-4 | **COMPLEMENTARY THERAPIES**

Herbal Therapy with Aloe Vera Gel

Aloe vera gel is found in many lotions, sunscreens, and cosmetics. Aloe vera has antibacterial, antiinflammatory and antiviral actions. Clinical trials have shown that aloe vera accelerates healing of burns, abrasions, frostbite, and canker sores. Itching can also be decreased with the use of aloe vera. Parents often keep aloe vera in the home to treat mild injuries in children. Contact dermatitis is a rare side effect associated with aloe vera.

Source: Kemper, K., Gardiner, P., & Coles, D. (2001). The skinny on herbal remedies for dermatologic disorders. *Contemporary Pediatrics, 7*, 103; Atherton, P. (1997, June–July). Aloe vera: Myth or medicine? *Positive Health*, 20; International Aloe Science Council. (2002). *The complete story of aloe vera.* Irving, TX: Author.

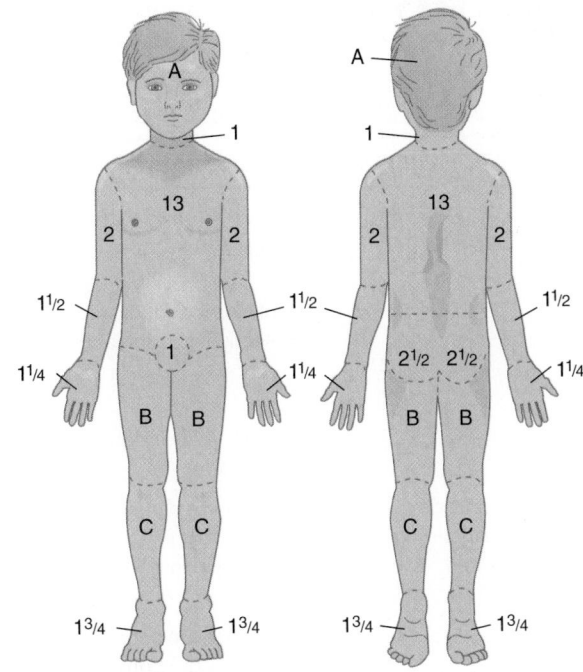

Relative Percentages of Areas Affected by Growth

Area	Age in years					
	0	1	5	10	11	Adult
A = ¹/₂ of head	9¹/₂	8¹/₂	6¹/₂	5¹/₂	4¹/₂	3¹/₂
B = ¹/₂ of one thigh	2³/₄	3¹/₄	4	4¹/₂	4¹/₂	4³/₄
C = ¹/₂ of one lower leg	2¹/₂	2¹/₂	2³/₄	3	3¹/₄	3¹/₂

Figure 21-15. ■ Classifications of burns in children. These charts determine percentage of skin surface area involved in pediatric burn injuries. (Adapted from Artz, C. P., & Moncrief, J. A. [1969]. *The treatment of burns* [2nd ed.]. Philadelphia: Saunders. With permission from Elsevier.)

calories and protein are increased to promote healing of skin tissue. Enteral feedings may begin within 6 hours of the burn injury. The LPN/LVN assesses the level of pain associated with procedures and administers pain medication according to the prescribed schedule to decrease pain during procedures. Continually evaluate effectiveness of pain medication. Comfort measures such as relaxation techniques, diversional activities, and therapeutic touch can be used in addition to pain medication. Demonstrate proper wound care and methods to prevent infection prior to discharge. Provide psychological support to the child and the family. Allow the child to talk about feelings, concerns, and fears. Provide referrals for social support, and encourage families to join community support groups. The Nursing Care Plan Chart on page 592 describes nursing care for a child with a burn.

NURSING CARE

PRIORITIES IN NURSING CARE

When caring for a child with a burn injury, priority of care may be determined by the classification of the burn itself. Moderate burns require dressing changes and teaching prior to discharge. Severe burns require hospitalization and extensive treatments. In general, the nurse assists with immediate care of the burn injury to maintain airway support, breathing, and circulation. Care focuses on fluid replacement, pain control, and prevention of infection. Psychological support for the child and family is paramount during the recovery process.

ASSESSING

The role of the LPN/LVN in burn care is one of continued data collection and monitoring the child for complications.

DIAGNOSING, PLANNING, AND IMPLEMENTING

The following nursing diagnoses can be used to plan and implement care of the burned child:

- Impaired Physical **M**obility related to joint stiffness and bed rest
- **P**ain related to tissue damage
- Deficient **F**luid Volume related to fluid shift and loss from damaged tissue
- Risk for **I**nfection related to loss of protective layers of the skin
- Imbalanced **N**utrition: Less Than Body Requirements related to increased need for calories and protein
- Disturbed **B**ody Image related to body disfigurement
- **A**nxiety (parent and child) related to burn injury and lengthy hospitalization

Possible outcomes for children with burn injuries may include:

- Child will remain free of secondary infections.
- Pain will be controlled.
- Nutrition will be adequate for weight gain and tissue repair.
- Child will verbalize feelings about the burn injury and identify sources of support.

NURSING CARE PLAN CHART

Child with a Burn

GOAL	INTERVENTION	RATIONALE	EXCEPTED OUTCOME
1. Impaired Skin Integrity related to exposure to extreme temperatures			
The child will demonstrate symptoms of healing from burns.	Keep child's pain level in control	*To minimize excessive movement that could compromise the integrity of the wound*	The child's wounds will have evidence of decreased erythema and inflammation.
	Apply topical medications and protective dressing as ordered	*Topical medications promote wound healing, and the dressing will protect the integrity of the wound, especially in early stages*	
	Provide a high-calorie, high-protein diet	*To promote wound healing*	
The family will provide assistance in maintaining the child's skin integrity.	Discuss with parents the interventions that will further protect skin integrity	*Teaching can increase the parents' involvement in the interventions that will promote skin integrity.*	The family will assist with pain relief, distraction, nutritional support, and dressing changes.
	Encourage the parents to provide distractions appropriate to the child's age and child's interest.	*Distraction methods are used to prevent scratching and rubbing of the wound and will also be used during medication application and dressing changes*	
2. Risk for Infection related to open wounds and altered immunologic response			
The child will have no symptoms of wound infection.	Remaining body hair can be shaved from around the wound borders and the wound must be cleaned with sterile technique per order	*Hair is a reservoir for harmful bacteria, and cleansing the wound routinely decreases bacteria*	The wound is without increased erythema and has no purulent drainage, and body temperature is maintained within normal limits.
	Maintain a strict policy of hand washing prior to contact with the child for any reason	*Hand washing reduces the presence of harmful bacteria*	
	Limit exposure to staff and visitors who have current infections	*The child should be protected from all forms of harmful bacteria*	
The family will understand the importance of preventing infection.	Discuss symptoms of infection such as disorientation, increased respiratory rate, fever, and chilling that should be reported promptly	*Educating parents about these symptoms will increase prompt reporting*	The family will verbalize signs and symptoms of infection, be able to state the risks associated with infection, and demonstrate preventative measures.
	Encourage parents to assist in limiting visitors and encouraging handwashing and the use of personal protective equipment	*These measures will further reduce the likelihood of exposure to harmful bacteria and give the parents a sense of participation in the child's care*	

The following nursing interventions should be implemented in caring for the child and family:

- Administer narcotics or other analgesics as needed prior to dressing changes. Keep the wound covered to decrease discomfort and prevent infection. Bed cradle may be used to keep linen off the wound. *Burns can be very painful and the child must be adequately medicated. Covering the wound decreases pain stimulation from contact with air and linen.*

- For minor burns, teach parents how to care for the wound and change the dressing (Figure 21-16 ■). *Minor burns are treated on an outpatient basis. Parents must understand how to protect the wound, how frequently to provide dressing changes, and how to recognize signs of infection should they occur.*

Figure 21-16. ■ Serious burns are most often treated in the ICU or in a specialized burn center. (**A**) Care of burns must be done with sterile technique to prevent introduction of infection to the compromised area. (**B**) The treated wound is covered with a sterile gauze.

- Follow doctor's orders and facility guidelines in changing dressings, whirlpool baths, debridement, and ointment application. *To promote healing, the eschar must be removed. Check facility policy to determine if this is an LPN/LVN function.*
- Strictly follow doctor's orders regarding care of skin graft and donor site. *A skin graft must remain fixed to underlying tissue until circulation is reestablished. Care must be taken to prevent injury to the graft site. The donor site should be kept clean and dry to promote healing.*
- Keep room temperature warm to prevent hypothermia. Avoid heat lamps. *When there is large destruction of skin, the body's thermoregulation mechanism is altered and the child develops hypothermia. Heat lamps should be avoided to prevent further burns.*
- Administer oral and IV fluids as ordered. Monitor intake and output and hematocrit. *Fluid shifts from vascular to interstitial space and leaks from damaged skin. Fluid balance must be monitored and maintained.*

- Administer high-protein nutrition, either oral or total parenteral nutrition (TPN), as ordered. *Proteins are needed for tissue repair.*
- Encourage activity within limitations of wound healing process. Books, games, and movies may be used for the child confined to bed. Physical therapy may be used to maintain and regain strength and movement. *Physical activity is necessary for muscle strength, growth, and positive mental outlook.*
- Use therapeutic communication techniques to help child and family cope with disfigurement. Refer family to RN and social worker as necessary. *The child may need support in dealing with altered body image. Parents may need support in dealing with guilt and change in child's appearance. Burn treatment is expensive, so the family may need support with financial obligations.*
- Teach the family how to care for the wound, skin graft, and donor site at home. *The healing of a burn generally takes several weeks or months to complete. The child may be discharged from the hospital and readmitted for surgery or follow-up treatment.*

EVALUATING

The child should be evaluated for infection and wound healing. Because immobility can cause pneumonia, contractures, and constipation, the child should be evaluated for these complications. Parents should be able to verbalize and demonstrate an understanding of home care.

Trauma to Skin from the Environment

SUNBURN

Overexposure to the sun's ultraviolet rays can damage the outer surface of the skin, resulting in a burn injury. A combination of low levels of melanin in children, a thin epidermal layer, and long periods of time spent in the sun places children at higher risk for sunburns. Children and adolescents who have had repeated sunburns or severe blistering from the sun are more likely to develop melanoma and basal cell carcinoma than those who have protected themselves from the sun's harmful rays.

In a relatively short time (30 minutes to 4 hours), sun exposure can cause the skin to become red and tender. If exposure is prolonged, edema, vesiculation, bullae, or blistering may result. Other symptoms of sunburn may include headache, fatigue, chills, and malaise.

Treatment includes symptomatic care. Increase oral fluids, cool compresses, and topical corticosteroid (only to intact skin) over the burned area to relieve pain and discomfort.

Prevention is the best medicine. Teach children and parents to apply sunscreen (SPF 15 or greater), to wear protective clothing, and to avoid sun exposure between 10 a.m. and 4 p.m. when the sun's rays are the strongest. These simple methods will greatly decrease the risk of developing melanoma later in life.

MELANOMA

Malignant melanoma is the most serious of all skin cancers. Although rare in children under the age of 14 years, it is increasing among adolescents. There is an increased risk of developing melanoma in children with dysplastic nevus syndrome, congenital nevi, or an immunodeficiency state. Melanoma arises from **melanocytes** (pigment-producing cells) in the dermis and epidermis. Damage to the pigment-producing cells is most often caused by a cumulative effect from the sun's ultraviolet rays. The use of tanning beds and excessive exposure to the sun has been associated with malignant melanoma.

Manifestations

Clinical manifestations include lesions (or moles) with color variations of brown, tan, or black; an irregular border; and a diameter greater than 6 mm (Figure 21-17 ■). The lesion may become ulcerated or may bleed.

Diagnosis

Diagnosis is made by inspection and palpation of the lesion. A biopsy of the lesion is done to determine malignancy. History assessment is collected to determine skin care practices relating to sun exposure.

A **B**

Figure 21-17. ■ **(A)** Benign juvenile melanoma on the nose of a child; this is a superficial skin tumor that is most common in children. Note symmetric shape and even brown tone. **(B)** Malignant melanoma. Note the asymmetric shape and black areas of the melanoma. (Phototake NYC)

Treatment

Medical treatment includes surgical removal of the lesion. Melanoma may spread to other parts of the body, so surrounding tissue is also removed. Chemotherapy may also be necessary.

clinical ALERT

It is important to teach children and parents to pay attention to moles and other markings. Teach the warning signs of melanoma, and stress that early attention is essential for a successful cure.

Nursing Considerations

Nursing care focuses on prevention, educating parents and children about the harmful effects the sun's ultraviolet rays, and teaching parents to seek medical attention if suspicious skin lesions or moles are noticed. Instruct the parents to apply sunscreen with SPF 15 or higher year-round when the child is outside and to avoid the sun during peak hours (10 a.m. to 4 p.m.). Teach that it is wise to cover up with long-sleeved shirts, long pants, and hats that protect the face when outside. Discourage use of tanning beds. Encourage parents and teach older children to inspect the skin for any suspicious lesions or moles and to report any changes in color, shape, or size to their pediatrician. The Health Promotion Issue on pages 596 and 597 discusses tanning and teens.

FROSTBITE

Overexposure to low environmental temperatures may cause skin and tissue damage known as **frostbite.** A combination of high concentration of water in skin cells and exposure to extremely low temperatures (below −2 °C) causes ice crystals to form in the tissue. Areas most commonly affected include the hands and feet (especially fingers and toes), as well as the cheeks, nose, and ears.

Manifestations

Skin may appear pale and white and have decreased sensation. If deeper tissues such as the dermis and subcutaneous tissue are involved, the skin first appears cyanotic with mottling and then becomes red and edematous. Blisters or bullae may appear after rewarming. If frostbite is severe, the skin tissue may become *necrotic* (dead). The client may lose tissue such as fingers, toes, tip of the nose, or earlobes.

Diagnosis

Diagnosis is made by inspection and palpation of the skin tissue that has been exposed to extremely low temperatures.

Treatment

Immediate medical treatment requires placing the child in a warmer environment and removing wet clothes. Rewarm the affected area slowly by submerging in warm water between 38 and to 40 °C (100.4 to 104 °F) for 10 to 15 minutes. Analgesics are given to decrease pain that is associated with the rewarming process. Cleanse the area with saline and cover with a sterile dressing.

Nursing Considerations

Nursing care focuses on rewarming the affected area while protecting the skin tissues from further injury. Monitor the affected area for increase in circulation and return of sensation. Assess the need for pain medication as sensation returns. If hospitalization is required, maintain sterile technique during dressing changes, follow prescribed antibiotic therapy regimens, and encourage proper nutrition to promote healing of skin tissue. Educate children to layer clothing and to wear hats, gloves, and an extra pair of warm socks when outside in cold temperatures. Instruct children to come inside when hands and feet feel numb or sting.

BITES

Children of all ages learn by playing and exploring the environment around them. Sometimes the environment can pose a health threat when children come into contact with animals, insects, or even snakes. Toddlers and young children sometimes experience human bites. Many times the bites may be harmless, but every bite warrants assessing, especially if the skin barrier has been damaged. Severe systemic problems may develop if the child encounters a severe reaction to the bite, which could progress to anaphylaxis (see Chapter 22 ⬤⬤).

Manifestations

Clinical manifestations for animal bites include redness, edema, and lacerations at the site of injury. The wound may drain and cellulitis may develop. Symptoms related to insect bites may depend on the insect itself and may cause either a local reaction or a systemic reaction. Some local reactions from insect bites include redness, itching, pain, hives, papules, and edema at the point of entry. Some systemic reactions include wheezing, urticaria, laryngeal or angioedema, and possibly anaphylaxis. Clinical manifestations for snake bites include burning at the puncture site, redness, ecchymosis, edema, dizziness, hypotension, tachycardia, sweating, and nausea and vomiting.

Diagnosis

Diagnosis is made by inspection and palpation of the skin tissue at the site of the animal or insect bite. Identification of the source of the bite (i.e., animal, insect, or snake) is helpful in diagnosis. Lab work is done for snake bites to determine whether the snake was venomous.

Treatment

Medical treatment involves irrigation of the wound and possible removal of dead tissue. Surgical repair or closure of the wound may be necessary. Antibiotics are prescribed to treat infection. If rabies cannot be ruled out from the animal, the child may need to receive human rabies immune globulin (HRIG) or human diploid cell rabies (HDCV) vaccine.

Nursing Considerations

Nursing care is focused on assessing local and systemic reactions to bites and stings. The source of the bite must be identified in order to determine whether the source is venomous or if the animal has rabies. Demonstrate to parents how to clean and dress wounds. Discuss ways to prevent insect bites and stings with the parents and child. Prevention methods include:

- Applying insect repellents containing DEET (diethyltoluamide)

clinical ALERT

Because of the thinness of the epidermis in children, DEET must be used with caution. Many manufacturers recommend applying DEET to a child's clothing, shoes, and hat rather than to the child's skin. Avoid repellents containing more than 10% DEET. If DEET is used on the skin, teach parents to have children wash with soap and water to remove DEET once they are inside.

- Wearing protective clothing when outdoors
- Covering the head with a hat
- Avoiding sweet-smelling lotions, creams, or perfumes that would attract insects
- Inspecting household pets for fleas and ticks. Pay attention to proper use of pet products and product warning labels
- Teach parents to observe for signs of infection and treat with antibiotics. Encourage children to avoid touching or handling strange animals, insects, or snakes

NURSING CARE
PRIORITIES IN NURSING CARE

Caring for a child who has experienced a trauma from outside sources requires an understanding of how the child interacts with his or her environment. Nursing care begins by identifying the source of the trauma, whether it stems from extreme environmental temperatures (sunburn or frostbite) or from animals, insects, or snakes. Children are curious about their surroundings. Nurses play an important role in promoting safety during play while educating children about hazards outside their homes.

HEALTH PROMOTION ISSUE

TEENS AND TANNING

Jesse, a 15-year-old female, comes to the pediatrician's office with her mom for a well visit. She has no history of health problems and is well currently, too. Jesse and her mom are experiencing some communication difficulties. Jesse challenges her mom's authority frequently. Jesse wants a membership to the tanning salon for her 16th birthday. Jesse states that she is unhappy with her pale skin and wants to be tanned. The nurse notes that Jesse is pale, freckled, has auburn hair, and has blue eyes. Jesse thinks tanning will make her more beautiful and is especially hopeful that she can get a tan before the prom. Her mom asks the nurse if there are any health risks related to the tanning salon.

DISCUSSION

The tanning salon industry is a $5 billion a year business with more than 28 million customers annually. The Food and Drug Administration has set forth guidelines related to the proper use of tanning beds. These guidelines regulate the amount of exposure in the first week of tanning and the gradual increase to a maximum exposure weekly. Studies have shown that more than 95% of tanning salon users do not follow the FDA guidelines but use the tanning beds without discretion.

Lights used by tanning salons emit mainly ultraviolet A radiation, which has been linked to more rapid changes in pigmentation and, with overexposure, to skin damage including loss of skin elasticity and premature aging. An adolescent is particularly at risk because the effects of ultraviolet damage are cumulative. So more exposure, over a long period of time, places the teenager at greater risk.

Tanning in salons has been linked to burns of the skin and the cornea. Suggested use of tanning salons includes covering sensitive areas of the skin and wearing eye protection. Exposure to the light emitted from a tanning bed may cause photosensitivity. Not all skin types respond in the desired manner to this light. Rashes and urticaria may occur. Tanning salons are linked with both melanoma and nonmelanoma skin cancers. It appears that excessive tanning damages the skin's DNA, which in turn blocks the immunosuppressant characteristics of the skin. Tanning, whether in the natural sunlight or from artificial lamps, accelerates aging of the skin. This effect includes wrinkling of exposed skin and loss of moisture.

Psychologically, tanning in salons can be addictive. A report by the *Journal of the American Academy of Dermatology* found that people felt more relaxed and less tense following exposure to ultraviolet lamps. They compared the emotions of these people to others who were exposed to a tanning bed where the lamp did not contain an ultraviolet lamp, but a placebo lamp. It is thought that tanning may stimulate secretion of endorphins and produce feelings of well-being.

PLANNING AND IMPLEMENTATION

The nurse should use this opportunity to thoroughly assess Jesse's skin health. What is the texture of her skin? What is her coloring? Fair-skinned, freckled individuals are at greater risk for skin cancer. Does she have any unusual moles, lumps, or discolored areas? This assessment could also be an opportunity for the nurse to teach Jesse how to conduct a skin self-assessment. Encourage Jesse to see a dermatologist for a baseline assessment. She should perform the skin self-assessment monthly. Teach Jesse to examine all of her skin, including those hard-to-visualize places. It may be necessary to perform the examination with a mirror and a light source to increase visibility. Moles need to be assessed for changes related to symmetry, border, color, and diameter. Moles that are asymmetrical or have irregular borders should be considered suspicious. Moles that have more than one shade of brown, black, or tan need to be assessed by a dermatologist. Moles that are ¼ of an inch in diameter or larger are also suspicious for melanoma. Jesse should also be aware of any mole that suddenly gets larger or becomes elevated. A mole that is crusty, oozes, or bleeds needs to be reported promptly to the physician. Itching, pain, and tenderness in the area of a mole are also reportable symptoms.

The nurse has the opportunity to teach Jesse about the risks of tanning salons. Each risk should be explained in a clear, concise manner. Adolescents have a tendency to not believe bad things will happen to them. Color pictures of the skin effects caused by exposure to ultraviolet light can help Jesse clearly understand the hazards. Teenagers may be particularly affected by accelerated aging caused by exposure to tanning salons.

This situation provides the perfect opportunity for the nurse to teach Jesse about protection from the harmful effects of the sun. The sun is most powerful during the hours of 1000 to 1600. Jesse should limit her exposure to the sun during these hours and always liberally apply a sunscreen with a sun protection factor of at least 15. Liberal application of sunscreen is equal to 1 ounce of sunscreen per application. Read the labels of sunscreens and choose one that blocks both UVA and UVB rays. The sunscreen should contain avobenzone, titanium dioxide, and transparent or microdis-

persed zinc oxide in the ingredient list. Sunscreen should be reapplied every few hours, or more often when swimming or perspiring heavily. Jesse should avoid the use of tan-accelerating products, as they will increase her risk of health hazards from exposure to ultraviolet light.

Certain medications could also accelerate the hazardous effects of ultraviolet light. Some of these medications are tetracycline, sulfa drugs, antiinflammatory medications, and diuretics. The nurse should teach Jesse that she should avoid exposure to the sun or tanning beds when she is taking any of these medications.

General teaching about skin health should be provided to Jesse so that she can develop healthy habits early in life. The skin, especially that on the face, should be washed two times a day with a mild, nonabrasive soap and warm water. Rinsing with cool water helps to close the pores. Immediately following bathing, a quality moisturizer should be applied. Even if Jesse's skin is oily, a mild moisturizer will be of benefit. In order to nourish her skin, Jesse's diet should contain a variety of fruits, vegetables, protein, and whole grains. She should also drink 8 to 10 glasses of water daily. Jesse should understand that regular exercise improves circulation, skin tone, and color. Adequate rest nightly provides a healthy glow to the skin. The nurse should also relate to Jesse that smoking

increases the aging process of the skin and should be avoided.

The nurse could suggest Jesse use self-tanning lotions or creams to achieve a bronze appearance without the risks of UVA exposure. Self-tanning products contain dihydroxyacetone (DHA). This substance is a sugar that interacts with dead surface cells in the epidermis, adding temporary color to the skin and making it somewhat darker. As the dead cells slough off, the color will fade, usually within a week. The nurse should remind Jesse that these products do not offer any protection from the harmful rays of the sun, and SPF protection still needs to be applied with exposure to the sun.

SELF-REFLECTION

Look at the models in a variety of fashion magazines. Do they appear to have a tan? What about actresses in television shows or movies? Are they tanned? If so, what message does this give to impressionable youth? Are you comfortable with your skin color, or do you try to artificially change it? List the ways you have compromised your skin health. What changes could you make in skin care regimen that could protect your skin from sun damage?

SUGGESTED RESOURCES

For the Nurse

Boe, K., & Tillotson, E. (2006). Encouraging sun safety for children and adolescents. *Journal of School Nursing, 22*(30), 136–141.

Cokkinides, V., Weinstock, M., Glanz, K., Albano, J., Ward, E., & Thun, M. (2006). Trends in sunburn, sun protection practices and attitudes toward sun exposure protection and tanning among U.S. adolescents: 1998–2004. *Pediatrics, 118*(3), 853–864.

For the Client

McNally, R. (Ed.). (2003). *Skin health information for teens: Health tips about dermatological concerns and skin cancer risks.* Detroit, MI: Omnigraphics.

ASSESSING

Identify the source of the injury: a fire or electrical source, a bite from animals or insects, overexposure to sun, or a cold injury due to low environmental temperatures. Assess for allergic reactions, either local or systemic. Note color, texture, and turgor of skin tissue. Assess for presence of lesions, lacerations, scrapes, puncture wounds, or blistering resulting from injury. Document the location of injury on the skin's surface and note the amount of body surface area involved. Assess the child's psychological response to the trauma and note coping mechanisms.

DIAGNOSING, PLANNING, AND IMPLEMENTING

The following nursing diagnoses may be used in planning nursing care for the child with skin conditions related to environment or trauma. (Some previously mentioned nursing diagnoses for burn clients will not be repeated here.)

- **H**yperthermia related to ultraviolet rays from the sun
- **H**ypothermia related to overexposure to low environmental temperature
- Risk for **I**nfection related to interruption of skin barrier due to animal bites, burns, or frostbite
- Acute **P**ain related to rewarming of skin from frostbite or from uncomfortable procedures for burn injuries
- Impaired **S**kin Integrity related to environmental trauma
- Disturbed **B**ody Image related to altered skin structures due to trauma

Typical outcomes for a child with conditions related to environment or trauma:

- Expresses understanding for decreased exposure to harmful environmental conditions.
- Skin remains intact and free of infection.
- Decreased pain level reported.
- Improved self image and self-esteem as evidenced by returning to normal social activities.

Nursing interventions related to children with conditions related to environment or trauma follow. Some nursing interventions related to children with a burn injury have been discussed and will not be repeated here.

- Assess for signs of infection resulting from injury. *Prompt treatment is necessary to prevent spread of infection.*
- Demonstrate proper procedures to clean and dress wounds. *Prevents spread of infection and promotes healing.*
- Administer analgesics for pain. Procedures for burn injuries and the rewarming process for frostbite can be very painful. *Analgesics promote comfort during procedures and allow the child to rest.*
- Monitor for signs of local or systemic allergic reactions related to insect or snake bites. *Systemic reactions include wheezing, urticaria, tachycardia, nausea and vomiting, laryngeal or angioedema, hypotension, dizziness, or anaphylactic shock.*
- Educate child to protect skin from harmful ultraviolet rays. *Decreased exposure to the sun will protect the skin from sunburn, which could be severe and could compromise skin integrity. Severe burns that blister may increase risk of developing melanoma.*
- Educate parents to dress their child appropriately when playing outside in cold weather. *Overexposure to environmental temperatures for a prolonged period of time may cause damage to skin tissue.*
- Provide a safe environment for the child to express feelings about disfigurement due to skin trauma. *Positive communication and acceptance will allow the child to feel secure and able to express emotions related to disfigurement.*

EVALUATING

The LPN/LVN evaluates skin tissue for signs of infection. Pain medication is evaluated for effectiveness. Watch for local or systemic allergic reactions to insect or snake bites. Monitor the family's ability to support and care for injuries related to trauma. Evaluate the child's ability to cope with altered appearance due to trauma. Evaluate the family's ability to dress the child appropriately during cold winter months.

Note: The reference and resource listings for this and all chapters have been compiled at the back of the book.

Chapter Review

 ## KEY TERMS by Topic

Use the audio glossary feature of either the CD-ROM or the Companion Website to hear the correct pronunciation of the following key terms.

Anatomy and Physiology
epidermis, melanin, dermis, arrector pili

Congenital Lesions
mongolian spot, telangiectactic nevi, stork bites, milia

Inflammatory Disorders
erythema toxicum neonatorum, dermatitis, irritant, contact dermatitis, diaper dermatitis, seborrheic dermatitis, comedones

Parasitic Infestations
pediculosis, nits, crabs, scabies

Skin Infections
cryotherapy, impetigo, cellulitis

Fungal Infections
ringworm, tinea capitis, tinea corporis, tinea pedis, tinea cruris, thrush

Burns
thermal burns, chemical burns, electrical burns, radiation burns, eschar

Trauma and Environment
melanocytes, frostbite

KEY Points

- Main functions of the skin include protecting the body from pathogens, temperature regulation, preventing dehydration, providing sensory receptors for pain, touch, pressure, and temperature, and aiding in production of vitamin D.

- The integumentary system includes the skin and its associated structures: hair, nails, sebaceous and sweat glands, blood vessels, nerve endings, and sensory organs.

- Contact dermatitis can stem from allergens (poison ivy, poison oak, latex, or nickel) or repeated exposure to irritants (detergents, bleaches, soaps, lotions, urine and stool).

- Breastfed infants are not as prone to diaper dermatitis.

- Seborrheic dermatitis, known as "cradle cap" in babies, may be a result of changes in sebaceous glands. Treatment includes daily shampooing with a nonmedicated shampoo.

- Eczema, a chronic inflammatory skin disorder with unknown cause, has been associated with an immune dysfunction of the skin. Eczema flare-ups are more common during the winter months when the air is dry. Eczema is not a contagious condition.

- Acne is a common skin condition affecting many adolescents. Treatment may be topical or systemic, depending on the severity of the condition. Nursing care involves attention to the emotional as well as the physical effects of the disorder.

- Impetigo, a superficial skin infection caused by streptococci or staphylococci, is highly contagious and can be transferred between children and adults. Poor sanitation and close living conditions place children at risk for contracting impetigo.

- Cellulitis is a bacterial infection of the dermis and subcutaneous tissue. Onset is usually rapid. Cellulitis requires medical attention; if it is not treated, it may result in septicemia.

- Dermatophytes are fungi that mainly affect the surface of the skin, hair, and nails. Tinea (ringworm) is a term used to describe a group of fungal infections of the skin that are transmitted from human to human or from animals to humans.

- Oral candidiasis (thrush) is usually found in a child with a depressed immune system. It appears as white plaques on the tongue, palate, and/or buccal mucosa that bleed easily.

- Pediculosis is infestation with lice, a parasite that lives on the outside of a human host. Head lice are commonly found on the back of the scalp, where the female louse lays eggs (viable nits) that hatch within 8 to 10 days. Nursing care for head lice focuses on methods to kill the parasite and alleviate itching.

- Burns are assessed for burn depth (thickness) and burn area (percentage of body surface area, BSA). Minor burns may be treated on an outpatient basis. Major burns require hospitalization and possible skin grafting.

- Melanoma arises from melanocytes (pigment-producing cells) in the dermis and epidermis. Usually these cells are damaged by overexposure to the sun's ultraviolet rays over a prolonged period of time.

- Nursing care for frostbite focuses on rewarming the affected area while protecting the skin tissues from further injury. The affected area is monitored for increase in circulation and return of sensation.

- Nursing care for bites focuses on assessing the local and systemic reactions to bites that may be venomous or rabid, and teaching about how to prevent future instances of trauma.

 ## EXPLORE MediaLink

Additional interactive resources for this chapter can be found on the Companion Website at www.prenhall.com/adams.

Click on Chapter 21 and "Begin" to select the activities for this chapter.

For chapter-related NCLEX®-style questions and an audio glossary, access the accompanying CD-ROM in this book.

Animations:
Eczema

FOR FURTHER Study

The chain of infection is illustrated in Figure 10-1.

For an illustration of interstitial space, see Figure 11-3.

For information about child abuse, see also Chapter 16.

See Chapter 18 and Table 18-7 for more information about herpes.

Anaphylaxis, oral candidiasis, and contact dermatitis are discussed in Chapter 22.

Critical Thinking Care Map

Caring for a Child with Eczema
NCLEX-PN® Focus Area: Physiological Integrity: Basic Care and Comfort

Case Study: Sarah's mother calls the pediatrician's office and reports that her 12-year-old daughter has been scratching the skin around her neck and behind her knees for the past 3 days and is unable to rest at night because of constant itching. The area now looks very red and scaly with yellow, crusted sores.

Nursing Diagnosis: Risk for Impaired **S**kin Integrity related to irritants and itching

COLLECT DATA

Subjective	Objective
_____	_____
_____	_____
_____	_____
_____	_____
_____	_____
_____	_____

Would you report this? Yes/No

If yes, to: _____

Nursing Care

_____

_____

_____

_____

_____

_____

_____

_____

_____

_____

_____

How would you document this? _____

_____

_____

Compare your documentation to the sample provided in Appendix I.

Data Collected
(use only those that apply)

- Temperature 98.8 °F
- Ruptured papules with yellow crust behind knees
- Enjoys playing with her baby brother
- Mother states they have had a lot of fish over the last week
- Stopped attending youth group with friends
- Menses began 2 months ago
- Mother states child is now wearing a small amount of makeup
- Lesions on neck are dry and scaly
- Child reports her skin itches and the sores leak fluid more during winter
- Child states she likes milk and cookies
- Mother states the child doesn't shower after swimming
- Child states she sleeps late on weekends

Nursing Interventions
(use only those that apply; list in priority order)

- Administer antipyretics.
- Obtain a thorough nutrition history.
- Hydrate skin with lotions and creams.
- Encourage wool clothing during winter months.
- Encourage showering after swimming.
- Administer oral antihistamines.
- Instruct to keep fingernails short.
- Encourage child to wear loose-fitting clothing.
- Keep environmental temperatures cool.
- Apply wet compresses to lesions that are crusted.
- Encourage a regular exercise program.

NCLEX-PN® Exam Preparation

TEST-TAKING TIP To avoid jumping to a conclusion too soon, cover the answers first, read the question slowly and think what the question is asking you to do. Is the question asking you to assess, plan, implement, or evaluate care? Then select the answer(s) that best fits the task.

1 The nurse is reviewing a list of instructions with a parent for an infant with oral candidiasis. Select all instructions that should be included on the list.

1. Swab oral mucosa with oral nystatin.
2. Clean bottle nipples in cool water.
3. Disinfect all toys.
4. Place stuffed animals in a plastic bag for 5 days.
5. Report rash in the diaper area.

2 A 12-year-old is receiving oral antibiotics because of a deep cut behind his left knee after falling off his bicycle. The child has returned for a follow-up visit. Which of the following assessment findings should be reported immediately to the nursing supervisor?

1. Lymphangitis
2. Last tetanus shot 6 months ago
3. Limps when walking
4. Pedal pulse of 76

3 Which of the following assessment findings is characteristic of port wine stains?

1. Color is deep yellow to orange in appearance
2. Does not blanch
3. Located on the folds of the neck
4. Laser treatments may be needed

4 The environmental temperature should be kept cool and _____ for children with eczema.

5 When taking a family history, the nurse discovers that both parents have a history of asthma. Which of the following skin disorders has been associated with asthma?

1. Eczema
2. Intertrigo
3. Diaper dermatitis
4. Tinea infections

6 The nurse is caring for an infant with seborrheic dermatitis. Which of the following symptoms would the nurse expect?

1. Red blisters on the buttocks
2. Yellow scaly patches on scalp
3. Erythematous papules on back of neck
4. Erythema in the folds of the skin

7 The nurse is discussing treatments for a 16-year-old with acne. Which of the following statements is correct about acne treatments?

1. "Oil-based skin products are best."
2. "Avoid using sunscreen while taking acne medication."
3. "It may take up to 3 months to see improvement in the skin."
4. "Tetracycline is contraindicated for adolescents with acne."

8 Which of the following nursing interventions is recommended for a child with impetigo?

1. Apply nystatin to open lesions.
2. Elevate extremities that have lesions.
3. Place toys in a plastic bag for 2 weeks.
4. Soak and remove crust on lesions several times a day.

9 Which of the following prevention methods should be followed to decrease the risk of melanoma? Use all that apply.

1. Avoid late afternoon sun between 4 p.m. and 6 p.m.
2. Apply sunscreen of SPF 15 or greater.
3. Use a tanning bed instead of the sun for tanning.
4. Report moles that are black with irregular borders.
5. Wear long-sleeved cotton clothing when outside.

10 A teenager is complaining that between his toes are red, scaly areas with deep fissures that itch and are painful. What should the nurse recommend the teenager do to avoid this skin condition in the future?

1. Wear flip-flops at all times in the locker room.
2. Apply Elimite cream on toes for 2 weeks.
3. Nothing; this is common among teenagers.
4. Wear tight-fitting wool socks.

Chapter 22

Care of the Child with Immune Disorders

HEALTH PROMOTION ISSUE:
Disclosing HIV Status: A Difficult Task for Teens

NURSING CARE PLAN CHART:
Child with Juvenile Rheumatoid Arthritis

NURSING PROCESS CARE PLAN:
Child with an Organ Transplant

CRITICAL THINKING CARE MAP:
Caring for a Client with AIDS

BRIEF Outline

Anatomy and Physiology

Brief Assessment Review

Congenital Immune Disorders

HIV and AIDS

Juvenile Rheumatoid Arthritis

Systemic Lupus Erythematosus (SLE)

Organ Transplantation

Allergies

Immunotherapy

Nursing Care

LEARNING Outcomes

After completing this chapter, you will be able to:
1. Define key terms.
2. Discuss the anatomy and physiology of the pediatric immunological system.
3. Describe immunological disorders to include HIV, AIDS, juvenile rheumatoid arthritis, and allergies.
4. Discuss clinical manifestations, diagnostic procedures, medical management, and nursing interventions related to immunological disorders.
5. Describe the care of children requiring organ transplants.

The immune system provides the child vital protection against many diseases. A functioning immune system allows the child to coexist with other children and adults and to avoid or minimize these diseases. On the other hand, when the immune system does not function properly, diseases and conditions such as allergies, juvenile arthritis, or possibly AIDS could affect the child. This chapter will review the anatomy and physiology of the immune system and discuss a variety of disorders related to the immune system.

Anatomy and Physiology

The primary role of the immune system is to recognize and eliminate foreign substances. The foreign substances are called **antigens.** When the immune system recognizes these antigens, **antibodies** or proteins are produced. The antibodies will now be available to attack the antigen should it invade the body in the future. This process is called the **immune response.**

Natural immunity is present at birth and lasts about 3 to 6 months. It includes:

- Intact skin, which prevents foreign substances from entering the body
- Body pH, which maintains an environment that is hostile to antigens
- Antibodies against certain antigens, which were passed to the child during pregnancy and breastfeeding
- Body processes of inflammation and phagocytosis, which fight antigens

Acquired immunity is developed over a period of time after birth by exposure to foreign substances. Acquired immunity is developed through humoral immunity and cell-mediated immunity.

Humoral immunity destroys bacteria, viruses, parasites, allergens, and other foreign substances by producing antibodies called **immunoglobulins.** The types of immunoglobulins and their basic functions are described in Table 22-1 ■. The production of immunoglobulins begins in early infancy but is not complete until age 6 or 7. The body's first response to antigens is called the **primary immune response.** Figure 22-1 ■ illustrates the events in the body's primary immune response. This first response produces antibodies within 3 days. It is important to note that the individual does not show symptoms when this first exposure and response occur. However, the primary response prepares the body to respond quickly to respond to second or repeated exposure.

The **secondary immune response** occurs when the child is exposed to the antigen in the future. Within

TABLE 22-1	
Types of Immunoglobulin (Ig) and Functions	
IMMUNOGLOBULIN	ACTION
IgM	First antibody produced with primary immune response
	Mediates *cytotoxic* (cell-killing) response
	Activates *complement* serum protein complex that is activated by the antigen-antibody complex in an immune reaction
IgG	Only immunoglobulin to cross placenta
	Active against bacteria, bacterial toxins, and viruses
	Activates complements
IgA	Prevents binding of viruses to cells of respiratory and GI tracts
IgD	Function not fully understood
IgE	Primarily responsible for allergic reactions

Source: Adapted from Ball, J., & Bindler, R. (2006). *Child health nursing: Partnering with children and families.* Upper Saddle River, NJ: Prentice Hall, Table 27-2, p. 959.

24 hours, the previously produced antibodies provide protection for the child.

Cell-mediated immunity provides the child protection against bacteria, viruses, fungi, and tumors. This process develops early in the child's life. Cell-mediated immunity is also the process that causes rejection of organs that have been transplanted. The thymus produces lymphocytes, which directly attack the foreign substances. Figure 22-2 ■ (lower left portion) illustrates the actions of the thymus. T lymphocytes, B lymphocytes, and natural killer (NK) cells play an important role in cell-mediated immunity.

Immunizations provide **active immunity.** In active immunity, an antigen is given, and antibodies are produced (see Figure 22-1) to provide immunity if the body is exposed in the future. Active immunity is the mechanism by which immunizations provide protection against childhood diseases that used to claim thousands of infants' lives. **Passive immunity** is provided by administering immunoglobulins to protect children against diseases to which they may have been exposed already. For example, a child with Kawasaki syndrome (see Chapter 13 ⬭) is given large doses of

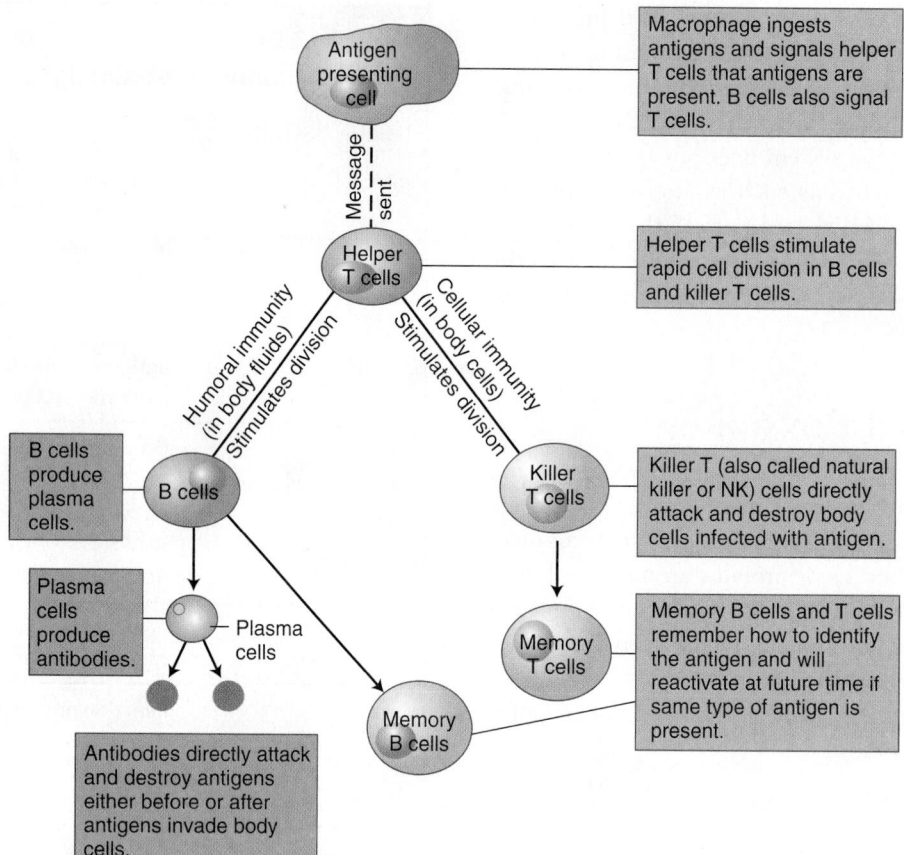

Figure 22-1. ■ Primary immune response.

immunoglobulins for a period of time to counter the effects of the disease. For more information about immunizations, and the childhood and adolescent immunization schedule, see Figure 6-3 ⚬⚬.

Brief Assessment Review

HISTORY

- Inquire about recent illnesses and infections. Ask especially about unexplained fevers.
- Does the child suffer from allergy symptoms?
- Inquire about stiffness or pain in the joints.
- Inquire about the child's appetite.
- Review immunization record.

PHYSICAL

- Obtain height and weight.
- Obtain vital signs.
- Inspect the oral cavity. (With immunosuppression, there may be thrush.)
- Inspect the skin for lesions.
- Assess range of motion in joints.
- Palpate the lymph nodes (see Figures 14-2 and 14-3 ⚬⚬).

Congenital Immune Disorders

SEVERE COMBINED IMMUNODEFICIENCY DISORDER

In severe combined immunodeficiency disorder (SCID), both humoral and cellular immunity is absent. There is a lack of functioning T cells and B cells. In infants with SCID, genetic mutations lead to impaired lymphoid development. B lymphocytes may appear in normal numbers but do not function effectively. Natural killer cells are few. Infants often become symptomatic (highly susceptible to infection) by 3 months of age, as maternal antibodies are lost. Resistant oral candidiasis may be the first infection noted. Treatment involves intravenous immunoglobulin, hematopoietic stem cell transplant with a histocompatible donor, and prophylactic antibiotics. Enzyme replacement therapy is helpful in certain cases.

clinical ALERT

Children with T-cell deficiencies may experience graft-versus-host reaction with normal blood transfusions. They must be given irradiated blood products that are negative for cytomegalovirus in order to avoid this risk.

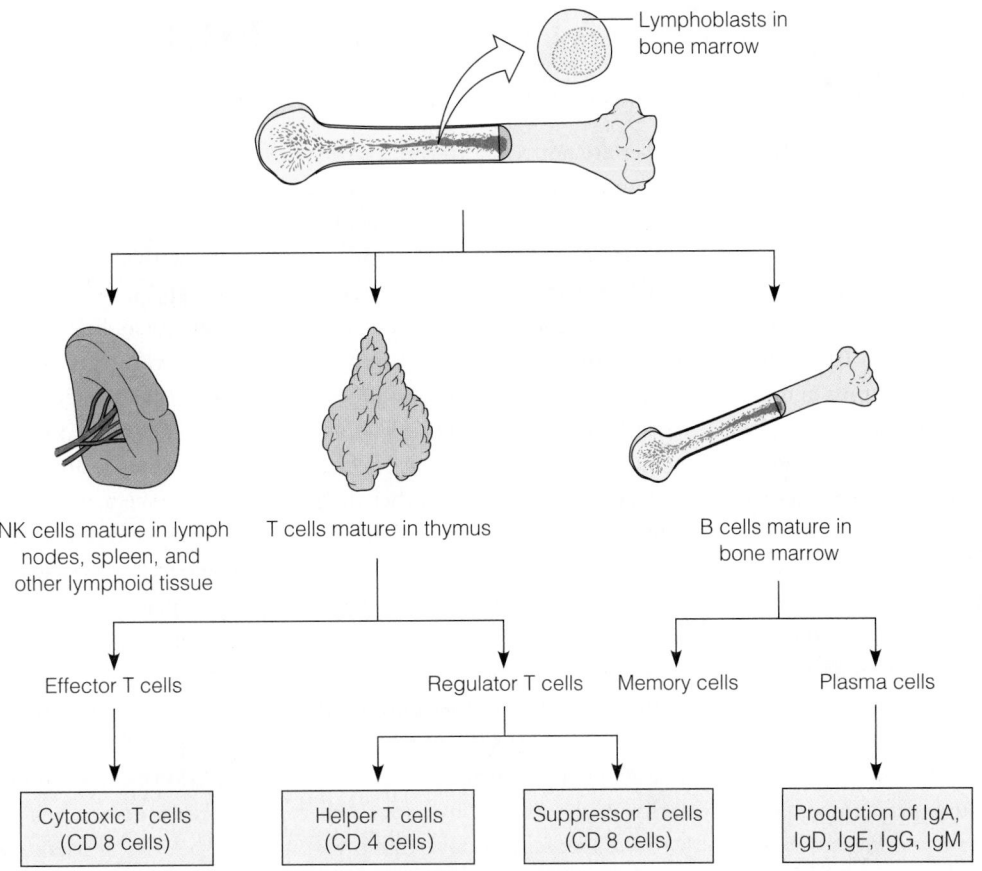

Figure 22-2. ■ The development and differentiation of lymphocytes shows how cell-mediated immunity works.

COMMON VARIABLE IMMUNODEFICIENCY

In common variable immunodeficiency (also called *acquired hypogammaglobulinemia*) there is a low level of circulating immunoglobulins of all classes. This disorder appears equally in male and female adolescents or young adults. Clients present with susceptibility to infection. Treatment is by regular administration of immunoglobulins and antibiotics to protect against infection.

HIV and AIDS

Human immunodeficiency virus (HIV) is a retrovirus that causes the end-stage condition acquired immunodeficiency syndrome (AIDS). AIDS is characterized by a defect in cell-mediated immunity that makes it difficult or sometimes impossible for the affected child to fight infection. In 2004, approximately 9,443 children under the age of 13 in the United States were living with AIDS.

HIV is transmitted to children primarily through perinatal transmission. During pregnancy, the virus can cross the placenta and infect the fetus. During birth, the newborn can be infected by exposure to maternal blood, amniotic fluid, or genital tract secretions. In the postpartum period, the newborn can contract the disease by exposure to breast milk of the HIV-positive mother.

Adolescents typically contract HIV through unprotected sexual activity and intravenous drug use. See the Health Promotion Issue on pages 606 and 607.

Because of the risk of perinatal transmission, the CDC has recommended HIV screening as a routine part of prenatal care. Women who refuse to be tested should be questioned about the reasons for refusal, and counseling should be provided. The screening test should be offered again later in the pregnancy. The woman may be reluctant to find out the diagnosis. However, the nurse should teach the client that risk for perinatal transmission is significantly reduced if the mother receives zidovudine (AZT) therapy during pregnancy and if the infant is delivered by cesarean section.

Infection with the virus during the perinatal period shortens the time between seroconversion and the condition of AIDS. The time frame between exposure and seroconversion and disease development can be within 2 years of birth.

Manifestations

Clinical manifestations include chronic otitis media, fever, skin irritation, failure to thrive, lack of weight gain, chronic diarrhea, hepatosplenomegaly, lymphadenopathy, and oral candidiasis. Although rare, Kaposi's sarcoma can develop. Kaposi's is manifested as purple papules that begin on the feet and spread across the skin.

MediaLink ● HIV/AIDS

DISCLOSING HIV STATUS: A DIFFICULT TASK FOR TEENS

Marilyn, age 16, came to the family practice office because she was constantly feeling tired. She also noticed that she had been losing weight over the past few months. The nurse took a careful health history, which included a past sexual history. Marilyn had a prescription for birth control pills and stated that she was sexually active with three to four sexual encounters monthly. She furthered stated that she was faithful to take her pills daily and that she knew each of the guys she had sex with, but they rarely used a condom.

Marilyn's mother accompanied her to the office this morning and is aware of her sexual activity. After discussing the health history with the nurse practitioner, the nurse drew an ELISA screen to test for HIV and the nurse practitioner performed a pelvic exam and Pap smear. A follow-up appointment was scheduled for Marilyn. The nurse taught Marilyn the importance of avoiding sexual contact until the lab results can be interpreted.

At the follow-up visit, the nurse practitioner tells Marilyn that the ELISA test is positive and that her Pap smear was negative. The nurse tells Marilyn that another ELISA test is necessary and gains consent to draw the specimen. Marilyn wants to know what this means. The nurse explains that two separate specimens must be drawn to confirm a diagnosis of HIV infection.

When the second ELISA results are obtained, Marilyn is told that she is infected with HIV. She is immediately stunned and states that there is no way that she could have contracted the virus. She states that she used her birth control pills faithfully and knew all of her partners well enough to know that they are not HIV positive.

The nurse patiently listens to Marilyn, while her mother is softly crying with her head in her hands. The nurse understands that Marilyn and her mother are not ready to receive the necessary information about her diagnosis. She makes an appointment with them in 2 days. She does discuss with Marilyn the importance of abstaining from sexual contact until they have had a chance to discuss the issue further.

Upon the return visit, Marilyn states that she has had time to think about the diagnosis. She does not want anybody to know about her diagnosis other than her mother. When the nurse explains the necessity of disclosing her diagnosis to her past partners, Marilyn becomes angry and states that she will not talk with them and that she hopes each of them has the virus and becomes gravely ill.

Marilyn also asks the nurse to tell her more about the treatment required. Marilyn had been told by a friend that there was medicine to take that prevented you from passing the virus on to others. This was the medicine Marilyn wanted to take. Marilyn stated she did not plan to curtail her sexual activity and knew that her partners would not agree to wear a condom. In fact, if she asked them to, they would know that something was wrong and she did not plan to tell anybody that she was HIV positive.

The nurse discusses Marilyn's case with the nurse practitioner. Together they work on a plan to accurately inform Marilyn and her mother about the disease, its treatment, and the lifestyle changes that are necessary.

DISCUSSION

Adolescents are physically developing into adulthood. Puberty marks the beginning of their sexual maturity. The hormones of adolescence increase the sex drive and cause teens to be preoccupied with the opposite sex. Physically they are capable of having sexual intercourse, but emotionally and cognitively, their stage of development causes them often to demonstrate risky behaviors related to sexuality.

Acceptance among peers is of utmost importance to teens. They want to be accepted and not stand out as different. These feelings cause a fear of rejection. Teens place extreme emphasis on their outward appearance. They may choose very specific (and sometimes extreme) types of clothing and hairstyles in order to be part of a group of teens. Fear of rejection can also cause teens to make decisions about their behavior that may not be wise. If friends want them to go somewhere or do something that is not typically allowed, they may risk the parental consequences instead of risking their peers' rejection.

Because their cognitive development allows them to think abstractly, teens begin to feel that they are invincible, possibly immortal. They can easily begin to feel that they are wise and do not need the advice and direction offered by authority figures. This is a hazard of adolescence, that teens seek independence but are not yet mature enough to know and consider all of the ramifications of their decisions.

Teens who have been diagnosed with HIV fear rejection from friends, family members, and even strangers if they disclose their diagnosis. They do not want to be labeled as sick or unclean. They fear that people will shun them.

Some teens may initially deny their diagnosis, hoping that it will go away. Some can even create a magical thinking scenario where they never deal in reality with the disease process. However, teens who try to pretend to others are rarely able to pretend to themselves. Oftentimes, feelings of despair, anxiety, and depression can overwhelm teens who are attempting to ignore their diagnosis.

Teens who are struggling with the diagnosis and the decision to disclose this information need support from a caring health care professional who can guide them into correct thinking and decision making. The nurse can play an important role in listening to the teen's concerns and giving appropriate information. The nurse can also help teens prepare themselves to disclose their diagnosis (when they are ready) by assisting with the right words to use and by helping them decide on the right timing for disclosure.

The nurse can discuss the benefits of nondisclosure with the teen. By disclosing the diagnosis to only a few trusted individuals, the teen can ensure that privacy is maintained and that the condition will not be discussed by those the teen does not want to tell. Nondisclosure prevents acquaintances from making judgments.

Nondisclosure also has risks that need to be discussed. Teens who do not admit to their diagnosis are less likely to follow the medical regime. Lack of proper medical treatment can further complicate the condition. Teens who choose to keep their diagnosis from friends and family lose the advantage of social support from these individuals.

Besides this risk to the infected teen, nondisclosure also allows further spread of the virus. Past partners have the right to know about their exposure and the necessity of seeking testing for themselves. Future partners have the right to be informed about their probable exposure, if they have sex without adequate protection.

Many websites and AIDS hotlines can provide teens a safe place to disclose their diagnosis. These sites allow teens an opportunity to practice how they will tell about their condition and to receive feedback from other teens who have struggled with the same decisions.

PLANNING AND IMPLEMENTATION

The nurse develops an extensive teaching plan for Marilyn that includes classroom learning, written materials, videos, peer counseling, and regular follow-up visits to the family practice clinic. The following content outline was developed:

- General knowledge about HIV/AIDS
- Transmission of HIV/AIDS
- Medical treatment of the disease
- The importance of social support
- How to discuss her condition with others

Marilyn needs to understand that there is no current cure for HIV/AIDS but that early intervention and continued treatment can increase the quality of life. Transmission of the virus can occur through contact with body fluids. This can occur during oral-penile contact, oral-vaginal contact, vaginal-penile contact, penile-rectal contact, substance abuse with needles and syringes, contact with blood such as sharing razors or toothbrushes, handling used feminine hygiene products, and so on. Marilyn should be encouraged to use condoms with each sexual encounter. She should understand that this will be necessary for the remainder of her life.

Marilyn needs to understand her prescribed medical regime. She needs to know about each drug, its side effects, and specific information about taking these drugs correctly. She needs to understand when to report symptoms of complications. She should have phone numbers to reach the health care provider any time of the day or night.

Marilyn will need emotional support to help her avoid feelings of rejection and isolation. The nurse can help Marilyn identify those people in her life who can lend her positive support. Those who might give negative feedback must also be identified. The nurse can assist Marilyn with how to discuss her condition with others. Role playing is an effective tool to use. The nurse can allow Marilyn to practice telling people about her diagnosis. The nurse may also be able to refer Marilyn to support groups with teens her age who can assist Marilyn in developing ways to tell her trusted friends and family.

As Marilyn becomes confident in managing her disease, she may feel the desire to help others who are HIV positive. The nurse should assess for this readiness and encourage Marilyn to use the things she learned to help others. The nurse can refer Marilyn to agencies that provide services to teens with a diagnosis of HIV.

SELF-REFLECTION

What medical secret have you kept for yourself or possibly for a family member or friend? Why was it important to keep that secret? What were the benefits of keeping this secret? What were the risks of keeping this secret?

SUGGESTED RESOURCES

For the Nurse

Diiorio, C., McCarty, F., Denzmore, P., & Landis, A. (2007). The moderating influence of mother-adolescent discussion on early and middle African-American adolescent sexual behavior. *Research in Nursing and Health, 30*(2), 193–202.

Wiener, L., Battles, H., & Wood, L. (2007). A longitudinal study of adolescents with perinatally or transfusion acquired HIV infection: Sexual knowledge, risk reduction, self-efficacy and sexual behavior. *AIDS and Behavior, 11*(3), 471–478.

For the Client

Goldman, L. (2001). *Breaking the silence: A guide to help children with complicated grief* (2nd ed.). New York: Brunner-Routledge.

Figure 22-3. ■ Oral thrush is a common finding in clients with HIV. (Visuals Unlimited).

Oral candidiasis or **thrush** is a chronic condition caused most commonly by the fungus *Candida albicans*. Thrush is seen as white patches on the oral and pharyngeal mucosa (Figure 22-3 ■) that may bleed easily. The fungal infection can also be found in the diaper region, under the arms or neck. Fluconazole or itraconazole is the treatment of choice for oral candidiasis. These medications are applied directly to the affected tissue. Candidiasis is also discussed in relation to vaginitis in Chapter 18 ⬤.

Diagnosis

The presence of HIV is determined with the polymerase chain reaction (PCR) test or the enzyme-linked immunosorbent assay (ELISA). This blood test (ELISA) may initially be negative, especially in the newborn. Testing is repeated as necessary and HIV is confirmed following two positive tests. A newer test, called the OraQuick Advance HIV1/2 Antibody Test, uses oral fluids obtained by swabbing the upper and lower gums. Results are available in 20 minutes, and positive results have been found to be 99% accurate.

Treatment

During pregnancy, HIV-positive mothers are treated with the antiretroviral agent zidovudine (AZT) to prevent transmission to the fetus. Most obstetricians will perform a cesarean section to further reduce the fetus's risk of exposure to the virus. After birth, the newborn is also treated with AZT to reduce the risk of transmission. Newborns can be treated prophylactically with antibiotics and immune globulin to prevent bacterial infections. In children where HIV is confirmed, antiretroviral therapy is used, usually combining several drugs (Table 22-2 ■).

Nursing Considerations

The nursing care of children with HIV/AIDS primarily involves reducing infection and transmission and promoting adequate growth and development. To reduce infection, the nurse must use proper sterile technique when performing invasive procedures as is appropriate for all clients. Invasive procedures should be avoided if possible.

Mothers who are HIV positive must avoid breastfeeding. The family should be taught proper hand washing techniques to prevent spread of infection. The family also

---

TABLE 22-2

Pharmacology: Antiretroviral Agents Used to Treat HIV

DRUG (GENERIC AND COMMON BRAND NAME)	USUAL ROUTE/DOSE	CLASSIFICATION AND PURPOSE	SELECTED SIDE EFFECTS	DON'T GIVE IF
Zidovudine (Retrovir)	100–180 mg/m^2 q6h PO for children 3 months to 13 years	Nucleoside reverse transcriptase inhibitors used to suppress viral load	Fever, malaise, myalgia, headache, nausea, vomiting, anorexia, cough, rash	Client is anemic or has a granulocyte count above 750/mm^3
Ritonavir (Norvir)	400–600 mg/m^2 PO BID for children 2–16 years	Protease inhibitors used in combination with other antiretroviral agents to suppress viral load	Weakness, nausea, diarrhea, vomiting	Client has suppressed liver function
Delavirdine mesylate (Rescriptor)	400 mg PO TID for children greater than 16 years	Nonnucleoside reverse transcriptase inhibitors used in combination with other antiretroviral agents to suppress viral load	Rash, headache, dizziness, chest pain	Client is currently being administered an antacid. Client has fever, blistering rash, oral lesions, conjunctivitis, muscle or joint pain

must understand the importance of avoiding other children and individuals with infections of all types, because the child with HIV is more susceptible to any infection (Box 22-1 ■). Diseases such as tuberculosis can be devastating. The importance of immunizations should be emphasized to the family. See Chapter 6 ⚭ for the immunization schedule.

Promoting adequate respiration and nutrition will also be important to assist the child with HIV/AIDS to avoid infection. The nurse can encourage the child to perform deep breathing exercises. The diet of these children should be assessed carefully for adequate nutritional content including calories, protein, vitamins and antioxidants. See Chapter 6 ⚭ for a nutritional assessment. Referral to a registered dietician may be necessary.

Because of the medical regime and frequent hospitalizations, children with HIV/AIDS are at risk for developmental delays. The nurse should assess physical and mental functioning and provide assistance to parents regarding activities to promote growth and development.

Juvenile Rheumatoid Arthritis

Juvenile rheumatoid arthritis (JRA) is a chronic disorder causing joint inflammation. It is **autoimmune** in nature, meaning that in this disorder, the body attacks itself, perceiving its own cells as foreign substances. In JRA, tissues surrounding joints may also be affected. Periods of remission are common in children. In fact, 70% of children will have permanent remission by the time they become adults.

Manifestations

Symptoms include systemic changes as well as musculoskeletal changes. The child presents with fever, rash, **lymphadenopathy** (enlarged lymph nodes), **splenomegaly** (enlarged spleen), and **hepatomegaly** (enlarged liver), indicating a systemic inflammatory process. The child may have a limp or favor one extremity over the other. Pain, stiffness, swelling, and loss of movement may be seen in one or more large joints such as the knees.

Diagnosis

JRA is diagnosed usually by presentation of clinical symptoms. Laboratory findings include positive rheumatoid factor, human leukocyte antigen B27, and antinuclear antibody.

Treatment

The medical management of JRA includes medication and physical therapy. The priorities of care are to relieve pain and prevent joint contractures. On occasion surgery is performed to reduce pain and improve joint function. Salicylates (aspirin) or nonsteroidal antiinflammatory drugs (NSAIDs) are used to reduce inflammation. These drugs can cause gastrointestinal upset, and the child should be monitored closely for side effects.

Physical therapy is essential in the treatment plan. Range-of-motion exercises, hydrotherapy, and muscle strengthening exercise help to prevent contractures (Figure 22-4 ■). Warm compresses are used to relieve discomfort and swelling. The child should be provided with adequate nutrition to promote healing (Box 22-2 ■).

Nursing Considerations

The care of the child with JRA usually takes place in the community. The family must be taught the importance of medication management, side effects, and need for physical therapy. The child should remain in school and have contact with peers as much as possible. Activities should be planned to enable the child to develop a positive self-image. Referral should be made for home care. The American Juvenile Rheumatoid Arthritis Association can be a valuable resource for families.

The child should be routinely evaluated for decreased pain and swelling in joints, increased mobility, and side effects of medication. With adequate treatment, the prognosis is favorable for complete recovery. The Nursing Care Plan

A

B

Figure 22-4. ■ (**A**) Stretching exercises are an important part of physical therapy for a child who has juvenile rheumatoid arthritis. (**B**) Swimming is very helpful for maintaining joint function in children with JRA.

Chart on page 611 further describes nursing care for children with juvenile rheumatoid arthritis.

Systemic Lupus Erythematosus (SLE)

SLE is an autoimmune disease of the connective tissue and blood vessels that causes inflammation in any organ of the body. According to the Arthritis Foundation, 25,000 children and adolescents in the United States have SLE. It occurs more frequently than leukemia, cystic fibrosis, or muscular dystrophy. There is a higher incidence of SLE in African American, Asian, and Hispanic children in the United States.

BOX 22-2 | NUTRITION THERAPY

Foods for Children with Juvenile Rheumatoid Arthritis

Inflammation caused by juvenile rheumatoid arthritis can be quite painful for children. Certain foods may have natural anti-inflammatory properties and promote joint health in those with this disorder. Pineapple contains the enzyme bromelain, which is associated with reducing inflammation. Flavonoids such as blueberries, tomatoes, broccoli, and apples decrease inflammation and strengthen connective tissues. Salmon, trout, and tuna contain omega-3 fatty acids, which relieve stiffness and pain in the joints. Ginger contains shogaols and gingerols, which are antioxidants and antiinflammatories. Ginger can be added to foods and found in beverages in many health food stores.

Certain foods also can increase inflammation in the joints. Children with rheumatoid arthritis should limit or avoid dairy products, eggs, hydrogenated oils, refined sugars, white flour, soy, corn and wheat products, caffeine, potatoes, green pepper, and eggplant.

Manifestations

The child with SLE may have an erythematous butterfly rash across the nose, cheeks, and cheekbones (called a *malar rash*). Figure 22-5 ■ shows this characteristic rash. Many SLE clients are photosensitive. Exposure to sun causes a diffuse maculopapular rash (see Figure 21-3 ⊕ for skin lesions). The disease is characterized in most children by swollen and painful joints. They may experience alopecia, *Raynaud's phenomenon* (pallor, numbness, and pain in the extremities, usually caused by exposure to cold), mouth ulcers, anemia, headache, memory loss, weight loss, fatigue, and low-grade fever. If the kidneys become inflamed, the child may develop nephritis. When the brain is inflamed,

Figure 22-5. ■ Butterfly rash of systemic lupus erythematosus.

NURSING CARE PLAN CHART

Child with Juvenile Rheumatoid Arthritis

GOAL	INTERVENTION	RATIONALE	EXPECTED OUTCOME
1. Chronic Pain related to inflammation of the joints			
The child will demonstrate reduced pain.	Administer antiinflammatories as prescribed and teach the child to self-administer these medications	*Antiinflammatories suppress the inflammatory process*	The child will verbalize reduced pain using a pain scale and be able to accomplish tasks of daily living.
	Apply heat to the joints via warm baths or heating pads.	*Heat is effective in reducing pain and joint stiffness*	
	Review the child's activity level and assist with planning activities	*Preventing the overuse of joints can reduce inflammation and the associated pain*	
The family will assist with pain reduction activities.	Provide nutritional planning	*Excess weight can cause strain on the joints and increase pain*	The family will assist with medication administration, and diet planning and implementation and will provide nonpharmacologic pain relief methods
	Teach parents to provide pharmacologic and non-pharmacologic pain relief methods	*The balance of pain relief methods is often most effective*	
2. Impaired Physical Mobility related to joint stiffness and pain			
The child will have increased mobility.	Determine level of current flexibility and limited mobility	*In order to develop an appropriate plan, knowledge of the extent of impairment is necessary*	The child's joints will remain flexible and without contractures. The child will be able to ambulate appropriately.
	Attend initial physical therapy session	*Learning about the exercises that are prescribed will assist the nurse in enforcing the exercises*	
	Position the child during rest periods	*Proper positioning decreases stress to the joints*	
The family will provide assistance with mobility restoration.	Encourage the family to assess their home for hazards or impediments to mobility	*The home should be free of structures such as excessive steps that could complicate the child's mobility*	The family will participate in physical therapy and positioning use appropriate assistive devices.
	Refer the family to home health care agencies	*These agencies can supply assistive devices that would increase the child's mobility*	

seizures and mood changes can occur. An inflamed heart may manifest as pericarditis or myocardial infarction. Inflammation of the lungs results in pleuritis. The disease is characterized by periods of exacerbation (brought on by sun exposure, stress, or infection) and remission.

Diagnosis

Diagnosis of SLE is made by observing for the physical findings and the presence of positive antinuclear antibodies (ANAs), anti-double stranded DNA antibodies (anti-DNA), and antiphospholipid antibodies. The complete

blood count (CBC) will show decreased RBCs, platelets, and white blood cells (WBCs). The urinalysis may show the presence of blood, protein, and cast cells. A kidney biopsy may be necessary. To determine the extent of involvement of other organs, x-rays, ECG, echogram, EEG, MRI, or CT scans may be necessary.

Treatment

Medications used to treat SLE include NSAIDs such as Naprosyn, Advil, or Tolectin to help control the discomfort associated with inflammation. Antimalarials such as

Plaquenil (hydroxychloroquine) are prescribed to help control the skin rash of SLE. The most commonly used medications for SLE are corticosteroids. Immunosuppressants such as Imuran and Cytoxan may be prescribed. Long-term prognosis depends on how severely internal organs are involved. The 5-year survival rate for children is 78% to 92% (Stichweh, Arce, & Pascual, 2004).

Nursing Considerations

The nurse should teach the child and the family to take corticosteroids properly. Be sure the child understands the possible side effects, including hunger leading to weight gain, mood changes, worsening acne, jitteriness, and insomnia. Corticosteroids may also cause hypertension, immunosuppression, growth retardation, and hyperglycemia. Caution the child and family to report these side effects. Emphasize that stopping corticosteroid administration abruptly can be dangerous.

Infection prevention is a priority nursing intervention. Children with SLE should understand the signs and symptoms of infections and be instructed to report them promptly to their health care provider. These children should also be diligent about keeping immunizations up-to-date. Children with SLE, particularly adolescents, may struggle with disturbed body image (Box 22-3 ■). This is primarily due to symptoms such as rash and alopecia. The nurse can help the child explore feelings and develop ways to manage them.

The child must be taught the importance of protecting the skin from sun exposure. The nurse can help the child understand the importance of using sunscreen daily, wearing appropriate clothing including a hat, and decreasing the time spent outdoors. The nurse must help the child with SLE and family to assess the diet to help combat growth retardation or the side effects of steroid use (including weight gain). The child's diet should include fruits and vegetables and be low in salt and sugar.

BOX 22-3 **LIFE SPAN CONSIDERATIONS**

Teens and Maculopapular Rash

The malar and maculopapular rashes of systemic lupus erythematosus can be very disturbing to children and teens. The nurse must help the child to understand that the maculopapular rash can be avoided by avoiding exposure to sunlight. The teen may need assistance with facial products that do not worsen the rash. Referral to a dermatologist may be necessary. The nurse should also assist the child or teen with SLE to voice their emotional concerns related to the appearance of their skin.

Organ Transplantation

Transplanting organs and tissues dates back to the fourth century BC, when a Chinese surgeon is said to have successfully switched the hearts of two clients. The first blood transfusion in 1667 is said to have occurred when a physician transfused the blood of a lamb into a 15-year-old boy with a malignant fever. The first human-to-human blood transfusion occurred in 1818, when a husband donated blood for his wife who was dying of blood loss following childbirth. The first bone transplant took place in 1668, when Russian scientists replaced a man's skull with that of a dog. Today, surgeons are able to transplant most major organs and tissues with human organs and tissue, animal organs and tissue, and manufactured organs. However, it is important to recognize that religious groups vary in their support of or opposition to organ donation (Box 22-4 ■). Parents might refuse to consider such surgery for their children.

ORGAN DONATION

Donors for organs and tissues can come from both living and deceased individuals, or from animals. Blood, skin, marrow, and kidneys can be donated from a living human or (in the case of skin) from the needy recipient. An **autogenous graft** is a skin graft in which skin is transplanted from one site to another site in the same recipient. A **xenograft** is an organ or tissue obtained from an animal for transplantation into a human. Major organs necessary for life, such as the heart, lung, liver, kidneys, corneas, bone, and pancreas, are harvested from individuals who are classified as brain dead and incapable of sustaining life on their own, or from recently deceased individuals. Declaration of brain death in the client is confirmed by clinical signs and medical testing. Clinical signs of brain death include diagnosis of an irreversible condition, apnea with an arterial $PaCO_2$ of at least 60 mm Hg, lack of response to deep stimuli, no spontaneous movement, lack of gag or corneal reflex, lack of oculocephalic reflex or doll's eye maneuver, and absence of toxic or metabolic disorders. Medical testing used to confirm brain death includes cerebral blood flow studies and electroencephalogram. Common causes for organ transplantation are shown in Table 22-3 ■.

Donor Screening and Donor Consent

Donors must be screened for compatibility. Individuals who abuse intravenous drugs; have severe hypertension; have preexisting infections of HIV, hepatitis B or C, syphilis, tuberculosis or septicemia; have a malignancy; and some with diabetes mellitus are not candidates for organ donation. It is best to obtain the client's consent for organ donation. However, if this is not possible because of the nature of the illness or injury, a family member can give consent for organ donation. This is emotionally easier for the family if they know the child's wishes. A donor card, provided by the

BOX 22-4   CULTURAL PULSE POINTS

Religious Beliefs Related to Organ Donation

- The **Amish** will consent to organ transplant but believe that it is God who ultimately heals.
- **Baptists** have adopted resolutions to encourage physicians to use organ transplantation to save lives and to encourage the public to be willing to donate their organs and tissues.
- **Buddhists** call organ transplantation a matter of individual conscience and an act of compassion.
- **Christian Scientists** rely on spiritual rather than medical healing. They do not have any specific statements regarding organ transplantation and consider this issue a matter of personal choice.
- **Episcopalians** promote organ and tissue transplantation and donation. The church relates this act of kindness to the life of Jesus Christ, who gave his life so that others may live.
- **Hindus** believe that organ transplantation is an individual decision and that it is ethical to use body parts to alleviate the suffering of other humans.
- **Jehovah's Witnesses** allow organ transplantation as long as all of the blood is drained from the organ or tissues prior to transplantation and any blood transfused is autologous blood, taken from the organ recipient prior to surgery.
- **Judaism** encourages organ transplantation. In 1992, the Rabbinical Council of America (Orthodox) stated that the pikuach nefest, an ancient requirement to save lives if possible, promotes organ donation despite Jewish laws that forbid mutilation of the body.
- **Lutheran** doctrine states that organ donation is a humanitarian act and an expression of sacrificial love for one's neighbor.
- **Roman Catholics** consider organ transplantation an act of charity. In 1990, Pope John Paul II made a statement in favor of organ donation in the form of living tissues or from those who are deceased.
- **Seventh-Day Adventists** strongly promote organ transplantation and the religion runs transplant hospitals. One example is Loma Linda University Medical Center in Southern California, which specializes in pediatric heart transplantation.
- **United Methodists** encourage organ donation and transplantation. Their 1992 resolution further states that prior to harvesting the organs, death must be determined by a reliable source and there should be no measure to hasten death. The religious organization encourages their pastors to discuss organ donation as a routine part of their hospice care.

TABLE 22-3

Common Causes for Organ Transplantation

ORGAN TRANSPLANTED	COMMON CAUSES
Heart and heart valves	Coronary artery disease, cardiomyopathy, valvular disease, congenital defects, viral infections
Intestine	Short bowel syndrome, Crohn's disease, inflammatory bowel disease, congenital defects, trauma
Kidney	Diabetes, hypertension, renal failure
Liver	Hepatitis C, alcoholism
Lung	Cystic fibrosis, primary pulmonary hypertension, idiopathic pulmonary fibrosis, chronic obstructive pulmonary disease
Pancreas	Type I diabetes
Blood	Surgery, trauma, burns, incompatibility such as Rh factor
Bone, tendons, marrow, stem cells	Cancer, arthritis, trauma. Marrow is used for sickle cell anemia, aplastic anemia, leukemia, Hodgkin's disease, lymphoma
Cornea	Corneal damage, keratoconus
Skin	Burns, trauma, cancer, foot ulcers due to diabetes
Arteries and veins	Atherosclerosis, trauma, aneurysms

Nursing Considerations

The recipient of organ donation requires careful preoperative and postoperative care. Preoperatively the child will need to be evaluated physically and emotionally to determine their level of readiness of the surgery. Children often are very direct in their questions. Table 22-4 ■ provides possible nursing responses to common questions children might ask. Most of these families have been waiting a long time for an organ to become available. They may be so excited that an organ has been found that they fail to consider that the organ may not function properly. Immunosuppressive drugs may be required to suppress the immune response and prevent rejection of the organ. Immunosuppressive agents are usually used in combination,

hospital or found at an organ donation website, can communicate the child's wishes concerning organ donation.

Living donors, those donating organs such as kidneys, need psychological care to determine if they are emotionally stable enough to donate the organ. It must be documented that they understand the associated risks. Follow-up care is also important to assist the donor in coping with feelings of fear and isolation during physical recovery.

TABLE 22-4

Questions a Child Might Ask About Organ Transplantation

QUESTION	NURSING RESPONSE
What is a transplant?	A transplant is a surgery to take out your old, diseased organ and replace it with a healthy one.
Why do I need a new organ?	Your (heart, lung, kidney, etc.) is not working right. To keep you from getting sicker, you need a new organ.
Where do these organs come from?	Some organs that are transplanted come from a friend or family member or even a stranger. These organs are ones that the person can live without. Some organs come from people who have died and have asked that their organs be used to help others.
Will I live at the hospital while I'm waiting for my organ?	No, you can live at home while you wait for the right organ to help you. You may have to get to the hospital quickly, though, when there is an organ found for you.
Will my life be better after the transplant?	Most children who have a transplant will get better soon. Right after the surgery you will need to take medicine and rest. Soon you should be able to go back to school. Your family and your doctor will keep a close watch over you.

and the regime varies according to the agency and the type of organ to be transplanted. The child's physical condition is documented through a variety of medical and laboratory tests. The nurse also helps maintain the carefully controlled environment that is used to protect the organ recipient from exposure to microorganisms.

Postoperative care also includes both emotional and physical care. Some research studies have linked organ transplantation with posttraumatic stress syndrome for both the parents and recipients of organ donation. Fear of rejection of the organ is a common concern among organ recipients. Following surgery, the nurse will be responsible for evaluating the return and maintenance of the function of the organ that was transplanted. For instance, the child who was a recipient of a kidney should be evaluated for urinary function and fluid and electrolyte balance. The child who was a recipient of a heart should be evaluated for cardiac status.

Rejection of the transplanted organ is a major issue in the postoperative period. The rejection can occur immediately, within minutes or hours, or within days or months. The nurse must constantly monitor for signs of rejection.

clinical ALERT

Signs of rejection include laboratory values outside of the normal range and lack of improvement of clinical symptoms related to the disease process prior to surgery.

Rejection may require removal of the transplanted organ or additional immunosuppressive therapy. Infection is also a particular hazard following organ transplantation therapy. The nurse must be diligent in observing for clinical symptoms of infection and reporting them promptly.

Allergies

An **allergy** is an altered reaction to an antigen or allergen. Common allergens include pet fur, cockroaches, cow's milk, dust, egg whites, medications, mites, mold, pollen, peanuts, seafood, shellfish, soy, tree nuts, and wheat. Reactions to an allergen do not occur until a repeated exposure takes place.

Manifestations

Clinical manifestations of allergies can be mild (Figure 22-6 ■), severe, or life threatening. Table 22-5 ■ outlines the type of reactions.

Diagnosis

Careful history taking is required to assist the diagnosis of allergies. Intradermal skin testing (Figure 22-7 ■) can be done to identify specific antigens. Food allergens can be identified by removing foods one at a time and observing for the allergic reaction. Once the allergen or allergens is identified, the allergen must be avoided.

Treatment

Oral antihistamines can be administered to decrease the symptoms of allergic reactions. If the child is allergic to medications, desensitization may allow the child to take medications that may be necessary for treatment of diseases. **Desensitization** is the process of administering doses of medication in increasing increments in an effort to avoid the allergic reaction. For example, penicillin is a medication that causes frequent allergic reactions in children. Penicillin is necessary for treatment of several infections. Desensitization may allow the child to be

A

B

Figure 22-6. ■ (**A**) Inflammation of the skin caused by the metal salts in jewelry. (**B**) Inflammation of the lip caused by allergic reaction to peanuts. (**A.** Biophoto Associates/Photo Researchers, Inc. **B.** Photo Researchers Inc.)

treated with penicillin when they encounter certain infections.

Nursing Considerations

The nurse can be instrumental in providing the child and the family with assistance in how to avoid allergens.

Figure 22-7. ■ Skin testing to determine the source of allergic reaction. (Phototake NYC).

CHILD WITH LIFE-THREATENING ALLERGIES

This may require removing pets from the home, controlling dust, placing plastic covers on beds and pillows, removing carpet, using high-efficiency air filters, and controlling and removing mold. The child who is allergic to bee or wasp stings must understand the use of premeasured, single-dose epinephrine or EpiPen (Figure 22-8 ■). A prescription is required and the EpiPen should be available at school, day care, and home. The nurse can teach the child to use the EpiPen properly. The child should also understand the care of the EpiPen. Care of the EpiPen includes storing it out of direct sunlight or extreme temperatures and

MediaLink Allergic Rhinitis

TABLE 22-5

Types of Allergic Reactions

TYPES	EXAMPLES	OCCURS	CLINICAL MANIFESTATIONS
Type I—localized or systemic	Hay fever, pet fur, insect bite	Within seconds or minutes of exposure	Rhinitis, sneezing, **urticaria** (hives), wheezing, vomiting, diarrhea, anaphylaxis
Type II—tissue specific	Reaction to blood transfusion, hemolytic disease of the newborn	Within 15 to 30 minutes of exposure	Symptoms vary but include fever and dyspnea
Type III—immune complex	Serum sickness, acute glomerulonephritis	Within 6 hours of exposure	Urticaria, fever, joint pain
Type IV—delayed	Tuberculin skin test, contact dermatitis, allograft tissue rejection	Within several hours after exposure	Symptoms vary but include fever, erythema, pruritus

Figure 22-8. ■ Parents and older children need instruction in use of the EpiPen, which should be carried with the child at all times. (Pearson Education/PH College).

checking the expiration date frequently. See Table 22-6 ■ for communicating with families with children who have life-threatening allergies.

LATEX ALLERGY

Latex allergy is an IgE-mediated response to repeated exposure to latex. (IgE is a type of immunoglobulin that is primarily responsible for allergic reactions.) Reactions to latex can be type I (local or systemic) or type IV (delayed hypersensitivity). Clients who have sensitivities/allergies to bananas, avocados, potatoes, chestnuts, and tropical fruits can also be at risk for developing an allergy to latex. Latex can be found in several health care products such as gloves, drains, adhesives, and catheters. Fortunately, nonlatex products are available. Latex substitutes must be used when the allergy is identified.

Immunotherapy

Immunotherapy is the prevention and treatment of disease using the administration of allergens, immunostimulants, immunosuppressants, interferon, and immune globulin. Immune globulin can be given IM or IV. Both of these routes can be useful when treating children following exposure to diseases such as hepatitis A or B, rubella, rubeola, and varicella. It is also useful in treating Kawasaki's syndrome (see Chapter 13 ○○), AIDS, and idiopathic thrombocytopenic purpura (see Chapter 14 ○○).

Children should be carefully assessed for hypersensitivity reaction or infusion reaction. Manifestations of hypersensitivity reaction and infusion reaction are listed in Box 22-5 ■.

BOX 22-5 | **ASSESSMENT**

Hypersensitivity Reaction and Infusion Reaction

Hypersensitivity Reaction
Hypersensitivity reaction is characterized by fever, chills, and **anaphylactic shock** (a systemic reaction to an allergen that occurs within minutes or up to 2 hours after exposure). Anaphylaxis is characterized by itching, hives, soft-tissue edema (such as swelling of lips and tongue), cough, dyspnea, pallor, perspiration, and tachycardia. These symptoms, if not treated promptly, can lead to respiratory distress and death.

Infusion Reaction
Infusion reaction is characterized by nausea, flushing, chills, headache, chest tightness, wheezing, skeletal and back pain, abdominal cramps, and anaphylaxis. The nurse monitors the client carefully during infusion of blood products. Infusion is stopped immediately if any signs of infusion reaction appear.

TABLE 22-6

Communicating Across the Life Span: Child with Life-threatening Allergies

	TODDLER	PRESCHOOLER	SCHOOL-AGE CHILD	ADOLESCENT
Nurse	To the parent: Everyone who cares for your child must be observant and watch for situations in which the child can get stung by a bee or wasp. The caregivers will also have to know how to administer epinephrine.	To the parent: You will need to purchase several EpiPens. Keep one in the car, one in your purse or backpack, one in the office at the day care, and one that can be packed when the child spends the night away from home at his grandmother's.	To the child: Let's review how to give yourself an injection with the EpiPen. Why don't you try it here on this orange? Do you know when you should give yourself this shot?	To the teen: You should be able to do any outdoor activity. Your allergy should not prevent you from camping or boating and hiking. Just be sure to carry your EpiPen with you.
Client/Parent	I don't feel comfortable teaching them. Can I bring them to the office and let you teach them how to give the shot?	Can you check to see if my insurance company will pay for these? Do they last forever, or will I need to check the expiration date?	I should give myself this shot immediately when a bee or wasp stings me.	That's a relief. I thought I'd be stuck inside the rest of my life.

NURSING CARE

PRIORITIES IN NURSING CARE

When caring for children with immune disorders, nursing care should be focused on gathering a thorough history of the child's condition. This is especially important when determining what allergen is causing the allergic reaction. Preventing infection through the use of aseptic and sterile technique and reverse isolation is important for the child with HIV/AIDS and organ transplantation. Children with JRA are often in pain and therefore intolerant to activity. The nurse should provide comfort measures and assistance with activities of daily living. Long-term illnesses such as HIV/AIDS, conditions requiring organ transplant, and JRA are emotionally taxing on both the children and their families. The nurse must encourage the expression of feelings and concerns related to the disease process and the healthcare required.

ASSESSING

In children with immune disorders, the nurse collects data about signs and symptoms of infection including fever, decreased breath sounds, fatigue, and skin irritation or lesions. Nutritional status, height and weight (see Procedures 8-7 and 8-8 ⬤⬤ ; see also Chapter 7 ⬤⬤) will give the nurse an indication of the child's general condition. Following organ transplantation, the nurse observes for signs and symptoms of organ rejection. For the child with JRA, joint mobility and joint pain are checked and recorded. The nurse must also assess the caregiver for signs and symptoms of role strain. Manifestations of role strain include physical symptoms of GI upset, headaches and insomnia; emotional symptoms of stress, anger and anxiety; and socioeconomic symptoms of withdrawal from social activities and diminished work productivity.

DIAGNOSING, PLANNING, AND IMPLEMENTING

Possible nursing diagnoses for children with immune disorders include:

- Imbalanced **N**utrition: Less than Body Requirements related to chronic immune disorders
- Impaired **S**kin Integrity related to altered immune status
- Delayed **D**evelopment related to physical disability and chronic immune disorder
- **A**ctivity Intolerance related to chronic pain
- Risk for **I**nfection related to suppressed immune system
- Risk for **C**aregiver Role Strain related to stress concerning child's immune disorder

Outcomes for children with immune disorders include that the child will:

- Maintain weight and body mass WNL.
- Demonstrate intact skin and mucous membranes.
- Achieve milestones related to physical, cognitive, and psychosocial development as expected.
- Participate in physical activity within symptoms of intolerance.
- Be free of symptoms of infection

The caregiver will:

- Demonstrate balance in providing care to the child.

Nursing interventions for children who have immune disorders include the following actions:

- Provide small frequent meals with items that are pleasing to the child. *Smaller meals are tolerated better. The child will be more likely to eat if offered a choice of foods.*
- Create a pleasant environment for mealtime. *The environment is essential for the child to enjoy their food and maintain adequate intake.*
- Protect the skin from injury by frequent position changes, pressure-reducing mattress and clean, wrinkle-free linens. *These measures reduce pressure and friction and therefore protect skin integrity.*
- Encourage ambulation as tolerated, including passive and active ROM exercises. *These measures will increase circulation and muscle tone and also strengthen muscles and joints.*
- Offer age-appropriate toys. *The correct toys will stimulate appropriate development.*
- Conduct and document frequent assessment of the child's developmental level. *This strategy will allow caregivers to intervene quickly if developmental delays are noted.*
- Refer and support the use of physical therapy. *This service will assist the child in maintaining joint function and preventing contractures.*
- Assist with activities of daily living, being careful to encourage the child's continued participation. *Assistance will help the child avoid fatigue. Continued participation will aid in building muscle strength and activity tolerance.*
- Provide protection from individuals who have current infections. *Children with immune disorders need protection from infections.*
- Follow universal precautions and proper hand washing techniques. *Provides protection from nosocomial infections.*
- Encourage family members to express feelings and concerns. *Expression of feelings will assist with decreasing anxiety.*
- Refer family members to community resources. *Additional support services can relieve some of the caregiver's burden.*

EVALUATING

The child with immune disorders should be evaluated for adequate nutritional status, skin integrity, appropriate growth and development, tolerance to activity, and risk for infection. Caregivers who manage the care of children with immune disorders should be evaluated for excessive stress and ineffective coping.

NURSING PROCESS CARE PLAN
Child with an Organ Transplant

Riley, age 4, is diagnosed with cardiomyopathy. She is awaiting transplantation of a heart. Her mother is concerned because her sister's son, who is also 4, speaks using short sentences and loves to skip and hop. Riley uses short phrases to communicate and can walk well, but doesn't skip or hop. Riley's mother wants to know if she should be worried.

Assessment. The following data should be collected as soon as possible:

- Perform a developmental screening to determine Riley's developmental level in each of the following areas: physical, gross motor, fine motor, language, socialization, cognition, and family relationship.
- Determine Riley's mother's knowledge related to developmental levels.
- Determine Riley's mother's expectations for Riley's future.

Nursing Diagnosis. The following important nursing diagnosis (among others) is established for this client:

- Risk for Delayed **D**evelopment related to chronic illness (cardiomyopathy)

Expected Outcomes

- Riley will achieve developmental milestones in each of the following areas: physical, gross motor, fine motor, language, socialization, cognition and family relationship.

Planning and Implementation

- Instruct Riley's parents about normal development of the 4-year-old child. *Knowledge of developmental milestones will keep Riley's parents expectations of achievements appropriate.*
- Teach them activities to promote normal development. *Knowledge of these activities can help them encourage developmental achievements.*
- Suggest age-appropriate toys. *Toys that are developmentally correct will encourage achievement of milestones.*
- Encourage Riley's parents to promote normal development despite her illness. *Enforces the importance of developmental growth.*
- Assist Riley's parents in establishing a method for positive rewards and feedback when Riley accomplishes developmental milestones. *Rewards and feedback serve as methods of encouragement.*
- Suggest a follow-up plan to monitor Riley's developmental progress. *Riley's progress and parental participation should be monitored to evaluate the current plan of care and make appropriate changes.*

Evaluation. Riley and her parents implement a plan to monitor and promote her developmental progress. They have implemented activities to encourage Riley in motor skills, language, socialization and cognition. Spending specific time together promotes family relationships as well. They are keeping monthly pediatric visits to monitor their success.

Critical Thinking in the Nursing Process

1. Develop a plan for promoting Riley's motor skills.
2. Develop a plan for promoting Riley's language skills.
3. List at least five toys that will aid in promoting Riley's developmental progress.

Note: Discussion of Critical Thinking questions appears in Appendix I.

Note: The reference and resource listings for this and all chapters have been compiled at the back of the book.

Chapter Review

 KEY TERMS by Topic

Use the audio glossary feature of either the CD-ROM or the Companion Website to hear the correct pronunciation of the following key terms.

Anatomy and Physiology
antigens, antibodies, immune response, natural immunity, acquired immunity, humoral immunity, immunoglobulins, primary immune response, secondary immune response, cell-mediated immunity, active immunity, passive immunity

HIV and AIDS
oral candidiasis, thrush

Juvenile Rheumatoid Arthritis
autoimmune, lymphadenopathy, splenomegaly, hepatomegaly

Organ Transplantation
autogenous graft, xenograft

Allergies
allergy, urticaria, desensitization

Immunotherapy
anaphylactic shock

KEY Points

- The primary role of the immune system is to recognize and eliminate foreign substances.

- There are two types of immunity: natural and acquired.

- The child can contract HIV via the placenta during pregnancy, by exposure at birth, or through breast milk. The adolescent can be exposed to the virus by sexual contact.

- The child who develops AIDS is immunocompromised. The nurse must be diligent in assisting children and their families in preventing infections.

- Both JRA and SLE cause inflammation and therefore discomfort and pain in affected children. The nurse must assist the child in maintaining mobility and preventing pain.

- Corticosteroid therapy is commonly prescribed for treatment of SLE. The side effects of these medications include hunger leading to weight gain, mood changes, worsening acne, jitteriness, insomnia, hypertension, immunosuppression, growth retardation, and hyperglycemia.

- Kidneys, hearts, bone marrow, tissues, corneas, and other organs can be transplanted in children. The nurse can assist in preparing the child for organ transplantation and providing postoperative care to prevent rejection of the organ.

- Common allergies in children include pet fur, cockroaches, cow's milk, dust, egg whites, medications, mites, mold, pollen, peanuts, seafood, shellfish, soy, tree nuts, and wheat.

- Careful history taking is required to assist the diagnosis of allergies.

- Anaphylactic shock is a systemic reaction to an allergen that occurs within minutes or up to 2 hours after exposure. Anaphylaxis is characterized by itching, *urticaria* (hives), soft-tissue edema, cough, dyspnea, pallor, perspiration, and tachycardia. These symptoms, if not treated promptly, can lead to respiratory distress and death.

 EXPLORE Media Link

Additional interactive resources for this chapter can be found on the Companion Website at www.prenhall.com/adams.

Click on Chapter 22 and "Begin" to select the activities for this chapter.

For chapter-related NCLEX®-style questions and an audio glossary, access the accompanying CD-ROM in this book.

Animations:

HIV

HIV/AIDS

Allergic rhinitis

FOR FURTHER Study

For a nutritional assessment and childhood immunization, see Chapter 6.

See Chapter 7 for care of the hospitalized or chronically ill child.

Nutritional status, height assessment, and weight assessment are provided in Procedures 8-7 and 8-8.

See Chapter 10 for information on infectious diseases.

Kawasaki's syndrome is discussed in Chapter 13.

For instructions for palpating lymph nodes, and for further discussion on AIDS and idiopathic thrombocytopenic purpura, see Chapter 14.

Candidiasis is discussed with vaginitis in Chapter 18.

Skin lesions are discussed further in Chapter 21.

See Appendix II for the childhood immunization schedule.

Critical Thinking Care Map

Caring for a Client with AIDS
NCLEX-PN® Focus Area: Safety and Infection

Case Study: Joe, age 15, recently had two positive polymerase chain reaction tests and was told that he was HIV positive. The condition and its implications were explained to Joe by the nurse. The nurse's teaching focused on preventing infection, promoting nutritional health, and providing knowledge about the disease process and the prescribed treatment. Immediately following the nurse's discussion, Joe said he wanted to continue going to high school and was sure that his friends weren't at risk for contracting the virus.

Nursing Diagnosis: Risk for Infection related to immunocompromised status

COLLECT DATA

Subjective	Objective
_____	_____
_____	_____
_____	_____
_____	_____
_____	_____
_____	_____

Would you report this? Yes/No

If yes, to: _____

Nursing Care

_____
_____
_____
_____
_____
_____
_____
_____
_____

How would you document this? _____
_____
_____
_____

Compare your documentation to the sample provided in Appendix I.

Data Collected
(use only those that apply)

- Note anxious behaviors such as wringing hands and pacing
- "I feel really tired."
- Lab results to include CBC, blood or wound cultures, serum protein and albumin
- "I'm very strict about my diet. It is low fat and low calorie."
- Intake and output
- Weight
- "I really don't like to take medicine. Can't I just take it when I think about it?"
- Skin turgor
- "My best friend has the flu."
- Vital signs
- "I'd feel like a nerd if I wore that mask to school."
- Skin assessment for wounds and wound drainage.

Nursing Interventions
(use only those that apply; list in priority order)

- Refer Joe to a nutritionist to plan an alternative diet.
- Instruct Joe in hand washing and other techniques to avoid contamination with harmful bacteria or viruses.
- Monitor intake and output by encouraging Joe to keep a food and fluid diary.
- Monitor Joe's weight at follow-up visits to determine nutritional status.
- Make frequent follow-up appointments with Joe to monitor lab values.
- Teach Joe and his parents to recognize symptoms of infections, colds, and flu in himself, family members, friends, or others he may come in contact with.
- Teach Joe about the long-term effects of life as an HIV-positive client.
- Use a pretest and posttest to determine Joe's level of understanding of his diagnosis and treatment regime.
- Make sure Joe and his parents understand the proper handling, storage, and preparation of food.
- Review immunization schedule and recommend required immunizations as appropriate.

TEST-TAKING TIP The process of elimination often gives a clue to the correct answer. If the question asks for one answer only, and if three of the answers are similar, the correct answer is likely to be the one dissimilar option.

1 A nurse is assigned to care for an adolescent with a latex allergy diagnosis. The nurse is taking the client's history and in order to determine the client's risk factors associated with latex allergies asks about an allergy to which foods? Choose all that apply

1. Cheese
2. Potatoes
3. Milk
4. Avocadoes
5. Yogurt
6. Bananas

2 The nurse is working at a health care clinic and is scheduled to give immunizations today. The nurse knows that the immunizations provide:

1. Protection from all communicable diseases.
2. Natural immunity from diseases.
3. Nonhumoral immunity from diseases.
4. Acquired immunity from diseases.

3 A young mother who is HIV positive has followed all of the recommended prenatal precautions and has just delivered a female child by cesarean section. After the infant is examined, the physician states that the infant has no outward symptoms of HIV. The nurse realizes the mother needs more education about the possibility of HIV transmission to her infant when she states:

1. "I know there is still the potential my child will have HIV."
2. "I will be breastfeeding my infant since she does not appear to have HIV."
3. "I realize we all must learn to wash our hands before and after caring for the baby."
4. "I understand my baby will be treated with AZT to reduce the risk of HIV transmission."

4 A 10-year-old child has been diagnosed with juvenile rheumatoid arthritis (JRA). The nurse realizes this is a chronic autoimmune disorder that causes joint inflammation. What symptom listed below is not associated with this disease?

1. Fever
2. Rash
3. Lymphadenopathy
4. Rhinitis

5 The type of immunity that protects the child against bacteria, viruses, fungi, and tumors and which is also responsible for the process that causes rejection of organs that have been transplanted is called:

1. Primary immunity
2. Lymph-mediated immunity
3. Acquired immunity
4. cell-mediated immunity

6 The nurse is caring for a pediatric client after a kidney transplant. The nurse knows this client has the potential for organ rejection and monitors the following closely:

1. Urinary function, fluid and electrolyte balance
2. Cardiac function, range of motion and edema
3. $PaCO_2$ more than 60 mm Hg, respirations more than 30
4. Thrombophlebitis and periorbital edema

7 In a pediatric clinic the mother of a 3-month-old child tells the nurse the child doesn't gain weight, has constant ear infections, fever, mouth infection (oral candidiasis), and diarrhea. On examination, the physician confirms that the child also has hepatosplenomegaly. The nurse suspects the child has a diagnosis of:

1. Juvenile rheumatoid arthritis
2. Latex allergies
3. Human immunodeficiency virus (HIV)
4. Chronic otitis media

8 The nurse realizes the following nursing interventions should be instituted for a child with a suspected diagnosis of HIV:

1. Avoidance of infection and proper nutrition
2. Antibiotic therapy and careful skin care
3. Exercise regime and range of motion
4. Administration of oral antihistamines and penicillin

9 The nurse is attempting to explain humoral immunity to a child's mother who has inquired about her child's ability to fight off illness during a well-baby visit to the clinic. The nurse tells the mother the following about humoral immunity so the mother will understand:

1. "Humoral immunity is present at birth and protects the child from everything."
2. "Humoral immunity occurs after the age of 10."
3. "Humoral immunity destroys bacteria, viruses, and allergens."
4. "Humoral immunity takes place at the same time as puberty."

10 You are caring for an adolescent with a known sensitivity to latex. In preparing for his care, you select nursing interventions to care for this client to prevent an allergic response to latex. Choose all that apply.

1. Use only nonlatex gloves.
2. Remove all latex materials from the room.
3. Use medications that are stored in glass.
4. Use only manual blood pressure cuffs.
5. Noninvasive latex products can be kept in the room.
6. A latex-free cart should be kept in or near the client's room.

Answers for NCLEX-PN® Review and Critical Thinking questions appear in Appendix I.

Thinking Strategically About...

You are employed by a pediatrician. Your responsibilities include obtaining client health histories, taking vital signs, weighing and measuring clients, vision and hearing screening, obtaining lab specimens, administering medications, assisting in procedures, and providing client teaching and discharge instructions. Today, there are 18 children scheduled.

CASE 1 SCENARIO

The first client of the day is Jeremy. He is 12 years old. He weighs 120 lb and is 5 ft tall. His vital signs are T 98.6, P 62, R 16, BP 106/76. Jeremy's mother relates that he is frequently fatigued. He is thirsty all the time, even during the night. He is also urinating many times a day and is always hungry. A review of the family history reveals that Jeremy's father has type I diabetes mellitus.

After conferring with the physician, you obtain a urine specimen and a blood specimen. A reagent strip is used to test the urine for glucose. The urine test is positive for glucose. Blood glucose reveals 210 mg/dL.

CRITICAL THINKING

Jeremy's mother tells you she just doesn't know what to do about her son and she is very worried. When considering the Essential Intellectual Traits (Box 2-3 🔗), determine which trait applies to Jeremy's mother's current level of thinking.

The test results reveal that Jeremy does have diabetes mellitus. You are responsible for teaching Jeremy to self-administer his insulin, but he is afraid of "shots." What measures could you take to minimize the pain of injections?

COLLABORATIVE CARE

Jeremy and his parents will need to adjust his diet in order to manage his disease appropriately. Describe the report of Jeremy's condition you will give when you contact the nutritionist.

Jeremy's mother is concerned about how she will manage Jeremy's care and keep him healthy. What resources would you want to suggest to Jeremy's mother?

CASE 2 SCENARIO

Jackson, 4 years old, is admitted to the pediatric unit with a diagnosis of gastroenteritis. For the past 48 hours, Jackson has been vomiting and having diarrhea. He has been unable to keep any food or beverage down. Over the past few hours, he has been irritable and sleepy. You take his vital signs and review his admission orders. The physician orders an electrolyte profile, complete blood count, and urinalysis. He also orders an IV of D5 ½ NS to infuse at 1,000 mL in 8 hours,

daily weight, and full liquid diet. Phenergan 12.5 mg, rectal suppository every 4 hours is ordered for nausea.

DATA COLLECTED

Jackson's admission vital signs are T 99.9, P 110, R 18, BP 90/60. Skin turgor is poor. Hematocrit is increased. Urine-specific gravity is increased. Current weight: 45 lb.

DELEGATING

Which of the previous orders could be delegated to the certified nursing assistant?

MANAGEMENT OF CARE

Calculate the infusion rate for the previous order using a drop factor of 10 drops/mL.

COMMUNICATION AND CLIENT TEACHING

Jackson improves and is ready for discharge. His mother asks the nurse what foods are appropriate if Jackson should have a stomach virus again. Develop a teaching plan to provide this nutritional information.

CASE 3 SCENARIO

Janice is a 17-year-old who is admitted to the emergency room following a motor vehicle crash. Janice has facial abrasions and a fractured right clavicle. She is being evaluated for an abdominal injury due to the impact of the seatbelt.

DATA COLLECTED

Janice is oriented to person, time, and place. She complains of shoulder and abdominal pain, 6 on a scale of 10. She is able to move the fingers of her right hand. The abrasions are not actively bleeding. Vital signs include T 98.6, P 110 and thready, R 14, BP 100/70. Her skin is pale and moist. Her bowel sounds are decreased in all four quadrants.

TIME MANAGEMENT AND PRIORITIES IN NURSING CARE

List in order the nursing interventions that need to be implemented for Janice.

DOCUMENTING AND REPORTING

What findings about Janice are important to document? Which are important to report to the physician?

CULTURAL CARE STRATEGIES

Janice's admission information reveals she is a Jehovah's Witness. How will this affect care management? What strategies are appropriate if she needs blood replacement?

Appendix I
Answers and Critical Thinking Discussion

Chapter 1

NCLEX-PN® ANSWERS

(1) 3. Outcome 4. Primary nursing care encompasses prevention activities, such as scoliosis screening. A sprained leg is also an existing condition so care is not preventive. Diabetes monitoring is tertiary care for an ongoing condition. An eye infection is an existing condition, so is not primary care. (2) 4. Outcome 4. Tertiary care is the management of chronic, long-term health care problems such as clients with permanent tracheostomies. Antibiotic therapy is often used for acute conditions, so this is not correct. Monitoring hematocrit is a primary (preventive) action in pregnancy. (3) 1, 2, 3. Outcome 5. While the role of the LPN/LVN varies from state to state, generally administering PO meds, supervising UAP, and collecting data are allowable. Some states do not allow LPNs to administer blood or blood products. LPNs/LVNs contribute data toward the nursing diagnoses but the RN develops them. (4) 1. Outcome 2. The statement "Your child will go home to complete recovery as soon as she is stable, so it is important for you to know about wound care." is correct. Children recuperate more quickly in their home environments, so they are sent home as soon as their condition is stable. Parents are educated to take care of their children and to be aware of signs of complications. "Your child will go home 2 weeks after surgery; this will give us time to watch the wound heal" reflects an outdated attitude from when children were kept in the hospital for longer periods of time. "We will keep your child here until we are sure there will be no complications" again reflects the attitude that the child must stay in the hospital until completely recovered. "If the wound is puffy, red, and warm to the touch when you are changing the dressing at home, lance it with a sterilized sewing needle," suggests that the parent would not only watch for complications, but also treat them; this is incorrect. (5) 2. Outcome 2. The LPN/LVN who uses the term *client* believes that this term reflects those who are active participants in their own care. Therefore the statement "My client would like to ask the doctor some questions now" is correct. "My patient in room 212 needs something for pain" is incorrect because this reflects the belief that the person is ill and in need of others to make decisions. "Don't worry, the doctor will be able to make decisions for you" is incorrect because it does not support the belief that clients are active participants in their own care.

The statement "I will help the teenage mother in the next room feed her baby" is incorrect because the term *client* should be used to describe people who are active participants in their own care. (6) 5, 8, 2, 7, 1, 4, 3, 6. Outcome 4. The following steps are the correct order for implementing research into practice. 1. Review current literature. 2. Gather data that provides rationales for a proposed change in practice. 3. Create a presentation presenting the risks and benefits to support a change in practice. 4. Develop clinical practice guidelines and a time frame for possible implementation. 5. Develop a plan to evaluate client outcomes. 6. Invite practitioners and administrators to discuss the proposed new practice guidelines. 7. Document approved changes to the clinical guidelines. 8. Publish positive client outcomes relating to the new clinical practice guidelines. (7) 1. Outcome 5. To function in the role of an LPN/LVN, every LPN/LVN should be knowledgeable of his or her own individual state's nurse practice acts. The Association of Women's Health, Obstetric and Neonatal Nurses is incorrect because it is not a governing body to authorize practice for LPNs/LVNs. The Nurse's Association of the American College of Obstetricians and Gynecologists is incorrect because it does not authorize practice for LPNs/LVNs. The American Nurses Association is incorrect because it is not a governing body to authorize practice for LPNs/LVNs. (8) 2. Outcome 5. Prioritizing care is part of the LPN/LVN role. It is correct for the nurse to place priority on a child receiving oxygen for croup. This situation is an assessment of airway, which is the top priority in nursing care. Acrocyanosis is quite normal in a 1-hour-old newborn and is not life-threatening. Although the 7-year-old in Buck's traction could be experiencing circulation problems, this priority still falls beneath airway assessment. Jaundice in a 2-day-old newborn is quite common and is not a top priority. (9) 2. Outcome 5. Contacting the nursing supervisor first is correct because the LPN/LVN is responsible for informing the RN if any changes occur in the health status of the client. Contacting the unlicensed assistive personnel is incorrect because UAP do not make decisions for client care. The child's father may be contacted, but this is not the first contact. The pediatrician may be notified, but not initially. (10) 3. Outcome 5. Teaches the client about reasonable expectations for toilet training is correct because health promotion teaching is an important role for the LPN/LVN. Establishing a nursing diagnosis for a client recovering from surgery for umbilical hernia is incorrect because LPN/LVNs only assist RNs in writing and updating nursing diagnoses. Independently planning care for clients in the home setting is the role of the RN. Only physicians and advanced practice nurses prescribe medications.

CARE PLAN HINTS

1. Parents may object to immunizations because of philosophical or religious reasons. They may also have some concerns about governmental control over their health. They may believe that immunizations are not safe, or they may desire to have an all-natural approach to their health care.
2. In the 1900s polio was epidemic and frequently resulted in paralysis or death. A vaccine for polio was introduced in 1951. By 1967, polio was reduced by 99% and by 1991 it was eradicated from the Western hemisphere.
3. Once proper teaching has been done, the decision to vaccinate is in the parent's hands. If the family refused immunizations, the nurse would need to provide additional teaching on disease recognition and reporting. The family should be treated with respect.

Chapter 2

NCLEX-PN® ANSWERS

(1) 3. Outcomes 5 and 6. Application of a fetal scalp electrode is a clinical skill not taught in a basic nursing education course. In many states, it is not an allowable skill for the LPN. Reporting to the RN is the best response. Response 4 is rude and does not promote collaborative care. (2) 4. Outcome 6. Right supervision includes the tasks of monitoring, evaluating, intervening when necessary, and providing feedback, if appropriate. The decision about the right task is made before delegation occurs. The decision about the right circumstances is made earlier. The decision about the right direction is made before teaching the person the task. (3) 4. Outcome 6. Delegation is transferring to a competent individual the authority to perform a nursing task. Only the CNA with experience meets these criteria. An inexperienced person should not be given this task. An experienced person with diabetes is not the appropriate choice if the person is not on staff. The client's husband probably would know the procedure but is not on staff. (4) 3. Outcome 6. Insulin is a drug that is regulated by some nurse practice acts to be a task designated for the registered nurse. The UAP should never give medications or directly contact the physician without notification of the LPN. The client's husband, in an acute care setting, should not be given the task of administering medication. (5) 2. Outcome 6. The CNA has incorrectly instructed the client regarding collection of a 24-hour urine specimen. It is the responsibility of the supervising LPN to review the procedure with her to ensure that she can perform it correctly next time. The CNA would not be praised; the first voided specimen is discarded. The CNA needs instruction, not reassignment. The CNA would not receive a raise. (6) 1. Outcome 4. Relevance is correct; it is important for the LPN/LVN to collect as much information about the client to determine what is relevant (such as backache, because it is important to rule out serious injury or infection). Clarity is incorrect because it is used to eliminate confusion by gathering more information. Accuracy is incorrect because it refers to the correctness of the data being examined. Precision is incorrect because it searches for the exactness of the data to determine precise information. (7) Deductive. Outcome 4. Deductive reasoning allows the nurse to take a statement about a client (child with stomachache) and to realize that certain conditions may accompany the stomachache: nausea, viral symptoms, or constipation. (8) 3. Outcome 3. Implications of actions is correct; the LPN/LVN exercises sound judgment by considering the consequences of the action prior to providing care. Point of view is incorrect; this refers to the LPN/LVN considering different perspectives of a situation versus the effects of the actions. Assumptions is incorrect. Assumptions refer to ideas that are taken for granted. Concepts is incorrect; this allows the LPN/LVN to use theories and laws from other disciplines to understand nursing problems. (9) 2, 3 and 5. Outcome 4. Statements that reflect the use of clarity as an intellectual standard to assist the nurse in verifying accuracy in order to clarify a problem are: "How would you describe the sensation you feel?" Give me an example of how it feels." "Tell me more about your pain." The statement "Could you be more specific about the type of pain you have?" is incorrect because it is an example of precision. Precision helps gain scientific exactness for precise information. The statement, "Are there any related factors that might contribute to your pain?" strives for depth, not clarity. (10) 2. Outcome 5. Proper training has not been completed by the LPN/LVN is correct. The LPN/LVN must be trained on all new equipment prior to use, and the training must be documented in the LPN's/LVN's file. Unlicensed assistive personnel can hang the fluids is incorrect; only licensed personnel can hang IV fluids. Only RNs can hang IV fluids is incorrect, since LPNs/LVNs are also licensed to hang IV fluids. Certified nursing assistants is incorrect; they are not licensed to hang IV fluids.

CRITICAL THINKING CARE MAP

Subjective Data   Mother states infant rarely hungry

Objective Data   Decreased urine output (4 diapers daily when typical should be 6 to 8). Dry mucous membranes. Lethargy. Intake of 5 ounces every 5 to 6 hours.

Report   Yes, to the registered nurse

Interventions

- Obtain vital signs every 1 to 2 hours.
- Contact the registered nurse to report findings.
- Teach parents to obtain and record vital signs.
- Teach parents the importance of adequate fluid intake during the use of the BiliBlanket.
- Teach parents the symptoms of dehydration.
- Closely monitor vital signs.
- Provide fluid replacement per order.

Documentation (date/time) 1200 4-day-old male infant, lethargic, dry mucous membranes. Mother reports 4 wet diapers daily. States oral intake 5 ounces formula, q 5 to 6 hours. Mother states infant is rarely hungry. T 99, P 150, R 42. Report called to supervising RN. S. Smith LPN

Chapter 3

NCLEX-PN® ANSWERS

(1) 4. Outcome 5. Reporting possible child abuse is a legal obligation of health care professionals. (2) 3. Outcome 6. It is vital for the nurse to provide nonjudgmental care. Her opinion of the situation cannot affect her nursing care. (3) 3. Outcome 3. Discussing health care issues with health care personnel involved in the direct care of a client is allowable. (4) 2. Outcome 7. In many states, reproductive rights of minors dictate that they may receive contraceptive information without parental consent. (5) 2. Outcome 6. Life and death decisions should be made by the family, with only support from health care professionals. (6) 4. Outcome 4. Giving the child control in aspects of her health care is important. However, choosing whether to have an IV and where to place it is not an issue she can control. She can choose to take a familiar object into the surgical suite with her. (7) 2. Outcome 3. Informed consent is essential for participation in medical research. (8) 1, 2, 5. Outcome 3. Health care personnel can expect families and clients to provide adequate information, seek knowledge, and participate actively in treatment. (9) 1. Outcome 4. Identifying information on the crib card is visible to the public and may compromise client privacy. (10) WIC. Outcome 2. Women, Infants and Children is the federal agency that provides food for mothers of infants and young children.

CARE PLAN HINTS

1. Typically most states recognize the rights of parents to make health care decisions for minor children, unless the child is emancipated.
2. The nurse should discuss with Jean the importance of disclosing this information to her parents and create a safe environment where this communication can take place.

3. The family should fully understand the illness and prescribed treatment as well as prognosis. Spiritual counseling would be helpful if desired by the family. Support groups of families who are experiencing long-term illnesses may be of assistance.

CRITICAL THINKING CARE MAP

Subjective Data

- States lack of sleep times 3 days
- 24-hour diet recall: six soft drinks
- States unable to care for a baby
- States family incapable of financially supporting another family member
- "My boyfriend says I have to abort the baby or he won't have anything to do with me."
- Concerned father will be physically abusive if he finds out she is pregnant

Objective Data

- Crying
- No eye contact with nurse

Report Yes, to the supervising nurse

Interventions

- Encourage client to express feelings and concerns openly.
- Address client in a nonjudgmental fashion.
- Explore options available to this client and the pros and cons of each.
- Encourage client to engage parents in decision-making process.
- Explore client's past successes in difficult circumstances.
- Encourage client to explore personal strengths.

Documentation (date) 0830 G1, 15-year-old female reported to school health nurse, crying. States 12 weeks pregnant. States parents do not know of pregnancy and she is unsure what to do. Feels there is no solution to this dilemma and has no hope. States fearful of father's reaction to the news of pregnancy, specifically concerned about his physical reaction. States boyfriend is encouraging her to abort the baby. States no sleep times 3 days. 24-hour diet recall: six soft drinks. Data reported to supervising RN. S. Metcalf LPN

Chapter 4

NCLEX-PN® ANSWERS

(1) 2. Outcome 5. A genogram is used to understand the relationships of family members to each other. The nurse is trying to assess the dynamic of this family so a genogram is the tool used for this type of assessment. Relationships to the community are described in an

ecomap. Genetic links would help in understanding inherited traits, not family dynamic. Physical characteristics do not help in understanding the family dynamic. (2) Ecomap. Outcome 5. An ecomap is a diagram used to demonstrate the interactions of a family within the community. (3) 2. Outcome 4. The mother's behavior of not maintaining eye contact is consistent with her Chinese culture which demonstrates respect to those in authority. Asking the woman to look at the doctor is counter to her cultural upbringing. Addressing the father only may be important in patriarchal families but is not the issue here. Avoiding eye contact does not always signify guilt. (4) 1, 2, and 5. Outcome 6. The nurse knows that an environmental assessment includes collecting and observing data regarding the physical aspects of the client's environment that would affect the health and well-being of the family. The exterior color of the house does not relate to safety. The number of televisions and their locations do not affect the health and safety of the family. (5) 3. Outcome 4. The nurse respects and supports the client's spiritual beliefs. Talking about medicine directly contradicts the mother's belief. Challenging the request does not show respect for the mother's beliefs and may increase conflict. Response 4 implies that you disagree with the mother. (6) 2. Outcome 4. Cultural and religious beliefs can affect the client's health, and nursing care should be planned with these aspects in mind. The nurse should base the client's care, as much as possible, on the client's culture or religious preferences. Reimbursement is not based on cultural and religious beliefs. Response 4 is a true statement but has nothing to do with care of the client. (7) 2. Outcome 6. Having close, supportive family during a time of loss is an important factor in helping parents deal with their grieving. Parents experiencing the loss of a child do need help with coping mechanisms to help them through their loss. The fact that they mention people have been telling them they need help is an indicator that they do need assistance with coping with their loss, and response 1 indicates denial. Response 3 is one of blame and anger indicating intervention is needed. Moving will only prolong the family's grieving process and slow healing. (8) 3. Outcomes 7 and 8. The LPN or LVN should notify the supervising registered nurse about the family's stress so appropriate actions can be taken. The RN would be the appropriate person to meet with the family as a group and determine what steps need to be taken or which referrals need to be made. Based on this assessment, the RN would set up a meeting with a family counselor. Ignoring the problem won't help the family resolve their issues. (9) 2. Outcome 6. The nurse has a responsibility to determine aspects of family functioning that may negatively affect the client's health. The

response in option 1 may make the family think they are being compared to other families and may decrease communication between the family and the nurse. Response 3 will upset the family and close the avenues of communication. The nurse is not trained to search out wrongdoing but rather to render client care. (10) 3 and 5. Outcomes 6 and 8. Contacting social services and consulting with the registered nurse will produce reliable local resources for the client. Web searches and using the Yellow Pages may not produce reliable local resources that can be trusted. Surveying other clients may also not be a source of reliable information because circumstances differ from family to family and community to community.

CARE PLAN HINTS

1. The ecomap should include Jean's parent's workplaces, their professional organizations, the family's civic affiliations, their religious affiliations, Jean's school, extended family, and sports activities.
2. With Jean's amputation, access to the home and safety hazards should be assessed.
3. It would be important to assess Jean's school for access. The nurse could also look for a support group of young amputees. Jean's parents may benefit from a support group of others who have experienced traumatic events.

CRITICAL THINKING CARE MAP

Subjective Data Complaint of daily stomachache; Refuses to go to school; Parents recently divorced; Parental relationship strained; Some days spent with mother, some spent with father; Father has new female relationship

Objective Data Sam's responses barely audible; Dark circles under eyes

Report Yes, these data should be reported to the registered nurse.

Interventions Evaluate family strengths and weaknesses. Encourage Sam and his mother to express concerns and fears. Explore negative feelings of anger, worry, sorrow, etc. Encourage each family member to seek to understand the other's feelings. Assist the family in setting realistic goals. Refer to community resources as needed.

Documentation (date) 1000 7-year-old male for office visit accompanied by mother who reports complaints of lack of appetite, excessive sleeping, frequent stomachaches and refusal to go to school. Mother also reports the family has recently gone through a divorce, there is unrest in the family, new living arrangements, and new caregivers introduced to the child. Dark circles noted under the child's eyes bilaterally. Verbal responses to questions barely audible. D. Adams LPN

Chapter 5

NCLEX-PN® ANSWERS

(1) 4. Outcomes 2 and 4. The nurse can promote autonomy in a toddler by encouraging the child to do things for herself when she is capable and ready. Helping the toddler complete tasks encourages dependency. Providing opportunities for the toddler to play with other children encourages socialization. Helping the toddler learn the difference between right and wrong is good but does not address or encourage autonomy. (2) 3. Outcome 3. Playing with puppets can help develop the child's imagination and cognitive skills and help her express her feelings. Reading books may be beyond the 5-year-old's skill level. Watching TV is a passive activity and can lead to increased boredom. Painting by number with oil paints may be too advanced for a 5-year-old child, would take time, and might prove messy for the hospital room. (3) 1. Outcome 3. Five-year-olds often engage in magical thinking and make-believe, which helps develop their imaginations. Thinking abstractly is a more advanced cognitive task. Understanding conversation about matter is too advanced for a 5-year-old. Comprehending another person's perspective is a cognitive behavior of older children. (4) 4. Outcomes 2 and 7. Two-year-olds begin to experience improved balance and coordination and can typically balance on one foot for a few seconds. Riding a bicycle is more normal in an older child. Jumping rope is a skill of older children. Skipping on alternate feet is a skill displayed in normally developed older children who do not have physical restrictions. (5) 3. Outcomes 4 and 7. Participation in sports is a good idea for an 8-year-old child if the sport is geared to the child's abilities and interests. Organized sports such as soccer are appropriate for this age group and encourage healthy competition, which can be beneficial in establishing a positive self-image. Competition is not harmful to self-image unless it becomes excessive. Girls and boys should be encouraged to be on the same team to learn about teamwork with the other gender; also, girls are usually taller than boys in this age group. (6) Peers. Outcome 7. Adolescents are more influenced by their peers than by anyone else at this stage of their development. (7) 2. Outcome 7. The nurse should talk with the child about the disruptive behavior to assess the cause and identify possible achievable solutions that can be implemented. Meeting with the teachers doesn't determine the cause of the behavior. Talking with the other children about the disruptive child breaks confidentiality, will alienate the child from the group, and will discourage the child from confiding in the nurse. The child's parents will also have to deal with the problem, but telling them they have to take care of the problem does not get to the root of what is actually causing the behavior. (8) Empty nest syndrome. Outcomes 4 and 7. Empty nest syndrome occurs when children have moved out of the house and the mother is no longer giving daily attention to her children. A great sense of loss can occur. The nurse can encourage the mother to become involved in outside activities and tell her that what she is experiencing is normal. (9) 4. Outcomes 2 and 7. The nurse should give explanations about the surgery to the child just before the scheduled procedure. Providing instruction the evening before the procedure may produce unwarranted worry by the child and parents and they may forget by morning what was discussed. Parents do not have to leave the room when the preoperative medication is given, nor should they be asked to hold the child down while medication is given. Parental presence will decrease anxiety and may be a comfort to the child. The nurse should explain what is being done and how the parents can help. (10) 2. Outcome 4. The nurse understands that the client in this situation is the 18-year-old and addresses his concerns with this statement. The nurse also recognizes that the grandfather is displaying acceptance instead of anger over his impending death. Response 1 may produce guilty feelings in the young adult who may perceive that his grandfather is putting on an act for him. Response 3 may be true but ignores his statement and concern for his grandfather. It is good to state that the staff will keep the grandfather comfortable, but saying it will be over soon may raise anxieties rather than help the boy.

CARE PLAN HINTS

1. The nurse should ask the mother the following: Has Jim seen a doctor since his birth? Has she tried to offer him solid foods? Does he cry between feedings or does he appear hungry after a bottle? Does she have any support with his care (emotional or physical)? Has anyone talked about normal activity and diet for a 9-month-old?

2. It would help to know if she lives alone and if she has the ability to obtain health care and proper nutrition for the baby. The nurse should also wonder why the first well-baby check is at 9 months.

3. With a birth weight of 7 lb, Jim should have doubled his weight by 5 to 6 months. His nutrition is inadequate. He is not reaching normal developmental milestones in a timely manner, and it appears that he has little stimulation and has limited opportunities for socialization. Social Services need to be notified for child protection; at the very least, the mother needs to be assisted with some parenting skills.

CRITICAL THINKING CARE MAP

Subjective Data Mother states: turns front to back, puts toys in mouth.

Objective Data 4 months old, VS: T98.0 F, P120, R 30, Wt. 15 lbs, Ht. 22½ inches, head circumference 16 inches,

Observed mother not providing safe environment for the child.

Report Yes; physical data are within normal limits. However, issues related to safety and possible physical harm to the infant should be reported to the nurse supervisor.

Interventions Teach need for close supervision because the child is becoming mobile. Instruct mother on toys for age of the child. Teach parent to avoid foods that could cause choking (raisins, peanuts, whole grapes). Instruct mother to keep activated charcoal in the first aid kit.

Documentation (date/time) 4-mo-old infant, well developed weight and length within normal limits; developmental milestones appropriate for age. Mother reports that child is rolling over. While in examining room, mother stepped away from exam table, leaving child unsupervised. Mother cautioned about leaving child unattended now that she is rolling over. Report given to supervising RN. N. Geiber, LVN

Chapter 6

NCLEX-PN® ANSWERS

(1) Answer is 0.5 mL. Outcome 2. (2) 1. Outcome 2. Primary preventions for a newborn are those that keep the client from developing health problems in the future. Immunizations prevent childhood diseases, so the nurse would discuss immunization schedules with the parents. Bimonthly visits with the pediatrician are not indicated unless there are problems or if this is the routine the physician requests. Treating a diaper rash is not primary prevention because a problem already exists. Changing the formula does not fall under the category of primary prevention. (3) 2. Outcome 2. Secondary prevention methods are interventions designed to detect problems in the early stages. Pap smears are necessary for those females who are sexually active; they detect some STIs and cervical cancer. Pregnancy tests are performed when pregnancy is suspected. Attending an abstinence support group would not protect the client from the physical risks already encountered. Increasing iron in the diet does not fall under the category of secondary prevention for sexual activity. (4) 2. Outcome 2. Tertiary prevention includes treatments used to keep the existing diseases from getting worse or progressing and from developing complications. Administering antibiotics for otitis media is an example of tertiary prevention. Hearing screening is diagnostic. Keeping children from interacting with other children for 48 hours is an example of preventative intervention. Reading books to a child does not fall under a preventative category. (5) 4. Outcome 1. A bright music box attached to the outside of the crib provides a visual stimulus for the

newborn. Choking and suffocation are safety hazards for the newborn, so balloons and ribbons are dangerous. Infants are not well-coordinated, so they may not be able to hold plastic keys. (6) 1, 4, and 5. Outcomes 1 and 4. The nurse has the opportunity to teach the mother about proper nutrition for her infant. Soft, easy-to-swallow foods such as rice cereal, pureed bananas, and vegetable puree and easily digestible foods are appropriate for a 6-month-old child. Because of absence of teeth, Cheerios may pose a choking threat to the child. Because of the immature digestive tract and lack of teeth, hot dogs are a bad choice. (7) 4. Outcome 2. The nurse should document the date of the injection, name and dosage of the vaccine, lot number and expiration date, and site and route of administration. Taking the temperature and blood pressure is not necessary or warranted for administering this type of vaccine in a healthy child. (8) 2. Outcomes 1, 2, and 3. The nurse has the opportunity to teach the client about dangers associated with smoking. When the nurse senses that the client will not cease smoking, the nurse should clearly and in a nonjudgmental manner encourage the client to reduce the number of cigarettes she smokes on a daily basis. Contacting social services does not address the smoking problem. The nicotine patch may have the same harmful effects as smoking. Informing the client that she will have to deal with lung cancer later in life does not address the present smoking problem and may shut off communication with the client. (9) 1. Outcomes 3 and 4. The nurse has the opportunity to teach the client about health promotion activities related to proper nutrition and understands that the client's mother is a single parent who is rarely at home. Lack of parental attention is one of the factors that contribute to a child's overeating and obesity. The choice of smoothies does not contribute to obesity. Academic achievement does not correlate with obesity. These family statistics are not contributing factors to obesity. (10) 1. Outcome 2. Narcotics can cause pinpoint pupils, drowsiness, euphoria, and respiratory depression, so the nurse must be cognizant of these signs and symptoms of narcotic use/abuse. Amphetamines tend to cause hyperactivity, not drowsiness. Depressants do not cause pinpoint pupils. Hallucinogens do not cause drowsiness.

CARE PLAN HINTS

1. Corrosive cleaners, insect and rodent poisons, fertilizers, and cat litter.
2. Hazardous substances should be placed in a locked cabinet out of reach of children. Children can be taught how to recognize hazardous substances by placing Mr. Yuk stickers on the substances. Parental supervision at all times is vital in areas where these substances are stored.

3. The parent is likely to experience guilt and sorrow that the child was injured. They may blame themselves for not watching the child more closely or not properly storing the hazardous substances. The parent may also fear that the child will become injured again.

CRITICAL THINKING CARE MAP

Subjective Data   Skips breakfast, Chips and cola for lunch, Chicken fingers, fries, and sweet tea for supper

Objective Data   Current weight 100 pounds, Previous weight 110 pounds

Report   Yes. To: Supervising nurse

Interventions   Explain importance of nutrition during adolescence. Use the food pyramid to discuss essential nutrients. Present a sample daily meal plan. Discuss ways to overcome difficulties related to food preparation and food acquisition. Refer to a dietitian prn.

Documentation   [date] 1500 14-year-old female to school clinic for initial assessment. Weight 100 pounds. Previous records show weight 110 pounds. States does not eat breakfast, has chips and cola for lunch, and chicken fingers, fries and sweet tea for supper. States this is a typical diet. Discussed findings with supervising nurse. Plan of care developed to improve nutritional status.

A. Green, LVN

UNIT I Thinking Strategically About …

CASE SCENARIO

CRITICAL THINKING

1. To add depth, the nurse would ask how Marie feels about the responsibility of the baby. What coping strategies does she plan to use in times of stress? To what resources does Marie have access?
2. To add breadth, the nurse would ask about the need for any alterations to permit access to and through Juan's house (e.g., need for ramps to be installed, doorways to be enlarged to accommodate wheelchair, hand railings to the tub and toilet, pathways to be cleared).
3. Obtain Jenny's length and weight and compare to previous documented values. Calculate Jenny's 24-hour caloric intake.

COLLABORATIVE CARE

- Marie should be referred to WIC (Women, Infants and Children), a federal program that provides nutritious foods and education to low-income pregnant, postpartum, and lactating women and to infants and children up to age 5.

MANAGEMENT OF CARE AND PRIORITIES

1. Visit Marie first, then Jenny, and finally complete the environmental assessment on Juan's house.
2. Visiting Marie would be the first priority because she is unsure of her ability to care for the infant and could accidentally harm or neglect him. Jenny is stable and has parents or CNA providing care. They could summon help if needed. An environmental assessment of Juan's house must be completed by afternoon.

DELEGATING

- When assessing Jenny, the LPN would identify areas of poor care, such as lack of hygiene, odor, or body position not in alignment. If there is evidence of poor care, further instruction in proper technique and follow-up supervision of the CNA would be warranted.

COMMUNICATION AND CLIENT TEACHING

1. The LPN would talk with the CNA regarding the needed care and watch the CNA perform the care. If the CNA's technique is not appropriate, further instruction and supervision would be needed.
2. Juan's family should be instructed in how to get the wheelchair up and down ramps, and in the importance of keeping clutter off the floor.

DOCUMENTING AND REPORTING

- If you believe Marie is at a high risk for neglecting the infant, you should stay in the house and call your supervising RN on the telephone.

CULTURAL STRATEGIES

- In Hispanic households, the male is usually the head of the house and would make the decisions regarding health care. Hispanic families should be assessed for the use of *curanderos* (healers), as well as for use of herbs or home remedies that may interfere with medical treatment.

Chapter 7

NCLEX-PN® ANSWERS

(1) 2. Outcome 2. Ten-month-olds are unsure of new environments and unfamiliar people. They are beginning to develop separation anxiety and fear of strangers. It will be several months before the negativism of the toddler becomes apparent. There is nothing in the question to indicate hostility or jealousy. (2) 1. Outcome 5. The question is about a mist tent at night. The size of the child's room must be evaluated to be sure the equipment will fit in the room. Provisions for the mist tent must be made before the child is discharged in order to have continuity of care. Although the other choices might be important, they do not pertain to this question. (3) 3. Outcome 5. As long as the child is not

contagious, she should be allowed to attend school. Skipping or altering the time of administration of antibiotics can affect their effectiveness. The school personnel can be taught to administer medication safely. (4) Home. Outcome 7. The 3-year-old needs as much stability as possible in an unfamiliar environment. Keeping the routine similar to the home environment provides stability. (5) 2. Outcomes 3 and 7. Allowing for the family's request promotes culturally sensitive care; rituals should not interfere with the rights of other clients. It is important that the nurse show respect for cultural beliefs related to healing. The ritual may be against policy, but that is not the first response to make. Burning may be prohibited, but the request should be discussed with the charge nurse or administrator. (6) 3. Outcome 6. The nurse must assess the mother's condition to determine whether she is experiencing caregiver strain. Help may be needed to provide a safe environment for the child if the mother is too tired to care for her child. Explaining the cause of diarrhea does not deal with the mother's exhaustion. The mother needs help to cope; moving the child to a nursing home for this would be an extreme reaction. Reporting diarrhea would not be the first action and might not be needed. (7) 5, 3, 2, 4, 1 Outcomes 5, 6, and 8. Change of position is most important; the child will need frequent position changes to prevent pressure ulcers. The child will need to be transferred regularly from bed to wheelchair, so ensuring safe transfer is second. Third is the importance of bathing the child soon after soiling. This may occur (perhaps not often), but skin breakdown can occur if urine and feces are not removed promptly. Safety in case of an emergency is a crucial part of teaching. Kindergarten is the lowest priority at this time. (8) 1. Outcomes 2, 3, 4, and 7. The safest way to transport a 9-month-old is in a crib with the side rails up. A stretcher belt is not a secure hold for an infant. It is better to separate the infant from the mother prior to entering the surgical area, to allow some time for adjustment. An infant could fall from a youth bed. (9) 1. Outcome 7. A private room would be required to allow for all the equipment that will be needed to care for this totally dependent child. A sitter may be required 24 hours a day, and extra room will be needed. An elderly roommate might frighten the child. A private room will also prevent the child from disturbing other residents. A room close to the nurses' station would be best for client safety. (10) 4. Outcomes 2 and 4. The 16-year-old should be allowed privacy during questioning. Any use of illicit drugs could interfere with anesthesia and pain medication and is a priority to assess.

CARE PLAN HINTS

1. The nurse should tell the child that he should feel better every day. It will be up to the doctor to say when he can play T-ball again, but it will be several weeks. Showing him a calendar will help him have a better idea of the time frame.

2. It is unlikely that the umbilical hernia will recur as long as the surgical repair heals well.

3. If Timmy exhibits signs of an infection (fever, elevated WBC count, nausea and vomiting) there is a possibility that surgery will be postponed.

CRITICAL THINKING CARE MAP

Subjective Data   Does not like school; Enjoys reading fiction stories; States pain in both hips; States he misses playing football

Objective Data   Is in 4th grade

Report   Yes, to the RN planning care. They are important observations related to his cognitive development.

Interventions   Orient to environment and facility routine. *Orientation to the environment and routine will help decrease fear and let client know what is expected of him.*

Tell him he must attend classes to keep up with his schoolwork. *Even though he does not like school, getting behind will make school more difficult.*

Insist he performs ADLs with minimal assistance. *Insisting that he do everything he can for himself will help prevent regression to a lower level of development.*

Documentation   (date/time) 10-year-old child admitted to room 24 of the rehabilitation unit. Oriented to room, bathroom, dining room, and physical therapy department. Oriented to facility routine including meals, physical therapy times, school activities, and visiting hours. States he does not like school, but likes to read fiction stories. Informed that he will be able to read for pleasure after his schoolwork is completed daily. D. Jones RN notified of likes and dislikes. P. Stromberg, LPN

Chapter 8

NCLEX-PN® ANSWERS

(1) 1, 2, 4, and 5. Outcome 2. Children's head circumference may be routinely measured until 36 months of age. In older children with head injuries or brain injuries, the circumference may be taken beyond this age, but it does not generally need to be taken once the bones of the skull have hardened. (2) 3. Outcomes 2 and 3. Infants are not able to control urine output. To assess the volume of urine accurately, the nurse uses an external collection bag to measure the urine output in infants. Inserting an indwelling catheter may cause injury in infants and the tubing is difficult to affix to the infant's leg. Weighing the diaper and infant are not reliable methods of determining urinary

output. (3) 1. Outcomes 3 and 4. The linens must be changed frequently for a child in an oxygen (mist) tent because of the condensation that is created. The condensation causes the child's gown, sheets, and everything in the tent to become damp. Plastic toys appropriate for the child's age should be in the tent; stuffed animals and blankets will become damp from the condensation. To receive the benefits from the mist tent, the child should be in the tent as much as possible. The air inside the tent is usually cool; fans would dissipate the moisture and the benefits of the mist would be lost. (4) 4. Outcomes 2 and 3. The vastus lateralis is the preferred site for an IM injection for an infant because it has enough muscle to "take" the needle and the injected material. The deltoid, dorsogluteal, and rectus femoris sites are not as fully developed as the vastus lateralis, so injury could result. (5) 1. Outcome 3. The nurse suctions secretions from the mouth first, then the nose, to remove the secretions. Suctioning the mouth first prevents mucus from being transferred from nose into mouth. The LPN/LVN would not insert an endotracheal or feeding tube. (6) 2, 4, and 5. Outcome 3. Restraints should be used as a last resort and for the shortest amount of time necessary. The nurse follows facility policy regarding the use of restraints. (7) 3. Outcome 3. The nurse uses a gloved index or little finger to insert the suppository into the anus in infants. The suppository is inserted no more than ½ inch into the anus in infants to avoid perforation of delicate tissue in the anal canal. Suppositories are sometimes needed in infants. (8) 1. Outcomes 2 and 4. The normal pulse range for a 2-year-old is 80 to 140, and normal respiration range is 20 to 40. P 120, R 35 is within normal range for a 2-year-old child. P 125, R 38 is within normal range for a 2-year-old child. P 140, R 40 is at the top end of normal. (9) 1. Outcomes 2 and 4. P 100, BP 130/90 indicates a rapid pulse rate and elevated blood pressure reading for this client. Normal pulse for an adolescent is 50 to 90 and normal blood pressure is 120/80. P 70, BP 119/80; P 60, BP 110/78; and P 90, BP 115/70 are within normal range for a normally developed nonobese 15-year-old female client. (10) 4. Outcomes 2 and 3. The nurse assesses the painful areas last. Assessing the painful areas first or causing additional pain can cause a change in the child's vital signs. Head to toe is often not the best approach for children. Emotional factors may affect the pain, but this is not the best answer. The client may need to be laid on a table, but outcome 4 is the most appropriate answer.

CARE PLAN HINTS

1. Keri can be allowed to say "ouch" or "that hurts" when the nurse is giving an injection. Music is appropriate for her. She also can play with stuffed animals or dolls. Watching nonviolent cartoons will allow her to be distracted from her pain.

2. The nurse should anticipate this question and discuss the possible answers with her father. It is important to be honest with Keri without giving her too many details. If possible, once Keri and her mom are stable, the nurse could arrange a visit.

3. Discuss with Keri's father which terms are typically used for injuries in the family, such as "boo-boo" or "ouchy." Use these with Keri in discussing her pain. Pain in the toddler can be expressed by crying, aggressive behavior, grinding teeth, or rubbing the affected site. Some children may demonstrate regressive behavior.

CRITICAL THINKING CARE MAP

Subjective Data   Yelling "no, no, no"

Objective Data   Crying, kicking and screaming, Face red, Carotid pulse 120 bpm

Report   Yes, to the physician in order to obtain an order for mummy restraints.

Interventions   Obtain physician's order for mummy restraints. Enlist assistance of a colleague during procedure. Assess restraints every 15 minutes. Provide emotional care during and after procedure. Remove restraints immediately after procedure.

Documentation   (date) 0800 18-month-old male crying, kicking, and screaming, "No, no, no." Face noted to be red. Dr. notified of child's anxiety and that safety was compromised. Order received for mummy restraints. S. Smith LPN

(date) 0830 Mummy restraints applied per protocol with assistance from M. Jones LPN. Nasogastric tube inserted without difficulty. Carotid pulse 120 bpm. S. Smith LPN

(date) 0855 Mummy restraints removed. Carotid pulse 120 bpm. Emotional care provided. Transported client to father's arms. S. Smith LPN

Chapter 9

NCLEX-PN® ANSWERS

(1) 2. Outcome 2. The sudden death of a child may leave unresolved issues for the parents to resolve. Parents often feel guilty about things they have not done or said to the child. Parents won't have had the time to engage in anticipatory grief if the child dies unexpectedly. Immediate detachment would not be a normal response. Uncomplicated grief responses also would not be normal in this situation and would require additional investigation or intervention. (2). 3. Outcome 3. It is important for the nurse to be aware of the discussions that have gone on between the child and parents before answering these questions. The family may

need help and support from the nurse in how to deal with answering questions about death with the dying child. It is true but evasive to say everyone will die. It is false to say only old people die. It is not appropriate to shift the responsibility for answering to the physician. (3) 1. Outcome 2. The client is trying to open up communication with the nurse, and the correct answer encourages this. Asking "where" blocks conversation. Telling the client what to think is not appropriate. Agreeing that most people do not want to die cuts off further conversation. (4) 3. Outcomes 2 and 3. Allowing the grieving process is essential for good mental health after experiencing a loss. It is not healthy to grieve alone. American culture is somewhat supportive of grieving, though it has more limits than other cultures. (5) 4. Outcome 2. Because the client knew of the scheduled amputation, her grief is anticipatory. She has not yet had the loss. Complicated grief occurs when a person does not resolve grief within about 6 months. Perceived grief is not a nursing description. Bereavement occurs after a loss. (6) 2. Outcomes 2 and 3. The preschool child generally views death as a temporary event and often asks where the person went and when he or she is returning. The school-aged child first develops the concept that death is a permanent happening. Preteens understand the permanence of death. Teens know that death is permanent. (7) 2. Outcome 5. The Living Will allows the client to express his or her wishes, while still mentally capable, regarding care at the time of death or in the event of a serious injury/disease. Because this client is a minor, he should be encouraged to discuss preparing a Living Will and his wishes with his family in order to prepare for his death. Health care workers cannot make a decision to withhold fluids and meds. Living Wills may be state-specific. They prevent court decisions by clarifying the client's wishes ahead of time. (8) 1, 2, 5, and 6. Outcome 4. Loss of bowel and bladder control, increased throat secretions, rapid respirations (tachypnea), and mottling can be signs of impending death. Other signs that can occur are a decrease in blood pressure and a decreased awareness of surroundings. Increased blood pressure signals a return to health. Dying people have a decreased awareness of their surroundings. (9) 2. Outcome 3. This response is representative of therapeutic communication and fosters trust in the nurse. Telling clients to get on with their lives blocks a healthful process. The couple may be able to have other children, but this response does not help them in their grief. Asking the couple to stop crying blocks therapeutic communication and the couple's healing. (10) 5, 4, 2, 1, and 3. Outcomes 3 and 5. After the death of a child, the parents become the client and will require nursing care. Holding them, if this is comfortable for them, and allowing them to cry gives them the emotional support they need at

this time. The nursing supervisor and physician should be notified of the child's death and time of death as soon as the parents are in control. The child's body will need to be prepared by providing post-mortem care per facility policy. The mortician would be notified when the family is ready for the body to be removed. All charting must be completed before the body is removed.

CARE PLAN HINTS

1. Timmy should be medicated for pain even if his respirations slow. Although prescribed medication may continue to slow his respirations and speed up the dying process, maintaining therapeutic blood levels of pain medication is important to provide comfort and alleviate suffering.
2. "I don't know. I know this is very difficult. Can you share with me how you are feeling?"
3. Timmy's grandmother should be encouraged to share her feelings about the loss of her grandson as well as the pain her daughter is experiencing.

CRITICAL THINKING CARE MAP

Subjective Data   States she will be relieved when Teresa is gone; Asking every 10 minutes "how much longer?"

Objective Data   Crying quietly; Identifies signs of impending death

Report   No, they are signs of healthy grieving.

Interventions   Ask mother if other family should be called. Ask mother if clergy should be called. Ask mother to help turn Teresa. Encourage mother to express feelings.

Documentation   (date/time) Unresponsive to verbal or tactile stimuli. Resp. irregular. Legs mottling. Mother at beside, crying quietly. Mother identifies signs of impending death, and questions "how much longer?" Mother states she will be glad when this is over. Offered to call family and clergy. Mother encouraged to express feelings. Mother assisted with morning care. K. Shewmaker, LPN

Chapter 10

NCLEX-PN® ANSWERS

(1) 1. Outcomes 2 and 4. Passive immunity is passed from the mother to the infant through the placenta and offers short-term protection from some organisms, so outcome 1 is incorrect as stated. Active immunity does provide antibodies to specific organisms. Active immunity gives long-term protection. (2) 1. Outcome 3. Infants are born with immature immune systems. By the age of 1, children have adult levels of immunoglobulin M antibodies to help them fight off diseases. Neutrophils are white blood cells that assist in the destruction of bacteria. The child's immune

system is not mature at birth. Wearing gloves will not prevent disease transmission in children. (3) 2. Outcome 3. Infants who were exposed to the varicella virus in utero may be born with congenital varicella syndrome. The syndrome is characterized by intrauterine growth retardation (IUGR), skin scarring, limb hypoplasia (underdevelopment), eye defects, brain defects, and death. Asthma, rash, and otitis media are associated with eczema. Polydactyly, pneumocephalus, and rhinitis are not the outcomes of exposure to varicella virus. Urticaria, seborrhea, and psoriasis are skin conditions and are not associated with exposure. (4) 4. Outcome 6. The nurse instructs the mother to place an ice pack on the injection site to reduce redness and swelling. The mother should be instructed to use only approved covered ice packs and not put ice directly on the skin because this can cause skin damage. The mother is right in reporting the reaction and not ignoring it. Rushing the child to the hospital is not necessary unless the child exhibits a severe reaction. Applying vinegar to the site will not help decrease redness and swelling from an immunization. (5) 3. Outcomes 5 and 6. The MMR vaccine contains very small amounts of neomycin. Persons with a documented allergy to neomycin should not be given the MMR vaccine. Administering the vaccine could cause an allergic reaction. Administering a smaller dose does not guarantee safety against allergic reaction. It does not change the allergy issue to give the immunization at a later date. (6) 3. Outcome 6. The nurse tells the mother that the cause of roseola is unknown but that contact with respiratory secretions is the suspected mode of transmission. Roseola is not transmitted through uncooked foods. Roseola is not contracted through bodily fluids. Roseola is not transmitted through unpasteurized milk. (7) 4. Outcome 6. The nurse instructs the parents that they should contact the physician if abdominal pain, left upper quadrant pain, or left shoulder pain occurs; any of these may indicate an impending or complete splenic rupture. Persons with infectious mononucleosis are contagious and must be instructed to remain at home to avoid spreading the disease. The child may have a low-grade fever, and this doesn't have to be reported to the physician. The parents will be instructed that the child cannot participate in vigorous activities or sports because of the susceptibility of the spleen to rupture, but it is not necessary to keep the child supine. (8) 4. Outcomes 5 and 6. The nurse tells the parents that the avian flu, also called the bird flu or H5N1, can be transmitted from birds to humans. There is currently not a human immunity to this disease. There is no proven vaccine available. The avian flu is not transmitted through pork. (9) 1, 2, 3, and 4. Outcome 4. Universal precautions are not the same as transmission-based precautions. (10) 1, 2, 3, 5, and 6. Outcomes 2 and 4. Immunizing with the HBV vaccine is not a standard precaution, although the HBV vaccine series is recommended for all health care workers.

CARE PLAN HINTS

1. Aunt Betty should be informed about the routes of transmission of chickenpox and the period of communicability. She should understand that in order to prevent infection she must not come in contact with Molly until her most recent outbreak of lesions has begun to form crusts. Aunt Betty should also understand the risks associated with transmission to the fetus in the first 20 weeks of pregnancy including intrauterine growth retardation (IUGR), skin scarring, limb hypoplasia (underdevelopment), eye defects, brain defects, and death.

2. The nurse must initially recognize this parental behavior as dangerous to the child. The child would be incapable of getting out of bed to go to the bathroom or to escape in case of fire. This action is considered child abuse. The nurse must report this parental action to the supervising nurse or physician, who will then report this act of child abuse to the proper state officials.

3. Chickenpox lesions that become infected develop tenderness, erythema, and purulent drainage. Cellulitis has a sudden onset. Symptoms include edema and erythema of the area. The area is warm to the touch. The child may also have a fever, chills, and malaise.

CRITICAL THINKING CARE MAP

Subjective Data   Screaming loudly; Crying inconsolably

Objective Data   R 12 and labored; Clutches toy stuffed frog while sobbing loudly; Clenched fists; Tightened jaw; Immediately hides head in mother's lap when nurse with mask approaches

Interventions   Stand further than 3 feet away from Wendy, remove the mask, and greet Wendy pleasantly each time the nurse enters the room. Replace mask. Repeat several times prior to moving close to Wendy. Provide the child a surgical mask to try on. Provide Wendy with a mask to put on her frog. Avoid approaching Wendy or touching her unless she is being held by her adoptive mother or father. Provide Wendy with age-appropriate diversional activities such as blocks.

Report   Yes, to the supervising nurse

Documentation   (date/time) 2-year-old female, recently adopted from Russia, diagnosed with diphtheria. Placed in private room, on droplet precautions. Adoptive mother and father at bedside. Immediate reaction to masked nurse entering the room witnessed. Screaming loudly. Crying inconsolably. Fists clenched and jaw tightened. Reported behaviors to supervising nurse. Developed plan of care to relieve fear. S. Shipman LVN

Answers for UNIT II Thinking Strategically About ...

CASE SCENARIO

CRITICAL THINKING

- Your role would be to provide emotional support to the parents. They obviously trust you. You can also serve as a resource person for the information that is being presented to them. Often when individuals are distressed they do not hear the details being presented to them.

COLLABORATIVE CARE

- Shelby's parents could benefit from a bereaved parents support group. In this group they could learn coping techniques and be able to discuss their grief with individuals who are experiencing similar reactions.

DELEGATING

- Shelby will need frequent hygiene, including oral hygiene. Also vital signs may be monitored more closely to determine Shelby's condition.

MANAGEMENT OF CARE

- Shelby's care should include positioning, hygiene and pain relief. Non-pharmacologic pain relief measures such as soft music in the room should accompany the use of pharmacologic methods. Encourage Shelby to talk about her fears and concerns with you but also with her parents. Often the last communication with a child becomes a precious memory for parents.

COMMUNICATION AND CLIENT TEACHING

- Explain briefly that as Shelby's body declines her heart will slow, decreasing circulation to her vital organs. This will cause her to slowly become less responsive. Help Shelby's parents understand the comfort measure that you will employ to assist Shelby with any pain she may experience.

TIME MANAGEMENT AND PRIORITIES IN NURSING CARE

- Discuss your assignments with the charge nurse. Delegate as much care as possible to the CNA and request to be able to stay with Shelby's parents as Shelby dies. Also discuss with Shelby's parents about your other responsibilities so they will understand the times you must leave the room.

DOCUMENTING AND REPORTING

- As Shelby dies, a decline in her vital signs becomes evident. Her level of responsiveness decreases. Urine production ceases. The skin becomes mottled. Periods of apnea may occur and gradually become longer apart. Respiration may also become noisy. These symptoms should be reported to the charge nurse and physician.

SPIRITUAL/CULTURAL CARE STRATEGIES

- To assist Shelby's parents with their spiritual need, you should contact the hospital chaplain and request his presence. Until he arrives, you can find out if Shelby's parents have any particular religious or spiritual rituals that they may find comforting, such as prayer or reading of spiritual writings. If they identify a ritual, assist them in performing this ritual.

Chapter 11

NCLEX-PN® ANSWERS

(1) 3. Outcomes 2 and 4. Normal hematocrit range for a 2-year-old child is 29% to 40%. This child's hematocrit is slightly below the normal range, indicating FVE. Normal urine specific gravity (SG) is 1.005–1.030 mEq/L, so this is normal. BUN ranges from 5 to 20 mg/dL, so this child's is normal. Sodium level is within normal limits of 135–145 mEq/L. (2) 1. Outcome 2. The nurse caring for a child with a diagnosis of hypernatremia would expect to see thirst and neurologic symptoms displayed in the client. Anemia is not a sign of hypernatremia. Anorexia is not associated with hypernatremia. Constipation is not the issue; diarrhea is. (3) 1. Outcome 5. The nurse caring for a child with a diagnosis of hyperkalemia knows that this electrolyte imbalance can adversely affect cardiac and respiratory status. The nurse monitors the child's pulse and respiratory rate and rhythm to detect early changes. Changes in blood glucose levels likely have to do with diabetic changes. Edema often signifies fluid volume excess. Urinary output is monitored with fluid imbalances. (4) Muscle weakness. Outcomes 2 and 4. Muscle weakness is a sign that hyponatremia is worsening. (5) 3. Outcome 5. The nurse should get a baseline assessment done and monitor the child for signs of increasing weakness which can be a precursor for decreased level of consciousness (LOC) in children with the diagnosis of hypercalcemia. Urinary calculi are not a parameter that needs to be closely watched. LOC is an advanced sign, not an early sign. The nurse would administer diuretics, but monitoring for weakness is priority. (6) 1. Outcomes 2 and 5. This response indicates the parents do not understand that vomiting is a recordable output and is important to record in clients with a diagnosis of dehydration. Additional instruction is needed. Fluid output can be measured by weighing diapers. Parents need to record all fluid intake. Diarrhea is one route of fluid loss. (7) 4. Outcome 5. The nurse anticipates weighing the client daily, maintaining strict I & O, and taking vital signs as ordered. Because the client is seriously dehydrated, he or she will be receiving IV fluid: The nurse will not see an order for fluids as wanted. (8) 2. Outcomes 2 and 4.

The nurse is aware that decreased PCO_2 is one of the indications of respiratory alkalosis (normal is 35–45 mm Hg). A pH of 7.4 is normal. Normal sodium in a child is 135–145 mEq/L, so this is normal. Normal potassium is 3.5–5.5 mEq/L, so this also is normal. (9) 3. Outcome 5. The nurse confirms her suspicions when she assesses the client's pulse and finds it is weak and thready. Bounding, strong pulse signifies an excess of fluid. Decreased blood pressure occurs with fluid deficit. An edematous tongue would not signify deficient fluid. (10) 3.2. Outcome 5. Convert the weight in pounds and ounces to a decimal by dividing the ounces by 16:

Weight at birth: 7 lb 12 oz = 7 12/16 lb = 7.75 lb
Three days after birth: 7 lb 8 oz = 7 8/16 lb = 7.5 lb

Subtract the current weight 7.50 lb from the previous weight 7.75 lb

$$\begin{array}{r} 7.75 \text{ lb} \\ - 7.50 \text{ lb} \\ \hline 0.25 \text{ lb} \end{array}$$

Divide the weight lost by the previous weight to obtain the percentage of weight loss:

$$0.25 \text{ lb}/7.75 = 3.2\%$$

CARE PLAN HINTS

1. Hypovolemic shock is recognized by confusion progressing to stupor or coma; tachypnea progressing to apnea; oliguria progressing to anuria; poor capillary refill progressing to weak, thready pulse; and hypotension.

2. Infants can have intolerance to formulas. However, this intolerance is not exhibited with symptoms of lethargy and irritability. The most common symptoms for formula intolerance are diarrhea, flatus, and abdominal pain shortly after feeding and mucus in the stools. Wesley may need to receive only oral rehydration solutions for 24 hours and then his normal formula could be resumed.

3. The harmful organism causing diarrhea can be found on toys, clothing, and furniture. After changing diapers and handling soiled linens and clothing, Wesley's mother and other caregivers should wash their hands thoroughly. During periods of illness, toys should not be shared and should be cleaned thoroughly.

CRITICAL THINKING CARE MAP

Subjective Data LPN states, "This rate is twice the rate ordered by the physician."

Objective Data Generalized edema; Moist lung sounds; Pulse 110 bpm, bounding; Hematocrit, 40%; Urine specific gravity, 1.000; Sodium, 133 mEq/L

Interventions Monitor intravenous fluid rate. Monitor and document intake and output. Monitor lab values and report imbalances. Monitor vital signs. Weigh the infant daily and document. Observe for edema of the extremities, face, and neck. Observe closely for symptoms of pulmonary edema including restlessness, tachypnea, labored breathing, a full and bounding pulse or a weak and thready pulse, possible crackles on lung auscultation, and profuse diaphoresis. Position the child to facilitate breathing and notify the physician immediately if symptoms are present.

Report Yes, this condition needs to be reported immediately, first to the supervising RN and then to the physician.

Documentation (date/time) 72-hour-old, term female infant lying prone under bili lights. Eye protection in place. IV to right wrist infusing LR @ 30 mL/hr per pump. IV rate ordered @ 15 mL/hr. Pulse 110 bpm, bounding. Generalized edema noted. Lungs sounds, moist bilaterally to auscultation. IV rate decreased to 15 mL/hr. Nursing supervisor and physician notified. L. Wiley LVN

Chapter 12

NCLEX-PN® ANSWERS

(1) 4. Outcome 4. The nurse must ensure that respiratory pathogens are not transmitted from the infant with RSV to the general population. Sterile gloves and double-bagging diapers would not prevent the spread of respiratory virus. The baby should not be allowed to go to the play room. Respiratory pathogens are transmitted through the air; therefore, the person feeding the infant should wear a mask. When burping the infant, respiratory secretions can be mixed with formula, contaminating the nurse's hands and uniform. (2) 1. Outcome 4. When a mist tent is used to administer oxygen, the bedding and clothing become moist from condensation. The bedding and clothing must be kept dry to prevent the child from chilling. Children this age become restless but must remain in the tent to ensure that the child receives the most benefit from the mist tent. Electrical appliances that could pose a fire hazard and danger to the child would not be placed in the child's mist tent. Other objects, such as favorite toys or blankets, can be placed in the tent to provide a source of comfort to the child. Common sense must be used, however, because the items in the tent may become damaged from the moisture. The tent should remain closed for the child to receive full benefit of the mist. (3) 2. Outcome 3. A fish is the best choice because they have very low incidences of allergic reactions and are low maintenance. Cat and dog dander, as well as bird feathers, can cause allergic asthma. (4) 1. Outcomes 2 and 3. The purpose of postural drainage is to drain mucus from the lungs. When

Appendix I   635

the mucus is removed, the lungs are better able to expand fully. Some bacteria will be removed with the mucus, but antibiotics will be necessary to treat the lung infection. Postural drainage does not dilate the bronchi or provide more room for lung expansion. (5) 2. Outcomes 3 and 4. Epiglottitis can result in airway obstruction. Anticipating this possible emergency situation, the nurse should plan ahead and have tracheostomy equipment available. The nurse would not routinely notify the respiratory therapist of an admission of epiglottitis. The physician may order that the child remain NPO, but the nurse would not order this. Antibiotics are ordered by the physician. (6) 1. Outcome 3. Halitosis is common following a tonsillectomy until the scab comes off. Increased pulse and restlessness are signs of bleeding. Crying could cause bleeding from the surgical site, so the nurse should encourage the parents to try to keep the child from crying. (7) 4. Outcome 4. Orange juice is acidic and could irritate the throat causing pain and bleeding. Popsicles®, Jell-O®, and pudding are cooling to the throat and may provide some relief from pain. (8) 3, 1, 4, 5, 2. Outcomes 3 and 4. It is important for the nurse to stay with the client with breathing difficulty to relieve anxiety and to be available should the child's condition deteriorate. Inhalers are frequently ordered to treat asthma, and the client needs instruction on their use. While the child is in the hospital, the parents should identify possible allergy triggers and eliminate them from the home if possible. The child and parents need to know that a good warm-up may prevent an asthma attack. The child will need follow-up care following discharge. (9) 4. Outcome 4. Using a plastic syringe (without a needle) is the most accurate measurement. It also allows parental control in giving the liquid to the child. Small amounts can be squirted into the child's mouth. Having the child drink the medication from a cup could result in spillage. (10) 9.75 mL. Outcome 4. Order is for 0.2 mg/kg. Convert pounds to kilograms. 43 lb = 19.5 kg. Multiply 0.2 mg times 19.5 kg = 3.9 mg per dose for this child. Available medication supply 2 mg/5 mL.

$$\frac{2 \text{ mg}}{5 \text{ mL}} = \frac{3.9 \text{ mg}}{X \text{ mL}}$$

Cross-multiply: 2X = 19.5. Divide 19.5 by 2 = 9.75 mL needed to provide 0.2 mg/kg (3.9 mg) of medication.

CARE PLAN HINTS

1. Blowing on a pinwheel, blowing bubbles, and blowing up balloons.
2. What were you doing prior to the asthma attack? Do you have any animals in the home? Are there any blooming plants in or around the house? What kind of pillows do you use? Have you eaten any new foods today?

3. While playing with dolls, the nurse can play the role of a sick child. The nurse's doll can say how she might feel, and ask Jimmy to tell how he feels.

CRITICAL THINKING CARE MAP

Subjective Data   Sleepy, Withdrawn, Crying

Objective Data   T 103.2, P 148, R 40: Nonproductive cough; Labored breathing; Lung sounds wheezy; Circumoral cyanosis; Weight gain

Report   Yes, to RN in charge

Interventions   Suction airway prn. *The airway always is a high priority.* Administer IV medication as ordered. *This may not be an LPN/LVN function in some states, but the LPN/LVN is responsible to notify RN that it must be done.* Offer 1000 mL clear liquids. *Increased fluids help thin secretions.* Provide mist tent. *This decreases swelling and thins secretions.* Administer expectorant cough syrup as ordered. *Expectorants thin secretions.* Provide droplet precautions. *They prevent spread of infection until cultures are obtained.*

Documentation (date/time) VS: T103.2, P148, R40. Lung sounds wheezy bilaterally, respirations labored. Circumoral cyanosis present. Airway suctioned, small amount white mucus. Expectorant given as ordered. Explained droplet precautions to mother. Charge RN notified. M. Jones, LVN

Chapter 13

NCLEX-PN® ANSWERS

(1) 3. Outcome 4. If the child vomits the diuretic, the parents should report this to the physician and not randomly give another tablet, because another dose of medication can cause severe potassium deficits in the child due to the potassium being excreted in the urine from the diuretic. Options 1, 2, and 4 indicate the parent has understood the instruction about diuretics. Diuretics should be given at the same time each day so the body gets accustomed to the effects. Diuretics help to excrete excess fluid from the kidneys. Children have to be monitored closely when taking diuretics and the parents should be aware of the signs of overdosage. (2) 4. Outcomes 3 and 4. Kawasaki's syndrome is an acute systemic inflammatory disease also known as mucocutaneous lymph node syndrome. Option 1 describes CHF, a circulatory deficit with decreased cardiac output. Congenital disorders that affect both the systemic and the pulmonic circulations are referred to as mixed congenital defects. Acute rheumatic fever (ARF) is an inflammatory disorder that can follow a group A beta-hemolytic *Streptococcus* infection of the throat. (3) 2, 4. Outcomes 3 and 4. In the subacute phase of Kawasaki's syndrome, the client has sloughing off of the skin on the lips, hands, and feet, as well as joint pain; other possible manifestations are thrombosis, large aneurysms of the coronary arteries, and

myocardial infarction. In the acute phase, the child can have swollen hands and feet, conjunctival hyperemia, and enlarged cervical lymph nodes. (4) 1. Outcomes 3 and 4. Rheumatic fever is confirmed by the presence of anti-streptolysin O titer. Kawasaki's syndrome is made by evaluating the child's symptoms, and blood work such as erythrocyte sedimentation rate. A glucose tolerance test would not be run for a suspected diagnosis of Kawasaki's syndrome. Red blood count tests are often run routinely with other blood tests and to determine a baseline, but is not a diagnostic test for Kawasaki's syndrome. (5) 3. Outcomes 3, 4, and 5. Crackles heard on auscultation indicate an accumulation of fluid in the lungs and are an alert for the nurse caring for a child with a diagnosis of CHF. A sunken fontanel indicates dehydration in an infant. Brady-cardia, a slow heart rate, is not indicative of CHF. A capillary refill of 2 seconds is a normal, acceptable finding. (6) 3. Outcomes 2, 3, and 4. Tetralogy of Fallot includes four defects: right ventricular hypertrophy, pulmonary stenosis, ventricular septal defect, and overriding aorta. The other options do not describe the four defects for this condition. (7) 4. Outcomes 3 and 4. Strong, bounding pulses in the upper extremities and thready, weak pulses in the legs, along with CHF, are possible findings in the client with coarctation of the aorta. The other options are distractors in the selection process. The nurse must be familiar with possible findings in the client who has coarctation of the aorta with CHF. (8) 1. Outcome 4. Prostaglandin E1 is given temporarily to maintain cardiac output and oxygen saturation. Antibiotics would be given to prevent endocarditis, which is an inflammation of the endocardium. The nurse would not give this medication prophylactically to prevent infection before surgery because it does not have antibiotic properties. Prostaglandin E1 would not be given to prevent the progression of central nervous system involvement. (9) 1. Outcome 4. Aspirin is given to decrease fever and inflammation, and IV immunoglobulin is given to decrease the occurrence of lesions and aneurysms that can form in Kawasaki's syndrome. Cephalosporin and furosemide, an antibiotic and diuretic, would not be given for this condition, nor would glucagon (a glucose-elevating agent) or phenobarbital (an antiseizure medication). Digoxin, a cardiac glycoside, and cisplatin, a medication given for certain cancers, would not be administered to a child with Kawasaki's disease. (10) 1, 3, 4, 6. Outcomes 4 and 5. A low fat, low-cholesterol diet, regular exercise plan, consultation with a dietitian, and cholesterol-lowering medications are all appropriate interventions for a child with a diagnosis of hyperlipidemia. Pain medications are not given for hyperlipidemia. Anticoagulants are not an appropriate medication for this disorder.

CARE PLAN HINTS

1. Encourage the use of salt substitutes. Avoid smoked or cured meats. Avoid salted snack foods. Most cheese and peanut butters contain excessive sodium. Frozen vegetables contain less sodium than canned varieties. Sodas are typically high in sodium.
2. Encourage Branson's family to purchase an automatic blood pressure cuff. Give them guidelines for choosing the right size. Calibrate the cuff with a manual sphygmomanometer. Demonstrate to Branson the proper method of obtaining a blood pressure reading. Have Branson do return demonstrations to verify his understanding. Teach Branson to take his blood pressure daily, prior to administering his blood pressure medication. Provide Branson a documentation record to keep track of his daily blood pressure. Teach him when to report elevated blood pressure readings.
3. Encourage Branson and his parents to pursue allergy testing to determine the exact cause of his symptoms. Once the allergens have been identified, diligence in avoiding these allergens may allow Branson to reduce his intake of antihistamines.

CRITICAL THINKING CARE MAP

Subjective Data "I'm just not hungry. Nothing tastes good." "The medication caused diarrhea and we didn't finish the prescription." Reports joint pain a 6 on a scale of 10. Takes Tylenol 4–6 hours for joint pain.

Objective Data Right wrist enlarged. Winces when wrist and elbow are moved. Vital signs: T 101.1 °F, P 110, R 12, BP 110/60.

Report Yes, pain should be reported promptly to the supervising nurse or, depending on the degree of pain, directly to the physician.

Interventions Thoroughly assess the child's pain. Include location, characteristics, onset/duration, frequency, quality, intensity, precipitating factors, and relief methods. Teach the child and parent nonpharmacologic methods of pain relief such as gentle joint massage, ROM exercises, application of heat, control of environmental factors (lighting, noise, room temperature), and relaxation techniques. Teach the child and parent the proper administration of prescribed pharmacologic agents to include route, dosage, side effects, reportable symptoms, and drug interactions. Develop a plan to reevaluate the child's pain.

Documentation (date) 0900 Parent of 10-year-old female client called to report symptoms of rash, temp 101 °F, and sore and painful wrists and elbows. Recent medical history includes positive Strep culture Date, treated with prescription for penicillin. Instructed parent to bring client to office for 11:00 a.m. appointment. G. Hoover LPN

Chapter 14

NCLEX-PN® ANSWERS

(1) 1. Outcome 4. Sickle cell anemia is caused by a recessive trait that primarily affects African Americans. A demand or deficit of iron in the bloodstream may be indicative of iron-deficiency anemia. Thalassemia is an inherited disorder caused by abnormal hemoglobin synthesis. Sickle cell anemia is not associated with the lymphatic system but rather the hematologic system. (2) 1. Outcome 4. Iron deficiency is a symptom of iron-deficiency anemia. Fever, stress, and vomiting are symptoms of a sickle cell crisis. (3) 4. Outcome 4. Children of Mediterranean descent are at greatest risk for thalassemia. Children from the Middle East, Asia, or Africa may be prone to beta or alpha thalassemia. (4) 4. Outcome 4. In sickle cell anemia, the blood values reveal decreased Hgb and increased reticulocyte counts. The other options are distractors, which is why the nurse must be familiar with clinical manifestations of disorders of the hematologic system. (5) 3. Outcomes 3 and 4. Symptoms of Hodgkin's disease include nontender, firm enlarged lymph nodes, usually in the cervical and supraclavicular areas. Lymph nodes can be found in various areas in the body and can be enlarged at times, but they don't signify possible Hodgkin's disease. Tumors can also be found in different parts of the body but are not indicative of Hodgkin's disease. (6) 1. Outcome 5. Chemotherapy can deplete the white blood cells, which can make the child susceptible to infections. Public places present a challenge and would put the child at risk for infection. Giving the child vitamin C won't prevent infections, because the child is in a depleted state already. Eating well during chemotherapy is recommended but won't change the effects of chemotherapy, which can cause nausea and decreased appetite. The child will have to have frequent blood tests during the course of the chemotherapy to check the platelet and white blood cell levels. (7) 2. Outcomes 3, 4, and 5. ALL is the overproduction of immature lymphocytes. Acute myelogenous leukemia (AML) occurs when cancer cells develop in the bone marrow (*myeloid tissue*). ALL is not a hereditary or sex-linked disorder. ALL is not a malignancy in the lymphatic system. (8) 1, 2, 3, 5. Outcomes 2, 4, and 5. The nurse realizes that care must be taken to avoid the unnecessary invasive procedures to include insertion of a rectal thermometer and suppository because doing so may cause bleeding in children with hemophilia. The nurse knows that the use of salicylates should be avoided because these medications can cause bleeding tendencies in all clients but especially so in clients who are hemophiliacs. It is all right for the child with hemophilia to drink carbonated beverages. (9) 4. Outcomes 4 and 5. Laboratory data for the child with idiopathic thrombocytopenic purpura include decreased platelet count, decreased antiplatelet antibodies,

presence of antinuclear antibodies, and positive direct Coombs' test. Options 1, 2, and 3 don't necessarily describe any particular disorder. The nurse must be aware of the possible lab results that will be seen in a child with ITP. (10) 1, 2, 4, 6 and 7. Outcome 4. The child with iron-deficiency anemia may crave dirt, hair, starch, and chalk among other things as well. Children with iron-deficiency anemia do not crave olives and bananas.

CARE PLAN HINTS

1. This crisis may have been triggered by the stress surrounding preparations for the family trip. It may also have been triggered if Yolanda caught the cold virus from her brother.
2. The client's pain must be the focus. The nurse can provide interventions when pain is at a low level. When position changes are necessary, the nurse can try to perform more than one task that involves movement at the same time.
3. Warm compresses can provide a measure of relief. Massage may be useful. Distraction can be a good tool with this age group.

CRITICAL THINKING CARE MAP

Subjective Data   States wants to see her friends as soon as possible and go to the movies. "The doctor said I could go about my normal life." Mother reports that Mandy's best friend has the flu.

Objective Data   Vital signs: T 99.0 F, P59, R 12, BP 120/80. WBC count 5000 mm^3

Report   Yes, to the registered nurse.

Interventions   Teach good hand washing habits. Screen visitors for those that may be ill. Avoid large crowds. Monitor white blood cell count. Encourage well-balanced diet high in protein. Teach client to monitor for symptoms of infection such as fever, redness, cold symptoms, etc.

Documentation   (date) 1500 15-year-old Black female for follow-up appointment after chemotherapy. Client states the doctor told her she could live a normal life and she wants to go to the movies with her friends. Client's mother is concerned because client's best friend has the flu. Vital signs: Temp 99.0, Pulse 59, Resp 12, BP 120/80. Labs drawn. WBC count 5000/mm^3. Vital signs and WBC reported to RN. Discussed methods of infection control with client and mother. A. Washington LPN.

Chapter 15

NCLEX-PN® ANSWERS

(1) 2. Outcomes 4 and 7. The restraints are in place to protect the child. If the restraints are removed, an adult must be present to prevent the child from dislodging the IV. If

the aunt is planning to leave the child unattended, the nurse must be notified and the restraint replaced. The restraints may be removed by the discretion of the nurse. A physician's order is not necessary to remove the restraints. The restraints do not need to be nor should they be kept on the child at all times. If there is a responsible adult in the room, the restraints may be removed by the nurse. They are reapplied by the nurse to prevent tissue damage and constricture that can occur by misapplication of the restraints. (2) 7.5 mL. Outcome 7. Order is 240 mg. Supply is 160 mg/5 mL. If there are 160 mg in 5 mL and you need 240 mg, how many milliliters will you need to administer the appropriate dosage for this child?

$$\text{Calculation: } \frac{160 \text{ mg}}{5 \text{ mL}} = \frac{240 \text{ mg}}{X \text{ mL}}$$

Cross-multiply: 160X = 1,200

X = 1,200 divided by 160

Solution: X = 7.5 mL needed to supply

240 mg of medication

(3) 2. Outcome 3. The father needs some time to adjust to his son's spinal anomaly. Simple answers to questions at this point are the best responses. More in-depth information will be given once the doctor has determined the extent of the defect. A full description with long-term complications is not appropriate initially, plus the father won't remember what is said because of his emotional state. Directing the father away from the defect will delay his acceptance. The nurse should be supportive, state the name of the defect if known, and not defray responses to the physician. (4) 1, 3, 5. Outcome 7. The nurse must look for physiologic responses to pain because the infant is unable to verbally express pain. These responses can include facial grimacing, tachycardia or bradycardia, pupil dilation, restlessness, or sleepiness. Bradypnea or slow breathing and flushing are not indicators of pain in an infant but may indicate other conditions. Tachypnea (rapid breathing) and anorexia are also not indicators of pain in an infant but may indicate other conditions. (5) 2.2 mL. Outcome 6. Convert pounds to kilograms. 7 lb 5 oz = 7 5/16 lb = 7.31 lb. Divide pounds by 2.2 (number of pounds in 1 kg). 7.31/2.2 = 3.32 kg. Multiply infant's weight in kilograms by dose ordered in milligrams. 3.32 × 20 = 66.4 mg. Calculate dosage: 66.4 mg divided by available concentration of 30 mg/mL = 2.2 mL dose to provide 20 mg. (6) 4. Outcome 6. Visual acuity at any age is done by testing one eye at a time, then testing both eyes at the same time. The exam is conducted in the following manner: Visual acuity is measured with the client standing or being held 20 feet away from the chart. The right eye is tested first with the left eye covered, and then the left eye is tested with the right eye covered. Both eyes are then tested together. The test can be done with or without corrective lenses. Holding the child further away or closer than 20 feet (such as is suggested in options 1 and 3) may result in an incorrect visual acuity diagnosis. (7) 2. Outcomes 3, 4, and 7. Reye's syndrome has been linked to the use of salicylates when caring for cold and flu symptoms. Products that do not contain salicylates should be used for these conditions. When the father checks the label on Pepto-Bismol® and Triaminicin, he will see that they contain salicylates and remember that use of salicylates is linked to Reye's syndrome. Reye's syndrome is not caused by bacteria. (8) 3. Outcomes 4 and 7. For a lumbar puncture, the nurse would place the client in a lateral side-lying position, the knees flexed to the abdomen and the back bowed or arched at the edge of the examination table or bed with the chin resting on the chest. The nurse positions the client and maintains position stability during the procedure to prevent injury. The prone knee-chest position would not be an appropriate position for this procedure because it would not open up the lumbar spaces. The supine position would not provide access to the client's back for the procedure. It is not possible to immobilize the client on a backboard for this procedure because of the rigidity of the backboard. The nurse has to be in contact with the client during the procedure to maintain safety. (9) 1 and 3. Outcomes 3, 4, and 7. Seizure precautions are instituted for clients with closed head injuries and suspected concussions. Specific seizure precautions vary slightly from one agency to another but, in general, they have a common theme. Airway, oxygen, and suctioning equipment are kept at the bedside. The side rails are padded to prevent injury from seizure activity. An IV access should be in place already from the ER to administer antiseizure medications. Use of padded tongue blades is highly controversial because of the injury they can cause, and they should never be taped to the bed of a pediatric client. (10) 4. Outcome 3. CP is a chronic disability caused by an abnormality in the pyramidal or extrapyramidal motor system. The client with CP has difficulty with muscle control as a result of this abnormality. This disease is not caused by an infection of the central nervous system. Cerebral palsy is not caused by a virus that causes an inflammation of the brain, nor does it result in severe mental retardation. There are many false notions about CP in the lay community; therefore the nurse must be familiar with the causes of CP to answer the parent's questions.

CARE PLAN HINTS

1. Cerebral palsy clients may have difficulty speaking and communicating. Ambulation may be difficult and require ambulation aids.

2. Students may not have had any experience with cerebral palsy clients. They may not understand the disorder and may make unkind comments. It may be difficult for Daniel to make friends.

3. Before school starts, the school nurse could have Daniel meet fellow students who have similar disabilities. Students without disabilities who have previously exhibited empathy could also meet with Daniel before school. The school nurse could also monitor Daniel's interactions with students and quickly address negative interactions.

CRITICAL THINKING CARE MAP

Subjective Data   Mom states, "Several children in her class at day care are sick with the same thing." Mom states, "She is very irritable."

Objective Data   Vital signs: T. 101.4; P 70; R 12; BP 90/60. Weight: 29 pounds. Emesis: 30 mL green vomitus × 1.

Report   Yes, to the physician or charge nurse

Interventions   Monitor vital signs for subtle changes. Monitor CBC values for signs of infection. Review immunization record. Teach mom signs and symptoms of infection and when to seek medical attention. Discuss ways to prevent transmission of bacteria including handwashing techniques and isolating child from other sick children.

Documentation   (date) 0900 4-year-old female presented to the office with T. 101.4 tympanic; P 70 regular; R 12, even and unlabored; BP 90/60 right arm. Mother states the child has not had an appetite, has had several episodes of vomiting and complains of neck pain. 30 mL green emesis noted. B. Razell LPN

Chapter 16

NCLEX-PN® ANSWERS

(1) 2. Outcome 3. Autism is marked in the child by the presence of repetitive behaviors such as hand movements or rocking. It is not abnormal for a 4-year-old child to converse without shyness. A normally developed 4-year-old would not be able to work through difficult math problems without assistance. Four-year-old children have learned some lessons about socialization and have learned to share toys and other items. (2) 1. Outcomes 3, 5, and 6. There is no cure for autism. There are some cases that have shown that with intensive interventions prior to age 5, some changes in behavior may be possible, but there are no guarantees. Autistic children have to be under constant supervision to maintain their safety. Eye contact with autistic children is important as it has been shown to help autistic children focus. (3) 3. Outcomes 5 and 6. Newborns with FAS have three types of characteristics: growth retardation, CNS abnormalities, and craniofacial abnormalities.

Hepatosplenomegaly, intussusception, and dysphagia are not signs and symptoms of FAS. Hepatotoxemia, portal hypertension, and jejunoileitis are also not linked to FAS, nor are club foot, hemophilia, and hepatitis. (4) 4. Outcome 3. Symptoms of substance abuse vary, depending on the specific substance(s) being abused. Physical symptoms might include dilated or pinpoint pupils, bloodshot eyes, bruising or needle marks, runny nose, and shaking hands. As a rule, psoriasis is not a symptom of drug/substance abuse. (5) 3. Outcomes 3 and 5. Common side effects of Adderall are irritability, euphoria, palpitations, insomnia, and restlessness. The nurse knows the common side effects of this medication and would not call the physician. The child is exhibiting common side effects of Adderall, so it would not warrant preparing for a code situation. Drug manufacturers are notified of abnormal, unreported side effects of their medications. (6) 2. Outcomes 3 and 5. Sexual abuse in children can be characterized by physical symptoms, mood changes, cognitive impairment, sexual symptoms, and lack of coping skills. Physical symptoms include a vaginal discharge, possibly with a strong odor; vaginal or anal bleeding or bruising (underpants or diaper may be blood stained); genital irritation such as redness, pain, itching, or burning; recurrent urinary tract infections; sexually transmitted infections and a positive pregnancy test, particularly at a young age; enuresis; and encopresis. Anorexia nervosa is not a key indicator of sexual abuse. Sometimes children are fearful of authority figures if they have been abused, but this is not a key indicator for sexual abuse in a child. The nurse would look for other indicators as described in the correct answer option. A diagnosis of diarrhea would not alert the nurse to suspecting sexual abuse in a child. (7) 4. Outcomes 3, 5, and 6. Bulimia is characterized by binge eating and purging. With anorexia nervosa, the adolescent may not only decrease the caloric intake, but also indulge in strenuous exercise programs in order to lose weight. Often, because of malnutrition, the client's fluid and electrolyte levels are unbalanced, which can lead to life-threatening arrhythmias. (8) 2. Outcomes 4, 5, and 6. Threats of suicide should be taken seriously. The teen in this situation should not be left alone and should be referred immediately to a qualified professional. Using therapeutic communication skills, the nurse should question the teen about depression and thoughts of suicide. If the teen admits suicidal thoughts, the plan for suicide should be explored, including method and opportunity. The more lethal the method and the more realistic the opportunity, the higher the probability the teen will attempt suicide. All teens do not go through this phase so this option is incorrect. The mother should not let her daughter lie down or leave her alone for any length of time. The last option does not reflect professionalism but rather denotes judgment, distracting from the issue. (9) 1, 2, 4, 5, 6. Outcome 5. Clients requesting bariatric surgery must have tried and failed at weight management alternatives for more than 6 months. The client must be physiologically mature and agree to a psychological evaluation before and after surgery. Female clients who are planning on bariatric surgery must avoid pregnancy for more than 1 year postoperatively to assure the tissue has healed and there is no potential for injury. No weight criterion has been set for bariatric surgery, but the client must be severely obese. The client's frame and height are taken into consideration. (10) 1, 2, 4, 5. Outcomes 2, 3, 5, and 6. Immature neck muscles make infants susceptible to injury when shaken. The jarring motion that occurs when an infant is shaken causes tearing of the nerve fibers in the brain and can lead to seizures, lethargy, respiratory difficulties, vision impairment, or loss of hearing. One-third of infants with shaken baby syndrome die from their injuries.

CARE PLAN HINTS

1. The media, including printed advertisements and television, present thinness as the most desirable body type. Clothing is displayed on thin models. Makeover programs include body restructuring to a state of thinness. The diet industry is one of the most lucrative in the United States. All of these aspects give the impression that body types other than thin are less than desirable.
2. The family must provide consistent, sometimes firm support. They need to consider themselves part of the problem and part of the solution. Family counseling is suggested.
3. Meghan's friends may contribute to the problem if they, too, are focused on staying thin. Including them in counseling, discussing the hazards of extreme weight loss, and encouraging them to develop healthy nutritional habits could assist Meghan in her recovery.

CRITICAL THINKING CARE MAP

Subjective Data Mother's report of lack of peer interaction. Teacher's report of lack of peer interaction. Jackson states that he has no friends.

Objective Data Jackson plays on the playground alone on the monkey bars. When buddies are picked for a class activity, Jackson is not picked. Jackson is observed attempting to talk to a group of boys in the lunchroom without success.

Report Yes, difficulties in social interactions can lead to social isolation if not managed properly. The supervising nurse would receive this report.

Interventions Involve Jackson's parents and his teacher in developing a plan to improve social interactions between Jackson and his peers. Use role-play to observe the social interaction between Jackson and his peers. Plan an opportunity to observe Jackson in a social interaction during school hours. Assist Jackson in developing social skills such as appropriate verbal and nonverbal communication, respect for other's privacy, and interpreting reactions from peers honestly. Develop a plan for positive feedback that rewards Jackson for appropriate social interaction. Help Jackson's mother develop a plan for additional opportunities to interact socially with other children.

Documentation (Date 1) 1500 Six-year-old male and mother in for follow-up visit after initial ADHD evaluation.
(Date 2) Discussed adaptation to medication and resolution of previous problems identified. Mother states that child is not interacting socially with peers at school and this is concerning to her. Report given to supervising nurse and plan of care developed to assist child in improving social interaction. Follow-up visit scheduled in 4 weeks. O. Ames LPN

Chapter 17

NCLEX-PN® ANSWERS

(1) 3. Outcomes 4 and 5. Option 3 not only provides reassurance that Timmy will be okay, but also provides teaching to the parent because there is no guarantee that Timmy will never have another bowel obstruction. The other options provide false information to the parent. (2) 1, 5. Outcome 4. The nurse knows that the child with a diagnosis of rickets needs extra calcium in the diet. Milk products are high in calcium and fortified with vitamin D. Salmon and sardines are high in calcium. Jell-O®, whole grain cereal, bread, and citrus fruits do not provide the calcium needed for a child with this disorder. Ice cream and pudding may provide some calcium, but they don't provide sufficient amounts for a child with this disorder. (3) 3. Outcome 4. Projectile vomiting is the highest priority because of the risk of dehydration and aspiration. Anorexia, infrequent bowel movements, and colicky abdominal cramps can also be seen with pyloric stenosis, but are not the priority. (4) 1, 2, 3. Outcomes 4 and 5. Following surgery for cleft palate, placing any hard object into the mouth (oral thermometer, spoon, or cup) could traumatize the incisional site and must therefore be avoided. A dropper can be used to provide nutrients without traumatizing the incision. A syringe can be used to provide medication or feedings. (5) 4. Outcomes 3 and 4. In this disease, the colon has a segment with limited nerve supply preventing movement of substances through the colon. Frequent evacuation of solids, liquids, and gas is not possible in Hirschsprung's disease because of the limited nerve supply. Excessive passage of meconium would

not occur with this disease. Excessive peristaltic movements within the GI tract are not possible with this disease. (6) 2. Outcomes 4 and 5. By positioning the infant upright after eating, gravity will help keep gastric contents from entering the esophagus. It is not necessary for the mother to discontinue breastfeeding or to administer continuous nasogastric feedings. The feedings should not be decreased for this disorder. (7) 3. Outcomes 3, 4, and 5. Passage of brown stool is common in the early stage of intussusception. The child will still need the barium enema for accurate diagnosis of intussusception. The nurse would note the bowel movement (amount and type) in the client's chart but would not notify the physician or measure the client's abdominal girth. The nurse would already have taken the client's vital signs as part of the nursing assessment. (8) 2. Outcomes 3 and 4. Infants need a nurturing, loving family that can independently provide care. Hospital staff should not be the main source of care. The infant should gain weight while hospitalized. Developmental milestones will take time to change. (9) 1. Outcome 5. Knowing what kind of poison was taken and what treatment was provided is most important for follow-up medical treatment. It is important to determine drug allergies, but emergency drugs rarely cause allergy, so this is not the highest priority in this situation. The type of poison ingested determines what type of emetic, if any, is to be given. (10) 2. Outcome 5. The nurse must first assess the client's abdomen before calling the doctor or parents. Giving a laxative or applying heat is contraindicated in case appendicitis or an acute abdomen is the cause of the pain.

CARE PLAN HINTS

1. Some pain medication can cause drowsiness, and GI distress when taken without food. John will take formula better when there is less discomfort. It is important to observe John's reaction to medication and feeding and adjust feeding and medication schedules as needed.

2. John can be fed with a paper cup. Place a small amount of formula (or breast milk) in a paper cup. Tip the cup slowly to encourage him to drink a little at a time.

3. He will have 6–8 wet diapers a day. His mucous membranes will be moist. His anterior fontanel will be flat. His weight will be within normal limits.

CRITICAL THINKING CARE MAP

Subjective Data Mother reports no fluid or solid intake in the past 48 hours. Mother reports infant is lethargic.

Objective Data Current weight: 12 pounds. Previous weight: 16 pounds. Mucous membranes pale. Vomiting × 6/day. Diarrhea × 10/day. Hyperactive bowels sounds in all four quadrants.

Report Yes, to the pediatrician.

Interventions Obtain a thorough nutrition history. Assess for possible causes of vomiting and diarrhea. Assess for signs and symptoms of dehydration. Develop a plan with the parents for nutritional and fluid replacement. Administer antiemetics as ordered. Monitor lab values carefully. Weigh daily.

Documentation (date) 0900 Mother of 7-month-old male infant calls the office to report vomiting and diarrhea of her child × 2 days. She states he has not had any fluid and is lethargic. Appointment made for 1000. Report given to Dr. Smithson. K. Young LPN

Chapter 18

NCLEX-PN® ANSWERS

(1) 3. Outcomes 4 and 5. The nurse knows that the child's urine will be blood-tinged following surgical repair of epispadias and would not call the physician unless bleeding increases or the child's condition deteriorates. A blood transfusion is not necessary for blood-tinged urine in the collection bag. The catheter won't be removed until the urine is clear and the child is able to urinate. (2) 4. Outcomes 3, 4, and 5. Infants with hypospadias are not circumcised right away to preserve the foreskin to use for surgical repair. Frequent blood tests are not necessary for an infant with a diagnosis of hypospadias. The infant will be able to urinate without being catheterized. The infant will be diapered with no other special supports.(3) 1. Outcomes 3 and 4. Symptoms of UTI are fever, nausea and vomiting, anorexia, strong-smelling urine, abdominal pain, dysuria, and hematuria. Oliguria, seizures, proteinuria, hypoalbuminemia, hyperlipidemia, and hyperproteinuria are not signs and symptoms of UTI. (4) 3. Outcome 4. Organisms related to the diagnosis of glomerulonephritis are group A beta-hemolytic *Streptococcus*, *Staphylococcus*, *Pneumococcus,* and coxsackievirus. Low pH levels and glucosuria are not indicative of glomerulonephritis. Gross or microscopic hematuria can also be a sign of glomerulonephritis as well as other urinary disorders, but the laboratory finding of *Streptococcus* alerts the nurse to the diagnosis. (5) 4. Outcome 4. Uremic syndrome occurs in end-stage renal disease, in which all body systems become affected when waste is not eliminated. Hypospadias, where the urethra is on the ventral surface of the penis, is not associated with the symptoms listed. Bladder exstrophy, noted by extrusion of the posterior bladder wall through the lower abdominal wall, is also not associated with the symptoms listed. Epispadias, an opening of the urethra on the *dorsal* (upper) surface of the penis, does not have the signs and symptoms that are listed in the options. (6) 4. Outcomes 3, 4, and 5. Because of the highly metastatic nature of Wilms'

tumors, the abdomen should not be palpated in a client with this condition. Obtaining a urine sample and vital signs are appropriate nursing interventions for a client with Wilms' tumor. (7) 3. Outcomes 4 and 5. The bladder is exposed to the outside in bladder exstrophy. The highest *priority* diagnosis with this condition is impaired tissue integrity, which is related to the exposed bladder tissue. Potential for infection is a possibility with bladder exstrophy, as is alteration in comfort and a need for parental teaching about this condition, but impaired tissue integrity is the highest priority for this diagnosis. (8) 3. Outcomes 2, 3, and 4. Bladder exstrophy is a condition in which the bladder extrudes to the outside of the abdomen through a lower abdominal wall defect. This condition is not inherited from either parent, nor is it located in the renal pelvis. Bladder exstrophy is not due to low folic acid intake by the mother during pregnancy, but rather is a physiological defect as described. (9) 1, 2, 3, 5, and 6. Outcomes 3 and 4. Nephrotic syndrome is characterized by hypoalbuminemia, proteinuria, edema, hyperlipidemia, and decreased immunity. Uremic frost is not a symptom of this condition. (10) 1, 2, 3, 4. Outcomes 2, 3, 4, and 5. The nurse teaches the parents of a 2-year-old child with a diagnosis of UTI that they should cleanse the perineum during each diaper change, that they should wipe the child's perineum from front to back, avoid bubble baths, and avoid putting the child in commercial hot tubs. The parents can use disposable or cloth diapers, as this doesn't affect the UTI, except that the diapers should be changed more often to prevent further infection and irritation.

CARE PLAN HINTS

1. Fluid-filled edematous tissue is at greater risk for impaired skin integrity. Turning James will reduce pressure on the tissue and prevent dependent edema as well.
2. An objective measurement of urine output is necessary to document a balance or imbalance of intake and output. When a child is unable to urinate in a measured container, the nurse may record weights of the diaper to document output.
3. The nurse should carefully assess whether the family understands James's medical condition and treatment. Their physical comfort during hospitalization is important. The nurse should also provide them an opportunity to express fears and concerns about James's condition.

CRITICAL THINKING CARE MAP

Subjective Data "Casey has had sex, and that's why she has these symptoms." "I have not ever had sex with anyone."

Objective Data Intact hymen. Mrs. Friedman is waving arms and pacing in examination room.

Report Yes, The data gathered need to be reported to the supervising nurse. The mother's misunderstanding could result in ineffective treatment for her daughter's vaginitis and it could damage their interpersonal relationship.

Interventions Assess Mrs. Friedman's knowledge level regarding vaginitis. Explain the physiology and causes of vaginitis. Describe the signs and symptoms of vaginitis. Explain medical treatment of vaginitis. Describe methods of preventing vaginitis. Present teaching in a nonjudgmental manner.

Documentation (date/time) 14-year-old female accompanied by mother to clinic with report of vulvar pain, edema, and pruritis. Mother states, "I'm sure she had sex. What am I going to do about that?" Client denies sexual intercourse. Procedure for pelvic examination described to client. She voiced understanding. Dr. Lewis assisted with pelvic examination and vaginal specimen obtained. Specimen sent to lab. H. Gregg LVN

Chapter 19

NCLEX-PN® ANSWERS

(1) 2. Outcomes 5 and 6. When children are more active, they need more calories to supply the needed energy. Lack of calories will result in hypoglycemia. It is easier to maintain the blood glucose level with dietary changes than to alter the insulin dose. Decreasing food intake will not help the situation but will result in hypoglycemia. Increasing or decreasing the insulin dosage is not appropriate without a physician order or ordered sliding scale. (2) 3. Outcomes 5 and 6. The adolescent is developing a sense of body image, the ability to think abstractly, and a self-image. Allowing and encouraging the adolescent to make decisions about the management of his or her diabetes fosters healthy development. The nurse knows the adolescent has to understand diabetes mellitus and therefore would not allow or teach the client to select the diet without restriction. The nurse encourages activity for good health and in order for the adolescent to feel as if he or she does not have physical restrictions. The nurse understands that the adolescent has to be in control and realizes that control of the disease is the priority, not maintaining a strict routine. (3) 4. Outcomes 4 and 5. Ketoacidosis is a life-threatening complication that should not occur when diabetes is diagnosed and brought under control in a timely manner. The nurse knows that if the child's diabetes is under control, diabetic ketoacidosis is not an expected outcome of the disease. The condition cannot be treated at home but must be treated in a medical facility. Diabetic ketoacidosis is not rare in children, but can occur when

the disease gets out of control. (4) 1. Outcomes 5 and 6. The nurse knows that self-administering shots can take time to learn and master. If the client is unable to give the injection, the nurse must administer the drug and allow her to practice injecting an orange or mannequin and try again the next time. Forcing the client to give the shot will increase her anxiety and decrease the trust between the client and nurse. Referring the client to the physician does not help the client learn how to give herself shots. The insulin must be given at the time ordered. (5) 1. Outcome 4. Corticosteroids cause weight gain, delayed growth, delayed puberty, fat deposits, and moon face. Delayed growth, weight loss, fat deposits, rapid growth, and precocious puberty are not side effects of corticosteroids. (6) 3, 2, 5, 4, 1. Outcome 5. The symptoms listed in this situation for a diabetic adolescent indicate a diagnosis of hyperglycemia due to the increased glucose/decreased insulin in the client's system from the automobile accident. The nurse prioritizes the following interventions based on the client's diagnosis. The nurse obtains a blood glucose level in order to determine how much insulin to give, which is based on a sliding scale. Because the client has increased urine output, there will be a need to increase fluid intake. The nurse starts an intake and output record before beginning the intervention of increasing fluid intake. The primary care provider needs to be made aware of the change in the client's condition. (7) 3. Outcome 3. The age at which an adolescent girl starts puberty is often similar to when the mother started puberty. The nurse asks the mother this question to assess familial traits. Telling the mother not to worry avoids the mother's concern about her daughter's development. Telling the mother to get ready for her daughter to start puberty does not address the mother's concern. Neither does telling her to teach her daughter about menstruation. (8) Hypocalcemia. Outcome 4. When the thyroid is removed, the parathyroid glands can inadvertently be removed or traumatized. Because the parathyroid glands work with the thyroid to regulate blood calcium, removal or trauma can result in hypocalcemia or low calcium levels. (9) 1. Outcome 4. Diabetes insipidus should be suspected when the child's specific gravity is below 1.005. This value should be reported because it indicates the need for further testing. The other options do not indicate a diagnosis of diabetes insipidus. (10) 4. Outcome 4. If type II diabetes mellitus is not controlled with oral medication, insulin may be necessary. Oral hypoglycemic medication does not replace insulin in clients with this disorder. Exercise is necessary for this client, so walking 3 miles is an appropriate response. The client needs to replace desserts in his diet with fruit. Drinking diet soda once a day is permitted.

CARE PLAN HINTS

1. The nurse can teach about a well-balanced diet that is high in calcium. Calcium will be needed for bone growth. Also, active exercise daily will promote bone growth.
2. Yes, because she has grown since birth, she would be expected to continue to grow at a rate slower than normal.
3. Allow her to make some choices and have some control. Suggest she choose the injection site. Place a Band-Aid® of her choice on the site. Have her give a "shot" to her doll.

CRITICAL THINKING CARE MAP

Subjective Data   Hungry, irritable

Objective Data   Sweating, tremors, pulse 102

Report   Yes, to the health care provider.

Interventions   Give orange juice with 1 packet sugar added. *Orange juice is high in sugar; adding more simple sugar will elevate the child's blood glucose (BG) within minutes. He is irritable, which indicates he is awake, and should be able to swallow. If BG can be elevated with fluids, it is better than starting an IV. If client is unable to take oral liquids, an IV would be necessary.* Monitor blood glucose every 30 minutes to 1 hour, and then every hour. *Frequent monitoring of BG is necessary to evaluate effectiveness of treatment. BG should return to normal within 30 minutes. If condition worsens, more frequent monitoring and additional treatment will be necessary.* Obtain a thorough nutrition history. *This is necessary to determine cause of this episode of hypoglycemia and to determine knowledge deficit.* Review causes, signs, and treatment of hypoglycemia. *Because client is a newly diagnosed diabetic, a review of content is necessary to ensure his understanding of his disorder, the signs of complications, and what he can do to prevent or alleviate the problem.*

Documentation   (date/time) 11-year-old admitted with irritability & hunger. T 98, P 102, R 24 BP 102/66. Skin pale and diaphoretic. States he became weak and sweaty during soccer practice. States he did not have a snack before practice. BG 48 mg/dL. 240 mL orange juice with 1 packet sugar given. Dietary intake included breakfast of eggs, toast, and banana; lunch of meat sandwich and lettuce salad. Signs, causes, and treatment of hypoglycemia reviewed. Report given to D. Wildman CRNP. A. Allen LPN

Chapter 20

NCLEX-PN® ANSWERS

(1) 2. Outcomes 4 and 5. The real issue here is the child's feelings. Response 2 acknowledges the client's feelings and encourages her to address the issue. The brace must be worn 23 hours a day in order to be effective, and another brace would not help the client's condition. It would not be appropriate for the nurse to suggest that the client take off the brace while attending school. (2) 3. Outcomes 3 and 4.

Osteosarcoma is found in the femur, tibia, and humerus and characterized by pain, swelling, and ambulation difficulties. If the client has swelling in the clavicle, difficulty using the hands, or stiffness in the back, it would not be associated with the diagnosis of osteosarcoma. (3) 3. Outcome 5. Teenagers who have had a limb amputated may develop signs of disturbed body image, such as hiding or overexposing the limb, refusing to look at or touch the limb, or exhibiting preoccupation with loss of the limb. The nurse knows that the client will be curious about the appearance of the limb, and it is helpful if the nurse is present when the client sees the amputation for the first time. Also important for the client is for the nurse to prepare the client for what may be seen when the bandages are taken off. Discussing what it will be like living without a limb is a step toward acceptance, and the nurse helps the client through this process by listening and clarifying. Talking about his surgery with his friend is a healthy coping mechanism and should be encouraged. (4) 1. Outcomes 4 and 5. The nurse first needs to explore the father's understanding of the disorder. Generally, in children with developmental dysplasia, triple diapers are used for several months, so the nurse should suspect the father has not comprehended the information if he responds as stated. Just telling him he is wrong is poor communication that could put him on the defensive. Infants do not need to be medicated so that they can wear triple diapers. (5) 4. Outcomes 4 and 5. Synthetic casts are preferred because they dry more quickly, are lighter, and allow for greater mobility than a plaster cast. Synthetic casts are weaker than plaster casts. (6) Resistance *or* hip click. Outcomes 3 and 4. The physician assesses the infant's hips while performing the Ortolani-Barlow maneuver for resistance, or a clicking sound, which indicates hip dislocation. (7) 2. Outcomes 4 and 5. Nothing should be placed on the traction ropes because of the risk of disrupting the traction. The nurse ensures that the weights are hanging freely so that the proper traction is maintained. If the child is old enough, the nurse explains that the weights have to be left alone and should not be touched. With younger children, the weights are kept out of the child's reach, and the nurse also explains this to the parents. The nurse makes sure the weights are situated in the pulleys. (8) 1. Outcomes 4 and 5. When assessing for capillary refill, the normal findings are that the compressed nail bed returns to normal color in less than 3 seconds. This finding is within normal limits. The nurse would not suggest the cast be removed or notify the physician. The leg may already be elevated to reduce swelling, and since the capillary refill is normal, elevating the leg higher is not an appropriate nursing intervention. (9) 1, 2, 3, 4, 5. Outcome 5. When teaching the parents of a child with a newly applied cast, the nurse tells them they should observe the cast for any drainage, and call the physician if the child complains of numbness or tingling in the extremity or if the extremity looks blue or extremely pale, as this may indicate that the cast is too tight and constricting the circulation or that there is extreme swelling under the cast. The nurse also tells the parents that the extremity should be elevated for the first 24 to 48 hours to decrease swelling. The use of powder inside the cast is not recommended because it can cause skin irritation. (10) 1. Outcomes 4 and 5. The Milwaukee brace should be worn for 23 hours a day. The mother will have to assess the area around the brace and provide skin care to prevent breakdown. The mother can be very helpful in working with her daughter in learning how to perform the activities of daily living with the brace on.

CARE PLAN HINTS

1. Many individuals play all types of sports with a prosthesis. Running, team sports such as baseball, and golf are possible. Jake should be encouraged to try whatever he would like to try.

2. A balanced diet is essential to Jake's energy level. His diet should be high in protein and low in sugar. It should contain adequate whole foods such as fruits and vegetables. He should have an adequate intake of water as well. Energy conservation is essential as well. His room and his living quarters should be arranged to allow him to decrease excess walking. Exercising the major muscle groups will also increase endurance.

3. The nurse could respond by saying, "Tell me more about your fears about having people stare. (Allow Jake to respond.) Are you afraid they will say mean things or laugh at you? Remember that people in general are far from perfect and usually stare because they don't understand what all you've been through." Another response the nurse could give is, "I guess it would be scary to see people's heads turning as you walk by. They could be thinking 'My, what an amazing young man that is.' It also would be okay if you look them directly in the eye and smile. You could even ask them if they'd like to hear your amazing story of survival. You do have a great story to tell."

CRITICAL THINKING CARE MAP

Subjective Data States, "It hurts real bad."

Objective Data Crying, non-weight-bearing, ankle swollen and bruised, pedal pulses present.

Report Yes, to the physician.

Interventions Instruct to support cast on pillows until dry. Instruct not to put anything inside cast. Instruct regarding signs of impaired circulation. Ice pack to ankle. Teach crutch walking.

Documentation (date) 0800 States "fell while roller blading and ankle hurts real bad." Non-weight-bearing on left leg upon admission. Left ankle swollen and bruised. Pedal pulses present. Dr. notified. Provided written and verbal instruction in cast care prior to discharge. M. Fowler, LPN

Chapter 21

NCLEX-PN® ANSWERS

(1) 1, 3, 5. Outcome 4. For a child with the fungal infection candidiasis, the following instructions should be given to the parent: Swab oral mucosa with oral nystatin, disinfect all toys, and report a rash in the diaper area. The option to clean bottle nipples in cool water is incorrect as bottle nipples should be cleaned in boiling water for 20 minutes to rid the nipples of the candidiasis. Placing stuffed animals in a plastic bag for 5 days is not necessary, nor will it rid the toys of the infection. (2) 1. Outcome 5. The nurse should immediately report lymphangitis, which indicates the infection is spreading and could lead to septicemia. The tetanus shot was within the last 6 months, so another shot is not needed. Limping would be expected, especially because the wound is deep and located behind the knee where bending or flexing the leg would produce pain. A pedal pulse of 76 is within normal limits for a child of this age. (3) 2. Outcome 3. Port-wine stains are a large, congenital vascular nevus with a purplish color that can be found on any part of the body and do not blanch when palpated. These discolorations are noticeable, so if a port wine stain is located on the neck, it is larger and visible beyond the folds of the neck. Physicians have tried many ways to treat port wine stains, including radiation, freezing, dermabrasion, and sclerotherapy. Laser treatment is currently the only method that destroys the capillaries in the skin without causing damage to the rest of the skin, but it is not always effective for port-wine stains. (4) Humid. Outcome 4. To prevent the skin from becoming dry and irritated, the temperature should be kept cool with constant humidity levels. (5) 1. Outcome 4. A family history of asthma has been linked to children with eczema. Intertrigo, diaper dermatitis, and tinea infections are not linked to a family history of asthma. (6) 2. Outcome 4. Red blisters on the buttocks, erythematous papules on the back of the neck, and erythema in the folds of the skin are not signs of seborrheic dermatitis. Yellow, scaly patches on scalp and forehead are indicative of seborrheic dermatitis. (7) 3. Outcome 4. It is important that the client understands that the results may not be seen right away and that acne treatments may be needed for 3 months to see an improvement. Oil-based skin products are not recommended because they can exacerbate the

condition. Sunscreen is necessary because some medications may cause skin sensitivity. Tetracycline is a common prescription medication for acne, and the physician will determine whether the client is a candidate for its use. (8) 4. Outcome 4. The crust from the impetigo lesions should be washed and removed several times a day. It is not recommended to apply nystatin to open impetigo lesions. Elevation of the extremities in persons with impetigo will not cure the infestation. Impetigo can be spread through contact with toys, so the family is advised to isolate the child's toys so that other children are not infected. Placing the toys in a plastic bag for 2 weeks is not necessary. (9) 2, 4, 5. Outcome 4. Prevention methods for melanoma include applying sunscreen of SPF 15 or greater, reporting moles that are black with irregular borders, and wearing long-sleeved cotton clothing when outside. Clients should be advised to avoid being in the direct sunlight during the peak hours from 10 a.m. to 4 p.m. Tanning beds can cause as much damage to the skin as the effects of direct sunlight, so clients should be advised of the potential damage of both tanning beds and the sun. (10) 1. Outcome 4. Shower shoes should be worn at all times in public showers and locker rooms. The question addresses what the client must do to avoid this condition commonly known as athlete's foot, which is annoying and contagious. Applying creams is recommended for the acquired condition. Doing nothing is not an appropriate response to the client. Wearing tight-fitting wool socks will not help the client avoid contracting this condition.

CARE PLAN HINTS

1. The wound has become infected, and the infection is spreading. Lymphangitis is inflammation of the lymphatic channels or vessels that occurs with infections of deep skin tissues. Lymphangitis could lead to septicemia.
2. The nurse may respond by saying, "Lucy, the medication in your IV is stronger and will help fight the infection in your leg to keep it from spreading."
3. The nurse could respond by saying, "Lucy will be more comfortable if she rests her leg and elevates it on some pillows. You could apply warm compresses to her leg to increase circulation and promote healing. Lucy might also enjoy having a friend over to watch TV, because cellulitis is not contagious."

CRITICAL THINKING CARE MAP

Subjective Data
- Mother states they have had a lot of fish over the last week
- Stopped attending youth group with friends
- Mother states child is now wearing a small amount of make-up

- Child reports her skin itches and the sores leak fluid more during the winter
- Child states she likes milk and cookies
- Mother states the child doesn't shower after swimming

Objective Data
- Lesions on neck dry and scaly
- Ruptured papules with yellow crust behind knees

Report   Yes, to the pediatrician.

Interventions
- Apply wet compresses to lesions that are crusted
- Hydrate skin with lotions and creams
- Encourage showering after swimming
- Administer oral antihistamines
- Obtain a thorough nutrition history
- Keep environmental temperatures cool.
- Instruct to keep fingernails short
- Encourage child to wear loose-fitting clothing

Documentation   (date) 1330 Mother of 12-year-old female calls the pediatrician's office reporting skin on neck and behind knees are red and have crusted open lesions that itch × 3 days. She states she is unable to rest and is scratching the areas all of the time. Appointment made for 1600. Report given to Dr. Peterson. S. Vargus, LPN

Chapter 22

NCLEX-PN® ANSWERS

(1) 2, 4, 6. Outcome 4. Clients who have sensitivities/allergies to bananas, avocados, potatoes, chestnuts, and tropical fruits can be at risk for developing an allergy to latex. The possible cause for this is a cross-reaction between the food and the latex allergen. Potatoes, milk, and yogurt have not been linked to latex sensitivities/allergies. (2) 4. Outcome 4. Immunizations provide acquired immunity from diseases by causing the formation of specific antibodies. No immunization protects against all diseases. Natural immunity is the condition present at birth and is part of acquired immunity. Nonhumoral immunity does not describe the role of immunizations. (3) 2. Outcome 3. Mothers who are HIV positive must avoid breastfeeding their infants. The mother demonstrates proper understanding of potential transmission of HIV by stating that she realizes the infant may still have the potential of having HIV; that hand washing is imperative before and after caring for the infant; and that the infant will be treated with AZT to reduce the risk of HIV transmission. (4) 4. Outcomes 3 and 4. Rhinitis is not associated with juvenile rheumatoid arthritis. Fever, rash, and lymphadenopathy are symptoms associated with JRA. (5) 4. Outcome 2. Cell-mediated immunity provides protection against bacteria, viruses, fungi, and tumors. This process develops early in the child's life.

Cell-mediated immunity is also the process that causes rejection of organs that have been transplanted. Primary and lymph-mediated immunity are not accurate terms. Acquired immunity includes cell-mediated immunity, but is not the best answer. (6) 1. Outcome 5. Urinary dysfunction and fluid and electrolyte imbalances are indicators of potential problems in the kidney transplant recipient. The nurse would not expect to see a disruption in cardiac or respiratory function, range of motion, or edema following this procedure. Thrombophlebitis and periorbital edema are not signs of organ rejection. (7) 3. Outcomes 3 and 4. The nurse suspects, with the symptoms described and results from the examination, that the client may have HIV. Of course, further evaluation will be needed to determine a definitive diagnosis so treatment can begin. The symptoms and result of the examination do not point to juvenile rheumatoid arthritis, latex allergies, or chronic otitis media. (8) 1. Outcome 4. Nursing interventions for children with HIV are avoidance of contact with persons with infections, colds, flu, and so forth, and proper nutrition. Antibiotic therapy and careful skin care are not nursing interventions for HIV, nor is starting an exercise regime and range of motion. Administration of oral antihistamines and penicillin are not indicated for this disease. (9) 3. Outcome 2. Humoral immunity destroys bacteria, viruses, parasites, allergens, and other foreign substances in the bloodstream by producing antibodies called immunoglobulins. This production of immunoglobulins begins in early infancy but is not complete until approximately age 6 or 7. Humoral immunity does not protect the child from everything. This statement is too broad and nonspecific. (10) 1, 2, 4, 6. Outcomes 3 and 4. When caring for the client with known latex allergies, the nurse knows to use only products that do not contain latex. All latex products must be removed from the client's room and, because regular blood pressure cuffs contain latex, specialized cuffs should be used. The latex-free cart should be kept available in or near the client's room.

CARE PLAN HINTS

1. Motor skill for a 4-year-old include hopping and skipping on one foot; catching and throwing a ball overhand; walking downstairs; using scissors; lacing shoes; copying a square; and adding three parts to a stick figure. Riley's parents can spend time daily demonstrating hopping and skipping and getting Riley to try the skill. They can also allot time daily to play catch with a ball. Paper and scissor activities would be another appropriate activity.

2. Language skills for a 4-year-old include a vocabulary of more than 1,500 words, using sentences of four or five words, asking frequent questions, singing simple songs,

and naming one or more colors. Riley's parents should encourage her to use new words to express herself. They can play children's CDs while riding in the car. Flash cards can be used to help Riley learn her colors.

3. Toys that would assist Riley include a medium sized, light-weight ball; a rope for her to jump over; a craft kit to include scissors, paper, chunky crayons, and tracing paper; a collection of CDs with simple children's songs; and homemade or purchased flashcards depicting colors.

CRITICAL THINKING CARE MAP

Subjective Data "I feel really tired." "I'd feel like a nerd if I wore that mask to school." "My best friend has the flu."

Objective Data Vital signs. Lab results to include CBC, blood or wound cultures. Serum protein and albumin. Skin assessment for wounds and wound drainage.

Report Yes. The nurse needs to report these findings because they further compromise Joe's condition, and interventions need to be planned and implemented to assist Joe in preventing infection.

Interventions Instruct Joe in hand washing and other techniques to avoid contamination with harmful bacteria or viruses. Review immunization schedule and recommend required immunizations as appropriate. Teach Joe and his parents to recognize symptoms of infections, colds, and flu in himself, family members, friends, or others he may come in contact with. Make sure Joe and his parents understand the proper handling, storage, and preparation of food. Make frequent follow-up appointments with Joe to monitor lab values.

Documentation (date/time). 15-year-old male with positive HIV test. Vital signs: Temp 99.2 degrees F, Pulse 66, Resp 14, BP 110/74. CBC drawn, awaiting results. Skin warm, dry, pink and without lesions. States "I'm really tired all the time." Teaching done re: infection prevention, therapeutic regime and information given about HIV and AIDS and the consequences. Following teaching, states "I'd feel like a nerd if I wore that mask to school." and "My best friend has the flu." Understanding of teaching is in question. Report given to charge nurse. Teaching plan revised. K. Anderson LPN.

UNIT III Thinking Strategically About ...

CASE 1 SCENARIO

CRITICAL THINKING

1. Jeremy's mother is exhibiting intellectual humility in her confession of not knowing everything she needs to about Jeremy's illness.

2. To minimize the pain of the injections, warm the insulin to room temperature (once open, it can be stored at room temperature); remove all air bubbles from the syringe prior to injection; allow alcohol to dry completely prior to the injection; assist the child in learning how to relax the muscle group to be used for the injection; praise him for his participation; observe the needle carefully for burrs; insert the needle swiftly in one motion; and hold the needle steady once it has penetrated the skin.

COLLABORATIVE CARE

1. The nutritionist will need Jeremy's complete health history, including all labs. To provide Jeremy and his family with an appropriate diet plan, the nutritionist will need to know Jeremy's height and weight, his typical diet, his likes and dislikes, what amount of exercise he engages in on a daily basis, and what medication regimen the physician has ordered.

2. The LPN should give Jeremy's mother reading material to reinforce teaching. Support groups can offer opportunities for exchange of information and assistance in problem solving.

CASE 2 SCENARIO

DELEGATING

- The following orders could be delegated to the certified nursing assistant: vital signs, daily weight, and assistance with diet.

MANAGEMENT OF CARE

- To find the infusion rate for an order D5 ½ NS to infuse at 1,000 mL in 8 hours using a drop factor of 10 drops/mL, convert 8 hours to minutes (480 minutes). Find the total number of drops in 1,000 mL (10,000). Divide the total number of drops by the total number of minutes to find the number of drops per minute.

$$\frac{10,000 \text{ drops/mL}}{480 \text{ minutes}} = 21 \text{ drops/minute}$$

COMMUNICATION AND CLIENT TEACHING

- Develop a teaching plan to provide nutritional information. The LPN can teach Jackson's mother to progress the diet slowly. Once vomiting has slowed, small sips of water can be offered to Jackson. Gelatin and clear broth can be added next. Once Jackson can keep these liquids down, his mother can offer him bland carbohydrates such as plain toast, rice, or crackers. Small bites of banana or spoonfuls of applesauce can be offered next.

CASE 3 SCENARIO

TIME MANAGEMENT AND PRIORITIES IN NURSING CARE

- Nursing interventions should be implemented for Janice in the following order: Assess carefully for symptoms of shock to include decreased blood pressure; rapid, thready pulse; rapid, shallow respirations; cool, pale, moist skin; thirst; restlessness; and changes in level of consciousness. Keep Janice's trunk and head flat with legs slightly elevated. Keep her warm with blankets. Do not give Janice anything to eat or drink. Provide emotional support.

DOCUMENTING AND REPORTING
- All information gathered is important to document. Symptoms of shock must be reported promptly to the physician.

CULTURAL CARE STRATEGIES
- Some followers of the Jehovah's Witness religion cannot accept blood or blood products. It is important to discuss the possibility of the need for blood replacement with the physician, nursing supervisor, and Janice's parents. If the parents will not give consent for the replacement, it is important that they understand the consequences if Janice does not receive the blood replacement. Some institutions may pursue a court order to be able to administer the blood without parental consent.

Appendix II
Growth Charts

Figure II-A. ■ Physical growth percentiles for length and weight—boys: birth to 36 months. (From CDC [2001]. http://www.cdc.gov/growthcharts)

Figure II-B. ■ Physical growth percentiles for length and weight—girls: birth to 36 months. (From CDC [2001]. http://www.cdc.gov/growthcharts)

2 to 20 years: Boys
Stature-for-age and Weight-for-age percentiles

NAME _____

RECORD # _____

Mother's Stature _____ Father's Stature _____

Date	Age	Weight	Stature	BMI*

*To Calculate BMI: Weight (kg) ÷ Stature (cm) ÷ Stature (cm) x 10,000
or Weight (lb) ÷ Stature (in) ÷ Stature (in) x 703

AGE (YEARS)

STATURE

WEIGHT

Revised and corrected November 21, 2000.
SOURCE: Developed by the National Center for Health Statistics in collaboration with
the National Center for Chronic Disease Prevention and Health Promotion (2000).
http://www.cdc.gov/growthcharts

CDC

Figure II-C. ■ Physical growth percentiles for stature and weight according to age—boys: 2 to 20 years. (From CDC [2001]. http:// www.cdc.gov/growthcharts)

2 to 20 years: Girls
Stature-for-age and Weight-for-age percentiles

NAME _____

RECORD # _____

Mother's Stature _____ Father's Stature _____

Date	Age	Weight	Stature	BMI*

*To Calculate BMI: Weight (kg) ÷ Stature (cm) ÷ Stature (cm) x 10,000
or Weight (lb) ÷ Stature (in) ÷ Stature (in) x 703

AGE (YEARS)

STATURE

WEIGHT

Revised and corrected November 21, 2000.
SOURCE: Developed by the National Center for Health Statistics in collaboration with
the National Center for Chronic Disease Prevention and Health Promotion (2000).
http://www.cdc.gov/growthcharts

CDC

Figure II-D. ■ Physical growth percentiles for stature and weight according to age—girls: 2 to 20 years. (From CDC [2001].
http://www.cdc.gov/ growthcharts)

Appendix III
Denver Developmental Screening

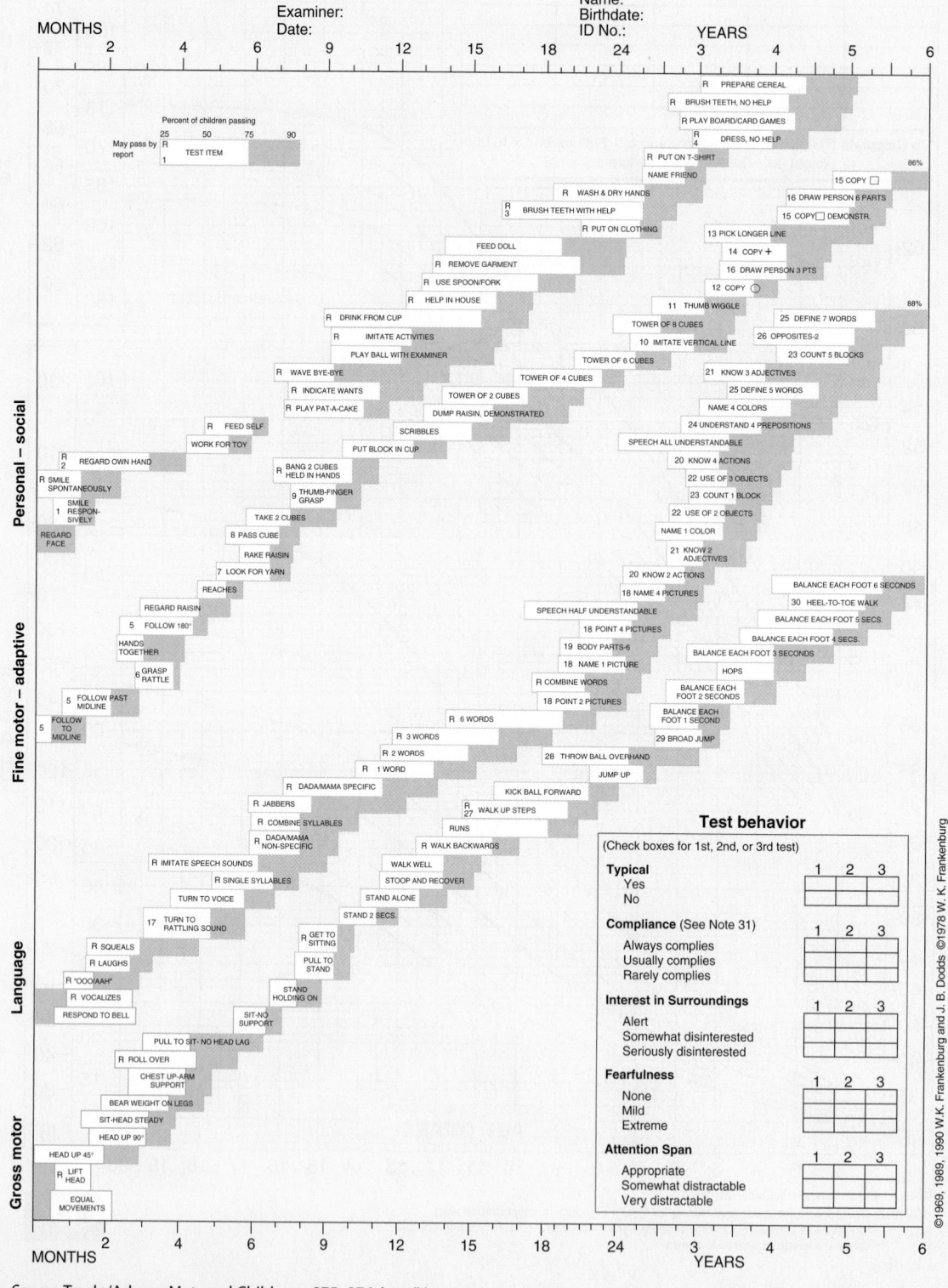

Source: Towle/Adams, Maternal Child, pgs. 875–876 App. IV

DIRECTIONS FOR ADMINISTRATION

1. Try to get child to smile by smiling, talking or waving. Do not touch him/her.
2. Child must stare at hand several seconds.
3. Parent may help guide toothbrush and put toothpaste on brush.
4. Child does not have to be able to tie shoes or button/zip in the back.
5. Move yarn slowly in an arc from one side to the other, about 8" above child's face.
6. Pass if child grasps rattle when it is touched to the backs or tips of fingers.
7. Pass if child tries to see where yarn went. Yarn should be dropped quickly from sight from tester's hand without arm movement.
8. Child must transfer cube from hand to hand without help of body, mouth, or table.
9. Pass if child picks up raisin with any part of thumb and finger.
10. Line can vary only 30 degrees or less from tester's line.
11. Make a fist with thumb pointing upward and wiggle only the thumb. Pass if child imitates and does not move any fingers other than the thumb.

12. Pass any enclosed form. Fail continuous round motions.
13. Which line is longer? (Not bigger.) Turn paper upside down and repeat. (pass 3 of 3 or 5 of 6).
14. Pass any lines crossing near midpoint.
15. Have child copy first. If failed, demonstrate.

When giving items 12, 14, and 15, do not name the forms. Do not demonstrate 12 and 14.

16. When scoring, each pair (2 arms, 2 legs, etc.) counts as one part.
17. Place one cube in cup and shake gently near child's ear, but out of sight. Repeat for other ear.
18. Point to picture and have child name it. (No credit is given for sounds only.)
    If less than 4 pictures are named correctly, have child point to picture as each is named by tester.

19. Using doll, tell child: Show me the nose, eyes, ears, mouth, hands, feet, tummy, hair. Pass 6 of 8.
20. Using pictures, ask child: Which one flies?... says meow?... talks?... barks?... gallops? Pass 2 of 5, 4 of 5.
21. Ask child: What do you do when you are cold?... tired?... hungry? Pass 2 of 3, 3 of 3.
22. Ask child: What do you do with a cup? What is a chair used for? What is a pencil used for?
    Action words must be included in answers.
23. Pass if child correctly places and says how many blocks are on paper (1, 5).
24. Tell child: Put block **on** table, **under** table, **in front of** me, **behind** me. Pass 4 of 4.
    (Do not help child by pointing, moving head or eyes.)
25. Ask child: What is a ball?... lake?... desk?... house?... banana?... curtain?... fence?... ceiling? Pass if defined in terms of use, shape, what it is made of, or general category (such as banana is fruit, not just yellow). Pass 5 of 8, 7 of 8.
26. Ask child: If a horse is big, a mouse is_____? If fire is hot, ice is_____? If sun shines during the day, the moon shines during the _____? Pass 2 of 3.
27. Child may use wall or rail only, not person. May not crawl.
28. Child must throw ball overhand 3 feet to within arm's reach of tester.
29. Child must perform standing broad jump over width of test sheet (8 1/2 inches).
30. Tell child to walk forward, ⊂⊃⊂⊃⊂⊃ → heel within 1 inch of toe. Tester may demonstrate.
    Child must walk 4 consecutive steps.
31. In the second year, half of normal children are non-compliant.

OBSERVATIONS:

Appendix IV
Common Conversions and Lab Values

Selected Common Conversions Between English and Metric Measurements

1 g = 1 mL (used when weighing diaper to determine fluid output)

1 grain = 60 mg

15 grains = 1 g

1 oz = 30 mL

1.2 lb = 1 kg (used when recording in metric or computing body mass index [BMI])

1 inch = 2.5 cm (used when recording in metric)

39 inches = 1 yd 3 inches

= 1 m (used when recording in metric)

Conversion Formulas for Temperature Readings

CELSIUS TO FAHRENHEIT
From °C up to °F:

$$°F = 1.8 \times °C + 32$$

First **multiply** °C by 1.8; then **add** 32.

FAHRENHEIT TO CELSIUS
From °F down to °C:

$$°C = (°F - 32) \text{ divided by } 1.8$$

First **subtract** 32 from °F; then **divide** by 1.8.

Normal Vital Sign Ranges by Age

AGE	TEMPERATURE IN DEGREES CELSIUS/ FAHRENHEIT	PULSE (AVERAGE AND RANGE)	RESPIRATIONS (AVERAGE AND RANGE)	BLOOD PRESSURE (mm Hg)
Newborns	36.8 (axillary)	130 (80–180)	35 (30–60)	73/55
1–3 years	37.7 (rectal)	120 (80–140)	30 (20–40)	90/55
6–8 years	37 (oral)	100 (75–120)	20 (15–25)	95/57
10 years	37 (oral)	70 (50–90)	19 (15–25)	102/62
Teen years	37 (oral)	70 (50–90)	18 (15–20)	120/80
Adult	37 (oral)	80 (60–100)	16 (12–20)	120/80
Older adult (greater than 70 years)	36 (oral)	80 (60–100)	16 (15–20)	Possible increased diastolic

Typical Laboratory Results for Infants and Children

COMPONENT TESTED	NORMAL LABORATORY VALUES
Hematocrit	Newborn: 44–65%; 1–3 years old: 29–40%; 4–10 years old: 31–43%
Urine specific gravity	Newborn: 1.001–1.020; Child: 1.005–1.030
Blood urea nitrogen	Infant: 5–15 mg/dL; Child: 5–20 mg/dL
Potassium	Infant: 3.6–5.8 mEq/L; Child: 3.5–5.5 mEq/L
Sodium	Infant: 134–150 mEq/L; Child: 135–145 mEq/L
Calcium	Newborn: 3.7–7.0 mEq/L or 7.4–14.0 mg/dL; Infant: 5.0–6.0 mEq/L or 10–12 mg/dL; Child: 4.5–5.8 mEq/L or 9–11.5 mg/dL
Blood Gases pH PaCO$_2$ HCO$_3$	Child: 7.36–7.44 Child: 35–45 mm Hg Child: 22–26 mEq/L

Note: Lab values may vary. Consult the laboratory at your health care agency.

Pediatric Lab Values for Oxygen Saturation

Normal	95–98%
Mild hypoxemia	90–95%
Moderate hypoxemia	85–90%
Severe hypoxemia	85% or lower

Lab Values for Urinalysis

CHARACTERISTIC	NORMAL VALUE
Bacteria	None to few organisms present
pH	4.50–8.0
Color	Clear, straw-colored, amber
Odor	Slight, nonoffensive odor
Glucose	Negative
Protein	Negative
Red blood cells	Negative on gross examination; 0–5 per high-powered field
White blood cells	Negative; fewer than 2 per high-powered field
Specific gravity	Newborn: 1.001–1.020; Child: 1.005–1.030
Ketones	Negative

Lab Values for Children with Renal Failure

LAB	NORMAL	FINDING IN RENAL FAILURE
Blood urea nitrogen	Infant: 5–15 mg/dL	Increased
	Child: 5–20 mg/dL	Increased
Serum creatinine	Newborn: 0.8–1.4 mg/dL	Increased
	Infant: 0.7–1.7 mg/dL	Increased
	2–6 years old: 0.3–0.6 mg/dL	Increased
	Greater than 6 years old: 0.4–1.2 mg/dL	Increased
Serum potassium	Infant: 3.6–5.8 mEq/L	Increased
	Child: 3.5–5.5 mEq/L	Increased
Serum sodium	Infant: 134–150 mEq/L	Increased or decreased
	Child: 135–145 mEq/L	Increased or decreased
Bicarbonate (HCO_3)	24–28 mEq/L	Decreased

Laboratory Values for Cholesterol

TEST	NORMAL	BORDERLINE LEVELS	HIGH LEVELS
Total cholesterol	Less than 170 mg/dL	170–199 mg/dL	More than 200 mg/dL
Low-density lipoproteins	Less than 110 mg/dL	110–129 mg/dL	More than 130 mg/dL
Triglycerides	100 mg/dL	100–150 mg/dL	More than 150 mg/dL
High-density lipoproteins	More than 35 mg/dL	Less than 35 mg/dL	

Appendix V
Standard Precautions for Infection Control

Excerpted from *Guideline for Isolation Precautions in Hospitals* (January 1996).

Background

Standard Precautions synthesize Blood/Body Fluid Precautions and guidelines for body substance isolation and apply them to all clients regardless of their diagnosis or presumed infection status. Standard Precautions apply to 1) blood; 2) all body fluids, secretions, and excretions except sweat, regardless of whether or not they contain visible blood; 3) nonintact skin; and 4) mucous membranes. Standard Precautions are designed to reduce the risk of transmission of microorganisms from both recognized and unrecognized sources of infection in hospitals.

II. Standard Precautions

A. *Handwashing*

Wash hands after touching blood, body fluids, secretions, excretions, and contaminated items, whether or not gloves are worn. Wash hands immediately after gloves are removed, between client contacts. Use an antimicrobial agent or a waterless antiseptic agent for specific circumstances (e.g., when hands are not visibly soiled, for control of outbreaks, etc.).

B. *Gloves*

Wear gloves (clean, nonsterile gloves are adequate) when touching blood, body fluids, secretions, excretions, and contaminated items. Put on clean gloves just before touching mucous membranes and nonintact skin. Change gloves between tasks and procedures on the same client after contact with material that may contain a high concentration of microorganisms. Remove gloves promptly after use and wash hands immediately to avoid transfer of microorganisms.

C. *Mask, Eye Protection, Face Shield*

Wear a mask and eye protection or a face shield to protect mucous membranes of the eyes, nose, and mouth during procedures that are likely to generate splashes or sprays of blood, body fluids, secretions, and excretions.

D. *Gown*

Wear a gown (a clean, nonsterile gown is adequate) to protect skin and to prevent soiling of clothing during procedures and client-care activities that are likely to generate splashes or sprays of blood, body fluids, secretions, or excretions.

E. *Client-Care Equipment*

Handle soiled equipment so as to prevent personal contamination of clothing and transfer of microorganisms. Ensure that reusable equipment is not used for the care of another client until it has been cleaned and reprocessed appropriately. Ensure that single-use items are discarded properly.

F. *Environmental Control*

Ensure that hospital procedures for the routine care, cleaning, and disinfection of environmental surfaces, beds, bedrails, bedside equipment, and other frequently touched surfaces are being followed.

G. *Linen*

Handle, transport, and process used linen soiled with blood, body fluids, secretions, and excretions in a manner that prevents skin and mucous membrane exposures and contamination of clothing, and that avoids transfer of microorganisms.

H. *Occupational Health and Bloodborne Pathogens*

1. Take care to prevent injuries when using needles, scalpels, and other sharp instruments or devices. Never recap used needles using both hands, or use any other technique that involves directing the point of a needle toward any part of the body; rather, use either a one-handed "scoop" technique or a mechanical device designed for holding the needle sheath. Do not remove used needles from disposable syringes by hand, and do not bend, break, or manipulate used needles by hand. Place all sharp items in appropriate puncture-resistant containers. Use mouthpieces, resuscitation bags, or other ventilation devices as an alternative to mouth-to-mouth resuscitation methods.

I. *Client Placement*

Place client who contaminates the environment or who does not (or cannot be expected to) assist in maintaining appropriate hygiene or environmental control in a private room.

Date last modified: April 1, 2005

Source: Department of Health and Human Services, Centers for Disease Control and Prevention.

Standard Precautions[†],[‡]

Use Standard Precautions for the care of all patients.

Airborne Precautions

In addition to Standard Precautions, use Airborne Precautions for patients known or suspected to have serious illnesses transmitted by airborne droplet nuclei. Examples of such illnesses include:

- Measles
- Varicella (including disseminated zoster)[†]
- Tuberculosis[‡]

Droplet Precautions

In addition to Standard Precautions, use Droplet Precautions for patients known or suspected to have serious illnesses transmitted by large particle droplets. Examples of such illnesses include:

- Invasive *Haemophilus influenzae* type B disease, including meningitis, pneumonia, epiglottitis, and sepsis
- Invasive *Neisseria meningitidis* disease, including meningitis, pneumonia, and sepsis

Other serious bacterial respiratory infections spread by droplet transmission, including:

- Diphtheria (pharyngeal)
- Mycoplasma pneumonia
- Pertussis
- Pneumonic plague
- Streptococcal (group A) pharyngitis, pneumonia, or scarlet fever in infants and young children

Serious viral infections spread by droplet transmission, including:

- Adenovirus[†]
- Influenza
- Mumps
- Parvovirus B19
- Rubella

Contact Precautions

In addition to Standard Precautions, use Contact Precautions for patients known or suspected to have serious illnesses easily transmitted by direct patient contact or by contact with items in the patient's environment. Examples of such illnesses include:

Gastrointestinal, respiratory, skin, or wound infections or colonization with multidrug-resistant bacteria judged by the infection control program, based on current state, regional, or national recommendations, to be of special clinical and epidemiologic significance

Enteric infections with a low infectious dose or prolonged environmental survival, including:

- *Clostridium difficile*
- For diapered or incontinent patients: enterohemorrhagic *Escherichia coli* O157:H7, *Shigella,* hepatitis A, or rotavirus

Respiratory syncytial virus, parainfluenza virus, or enteroviral infections in infants and young children

Skin infections that are highly contagious or that may occur on dry skin, including:

- Diphtheria (cutaneous)
- Herpes simplex virus (neonatal or mucocutaneous)
- Impetigo
- Major (noncontained) abscesses, cellulitis, or decubiti
- Pediculosis
- Scabies
- Staphylococcal furunculosis in infants and young children
- Zoster (disseminated or in the immunocompromised host)[†]
- Viral/hemorrhagic conjunctivitis
- Viral hemorrhagic infections (Ebola, Lassa, or Marburg)

Source: Centers for Disease Control and Prevention Fundamentals of Isolation Precautions.

[†]Certain infections require more than one type of precaution.

[‡]See Jensen, P., Lambert, L., Iademarco, M. (2005). Guidelines for preventing the transmission of *Mycobacterium tuberculosis* in health-care settings. *Morbidity and Mortality Weekly Report, 54*(RR17), 1–141.

Contents: *These precautions last reviewed and updated by CDC, April 1, 2005.*

Appendix VI
NANDA-Approved Nursing Diagnoses

Note: The initial letter of the key word in each NANDA diagnosis is in boldface.

Activity
  Activity Intolerance
  Risk for Activity Intolerance

Adaptive Capacity
  Decreased Intracranial Adaptive Capacity

Airway Clearance
  Ineffective Airway Clearance

Allergy Response
  Latex Allergy Response
  Risk for Latex Allergy Response

Anxiety
  Death Anxiety

Aspiration
  Risk for Aspiration

Attachment
  Risk for Impaired Attachment, Parent
  Risk for Impaired Attachment, Infant
  Risk for Impaired Attachment, Child

Blood Glucose
  Risk for Unstable Blood Glucose

Body Image
  Disturbed Body Image

Body Temperature
  Risk for Imbalanced Body Temperature

Bowel
  Bowel Incontinence

Breastfeeding
  Effective Breastfeeding
  Ineffective Breastfeeding
  Interrupted Breastfeeding

Breathing Pattern
  Ineffective Breathing Pattern

Cardiac Output
  Decreased Cardiac Output

Caregiver Role Strain
  Risk for Caregiver Role Strain

Comfort
  Readiness for Enhanced Comfort

Communication
  Readiness for Enhanced Communication
  Impaired Verbal Communication

Confusion
  Acute Confusion
  Chronic Confusion
  Risk for Acute Confusion

Constipation
  Perceived Constipation
  Risk for Constipation

Contamination
  Risk for Contamination

Coping
  Ineffective Community Coping
  Readiness for Enhanced Community Coping
  Defensive Coping
  Compromised Family Coping
  Disabled Family Coping
  Readiness for Enhanced Family Coping
  Readiness for Enhanced Individual Coping
  Ineffective Coping

Decision Making
  Readiness for Enhanced Decision Making
  Decisional Conflict (Specify)

Denial
  Ineffective Denial

Dentition
  Impaired Dentition

Development
  Risk for Delayed Development

Diarrhea

Disuse Syndrome
  Risk for Disuse Syndrome

Diversional Activity
  Deficient Diversional Activity

Dysreflexia
  Autonomic Dysreflexia
  Risk for Autonomic Dysreflexia

Energy Field
  Disturbed Energy Field

Environmental Interpretation Syndrome
  Impaired Environmental Interpretation Syndrome

Failure to Thrive
  Adult Failure to Thrive

Falls
  Risk for Falls

Family Processes
  Dysfunctional Family Processes: Alcoholism
  Interrupted Family Processes
  Readiness for Enhanced Family Processes

Fatigue

Fear

Fluid Balance
  Readiness for Enhanced Fluid Balance

Fluid Volume
  Deficient Fluid Volume
  Risk for Deficient Fluid Volume
  Excess Fluid Volume
  Risk for Imbalanced Fluid Volume

Gas Exchange
  Impaired Gas Exchange

Grieving
  Complicated Grieving
  Risk for Complicated Grieving

Growth
  Risk for Disproportionate Growth

Growth and Development
  Delayed Growth and Development

Health Behavior
  Risk-Prone Health Behavior
  Health Seeking Behaviors (Specify)

Home Maintenance
  Impaired Home Maintenance

Hope
  Readiness for Enhanced Hope

Hopelessness

Human Dignity
  Risk for Compromised Human Dignity

Hyperthermia

Hypothermia

Identity
  Disturbed Personal Identity

Immunization Status
  Readiness for Enhanced Immunization Status

Infant Behavior
  Disorganized Infant Behavior
  Risk for Disorganized Infant Behavior
  Readiness for Enhanced Organized Infant Behavior

Infant Feeding Pattern
  Ineffective Infant Feeding Pattern

Infection
  Risk for Infection

Injury
  Risk for Injury

Insomnia

Knowledge
  Deficient Knowledge (Specify)
  Readiness for Enhanced Knowledge (Specify)

Lifestyle
  Sedentary Lifestyle

Liver Function
  Risk for Impaired Liver Function

Loneliness
  Risk for Loneliness

Memory
  Impaired Memory

Mobility
  Impaired Bed Mobility
  Impaired Physical Mobility
  Impaired Wheelchair Mobility

Moral
  Moral Distress

Nausea

Neglect
  Unilateral Neglect

Neurovascular Dysfunction
  Risk for Peripheral Neurovascular Dysfunction

Noncompliance (Specify)

Nutrition
  Imbalanced Nutrition: Less than Body Requirements
  Imbalanced Nutrition: More than Body Requirements
  Risk for Imbalanced Nutrition: More than Body
    Requirements
  Readiness for Enhanced Nutrition

Oral Mucous Membrane
  Impaired Oral Mucous Membrane

Pain
  Acute Pain
  Chronic Pain

Parenting
  Impaired Parenting
  Readiness for Enhanced Parenting
  Risk for Impaired Parenting

Perioperative Positioning Injury
  Risk for Perioperative Positioning Injury

Poisoning
  Risk for Poisoning
Post-Trauma Syndrome
  Risk for Post-Trauma Syndrome
Power
  Readiness for Enhanced Power
Powerlessness
  Risk for Powerlessness
Protection
  Ineffective Protection
Rape-Trauma Syndrome
  Rape-Trauma Syndrome: Compound Reaction
  Rape-Trauma Syndrome: Silent Reaction
Religiosity
  Impaired Religiosity
  Readiness for Enhanced Religiosity
  Risk for Impaired Religiosity
Relocation Stress Syndrome
  Risk for Relocation Stress Syndrome
Role Conflict
  Parental Role Conflict
Role Performance
  Ineffective Role Performance
Self-Care
  Readiness for Enhanced Self-Care
Self-Care Deficit
  Bathing/Hygiene Self-Care Deficit
  Dressing/Grooming Self-Care Deficit
  Feeding Self-Care Deficit
  Toileting Self-Care Deficit
Self-Concept
  Readiness for Enhanced Self-Concept
Self-Esteem
  Chronic Low Self-Esteem
  Situational Low Self-Esteem
  Risk for Situational Low Self-Esteem
Self-Mutilation
  Risk for Self-Mutilation
Sensory Perception
  Disturbed Visual Sensory Perception (Specify)
  Disturbed Auditory Sensory Perception (Specify)
  Disturbed Kinesthetic Sensory Perception (Specify)
  Disturbed Gustatory Sensory Perception(Specify)
  Disturbed Tactile Sensory Perception (Specify)
  Disturbed Olfactory Sensory Perception (Specify)
Sexual Dysfunction
Sexuality Pattern
  Ineffective Sexuality Pattern

Skin Integrity
  Impaired Skin Integrity
  Risk for Impaired Skin Integrity
Sleep Deprivation
Sleep
  Readiness for Enhanced Sleep
Social Interaction
  Impaired Social Interaction
Social Isolation
Sorrow
  Chronic Sorrow
Spiritual Distress
  Risk for Spiritual Distress
Spiritual Well-Being
  Readiness for Enhanced Spiritual Well-Being
Stress Overload
Sudden Infant Death Syndrome
  Risk for Sudden Infant Death Syndrome
Suffocation
  Risk for Suffocation
Suicide
  Risk for Suicide
Surgical Recovery
  Delayed Surgical Recovery
Swallowing
  Impaired Swallowing
Therapeutic Regimen Management
  Ineffective Community Therapeutic Regimen
    Management
  Effective Therapeutic Regimen Management
  Ineffective Family Therapeutic Regimen Management
  Ineffective Therapeutic Regimen Management
  Readiness for Enhanced Therapeutic Regimen
    Management
Thermoregulation
  Ineffective Thermoregulation
Thought Processes
  Disturbed Thought Processes
Tissue Integrity
  Impaired Tissue Integrity
Tissue Perfusion
  Ineffective Renal Tissue Perfusion (Specify)
  Ineffective Cerebral Tissue Perfusion (Specify)
  Ineffective Cardiopulmonary Tissue Perfusion (Specify)
  Ineffective Gastrointestinal Tissue Perfusion (Specify)
  Ineffective Peripheral Tissue Perfusion (Specify)
  Ineffective Peripheral Tissue Perfusion

Appendix VII

Sign Language for Health Care Professionals

Ache (or pain)

Allergic*

Bathroom

Better

Congratulate (or praise)

Constipate*

Dizzy

Drink

Faint

Feel

Headache

Lie down

*Indicates signs that are in manually signed English. Those without an asterisk are American Sign Language.

Medicine

Name

Nauseous

No

Nurse

Pain

Please

Put on

Sick

Stay

Stomachache*

Thank you (or good)

Thirsty

Vomit

Want

Yes

Appendix VIII
Spanish Translations of English Phrases

This appendix provides some basic phrases you might need when working with families and children. It does not contain all possible ways to phrase questions, but it can be helpful when translators are not available. Most sentences are written for speaking to children and so are informal.

The appendix starts with introductory conversation. Then general nursing phrases or sentences are listed. There is a section for communicating with parents. Last, there are questions to ask if abuse is suspected or possible.

ESSENTIAL INTRODUCTORY PHRASES

Hello

I am a nurse.

I am a student nurse.

My name is _____.

What is your name?

Thank you

Please

Is someone here with you?

Does he (she) speak English?

Goodbye

GENERAL PHRASES

Is there anything that is worrying you?

I would like to take your blood pressure.

I would like to take your pulse.

I would like to take your temperature.

I would like to listen to your heart and lungs.

Please urinate in this cup and leave it in the bathroom.

Please stand up.

Please sit down.

Please lie down.

Are you having pain?

Do you need medicine for pain?

Do you need to urinate?

This is a bedpan to urinate in.

Can I help you to the bathroom?

Do you need to have a bowel movement?

I will help you.

I will stay with you.

FRASES INTRODUCTORAS ESENCIALES

Hola

Soy enfermera (enfermero).†

Soy estudiante de enfermería.

Mi nombre es _____.

Me llamo _____.

¿Cuál es su nombre? (formal, to parent)

¿Cómo te llamas? (informal, to child)

¿Cómo quieres ser llamada (llamado)?

Gracias

Por favor

¿Hay alquien aquí contigo?

¿Habla él (ella) inglés?

Adiós

FRASES GENERALES

¿Hay algo o alguna cosa que te preocupes?

Quisiera tomarle la presió arterial.

Quisiera tomarle el pulso.

Quisiera tomarle la temperatura.

Quisiera escucharle el corazon y los pulmones.

Puedes orinar en este vaso y dejarlo en el baño.

Por favor, levántete.

Por favor, siéntete.

Por favor, acuéstete.

¿Tienes dolores?

¿Necesitas medicina para el dolor?

¿Necesitas orinar?

Aquí tienes el bacín (la chata) (el pato) para orinar.

¿Te ayudo a ir al baño?

¿Necesitas mover el vientre (obrar)? Necesitas "Hacer caca"—coloquial

Te voy a ayudar.

Me quedaré contigo.

This is medicine for your pain. You will feel better soon.	Esta medicina es para el dolor. Va a sentirte mejor pronto.
Please turn on your left side.	Por favor voltéese al lado izquierdo.
Please turn on your right side.	Por favor voltéese al lado derecho.
Are you hungry?	¿Tienes hambre?
Are you thirsty?	¿Tienes sed?
Are you cold?	¿Tienes frío?
Are you tired?	¿Estás cansada (cansado)?

QUESTIONS OR COMMUNICATIONS WITH THE MOTHER OR FATHER

POSIBLES PREGUNTAS O COMUNICACIONES CON MADRES O PADRES

How big is my baby?	¿De qué tamaño es el (la) bebé?
How much does the baby weigh now?	¿Cuánto pesa el bebé ahora?
What is your doctor's name?	¿Cuál es el nombre de su doctor?
Your baby (child) is having some trouble now.	El bebé (hijo o hija) está pasando por algunos problemas.
Your baby (child) is OK.	El bebé (hijo o hija) está bien.
We are giving your baby (child) oxygen.	Le vamos a dar oxígeno al (a la) bebé (hijo o hija).
Your baby (child) is having problems breathing.	El (la) bebé (hijo o hija) tiene problemas al respirar.
Would you like to see your baby (child) now?	¿Quiere ver a su bebé (hijo or hija) ahora?

PHRASES RELATED TO CLIENT SAFETY

FRASES RELACIONADAS CON LA SEGURIDAD DEL CLIENTE

I would like to talk to you alone.	Quisiera hablar a solas contigo.
Are you safe at home?	¿Sufres de peligros en casa?
Are you afraid of your father (mother, person in your family)?	¿Te tienes miedo a tu padre (madre, alguien en tu familia)?
Has he or she hit, slapped, kicked, or punched you?	¿Te ha golpeado?
	¿Te ha abofeteado?
	¿Te ha pateado?
	¿Te ha dado puñetazos?
How many times?	¿Cuántas veces?

†In Spanish, nouns that end in *a* indicate female gender; nouns that end in *o* indicate male gender.

References and Resources

CHAPTER 1

American Academy of Pediatrics. (2005). The changing concept of sudden infant death syndrome: Diagnostic coding shifts, controversies regarding the sleeping environment, and new variables to consider in reducing risk. *Pediatrics, 116*(5), 1245–1255.

American Nurses Association (ANA). (1998). *Standards of clinical practice* (2nd ed.). Washington, DC: American Nurses Publishing.

American Nurses Association (ANA). (1991). *Nursing's agenda for health care reform.* Washington, DC: Author.

American Nurses Association (ANA). (1980). *Nursing: A social policy statement.* Kansas City, MO: Author.

Brady-Fryer, B., Wiebe, N., & Landeer, J. (2004). Pain relief for neonatal circumcision. *The Cochrane Library*, issue 4.

Clifford, P. A., String, M., Christensen, H., & Mountain, D. (2004). Pain assessment and intervention for term newborns. *Journal of Midwifery and Women's Health, 49*(6), 514–519.

Gennaro, S., Hodnett, E., & Kearney, M. (2001). Making evidence-based practice a reality in your institutions: Evaluating the evidence and using the evidence to change clinical practice. *The American Journal of Maternal/Child Nursing, 26*(5), 236–250.

Henry, P. R., Haubold, K., & Dobrzykowski, T. (2004). Pain in the healthy full-term neonate: Efficacy and safety of interventions. *Newborn Infant Nursing Review, 4*(2), 126–130.

Krepper, R., Young, A., Cummings, E. (1994). Pediatric home healthcare: A paradox. *Home Health Care Nurse, 12*(4), 15–19.

Leininger, M., McFarland, M., McFarlane, M. (2002). *Transcultural nursing* (3rd ed.). New York: McGraw-Hill Professional.

National Council of State Boards of Nursing, Incorporated. (1995). *Delegation: Concepts and decisional-making process.* Chicago: Author.

North American Nursing Diagnosis Association (NANDA). (2008). *NANDA nursing diagnoses: Definitions and classification, 2008–2009.* Philadelphia: Elsevier.

Ramont, R. P., Niedringhaus, D. M., & Towle, M. A. (2006). *Comprehensive nursing care.* Upper Saddle River, NJ: Prentice Hall.

Razums, I., Dalton, M., & Wilson, D. (2004). Practice applications of research. Pain management for newborn circumcision. *Pediatric Nursing, 30*(5), 414–417.

U.S. Department of Health and Human Services. (1991). *Healthy People 2000.* Washington, DC: U.S. Government Printing Office.

U.S. Department of Health and Human Services. (2000). *Healthy People 2010* (2nd ed.). Washington, DC: U.S. Government Printing Office.

Zotti, M. E., Brown, P., & Stotts, C. (1996). Community-based nursing versus community health nursing: What does it all mean? *Nursing Outlook, 44*, 211.

CHAPTER 2

Estabrooks, C. (1998). Will evidence-based nursing practice make practice perfect? *Canadian Journal of Nursing Research, 30*(1), 15–36.

National Council of State Boards of Nursing, Incorporated. (1995). *Delegation: Concepts and decisional-making process.* Chicago: Author.

Paul, R., & Elder, L. (2005). *The miniature guide to critical thinking concepts & tools.* Dillon Beach, CA: Foundation for Critical Thinking.

Pravikoff, D., Ranner, A., & Pierce, S. (2005). Readiness of U.S. nurses for evidence-based practice. *American Journal of Nursing, 105*(9), 40–51.

Spratley E., Johnson, A., Sochalski, J., Fritz, M., Spencer, W. (2001). *The registered nurse population March 2000: Findings from the National Sample Survey of Registered Nurses.* Rockville, MD: U.S. Department of Health and Human Services.

CHAPTER 3

American Association of Colleges of Nursing. (1999). *Nursing educational agenda for the 21st century.* Washington, DC: Author.

American Nurses Asociation. (1998). *Standards of clinical nursing practice* (2nd ed.). Silver Spring, MD: Author.

American Nurses Association. (2000). *New position statement adolescent health task force.* Washington, DC: Author.

Anderson, M. A. (2001). *Nursing leadership: Management and professional practice for the LPN/LVN* (2nd ed.). Philadelphia: FA Davis.

Centers for Disease Control. (2000). Building data systems for monitoring and responding to violence against women. *Weekly Report on Domestic Violence, 49*, (RR11). Retrieved June 28, 2006, from the Internet.

Centers for Disease Control. (2005). National surveillance data for Chlamydia, gonorrhea, and syphilis. *Trends in Reportable Sexually Transmitted Diseases in the United States, 2005.* Retrieved April 10, 2007, from http://www.cdc.gov.

Coty, E., Davis, J., & Angell, L. (2002). Documentation: *The language of nursing.* Upper Saddle River, NJ: Prentice Hall.

Guttmacher Institute. (2007, April). *An overview of minors' consent laws.* Guttmacher Institute State Policies in Brief. Accessed online.

Joint Commission on Accreditation of Healthcare Organizations. (2000). *2000 accreditation manual for hospitals.* Chicago: Author.

Miller, F., Emanuel, E., Rosenstein, D., & Straus, S. (2004). Ethical issues concerning research in complementary and alternative medicine. *Journal of the American Medical Association, 291*(5), 599–604.

National Association for Practical Nurse Education and Service. (1998). *Code of Ethics for licensed practical/vocational nurses.* Silver Spring, MD: Author.

Ramont, R. P., Niedringhaus, D. M., Towle, M. A. (2008). *Fundamental nursing care.* (2nd ed.). Upper Saddle River, NJ: Prentice Hall.

Thompson, J. B., Thompson, H. O. (1981). *Ethics in nursing.* New York: Macmillan.

National Federation of Licensed Practical Nurses. (1998). *Nursing practice standards for the licensed practical/vocational nurse.* Garner, NC: Author.

Richardson, J. (2001) Integrating complementary therapies into health care education: A cautious approach. *Journal of Clinical Nursing, 10*(6), 792.

Simpson, R. L. (1994). Ensuring patient data privacy, confidentiality, and security. *Nursing Management, 25*(7), 18–20.

U.S. Department of Health and Human Services. (1992). *Healthy people 2000.* Rockville, MD: Author.

U.S. Department of Health and Human Services. (2000). *Healthy people 2010.* Rockville, MD: Author.

Wilkinson, J. M. (2007). *Nursing process and critical thinking* (4th ed.). Upper Saddle River, NJ: Prentice Hall.

CHAPTER 4

American Association of Retired People. *Help for grandparents raising grandchildren.* Retrieved April 11, 2007 from the Internet.

Duvall, E. (1977). *Marriage and family development* (5th ed.). Philadelphia: Lippincott.

Friedman, M. (1992). *Family nursing theory and assessment*. New York: Appleton-Century-Crofts.

Giger J., & Davidhizar, R. (Eds.). (1995). *Transcultural nursing: Assessment and interventions* (2nd ed.). St. Louis, MO: Mosby.

Ramont, R. R., Niedringhaus, D. M., & Towle, M.A. (2006). *Comprehensive nursing care*. Upper Saddle River, NJ: Prentice Hall.

Simmons, R., & O'Neil, G. (2001) *Households and families: 2000*. Census Brief 2000. U.S. Census Bureau, U.S. Department of Commerce, Economics and Statistics Administration. Retrieved March 17, 2007, from the Internet.

Simmons, T., & Dye, J. L. (2003). *Grandparents living with grandchildren: 2000*. Census Brief 2000. Washington, DC: U.S. Department of Commerce, Economics and Statistics Administration.

CHAPTER 5

Andrews, M.M., and Boyle, J.S. (2002). *Transcultural concepts in nursing care* (4th ed.). Philadelphia: Lippincott Williams & Wilkins.

Ball, J., & Bindler, R. (2003). *Pediatric nursing caring for children* (3rd ed.). Upper Saddle River, NJ: Prentice Hall.

Carter, B., & McGoldrick, M. (1999). *The expanded family life cycle–Individual, family, and social perspectives* (3rd ed.). Needham Heights, MA: Allyn & Bacon.

Cox, H., Hinz, M., Lubno, M.A., Scott-Tilley, D., Newfield, S., McCarthy Slater, M., & Sridaromont, K. (2002). *Clinical applications of nursing diagnosis: Adult, child, women's, psychiatric, gerontic, and home health considerations* (4th ed.). Philadelphia, F.A. Davis.

Criddle, L., & Muir, N. (2006). *Look both ways: Help protect your family on the Internet*. Redmond, WA: Microsoft.

Eby, L. (2005). *Mental health nursing care*. Upper Saddle River, NJ: Prentice Hall.

Gralla, P. (2006). *The complete idiot's guide to Internet privacy and security*. Indianapolis, IN: Alpha.

Leavitt, J., & Linford, S. (2006). *Faux Paw's adventures in the Internet: Keeping children safe online*. New York: Wiley.

London, M. L., Ladewig, P. W., & Ball, J. W. (2003). *Maternal-newborn & child nursing: Family-centered care*. Upper Saddle River, NJ: Prentice Hall.

Marshall, W. A., & Tanner, J. M. (1969). Variations in the pattern of pubertal changes in girls. *Archives of Disease in Childhood*, 445(235); 291–303.

Marshall, W. A., & Tanner, J. M. (1970). Variations in the pattern of pubertal changes in boys. *Archives of Disease in Childhood*, 45(239); 13–23.

NAC Corner statistics and tips for our young messengers. (2007, March). *i-Parent Times*. Retrieved April 17, 2007 from the Internet.

National Center for Missing and Exploited Children. *Child safety on the information highway*. Office of Juvenile Justice and Delinquency Prevention. Washington, DC: U.S. Department of Justice. Retrieved April 17, 2007 from the Internet.

Olds, S. B., London, M. L., Ladewig, P. W., & Davidson, M. R. (2004). *Maternal-newborn nursing & women's health care* (7th ed.). Upper Saddle River, NJ: Prentice Hall.

Ramont, R. R., Niedringhaus, D. M., & Towle, M. A. (2006). *Comprehensive nursing care*. Upper Saddle River, NJ: Prentice Hall.

Roddel, V. (2007). *Internet safety family guide*. Rochester, NY: Lulu.

Tanner, J. M. (1962). *Growth of adolescents*. Oxford: Blackwell.

Tanner, J. M. (1966). *Growth at adolescence*. New York: Appleton.

CHAPTER 6

Abraham, K. (2004). Recognizing and treating childhood obesity. *American Journal of Nurse Practitioners*, 8(9), 31–32, 35–38.

Abrams, S. A. (2001). Calcium turnover and nutrition through the life cycle. *Proceedings of the Nutrition Society*, 60(2), 283–289.

American Academy of Pediatric Dentistry. (2003). *Clinical guidelines of fluoride therapy*. Chicago: Author.

American Academy of Pediatrics. (2000). Recommendations for preventive pediatric health care. *Pediatrics*, 105(3), 645–646.

American Academy of Pediatrics. (2001). The use and misuse of fruit juice in pediatrics. *Pediatrics*, 107(5), 1210–1213.

American Academy of Pediatrics. (2006). *Car safety seats: A guide for families*. Author.

Anderson, R. N., & Smith, B. L. (2005). Deaths: Leading causes for 2002. *National Vital Statistics Report*, 53(17). Hyattsville, MD: National Center for Health Statistics.

Breastfeeding and the use of human milk. (2005). *Pediatrics*, 115(2), 496–506.

Carmona, R. (2003). Reshaping America's healthcare for the future. Washington, DC: Joint Economic Committee of U. S. Congress.

Centers for Disease Control and Prevention. Recommended childhood and adolescent immunization schedule, United States 2006. Atlanta, GA: Author.

Consumer Product Safety Commission (CPSC). (2003, April). CPSC amends age guidelines. *CPSC Monitor*, 50.

de Young, S. (2002). *Teaching strategies for nurse educators*. Upper Saddle River, NJ: Prentice Hall.

Fuller, C. (2001). *Opening your child's nine learning windows*. Grand Rapids, MI: Zondervan.

Guidance for effective discipline. (2004). *Pediatrics*, 114(4), 1126.

Hay, W., Hayward, A., Levin, M., & Sondheimer, J. (2002). *Current pediatric diagnosis and treatment* (16th ed.). New York: McGraw-Hill.

National Center for Education in Maternal and Child Health. (2001). Bright futures at Georgetown University. Washington, DC: Georgetown University Public Policy Institute.

National Safety Council. (2004). *Child passenger safety: Fact sheet*. Washington, DC: Author.

O'Neil, J., Kelly, T., & Kirby, J. (1995). *350 tested strategies to prevent crime: A resource for municipal agencies & community groups*. Washington, DC: National Crime Prevention Council.

Pediatric Nutrition Practice Group of the American Dietetic Association. (2003). *Infant feedings: Guidelines for preparation of formula and breast milk in health care facilities*. Chicago, IL: American Dietetic Association.

U.S. Department of Agriculture, Center for Nutrition Policy and Promotion. (2005, April). *My pyramid: Steps to a healthier you*. CNPP-15. Retrieved September 17, 2006, from www.mypyramid.gov/downloads/miniposter.pdf.

U.S. Department of Health and Human Services. (1979). *Healthy people*. Washington, DC: U.S. Government Printing Office.

U.S. Department of Health and Human Services. (1980). *Promoting health/preventing illness: Objectives for the nation*. Washington, DC: U.S. Government Printing Office.

U.S. Department of Health and Human Services. (1991). *Healthy people 2000*. Washington, DC: U.S. Government Printing Office.

U.S. Department of Health and Human Services. (2000). *Healthy people 2010*. Washington, DC: U.S. Government Printing Office.

Wilkinson, B. (1983). *The 7 laws of the learner: How to teach almost anything to practically anyone*. Portland, OR: Multnomah Press.

CHAPTER 7

Bindler, R., & Howry, L. (2005). *Pediatric drug guide with nursing implications*. Upper Saddle River, NJ: Prentice Hall.

Carney, K. L. (1998). *What is cancer anyway?* New York: Dragonfly.

Elkins, P. & Roberts, M. (1984). A preliminary evaluation of hospital preparation of nonpatient children: Primary prevention in a "let's pretend hospital". *Child Health Care*, 13(1), 31–36.

Heamann, D. (1994). Let's Pretend: a hospital teaches children about health care. *Nursing Forum, 29*(4), 5–9.

Let's Pretend Hospital. Search Internet websites for sponsoring agency reports of their experiences.

McDaniel, L. (1993). *Let him live (one last wish)*. Boston: Laurel Leaf.

Newachek, P. A., McManus, M., Fix, H. B., Hung, Y. Y., & Halfon, N. (2000). Access to health care for children with special health needs. *Pediatrics, 105*(4), 760–766.

Richmond, C. (1996). *Chemo Girl: Saving the world one treatment at a time.* New York: Jones & Bartlett.

Smith, S., Duell, D., and Martin, B. (2004). *Clinical nursing skills: Basic to advanced skills* (6th ed.). Upper Saddle River, NJ: Prentice Hall.

CHAPTER 8

Ball, J., Bindler, R. (2006). *Child health nursing: Partnering with children and families.* Upper Saddle River, NJ: Prentice Hall.

Bindler, R., & Howry, L. (2005). *Pediatric drug guide with nursing implications.* Upper Saddle River, NJ: Prentice Hall.

Bindler, R. C., Ball, J. W., London, M. L., & Ladewig, P. W. (2003). *Clinical skills manual for maternal–newborn and child nursing.* Upper Saddle River, NJ: Prentice Hall.

Blackwell, P., & Baker, B. (2002). Estimating communication competence of infants and toddlers. *Journal of Pediatric Health Care, 16*(1), 19–35.

Humphries, J. (2002). The school health nurse and health education in the classroom. *Nursing Standard, 16*(17), 42–45.

Sydnor-Greenberg, N., & Dokken, D. (2001). Communication in health-care: Thought on the child's perspective. *Journal of Child and Family Nursing, 4*(3), 225–230.

CHAPTER 9

Eby, Linda. (2005). *Mental health nursing care.* Upper Saddle River, NJ: Prentice Hall.

Farrell, M. M., & Levine, D. L. (1993). Brain death in the pediatric patient: Historical, sociological, medical, religious, cultural, legal and ethical considerations. *Critical Care Medicine, 21*(12), 1951–1965.

Faulkner, K. W. (1997). Talking about death with a dying child. *American Journal of Nursing, 97*(6), 67–69.

Gootman, M. E. (1994). *When a friend dies: A book for teens about grieving and healing.* Minneapolis: Free Spirit Publishing.

Greenlee, S. (1992). *When someone dies.* Atlanta: Peachtree Publishing. (Ages 9–12)

How to relieve pain without medicine. (2004, November 15). *Pain/Anesthetics News.* Retrieved April 2, 2007 from the Internet.

Kübler-Ross, E. (1969). *On death and dying.* New York: Macmillan.

Koch D'Agostino, C. (1998, September). Issues in pediatric organ donation. *Jacksonville Medicine/Northeast Florida Medicine.* Retrieved September 25, 2006 from the Internet.

LeMone, P., & Burke, K. (2004). *Medical surgical nursing critical thinking in client care* (3rd ed.). Upper Saddle River, NJ: Pearson Education.

London, M. L., Ladewig, P. W., Ball, J. W., & Bindler, R. C. (2003). *Maternal–newborn & child nursing.* Upper Saddle River, NJ: Prentice Hall.

National Association of School Psychologists. (2001). *Helping children cope with loss, death, and grief: Response to a national tragedy.* Retrieved September 19, 2006 from the Internet.

National Organ Procurement and Transplantation Network. (1998, Spring). *UNOS Update.*

Spector, R. E. (2000). Cultural diversity in health and illness (5th ed., pp. 137–138, 144–149). Upper Saddle River, NJ: Prentice Hall Health.

Wolfelt, A. (2001). *Healing your grieving heart for kids.* Ft. Collins, CO: Companion.

Worden, J. W. *Talking to Children About Death.* Compiled from keynote addresses by J. W. Worden, Ph.D., at 1991 ADEC Annual Meeting.

Worden, J. W. (1996). *Children and grief: When a parent dies.* New York: Gilford Press.

CHAPTER 10

Allen, P. (2006). Avian influenza pandemic: Not if, but when. *Pediatric Nursing, 32*(1), 76–81.

American Academy of Pediatrics. (2003). *Red book: Report of the Committee on Infectious Diseases* (26th ed.). Elk Grove Village, IL: Author.

Aultshuler, L. (2006). *The bird-flu primer: The guide to being prepared and surviving an avian flu pandemic.* San Francisco: Sterling & Ross Publishers, Inc.

Ball, J., & Bindler, R. (2006). *Child health nursing: Partnering with children & families.* Upper Saddle River, NJ: Prentice Hall.

Bindler, R. M., & Howry, L. B. (1997). *Pediatric drugs and nursing implications* (2nd ed.). Stamford, CT: Appleton & Lange.

D'Amico, D., & Barbarito, C. (2007). *Health & Physical Assessment in Nursing.* Upper Saddle River, NJ: Prentice Hall.

Fleming, K., & Randle, J. (2006). Toys—friend or foe? A study of infection risk in a paediatric intensive care unit. *Paediatric Nursing, 18*(4), 14–18.

Kee, J. (2005). *Laboratory and diagnostic tests with nursing implications* (7th ed.). Upper Saddle River, NJ: Prentice Hall.

Peck, P. (2006, February 13). FDA approves diarrhea vaccine for infants. *MedPage Today.*

Prymula, R. (2006). Pneumocccocal capsular polysaccharides conjugated to protein D for prevention of acute otitis media caused by both *Streptococcus pneumoniae* and *Haemophilus influenze:* A randomized double-blind efficacy study. *Lancet, 367*(9509), 740–748.

Ray, M., & Walker-Jenkins, A. (2006). Confronting bird flu: Will pandemic avian flu be the next public health threat? *Lifelines, 10*(1), 21–29.

Rosenfeld, I. (2006, April 6). New vaccines that protect the young. *Parade Magazine,* 20.

Sheff, B. (2006). Avian influenza: Poised to launch a pandemic? *Nursing 2006, 36*(1), 51–53.

Smith, S., Duell, D., & Martin, B. (2004). *Clinical nursing skills: Basic to advanced skills* (6th ed.). Upper Saddle River, NJ: Prentice Hall.

Wilkinson, J. (2000). *Nursing Diagnosis Handbook* (7th ed.). Upper Saddle River, NJ: Prentice Hall.

Wilson, B., Shannon, M., & Stang, C. (2006). *Nurses' drug guide.* Upper Saddle River, NJ: Prentice Hall.

CHAPTER 11

Atherly-John, Y., Cunningham, S., & Crain, E. (2002). A randomized trial of oral vs. intravenous rehydration in a pediatric emergency department. *Archives of Pediatric and Adolescent Medicine, 156,* 1240–1243.

Ball, J. W., & Bindler, R. C. (2003). *Pediatric nursing: Caring for children* (3rd ed.). Upper Saddle River, NJ: Prentice Hall.

Dale, J. (2004). Oral rehydration solutions in the management of acute gastroenteritis among children. *Journal of Pediatric Health Care, 18*(4), 211–212.

Fluid & electrolytes made incredibly easy. (2005). Philadelphia: Springhouse.

Hogan, M. A., & Wane, D. (2003). *Fluids, electrolytes, and acid–base balance, reviews and rationales.* Upper Saddle River, NJ: Prentice Hall.

Kee, J. (2005). *Laboratory and diagnostic tests with nursing implications* (7th ed.). Upper Saddle River, NJ: Prentice Hall.

Le, D., & Macnab, A. J. (2001). Self strangulation by hanging from cloth towel dispensers in Canadian schools. *Injury Prevention, 7*(3), 231–233.

Martin, A. (2006). The choking game: Important information for camp nurses. *Compasspoint, 16*(2): 22–23.

Santosham, M. (2002). Oral rehydration therapy. *Archives of Pediatric and Adolescent Medicine, 156,* 1177–1179.

Shapiro, L. (2004). *The secret language of children: How to understand what your kids are really saying.* Naperville, IL: Sourcebooks.

Smith, S., Duell, D., & Martin, B. (2004). *Clinical nursing skills: Basic to advanced skills* (6th ed.). Upper Saddle River, NJ: Prentice Hall.

Waller, M., Hallfors, D., Halpern, C., Iritani, B., Ford, C., and Guo, B. (2006). Gender differences in associations between depressive symptoms and patterns of substance use and risky sexual behavior among a nationally representative sample of U.S. adolescents. *Archives of Women's Mental Health, 9*(3), 139–150.

Wilson, B., Shannon, M., & Stang, C. (2006). *Nurses' drug guide.* Upper Saddle River, NJ: Prentice Hall.

CHAPTER 12

Aligne, C. A., Auinger, P., Byrd, R. S., & Weitzman, M. (2000.) Risk factors for pediatric asthma. *American Journal of Respiratory and Critical Care Medicine, 162*(3), 873–877.

American Academy of Pediatrics. (2006). 2005 American Heart Association guidelines for cardiopulmonary resuscitation and emergency cardiovascular care of pediatric and neonatal patients: Neonatal resuscitation guidelines. *Pediatrics, 117*(5), 1029–1038.

Baroi, M., Anderson, Y, & Mischler, E. (1997) Cystic fibrosis newborn screening: Impact of early screening results on parenting stress. *Pediatric Nursing, 23*(2), 143–151.

Bindler, R., & Howry, L. (2005). *Pediatric drug guide with nursing implications.* Upper Saddle River, NJ: Prentice Hall.

Clinical Practice Guideline: Diagnosis and management of childhood obstructive sleep apnea syndrome. (2002, April 4). *Pediatrics, 109*(4), 704–712.

Gutierrez, K., & Queener, S. F. (2003). *Pharmacology for nursing practice.* St. Louis: Mosby (pp. 850–851).

Marcus, C. L., Chapman, D., Ward, S. D., & McColley, S. A. (2002). Clinical practice guideline: Diagnosis and management of childhood obstructive sleep apnea syndrome. *Pediatrics, 109*(4), 704–712.

Paradise, J. L. (2002). Tonsillectomy and adenotonsillectomy for recurrent throat infection in moderately affected children. *Pediatrics, 110*(1), 7–15.

Ramilo, O., & Jafri, H. (2004). RSV can increase the risk of asthma. *Journal of Infectious Diseases. 200,* 1856–1865.

Ray, R. M., Bower, C. M. (2005). Pediatric obstructive sleep apnea: The year in review. *Current Opinions in Otolaryngology, and Head and Neck Surgery 13*(6), 360–365.

Temple, R. H., Timms, M. S. (2001). Pediatric coblation tonsillectomy. *Int J Pediatric Otorhinolaryngology, 61,* 195–198.

CHAPTER 13

Ball, J. & Bindler, R. (2006). *Child health nursing: Partnering with children & families.* Upper Saddle River, NJ: Prentice Hall.

Connor, J. A. (2002). Alternations in cardiovascular function in children. In K. L. McCance & S. E. Huether (Eds.), *Pathophysiology: The biologic basis for disease in adults and children* (4th ed., pp. 1048–1081). St. Louis: Mosby.

D'Amico, D., & Barbarito, C. (2007). *Health & physical assessment in nursing.* Upper Saddle River, NJ: Prentice Hall.

Kavey, R. E., Daniels, S. R., Lauer, R. M., Atkins, D. L., Hayman, L. L., & Taubert, K. (2003). American Heart Association guidelines for primary prevention of atherosclerotic cardiovascular disease beginning in childhood. *Circulation, 107*(11), 1562–1566.

Kee, J. (2005). *Laboratory and diagnostic tests with nursing implications.* (7th ed.). Upper Saddle River, NJ: Prentice Hall.

Mussatto, K. A., & Tweddell, J. S. (2005). Quality of life following surgery for congenital cardiac malformations in neonates and infants. *Cardiology in the Young, 15*(suppl. 1), 174–178.

Mussatto, K A., & Wernovsky, G. (2005). Challenges facing the child, adolescent and young adult after the arterial switch surgery. *Cardiology in the Young, 15*(suppl. 1), 111–121.

National High Blood Pressure Working Group on High Blood Pressure in Children and Adolescents. (2004). The fourth report on the diagnosis, evaluation, and treatment of high blood pressure in children and adolescents. *Pediatrics, 114*(2), 555–576.

Rempel, G. R. (2004). Technological advances in pediatrics: Challenges for parents and nurses. *Journal of Pediatric Nursing, 19*(1), 13–24

Rempel, G. R., Cender, L. M., Lynam, M. J., Sandor, G. G., & Farquharson, D. (2004). Parents' perspectives on decision making after antenatal diagnosis of congenital heart disease. *Journal of Obstetric, Gynecologic, and Neonatal Nursing, 33*(1), 64–70.

Smith, S., Duell, D., & Martin, B. (2004). *Clinical nursing skills: Basic to advanced skills,* (6th ed.). Upper Saddle River, NJ: Prentice Hall.

Soetenga, D., & Mussatto, K. A. (2004). Management of infants with hypoplastic left heart syndrome: Integrating research into nursing practice. *Critical Care Nurse, 24*(6), 46–66.

Taubert, K. (1994). Seven-year national survey of Kawasaki's syndrome and acute rheumatic fever. *Pediatric Infectious Disease Journal, 13,* 704–708.

Wilkinson, J. (2000). *Nursing Diagnosis Handbook* (7th ed.). Upper Saddle River, NJ: Prentice Hall.

Wilson, B., Shannon, M., & Stang, C. (2006). *Nurses' drug guide.* Upper Saddle River, NJ: Prentice Hall.

CHAPTER 14

Ball, J., & Bindler, R. (2006). *Child health nursing: Partnering with children & families.* Upper Saddle River, NJ: Prentice Hall.

D'Amico, D., & Barbarito, C. (2007). *Health & physical assessment in nursing.* Upper Saddle River, NJ: Prentice Hall.

Hoffman, M., Harger, A., & Lenkowski, A. (2006). Cutaneous wound healing is impaired in hemophilia B. *Blood, 108*(9), 3053–3060.

Kee, J. (2005). *Laboratory and diagnostic tests with nursing implications* (7th ed.). Upper Saddle River, NJ: Prentice Hall.

Lemone, P., & Burke, K. (2004). *Medical-surgical nursing: critical thinking in client care* (3rd ed.). Upper Saddle River, NJ: Prentice Hall.

London, M., Ladewig, P., Ball, J., & Bindler, R. (2007). *Maternal and child nursing care.* (2nd ed.). Upper Saddle River, NJ: Pearson Education.

National Hemophilia Foundation (n. d.). *Future therapies.* Retrieved January 8, 2007, from http://www.hemophilia.org.

Pui, C. H., Campana, D., & Evans, W. E. (2001). Childhood acute lymphoblastic leukaemia—current status and future perspectives. *Lancet Oncology, 2*(10), 597–607.

Pui, C. H., Sandlund, J. T., Pei, D., Rivera, G., Howard, S.R., Ribeiro, R., et al. (2001-7, 2003). Results of therapy for acute lymphoblastic leukemia in black and white children. *Journal of the American Medical Association, 290* (15), 2001–2007.

Ries, L. A. G., Smith, M. A., Gurney, J. G., Linet, M., Tamra, T., Young, J. L., et al. (Eds). (1999). *Cancer incidence and survival among children and adolescents: United States SEER Program 1975–1995* (NIH Pub. No. 99-4649). Bethesda, MD: National Cancer Institute, SEER Program.

Smith, S., Duell, D., & Martin, B. (2004). *Clinical nursing skills: Basic to advanced skills* (6th ed.). Upper Saddle River, NJ: Prentice Hall.

Wilkinson, J. (2000). *Nursing Diagnosis Handbook* (7th ed.). Upper Saddle River, NJ: Prentice Hall.

Wilson B., Shannon, M., & Stang, C. (2006). *Nurses' drug guide.* Upper Saddle River, NJ: Prentice Hall.

CHAPTER 15

Acello, B. (2005). *The long-term care nursing desk reference.* Marblehead, MA: HCPro.

Addington-Hall, J., Higginson, I. (eds.). (2001). *Palliative care for non-cancer patients.* London: Oxford University Press.

American Academy of Pediatrics (AAP) Committee on Fetus and Newborn & American College of Obstetricians and Gynecolgists (ACOG) Committee on Obstetrics (2002). *Guidelines for perinatal care* (5th ed.). Evanston, IL: Author.

American Academy of Pediatrics Committee on Quality Improvement, Subcommitee on Febrile Seizures. (1999). Practice parameter: Long-term treatment of the child with simple febrile seizures. *Pediatrics*, 103(6, Pt. 1), 1307–1309.

American Association of Mental Retardation (2002). The AAMR Definition of Mental Retardation. Retrieved May 6, 2007 from the Internet.

Ball, J., & Bindler, R. (2006). *Child health nursing: Partnering with children & families.* Upper Saddle River, NJ: Prentice Hall.

Crist, W. M. (2000). Neoplastic disease and tumors. In R. E. Behrman, R. M. Kliegman, & H. B. Jenson (Eds.), *Nelson textbook of pediatrics* (16th ed., p. 1531). Philadelphia: Saunders.

D'Amico, D., & Barbarito, C. (2007). *Health and physical assessment in nursing.* Upper Saddle River, NJ: Prentice Hall.

Halloran, D. (2005). Hearing screening at well child visits. *Archives of Pediatric and Adolescent Medicine, 159*, 949–955.

International Dyslexia Association. (2002). *Just the facts: Definition of dyslexia.* Retrieved May 6, 2007 from the Internet.

Johnson, A. N. (2002). Update on newborn hearing screening programs. *Pediatric Nursing*, 22(3), 267–270.

Joseph, D. (2001). *Spina Bifida Association fact sheet: Urologic care and management.* Retrieved May 6, 2007 from the Internet.

Kee, J. (2005). *Laboratory and diagnostic tests with nursing implications* (7th ed.). Upper Saddle River, NJ: Prentice Hall.

LeMone, P., & Burke, K. (2004). *Medical-surgical nursing* (3rd ed.). Upper Saddle River, NJ: Prentice Hall.

Marx, R., & Davidson, S. (2003). *Facing the ultimate loss: Coping with the death of a child.* Belgium, WI: Champion.

Millar, J. (2006). Evaluation and treatment of the child with febrile seizures. *American Family Physician*, 73(10), 1761–1764.

Niemala, M., Pihakari, O., Pokka, T., & Uhari, M. S. (2000). Pacifier as a risk factor for acute otitis media: A randomized, controlled trial of parental counseling. *Pediatrics, 106*, 483–488.

Olson, S. L. (1998). Bedside musical care: Applications in pregnancy, childbirth, and neonatal care. *JOGNN*, 27(5), 569–575.

Peck, P. (2005, November 8). Listen up: Cradle to grave, many Americans can't hear what is being said. *MedPage Today.*

Peck, P. (2005, November 8). Sound vs. silence may divide those with hearing loss. *MedPage Today.*

Pepino, M., & Mennella, J. (2005). Sucrose-induced analgesia is related to sweet preferences in children but not in adults. *Pain, 119*, 210–218.

Rice, E. (ed.). (2005). *If they could only hear me: A collection of personal stories about ALS and the families that have been affected.* Charleston, SC: BookSurge Publishers.

Shachtman, T. (2006, February). Medical sleuth. *Smithsonian*, 23–30.

Smith, S., Duell, D. & Martin, B. (2004). *Clinical nursing skills: Basic to advanced skills* (6th ed.). Upper Saddle River, NJ: Prentice Hall.

Stempien, L. (2000). Intrathecal baclofen pump use for spasticity: A clinical survey. *American Journal of Physical Medicine and Rehabilitation*, 79(6), 536–541.

Wilson, B., Shannon, M. & Stang, C. (2006). *Nurses' drug guide.* Upper Saddle River, NJ: Prentice Hall.

Wismer Fries, A., Ziegler, T., Kurian, J., Jacoris, S., & Pollack, S. (2005). Early experience in humans is associated with changes in nuropeptides critical for regulating social behavior. *Proceedings of the National Academy of Sciences of the United States of America, 103*, 17237–17240.

CHAPTER 16

American Academy of Child and Adolescent Psychiatry. (1998). Practice parameters for the assessment and treatment of children and adolescents with depressive disorders. *Journal of the American Academy of Child and Adolescent Psychiatry*, 37, (01).

Ball, J. W., & Bindler, R. C. (2006). *Child health nursing: Partnering with children & families.* Upper Saddle River, NJ: Prentice Hall.

D'Amico, D., & Barbarito, C. (2007). *Health & physical assessment in nursing.* Upper Saddle River, NJ: Prentice Hall.

Faraone, S. (2002). Adoption study of ADHD. *Journal of the American Academy of Child and Adolescent Psychiatry* 41(12), 1390–1391.

Findling, R., McNamara, N., O'Riordan, M., Reed, M., Demeter, C., Branicky, L., et al. (2003). An open-label pilot study of St. John's wort in juvenile depression. *Journal of American Academy of Child and Adolescent Psychiatry*, 42(8), 908–914.

Flora, D. (2006). Changes in drug use during young adulthood: The effect of parent alcoholism and transition into marriage. *Psychology of Addiction Behaviors* 19(4), 352–362.

Glewe, G. (2005). Bullying, psychosocial adjustment, and academic performance in elementary school. *Archives of Pediatric and Adolescent Medicine, 159*, 1026–1031.

Inge, T. H., Krebs, N. F., Garcia, V. F., Skelton, J. A., Guice, K. S., Strauss, R. S., et al. (2004). Bariatric surgery for severely overweight adolescents: Concerns and recommendations. *Pediatrics*, 114(1):217–223.

Keck, P., McElroy, S. (2003). New approach in managing bipolar depression. *Journal of Clinical Psychiatry* 61(suppl 1), 13–18.

Merten, S. (2005). Neonatal security: It takes a community. *Nursing Management* 36(8), 41–44.

Rabun, J., Jr. (2005). Guidelines on prevention of & response to infant abductions (8th ed.). National Center for Missing and Exploited Children. Alexandria, VA: U. S. Department of Justice.

Shogan, M. G. (2002). Emergency management plan for newborn abductions. *JOGNN*, 31(3), 340–346.

Simpson, T., & Ivey, J. (2005). Pediatric management problems. *Pediatric Nursing*, 31(4), 312–313.

U.S. Department of Health and Human Services. (2006). *Healthy people 2010.* Washington, DC: Author. Retrieved April 22, 2006, from http://www.healthypeople.gov/, accessed 4/22/06.

Vlam, S. (2006). Attention deficit hyperactivity disorder. Nurses are important members of the team. *Journal of Pediatric Nursing* 21(3), 171–174.

CHAPTER 17

Ariza, A. J., Chen, E. H., Binns, H. J., & Christoffel, K. K. (2004). Risk factors for overweight in five- to six-year-old Hispanic-American children: A pilot study. *Journal of Urban Health, 81*, 150–161.

Ball, J., Bindler, R. (2006). *Child health nursing: Partnering with children and families*. Upper Saddle River, NJ: Prentice Hall.

Bindler, R., & Howry, L. (2005). *Pediatric drug guide with nursing implications*. Upper Saddle River, NJ: Prentice Hall.

Binns, H., & Ariza, A. (2004). Guidelines help clinicians identify risk factors for overweight in children. *Pediatric Annals, 33*, 18–22.

Bowman, S., Gortmaker, S., Ebbeling, C., Pereira, M., & Ludwig, D. (2004). Effects of fast-food consumption on energy intake and diet quality among children in a national household survey. *Pediatrics, 113*(1), 112–118.

Freeland-Graves, J., & Nitzke, S. (2002). Position of the American Dietetic Association: Total diet approach to communicating food and nutrition information. *Journal of the American Dietetic Association, 102*, 100–108.

Hassink, S. (ed.). (2006). A parent's guide to childhood obesity: A roadmap to health. Washington, DC: American Academy of Pediatrics.

Kalliomäki, M., Salminen, S., Poussa, T., Arvilommi, H., & Isolauri, E. (2003). Probiotics and prevention of atopic disease: 4 year follow-up of randomized placebo-controlled trial. *Lancet, 361*(9372), 1869–1871.

Moran, R. (1999, February 15). Evaluation and treatment of childhood obesity. *American Family Physician*.

Nestle, M. (2002). *Food politics: How the food industry influences nutrition and health*. Berkeley: University of California Press.

North American Society of Pediatric Gastroenterology, Hepatology and Nutrition (NASPGHAN). (2001). Pediatric gastroesophageal reflux: Clinical practice guideline summary. *Journal of Pediatric Gastroenterology and Nutrition, 32*(suppl. 2), 1–13.

Okie, S. (2006). Fed up: Winning the war against childhood obesity. Washington, D.C.: National Academics Press.

Pick, M. (2006). *Probiotics—For life!* Portland, ME: Women to Women. Retrieved September 17, 2006, from http://www.womentowomen.com/digestionandgihealth/probiotics.asp.

Taveras, E., Berkey, C., Rifas-Shiman, S., Ludwig, D., Rockett, H., Field, A., Colditz, G., & Gillman, M. (2005). Association of consumption of fried food away from home with body mass index and diet quality in older children and adolescents. *Pediatrics, 116*(4), e518–e524.

Wong, W. Y., Eskes, T. K., Kuihpers-Jagtman, A. M., Spauwen, P. H., Steegers, E. A., Thomas, C, M., Hamel, B. C., Blom, H. J., and Steegers-Theunissen, R. P., (1999). Nonsyndromic orofacial clefts: Association with maternal hyperhomocysteinemia. *Teratology, 60*, 253–257.

Yuan, M., Konstantopoulos, N., Lee, J., Shulman, G., et al. (2001). Reversal of obesity- and diet-induced insulin resistance with salicylates or targeted disruption of Ikk3. *Science, 293*, 1673–1677.

CHAPTER 18

Ball, J. W., & Bindler, R. C. (2006). *Child health nursing: Partnering with children and families*. Upper Saddle River, NJ: Prentice Hall.

Campoy, S. (2005). Pharmacology and chronic kidney disease: How chronic kidney disease and its complications alter drug response. *American Journal of Nursing, 105*(9), 60–71.

Centers for Disease Control and Prevention. (2006). *Human papillomavirus (HPV), cervical cancer, and HPV vaccine and recommendations: A current issues in immunization NetConference* (Course number EV0378). Retrieved April 27, 2007.

Condon, M. (2004). *Women's health: Body, mind, spirit: An integrated approach to wellness and illness*. Upper Saddle River, NJ: Prentice Hall.

D'Amico, D., & Barbarito, C. (2007). *Health and physical assessment in nursing*. Upper Saddle River, NJ: Prentice Hall.

Frazer, I., Ferris, D., Ferenczy, A., & Villa, L. (2006). Advances in prevention of cervical cancer and other human papillomavirus-related diseases. *Pediatric Infectious Disease Journal, 25*(2), S65–81.

Greydanus, D. (2003). *American Academy of Pediatrics: Caring for your teenager*. New York: Bantam.

Kee, J. (2005). *Laboratory and diagnostic tests with nursing implications* (7th ed.). Upper Saddle River, NJ: Prentice Hall.

Legg, V. (2005). Complications of chronic kidney disease. *American Journal of Nursing, 105*(6), 40–49.

Lichtman, R. (2005). *Gynecology: Well-woman care* (2nd ed.). Upper Saddle River, NJ: Prentice Hall.

London, M. L., Ladewig, P. W., Ball, J. W., & Bindler, R. C. (2007). *Maternal and child nursing care* (2nd ed.). Upper Saddle River, NJ: Prentice Hall.

Lopez, R. I. (2003). *The teen health book: A parent's guide to adolescent health and well-being*. New York: WW Norton.

Mercer, R. (2003, February). Dry at night: Treating nocturnal enuresis. *Advances for Nurse Practitioners*, 26–32.

National Kidney and Urologic Diseases Clearinghouse. (2003). *How can urinary tract infection be prevented?* Bethesda, MD: Author. Retrieved September 5, 2006, from the Internet.

National Kidney and Urologic Disease Clearinghouse. (2005). Urinary tract infections in children. NIH Publication No. 06-4246. Bethesda, MD: Author.

National Women's Health Information Center. (2003). *A lifetime of good health: Your guide to staying healthy*. Washington, DC: U.S. Department of Health and Human Services.

The Pennsylvania State University Health Services. (2005, September 30). *What happens during a pelvic exam*. Retrieved September 17, 2006, from the Internet.

Reichert, G. (1998). Female circumcision: What you need to know about genital mutilation. *Lifelines, 2*(3), 28–34.

Reisser, P. (2002). *Teen health guide*. Colorado Springs, CO: Focus on the Family.

Schmidt, J. (2007). HPV vaccine: Implications for nurse and patients. *Nursing for Women's Health, 11*(1), 83–87.

Smith, S., Duell, D., & Martin, B. (2004). *Clinical nursing skills: Basic to advanced skills* (6th ed.). Upper Saddle River, NJ: Prentice Hall.

Varney Burst, H. (2004). *Varney's midwifery* (4th ed.). Sudbury, MA: Jones and Bartlett.

WebMD. *A–Z health guide from WebMD: Medical tests*. Retrieved September 17, 2006, from the Internet.

Wilkinson, J. (2000). *Nursing diagnosis handbook* (7th ed.). Upper Saddle River, NJ: Prentice Hall.

Wilson, B., Shannon, M., & Stang, C. (2006). *Nurses' drug guide*. Upper Saddle River, NJ: Prentice Hall.

Youngkin, E., & Davis, M. (2004). *Women's health: A primary care clinical guide* (3rd ed.). Upper Saddle River, NJ: Prentice Hall.

CHAPTER 19

American Academy of Pediatrics Section on Endocrinology and Committee on Genetics. (2000). Technical report: Congenital adrenal hyperplasia. *Pediatrics, 106*(6), 1511–1518.

American Diabetes Association. (2000). Type 2 diabetes in children and adolescents. *Diabetes Care, 23*(3), 381–389.

Jacobson-Dickman, E., & Levitsky, L. (2005). Oral agents in managing diabetes mellitus in children and adolescents. *Pediatric Clinics of North America, 52*(6),1689–703.

Kidson, W. (1998). Polycystic ovary syndrome: A new direction in treatment. *Medical Journal of Australia, 169*, 537–540.

Largo, R. S., Gnatuk, C. L., Kunselman, A. R., & Dunaif, A. (2005). Change in glucose tolerance over time in women with polycystic ovarian syndrome: A controlled study. *Journal of Clinical Endocrinology and Metabolism, 90*(6), 3236–3242.

London, M., Ladewig, P., Ball, J., & Bindler, R. (2007). *Maternal and child nursing care*. (2nd ed.). Upper Saddle River, NJ: Pearson Education.

Ries, L. A. G., Melbert, D., Krapcho, M., Mariotto, A., Miller, B. A., Feuer, E. J., et al. (Eds). (2007). *SEER cancer statistics review, 1975–2004*. National Cancer Institute, Bethesda, MD. Retrieved May 6, 2007 from the Internet. Based on November 2006 SEER data submission.

Robinson, D., & Drumm, L. (2001). Maple syrup urine disease: A standard of nursing care. *Pediatric Nursing, 27*(3), 255–264, 270.

CHAPTER 20

American Academy of Pediatrics, Committee on Sports Medicine and Fitness. (2001). Strength training by children and adolescents. *Pediatrics, 107*(6), 1470–1472.

Anrig, C. (2004). Relief versus wellness care in the family practice. *Dynamic Chiropractic, 22*(7), 1.

Anrig, C. (2005). The backpack dilemma: Function vs. fashion. *Dynamic Chiropractic, 23*(18), 1.

Antonio, J., & Stout, J. (2004). *Fit kids for life: A parent's guide to optimal nutrition and training for young athletes*. Laguna Beach, CA: Basic Health Publications.

Ball, J., & Bindler, R. (2006). *Child health nursing: Partnering with children & families*. Upper Saddle River, NJ: Prentice Hall.

Benjamin, H., Glow, K. (2003). Strength training for children and adolescents. What can physicians recommend? *The Physician and Sports Medicine, 31*(9), 1.

D'Amico, D., & Barbarito, C. (2007). *Health & physical assessment in nursing*. Upper Saddle River, NJ: Prentice Hall.

Fallon, J. M. (1997). The role of the chiropractic adjustment in the care and treatment of 332 children with otitis media. *Journal of Clinical Chiropractic Pediatrics 2*, 167–183.

Hart, E. S. (2003, April 22). Boston brace: The role of bracing in the treatment of idiopathic scoliosis. *Massachusetts General Hospital Orthopaedic Surgery*.

Kee, J. (2005). *Laboratory and diagnostic tests with nursing implications*. (7th ed.). Upper Saddle River, NJ: Prentice Hall.

Lee, A. C., Li, D. H., & Kemper, K. J. (2000). Chiropractic care for children. *Archives of Pediatrics and Adolescent Medicine, 154*, 401–407.

Macias, B., Murthy, G., Chambers, H., & Hargens, A. (2005). High contact pressure beneath backpack straps of children contributes to pain. *Archives of Pediatrics and Adolescent Medicine, 159*(12), 1186–1187.

National Center for Health Statistics. (2001). Sports-related injuries cause 2.6 million visits annually by children and young adults to emergency rooms. Hyattsville, MD: Author.

National Clearinghouse on Child Abuse and Neglect Information. (2003). Recognizing child abuse and neglect: Signs and symptoms. Washington, DC: Department of Health and Human Services.

Sheir-Neiss, G. I., Kruse, R. W., Rahman, T., et al. (2003). The association of backpack use and back pain in adolescents. *Spine, 28*(9), 922–930.

Shields, B., and Smith, G. (2006). "Cheerleading Related Injuries to Children 5 to 18 Years of Age: United States 1990–2002. *Pediatrics, 120*, 122–129.

Smith, S., Duell, D., & Martin, B. (2004). *Clinical nursing skills: Basic to advanced skills* (6th ed.). Upper Saddle River, NJ: Prentice Hall.

Wilkinson, J. (2000). *Nursing Diagnosis Handbook* (7th ed.). Upper Saddle River, NJ: Prentice Hall.

Wilson, B., Shannon, M., & Stang, C. (2006). *Nurses' drug guide*. Upper Saddle River, NJ: Prentice Hall.

CHAPTER 21

American Academy of Dermatology. (2001, Fall). *Piercing perils tattoo taboo. Dermatology Insights*. Retrieved May 6, 2007 from the Internet.

Atherton, P. (1997). Aloe vera: Myth or medicine? *Positive Health, 20*. Accessed on the Internet.

Ball, J., & Bindler, R. (2006). *Child health nursing: Partnering with children & families*. Upper Saddle River, NJ: Prentice Hall Publishers.

Boe, K., Tillotson, E. (2006). Encouraging sun safety for children and adolescents. *Journal of School Nursing, 22*(30), 136–141.

Children's Hospital Boston. (2006). *Body piercing: A guide for teens*. Center for Young Women's Health, Children's Hospital Boston. Retrieved May 6, 2007 from the Internet.

Cokkinides, V., Weinstock, M., Glanz, K., Albano, J., Ward, E., & Thun, M. (2006). Trends in sunburn, sun protection practices and attitudes toward sun exposure protection and tanning among U.S. adolescents: 1998–2004. *Pediatrics, 188*(3), 853–864.

Dillon, P. (2003). *Nursing health assessment. A critical thinking case studies approach*. Philadelphia: FA Davis.

Flinders, D., & De Schweinitz, P. (2004). Pediculosis and scabies. *American Family Physician, 69*, 341.

Hatfield, N. (2003). *Introductory pediatric nursing*. Philadelphia: Lippincott.

International Aloe Science Council. (2002). *The complete story of aloe vera*. Irving, TX: Author.

Kemper, K., Gardiner, P., & Coles, D. (2001). The skinny on herbal remedies for dermatologic disorders. *Contemporary Pediatrics, 7*, 103.

La Leche League. (2005, March). *FAQ on tattoos and breastfeeding*. Retrieved May 6, 2007 from the Internet.

McNally, R. (ed.). (2003). *Skin health information for teens: Health tips about dermatological concerns and skin cancer risks*. Detroit, MI: Omnigraphics, Inc.

National Institute of Arthritis and Musculoskeletal and Skin Disorders. (2003). *Handout on Health: Atopic dermatitis*. Bethesda, MD: NIAMS.

Potts, N., & Mandleco, B. (2002). *Pediatric nursing: Caring for children and their families*. New York: Delmar.

CHAPTER 22

Ball, J. & Bindler, R. (2006). *Child health nursing: Partnering with children & families*. Upper Saddle River, NJ: Prentice Hall.

D'Amico, D., & Barbarito, C. (2007). *Health & Physical Assessment in Nursing*. Upper Saddle River, NJ: Prentice Hall.

Diiorio, C., McCarty, F., Denzmore, P., & Landis, A. (2007). The moderating influence of mother-adolescent discussion on early and middle African-American adolescent sexual behavior. *Research in Nursing and Health, 30*(2), 193–202.

Ignatavicius, D. D., Workman, M. L., & Mishler, M. A. (1995). *Medical-surgical nursing: A nursing process approach* (2nd ed.). Philadelphia: Saunders.

Kee, J. (2005). *Laboratory and diagnostic tests with nursing implications* (7th ed.). Upper Saddle River, NJ: Prentice Hall.

North American Nursing Diagnosis Association (NANDA). (2008). *NANDA nursing diagnoses: Definitions and classification, 2008–2009*. Philadelphia: Elsevier.

Smith, S., Duell, D., & Martin, B. (2004). *Clinical nursing skills: Basic to advanced skills* (6th ed.). Upper Saddle River, NJ: Prentice Hall.

Stichweh, D., Arce, E., & Pascual, V. (2004). Update on pediatric systemic lupus erythematosus. *Current Opinion in Rheumatology, 16*, 577–587.

Wiener, L., Battles, H., & Wood, L. (2007). A longitudinal study of adolescents with perinatally or transfusion acquired HIV infection: Sexual knowledge, risk reduction, self-efficacy and sexual behavior. *AIDS and Behavior, 11*(3), 471–478.

Wilkinson, J. *Nursing diagnosis handbook* (8th ed.). (2005). Upper Saddle River, NJ: Prentice Hall.

Wilson, B. E., Shannon, M. T., & Stang, C. L. (2006). *Prentice Hall nurses' drug guide 2006*. Upper Saddle River, NJ: Prentice Hall.

Glossary

(Note: Glossary terms may appear in more than one chapter. Boldface numbers after the glossary term indicate the chapter(s) in which the term is defined. Other words or terms that may require definitions are italicized in the text and are defined there.)

A

Abortion: the termination of a pregnancy before the fetus is viable **(3)**

Accuracy: correctness **(2)**

Acetabulum: hip socket **(20)**

Acetone breath: breath with odor of nail polish remover or rotting apples, indicating diabetic ketoacidosis **(19)**

Acidosis: condition that develops when there is an increase of hydrogen ion concentration; body pH less than 7.36 **(11)**

Acquired immunity: immunity that is developed over a period of time after birth by exposure to foreign substances; developed through humoral immunity and cell-mediated immunity **(22)**

Acquired immunodeficiency syndrome (AIDS): a life-threatening, end-stage infection with HIV **(18)**

Active immunity: process in which the body reacts rapidly by producing a specific antibody to stop or slow the growth of an antigen until white blood cells can destroy it. The body will recognize and respond faster on future exposure to the antigen. **(10, 22)**

Active transport: movement of solutes across the cell membrane by means of metabolic activity and carrier cells **(11)**

Acute: having a rapid onset, severe symptoms, and a short course **(14)**

Acute conjunctivitis: (also known as *pinkeye*) inflammation of the conjunctiva caused by allergies, bacteria, or viruses **(15)**

Acute lymphoblastic leukemia: overproduction of immature lymphocytes **(14)**

Acute myelogenous leukemia: condition that occurs when cancer cells develop in the bone marrow (*myeloid tissue*) **(14)**

Acute renal failure: sudden onset of diminished kidney function, resulting in the imbalance of fluids and electrolytes **(18)**

Adaptability: the ability to change when faced with problems **(4)**

Afterload: resistance against which the ventricles pump **(13)**

Agglutination: after vasoconstriction, the clumping together of red blood cells **(14)**

Airborne precautions: precautions that protect others from diseases that can be transmitted by the airborne route **(10)**

Airborne transmission: transmission of harmful organisms suspended in the air **(10)**

Algor mortis: gradual decrease of the body's temperature after death **(9)**

Alkalosis: condition that develops when there is a decrease of hydrogen ion concentration; body's pH more than 7.44 **(11)**

Allergy: altered reaction to an antigen or allergen **(22)**

Allogeneic donor: donor who is a relative, usually a sibling **(14)**

Alveoli: glandular cells that are arranged in grapelike clusters, as in the lung **(12)**

Amblyopia: (also known as *lazy eye*) reduction of vision in one eye **(15)**

Anabolism: the liver's process of building compounds necessary for normal body functions **(17)**

Anaphylactic shock: systemic reaction to an allergen that occurs within minutes or up to 2 hours after exposure **(22)**

Anemia: decrease in the number of red blood cells and a decrease in hemoglobin or both **(14)**

Anions: negatively charged electrolytes **(11)**

Anorexia nervosa: eating disorder characterized by weight loss, emaciation, and an exaggerated fear of gaining weight **(16)**

Antibodies: protein substances produced in the blood or tissues in response to a specific antigen **(22)**

Antigen: foreign substance that, when introduced into the body, stimulates the production of an antibody **(22)**

Antigenic drift: minor genetic changes that occur to the virus as it replicates within host cells **(10)**

Antigenic shift: abrupt or major change in a virus that makes it capable of infecting humans **(10)**

Apnea: brief period of absence or cessation of breathing **(12)**

Appendicitis: inflammation of the vermiform appendix, a small sac at the end of the cecum **(17)**

Arrector pili: an involuntary muscle that raises hair vertically in response to cold or fear **(21)**

Arthralgia: swelling and pain in the joints **(14)**

Ascites: an abnormal accumulation of serous fluid in the abdominal cavity **(18)**

Asperger's syndrome: disorder similar to autism in which the child exhibits social isolation, communication difficulties, clumsiness, and a focused area of interest and attention **(16)**

Assault: sudden, violent physical attack on someone **(16)**

Assisted suicide: (also known as *voluntary euthanasia*) situation in which the dying individual desires control over the time and manner of death **(9)**

Associative play: learning to share and work together on a project **(6)**

Assumptions: ideas taken for granted **(2)**

Asthma: chronic inflammatory disorder of the tracheobronchial tree **(12)**

Astigmatism: uneven focusing of light resulting in blurred images **(15)**

Atelectasis: congenital condition characterized by the incomplete expansion of the lungs at birth **(12)**

Aura: recognizable sensation that signals a seizure is about to occur **(15)**

Autism: complex developmental disability that typically appears during the first 3 years of life and is the result of a neurologic disorder that affects the normal functioning of the brain, affecting development in the areas of social interaction and communication skills **(16)**

Autogenous graft: skin graft in which skin is transplanted from one site to another in the same recipient **(22)**

Autoimmune: immune response by the body against itself **(22)**

Autologous donor: person who donates for his or her own later use **(14)**

Autonomic reflexes: reflexes that control cardiac and smooth muscles and glands **(15)**

Autopsy: (also known as *postmortem examination*) examination of the body after death to determine more details about the cause of death, the disease, or other data **(9)**

Avian flu: (also known as *bird flu* or *H5N1*) illness caused by influenza viruses that occur naturally among wild birds and are deadly to domestic birds, and which, if transmitted to humans, could spark a pandemic **(10)**

Axon: fiber carrying the impulse away from a nerve cell body **(15)**

B

Babinski's reflex: reflex elicited by stroking the lateral side of the newborn's foot from heel to toe; the big toe should dorsiflex and the other toes should flare **(8)**

Balanoposthitis: inflammation or infection of the glans penis **(18)**

Balloon atrial septostomy: (also known as *Rashkind procedure*) procedure in which an enlargement of the existing opening in the cardiac septum is made, allowing better mixing of oxygenated blood from the lungs with the systemic blood **(13)**

Bariatric surgery: surgery to reduce stomach size **(16, 17)**

Biliary atresia: failure of the bile ducts outside the liver to form properly **(17)**

Binuclear family: both parents share custody of the children **(4)**

Bioterrorism: release of deadly infectious agents for the purpose of causing chaos and fear **(10)**

Bipolar disorder: (also known as *manic depression*) disorder involving mood swings between mania and depression **(16)**

Bladder exstrophy: a defect in which there is an absence of part of the abdominal wall and anterior wall of the bladder, causing the posterior wall of the bladder to protrude through the defect **(18)**

Blended family: a family in which one or both spouses have had a previous marriage and children from that marriage **(4)**

Boundary: an imaginary border beyond which the members of the system come in contact with others outside the system **(4)**

Breadth: scope **(2)**

Bronchopulmonary dysplasia (BPD): chronic lung disease that affects infants with respiratory distress syndrome, congenital heart defects, meconium aspiration, or other conditions that result from assisted mechanical ventilation **(12)**

Brushfield spots: white speckles on the edge of the iris **(15)**

Buccal space: area inside the cheek by the second molars **(17)**

"Buffalo hump": fat deposits on the back between the shoulders **(19)**

Bulimia: binge eating and purging **(16)**

Buphthalmos: enlargement of the eyeball **(15)**

C

Candidiasis: (also known as *Monilia* or *yeast infection*) infection with a common organism causing vaginitis **(18)**

Cardiac output: total volume of blood forced out of the ventricles in 1 minute **(13)**

Cardiac region: area around the cardiac sphincter **(17)**

Cardiac sphincter: ring surrounding the opening between the esophagus and the stomach that prevents food and gastric acid from being pushed from the stomach into the esophagus **(17)**

Cardiomegaly: enlargement of the heart **(13)**

Carditis: inflammation of the heart **(13)**

Care plan: organized, prioritized plan for addressing nursing diagnoses and helping the client reach measurable, identified outcomes (or goals) **(1)**

Catabolism: the liver's process of breaking down compounds **(17)**

Cataracts: opacities of the lens of one or both eyes **(15)**

Cations: positively charged electrolytes **(11)**

Celiac disease: gluten-sensitive enteropathy or sprue; a chronic malabsorption syndrome in which one is unable to digest gluten, a protein found in wheat, barley, rye, and oats **(17)**

Cell body: part of the cell that contains the nucleus and cytoplasm **(15)**

Cell-mediated immunity: immunity that provides protection against bacteria, viruses, fungi, and tumors; the process that causes rejection of organs that have been transplanted **(22)**

Cellulitis: bacterial infection of the dermis and subcutaneous tissue **(21)**

Cephalhematoma: accumulation of blood between the periosteum and the skull bone **(9)**

Cephalocaudal: proceeding from head to toe **(5, 15)**

Cervical dysplasia: abnormal changes in the tissue of the cervix **(18)**

Chancre: painless open sore **(18)**

Chelation therapy: the administration of a chemical that binds to lead to increase the rate of excretion **(17)**

Chemical burns: burns caused by strong acids or alkali, such as the chemical found in cleansers containing lye, toilet cleaners, or preparations used to open clogged drains **(21)**

Cheyne-Stokes respiration: period of progressive depth of breathing followed by period of apnea **(9, 12)**

Child exploitation: unethical use of a child for one's own profit **(16)**

Child life specialist: trained professional who plans therapeutic activities for the child who is ill or hospitalized **(7)**

Child molestation: sexual involvement other than intercourse with children **(16)**

Child pornography: photography or visual representation of children nude or in sexual acts **(16)**

Chlamydia: a sexually transmitted infection caused by *Chlamydia trachomatis* **(18)**

Chordee: congenital anomaly that causes a ventral curvature of the penis, which is caused by fibrous tissues along the corpus spongiosum **(18)**

Chorea: involuntary, spasmodic movements of the limbs and face **(13)**

Chronic renal failure: progressive, irreversible loss of kidney function **(18)**

Chronic: of long duration, with little change or slow progression **(7)**

Chyme: semiliquid substance of digestive acid and enzymes **(17)**

Circumoral: around the mouth **(13)**

Circumoral cyanosis: bluish discoloration of the skin around the mouth **(12)**

Clarity: clearness **(2)**

Cleft lip: condition that results from failure of the upper lip to join medially; can be unilateral or bilateral **(17)**

Cleft palate: condition that results from failure of the medial nasal and maxillary processes to join, leaving an opening between the roof of the mouth and the floor of the nasal passage **(17)**

Closed head injury: result of head trauma, from either an external force, such as a blow to the head, or an internal force, such as shaking the infant hard enough for the brain to strike the inside of the skull **(15)**

Closed reduction: reduction of a fractured bone by manually moving the bones into alignment **(20)**

Clubbing: enlargement of the end of the fingers associated with disorders that cause cyanosis **(13)**

Coarctation: narrowing or constricting, especially of the aorta or of a blood vessel **(13)**

Cochlear implants: implanted devices that can help children who are deaf to hear **(15)**

Cognitive development: intellectual ability of an individual **(5)**

Cohabitating family: unmarried partners with or without children **(4)**

Comedones: whiteheads and blackheads **(21)**

Comfort measures only: order written to indicate that the goal of treatment is a comfortable, dignified death and that further life-sustaining measures are not indicated **(9)**

Communal family: a family that includes adults and children who may or may not be related **(4)**

Communicable diseases: diseases transmitted from one person to another by way of direct contact with body fluids **(10)**

Community-based nursing: philosophy of nursing that care should be provided to individuals, families, and groups wherever they are, including where they live, work, play, pray, or go to school **(1)**

Compartment syndrome: condition that occurs when increased pressure in a limited space compromises circulation and nerve innervation, possibly leading to necrosis **(20)**

Competent individual: person who has received training, including instruction and clinical practice, to perform certain tasks and who can demonstrate safe performance **(2)**

Complicated grief: (also known as *dysfunctional grief*) condition of grief in which an individual cannot accept what has happened or move on with life **(9)**

Concepts: ideas; theories, laws, and principles **(2)**

Conchae: three shelflike structures protruding into the nasal cavity from the sides **(12)**

Conclusions: decisions based on prior thought **(2)**

Concrete operations period: period in which child interacts primarily with the local environment **(5)**

Concussion: injury that causes temporary neurologic impairment but no permanent damage to brain tissue; may be caused by blunt injury to the head or by shaking an infant or child **(15)**

Confidence in reason: trust in the outcome of logical thought **(2)**

Confidentiality: ethical principle or legal right that a health professional will keep private any privileged information **(3)**

Congenital condition: condition present at birth **(7)**

Conization: removal of a cone-shaped wedge of tissue from the cervix **(18)**

Conjunctival hyperemia: increased amount of blood in the conjunctiva **(13)**

Conscious sedation: the administration of IV medication to produce an impaired level of consciousness **(7)**

Consolidation: creation of a solid or firm, inelastic lung **(12)**

Contact dermatitis: skin inflammation from allergens (poison ivy, poison oak, latex, and/or nickel) or repeated exposure to irritants (detergents, bleaches, soaps, lotions, urine, and stool) **(21)**

Contact precautions: precautions that protect individuals from skin or inanimate objects that are infected with harmful organisms **(10)**

Contractility: ability of the ventricles to stretch **(13)**

Convalescent period: time frame from the beginning of the resolution of symptoms to restoration of wellness **(10)**

Cooperative play: organized play such as games at school or sports **(6)**

Coprolalia: uncontrollable use of obscene language **(16)**

Copropraxia: involuntary obscene gestures **(16)**

Coryza: (also known as *rhinitis* or *nasopharyngitis*) inflammation of the nasal mucosa, often caused by a viral infection such as the common cold **(12)**

Crabs: pubic lice **(21)**

Crackles: coarse sounds in breathing; formerly called rales **(12)**

Critical thinking: process of analyzing one's own thinking and improving how one thinks or solves problems **(2)**

Crohn's disease: random inflammation of the entire gastrointestinal tract that involves all layers of bowel wall **(17)**

Croup: term used to represent a group of respiratory illnesses that result from inflammation and swelling of the larynx, trachea, and large bronchi; the causative agent can be either viral or bacterial **(12)**

Cryotherapy: freezing with liquid nitrogen **(21)**

Cryptorchidism: a condition in which one or both of the testicles fail to descend into the scrotum **(18)**

Cult family: group in which a leader makes all decisions and controls the actions of all those who live there **(4)**

Cultural competence: set of skills, knowledge, and attitudes that includes awareness and acceptance of differences, awareness of one's own cultural values, understanding of the dynamics of difference, development of cultural knowledge, and ability to adapt practice skills to fit the cultural context of the client or patient **(1)**

Cultural proficiency: quality obtained when cultural competence components become second nature to the nurse **(1)**

Culture theory: factors of culture that should be considered when working with families **(4)**

Culture: a style of behavior patterns, beliefs, and products of human work of a given community or population **(4)**

Cushing's syndrome: hyperfunction of the adrenal cortex **(19)**

Cystitis: bladder infection **(18)**

Cysts: fluid-filled sacs **(18)**

D

Date rape: sexual intercourse during a social outing without consent, occurring as a result of threat or physical force **(16)**

Deductive reasoning: process of taking a generalized idea and figuring out what specifics to expect from it **(2)**

Deep sedation: controlled state of depressed consciousness or unconsciousness in which the child is unable to maintain protective reflexes **(7)**

Defense mechanisms: ways of protecting the ego from threatening impulses or painful realities of life experiences **(5)**

Dehydration: a condition of deficient fluid volume in the intravascular and interstitial fluid compartments **(11)**

Delegation: transfer to a competent individual of the authority or right to perform selected nursing tasks in a selected situation **(1, 2)**

Demandingness: a state relating to the demands that parents make on the children, their expectations for mature behavior, the discipline and supervision they provide, and their willingness to confront behavioral problems **(4)**

Dendrite: extension of a nerve cell that conducts the electrical impulses toward the cell body **(15)**

Depression: prolonged feeling of sadness or hopelessness that interferes with normal activities of life **(16)**

Depth: complexities of an issue **(2)**

Dermatitis: inflammation of the dermis or skin **(21)**

Dermis: inner thicker layer of the skin that contains most of the associated structures **(21)**

Desensitization: process of administering doses of medication in increasing increments in an effort to avoid the allergic reaction **(22)**

Desired outcomes: general goals for a client **(1)**

Desquamation: to shed, peel, or come off in scales, as in skin **(10)**

Development: process of maturation including the refinement of body systems, thought processes, and judgment **(5)**

Diabetes mellitus: disorder of carbohydrate, protein, and fat metabolism, the most common metabolic disorder in children **(19)**

Diabetic ketoacidosis: an increase in ketone bodies in the urine, caused by an increased rate of free fatty acid metabolism by the liver **(19)**

Dialysis: mechanical process of removing wastes from blood or lymph through the processes of diffusion, osmosis, and ultrafiltration; once the blood or lymph is filtered, it is returned to the body **(18)**

Diaper dermatitis: dermatitis caused by irritation from urine and/or stool **(21)**

Diaphragm: large muscle dividing the chest and abdominal cavities **(12)**

Diaphysis: main section of a long bone, contains the medullary cavity **(20)**

Diffusion: process in which solutes move across the cell membrane from an area of higher concentration to an area of lower concentration **(11)**

Diplopia: double vision **(15)**

Disequilibrium syndrome: complication caused by cerebral edema; symptoms include fatigue, nausea, vomiting, tremors (which can progress to delirium), seizures, and coma **(18)**

Diverticulum: out-pouch in the ileum, usually near the ileocecal valve **(17)**

Down syndrome: most common chromosomal abnormality, results from trisomy 21; signs include *microcephaly* (small head), wide short neck, epicanthal folds, and short broad hands with a simian line; associated with increased incidence of congenital heart defects, mental retardation, diabetes, and hearing loss **(15)**

Droplet method: indirect method of transmission of harmful organisms **(10)**

Droplet precautions: are implemented to prevent the spread of infection by the droplet route **(10)**

Drowning: loss of life within 24 hours following submersion in water or other liquid **(15)**

Dysfunctional grief: (also known as *complicated grief*) condition of grief in which an individual cannot accept what has happened or move on with life **(9)**

Dyslexia: specific, common learning disability that is neurologic in origin **(15)**

Dysphagia: difficulty swallowing **(12)**

Dysphonia: muffled or hoarse voice **(12)**

Dyspnea: difficulty breathing **(12)**

Dysuria: painful urination **(18)**

E

Ecchymosis: bruising **(14)**

Echolalia: words repeated over and over again **(16)**

Ecomap: a diagram of the interactions of family members to the immediate environment **(4)**

Ego: realistic part of the personality that searches for acceptable methods of meeting pleasure needs **(5)**

Egocentrism: the tendency to view things only from one's own point of view **(5)**

Electrical burns: burns caused by contact with exposed electric wires **(21)**

Electrolytes: solutes within the body fluid; also called minerals or salts **(11)**

Emancipated minors: those minors responsible for their own health care decisions and expenses **(3)**

Emulsifier: a substance that breaks down large molecules of fat into smaller molecules of fat **(17)**

Encephalitis: inflammation of the brain, most often caused by a viral infection **(15)**

Encopresis: condition in which child delays defecation or experiences frequent soiling of feces **(16)**

Endometriosis: the presence of endometrium elsewhere than in the lining of the uterus; causes premenstrual pain and dysmenorrhea **(18)**

End-stage renal disease: condition in which kidney function is less than 10%; person requires dialysis or kidney transplantation to survive **(18)**

Enucleation: removal of the eye and placement of a prosthesis **(15)**

Enuresis: urinary incontinence occurring in a child who is capable of obtaining bladder control **(18)**

Epicanthal folds: folds of skin over the inner canthus of the eye, common in children with Down syndrome **(15)**

Epidermis: outer thin layer of the skin consisting of several layers **(21)**

Epiglottitis: inflammation of the epiglottis caused by a bacterial infection of the pharynx and soft tissue of the larynx **(12)**

Epilepsy: chronic disorder characterized by repeated seizure activity **(15)**

Epiphora: watering of the eyes **(15)**

Epiphyseal plate: growth plate; portion of the bone that remains open until late adolescence **(20)**

Epiphysis: attachment site for muscles, considered the site for ossification **(20)**

Epispadias: condition that occurs when the urethra opens on the dorsal (upper) surface of the penis **(18)**

Epistaxis: nosebleed **(12)**

Equines: midfoot **(20)**

Erythema marginatum: a red skin rash that sometimes occurs with rheumatic fever **(13)**

Erythema migrans: early symptom of Lyme disease; a red rash with a bull's eye appearance at the site of the bite **(10)**

Erythrocytes: red blood cells (RBCs) **(14)**

Erythropoiesis: formation or production of red blood cells **(14)**

Eschar: dead matter that is sloughed off the surface of the skin, especially after a burn **(12, 21)**

Esophageal atresia: a potentially life-threatening defect in which the esophagus ends in a blind pouch before reaching the stomach **(12, 17)**

Esotropia: turning of the eye inward **(15)**

Ethics: system of values and ideas that shape a sense of right and wrong **(3)**

Ethnicity: a group with a common ancestry, race, religion, and culture **(4)**

Eupnea: normal breathing pattern **(12)**

Euthanasia: act of compassionately putting to death a person suffering from incurable or distressing disease **(9)**

Exhibitionism: exposing the genitals to strangers **(16)**

Exophthalmos: prominent or bulging eyes **(19)**

Exotropia: turning outward of the eye **(15)**

Extended family: a network of relatives and/or close friends who take an active role in the emotional support of the family **(4)**

F

Failure to thrive (FTT): general term used to describe the child who fails to gain weight or loses weight for unknown reasons **(17)**

Fair-mindedness: consciously treating all points of view equally, without reference to one's own points of view **(2)**

Fairness: impartiality **(2)**

Family: two or more individuals who come together for the purpose of nurturing **(4)**

Family assessment: an ongoing process of examining relationships and functioning of members of the family **(4)**

Family-centered care: treatment to a designated client with recognition that the family system or unit may also need intervention **(4)**

Family development theory: analytical description of the changes the family undergoes over time **(4)**

Family role: expectations or behaviors associated with a person's position in the family **(4)**

Family system: a group of individuals (as defined by its members) who establish a relationship for the benefit of nurturing, supporting, educating, and providing for the needs of each individual **(4)**

Family systems theory: analysis of family systems and boundaries between the family and the world **(4)**

Febrile seizure: a generalized seizure that usually occurs when a child's temperature rises rapidly to above 102 °F (39 °C) **(15)**

Fecalith: a hard mass of feces **(17)**

Fibroadenoma: a freely movable rounded mass with well-defined borders and a solid rubbery texture **(18)**

Fibrocyst: fluid-filled mass **(18)**

Fibromyalgia: disorder characterized by widespread musculoskeletal pain and fatigue **(15)**

Fibrosis: replacement of inflamed or damaged tissue with connective or scar tissue **(18)**

Filtration: process by which solvents and solutes are pushed across a cell membrane from an area of higher pressure to an area of lower pressure **(11)**

Fissures: cracks or lines present on skin tissues **(13)**

Focal seizures: seizures caused by abnormal electrical activity in a specific area of the brain, most commonly in the temporal, frontal, or parietal lobes of the cerebrum **(15)**

Fomites: inanimate objects that transmit harmful bacteria indirectly **(10)**

Formal operation period: period when the child gradually completes intellectual development necessary to function as an adult **(5)**

Forschheimer spots: erythematous pinpoint lesions of the soft palate, sometimes occurring with rubella **(10)**

Fracture: condition that results from an injury and causes the continuity of the bone to be altered **(20)**

Frostbite: skin and tissue damage caused by overexposure to low environmental temperatures **(21)**

Fulminating hepatitis: progressive, total destruction of the liver **(17)**

Fundus: rounded top of an organ, such as the uterus or the stomach **(17)**

G

Ganglia: groups of nerve cell bodies located in the PNS **(15)**

Gastroenteritis: inflammation of the stomach; may be caused by bacteria, such as *Escherichia coli* or salmonella; virus, such as rotavirus; as well as toxins and allergies **(17)**

Gastroesophageal reflux disease: condition caused by a relaxation of the cardiac sphincter **(17)**

Generalized anxiety disorder: (also known as *overanxious disorder*) disorder in which the child is prone to excessive worry about the future **(16)**

Generalized seizures: seizures that result from diffuse electrical activity that begins in one area of the brain and spreads to involve the entire cerebral cortex and brainstem **(15)**

Genital warts: (also known as *condylomata acuminata*) a sexually transmitted infection with human papilloma virus **(18)**

Genitourinary system: consists of structures of the urinary system and the reproductive system **(18)**

Genogram: a diagram of relationships of members of the family **(4)**

Genu valgum: (also known as *knock knees*) inward slant of the thigh **(20)**

Genu varum: (also known as *bowlegs*) legs bowed outward at the knee (or below the knee) **(20)**

Gingiva: mucous membrane covering the front of the mouth and the inside of the lips **(17)**

Glaucoma: condition caused by increased intraocular pressure (IOP) due to inadequate drainage of the aqueous humor **(15)**

Glomerulonephritis: inflammation of the glomeruli **(18)**

Goiter: painless enlargement of thyroid gland **(19)**

Goniotomy: surgical technique by which the flow of aqueous humor is increased from the anterior chamber **(15)**

Gonorrhea: a sexually transmitted infection caused by *Neisseria gonorrhoeae* **(18)**

Gower's maneuver: a classic symptom of muscular dystrophy in which the child uses the upper extremities to lift up from the floor **(20)**

Graves' disease: autoimmune disorder in which antibodies attack the thyroid gland **(19)**

Greater curvature: outer curved area of the stomach **(17)**

Greenstick fracture: fracture in which one side of the bone is broken and the other side is bent **(20)**

Grief: feeling of extreme sadness resulting from a loss **(9)**

Growth: process of increasing in physical size **(5)**

Growth hormone deficiency: decrease in growth hormone that results from inheritance, genetic mutation, injury, or disease of the hypothalamus or pituitary gland **(19)**

Guillain-Barré syndrome: (also known as *postinfectious polyneuritis*) relatively rare disorder characterized by ascending and then descending paralysis **(15)**

H

Health: sense of physical, psychological, emotional, and spiritual well-being, not just the absence of disease **(6)**

Health promotion: encouraging lifestyle changes that result in the individual becoming healthier **(6)**

Hematology: study of blood and blood-forming tissues **(14)**

Hematomas: accumulations of blood under the skin **(15)**

Hematopoiesis: process in which blood cells are produced in the bone marrow **(14, 20)**

Hematuria: blood in the urine **(18)**

Hemolysis: destruction or dissolution of red blood cells, with subsequent release of hemoglobin **(14)**

Hemophilia: rare hereditary gender-linked disorder causing a deficiency in a specific blood clotting factor **(14)**

Hemoptysis: bloody sputum **(18)**

Hemosiderin: the by-product of hemolysis **(14)**

Hemosiderosis: iron overload, the buildup of iron in tissues and organs **(14)**

Hemothorax: presence of bloody fluids in the chest cavity **(12)**

Hepatitis: inflammation of the liver caused by a viral infection **(17)**

Hepatomegaly: enlarged liver **(13, 17, 22)**

Hernia: protrusion of intestines through a weakness in the abdominal or pelvic muscles **(17)**

Heterochromia: different-colored eyes **(15)**

Hip spica cast: cast covering the upper thighs and lower torso **(20)**

Hirschsprung's disease: (also known as *megacolon*) a condition in which the autonomic parasympathetic ganglion that normally causes peristalsis in the intestine is absent **(17)**

Hirsutism: excessive hair growth **(18)**

Holistic: inclusive of the physical, psychological, and spiritual aspects of the person **(1)**

Holistic health: aspects of a person's condition that include the physical, psychological, and spiritual aspects of the person **(16)**

Homeostasis: state of balance of fluids and electrolytes within the body **(11)**

Hormones: main regulators of growth and development, metabolism, and reproduction **(19)**

Hospice care: movement of care based on the holistic concepts of palliative care that emphasize quality of life rather than cure **(9)**

Human immunodeficiency virus (HIV): a retrovirus that attacks and destroys the body's immune system **(18)**

Humoral immunity: immunity that destroys bacteria, viruses, parasites, allergens, and other foreign substances by producing antibodies called immunoglobulins **(22)**

Hydronephrosis: distension of the renal pelvis caused by increased pressure due to urinary backup **(18)**

Hydrophobia: in rabies, a reflex contraction at the sight of liquid accompanied by painful contractures in the muscles used for swallowing **(10)**

Hymen: a thin membrane that partially covers the vaginal orifice **(18)**

Hypercalcemia: condition characterized by an increase in serum calcium above normal levels **(11)**

Hyperkalemia: condition that occurs when there is an increase above normal range in serum potassium levels **(11)**

Hyperlipidemia: condition characterized by increased total cholesterol, low-density lipoproteins, and triglycerides accompanied by decreased high-density lipoproteins **(13, 18)**

Hypernatremia: state of sodium excess related to the body's water **(11)**

Hyperopia: farsightedness **(15)**

Hypertonic dehydration: fluid and sodium loss in which relatively more fluid than sodium is lost (as in diabetes) **(11)**

Hypertropia: (also known as *anoopsia*) vertical deviation of one of the eyes **(15)**

Hyperventilation: deep, rapid respirations **(12)**

Hypervolemia: abnormally increased volume of blood; fluid volume excess (FVE); occurs with retention of fluid and sometimes sodium in the extracellular compartment **(11)**

Hyphema: hemorrhage into the anterior chamber of the eye **(15)**

Hypoalbuminemia: abnormally low level of albumin in the blood **(18)**

Hypocalcemia: condition characterized by serum calcium levels below normal levels **(11)**

Hypokalemia: condition that occurs when there is a decrease below normal range in serum potassium levels **(11)**

Hyponatremia: state of sodium deficit related to the body's water **(11)**

Hypopituitarism: condition in which there is a decreased function of the pituitary gland resulting in GHD **(19)**

Hypospadias: condition that occurs when the urethra opens on the ventral (lower) surface of the penis **(18)**

Hypotonic dehydration: fluid and sodium loss in which relatively more sodium than fluid is lost (as, for example, in renal disease) **(11)**

Hypoventilation: slow, shallow respirations **(12)**

Hysterectomy: removal of the uterus **(18)**

I

Id: basic energy that drives the individual to seek pleasure **(5)**

Idiopathic thrombocytopenic purpura: (also called ITP) bleeding disorder of unknown cause that leads to a decrease in the number of platelets **(14)**

Illness: state of disease or sickness; may be physical or psychological; may be acute, chronic, or terminal **(7, 10)**

Illness prevention: specific behaviors that can prevent illness and limit injury **(6)**

Immune response: bodily defense reaction that recognizes an antigen and produces antibodies specific against that antigen **(22)**

Immunization: process of inducing resistance to communicable diseases **(10)**

Immunoglobulins: any of a group of large glycoproteins that are secreted by plasma cells and that function as antibodies in the immune response by binding with specific antigens **(22)**

Impetigo: superficial skin infection that appears on the face, hands, neck, or extremities, caused by streptococci or staphylococci **(21)**

Implications: consequences **(2)**

Incest: sexual intercourse between close blood relatives that may or may not be consensual **(16)**

Incubation period: time between the entry of a pathogen into a reservoir and the onset of clinical signs and symptoms **(10)**

Individualized education plan (IEP): plan for meeting educational requirements of a child with special needs **(7)**

Inductive reasoning: process of making generalized statements from a limited set of facts **(2)**

Inferences: deductions **(2)**

Information: knowledge gained through research or observation **(2)**

Informed consent: written approval for a treatment or procedure, following explanation of pros and cons by the physician or other professional who is performing the procedure **(3)**

Inotropic: affecting the contraction of muscle, especially heart muscle **(13)**

Insulin resistance: condition in which the body produces enough insulin but is unable to use it effectively **(19)**

Intellectual autonomy: having a rational control over one's ideas and beliefs **(2)**

Intellectual courage: facing and fairly addressing ideas, beliefs, or viewpoints that might, on a superficial level, seem absurd or false, or toward which we might have negative emotions **(2)**

Intellectual empathy: imagining oneself in the place of others in order to better understand them **(2)**

Intellectual humility: having a consciousness that one's knowledge base, prejudices, biases, and point of view have limitations **(2)**

Intellectual integrity: being true and consistent with intellectual standards, holding oneself to the same standards of proof as one holds those with opposing views, and honestly admitting when one is inconsistent in one's thoughts and actions **(2)**

Intellectual standards: concepts that guide the critical thinker to better and better reasoning **(2)**

Intercostal muscles: muscles between the ribs **(12)**

Interpretations: ways of clarifying the meaning **(2)**

Interstitial: related to spaces within a structure, such as the spaces within a tissue or organ **(11)**

Interventions: nursing actions to assist the client toward an improvement in health **(1)**

Intracranial pressure: the force exerted within the cranial cavity by the brain, blood, and CSF **(15)**

Intraductal papillomas: tumors growing in a mammary duct, most commonly occurring during menopause **(18)**

Intussusception: condition that occurs when one portion of the intestine telescopes into another portion **(17)**

Iron-deficiency anemia: condition that results when the demand for stored iron is greater than what the body can supply **(14)**

Irritant: source of irritation as a foreign substance **(21)**

Isogeneic donor: (also called syngeneic donor) donor who is an identical twin **(14)**

Isotonic dehydration: loss of fluid and sodium in equal proportions (as from vomiting); common dehydration in children **(11)**

K

Ketoacidosis: condition that occurs when glucose storage is depleted and fat storage must be used for energy needs **(11)**

Koplik's spots: small, irregular red spots with a bluish-white center appearing on the buccal mucosa in association with measles **(10)**

Kussmaul respiration: rapid and deep, labored breathing **(10, 11, 19)**

Kwashiorkor: deficiency in protein in the diet resulting in muscle wasting **(17)**

Kyphosis: (also known as *hunchback*) excessive convex curvature of the thoracic spine **(20)**

L

Lactose intolerance: congenital or acquired disorder in which the person fails to produce lactase, an enzyme needed in the digestion of lactose **(17)**

Latch-key children: school-age children who come home from school to an empty house and may remain unsupervised until parents return from work **(6)**

Lesser curvature: inner curved area of the stomach **(17)**

Leukemia: cancer of the blood-forming organs **(14)**

Leukocytes: white blood cells (WBC) **(14)**

Leukokoria: reflection in the child's eye. This sign is called the cat's-eye reflex **(15)**

Ligation: obstruction of a vessel or duct using a suture or wire ligature **(13)**

Lingual frenulum: thin membrane that attaches the tongue to the floor of the mouth **(17)**

Livor mortis: discoloration that results after blood circulation has ceased and red blood cells break down, releasing hemoglobin; appears in the lowest or dependent areas of the body **(9)**

Logan clamp: metal bow taped to both sides of the suture line **(17)**

Logical: reasonable **(2)**

Lordosis: (also known as *sway back*) excessive concave curvature of the lumbar spine **(20)**

Loss: feeling, either real or perceived, that is experienced when something important is removed from the body or the environment **(9)**

Lumpectomy: removal of a lump (usually cancerous) from a woman's breast **(18)**

Lymphadenopathy: enlarged lymph nodes **(22)**

M

Magical thinking: the child believes that ideas and mental images become reality **(5)**

Mammography: imaging exam of the breast with x-rays, ultrasound, or nuclear magnetic resonance **(18)**

Mammoplasty: breast reconstruction **(18)**

Mantoux test: skin test in which a small amount of tuberculin is injected under the skin to determine prior exposure to tuberculosis **(12)**

Mastectomy: removal of the breast **(18)**

Maturation: process of becoming fully developed **(5)**

Mature minor act: an act that permits adolescents age 14 or 15 to make decisions about their treatment **(3)**

Meconium: the first fetal stool **(12)**

Meconium aspiration: aspiration of amniotic fluid contaminated with meconium by a fetus in hypoxic distress **(12)**

Mediastinal shift: a shift in organs caused by pressure from the intact lung **(12)**

Megacolon: (also known as *Hirschsprung's disease*) a condition in which the autonomic parasympathetic ganglion that normally causes peristalsis in the intestine is absent **(17)**

Melanin: pigment that adds color to the skin **(21)**

Melanocytes: pigment-producing cells **(21)**

Melena: tarry stool **(14)**

Menarche: the beginning of the menstrual cycle **(5)**

Meningitis: inflammation of the meninges by either a bacteria or a virus **(15)**

Meningocele: herniation of the meninges through the vertebral defect **(15)**

Mental retardation: disability characterized by significant limitations both in intellectual functioning and in adaptive behavior as expressed in conceptual, social, and practical adaptive skills **(15)**

Metabolic acidosis: condition involving an excess of acids in the body **(11)**

Metabolic alkalosis: condition that results from a loss of metabolic acid or an excess of bicarbonate **(11)**

Metaphysis: zone of growth between the epiphysis and diaphysis during development of a bone, responsible for converting new cartilage into bone **(20)**

Milia: white pinpoint spots on a newborn that resemble whiteheads **(21)**

Miscarriage: (also known as *spontaneous abortion*) nonelective abortion that occurs within the first 20 weeks of pregnancy **(3)**

Mongolian spot: dark discolored area found over the lower back and sacrum of infants of Black, Hispanic, South Asian, or East Asian descent; over time, skin tones darken to become the same color as the Mongolian spot **(21)**

Monilia: (also known as *Candidiasis* or *yeast infection*) a common organism causing vaginitis **(18)**

"Moon face": round cheeks and double chin associated with Cushing's syndrome **(19)**

Morbidity: prevalence of a specific disease or disorder in the population at a specific period of time **(1)**

Moro reflex: (also known as *startle* reflex) reflex that occurs when newborns have a sense of falling, in which newborn quickly extends (abducts) the arms with fingers flared and thumb and first finger forming a "C," then adducts in an embracing motion; the lower extremities may extend and flex; a slight tremor may be noted **(8)**

Mortality: number of deaths over a given period of time for a given population **(1)**

Motility disorders: conditions that prevent gastrointestinal contents from moving through the system in a normal manner **(17)**

Mottled: bluish or purplish marbled appearance of the skin **(9)**

Muscular dystrophy: a group of inherited diseases that cause muscle degeneration and wasting **(20)**

Myelin sheath: lipoprotein covering of the axon **(15)**

Myelination: development of the myelin sheath around the nerve fiber **(15)**

Myelomeningocele: a herniation of the spinal nerves and cord, as well as the meninges, through the vertebral defect **(15)**

Myomectomy: removal of tumor and surrounding myometrium **(18)**

Myopia: nearsightedness **(15)**

Myringotomy: surgical procedure in which a small plastic tube is inserted through the tympanic membrane to facilitate drainage of fluid and ventilation of the middle ear **(15)**

N

Nasopharyngitis: (also known as *rhinitis* or *coryza*) inflammation of the nasal mucosa, often caused by a viral infection such as the common cold **(12)**

Natural immunity: immunity that is present at birth and lasts about 3 to 6 months **(22)**

NCLEX-PN® focus area: one of 11 areas of Client Needs around which the NCLEX-PN® test is constructed **(2)**

Near-drowning: suffocation from submersion in liquid that is survived in the first 24 hours following the incident; most often associated with asphyxia and aspiration **(15)**

Negative feedback: mechanism in blood levels of most hormones where high levels of a hormone in the blood inhibit (switch off) hormone production and low levels trigger (switch on) hormone production **(19)**

Nephroblastoma: (also known as *Wilms' tumor*) highly metastatic cancerous tumor of the kidney **(18)**

Nephrolithiasis: kidney stones **(18)**

Nephrotic syndrome: clinical state characterized by edema, proteinuria, hypoalbuminemia, hyperlipidemia, and altered immunity **(18)**

Neural tube: fetal tissue that develops into the central nervous system **(15)**

Neurologic trauma: any injury to the head or spinal cord due to force, anoxia, or penetration **(15)**

Neurons: nerve cells that transmit impulses from one part of the body to another **(15)**

Nits: louse eggs **(21)**

Nociceptor: sensory receptor that detects and differentiates pain sensation **(15)**

Nonorganic failure to thrive: a disorder characterized by inadequate growth in height and weight **(16)**

Nosocomial infection: infection acquired in a health care setting **(10)**

Nuclear family: members of a single-family unit **(4)**

Nursing diagnoses: names for client conditions that nurses are qualified and trained to treat independently; they have been defined and developed by the North American Nursing Diagnosis Association (NANDA) **(1)**

Nystagmus: involuntary movement of the eyes **(15)**

O

Obesity: excessive weight and accumulation of body fat **(16, 17)**

Object permanence: an understanding that unseen objects still exist **(5)**

Objective data: data that can be observed and measured by the senses or by mechanical instruments **(1)**

Obsessive-compulsive disorder: disorder characterized by ritualistic thoughts or actions that interfere with activities of daily living **(16)**

Obstructive uropathy: condition in which the structure or function of the urinary system is altered, resulting in obstruction of urine flow **(18)**

Open reduction: reduction of a fractured bone by surgically aligning the bone and stabilizing the ends with nails, plates, or screws **(20)**

Oral candidiasis: (also known as *thrush*) chronic condition caused most commonly by the fungus *Candida albicans* **(22)**

Orchiectomy: removal of one testis and spermatic cord **(18)**

Ordinal position: a person's ranking by order of birth in the family **(5)**

Orthopnea: dyspnea or difficulty breathing that is relieved by sitting or standing **(12)**

Orthoptics: eye exercises **(15)**

Osmosis: movement of fluid (the solvent) across the cell membrane from an area of lesser solute concentration to an area of greater solute concentration; causes the concentration of solutes on both sides of the cell membrane to become equal **(11)**

Ossification: the hardening or calcification of soft tissue into a bonelike material, marking the transition from embryo to fetus **(20)**

Otalgia: ear pain **(15)**

Otitis media: inflammation of the middle ear that may be accompanied by fluid in the middle ear **(15)**

Ovarian cancer: the most lethal of female reproductive cancers; it remains asymptomatic until the cancer has spread to surrounding tissue or has been transported by the lymphatic system to other parts of the body **(18)**

P

Palliative care: (also known as *palliative management*) care in which the goal is relief from suffering, not cure **(9)**

Palliative management: (also known as *palliative care*) care that involves a shift in treatment goals from cure to providing relief from suffering **(9)**

Palmar grasp reflex: reflex that occurs when a finger or small object is placed in the newborn's hand; newborns grasp the finger tightly enough to be lifted from the bed **(8)**

Pancytopenia: a state of decreased RBCs **(14)**

Pandemic flu: global outbreak of virulent human influenza **(10)**

Papillae: small, raised bumps covering the tongue **(17)**

Parallel play: side-by-side play, typical of toddlers **(5, 6)**

Paraphimosis: inability to return the foreskin over the glans, causing constriction of the penis **(18)**

Parasympathetic nervous system: part of the autonomic nervous system that controls bodily processes in nonstressful situations; clinical manifestations include constriction of pupils, decreased heart rate, constriction of bronchioles, and increased peristalsis **(15)**

Parenchyma: functional part of an organ **(17)**

Parotid gland: largest of the salivary glands, located below and in front of the ears at the angle of the jaw **(17)**

Passive immunity: immunity provided by administering immunoglobulins to protect children against diseases to which they may have been exposed already **(10, 22)**

Pathogens: harmful organisms **(10)**

PCA pump: patient-controlled analgesia device, which allows the client to control the amount and timing of medication up to a preset amount **(7)**

Pediatrics: the medical science related to diagnosis and treatment of childhood illness **(1)**

Pediculosis: infestation with parasites (lice) that live on the outside of a human host **(21)**

Pedophile: person who has sexual interest in children **(16)**

Peer pressure: influencing a person to follow the desire or behavior of the group **(6)**

Percentile: measure of what portion of the overall population is the same **(5)**

Periorbital edema: edema around the eyes **(18)**

Peristalsis: wavelike contraction of the smooth muscle that lies underneath the mucous membrane **(17)**

PERRLA: pupils equally round and react to light and accommodation **(15)**

Petechiae: pinpoint hemorrhages **(14)**

Phenylketonuria: congenital disorder that results in toxic accumulation of phenylalanine and its metabolites; can lead to mental retardation, and/or brain damage **(17)**

Phimosis: condition that occurs when the opening of the foreskin is small and unable to be retracted over the glans **(18)**

Photophobia: sensitivity to light **(15)**

Pica: ingestion of nonfood material **(14, 17)**

Plantar grasp reflex: reflex that occurs when the sole of the foot is touched; toes curl under as if newborns are trying to "grasp" with their feet **(8)**

Plasma: clear, fluid portion of circulating blood **(11)**

Plicae: the inner lining of the small intestines **(17)**

Pneumonia: inflammation or infection of the bronchioles and alveoli in the lung **(12)**

Pneumothorax: air in the chest cavity that can result from chest trauma or spontaneous rupturing of alveoli **(12)**

Point of maximal impulse: site where the heart rate can be best heard **(13)**

Points of view: perspectives **(2)**

Poisoning: ingestion of a toxic substance **(17)**

Polycystic kidney: condition in which one or both kidneys are enlarged and contain fluid-filled cysts **(18)**

Polycystic ovary syndrome: condition that results from numerous follicular cysts **(18)**

Polydipsia: excessive thirst **(19)**

Polyphagia: excessive hunger **(19)**

Polyuria: excessive urine output **(19)**

Portal of entry: method in which a harmful organism enters a new host **(10)**

Portal of exit: method in which a harmful organism leaves the reservoir **(10)**

Positive feedback: mechanism in which increase in one substance causes an increased response until some major event occurs that causes a decrease in the substance **(19)**

Postictal: following a seizure **(15)**

Postinfectious polyneuritis: (Guillain-Barré syndrome) relatively rare disorder characterized by ascending and then descending paralysis **(15)**

Postmortem examination: (also known as *autopsy*) examination of the body after death to determine more details about the cause of death, the disease, or other statistical data **(9)**

Precision: scientific exactness **(2)**

Precocious puberty: the presence of any secondary sex characteristics before the age of 8 in girls and before the age of 9 in boys **(19)**

Preload: volume of blood in the ventricles at the end of the diastole **(13)**

Preoperational: pertaining to a level at which the child learns to interact with others in the environment **(5)**

Primary care: care that includes preventive activities such as immunizations, well-child checkups, and routine physical examinations **(1)**

Primary immune response: body's first response to antigens **(22)**

Primary prevention: keeping health problems from beginning **(6)**

Prodromal period: stage of an infectious process that occurs just prior to the onset of clinical symptoms **(10)**

Prostaglandins: potent hormonelike substances that mediate physiologic functions such as control of blood pressure, contraction of smooth muscle, and modulation of inflammation **(19)**

Proteinuria: protein in the urine **(18)**

Proximodistal: from the center of the body to the periphery and from general to specific **(5)**

Pruritis: itching **(17)**

Pseudohermaphroditism: (also known as *ambiguous genitalia*) rare condition in which determining the gender of the child is difficult **(18, 19)**

Psychosexual: related to emotional, mental, physiologic, and behavioral components of sex or sexual development **(5)**

Psychosocial health: aspects of health, including mental, emotional, social, and spiritual stability **(16)**

Puberty: a period of transition and sexual maturation **(5)**

Pulmonary stenosis: narrowing of the pulmonary valve **(13)**

Purging: induction of vomiting, abuse of laxatives or diuretics, or both **(16)**

Purpose: an end, aim, or result **(2)**

Purpura: rash in which blood cells leak into the skin **(14)**

Pyelonephritis: kidney infection **(18)**

Pyeloplasty: removal of the obstructed ureter segment and replacement into the renal pelvis **(18)**

Pyloric stenosis: progressive hypertrophy of the pyloric sphincter resulting in obstruction **(17)**

Pyloroplasty: surgical widening of the pyloric canal to facilitate emptying of gastric contents into the duodenum **(17)**

Pylorus: passage at the lower end of the stomach that opens into the duodenum **(17)**

R

Race: biologic deviations as shown in physical features **(4)**

Radiation burns: burns caused by exposure to radiation, the most common type being sunburn **(21)**

Rape: forced sexual intercourse including vaginal, anal, or oral penetration **(16)**

Rashkind procedure: (also known as *balloon atrial septostomy*) procedure in which an existing opening in the cardiac septum is enlarged, allowing better mixing of oxygenated blood (from the lungs) with the systemic blood **(13)**

Reanastomosis: reconnection of a divided vessel **(17)**

Reasoning: process of forming conclusions, judgments, or inferences from facts or assumptions **(2)**

Rebound tenderness: following palpation, the increase in discomfort when abdominal pressure is released **(17)**

Reduction mammoplasty: reduction in the size of the breast by removing fat tissue with an attempt to leave the mammary glands intact **(18)**

Relevance: connection to the matter in hand **(2)**

Religion: the belief in a superhuman power recognized as creator and governor of the universe **(4)**

Remission: lack of evidence of any clinical symptoms of a disorder **(14)**

Renal failure: inability of the kidneys to remove liquid waste from the blood **(18)**

Reportable disease: disease that poses a public health hazard **(3)**

Reservoir: site where harmful organisms grow and reproduce **(10)**

Residual volume: (of food) amount of the feeding that remains in the client's stomach **(8)**

Respiratory acidosis: an accumulation of carbon dioxide caused by states of hypoventilation, altered perfusion, or inadequate respiratory diffusion **(11)**

Respiratory alkalosis: condition characterized by a low level of carbon dioxide in the blood **(11)**

Respiratory syncytial virus (RSV): RNA-containing virus that causes bronchiolitis and bronchopneumonia in children **(12)**

Responsiveness: a state relating to how much parents foster individuality, self-assertion, and self-regulation and how responsive they are to special needs and demands **(4)**

Reverse isolation: precaution used for individuals who are immunocompromised to protect them from harmful organisms that may be brought in from outside **(10)**

Reye's syndrome: acute encephalitis characterized by an onset of symptoms 1 to 3 weeks following a viral infection **(15)**

Rhinitis: (also known as *nasopharyngitis* or *coryza*) inflammation of the nasal mucosa, often caused by a viral infection such as the common cold; classic symptoms include redness and swelling of the nasal and pharyngeal mucosa **(12)**

Rhonchi: coarse rattling sounds, usually caused by secretion in a bronchial tube, common in the child with respiratory disorders **(12)**

Rickets: condition caused by a vitamin D deficiency preventing the proper absorption and utilization of calcium and phosphorus **(17)**

Rigor mortis: stiffening of the body that occurs about 2 to 4 hours after death **(9)**

Ringworm: (also known as *tinea*) group of fungal infections of the skin that are transmitted from human to human or from animal to human **(21)**

Rooting reflex: reflex that occurs when the newborn's cheek is stroked and the infant turns the head in that direction **(8)**

Rugae: folds, creases, or wrinkles, as in the lining of the mucous membranes in the vagina **(17)**

S

Scabies: infestation caused by the mite *Sarcoptes scabiei* **(21)**

Scurvy: condition caused by a lack of vitamin C in the diet **(17)**

Seasonal flu: (also known as *common flu*) respiratory illness that can be transmitted from person to person, generally caused by influenza A or B **(10)**

Seborrheic dermatitis: "cradle cap," condition in newborns that causes dandruff and that may be a result of changes in sebaceous glands **(21)**

Secondary care: care that refers to relatively serious or complicated care **(1)**

Secondary immune response: body's response to a second exposure to an antigen **(22)**

Secondary prevention: early detection and screening for health problems **(6)**

Seizures: periods of sudden discharge of electrical activity in the brain that cause involuntary muscle activity, change in level of consciousness (LOC), or altered behavior and sensory manifestation **(15)**

Sensorimotor: first level of cognitive development in which baby and young child begin interaction with the environment by reflex response, from birth to 2 years of age **(5)**

Separation anxiety: feelings of anger, fear, grief, or revenge in association with a closely related person **(5, 7)**

Separation anxiety disorder: (also known as *anaclitic depression*) fear of separation from individuals or locations **(16)**

Septum: wall **(13)**

Sexual abuse: sexual acts that are imposed on children who cannot protect themselves because of their lack of emotional or cognitive development **(16)**

Shaken-baby syndrome: syndrome in infants in which brain injury is caused by shaking of such violence that the child's brain rebounds against the skull **(16)**

Sickle cell anemia: hereditary disorder affecting the formation of hemoglobin **(14)**

Sickle cell crisis: acute episode of severe symptoms of sickle cell anemia **(14)**

Sickling: changing of the RBC's shape **(14)**

Significance: importance **(2)**

Simian crease: horizontal crease extending across the entire palm **(15)**

Single-parent family: either a mother or a father who raises the children alone **(4)**

Solute: substance dissolved in a solution or fluid **(11)**

Solution: substance formed when one or more solutes are dissolved in a solvent **(11)**

Solvent: liquid in which a substance or solute is dissolved **(11)**

Somatic reflexes: reflexes that control skeletal muscle contractions **(15)**

Spanking: one or two flat-handed swats on a child's wrist or buttocks **(6)**

Spina bifida: incomplete closure of the vertebra and neural tube **(15)**

Splenomegaly: enlarged spleen **(17, 22)**

Sprain: condition that occurs when the ligament associated with a joint is torn following trauma to the joint **(20)**

St. Vitus's dance: chorea associated with rheumatic fever occurring chiefly in children and associated with rheumatic fever **(13)**

Staging: process of naming the extent of the spread of cancer **(14)**

Standard precautions: combination of universal precautions and body substance isolation techniques that apply to all clients in a hospital **(10)**

Startle reflex: *See* Moro reflex **(8)**

Stasis: pooling of urine or other body fluids **(18)**

Status epilepticus: continuous seizure for more than 30 minutes accompanied by loss of consciousness **(15)**

Statutory rape: sexual intercourse that occurs between a minor and an adult with consent given by the minor **(16)**

Steatorrhea: fat in the stool **(12, 17)**

Stepfamily: a new marriage that creates family relationships between people who were previously in different families **(4)**

Stepping reflex: reflex obtained by holding newborns with the feet touching the table; newborns will step as if walking **(8)**

Stereotyping: not allowing for individual or group diversity **(4)**

Stereotypy: rigid and obsessive behaviors **(16)**

"Stork bites": (also known as *telangiectatic nevi*) dark red spots on the eyelids, forehead, or nape of the neck, that usually fade in time **(21)**

Strabismus: lack of coordination of the visual axes of the eye; eyes do not stay parallel to each other but may diverge in any direction **(15)**

Strain: minor injury to the muscle or tendon **(20)**

Stridor: high-pitched inspiratory crowing sound caused by severely narrowed airways **(12)**

Stroke volume: amount of blood forced out by the ventricles during a heart contraction **(13)**

Subjective data: knowledge gained from an understanding of the client's or group's subjective or personal experience **(1)**

Sublingual glands: glands that open into the floor of the mouth **(17)**

Submandibular glands: glands that lie behind the mandible and secrete saliva into the submandibular ducts **(17)**

Sucking reflex: sucking movements of an infant's lips elicited when the newborn's lips are touched **(8)**

Suicide: taking of one's own life **(16)**

Superego: moral system that contains learned values and conscience **(5)**

Supervision: the act of giving directions to workers and inspecting the tasks performed **(2)**

Surfactant: a substance that decreases the surface tension of fluid inside the alveoli, allowing the lungs to expand **(12)**

Susceptible host: individual at risk for contracting the disease caused by the harmful organism **(10)**

Sympathetic nervous system: part of the autonomic nervous system that provides assistance to a person in a stressful or life-threatening situation, causing physical changes that allow the person to respond quickly to danger **(15)**

Syngeneic donor: (also called isogeneic donor) donor who is an identical twin **(14)**

Syphilis: sexually transmitted infection caused by *Treponema pallidum* **(18)**

System: an organized group of entities which can perform a particular function in the face of change from within or without **(4)**

T

Tachypnea: rapid respiration **(12)**

Talipes: clubfoot; a congenital unilateral or bilateral twisting of the foot, usually inward **(20)**

Telangiectatic nevi: (also known as *stork bites*) dark red spots on the eyelids, forehead, or nape of the neck; usually fade in time **(21)**

Tenesmus: painful straining to defecate **(18)**

Terminal: final, fatal **(7)**

Tertiary care: management of chronic, terminal, complicated, long-term health care problems **(1)**

Tertiary prevention: disease treatment to prevent further health problems **(6)**

Therapeutic play: play that allows the individual to deal with fears associated with the health care experience **(7)**

Thermal burns: burns caused by flame or hot objects such as coffee, grease, or stoves **(21)**

Thrombocyte: (also known as a *platelet*) assists the body's clotting mechanism **(14)**

Thrush: (also known as *oral candidiasis*) fungal infection of the mouth that is caused by *Candida albicans* **(21, 22)**

Tics: sudden, rapid, involuntary movements of head, eyes, and upper body **(16)**

Tinea capitis: scalp fungus **(21)**

Tinea corporis: fungal infection that creates a circular reddened patch on the skin with raised borders **(21)**

Tinea cruris: (also known as *jock itch*) fungal infection that causes the skin in the groin area to become red and scaly, with raised papules or vesicles forming a circular rash **(21)**

Tinea pedis: (also known as *athlete's foot*) fungal infection that causes the skin between the toes and on the soles of the feet to become red, with deep scaly fissures that are painful and itchy **(21)**

Tinnitus: ringing or other sound in the ears **(15)**

Tonic-clonic movements: movements involved in seizures in children; sustained contractions of skeletal muscles that occur involuntarily. These contractions are followed by the clonic phase where muscles contract and are following by periods of relaxation **(15)**

Tonometer: instrument used to measure intraocular pressure (IOP) **(15)**

Tonsillectomy: surgical removal of the tonsils **(12)**

Tonsillitis: inflammation of the palatine and pharyngeal tonsils **(12)**

Torticollis: (also known as *wry neck*) tilt of the head caused by rotation of the cervical spine **(20)**

Toxoid: toxin that has been treated to destroy harmful effects while maintaining its capability of forming antibodies against the toxin **(10)**

Tracheoesophageal fistula: potentially life-threatening defect when a connection between the trachea and esophagus is present **(12, 17)**

Transmission: means by which an infectious agent travels from a portal of exit to a portal of entry **(10)**

Transmission-based precautions: precautions that include standard precautions plus airborne precautions, droplet precautions, or contact precautions **(10)**

Transposition of the great arteries: congenital condition in which the aorta is attached to the right ventricle, and the pulmonary artery is attached to the left ventricle, causing the blood to be insufficiently oxygenated **(13)**

Trichomoniasis: a sexually transmitted infection caused by *Trichomonas vaginalis* **(18)**

Tripod position: position with person sitting upright, leaning forward with the chin thrust forward, mouth open, and tongue protruding **(12)**

Tuberculosis (TB): infection of the respiratory system by the acid-fast bacillus *Mycobacterium tuberculosis* **(12)**

U

Universal precautions: set of precautions designed to prevent transmission of blood-borne pathogens when providing first aid or health care **(10)**

Uremic frost: urea crystals deposited on the skin **(18)**

Uremic syndrome: condition that develops in end-stage renal disease characterized by nausea, vomiting, anorexia, uremic breath odor, anemia, uremic frost, pruritis, malaise, headache, confusion, tremors, pulmonary edema, dyspnea, and congestive heart failure **(18)**

Urticaria: hives; a vascular reaction, marked by the development of wheals **(22)**

V

Vaccines: a product that contains killed, live, recombinant, or conjugated microorganisms and that is administered parenterally to induce immunity **(10)**

Vacutainer®: hollow, plastic device with a shielded or blunted needle on one end and a sharp needle on the other end that enters the vein; the device facilitates the collection of blood specimens **(8)**

Vaginitis: inflammation of the vagina that may be accompanied by vulvar pain, foul odor, pruritus, and vaginal discharge or bleeding **(18)**

Valve ablation: removal of a faulty valve **(18)**

Varus: hindfoot **(20)**

Vaso-occlusion: sickle cells obstructing circulation **(14)**

Vesicoureteral reflux: defect of the vesicoureteral valve that allows urine to flow back toward the kidneys **(18)**

Viability: ability to live outside the uterus, usually 24 weeks **(12)**

Villi: (singular, *villus*) fingerlike projections **(17)**

Volvulus: abnormal twisting of the intestine causing obstruction **(17)**

W

Wilms' tumor: (also known as *nephroblastoma*) highly metastatic cancerous tumor of the kidney **(18)**

X

Xenograft: organ or tissue obtained from an animal for transplantation into a human **(22)**

Index

(*Note*: Figures and tables, denoted by *f* and *t*, are generally cited only when they appear outside the text discussion.)

A

AAP. *See* American Academy of Pediatrics (AAP)
ABCDE (asymmetry, border irregularity, color variation, diameter, elevation) mnemonic for lesion malignancy, 574
ABCs (airway, breathing, circulation), monitoring, with burn victims, 590
Abdominal circumference, measuring, 182, 183–184
Abortion
  legal and ethical issues, 40
  thalassemia, 369
Abt, Isaac, 4*t*
Abuse
  bullying, 441
  burns, 589, 590*f*
  cupping appearing as, 271, 271*f*
  emotional abuse and neglect, 441
  family violence, 437–447, 440*f*, 441*t*, 444*f*, 444*t*, 445*t*, 446*f*
  fractures, 558
  infant abduction, preventing, 438–439
  nonorganic failure to thrive, 441–442
  nursing care, 446–447
  physical abuse, 437, 440, 440*f*, 441*t*, 443
  potential, assessing, 62, 63
  reporting, 4*t*, 37, 37*f*, 64, 437
  sexual abuse, 442–443
  shaken baby syndrome, 440
  substance abuse, 444–446, 444*f*, 444*t*, 445*t*, 446*f*
Acceptance, in grief process, 231
Accommodator learning, 100, 101
Accuracy, in critical thinking, 19
Accutane (isotretinoin), 580
Acel-Immune (DTaP, Tripedia), 104*f*, 104*t*, 256*t*
Acetaminophen (Tylenol)
  communicable diseases, 259
  newborn male circumcision, 10
  poisonings, 475*t*
Acetone breath, 535
Acid-base disorders. *See also* Fluid, electrolyte, and acid-base disorders, care of child with
  Health Promotion Issue, 302–303
  metabolic acidosis, 301, 304
  metabolic alkalosis, 304
  nursing care, 304–305
  nursing care plan chart, 305–306
  principles related to, 288*t*, 298–300, 298*f*, 299*f*
  respiratory acidosis, 300, 301*f*, 302–303
  respiratory alkalosis, 300–301, 305–306

Acidophilus, 461
Acidosis, defined, 298
Acids, as poisons, 475*t*
Acne vulgaris, 580, 580*f*, 581
Acquired heart diseases
  congestive heart failure, 348, 348*f*
  heart health in children, promoting, 352–353
  hyperlipidemia, 349–350, 350*f*
  hypertension, systemic, 348–349, 349*t*, 357
  Kawasaki's syndrome, 350–351, 350*f*
  rheumatic fever, acute, 354, 355, 359
Acquired hypogammaglobulinemia (common variable immunodeficiency), 605
Acquired immunity, 603
Acquired immunodeficiency syndrome (AIDS). *See also* Human immunodeficiency virus (HIV)
  immune disorders, 605, 609, 620
  sexually transmitted infections, 505
ACTH (adrenocorticotropic hormone), 523*t*
Activated charcoal, 476*t*
Active immunity, 252, 603
Active transport of solutes, 281, 283*f*
Activity. *See* Exercise and activity
Acute lymphoblastic leukemia, 372, 372*f*
Acute myelogenous leukemia, 372–373, 373*f*
Acute postinfectious glomerulonephritis, 489–491, 491*f*
Acute poststreptococcal glomerulonephritis, 489
Acute renal failure, 492–495, 493*f*, 493*t*, 495*f*
Acyclovir, 503*t*
Adapalene (Differin), 580
Adaptability of families, 52
ADD (attention deficit disorder), 428–429, 429*t*
Adderall (amphetamine sulfate), 428, 429*t*
Addison's disease (adrenal insufficiency), 532
Adenohypophysis (anterior pituitary gland), 522*f*, 523*t*
ADH. *See* Antidiuretic hormone (ADH)
ADHD (attention deficit/hyperactivity disorder), 428–429, 429*t*, 450
Admission to hospitals
  admission forms, 137, 138*f*
  process of, 144–146, 145*t*, 146*f*
Adolescents
  abusive home, removal from, 441*t*
  caloric intake, 115*t*
  cancer diagnosis, talking with children about, 371*t*
  cardiac testing, preparing a child for, 344*t*
  cast care instructions, 564*t*
  choking hazards, communicating about, 319*t*
  disasters, effects on, 447
  dying, understanding of, 232, 232*f*, 232*t*
  families with, 54*t*
  health promotion, 126

herpes lesions, 586*t*
hospitalized children, 144
hypovolemia, communicating about, 296*t*
legal and ethical issues affecting, 39–40
life-threatening allergies, 616*t*
menstruation, preparing for, 508*t*
nutrition, 127, 128*f*
ostomy, communicating about, 464*t*
physical growth and development, 85–87, 86*t*, 87*f*, 87*t*, 92*t*
psychosocial health, 126–127, 127*f*
routes of drug administration, 216*t*
sexuality and pregnancy, 127, 129
thyroid replacement, side effects of, 529*t*
visual impairment, communicating about, 408*t*
Adrenal glands
  adrenal crisis, 531
  disorders of, 531–532
  location, secretions, and effects, 522*f*, 524*t*
Adrenal insufficiency (Addison's disease), 532
Adrenalin. *See* Epinephrine
Adrenocortical hyperplasia (congenital adrenal hyperplasia), 531–532
Adrenocorticotropic hormone (ACTH), 523*t*
Adriamycin, 371*t*
Adults
  abuse, potential for, assessing, 63
  physical growth and development, 87, 90, 90*f*
Adults, older
  physical growth and development, 90–91
  stages of family development, 55*t*
Advance directives, 37, 38*f*, 240–241
Advil (ibuprofen), 611
Aerosol medications, administering, 216
African heritage, people with
  bone density, 546
  cyanosis, 343
  female circumcision, 505
  major cultural groups and traits, 56
  sickle cell anemia, 367–368
  systemic lupus erythematosus, 610
  thalassemia, 369
  U.S. infant, neonatal, and postneonatal mortality, 8, 8*t*
Afterload, cardiovascular, 343
Agglutination, 362
Aggressive behavior, 431
Agranulocytes, 362
AIDS. *See* Acquired immunodeficiency syndrome (AIDS)
Airborne precautions, 253
Airborne transmission of pathogens, 251
Airway
  airway insertion, assisting with, 203*t*, 208–209, 209*f*
  burn victims, 590
  clearance procedures, 202–205, 203*f*, 203*t*

Body mass index (BMI)
  calculating, 180–181
  heart health promotion, 352
Body surface area, estimating, 590, 591f
Bolus IV administration, 223
Bone marrow aspiration, 376
Bone marrow transplant (hematopoietic stem
    cell transplantation), 373, 376–377
Bones. See Musculoskeletal disorders;
    Musculoskeletal system
Books for hospitalized children, 144, 145t
Bordetella pertussis, 262t
Borrelia burgdorferi, 269, 270
Boston braces, 552
Bottle feeding babies
  nutrition, 107, 108f, 108t, 110
  propping the bottle, 113
Botulism, 252
Boundaries, defined, 52
Bow-legs (genu varum), 547, 547f
Bowel strangulation, 461
Braces, children with, 551, 552
Bradycephaly, 405
Brain
  development, anatomy, and physiology,
      383–384, 383f, 384f
  sickle cell anemia, 368t
  tumors, 402–403, 402f, 402t, 403t
Brain death, criteria for, 245
Brainstem, 384, 384f
Brainstem gliomas, 402f, 403t
Brazelton, T. Berry, 106
Breadth of an issue, 19, 20
Breastfeeding
  health promotion, 107–110,
      108f, 108t, 109f
  HIV, 608
Breasts
  breast implants, 512
  breast self-examination, 510–511, 511f
  cancer, 511–512, 512t
  mammography, 510
  nonmalignant disorders, 510–511
  surgery, 512
Breathing, by burn victims, 590
Breathing exercises, 375
Breck feeders, 458
Breckinridge, Mary, 4t
Brennamen, Joseph, 4t
Bronchi, 312, 312f
Bronchioles, 327
Bronchiolitis, 327–328
Bronchitis, 263t
Bronchopulmonary dysplasia, 322–323
Brudzinski's sign
  meningitis, 397, 397f
  polio, 263t
Brushfield spots, 405
Bryant traction, 559f
Buccal space, 453
Buck traction, 559f
Buddhists
  death-related practices, 246

mourning and after-death rites, 238t
organ donation, 613
"Buffalo hump," 531
Buffer system, in acid-base balance, 299, 299f
Bulb syringes, 202–203, 203f, 204
Bulimia, 434–435, 434f. See also Eating
    disorders
Bullae, 574, 575f
Bull's-eye rash, 269, 269f
Bullying, 441
BUN (blood urea nitrogen), 288t, 493t
Buphthalmos, 413
Buproprion hydrochloride (Wellbutrin), 429t
Buretrol devices, 222, 222f
Burns
  abuse, possibility of, 589, 590f
  body surface area affected, 590, 591f
  depth, 589–590
  integumentary disorders, 589–593, 590f,
      591f, 593f
  nursing care, 591–593, 593f
  physical injury and safety guidelines, 113
  toddlers, 122, 122f
  types of, 589, 590f
Burping newborns, 109, 110, 110f
Butterfly (malar) rash, 610, 610f, 612

C

Calcitonin, 523t
Calcium, dietary, 546
Calcium disodium ethylenediamine tetraacetate
    (CaNa$_2$EDTA), 476
Calcium levels
  imbalance of, 295–296, 295f, 295t, 299t
  normal values, 288t
  regulation of, 282
Caloric intake, by age group, 115t
CAM. See Complementary and alternative
    therapies (CAM); Complementary
    Therapies
Camphylobacter jejuni, 399
CaNa$_2$EDTA (calcium disodium
    ethylenediamine tetraacetate), 476
Cancer
  ABCDE (asymmetry, border irregularity,
      color variation, diameter, elevation)
      mnemonic for lesion malignancy, 574
  acute lymphoblastic leukemia, 372, 372f
  acute myelogenous leukemia, 372–373, 373f
  brain tumors, 402–403, 402f, 402t, 403f
  breast, 511–512, 512t
  cervical, 514, 515f
  chemotherapy, nursing care plan chart for, 376
  hematopoietic stem cell transplantation, 373,
      376–377
  Hodgkin's lymphoma, 46, 370–371, 370f,
      371t, 380
  Kaposi's sarcoma, 605
  leukemia, 372–373, 372f, 373f, 374–375
  melanoma, 594, 594f, 596–597
  musculoskeletal tumors, 565–566, 565f,
      566f, 567
  neuroblastoma, 403

non-Hodgkin's lymphoma, 371–372
ovarian, 515
testicular, 502
thyroid, 530–531
tumor sites by age group, 402t
Wilms' tumor, 495–496, 495t
Candida albicans
  diaper dermatitis, 578
  thrush, 587, 608
  vaginitis, 508, 509
Candida infections (candidiasis, monilia, yeast
    infection)
  diaper dermatitis, 578
  penile, 505
  thrush (oral candidiasis), 587, 608, 608f
  vaginitis, 505, 508, 509, 533
"Canker sores," 585
Capillary blood pressure, 281
Capillary blood specimens, 189
Capillary (strawberry) hemangiomas, 574,
    575–576, 576f
Car seats, 113, 114, 114f, 115t, 122
Carbamazepine (Tegretol)
  bipolar disorder, 431
  seizures, 394t
Carbolic acid, 3t
Carbon dioxide partial pressure (PaCO$_2$),
    288t, 299
Carbonic acid, 298, 298f
Cardiac output, 343
Cardiac region of the stomach, 453
Cardiac sphincter, 453
Cardiogenic shock, 348, 348f
Cardiomegaly, 348
Cardiopulmonary resuscitation (CPR),
    319–320, 321f
Cardiovascular disorders, care of child with,
    340–360. See also Cardiovascular
    system
  acquired heart diseases, 348–354, 348f,
      349t, 350f, 355
  acute rheumatic fever, 354, 355, 359
  atrial septal defect, 344–345, 344f, 344t,
      345f
  chapter review, 358
  coarctation of the aorta, 347, 347f
  congenital anomalies and defects, 343–348,
      344f, 344t, 345f, 346f, 347f
  congestive heart failure, 348, 348f
  critical thinking care map, 359
  health promotion issue, 352–353
  hyperlipidemia, 349–350, 350f
  hypertension, systemic, 348–349, 349t,
      357
  Kawasaki's syndrome, 350–351, 350f
  NCLEX-PN® exam preparation, 360
  nursing care, 354–357, 355f
  nursing process care plan, 357
  patent ductus arteriosus, 344f, 345, 345f
  tetralogy of Fallot, 346, 346f
  transposition of the great vessels, 347–348,
      347f
  ventricular septal defect, 344f, 345–346

F

Face masks for oxygen, 206f
Failure to thrive, 473
Fair-mindedness, 24
Fairness in critical thinking, 19, 20
Families. *See also* Dying child, care of family
        with; Families, introduction to care of
    assessment techniques and tools, 57, 60–62,
        60f, 61f, 62f, 63
    defined, 51
    family assessment, defined, 60
    family-centered care, 51
    family development theory, 53–55, 53–55t
    family roles, 57
    family structure, 72
    family systems, defined, 52
    family systems theory, 52–53
    family units, 51–52, 51f, 52f
    hospitalized children, 137, 139, 139f, 140t
    of patients, as clients, 5
    therapy for, 448
Families, introduction to care of, 50–68
    chapter review, 66
    critical thinking care map, 67
    family assessment techniques and tools, 57,
        60–62, 60f, 61f, 62f, 63
    family units, 51–52, 51f, 52f
    NCLEX-PN® exam preparation, 68
    nursing care, 63–64
    nursing process care plan, 64–65
    role of LPN/LVN, 62
    roles and functions of the family, 57, 57t,
        58–59
    stress, families under, 62–63
    theoretical framework for working with
        families, 52–57, 53–55t
Famotidine (Pepcid), 466
Fantasy, 76t
Fasting, 286, 288
Fatigue, 374–375, 540
Febrile seizures, 391–392
Fecaliths, 462
Federal programs affecting children, 33–34,
        33f, 33t
Female reproductive disorders
    breast disorders, 510–512, 511f, 512f
    breast self-examination, 510–511, 511f
    female circumcision, 505
    imperforate hymen, 505
    menstrual disorders, 505, 508, 508t, 509f
    ovarian disorders, 514–515
    Pap smear, young woman's first, 506–507
    uterine disorders, 513–514, 513f, 514t, 515f
    vaginitis, 508–510, 519
Females. *See also* Female reproductive disorders
    abuse, potential for, 63
    reproductive system, 499–500, 499f
Feosol (ferrous sulfate), 366t
Feostat (ferrous fumarate), 366t
Fergon (ferrous gluconate), 366t
Ferrous fumarate (Feostat), 366t
Ferrous gluconate (Fergon), 366t

Ferrous sulfate (Feosol), 366t
Fetal alcohol syndrome, 446, 446f
Fetal research, 40
"Fever blisters," 585
Fibroadenoma, 511
Fibroblast cells, 582
Fibrocystic breast disease, 510–511
Fibrocysts, 511
Fibroid uterine tumors, 513, 513f
Fibromyalgia, 396
Fibrosis, 510
Fifth disease (erythema infectiosum), 260f,
        266–267t
Filtration of solvents and solutes, 281, 283f
Fine motor skills
    adolescents, 86t
    infants, 77–79t
    preschool children, 84t
    school-age children, 85t
    toddlers, 82t
Fire safety, 122, 123
Fissures
    Kawasaki's syndrome, 350, 350f
    skin lesions, 574, 575f
5% dextrose in water IV solution (D₅W), 290
Five Ps (paresthesia, pain/pressure, pallor,
        paralysis, pulselessness) of neurovascular
        status, 560, 563
Five Rules of Delegation, 28
Flagyl (metronidazole), 503t, 505, 509
Flonase (fluticasone), 333t
Fluconazole, 587, 608
Fluid, electrolyte, and acid-base disorders, care
        of child with, 280–309. *See also* Acid-
        base disorders
    calcium imbalance, 288t, 295–296, 295f,
        295t
    chapter review, 307
    critical thinking care map, 308
    dehydration, 283, 286–290, 286f, 287–288t,
        287f, 288t, 289f
    fluid balance assessment, 282, 284t, 285,
        285f
    hypervolemia, 290–291, 291f
    NCLEX-PN® exam preparation, 309
    nursing care, 296–297, 296t
    nursing process care plan, 297–298
    potassium imbalance, 288t, 293–295, 293f,
        294t
    principles related to, 281–282, 282f, 283f
    sodium imbalance, 291–293
    water percentage in body, 281, 281f
Fluid deprivation test, 527–528
Fluid intake
    fatigue of chemotherapy, 374
    fluid balance, 282
    IV fluid replacement, 290, 290f
    oral replacement, 288–290
    restricting, 292
    voluntary restrictions, 288
Fluoxetine hydrochloride (Prozac), 431
Fluticasone (Flonase), 333t
Focal seizures, 393–394

Folate, 458
Follicle-stimulating hormone (FSH), 523t
Fomites, 251
Fontanels
    fluid and electrolyte status, 284t, 288t
    newborns, 384, 384f
Food allergies, 616
Football hold for breastfeeding, 107, 109f
Foramen ovale, 347f
Foreign body obstructed airway, 318–320,
        319t, 320f, 321f
Foreign object in ear, 416
Formal operations period of cognitive
        development, 72t, 73
Forscheimer spots, 264t
Fractures
    abuse, 558
    cast care, 560–561, 561f, 564
    client teaching, 563, 564t
    critical thinking care map, 569
    crutches, 562, 562f
    musculoskeletal trauma, 558–560
    Salter-Harris classification system, 559, 559f
    traction, 559, 559f, 562–563, 563f
    types of, 558f
Francisella tularensis, 252
Free association, 75
French-Canadians, 526
Freud, Sigmund, 75, 75f
Frontier School of Midwifery, 4t
Frontier School of Midwifery and Family
        Nursing, 4t
Frostbite, 594–595
FSH (follicle-stimulating hormone), 523t
Fulminating hepatitis, 478
Fundus of the stomach, 453
Fungal skin infections, 586–587, 587f

G

Gag reflex, 198
Galactosemia, 525
Ganglia, 383
Gardasil (HPV vaccine), 504, 514
Garlic, 315
GAS. *See Streptococcus* group A (GAS)
        infections
Gastric lavage, 476t
Gastroenteritis, 461, 482
Gastroesophageal reflux disease (GERD),
        464, 466
Gastrointestinal disorders, care of child with,
        452–483. *See also* Gastrointestinal
        system
    appendicitis, 461–462, 462f
    celiac disease, 470
    chapter review, 481
    cleft lip and palate, 455, 458–459, 458f
    colic, 467–468
    congenital defects, 455, 458–461, 458f,
        459f, 460f
    critical thinking care map, 482
    esophageal atresia, 459–460, 459f
    gastroenteritis, 461, 482

N

Nails, 572
NANDA (North American Nursing Diagnosis Association), 5
Naprosyn. *See* Naproxen (Naprosyn)
Naproxen (Naprosyn)
  musculoskeletal disorders, 557*t*
  systemic lupus erythematosus, 611
Narcan, 476
Nasal flaring, 313*f*, 332
Nasal medications, administering, 215–216
Nasal oxygen cannulas, 206*f*
Nasopharyngeal airways, 209, 209*f*
Nasopharyngitis, 315
National Center for Missing and Exploited Children, 438
National Childhood Vaccine Injury Act (1986), 104
National Council of State Boards of Nursing, 25
National Institutes of Health, 36
National League for Nurses (NLN), 9, 12
National Marrow Donor Program, 373
National School Lunch Program, 33, 33*t*
Native Alaskans, 531
Native American heritage, people with
  cleft lip and palate, 458
  mourning and after-death rites, 238*t*
  touch, use of as nonverbal support, 225
Natural immunity, 603
Natural killer (NK) cells, 603, 605*f*
Naturopathy, 15
NCLB (No Child Left Behind), 33*t*
NCLEX-PN® exam preparation
  cardiovascular disorders, 360
  communicable diseases, child with, 277
  critical thinking in pediatric care, 31
  dying child, care of family with, 249
  endocrine disorders, 544
  families, nursing care of, 68
  fluid, electrolyte, and acid-base disorders, 309
  gastrointestinal disorders, 483
  genitourinary disorders, 520
  hematologic and lymphatic disorders, 381
  hospitalized and chronically ill children, 162
  illness prevention, health promotion, and nutrition in children, 133
  immune disorders, 621
  integumentary disorders, 601
  legal and ethical issues in pediatric nursing, 49
  life span growth and development, 96
  musculoskeletal disorders, 570
  neurologic and sensory disorders, 424
  pediatric nursing in the community, 17
  procedures for the pediatric client, 228
  psychosocial disorders, 451
  respiratory disorders, 339
NCLEX-PN® focus areas
  critical thinking care maps, 22, 23
  health promotion and maintenance, 67

physiologic adaptation, 308
physiologic integrity, 30, 161, 359, 569
physiologic integrity: basic care and comfort, 482
physiological integrity, 338, 519, 543
physiological integrity: basic care and comfort, 132, 600
physiological integrity: reduction of risk potential, 380
psychosocial integrity, 248, 450
safe and effective care environment, 227
safe and effective care environment: coordinated care, 48
safety, 95, 423
safety and infection, 620
safety and infection control, 276
Near-drowning, 401–402, 401*f*
Necator americanus, 474*t*
Negative feedback mechanisms of hormones, 522, 522*f*
Neglect
  emotional, 441
  reporting, 64
Neighborhoods, assessment of, 61, 62*f*
Neisseria gonorrhoeae, 503, 503*t*
Neisseria meningitidis, 397
Neonatal Infant Pain Scale (NIPS), 10
Neonatal respiratory distress syndrome, 313*f*, 321–322, 322*f*
Neonatal Resuscitation Program, 319
Neonates
  foreign body obstructed airway, 319
  mortality rates, 8*t*
  music therapy, 385
  stimulation, 4*t*
Nephroblastoma (Wilms' tumor), 495–496, 495*t*
Nephrogenic diabetes insipidus, 527, 528
Nephrolithiasis, 487
Nephrotic syndrome, 491–492, 492*f*, 498–499
Nervous system. *See also* Neurologic and sensory disorders, care of child with; Neurologic disorders
  anatomy and physiology, 383–386, 383*f*, 384*f*, 385*f*, 386*f*
  assessment, 386–388, 387*t*
  central nervous system, 383–385, 383*f*, 384*f*, 385*f*
  diabetes mellitus, effects of, 533*f*
  malnutrition, 472*f*
  medication, effect on children, 211*t*
  pain, 388–389, 388*f*
  peripheral nervous system, 385–386, 386*f*
  premenstrual syndrome, effects of, 509*f*
  prenatal development, 383–384
Neural tube defects, 389–390, 389*f*
Neuroblastoma, 403
Neurohypophysis (posterior pituitary gland), 522*f*, 523*t*
Neurologic and sensory disorders, care of child with, 382–424. *See also* Nervous system; Neurologic disorders; Senses and sensory ability; Sensory disorders

chapter review, 422
critical thinking care map, 423
NCLEX-PN® exam preparation, 424
Neurologic disorders. *See also* Nervous system; Neurologic and sensory disorders, care of child with
  amyotrophic lateral sclerosis, 391, 392–393
  brain tumors, 402–403, 402*f*, 402*t*, 403*t*
  cerebral palsy, 395–396, 396*f*, 421
  concussion, 401
  congenital, 389–391, 389*f*, 390*f*
  Down syndrome, 405–406, 406*f*
  drowning and near-drowning, 401–402, 401*f*
  fibromyalgia, 396
  fluid and electrolyte status, 284*t*, 287*f*
  Guillain-Barré syndrome, 399
  health promotion issue, 392–393
  hematoma, 399–401, 399*f*, 400*f*
  hydrocephalus, 390–391, 390*f*
  meningitis and encephalitis, 397–398, 397*f*, 398*t*, 423
  mental retardation, 403–406, 406*f*
  nervous system infections, 397–399, 397*f*, 398*t*
  neuroblastoma, 403
  neurologic deterioration, rapidity of, 420
  nursing care, 420
  nursing process care plan, 421
  Reye's syndrome, 398
  seizures, 391–395, 394*t*, 395*f*
  spina bifida, 389–390, 389*f*
  trauma, 399–402, 399*f*, 400*f*, 401*f*
Neurons, 383, 383*f*
Newborns. *See* Neonates
Newborns' and Mothers' Health Protection Act (1996), 4*t*
Nexium (esomeprazole), 466
Nicotine, 445*t*
90-90 traction, 559*f*
NIPS (Neonatal Infant Pain Scale), 10
Nissen fundoplication, 466
Nits, 581, 582*f*
Nix (permethrin), 582
NK (natural killer) cells, 603, 605*f*
NLN (National League for Nurses), 9, 12
No Child Left Behind (NCLB), 33*t*
Nociceptors, 388
Nodules, 574, 575*f*
Nolvadex (tamoxifen), 512
Non-Hodgkin's lymphoma, 371–372
Non-steroidal anti-inflammatory agents (NSAIAs)
  juvenile rheumatoid arthritis, 609
  patent ductus arteriosus, 345
  sprains, 556, 557*t*
  systemic lupus erythematosus, 611
Nonorganic failure to thrive, 441–442
Noradrenalin (norepinephrine), 524*t*
Norepinephrine (noradrenalin), 524*t*
Normal saline IV solution, 290
North American Nursing Diagnosis Association (NANDA), 5

urethral malposition, 487
urinary tract infections, 489
vaginitis, 509–510
warts, 584
Wilms' tumor, 496
Nursing diagnoses, in nursing process care
    plans
  child dying at home, 242
  child undergoing hospitalization for surgery,
      153
  child with amputation, 567
  child with an organ transplant, 618
  child with bilateral cleft lip, 480
  child with cerebral palsy, 421
  child with chickenpox, 273
  child with hypertension, 357
  child with nephrotic syndrome, 498
  client with anorexia nervosa, 436
  client with asthma, 336
  client with cellulitis, 589
  client with diarrhea, 298
  client with fractured arm, 225
  client with growth hormone deficiency, 539
  client with Hodgkin's lymphoma, 46
  client with sickle cell anemia, 378
  described, 5–6
  family desiring alternative therapies, 7
  infant with delayed growth and
      development, 92
  pediatric client with unintentional
      poisoning, 130
  stressful family situation, 65
Nursing practice, essential features of, 5
Nursing process
  LPN/LVN participating in, 13
  pediatric care, 5–6, 6f
Nursing Process Care Plans
  child dying at home, 242–243
  child undergoing hospitalization for surgery,
      153
  child with amputation, 567
  child with an organ transplant, 618
  child with bilateral cleft lip, 480
  child with cerebral palsy, 421
  child with chickenpox, 272–273
  child with hypertension, 357
  child with nephrotic syndrome, 498–499
  client with anorexia nervosa, 436
  client with asthma, 336
  client with cellulitis, 588–589
  client with diarrhea, 297–298
  client with fractured arm, 225
  client with growth hormone deficiency, 539
  client with Hodgkin's lymphoma, 46, 46f
  client with sickle cell anemia, 378
  family desiring alternative therapies, 7
  infant with delayed growth and
      development, 92–93
  pediatric client with unintentional
      poisoning, 130
  stressful family situation, 64–65
Nursing's Agenda for Health Care Reform (ANA
    and NLN), 9, 12

Nutrition and diet. *See also* Illness prevention,
    health promotion, and nutrition in
    children; Nutrition Therapy
  adolescents, 127, 128f
  caloric intake by age group, 115t
  childhood obesity and fast foods, 456–457
  children, feeding, 195, 196
  fasting, 286, 288
  fatigue of chemotherapy, 374
  fluid and electrolyte status, 284t
  fluid intake, restricting, 292
  food allergies, 616
  gastroesophageal reflux disease, 466
  health promotion, 107–111, 108f, 108t,
      109f, 110f, 112f
  hyperlipidemia, 350
  infants, 115–116, 115t
  iron absorption, food for, 366
  malabsorption or inborn metabolic disorders,
      470, 471
  metabolic X syndrome, 541
  My Pyramid, 111, 112f
  nutrition disorders, 473
  oral fluid replacement, 288–290
  poor, preventing, 110–111, 112f
  school-age children, 125–126
  toddlers, 120–121, 121f, 123–124
  tonsillectomy, 317, 318
  tube feeding, 195–200, 197f,
      198f, 199f
Nutrition Therapy
  commercial rehydration agents, 290
  foods for children with juvenile rheumatoid
      arthritis, 610
  low-salt, low-protein diet, 528
  potassium, foods high in, 294
Nystagmus, 413
Nystatin, 509, 587

O

Obesity
  defined, 432, 473
  preventing, 110–111
  psychological disorders, 432–433
Object permanence, 73
Objective data, 5
Obsessive-compulsive disorder (OCD), 430
Obstructive uropathy, 487–488, 487f
Occult blood, specimen for, 192
OCD (obsessive-compulsive disorder), 430
Office of Alternative Medicine, National
    Department of Health, 4t
Omeprazole (Prilosec), 466
Omphalocele, 460, 460f
Oncovin (vincristine), 371t
Open fractures, 558f
Open reduction of fractures, 559
Ophthalmic medications, administering,
    213–214, 214f
Opisthotonos, 397f, 398t
Oral candidiasis (thrush), 587, 608, 608f
Oral care as comfort measure, 240
Oral contraceptives, 514t, 541

Oral health
  adolescents, 127
  infants, 116, 116f
  oral care, 240
  school-age children, 126
  toddlers, 121, 123–124
Oral hypoglycemic medications, 538, 538t,
    541
Oral Maintenance Solution, 290
Oral medications, administration of, 212–213,
    216t
Oral stage of psychosexual development, 76t
Oral temperature, measuring, 168, 168f
OraQuick Advance HIV 1/2 Antibody Test,
    608
Orchiopexy, 502
Orchitis, 264t, 502
Ordinal position, defined, 71
Organ donation
  cultural traditions, 238t
  dying children, 234–235
  source of, 612
Organ Procurement Organization, 234–235
Organ transplantation
  causes for, 613t
  cultural traditions, 613
  immune system, 612–614
  nursing process care plan, 618
  questions about, 613, 614t
  rejection, 614
  reverse isolation, 253
Organogenesis, 384
Oropharyngeal airways, 209, 209f
Orthodox Jews, 246
Orthomyxoviridae, 266t
Orthopnea, defined, 313
Orthoptics, 412
Ortolani-Barlow maneuver, 548, 548f
Osgood-Schlatter disease, 557–558, 558f
Osmosis, 281, 283f
Osteomalacia, 546
Osteomyelitis, 563–564, 564f
Osteosarcoma, 565, 565f, 566f, 567
Ostomies, 463–464, 464f, 464t, 465–466,
    466f
Otalgia, 416
Otic medications, administering, 213,
    214–215, 215f
Otitis media
  bottle propping, 113
  Haemophilus influenzae type B, 263t
  pneumococcal infections, 265t
  sensory disorders, 416–417, 417f
  upper respiratory infections, 315
  vaccine, 259
Outcomes, expected, in nursing care plan
    charts
  child and the surgical experience, 154–155
  child undergoing chemotherapy, 376
  child who is physically abused, 443
  child with a burn, 592
  child with diabetes mellitus, 534–535
  child with influenza, 274

Significance of information in critical thinking, 19, 21
Silver nitrate solution, 3t
Simethicone (Mylicon), 467
Simian creases, 405
Single-parent families, 51
Singulair (montelukast), 333t
Sinuses
    anatomy and physiology, 311–312
    sinusitis, 263t
SIRES (stabilize, identify, reverse, eliminate, support) mnemonic for poisonings, 475
Six Rights and Three Checks of Medication Administration, 44
Sixth disease (exanthem subitum, roseola), 267t
Skeleton, 546–547, 546f, 547f. See also Musculoskeletal disorders; Musculoskeletal system
Skin. See also Integumentary disorders; Integumentary system
    dark, and assessing cyanosis, 343
    functions of, 572
    Kawasaki's syndrome, 350, 351
    medication, effect on children, 210t
    sickle cell anemia, 368t
    soothing itchy, 272
Skin stimulation as comfort measure, 240
SLE. See Systemic lupus erythematosus (SLE)
Sleep
    positioning infants to prevent SIDS, 323
    sleeping with infants, 114
Small intestine, 453f, 454
Smallpox, 252
Smoking. See Tobacco and smoking
Snake bites, 595
Snellen E or picture chart, 411–412, 412f
Snellen letter chart, 410–411, 411f
Sodium, dietary, 528
Sodium as electrolyte, 282
Sodium bicarbonate
    hyperkalemia, 295
    metabolic acidosis, 301
Sodium levels
    imbalance of, 283f, 291–291
    normal values, 288t, 493t
Sodium polystyrene sulfonate (Kayexalate), 294t
Sodium-potassium pump, 281, 283f, 291
Solumedrol (prednisone), 333t
Solutes, 281
Solutions, 281
Solvents, 281
Somatic reflexes, 385
Somatostatin, 524t
Southeast Asian heritage, people with. See also Asian heritage, people with
    communicable diseases, 271
    illness and death, practices related to, 237
Space, personal, 56
Spanking, 106
Specimen collection
    blood, 188–190, 189f

spinal fluid, 194–195, 195f
sputum, 193–194, 194f
stool, 192, 192f
urine, 190–191, 191f
wound or throat culture, 192–193, 193f
Spider angiomas, 574
Spina bifida, 389–390, 389f
Spinal cord
    injury, 400
    nervous system, 384, 385f
Spiral fractures, 558f
Spiritual care strategies, 278
Spleen
    sickle cell anemia, 368, 368t
    splenomegaly, 477, 609
Splenic sequestration, 368
Sprains, 556, 557t
Sprue (celiac disease), 470
Sputum specimen collection, 193–194, 194f
St. John's wort (Hypericum perforatum, Klamathweed), 432
St. Louis encephalitis virus, 398
St. Vitus's dance (Sydenham chorea), 354
Staging
    Hodgkin's lymphoma, 370
    Wilms' tumor, 495t
Standard precautions
    disease transmission, 253
    hepatitis, 477
Staphylococcus aureus
    cellulitis, 585
    communicable diseases, 258
    osteomyelitis, 563
Staphylococcus epidermidis, 258
Staphylococcus infections
    glomerulonephritis, 489
    impetigo, 584
    styes, 408
Startle (Moro) reflex, 184f, 185
Stasis of urine, 487
State Children's Health Insurance Program (SCHIP), 33t
Status asthmaticus, 332
Status epilepticus, 393
Statutory rape, 442
Steatorrhea, 324, 470
Stem cells
    bone marrow transplant, 373, 376–377
    legal and ethical issues, 40
    severe combined immunodeficiency disorder, 604
Stepfamilies, 52
Stepping reflex, 185
Stereotyping, 55
Stereotypy, 427
Still's disease (juvenile rheumatoid arthritis), 556, 609–610, 610f, 611
Stimate. See Desmopressin acetate (DDAVP, Stimate)
Stimulation of neonates, 4t
STIs (sexually transmitted infections). See Sexually transmitted infections (STIs)
Stocking patterned burns, 589, 590f

Stomach, 453–454, 453f
Stomatitis, 371
Stool
    meconium, 107, 108f, 324, 455
    melena, 365
    newborns, 107, 108f
    specimens, obtaining, 192, 192f
    steatorrhea, 324, 470
Stork bites (telangiectactic nevi), 575
Strabismus
    retinoblastoma, 408
    visual acuity, 412, 412f
Strains, 556–557
Strangers, teaching toddlers about, 122–123
Strattera (atomoxetine hydrochloride), 428, 429t
Stratum corneum, 572, 572f
Stratum germinatum, 572, 572f
Strawberry (capillary) hemangiomas, 574, 575–576, 576f
Strength training, 554
Streptococcus group A beta-hemolytic infections
    acute postinfectious glomerulonephritis, 489
    cellulitis, 585
    rheumatic fever, acute, 354
Streptococcus group A (GAS) infections
    common communicable diseases, 267–268t
    nasopharyngitis, 315
Streptococcus group B (GBS) infections, 268t
Streptococcus infections
    impetigo, 584
    vaginitis, 508
Streptococcus pneumoniae infections
    cellulitis, 585
    meningitis, 397
    otitis media, 259
    pneumococcal infections, 265t
Stress, families under, 62–63, 64–65
Stridor, 313
Stroke volume, 342
Strong Families/Safe Children (SF/SC), 33t
Styes, 408
Subcutaneous injections, administering, 216, 216t, 217, 218f, 220
Subcutaneous layer of skin (superficial fascia), 572f, 573, 573f
Subdural hematoma, 399, 399f
Subjective data, 5
Sublingual glands, 453, 453f
Sublingual medications, 216t
Submandibular glands, 453, 453f
Substance abuse
    commonly abused drugs and their effects, 445t
    psychological disorders, 444–446, 444f
    stages of, 444t
Succimer (DMSA), 476
Sucking
    newborn male circumcision, pain relief for, 10
    reflex, 185
Sucrose, oral, for pain relief, 10
Sudden infant death syndrome (SIDS), 8, 323

Sudoriferous glands (sweat glands), 572*f*, 573, 573*f*
Suicidal ideation, 432
Suicide
  antidepressant medications, 431
  psychological disorders, 432
Sulfate as electrolyte, 282
Sulfonylurea (Glyburide), 538*t*
Summer Food Service Breakfast Program (SFSBP), 33*t*
Sun exposure
  melanoma, 594
  sunburn, 593–594
  systemic lupus erythematosus, 610, 612
  tanning beds, 596–597
Sunna, 505
Superego, 75, 75*f*
Superficial fascia (subcutaneous layer of skin), 572*f*, 573, 573*f*
Supervision of delegated tasks, 28
Support groups
  referral to, 41
  staff, for, 41
Surfactant, 311
Surgery
  appendicitis, 461–462, 462*f*
  atrial septal defects, 345
  bariatric surgery, 433, 473
  biliary atresia, 477
  breasts, 512
  cataracts, 414
  cleft lip and palate, 458–459, 458*f*
  conscious sedation, 150, 150*t*
  cryptorchidism, 502
  fluid and electrolyte status, 284*t*
  gastroesophageal reflux disease, 466
  Hirschsprung's disease, 470
  imperforate anus, 460
  infection, signs of, 498
  inflammatory bowel disease, 463–464, 464*f*, 464*t*, 465–466, 466*f*
  intussusception, 469
  Meckel's diverticulum, 469
  melanoma, 594
  musculoskeletal tumors, 565, 565*f*, 566, 566*f*, 567
  myringotomy, 416
  nursing care plan charts, 154–155
  nursing process care plans, 153
  obstructive uropathy, 488
  omphalocele, 460
  patent ductus arteriosus, 345
  postoperative care, 148–150, 149*f*
  postoperative infection, preventing, 487
  preoperative care, 147–148, 147*f*, 148*f*, 148*t*
  retinoblastoma, 409
  spina bifida, 389–390
  tetralogy of Fallot, 346
  thyroid cancer, 531
  thyroidectomy, 530
  transposition of the great arteries, 347

urethral malposition, 486–487, 487*f*
ventricular septal defect, 346
ventriculoperitoneal shunts, 390*f*, 391
Wilms' tumor, 495
Surma, 477
Sutures, cranial, 384*f*
Swayback (lordosis), 553, 553*t*
Sweat glands (sudoriferous glands), 572*f*, 573, 573*f*
Sweat test (pilocarpine iontophoresis), 324, 325*f*, 325*t*
Sydenham chorea (St. Vitus's dance), 354
Sympathetic nervous system
  anatomy and physiology, 385–386, 386*f*
  tumors, 403
Syngeneic donors for stem cells, 373
Synthroid (levothyroxin), 529
Syphilis, 503–504, 503*t*, 504*f*
Systemic lupus erythematosus (SLE)
  autoimmune disease, 610–612, 610*f*
  secondary nephrotic syndrome, 491
Systems, defined, 52

T

T lymphocytes (T cells)
  cell-mediated immunity, 603, 605*f*
  communicable disease, 252
  deficiencies, and graft-*versus*-host reaction, 604
T_4 (thyroxine), 523*t*
T_3 (triiodothyronine), 523*t*
Tachypnea, 330
Tagamet (cimetidine), 466
Talipes (clubfoot), 549, 549*f*
Tamofen (tamoxifen), 512*t*
Tamone (tamoxifen), 512*t*
Tamoxifen (Tamofen, Tamone, Nolvadex), 512, 512*t*
Tanner's stages of sexual maturity, 85, 87*t*, 499
Tasks
  delegation of, 25, 27–28, 27*f*
  family and parental, 53–55*t*
Tattoos, 583
Tay-Sachs disease, 525–526
Tears, artificial, 240
Tebrazid (pyrazinamide), 330, 331*t*
Technology, legal and ethical issues, 40
Teenagers. *See* Adolescents
Teeth
  bottle propping, 113
  deciduous, eruption of, 80, 81*f*
  infants, 116, 116*f*
  school-age children, 126
  toddlers, 123–124
Tegretol (carbamazepine)
  bipolar disorder, 431
  seizures, 394*t*
Telangiectactic nevi (stork bites), 575
Temperature, body, measuring, 165–169, 166*t*, 167*f*, 168*f*, 169*f*
Tenesmus, 513

TENS (transelectrical nerve stimulation), 152
Teratogens
  Accutane, 580
  Flagyl (metronidazole), 505
Tertiary care, in community-based nursing, 12
Tertiary circular reactions, 73
Tertiary illness prevention, 99
Tertiary syphilis, 504
Testes
  endocrine glands, 522*f*, 524*t*
  testicular cancer, 502
  testicular self-examination, 502, 502*f*
  testicular torsion, 501, 501*f*
Testimony, providing, 41
Testosterone, 524*t*, 540, 541
Tetanus bacillus, 261*t*
Tetanus (lockjaw), 261*t*
Tetanus toxoid, 256*t*
Tetracycline, 580
Tetralogy of Fallot, 346, 346*f*
Thalassemia, 369–370
Theodur. *See* Theophylline
Theophylline
  asthma, 333*t*
  St. John's wort, 432
Theoretical framework for working with families, 52–57, 53–55*t*
Therapeutic play, 137. *See also* Play therapy
Therapeutic touch. *See* Touch, therapeutic
Thermal burns, 589, 590*f*
Thinking Strategically
  care of the ill child, 278
  pediatric disorders, 622
  pediatric nursing, introduction to, 134
Thirst, 288*t*
Thoracic duct, 363
Thought, elements of, 21–22
3-day measles (rubella, German measles). *See* Rubella (German measles, 3-day measles)
Throats
  fluid and electrolyte status, 284*t*
  sample, obtaining for culture, 192–193, 193*f*
Thrombocytes (platelets), 362, 362*f*
Thrush (oral candidiasis), 587, 608, 608*f*
Thymosin, 523*t*
Thymus gland, 522*f*, 523*t*
Thyroid gland
  cancer, 530–531
  disorders, 528–531, 529*f*, 529*t*
  location, secretions, and effects, 522*f*, 523*t*
  metabolic X syndrome, 540, 541
Thyroid-stimulating hormone (TSH), 523*t*
Thyroxine (T_4), 523*t*
Tick bites, 269, 270
Tickborne typhus (Rocky Mountain spotted fever, Sao Paulo typhus), 269–270, 269*f*
Time, sense of, 57
Time management, 278, 622
Time-outs, 106, 107*f*
Tinea capitis, 586, 587*f*
Tinea corporis, 586, 587*f*
Tinea cruris, 586

Variola major virus, 252
Varus, 549, 549f
Vasoocclusion, 368
Vastus lateralis muscles, 217, 218f, 219
Venous specimens, obtaining, 189–190, 189f
Ventolin (albuterol), 333t
Ventral surface of the penis, 486, 486f
Ventricular septal defect, 344f, 345–346
Ventriculoperitoneal shunts, 390f, 391
Ventrogluteal muscles, 217, 218f, 219
Versed (midazolam), 150t
Vesicles, 574, 575f, 582
Vesicoureteral reflux, 488
VFC (Vaccination Funding for Children), 33t
Viability of fetus, 311
Vibration as comfort measure, 240
Villi of the small intestine, 454
Vinblastine, 371t
Vincristine (Oncovin), 371t
Visceral larva migrans (toxocariasis), 474t
Visual impairment
    blindness prevention, with silver nitrate solution, 3t
    eye disorders, 410, 410f, 412–414, 412f, 413f, 414f
    oxygen use in premature infants, 322
Visual learners, 100
Visualization therapy, 375
Vital signs, obtaining
    Apgar score, 174–175, 174t
    blood pressure, 166t, 172–174, 173f
    normal ranges by age, 166t
    pain, 175–178, 175f

pulse, 166t, 169, 169f, 170–171, 170f
respirations, 166t, 169, 171–172
temperature, 165–169, 166t, 167f, 168f, 169f
Vitamin C
    iron absorption, 366
    scurvy, 473
Vitamin D
    osteomalacia, 546
    rickets, 473
Vitamin E
    heart health, 349
Voluntary euthanasia, 241
Volvulus, 469, 469f
Von Bertalanffy, Ludwig, 52

W

Wall-eye, 412
Warts (papillomavirus), 583–584, 584f
Watson, Jean, 5
Weight, body
    fluid and electrolyte status, 284t
    fluid balance, monitoring, 282
    measuring, 180–181, 181f
    metabolic X syndrome, 540, 541
    weight gain, with hypervolemia, 290
    weight loss, calculating, 286, 289
Weight training, 554
Well-child visits, 99–101, 102t
Wellbutrin (buproprion hydrochloride), 429t
West Nile virus, 398
Western blot test, 269
Western equine virus, 398
Wheals, 574, 575f

White blood cells (leukocytes), 362, 362f
White House Conference on Children and Youth Protection charter, 4t
Whooping cough (pertussis), 262t
WIC (Women, Infants and Children) program, 4t, 33, 33t
Wilms' tumor (nephroblastoma), 495–496, 495t
The Womanly Art of Breastfeeding (La Leche League), 4t
Women. See Female reproductive disorders; Females
Women, Infants and Children (WIC) program, 4t, 33, 33t
Wong Pain Rating Scale, 175f
Wound specimens for culture, 192–193, 193f
Wry neck (torticollis), 553, 553f

X

Xenografts, 612
Xopenex (levalbuterol), 333t

Y

Yeast infections. See Candida infections (candidiasis, monilia, yeast infection)
Yellen (Gomco) clamps, 501
Yersinia pestis, 252
Yoga, 375

Z

Zidovudine (AZT, Retrovir), 605, 608, 608t
Zinc oxide cream, 578
Zoloft (sertraline hydrochloride), 431

SINGLE PC LICENSE AGREEMENT AND LIMITED WARRANTY

Pearson Education, Inc.

**YOU SHOULD CAREFULLY READ THE TERMS AND CONDITIONS BEFORE USING THE CD-ROM PACKAGE.
USING THIS CD-ROM PACKAGE INDICATES YOUR ACCEPTANCE OF THESE TERMS AND CONDITIONS.**

Pearson Education, Inc. provides this program and licenses its use. You assume responsibility for the selection of the program to achieve your intended results, and for the installation, use, and results obtained from the program. This license extends only to use of the program in the United States or countries in which the program is marketed by authorized distributors.

LICENSE GRANT

You hereby accept a nonexclusive, nontransferable, permanent license to install and use the program ON A SINGLE COMPUTER at any given time. You may copy the program solely for backup or archival purposes in support of your use of the program on the single computer. You may not modify, translate, disassemble, decompile, or reverse engineer the program, in whole or in part.

TERM

The License is effective until terminated. Pearson Education, Inc. reserves the right to terminate this License automatically if any provision of the License is violated. You may terminate the License at any time. To terminate this License, you must return the program, including documentation, along with a written warranty stating that all copies in your possession have been returned or destroyed.

LIMITED WARRANTY

THE PROGRAM IS PROVIDED "AS IS" WITHOUT WARRANTY OF ANY KIND, EITHER EXPRESSED OR IMPLIED, INCLUDING, BUT NOT LIMITED TO, THE IMPLIED WARRANTIES OR MERCHANTABILITY AND FITNESS FOR A PARTICULAR PURPOSE. THE ENTIRE RISK AS TO THE QUALITY AND PERFORMANCE OF THE PROGRAM IS WITH YOU. SHOULD THE PROGRAM PROVE DEFECTIVE, YOU (AND NOT PRENTICE-HALL, INC. OR ANY AUTHORIZED DEALER) ASSUME THE ENTIRE COST OF ALL NECESSARY SERVICING, REPAIR, OR CORRECTION. NO ORAL OR WRITTEN INFORMATION OR ADVICE GIVEN BY PRENTICE-HALL, INC., ITS DEALERS, DISTRIBUTORS, OR AGENTS SHALL CREATE A WARRANTY OR INCREASE THE SCOPE OF THIS WARRANTY.

SOME STATES DO NOT ALLOW THE EXCLUSION OF IMPLIED WARRANTIES, SO THE ABOVE EXCLUSION MAY NOT APPLY TO YOU. THIS WARRANTY GIVES YOU SPECIFIC LEGAL RIGHTS AND YOU MAY ALSO HAVE OTHER LEGAL RIGHTS THAT VARY FROM STATE TO STATE.

Pearson Education, Inc. does not warrant that the functions contained in the program will meet your requirements or that the operation of the program will be uninterrupted or error-free.

However, Pearson Education, Inc. warrants the diskette(s) or CD-ROM(s) on which the program is furnished to be free from defects in material and workmanship under normal use for a period of ninety (90) days from the date of delivery to you as evidenced by a copy of your receipt.

The program should not be relied on as the sole basis to solve a problem whose incorrect solution could result in injury to person or property. If the program is employed in such a manner, it is at the user's own risk and Pearson Education, Inc. explicitly disclaims all liability for such misuse.

LIMITATION OF REMEDIES

Pearson Education, Inc.'s entire liability and your exclusive remedy shall be:

1. the replacement of any diskette(s) or CD-ROM(s) not meeting Pearson Education, Inc.'s "LIMITED WARRANTY" and that is returned to Pearson Education, or

2. if Pearson Education is unable to deliver a replacement diskette(s) or CD-ROM(s) that is free of defects in materials or workmanship, you may terminate this agreement by returning the program.

IN NO EVENT WILL PRENTICE-HALL, INC. BE LIABLE TO YOU FOR ANY DAMAGES, INCLUDING ANY LOST PROFITS, LOST SAVINGS, OR OTHER INCIDENTAL OR CONSEQUENTIAL DAMAGES ARISING OUT OF THE USE OR INABILITY TO USE SUCH PROGRAM EVEN IF PRENTICE-HALL, INC. OR AN AUTHORIZED DISTRIBUTOR HAS BEEN ADVISED OF THE POSSIBILITY OF SUCH DAMAGES, OR FOR ANY CLAIM BY ANY OTHER PARTY.

SOME STATES DO NOT ALLOW FOR THE LIMITATION OR EXCLUSION OF LIABILITY FOR INCIDENTAL OR CONSEQUENTIAL DAMAGES, SO THE ABOVE LIMITATION OR EXCLUSION MAY NOT APPLY TO YOU.

GENERAL

You may not sublicense, assign, or transfer the license of the program. Any attempt to sublicense, assign or transfer any of the rights, duties, or obligations hereunder is void.

This Agreement will be governed by the laws of the State of New York.

Should you have any questions concerning this Agreement, you may contact Pearson Education, Inc. by writing to:

Director of New Media
Higher Education Division
Pearson Education, Inc.
One Lake Street
Upper Saddle River, NJ 07458

Should you experience problems using this CD-ROM, you can get support by filling out the web form located at http://247. prenhall.com

YOU ACKNOWLEDGE THAT YOU HAVE READ THIS AGREEMENT, UNDERSTAND IT, AND AGREE TO BE BOUND BY ITS TERMS AND CONDITIONS. YOU FURTHER AGREE THAT IT IS THE COMPLETE AND EXCLUSIVE STATEMENT OF THE AGREEMENT BETWEEN US THAT SUPERSEDES ANY PROPOSAL OR PRIOR AGREEMENT, ORAL OR WRITTEN, AND ANY OTHER COMMUNICATIONS BETWEEN US RELATING TO THE SUBJECT MATTER OF THIS AGREEMENT.

Guide to Special Features

CLIENT TEACHING

CRITICAL THINKING CARE MAPS

CULTURAL PULSE POINTS

HEALTH PROMOTION ISSUES

Guide to Special Features

NURSING CARE CHECKLISTS

NURSING CARE PLAN CHARTS

NURSING PROCESS CARE PLANS

PROCEDURES

localized variant of *Henoch-Schönlein purpura*, also characterized by IgA deposition in the mesangium. In contrast to Berger disease, which is purely a renal disorder, Henoch-Schönlein purpura is a systemic syndrome involving the skin (purpuric rash), gastrointestinal tract (abdominal pain), joints (arthritis), and kidneys.

Pathogenesis. Accumulating evidence suggests that IgA nephropathy is associated with an abnormality in IgA production and clearance. IgA, the main immunoglobulin in mucosal secretions, is at low levels in normal serum but increased in 50% of patients with IgA nephropathy. Patients with IgA nephropathy have increased production of this immunoglobulin in the marrow. In addition, circulating IgA-containing immune complexes are present in some patients. A genetic influence is suggested by the occurrence of this condition in families and in HLA-identical siblings, and by the increased frequency of certain HLA and complement phenotypes in some populations. Studies also suggest an abnormality in glycosylation of the IgA immunoglobulin, a process that would reduce plasma clearance of IgA, thus favoring deposition in the mesangium. The prominent mesangial deposition of IgA suggests entrapment of IgA immune complexes in the mesangium, and the absence of C1q and C4 in glomeruli points to activation of the alternative complement pathway. Taken together, these clues suggest a genetic or acquired abnormality of immune regulation, leading to increased IgA synthesis in response to respiratory or gastrointestinal exposure to environmental agents (e.g., viruses, bacteria, food proteins). IgA and IgA complexes are then entrapped in the mesangium, where they activate the alternative complement pathway and initiate glomerular injury. In support of this scenario, IgA nephropathy occurs with increased frequency in patients with celiac disease, in whom intestinal mucosal defects are seen, and in liver disease where there is defective hepatobiliary clearance of IgA complexes (*secondary IgA nephropathy*).

Figure 14-11   ■

IgA nephropathy showing characteristic immunofluorescence deposition of IgA, principally in mesangial regions.

course is highly variable. Many patients maintain normal renal function for decades. Slow progression to chronic renal failure occurs in 25% to 50% of cases during a period of 20 years.

Hereditary Nephritis

Hereditary nephritis refers to a group of hereditary familial renal diseases associated primarily with glomerular injury. The best-studied entity is *Alport syndrome*, in which nephritis is accompanied by nerve deafness and various eye disorders, including lens dislocation, posterior cataracts, and corneal dystrophy. Males tend to be affected more frequently and more severely than females and are more likely to develop renal failure. Patients present at age 5 to 20 years with gross or microscopic hematuria and proteinuria, and overt renal failure occurs between 20 and 50 years of age. The inheritance is heterogeneous, being X-linked, autosomal recessive, or autosomal dominant in most pedigrees.

MORPHOLOGY

Histologically, the lesions vary considerably. The glomeruli may be normal or may show mesangial widening and segmental inflammation confined to some glomeruli (focal GN); diffuse mesangial proliferation (mesangioproliferative); or (rarely) overt crescentic GN. The characteristic immunofluorescence picture is of **mesangial deposition of IgA,** often with C3 and properdin and smaller amounts of IgG or IgM (Fig. 14–11). Early complement components are usually absent. Electron microscopy confirms the presence of electron-dense deposits in the mesangium.

MORPHOLOGY

Histologically, there is segmental glomerular proliferation or sclerosis, or both, and an increase in mesangial matrix. In some kidneys, interstitial cells take on a foamy appearance, owing to accumulation of neutral fats and mucopolysaccharides **(foam cells).** With progression, there is increasing glomerulosclerosis, vascular narrowing, tubular atrophy, and interstitial fibrosis. With the electron microscope, the basement membrane of glomeruli appears thin and attenuated; with increasing age, progressive proteinuria, and renal insufficiency, the basement membrane of glomeruli and tubules shows irregular foci of thickening or attenuation with pronounced splitting and lamination of the lamina densa, yielding a "basket-weave" appearance.

Clinical Course. The disease affects children and young adults. More than half of the patients present with gross hematuria after an infection of the respiratory or, less commonly, gastrointestinal or urinary tract; 30% to 40% have only microscopic hematuria, with or without proteinuria; and 5% to 10% develop a typical acute nephritic syndrome. The hematuria typically lasts for several days and then subsides, only to return every few months. The subsequent

The basement membrane defect has been traced in patients with X-linked disease to mutations in the gene encoding the $\alpha5$ chain of collagen type IV, interfering with the structure and permeability of the GBM. Male patients usually present with persistent hematuria, which is most often asymptomatic and follows a benign course. Additional mutations in an $\alpha6$ collagen chain occur in some patients.

Autosomal recessive forms of hereditary nephritis have been linked to homozygous defects in the genes that encode $\alpha3$ and $\alpha4$ type IV collagen. These genes are located head to head on chromosome 2. In a few instances, a heterozygous defect in these is associated with persistent, often familial hematuria and a benign course (so-called benign familial hematuria).

CHRONIC GLOMERULONEPHRITIS

Having discussed various forms of glomerular disease, we should now turn to one of their unfortunate outcomes, chronic CrGN. It is an important cause of end-stage renal disease presenting as chronic renal failure. Thirty percent to 50% of all patients who require chronic hemodialysis or renal transplantation have the diagnosis of chronic CrGN.

By the time chronic CrGN is discovered, the glomerular changes are so far advanced that it is difficult to discern the nature of the original lesion. It probably represents the end stage of a variety of entities, prominent among which are RPGN, FSG, MGN, and MPGN. It has been estimated that perhaps 20% of cases arise with no history of symptomatic renal disease. Although chronic CrGN may develop at any age, it is usually first noted in young and middle-aged adults.

MORPHOLOGY

Classically, the kidneys are symmetrically contracted and their surfaces are red-brown and diffusely granular.

Microscopically, the feature common to all cases is advanced scarring of the glomeruli and Bowman's spaces, sometimes to the point of complete replacement or hyalinization of the glomeruli (Fig. 14–12). This obliteration of the glomeruli is the end point of many diseases, and it is impossible to ascertain from such kidneys the nature of the earlier lesion.

The obstruction to blood flow between afferent and efferent arterioles secondary to glomerular damage must of necessity have an impact on the other elements of the kidney. There is, then, marked interstitial fibrosis, associated with atrophy and replacement of many of the tubules in the cortex. The small and medium-sized arteries are frequently thick walled, with narrowed lumina, secondary to hypertension. Lymphocytic (and, rarely, plasma cell) infiltrates are present in the interstitial tissue. As damage to all structures progresses, it may become difficult to ascertain whether the primary lesion was glomerular, vascular, or interstitial. Such markedly damaged kidneys are designated "end-stage kidneys."

Figure 14–12 ■

Chronic glomerulonephritis. A Masson trichrome preparation shows complete replacement of virtually all glomeruli by blue-staining collagen. (Courtesy of Dr. M. A. Venkatachalam, Department of Pathology, University of Texas Health Sciences Center, San Antonio, TX.)

Clinical Course. Most often, chronic GN develops insidiously and is discovered only late in its course, after the onset of renal insufficiency. Very frequently, renal disease is first suspected with the discovery of proteinuria, hypertension, or azotemia on routine medical examination. In some patients the course is punctuated by transient episodes of either the nephritic or the nephrotic syndrome. Some of these patients may seek medical attention for the edema. As the glomeruli become obliterated, the avenue for protein loss is progressively closed and the nephrotic syndrome thus becomes less common with more advanced disease. Some proteinuria, however, is constant in all cases. Hypertension is very common, and its effects may dominate the clinical picture. Although microscopic hematuria is usually present, grossly bloody urine is infrequent at this stage.

Without treatment, the prognosis is poor; relentless progression to uremia and death is the rule. The rate of progression is extremely variable, however, and 10 years or more may elapse between onset of the first symptoms and terminal renal failure requiring renal replacement. Renal dialysis and renal transplantation, of course, alter this course and allow long-term survival.

● DISEASES AFFECTING TUBULES AND INTERSTITIUM

Most forms of tubular injury also involve the interstitium, so the two are discussed together. Under this heading we present diseases characterized by (1) inflammatory involvement of the tubules and interstitium (interstitial nephritis) and (2) ischemic or toxic tubular injury, leading to *acute tubular necrosis* and *acute renal failure*.

Tubulointerstitial Nephritis

Tubulointerstitial nephritis (TIN) refers to a group of inflammatory diseases of the kidneys that primarily involve the interstitium and tubules. The glomeruli may be spared altogether or affected only late in the course. In most cases of TIN caused by bacterial infection, the renal pelvis is prominently involved—hence the more descriptive term *pyelonephritis* (from *pyelo*, "pelvis"). The term *interstitial nephritis* is generally reserved for cases that are noninfectious in origin. These include tubular injury resulting from drugs, metabolic disorders such as hypokalemia, physical injury such as from irradiation, and immune reactions. On the basis of clinical features and the character of the inflammatory exudate, TIN, regardless of the etiologic agent, can be divided into acute and chronic categories. In the following section we present pyelonephritis first, followed by other, noninfectious forms of interstitial nephritis.

ACUTE PYELONEPHRITIS

Acute pyelonephritis, a common suppurative inflammation of the kidney and the renal pelvis, is caused by bacterial infection. It is an important manifestation of urinary tract infection (UTI), which implies involvement of the lower (cystitis, prostatitis, urethritis) or upper (pyelonephritis) urinary tract, or both. As we shall see, pyelonephritis is almost always associated with infection of the lower urinary tract. The latter, however, may remain localized without extending to involve the kidney. UTIs are extremely common clinical problems.

Pathogenesis. The principal causative organisms are the enteric gram-negative rods. *Escherichia coli* is by far the most common one. Other important organisms are species of *Proteus*, *Klebsiella*, *Enterobacter*, and *Pseudomonas*; these are usually associated with recurrent infections, especially in patients who undergo urinary tract manipulations or have congenital or acquired anomalies of the lower urinary tract (see later). Staphylococci and *Streptococcus faecalis* may also cause pyelonephritis, but they are uncommon.

There are two routes by which bacteria can reach the kidneys: through the bloodstream (hematogenous) and from the lower urinary tract (ascending infection). Although *hematogenous spread* is the far less common of the two, acute pyelonephritis may result from seeding of the kidneys by bacteria in the course of septicemia or infective endocarditis (Fig. 14–13). *Ascending infection* from the lower urinary tract is the most important and common route by which the bacteria reach the kidney. The first step in the pathogenesis of ascending infection appears to be adhesion of bacteria to mucosal surfaces, followed by colonization of the distal urethra (and the introitus in females). From here the organisms must gain access to the bladder, by expansive growth of the colonies and by moving against the flow of urine. This may occur during urethral instrumentation, including catheterization and cystoscopy, which are important predisposing factors in the pathogenesis of UTIs. In the absence of instrumentation, UTI most commonly affects females. Because of the close proximity of the urethra to the rectum, colonization by the enteric bacteria is favored. Furthermore, the short urethra, and trauma to the urethra during sexual intercourse, facilitate the entry of bacteria into the urinary bladder. Ordinarily, bladder urine is sterile and remains so, owing to antimicrobial properties of the bladder mucosa and to the flushing action associated with periodic voiding of

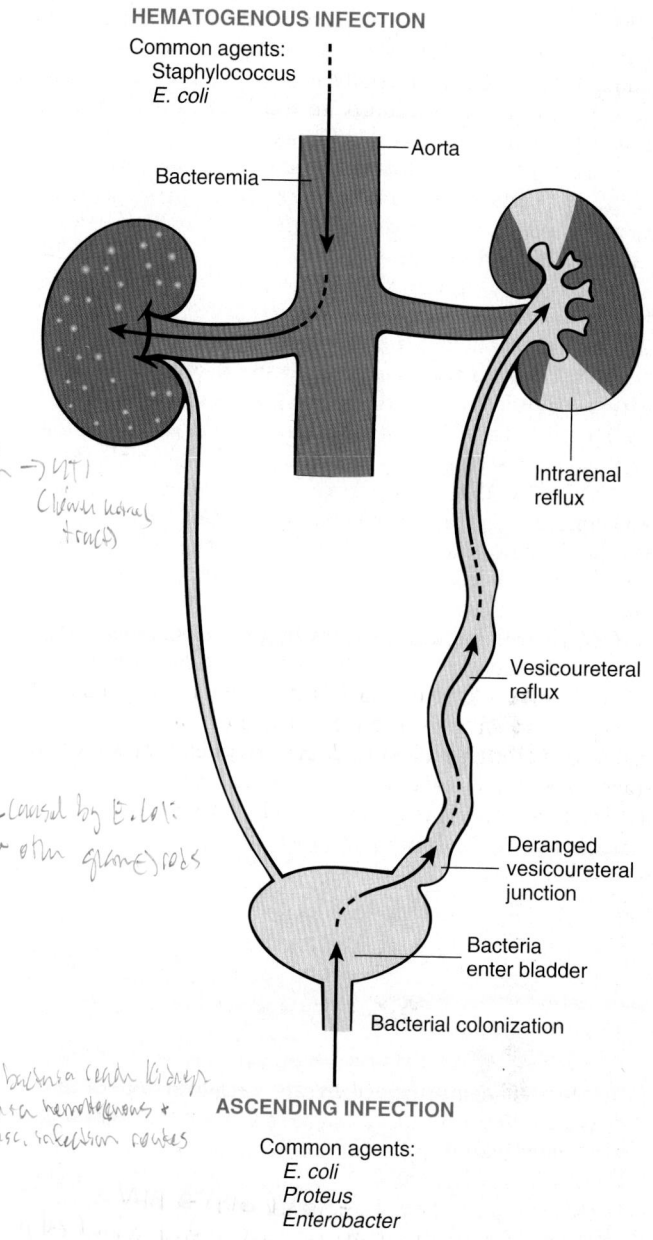

HEMATOGENOUS INFECTION
Common agents:
  Staphylococcus
  E. coli

— Aorta
Bacteremia —

Intrarenal reflux

Vesicoureteral reflux

Deranged vesicoureteral junction

Bacteria enter bladder

Bacterial colonization

ASCENDING INFECTION
Common agents:
  E. coli
  Proteus
  Enterobacter

Figure 14–13 ■

Schematic representation of pathways of renal infection. Hematogenous infection results from bacteremic spread. More common is ascending infection, which results from a combination of urinary bladder infection, vesicoureteral reflux, and intrarenal reflux.

urine. With outflow obstruction or bladder dysfunction, however, the natural defense mechanisms of the bladder are overwhelmed, setting the stage for UTI. Obstruction at the level of the urinary bladder results in incomplete emptying and increased residual volume of urine. In the presence of stasis, bacteria introduced into the bladder can multiply undisturbed, without being flushed out or destroyed by the bladder wall. From the contaminated bladder urine, the bacteria ascend along the ureters to infect the renal pelvis and parenchyma. Accordingly, UTI is particularly frequent among patients with urinary tract obstruction, as may occur with benign prostatic hypertrophy and uterine prolapse.

- because is when onto the pelvis due to incompetence of vesicoureteral orifice → vesicoureteral reflux

- yellow nodular abscesses on the surface
- abscess formation within the renal parenchyma
- neutrophils → white casts in urine

528 ■ Chapter 14 THE KIDNEY AND ITS COLLECTING SYSTEM

Although obstruction is an important predisposing factor in the pathogenesis of ascending infection, it is the *incompetence of the vesicoureteral orifice* that allows bacteria to ascend the ureter into the pelvis. The normal ureteral insertion into the bladder is a competent one-way valve that prevents retrograde flow of urine, especially during micturition, when the intravesical pressure rises. An incompetent vesicoureteral orifice allows the reflux of bladder urine into the ureters (*vesicoureteral reflux [VUR]*). VUR is present in 35% to 45% of young children with UTI. It is usually a congenital defect that results in incompetence of the ureterovesical valve. VUR can also be acquired in patients with flaccid bladder resulting from spinal cord injury. The effect of VUR is similar to that of an obstruction in that after voiding there is residual urine in the urinary tract, which favors bacterial growth. Furthermore, VUR affords a ready mechanism by which the infected bladder urine can be propelled up to the renal pelves and farther into the renal parenchyma through open ducts at the tips of the papillae (*intrarenal reflux*).

Besides the various predisposing factors already discussed (obstruction, VUR, pregnancy, and instrumentation of the urinary tract), diabetes tends to increase the risk of serious complications of pyelonephritis, including septicemia, necrotizing papillitis, and recurrence of infection.

Figure 14–14 ■

Acute pyelonephritis. The cortical surface is studded with focal pale abscesses, more numerous in the upper pole and middle region of the kidney; the lower pole is relatively unaffected. Between the abscesses there is dark congestion of the renal surface.

MORPHOLOGY

One or both kidneys may be involved. The affected kidney may be normal in size or enlarged. **Characteristically, discrete, yellowish, raised abscesses are grossly apparent on the renal surface** (Fig. 14–14). They may be widely scattered or limited to one region of the kidney, or they may coalesce to form a single large area of suppuration.

The characteristic histologic feature of acute pyelonephritis is suppurative necrosis or abscess formation within the renal parenchyma. In the early stages the suppurative infiltrate is limited to the interstitial tissue, but later abscesses rupture into tubules. Large masses of neutrophils frequently extend within involved nephrons into the collecting ducts, giving rise to the characteristic white cell casts found in the urine. Typically, the glomeruli appear to be resistant to the infection.

When the element of obstruction is prominent, the suppurative exudate may be unable to drain and thus fills the renal pelvis, calyces, and ureter, producing **pyonephrosis.**

A second (and fortunately infrequent) form of pyelonephritis is necrosis of the renal papillae, known as **necrotizing papillitis** or **papillary necrosis.** This is particularly common among diabetics who develop acute pyelonephritis and may also complicate acute pyelonephritis when there is significant urinary tract obstruction. It is also seen with the chronic interstitial nephritis associated with analgesic abuse (described later). This lesion consists of a combination of ischemic and suppurative

necrosis of the tips of the renal pyramids (renal papillae). **The pathognomonic gross feature of necrotizing papillitis is sharply defined gray-white to yellow necrosis of the apical two thirds of the pyramids.** One papilla or several or all papillae may be affected. Microscopically, the papillary tips show characteristic coagulative necrosis, with surrounding neutrophilic infiltrate.

When the bladder is involved in a UTI, as is often the case, **acute** or **chronic cystitis** results. In long-standing cases associated with obstruction, the bladder may be grossly hypertrophic, with trabeculation of its walls, or it may be thinned and markedly distended from retention of urine.

Clinical Course. Acute pyelonephritis is often associated with predisposing conditions, some of which were covered in the discussion of pathogenetic mechanisms. These include the following:

- *Urinary obstruction*, either congenital or acquired.
- *Instrumentation* of the urinary tract, most commonly catheterization.
- *Vesicoureteral reflux.*
- *Pregnancy.* Four percent to 6% of pregnant women develop bacteriuria sometime during pregnancy, and 20% to 40% of these eventually develop symptomatic urinary infection if not treated.
- *Patient's sex and age.* After the first year of life (when congenital anomalies in males commonly become evident) and up to around age 40 years, infections are

[handwritten margin notes at top: - Sudden onset, pain at costovertebral angle, chills/fever/malaise - bacteriuria, urethral irritation, benign & self-limited - necrotizing papillitis → poorer prognosis]

much more frequent in females. With increasing age, the incidence in males rises, owing to the development of prostatic hyperplasia and frequent instrumentation.

- ■ *Preexisting renal lesions*, causing intrarenal scarring and obstruction.
- ■ *Diabetes mellitus*, in which acute pyelonephritis is caused by more frequent instrumentation, the general susceptibility to infection, and the neurogenic bladder dysfunction exhibited by patients.
- ■ *Immunosuppression and immunodeficiency.*

When uncomplicated acute pyelonephritis is clinically apparent, the onset is usually sudden, with pain at the costovertebral angle and systemic evidence of infection, such as chills, fever, and malaise. *Urinary findings include pyuria and bacteriuria.* In addition, there are usually indications of bladder and urethral irritation (dysuria, frequency, urgency). Even without antibiotic treatment, the disease tends to be benign and self-limited. The symptomatic phase of the disease usually lasts no longer than a week, although bacteriuria may persist much longer. In cases with predisposing influences, the disease may become recurrent or chronic, particularly when it is bilateral. The development of necrotizing papillitis is associated with a much poorer prognosis. These patients have evidence of overwhelming sepsis and, often, renal failure.

CHRONIC PYELONEPHRITIS AND REFLUX NEPHROPATHY

[handwritten note: - interstitial inflammation & scarring of renal parenchyma & gross scarring & deformity of pelvicalyceal system]

Chronic pyelonephritis is defined here as a *morphologic entity in which predominantly interstitial inflammation and scarring of the renal parenchyma is associated with grossly visible scarring and deformity of the pelvicalyceal system.* Chronic pyelonephritis is an important cause of chronic renal failure. It can be divided into two forms: chronic obstructive pyelonephritis and chronic reflux-associated pyelonephritis.

Chronic Obstructive Pyelonephritis. We have seen that obstruction predisposes the kidney to infection. Recurrent infections superimposed on diffuse or localized obstructive lesions lead to recurrent bouts of renal inflammation and scarring, which eventually cause chronic pyelonephritis. *[handwritten: - recurrent infections superimposed on obstructive lesions]* The disease can be bilateral, as with congenital anomalies of the urethra (posterior urethral valves), resulting in fatal renal insufficiency unless the anomaly is corrected; or unilateral, such as occurs with calculi and unilateral obstructive anomalies of the ureter.

Chronic Reflux-Associated Pyelonephritis (Reflux Nephropathy). This is the more common form of chronic pyelonephritic scarring and results from superimposition of a UTI on congenital vesicoureteral reflux and intrarenal reflux. *[handwritten: - UTI superimposed on congenital vesicoureteral reflux and intrarenal reflux]* Reflux may be unilateral or bilateral; thus, the resultant renal damage either may cause scarring and atrophy of one kidney or may involve both and lead to chronic renal insufficiency. Whether vesicoureteral reflux causes renal damage in the absence of infection (sterile reflux) is uncertain, because it is difficult clinically to rule out remote infections in a patient first seen with pyelonephritic scarring.

MORPHOLOGY

One or both kidneys may be involved, either diffusely or in patches. Even when involvement is bilateral, the kidneys are not equally damaged and therefore are not equally contracted. This uneven scarring is useful in differentiating chronic pyelonephritis from the more symmetrically contracted kidneys caused by vascular sclerosis (often referred to as "benign nephrosclerosis") and chronic GN. The hallmark of chronic pyelonephritis is scarring involving the pelvis or calyces, or both, leading to papillary blunting and marked calyceal deformities (Fig. 14–15).

The microscopic changes are largely nonspecific, and similar alterations may be seen with other tubulointerstitial disorders such as analgesic nephropathy. The parenchyma shows the following features:

- ■ Uneven interstitial fibrosis and an inflammatory infiltrate of lymphocytes, plasma cells, and occasionally neutrophils.
- ■ Dilation or contraction of tubules, with atrophy of the lining epithelium. Many of the dilated tubules contain pink to blue, glassy-appearing

[handwritten margin notes beside figure: ✱ uneven scarring involving the pelvis or calyces leading to papillary blunting & marked calyceal deformities - lymphocytes, plasma cells, & neutrophils • colloid cysts ↓ "thyroidization" • glomerulosclerosis]

Figure 14–15   ■

Typical coarse scars of chronic pyelonephritis associated with vesicoureteral reflux. The scars are usually polar and are associated with underlying blunted calyces.

PAS-positive casts known as colloid casts that suggest the appearance of thyroid tissue, hence the descriptive term thyroidization. Often, neutrophils are seen within tubules.
■ Chronic inflammatory infiltration and fibrosis involving the calyceal mucosa and wall.
■ Vascular changes similar to those of hyaline or proliferative arteriolosclerosis caused by the frequently associated hypertension.
■ Although glomeruli may be normal, in most cases, glomerulosclerosis is seen in areas of better-preserved renal parenchyma. Such changes represent secondary FSG caused by hemodynamic adjustments (described earlier under Renal Ablation Glomerulopathy).

Figure 14–16 ■

Drug-induced interstitial nephritis, with prominent eosinophilic and mononuclear infiltrate. (Courtesy of Dr. H. Rennke, Department of Pathology, Brigham and Women's Hospital, Boston.)

Clinical Course. Many patients with chronic pyelonephritis come to medical attention—relatively late in the course of the disease—because of the gradual onset of renal insufficiency or because signs of kidney disease are noticed on routine laboratory tests. Often the renal disease is heralded by the development of hypertension. Ultrasonography can be used to determine the size and shape of the kidneys. Pyelograms are characteristic: they show the affected kidney to be asymmetrically contracted, with some degree of blunting and deformity of the calyceal system (caliectasis). Renal cortical scanning with radioactive technetium can also detect early scarring. The presence or absence of significant bacteriuria is not particularly helpful diagnostically; its absence certainly should not rule out chronic pyelonephritis. If the disease is bilateral and progressive, tubular dysfunction occurs with loss of concentrating ability, manifested by polyuria and nocturia.

As noted earlier, some patients with chronic pyelonephritis or reflux nephropathy ultimately develop glomerular lesions of FSG. These are associated with proteinuria and eventually lead to progressive chronic renal failure. Such glomerular lesions may be caused by adaptive responses that occur in glomeruli as a result of reductions of renal mass, as discussed earlier.

DRUG-INDUCED INTERSTITIAL NEPHRITIS

In this era of antibiotics and analgesics, drugs have emerged as important causes of renal injury. Two forms of tubulointerstitial nephritis caused by drugs are discussed below.

Acute Drug-Induced Interstitial Nephritis

This is an adverse reaction to any of an increasing number of drugs. Acute tubulointerstitial nephritis most frequently occurs with synthetic penicillins (methicillin, ampicillin), other synthetic antibiotics (rifampin), diuretics (thiazides), nonsteroidal anti-inflammatory agents (phenylbutazone), and miscellaneous drugs (phenindione, cimetidine). The disease begins about 15 days (range, 2 to 40 days) after exposure to the drug and is characterized by *fever, eosinophilia* (which may be transient), *a rash* in about 25% of patients, and *renal abnormalities.* Renal findings include hematuria, minimal or no proteinuria, and leukocyturia (in-cluding eosinophils). *A rising serum creatinine level or acute renal failure with oliguria develops in about 50% of cases,* particularly in older patients. It is important to recognize drug-induced renal failure, because withdrawal of the offending drug is followed by recovery, although it may take several months for renal function to return to normal.

MORPHOLOGY

The abnormalities are in the interstitium, which shows pronounced edema and infiltration by mononuclear cells, principally lymphocytes and macrophages (Fig. 14–16). Eosinophils and neutrophils may be present, often in large numbers. With some drugs (e.g., methicillin, thiazides, rifampin), interstitial granulomas with giant cells may be seen. The glomeruli are normal except in some cases caused by nonsteroidal anti-inflammatory agents when minimal change disease and the nephrotic syndrome develop concurrently.

Pathogenesis. Many features of the disease suggest an immune mechanism. Clinical evidence of hypersensitivity includes the latent period, the eosinophilia and rash, the fact that the onset of nephropathy is not dose related, and the recurrence of hypersensitivity after re-exposure to the same or a cross-reactive drug. IgE serum levels are increased in some patients, suggesting type I hypersensitivity. The mononuclear or granulomatous infiltrate, together with positive skin tests to drug haptens, suggests a type IV hypersensitivity reaction.

The most likely sequence of pathogenetic events is that the drugs act as haptens that, during secretion by tubules, covalently bind to some cytoplasmic or extracellular component of tubular cells and become immunogenic. The resultant injury is then caused by IgE- and cell-mediated immune reactions to tubular cells or their basement membranes.

Analgesic Nephropathy

Patients who consume large quantities of analgesics may develop chronic interstitial nephritis, *often associated with renal papillary necrosis*. Although at times ingestion of single types of analgesics has been incriminated, most patients who develop this nephropathy consume mixtures containing some combination of phenacetin, aspirin, acetaminophen, caffeine, and codeine for long periods. Aspirin and acetaminophen are the major culprits. While they can cause renal disease in apparently healthy individuals, preexisting renal disease seems to be a necessary precursor to analgesia-induced renal failure.

Pathogenesis. The pathogenesis of the renal lesions is not entirely clear. Papillary necrosis is the initial event, and the interstitial nephritis in the overlying renal parenchyma is a secondary phenomenon. Acetaminophen, a phenacetin metabolite, injures cells by both *covalent binding* and *oxidative damage*. The ability of aspirin to inhibit prostaglandin synthesis suggests that this drug may induce its potentiating effect by inhibiting the vasodilatory effects of prostaglandin and predisposing the papilla to ischemia. Thus, the papillary damage may be caused by a combination of direct toxic effects of phenacetin metabolites as well as ischemic injury to both tubular cells and vessels.

MORPHOLOGY

The necrotic papillae appear yellowish brown, owing to the accumulation of breakdown products of phenacetin and other lipofuscin-like pigments. Later on, the papillae may shrivel, be sloughed off, and drop into the pelvis. Microscopically, the papillae show coagulative necrosis associated with loss of cellular detail but preservation of tubular outlines. Foci of dystrophic calcification may occur in the necrotic areas. The cortex drained by the necrotic papillae shows tubular atrophy, interstitial scarring, and inflammation. The small vessels in the papillae and urinary tract submucosa exhibit characteristic PAS-positive basement membrane thickening (analgesic microangiopathy).

Common clinical features of analgesic nephropathy include chronic renal failure, hypertension, and anemia. The anemia results in part from damage to red cells by phenacetin metabolites. Cessation of analgesic intake may stabilize or even improve renal function. A complication of analgesic abuse is the increased incidence of *transitional cell carcinoma* of the renal pelvis or bladder in patients who survive the renal failure.

Acute Tubular Necrosis

Acute tubular necrosis (ATN) is a clinicopathologic entity characterized morphologically by destruction of tubular epithelial cells and clinically by acute suppression of renal function. It is the most common cause of acute renal failure. Acute renal failure signifies an acute suppression of renal function, with urine flow falling within 24 hours to less than 400 mL (oliguria). Other causes of acute renal failure

include (1) severe glomerular diseases such as RPGN, (2) diffuse renal vascular diseases such as polyarteritis nodosa and acute thrombotic angiopathies, (3) acute papillary necrosis associated with acute pyelonephritis, (4) acute drug-induced interstitial nephritis, and (5) diffuse cortical necrosis. Here we discuss ATN; the other causes of acute renal failure are discussed elsewhere in this chapter.

ATN is a reversible renal lesion that arises in a variety of clinical settings. Most of these, ranging from severe trauma to acute pancreatitis to septicemia, have in common a period of inadequate blood flow to the peripheral organs, usually in the setting of marked hypotension and shock. The pattern of ATN associated with shock is called *ischemic ATN*. Mismatched blood transfusions and other hemolytic crises, as well as myoglobinuria, also produce a picture resembling ischemic ATN. A second pattern, called *nephrotoxic ATN*, is caused by a variety of poisons, including heavy metals (e.g., mercury); organic solvents (e.g., carbon tetrachloride); and a multitude of drugs such as gentamicin, other antibiotics, and radiographic contrast agents. Because of the many precipitating factors, ATN occurs quite frequently. Moreover, its reversibility adds to its clinical importance because proper management means the difference between full recovery and death.

Pathogenesis. The critical events in both ischemic and nephrotoxic ATN are believed to be (1) tubular injury and (2) persistent and severe disturbances in blood flow, as depicted in Figure 14–17.

■ Tubular epithelial cells are particularly sensitive to anoxia and are also vulnerable to toxins. Several factors predispose the tubules to toxic injury, including a vast electrically charged surface for tubular reabsorption, active transport systems for ions and organic acids, and the capability for effective concentration. Ischemia causes numerous structural alterations in epithelial cells. *Loss of cell polarity* appears to be a functionally important (reversible) early event. This leads to redistribution of membrane proteins (e.g., Na^+,K^+-ATPase) from the basolateral to the luminal surface of tubular cells, resulting in increased sodium delivery to distal tubules. The latter, through a tubuloglomerular feedback system, causes vasoconstriction. Further damage to the tubules and the resultant tubular debris could block urine outflow and eventually increase intratubular pressure, thereby decreasing the GFR. Additionally, fluid from the damaged tubules could leak into the interstitium, resulting in increased interstitial pressure and collapse of the tubule. Ischemic tubular cells also express cytokines and adhesion molecules that serve to recruit and immobilize leukocytes that can participate in tissue injury.

■ Ischemic renal injury is also characterized by severe hemodynamic alterations that cause reduced GFR. The major one is intrarenal *vasoconstriction*, which results in both reduced glomerular plasma flow and reduced oxygen delivery to the functionally important tubules in the outer medulla (thick ascending limb and straight segment of the proximal tubule) (see Fig. 14–17). Although a number of vasoconstrictor pathways have been implicated in this phenomenon (e.g., renin-angiotensin, norepinephrine), some triggered by the increased distal sodium delivery, the current opinion is that vasoconstriction is mediated by

Figure 14–17

Postulated sequence in acute renal failure (see text). NO, nitric oxide; GFR, glomerular filtration rate; PGI$_2$, prostaglandin I$_2$ (prostacyclin). (Modified from Brady HR, et al: Acute renal failure. In Brenner BM [ed]: Brenner and Rector's The Kidney, 5th ed, vol II. Philadelphia, WB Saunders, 1996, p 1210.)

sublethal endothelial injury, leading to increased release of the endothelial vasoconstrictor *endothelin* and decreased production of the vasodilator *nitric oxide*. Finally, there is also some evidence of a direct effect of ischemia or toxins on the glomerulus, causing a reduced glomerular ultrafiltration coefficient, possibly owing to a reduction in the effective filtration surface.

If the patient survives for a week, epithelial regeneration becomes apparent in the form of a low cuboidal epithelial covering and mitotic activity in the persisting tubular epithelial cells. Except where the basement membrane is destroyed, regeneration is total and complete.

MORPHOLOGY

Ischemic ATN is characterized by necrosis of short segments of the tubules. Most of the lesions are seen in the straight portions of the proximal tubule and the ascending thick limbs, but no segment of the proximal or distal tubules is spared. Tubular necrosis is often subtle, requiring careful histologic examination; it is usually associated with the difficult-to-discern rupture of the basement membrane **(tubulorrhexis).** A striking additional finding is the presence of proteinaceous casts in the distal tubules and collecting ducts. They consist of Tamm-Horsfall protein (secreted normally by tubular epithelium) along with hemoglobin and other plasma proteins. When crush injuries have produced ATN, the casts are composed of myoglobin. The interstitium usually discloses generalized edema along with a mild inflammatory infiltrate consisting of polymorphonuclear leukocytes, lymphocytes, and plasma cells. The histologic picture in **toxic ATN** is basically similar, with some differences. Necrosis is most prominent in the proximal tubule, and the tubular basement membranes are generally spared.

Clinical Course. The clinical course of ATN may be divided into initiating, maintenance, and recovery stages. The *initiating* phase, lasting about 36 hours, is usually dominated by the inciting medical, surgical, or obstetric event in the ischemic form of ATN. The only indication of renal involvement is a slight decline in urine output with a rise in blood urea nitrogen. At this point, oliguria could be explained on the basis of a transient decrease in blood flow to the kidneys.

The *maintenance* phase begins anywhere from the second to the sixth day. Urine output falls dramatically, usually to between 50 and 400 mL/day. Sometimes it declines to only a few milliliters per day, but complete anuria is rare. Oliguria may last only a few days or may persist as long as 3 weeks. The clinical picture is dominated by the signs and symptoms of uremia and fluid overload. In the absence of careful supportive treatment or dialysis, patients may die during this phase. With good care, however, survival is the rule.

The *recovery* is ushered in by a steady increase in urine volume, reaching up to about 3 L/day over the course of a few days. Because tubular function is still deranged, serious electrolyte imbalances may occur during this phase. There also appears to be increased vulnerability to infection. For these reasons, about 25% of deaths from ATN occur during this phase.

During the final phase, there is a gradual return of the patient's well-being. Urine volume returns to normal; however, subtle functional impairment of the kidneys, particularly of the tubules, may persist for months. With modern methods of care, patients who do not die from the underlying precipitating problem have a 90% to 95% chance of recovering from ATN.

DISEASES INVOLVING BLOOD VESSELS

Nearly all diseases of the kidney involve the renal blood vessels secondarily. Systemic vascular disease, such as various forms of arteritis, also involves renal blood vessels, and often the effects on the kidney are clinically important. These were considered in Chapter 10. The kidney is intimately involved in the pathogenesis of both essential and secondary hypertension, as discussed in detail in Chapter 10. Here we shall cover the two renal lesions associated with benign and malignant hypertension.

Benign Nephrosclerosis

Benign nephrosclerosis, the term used for the renal changes in benign hypertension, is always associated with hyaline arteriolosclerosis. Some degree of benign nephrosclerosis, albeit mild, is present at autopsy in many persons older than 60 years of age. The frequency and severity of the lesions are increased in young age groups in association with hypertension and diabetes mellitus.

The kidneys are symmetrically atrophic, each weighing 110 to 130 g, with a surface of diffuse, fine granularity that resembles grain leather.

MORPHOLOGY

Microscopically, the basic anatomic change is hyaline thickening of the walls of the small arteries and arterioles, known as **hyaline arteriolosclerosis**. This appears as a homogeneous, pink hyaline thickening, at the expense of the vessel lumina, with loss of underlying cellular detail (Fig. 14–18). The narrowing of the lumina results in markedly decreased blood flow through the affected vessels and thus produces ischemia in the organ served. All structures of the kidney show ischemic atrophy. In far-advanced cases of benign nephrosclerosis the glomerular tufts may become obliterated by homogeneous hyalinization. Diffuse tubular atrophy and interstitial fibrosis are present. Often there is a scant interstitial lymphocytic infiltrate. The larger blood vessels (interlobar and arcuate arteries) show reduplication of internal elastic lamina along with fibrous thickening of the media (fibroelastic hyperplasia) and the subintima.

Figure 14–18 ■

Benign nephrosclerosis. High-power view of two arterioles with hyaline deposition, marked thickening of the walls, and a narrowed lumen. (Courtesy of Dr. M. A. Venkatachalam, Department of Pathology, University of Texas Health Sciences Center, San Antonio, TX.)

It should be remembered that many renal diseases cause hypertension, which in turn may lead to benign nephrosclerosis. Thus, this renal lesion is often seen superimposed on other primary kidney diseases. Similar changes in arteries and arterioles are seen in patients with chronic thrombotic angiopathies.

Because this renal lesion alone rarely causes severe damage to the kidney, it very infrequently leads to uremia and death. Nonetheless, there is usually some functional impairment, such as loss of concentrating ability or a variably diminished GFR. A mild degree of proteinuria is a constant finding. Usually these patients die of hypertensive heart disease or cerebrovascular accidents rather than of renal disease.

Malignant Hypertension and Malignant Nephrosclerosis

Malignant hypertension is far less common than benign hypertension, occurring in only a very small percentage of patients with elevated blood pressure. It may arise de novo (i.e., without preexisting hypertension), or it may appear suddenly in a person who had mild hypertension.

Pathogenesis. The basis for this turn for the worse in hypertensive subjects is unclear, but the following sequence of events is suggested. The initial event appears to be some form of vascular damage to the kidneys. This most commonly results from long-standing benign hypertension, with eventual injury to the arteriolar walls, or it may spring from arteritis. In either case, the result is increased permeability of the small vessels to fibrinogen and other plasma proteins, endothelial injury, and platelet deposition. This leads to the appearance of *fibrinoid necrosis* of arterioles and small arteries and intravascular thrombosis. Mitogenic factors from platelets (e.g., platelet-derived growth factor) and plasma cause intimal smooth hyperplasia of vessels, resulting in the hyperplastic arteriolosclerosis typical of malignant hypertension and further narrowing of the lumina. The kidneys become markedly ischemic. With severe involvement of the renal afferent arterioles, the renin-angiotensin system receives a powerful stimulus, and indeed *patients with malignant hypertension have markedly elevated levels of plasma renin*. This then sets up a self-perpetuating cycle in which angiotensin II causes intrarenal vasoconstriction, and the attendant renal ischemia perpetuates renin secretion. Aldosterone levels are also elevated, and salt retention undoubtedly contributes to the elevation of blood pressure. The consequences of the markedly elevated blood pressure on the blood vessels throughout the body are known as *malignant arteriolosclerosis*, and the renal disorder is referred to as *malignant nephrosclerosis*.

arrangement of cells whose origin is believed to be intimal smooth muscle, although this issue is not finally settled. This lesion, called **hyperplastic arteriolosclerosis,** causes marked narrowing of arterioles and small arteries, to the point of total obliteration. Necrotizing arteriolitis may extend to involve the glomeruli **(necrotizing glomerulitis).** Microthrombi may be seen within the glomeruli as well as necrotic arterioles. Identical lesions are seen in patients with acute thrombotic angiopathies.

Clinical Course. The full-blown syndrome of *malignant hypertension is characterized by diastolic pressures greater than 120 mm Hg, papilledema, encephalopathy, cardiovascular abnormalities, and renal failure*. Most often, the early symptoms are related to increased intracranial pressure and include headaches, nausea, vomiting, and visual impairments, particularly the development of scotomas, or spots before the eyes. At the onset of rapidly mounting blood pressure there is marked proteinuria and microscopic, or sometimes macroscopic, hematuria but no significant alteration in renal function. Soon, however, renal failure makes its appearance. The syndrome is a true medical emergency that requires prompt and aggressive antihypertensive therapy before the irreversible renal lesions develop. About 50% of patients survive at least 5 years, and further progress is still being made. Ninety percent of deaths are caused by uremia and the other 10% by cerebral hemorrhage or cardiac failure.

Thrombotic Microangiopathies

As described in Chapter 12, these represent clinical syndromes characterized morphologically by widespread thrombosis in the microcirculation, and clinically by *microangiopathic hemolytic anemia, thrombocytopenia,* and, in certain instances, *renal failure*. The diseases include (1) childhood hemolytic-uremic syndrome (HUS), (2) various

MORPHOLOGY

The kidney may be essentially normal in size or slightly shrunken, depending on the duration and severity of the hypertensive disease. Small, pinpoint petechial hemorrhages may appear on the cortical surface from rupture of arterioles or glomerular capillaries, giving the kidney a peculiar flea-bitten appearance.

The microscopic changes reflect the pathogenetic events described earlier. Damage to the small vessels is manifested as **fibrinoid necrosis** of the arterioles (Fig. 14–19A). The vessel walls appear to take on a homogeneous, granular eosinophilic appearance masking underlying detail. Also, there is often a sprinkling of inflammatory cells, giving rise to the term **necrotizing arteriolitis.** The inflammation is presumably secondary to vascular damage. A different response is seen in the interlobular arteries and larger arterioles, where the proliferation of intimal cells produces an onion-skin appearance (Fig. 14–19B). This name is derived from the concentric

Figure 14–19

Malignant hypertension. *A,* Fibrinoid necrosis of afferent arteriole. (PAS stain.) *B,* Hyperplastic arteriolitis (onion-skin lesion). (Courtesy of Dr. H. Rennke, Department of Pathology, Brigham and Women's Hospital, Boston.)

forms of adult HUS, and (3) thrombotic thrombocytopenic purpura (TTP). Although clinically overlapping, HUS and TTP are pathogenetically distinct. Central to the pathogenesis of HUS is *endothelial injury and activation*, with resultant intravascular thrombosis. TTP is now known to be caused by an acquired defect in proteolytic cleavage of von Willebrand factor multimers (Chapter 12).

Childhood HUS is the best characterized of the renal syndromes. As many as 75% of cases follow intestinal infection with verocytotoxin-producing *E. coli*, such as occurs in epidemics caused by ingestion of infected ground meat (e.g., hamburgers) and infections with Shiga toxin–producing bacteria. (Verocytotoxins are so called because they cause damage to vero cells in culture.) *The disease is one of the main causes of acute renal failure in children.* It is characterized by the sudden onset, usually after a gastrointestinal or flulike prodromal episode, of bleeding manifestations (especially hematemesis and melena), severe oliguria, hematuria, microangiopathic hemolytic anemia, and (in some patients) prominent neurologic changes.

The pathogenesis of this syndrome is related to the effects of verocytotoxin on endothelium, causing increased adhesion of leukocytes, increased endothelin production and loss of endothelial nitric oxide (both favoring vasoconstriction), and (in the presence of cytokines, such as tumor necrosis factor) endothelial lysis. The resultant endothelial damage enhances thrombosis, most prominent in interlobular and afferent arterioles and glomerular capillaries, as well as vasoconstriction, resulting in the characteristic microangiopathy.

If the renal failure is managed properly with dialysis, most patients recover in a matter of weeks. The long-term (15- to 25-year) prognosis, however, is not uniformly favorable, because about 25% of children eventually develop renal insufficiency.

CYSTIC DISEASES OF THE KIDNEY

Cystic diseases of the kidney are a heterogeneous group comprising hereditary, developmental but nonhereditary, and acquired disorders. As a group, they are important for several reasons: (1) they are reasonably common and often present diagnostic problems for clinicians, radiologists, and pathologists; (2) some forms, such as adult polycystic disease, are major causes of chronic renal failure; and (3) they can occasionally be confused with malignant tumors. Here we shall briefly mention simple cysts, the most common form, and discuss in some detail polycystic kidney disease.

Simple Cysts

These generally innocuous lesions occur as multiple or single cystic spaces that vary in diameter within a wide range. Commonly, they are 1 to 5 cm in diameter; translucent; lined by a gray, glistening, smooth membrane; and filled with clear fluid. Microscopically, these membranes are composed of a single layer of cuboidal or flattened cuboidal epithelium, which in many instances may be completely atrophic. The

cysts are usually confined to the cortex. Rarely, large massive cysts up to 10 cm in diameter are encountered.

Simple cysts are a common postmortem finding that has no clinical significance. The main importance of cysts lies in their differentiation from kidney tumors, when they are discovered either incidentally or because of hemorrhage and pain. Radiographic studies show that, in contrast to renal tumors, renal cysts have smooth contours, are almost always avascular, and give fluid rather than solid signals on ultrasonography.

Dialysis-associated acquired cysts occur in the kidneys of patients with end-stage renal disease who have undergone prolonged dialysis. They are present in both cortex and medulla and may bleed, causing hematuria. Occasionally, renal adenomas or even adenocarcinomas arise in the walls of these cysts.

Autosomal Dominant (Adult) Polycystic Kidney Disease

Adult polycystic kidney disease (APKD) is characterized by multiple expanding cysts of both kidneys that ultimately destroy the intervening parenchyma. It is seen in approximately 1 in 500 to 1000 persons and accounts for 10% of cases of chronic renal failure. This disease is genetically heterogeneous. It can be caused by inheritance of at least two autosomal dominant genes of very high penetrance. In 90% of families, *PKD1*, the defective gene, is on the short arm of chromosome 16. This gene encodes a large (430-kD) and complex cell membrane–associated protein, called *polycystin-1*, that is mainly extracellular. The polycystin molecule has regions of homology to proteins known to be involved in cell-cell or cell-matrix adhesion (e.g., lectin-like domains, fibronectin-like domains). How mutations in this protein cause cyst formation is at present unclear, but it is thought that the resultant defects in cell-matrix interactions may lead to alterations in growth, differentiation, and matrix production by tubular epithelial cells and to cyst formation. It is interesting to note that whereas germ-line mutations of the *PKD1* gene are present in all renal tubular cells of affected patients, cysts develop in only some tubules. This is explained by the fact that both alleles of *PKD1* must be lost for cysts to develop. Thus, as with tumor supressor genes, a second "somatic hit" is required for expression of the disease. The *PKD2* gene, implicated in 10% of all cases, resides on chromosome 4 and encodes *polycystin-2*, a 968–amino acid protein. Although structurally distinct, polycystins 1 and 2 are believed to act together by forming heterodimers. Thus, mutation in either gene gives rise to the same phenotype.

MORPHOLOGY

The kidneys may achieve enormous size, and weights of up to 4 kg for each kidney have been recorded. These very large kidneys are readily palpable abdominally as masses extending into the pelvis. On gross examination the kidney seems to be composed solely of a mass of cysts of varying sizes up to 3 or 4 cm in diameter with no intervening

Figure 14-20 ■

Autosomal dominant adult polycystic kidney, viewed from the external surface (*A*) and bisected (*B*). The kidney is markedly enlarged (note the centimeter rule) with numerous dilated cysts.

parenchyma. The cysts are filled with fluid, which may be clear, turbid, or hemorrhagic (Fig. 14–20).

Microscopic examination reveals some normal parenchyma dispersed among the cysts. Cysts may arise at any level of the nephron, from tubules to collecting ducts, and therefore they have a variable, often atrophic lining. Occasionally, Bowman's capsules are involved in the cyst formation, and in these cases glomerular tufts may be seen within the cystic space. The pressure of the expanding cysts leads to ischemic atrophy of the intervening renal substance. Evidence of superimposed hypertension or infection is common.

Clinical Course. Polycystic kidney disease in adults usually *does not produce symptoms until the fourth decade*, by which time the kidneys are quite large. The most common complaint of the patient is *flank pain* or at least a heavy, dragging sensation. Acute distention of a cyst, either by intracystic hemorrhage or by obstruction, may cause excruciating pain. Sometimes attention is first drawn to the lesion by palpation of an abdominal mass. *Intermittent gross hematuria* commonly occurs. The most important complications, because of their deleterious effect on already marginal renal function, are *hypertension and urinary infection.* Hypertension of varying severity develops in about 75% of patients. Saccular aneurysms of the circle of Willis (Chapter 23) are present in 10% to 30% of patients, and these individuals have a high incidence of subarachnoid hemorrhage. Asymptomatic liver cysts occur in one third of patients.

Although the disease is ultimately fatal, the outlook is generally better than with most chronic renal diseases. The condition tends to be relatively stable and progresses very slowly. End-stage renal failure occurs at about age 50, but there is wide variation in the course of this disorder, and nearly normal life spans are reported. Those who develop renal failure are treated by renal transplantation. Death usually results from uremia or hypertensive complications.

Autosomal Recessive (Childhood) Polycystic Kidney Disease

This rare developmental anomaly is genetically distinct from adult polycystic kidney disease, having autosomal recessive inheritance. Perinatal, neonatal, infantile, and juvenile subcategories have been defined, depending on time of presentation and the presence of associated hepatic lesions. All result from mutations in an unidentified gene localized to chromosome 6p. The first two are most common; serious manifestations are usually present at birth, and young infants may die quickly from pulmonary or renal failure. Kidneys exhibit numerous small cysts in the cortex and medulla that give the kidney a spongelike appearance. Dilated, elongated channels at right angles to the cortical surface completely replace the medulla and cortex. The cysts have a uniform lining of cuboidal cells, reflecting their origin from the collecting tubules. The disease is invariably bilateral. In almost all cases, there are multiple epithelium-lined cysts in the liver as well as proliferation of portal bile ducts. Patients who survive infancy develop liver cirrhosis (congenital hepatic fibrosis).

URINARY OUTFLOW OBSTRUCTION

Renal Stones

Urolithiasis is calculus formation at any level in the urinary collecting system, but most often the calculi arise in the kidney. They occur frequently, as evidenced by the finding of stones in about 1% of all autopsies. Symptomatic

[handwritten notes at top of page]
- Magnesium stones → in pts w/persistent alkaline flow UTIs
- Proteus vulgaris & staphylococci → urea splitting bacteria that predispose to urolithiasis
- uric acid stones → uric uric acid, favors stone formation
- cysteine stones → due to genetic defect in transport → ↑excretion of cysteine urine

Table 14-4. PREVALENCE OF VARIOUS TYPES OF RENAL STONES

Stone	Percentage of All Stones
Calcium oxalate (phosphate)	75
Idiopathic hypercalciuria (50%)	
Hypercalcemia and hypercalciuria (10%)	
Hyperoxaluria (5%)	
Enteric (4.5%)	
Primary (0.5%)	
Hyperuricosuria (20%)	
No known metabolic abnormality	
(15%–20%)	
Struvite (Mg, NH_3, Ca, PO_4)	10–15
Renal infection	
Uric acid	6
Associated with hyperuricemia	
Associated with hyperuricosuria	
Idiopathic (50% of uric acid stones)	
Cystine	1–2
Others or unknown	±10

urolithiasis is more common in males. A familial tendency toward stone formation has long been recognized.

Pathogenesis. About 75% of renal stones are composed of either calcium oxalate or calcium oxalate mixed with calcium phosphate. Another 15% are composed of magnesium ammonium phosphate, and 10% are either uric acid or cystine stones. In all cases, there is an organic matrix of mucoprotein that makes up about 2.5% of the stone by weight (Table 14–4).

The cause of stone formation is often obscure, particularly in the case of calcium-containing stones. Probably involved is a confluence of predisposing conditions. *The most important cause is increased urine concentration of the stone's constituents, so that it exceeds their solubility in urine (supersaturation).* As shown in Table 14–4, 50% of the patients who develop *calcium stones* have hypercalciuria that is not associated with hypercalcemia. Most in this group absorb calcium from the gut in excessive amounts (absorptive hypercalciuria) and promptly excrete it in the urine, and some have a primary renal defect of calcium reabsorption (renal hypercalciuria). In 5% to 10% of patients there is hypercalcemia (due to hyperparathyroidism, vitamin D intoxication, or sarcoidosis) and consequent hypercalciuria. In 20% of this subgroup, there is excessive excretion of uric acid in the urine, which favors calcium stone formation; presumably the urates provide a nidus for calcium deposition. In 5% there is hyperoxaluria or hypercitraturia, and in the remainder there is no known metabolic abnormality.

The causes of the other types of renal stones are better understood. *Magnesium ammonium phosphate (struvite) stones* almost always occur in patients with a persistently alkaline urine due to UTIs. In particular, the urea-splitting bacteria, such as *Proteus vulgaris* and the staphylococci, predispose the patient to urolithiasis. Moreover, bacteria may serve as particulate nidi for the formation of any kind of stone. In avitaminosis A, desquamated squames from the metaplastic epithelium of the collecting system act as nidi.

Gout and diseases involving rapid cell turnover, such as the leukemias, lead to high uric acid levels in the urine and the possibility of *uric acid stones*. About half of the patients with uric acid stones, however, have neither hyperuricemia nor increased urine urate but an unexplained tendency to excrete a persistently acid urine (under pH 5.5), favoring stone formation. *Cystine stones* are almost invariably associated with a genetically determined defect in the renal transport of certain amino acids, including cystine. In contrast to magnesium ammonium phosphate stones, both uric acid and cystine stones are more likely to form when the urine is relatively acidic.

Urolithiasis may also conceivably result from the lack of influences that normally inhibit mineral precipitation. Inhibitors of crystal formation in urine include pyrophosphate, mucopolysaccharides, diphosphonates, and a glycoprotein called *nephrocalcin*, but no deficiency of any of these substances has been consistently demonstrated in patients with urolithiasis.

MORPHOLOGY

Stones are unilateral in about 80% of patients. Common sites of formation are renal pelves and calyces and the bladder. Often, many stones are found in one kidney. They tend to be small (average diameter 2 to 3 mm) and may be smooth or jagged. Occasionally, progressive accretion of salts leads to the development of branching structures known as **staghorn calculi,** which create a cast of the renal pelvis and calyceal system. These massive stones are usually composed of magnesium ammonium phosphate.

[handwritten margin notes]
- Stones are unilateral
- renal pelvis, calyces
- can lead to staghorn calculi

Clinical Course. Stones may be present without producing either symptoms or significant renal damage. This is particularly true with large stones lodged in the renal pelvis. Smaller stones may pass into the ureter, producing a typical intense pain known as *renal or ureteral colic,* characterized by paroxysms of flank pain radiating toward the groin. Often at this time there is *gross hematuria.* The clinical significance of stones lies in their capacity to obstruct urine flow or to produce sufficient trauma to cause ulceration and bleeding. In either case, they *predispose the patient to bacterial infection.* Fortunately, in most cases the diagnosis is readily made radiologically.

[handwritten margin notes]
- gross hematuria
- can lead to infection
- renal/ureteral colic → flank pain radiating to groin

Hydronephrosis

Hydronephrosis refers to dilation of the renal pelvis and calyces, with accompanying atrophy of the parenchyma, caused by obstruction to the outflow of urine. The obstruction may be sudden or insidious, and it may occur at any level of the urinary tract, from the urethra to the renal pelvis. The most common causes are as follows:

A. *Congenital:* Atresia of the urethra, valve formations in either ureter or urethra, aberrant renal artery compressing the ureter, renal ptosis with torsion, or kinking of the ureter

[handwritten note at bottom]
- hydronephrosis → dilation of the renal pelvis & calyces w/accompanying parenchymal atrophy caused by obstruction to the outflow of urine

B. *Acquired*

1. Foreign bodies: Calculi, necrotic papillae
2. Tumors: Benign prostatic hypertrophy, carcinoma of the prostate, bladder tumors (papilloma and carcinoma), contiguous malignant disease (retroperitoneal lymphoma, carcinoma of the cervix or uterus)
3. Inflammation: Prostatitis, ureteritis, urethritis, retroperitoneal fibrosis
4. Neurogenic: Spinal cord damage with paralysis of the bladder
5. Normal pregnancy: Mild and reversible

Bilateral hydronephrosis occurs only when the obstruction is below the level of the ureters. If blockage is at the ureters or above, the lesion is unilateral. Sometimes obstruction is complete, allowing no urine to pass; usually it is only partial.

Even with complete obstruction, glomerular filtration persists for some time, and the filtrate subsequently diffuses back into the renal interstitium and perirenal spaces, whence it ultimately returns to the lymphatic and venous systems. Because of the continued filtration, the *affected calyces and pelvis become dilated*, often markedly so. The unusually high pressure thus generated in the renal pelvis, as well as that transmitted back through the collecting ducts, causes compression of the renal vasculature. Both arterial insufficiency and venous stasis result, although the latter is probably more important. The most severe effects are seen in the papillae, because they are subjected to the greatest increases in pressure. Accordingly, *the initial functional disturbances are largely tubular, manifested primarily by impaired concentrating ability.* Only later does glomerular filtration begin to diminish. Experimental studies indicate that serious irreversible damage occurs in about 3 weeks with complete obstruction, and in 3 months with incomplete obstruction. However, functional impairment can be demonstrated only a few hours after ureteral ligation. The obstruction also triggers an interstitial inflammatory reaction, leading eventually to interstitial fibrosis.

filtration is compromised relatively early, and as a consequence, renal function may cease while dilation is still comparatively slight. Depending on the level of the obstruction, one or both ureters may also be dilated **(hydroureter).**

Microscopically, the early lesions show tubular dilation, followed by atrophy and fibrous replacement of the tubular epithelium with relative sparing of the glomeruli. Eventually, in severe cases the glomeruli also become atrophic and disappear, converting the entire kidney into a thin shell of fibrous tissue. With sudden and complete obstruction, there may be coagulative necrosis of the renal papillae, similar to the changes of necrotizing papillitis. In uncomplicated cases, the accompanying inflammatory reaction is minimal. Complicating pyelonephritis, however, is common.

Clinical Course. *Bilateral* complete obstruction produces anuria, which is soon brought to medical attention. When the obstruction is below the bladder, the dominant symptoms are those of bladder distention. Paradoxically, incomplete bilateral obstruction causes polyuria rather than oliguria, as a result of defects in tubular concentrating mechanisms, and this may obscure the true nature of the disturbance. Unfortunately, *unilateral* hydronephrosis may remain completely silent for long periods unless the other kidney is for some reason not functioning. Often the enlarged kidney is discovered on routine physical examination. Sometimes the basic cause of the hydronephrosis, such as renal calculi or an obstructing tumor, produces symptoms that indirectly draw attention to the hydronephrosis. Removal

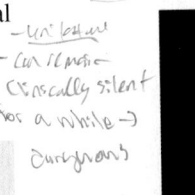

MORPHOLOGY

Bilateral hydronephrosis (as well as unilateral hydronephrosis when the other kidney is already damaged or absent) leads to renal failure, and the onset of uremia tends to abort the natural course of the lesion. In contrast, **unilateral** involvements display the full range of morphologic changes, which vary with the degree and speed of obstruction. With subtotal or intermittent obstruction, the kidney may be massively enlarged (lengths in the range of 20 cm) and the organ may consist almost entirely of the greatly distended pelvicalyceal system. The renal parenchyma itself is compressed and atrophied, with obliteration of the papillae and flattening of the pyramids (Fig. 14-21). On the other hand, **when obstruction is sudden and complete, glomerular**

Figure 14-21

Hydronephrosis of the kidney, with marked dilation of the pelvis and calyces and thinning of renal parenchyma.

of obstruction within a few weeks usually permits full return of function; however, with time the changes become irreversible.

TUMORS

Many types of benign and malignant tumors occur in the urinary tract. In general, benign tumors such as small (less than 0.5 cm) cortical papillary adenomas or medullary fibromas (interstitial cell tumors) have no clinical significance. The most common malignant tumor of the kidney is renal cell carcinoma, followed in frequency by nephroblastoma (Wilms tumor) and by primary tumors of the calyces and pelvis. Other types of renal cancer are rare and need not be discussed here. *Tumors of the lower urinary tract are about twice as common as renal cell carcinomas.* They are described at the end of this section.

Renal Cell Carcinoma

These tumors are derived from the renal tubular epithelium, and hence they are located predominantly in the cortex. Renal carcinomas represent 80% to 85% of all primary malignant tumors of the kidney, and 2% to 3% of all cancers in adults. This translates into about 30,000 cases per year; 40% of patients die of the disease. Carcinomas of the kidney are most common from the sixth to seventh decades, and men are affected about twice as commonly as women. The risk of developing these tumors is higher in smokers and those who have occupational exposure to cadmium. Smokers who are exposed to cadmium have a particularly high incidence of renal cell carcinomas. The risk of developing renal cell cancer is increased 30-fold in individuals who develop acquired polycystic disease as a complication of chronic dialysis. The role of genetic factors in the causation of these cancers is discussed later.

In the past, renal cell cancers were classified on the basis of morphology and growth patterns. However, recent advances in the understanding of the genetic basis of renal carcinomas have led to a new classification based on the molecular origins of these tumors. The three most common forms are as follows:

■ *Clear cell carcinomas.* These are the most common type, accounting for 70% to 80% of renal cell cancers. Histologically, they are made up of cells with clear or granular cytoplasm. Whereas the majority of them are sporadic, they also occur in familial forms or in association with von Hippel-Lindau (VHL) disease. It is the study of VHL disease that has provided molecular insights into the causation of clear cell carcinomas. VHL is an autosomal dominant disease characterized by predisposition to a variety of neoplasms, but particularly to hemangioblastomas of the cerebellum and retina. Hundreds of bilateral renal cysts and bilateral, often multiple, clear cell carcinomas develop in 40% to 60% cases. Patients with the VHL syndrome inherit a germ-line mutation of the *VHL* gene on chromosome 3p25 and lose the second allele by somatic mutation. Thus, the loss of both copies of this tumor suppressor gene gives rise to clear cell carcinoma. The *VHL* gene is also involved in sporadic clear cell carcinomas. Cytogenetic abnormalities giving rise to loss of chromosomal segment 3p14 to 3p26 are often seen in sporadic renal cell cancers. This region harbors the *VHL* gene (3p25.3). The second, nondeleted allele is inactivated by a somatic mutation or hypermethylation in 80% of sporadic cases. Thus, homozygous loss of the *VHL* gene seems to be the common underlying molecular abnormality in both sporadic and familial forms of clear cell carcinomas.

■ *Papillary renal cell carcinomas.* These comprise 10% to 15% of all renal cancers. As the name indicates, they show a papillary growth pattern. These tumors are frequently multifocal and bilateral and appear as early stage tumors. Like clear cell carcinomas they occur in familial and sporadic forms, but unlike these tumors, papillary renal cancers have no abnormality of chromosome 3. The culprit in the case of papillary renal cell cancers is the *MET* protooncogene, located on chromosome 7q31. The *MET* gene is a tyrosine kinase receptor for the growth factor called hepatocyte growth factor (also called scatter factor). It is an overdose of *MET* gene due to twofold to threefold gains in chromosome 7 that seem to spur abnormal growth in the proximal tubular epithelial cell precursors of papillary carcinomas. In keeping with this, trisomy of chromosome 7 is seen commonly in the familial cases. In these patients, along with overdose there are activating mutations of the *MET* gene. By contrast, in sporadic cases there is trisomy of chromosome 7 but there is no mutation of the *MET* gene. Sporadic cases also have trisomies of chromosomes 16 and 17 and loss of the Y chromosome. No specific oncogenes have been ascribed to these other chromosomes.

■ *Chromophobe renal carcinomas.* These are the least common, representing 5% of all renal cell carcinomas. They arise from either cortical collecting ducts or their intercalated cells. Their name derives from the fact that the tumor cells stain more darkly (i.e., less clear) than cells in clear cell carcinomas. These tumors are unique in having multiple losses of entire chromosomes, including chromosome 1, 2, 6, 10, 13, 17, and 21. Thus, they show extreme hypodiploidy. Because of multiple losses, the "critical hit" has not been determined. In general, chromophobe renal cancers have a good prognosis.

MORPHOLOGY

Clear cell cancers (the most common form) are usually solitary and large when symptomatic (spherical masses 3 to 15 cm in diameter), but increased use of high-resolution radiographic techniques for investigation of unrelated problems has led to the detection of even smaller lesions. They may arise anywhere in the cortex. The cut surface of clear cell renal cell carcinomas is yellow to orange to gray-white, with prominent areas of cystic softening or of hemorrhage, either fresh or old (Fig. 14-22). The margins of the tumor are well defined. However, at times small processes project into the surrounding parenchyma and small satellite nodules are found in the surrounding substance, providing clear evidence of the aggressiveness of these lesions. As the tumor enlarges, it may fungate through the walls of the collecting system, extending through the calyces and pelvis as far as the ureter. Even more frequently, the tumor invades the renal vein and grows as a solid column within this vessel, sometimes extending in serpentine fashion as far as the inferior vena cava and even into the right side of the heart. Occasionally, there is direct invasion into the perinephric fat and adrenal gland. Papillary renal cell carcinomas tend to be bilateral and multiple. They may also show gross evidence of necrosis, hemorrhage, and cystic degeneration, but they are less vibrantly orange-yellow, owing to a lower lipid content. Chromophobe type renal cell carcinomas tend to be grossly tan-brown.

Depending on the amounts of lipid and glycogen present, **the tumor cells of clear cell renal cell carcinoma may appear almost vacuolated or may be solid.** The classic vacuolated (lipid-laden), or clear, cells are demarcated only by their cell membranes. The nuclei are usually small and round (Fig. 14-23). At the other extreme are granular cells, resembling the tubular epithelium, which have small, round, regular nuclei enclosed within granular pink cytoplasm. Some tumors exhibit marked degrees of anaplasia, with numerous mitotic figures and markedly enlarged, hyperchromatic, pleomorphic nuclei. Between the extremes of clear cells and solid, granular cells, all intergradations may be found. The cellular arrangement, too, varies widely. The cells may form abortive tubules or may cluster in cords or disorganized masses. The stroma is usually scant but highly vascularized.

Papillary renal cell carcinomas exhibit varying degrees of papilla formation with fibrovascular cores. The cells can have clear or, more commonly, pink cytoplasm. **Chromophobe type renal cell carcinoma** cells usually have clear, flocculent cytoplasm with very prominent, distinct cell membranes. The nuclei are surrounded by halos of cleared cytoplasm. Ultrastructurally, large numbers of characteristic macrovesicles are seen.

Clinical Course. Renal cell carcinomas have several peculiar clinical characteristics that create especially difficult and challenging diagnostic problems. The symptoms vary, but the *most frequent presenting manifestation is hematuria, occurring in more than 50% of cases.* Macroscopic hematuria tends to be intermittent and fleeting, superimposed on a steady microscopic hematuria. Less commonly (because of wide use of imaging studies for unrelated conditions),

Figure 14-22

Renal cell carcinoma: typical cross-section of yellowish, spherical neoplasm in one pole of the kidney. Note the tumor in the dilated, thrombosed renal vein.

the tumor may declare itself simply by virtue of its size, when it has grown large enough to produce flank pain and a palpable mass. Extrarenal effects are fever and polycythemia, both of which may be associated with a renal cell carcinoma but which, because they are nonspecific, may be misinterpreted for some time before their true significance is appreciated. Polycythemia affects 5% to 10% of patients with this disease. It results from elaboration of erythropoietin by the renal tumor. Uncommonly, these tumors produce a variety of hormone-like substances, resulting in hypercalcemia, hypertension, Cushing syndrome, or feminization or masculinization. These, as will be recalled from Chapter 6, are paraneoplastic syndromes. In many patients the primary tumor remains silent and is discovered

Figure 14-23

High-power detail of the clear cell pattern of renal cell carcinoma.

only after its metastases have produced symptoms. The prevalent locations for metastases are the lungs and the bones. It must be apparent that renal cell carcinoma presents in many fashions, some quite devious, *but the triad of painless hematuria, long-standing fever, and dull flank pain is characteristic.*

Wilms Tumor

Although Wilms tumor occurs infrequently in adults, it is the third most common organ cancer in children younger than the age of 10 years. It is therefore one of the major cancers of children. These tumors contain a variety of cell and tissue components, all derived from the mesoderm. Wilms tumor, like retinoblastoma, may arise sporadically or be familial, with the susceptibility to tumorigenesis inherited as an autosomal dominant trait. This tumor is discussed in greater detail in Chapter 7 along with other tumors of childhood.

Tumors of the Urinary Bladder and Collecting System (Renal Calyces, Renal Pelvis, Ureter, and Urethra)

The entire urinary collecting system from renal pelvis to urethra is lined with transitional epithelium, so its epithelial tumors assume similar morphologic patterns. Tumors in the collecting system above the bladder are relatively uncommon; those in the bladder, however, are an even more frequent cause of death than are kidney tumors. Nevertheless, in the individual case, a small lesion in the ureter, for example, may cause urinary outflow obstruction and have greater clinical significance than a much larger mass in the capacious bladder. We shall consider first the range of histologic patterns *as they occur in the urinary bladder*, and then their clinical implications.

MORPHOLOGY

Tumors arising in the urinary bladder range from small benign papillomas to large invasive cancers (Fig. 14-24). The very rare benign **papillomas** are 0.2- to 1.0-cm frondlike structures having a delicate fibrovascular core covered by multilayered, well-differentiated transitional epithelium. In some of these lesions, the covering epithelium appears as normal as the mucosal surface whence these tumors arise; such lesions are usually solitary, almost invariably noninvasive, and benign and rarely recur once removed.

The classification and nomenclature of bladder cancers have undergone revision. Traditionally, bladder carcinomas have been called transitional cell carcinomas, but the term **urothelial neoplasms** is preferred by the International Society of Urologic Pathology (ISUP) consensus classification. **Urothelial (transitional) cell carcinomas** range from papillary to flat, noninvasive to invasive, and extremely well

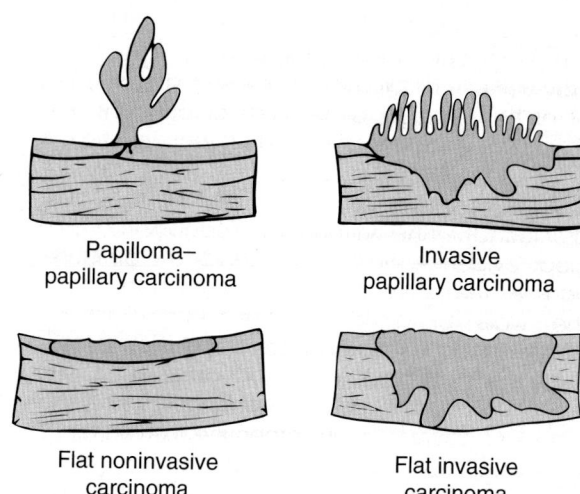

Papilloma–
papillary carcinoma

Invasive
papillary carcinoma

Flat noninvasive
carcinoma

Flat invasive
carcinoma

Figure 14–24 ■

Four morphologic patterns of bladder tumor.

---

differentiated (grade I, Fig. 14-25) to highly anaplastic aggressive cancers (grade III). Grade I carcinomas (ISUP, low malignant potential) are always papillary and are rarely invasive, but they may recur after removal. Whether the regrowth is a true recurrence or a second primary growth is uncertain. Increasing degrees of cellular atypia and anaplasia are encountered in papillary exophytic growths, accompanied by increase in size of the lesion and evidence of invasion of the submucosal or muscular layers. These tumors are unequivocally urothelial cell carcinomas, grade II or grade III. Grade III cancers can be papillary or occasionally flat, may cover larger areas of the mucosal surface, invade deeper, and have a shaggier necrotic surface. (The grade I and grade III transitional carcinomas correspond roughly to urothelial carci-

Figure 14–25 ■

Grade I papillary transitional cell carcinoma of the bladder. The delicate papilla is covered by orderly transitional epithelium.

noma, low grade and high grade, respectively.) Occasionally, these cancers show foci of squamous cell differentiation, but only 5% of bladder cancers are true **squamous cell carcinomas.** Carcinomas of grades II and III infiltrate surrounding structures, spread to regional nodes, and, on occasion, metastasize widely.

In addition to overt carcinoma, an **in situ stage of bladder carcinoma** can be recognized, often in patients with previous or simultaneous papillary or invasive tumors. Indeed, wide areas of atypical hyperplasia and dysplasia may be present. It is now thought that these epithelial changes and cancers in situ are caused by the generalized influence of a putative carcinogen on urothelium and that they may be the precursors of invasive carcinomas in some patients. However, despite the presence of wide areas of epithelial lesions, the bladder tumors, even when multiple, are monoclonal in origin. Apparently, clonal descendants of a single transformed cell can seed multiple areas of the mucosa.

Clinical Course. *Painless hematuria is the dominant clinical presentation* of all these tumors. Because most arise in the bladder, we shall consider these first. They affect men about three times as frequently as women and usually develop between the ages of 50 and 70 years. Although most occur in persons with no known history of exposure to industrial solvents, bladder tumors are 50 times more common in those exposed to β-naphthylamine. Cigarette smoking, chronic cystitis, schistosomiasis of the bladder, and certain drugs (cyclophosphamide) are also believed to induce higher attack rates.

The clinical significance of bladder tumors depends on their histologic grade and differentiation and, most importantly, on the depth of invasion of the lesion. Except for the clearly benign papillomas, all tend stubbornly to recur after removal and tend to kill by infiltrative obstruction of ureters rather than by metastasis. Lesions that invade the ureteral or urethral orifices cause urinary tract obstruction. In general, with low-grade shallow lesions, the prognosis after removal is good, but when deep penetration of the bladder wall has occurred, the 5-year survival rate is less than 20%. Overall 5-year survival is 57%.

Although papillary and cancerous neoplasms of the lining epithelium of the collecting system occur much less frequently in the renal pelvis than in the bladder, they nonetheless make up 5% to 10% of primary renal tumors. Painless hematuria is the most characteristic feature of these lesions, but in their critical location they produce pain in the costovertebral angle as hydronephrosis develops. Infiltration of the walls of the pelvis, calyces, and renal vein worsens the prognosis. Despite removal of the tumor by nephrectomy, less than 50% of patients survive for 5 years. Cancer of the ureter is fortunately the rarest of the tumors of the collecting system. The 5-year survival rate is less than 10%.

BIBLIOGRAPHY

Asplin JR, Favus MJ, Coe FL: Nephrolithiasis. In Brenner BM (ed): Brenner and Rector's Kidney, 6th ed. Vol 2. Philadelphia, WB Saunders, 2000, p1774. (A detailed account of causes and manifestations of renal stones.)

Doublier S, et al: Nephrin redistribution on podocytes is a potential mechanism for proteinuria in patients with primary acquired nephrotic syndrome. Am J Pathol 158:1723, 2001. (A report implicating nephrin in many forms of nephrotic syndrome.)

Epstein JI, et al: The World Health Organization/International Society of Urologic Pathology consensus classification of urothelial (transitional cell) neoplasms of the urinary bladder. Am J Surg Pathol 22:1435, 1998. (A modified classification of bladder cancer.)

Floege J, Feehally J: IgA nephropathy: recent developments. J Am Soc Nephrol 11:2395, 2000. (An update on the pathogenesis of this disease.)

Fored CM, et al: Acetaminophen, aspirin, and chronic renal failure. N Engl J Med 345:1801, 2001. (An important paper that analyzes the factors underlying analgesic nephropathy.)

Garin EH: Circulating mediators of proteinuria in idiopathic minimal lesion nephrotic syndrome. Pediatr Nephrol 14:872, 2000. (A review of evidence linking circulating factors with lipoid nephrosis.)

Grantham JJ: Polycystic kidney disease: from the bedside to the gene and back. Curr Opin Nephrol Hypertension 10:533, 2001. (An excellent update on the genetics and pathogenesis of polycystic kidney disease.)

Hrick DE, et al: Glomerulonephritis. N Engl J Med 339:888, 1998. (A broad-ranging review of the proliferative forms of glomerulonephritides.)

Lameire N, Vanholder R: Pathophysiologic features and prevention of human and experimental acute tubular necrosis. J Am Soc Nephrol 12(Suppl 17):S20, 2001. (A review of acute tubular necrosis with implications for treatment.)

Manthey DE, Teichman J: Nephrolithiasis. Emerg Med Clin North Am 19:633, 2001. (A clinically oriented review of renal stones.)

Miller O, Hemphill RR: Urinary tract infection and pyelonephritis. Emerg Med Clin North Am 19:655, 2001. (An excellent review of acute urinary tract infections.)

Nordstrand A, et al: Pathogenetic mechanisms in acute poststreptococcal glomerulonephritis. Scand J Infect Dis 31:523, 1999. (A good discussion of the immunologic mechanisms involved in this entity.)

Phillips JL, et al: The genetic basis of renal epithelial tumors: advances in research and its impact on prognosis and therapy. Curr Opin Urol 11:463, 2001. (An update on the molecular pathogenesis of renal cancer.)

Reuter VE, Prestic JC: Contemporary approach to the classification of renal epithelial tumors. Semin Oncol 27:124, 2000. (A nice discussion of morphology, clinical features, and genetic attributes of renal cell cancer.)

Somlo S, Mundel P: Getting a foothold in nephrotic syndrome. Nat Genet 24:333, 2000. (Molecular basis of nephrotic syndrome, as revealed by study of mutations in slit diaphragm protein.)

Tryggvason K, Wartioovaara J: Molecular basis of glomerular permselectivity. Curr Opin Nephrol Hypertens 10:543, 2001. (An excellent and brief review of the molecular architecture of slit diaphragms and control of glomerular permeability.)

15

The Oral Cavity and the Gastrointestinal Tract

JAMES M. CRAWFORD, MD, PhD
VINAY KUMAR, MD

■ Oral Cavity

Diseases of the oral cavity can be broadly divided into two groups: those affecting the soft tissues (including the salivary glands) and those that involve the teeth. Only the more common conditions affecting the soft tissues are considered in this chapter. Excluded are extraoral diseases that sometimes involve the mouth and pharynx, such as diphtheria, lichen planus, and leukemia, as well as dental disorders.

ULCERATIVE AND INFLAMMATORY LESIONS

Although several ulcerative and inflammatory conditions are discussed here, it is important to remember that mechanical trauma and cancer may produce ulcerations in the oral cavity and must be considered in the differential diagnosis.

Aphthous Ulcers (Canker Sores). These lesions are extremely common, small (usually less than 5 mm in diameter), painful, shallow ulcers. Characteristically, they take the form of rounded, superficial erosions, often covered with a gray-white exudate and having an erythematous rim. They appear singly or in groups on the nonkeratinized oral mucosa, particularly the soft palate, buccolabial mucosa, floor of the mouth, and lateral borders of the tongue. They are more common in the first 2 decades of life and are often apparently triggered by stress, fever, ingestion of certain foods, and activation of inflammatory bowel disease. In patients who are not immunosuppressed or do not have known viral infection such as with herpesvirus, an autoimmune basis is

suspected. The canker sores are self-limited and usually resolve within a few weeks, but they may recur in the same or a different location in the oral cavity. Frequent episodes—four times or more per year—earn the moniker of recurrent aphthous stomatitis.

Herpesvirus Infection. Herpetic stomatitis is an extremely common infection caused by herpes simplex virus (HSV) type 1. The pathogen is transmitted from person to person, most often by kissing; by middle life over three fourths of the population have been infected. In most adults, the primary infection is asymptomatic, but the virus persists in a dormant state within ganglia about the mouth (e.g., trigeminal). With reactivation (fever, sun or cold exposure, respiratory tract infection, trauma), solitary or multiple small (less than 5 mm in diameter) vesicles containing clear fluid appear. They occur most often on the lips or about the nasal orifices and are well known as "cold sores" or "fever blisters." They soon rupture, leaving shallow, painful ulcers that heal within a few weeks, but recurrences are common. Histologically, the vesicles begin as an intraepithelial focus of intercellular and intracellular edema. The infected cells become ballooned and develop intranuclear acidophilic viral inclusions. Sometimes adjacent cells fuse to form giant cells or polykaryons. Necrosis of the infected cells and the focal collections of edema fluid account for the intraepithelial vesicles seen clinically (Fig. 15–1). Identification of the inclusion-bearing cells or polykaryons in smears of blister fluid constitutes the diagnostic *Tzanck test* for HSV infection; antiviral agents may accelerate healing.

When primary infection with HSV type 1 occurs in a prepubescent child or immunocompromised adult, a more

Figure 15-1

Herpesvirus pharyngitis. *A,* Herpesvirus blister in mucosa. *B,* High-power view of cells from blister in *A,* showing glassy intranuclear herpes simplex inclusion bodies.

virulent disseminated eruption is likely, marked by multiple vesicles throughout the oral cavity, including the pharynx (herpetic gingivostomatitis). In the worst case, viremia may seed the brain (encephalitis) or produce disseminated visceral lesions. HSV type 1 may localize in many other sites, including the conjunctivae (keratoconjunctivitis) and the esophagus when a nasogastric tube is introduced through an infected oral cavity. HSV type 2 (the agent of herpes genitalis), on the other hand, is transmitted sexually and produces vesicles on the genital mucous membranes and external genitalia that have the same histologic characteristics as those that occur about the mouth.

Fungal Infection. *Candida albicans* is a normal inhabitant of the oral cavity found in 30% to 40% of the population; it causes disease only when there is some impairment of the usual protective mechanisms. Oral candidiasis (thrush, moniliasis) is a common fungal infection among persons rendered vulnerable by diabetes mellitus, anemia, antibiotic or glucocorticoid therapy, immunodeficiency, or debilitating illnesses such as disseminated cancer. Patients with the acquired immunodeficiency syndrome (AIDS) are at particular risk. Typically, *oral candidiasis takes the form of an adherent white, curdlike, circumscribed plaque anywhere within the oral cavity* (Fig. 15-2). The pseudomembrane can be scraped off to reveal an underlying granular erythematous inflammatory base. Histologically, the pseudomembrane is composed of a myriad of fungal organisms superficially attached to the underlying mucosa. In milder infections there is minimal ulceration, but in severe cases the entire mucosa may be denuded. The fungi can be identified within these pseudomembranes as boxcar-like chains of tubular cells producing pseudohyphae from which bud ovoid yeast forms, typically 2 to 4 μm in greatest diameter.

In the particularly vulnerable host, candidiasis may spread into the esophagus, especially when a nasogastric tube has been introduced, or it may produce widespread visceral lesions when the fungus gains entry into the bloodstream. Disseminated candidiasis is a life-threatening infection that must be treated aggressively. For poorly understood reasons,

local candidal lesions may appear in the vagina, not only in predisposed persons but also in apparently healthy young women, particularly ones who are pregnant or using oral contraceptives or using broad-spectrum antibiotics.

Acquired Immunodeficiency Syndrome (AIDS). AIDS and less advanced forms of human immunodeficiency virus (HIV) infection are often associated with lesions in the oral cavity. They may take the form of candidiasis, herpetic vesicles, or some other microbial infection (producing gingivitis or glossitis). Of particular interest are the intraoral lesions of Kaposi sarcoma and hairy leukoplakia. Kaposi sarcoma, as described in Chapters 5 and 10, is a multifocal, systemic disease that eventually evolves into highly vascular

Figure 15-2

Oral candidiasis ("thrush"). A white plaquelike membrane coats the gingival mucosa of the left lower jaw in an edentulous young patient. This pseudomembrane is composed of a layer of candidal pseudohyphae (not shown). (Courtesy of Dr. Harvey P. Kessler, Department of Oral Surgery, College of Dentistry, University of Florida, Gainesville, FL.)

tumor nodules. Although Kaposi sarcoma may occur in the absence of HIV infection, it affects about 25% of AIDS patients, particularly homosexual or bisexual males. More than 50% of those afflicted develop intraoral purpuric discolorations or violaceous, raised, nodular masses; sometimes this involvement constitutes the presenting manifestation.

Hairy leukoplakia is an uncommon lesion seen virtually only in persons infected with HIV. It constitutes white confluent patches, anywhere on the oral mucosa, that have a "hairy" or corrugated surface resulting from marked epithelial thickening. It is caused by Epstein-Barr virus infection of epithelial cells. Occasionally, the development of hairy leukoplakia calls attention to the existence of the underlying HIV infection.

Figure 15-3 ■

A, Leukoplakia of the tongue in a smoker. Microscopically, this lesion showed severe dysplasia with transformation to squamous cell carcinoma in the posterior elevated portion *(arrow). B,* Leukoplakia caused by marked epithelial thickening and hyperkeratosis.

LEUKOPLAKIA

As generally used, the term *leukoplakia refers to a whitish, well-defined mucosal patch or plaque caused by epidermal thickening or hyperkeratosis.* The term is not applied to other white lesions, such as those caused by candidiasis, lichen planus, or many other disorders.

The plaques are more frequent among older men and are most often on the vermilion border of the lower lip, buccal mucosa, and the hard and soft palates and less frequently on the floor of the mouth and other intraoral sites. They appear as localized, sometimes multifocal or even diffuse, smooth or roughened, leathery, white, discrete areas of mucosal thickening. On microscopic evaluation they vary from banal hyperkeratosis without underlying epithelial dysplasia to mild to severe dysplasia bordering on carcinoma in situ (Fig. 15-3). Only histologic evaluation distinguishes among these changes. The lesions are of unknown cause except that there is a *strong association with the use of tobacco,* particularly pipe smoking and smokeless tobacco (pouches, snuff, chewing). Less strongly implicated are *chronic friction,* as from ill-fitting dentures or jagged teeth; *alcohol abuse;* and irritant foods. More recently, human papillomavirus antigen has been identified in some tobacco-related lesions, raising the possibility that the virus and tobacco act in concert in the induction of these lesions.

Oral leukoplakia is an important finding because 3% to 6% (depending somewhat on location) undergo transformation to squamous cell carcinoma (see Fig. 15-3A). It is impossible to distinguish the innocent lesion from the ominous one on visual inspection. The transformation rate is greatest with lip and tongue lesions and lowest with those on the floor of the mouth. Those lesions that display significant dysplasia on microscopic examination have a greater probability of cancerous transformation.

Three somewhat related lesions must be differentiated from the usual oral leukoplakia. Hairy leukoplakia, described earlier and seen virtually only in patients with AIDS, has a corrugated or "hairy" surface rather than the white, opaque thickening of oral leukoplakia and has not been related to the development of oral cancer. Verrucous leukoplakia exhibits a corrugated surface caused by excessive hyperkeratosis. This seemingly innocuous form of leukoplakia recurs and insidi-

ously spreads over time, resulting in a diffuse warty-type of oral lesion that may yet harbor squamous cell carcinoma. *Erythroplasia* refers to red, velvety, often granular, circumscribed areas that may or may not be elevated, having poorly defined, irregular boundaries. Histologically, erythroplasia almost invariably reveals marked epithelial dysplasia (the malignant transformation rate is more than 50%), so recognition of this lesion becomes even more important than identification of oral leukoplakia.

CANCERS OF THE ORAL CAVITY AND TONGUE

The overwhelming preponderance of oral cavity cancers are squamous cell carcinomas. Although they represent only about 3% of all cancers in the United States, they are disproportionately important. Almost all are readily accessible to biopsy and early identification, but about half result in death within 5 years and indeed may have already metastasized by the time the primary lesion is discovered. These cancers tend to occur later in life and are rare before age 40. The various influences thought to be important in development of these cancers are summarized in Table 15-1.

Table 15–1. RISK FACTORS FOR ORAL CANCER

Factor	Comments
Leukoplakia, erythroplasia	See text discussion
Tobacco use	Best-established influence, particularly pipe smoking and smokeless tobacco
Human papillomavirus types 16, 18, and 33	Identified by molecular probes in one half to one third of cases; early involvement in carcinogenesis is hypothesized
Alcohol abuse	Less strong influence than tobacco
Protracted irritation	Weakly associated

Figure 15–4

Oral squamous cell carcinoma. Invasive tumor islands show formation of keratin pearls.

MORPHOLOGY

The three predominant sites of origin of oral cavity carcinomas are (in order of frequency) the (1) vermilion border of the lateral margins of the lower lip, (2) floor of the mouth, and (3) lateral borders of the mobile tongue. Early lesions appear as pearly white to gray, circumscribed thickenings of the mucosa closely resembling leukoplakic patches. They then may grow in an exophytic fashion to produce readily visible and palpable nodular and eventually fungating lesions, or they may assume an endophytic, invasive pattern with central necrosis to create a cancerous ulcer. The squamous cell carcinomas are usually moderately to well-differentiated keratinizing tumors (Fig. 15–4). Before the lesions become advanced it may be possible to identify epithelial atypia, dysplasia, or carcinoma in situ in the margins, suggesting origin from leukoplakia or erythroplasia. Spread to regional nodes is present at the time of initial diagnosis only rarely with lip cancer, in about 50% of cases of tongue cancer, and in more than 60% of those with cancer of the floor of the mouth. More remote spread to tissues or organs in the thorax or abdomen is less common than extensive regional spread.

Clinical Features. These lesions may cause local pain or difficulty in chewing, but many are relatively asymptomatic and so the lesion (very familiar to the exploring tongue) is ignored. As a result, a significant number are not discovered until beyond cure. The overall 5-year survival rates after surgery and adjuvant radiation and chemotherapy are about 40% for cancers of the base of the tongue, pharynx, and floor of the mouth without lymph node metastasis, compared with under 20% for those with lymph node metastasis. When these cancers are discovered at an early stage, 5-year survival can exceed 90%.

SALIVARY GLAND DISEASES

Although diseases primary to the major salivary glands are in general uncommon, the parotids bear the brunt of these involvements. Among the many possible disorders, attention is restricted here to sialadenitis and salivary gland tumors.

Sialadenitis

Inflammation of the major salivary glands may be of viral, bacterial, or autoimmune origin. Dominant among these causations is the infectious viral disease *mumps*, which may produce enlargement of all the major salivary glands but predominantly the parotids. Although a number of viruses may cause mumps, the dominant cause is a paramyxovirus, an RNA virus related to the influenza and parainfluenza viruses. It usually produces a diffuse, interstitial inflammation marked by edema and a mononuclear cell infiltration and, sometimes, by focal necrosis. Although childhood mumps is self-limited and rarely leaves residua, mumps in adults may be accompanied by pancreatitis or orchitis; the latter sometimes causes permanent sterility.

Bacterial sialadenitis most often occurs secondary to ductal obstruction resulting from stone formation *(sialolithiasis)*, but it may also arise after retrograde entry of oral cavity bacteria under conditions of severe systemic dehydration such as the postoperative state. Patients with chronic, debilitating medical conditions, compromised immune function, or on medications contributing to oral or systemic dehydration are at increased risk for acute bacterial sialadenitis. The sialadenitis may be largely interstitial or cause focal areas of suppurative necrosis or even abscess formation.

Chronic sialadenitis arises from decreased production of saliva with subsequent inflammation. The dominant cause is *autoimmune sialadenitis*, which is almost invariably bilateral. This is seen in Sjögren syndrome, discussed in Chapter 5. All of the salivary glands (major and minor), as well as the lacrimal glands, may be affected in this disorder, which induces dry mouth *(xerostomia)* and dry eyes *(keratoconjunctivitis sicca).* The combination of salivary and lacrimal gland inflammatory enlargement, which is usually painless, and xerostomia, whatever the cause, is sometimes referred to by the eponymic term *Mikulicz syndrome.* The causes include sarcoidosis, leukemia, lymphoma, and idiopathic lymphoepithelial hyperplasia.

Salivary Gland Tumors

The salivary glands give rise to a diversity of tumors that belies their small size. About 80% of tumors occur within the parotid glands and most of the others in the submandibular glands. Males and females are affected about equally, usually in the sixth or seventh decade of life. In the parotids 70% to 80% of these tumors are benign, whereas in the submaxillary glands only half are benign. Thus, it is evident that *a neoplasm in the submaxillary glands is more ominous than one in the parotids.* The dominant tumor arising in the parotids is the benign pleomorphic adenoma, which is sometimes called a mixed tumor of salivary gland origin. Much less frequent is the papillary cystadenoma lymphomatosum (Warthin tumor). Collectively, these two types account for three fourths of parotid tumors. Whatever the type, they present clinically as a mass causing a swelling at the angle of the jaw. Among the diverse cancers of parotid glands, the two dominant types are (1) malignant mixed tumors arising either de novo or in preexisting, benign, pleomorphic adenomas and (2) mucoepidermoid carcinoma (containing adenocarcinomatous and squamous cell carcinomatous features). Only the benign pleomorphic adenoma and Warthin tumor are sufficiently common to merit description.

Pleomorphic Adenoma (Mixed Tumor of Salivary Glands). This tumor accounts for over 90% of benign tumors of the salivary glands. It is a slow-growing, well-demarcated, apparently encapsulated lesion rarely exceeding 6 cm in greatest dimension. Most often arising in the superficial parotid, it usually causes painless swelling at the angle of the jaw and can be readily palpated as a discrete mass. It is nonetheless often present for years before being brought to medical attention. Despite its encapsulation, histologic examination often reveals multiple sites where the tumor penetrates the capsule. Adequate margins of resection are thus necessary to prevent recurrences. This may require sacrifice of the facial nerve, which courses through the parotid gland. On average, about 10% of excisions are followed by recurrence.

MORPHOLOGY

The characteristic histologic feature is heterogeneity. The tumor cells form ducts, acini, tubules, strands, or sheets of cells. The epithelial cells are small and dark and range from cuboidal to spindle forms. These epithelial elements are intermingled with a loose, often myxoid connective tissue stroma sometimes containing islands of apparent chondroid or, rarely, bone (Fig. 15–5). Immunohistochemical evidence suggests that all of the diverse cell types within these tumors, including those within the stroma, are of myoepithelial derivation. When primary or recurrent benign tumors are present for many (10 to 20) years, malignant transformation may occur, referred to then as a **malignant mixed**

Figure 15–5 ■

Pleomorphic adenoma. *A,* A well-demarcated tumor in the parotid gland. *B,* Low-power view showing a well-demarcated tumor with normal parotid acini below. *C,* High-power view showing amorphous myxoid stroma resembling cartilage, with interspersed islands and strands of myoepithelial cells. (Courtesy of E. Lee, MD, Department of Pathology, University of Texas Southwestern Medical Center, Dallas.)

salivary gland tumor. Malignancy is less common in the parotid gland (15%) than in the submandibular glands (40%).

Warthin Tumor (Papillary Cystadenoma Lymphomatosum, Cystadenolymphoma). This infrequent benign tumor occurs virtually only in the region of the parotid gland and is thought to represent heterotopic salivary tissue trapped within a regional lymph node during embryogenesis. This tumor is generally a small, well-encapsulated, round to ovoid mass that on transection often reveals mucin-containing cleftlike or cystic spaces within a soft gray background. Microscopically, it exhibits two characteristic features: (1) a two-tiered epithelial layer lining the branching, cystic, or cleftlike spaces; and (2) an immediately subjacent, well-developed lymphoid tissue sometimes forming germinal centers. A recurrence rate of about 10% is attributed to incomplete excision, multicentricity, or a second primary tumor. Malignant transformation is rare; about half of reported cases have had prior radiation exposure.

Esophagus

Lesions of the esophagus run the gamut from bland esophagitis to highly lethal cancers, yet they evoke a similar and remarkably limited range of symptoms. All produce *dysphagia* (difficulty in swallowing), which is attributed either to deranged esophageal motor function or to narrowing or obstruction of the lumen. *Heartburn* (retrosternal burning pain) usually reflects regurgitation of gastric contents into the lower esophagus. Less commonly, *hematemesis* (vomiting of blood) and *melena* (blood in the stools) are evidence of severe inflammation, ulceration, or laceration of the esophageal mucosa. Massive hematemesis may reflect life-threatening rupture of esophageal varices.

ANATOMIC AND MOTOR DISORDERS

Both esophageal anatomy and motor function may be affected secondarily by many esophageal disorders. Anatomic disorders encountered infrequently are summarized in Table 15–2. The more common conditions are described here.

Hiatal Hernia

In hiatal hernia, separation of the diaphragmatic crura and widening of the space between the muscular crura and the esophageal wall permits a dilated segment of the stomach to protrude above the diaphragm. Two anatomic patterns are recognized (Fig. 15–6): the axial, or sliding, hernia and the nonaxial, or paraesophageal, hernia. The *sliding hernia* constitutes 95% of cases; protrusion of the stomach above the diaphragm creates a bell-shaped dilation, bounded below by the diaphragmatic narrowing. In *paraesophageal hernias*, a separate portion of the stomach, usually along the greater curvature, enters the thorax through the widened foramen. The cause of this deranged anatomy is obscure.

On the basis of radiographic studies, hiatal hernias are reported in 1% to 20% of adult subjects, increasing in incidence with age. Only about 9% of these adults, however,

■

Table 15–2.   SELECTED ANATOMIC DISORDERS OF THE ESOPHAGUS

Disorder	Clinical Presentation and Anatomy
Stenosis	Adult with progressive dysphagia to solids and eventually to all foods; a lower esophageal narrowing, which is usually the result of chronic inflammatory disease, including gastroesophageal reflux
Atresia, fistula	Newborn with aspiration, paroxysmal suffocation, pneumonia; esophageal atresia (absence of a lumen) and tracheoesophageal fistula may occur together
Webs, rings	Episodic dysphagia to solid foods; a (presumably) acquired mucosal web or mucosal and submucosal concentric ring partially occluding the esophagus
Diverticula	Episodic food regurgitation, especially nocturnal, sometimes pain is present; an acquired outpouching of the esophageal wall

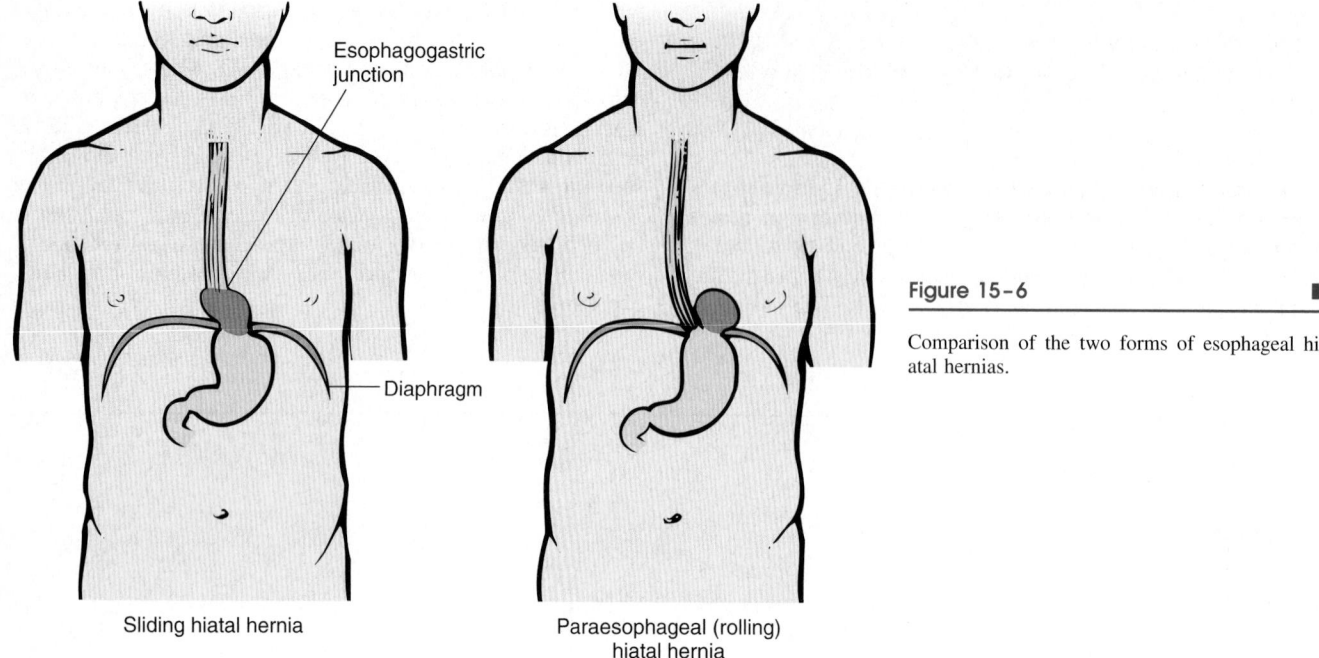

Esophagogastric
junction

Diaphragm

Sliding hiatal hernia

Paraesophageal (rolling)
hiatal hernia

Figure 15-6 ■

Comparison of the two forms of esophageal hiatal hernias.

suffer from heartburn or regurgitation of gastric juices into the mouth. These symptoms more likely result from incompetence of the lower esophageal sphincter than from the hiatal hernia per se and are accentuated by positions favoring reflux (bending forward, lying supine) and obesity. Although most patients with sliding hiatal hernias do not have reflux esophagitis (discussed later), those with severe reflux esophagitis are likely to have a sliding hiatal hernia. Other complications affecting both types of hiatal hernias include mucosal ulceration, bleeding, and even perforation. Paraesophageal hernias rarely induce reflux, but they can become strangulated or obstructed.

Achalasia

The term *achalasia* means "failure to relax" and in the present context denotes incomplete relaxation of the lower esophageal sphincter in response to swallowing. This produces functional obstruction of the esophagus, with consequent dilation of the more proximal esophagus. Manometric studies show three major abnormalities in achalasia: (1) aperistalsis, (2) partial or incomplete relaxation of the lower esophageal sphincter with swallowing, and (3) increased resting tone of the lower esophageal sphincter. It is now generally accepted that in primary achalasia there is loss of intrinsic inhibitory innervation of the lower esophageal sphincter and smooth muscle segment of the esophageal body. Secondary achalasia may arise from pathologic processes that impair esophageal function. The classic example is Chagas disease, caused by *Trypanosoma cruzi*, which causes destruction of the myenteric plexus of the esophagus, duodenum, colon, and ureter. In most instances, however, achalasia occurs as a primary disorder of uncertain etiology. Autoimmunity and previous viral infection have been hypothesized but remain unproven.

In primary achalasia there is progressive dilation of the esophagus above the level of the lower esophageal sphincter. The wall of the esophagus may be of normal thickness, thicker than normal because of hypertrophy of the muscularis, or markedly thinned by dilation. The myenteric ganglia are usually absent from the body of the esophagus but may or may not be reduced in number in the region of the lower esophageal sphincter. Inflammation in the location of the esophageal myenteric plexus is pathognomonic of the disease. Although achalasia is not a mucosal disease, stasis of food may produce mucosal inflammation and ulceration proximal to the lower esophageal sphincter.

Achalasia is characterized clinically by progressive dysphagia and inability to completely convey food to the stomach. Nocturnal regurgitation and aspiration of undigested food may occur. It usually becomes manifest in young adulthood, but it may appear in infancy or childhood. The most serious aspect of this condition is the hazard of developing esophageal squamous cell carcinoma, reported to occur in about 5% of patients and typically at an earlier age than in those without achalasia.

Lacerations (Mallory-Weiss Syndrome)

Longitudinal tears in the esophagus at the esophagogastric junction are termed *Mallory-Weiss tears*. They are encountered in chronic alcoholics after a bout of severe retching or vomiting, but they may also occur during acute illnesses with severe vomiting. The presumed pathogenesis is inadequate relaxation of the musculature of the lower esophageal sphincter during vomiting, with stretching and tearing of the esophagogastric junction at the moment of propulsive expulsion of gastric contents. This thinking is supported by the fact that a hiatal hernia is found in more than 75% of patients with Mallory-Weiss tears. Interestingly, almost half of patients presenting with upper gastrointestinal bleeding attributable to a Mallory-Weiss tear have no antecedent history of nausea, retching, abdominal pain, or vomiting. One must hypothesize that normal variability in intra-abdominal pressure can be transduced through a hiatal hernia, occasionally leading to a Mallory-Weiss tear. Tears may involve only the mucosa or may penetrate the wall. Infection of the defect may lead to an inflammatory ulcer or to mediastinitis.

Esophageal lacerations account for 5% to 10% of upper gastrointestinal bleeding episodes. Most often bleeding is not profuse and ceases without surgical intervention, but life-threatening hematemesis may occur. Even with severe blood loss, supportive therapy with vasoconstrictive medications, transfusions, and sometimes balloon tamponade, is usually all that is required. Healing is usually prompt, with minimal to no residua.

Varices

One of the few potential sites for communication between the intra-abdominal splanchnic circulation and the systemic venous circulation is through the esophagus. When portal venous blood flow into the liver is impeded by cirrhosis or other causes, the resultant portal hypertension induces the formation of collateral bypass channels wherever the portal and systemic systems communicate. Portal blood flow is thereby diverted through the coronary veins of the stomach into the plexus of esophageal subepithelial and submucosal veins, thence into the azygos veins and the superior vena cava. The increased pressure in the esophageal plexus produces dilated tortuous vessels called varices. *Patients with cirrhosis develop varices at a rate of 5% to 15% per year, so that varices are present in approximately two thirds of all cirrhotic patients.* They are most often associated with alcoholic cirrhosis.

Figure 15-7 ■

Esophageal varices: a view of the everted esophagus and gastroesophageal junction, showing dilated submucosal veins (varices). The blue-colored varices have collapsed in this postmortem specimen.

MORPHOLOGY

Varices appear primarily as tortuous dilated veins lying primarily within the submucosa of the distal esophagus and proximal stomach. The net effect is irregular protrusion of the overlying mucosa into the lumen, although varices are collapsed in surgical or postmortem specimens (Fig. 15-7). When the varix is unruptured, the mucosa may be normal, but often it is eroded and inflamed because of its exposed position, further weakening the tissue support of the dilated veins.

Variceal rupture produces massive hemorrhage into the lumen, as well as suffusion of blood into the esophageal wall. Varices produce no symptoms until they rupture. Among patients with advanced cirrhosis of the liver, half the deaths result from rupture of a varix, either as a direct consequence of the hemorrhage or from the hepatic coma triggered by the hemorrhage. However, even when varices are present, they account for less than half of all episodes of hematemesis. Bleeding from concomitant gastritis, peptic ulcer, or esophageal laceration accounts for most of the remainder.

The factors leading to initial rupture of a varix are unclear: silent erosion of overlying thinned mucosa, increased tension in progressively dilated veins, and vomiting with increased intra-abdominal pressure are likely to be involved. One half of patients are found to have coexistent hepatocellular carcinoma, suggesting that a progressive decrease in hepatic functional reserve from tumor growth enhances the likelihood of variceal rupture. Once begun, variceal hemorrhage subsides spontaneously in only 50% of cases; endoscopic injection of thrombotic agents (sclerotherapy) or balloon tamponade is often required. When varices bleed, 20% to 30% of patients die during the first episode. Among those who survive, rebleeding occurs in approximately 70% within 1 year, with a similar rate of mortality for each episode.

ESOPHAGITIS

Injury to the esophageal mucosa with subsequent inflammation is a common condition worldwide. The inflammation may have many origins: prolonged gastric intubation, uremia, ingestion of corrosive or irritant substances, and radiation or chemotherapy, among others. In northern Iran, the prevalence of esophagitis is over 80%; it is also extremely high in regions of China. The basis of this prevalence is unknown. *The overwhelming preponderance of cases in Western countries are attributable to reflux of gastric contents (reflux esophagitis).* Gastroesophageal reflux disease, as it is known clinically, affects about 0.5% of the US adult population and has recurrent heartburn as its dominant symptom. There are many presumed contributory factors:

- Decreased efficacy of esophageal antireflux mechanisms
- Inadequate or slowed esophageal clearance of refluxed material
- The presence of a sliding hiatal hernia
- Increased gastric volume, contributing to the volume of refluxed material
- Impaired reparative capacity of the esophageal mucosa by prolonged exposure to gastric juices

Any one of these influences may assume primacy in an individual case, but more than one is likely to be involved in most instances.

MORPHOLOGY

The anatomic changes depend on the causative agent and on the duration and severity of the exposure. Mild esophagitis may appear macroscopically as simple hyperemia, with virtually no histologic abnormality. In contrast, the mucosa in severe esophagitis exhibits confluent epithelial erosions or total ulceration into the submucosa. Three histologic features are characteristic of uncomplicated **reflux esophagitis** (Fig. 15–8), although only one or two may be present: (1) eosinophils, with or without neutrophils, in the epithelial layer; (2) basal zone hyperplasia; and (3) elongation of lamina propria papillae. Intraepithelial neutrophils are markers of more severe injury.

Clinical Features. The dominant manifestation of reflux disease is heartburn, sometimes accompanied by regurgitation of a sour brash. Rarely, chronic symptoms are punctuated by attacks of severe chest pain mimicking a heart attack. *The severity of symptoms is not related closely to the presence and degree of anatomic esophagitis.* Although largely limited to adults older than age 40, reflux esophagitis

is occasionally seen in infants and children. The potential consequences of severe reflux esophagitis are bleeding, development of stricture, and Barrett esophagus, with its predisposition to malignancy.

BARRETT ESOPHAGUS

Barrett esophagus is a complication of long-standing gastroesophageal reflux, occurring in up to 10% of patients with persistent symptomatic reflux disease, as well as in some patients with asymptomatic reflux. *Barrett esophagus is defined as the replacement of the normal distal stratified squamous mucosa by metaplastic columnar epithelium containing goblet cells.* Prolonged and recurrent gastroesophageal reflux is thought to produce inflammation and eventually ulceration of the squamous epithelial lining. Healing occurs by ingrowth of stem cells and re-epithelialization. In the microenvironment of an abnormally low pH in the distal esophagus caused by acid reflux, the cells differentiate into columnar epithelium. Metaplastic columnar epithelium is thought to be more resistant to injury from refluxing gastric contents. Barrett esophagus affects males more often than females (ratio of 4:1) and is much more common in whites than in other races. Genetic factors are suggested by clustering in families.

Ulcer and stricture may develop as a complication of Barrett esophagus. However, the chief clinical significance of Barrett esophagus relates to the development of adenocarcinoma. Patients with Barrett esophagus have a 30- to 40-fold greater risk of developing esophageal adenocarcinoma compared with normal populations. Hence, periodic screening with esophageal biopsy is recommended for these patients.

MORPHOLOGY

Barrett esophagus is apparent as a salmon-pink, velvety mucosa between the smooth, pale pink esophageal squamous mucosa and the more lush light brown gastric mucosa (Fig. 15–9A). It may exist as tongues extending up from the gastroesophageal junction, as an irregular circumferential band displacing the squamocolumnar junction cephalad, or as isolated patches (islands) in the distal esophagus. The length of the changes is not as important as the presence in the anatomic esophagus of metaplastic mucosa containing goblet cells. **Microscopically, the esophageal squamous epithelium is replaced by metaplastic columnar epithelium,** as depicted in Figure 15–9B. **Barrett mucosa may be quite focal and variable from one site to the next, often necessitating repeated endoscopy and biopsy for definitive diagnosis.** Critical to the pathologic evaluation of patients with Barrett mucosa is the recognition of dysplastic changes in the mucosa that may be precursors of cancer.

Figure 15–8 ■

Reflux esophagitis showing the superficial portion of the mucosa. Numerous eosinophils *(arrows)* are present within the mucosa, and the stratified squamous epithelium has not undergone complete maturation owing to ongoing inflammatory damage.

Figure 15-9 ■

Barrett esophagus. *A,* Endoscopic view showing red velvety gastrointestinal-type mucosa extending from the gastroesophageal orifice. Note paler squamous esophageal mucosa. *B,* Microscopic view showing mixed gastric- and intestine-type columnar epithelial cells in glandular mucosa. (*A,* Courtesy of Dr. F. Farraye, Brigham and Women's Hospital, Boston.)

ESOPHAGEAL CARCINOMA

Benign tumors may arise in the esophagus from both the squamous mucosa and underlying mesenchyme. However, these are overshadowed by cancer of the esophagus, of which there are two types: squamous cell carcinomas and adenocarcinomas. Worldwide, squamous cell carcinomas constitute 90% of esophageal cancers, but in the United States there has been an exponential increase in the incidence of adenocarcinomas associated with Barrett esophagus. Currently, this form of cancer has surpassed squamous cell carcinoma in incidence. In the United States, most cases occur in adults older than the age of 50 with a male-to-female ratio of 3:1. Adenocarcinoma arising in Barrett esophagus is more common in whites than in blacks. By contrast, squamous cell carcinomas

are more common in blacks worldwide. There are striking and puzzling differences in the geographic incidence of esophageal carcinoma. In the United States, there are about 6 new cases per 100,000 population per year, accounting for 1% to 2% of all cancer deaths. In regions of Asia extending from the northern provinces of China to the Caspian littoral in Iran, the prevalence is well over 100 per 100,000, and 20% of cancer deaths are caused by esophageal carcinoma (mainly squamous cell type), with females being affected more often than males. These epidemiologic contrasts must contain causative clues that remain to be deciphered.

Etiology and Pathogenesis. The environmental and dietary factors associated with *squamous cell carcinoma* are presented in Table 15–3. An important contributing factor is retarded passage of food through the esophagus, prolonging mucosal exposure to potential carcinogens such as those contained in tobacco and alcoholic beverages. There is a well-defined predisposing role for chronic esophagitis, itself associated with alcohol and tobacco. However, different influences must underlie the very high incidence of this tumor among the orthodox Moslems of Iran, who neither drink nor smoke. Other environmental factors are invoked, particularly diet, without much direct causal evidence. Strong association with human papillomavirus is noted in high-incidence areas. The role of genetic predisposition is extremely ill defined, but the rare genetic syndrome of tylosis, characterized by excess keratin formation in the skin of the palm and soles, carries an almost certain probability of the development of esophageal cancer. *Barrett esophagus is the only recognized precursor of esophageal adenocarcinoma.*

Links have been drawn between the previously mentioned risk factors and molecular changes. For example, the tumor suppressor gene *TP53* is abnormal in up to 50% of squamous cell carcinomas and is correlated with the use of tobacco and alcohol. The frequency of *TP53* mutations in Barrett esophagus increases with increasing degrees of mucosal dysplasia. Abnormalities affecting the *p16/CDKN2A* tumor suppressor gene are also noted. However, notably infrequent in the esophageal dysplasia-carcinoma sequence are mutations in *K-RAS*, unlike the colorectal adenoma-carcinoma sequence.

■

Table 15-3. RISK FACTORS FOR SQUAMOUS CELL CARCINOMA OF THE ESOPHAGUS

Esophageal Disorders

Long-standing esophagitis
Achalasia
Plummer-Vinson syndrome (esophageal webs, microcytic hypochromic anemia, atrophic glossitis)

Life Style

Alcohol consumption
Tobacco abuse

Dietary

Deficiency of vitamins (A, C, riboflavin, thiamine, pyridoxine)
Deficiency of trace metals (zinc, molybdenum)
Fungal contamination of foodstuffs
High content of nitrites/nitrosamines

Genetic Predisposition

Tylosis (hyperkeratosis of palms and soles)

MORPHOLOGY

Squamous cell carcinomas are usually preceded by a long prodrome of mucosal epithelial dysplasia followed by carcinoma in situ and, ultimately, by the emergence of invasive cancer. Early overt lesions appear as small, gray-white, plaquelike thickenings or elevations of the mucosa. In months to years, these lesions become tumorous, taking one of three forms: (1) polypoid exophytic masses that protrude into the lumen; (2) necrotizing cancerous ulcerations that extend deeply and sometimes erode into the respiratory tree, aorta, or elsewhere (Fig. 15-10); and (3) diffuse infiltrative neoplasms that impart thickening and rigidity to the wall and narrowing of the lumen. Whichever the pattern, about 20% arise in the cervical and upper thoracic esophagus, 50% in the middle third, and 30% in the lower third.

Adenocarcinomas appear to arise from dysplastic mucosa in the setting of Barrett esophagus. Unlike squamous cell carcinomas, they are usually in the distal one third of the esophagus and may invade the subjacent gastric cardia. Initially appearing as flat or raised patches on an otherwise intact mucosa, they may develop into large nodular masses or exhibit deeply ulcerative or diffusely infiltrative features. Microscopically, most tumors are mucin-producing glandular tumors exhibiting intestinal-type features, in keeping with the morphology of the preexisting metaplastic mucosa. The occasional development of tumors of other alimentary cell types supports the concept that Barrett epithelium arises from multipotential cells.

Figure 15-10 ■

Large ulcerated squamous cell carcinoma of the esophagus.

Clinical Features. Esophageal carcinoma is insidious in onset and produces dysphagia and obstruction gradually and late. Weight loss, anorexia, fatigue, and weakness appear, followed by pain, usually related to swallowing. Diagnosis is usually made by imaging techniques and endoscopic biopsy. Because these cancers extensively invade the rich esophageal lymphatic network and adjacent structures, surgical excision rarely is curative. Thus, there is emphasis on routine screening procedures, particularly for those with manifestations of chronic esophagitis or known Barrett esophagus. Esophageal cancer detected when confined to the mucosa or submucosa is amenable to surgical treatment.

■ Stomach

Gastric disorders frequently cause clinical disease, ranging from bland chronic gastritis to the anything but bland gastric carcinoma. Gastric infection with *Helicobacter pylori* represents perhaps the most common gastrointestinal infection. Occasionally, congenital anomalies are encountered, which are summarized in Table 15-4.

In keeping with the limited sensory apparatus of the alimentary tract, gastric disorders give rise to symptoms similar to esophageal disorders, primarily *heartburn* and *vague epigastric pain*. With breach of the gastric mucosa and bleeding, *hematemesis* or *melena* may ensue. Unlike esophageal bleeding, however, blood quickly congeals and turns brown

Table 15-4. CONGENITAL GASTRIC ANOMALIES

Condition	Comment
Pyloric stenosis	1 in 300 to 900 live births Male to female ratio 3:1 Pathology: muscular 　hypertrophy of pyloric 　smooth muscle wall Symptoms: persistent, nonbilious 　projectile vomiting in young 　infant
Diaphragmatic hernia	Rare Pathology: herniation of 　stomach and other abdominal 　contents into thorax through 　a diaphragmatic defect Symptoms: acute respiratory 　embarassment in newborn
Gastric heterotopia	Uncommon Pathology: a nidus of gastric 　mucosa in the esophagus 　or small intestine ("ectopic rest") Symptoms: asymptomatic, 　or an anomalous peptic 　ulcer in adult

in the acid environment of the stomach lumen. Vomited blood hence has the appearance of coffee grounds.

GASTRITS

This diagnosis is both overused and often missed—overused when it is applied loosely to any transient upper abdominal complaint in the absence of validating evidence and missed because most patients with chronic gastritis are asymptomatic. *Gastritis is simply defined as inflammation of the gastric mucosa.* By far the majority of cases are *chronic gastritis*, but occasionally, distinct forms of *acute gastritis* are encountered.

Chronic Gastritis

Chronic gastritis is defined as the presence of chronic mucosal inflammatory changes leading eventually to mucosal atrophy and epithelial metaplasia. It is notable for distinct causal subgroups and for patterns of histologic alterations that vary in different parts of the world. In the Western world, the prevalence of histologic changes indicative of chronic gastritis exceeds 50% in the later decades of adult life.

Pathogenesis. By far the most important etiologic association is chronic infection by the bacillus *Helicobacter pylori* (Fig. 15–11). This organism is a worldwide pathogen that has the highest infection rates in developing countries. Prevalence of infection among adults in Puerto Rico exceeds 80%; American adults older than age 50 exhibit

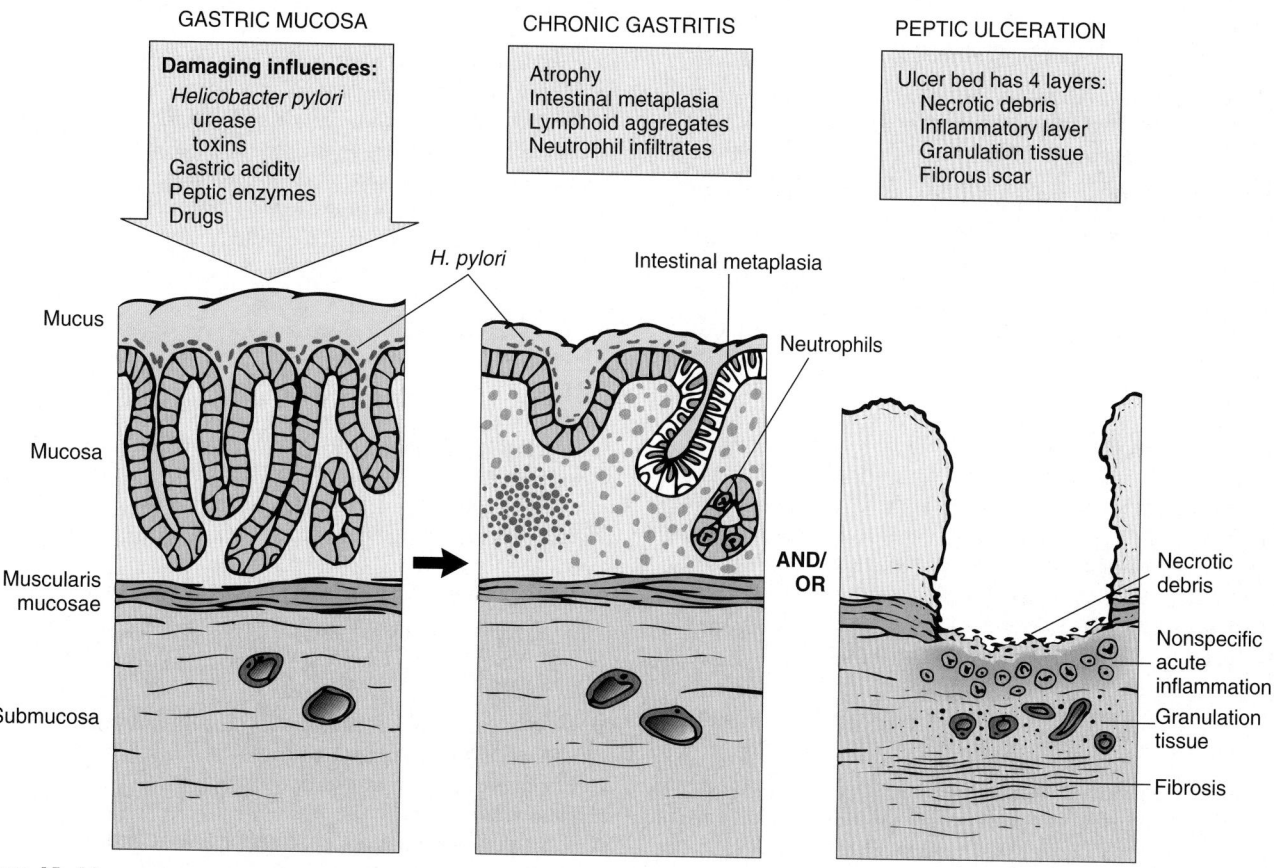

Figure 15-11

Schematic presentation of the presumed action of *Helicobacter pylori* in the development of chronic gastritis and peptic ulceration. The histologic features of the two disease conditions are depicted.

prevalence rates approaching 50%. In areas where the infection is endemic, it seems to be acquired in childhood and persists for decades. Most individuals with the infection also have the associated gastritis but are asymptomatic.

H. pylori is a noninvasive, non–spore-forming, S-shaped gram-negative rod measuring approximately 3.5×0.5 μm. The mechanisms by which *H. pylori* causes tissue injury are discussed in detail in the section on peptic ulcer. Suffice it to say that gastritis develops owing to the combined influence of bacterial enzymes and toxins and release of noxious chemicals by the recruited neutrophils. Patients with chronic gastritis and *H. pylori* usually improve symptomatically when treated with antimicrobial agents and relapses are associated with reappearance of this organism. Improvement in the underlying chronic gastritis may take much longer.

Other forms of chronic gastritis are much less common in the United States. A notable form is *autoimmune gastritis*, which results from autoantibodies to the gastric gland parietal cells, in particular to the acid-producing enzyme H^+,K^+-ATPase. The autoimmune injury leads to gland destruction and mucosal atrophy, with concomitant loss of acid and intrinsic factor production. The resultant deficiency of intrinsic factor leads to pernicious anemia, discussed in Chapter 12. This form of gastritis is seen most often in Scandinavia, in association with other autoimmune disorders such as Hashimoto thyroiditis and Addison disease.

Figure 15-12 ■

Helicobacter pylori gastritis. A Steiner silver stain demonstrates the numerous darkly stained *Helicobacter* organisms along the luminal surface of the gastric epithelial cells. Note that there is no tissue invasion by bacteria.

MORPHOLOGY

Regardless of the cause or histologic distribution of chronic gastritis, the inflammatory changes consist of a lymphocytic and plasma cell infiltrate in the lamina propria, occasionally accompanied by neutrophilic inflammation of the neck region of the mucosal pits. The inflammation may be accompanied by variable gland loss and mucosal atrophy. When present, *H. pylori* organisms are found nestled within the mucus layer overlying the superficial mucosal epithelium (Fig. 15-12). In the autoimmune variant, loss of parietal cells is particularly prominent. Two additional features are of note. **Intestinal metaplasia** refers to the replacement of gastric epithelium with columnar and goblet cells of intestinal variety. This is significant, because gastrointestinal-type carcinomas (see later) appear to arise from **dysplasia** of this metaplastic epithelium. Second, *H. pylori*-induced proliferation of **lymphoid tissue** within the gastric mucosa has been implicated as a precursor of gastric lymphoma.

Clinical Features. Chronic gastritis usually causes few or no symptoms; upper abdominal discomfort and nausea and vomiting can occur. When severe parietal cell loss occurs in the setting of autoimmune gastritis, hypochlorhydria or achlorhydria (referring to levels of gastric luminal hydrochloric acid) and hypergastrinemia are characteristi-

cally present. Individuals with chronic gastritis from other causes may be hypochlorhydric, but because parietal cells are never completely destroyed, these patients do not develop achlorhydria or pernicious anemia. Serum gastrin levels are usually within the normal range or only modestly elevated. Most important is the relationship of chronic gastritis to the development of peptic ulcer and gastric carcinoma. Most patients with a peptic ulcer, whether duodenal or gastric, have *H. pylori* infection. The long-term risk of gastric carcinoma for persons with *H. pylori*–associated chronic gastritis is increased about fivefold relative to the normal population. For autoimmune gastritis, the risk for cancer is in the range of 2% to 4% of affected individuals, which is well above that of the normal population.

Acute Gastritis

Acute gastritis is an acute mucosal inflammatory process, usually of a transient nature. The inflammation may be accompanied by hemorrhage into the mucosa and, in more severe circumstances, by sloughing of the superficial mucosal epithelium *(erosion)*. This severe erosive form of the disease is an important cause of acute gastrointestinal bleeding.

Pathogenesis. The pathogenesis is poorly understood, in part because normal mechanisms for gastric mucosal protection are not totally clear. Acute gastritis is frequently associated with the following:

- Heavy use of nonsteroidal anti-inflammatory drugs (NSAIDs), particularly aspirin
- Excessive alcohol consumption
- Heavy smoking
- Treatment with cancer chemotherapeutic drugs
- Uremia
- Systemic infections (e.g., salmonellosis)
- Severe stress (e.g., trauma, burns, surgery)

- Ischemia and shock
- Suicide attempts with acids and alkali
- Mechanical trauma (e.g., nasogastric intubation)
- After distal gastrectomy with reflux of bilious material

One or more of the following influences are thought to be operative in these varied settings: disruption of the adherent mucous layer, stimulation of acid secretion with hydrogen ion back-diffusion into the superficial epithelium, decreased production of bicarbonate buffer by superficial epithelial cells, reduced mucosal blood flow, and direct damage to the epithelium. Not surprisingly, mucosal insults can act synergistically. Finally, acute infection with *H. pylori* induces neutrophilic inflammation of the gastric mucosa, but this event usually escapes the notice of the patient.

MORPHOLOGY

There is a spectrum of severity ranging from extremely localized (as occurs in NSAID-induced injury) to diffuse and from superficial inflammation to involvement of the entire mucosal thickness with hemorrhage and focal erosions. Concurrent erosion and hemorrhage is readily visible by endoscopy and is termed **acute erosive gastritis**. All variants are marked by mucosal edema and an inflammatory infiltrate of neutrophils and possibly by chronic inflammatory cells. Regenerative replication of epithelial cells in the gastric pits is usually prominent. Provided that the noxious event is short lived, acute gastritis may disappear within days with complete restitution of the normal mucosa.

Clinical Features. Depending on the severity of the anatomic changes, acute gastritis may be entirely asymptomatic, may cause variable epigastric pain with nausea and vomiting, or may present as overt hematemesis, melena, and potentially fatal blood loss. Overall, *it is one of the major causes of hematemesis, particularly in alcoholics.* Even in certain other settings, the condition is quite common; as many as 25% of persons who take daily aspirin for rheumatoid arthritis develop acute gastritis at some time in their course, many with occult or overt bleeding. The risk of gastric bleeding from NSAID-induced gastritis is dose related, thus increasing the likelihood of this complication in patients requiring long-term use of such drugs.

GASTRIC ULCERATION

Ulcers are defined as a breach in the mucosa of the alimentary tract that extends through the muscularis mucosae into the submucosa or deeper. This is to be contrasted to *erosions,* in which there is a breach in the epithelium of the mucosa only. Erosions may heal within days, whereas healing of ulcers takes much longer. Although ulcers may occur anywhere in the alimentary tract, none are as prevalent as the peptic ulcers that occur in the duodenum and stomach.

Peptic Ulcers

Peptic ulcers are chronic, most often solitary, lesions that occur in any portion of the gastrointestinal tract exposed to the aggressive action of acid-peptic juices. At least 98% of peptic ulcers are either in the first portion of the duodenum or in the stomach, in a ratio of about 4:1.

Epidemiology. Peptic ulcers are remitting, relapsing lesions that are most often diagnosed in middle-aged to older adults, but they may first become evident in young adult life. They often appear without obvious precipitating influences and may then heal after a period of weeks to months of active disease. *Even with healing, however, the propensity to develop peptic ulcers remains.* Thus, it is difficult to obtain accurate data on the prevalence of active disease. Best estimates suggest that in the American population, about 2.5% of males and 1.5% of females have peptic ulcers. For both men and women in the United States, the lifetime risk of developing peptic ulcer disease is about 10%.

Genetic or racial influences appear to play little or no role in the causation of peptic ulcers. Duodenal ulcers are more frequent in patients with alcoholic cirrhosis, chronic obstructive pulmonary disease, chronic renal failure, and hyperparathyroidism. With respect to the last two conditions, hypercalcemia, whatever its cause, stimulates gastrin production and, therefore, acid secretion.

Pathogenesis. There are two key facts. First, *the fundamental requisite for peptic ulceration is mucosal exposure to gastric acid and pepsin.* Second, *there is a very strong causal association with H. pylori infection.* Despite the clarity of these two statements, the actual pathogenesis of mucosal ulceration remains murky. It is best perhaps to consider that peptic ulcers are induced by an imbalance between the gastroduodenal mucosal defenses and the countervailing aggressive forces that overcome such defenses, as depicted in Figure 15–13. Both sides of the imbalance are considered.

The array of *host mechanisms* that prevent the gastric mucosa from being digested like a piece of meat include the following:

- Secretion of mucus by surface epithelial cells
- Secretion of bicarbonate into the surface mucus, to create a buffered surface microenvironment
- Secretion of acid- and pepsin-containing fluid from the gastric pits as "jets" through the surface mucus layer, entering the lumen directly without contacting surface epithelial cells
- Rapid gastric epithelial regeneration
- Robust mucosal blood flow, to sweep away hydrogen ions that have back-diffused into the mucosa from the lumen and to sustain the high cellular metabolic and regenerative activity
- Mucosal elaboration of prostaglandins, which help maintain mucosal blood flow

Among the "aggressive forces," *H. pylori* is very important, because this infection is present in 70% to 90% of patients with duodenal ulcers and in about 70% of those with gastric ulcers. Furthermore, antibiotic treatment of *H. pylori*

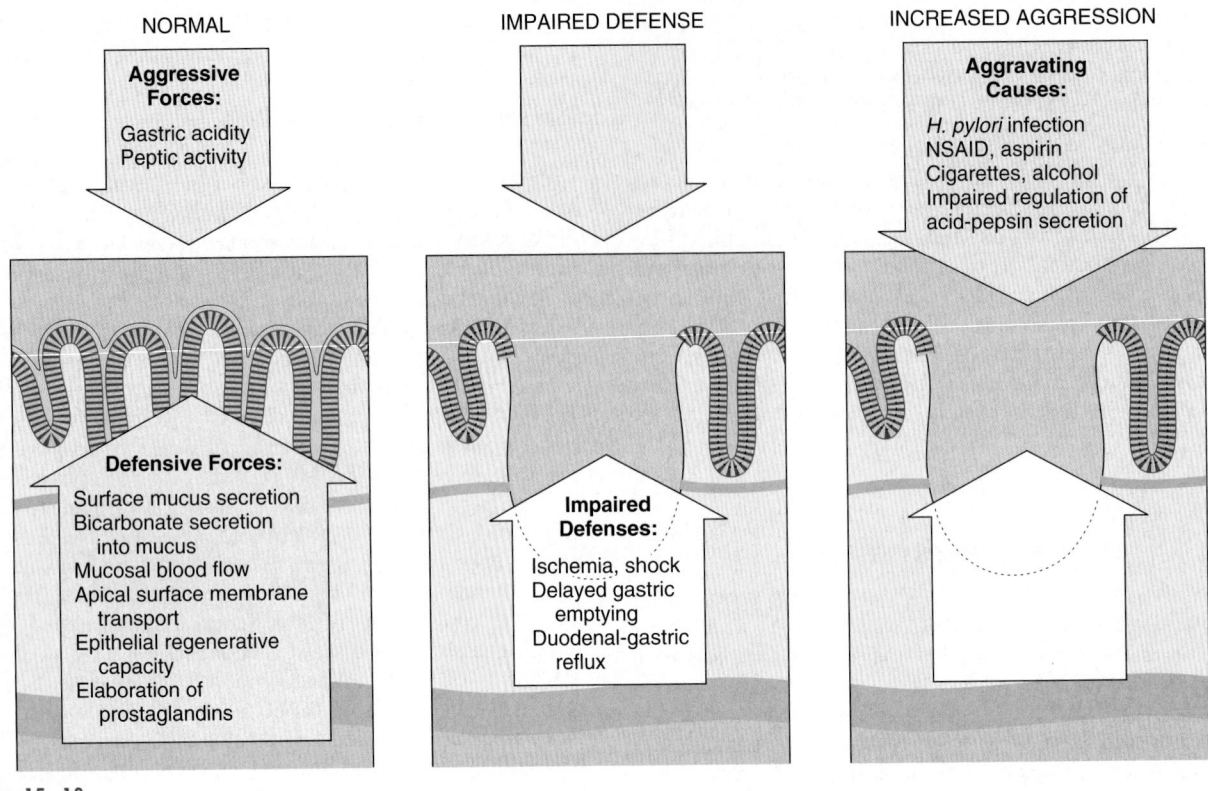

Figure 15-13

Diagram of aggravating causes of, and defense mechanisms against, peptic ulceration.

infection promotes healing of ulcers and tends to prevent their recurrence. Hence, much interest is focused on the possible mechanisms by which this tiny noninvasive spiral organism tips the balance of mucosal defenses. The possible mechanisms are as follows:

■ Although *H. pylori* does not invade the tissues, it induces an intense inflammatory and immune response. There is increased production of proinflammatory cytokines such as interleukin (IL)-1, IL-6, tumor necrosis factor (TNF), and, most notably, IL-8. This cytokine is produced by the mucosal epithelial cells, and it recruits and activates neutrophils.

■ Several bacterial gene products are involved in causing epithelial cell injury and induction of inflammation. *H. pylori* secretes a urease that breaks down urea to form toxic compounds such as ammonium chloride and monochloramine. The organisms also elaborate phospholipases that damage surface epithelial cells. Bacterial proteases and phospholipases break down the glycoprotein-lipid complexes in the gastric mucus, thus weakening the first line of mucosal defense. Epithelial injury is also caused by a vacuolating toxin (VacA). Another toxin, encoded by the cytotoxin-associated gene A (CagA), is a powerful stimulus for the production of IL-8 by the epithelial cells.

■ *H. pylori* enhances gastric acid secretion and impairs duodenal bicarbonate production, thus reducing luminal pH in the duodenum. This altered milieu seems to favor gastric metaplasia (the presence of gastric epithelium) in the first part of the duodenum. Such metaplastic foci provide areas for *H. pylori* colonization.

■ Several *H. pylori* proteins are immunogenic, and they evoke a robust immune response in the mucosa. Both activated T cells and B cells can be seen in chronic gastritis caused by *H. pylori*. The B lymphocytes aggregate to form follicles. The role of T and B cells in causing epithelial injury is not established, but T-cell–driven activation of B cells may be involved in the pathogenesis of gastric lymphomas.

Only 10% to 20% of individuals worldwide infected with *H. pylori* actually develop peptic ulcer. Hence, a key enigma is why most are spared and some are susceptible. Perhaps there are unknown interactions with *H. pylori* and the mucosa that occur only in some individuals. Emerging evidence also strongly implicates bacterial factors. Thus, strains producing VacA and CagA cause more intense tissue inflammation and cytokine production. Recent molecular analyses are beginning to uncover subtle genetic differences between different strains and their pathogenecity. *Suffice it to say that while the link between H. pylori infection and gastric and duodenal ulcers is well established, variability in host-pathogen interactions leading to ulceration remains to be deciphered.*

NSAIDs are the major cause of peptic ulcer disease in patients who do not have *H. pylori* infection. The gastroduodenal effects of NSAIDs range from acute erosive gastritis and acute gastic ulceration to peptic ulceration in 1% to 3% of users. Because NSAIDs are among the most commonly used medications, the magnitude of gastroduodenal toxicity caused by these agents is quite large. Risk factors for NSAID-induced gastroduodenal toxicity are increasing age, higher dose, and prolonged usage. Thus, those who take these drugs for chronic rheumatic conditions are at particularly high risk. Suppression of mucosal prostaglandin synthesis is the key to NSAID-induced peptic ulceration. Inhibition of prostaglandin synthesis increases secretion of hydrochloric acid and reduces bicarbonate and mucin production. Loss of mucin degrades the mucosal barrier that normally prevents acid from reaching the epithelium. Synthesis of glutathione, a free radical scavenger, is also reduced. Some NSAIDs can penetrate the gut mucosal cells as well. By mechanisms not clear, some NSAIDs also impair angiogenesis, thus impeding the healing of ulcers. Whether coexisting *H. pylori* infection affects NSAID-induced ulceration is not entirely settled.

Other events may act alone or in concert with *H. pylori* and NSAIDs to promote peptic ulceration. Cigarette smoking impairs mucosal blood flow and healing. Alcohol has not been proved to directly cause peptic ulceration, but alcoholic cirrhosis is associated with an increased incidence of peptic ulcers. Corticosteroids in high dose and with repeated use promote ulcer formation. Finally, even in the era of *H. pylori*, there are compelling arguments that personality and psychological stress are important contributing factors, although data on cause and effect are lacking.

Finally, mention should be made of the *Zollinger-Ellison syndrome* (Chapter 20). This is associated with multiple peptic ulcerations in the stomach, duodenum, and even jejunum, owing to excess gastrin secretion by a tumor and, hence, excess gastric acid production.

Figure 15-15   ■

Medium-power detail of the base of a nonperforated peptic ulcer, demonstrating the layers of necrosis (N), inflammation (I), granulation tissue (G), and scar (S) moving from the luminal surface at the top to the muscle wall at the bottom.

MORPHOLOGY

All peptic ulcers, whether gastric or duodenal, have an identical gross and microscopic appearance. **By definition, they are defects in the mucosa that penetrate at least into the submucosa, and often into the muscularis propria or deeper. Most are round, sharply punched-out craters 2 to 4 cm in diameter** (Fig. 15-14); those in the duodenum tend to be smaller, and occasional gastric lesions are significantly larger. Favored sites are the anterior and posterior walls of the first portion of the duodenum and the lesser curvature of the stomach. The location within the stomach is dictated by the extent of the associated gastritis: antral gastritis is most common, and the ulcer is often along the lesser curvature at the margin of the inflamed area and the upstream acid-secreting mucosa of the corpus. Occasional gastric ulcers occur on the greater curvature or anterior or posterior walls of the stomach, the very same locations of most ulcerative cancers.

Classically, **the margins of the crater are perpendicular and there is some mild edema of the immediately adjacent mucosa, but unlike ulcerated cancers there is no significant elevation or beading of the edges.** The surrounding mucosal folds may radiate like wheel spokes. The base of the crater appears remarkably clean, owing to peptic digestion of the inflammatory exudate and necrotic tissue. Infrequently, an eroded artery is visible in the ulcer (usually associated with a history of significant bleeding). If the ulcer crater penetrates through the duodenal or gastric wall, a localized or generalized peritonitis may develop. Alternatively, the perforation is sealed by an adjacent structure such as adherent omentum, liver, or pancreas.

The histologic appearance varies with the activity, chronicity, and degree of healing. In a chronic, open ulcer, four zones can be distinguished (Fig. 15-15):

Figure 15-14   ■

Peptic ulcer of the duodenum. Note that the ulcer is small (2 cm) with a sharply punched-out appearance. Unlike cancerous ulcers, the margins are not elevated. The ulcer base shows a small amount of blood but is otherwise clean. Compare with the ulcerated carcinoma in Figure 15-17.

(1) the base and margins have a thin layer of necrotic fibrinoid debris underlain by (2) a zone of active nonspecific inflammatory infiltration with neutrophils predominating, underlain by (3) granulation tissue, deep to which is (4) fibrous, collagenous scar that fans out widely from the margins of the ulcer. Vessels trapped within the scarred area are characteristically thickened and occasionally thrombosed, but in some instances they are widely patent. With healing, the crater fills with granulation tissue, followed by re-epithelialization from the margins and more or less restoration of the normal architecture (hence the prolonged healing times). Extensive fibrous scarring remains.

Chronic gastritis is extremely common among patients with peptic ulcer disease, and *H. pylori* infection is almost always demonstrable in those patients with gastritis. Similarly, patients with NSAID-associated peptic ulcers do not have gastritis unless there is coexistent *H. pylori* infection. This feature is helpful in distinguishing peptic ulcers from acute gastric ulceration (discussed later), because gastritis in adjacent mucosa is generally absent in the latter condition.

Clinical Features. Most peptic ulcers cause epigastric gnawing, burning, or boring pain, but a significant minority first come to light with complications such as hemorrhage or perforation. The pain tends to be worse at night and occurs usually 1 to 3 hours after meals during the day. Classically, the pain is relieved by alkalis or food, but there are many exceptions. Nausea, vomiting, bloating, belching, and significant weight loss (raising the specter of some hidden malignancy) are additional manifestations.

Bleeding is the chief complication, occurring in up to one third of patients, and may be life-threatening. Perforation occurs in far fewer patients but accounts for the greater portion of the 3000 deaths from this disease per year in the United States. Obstruction of the pyloric channel is rare. Malignant transformation is unknown with duodenal ulcers and is very rare with gastric ulcers. The latter event is always open to the possibility that carcinoma was present from the outset.

Peptic ulcers are notoriously chronic, recurrent lesions—they more often impair the quality of life than shorten it. When untreated, the average individual requires 15 years for healing of a peptic ulcer. Nevertheless, with present-day therapies (including antibiotics active against *H. pylori*), most ulcer victims can be helped if not cured, and they usually escape the surgeon's knife.

Acute Gastric Ulceration

Focal, acutely developing gastric mucosal defects may appear after severe stress and are designated *stress ulcers*. Generally, there are multiple lesions located mainly in the stomach and occasionally in the duodenum. Stress ulcers are most commonly encountered in the following conditions:

■ Severe trauma, including major surgical procedures, sepsis, or grave illness of any type

■ Extensive burns (the ulcers are then referred to as Curling ulcers)
■ Traumatic or surgical injury to the central nervous system or an intracerebral hemorrhage (the ulcers are then called Cushing ulcers)
■ Chronic exposure to gastric irritant drugs, particularly NSAIDs and corticosteroids

The pathogenesis of these lesions is uncertain and may vary with the setting. The systemic acidosis that can accompany severe trauma and burns, for example, may contribute to mucosal compromise presumably by lowering the intracellular pH of mucosal cells already rendered hypoxic by impaired mucosal blood flow. With cranial lesions, direct stimulation of vagal nuclei by increased intracranial pressure is proposed, because gastric acid hypersecretion has been documented in these patients.

MORPHOLOGY

Acute stress ulcers are usually circular and small (less than 1 cm in diameter). The ulcer base is frequently stained a dark brown by the acid digestion of extruded blood. Unlike chronic peptic ulcers, acute stress ulcers are found anywhere in the stomach. They may occur singly, but more often they are multiple, located throughout the stomach and duodenum (Fig. 15-16). Microscopically, acute stress ulcers are abrupt lesions, with essentially unremarkable adjacent mucosa. They range in depth from very superficial lesions (erosion) to deeper lesions that involve the entire mucosal thickness (true ulceration). The shallow erosions are, in essence, an extension of acute erosive gastritis. The deeper lesions comprise well-defined ulcerations but are not precursors of chronic peptic ulcers. Even the deeper lesions do not penetrate the muscularis propria.

Clinical Features. A high percentage of patients admitted to hospital intensive care units with sepsis, severe

Figure 15-16 ■

Multiple stress ulcers of the stomach, highlighted by the dark digested blood in their bases.

burns, or trauma acutely develop superficial gastric erosions or ulcers. These may be of limited clinical consequence or life-threatening. Although prophylactic antacid regimens and blood transfusions may blunt the impact of stress ulceration, the single most important determinant of clinical outcome is the ability to correct the underlying condition. The gastric mucosa can recover completely if the patient does not die from the primary disease.

TUMORS

As with the remainder of the gastrointestinal tract, tumors arising from the mucosa predominate over mesenchymal tumors. These are broadly classified into polyps and carcinoma.

Gastric Polyps

The term "polyp" is applied to any nodule or mass that projects above the level of the surrounding mucosa. Occasionally, a lipoma or leiomyoma arising in the wall of the stomach may protrude from under the mucosa to produce an apparent polypoid lesion. However, the use of the term "polyp" in the gastrointestinal tract is generally restricted to mass lesions arising in the mucosa. Gastric polyps are uncommon and are found in about 0.4% of adult autopsies, as compared with colonic polyps, which are seen in 25% to 50% of older persons. In the stomach, these lesions are most frequently (1) hyperplastic polyps (80% to 85%), (2) fundic gland polyps (about 10%), and (3) adenomatous polyps (about 5%). All three types arise in the setting of chronic gastritis and so are seen in the same patient populations. Hyperplastic and fundic gland polyps are essentially innocuous. In contrast, there is a definite risk of an adenomatous polyp harboring adenocarcinoma, which increases with polyp size.

MORPHOLOGY

Hyperplastic polyps arise from an exuberant reparative response to chronic mucosal damage and hence are composed of a hyperplastic mucosal epithelium and an inflamed edematous stroma. They are not true neoplasms. Fundic gland polyps are small collections of dilated corpus-type glands thought to be small hamartomas. On the other hand, the less common adenomas contain dysplastic epithelium. As with colonic adenomas, to be described later, adenomas are true neoplasms.

Gastric Carcinoma

Among the malignant tumors that occur in the stomach, carcinoma is overwhelmingly the most important and the most common (90% to 95%). Next in order of frequency are lymphomas and carcinoids (4% and 3%, respectively, discussed later in this chapter) and mesenchymal spindle cell tumors (2%).

Epidemiology and Classification. Gastric carcinoma is a worldwide disease with a widely varying incidence. Japan, Colombia, Costa Rica, and Hungary have a particularly high incidence. Nevertheless, in most countries there has been a steady decline in both the incidence and the mortality of gastric cancer. Yet it remains among the leading killer cancers, representing 3% of all cancer deaths in the United States. This is attributable to its discouraging 5-year survival rate, which remains at less than 20%.

Gastric cancers exhibit two morphologic types, denoted *intestinal* and *diffuse*. The *intestinal variant* is thought to arise from gastric mucous cells that have undergone intestinal metaplasia in the setting of chronic gastritis. This pattern of cancer tends to be better differentiated and is the more common type in high-risk populations. *Intestinal-type carcinoma is the pattern that is progressively diminishing in frequency in the United States.* In contrast, the *diffuse variant* is thought to arise de novo from native gastric mucous cells, is not associated with chronic gastritis, and tends to be poorly differentiated. Most importantly, diffuse gastric carcinoma has not significantly changed in frequency in the past 60 years and now constitutes approximately half of gastric carcinomas in the United States. Whereas the intestinal-type carcinoma occurs primarily after age 50 years with a 2:1 male predominance, the diffuse carcinoma occurs at an earlier age with no male predominance. It would almost appear that there are two quite distinct forms of gastric carcinoma.

Pathogenesis. The major factors thought to affect the genesis of this form of cancer are environmental, as summarized in Table 15–5. Several points are worthy of emphasis. Risk factors for the increasingly more common diffuse carcinoma are largely unknown, although germ-line mutations in E-cadherin leading to an autosomal dominant inheritance of diffuse gastric carcinoma have been reported. The predisposing influences for the intestinal-type adenocarcinoma are many, but their relative importance is changing. For example, dietary factors have changed drastically in recent years with the increased use of refrigeration worldwide, markedly decreasing

Table 15–5. RISK FACTORS FOR GASTRIC CARCINOMA

Intestinal-Type Adenocarcinoma

Diet
  Nitrites derived from nitrates (found in food and drinking water, and used as preservatives in prepared meats) may undergo nitrosation to form nitrosamines and nitrosamides
  Smoked foods and pickled vegetables
  Excessive salt intake
  Decreased intake of fresh vegetables and fruits: antioxidants present in these foods may be protective by inhibition of nitrosation
Chronic gastritis with intestinal metaplasia
  Infection with *Helicobacter pylori*
  Pernicious anemia
Altered anatomy
  After subtotal distal gastrectomy

Diffuse Carcinoma

Risk factors undefined, except for a rare inherited mutation of E-cadherin
Infection with *Helicobacter pylori* and chronic gastritis often absent

the need for food preservation by the use of nitrates, smoking, and salt. Chronic gastritis associated with *H. pylori* infection remains a major risk factor for gastric carcinoma. A recent prospective study from Japan has underscored the relationship between *H. pylori* infection and gastric cancer. The risk is particularly high in those with chronic gastritis limited to the gastric antrum. These patients develop severe gastric atrophy, intestinal metaplasia, and ultimately dysplasia and cancer. Of note, patients with *H. pylori*–associated duodenal ulcers are largely protected from developing gastric cancer. The mechanism by which *H. pylori* causes neoplastic transformation is not entirely clear. Perhaps chronic inflammation generates DNA-damaging free radicals, and the resulting mutations lead to hyperproliferation that is not balanced by apoptosis. Much remains to be known.

Figure 15–17 ■

Ulcerative gastric carcinoma. The ulcer is large with irregular, heaped-up margins. There is extensive excavation of the gastric mucosa with a necrotic gray area in the deepest portion. Compare with the benign peptic ulcer in Figure 15–14.

MORPHOLOGY

The location of gastric carcinomas within the stomach is as follows: pylorus and antrum, 50% to 60%; cardia, 25%; and the remainder in the body and fundus. The lesser curvature is involved in about 40% and the greater curvature in 12%. **Thus, a favored location is the lesser curvature of the antropyloric region.** Although less frequent, an ulcerative lesion on the greater curvature is more likely to be malignant.

Gastric carcinoma is classified on the basis of depth of invasion, macroscopic growth pattern, and histologic subtype. The morphologic feature having the greatest impact on clinical outcome is the **depth of invasion. Early gastric carcinoma is defined as a lesion confined to the mucosa and submucosa, regardless of the presence or absence of perigastric lymph node metastases. Advanced gastric carcinoma is a neoplasm that has extended below the submucosa into the muscular wall** and has perhaps spread more widely. Gastric mucosal **dysplasia** is the presumed precursor lesion of early gastric cancer, which then in turn progresses to "advanced" lesions.

The three macroscopic growth patterns of gastric carcinoma, which may be evident at both the early and advanced stages, are (1) **exophytic,** with protrusion of a tumor mass into the lumen; (2) **flat or depressed,** in which there is no obvious tumor mass within the mucosa; and (3) **excavated,** whereby a shallow or deeply erosive crater is present in the wall of the stomach. Exophytic tumors may contain portions of an adenoma. Flat or depressed malignancy presents only as regional effacement of the normal surface mucosal pattern. Excavated cancers may mimic, in size and appearance, chronic peptic ulcers, although more advanced cases exhibit heaped-up margins (Fig. 15–17). Uncommonly, a broad region of the gastric wall, or the entire stomach, is extensively infiltrated by malignancy. The rigid and thickened stomach is termed a *leather bottle stomach,* or **linitis plastica;**
metastatic carcinoma from the breast and lung may generate a similar picture.

The histologic appearances of gastric cancer have been variously subclassified, but the two most important types are the intestinal type and diffuse type (Fig. 15–18). The **intestinal variant** is composed of malignant cells forming neoplastic intestinal glands resembling those of colonic adenocarcinoma. The **diffuse variant** is composed of gastric-type mucous cells that generally do not form glands but rather permeate the mucosa and wall as scattered individual "signet-ring" cells or small clusters in an "infiltrative" growth pattern.

Whatever the histologic variant, all gastric carcinomas eventually penetrate the wall to involve the serosa, spread to regional and more distant lymph nodes, and metastasize widely. For obscure reasons, the earliest lymph node metastasis may sometimes involve a supraclavicular lymph node (Virchow's node). Another somewhat unusual mode of intraperitoneal spread in females is to both the ovaries, giving rise to the so-called **Krukenberg tumor** (Chapter 19).

Clinical Features. Early gastric carcinoma is generally asymptomatic and can be discovered only by repeated endoscopic examinations in persons at high risk, as is the practice in Japan. Advanced carcinoma also may be asymptomatic, but it often first comes to light because of abdominal discomfort or weight loss. Uncommonly, these neoplasms cause dysphagia when they are located in the cardia or obstructive symptoms when they arise in the pyloric canal. The only hope for cure is early detection and surgical removal, because the most important prognostic indicator is stage of the tumor at the time of resection.

Figure 15–18   ■

Gastric cancer. *A,* Intestinal type demonstrating gland formation by malignant cells, which are invading the muscular wall of the stomach. (H & E.) *B,* Diffuse type demonstrating individual red, mucin-containing malignant cells in the lamina propria of an intact mucosa. (Mucicarmine stain.)

Small and Large Intestines

Many conditions, such as infections, inflammatory diseases, and tumors, affect both the small and large intestines. These two organs are therefore considered together. Collectively, disorders of the intestines account for a large portion of human disease.

DEVELOPMENTAL ANOMALIES

These deviations from the norm are uncommon, but sometimes dramatic, sources of clinical disease. In the small intestine the major anomalies are as follows:

■ *Atresia or stenosis*, the former being complete failure of development of the intestinal lumen and the latter representing only narrowing. Both defects usually involve only a segment of bowel.
■ *Duplication* usually takes the form of well-formed saccular to tubular cystic structures, which may or may not communicate with the lumen of the small intestine.
■ *Meckel diverticulum* is the most common and innocuous of the anomalies. It results from failure of involution of the omphalomesenteric duct, leaving a persistent blind-ended tubular protrusion up to 5 to 6 cm long (Fig. 15–19). The diameter is variable, sometimes approximating that of the

small intestine itself. Such diverticula are usually in the ileum within about 2 feet (85 cm) of the cecum and are composed of all layers of the normal small intestine. They generally are asymptomatic, except when they permit

Figure 15–19   ■

Meckel diverticulum. The blind pouch is located on the antimesenteric side of the small bowel.

bacterial overgrowth that depletes vitamin B_{12}, producing a syndrome similar to pernicious anemia. Rarely, pancreatic rests are found in a Meckel diverticulum, and in about half of the cases there are heterotopic islands of functioning gastric mucosa. Peptic ulceration in the adjacent intestinal mucosa sometimes is responsible for mysterious intestinal bleeding or symptoms resembling acute appendicitis.

■ In *omphalocele*, a congenital defect of the periumbilical abdominal wall leaves behind a membranous sac, into which the intestines herniate.

In the *large intestine*, the major anomalies are

■ *Malrotation* of the developing bowel, preventing the intestines from assuming their normal intra-abdominal positions. The cecum, for example, may be found anywhere in the abdomen, including the left upper quadrant, rather than in its normal position in the right lower quadrant. The large intestine is predisposed to volvulus (discussed later). Confusing clinical syndromes may arise when appendicitis presents as left upper quadrant pain.

■ *Hirschsprung disease*, leading to congenital megacolon.

Hirschsprung Disease: Congenital Megacolon

Distention of the colon to greater than 6 or 7 cm in diameter (megacolon) occurs as a congenital and as an acquired disorder. Hirschsprung disease (congenital megacolon) results when, during development, the caudad migration of neural crest–derived cells along the alimentary tract arrests at some point before reaching the anus. Hence, an aganglionic segment is left that lacks both the Meissner submucosal and Auerbach myenteric plexuses. This causes functional obstruction and progressive distention of the colon proximal to the affected segment. In most instances, only the rectum and sigmoid are aganglionic, but in about a fifth of cases a longer segment, and rarely the entire colon, is affected.

Genetically, Hirschsprung disease is heterogeneous, and several different defects that lead to the same outcome have been identified. Approximately 50% of cases result from mutations in *RET* gene and RET ligands, as this signaling pathway is required for development of the myenteric nerve plexus. Many of the remaining cases arise from mutations in endothelin 3 and endothelin receptors. Hirschsprung disease occurs in approximately 1 in 5000 to 8000 live births; it predominates in males in a ratio of 4:1. It is much more frequent in those with other congenital anomalies such as hydrocephalus, ventricular septal defect, and Meckel diverticulum.

MORPHOLOGY

The critical lesion is the lack of ganglion cells, and of ganglia, in the muscle wall and submucosa of the affected segment. The affected segment is not distended—it is the up-stream, properly innervated segment that undergoes dilation. Thus, when only the distal colon is affected, the remainder of the colon becomes massively distended, sometimes achieving a diameter of 15 to 20 cm. The wall may be thinned by distention or in some cases is thickened by compensatory muscle hypertrophy. The mucosal lining of the distended portion may be intact or have shallow, so-called **stercoral** ulcers produced by impacted, inspissated feces.

Clinical Features. In most cases a delay occurs in the initial passage of meconium, which is followed by vomiting in 48 to 72 hours. When a very short distal segment of the rectum alone is involved, the obstruction may not be complete and may not produce manifestations until later in infancy, in the form of alternating periods of obstruction and passage of diarrheal stools. The principal threat to life is superimposed enterocolitis with fluid and electrolyte disturbances. More rarely, the distended colon perforates, usually in the thin-walled cecum. The diagnosis is established by documenting the absence of ganglion cells in the nondistended bowel segment.

Acquired megacolon may result from (1) Chagas disease, in which the trypanosomes directly invade the bowel wall to destroy the plexuses, (2) organic obstruction of the bowel by a neoplasm or inflammatory stricture, (3) toxic megacolon complicating ulcerative colitis or Crohn disease (discussed later), or (4) a functional psychosomatic disorder. Except for the trypanosomal Chagas disease, in which the inflammatory involvement of the ganglia is evident, the remaining forms of megacolon are not associated with any deficiency of mural ganglia.

VASCULAR DISORDERS

Ischemic Bowel Disease

Ischemic lesions may be restricted to the small or large intestine or may affect both, depending on the particular vessel or vessels involved. Acute occlusion of one of the three major supply trunks of the intestines—celiac, superior, and inferior mesenteric arteries—may lead to infarction of extensive segments of intestine. However, insidious loss of one vessel may be without effect, owing to the rich anastomotic interconnections between the vascular beds. Lesions within the end-arteries that penetrate the gut wall produce small, focal ischemic lesions. As illustrated in Figure 15–20, the severity of injury ranges from *transmural infarction* of the gut, involving all visceral layers, to *mural infarction* of the mucosa and submucosa, sparing the muscular wall, to *mucosal infarction*, if the lesion extends no deeper than the muscularis mucosae.

Almost always, transmural infarction implies acute occlusion of a major mesenteric artery. Mural or mucosal infarction more often results from either physiologic hypoperfusion or more localized anatomic defects and may be acute or chronic. Mesenteric venous thrombosis is a less frequent cause of vascular compromise. The predis-

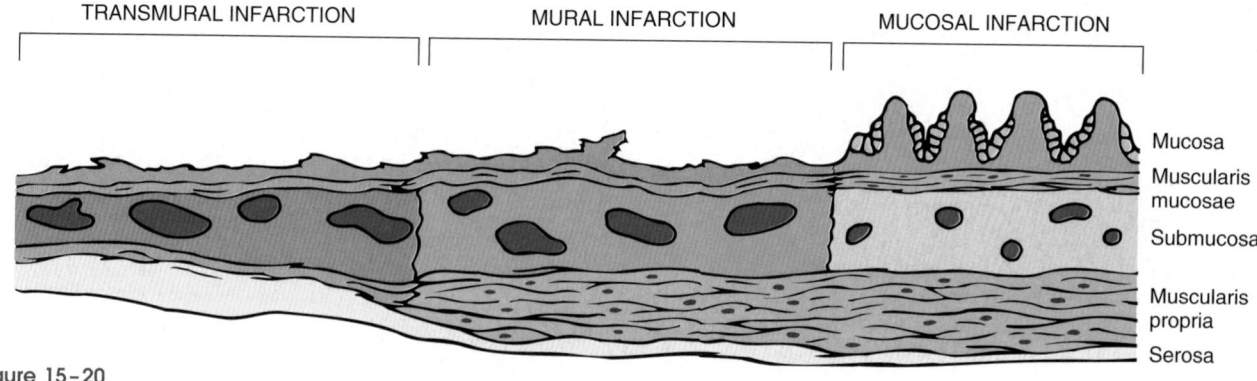

Figure 15-20

Acute ischemic bowel disease. Schematic of the three levels of severity, diagrammed for the small intestine.

posing conditions for all three forms of ischemia are as follows:

■ *Arterial thrombosis:* severe atherosclerosis (usually at the origin of the mesenteric vessel), systemic vasculitis, dissecting aneurysm, angiographic procedures, aortic reconstructive surgery, surgical accidents, hypercoagulable states, and oral contraceptives

■ *Arterial embolism:* cardiac vegetations (as with endocarditis, or myocardial infarction with mural thrombosis), angiographic procedures, and aortic atheroembolism

■ *Venous thrombosis:* hypercoagulable states induced, for example, by oral contraceptives or antithrombin III deficiency, intraperitoneal sepsis, the postoperative state, vascular-invasive neoplasms (particularly hepatocellular carcinoma), cirrhosis, and abdominal trauma

■ *Nonocclusive ischemia:* cardiac failure, shock, dehydration, vasoconstrictive drugs (e.g., digitalis, vasopressin, propranolol)

■ *Miscellaneous:* radiation injury, volvulus, stricture, and internal or external herniation

MORPHOLOGY

Transmural intestinal infarction may involve a short or long segment, depending on the particular vessel affected and the patency of the anastomotic supply. Whether the occlusion is arterial or venous, the infarction always has a dark red hemorrhagic appearance because of reflow of blood into the damaged area (Fig. 15-21). The ischemic injury usually begins in the mucosa and extends outward; within 18 to 24 hours there is a thin, fibrinous exudate over the serosa. With arterial occlusion the demarcation from adjacent normal bowel is fairly sharply defined, but with venous occlusion the margins are less distinct. Histologically, the changes are those that would be anticipated, with marked edema, interstitial hemorrhage, necrosis, and sloughing of the mucosa. Within 24 hours intestinal bacteria produce outright gangrene and sometimes perforation of the bowel.

Mural and mucosal infarctions characteristically are marked by multifocal lesions interspersed with spared areas. Their location depends in part on the extent of preexisting atherosclerotic narrowing of the arterial supply; lesions can be scattered over large regions of the small or large intestines. Affected foci may or may not be visible from the serosal surface, because by definition the ischemia does not affect the entire thickness of the bowel. When the bowel is opened, hemorrhagic edematous thickening of the mucosa, sometimes with superficial ulcerations, is seen. Histologic features are those of acute injury: edema, hemorrhage, and outright necrosis of the affected tissue layers (Fig. 15-22). Inflammation develops at the margins of the lesions, and an inflammatory fibrin-containing exudate **(pseudomembrane),** usually secondary to bacterial superinfection, may coat the affected mucosa. Alternatively, **chronic vascular insufficiency may produce a chronic inflammatory and ulcerative condition, mimicking idiopathic inflammatory bowel disease** (discussed later).

Figure 15-21

Infarcted small bowel, secondary to acute thrombotic occlusion of the superior mesenteric artery.

Figure 15-22 ■

Mucosal infarction of the small bowel. The mucosa is hemorrhagic, and there is no epithelial layer. The remaining layers of the bowel are intact.

Clinical Features. Ischemic bowel injury is most common in the later years of life. With the transmural lesions, there is the sudden onset of abdominal pain, often out of proportion to the physical signs. Sometimes the pain is accompanied by bloody diarrhea. The onset of pain tends to be more sudden with mesenteric embolism than with arterial or venous thrombosis. Because this condition may progress to shock and vascular collapse within hours, the diagnosis must be made promptly, and making it requires a high index of suspicion in the appropriate setting (e.g., recent major abdominal surgery, recent myocardial infarction, atrial fibrillation, or manifestations suggestive of some form of vegetative endocarditis). The mortality rate with infarction of the bowel approaches 90%, largely because the window of time between onset of symptoms and perforation caused by gangrene is so small.

In contrast, mural and mucosal ischemia may appear only as unexplained abdominal distention or gastrointestinal bleeding, sometimes accompanied by the gradual onset of abdominal pain or discomfort. Suspicion is raised if the patient has experienced conditions that favor acute hypoperfusion of the bowel, such as an episode of severe cardiac decompensation or shock. Mucosal and mural infarction are not by themselves fatal, and, indeed, if the cause or causes of hypoperfusion can be corrected, the lesions may heal.

Angiodysplasia

Tortuous dilations of submucosal and mucosal blood vessels are seen most often in the cecum or right colon, usually only after the sixth decade of life. They are prone to rupture and bleed into the lumen. *Such lesions account for 20% of significant lower intestinal bleeding.* The hemorrhage may be chronic and intermittent and only cause severe anemia, but rarely it is acute and massive.

These lesions sometimes are part of a systemic disorder such as hereditary hemorrhagic telangiectasia (Osler-Weber-Rendu syndrome) or limited scleroderma, sometimes called the CREST syndrome (Chapter 5). Most often, they are isolated lesions thought to develop over decades as the result of mechanical factors operative in the colonic wall. As penetrating veins pass through the muscularis they are subject to intermittent occlusion during peristaltic contractions, but the thicker-walled arteries remain patent, thus producing venous distention and ectasia.

Hemorrhoids

Hemorrhoids are variceal dilations of the anal and perianal submucosal venous plexuses. They are common after age 50 and develop in the setting of persistently elevated venous pressure within the hemorrhoidal plexus. Common predisposing conditions are straining at stool in the setting of chronic constipation and the venous stasis of pregnancy in younger women. More rarely, hemorrhoids may reflect portal hypertension, usually resulting from cirrhosis of the liver (Chapter 16).

Varicosities in the superior and middle hemorrhoidal veins appear above the anorectal line and are covered by rectal mucosa *(internal hemorrhoids)*. Those that appear below the anorectal line represent dilations of the inferior hemorrhoidal plexus and are covered by anal mucosa *(external hemorrhoids)*. Both are thin-walled, dilated vessels that commonly bleed, sometimes masking bleeding from far more serious proximal lesions. They may become thrombosed, particularly when subject to trauma from passage of stool. Finally, internal hemorrhoids may prolapse during straining at stool and then become trapped by the compressive anal sphincter, leading to sudden, extremely painful, edematous hemorrhagic enlargement or strangulation.

DIARRHEAL DISEASES

Diarrheal diseases of the bowel make up a veritable Augean stable of entities. Many are caused by microbiologic agents; others arise in the setting of malabsorptive disorders and idiopathic inflammatory bowel disease (discussed in a subsequent section). Consideration will first be given to the conditions known as *diarrhea* and *dysentery*.

Diarrhea and Dysentery

Although a precise definition of diarrhea is elusive, an increase in stool mass, stool frequency, or stool fluidity is perceived as diarrhea by most patients. For many individuals, this consists of daily stool production in excess of 250 g, containing 70% to 95% water. Over 14 L/day of fluid may be lost in severe cases of diarrhea, equivalent to the circulating blood volume! Diarrhea is often accompanied by pain, urgency, perianal discomfort, and incontinence. *Low-volume, painful, bloody diarrhea is known as dysentery.*

Diarrheal disorders are categorized as follows:

■ *Secretory diarrhea:* net intestinal fluid secretion that is isotonic with plasma and persists during fasting
■ *Osmotic diarrhea:* excessive osmotic forces exerted by luminal solutes that abate with fasting

Table 15-6. MAJOR CAUSES OF DIARRHEAL ILLNESSES

Secretory Diarrhea

Infectious: viral damage to surface epithelium
   Rotavirus
   Norwalk virus
   Enteric adenoviruses
Infectious: enterotoxin-mediated
   Vibrio cholerae
   Escherichia coli
   Bacillus cereus
   Clostridium perfringens
Neoplastic: tumor elaboration of peptides or serotonin
Excessive laxative use

Osmotic Diarrhea

Lactulose therapy (for hepatic encephalopathy, constipation)
Prescribed gut lavage for diagnostic procedures
Antacids ($MgSO_4$ and other magnesium salts)

Exudative Diseases

Infectious: destruction of the epithelial layer
   Shigella spp.
   Salmonella spp.
   Campylobacter spp.
   Entamoeba histolytica
Idiopathic inflammatory bowel disease

Malabsorption

Defective intraluminal digestion
Defective mucosal cell absorption
Reduced small intestinal surface area
Lymphatic obstruction
Infectious: impaired mucosal cell absorption
   Giardia lamblia

Deranged Motility

Decreased intestinal retention time
   Surgical reduction of gut length
   Neural dysfunction, including irritable bowel syndrome
   Hyperthyroidism
Decreased motility (increased intestinal retention time)
   Surgical creation of a "blind" intestinal loop
   Bacterial overgrowth in the small intestine

■ *Exudative diseases:* output of purulent, bloody stools that persists on fasting; stools are frequent but may be small or large volume
■ *Malabsorption:* output of voluminous, bulky stools with increased osmolarity owing to unabsorbed nutrients and excess fat (steatorrhea); it usually abates on fasting
■ *Deranged motility:* highly variable features regarding stool output, volume, and consistency; other forms of diarrhea must be excluded

The major causes of diarrhea are presented in Table 15-6; selected entities are discussed here. It is important to bear in mind that multiple mechanisms may be operative in the same patient.

Infectious Enterocolitis

Intestinal diseases of microbial origin are marked principally by diarrhea and sometimes by ulceroinflammatory changes in the small or large intestine. *Infectious enterocolitis is a global problem of staggering proportions, causing 2.9 million deaths annually worldwide and accounting for up to one half of deaths in children younger than 5 years of age in some countries.* Although far less prevalent in industrialized nations, infectious enterocolitis is still responsible for approximately 1.5 episodes of diarrhea per person (child and adult) per year, second only to the common cold in frequency. About 500 infants and young children die of diarrheal disease annually in the United States. Moreover, the most common health problem encountered by the more than 300 million people who travel internationally per year is diarrhea.

Among the most common offenders are rotavirus, caliciviruses, and enterotoxigenic *Escherichia coli*. However, many pathogens can cause diarrhea; the major offenders vary with the age, nutrition, and immune status of the host, environment (living conditions, public health measures), and special predispositions such as foreign travel, exposure to more virulent organisms while hospitalized, and wartime dislocation. In 40% to 50% of cases, the specific agent cannot be isolated.

Worldwide, intestinal parasitic disease and protozoal infections are also major causes of chronic or recurrent infectious enterocolitis. Collectively, they affect more than one half of the world's population, because they are endemic in less developed nations. Of the various lower alimentary tract infections, only selected examples are described here.

Viral Gastroenteritis. At the very least, viral infection of superficial epithelium in the small intestine destroys these cells and their absorptive function. Repopulation of the small intestinal villi with immature enterocytes and relative preservation of crypt secretory cells leads to net secretion of water and electrolytes, compounded by an osmotic diarrhea from incompletely absorbed nutrients. Recent evidence indicates that intrinsic viral factors such as the nonstructural protein 4 (NSP4) of rotavirus may have a direct diarrheal effect, occurring before destruction of enterocytes by viral virulence factors.

Symptomatic disease is caused by several distinct groups of viruses:

■ *Rotavirus* accounts for an estimated 130 million cases and 0.9 million deaths worldwide per year. The affected population is children 6 to 24 months of age; spread is by fecal-oral contamination.
■ *Caliciviruses* are responsible for most cases of nonbacterial foodborne epidemic gastroenteritis in older children and adults. Infection in young children is unusual. These were previously referred to as the Norwalk family of viruses.
■ Additional viruses accounting for infectious diarrhea in children, almost always by person-to-person contact, include several subtypes of *adenovirus* (Ad40 and Ad41) and *astrovirus.*

Bacterial Enterocolitis. Several mechanisms underlying bacterial diarrheal illness were discussed briefly in Chapter 9 but are worthy of emphasis at this time:

■ *Ingestion of preformed toxin*, present in contaminated food. Major offenders of food poisoning are *Staphylococcus aureus*, *Vibrio* species, and *Clostridium perfringens*. One may also ingest preformed neurotoxins, exemplified by *Clostridium botulinum.*
■ *Infection by toxigenic organisms*, which proliferate within the gut lumen and elaborate an enterotoxin.

■ *Infection by enteroinvasive organisms*, which proliferate, invade, and destroy mucosal epithelial cells.

The latter two mechanisms involve bona fide bacterial replication in the gut and depend on three key bacterial properties:

1. *The ability to adhere to the mucosal epithelial cells.* To produce disease, ingested organisms must adhere to the mucosa; otherwise they are swept away by the fluid stream. Adherence is often mediated by plasmid-coded *adhesins*—rigid, wiry proteins expressed on the surface of the organism.
2. *The ability to elaborate enterotoxins.* Enterotoxigenic organisms produce polypeptides that cause diarrhea. The polypeptides may be secretagogues, which activate secretion without inducing cell damage; cholera toxin, elaborated by *Vibrio cholerae*, is the prototype toxin of this type. Alternatively, they may be cytotoxins, which cause direct epithelial cell necrosis, as exemplified by Shiga toxin.
3. *The capacity to invade.* Enteroinvasive organisms such as *Shigella* possess a large virulence plasmid that confers the capacity for epithelial cell invasion. This is followed by intracellular proliferation, cell lysis, and cell-to-cell spread. Other organisms such as *Salmonella typhi* and *Yersinia enterocolitica* pass through mucosal epithelial cells en route to lymphatics and the bloodstream.

The major bacteria giving rise to *bacterial enterocolitis* are presented in Table 15–7.

MORPHOLOGY

Given the multitude of bacterial pathogens, the pathologic manifestations of small intestinal and colonic bacterial disease are quite variable. **Most bacterial infections exhibit a general nonspecific pattern of damage to the surface epithelium, with an increased mitotic rate in mucosal crypts and decreased maturation of surface epithelial cells. There follows hyperemia and edema of the lamina propria and variable neutrophilic infiltration into the lamina propria and epithelial layer.** In more severe infections with cytotoxin-producing or enteroinvasive bacteria, progressive destruction of the mucosa leads to erosion, ulceration, and severe submucosal inflammation. Notable features of particular infections include the following:

■ *Escherichia coli* (a particularly versatile organism):

  ■ Enterotoxigenic strains (ETEC) affect the small intestine, with histologic features similar to *Vibrio cholerae* (described later).
  ■ The Shiga toxin–producing strain (STEC) O157:H7 produces most severe disease in the right colon, with hemorrhage and ulceration.
  ■ Enteropathogenic strains (EPEC) affect the small intestine, producing villus blunting.

Table 15–7. MAJOR CAUSES OF BACTERIAL ENTEROCOLITIS

Organism	Pathogenic Mechanism	Source	Clinical Features
Escherichia coli			Traveler's diarrhea, including:
ETEC	Cholera-like toxin, no invasion	Food, water	Watery diarrhea
STEC	Shiga toxin, no invasion	Undercooked beef products	Hemorrhagic colitis, hemolytic-uremic syndrome (Chapter 14)
EPEC	Attachment, enterocyte effacement, no invasion	Weaning foods, water	Watery diarrhea, infants and toddlers
EIEC	Invasion, local spread	Cheese, water, person-to-person	Fever, pain, diarrhea, dysentery
EAEC	Aggregative adherence, fimbriae, toxins	Sporadic outbreaks	Acute or persistent diarrhea (>14 days) in children younger than 2 years
Salmonella spp.	Invasion, translocation, lymphoid inflammation, dissemination	Milk, beef, eggs, poultry	Fever, pain, diarrhea or dysentery, bacteremia, extraintestinal infection, common-source outbreaks
Shigella spp.	Invasion, local spread	Person-to-person, low-inoculum	Fever, pain, diarrhea, dysentery, epidemic spread
Campylobacter	?Toxins, invasion	Milk, poultry, animal contact	Fever, pain, diarrhea, dysentery, food sources, animal reservoirs
Yersinia enterocolitica	Invasion, translocation, lymphoid inflammation, dissemination	Milk, pork	Fever, pain, diarrhea, mesenteric lymphadenitis, extraintestinal infection, food sources
Vibrio cholerae, other *Vibrio* species	Enterotoxin, no invasion	Water, shellfish, person-to-person spread	Watery diarrhea, cholera, pandemic spread
Clostridium difficile	Cytotoxin, local invasion	Nosocomial environmental spread	Fever, pain, bloody diarrhea, after antibiotic use, nosocomial acquisition
Clostridium perfringens	Enterotoxin, no invasion	Meat, poultry, fish	Watery diarrhea, food sources, "pigbel"
Mycobacterium tuberculosis	Invasion, mural inflammatory foci with necrosis and scarring	Contaminated milk, swallowing of coughed-up organisms	Chronic abdominal pain, complications of malabsorption, stricture, perforation, fistulae, hemorrhage

EAEC, enteroaggregative *E. coli;* EIEC, enteroinvasive *E. coli;* EPEC, enteropathogenic *E. coli;* ETEC, enterotoxigenic *E. coli;* STEC, Shiga toxin–producing *E. coli.*

Figure 15-23 ■

Pseudomembranous colitis. Plaques of yellow fibrin and inflammatory debris are adherent to a reddened colonic mucosa.

- Enteroinvasive strains (EIEC) affect the colon, with histologic features similar to *Shigella*.
- Enteroaggregative strains (EAEC) also affect the colon and exhibit a "stacked brick" pattern of adherence in tissues.

- *Salmonella* species are a major cause of common-source outbreaks of enterocolitis, producing localized mucosal disease primarily in the ileum and colon (as with *S. enteritidis*, *S. typhimurium*, and others). *S. typhimurium* is the archetypal organism that invades Peyer patches and produces local ulceration over massively enlarged lymphoid tissue. Life-threatening systemic illness is the hallmark of *S. typhi*, whereby small intestinal invasion leads to systemic dissemination **(typhoid fever)**. Typhoid fever is a protracted disease featuring **bacteremia** (first week), widespread reticuloendothelial involvement with **splenomegaly** and **foci of necrosis in the liver** (second week), and **ulceration of Peyer patches with intestinal bleeding and ulceration** (third week). **Gallbladder colonization** produces a chronic carrier state; chronic infection also may affect the joints, bones, meninges, and other sites.
- *Shigella* affects primarily the distal colon, producing acute mucosal inflammation and erosion.
- *Campylobacter jejuni* (and other species) affects the small intestine, appendix, and colon, producing multiple superficial ulcers, mucosal inflammation, and exudates.
- *Yersinia enterocolitica* and *Y. pseudotuberculosis* affect the ileum, appendix, and colon. Peyer patch invasion leads to mesenteric lymph node enlargement with necrotizing granulomas. Systemic spread may lead to peritonitis, pharyngitis, and pericarditis.
- *Vibrio cholerae* (cholera) affects the small intestine, especially more proximally. The mucosa is essentially intact, with only mucus-depleted crypts.
- *Clostridium difficile* is a normal gut organism, but cytotoxin-producing strains may overgrow after systemic antibiotic use. A distinctive **pseudomembranous colitis** is produced, which derives its name from the plaquelike adhesion of fibrinopurulent debris and mucus to the damaged superficial mucosa (Fig. 15-23). These are not true "membranes," because the coagulum is not an epithelial layer.
- *Clostridium perfringens* exhibits features similar to *V. cholerae*, but with some epithelial damage. Some strains produce a severe necrotizing enterocolitis with perforation **(pigbel)**.
- Ingested *Mycobacterium tuberculosis* incites chronic inflammation and granuloma formation in mucosal lymphoid tissue—particularly Peyer patches in the terminal ileum—and regional lymph nodes (Chapter 13).

Protozoal Infection. *Entamoeba histolytica* is a dysentery-causing protozoal parasite spread by fecal-oral contamination. Amebae invade the crypts of colonic glands and burrow down into the submucosa (Fig. 15-24); the organisms then fan out laterally to create a flask-shaped ulcer with a narrow neck and broad base. There may be very little inflammatory infiltrate within the ulcer. In about 40% of patients with amebic dysentery, parasites penetrate portal vessels and embolize to the liver to produce solitary, or less often multiple, discrete hepatic abscesses, some exceeding 10 cm in diameter. Some patients may present with amebic liver abscesses, without a clinical history of amebic dysentery. As with the intestinal lesions, there is a scant inflammatory reaction at the margin. The liquefied tissue in the fibrin-lined cavity may be dark-chocolate colored because of hemorrhage. Occasional amebic abscesses are encountered in the lung, heart, kidneys, and even brain. Such abscesses remain long after the acute intestinal illness has passed.

Figure 15-24 ■

Amebiasis of the colon with three *Entamoeba histolytica* trophozoites within the submucosa.

Figure 15-25 ■

Giardia lamblia. Trophozoite *(arrow)* of the organism immediately adjacent to the duodenal surface epithelium; note the double nuclei. The other luminal material is mucus (bluish) and an erythrocyte displaced by the biopsy procedure. (H & E.)

Giardia lamblia is an intestinal protozoan spread by feces-contaminated water. *Giardia* attach to the small intestinal mucosa but do not appear to invade (Fig. 15–25). Small intestinal morphology may range from virtually normal to marked blunting of the villi with a mixed inflammatory infiltrate in the lamina propria. A malabsorptive diarrhea appears to result from mucosal cell injury by mechanisms that are not understood.

Cryptosporidiosis has emerged as an important cause of diarrhea in animals and humans worldwide. It is the major cause of childhood diarrhea and accounts for up to 20% of all cases of childhood diarrhea in developing countries. It is also a potentially fatal complication of AIDS. Waterborne contamination and an increased population at risk for zoonotic contamination have contributed to the increase in this disease.

Clinical Features. The clinical features of viral and protozoal infection have been briefly noted already. At the risk of oversimplification, bacterial enterocolitis takes the following forms:

■ *Ingestion of preformed bacterial toxins.* Symptoms develop within a matter of hours; explosive diarrhea and acute abdominal distress herald an illness that passes within a day or so. Ingested systemic neurotoxins, as from *C. botulinum*, may produce rapid, and fatal, respiratory failure.
■ *Infection with enteric pathogens.* With ingestion of enteric pathogens, an incubation period of several hours to days is followed by *diarrhea and dehydration* if the primary pathogenic mechanism is a secretory enterotoxin or *dysentery* if the primary mechanism is a cytotoxin or an enteroinvasive process. Traveler's diarrhea (e.g., Montezuma's revenge, turista) usually occurs after ingestion of feces-contaminated food or water; it begins abruptly and subsides within 2 to 3 days.
■ *Insidious infection. Yersinia* and *Mycobacterium* may also present as subacute diarrheal illnesses mimicking Crohn disease. All enteroinvasive organisms can mimic, or even precipitate, acute onset of idiopathic inflammatory bowel disease (discussed later).

In general, bacterial enterocolitis is a more severe illness than viral disease. The complications of bacterial enterocolitis result from massive fluid loss or destruction of the intestinal mucosal barrier and include dehydration, sepsis, and perforation. In the most severe cases, death ensues rapidly without quick intervention, particularly in the very young.

A distressing gastrointestinal emergency in neonates, particularly those who are premature or of low birth weight, is *necrotizing enterocolitis.* This acute, necrotizing inflammation of the small and large intestines is thought to result from a combination of functional immaturity of the neonatal gut, colonization and invasion by pathogenic organisms, and secondary ischemic injury. A small portion of terminal ileum and ascending colon may be affected, or the entire small and large intestines may be involved. The injury is initially mucosal, but in severe cases the entire bowel wall becomes hemorrhagic and gangrenous, necessitating surgical resection. In a typical case, there is abdominal distention, tenderness, ileus, and diarrhea with occult or frank blood. Onset of gangrene and perforation are immediately life-threatening.

Malabsorption Syndromes

Malabsorption is characterized by suboptimal absorption of fats, fat-soluble and other vitamins, proteins, carbohydrates, electrolytes and minerals, and water. At the most basic level, it is the result of disturbance of at least one of these normal digestive functions:

1. *Intraluminal digestion,* in which proteins, carbohydrates, and fats are enzymatically broken down. The process begins in the mouth with saliva, receives a major boost from gastric peptic digestion, and continues in the small intestine, assisted by pancreatic enzyme secretion and the emulsive action of bile.
2. *Terminal digestion,* which involves the hydrolysis of carbohydrates and peptides by disaccharidases and peptidases, respectively, in the brush border of the small intestinal mucosa.
3. *Transepithelial transport,* in which nutrients, fluid, and electrolytes are transported across the epithelium of the small intestine for delivery to the intestinal vasculature. Absorbed fatty acids are converted to triglycerides and are assembled with cholesterol and apoprotein B into chylomicrons for delivery to the intestinal lymphatic system.

A host of disorders interrupt the just-described sequence either directly or indirectly (Table 15–8). The malabsorptive disorders most commonly encountered in the United States are pancreatic insufficiency, celiac disease, and Crohn disease.

Excessive growth of normal bacteria within the proximal small intestine *(bacterial overgrowth)* also impairs intraluminal digestion and can damage mucosal epithelial cells. Immunologic deficiencies, inadequate gastric acidity, and intestinal stasis, as from surgical alteration of small intestinal anatomy, predispose to bacterial overgrowth. The intestinal mucosa in bacterial overgrowth either is normal or is minimally damaged.

Typical features of defective intraluminal digestion are an *osmotic diarrhea* from undigested nutrients, as with pancreatic insufficiency, and *steatorrhea*—excess output of

Table 15-8. THE MAJOR MALABSORPTION SYNDROMES

Defective Intraluminal Digestion

Digestion of fats and proteins
  Pancreatic insufficiency, due to pancreatitis or cystic fibrosis
  Zollinger-Ellison syndrome, with inactivation of pancreatic enzymes by excess gastric acid secretion
Solubilization of fat, due to defective bile secretion
  Ileal dysfunction or resection, with decreased bile salt uptake
  Cessation of bile flow from obstruction, hepatic dysfunction
Nutrient preabsorption or modification by bacterial overgrowth

Primary Mucosal Cell Abnormalities

Defective terminal digestion
  Disaccharidase deficiency (lactose intolerance)
  Bacterial overgrowth, with brush border damage
Defective transepithelial transport
  Abetalipoproteinemia

Reduced Small Intestinal Surface Area

Gluten-sensitive enteropathy (celiac disease)
Short-gut syndrome, following surgical resections
Crohn disease

Lymphatic Obstruction

Lymphoma
Tuberculosis and tuberculous lymphadenitis

Infection

Acute infectious enteritis
Parasitic infestation
Tropical sprue
Whipple disease *(Tropheryma whippelii)*

Iatrogenic

Subtotal or total gastrectomy
Distal ileal resection or bypass

---

undigested fat in stool. The latter can arise either from inadequate action of pancreatic lipases or from inadequate solubilization of fat by hepatic bile secreted into the gut lumen.

The classic example of defective mucosal cell absorption is *lactose intolerance.* The inherited deficiency of disaccharidase is rare but is of great consequence because in infants it produces milk intolerance, leading to diarrhea, weight loss, and failure to thrive. The acquired deficiency is common among adults, particularly North American blacks. Aside from the need to avoid milk products, the disorder is of minimal consequence. The intestinal mucosa is morphologically normal. Diagnosis is most readily made by measurement of breath hydrogen level, which reflects bacterial overgrowth in the presence of excess intraluminal carbohydrate.

The rare autosomal recessive deficiency of apolipoprotein B *(abetalipoproteinemia)* renders the mucosal epithelial cell unable to export lipid, because this protein is synthesized by these cells for assembly of dietary lipids into chylomicrons for export to intestinal lymphatics. Hence, mucosal absorptive cells contain vacuolated lipid inclusions, but the mucosa is otherwise normal. This deficiency causes diarrhea and steatorrhea in infancy and significant failure to thrive. There are systemic lipid membrane abnormalities as well, readily observed in circulating erythrocytes as a characteristic burr cell transformation termed *acanthocytosis.*

Gluten-sensitive enteropathy, also known as celiac disease, is the prototype of a noninfectious cause of malabsorption resulting from a reduction in small intestinal absorptive surface area. The basic disorder in celiac disease is sensitivity to gluten, the component of wheat and related grains (oat, barley, and rye) that contains the water-insoluble protein gliadin. Gliadin peptides are efficiently presented by celiac disease–specific HLA-DQ2- and HLA-DQ8-positive antigen-presenting cells in the lamina propria of the small intestine to CD4+ T cells, thereby driving an immune response to gluten. There is hence a strong genetic susceptibility, with 95% of patients having an HLA-DQ2 haplotype and most of the remainder having HLA-DQ8. Early exposure of the immature immune system of the infant to high levels of gliadin is a prominent cofactor for manifestation of clinically overt celiac disease later in life. The small intestinal mucosa, when exposed to gluten, accumulates large numbers of B cells and plasma cells sensitized to gliadin; accumulation of lymphocytes in gastric and colonic mucosa also may occur. In addition to filling the lamina propria, lymphocytes also cross into the epithelial space, with accompanying damage to surface enterocytes. Total flattening of mucosal villi (and hence loss of surface area) is the outcome, affecting the proximal more than the distal small intestine.

With an estimated prevalance of 1 in 3000, it was considered uncommon in the United States. However, with new serologic tests, it is now believed to be very common, affecting 1 in 300 persons both in Europe and in the United States. Many patients have subclinical disease. Patients with celiac disease have increased levels of serum antibodies to a variety of antigens, including gluten and IgA antiendomysial autoantibodies. The antiendomysial autoantibodies are directed against tissue transglutaminase, a ubiquitous enzyme capable of deamidating gliadin peptides. This enhances their presentation by HLA-DQ2, thereby eliciting a proliferative response of gliadin-specific T-cell clones.

The age of presentation with symptomatic diarrhea and malnutrition varies from infancy to midadulthood; removal of gluten from the diet is met with dramatic improvement. There is, however, a low long-term risk of malignant disease on the order of a two-fold increase over the usual rate. Intestinal lymphomas, especially T-cell lymphomas, are disproportionately represented; other malignancies include gastrointestinal and breast carcinomas.

Tropical sprue and *Whipple disease* are two disorders that exemplify malabsorption syndromes arising from intestinal infection. Tropical sprue resembles celiac disease in symptomatology but occurs almost exclusively in persons living in or visiting the tropics. No specific causal agent has been clearly identified, but the appearance of malabsorption within days or a few weeks of an acute diarrheal enteric infection strongly implicates an infectious process, as does prompt response to broad-spectrum antibiotic therapy. Small intestinal changes vary from near normal to a severe diffuse enteritis with villus flattening. In contrast to celiac disease, injury is seen at all levels of the small intestine.

Whipple disease is a rare, systemic infection that may involve any organ of the body but principally affects the intestine, central nervous system, and joints. The hallmark of Whipple disease is a small intestinal mucosa laden with distended periodic acid–Schiff (PAS)-positive macrophages in the lamina propria. The causal organism is a gram-positive and culture-resistant actinomycete, *Tropheryma whippelii*. Although not an obligate intracellular pathogen, phagocytosed organisms and degenerated fragments thereof persist in lamina propria macrophages for years. Similar macrophages are found in the brain, the synovium of affected joints, and elsewhere. At each of these sites, inflammation is essentially absent. Occurring principally in males in the fourth to fifth decades of life, Whipple disease causes a malabsorptive syndrome occasionally accompanied by lymphadenopathy, hyperpigmentation, polyarthritis, and obscure central nervous system complaints. Response to antibiotic therapy is usually prompt, although some patients have a protracted course.

Clinical Features. Clinically, the malabsorption syndromes resemble each other more than they differ. The passage of abnormally bulky, frothy, greasy, yellow or gray stools is a prominent feature of malabsorption, accompanied by weight loss, anorexia, abdominal distention, borborygmi and flatus, and muscle wasting. The consequences of malabsorption affect many organ systems:

■ *Hematopoietic system:* anemia from iron, pyridoxine, folate, or vitamin B_{12} deficiency (vitamin B_{12} is normally absorbed in the ileum) and bleeding from vitamin K deficiency (a fat-soluble vitamin)
■ *Musculoskeletal system:* osteopenia and tetany from defective calcium, magnesium, vitamin D, and protein absorption
■ *Endocrine system:* amenorrhea, impotence, and infertility from generalized malnutrition; and hyperparathyroidism from protracted calcium and vitamin D deficiency
■ *Skin:* purpura and petechiae from vitamin K deficiency; edema from protein deficiency; dermatitis and hyperkeratosis from deficiencies of vitamin A (also fat soluble), zinc, essential fatty acids, and niacin; mucositis from vitamin deficiencies
■ *Nervous system:* peripheral neuropathy from vitamin A and B_{12} deficiencies

IDIOPATHIC INFLAMMATORY BOWEL DISEASE

Crohn disease (CD) and ulcerative colitis (UC) are chronic relapsing disorders of unknown origin. These diseases share many common features and are collectively known as idiopathic inflammatory bowel disease (IBD). *CD may affect any portion of the gastrointestinal tract from esophagus to anus but most often involves the small intestine and colon; about half of cases exhibit noncaseating granulomatous inflammation. UC is a nongranulomatous disease limited to the colon.* Before considering these diseases separately, the pathogenesis of these two forms of IBD will be considered.

Etiology and Pathogenesis. The normal intestine is in a steady state of "physiologic" inflammation, representing a dynamic balance between (1) factors that activate the host immune system, such as luminal microbes, dietary antigens, and endogenous inflammatory stimuli; and (2) host defenses that down-regulate inflammation and maintain the

integrity of the mucosa. The search for the cause or causes of loss of this balance in CD and UC has revealed many parallels, not the least of which is that *both diseases remain unexplained* and are thus best designated as *idiopathic.* Although CD and UC share important pathophysiologic features, there are sufficient differences to justify regarding them as two separate diseases. Attempts to explain their origin have included investigation of the following:

■ *Genetic predisposition.* There is little doubt that genetic factors are important in the occurrence of IBD. First-degree relatives are 3 to 20 times more likely to develop the disease, and monozygotic twins exhibit 30% to 50% concordance rates for CD (less so for ulcerative colitis). Genome-wide scans of affected patients suggest that several loci on chromosomes 3, 7, 12, and 16 are involved. Most exciting is the recent discovery of the IBD1 locus on chromosome 16. The product of the implicated gene, *NOD2*, activates nuclear factor kappa B (NFκB) in macrophages in response to bacterial lipopolysaccharide and thus may be involved in regulating the immune-inflammatory response. In keeping with an underlying immunologic dysfunction, both CD and UC have been linked to specific major histocompatibility complex class II alleles. Interestingly, UC has been associated with the HLA-DR2 (in Japanese), whereas CD seems to be linked to specific HLA-DR1 and -DQw5 alleles. These associations indicate that the CD and UC are genetically distinct.
■ *Immunologic factors.* Accumulating evidence suggests that both UC and CD are associated with profound derangement of mucosal immunity. The most compelling evidence to support this hypothesis comes from animal models of IBD. "Knockout" mice in which genes for cytokines (IL-2, IL-10, TNF), cytokine receptors (IL-2Rα, IL-10R), or T-cell receptors are deleted develop inflammation of the gut resembling IBD. An important conclusion to be drawn from these studies is that a variety of forms of immune dysregulation can lead to bowel inflammation. In keeping with this, a very large number of immunologic abnormalities have been noted in patients with CD and UC. Although both activated T and B cells can be found in the mucosa, it appears that T cells are the driving force in IBD. Autoantibodies such as antineutrophil cytoplasmic antibodies (ANCA), seen in some patient with UC, are considered secondary to the disease.
■ *Microbial factors.* The sites affected by IBD—the distal ileum and the colon—are awash in bacteria. While there is no evidence that these diseases are caused by microbes, it is quite likely that microbes provide the antigenic trigger to a fundamentally dysregulated immune system. This concept is strengthened by the observations that in murine models, IBD develops in the presence of normal gut flora but not in germ-free mice.

To summarize, IBD is a heterogeneous group of diseases characterized by an exaggerated and destructive mucosal immune response. The tissue injury in IBD is likely to be initiated by diverse genetic and immunologic pathways that are modified by environmental influences, including microbes and their products.

Inflammation is the final common pathway for the pathogenesis of IBD. Both the clinical manifestations of IBD and the morphologic changes are ultimately the result of activation of inflammatory cells—neutrophils initially and mononuclear cells later in the course. The products of these inflammatory cells cause nonspecific tissue injury. *Inflammation causes (1) impaired integrity of the mucosal epithelial barrier, (2) loss of surface epithelial cell absorptive function, and (3) activation of crypt epithelial cell secretion.* The inflammation ultimately causes outright mucosal destruction, which leads to obvious loss of mucosal barrier and absorptive function. Collectively, these events give rise to the intermittent bloody diarrhea that is characteristic of these diseases. Most current therapeutic interventions act entirely or partly through nonspecific down-regulation of the immune system.

Crohn Disease

This disease may affect any level of the alimentary tract, from mouth to anus. Active cases of CD are often accompanied by extraintestinal complications of immune origin, such as iritis and uveitis, sacroiliitis, migratory polyarthritis, erythema nodosum, hepatic pericholangitis and sclerosing cholangitis (bile duct inflammatory disorders), and obstructive uropathy with attendant nephrolithiasis and predisposition to urinary tract infections. Systemic amyloidosis is a rare late consequence. Thus, *CD must be viewed as a systemic inflammatory disease with predominant gastrointestinal involvement.*

Epidemiology. Worldwide in distribution, CD is much more prevalent in the United States, Great Britain, and Scandinavia than in Central Europe and is rare in Asia and Africa. In the United States, its annual incidence is 3 to 5 per 100,000 population, which is slightly less frequent than the incidence of ulcerative colitis. The incidence and prevalence of CD has been steadily rising in the United States and Western Europe. It occurs at any age, from young childhood to advanced age, but the peak incidence is between the second and third decades of life, with a minor peak in the sixth and seventh decades. Females are affected slightly more often than males. Whites appear to develop the disease two to five times more often than do nonwhites. In the United States, CD occurs three to five times more often among Jews than among non-Jews.

MORPHOLOGY

In CD, there is gross involvement of the small intestine alone in about 30% of cases, of small intestine and colon in 40%, and of the colon alone in about 30%. CD may involve the duodenum, stomach, esophagus, and even mouth, but these sites are distinctly uncommon. **When fully developed, CD is characterized by (1) sharply delimited and typically transmural involvement of the bowel by an inflammatory process with mucosal damage, (2) the presence of non-caseating granulomas in 40% to 60% of cases, and (3) fissuring with formation of fistulae.** In diseased segments, the serosa becomes granular and dull gray and often the mesenteric fat wraps around the

bowel surface **("creeping fat"). The intestinal wall is rubbery and thick, the result of edema, inflammation, fibrosis, and hypertrophy of the muscularis propria.** As a result, the lumen is almost always narrowed; in the small intestine this is evidenced radiographically as the "string sign," a thin stream of barium passing through the diseased segment. Strictures may occur in the colon but are usually less severe. **A classic feature of CD is the sharp demarcation of diseased bowel segments from adjacent uninvolved bowel. When multiple bowel segments are involved, the intervening bowel is essentially normal ("skip" lesions).**

In the intestinal mucosa, early disease exhibits focal mucosal ulcers resembling canker sores (aphthous ulcers), edema, and loss of the normal mucosal texture. With progressive disease, ulcers coalesce into long, serpentine linear ulcers, which tend to be oriented along the axis of the bowel (Fig. 15-26). Because the intervening mucosa tends to be relatively spared, it acquires a coarsely textured, cobblestone appearance. **Narrow fissures develop between the folds of the mucosa,** often penetrating deeply through the bowel wall all the way to the serosa. This may lead to adhesions with adjacent loops of bowel. Further extension of fissures leads to **fistula or sinus tract formation,** either to an adherent viscus, to the outside skin, or into a blind cavity to form a localized abscess.

Figure 15-26 ■

Crohn disease of the ileum showing narrowing of the lumen, bowel wall thickening, serosal extension of mesenteric fat ("creeping fat"), and linear ulceration of the mucosal surface *(arrowheads).*

Figure 15-27 ■

Crohn disease of the colon showing a deep fissure extending into the muscle wall, a second, shallow ulcer *(upper right)*, and relative preservation of the intervening mucosa. Abundant lymphocyte aggregates are present, evident as dense blue patches of cells at the interface between mucosa and submucosa.

By microscopic examination, the mucosa exhibits several characteristic features (Fig. 15-27): (1) **inflammation,** with neutrophilic infiltration into the epithelial layer and accumulation within crypts to form **crypt abscesses**; (2) **ulceration,** which is the usual outcome of active disease; and (3) **chronic mucosal damage** in the form of architectural distortion, atrophy, and metaplasia (including rudimentary gastric metaplasia in the intestine). **Granulomas may be present anywhere in the alimentary tract, even in patients with CD limited to one bowel segment. However, the absence of granulomas does not preclude a diagnosis of CD.** In diseased segments, the muscularis mucosae and muscularis propria are usually markedly thickened, and fibrosis affects all tissue layers. Lymphoid aggregates scattered through the various tissue layers and in the extramural fat also are characteristic.

Particularly important in patients with long-standing chronic disease are dysplastic changes appearing in the mucosal epithelial cells. These may be focal or widespread, tend to increase with time, and are thought to be related to a five-fold to six-fold increased risk of carcinoma, particularly of the colon.

Clinical Features. The presentation of CD is highly variable and ultimately unpredictable. The dominant manifestations are recurrent episodes of diarrhea, crampy abdominal pain, and fever lasting days to weeks. These manifestations usually begin insidiously, but in some instances, particularly in young persons, the onset of the pain is so abrupt and the diarrhea so mild that abdominal exploration is performed with a diagnosis of appendicitis. Some melena is present in about 50% of cases with colon involvement; it is usually mild but sometimes massive. In most patients, after an initial attack, the manifestations remit either spontaneously or with therapy, but characteristically they are followed by relapses, and intervals between successive attacks grow shorter. In 10% to 20% of patients the symptom-free interval after the initial attack may last for decades, and for a very fortunate few the first attack is the last. Alternatively, about 20% of patients experience continuously active disease following their diagnosis. For the majority, the course fluctuates between years of remission and years with clinically active disease. Superimposed on this course are the potential development of malabsorption and some of the extraintestinal manifestations mentioned earlier.

The debilitating consequences of CD include (1) *fistula formation* to other loops of bowel, the urinary bladder, vagina, or perianal skin; (2) *abdominal abscesses* or peritonitis; and (3) *intestinal stricture* or obstruction, necessitating surgical intervention. Rare but devastating events are massive intestinal bleeding, toxic dilation of the colon, or carcinoma of the colon or small intestine. Although the increased risk for carcinoma is significant, it is substantially less than that associated with ulcerative colitis.

Ulcerative Colitis

Ulcerative colitis (UC) is an ulceroinflammatory disease affecting the colon but limited to the mucosa and submucosa except in the most severe cases. UC begins in the rectum and extends proximally in a continuous fashion, sometimes involving the entire colon. Like CD, UC is a systemic disorder associated in some patients with migratory polyarthritis, sacroiliitis, ankylosing spondylitis, uveitis, erythema nodosum, and hepatic involvement (pericholangitis and primary sclerosing cholangitis). There are several important differences between UC and CD:

- In UC, well-formed granulomas are absent.
- UC does not exhibit skip lesions.
- The mucosal ulcers in UC rarely extend below the submucosa, and there is surprisingly little fibrosis.
- Mural thickening does not occur in UC, and the serosal surface is usually completely normal.
- Patients with UC are at greater risk for carcinoma.

Some of the distinctive features of CD and UC are depicted in Figure 15-28 and compared in Table 15-9.

Epidemiology. UC is somewhat more common than CD in the United States and Western countries, with an incidence of around 7 per 100,000 population, but it is infrequent in Asia, Africa, and South America. As with CD, the

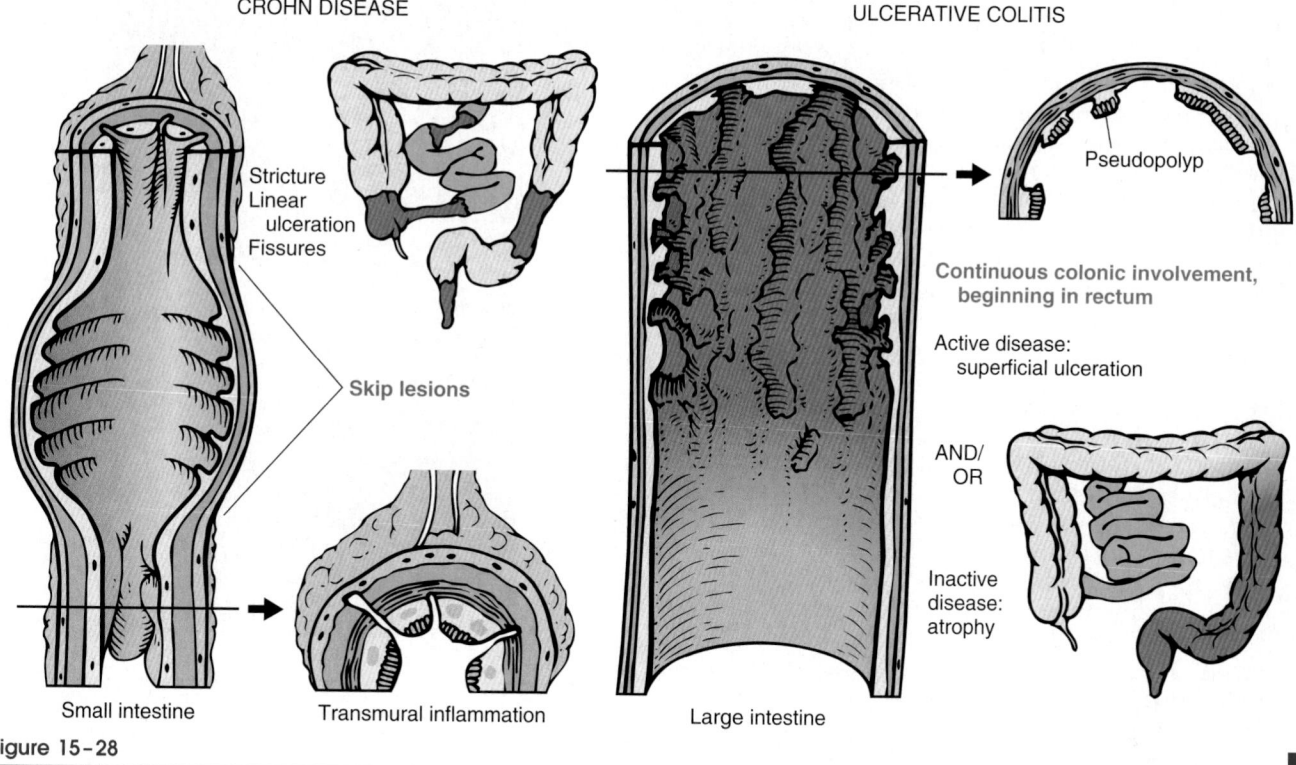

CROHN DISEASE   ULCERATIVE COLITIS

Pseudopolyp

Stricture
Linear
ulceration
Fissures

Continuous colonic involvement,
beginning in rectum

Active disease:
superficial ulceration

Skip lesions

AND/
OR

Inactive
disease:
atrophy

Small intestine   Transmural inflammation   Large intestine

Figure 15–28

The distribution patterns of Crohn disease and ulcerative colitis are compared, as well as the different conformations of the ulcers and wall thickenings.

incidence of this condition has risen in recent decades. In the United States it is more common among whites than among nonwhites and exhibits no particular sex predilection. The disease may arise at any age, with a peak inci-

dence between ages 20 and 25 years. Individuals with UC and ankylosing spondylitis have an increased frequency of HLA-B27, but this association is related to the spondylitis and not to UC.

Table 15–9.   DISTINCTIVE FEATURES OF CROHN DISEASE AND ULCERATIVE COLITIS*

Feature	Crohn Disease (Small intestine)	Crohn Disease (Colon)	Ulcerative Colitis
Macroscopic			
Bowel region	Ileum ± colon†	Colon ± ileum	Colon only
Distribution	Skip lesions	Skip lesions	Diffuse
Stricture	Early	Variable	Late/rare
Wall appearance	Thickened	Variable	Thin
Dilation	No	Yes	Yes
Microscopic			
Pseudopolyps	None to slight	Marked	Marked
Ulcers	Deep, linear	Deep, linear	Superficial
Lymphoid reaction	Marked	Marked	Mild
Fibrosis	Marked	Moderate	Mild
Serositis	Marked	Variable	Mild to none
Granulomas	Yes (40% to 60%)	Yes (40% to 60%)	No
Fistulae/sinuses	Yes	Yes	No
Clinical			
Fat/vitamin malabsorption	Yes	Yes, if ileum	No
Malignant potential	Yes	Yes	Yes
Response to surgery‡	Poor	Fair	Good

*Not all features present in a single case.
†Crohn disease can occur elsewhere in the small intestine as well.
‡Based on likelihood of disease recurrence after surgical removal of a diseased segment.

MORPHOLOGY

At the time of diagnosis, UC involves the rectum or rectosigmoid colon only in about 50% of cases; presentation with pancolitis occurs much less frequently. Colonic involvement is continuous from the distal colon, so that "skip lesions" are not encountered. Active disease denotes ongoing inflammatory destruction of the mucosa, with macroscopic hyperemia, edema, and granularity with friability and easy bleeding. With severely active disease, there is extensive and broad-based ulceration of the mucosa in the distal colon or throughout its length (Fig. 15-29). Isolated islands of regenerating mucosa bulge upward to create **pseudopolyps**. Often the undermined edges of adjacent ulcers interconnect to create tunnels covered by tenuous mucosal bridges. As with CD, the ulcers of UC are frequently aligned along the axis of the colon, but rarely do they replicate the linear serpentine ulcers of CD. In rare cases, the muscularis propria is so compromised as to permit perforation and pericolonic abscess formation. Exposure of the muscularis propria and neural plexus to fecal material also may lead to complete shutdown of neuromuscular function. When this occurs, the colon progressively swells and becomes gangrenous **(toxic megacolon)**. With indolent chronic disease or with healing of active disease, progressive mucosal atrophy leads to a flattened and attenuated mucosal surface.

The pathologic features of UC are those of mucosal inflammation, ulceration, and chronic mucosal damage (Fig. 15-30). First, **a diffuse, predominantly mononuclear inflammatory infiltrate in the lamina propria is almost universally present,** even at the time of clinical presentation. Neutrophilic infiltration of the epithelial layer may produce collections of neutrophils in crypt lumina **(crypt abscesses).** These are not specific for UC and may be observed in CD or any active inflammatory colitis. Unlike CD, there are no granulomas, although rupture of crypt abscesses may incite a foreign body reaction in the lamina propria. Second, **further destruction of the mucosa leads to outright ulceration, extending into the submucosa and sometimes leaving only the raw, exposed muscularis propria.** Third, with remission of active disease, **granulation tissue fills in the ulcer craters,** followed by regeneration of the mucosal epithelium. **Submucosal fibrosis and mucosal architectural disarray and atrophy remain as residua of healed disease.**

The most serious complication of UC is the development of colon carcinoma. Two factors govern the risk: duration of the disease and its anatomic extent. It is believed that with 10 years of disease limited to the left colon the risk is minimal, and at 20 years the risk is on the order of 2%. With pancolitis, the risk of carcinoma is 10% at 20 years and 15% to 25% by 30 years. Overall, the annual incidence of colon cancer in patients with UC of more than 10 years' duration is 0.8% to 1%.

Figure 15-29 ■

Ulcerative colitis. The pale, irregular regions comprise ulcerations that have in many instances coalesced, leaving virtual islands of residual mucosa. A tendency toward pseudopolyp formation is already evident. The darker material is adherent mucus stained by feces.

Clinical Features. UC is a chronic relapsing and remitting disorder marked by attacks of bloody mucoid diarrhea that may persist for days, weeks, or months and then subside, only to recur after an asymptomatic interval of months to years or even decades. Presentation is usually insidious, with cramps, tenesmus, and colicky lower abdominal pain

Figure 15-30 ■

Ulcerative colitis. Low-power micrograph showing marked chronic inflammation of the mucosa with atrophy of colonic glands, moderate submucosal fibrosis, and a normal muscle wall.

that is relieved by defecation. Some patients manifest fever and weight loss. Grossly bloody stools are more common with UC than with CD, and the blood loss may be considerable. In the fortunate patient, the first attack is the last, representing about 10% of patients. At the other end of the spectrum, the explosive initial attack may lead to such serious bleeding and fluid and electrolyte imbalance as to constitute a medical emergency. For the most part, however, the vast majority of patients experience a relapsing course. Intercurrent infectious illnesses, as with enterotoxin-forming *Clostridium difficile*, may first bring UC to light; they do not precipitate the disease.

Extraintestinal manifestations, particularly migratory polyarthritis, are more common with UC than with CD. Uncommon but *life-threatening complications* include severe diarrhea and electrolyte derangements, massive hemorrhage, severe colonic dilation (toxic megacolon) with potential rupture, and perforation with peritonitis. Inflammatory strictures of the colorectum, while uncommon, must be differentiated from cancer.

Diagnosis can usually be made by endoscopic examination and biopsy. Specific infectious causes must always be ruled out. The most feared long-term complication of UC is cancer. The sequential mucosal changes from dysplasia to invasive carcinoma provide the rationale for surveillance programs of repeated colonoscopies and multiple biopsies aimed at detecting dysplasia for possible prophylactic colectomy.

COLONIC DIVERTICULOSIS

A diverticulum is a blind pouch leading off the alimentary tract, lined by mucosa, that communicates with the lumen of the gut. Congenital diverticula have all three layers of the bowel wall (mucosa, submucosa, and most notably the muscularis propria) and are distinctly uncommon. The prototype is *Meckel diverticulum*, described earlier.

Virtually all other diverticula are acquired and either lack or have an attenuated muscularis propria. *Acquired diverticula may occur anywhere in the alimentary tract, but by far the most common location is the colon*, giving rise to *diverticular disease* of the colon, also called *diverticulosis.* The colon is unique in that the outer longitudinal muscle coat is not complete but is gathered into three equidistant bands (the taeniae coli). Where nerves and arterial vasa recta penetrate the inner circular muscle coat alongside the taeniae, focal defects in the muscle wall are created. The connective tissue sheaths accompanying these penetrating vessels provide potential sites for herniations.

Colonic diverticulosis is relatively infrequent in native populations of non-Western countries. Although unusual in Western adults younger than 30 years of age, in those older than the age of 60 the prevalence approaches 50%. This disparity is attributed to the consumption of a refined, low-fiber diet in Western societies, resulting in reduced stool bulk with increased difficulty in passage of intestinal contents. Exaggerated spastic contractions of the colon isolate segments of the colon (segmentation) in which the intraluminal pressure becomes markedly elevated, with consequent herniation of the bowel wall through the anatomic points of weakness. Thus, *two factors are thought to be important in the genesis of diverticular protrusions: (1) exaggerated peristaltic contractions with abnormal elevation of intraluminal pressure and (2) focal defects peculiar to the normal muscular colonic wall.*

MORPHOLOGY

Most colonic diverticula are **small flasklike or spherical outpouchings, usually 0.5 to 1 cm in diameter** (Fig. 15–31A). They are located in the sigmoid colon in approximately 95% of patients. Infrequently, more proximal levels and sometimes

Figure 15–31

Diverticulosis. *A,* Section through the sigmoid colon showing multiple saclike diverticula protruding through the muscle wall into the mesentery. The muscularis between the diverticular protrusions is markedly thickened *(arrowheads). B,* Low-power micrograph of diverticulum of the colon showing protrusion of mucosa and submucosa through the muscle wall. A dilated blood vessel at the base of the diverticulum was a source of bleeding; some blood clot is present within the diverticular lumen.

the entire colon are affected. Isolated cecal diverticula also occur. The exaggerated peristalsis often induces muscular hypertrophy in affected segments, with unusually prominent taenia coli and circular muscle bundles. Most diverticula penetrate between the bundles of circular muscle fibers adjacent to the mesenteric and lateral taeniae at sites of penetrating blood vessels. They frequently dissect into the appendices epiploicae and therefore may be inapparent on casual external inspection.

In the uninflamed state the walls are usually very thin, made up largely of mucosa and submucosa enclosed within fat or an intact peritoneal covering (Fig. 15–31B). Inflammatory changes may supervene to produce both diverticulitis and peridiverticulitis. Perforation may lead to localized peritonitis or abscess formation. When multiple closely adjacent diverticula become inflamed, the bowel wall may be encased by fibrous tissue, with narrowing of the lumen producing a remarkable resemblance to a cancerous stricture.

Clinical Features. In most persons, diverticular disease is asymptomatic and is discovered only at autopsy or by chance during a laparoscopy or barium enema for some other problem. In only about a fifth of the cases does intermittent cramping or sometimes continuous left-sided lower quadrant discomfort appear, with a sensation of never being able to completely empty the rectum. Superimposed diverticulitis accentuates the symptoms and produces left lower quadrant tenderness and fever. Other, less common complications include minimal chronic intermittent bleeding or, rarely, brisk hemorrhage, perforation with pericolic abscess, or fistula formation.

The treatment of this condition merits brief mention because it bears on its pathogenesis. A high-fiber diet is recommended on the theory that the increased stool bulk reduces the exaggerated peristalsis as the source of discomfort. Whether a high-fiber diet prevents disease progression or protects against superimposed diverticulitis is unclear.

BOWEL OBSTRUCTION

The major causes of intestinal obstruction are listed in Table 15–10. Although any part of the gut may be involved, because of its narrow lumen, the small bowel is most commonly affected. Four entities—hernias, intestinal adhesions, intussusception, and volvulus—account for at least 80% of the cases.

A weakness or defect in the wall of the peritoneal cavity may permit protrusion of a pouchlike, serosa-lined sac of peritoneum, called a *hernial sac.* The usual sites of weakness are anteriorly at the inguinal and femoral canals, at the

Table 15–10.   MAJOR CAUSES OF INTESTINAL OBSTRUCTION

Mechanical Obstruction

Hernias, internal or external
Adhesions
Intussusception
Volvulus
Tumors
Inflammatory strictures
Obstructive gallstones, fecaliths, foreign bodies
Congenital stricture, atresias
Congenital bands
Meconium in cystic fibrosis
Imperforate anus

Pseudo-obstruction

Paralytic ileus (e.g., postoperative)
Vascular: bowel infarction
Myopathies and neuropathies (e.g., Hirschsprung disease)

umbilicus, and in surgical scars. Rarely, retroperitoneal hernias may occur, chiefly about the ligament of Trietz. *Hernias are of concern because segments of viscera frequently intrude and become trapped in them (external herniation).* This is particularly true with inguinal hernias, which have narrow orifices and large sacs. The most frequent intruders are small bowel loops, but portions of omentum or large bowel also may become trapped. Pressure at the neck of the pouch may impair venous drainage of the trapped viscus. The ensuing stasis and edema increase the bulk of the herniated loop, leading to permanent trapping *(incarceration).* Further compromise of its blood supply and drainage leads to infarction of the trapped segment *(strangulation).*

Surgical procedures, infection, and even endometriosis often cause localized or general peritoneal inflammation (peritonitis). With healing, *adhesions* may develop between bowel segments or the abdominal wall and the operative site. These fibrous bridges can create closed loops through which the intestines may slide and become trapped *(internal herniation).* The sequence of events is much the same as with external hernias.

Intussusception denotes telescoping of a proximal segment of bowel into the immediately distal segment. In children, intussusception sometimes occurs without apparent anatomic basis, perhaps related to excessive peristaltic activity. In adults, such telescoping often points to an intraluminal mass (e.g., tumor) that becomes trapped by a peristaltic wave and pulls its point of attachment along with it into the distal segment. Not only does intestinal obstruction ensue, but the vascular supply may be so compromised as to cause infarction of the trapped segment.

Volvulus refers to twisting of a loop of bowel or other structure (e.g., ovary) about its base of attachment, constricting the venous outflow and sometimes the arterial supply as well. Volvulus affects the small bowel most often and rarely the redundant sigmoid. Intestinal obstruction and infarction may follow.

TUMORS OF THE SMALL AND LARGE INTESTINES

Epithelial tumors of the intestines are a major cause of morbidity and mortality worldwide. The colon, including the rectum, is host to more primary neoplasms than any other organ in the body. Colorectal cancer ranks second only to bronchogenic carcinoma among the cancer killers. About 5% of Americans will develop colorectal cancer, and 40% of this population will die of the disease. Adenocarcinomas constitute the vast majority of colorectal cancers and represent 70% of all malignancies arising in the gastrointestinal tract. Curiously, the small intestine is an uncommon site for benign or malignant tumors despite its great length and its vast pool of dividing mucosal cells. The classification of intestinal tumors is the same for the small and large bowel and is summarized in Table 15–11.

Before embarking on our discussion, several concepts pertaining to terminology must be emphasized (Fig. 15–32):

- A *polyp* is a tumorous mass that protrudes into the lumen of the gut; traction on the mass may create a stalked, or *pedunculated*, polyp. Alternatively, the polyp may be *sessile*, without a definable stalk.
- Polyps may be formed as the result of abnormal mucosal maturation, inflammation, or architecture. These polyps are *non-neoplastic* and do not have malignant potential; an example is the hyperplastic polyp.
- Those polyps that arise as the result of epithelial proliferation and dysplasia are termed *adenomatous polyps* or *adenomas. They are true neoplastic lesions ("new growth") and are precursors of carcinoma.*
- Some polypoid lesions may be caused by submucosal or mural tumors. However, as with the stomach, the term *polyp,* unless otherwise specified, refers to lesions arising from the epithelium of the mucosa.

Non-neoplastic Polyps

The overwhelming majority of intestinal polyps occur sporadically, particularly in the colon, and increase in frequency with age. Non-neoplastic polyps represent about 90% of all epithelial polyps in the large intestine and are found in more than half of all persons age 60 years or older. Most are *hyperplastic polyps*, which are small (less than 5 mm in diameter), nipple-like, hemispherical, smooth protrusions of the mucosa. They may occur singly but are more often multiple. Although they may be anywhere in the colon, well over half are found in the rectosigmoid region. Histologically, they contain abundant crypts lined by well-differentiated goblet or absorptive epithelial cells, separated by a scant lamina propria. Although the vast majority of hyperplastic polyps have *no malignant potential*, it is now being recognized that some so-called hyperplastic polyps on the right side of the colon may be precursors of colorectal carcinomas. As discussed later, they show microsatellite instability and can give rise to colon cancers by the mismatch repair pathway.

Juvenile polyps are essentially hamartomatous proliferations, mainly of the lamina propria, enclosing widely

---

Table 15–11. TUMORS OF THE SMALL AND LARGE INTESTINES

Non-neoplastic (Benign) Polyps

Hyperplastic polyps
Hamartomatous polyps
   Juvenile polyps
   Peutz-Jeghers polyps
Inflammatory polyps
Lymphoid polyps

Neoplastic Epithelial Lesions

Benign polyps
   Adenoma*
Malignant lesions
   Adenocarcinoma*
   Carcinoid tumor
   Anal zone carcinoma

Mesenchymal Lesions

Gastrointestinal stromal tumors (benign or malignant)
Other benign lesions
   Lipoma
   Neuroma
   Angioma
Kaposi sarcoma

Lymphoma

*Benign and malignant counterparts of the most common neoplasms in the intestines.

---

spaced, dilated cystic glands. They occur most frequently in children younger than 5 years old but also are found in adults of any age; in the latter group they may be called *retention polyps*. Irrespective of terminology, the lesions are

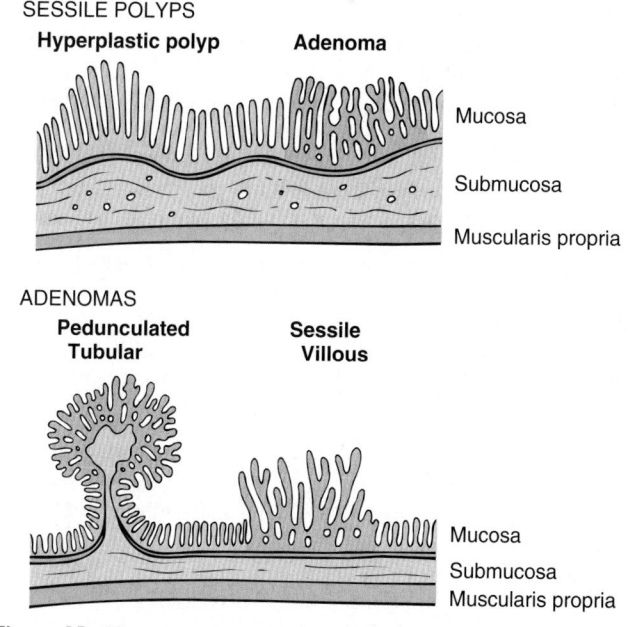

SESSILE POLYPS
Hyperplastic polyp   Adenoma

Mucosa
Submucosa
Muscularis propria

ADENOMAS
Pedunculated
Tubular   Sessile
                 Villous

Mucosa
Submucosa
Muscularis propria

Figure 15–32

Diagrammatic representation of two forms of sessile polyp (hyperplastic polyp and adenoma) and of two types of adenoma (pedunculated and sessile). There is only a loose association between the tubular architecture for pedunculated adenomas and the villous architecture for sessile polyps.

usually large in children (1 to 3 cm in diameter) but smaller in adults; they are rounded, smooth, or slightly lobulated and sometimes have a stalk up to 2 cm long. In general, they occur singly and in the rectum, and being hamartomatous they have no malignant potential. Juvenile polyps may be the source of rectal bleeding and in some cases become twisted on their stalks to undergo painful infarction.

Adenomas

Adenomas are neoplastic polyps that range from small, often pedunculated tumors to large lesions that are usually sessile. Because the incidence of adenomas in the small intestine is very low, this discussion focuses on those adenomas that arise in the colon. The prevalence of colonic adenomas is 20% to 30% before age 40, rising to 40% to 50% after age 60. Males and females are affected equally. There is a well-defined familial predisposition to sporadic adenomas, accounting for about a four-fold greater risk for adenomas among first-degree relatives, and also a four-fold greater risk of colorectal carcinoma in any patient with adenomas.

All adenomatous lesions arise as the result of epithelial proliferation and dysplasia, which may range from mild to so severe as to represent transformation to carcinoma. Furthermore, there is strong evidence that most sporadic invasive colorectal adenocarcinomas arise in preexisting adenomatous lesions. Adenomatous polyps are segregated into three subtypes on the basis of the epithelial architecture:

■ *Tubular adenomas:* mostly tubular glands, recapitulating mucosal topology
■ *Villous adenomas:* villous projections
■ *Tubulovillous adenomas:* a mixture of the above

Tubular adenomas are by far the most common; 5% to 10% of adenomas are tubulovillous, and only 1% are villous. Most tubular adenomas are small and pedunculated; villous adenomas tend to be large and sessile. Conversely, most pedunculated polyps are tubular, and large sessile polyps usually exhibit villous features.

The malignant risk with an adenomatous polyp is correlated with three interdependent features: polyp size, histologic architecture, and severity of epithelial dysplasia, as follows:

■ Cancer is rare in tubular adenomas smaller than 1 cm in diameter.
■ The likelihood of cancer is high (approaching 40%) in sessile villous adenomas more than 4 cm in diameter.
■ Severe dysplasia, when present, is often found in villous areas.

However, among these variables, *maximum diameter is the chief determinant of the risk of an adenoma's harboring carcinoma*; architecture does not provide substantive independent information.

MORPHOLOGY

Tubular adenomas may arise anywhere in the colon, but about half are found in the rectosigmoid, the proportion increasing with age. In about half of the instances they occur singly, but in the remainder two or more lesions are distributed at random. The smallest adenomas are sessile; lesions 0.3 cm in size can be identified at endoscopy. Among the larger tubular adenomas up to 2.5 cm in diameter, most have slender stalks 1 to 2 cm long and raspberry-like heads (Fig. 15-33A). Histologically, the stalk is covered by normal colonic mucosa but the head is composed of neoplastic epithelium, forming branching glands lined by tall, hyperchromatic, somewhat disorderly cells, which may or may not show mucin secretion (Fig. 15-33B). In some instances there are small foci of villous architecture. In the clearly benign lesion, the branching glands are well separated by lamina propria, and the level of dysplasia or cytologic atypia is slight. However, all degrees of dysplasia may be encountered, ranging up to cancer confined to the mucosa (**intramucosal carcinoma)** or **invasive carcinoma** extending into the submucosa of the stalk. A frequent finding in any adenoma is superficial erosion of the epithelium, the result of mechanical trauma.

Villous adenomas are the larger and more ominous of the epithelial polyps. They tend to occur in older persons, most commonly in the rectum and rectosigmoid, but they may be located elsewhere. They generally are sessile, up to 10 cm in diameter, velvety or cauliflower-like masses projecting 1 to 3 cm above the surrounding normal mucosa. The histology is that of frondlike villiform extensions of the mucosa covered by dysplastic, sometimes very disorderly, sometimes piled-up, columnar epithelium (Fig. 15-34). All degrees of dysplasia may be encountered, and invasive carcinoma is found in up to 40% of these lesions, the frequency being correlated with the size of the polyp.

Tubulovillous adenomas are composed of a broad mix of tubular and villous areas. They are intermediate between the tubular and the villous lesions in their frequency of having a stalk or being sessile, their size, the degree of dysplasia, and the risk of harboring intramucosal or invasive carcinoma.

Clinical Features. The smaller adenomas are usually asymptomatic, until such time that occult bleeding leads to clinically significant anemia. Villous adenomas are much more frequently symptomatic because of overt or occult rectal bleeding. The most distal villous adenomas may secrete sufficient amounts of mucoid material rich in protein and potassium to produce hypoproteinemia or hypokalemia. Adenomas of the small intestine may present with anemia or rarely intussusception or obstruction. Adenomas in the immediate vicinity of the ampulla of Vater may produce biliary obstruction. On discovery, all adenomas, regardless of their location in the alimentary tract, are to be considered potentially malignant; thus, in practical terms, prompt and adequate excision is mandated.

Figure 15-33   ■

A, Pedunculated adenoma showing a fibrovascular stalk covered by normal colonic mucosa and a head that contains abundant dysplastic epithelial glands, hence the blue color. *B,* A small focus of adenomatous epithelium in an otherwise normal (mucin-secreting, clear) colonic mucosa, showing how the dysplastic columnar epithelium (deeply stained) can populate a colonic crypt ("tubular" architecture).

Familial Polyposis Syndromes

Familial polyposis syndromes are uncommon autosomal dominant disorders. Their importance lies in the propensity for malignant transformation and in the insights that such transformation has provided in unraveling the molecular basis of colorectal cancer. In *familial adenomatous polyposis* (FAP), patients typically develop 500 to 2500 colonic adenomas that carpet the mucosal surface (Fig. 15–35); a minimum number of 100 is required for the diagnosis. Multiple adenomas may also be present elsewhere in the alimentary tract, including almost a 100% lifetime incidence of duodenal adenomas. Most polyps are tubular adenomas; occasional polyps have

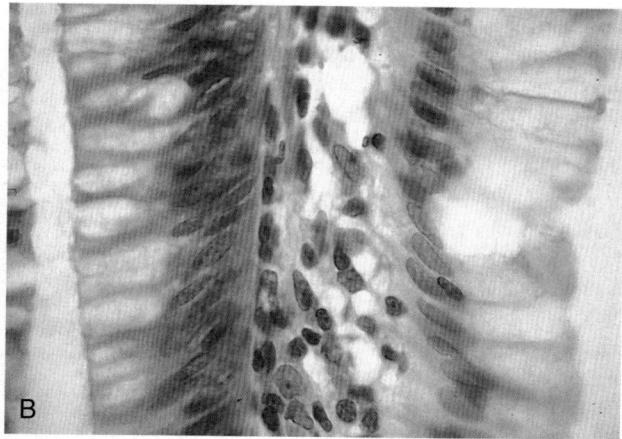

Figure 15-34   ■

A, Sessile adenoma with villous architecture. Each frond is lined by dysplastic epithelium. *B,* Portion of a villous frond with dysplastic columnar epithelium on the left and normal colonic columnar epithelium on the right.

Figure 15-35 ■

Familial adenomatous polyposis. The surface is carpeted by innumerable polypoid adenomas. (Courtesy of Dr. Tad Wieczorek, Brigham and Women's Hospital, Boston.)

villous features. Polyps usually become evident in adolescence or early adulthood. *The risk of colonic cancer is virtually 100% by midlife, unless a prophylactic colectomy is performed.* The genetic defect underlying FAP has been localized to the *APC* gene on chromosome 5q21, as discussed later; *Gardner syndrome* and the much rarer *Turcot syndrome* appear to share the same genetic defect as FAP. These syndromes differ from each other with respect to the occurrence of extraintestinal tumors in the latter two: osteomas, gliomas, and soft tissue tumors, to name a few.

Peutz-Jeghers polyps are uncommon hamartomatous polyps that occur as part of the rare autosomal dominant Peutz-Jeghers syndrome, characterized in addition by melanotic mucosal and cutaneous pigmentation. This syndrome is caused by germ-line mutations in the *LKB1* gene, which encodes a serine threonine kinase. Cowden syndrome is also characterized by hamartomatous polyps in the gastrointestinal tract, and by an increased risk of neoplasms of the thyroid, breast, uterus, and skin. This syndrome is caused by germ-line mutations in the *PTEN* (phosphatase and tensin homologue) tumor suppressor gene. This gene, mutated in a large number of human cancers, acts as a phosphatase and has the ability to regulate many intracellular signaling pathways. It acts as a growth inhibitor by interrupting signals from several tyrosine kinase receptors (e.g., epidermal growth factor receptor) and by favoring apoptoses through the BAD/BCL2 pathways (Chapter 6). Peutz-Jeghers and Cowden syndromes, like the other familial polyposis syndromes, are associated with an increased risk of both intestinal and extraintestinal malignancies.

Colorectal Carcinoma

A great majority (98%) of all cancers in the large intestine are adenocarcinomas. They represent one of the prime challenges to the medical profession, because they almost always arise in adenomatous polyps that are generally curable by resection. With an estimated 134,000 new cases per year and about 55,000 deaths, this disease accounts for nearly 15% of all cancer-related deaths in the United States.

Epidemiology. The peak incidence for colorectal cancer is 60 to 70 years of age; fewer than 20% of cases occur before the age of 50 years. When colorectal cancer is found in a young person, preexisting ulcerative colitis or one of the polyposis syndromes must be suspected. Adenomas are the presumed precursor lesion; the frequency with which colorectal cancer arises de novo from flat colonic mucosa remains undefined but appears to be low. Males are affected about 20% more often than females.

Colorectal carcinoma has a worldwide distribution, with the highest incidence rates in the United States, Canada, Australia, New Zealand, Denmark, Sweden, and other developed countries. Its incidence is substantially lower, up to 30-fold less, in India, South America, and Africa. The incidence in Japan, which formerly was very low, has now risen to the intermediate levels observed in the United Kingdom. Environmental factors, particularly dietary practices, are implicated in these striking geographic contrasts. The dietary factors receiving the most attention are (1) a low content of unabsorbable vegetable fiber, (2) a corresponding high content of refined carbohydrates, (3) a high fat content (as from meat), and (4) decreased intake of protective micronutrients such as vitamins A, C, and E. It is theorized that reduced fiber content leads to decreased stool bulk, increased fecal retention in the bowel, and an altered bacterial flora of the intestine. Potentially toxic oxidative byproducts of carbohydrate degradation by bacteria are therefore present in higher concentrations in the small stools and are held in contact with the colonic mucosa for longer periods of time. Moreover, high fat intake enhances the synthesis of cholesterol and bile acids by the liver, which in turn may be converted into potential carcinogens by intestinal bacteria. Refined diets also contain less of vitamins A, C, and E, which may act as oxygen radical scavengers. Intriguing as these scenarios are, they remain unproven. Indeed, recent studies have challenged the notion that a high-fiber diet offers protection against colorectal cancers.

Several recent epidemiologic studies suggest that use of aspirin and other NSAIDs exerts a protective effect against colon cancer. In the Nurses' Health Study, women who used four to six tablets of aspirin/day for 10 years or more had a decreased incidence of colon cancer. The basis of such chemoprevention is not fully understood. Possible mechanisms include induction of apoptosis in tumor cells and inhibition of angiogenesis. The latter effect seems to be mediated by inhibition of cyclooxygenase-2. This enzyme in the prostaglandin synthesis pathway (Chapter 2) seems to favor angiogenesis by enhancing production of vascular endothelial growth factor (VEGF). On the basis of these findings, the Federal Drug Administration has approved the use of cyclooxygenase-2 inhibitors as chemopreventive agents in patients with familial adenomatous polyposis syndrome.

The Adenoma-Carcinoma Sequence. The development of carcinoma from adenomatous lesions is referred to as the adenoma-carcinoma sequence and is documented by these observations:

■ Populations that have a high prevalence of adenomas have a high prevalence of colorectal cancer, and vice versa.

■ The distribution of adenomas within the colorectum is more or less comparable to that of colorectal cancer.

■ The peak incidence of adenomatous polyps antedates by some years the peak for colorectal cancer.

■ When invasive carcinoma is identified at an early stage, surrounding adenomatous tissue is often present.

■ The risk of cancer is directly related to the number of adenomas, and hence the virtual certainty of cancer in patients with familial polyposis syndromes.

■ Programs that assiduously follow patients for the development of adenomas, and remove all that are identified, reduce the incidence of colorectal cancer.

Colorectal Carcinogenesis. Study of colorectal carcinogenesis has provided fundamental insights into the general mechanisms of cancer evolution. Many of these principles were discussed in Chapter 6. Here we will discuss concepts specifically pertinent to carcinogenesis in the colon.

It is now believed that there are two pathogenetically distinct pathways for the development of colon cancer, both of which involve the stepwise accumulation of multiple mutations. However, the genes involved and the mechanisms by which the mutations accumulate are different.

The first pathway, sometimes called the *APC/β-catenin pathway,* is characterized by chromosomal instability that results in stepwise accumulation of mutations in a series of oncogenes and tumor suppressor genes. The molecular evolution of colon cancer along this pathway occurs through a series of morphologically identifiable stages. Initially, there is localized colon epithelial proliferation. This is followed by the formation of small adenomas that progressively enlarge, become more dysplastic, and ultimately develop into invasive cancers. This is referred to as the adenoma-carcinoma sequence (Fig. 15–36). The genetic correlates of this pathway are as follows:

■ *Loss of the* APC *tumor suppressor gene.* This is believed to be the earliest event in the formation of adenomas. Recall that in the FAP and Gardner syndromes, germline mutations in the *APC* gene give rise to hundreds of adenomas that progress to form cancers. Both copies of the *APC* gene must be lost for adenomas to develop. As discussed in Chapter 6, the functions of the APC protein are intimately linked to β-catenin. Normal APC promotes the degradation of β-catenin; with loss of APC function, the accumulated β-catenin translocates to the nucleus and activates the transcription of several genes, such as *MYC* and cyclin D1, that promote cell proliferation. *APC* mutations are present in 80% of sporadic colon cancers.

■ Mutation of K-RAS. The *K-RAS* gene encodes a signal transduction molecule that oscillates between an activated guanosine triphosphate–bound state and an inactive guanosine diphosphate–bound state. As discussed in Chapter 6, mutated *RAS* is trapped in an activated state that delivers mitotic signals and prevents apoptosis. The *K-RAS* mutation typically follows the loss of *APC*. It is mutated in fewer than 10% of adenomas less than 1 cm,

in 50% of adenomas larger than 1 cm, and in 50% of carcinomas.

■ *18q21 deletion.* Loss of a putative cancer suppressor gene on 18q21 has been found in 60% to 70% of colon cancers. Three genes have been mapped to this chromosome location: *DCC* (deleted in colon carcinoma), *DPC4/SMAD4* (deleted in pancreatic carcinoma), and *SMAD2.* It is not clear which of these genes is relevant in colon carcinogenesis. *DCC* encodes a cell adhesion–like molecule called netrin-1, which is involved in axonal guidance. *DPC/SMAD4* and *SMAD2* encode components of the transforming growth factor β (TGF-β) signaling pathway. Because TGF-β signaling normally inhibits the cell cycle, the loss of these genes may allow unrestrained cell growth.

■ *Loss of* TP53. Loss of this tumor suppressor gene is noted in 70% to 80% of colon cancers, yet similar losses are infrequent in adenomas, suggesting that mutations in *TP53* occur late in colorectal carcinogenesis. The critical role of *TP53* in cell cycle regulation was discussed in Chapter 6.

The adenoma-carcinoma sequence just described accounts for about 80% of sporadic colorectal cancers.

The second pathway is characterized by genetic lesions in *DNA mismatch repair genes* (Chapter 6). It is involved in 10% to 15% of sporadic cases. As in the *APC/β*-catenin schema, there is accumulation of mutations, but the involved genes are different, and, unlike in the adenoma-carcinoma sequence, there are no clearly identifiable morphologic correlates. Defective DNA repair caused by inactivation of DNA mismatch repair genes is the fundamental and the most likely initiating event in colorectal cancers that travel this road. Inherited mutations in one of five DNA mismatch repair genes (*MSH2, MSH6, MLH1, PMS1,* and *PMS2*) give rise to the hereditary nonpolyposis colon carcinoma (HNPCC). Of these genes, *MLH1* is the one most commonly involved in sporadic colon carcinomas. Loss of DNA mismatch repair genes leads to a hypermutable state in which simple repetitive DNA sequences, called *microsatellites,* are unstable during DNA replication, giving rise to widespread alterations in these repeats. The resulting *microsatellite instability* (MSI) is the molecular signature of defective DNA mismatch repair, and hence this pathway is often referred to as the MSI pathway. Most microsatellite sequences are in noncoding regions of the genes, and, hence, mutations in these genes are probably harmless. However, some microsatellite sequences are located in the coding or promoter region of genes involved in regulation of cell growth. Such genes include type II TGF-β receptor and *BAX.* TGF-β signaling inhibits the growth of colonic epithelial cells, and the *BAX* gene causes apoptosis. Loss of mismatch repair leads to the accumulation of mutations in these and other growth-regulating genes, culminating in the emergence of colorectal carcinomas.

Although there is no readily identifiable adenoma-carcinoma sequence that typifies tumors arising from defects in mismatch repair, it has been noted that some of the so-called hyperplastic polyps seen on the right side of the colon display microsatellite instability and may well be precancerous. Fully developed tumors that arise via the mismatch repair pathway do show some distinctive morphologic features, including proximal colonic location,

NORMAL COLON	MUCOSA AT RISK	ADENOMAS		CARCINOMA

Mucosa
Submucosa
Muscularis
propria

Germ-line (inherited) or somatic (acquired) mutations of tumor suppressor genes ("first hit")

Methylation abnormalities Inactivation of normal alleles ("second hit")

Protooncogene mutation

Homozygous loss of additional tumor suppressor genes

Additional mutations Gross chromosomal alterations

APC at 5q21	*APC*	*K-RAS* at 12p12	Loss of heterozygosity at 18q21 *TP53* at 17p53	Many genes

Figure 15–36 ■

Schematic of the morphologic and molecular changes in the adenoma-carcinoma sequence. It is postulated that loss of one normal copy of the tumor suppressor gene *APC* occurs early. Indeed, individuals may be born with one mutant allele, rendering them extremely likely to develop colon cancer. This is the "first hit" according to Knudson's hypothesis. The loss of the normal copy of *APC* follows ("second hit"). Mutations of the oncogene *K-RAS* seem to occur next. Additional mutations inactivate the tumor suppressor genes *DCC* and *TP53*, leading finally to the emergence of carcinoma, in which additional mutations occur. Although there seems to be a temporal sequence of changes, as shown, the accumulation of mutations, rather than their occurrence in a specific order, is more important.

mucinous histology, and infiltration by lymphocytes. In general, these tumors have a better prognosis than do stage-matched tumors that arise by the *APC*/β-catenin pathway.

MORPHOLOGY

About 25% of colorectal carcinomas are in the cecum or ascending colon, with a similar proportion in the rectum and distal sigmoid. An additional 25% are in the descending colon and proximal sigmoid; the remainder are scattered elsewhere. Hence, a substantial portion of cancers is undetectable by digital or proctosigmoidoscopic examination. Most often carcinomas occur singly and have frequently obliterated their adenomatous origins. When multiple carcinomas are present, they are often at widely disparate sites in the colon.

Although all colorectal carcinomas begin as in situ lesions, they evolve into different morphologic patterns. **Tumors in the proximal colon tend to grow as polypoid, exophytic masses that extend along one wall of the capacious cecum and ascending colon** (Fig. 15–37). Obstruction is uncommon. **When carcinomas in the distal colon are discovered, they tend to be annular, encircling lesions that produce so-called napkin-ring constrictions of the bowel and narrowing of the lumen** (Fig. 15–38); the margins of the napkin ring are classically heaped up. Both forms of neoplasm directly penetrate the bowel wall over the course of time (probably years) and may appear as firm masses on the serosal surface.

Regardless of their gross appearance, all colon carcinomas are microscopically similar. Almost all are adenocarcinomas that range from well-differentiated (Fig. 15–39) to undifferentiated, frankly anaplastic masses. Many tumors produce mucin, which is secreted into the gland lumina or into the interstitium of the gut wall. Because these secretions dissect through the gut wall, they facilitate extension of the cancer and worsen the prognosis. Cancers of the anal zone are predominantly squamous cell in origin.

Figure 15–37 ■

Carcinoma of the cecum. The exophytic carcinoma projects into the lumen but has not caused obstruction.

Figure 15–38   ■

Carcinoma of the descending colon. This circumferential tumor has heaped-up edges and an ulcerated central portion. The arrows identify separate mucosal polyps.

Clinical Features. Colorectal cancers remain asymptomatic for years; symptoms develop insidiously and frequently have been present for months, sometimes years, before diagnosis. Cecal and right colonic cancers most often are called to clinical attention by the appearance of fatigue, weakness, and iron deficiency anemia. Left-sided lesions may produce occult bleeding, changes in bowel habit, or crampy left lower quadrant discomfort. Although anemia in females may arise from gynecologic causes, it is a clinical maxim that *iron deficiency anemia in an older man means gastrointestinal cancer until proved otherwise.*

All colorectal tumors spread by direct extension into adjacent structures and by metastasis through the lymphatics and blood vessels. In order of preference, the favored sites for metastasis are the regional lymph nodes, liver, lungs, and bones, followed by many other sites including the serosal membrane of the peritoneal cavity. In general, the disease has spread beyond the range of curative surgery in 25% to 30% of patients. Carcinomas of the anal region are locally invasive and metastasize to regional lymph nodes and distant sites.

The detection and diagnosis of colorectal neoplasms relies on a variety of methods, beginning with digital rectal examination and fecal testing for occult blood loss. Barium enema, sigmoidoscopy, and colonoscopy usually require confirmatory biopsy for diagnosis. Computed tomography and other radiographic studies are usually employed to assess metastatic spread. Serum markers for disease, such as elevated blood levels of carcinoembryonic antigen, are of little diagnostic value, because they reach significant levels only after the tumor has achieved considerable size and has very likely spread. Moreover, "positive" carcinoembryonic antigen levels may be produced by carcinomas of the lung, breast, ovary, urinary bladder, and prostate, as well as such non-neoplastic disorders as alcoholic cirrhosis, pancreatitis, and ulcerative colitis. Because *APC* mutations occur early in colon cancers, molecular detection of *APC* mutations in epithelial cells, isolated from stools, is being evaluated as a diagnostic test.

The single most important prognostic indicator of colorectal carcinoma is the extent (stage) of the tumor at the time of diagnosis. The American Joint Commission on Cancer uses the TNM classification (Table 15–12). The challenge is to discover these neoplasms when curative resection is possible, preferably in their "infancy" when they are still adenomatous polyps.

Small Intestinal Neoplasms

Whereas the small bowel represents 75% of the length of the alimentary tract, its tumors account for only 3% to 6% of gastrointestinal tumors, with a slight preponderance of benign tumors. The number of deaths in the United States annually is under 1000, representing only about 1% of gastrointestinal malignancies. The most frequent benign tumors in the small intestine are stromal tumors of predominantly smooth muscle origin, adenomas, and lipomas, followed by various neurogenic, vascular, and hamartomatous epithelial lesions. Small intestinal adenocarcinomas and carcinoids have a roughly equal incidence. Gastrointestinal stromal tumors (GISTs) have received much attention recently because they have an activating mutation affecting *KIT*, a tyrosine kinase receptor. Because of this, they can be treated with the tyrosine kinase inhibitor STI-571 (Gleevec), originally developed for treatment of chronic myeloid leukeumia (Chapters 6 and 12).

Figure 15–39   ■

Invasive adenocarcinoma of colon showing malignant glands infiltrating the muscle wall.

Table 15-12. TNM STAGING OF COLON CANCERS

Tumor (T)

0 = none evident
is = in situ (limited to mucosa)
1 = invasion of submucosa
2 = invasion of muscularis propria
3 = invasion of subserosa or nonperitonealized pericolic fat
4 = invasion of contiguous structures

Lymph Nodes (N)

0 = none evident
1 = 1 to 3 positive pericolic nodes
2 = 4 or more positive pericolic nodes
3 = any positive node along a named blood vessel

Distant Metastasis (M)

0 = none evident
1 = any distant metastasis

5-Year Survival Rates

T1 = 97%
T2 = 90%
T3 = 78%
T4 = 63%
Any T; N1; M0 = 66%
Any T; N2; M0 = 37%
Any T; N3; M0 = data not available
Any M1 = 4%

ADENOCARCINOMA OF THE SMALL INTESTINE

These tumors grow in a napkin-ring encircling pattern or as polypoid fungating masses, in a manner similar to colonic cancers. Most small bowel carcinomas arise in the duodenum (including the ampulla of Vater). Cramping pain, nausea, vomiting, and weight loss are the common presenting signs and symptoms, but such manifestations generally appear late in the course of these cancers. Most have already penetrated the bowel wall, invaded the mesentery or other segments of the gut, spread to regional nodes, and sometimes metastasized to the liver and more widely by the time of diagnosis. Despite these problems, wide en bloc excision of these cancers yields a 5-year survival rate of about 70%. Duodenal lesions in the periampullary region may lead to obstructive jaundice early in their course.

CARCINOID TUMORS

Cells generating bioactive compounds, particularly peptide and nonpeptide hormones, are normally dispersed along the length of the gastrointestinal tract mucosa and play a major role in coordinated gut function. Although they are derived from epithelial stem cells in the mucosal crypts, they are designated *endocrine* because phenotypically they resemble endocrine cells in parenchymal organs (e.g., pancreatic islets). Endocrine cells are abundant in other organs, including the lungs, but the great preponderance of tumors arising from these cells are in the gut. A scattering of carcinoid tumors arises in the pancreas or peripancreatic tissue, lungs, biliary tree, and even liver. The term *carcinoid* is an old reference to "carcinoma-like,"

which has persisted through the decades. The peak incidence of these neoplasms is in the sixth decade, but they may appear at any age. They comprise less than 2% of colorectal malignancies but almost half of small intestinal malignant tumors.

Although all carcinoids are potentially malignant tumors, the tendency for aggressive behavior correlates with the site of origin, the depth of local penetration, and the size of the tumor. For example, *appendiceal and rectal carcinoids infrequently metastasize*, even though they may show extensive local spread. By contrast, 90% of ileal, gastric, and colonic carcinoids that have penetrated halfway through the muscle wall have spread to lymph nodes and distant sites at the time of diagnosis, especially those greater than 2 cm in diameter.

As with normal gut endocrine cells, the cells of carcinoid tumors can synthesize and secrete a variety of bioactive products and hormones. Although multiple factors may be synthesized by a single tumor, when a tumor secretes a predominant product to cause a clinical syndrome, it may be called by that name (e.g., gastrinoma, somatostatinoma, and insulinoma).

MORPHOLOGY

The appendix is the most common site of gut carcinoid tumors, followed by the small intestine (primarily ileum), rectum, stomach, and colon. In the appendix they appear as bulbous swellings of the tip, which frequently obliterate the lumen. Elsewhere in the gut, they appear as intramural or submucosal masses that create small, polypoid, or plateau-like elevations rarely more than 3 cm in diameter (Fig. 15–40A). The overlying mucosa may be intact or ulcerated, and the tumors may permeate the bowel wall to invade the mesentery. Those that arise in the stomach and ileum are frequently multicentric, but the remainder tend to be solitary lesions. **A characteristic feature is a solid, yellow-tan appearance on transection.** The tumors are exceedingly firm, owing to striking desmoplasia; and when these fibrosing lesions penetrate the mesentery of the small bowel they may cause sufficient angulation or kinking to cause obstruction. When present, visceral metastases are usually small, dispersed nodules and rarely achieve the size seen with the primary lesions. Notably, **rectal and appendiceal carcinoids almost never metastasize.**

Histologically, the neoplastic cells may form discrete islands, trabeculae, strands, glands, or undifferentiated sheets. Whatever their organization, the tumor cells are monotonously similar, having a scant, pink granular cytoplasm and a round-to-oval stippled nucleus. In most tumors, there is minimal variation in cell and nuclear size and mitoses are infrequent or absent (Fig. 15–40B). By electron microscopy (Fig. 15–40C), the cells in most tumors contain cytoplasmic, well-formed, membrane-bound secretory granules with osmophilic centers (dense-core granules). Most carcinoids can be shown to contain chromogranin A, synaptophysin,

Figure 15–40

Carcinoid tumor. *A,* Multiple protruding tumors are present at the ileocecal junction. *B,* The tumor cells exhibit a monotonous morphology, with a delicate intervening fibrovascular stroma. (H & E.) *C,* Electron micrograph showing dense-core bodies in the cytoplasm.

and neuron-specific enolase. Specific hormonal peptides may occasionally be identified by immunocytochemical techniques.

Clinical Features. Gastrointestinal carcinoids are frequently asymptomatic, including virtually all that arise in the appendix. Only rarely do carcinoids produce local symptoms secondary to angulation or obstruction of the small intestine. However, the secretory products of some carcinoids may produce a variety of syndromes or endocrinopathies. Gastric, peripancreatic, and pancreatic carcinoids can release their products directly into the systemic circulation and can produce the Zollinger-Ellison syndrome by excess elaboration of gastrin, Cushing syndrome caused by adrenocorticotropic hormone secretion, hyperinsulinism, and others. In some instances, these tumors may be less than 1.0 cm in size and extremely difficult to find, even during surgical exploration.

Some neoplasms are associated with a distinctive *carcinoid syndrome,* detailed in Table 15–13. The syndrome occurs in about 1% of all patients with carcinoids and in 20%

of those with widespread metastases. The precise basis of the carcinoid syndrome is uncertain, but most manifestations are thought to arise from elaboration of serotonin (5-hydroxytryptamine [5-HT]). Elevated levels of 5-HT and its metabolite, 5-hydroxyindoleacetic acid (5-HIAA), are present in the blood and urine of most patients with the classic syndrome; 5-HT is degraded in the liver to functionally inactive 5-HIAA. Thus, with gastrointestinal carcinoids, hepatic dysfunction resulting from metastases must be present for the development of the syndrome. The possibility that other secretory products such as histamine, bradykinin, and prostaglandins contribute to the manifestations of this syndrome has not been excluded.

The 5-year survival rate for carcinoids (excluding appendiceal) is approximately 90%. Even with small bowel tumors that have spread to the liver, it is better than 50%. However, widespread disease usually causes death.

GASTROINTESTINAL LYMPHOMA

Any segment of the gastrointestinal tract may be involved secondarily by systemic dissemination of non-Hodgkin lymphomas. However, up to 40% of lymphomas arise in sites other than lymph nodes, and the gut is the most common extranodal location; 1% to 4% of all gastrointestinal malignancies are lymphomas. By definition, primary gastrointestinal lymphomas exhibit no evidence of liver, spleen, or bone marrow involvement at the time of diagnosis; regional lymph node involvement may be present. Sporadic lymphomas are the most common form in the Western hemisphere and appear to arise from the B cells of mucosa-associated lymphoid tissue (MALT) (Chapter 12). This type of gastrointestinal lymphoma usually affects adults, lacks a sex predilection, and may arise anywhere in the gut: stomach (55% to 60% of cases), small intestine (25% to 30%), proximal colon (10% to 15%), and distal colon (up to 10%). The appendix and esophagus are only rarely involved. For most gastrointestinal lymphomas, no specific associations with predisposing diseases or pathologic lesions have been reported. However, it appears very

---

Table 15–13. CLINICAL FEATURES OF THE CARCINOID SYNDROME

Vasomotor disturbances
   Cutaneous flushes and apparent cyanosis (most patients)
Intestinal hypermotility
   Diarrhea, cramps, nausea, vomiting (most patients)
Asthmatic bronchoconstrictive attacks
   Cough, wheezing, dyspnea (about one third of patients)
Hepatomegaly
   Nodular, related to hepatic metastases (some cases)
Niacin deficiency (due to shunting of niacin to serotonin synthesis)
Systemic fibrosis
   Cardiac involvement
      Pulmonic and tricuspid valve thickening and stenosis
      Endocardial fibrosis, principally in right ventricle (bronchial
         carcinoids affect the left side)
   Retroperitoneal and pelvic fibrosis
   Collagenous pleural and intimal aortic plaques

likely that gastric MALT lymphomas arise in the setting of mucosal lymphoid activation, as a result of *Helicobacter*-associated chronic gastritis. With *H. pylori* infection, there is an intense activation of T and B cells in the mucosa. This leads to polyclonal B-cell hyperplasia and eventually to the emergence of a monoclonal B-cell neoplasm. Celiac disease (as discussed) is associated with a higher than normal risk of T-cell lymphomas.

Primary gastrointestinal lymphomas generally have a better prognosis than do those arising in other sites, because combined surgery, chemotherapy, and radiation therapy offer reasonable hopes of cure.

■ ■ ■ Appendix

Diseases of the appendix loom large in surgical practice; appendicitis is the most common acute abdominal condition the surgeon is called on to treat. Despite the preeminence of this diagnostic entity, a differential diagnosis must include virtually every acute process that can occur within the abdominal cavity, as well as some emergent conditions affecting organs of the thorax. On occasion, a tumor arises in the appendix, necessitating abdominal exploration.

ACUTE APPENDICITIS

Surveys indicate that approximately 10% of persons in the United States and other Western countries develop appendicitis at some time. No age is immune, but the peak incidence is in the second and third decades, although lately a second smaller peak is appearing among elderly persons. Males are affected more often than females in a ratio of 1.5:1.

Pathogenesis. Appendiceal inflammation is associated with obstruction in 50% to 80% of cases, usually in the form of a fecalith and, less commonly, a gallstone, tumor, or ball of worms *(Oxyuriasis vermicularis)*. With continued secretion of mucinous fluid, the build-up of intraluminal pressure presumably is sufficient to cause collapse of the draining veins. Obstruction and ischemic injury then favors bacterial proliferation with additional inflammatory edema and exudation, further embarrassing the blood supply. Nevertheless, a significant minority of inflamed appendices have no demonstrable luminal obstruction, and the pathogenesis of the inflammation remains unknown.

MORPHOLOGY

At the earliest stages, only a scant neutrophilic exudate may be found throughout the mucosa, submucosa, and muscularis propria. Subserosal vessels are congested, and often there is a modest perivascular neutrophilic infiltrate. The inflammatory reaction transforms the normal glistening serosa into a dull, granular, red membrane; this transformation signifies **early acute appendicitis** for the operating surgeon. At a later stage, a prominent neutrophilic exudate generates a fibrinopurulent reaction over the serosa (Fig. 15–41). As the inflammatory process worsens, there is abscess formation within the wall, along with ulcerations and foci of necrosis in the mucosa. This state constitutes **acute suppurative appendicitis.** Further appendiceal compromise leads to large areas of hemorrhagic green ulceration of the mucosa, and green-black gangrenous necrosis through the wall extending to the serosa, creating **acute gangrenous appendici-**

Figure 15–41 ■

Acute appendicitis. The inflamed appendix *(bottom)* is red, swollen, and covered with a fibrinous exudate. For comparison, a normal appendix is shown *(top)*.

tis that is quickly followed by rupture and suppurative peritonitis.

The histologic criterion for the diagnosis of acute appendicitis is neutrophilic infiltration of the muscularis propria. Usually, neutrophils and ulcerations are also present within the mucosa.

Clinical Features. Acute appendicitis is either the easiest or the most difficult of abdominal diagnoses. The classic case is marked by (1) mild periumbilical discomfort, followed by (2) anorexia, nausea, and vomiting, soon associated with (3) right lower quadrant tenderness, which in the course of hours is transformed into (4) a deep constant ache or pain in the right lower quadrant. Fever and leukocytosis appear early in the course. Regrettably, a large number of cases are not classic. The condition can be remarkably silent, particularly in the aged, or can fail to reveal localizing right-sided lower quadrant signs, as when the appendix is retrocecal or when there is malrotation of the colon. Moreover, the following disorders may present many of the clinical features of acute appendicitis: (1) mesenteric lymphadenitis after a viral systemic infection, (2) gastroenteritis with mesenteric adenitis, (3) pelvic inflammatory disease with tubo-ovarian involvement, (4) rupture of an ovarian follicle at the time of ovulation, (5) ectopic pregnancy, (6) Meckel diverticulitis, and other conditions as well. Thus, with conventional diagnostic techniques (starting with physical examination), an accurate diagnosis of acute appendicitis can be made only about 80% of the time. Newer preoperative imaging modalities may be increasing diagnostic accuracy to 95%. Regardless, *it is generally conceded that it is better to occasionally resect a normal appendix than to risk the morbidity and mortality (about 2%) of appendiceal perforation.*

TUMORS OF THE APPENDIX

Carcinoids (discussed earlier) are the most common form of neoplasia in the appendix. The only other lesions worthy of mention are mucocele of the appendix and mucinous neoplasms.

Mucocele refers to dilation of the lumen of the appendix by mucinous secretion. It is caused by non-neoplastic obstruction of the lumen and is usually associated with a fecalith in the lumen, permitting the slow accumulation of sterile mucinous secretions. Eventually, the distention induces atrophy of the mucin-secreting mucosal cells and the secretions stop. This condition is usually asymptomatic; rarely, a mucocele ruptures, spilling otherwise innocuous mucin into the peritoneum.

Mucinous neoplasms range from the benign *mucinous cystadenoma*, to *mucinous cystadenocarcinoma*, which invades the wall, to a form of disseminated intraperitoneal cancer called *pseudomyxoma peritonei*. The cystadenoma is histologically identical to analogous tumors in the ovary (Chapter 19). The malignant mucin-secreting neoplasms (cystadenocarcinomas) invade the wall, allowing tumor cells to implant throughout the peritoneal cavity, which becomes filled with mucin (pseudomyxoma peritonei).

BIBLIOGRAPHY

Oral Cavity

Ficarra G, Eversole LE: HIV-related tumors of the oral cavity. Crit Rev Oral Biol Med 5:159, 1994. (A discussion of risk conditions for squamous cell carcinoma, lymphoma, and Kaposi's sarcoma of the oral cavity.)

Forastiere A, et al: Head and neck cancer. N Engl J Med 345:1890, 2001. (A review of molecular and clinical features of cancers of head and neck, including oral cavity.)

Iezzoni JC, et al: The role of Epstein-Barr virus in lymphoepithelioma-like carcinomas. Am J Clin Pathol 103:308, 1995. (A discussion of virus-induced neoplasms throughout the alimentary tract, including oral cavity squamous cell carcinoma and lymphoma-like lesions.)

Simpson RH: Classification of salivary gland tumors—a brief histopathological review. Histol Histopathol 10:737, 1995. (A primer on the morphologic features of salivary gland tumors.)

Esophagus

Haggitt RC: Barrett's esophagus, dysplasia, and adenocarcinoma. Hum Pathol 25:982, 1994. (A comparison of histological and molecular features of dysplasia in Barrett's esophagus.)

Jankowski JA, et al: Molecular evolution of the metaplasia-dysplasia-adenocarcinoma sequence in the esophagus. Am J Pathol 154:965, 1999. (A review focusing on the abnormalities of oncogenes, tumor suppressor genes, and growth factors in the development of esophageal adenocarcinoma.)

Katzka DA, Rustagi AK: Gastroesophageal reflux disease and Barrett's esophagus. Med Clin North Am 84:1137, 2000. (An excellent discussion of these common conditions—both clinical and basic.)

McCormick PA: Pathophysiology and prognosis of oesophageal varices. Scand J Gastroenterol 29(Suppl 207):1, 1994. (A convincing discussion of the grave nature of this disease condition.)

Paterson WG: Etiology and pathogenesis of achalasia. Gastrointest Endosc Clin North Am 11:249, 2001.

Spechler SJ: Barrett's esophagus. N Engl J Med 346:836, 2002. (An excellent discussion that touches on clinical, histologic, and prognostic issues.)

Stomach

Appelman HD: Gastritis: terminology, etiology, and clinicopathological correlations: another biased view. Hum Pathol 25:1006, 1994. (An enlightened review of the many attempts to understand, and classify, chronic gastritis.)

Bjorkman DJ, Kimmey MB: Nonsteroidal anti-inflammatory drugs and gastrointestinal disease: pathophysiology, treatment and prevention. Dig Dis 13:199, 1995. (A review of the predominantly upper gastrointestinal tract disorders induced by these often-used pharmaceuticals.)

Dundan WG, et al: Virulence factors of *Helicobacter pylori*. Int J Med Microbiol 290:647, 2001. (An excellent summary of *Helicobacter*-elaborated toxins and enzymes.)

Fox JG, Wang TC: *Helicobacter pylori*—not a good bug after all. N Engl J Med 345:829, 2001. (An editorial that discusses the role of *H. pylori* in gastric cancer.)

Fuchs CS, Mayer RJ: Gastric carcinoma. N Engl J Med 333:32, 1995. (A review of epidemiology, pathology, and clinical features of gastric cancer.)

Israel DA, et al: *Helicobacter pylori* strain-specific differences in genetic content, identified by microarray, influence host inflammatory responses. J Clin Invest 107:611, 2001. (This paper relates molecular differences in *H. pylori* isolates to pathogenicity.)

Sepulveda AR: Molecular testing of *Helicobacter pylori*-associated chronic gastritis and premalignant gastric lesions: clinical implications. J Clin Gastroenterol 32:377, 2001. (An examination of both the molecular evolution of gastric cancer and the role of molecular analysis in clinical management.)

Werner M, et al: Gastric adenocarcinoma: pathomorphology and molecular pathology. J Cancer Res Clin Oncol 124:207, 2001. (Current concepts in gastric carcinogenesis.)

Small and Large Intestines

Andres PG, Friedman LS: Epidemiology and the natural course of inflammatory bowel disease. Gastroenterol Clin North Am 28:255, 1999. (Selected clinical and epidemiological update of inflammatory bowel disease.)

Farrell RJ, Kelley CP: Celiac sprue. N Engl J Med 346:180, 2002. (An excellent review of this common but under-recognized disorder.)

Fernhead NS, et al: The ABC of *APC*. Hum Mol Genet 10:721, 2001. (An excellent review and update on the APC/β-catenin pathway of colorectal cancers.)

Guerrant RL, et al: Diarrhea in developed and developing countries: magnitude, special settings, and etiologies. Rev Infect Dis 12(Suppl 1):S41, 1990. (An excellent analysis of the various etiologies and their prevalence.)

Gupta RA, Dubois R: Colorectal cancer prevention and treatment by inhibition of cyclooxygenase-2. Nature Rev Cancer 1:11, 2001. (An excellent discussion of the clinical evidence documenting chemopreventive actions of cyclooxygenase inhibitors, and the possible molecular basis of this action.)

Jass JR: Serrated route to colorectal cancer: back street or super highway? J Pathol 193:283, 2001. (A discussion of the evidence that some hyperplastic polyps can give rise to colon cancer by the mismatch repair pathway.)

Kulke MH, Mayer RJ: Carcinoid tumors. N Engl J Med 340:858, 1999. (An excellent clinical review of carcinoid tumors.)

Lee WS: Gastrointestinal infections in children in the Southeast Asia region: emerging issues. J Pediatr Gastroenterol Nutr 30:241, 2000. (Update on epidemiology of this worldwide disease.)

Levine JS: Intestinal ischemic disorders. Dig Dis 13:3, 1995. (A review of the clinical and pathophysiologic features, particularly those of severe disease.)

Müller HH, et al: Genetics of hereditary colon cancer—a basis for prevention? Eur J Cancer 36:1215, 2000. (Discussion of molecular basis of polyposis syndromes.)

Papadakis KA, Targan SR: Current theories on the causation of inflammatory bowel disease. Gastroenterol Clin 28:283, 1999. (A comprehensive discussion of the genetic and immunologic factors in IBD.)

Peltomäki P: Deficient DNA mismatch repair: a common etiologic factor for colon cancer. Hum Mol Genet 10:735, 2001. (A discussion of the molecular pathways that involve mismatch repair genes and give rise to colon cancer.)

Podolsky DK: Inflammatory bowel disease. N Engl J Med 325:929, 1008, 1991. (The definitive summary of both Crohn disease and ulcerative colitis, highlighting the similarities and differences.)

van Heel DA, et al: Crohn's disease: genetic susceptibility, bacteria, and innate immunity. Lancet 357:1902, 2001. (A commentary on the discovery of the *NOD2* gene as a susceptibility marker for Crohn disease.)

Wirtzfelt DA, et al: Hamartomatous polyposis syndromes: molecular genetics, neoplastic risk, and surveillance recommendations. Ann Surg Oncol 8:319, 2001. (A discussion of these uncommon diseases and their genetics.)

Young-Fadok TM, et al: Colonic diverticular disease. Curr Prob Surg 37:459, 2000. (An excellent review of pathogenesis and clinical management.)

Appendix

Birnbaum BA, Wilson SR: Appendicitis at the millennium. Radiology 215:337, 2000. (An excellent overview of pathophysiology and treatment.)

Gray GF Jr, Wackym PA: Surgical pathology of the vermiform appendix. Pathol Annu 21:111, 1986. (A review of the essential pathology of the appendix.)

Young RH, et al: Mucinous tumors of the appendix associated with mucinous tumors of the ovary and pseudomyxoma peritonei: a clinicopathological analysis of 22 cases supporting an origin in the appendix. Am J Surg Pathol 15:415, 1991. (A definitive discussion of mucinous tumors of the appendix and peritoneum.)

16

The Liver and the Biliary Tract

JAMES M. CRAWFORD, MD, PhD

The Liver

The Biliary Tract

DISORDERS OF THE GALLBLADDER
Cholelithiasis (Gallstones)
Cholecystitis
Acute Calculous Cholecystitis
Acute Acalculous Cholecystitis
Chronic Cholecystitis

DISORDERS OF EXTRAHEPATIC BILE DUCTS
Choledocholithiasis and Ascending
Cholangitis
Biliary Atresia
TUMORS
Carcinoma of the Gallbladder
Carcinoma of the Extrahepatic Bile Ducts,
Including Ampulla of Vater

The Liver

The right upper quadrant of the abdomen is dominated by the liver and its companion biliary tree and gallbladder. These structures are considered together not only because of their anatomic proximity and interrelated functions but also because diseases affecting these organs may have overlapping features. Discussion of the liver dominates because the liver plays by far the greater role in normal physiology and is afflicted by a wider variety of diseases.

Residing at the crossroads between the digestive tract and the rest of the body, the liver has the enormous task of maintaining the body's metabolic homeostasis. This includes the processing of dietary amino acids, carbohydrates, lipids, and vitamins; synthesis of serum proteins; and detoxification and excretion into bile of endogenous waste products and pollutant xenobiotics. Hepatic disorders have far-reaching consequences, given the critical dependence of other organs on the metabolic function of the liver. Liver injury and its manifestations tend to follow characteristic patterns, which are discussed first before specific diseases are described.

GENERAL PRINCIPLES

The liver is vulnerable to a wide variety of metabolic, toxic, microbial, and circulatory insults. In some instances, the disease process is primary to the liver. In others, the hepatic involvement is secondary, often to some of the most common diseases in humans, such as cardiac decompensation, alcoholism, and extrahepatic infections. The functional reserve of the liver masks to some extent the clinical impact of early liver damage. However, with progression of diffuse disease or strategic disruption of the circulation or bile flow, the consequences of deranged liver function become life-threatening.

Hepatic Injury

From a morphologic standpoint, the liver is an inherently simple organ, with a limited repertoire of responses to injurious events. Regardless of cause, five general responses are seen. These processes, and the morphologic terms used to describe them, are summarized in the following brief overview.

MORPHOLOGY

INFLAMMATION. Injury to hepatocytes associated with an influx of acute or chronic inflammatory cells into the liver is termed **hepatitis**. Although hepatocyte necrosis may precede the onset of inflammation, the converse is also true. Attack of viable antigen-expressing liver cells by sensitized T cells is a common cause of liver damage. Inflammation may be limited to portal tracts or may spill over into the parenchyma. When hepatocytes undergo destruction, scavenger macrophages quickly engulf the dead cells, generating clumps of inflammatory cells in an otherwise normal parenchyma. Foreign bodies, organisms, and a variety of drugs may incite a granulomatous reaction.

DEGENERATION. Damage from toxic or immunologic insult may cause hepatocytes to take on a swollen, edematous appearance **(ballooning degeneration)** with irregularly clumped cytoplasm and large, clear spaces. Alternatively, retained biliary material may impart a diffuse, foamy, swollen appearance to the hepatocyte **(foamy degeneration)**. Substances may accumulate in viable hepatocytes, including iron, copper, and retained biliary material. Accumulation of fat droplets within hepatocytes is known as **steatosis.** Multiple tiny droplets that do not displace the nucleus are known as **microvesicular steatosis** and appear in such conditions as alcoholic liver disease, Reye syndrome, and acute fatty liver of pregnancy (a potentially fatal cause of hepatic failure in the third trimester of pregnancy). A single large droplet that displaces the nucleus, **macrovesicular steatosis,** may be seen in the alcoholic liver or in the livers of obese or diabetic individuals.

CELL DEATH. Virtually any significant insult to the liver may cause hepatocyte destruction. In necrosis, poorly stained mummified hepatocytes remain, most commonly as the result of ischemia **(coagulative necrosis)**. Cell death that is toxic or immunologically mediated occurs via **apoptosis,** in which isolated hepatocytes become shrunken, pyknotic, and intensely eosinophilic. Alternatively, hepatocytes may osmotically swell and rupture, so-called **hydropic degeneration** or **lytic necrosis.**

In the setting of ischemia and a number of drug and toxic reactions, hepatocyte necrosis is distributed immediately around the central vein **(centrilobular necrosis)**. Pure midzonal and periportal necrosis is rare. Instead, with most other causes of hepatic injury, a variable mixture of inflammation and hepatocyte death is encountered. In immunologically mediated hepatocyte death, apoptosis may be limited to scattered cells within the hepatic parenchyma or to the interface between the periportal parenchyma and inflamed portal tracts **(interface hepatitis)**. With more severe inflammatory or toxic injury, apoptosis or necrosis of contiguous hepatocytes may span adjacent lobules in a portal-to-portal, portal-to-central, or central-to-central fashion **(bridging necrosis)**. Destruction of entire lobules **(submassive necrosis)** or most of the liver parenchyma **(massive necrosis)** is usually accompanied by hepatic failure. With disseminated candidal or bacterial infection, macroscopic abscesses may occur.

FIBROSIS. Fibrous tissue is formed in response to inflammation or direct toxic insult to the liver. Deposition of collagen has lasting consequences on hepatic patterns of blood flow and perfusion of hepatocytes. In the initial stages, fibrosis may develop within or around portal tracts or the central vein or may be deposited directly within the sinusoids. With time, fibrous strands link regions of the liver (portal-to-portal, portal-to-central, central-to-central), a process called **bridging fibrosis.**

Unlike all of the other lesions, which are reversible, **fibrosis is generally considered an irreversible consequence of hepatic damage,** but there is growing evidence that cessation of hepatic injury in some settings can lead to reversal of fibrosis. Best documented are regression of fibrosis in treated schistosomal hepatic infection and hereditary hemochromatosis (see later).

CIRRHOSIS. With continuing fibrosis and parenchymal injury, the liver is subdivided into nodules of regenerating hepatocytes surrounded by scar tissue, termed **cirrhosis.** This end-stage form of liver disease is discussed later in this section.

The liver has enormous functional reserve, and regeneration occurs in all but the most fulminant of hepatic diseases. Thus, in a normal individual, surgical removal of 75% of the liver produces minimal hepatic impairment, and regeneration restores liver mass within a few weeks. When massive hepatocellular necrosis occurs and leaves the connective tissue framework intact, almost perfect restitution can occur if the patient can survive the metabolic insult of liver failure.

The ebb and flow of hepatic injury may be imperceptible to the patient and detectable only by laboratory tests (Table 16–1). Alternatively, hepatic function may be so impaired as to be life-threatening. The major clinical consequences of liver disease are listed in Table 16–2 and are discussed next.

Jaundice and Cholestasis

Hepatic bile formation serves two major functions. Bile constitutes the primary pathway for the elimination of bilirubin, excess cholesterol, and xenobiotics that are insufficiently water soluble to be excreted into urine. Second, secreted bile salts and phospholipid molecules promote emulsification of dietary fat in the lumen of the gut. Because bile formation is one of the most sophisticated functions of the liver, it is also one of the most readily disrupted. Thus, *jaundice,* a yellow discoloration of skin and sclerae (icterus), occurs when systemic retention of bilirubin leads to elevated serum levels above 2.0 mg/dL, the normal in the adult being less than 1.2 mg/dL. *Cholestasis,* on the other hand, is defined as systemic retention of not only bilirubin but also other solutes eliminated in bile (particularly bile salts and cholesterol).

Table 16-1. LABORATORY EVALUATION OF LIVER DISEASE

Test Category	Serum Measurement
Hepatocyte integrity	Cytosolic hepatocellular enzymes* *Serum aspartate aminotransferase* (AST) *Serum alanine aminotransferase* (ALT) Serum lactate dehydrogenase (LDH)

Biliary excretory function	Substances secreted in bile*
	 Serum bilirubin
	   Total: unconjugated plus conjugated
	   Direct: conjugated only
	   Delta: covalently linked to albumin
	 Urine bilirubin
	 Serum bile acids
	 Plasma membrane enzymes*
	   (from damage to bile canaliculus)
	 Serum alkaline phosphatase
	 Serum γ-glutamyl transpeptidase
	 Serum 5′-nucleotidase

Hepatocyte function	Proteins secreted into the blood *Serum albumin†* *Prothrombin time** (factors V, VII, X, prothrombin, fibrinogen) Hepatocyte metabolism Serum ammonia* Aminopyrine breath test (hepatic demethylation) Galactose elimination (intravenous injection)

Most common tests are in italics.
*An elevation implicates liver disease.
†A decrease implicates liver disease.

Table 16-2. CLINICAL CONSEQUENCES OF LIVER DISEASE

Characteristic Signs	Hepatic dysfunction:
	   Jaundice and cholestasis
	   Hypoalbuminemia
	   Hyperammonemia
	   Hypoglycemia
	   Fetor hepaticus
	   Palmar erythema
	   Spider angiomas
	   Hypogonadism
	   Gynecomastia
	   Weight loss
	   Muscle wasting
	 Portal hypertension from cirrhosis:
	   Ascites
	   Splenomegaly
	   Hemorrhoids
	   Caput medusae—abdominal skin

Life-threatening Complications	Hepatic failure
	   Multiple organ failure
	   Coagulopathy
	   Hepatic encephalopathy
	   Hepatorenal syndrome
	 Portal hypertension from cirrhosis
	   Esophageal varices, risk of rupture
	 Malignancy with chronic disease
	   Hepatocellular carcinoma

BILIRUBIN AND BILE ACIDS

Bilirubin is the end product of heme degradation (Fig. 16–1). Most of the daily production (0.2 to 0.3 g) is derived from breakdown of senescent erythrocytes, with the remainder derived primarily from the turnover of hepatic hemoproteins and from premature destruction of newly formed erythrocytes in the bone marrow. The latter pathway is important in hematologic disorders associated with excessive intramedullary hemolysis of defective erythrocytes (ineffective erythropoiesis; Chapter 12). Whatever the source, heme oxygenase oxidizes heme to biliverdin, which is then reduced to bilirubin by biliverdin reductase. Bilirubin thus formed outside the liver in cells of the mononuclear phagocyte system (including the spleen) is released and bound to serum albumin. Hepatocellular processing of bilirubin involves (1) carrier-mediated uptake at the sinusoidal membrane, (2) cytosolic protein binding and delivery to the endoplasmic reticulum, (3) conjugation with one or two molecules of glucuronic acid by bilirubin uridine diphosphate-glucuronosyltransferase (UGT1A1), and (4) excretion of the water-soluble, nontoxic bilirubin glucuronides into bile. Most bilirubin glucuronides are deconjugated by gut bacterial β-glucuronidases and degraded to colorless urobilinogens. The urobilinogens, and the residue of intact pigment, are largely excreted in feces. Approximately 20% of the urobilinogens are reabsorbed in the ileum and colon, returned to the liver, and promptly re-excreted into bile. The small amount escaping this enterohepatic circulation is excreted in urine.

The brilliant yellow color of bilirubin makes it an easily identified component of hepatic bile. However, bilirubin excretion is but a minor cog in the hepatic machinery, which secretes 12 to 36 g of bile acids into bile per day. Bile acids are steroid molecules derived from cholesterol, with steroid ring hydroxyl groups and a side-chain carboxyl group. The polar groups make bile salts planar amphipathic molecules, enabling them to solubilize phospholipid and cholesterol in bile and dietary lipids in the gut lumen. The primary human bile acids are cholic acid and chenodeoxycholic acid, which are secreted as taurine and glycine conjugates. Ten percent to 20% of secreted bile acids are deconjugated in the intestines by bacterial action. Virtually all conjugated and deconjugated bile acids are reabsorbed (especially in the ileum) and returned to the liver for uptake, reconjugation, and resecretion. Fecal loss of bile acids (0.2 to 0.6 g/day) is matched by de novo hepatic synthesis of bile acids from cholesterol. The *enterohepatic circulation* of bile acids provides an efficient mechanism for maintaining a large endogenous pool of bile acids for secretory and digestive purposes.

PATHOPHYSIOLOGY OF JAUNDICE

Both unconjugated bilirubin and bilirubin glucuronides may accumulate systemically and deposit in tissues, giving rise to the yellow discoloration of jaundice. This is particularly evident in the yellowing of the sclerae (icterus). There are two important pathophysiologic differences between the two forms of bilirubin. *Unconjugated bilirubin is tightly complexed to serum albumin and is virtually insoluble in* water at physiologic pH. *This form cannot be excreted in the urine even when blood levels are high.* Normally, a very small amount of unconjugated bilirubin is present as an albumin-free anion in plasma. This fraction of unbound bilirubin may diffuse into tissues (particularly the brain in infants) and produce toxic injury. The unbound plasma fraction may increase in severe hemolytic disease or when protein-binding drugs displace bilirubin from albumin. Hence, hemolytic disease of the newborn (erythroblastosis fetalis) may lead to accumulation of unconjugated bilirubin in the brain, which can cause severe neurologic damage, referred to as *kernicterus* (Chapter 7). In contrast, *conjugated bilirubin is water soluble, nontoxic, and only loosely bound to albumin. Because of its solubility and weak association with albumin, excess conjugated bilirubin in plasma can be excreted in urine.* With prolonged conjugated hyperbilirubinemia, a portion of circulating pigment may become covalently bound to albumin. This "delta fraction" may persist in the circulation for weeks after correction of a cholestatic insult, owing to the plasma lifetime of albumin.

In the normal adult, serum bilirubin levels vary between 0.3 and 1.2 mg/dL, and the rate of systemic bilirubin production is equal to the rates of hepatic uptake, conjugation, and biliary excretion. Jaundice becomes evident when the serum bilirubin levels rise above 2.0 to 2.5 mg/dL; levels as high as 30 to 40 mg/dL can occur with severe disease. Jaundice occurs when the equilibrium between bilirubin production and clearance is disturbed by one or more of the following mechanisms (Table 16–3): (1) excessive production of bilirubin, (2) reduced hepatic uptake, (3) impaired conjugation, (4) decreased hepatocellular excretion, and (5) impaired bile flow (both intrahepatic and extrahepatic). The first three mechanisms produce unconjugated hyperbilirubinemia, and the latter two produce predominantly conjugated hyperbilirubinemia. More than one mechanism may operate to produce jaundice, especially in hepatitis, which may produce unconjugated and conjugated hyperbilirubinemia. In general, however, one mechanism predominates, so that knowledge of the predominant form of plasma bilirubin is of value in evaluating possible causes of hyperbilirubinemia.

Of the various causes of jaundice listed in Table 16–3, the most common are hemolytic anemias (Chapter 12), *hepatitis, and obstruction to the flow of bile* (discussed later in this chapter). Physiologic jaundice of the newborn and clinical jaundice resulting from inborn errors of metabolism merit brief consideration.

■ Because the hepatic machinery for conjugating and excreting bilirubin does not fully mature until about 2 weeks of

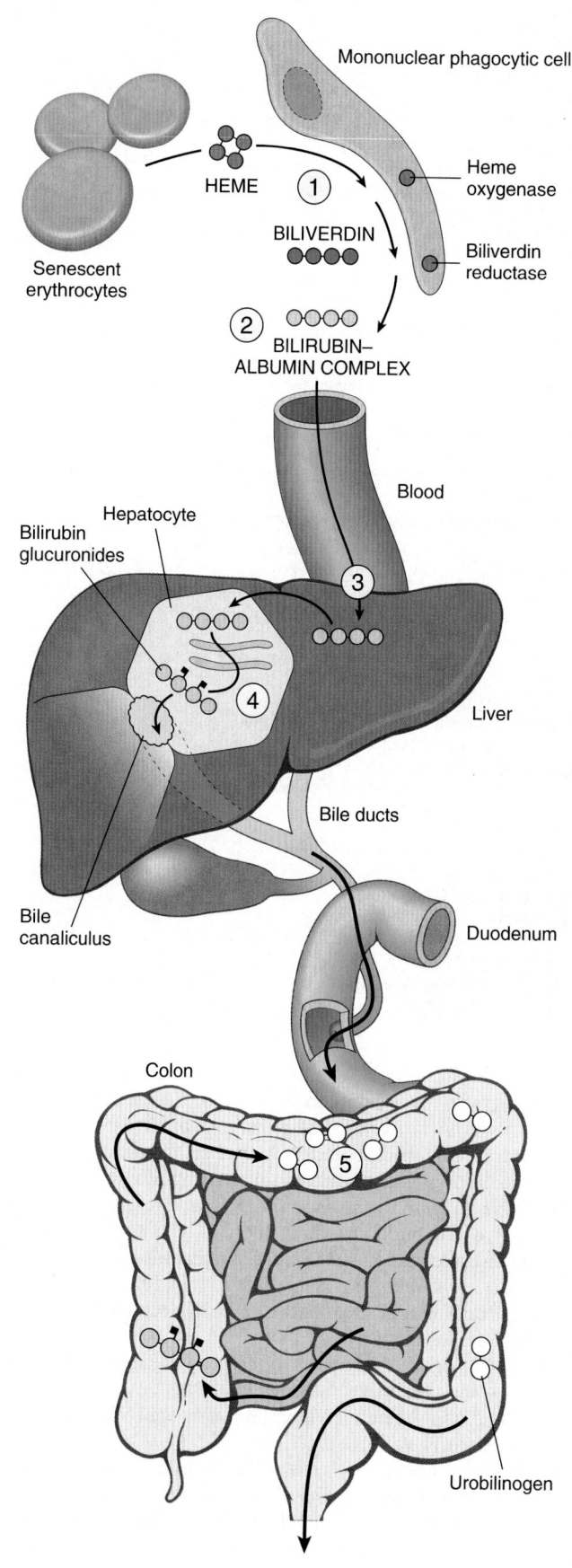

Figure 16–1   ■

Bilirubin metabolism and elimination. 1, Normal bilirubin production (0.2 to 0.3 g/day) is derived primarily from the breakdown of senescent circulating erythrocytes, with a minor contribution from degradation of tissue heme-containing proteins. 2, Extrahepatic bilirubin is bound to serum albumin and delivered to the liver. 3, Hepatocellular uptake and 4, glucuronidation by glucuronosyltransferase in the hepatocytes generates bilirubin monoglucuronides and diglucuronides, which are water soluble and readily excreted into bile. 5, Gut bacteria deconjugate the bilirubin and degrade it to colorless urobilinogens. The urobilinogens and the residue of intact pigments are excreted in the feces, with some reabsorption and re-excretion into bile.

■

Table 16-3. CAUSES OF JAUNDICE

Predominantly Unconjugated Hyperbilirubinemia

Excess production of bilirubin
  Hemolytic anemias
  Resorption of blood from internal hemorrhage (e.g., alimentary tract
    bleeding, hematomas)
  Ineffective erythropoiesis syndromes (e.g., pernicious anemia, thalassemia)
Reduced hepatic uptake
  Drug interference with membrane carrier systems
  Some cases of Gilbert syndrome
Impaired bilirubin conjugation
  Physiologic jaundice of the newborn (decreased UGT1A1 activity,
    decreased excretion)
  Breast milk jaundice (?increased deconjugation by β-glucuronidases)
  Genetic deficiency of bilirubin UGT1A1 activity (Crigler-Najjar
    syndromes types I and II)
  Gilbert syndrome (decreased expression of UGT1A1)
  Diffuse hepatocellular disease (e.g., viral or drug-induced hepatitis,
    cirrhosis)

Predominantly Conjugated Hyperbilirubinemia

Decreased hepatic excretion of bilirubin glucuronides
  Deficiency in canalicular membrane transporters (Dubin-Johnson
    syndrome, Rotor syndrome)
  Drug-induced canalicular membrane dysfunction (e.g., oral
    contraceptives, cyclosporine)
  Hepatocellular damage or toxicity (e.g., viral or drug-induced hepatitis,
    total parenteral nutrition, systemic infection)
Decreased intrahepatic bile flow
  Impaired bile flow through bile canaliculi (e.g., drug-induced
    microfilament dysfunction)
  Inflammatory destruction of intrahepatic bile ducts (e.g., primary biliary
    cirrhosis, primary sclerosing cholangitis, graft-versus-host disease,
    liver transplantation)
Extrahepatic biliary obstruction
  Gallstone obstruction of biliary tree
  Carcinomas of head of pancreas, extrahepatic bile ducts, ampulla of Vater
  Extrahepatic biliary atresia
  Biliary strictures and choledochal cysts
  Primary sclerosing cholangitis (extrahepatic)
  Liver fluke infestation

UGT1A1, bilirubin uridine diphosphate-glucuronosyltransferase.

age, almost every newborn develops transient and mild unconjugated hyperbilirubinemia, termed *neonatal jaundice* or *physiologic jaundice of the newborn*. Breast-fed infants tend to exhibit jaundice with greater frequency, possibly because of β-glucuronidases present in maternal milk.

■ *Crigler-Najjar syndrome type I* is a rare autosomal recessive condition in which there is a complete lack of the enzyme responsible for the conjugation of glucuronic acid to bilirubin. This syndrome is invariably fatal, causing death within 18 months of birth secondary to brain damage (kernicterus).

■ *Crigler-Najjar syndrome type II* is a less severe, nonfatal autosomal recessive disorder exhibiting a partial defect in the conjugating enzyme; the major consequence is extraordinarily yellow skin.

■ *Gilbert syndrome* is a relatively common, benign, somewhat heterogeneous inherited condition presenting as mild, fluctuating unconjugated hyperbilirubinemia. The primary cause is decreased hepatic levels of glucuronosyltransferase. Although this is attributed to a mutation of the responsible gene, additional polymorphisms may play a

role in the variable expression of this disorder. Affecting up to 7% of the population, the hyperbilirubinemia may go undiscovered for years and *does not have associated morbidity*.

■ *Dubin-Johnson syndrome* results from an autosomal recessive defect in the transport protein responsible for hepatocellular excretion of bilirubin glucuronides across the canalicular membrane. These patients exhibit conjugated hyperbilirubinemia. Other than having a darkly pigmented liver (from polymerized epinephrine metabolites, not bilirubin) and hepatomegaly, patients are otherwise without functional problems.

■ *Rotor syndrome* appears to be a variant of Dubin-Johnson syndrome in which the liver is not pigmented.

CHOLESTASIS

Cholestatic conditions, which result from hepatocellular dysfunction or intrahepatic or extrahepatic biliary obstruction, may also present as jaundice. However, sometimes *pruritus* is the presenting symptom, presumably related to the elevation in plasma bile acids and their deposition in peripheral tissues, particularly skin. *Skin xanthomas* (focal accumulations of cholesterol) sometimes appear, the result of hyperlipidemia and impaired excretion of cholesterol. A *characteristic laboratory finding is an elevated level of serum alkaline phosphatase*, an enzyme present in bile duct epithelium and in the canalicular membrane of hepatocytes. An isozyme is normally present in many other tissues such as bone, and so the increased levels must be verified as being hepatic in origin. Other manifestations of reduced bile flow relate to intestinal malabsorption, including inadequate absorption of the fat-soluble vitamins A, D, and K.

MORPHOLOGY

The morphologic features of cholestasis are similar for both nonobstructive and obstructive conditions. **Common to both forms is the accumulation of bile pigment within the hepatic parenchyma** (Fig. 16-2). Elongated green-brown plugs of bile are visible in dilated bile canaliculi. Rupture of canaliculi leads to extravasation of bile into the sinusoid, which is quickly phagocytosed by Kupffer cells. Droplets of bile pigment also accumulate within hepatocytes, which can take on a wispy appearance (feathery or **foamy degeneration**). **Obstruction to the biliary tree, either intrahepatic or extrahepatic, induces distention of upstream bile ducts by bile.** The bile stasis and back-pressure induce proliferation of epithelial cells and looping and reduplication of the ductules connecting bile ducts to the parenchyma, termed **bile ductular proliferation.** Associated portal tract findings include edema and periductal infiltrates of neutrophils. Prolonged obstructive cholestasis leads not only to foamy change of hepatocytes but also to focal destruction of the parenchyma, giving rise to **bile lakes** filled with cellular debris and pigment. **Unrelieved obstruction leads to portal tract fibrosis,**

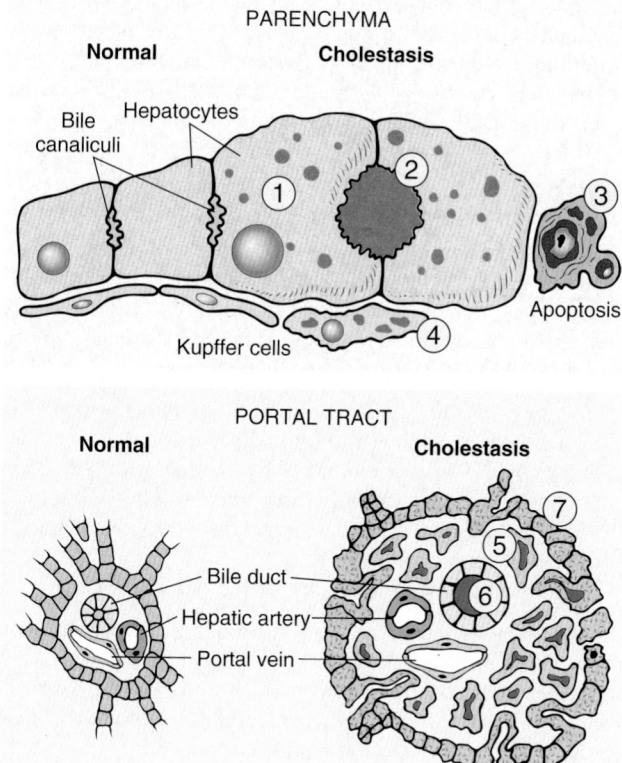

PARENCHYMA

Normal | **Cholestasis**

Bile canaliculi
Hepatocytes
Kupffer cells
Apoptosis

PORTAL TRACT

Normal | **Cholestasis**

Bile duct
Hepatic artery
Portal vein

Figure 16-2 ■

Schematic illustration of the morphologic features of cholestasis and comparison with normal liver. In the parenchyma *(top)*, cholestatic hepatocytes (1) are enlarged with dilated canalicular spaces (2). Apoptotic cells (3) may be seen, and Kupffer cells (4) frequently contain regurgitated bile pigments. In the portal tracts of obstructed livers *(bottom)*, there is also bile ductular proliferation (5), edema, bile pigment retention (6), and eventually neutrophilic inflammation (not shown). Hepatocytes immediately adjacent to portal tracts (7) are swollen and undergoing toxic degeneration.

which initially extends into and subdivides the parenchyma with relative preservation of hepatic architecture. Ultimately, an end-stage bile-stained, cirrhotic liver is created—biliary cirrhosis (discussed later).

Because extrahepatic biliary obstruction is frequently amenable to surgical alleviation, correct and prompt diagnosis is imperative. In contrast, cholestasis caused by diseases of the intrahepatic biliary tree or hepatocellular secretory failure (collectively termed *intrahepatic cholestasis*) cannot be benefited by surgery (short of transplantation), and the patient's condition may be worsened by an operative procedure. *There is thus some urgency in making a correct diagnosis of the cause of jaundice and cholestasis.*

Hepatic Failure

The most severe clinical consequence of liver disease is hepatic failure. This may be the result of sudden and massive hepatic destruction. More often, it is the end point of progressive damage to the liver, either by insidious destruction of hepatocytes or by repetitive discrete waves of parenchymal damage. Whatever the sequence, 80% to 90% of hepatic functional capacity must be eroded before hepatic failure ensues. In many cases, the balance is tipped toward decompensation by intercurrent diseases, which place demands on the liver. These include systemic infections, electrolyte disturbances, stress (major surgery, heart failure), and gastrointestinal bleeding.

The morphologic alterations that cause liver failure fall into three categories:

1. *Massive hepatic necrosis.* This is most often caused by fulminant viral hepatitis (hepatotropic or nonhepatotropic viruses). Drugs and chemicals also may induce massive necrosis and include acetaminophen, halothane, antituberculosis drugs (rifampin, isoniazid), antidepressant monoamine oxidase inhibitors, industrial chemicals such as carbon tetrachloride, and mushroom poisoning *(Amanita phalloides)*. The mechanism may be direct toxic damage to hepatocytes (e.g., acetaminophen, carbon tetrachloride, and mushroom toxins) but more often is a variable combination of toxicity and inflammation with immune-mediated hepatocyte destruction.
2. *Chronic liver disease.* This is the most common route to hepatic failure and is the end point of relentless chronic liver damage ending in cirrhosis. The many causes of cirrhosis are discussed later.
3. *Hepatic dysfunction without overt necrosis.* Hepatocytes may be viable but unable to perform normal metabolic function, as in acute fatty liver of pregnancy, tetracycline toxicity, and the very rare Reye syndrome.

Clinical Features. Regardless of cause, the clinical signs of hepatic failure are much the same. *Jaundice* is an almost invariable finding. Impaired hepatic synthesis and secretion of albumin leads to *hypoalbuminemia*, which predisposes to peripheral edema. *Hyperammonemia* is attributable to defective hepatic urea cycle function. *Fetor hepaticus* is a characteristic body odor variously described as "musty" or "sweet and sour" and occurs occasionally. It is related to the formation of mercaptans by the action of gastrointestinal bacteria on the sulfur-containing amino acid methionine and shunting of splanchnic blood from the portal into the systemic circulation (portosystemic shunting). On a longer-term basis, impaired estrogen metabolism and consequent hyperestrogenemia are the putative causes of *palmar erythema* (a reflection of local vasodilatation) and *spider angiomas* of the skin. Each angioma is a central, pulsating, dilated arteriole from which small vessels radiate. In the male, hyperestrogenemia also leads to *hypogonadism* and *gynecomastia.*

Hepatic failure is life-threatening for a number of reasons. First, with severely impaired liver function, patients are highly susceptible to failure of multiple organ systems. Thus, respiratory failure with pneumonia and sepsis combines with renal failure to claim the lives of many patients with hepatic failure. A *coagulopathy* develops, attributable to impaired hepatic synthesis of blood clotting factors II, VII, IX, and X. The resultant bleeding tendency may lead to massive gastrointestinal hemorrhage as well as petechial bleeding elsewhere. Intestinal absorption of blood places a metabolic load on the liver that worsens the severity of hepatic failure. The outlook of full-blown hepatic failure is grave: a rapid downhill course is usual, with death occurring within weeks to a few months in about 80%. A fortunate few can be tided over an acute episode until hepatocellular regeneration restores adequate hepatic function. Alternatively, liver transplantation may save the patient.

Two particular complications merit separate consideration, because they herald the most grave stages of hepatic failure.

HEPATIC ENCEPHALOPATHY

Hepatic encephalopathy is a feared complication of acute and chronic liver failure. Patients exhibit a spectrum of disturbances in consciousness, ranging from subtle behavioral abnormalities to marked confusion and stupor, to deep coma and death. These changes may progress over hours or days as, for example, in fulminant hepatic failure or, more insidiously, in a patient with marginal hepatic function from chronic liver disease. Associated fluctuating neurologic signs include rigidity, hyperreflexia, nonspecific electroencephalographic changes, and, rarely, seizures. Particularly characteristic is *asterixis*, which is a pattern of nonrhythmic, rapid extension-flexion movements of the head and extremities, best seen when the arms are held in extension with dorsiflexed wrists.

Hepatic encephalopathy is regarded as a metabolic disorder of the central nervous system and neuromuscular system. In most instances, there are only minor morphologic changes in the brain, such as edema and an astrocytic reaction. Two physiologic factors appear to be important in the genesis of this disorder: (1) severe loss of hepatocellular function and (2) shunting of blood around the chronically diseased liver. The net result is exposure of the brain to an altered metabolic milieu. In the acute setting, a key feature appears to be an elevated blood ammonia level, which impairs neuronal function and promotes generalized brain edema. In the chronic setting, deranged neurotransmission arises as a result of a number of adverse alterations in central nervous system amino acid metabolism.

HEPATORENAL SYNDROME

Hepatorenal syndrome refers to the appearance of renal failure in patients with severe liver disease, in whom there are no intrinsic morphologic or functional causes for the renal failure. Excluded by this definition are concomitant damage to both organs, as may occur with carbon tetrachloride exposure, certain mycotoxins, and the copper toxicity of Wilson disease. Also excluded are instances of advanced hepatic failure in which circulatory collapse leads to acute tubular necrosis and renal failure. Kidney function promptly improves if hepatic failure is reversed. Although the exact cause is unknown, evidence points to splanchnic vasodilatation and systemic vasoconstriction, leading to severe reduction of renal blood flow, particularly to the cortex. Onset of this syndrome is typically heralded by a drop in urine output, associated with rising blood urea nitrogen and creatinine values. *The ability to concentrate urine is retained, producing a hyperosmolar urine devoid of proteins and abnormal sediment that is surprisingly low in sodium (unlike renal tubular necrosis).*

The renal failure may hasten death in the patient with acute fulminant or advanced chronic hepatic disease. Alternatively, borderline renal insufficiency (serum creatinine of 2 to 3 mg/dL) may persist for weeks to months, as in cirrhotic patients whose ascites is refractory to diuretic therapy.

Cirrhosis

Cirrhosis is among the top 10 causes of death in the Western world. Although largely the result of alcohol abuse, other major contributors include chronic hepatitis, biliary disease, and iron overload. This end stage of chronic liver disease is defined by three characteristics:

1. *Bridging fibrous septa* in the form of delicate bands or broad scars replacing multiple adjacent lobules
2. *Parenchymal nodules* created by regeneration of encircled hepatocytes, varying from very small (<3 mm in diameter, micronodules) to large (several centimeters in diameter, macronodules)
3. Disruption of the architecture of the *entire liver*

The parenchymal injury and consequent fibrosis are diffuse, extending throughout the liver; focal injury with scarring does not constitute cirrhosis. Moreover, the fibrosis, once developed, is generally irreversible, although regression is observed in selected instances.

There is no satisfactory classification of cirrhosis save for specification of the presumed underlying etiology, which varies both geographically and socially. The following is the approximate frequency of etiologic categories in the Western world:

■ Alcoholic liver disease, 60% to 70%
■ Viral hepatitis, 10%
■ Biliary diseases, 5% to 10%
■ Hereditary hemochromatosis, 5%
■ Wilson disease, rare
■ α_1-Antitrypsin (AAT) deficiency, rare
■ Cryptogenic cirrhosis, 10% to 15%

Other infrequent types of cirrhosis are (1) the cirrhosis developing in infants and children with galactosemia or tyrosinosis; (2) drug-induced cirrhosis, as with α-methyldopa; and (3) syphilis. Severe sclerosis can occur in the setting of cardiac disease (sometimes called cardiac cirrhosis, discussed later). After all the categories of cirrhosis of known causation have been excluded, a substantial number of cases remain, referred to as cryptogenic cirrhosis. The magnitude of this "wastebasket" speaks eloquently to the difficulty in establishing an etiologic diagnosis once cirrhosis is well established.

Pathogenesis. The three major pathologic mechanisms that combine to create cirrhosis are hepatocellular death, regeneration, and progressive fibrosis. The many causes of hepatocellular destruction are discussed elsewhere in this chapter; regeneration is a normal host response. With regard to fibrosis, the normal liver contains interstitial collagens (types I, III, and IV) in portal tracts and around central veins, with occasional bundles in the parenchyma. A delicate reticulin framework of type IV collagen lies in the space between sinusoidal endothelial cells and hepatocytes (the space of Disse). In cirrhosis, types I and III collagen and other components of the extracellular matrix are deposited in all portions of the lobule and sinusoidal endothelial cells loose their fenestrations. Portal vein–to–hepatic vein and hepatic artery–to–portal vein vascular shunts also develop. These processes essentially convert sinusoids from fenestrated endothelial channels with free exchange of solutes between plasma and hepatocytes, to higher-pressure, fast-flow vascular channels without such solute exchange. In particular, the movement of proteins (e.g., albumin, clotting factors, lipoproteins) between hepatocytes and the plasma is markedly impaired.

The major source of excess collagen in cirrhosis appears to be the fat-storing perisinusoidal stellate cell, which lies in the space of Disse. Although they normally function as vitamin A and fat-storage cells, during the development of cirrhosis they become activated, lose their retinyl ester stores, and transform into myofibroblast-like cells. The stimuli for synthesis and deposition of collagen may come from several sources:

- Chronic inflammation, with production of inflammatory cytokines such as tumor necrosis factor (TNF), lymphotoxin, and interleukin 1
- Cytokine production by injured endogenous cells (Kupffer cells, endothelial cells, hepatocytes, and bile duct epithelial cells)
- Disruption of the extracellular matrix
- Direct stimulation of stellate cells by toxins

Clinical Features. All forms of cirrhosis may be clinically silent. When symptomatic they lead to nonspecific manifestations: anorexia, weight loss, weakness, and, in advanced disease, frank debilitation. Incipient or overt hepatic failure may develop, usually precipitated by imposition of a metabolic load on the liver, as from systemic infection or a gastrointestinal hemorrhage. The ultimate mechanism of death in most patients with cirrhosis is (1) progressive liver failure, (2) a complication related to portal hypertension, or (3) the development of hepatocellular carcinoma.

PORTAL HYPERTENSION

Increased resistance to portal blood flow may develop in a variety of circumstances, which can be divided into prehepatic, intrahepatic, and posthepatic causes. The major prehepatic conditions are occlusive thrombosis and narrowing of the portal vein before it ramifies within the liver. Massive splenomegaly also may shunt excessive blood into the splenic vein. The major posthepatic causes are severe right-sided heart failure, constrictive pericarditis, and hepatic vein outflow obstruction. *The dominant intrahepatic cause is cirrhosis, accounting for most cases of portal hypertension.* Far less frequent are schistosomiasis, massive fatty change, diffuse granulomatous diseases such as sarcoidosis and miliary tuberculosis, and diseases affecting the portal microcirculation, exemplified by nodular regenerative hyperplasia (discussed later).

Portal hypertension in cirrhosis results from increased resistance to portal flow at the level of the sinusoids and compression of central veins by perivenular fibrosis and expansile parenchymal nodules. Anastomoses between the arterial and portal systems in the fibrous bands also contribute to portal hypertension by imposing arterial pressure on the low-pressure portal venous system. The four major clinical consequences are (1) ascites, (2) the formation of

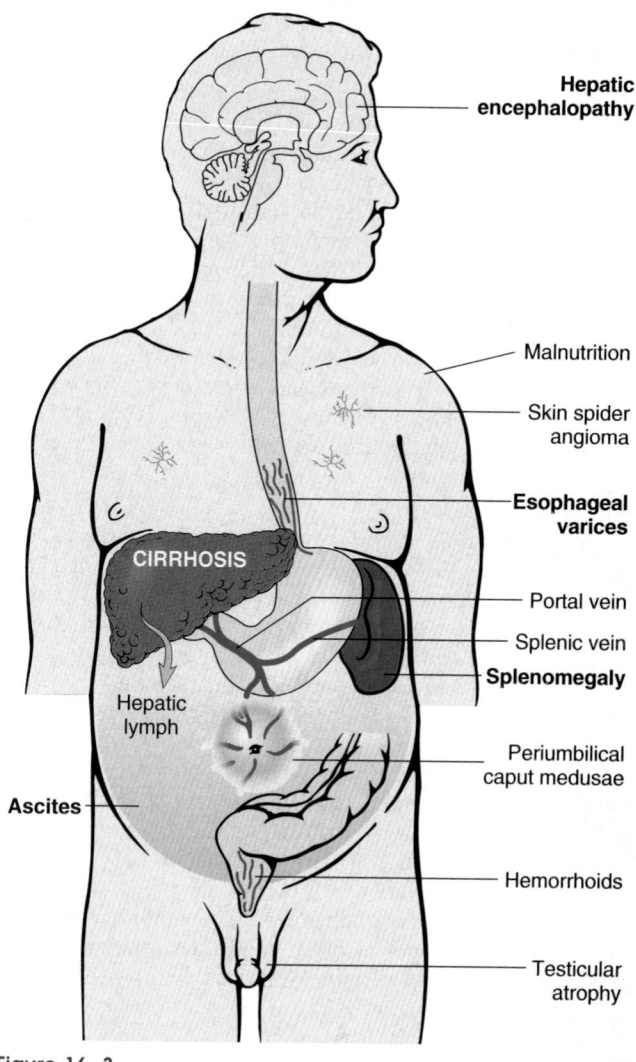

Figure 16–3   ■

Some clinical consequences of portal hypertension in the setting of cirrhosis. The most important manifestations are in boldface.

portosystemic venous shunts, (3) congestive splenomegaly, and (4) hepatic encephalopathy (discussed earlier). The manifestations of portal hypertension in the setting of cirrhosis are illustrated in Figure 16–3 and described next.

Ascites

Ascites refers to the collection of excess fluid in the peritoneal cavity. It usually becomes clinically detectable when at least 500 mL has accumulated, but many liters may collect and cause massive abdominal distention. It is generally a serous fluid having up to 3 g/dL of protein (largely albumin) as well as the same concentrations of solutes such as glucose, sodium, and potassium as in the blood. The fluid may contain a scant number of mesothelial cells and mononuclear leukocytes. Influx of neutrophils suggests secondary infection, whereas red cells point to possible disseminated intra-abdominal cancer. With long-standing ascites, seepage of peritoneal fluid through transdiaphragmatic lymphatics may produce hydrothorax, more often on the right side.

The pathogenesis of ascites is complex, involving one or more of the following mechanisms:

■ Sinusoidal hypertension, altering Starling forces and driving fluid into the space of Disse, which is then removed by hepatic lymphatics; this movement of fluid is also promoted by hypoalbuminemia.
■ Percolation of hepatic lymph into the peritoneal cavity: normal thoracic duct lymph flow approximates 800 to 1000 mL/day. With cirrhosis, hepatic lymphatic flow may approach 20 L/day, exceeding thoracic duct capacity. Hepatic lymph is rich in proteins and low in triglycerides, which is reflected in the protein-rich ascitic fluid.
■ Renal retention of sodium and water due to secondary hyperaldosteronism (Chapter 4), despite a total body sodium value greater than normal.

Portosystemic Shunts

With the rise in portal system pressure, bypasses develop wherever the systemic and portal circulation share capillary beds. Principal sites are veins around and within the rectum (manifest as hemorrhoids), the cardioesophageal junction (producing esophagogastric varices), the retroperitoneum, and the falciform ligament of the liver (involving periumbilical and abdominal wall collaterals). Although hemorrhoidal bleeding may occur, it is rarely massive or life-threatening. Much more important are the esophagogastric varices that appear in about 65% of patients with advanced cirrhosis of the liver and cause massive hematemesis and death in about half of them (Chapter 15). Abdominal wall collaterals appear as dilated subcutaneous veins extending from the umbilicus toward the rib margins (caput medusae) and constitute an important clinical hallmark of portal hypertension.

Splenomegaly

Long-standing congestion may cause congestive splenomegaly. The degree of enlargement varies widely (up to 1000 g) and is not necessarily correlated with other features of portal hypertension. Massive splenomegaly may secondarily induce a variety of hematologic abnormalities attributable to hypersplenism (Chapter 12).

INFLAMMATORY DISORDERS

Inflammatory disorders of the liver dominate the clinical practice of hepatology. Virtually any insult to the liver can kill hepatocytes and recruit inflammatory cells. Moreover, inflammatory diseases are frequently chronic, so that the practice of hepatology is largely populated by patients with chronic liver disease. Among inflammatory disorders, infection ranks supreme. The liver is almost inevitably involved in bloodborne infections, whether systemic or arising within the abdomen. Although discussed elsewhere, those in which the hepatic lesion is prominent include miliary tuberculosis, malaria, staphylococcal bacteremia, the salmonelloses, candidiasis, and amebiasis. However, the foremost primary hepatic infections are the viral hepatitides.

Viral Hepatitis

Systemic viral infections that can involve the liver include (1) infectious mononucleosis (Epstein-Barr virus), which may cause a mild hepatitis during the acute phase; (2) cytomegalovirus or herpesvirus infections, particularly in the newborn or immunosuppressed patient; and (3) yellow fever, which has been a major and serious cause of hepatitis in tropical countries. Infrequently, in children and immunosuppressed patients, the liver is affected in the course of rubella, adenovirus, or enterovirus infections. However, unless otherwise specified, the term *viral hepatitis* is reserved for infection of the liver caused by a small group of viruses having a particular affinity for the liver (Table 16–4). Because these viruses cause similar morphologic patterns of disease, the histologic changes in viral hepatitis are described together, but only after an introduction to the specific forms of viral hepatitis.

ETIOLOGIC AGENTS

Hepatitis A Virus (HAV)

Hepatitis A is a benign, self-limited disease with an incubation period of 2 to 6 weeks. *HAV does not cause chronic hepatitis or a carrier state and only rarely causes fulminant hepatitis. Case fatalities from HAV occur at a very low rate, about 0.1%, and appear to be more likely to occur in patients with preexisting liver disease from other causes such as hepatitis B virus or alcohol.* HAV occurs throughout the world and is endemic in countries with poor hygiene and sanitation, so that most natives of such countries have detectable anti-HAV by the age of 10 years. Clinical disease tends to be mild or asymptomatic and rare after childhood. In developed countries, the prevalence of seropositivity increases gradually with age, reaching 50% by age 50 years in the United States. Unfortunately, HAV infection in adulthood may create considerably greater morbidity than the innocuous childhood infection.

HAV is spread by ingestion of contaminated water and foods and is shed in the stool for 2 to 3 weeks before and 1 week after the onset of jaundice. HAV is not shed in any significant quantities in saliva, urine, or semen. Close personal contact with an infected individual during the period of fecal shedding, with fecal-oral contamination, accounts for most cases and explains the outbreaks in institutional settings such as schools and nurseries. Waterborne epidemics may occur in developing countries where people live in overcrowded, unsanitary conditions; the incidence of infectious particles in the water supply may exceed 35%, despite routine indicators of fecal pollution falling within acceptable limits. Among developed countries, sporadic infections may be contracted by the consumption of raw or steamed shellfish (oysters, mussels, clams), which concentrate the virus from sea water contaminated with human sewage. *Because HAV viremia is transient, bloodborne transmission of HAV occurs only rarely; therefore, donated blood is not specifically screened for this virus.*

HAV is a small, nonenveloped, single-stranded RNA picornavirus. The virus itself does not appear to be cytotoxic to hepatocytes, and hence the liver injury seems to result from immunologically mediated damage of infected

Table 16-4. THE HEPATITIS VIRUSES

	Hepatitis A Virus	Hepatitis B Virus	Hepatitis C Virus	Hepatitis D Virus	Hepatitis E Virus	Hepatitis G Virus
Year of Identification	1973	1965	1989	1977	1980	1995
Agent	27-nm iscosahedral capsid, ss RNA	42-nm enveloped dsDNA	30- to 60-nm enveloped ssRNA	35-nm enveloped ssRNA; replication defective	32- to 34-nm unenveloped ssRNA	ssRNA virus
Classification	Picornavirus	Hepadnavirus	Flavivirus	Unknown	Caliciviridae	Flavivirus
Transmission	Fecal-oral	Parenteral; close personal contact	Parenteral; close personal contact	Parenteral; close personal contact	Waterborne	Parenteral
Incubation Period (Weeks)	2–6	4–26	2–26	4–7 in superinfection with HBV	2–8	Unknown
Fulminant Hepatitis	0.1%–0.4%	<1%	Rare	3%–4% in coinfection	0.3%–3%; 20% in pregnant women	No
Carrier State	None	0.1%–1.0% of blood donors in United States and Western world	0.2%–1.0% of blood donors in United States and Western world	1%–10% in drug addicts and hemophiliacs	None	1%–4% of blood donors in United States (estimated)
Chronic Hepatitis	None	5%–10% of acute infections	>70%	<5% coinfection, 80% superinfection	None	None
Hepatocellular Carcinoma	No	Yes	Yes	No increase above hepatitis B virus	No	No

hepatocytes. As depicted in Figure 16–4, specific antibody against HAV of the IgM type appears in blood at the onset of symptoms, constituting a reliable marker of acute infection. Fecal shedding of the virus ends as the IgM titer rises. The IgM response declines in a few months, accompanied by the appearance of IgG anti-HAV. The latter persists for life, providing immunity against reinfection by all strains of HAV (hence the value of vaccination).

Hepatitis B Virus (HBV)

HBV can produce (1) acute hepatitis with recovery and clearance of the virus, (2) nonprogressive chronic hepatitis, (3) progressive chronic disease ending in cirrhosis, (4) fulminant hepatitis with massive liver necrosis, and (5) an asymptomatic carrier state, with or without progressive subclinical disease. HBV also plays an important role in the development of hepatocellular carcinoma. Figure 16–5 depicts the approximate frequencies of these outcomes.

Globally, liver disease caused by hepatitis B virus is an enormous problem with an estimated worldwide carrier rate of 350 million. It is estimated that HBV has infected over 2 billion of the individuals alive today at some point in their lives. Seventy-five percent of all chronic carriers live in Asia and the Western Pacific rim. In the United States there are 200,000 to 300,000 new infections per year. Unlike HAV, HBV remains in blood during the last stages of a prolonged incubation period (4 to 26 weeks) and during active episodes of acute and chronic hepatitis. It is also present in all physiologic and pathologic body fluids, with the exception of stool. HBV is a hardy virus and can withstand extremes of

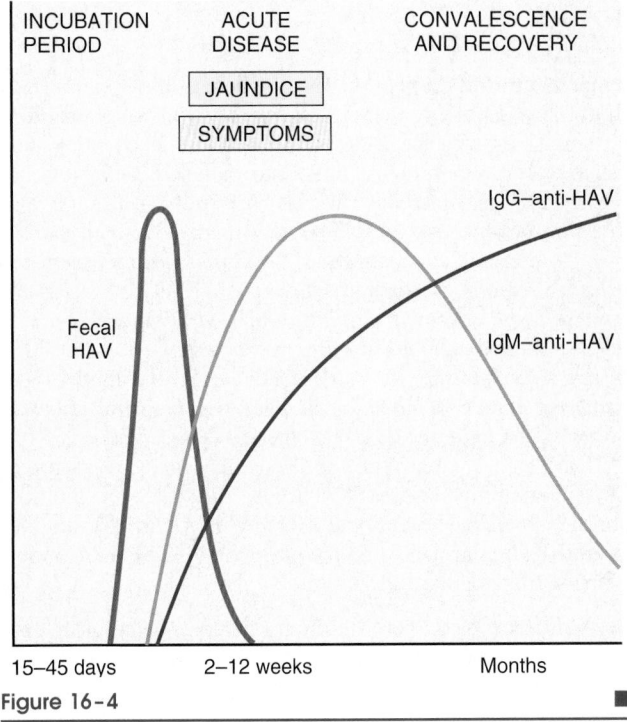

Figure 16-4

The sequence of serologic markers in acute hepatitis A infection. HAV, hepatitis A virus.

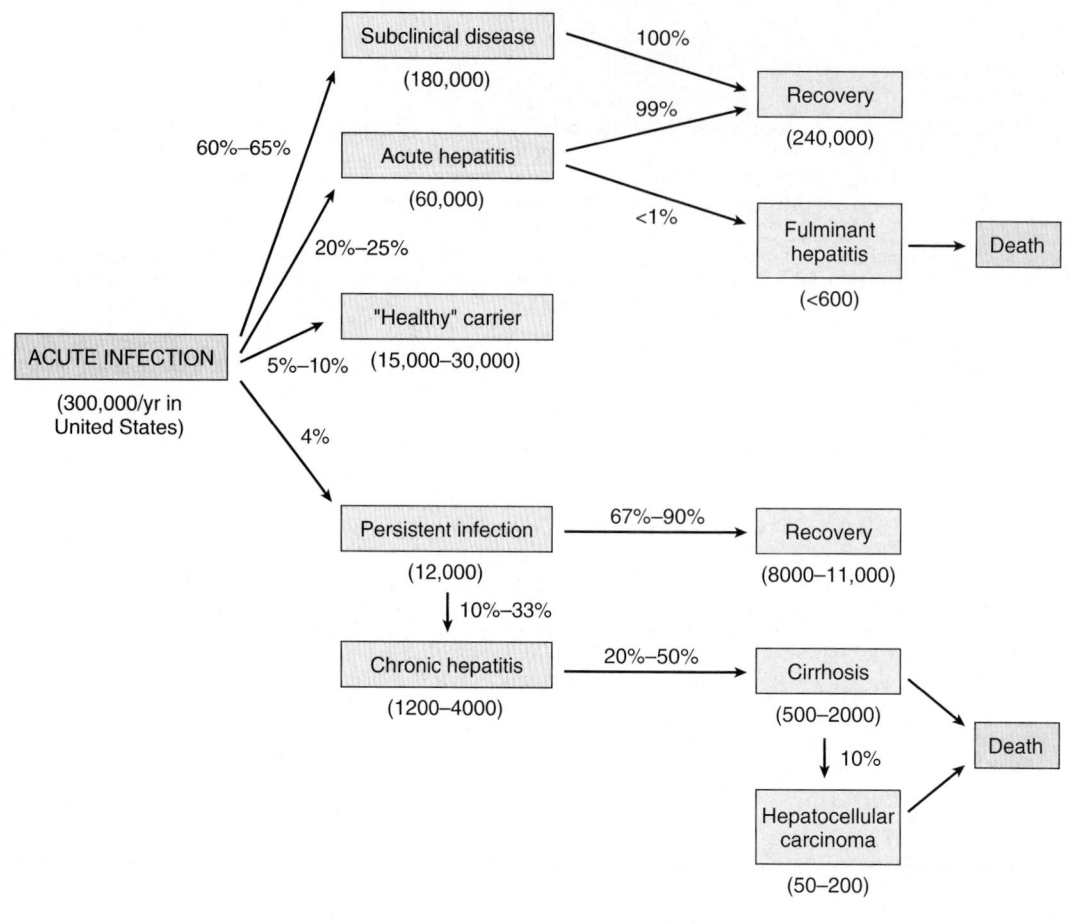

Figure 16–5

The potential outcomes of hepatitis B infection in adults, with their approximate annual frequencies in the United States. (Population estimates courtesy of John L. Gollan, MD, PhD, Brigham and Women's Hospital, Boston.)

temperature and humidity. Thus, whereas blood and body fluids are the primary vehicles of transmission, virus may also be spread by contact with body secretions such as semen, saliva, sweat, tears, breast milk, and pathologic effusions. *In regions of high endemicity, vertical transmission from mother to child during birth constitutes the main mode of transmission. In areas of low endemicity, horizontal transmission via transfusion, blood products, dialysis, needle-stick accidents among health care workers, intravenous drug abuse, and sexual transmission (homosexual or heterosexual) constitutes the primary mechanisms for HBV infection.* In one third of patients the source of infection is unknown. Perinatal infection produces the highest rate of chronic HBV infection.

HBV is a member of the Hepadnaviridae, a group of DNA-containing viruses that cause hepatitis in multiple animal species. The genome of HBV is a partially double-stranded circular DNA molecule having 3200 nucleotides, which codes for the following:

■ A nucleocapsid "core" protein (HBcAg, hepatitis B core antigen) and a longer polypeptide transcript with a pre-core and core region, designated HBeAg (hepatitis B "e" antigen). HBcAg is retained in the infected hepatocyte; HBeAg is secreted into blood, thereby providing an antigenic handle for the immune system.

■ Envelope glycoprotein (HBsAg, hepatitis B surface antigen), also immunogenic when present in blood.
■ DNA polymerase.
■ A protein from the X region (HBV X-protein), which acts as a promiscuous transcriptional transactivator of host genes and may play a role in the causation of hepatocellular carcinoma following its integration into the host genome.

Infected hepatocytes can synthesize and secrete massive quantities of noninfective surface protein (HBsAg), which appears in cells and serum as spheres and tubules 22 nm in diameter.

After exposure to the virus, the long asymptomatic 4- to 26-week incubation period (mean, 6 to 8 weeks) is followed by acute disease lasting many weeks to months. The natural course of acute disease can be followed by serum markers (Fig. 16–6).

■ HBsAg appears before the onset of symptoms, peaks during overt disease, and then declines to undetectable levels in 3 to 6 months.
■ HBeAg, HBV-DNA, and DNA polymerase appear in serum soon after HBsAg, and all signify active viral replication. Persistence of HBeAg is an important indi-

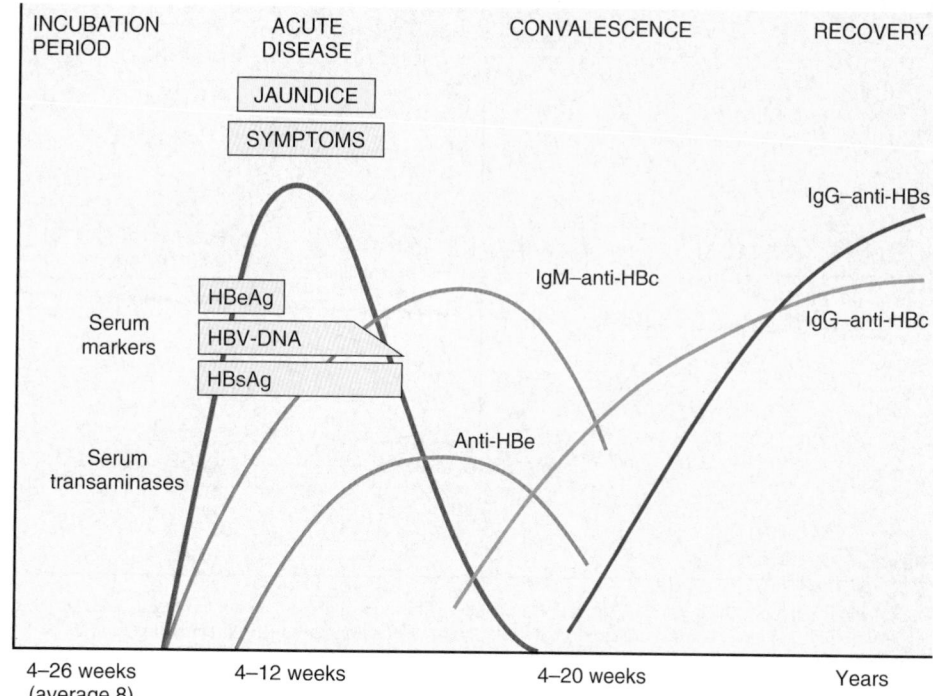

Figure 16-6   ■

The sequence of serologic markers in acute hepatitis B infection, showing resolution of active infection.

cator of continued viral replication, infectivity, and probable progression to chronic hepatitis.

■ IgM anti-HBc becomes detectable in serum shortly before the onset of symptoms, concurrent with the onset of elevated serum aminotransferase levels (indicative of hepatocyte destruction). Over months the IgM anti-HBc antibody is replaced by IgG anti-HBc.

■ The appearance of anti-HBe antibodies implies that an acute infection has peaked and is on the wane.

■ IgG anti-HBs does not rise until the acute disease is over and is usually not detectable for a few weeks to several months after the disappearance of HBsAg. Anti-HBs may persist for life, conferring protection; this is the basis for current vaccination strategies using noninfectious HBsAg.

HBV infections pass through two phases. During the *proliferative phase*, HBV-DNA is present in episomal form, with formation of complete virions and all associated antigens. Cell surface expression of viral HBsAg and HBcAg in association with MHC class I molecules leads to activation of cytotoxic CD8+ T lymphocytes. An *integrative phase* may follow, in which viral DNA may be incorporated into the host genome. With cessation of viral replication and the appearance of antiviral antibodies, infectivity ends and liver damage subsides. However, the risk of hepatocellular carcinoma persists. This may be caused in part by HBV X-protein–mediated dysregulation of growth (Chapter 6).

Occasionally, infectious variant strains of hepatitis B virus emerge that are incapable of HBeAg expression but are still capable of synthesizing HBcAg. The loss of circulating HBeAg, and hence anti-HBe formation, is associated with fulminant hepatitis. A second ominous development is the appearance of vaccine-induced escape mutants, which replicate in the presence of vaccine-induced immunity. The

quintessential example is replacement of arginine at amino acid 145 of HBsAg with glycine, which significantly alters recognition of HBsAg by anti-HBsAg antibodies.

There are several reasons to believe that HBV does not cause direct hepatocyte injury. Most important, many chronic carriers have virions in their hepatocytes with no evidence of cell injury. Hepatocyte damage is believed to result from damage to the virus-infected cells by CD8+ cytotoxic T cells.

Hepatitis C Virus (HCV)

HCV is also a major cause of liver disease. The worldwide carrier rate is estimated at 175 million persons (a 3% prevalence rate), and 2 to 3 million persons in the United States have persistent chronic infection. The number of newly acquired infections of HCV per year dropped from 180,000 in the mid 1980s to about 28,000 in the mid 1990s. This welcome change has resulted from the marked reduction in transfusion-associated hepatitis C (as a result of screening procedures) and a decline of infections in injection drug abusers (related to practices motivated by fear of human immunodeficiency virus [HIV] infection). However, the death rate from HCV will continue to climb, owing to the decades-long lag time between acute infection and liver failure. *The major routes of transmission are inoculations and blood transfusions, with intravenous drug use accounting for over 40% of cases in the United States.* Transmission via blood products is now fortunately rare, accounting for only 4% of all acute HCV infections. Occupational exposure among health care workers accounts for 4% of cases. The rates of sexual transmission and vertical transmission are low. Sporadic hepatitis of unknown source accounts for 40% of cases. *HCV has a higher rate of progression to chronic disease and eventual cirrhosis, estimated at 20%*

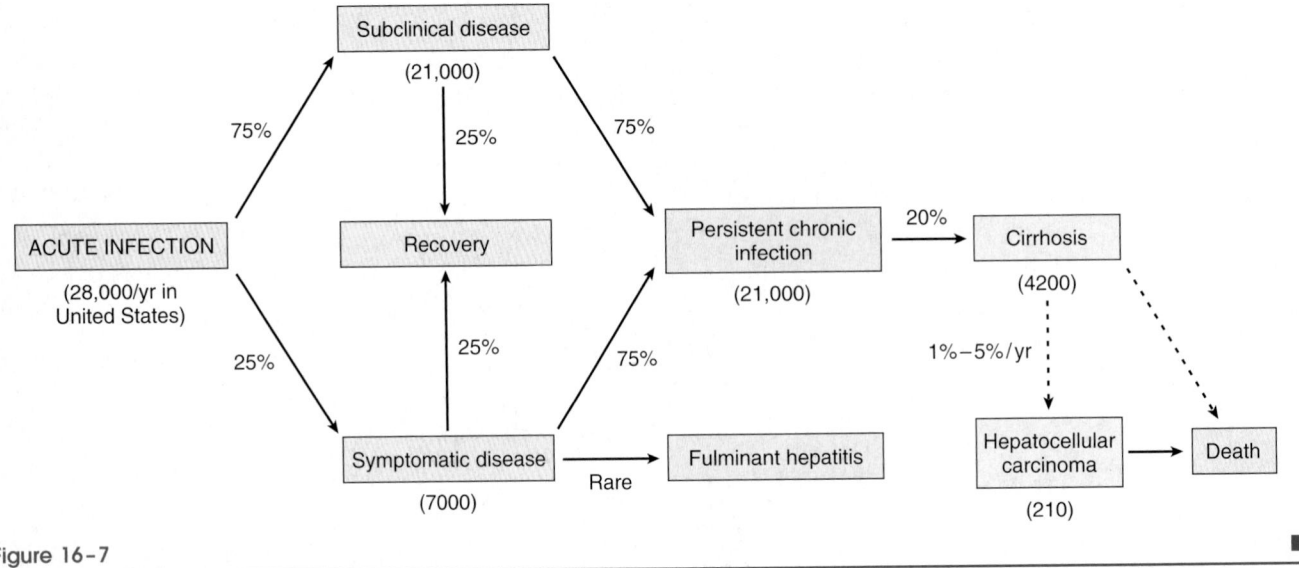

Figure 16-7

The potential outcomes of hepatitis C infection in adults, with their approximate annual frequencies in the United States. The population estimates are for newly detected infection; because of the decades-long lag time for progression from acute infection to cirrhosis, the actual annual death rate from hepatitis C is about 10,000 per year and is expected to exceed 22,000 deaths per year by 2008.

(Fig. 16–7). *Thus, HCV may in fact be the leading cause of chronic liver disease in the Western world.*

HCV is a positive-sense single-stranded RNA virus belonging to Flaviviridae, a class of viruses that includes the hepatitis G virus and the causative agents of dengue fever and yellow fever. It contains highly conserved 5' and 3' terminal regions that flank a nearly 9000-nucleotide sequence that is inherently unstable. Multiple types and subtypes have been documented, including within the same individual. This variability has seriously hampered efforts to develop an HCV vaccine, particularly because *elevated titers of anti-HCV IgG occurring after active infection do not seem to confer effective immunity to subsequent HCV infection, either from reactivation of an endogenous strain or by infection with a new strain.*

The incubation period for HCV hepatitis ranges from 2 to 26 weeks, with a mean of 6 to 12 weeks. HCV RNA is detectable in blood for 1 to 3 weeks and is accompanied by elevations in serum aminotransferase levels. The clinical course of acute HCV hepatitis is usually milder than that of HBV hepatitis and is asymptomatic in 75% of individuals. Although neutralizing anti-HCV antibodies develop within weeks to a few months, circulating HCV-RNA persists in a high percentage of patients. Hence, a characteristic feature of HCV infection is episodic elevations of serum aminotransferase levels, even in the absence of clinical symptoms, presumably reflecting recurrent bouts of hepatocellular necrosis. *Persistent infection is the hallmark of HCV infection, occurring in more than 75% of individuals with subclinical or asymptomatic acute infection* (see Fig. 16–7). Cirrhosis develops in 20% of persistently infected individuals: it can be present at the time of diagnosis or may develop over 5 to 20 years. Alternatively, patients may have documented chronic HCV infection for decades, without progressing to cirrhosis. Fulminant hepatitis is rare.

Hepatitis D Virus (HDV)

Also called hepatitis delta virus, HDV is a unique RNA virus that is replication defective, causing infection only when it is encapsulated by HBsAg. Thus, *although taxonomically distinct from HBV, HDV is absolutely dependent on HBV coinfection for multiplication.* Delta hepatitis thus arises in two settings (Fig. 16–8): (1) acute coinfection after exposure to serum containing both HDV and HBV and (2) superinfection of a chronic carrier of HBV with a new inoculum of HDV. In the first case, HBV infection must become established before HBsAg is available for the development of complete HDV virions. Most coinfected individuals can clear the viruses and recover completely. Fulminant hepatitis, and rarely chronic hepatitis, may occur. The course is different in superinfected individuals. In most cases, there is an acceleration of hepatitis, most often to more severe chronic hepatitis, occurring 4 to 7 weeks later. The carrier may have been previously asymptomatic ("healthy") or may have already had underlying chronic hepatitis (see Fig. 16–8).

Infection by HDV is worldwide, with prevalence rates ranging from 8% among HBsAg carriers in southern Italy to as high as 40% in Africa and the Middle East. Surprisingly, HDV infection is uncommon in Southeast Asia and China. In the United States, HDV infection is largely restricted to drug addicts and multiply transfused individuals (e.g., hemophiliacs), who exhibit prevalence rates of 1% to 10%. Other high-risk groups for HBV are at low risk for HDV infection for unclear reasons.

HDV is a double-shelled particle that by electron microscopy resembles HBV. The external coat antigen of HBsAg surrounds an internal delta antigen (HDV Ag). Associated with HDV Ag is a small circular molecule of single-stranded RNA. Although the relationship between HBV and HDV in the pathogenesis of liver disease remains unclear, HDV infection has an adverse influence on the clinical course.

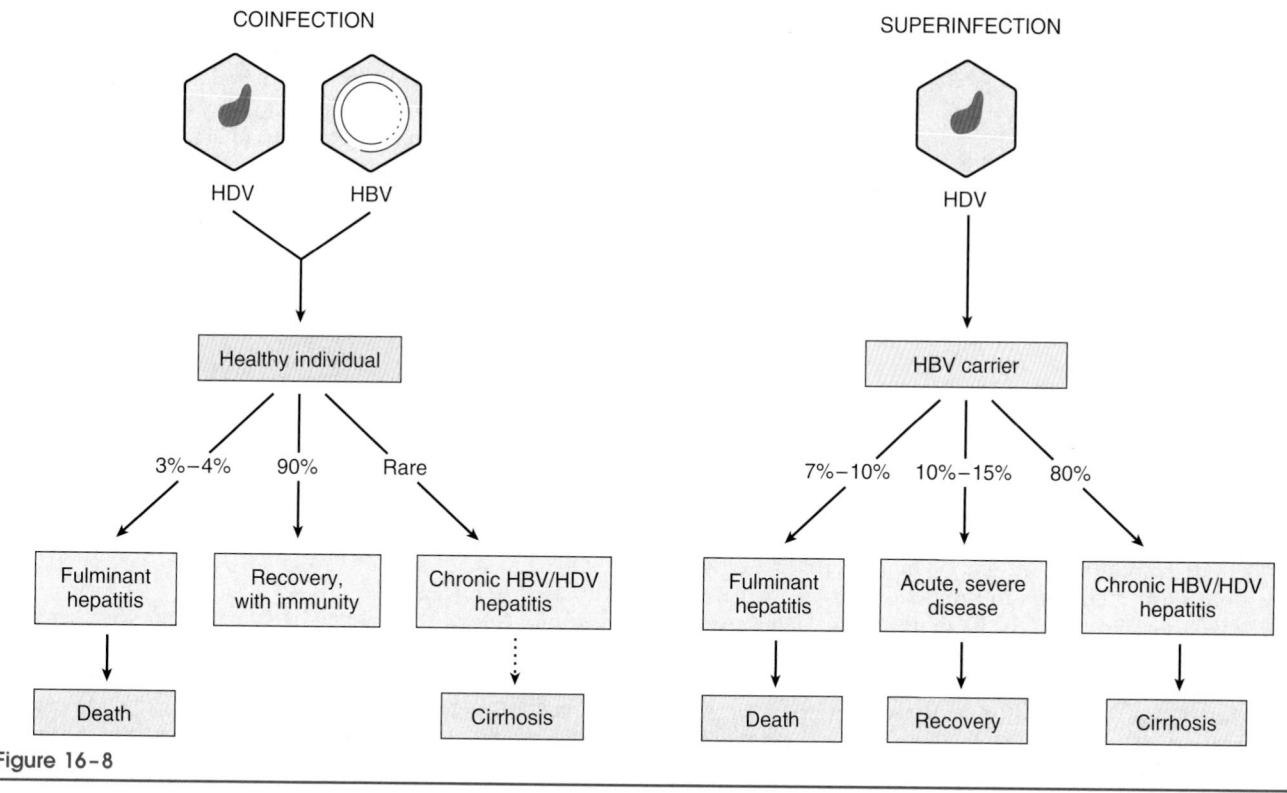

COINFECTION

SUPERINFECTION

Figure 16-8

The differing clinical consequences of the two patterns of combined hepatitis D virus (HDV) and hepatitis B virus (HBV) infection.

HDV RNA and the HDV Ag are detectable in the blood and liver just before and in the early days of acute symptomatic disease. *IgM anti-HDV is the most reliable indicator of recent HDV exposure,* but its appearance is transient. Nevertheless, acute coinfection by HDV and HBV is best indicated by detection of IgM against both HDV Ag and HBcAg (denoting new infection with hepatitis B). With chronic delta hepatitis arising from HDV superinfection, HBsAg is present in serum; and anti-HDV antibodies (IgM and IgG) persist in low titer for months or longer.

Hepatitis E Virus (HEV)

HEV hepatitis is an enterically transmitted, waterborne infection occurring primarily beyond the years of infancy. HEV is endemic in India, with prevalence rates of anti-HEV IgG antibodies approaching 40% in the Indian population. Epidemics have been reported from Asia, sub-Saharan Africa, and Mexico. Sporadic infection seems to be uncommon; it is seen mainly in travelers and accounts for over 50% of cases of sporadic acute viral hepatitis in India. In most cases, the disease is self-limited; HEV is not associated with chronic liver disease or persistent viremia. *A characteristic feature of the infection is the high mortality rate among pregnant women, approaching 20%.* The average incubation period after exposure is 6 weeks (range, 2 to 8 weeks).

HEV is a nonenveloped, single-stranded RNA virus that is best characterized as a calicivirus. A specific antigen (HEV Ag) can be identified in the cytoplasm of hepatocytes during active infection. Virus can be detected in stool by immunoelectron microscopy, and serum anti-HEV and HEV-RNA are detectable.

Hepatitis G Virus (HGV)

The handful of epidemics designated as "hepatitis F" occurred some years ago and have not produced an identifiable virus. In the meantime, the "alphabet train" moved forward, and hepatitis G virus, a flavivirus bearing similarities to HCV, was cloned in 1995. HGV is transmitted by contaminated blood or blood products and, possibly, via sexual transmission. The prevalence of HGV RNA in blood donors ranges from 1% to 4%, and in a report from Taiwan the incidence of new HGV infections among hemodialysis patients exceeds 2% per year. In up to 75% of infections, HGV is cleared from plasma; in the remainder of cases HGV infection becomes chronic. *The site of HGV replication is most likely in mononuclear cells; hence, HGV is inappropriately named, as it is not hepatotropic and does not cause elevations in serum aminotransferases. Although not proven definitively, extensive data do not indicate any pathologic effects of HGV, and the blood supply does not appear to need screening for HGV RNA.* Surprisingly, HGV infection seems to have a protective effect on patients coinfected with HIV. Studies suggest that HGV inhibits HIV replication in cultures of peripheral blood mononuclear cells.

CLINICAL SYNDROMES

A number of clinical syndromes may develop after exposure to hepatitis viruses:

■ *Carrier state:* without apparent disease, or with subclinical chronic hepatitis
■ *Asymptomatic infection:* serologic evidence only

- *Acute hepatitis:* anicteric or icteric
- *Chronic hepatitis:* with or without progression to cirrhosis
- *Fulminant hepatitis:* submassive to massive hepatic necrosis

Not all of the hepatotropic viruses provoke each of these clinical syndromes. With rare exception, HAV and HEV do not generate a carrier state or cause chronic hepatitis. Other infectious or noninfectious causes, particularly drugs and toxins, can lead to essentially identical syndromes. Therefore, serologic studies are critical for the diagnosis of viral hepatitis and the distinction among the various types.

The Carrier State

A "carrier" is an individual without manifest symptoms who harbors and therefore can transmit an organism. With hepatotropic viruses, there are (1) those who harbor one of the viruses but are suffering little or no adverse effects and (2) those who have nonprogressive liver damage but are essentially free of symptoms or disability. Both constitute reservoirs of infection. In the case of HBV, infection early in life, particularly through vertical transmission during childbirth, produces a carrier state 90% to 95% of the time. In contrast, only 1% to 10% of HBV infections acquired in adulthood yield a carrier state. Individuals with impaired immunity are particularly likely to become carriers. The situation is less clear with HDV, although there is a well-defined low risk of post-transfusion hepatitis D, indicative of a carrier state in conjunction with HBV. HCV can clearly induce a carrier state, which is estimated to affect 0.2% to 0.6% of the general US population.

Asymptomatic Infection

Not surprisingly, patients in this group are identified only incidentally on the basis of minimally elevated serum aminotransferases or after the fact by the presence of antiviral antibodies.

Acute Viral Hepatitis

Any one of the hepatotropic viruses can cause acute viral hepatitis. Whatever the agent, the disease is more or less the same and can be divided into four phases: (1) an incubation period, (2) a symptomatic preicteric phase, (3) a symptomatic icteric phase (with jaundice and scleral icterus), and (4) convalescence. The incubation period for the different viruses is provided in Table 16–4. Peak infectivity, attributed to the presence of circulating infectious viral particles, occurs during the last asymptomatic days of the incubation period and the early days of acute symptoms.

The preicteric phase is marked by nonspecific, constitutional symptoms. Malaise is followed in a few days by general fatigability, nausea, and loss of appetite. Weight loss, low-grade fever, headaches, muscle and joint aches, vomiting, and diarrhea are inconstant symptoms. About 10% of patients with acute hepatitis, most often those with hepatitis B, develop a serum sickness–like syndrome. This consists of fever, rash, and arthralgias, attributed to circulating immune complexes. The hepatitis-related origin of all these symptoms is suggested by elevated serum aminotransferase levels. Physical examination reveals a mildly enlarged, tender liver.

In some patients, the nonspecific symptoms are more severe, with higher fever, shaking chills, and headache, sometimes accompanied by right upper quadrant pain and tender liver enlargement. Surprisingly, as jaundice appears and these patients enter the icteric phase, other symptoms begin to abate. The jaundice is caused predominantly by conjugated hyperbilirubinemia and hence is accompanied by dark-colored urine related to the presence of conjugated bilirubin. With hepatocellular damage and consequent defect in bilirubin conjugation, unconjugated hyperbilirubinemia can also occur. The stools may become light colored, and the retention of bile salts may cause distressing skin itching (pruritus). An icteric phase is usual in adults (but not children) with HAV but is absent in about half the cases of HBV and is absent in most cases of HCV. In a few weeks to perhaps several months, the jaundice and most of the other systemic symptoms clear as convalescence begins.

Chronic Viral Hepatitis

Chronic hepatitis is defined as symptomatic, biochemical, or serologic evidence of continuing or relapsing hepatic disease for more than 6 months, with histologically documented inflammation and necrosis. Although the hepatitis viruses are responsible for most cases, there are many causes of chronic hepatitis (described later). They include Wilson disease, α_1-antitrypsin deficiency, chronic alcoholism, drugs (isoniazid, α-methyldopa, methotrexate), and autoimmunity.

In chronic hepatitis, *etiology rather than the histologic pattern is the single most important factor determining probability of developing progressive chronic hepatitis.* In particular, HCV is notorious for causing a chronic hepatitis evolving to cirrhosis in a significant percentage of patients (see Fig. 16–7), regardless of histologic features at the time of initial evaluation.

The clinical features of chronic hepatitis are highly variable and are not predictive of outcome. In some patients, the only signs of chronic disease are persistent elevations of serum aminotransferase levels. The most common overt symptom is fatigue, and less commonly malaise, loss of appetite, and bouts of mild jaundice. Physical findings are few, the most common being spider angiomas, palmar erythema, mild hepatomegaly, hepatic tenderness, and mild splenomegaly. Laboratory studies may reveal prolongation of the prothrombin time and, in some instances, hypergammaglobulinemia, hyperbilirubinemia, and mild elevations in alkaline phosphatase levels. Occasionally in cases of HBV and HCV, circulating antibody-antigen complexes produce immune-complex disease, in the form of vasculitis (subcutaneous or visceral, Chapter 10) and glomerulonephritis (Chapter 14). Cryoglobulinemia is found in up to 50% of patients with hepatitis C.

The clinical course is highly variable. Patients may experience spontaneous remission or may have indolent disease without progression for years. Conversely, some patients have rapidly progressive disease and develop cirrhosis within a few years. The major causes of death relate to cirrhosis, namely, liver failure, hepatic encephalopathy, or massive hematemesis from esophageal varices. Patients with long-standing HBV (particularly neonatal) or HCV infection are at a substantially increased risk for hepatocellular carcinoma.

Table 16-5.   KEY MORPHOLOGIC FEATURES OF VIRAL HEPATITIS

Carrier State

Essentially normal liver biopsy
HBV: "ground-glass" hepatocytes, "sanded" nuclei
HCV: chronic hepatitis usually present histologically

Acute Hepatitis

Enlarged, reddened liver; greenish if cholestatic
Parenchymal changes
  Hepatocyte injury: swelling (ballooning degeneration)
    Cholestasis: canalicular bile plugs
    HCV: mild fatty change of hepatocytes
  Hepatocyte necrosis: isolated cells or clusters
    Cytolysis (rupture) or apoptosis (shrinkage)
    If severe: bridging necrosis (portal-portal, central-central,
      portal-central)
    Lobular disarray: loss of normal architecture
  Regenerative changes: hepatocyte proliferation
  Sinusoidal cell reactive changes
    Accumulation of phagocytosed cellular debris in Kupffer cells
    Influx of mononuclear cells into sinusoids
Portal tracts
  Inflammation: predominantly mononuclear
  Inflammatory spillover into adjacent parenchyma, with
    hepatocyte necrosis

Chronic Hepatitis

Changes shared with acute hepatitis
  Hepatocyte injury, necrosis, and regeneration
  Sinusoidal cell reactive changes
Portal tracts
  Inflammation
    Confined to portal tracts, *or*
    Spillover into adjacent parenchyma, with necrosis of hepatocytes
      ("interface hepatitis"), *or*
    Bridging inflammation and necrosis
  Fibrosis:
    Portal deposition, *or*
    Portal and periportal deposition, *or*
    Formation of bridging fibrous septa
HCV: bile duct epithelial cell proliferation, lymphoid aggregate formation

Cirrhosis: the End-Stage Outcome

MORPHOLOGY

The general morphologic features of viral hepatitis are listed in Table 16-5 and are depicted schematically in Figure 16-9. The morphologic changes in acute and chronic viral hepatitis are shared among the hepatotropic viruses and can be mimicked by drug reactions. With acute hepatitis, hepatocyte injury takes the form of diffuse swelling **(ballooning degeneration),** so that the cytoplasm looks empty and contains only scattered wisps of cytoplasmic remnants. An inconstant finding is **cholestasis,** with bile plugs in canaliculi and brown pigmentation of hepatocytes. Fatty change is mild and is unusual except with HCV infection. Whether acute or chronic, HBV infection may generate **"ground-glass"** hepatocytes: a finely granular, eosinophilic cytoplasm shown by electron microscopy to contain massive quantities of HBsAg in

the form of spheres and tubules. Other HBV-infected hepatocytes may have **"sanded" nuclei,** owing to abundant intranuclear HBcAg.

Two patterns of hepatocyte **necrosis** are seen. In the first, rupture of cell membranes leads to **cytolysis.** The necrotic cells appear to have "dropped out," with collapse of the sinusoidal collagen reticulin framework where the cells have disappeared; scavenger macrophage aggregates mark sites of dropout. The second pattern of cell death, **apoptosis,** is more distinctive. Apoptotic hepatocytes shrink, become intensely eosinophilic, and have fragmented nuclei; effector T cells may still be present in the immediate vicinity. Apoptotic cells also are phagocytosed within hours by macrophages and hence may be difficult to find despite extensive ongoing apoptosis. In severe cases, confluent necrosis of hepatocytes may lead to **bridging necrosis** connecting portal-to-portal, central-to-central, or portal-to-central regions of adjacent lobules, signifying a more severe form of acute hepatitis. Hepatocyte swelling, necrosis, and regeneration produce compression of the vascular sinusoids and loss of the normal, more or less radial array of the parenchyma (so-called **lobular disarray).**

Inflammation is a characteristic and usually prominent feature of acute hepatitis. **Kupffer cells undergo hypertrophy and hyperplasia** and are often laden with lipofuscin pigment caused by phagocytosis of hepatocellular debris. **The portal tracts are usually infiltrated with a mixture of inflammatory cells.** The inflammatory infiltrate may spill over into the parenchyma to cause necrosis of periportal hepatocytes **(interface hepatitis).**

Finally, bile duct epithelium may become reactive and even proliferate, particularly in cases of HCV hepatitis, forming poorly defined ductular structures in the midst of the portal tract inflammation. Bile duct destruction, however, does not occur.

The histologic features of **chronic hepatitis** range from exceedingly mild to severe. Smoldering hepatocyte necrosis throughout the lobule may occur in all forms of chronic hepatitis. In the mildest forms, significant inflammation is limited to portal tracts and consists of lymphocytes, macrophages, occasional plasma cells, and rare neutrophils or eosinophils. **Lymphoid aggregates** in the portal tract are often seen in HCV infection. Liver architecture is usually well preserved. Continued **periportal necrosis** and **bridging necrosis** are harbingers of progressive liver damage. **The hallmark of irreversible liver damage is the deposition of fibrous tissue.** At first, only portal tracts exhibit increased fibrosis, but with time **periportal fibrosis** occurs, followed by linking of fibrous septa between lobules **(bridging fibrosis).**

Continued loss of hepatocytes and fibrosis results in cirrhosis, with fibrous septa and hepatocyte regenerative nodules. This pattern of cirrhosis is

ACUTE HEPATITIS

Portal tract

Inflammatory
infiltrate

Bile duct
reaction

Periportal
necrosis

Balllooning degeneration

Apoptosis

Macrophage
aggregates

Fatty change
(Hepatitis C)

Cholestasis

Apoptosis

Central vein

CHRONIC HEPATITIS

Portal tract

Lymphoid aggregates

Bridging necrosis

Central vein

Bridging fibrosis

Periportal necrosis

Periportal
fibrosis

"Ground-glass" cells
(Hepatitis B)

Apoptosis

Lymphocytes

Fatty change
(Hepatitis C)

Macrophage
aggregate

Central vein

Figure 16-9

Diagrammatic representation of the morphologic features of acute and chronic hepatitis.

characterized by irregularly sized nodules separated by variable but mostly broad scars (Fig. 16-10). The nodules are predominantly greater than 0.3 cm in diameter, earning the term **macronodular cirrhosis.** While such cirrhosis is characteristic of postviral cirrhosis, it is not specific to this etiology, because hepatotoxins (carbon tetrachloride, mushroom poisoning), pharmaceutical agents (acetaminophen, α-methyldopa), and even alcohol (discussed later) may give rise to macronodular cirrhosis. Notably, in 10% to 15% of cases an etiology for the cirrhosis cannot be identified.

Massive Hepatic Necrosis

Hepatic failure and its sequelae were discussed earlier. Fulminant hepatic failure denotes clinical hepatic insufficiency that progresses from onset of symptoms to hepatic encephalopathy within 2 to 3 weeks. A course extending up to 3 months is called subfulminant failure. *The histologic correlate of fulminant hepatic failure is massive hepatic necrosis.* Viral hepatitis accounts for 50% to 65% of all cases, with contributions from acute HBV, HDV-HBV, HAV, HCV, herpesvirus, and adenovirus. It is a serious complication of HEV infection

in pregnant women (see Table 16-4). Various drugs and chemicals are responsible for 25% to 30% of cases, by acting as direct hepatotoxins or by evoking idiosyncratic inflammatory reactions. Principally implicated are acetaminophen (in suicidal doses), isoniazid, antidepressants (particularly monoamine oxidase inhibitors), halothane, α-methyldopa, and the mycotoxins of the mushroom *Amanita phalloides.* Fortunately rare is the massive hepatic necrosis occurring in heat

Figure 16-10

Cirrhosis resulting from chronic viral hepatitis.

stroke. Other causes of fulminant hepatic failure (discussed later) in which hepatic necrosis is not the primary event include obstruction of the hepatic veins, Wilson disease, syndromes of micro vesicular steatosis (e.g., acute fatty liver of pregnancy), massive malignant infiltration, reactivation of chronic hepatitis B or superinfection with HDV, and autoimmune hepatitis.

Figure 16-11 ■

Massive necrosis, cut section of liver. The liver is small (700 g), bile stained, and soft. The capsule is wrinkled.

MORPHOLOGY

With massive hepatic necrosis, the distribution of liver destruction is extremely capricious: **the entire liver may be involved or only random areas are affected.** With massive loss of hepatic substance, the liver may shrink to as little as 500 to 700 g and become transformed into a limp, red organ covered by a wrinkled, too-large capsule. On transection (Fig. 16-11), necrotic areas have a muddy red, mushy appearance with blotchy bile staining. Microscopically, complete destruction of hepatocytes in contiguous lobules leaves only a collapsed reticulin framework and preserved portal tracts. There may be surprisingly little inflammatory reaction. Alternatively, with survival for several days there is a massive influx of inflammatory cells to begin the clean-up process (Fig. 16-12).

Patient survival for more than a week permits regeneration of surviving hepatocytes. Regeneration is initially in the form of strings of ductular structures, which mature into hepatocytes if given time. If the parenchymal framework is preserved, regeneration is orderly and native liver architecture is restored. With more massive destruction of confluent lobules, regeneration is disorderly, yielding nodular masses of liver cells. Scarring may occur in patients with a protracted course of submassive or patchy necrosis, representing a route for developing so-called macronodular cirrhosis, as noted earlier.

- Female predominance (70%)
- The absence of serologic markers of a viral etiology
- Elevated serum IgG levels (>2.5 g/dL)
- High titers of autoantibodies in 80% of cases
- An increased frequency of HLA-B8 or HLA-DRw3
- The presence of other forms of autoimmune diseases, seen in up to 60% of patients, including rheumatoid arthritis, thyroiditis, Sjögren syndrome, and ulcerative colitis

Fulminant hepatic failure may present as jaundice, encephalopathy, and fetor hepaticus, as described previously. Notably absent on physical examination are stigmata of chronic liver disease (e.g., gynecomastia, spider angiomas). Life-threatening extrahepatic complications include coagulopathy with bleeding, cardiovascular instability, renal failure, acute respiratory distress syndrome, electrolyte and acid-base disturbances, and sepsis. Overall mortality ranges from 25% to 90% in the absence of liver transplantation.

Autoimmune Hepatitis

Autoimmune hepatitis is a syndrome of chronic hepatitis in patients with a heterogeneous set of immunologic abnormalities. The histologic features are indistinguishable from chronic viral hepatitis. This disease may run an indolent or severe course and typically responds dramatically to immunosuppressive therapy. Salient features include

Figure 16-12 ■

Massive necrosis, microscopic section. Portal tracts and central veins are closer together than normal, owing to necrosis and collapse of the intervening parenchyma. The rudimentary ductal structures are the result of early hepatocyte regeneration. An infiltrate of chronic inflammatory cells is present.

Autoimmune hepatitis can be divided into three subtypes on the basis of the autoimmune antibodies. Type 1, constituting 80% to 85% of cases, is characterized by the presence of circulating antinuclear and/or anti–smooth muscle antibodies. Type 2, comprising a minority of about 5% of cases, is strongly associated with liver/kidney microsomal type 1 antibodies. Type 3, comprising the remainder of patients, is characterized by the presence of antibodies to soluble liver antigen. While there are differences in age at presentation (type 2 patients are younger), the relevance of this subclassification to clinical management remains unclear. Although autoimmune hepatitis presents with the entire spectrum of mild to severe chronic hepatitis, it is the symptomatic patients who tend to present with established severe liver damage. Response to immunosuppressive therapy is usually dramatic, although a full remission of disease is unusual. The overall risk of cirrhosis is 5%. In these patients, death is largely a consequence of cirrhosis, as occurs in other types of chronic liver diseases.

Liver Abscesses

In developing countries, liver abscesses are common; most result from parasitic infections, such as amebic, echinococcal, and (less commonly) other protozoal and helminthic organisms. In developed countries, parasitic liver abscesses are distinctly uncommon and many occur in immigrants. Instead, in the Western world, bacterial or fungal abscesses are more common, representing a complication of an infection elsewhere. The organisms reach the liver through one of the following pathways: (1) ascending infection in the biliary tract (ascending cholangitis); (2) vascular seeding, either portal or arterial; (3) direct invasion of the liver from a nearby source; or (4) a penetrating injury. Debilitating disease with immune deficiency is a common setting—for example, extreme old age, immunosuppression, or cancer chemotherapy with marrow failure.

Pyogenic (bacterial) hepatic abscesses may occur as solitary or multiple lesions, ranging from millimeters to massive lesions many centimeters in diameter. Bacteremic spread through the arterial or portal system tends to produce multiple small abscesses, whereas direct extension and trauma usually cause solitary large abscesses. Biliary abscesses, which are usually multiple, may contain purulent material in adjacent bile ducts. Gross and microscopic features are those of any pyogenic abscess. Occasionally, fungi or parasites rather than bacteria can be identified. On rare occasion, hepatic abscesses in the subdiaphragmatic region, particularly amebic ones, may extend into the thoracic cavity to produce empyema or a lung abscess.

Liver abscesses are associated with fever and, in many instances, with right upper quadrant pain and tender hepatomegaly. Jaundice is often the result of extrahepatic biliary obstruction. Although antibiotic therapy may control smaller lesions, surgical drainage is often necessary. Because diagnosis is frequently delayed, particularly in patients with serious coexistent disease, the mortality rate with large liver abscesses ranges from 30% to 90%. With early recognition and management, up to 80% of patients may survive.

DRUG- AND TOXIN-INDUCED LIVER DISEASE

As the major drug metabolizing and detoxifying organ in the body, the liver is subject to potential damage from an enormous array of therapeutic and environmental chemicals. Injury may result from direct toxicity, occur via hepatic conversion of a xenobiotic to an active toxin, or be produced by immune mechanisms, usually by the drug or a metabolite acting as a hapten to convert a cellular protein into an immunogen.

Principles of drug and toxic injury were discussed in Chapter 8. Here it suffices to recall that drug reactions may be classified as predictable (intrinsic) reactions or unpredictable (idiosyncratic) ones. Predictable drug reactions may occur in anyone who accumulates a sufficient dose. Unpredictable reactions depend on idiosyncrasies of the host, particularly the host's propensity to mount an immune response to the antigenic stimulus, and the rate at which the host metabolizes the agent. Major examples include chlorpromazine, an agent that causes cholestasis in those patients who are slow to metabolize it to an innocuous byproduct, and halothane, which can cause a fatal immune-mediated hepatitis in some patients exposed to this anesthetic on multiple occasions. A broad classification of offending agents is offered in Table 16–6. The injury may be immediate or take weeks to months to develop, and it may take the form of overt hepatocyte necrosis,

■

Table 16–6. DRUG- AND TOXIN-INDUCED HEPATIC INJURY

Hepatocellular Damage	Drug or Toxin
Microvesicular fatty change	Tetracycline, salicylates, yellow phosphorus, ethanol
Macrovesicular fatty change	Ethanol, methotrexate, amiodarone
Centrilobular necrosis	Bromobenzene, CCl_4, acetaminophen, halothane, rifampin
Diffuse or massive necrosis	Halothane, isoniazid, acetaminophen, α-methyldopa, trinitrotoluene, *Amanita phalloides* (mushroom) toxin
Hepatitis, acute and chronic	α-Methyldopa, isoniazid, nitrofurantoin, phenytoin, oxyphenisatin
Fibrosis-cirrhosis	Ethanol, methotrexate, amiodarone, most drugs that cause chronic hepatitis
Granuloma formation	Sulfonamides, α-methyldopa, quinidine, phenylbutazone, hydralazine, allopurinol
Cholestasis (with or without hepatocellular injury)	Chlorpromazine, anabolic steroids, erythromycin estolate, oral contraceptives, organic arsenicals
Vascular Disorders	
Veno-occlusive disease	Cytotoxic drugs, pyrrolizidine alkaloids (bush tea)
Hepatic or portal vein thrombosis	Estrogens, including oral contraceptives, cytotoxic drugs
Peliosis hepatitis	Anabolic steroids, oral contraceptives, danazol
Hyperplasia and Neoplasia	
Adenoma	Oral contraceptives
Hepatocellular carcinoma	Vinyl chloride, aflatoxin, Thorotrast
Cholangiocarcinoma	Thorotrast
Angiosarcoma	Vinyl chloride, inorganic arsenicals, Thorotrast

cholestasis, or insidious onset of liver dysfunction. Most important, *drug-induced chronic hepatitis is clinically and histologically indistinguishable from chronic viral hepatitis or autoimmune hepatitis, and hence serologic markers of viral infection are critical for making the distinction.* Among the agents listed in Table 16–6, predictable drug reactions are ascribed to acetaminophen (also called phenacetin), tetracycline, antineoplastic agents, *Amanita phalloides* toxin, carbon tetrachloride, and, to a certain extent, alcohol. Many others such as sulfonamides, α-methyldopa, and allopurinol cause idiosyncratic reactions.

A diagnosis of drug-induced liver disease may be made on the basis of a temporal association of liver damage with drug administration and, it is hoped, recovery on removal of the drug, combined with exclusion of other potential causes. Exposure to a toxin or therapeutic agent should always be included in the differential diagnosis of any form of liver disease.

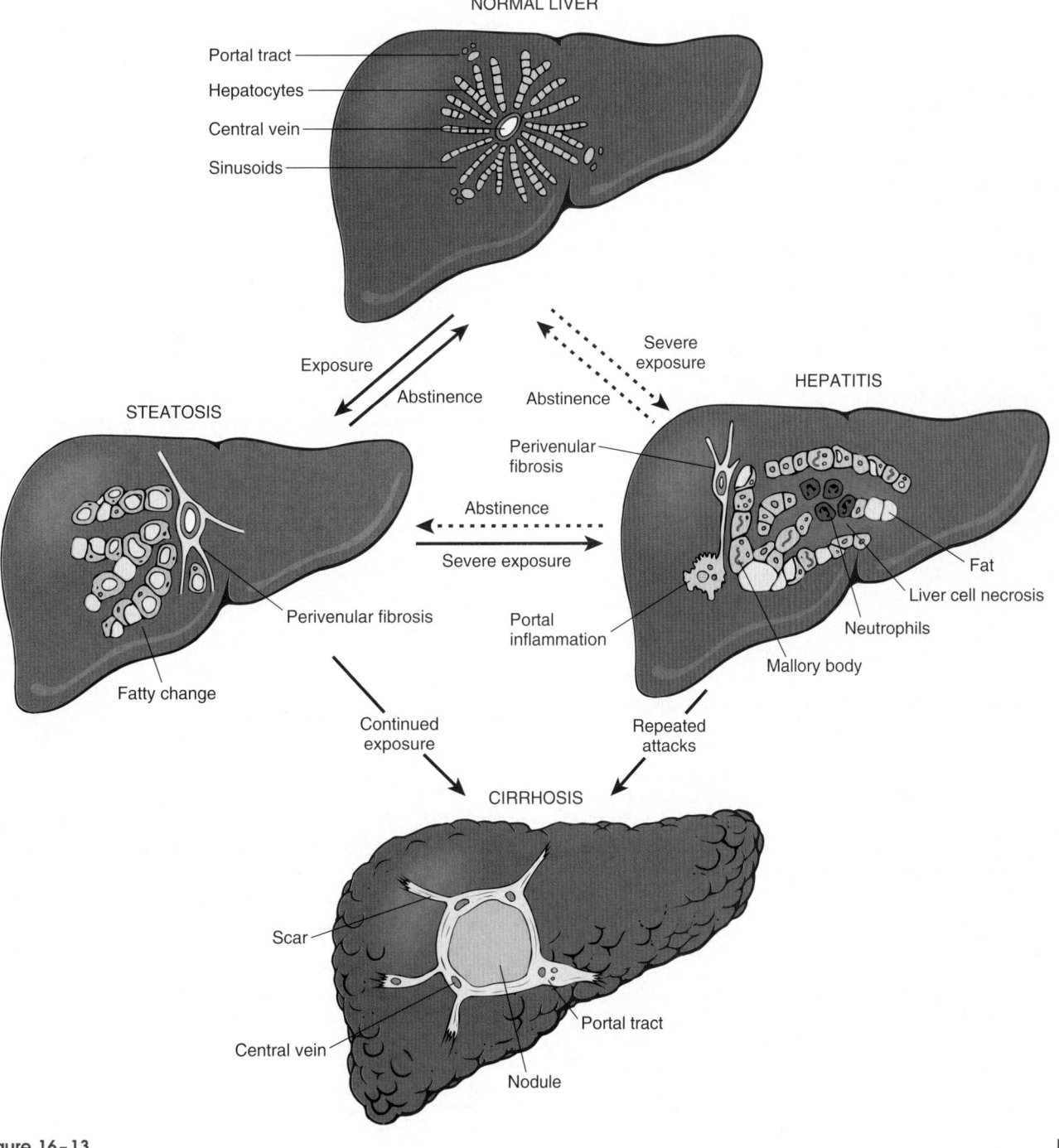

Figure 16–13

Alcoholic liver disease. The interrelationships among hepatic steatosis, hepatitis, and cirrhosis are shown, along with a depiction of key morphologic features at the microscopic level.

Alcoholic Liver Disease

Excessive ethanol consumption is the leading cause of liver disease in most Western countries. The following statistics attest to the magnitude of the problem in the United States:

■ More than 10 million Americans are alcoholics.
■ Alcohol abuse causes 100,000 to 200,000 deaths annually in the United States, the fifth leading cause of death. Of these deaths, 20,000 are attributable directly to end-stage cirrhosis; many more are the result of automobile accidents.
■ From 25% to 30% of hospitalized patients have problems related to alcohol abuse.

Chronic alcohol consumption has a variety of adverse effects, as pointed out in Chapter 8. Of great impact, however, are the three distinctive, albeit overlapping, forms of liver disease: (1) hepatic steatosis (fatty liver), (2) alcoholic hepatitis, and (3) cirrhosis, collectively referred to as alcoholic liver disease. At least 80% of heavy drinkers develop fatty liver (steatosis), 10% to 35% develop alcoholic hepatitis, and approximately 10% develop cirrhosis. Because the first two conditions may develop independently, they do not necessarily represent a continuum of changes. The morphology of the three forms of alcoholic liver disease is presented first, because this facilitates consideration of their pathogenesis. The various forms of alcoholic liver disease are depicted in Figure 16-13.

Figure 16-14

Alcoholic liver disease: macrovesicular steatosis, involving most regions of the hepatic lobule. The intracytoplasmic fat is seen as clear vacuoles. Some early fibrosis *(stained blue)* is present. (Masson trichrome.)

MORPHOLOGY

HEPATIC STEATOSIS (FATTY LIVER). After even moderate intake of alcohol, small **(microvesicular)** lipid droplets accumulate in hepatocytes. With chronic intake of alcohol, lipid accumulates to the point of creating large clear **macrovesicular** globules, compressing and displacing the nucleus to the periphery of the hepatocyte. This transformation is initially centrilobular, but in severe cases it may involve the entire lobule (Fig. 16-14). Macroscopically, the fatty liver of chronic alcoholism is large (up to 4 to 6 kg), soft, yellow, and greasy. Although there is little or no fibrosis at the outset, with continued alcohol intake fibrous tissue develops around the central veins and extends into the adjacent sinusoids. **Up to the time that fibrosis appears, the fatty change is completely reversible if there is abstention from further intake of alcohol.**

ALCOHOLIC HEPATITIS. This is characterized by the following:

■ **Hepatocyte swelling and necrosis.** Single or scattered foci of cells undergo swelling (ballooning) and necrosis. The swelling results from the accumulation of fat and water, as well as proteins that normally are exported.
■ **Mallory bodies.** Scattered hepatocytes accumulate tangled skeins of cytokeratin intermediate filaments and other proteins, visible as eosinophilic cytoplasmic inclusions in degenerating hepato-

cytes (Fig. 16-15). These inclusions are a characteristic but not specific feature of alcoholic liver disease, because they are also seen in primary biliary cirrhosis, Wilson disease, chronic cholestatic syndromes, and hepatocellular tumors.
■ **Neutrophilic reaction.** Neutrophils permeate the lobule and accumulate around degenerating hepatocytes, particularly those containing Mallory bodies. Lymphocytes and macrophages also enter portal tracts and spill into the parenchyma.
■ **Fibrosis.** Alcoholic hepatitis is almost always accompanied by a brisk sinusoidal and perivenular fibrosis; occasionally periportal fibrosis may predominate, particularly with repeated bouts of heavy alcohol intake. In some cases there is cholestasis and mild deposition of hemosiderin (iron) in hepatocytes and Kupffer cells. Macroscopically, the liver is mottled red with bile-stained areas. Although the liver may be normal or increased in size, it often contains visible nodules and fibrosis, indicative of evolution to cirrhosis.

ALCOHOLIC CIRRHOSIS. The final and irreversible form of alcoholic liver disease usually evolves slowly and insidiously. At first the cirrhotic liver is yellow-tan, fatty, and enlarged, usually weighing over 2 kg. Over the span of years it is transformed into a brown, shrunken, nonfatty organ, sometimes weighing less than 1 kg. Arguably, cirrhosis may develop more rapidly in the setting of alcoholic hepatitis, within 1 to 2 years. Initially, the developing fibrous septa are delicate and extend through sinusoids from central vein to portal regions as well as from portal tract to portal tract. Regenerative activity of entrapped parenchymal hepatocytes generates fairly uniformly sized nodules. As these nodules tend to be less than 0.3 cm in diameter, this pattern of cirrhosis is termed **micronodular cirrhosis** (vs. the

Figure 16–15

Alcoholic hepatitis. *A*, The cluster of inflammatory cells marks the site of a necrotic hepatocyte. A Mallory body is present in a second hepatocyte *(arrow)*. *B*, Eosinophilic Mallory bodies are seen in hepatocytes, which are surrounded by fibrous tissue. (H & E.)

macronodular cirrhosis described for viral hepatitis). With time, the nodularity becomes more prominent; scattered larger nodules create a "hobnail" appearance on the surface of the liver (Fig. 16–16). As fibrous septa dissect and surround nodules, the liver becomes more fibrotic, loses fat, and shrinks progressively. Residual regenerating parenchymal islands are engulfed by ever wider bands of fibrous tissue, and the liver is converted into a mixed micronodular and macronodular pattern (Fig. 16–17). Ischemic necrosis and fibrous obliteration of nodules eventually create broad expanses of tough, pale scar tissue. Bile stasis often develops; Mallory bodies are only rarely evident at this stage. Thus, **end-stage alcoholic cirrhosis** eventually comes to resemble, both macroscopically and microscopically, the cirrhosis developing from viral hepatitis and other causes.

Pathogenesis. Short-term ingestion of up to 80 g of ethanol per day (eight beers or 7 ounces of 80-proof liquor) generally produces mild, reversible hepatic changes, such as fatty liver. Daily ingestion of 160 g or more of ethanol for 10 to 20 years is associated more consistently with severe injury; chronic intake of 80 to 160 g/day is considered a borderline risk for severe injury. For reasons that may relate to decreased gastric metabolism of ethanol and differences in body composition, women appear to be more susceptible to hepatic injury than men. However, only 10% to 15% of alcoholics develop

Figure 16–16

Alcoholic cirrhosis showing the characteristic diffuse nodularity of the surface induced by the underlying fibrous scarring. The average nodule size is 3 mm in this close-up view. The greenish tint is caused by bile stasis.

Figure 16–17

Alcoholic cirrhosis. Nodules of varying sizes are entrapped in blue-staining fibrous tissue. (Masson trichrome.)

cirrhosis. Individual, possibly genetic, susceptibility must exist, but no reliable genetic markers of susceptibility have been identified. In addition, there is an inconstant relationship between hepatic steatosis and alcoholic hepatitis as precursors to cirrhosis. Moreover, cirrhosis may develop without antecedent evidence of steatosis or alcoholic hepatitis. In the absence of a clear understanding of the pathogenetic factors influencing liver damage, no "safe" upper limit for alcohol consumption can be proposed (despite the current popularity of red wines for amelioration of coronary vascular disease).

The pharmacokinetics and metabolism of alcohol were examined in Chapter 8. Pertinent to this discussion are the detrimental effects of alcohol and its byproducts on hepatocellular function:

■ Hepatocellular steatosis results from (1) the shunting of normal substrates away from catabolism and toward lipid biosynthesis, owing to generation of excess reduced nicotinamide-adenine dinucleotide by the two major enzymes of alcohol metabolism, alcohol dehydrogenase and acetaldehyde dehydrogenase (generating acetate); (2) impaired assembly and secretion of lipoproteins; and (3) increased peripheral catabolism of fat.

■ Induction of cytochrome P-450 leads to augmented transformation of other drugs to toxic metabolites. In particular, this can accelerate the metabolism of acetaminophen into highly toxic metabolites and increase the risk of liver injury even with therapeutic doses of this commonly used analgesic.

■ Free radicals are generated during oxidation of ethanol by the microsomal ethanol oxidizing system; the free radicals react with membranes and proteins.

■ Alcohol directly affects microtubular and mitochondrial function and membrane fluidity.

■ Acetaldehyde (the major intermediate metabolite of alcohol en route to acetate production) induces lipid peroxidation and acetaldehyde-protein adduct formation, further disrupting cytoskeletal and membrane function.

■ Neutrophil infiltration of the liver is common in alcoholic hepatitis, and it is thought that activated neutrophils release toxic oxygen metabolites. Elevated levels of interleukin 8, a chemoattractant of neutrophils, is seen in plasma of patients with alcoholic hepatitis.

■ Alcohol induces an immunologic attack on hepatocytes that are antigenically altered by alcohol or by acetaldehyde-induced alterations in hepatic proteins.

■ Because generation of acetaldehyde and free radicals is maximal in the centrilobular region of the parenchyma, this region is most susceptible to toxic injury.

■ Concurrent viral hepatitis, particularly hepatitis C, is a major factor that accelerates liver disease in alcoholics. The prevalence of hepatitis C in patients with alcoholic disease is about 30%.

In addition, alcohol can become a major caloric source in the diet, displacing other nutrients and leading to malnutrition and vitamin deficiencies (e.g., thiamine and vitamin B_{12}) in the alcoholic. This is compounded by impaired digestive function, primarily related to chronic gastric and intestinal mucosal damage, and pancreatitis. Alcohol-induced stimulation of fibrosis is multifactorial and remains poorly understood; possible mechanisms of hepatic fibrosis were discussed earlier in this chapter.

Clinical Features. *Hepatic steatosis* may become evident as hepatomegaly with mild elevation of serum bilirubin and alkaline phosphatase levels. Alternatively, there may be no clinical or biochemical evidence of liver disease. Severe hepatic compromise is unusual. Alcohol withdrawal and the provision of an adequate diet are sufficient treatment. For the occasional heavy drinker, mild hepatic steatosis is a common transient event in the metabolic disposition of excess alcohol.

It is estimated that 15 to 20 years of excessive drinking are necessary to develop alcoholic hepatitis. However, in such patients the clinical features of *alcoholic hepatitis* appear relatively acutely, usually after a bout of heavy drinking. Symptoms and laboratory abnormalities may be minimal or so severe as to constitute fulminant hepatic failure. Between these two extremes are the nonspecific symptoms of malaise, anorexia, weight loss, upper abdominal discomfort, tender hepatomegaly, and fever and the laboratory findings of hyperbilirubinemia, elevated alkaline phosphatase, and often a neutrophilic leukocytosis. Alanine aminotransferase (ALT) and aspartate aminotransferase (AST) levels are elevated but usually remain below 500 U/mL. The outlook is unpredictable; each bout of hepatitis carries about a 10% to 20% risk of death. With repeated bouts, cirrhosis appears in about one third of patients within a few years; alcoholic hepatitis also may be superimposed on cirrhosis. With proper nutrition and total cessation of alcohol consumption, alcoholic hepatitis may clear slowly. However, in some patients the hepatitis persists despite abstinence and progresses to cirrhosis.

The manifestations of *alcoholic cirrhosis* are similar to other forms of cirrhosis, presented earlier. Commonly, the first signs of cirrhosis relate to complications of portal hypertension. The stigmata of cirrhosis (e.g., an abdomen grossly distended with ascites, wasted extremities, caput medusae) may be the presenting features. Alternatively, a patient may first present with life-threatening variceal hemorrhage, dying as a result of either exsanguination or the hepatic encephalopathy precipitated by the metabolism of excess blood in the gastrointestinal tract. In other cases, insidious onset of malaise, weakness, weight loss, and loss of appetite precede the appearance of jaundice, ascites, and peripheral edema. Laboratory findings reflect the developing hepatic compromise, with elevated serum aminotransferase levels, hyperbilirubinemia, variable elevation of alkaline phosphatase, hypoproteinemia (globulins, albumin, and clotting factors), and anemia. Lastly, cirrhosis may be clinically silent, discovered only at autopsy or when stress such as infection or trauma tips the balance toward hepatic insufficiency.

The long-term outlook for alcoholics with liver disease is variable. The most important aspect of treatment is abstinence from alcohol. Five-year survival approaches 90% in abstainers who are free of jaundice, ascites, or hematemesis but drops to 50% to 60% in those who continue to imbibe. In the end-stage alcoholic, the immediate causes of death are (1) hepatic failure, (2) a massive gastrointestinal hemorrhage, (3) an intercurrent infection (to which these patients are predisposed), (4) hepatorenal syndrome after a bout of alcoholic hepatitis, and (5) hepatocellular carcinoma in 3% to 6% of cases.

Nonalcoholic Fatty Liver

Nonalcoholic fatty liver (NAFL) is a common but under-appreciated condition. It is an indolent disorder that features elevated serum aminotransferase levels and a low risk for development of hepatic fibrosis or cirrhosis. As the name denotes, this is a fatty liver occurring in individuals who do not drink alcohol. In some patients, the presence of parenchymal mixed inflammation with neutrophils and mononuclear cells, hepatocytes containing Mallory hyaline, and hepatocyte destruction earns the moniker of *nonalcoholic steatohepatitis (NASH)*. The single most consistent association for NAFL and the subgroup of NASH is obesity: up to a fifth of individuals exceeding their ideal body weight by 40% have NAFL, as opposed to less than a 3% incidence of NAFL in individuals who are not overweight. The other key associations for NAFL are type 2 diabetes mellitus and glucose intolerance, and hyperlipidemia.

Most patients with NAFL are asymptomatic, although some may have fatigue, malaise, right upper quadrant discomfort, or more severe symptoms of chronic liver disease. Liver biopsy is required for diagnosis. There is no proven therapy other than recommending weight loss in appropriate individuals. Fortunately, progression to cirrhosis is unusual. However, because NAFL is an underrecognized form of disease, it is hypothesized to be a significant contributor to the group of patients with "cryptogenic" cirrhosis.

INBORN ERRORS OF METABOLISM AND PEDIATRIC LIVER DISEASE

This distinct group of liver diseases, attributable to inborn errors of metabolism, includes hemochromatosis, Wilson disease, and α_1-antitrypsin deficiency, which may present in children or in adults. An additional set of diseases, referred to as neonatal hepatitis, appears in infancy and represents a diverse group of inherited and acquired conditions.

Hemochromatosis

Hereditary hemochromatosis refers to an HLA-linked autosomal recessive disease characterized by the excessive accumulation of body iron, most of which is deposited in the parenchymal organs such as the liver and pancreas. Acquired forms of hemochromatosis with known sources of excess iron are called *secondary iron overload* (Table 16–7).

As discussed in Chapter 12, the total body iron pool ranges from 2 to 6 g in normal adults; about 0.5 g is stored in the liver, 98% of which is in hepatocytes. In hereditary hemochromatosis, iron accumulates over the lifetime of an individual from excessive intestinal absorption. Total iron accumulation may exceed 50 g, over one third of which accumulates in the liver. Symptoms usually first appear in the fifth to sixth decades of life. Males predominate (ratio of 5 to 7:1) with slightly earlier clinical presentation, partly because physiologic iron loss (menstruation, pregnancy) retards iron accumulation in women. Fully developed cases exhibit (1)

Table 16–7. CLASSIFICATION OF IRON OVERLOAD

Hereditary Hemochromatosis
Secondary Iron Overload

Parenteral iron overload
  Transfusions
    Long-term hemodialysis
    Aplastic anemia
    Sickle cell disease
    Myelodysplastic syndromes
    Leukemias
  Iron-dextran injections
Ineffective erythropoiesis with increased erythroid activity
  β-Thalassemia
  Sideroblastic anemia
  Pyruvate kinase deficiency
Increased oral intake of iron
  African iron overload (Bantu siderosis)
Congenital atransferrinemia
Chronic liver disease
  Chronic alcoholic liver disease
  Porphyria cutanea tarda

micronodular cirrhosis (all patients), (2) diabetes mellitus (75% to 80% of patients), and (3) skin pigmentation (75% to 80%). However, with current laboratory testing and early diagnosis, approximately 75% of patients are asymptomatic and have neither cirrhosis nor diabetes at the time of diagnosis.

Pathogenesis. It may be recalled that the total body content of iron is tightly regulated, whereby the limited daily losses of iron are matched by gastrointestinal absorption since there is no excretory pathway for excess absorbed iron. *In hereditary hemochromatosis there is a primary defect in regulation of intestinal absorption of dietary iron, leading to net iron accumulation of 0.5 to 1.0 g/yr.* The hereditary hemochromatosis gene, *HFE*, is located on the short arm of chromosome 6 close to the HLA gene complex. It encodes a 343–amino acid protein that is similar in structure to major histocompatibility complex class I proteins. There are two common mutations in the *HFE* gene. The first is a mutation at nucleotide 845 in which adenine is substituted for guanine, resulting in a tyrosine substitution for cysteine at amino acid position 282 (C282Y). The second mutation is a guanine substitution for cytosine, resulting in an aspartate substitution for histidine at amino acid position 63 (H63D). This amino acid substitution is in the HLA-like peptide binding domain of the molecule.

The role of intact *HFE* in regulating iron uptake by the intestinal enterocyte, and in iron physiology overall, remains unclear. It interacts with transferrin receptor in the plasma membrane and can modulate transferrin receptor interaction with circulating transferrin-iron complexes. The disulfide bridge disrupted by the C282Y mutation is required for interaction with β_2-microglobulin, a circulating plasma protein that plays an undefined role in iron homeostasis. The mechanism for H63D alteration of *HFE* function is not yet known.

In white populations of northern European extraction, the frequency of the C282Y mutation in the *HFE* gene is approximately 12% and of H63D, approximately 25%. However, most hereditary hemochromatosis patients (83%) are homozygous for C282Y, because the penetrance of H63D is much lower. Compound C282Y/H63D heterozygotes or homozygotes for H63D comprise about 10% of hereditary hemochromatosis patients, and a small percentage of individuals with pedigree-documented hereditary hemochromatosis do not have mutations in *HFE*. Overall in the US population, the frequency of homozygous hereditary hemochromatosis attributable to either of these mutations is 0.45% (1 of every 220 persons), and heterozygosity is 10% (1 of every 10 persons), making hereditary hemochromatosis one of the most common inborn errors of metabolism.

Hereditary hemochromatosis manifests typically after 20 g of storage iron has accumulated. Regardless of source, excessive iron seems to be directly toxic to tissues by the following mechanisms: (1) lipid peroxidation by iron-catalyzed free radical reactions, (2) stimulation of collagen formation, and (3) direct interactions of iron with DNA, leading to lethal injury or predisposition to hepatocellular carcinoma. Whatever the actions of iron, they are reversible in cells not fatally injured, and removal of excess iron by therapy promotes recovery of tissue function.

The most common causes of secondary iron overload are the anemias associated with ineffective erythropoiesis, discussed in Chapter 12. In these disorders, the excess iron may result not only from transfusions but also from increased absorption. Transfusions alone, as in sickle cell and aplastic anemias, lead to systemic hemosiderosis in which parenchymal organ injury tends to occur only in extreme cases. Alcoholic cirrhosis is often associated with a modest increase in stainable iron within liver cells. However, this may represent alcohol-induced redistribution of iron, because total body iron is not significantly increased. A rather unusual form of iron overload resembling hereditary hemochromatosis occurs in sub-Saharan Africa, the result of ingesting large quantities of alcoholic beverage fermented in iron utensils such as steel drums (Bantu siderosis). A genetic predisposition to accumulating excess iron, unrelated to the *HFE* gene, has been identified in these African populations.

Lastly, neonatal hemochromatosis is a rare disorder characterized by neonatal liver failure with onset in utero. It is associated with massive iron accumulation in parenchymal organs, sparing the mononuclear phagocyte system. It is an important cause of neonatal liver failure, most likely representing the end point of diverse processes such as maternal alloimmune hepatitis or intrauterine infection. As it may recur in sequential pregnancies even when paternity has been different, there may be a mitochondrial basis of inheritance or an in utero environmental exposure. The prognosis of this condition is poor.

MORPHOLOGY

The morphologic changes in hereditary hemochromatosis are characterized principally by (1) the **deposition of hemosiderin** in the following organs (in decreasing order of severity): liver, pancreas, myocardium, pituitary, adrenal, thyroid and parathyroid glands, joints, and skin, (2) **cirrhosis,** and (3) **pancreatic fibrosis.** In the liver, iron becomes evident first as golden-yellow hemosiderin granules in the cytoplasm of periportal hepatocytes, which stain blue with the Prussian blue stain (Fig. 16–18). With

increasing iron load, there is progressive involvement of the rest of the lobule, along with bile duct epithelium and Kupffer cell pigmentation. Iron is a direct hepatotoxin, and inflammation is characteristically absent. At this stage, the liver is typically slightly larger than normal, dense, and chocolate brown. Fibrous septa develop slowly, leading ultimately to a micronodular pattern of cirrhosis in an intensely pigmented liver.

In normal individuals the iron content of unfixed liver tissue is less than 1000 μg/g dry weight. Adult patients with hereditary hemochromatosis exhibit over 10,000 μg/g dry weight of iron; hepatic iron concentrations in excess of 22,000 μg/g dry weight are associated with the development of fibrosis and cirrhosis.

The **pancreas** becomes intensely pigmented, has diffuse interstitial fibrosis, and may exhibit some parenchymal atrophy. Hemosiderin is found in the acinar and the islet cells and sometimes in the interstitial fibrous stroma. The **heart** is often enlarged and has hemosiderin granules within the myocardial fibers. The pigmentation may induce a striking brown coloration of the myocardium. A delicate interstitial fibrosis may appear. Although **skin** pigmentation is partially attributable to hemosiderin deposition in dermal macrophages and fibroblasts, most of the coloration results from increased epidermal melanin production. The combination of these pigments renders the skin slate-gray. With hemosiderin deposition in the **joint synovial linings,** an acute synovitis may develop. There is also excessive deposition of calcium pyrophosphate, which damages the articular cartilage and sometimes produces disabling polyarthritis, referred to as pseudogout. The **testes** may be small and atrophic but are usually not discolored.

Figure 16–18

Hereditary hemochromatosis. Hepatocellular iron deposition is blue in this Prussian blue–stained histologic section. The parenchymal architecture is normal.

Clinical Features. Hereditary hemochromatosis is more often a disease of males and rarely becomes evident before age 40. The principal manifestations include hepatomegaly, abdominal pain, skin pigmentation (particularly in sun-exposed areas), deranged glucose homeostasis or frank diabetes mellitus from destruction of pancreatic islets, cardiac dysfunction (arrhythmias, cardiomyopathy), and atypical arthritis. In some patients, the presenting complaint is hypogonadism (e.g., amenorrhea in the female and loss of libido and impotence in the male). It is thought that the hypogonadism is caused by derangement in the hypothalamic-pituitary axis. The classic clinical triad of cirrhosis with hepatomegaly, skin pigmentation, and diabetes mellitus may not develop until late in the course of the disease. Death may result from cirrhosis or cardiac disease. A significant cause of death is hepatocellular carcinoma, because treatment of iron overload does not remove the risk for this aggressive neoplasm.

Fortunately, hereditary hemochromatosis can be diagnosed long before irreversible tissue damage has occurred. Screening involves demonstration of very high levels of serum iron and ferritin, exclusion of secondary causes of iron overload, and liver biopsy if indicated. Also important is screening of family members of probands for *HFE* mutations. The natural course of the disease can be substantially altered by a variety of interventions, mainly phlebotomy and the use of iron chelators to drain off the excess iron.

Patients with hereditary hemochromatosis diagnosed in the subclinical, precirrhotic stage and treated by regular phlebotomy have a normal life expectancy. Heterozygotes may exhibit a mild increase in iron absorption and accumulation; there is some evidence that the heterozygous state may increase the severity of coexistent liver disease.

Wilson Disease

This autosomal recessive disorder of copper metabolism is marked by the *accumulation of toxic levels of copper in many tissues and organs, principally the liver, brain, and eye.* The gene for Wilson disease has a frequency of 1:200. The incidence of this disease is approximately 1:30,000; thus, it is much less common than hereditary hemochromatosis.

Normal copper physiology involves (1) absorption of ingested copper (2 to 5 mg/day); (2) plasma transport complexed to albumin; (3) hepatocellular uptake, followed by incorporation into an α_2-globulin to form ceruloplasmin; (4) secretion of ceruloplasmin into plasma, where it accounts for 90% to 95% of plasma copper; and (5) hepatic uptake of desialylated, senescent ceruloplasmin from the plasma, followed by lysosomal degradation and secretion of free copper into bile. In Wilson disease, the initial steps of copper absorption and transport to the liver are normal. However, absorbed copper fails to enter the circulation in the form of ceruloplasmin and biliary excretion of copper is markedly diminished. *The gene responsible for Wilson disease is* ATP7B, *located on chromosome 13. This codes for an ATP-dependent metal ion transporter that localizes to the Golgi region of hepatocytes. Defective function of this transporter leads to failure to excrete copper into bile, the*

primary route for copper elimination from the body. Copper thus accumulates progressively in the liver, apparently causing toxic liver injury by (1) promoting the formation of free radicals, (2) binding to sulfhydryl groups of cellular proteins, and (3) displacing other metals in hepatic metalloenzymes. Usually by 5 years of age, non–ceruloplasmin-bound copper spills over into the circulation, causing hemolysis and pathologic changes at other sites, such as brain, cornea, kidneys, bones, joints, and parathyroid glands. Concomitantly, urinary excretion of copper increases markedly. *The biochemical diagnosis of Wilson disease is based on a decrease in serum ceruloplasmin, increase in hepatic copper content, and increase in urinary excretion of copper.*

MORPHOLOGY

The liver often bears the brunt of injury in Wilson disease, with hepatic changes ranging from relatively minor to massive damage. **Fatty change** may be mild to moderate, with vacuolated nuclei (glycogen or water) and occasional hepatocyte focal necrosis. An **acute hepatitis** can mimic acute viral hepatitis, save possibly for the accompanying fatty change. A **chronic hepatitis** resembles chronic hepatitis of viral, drug, or alcoholic origin but may exhibit such distinguishing features as fatty change, vacuolated nuclei, and Mallory bodies. With progression of chronic hepatitis, **cirrhosis** develops. **Massive liver necrosis** is a rare manifestation that is indistinguishable from that caused by viruses or drugs. Excess copper deposition can often be demonstrated by special stains (e.g., rhodanine stain for copper, orcein stain for copper-associated protein). Because copper also accumulates in chronic obstructive cholestasis, and because histology cannot reliably distinguish Wilson disease from viral- and drug-induced hepatitis, demonstration of hepatic copper content in excess of 250 μg/g dry weight is most helpful for making a diagnosis.

In the **brain**, toxic injury primarily affects the basal ganglia, particularly the putamen, which demonstrates atrophy and even cavitation. Nearly all patients with neurologic involvement develop **eye lesions** called **Kayser-Fleischer rings** (green to brown deposits of copper in Descemet membrane in the limbus of the cornea)—hence the alternative designation of this condition as hepatolenticular degeneration.

Clinical Features. The age at onset and the clinical presentation of Wilson disease are extremely variable, but the disorder rarely manifests before age 6 years. The most common presentation is acute or chronic liver disease. Neuropsychiatric manifestations, including mild behavioral changes, frank psychosis, or a Parkinson disease–like syndrome, are the initial features in most of the remaining cases. Demonstration of Kayser-Fleischer rings or markedly elevated hepatic copper levels in a patient with a low serum ceruloplasmin level strongly favor the diagnosis. Early recognition and long-term copper chelation therapy (as with D-penicillamine) have dramatically altered the usual progressive downhill course. Patients with fulminant hepatitis and unmanageable cirrhosis require liver transplantation.

α_1-Antitrypsin Deficiency

α_1-Antitrypsin deficiency (AAT) is an autosomal recessive disorder marked by abnormally low serum levels of this protease inhibitor (Pi). The major function of AAT is the inhibition of proteases, particularly neutrophil elastase released at sites of inflammation. AAT deficiency leads to pulmonary emphysema, because a relative lack of this protein permits tissue-destructive enzymes to run amok (Chapter 13).

AAT is a small (394–amino acid) plasma glycoprotein synthesized predominantly by hepatocytes. The *AAT* gene, located on human chromosome 14, is very polymorphic, and at least 75 AAT forms have been identified. The most common allele is *PiM*, and the normal *PiMM* genotype occurs in 90% of individuals. Most allelic variants produce normal or mildly reduced levels of serum AAT. However, homozygotes for the Z allele (*PiZZ* genotype) have circulating AAT levels that are only 10% of normal levels. Expression of *AAT* alleles is autosomal codominant, and consequently *PiMZ* heterozygotes have intermediate plasma levels of AAT. The gene frequency of *PiZ* is 1.2% in the North American white population, yielding a *PiZZ* genotype frequency of approximately 1:7000.

The PiZ polypeptide contains a single amino acid substitution that results in misfolding of the nascent polypeptide in the hepatocyte endoplasmic reticulum. Because the mutant protein cannot be secreted by the hepatocyte, it accumulates in the endoplasmic reticulum and undergoes excessive lysosomal degradation. Curiously, all individuals with the *PiZZ* genotype accumulate AAT in the liver, but only 8% to 20% develop significant liver damage. A proposed explanation is a separate genetic tendency toward reduced intracellular protein degradation via the ubiquitin-proteasomal pathway, rendering susceptible individuals with *PiZZ* genotypes less able to degrade accumulated AAT protein within hepatocytes.

Figure 16–19 ■

α_1-Antitrypsin deficiency. Periodic acid–Schiff stain of liver, highlighting the characteristic red cytoplasmic granules. (Courtesy of Dr. I. Wanless, Toronto Hospital.)

Clinical Course. Ten percent to 20% of newborns with AAT deficiency exhibit cholestasis. In older children, adolescents, and adults, presenting symptoms may be related to chronic hepatitis, cirrhosis, or pulmonary disease. The disease may remain silent until cirrhosis appears in middle to later life. Hepatocellular carcinoma develops in 2% to 3% of *PiZZ* adults, usually but not always in the setting of cirrhosis. The treatment, and cure, for the severe hepatic disease is orthotopic liver transplantation.

Neonatal Hepatitis

As mentioned earlier, mild transient elevations in serum unconjugated bilirubin are common in normal newborns. Prolonged conjugated hyperbilirubinemia in the newborn, termed *neonatal cholestasis*, affects approximately 1 in 2500 live births. The major conditions causing it are extrahepatic biliary atresia (EHBA), discussed later, and a variety of other disorders collectively referred to as *neonatal hepatitis*. Neonatal hepatitis is not a specific entity, nor are the disorders necessarily inflammatory. Instead, the finding of "neonatal cholestasis" should evoke a diligent search for recognizable toxic, metabolic, and infectious liver diseases. Some of the major causes are listed in Table 16–8, noting that this is an abbreviated version of an extensive list that contains many unusual infections and inherited diseases.

Clinical presentation of infants with any form of neonatal cholestasis is fairly stereotypical, with jaundice, dark urine, light or acholic stools, and hepatomegaly. Variable degrees

---

MORPHOLOGY

Hepatocytes in AAT deficiency contain round to oval cytoplasmic globular inclusions of retained AAT, which are strongly positive in a periodic acid–Schiff (PAS) stain (Fig. 16-19). By electron microscopy they lie within smooth, and sometimes rough, endoplasmic reticulum. Hepatic injury associated with PiZZ homozygosity may range from marked cholestasis with hepatocyte necrosis in newborns, to childhood cirrhosis, or to a smoldering chronic inflammatory hepatitis or cirrhosis that becomes apparent only late in life.

Table 16-8. MAJOR CAUSES OF NEONATAL CHOLESTASIS

Bile duct obstruction
 Extrahepatic biliary atresia
Neonatal infection
 Cytomegalovirus
 Bacterial sepsis
 Urinary tract infection
 Syphilis
Toxic
 Drugs
 Parenteral nutrition
Metabolic diseases
 Amino acid
  Tyrosinemia
 Lipid
  Niemann-Pick disease
 Carbohydrate
  Galactosemia
 Bile acid metabolism
  Δ^4-3-oxosteroid 5β-reductase deficiency
 Miscellaneous
  α_1-Antitrypsin deficiency
  Cystic fibrosis
  Progressive familial intrahepatic cholestasis
Miscellaneous
 Shock/hypoperfusion
 Indian childhood cirrhosis
 Alagille syndrome (paucity of bile ducts)
Idiopathic neonatal hepatitis

of hepatic synthetic dysfunction, such as hypoprothrombinemia, may be present. Despite the long list of disorders associated with neonatal cholestasis, most are quite rare. *"Idiopathic" neonatal hepatitis represents 50% to 60% of cases; about 20% are caused by extrahepatic biliary atresia and 1.5% to AAT deficiency.* Differentiation of the two most common causes assumes great importance, because definitive treatment of biliary atresia requires surgical intervention, whereas surgery may adversely affect the clinical course of a child with idiopathic neonatal hepatitis. Fortunately, discrimination between neonatal hepatitis and biliary atresia can be made in about 90% of cases using clinical data and liver biopsy. Only in extrahepatic biliary obstruction are there histologic features of biliary obstruction (described later).

Reye Syndrome

Reye syndrome is a rare disease characterized by fatty change in the liver and encephalopathy. The most severe forms are fatal. It primarily affects children younger than 4 years of age, typically developing 3 to 5 days after a viral illness. The onset is heralded by pernicious vomiting and is accompanied by irritability or lethargy and hepatomegaly. Serum bilirubin, ammonia, and aminotransferase levels are essentially normal at this time. Although most patients recover, about 25% progress to coma, accompanied by elevations in the serum levels of bilirubin, aminotransferases, and particularly ammonia. Death occurs from progressive neurologic deterioration or liver failure. Survivors of more

serious illness may be left with permanent neurologic impairments. Therapy is entirely symptomatic and supportive. The pathogenesis of Reye syndrome is incompletely understood, but it seems to be caused by mitochondrial dysfunction, occurring alone or in combination with viral infection. Because Reye syndrome has been associated with salicylate administration during viral illnesses, treatment of febrile illness in children with aspirin is now strongly discouraged. There is, however, no evidence that salicylates play a causal role in this disorder. Although the case rate for Reye syndrome in the United States for individuals younger than 18 years of age is less than 1 per million per year, this disorder must remain in the differential diagnosis of postviral disorders in children.

MORPHOLOGY

The key pathologic finding in the **liver** is microvesicular steatosis. Electron microscopy of hepatocellular mitochondria reveals pleomorphic enlargement and electron lucency of the matrices, with disruption of cristae and loss of dense bodies. In the **brain,** cerebral edema is usually present. Astrocytes are swollen and mitochondrial changes similar to those seen in the liver may develop. Inflammation is notably absent, as is any evidence of viral infection. **Skeletal muscles, kidneys,** and **heart** may also reveal microvesicular fatty change and mitochondrial alterations, although more subtle than those of the liver.

OBSTRUCTIVE BILIARY TRACT DISEASE

Biliary tract disorders cannot always be divided into those that affect only the intrahepatic or only the extrahepatic portions, particularly because extrahepatic biliary disorders incite secondary changes within the liver. Accordingly, reference should be made to the subsequent section on the gallbladder and biliary tree, particularly biliary atresia, which affects both extrahepatic and intrahepatic bile ducts. In addition, hepatic bile ducts are frequently damaged as part of a more general liver disease, as in drug toxicity, viral hepatitis, and transplantation (both orthotopic liver transplantation and graft-versus-host disease after bone marrow transplantation). With these caveats, consideration will now be given to three disorders of bile ducts that culminate in cirrhosis, as summarized in Table 16-9.

Secondary Biliary Cirrhosis

Prolonged obstruction to the extrahepatic biliary tree results in profound damage to the liver itself. The most common cause of obstruction is extrahepatic cholelithiasis (gallstones, described later). Other obstructive conditions include biliary atresia, malignancies of the biliary tree and head of the pancreas, and strictures resulting from previous

Table 16-9. DISTINGUISHING FEATURES OF THE MAJOR OBSTRUCTIVE BILE DUCT DISORDERS

	Secondary Biliary Cirrhosis	Primary Biliary Cirrhosis	Primary Sclerosing Cholangitis
Etiology	Extrahepatic bile duct obstruction: biliary atresia, gallstones, stricture, carcinoma of pancreatic head	Possibly autoimmune; associated with other autoimmune conditions	Unknown, possibly autoimmune; 50%–70% of cases associated with inflammatory bowel disease
Sex Predilection	None	Female-to-male 10:1	Female-to-male 1:2
Symptoms and Signs	Pruritus, jaundice, malaise, dark urine, light stools, hepatosplenomegaly	Same as secondary biliary cirrhosis; insidious onset	Same as secondary biliary cirrhosis; insidious onset
Laboratory Findings	Conjugated hyperbilirubinemia, increased serum alkaline phosphatase, bile acids, cholesterol	Same as secondary biliary cirrhosis, plus elevated serum IgM and presence of autoantibodies, especially against mitochondrial pyruvate dehydrogenase	Same as secondary biliary cirrhosis, plus elevated serum IgM, hypergammaglobulinemia
Important Pathologic Findings Before Cirrhosis Develops	Prominent bile stasis in bile ducts, bile duct proliferation with surrounding neutrophils, portal tract edema	Dense lymphocytic infiltrate in portal tracts with granulomatous destruction of bile ducts	Periductal portal tract fibrosis, segmental stenosis of extrahepatic and intrahepatic bile ducts

surgical procedures. The initial morphologic features of cholestasis were described earlier and are entirely reversible with correction of the obstruction. However, secondary inflammation resulting from biliary obstruction initiates periportal fibrogenesis, which eventually leads to scarring and nodule formation, generating secondary biliary cirrhosis. Subtotal obstruction may promote secondary bacterial infection of the biliary tree (ascending cholangitis), which further contributes to the damage. Enteric organisms such as coliforms and enterococci are common culprits.

Primary Biliary Cirrhosis

Primary biliary cirrhosis is a chronic, progressive, and often fatal cholestatic liver disease, characterized by the destruction of intrahepatic bile ducts, portal inflammation and scarring, and the eventual development of cirrhosis and liver failure over years to decades. *The primary feature of this disease is a nonsuppurative, granulomatous destruction of medium-sized intrahepatic bile ducts;* cirrhosis appears only late in the course. This is primarily a disease of middle-aged women, with an age at onset between 20 and 80 years and peak incidence between 40 and 50 years of age. The onset is insidious, usually presenting as pruritus; jaundice develops late in the course. Over a period of two or more decades, the patients develop hepatic decompensation, including portal hypertension with variceal bleeding, and hepatic encephalopathy. For end-stage patients, liver transplantation offers the only hope for long-term survival.

Serum alkaline phosphatase and cholesterol levels are almost always elevated; hyperbilirubinemia is a late development and usually signifies incipient hepatic decompensation. A striking feature of the disease is autoantibodies, especially antimitochondrial antibodies in over 90% of patients. Particularly characteristic of primary biliary cirrhosis are antibodies to mitochondrial pyruvate dehydrogenase. Associated extrahepatic conditions include the sicca complex of dry eyes and

mouth (Sjögren syndrome), scleroderma, thyroiditis, rheumatoid arthritis, Raynaud phenomenon, membranous glomerulonephritis, and celiac disease. Many lines of evidence suggest an autoimmune cause for primary biliary cirrhosis involving lymphocyte-mediated destruction of bile duct epithelial cells, but the inciting factors remain unclear. Much attention has been given to the pathogenesis of this disorder. It is hypothesized that destruction of bile ducts is mediated by autoreactive T lymphocytes, perhaps reacting to an aberrantly expressed mitochondrial protein on the bile duct epithelial cell surface rather than in its normal location in the mitochondrion. The antimitochondrial antibodies are probably secondary to cell damage.

Primary Sclerosing Cholangitis

Primary sclerosing cholangitis is characterized by inflammation, obliterative fibrosis, and segmental dilation of the obstructed intrahepatic and extrahepatic bile ducts. Endoscopic retrograde cholangiography demonstrates characteristic "beading" of the contrast medium in radiographs of the intrahepatic and extrahepatic biliary tree. This change is attributable to the irregular strictures and dilations of affected bile ducts. Primary sclerosing cholangitis is commonly seen in association with inflammatory bowel disease (Chapter 15), particularly chronic ulcerative colitis, which coexists in approximately 70% of patients. Conversely, the prevalence of primary sclerosing cholangitis in patients with ulcerative colitis is about 4%. The disorder tends to occur in the third through fifth decades, most often after development of inflammatory bowel disease. Males are affected more often than females in a ratio of 2:1.

Symptoms at presentation include progressive fatigue, pruritus, and jaundice. Asymptomatic patients may come to attention only on the basis of a persistent elevation of serum alkaline phosphatase levels. Unlike primary biliary cirrhosis, autoantibodies are present in less than 10% of patients. Severely afflicted patients exhibit symptoms associated with chronic liver disease, including weight loss, ascites, variceal bleeding, and encephalopathy. This disease also follows a protracted course over many years. There does appear to be an increased risk for cholangiocarcinoma in this patient population. The cause is unknown, but hypothesized mechanisms include exposure to gut-derived toxins, autoimmune immunologic attack, and ischemic damage to the end-arterial supply of the biliary tree. The association with ulcerative colitis, linkage with certain HLA-DR alleles, and presence of P-ANCA (Chapter 10) antibodies in 80% of cases all suggest that this is an immunologically mediated disease. As with primary biliary cirrhosis, liver transplantation is the definitive treatment.

MORPHOLOGY

In all three conditions (primary and secondary biliary cirrhosis and primary sclerosing cholangitis), the end-stage liver exhibits extraordinary yellow-green pigmentation, associated with marked icteric discoloration of body tissues and fluids. On cut surface, the liver is hard, with a finely granular appearance (Fig. 16–20). The histology of **secondary biliary cirrhosis** is characterized by coarse fibrous septa that subdivide the liver in a jigsaw-like pattern. Embedded in the septa are distended large and small bile ducts, which contain inspissated pigmented material. There is extensive proliferation of smaller bile ductules and edema (Fig. 16–21), particularly at the interface between septa (formerly portal tracts) and the parenchyma. The complication of bacterial infection incites a robust neutrophilic infiltration of bile ducts; severe pylephlebitis (vein inflammation) and cholangitic abscesses may develop.

In contrast to secondary biliary cirrhosis, interlobular bile ducts are absent in the end stage of

Figure 16–21 ■

Portal tract bile ductular proliferation in the setting of biliary cirrhosis. A mixed inflammatory infiltrate is also present.

primary biliary cirrhosis. However, the morphology of this disease is most revealing in the precirrhotic stage. Interlobular bile ducts are destroyed by inflammation (the **florid duct lesion**), featuring intraepithelial infiltration of lymphocytes and accompanying granulomatous inflammation. There is a dense portal tract infiltrate of lymphocytes, macrophages, plasma cells, and occasional eosinophils (Fig. 16–22). The obstruction to intrahe-

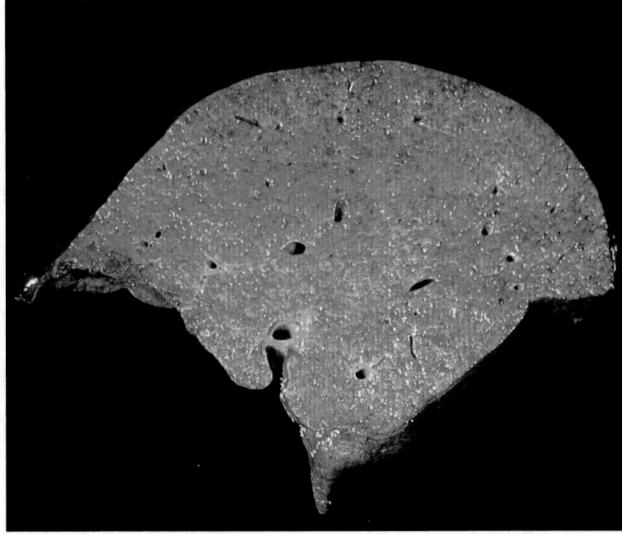

Figure 16–20 ■

Biliary cirrhosis. This sagittal section through the liver demonstrates the fine nodularity and bile staining of end-stage primary biliary cirrhosis.

Figure 16–22 ■

Primary biliary cirrhosis. A portal tract is markedly expanded by an infiltrate of lymphocytes and plasma cells. The granulomatous reaction to a bile duct undergoing destruction (florid duct lesion) is highlighted by the arrowheads.

Figure 16-23 ■

Primary sclerosing cholangitis. A bile duct undergoing degeneration is entrapped in a dense, onion-skin concentric scar.

patic bile flow leads to upstream bile ductular proliferation, inflammation and necrosis of the adjacent periportal hepatic parenchyma, and generalized cholestasis. Over years to decades, relentless portal tract scarring and bridging fibrosis leads to cirrhosis.

The characteristic feature of **primary sclerosing cholangitis** is a fibrosing cholangitis of bile ducts. Specifically, affected portal tracts exhibit concentric periductal onion-skin fibrosis and a modest lymphocytic infiltrate (Fig. 16-23). Progressive atrophy of the bile duct epithelium leads to obliteration of the lumen, leaving behind a solid, cordlike fibrous scar. In between areas of progressive stricture, bile ducts become ectatic and inflamed, presumably the result of downstream obstruction. As the disease progresses over years, the entire liver becomes markedly cholestatic and fibrotic. Ultimately, biliary cirrhosis develops, much like that seen with primary and secondary biliary cirrhosis.

HLA-DR alleles, and presence of P-ANCA (Chapter 10) antibodies in 80% of cases all suggest that this is an immunologically mediated disease. As with primary biliary cirrhosis, liver transplantation is the definitive treatment.

CIRCULATORY DISORDERS

Given the enormous flow of blood through the liver, it is not surprising that circulatory disturbances have considerable impact on the liver. These disorders can be grouped according to whether blood flow into, through, or from the liver is impaired (Fig. 16-24).

Impaired Blood Flow Into the Liver

HEPATIC ARTERY INFLOW

Liver infarcts are rare, thanks to the double blood supply to the liver. Interruption of the main hepatic artery does not always produce ischemic necrosis of the organ, because retrograde arterial flow through accessory vessels and the portal venous supply may sustain the liver parenchyma. The one exception is hepatic artery thrombosis in the transplanted liver, which generally leads to loss of the organ. Thrombosis or compression of an intrahepatic branch of the hepatic artery by polyarteritis nodosa (Chapter 10), embolism, neoplasia, or sepsis may result in a localized parenchymal infarct.

PORTAL VEIN OBSTRUCTION

Blockage of the portal vein may be insidious and well tolerated or may be a catastrophic and potentially lethal event; most cases fall somewhere in between. Occlusive disease of the portal vein or its major radicles typically produces abdominal pain and, in most instances, ascites and other manifestations of portal hypertension, principally esophageal varices that are prone to rupture. The ascites, when present, is often massive and intractable. Acute impairment of visceral blood flow leads to profound congestion and bowel infarction.

Extrahepatic portal vein obstruction may arise from the following:

■ Peritoneal sepsis (e.g., acute diverticulitis or appendicitis leading to pylephlebitis in the splanchnic circulation)
■ Lymphatic metastasis from abdominal cancers creating massive enlargement of hilar lymph nodes
■ Pancreatitis that initiates splenic vein thrombosis that propagates into the portal vein
■ Postsurgical thromboses after upper abdominal procedures
■ Banti syndrome, in which subclinical thrombosis of the portal vein (as from neonatal omphalitis or umbilical vein catheterization) produces a fibrotic, partially recanalized vascular channel presenting as splenomegaly or esophageal varices years after the occlusive event

Intrahepatic thrombosis of a portal vein radicle, when acute, does not cause ischemic infarction but instead results in a sharply demarcated area of red-blue discoloration (so-called infarct of Zahn). There is no necrosis, only hepatocellular atrophy and marked congestion in distended sinusoids. Vascular invasion by primary or secondary cancer in the liver can progressively occlude portal inflow to the liver; tongues of hepatocellular carcinoma can even occlude the main portal vein. Hepatoportal sclerosis is a chronic, generally bland condition of progressive portal tract sclerosis leading to impaired portal vein inflow. In those instances in which a cause can be identified, it may be a myeloproliferative disorder with associated hypercoagulability, peritonitis, or exposure to arsenicals.

Impaired Blood Flow Through the Liver

The most common intrahepatic cause of portal blood flow

Figure 16-24   ■

Hepatic circulatory disorders. The forms and clinical manifestations of compromised blood flow are contrasted.

periportal sinusoidal occlusion and parenchymal necrosis that may occur in the eclampsia of pregnancy. Subsequent suffusion of blood under the capsule may precipitate a fatal intra-abdominal hemorrhage (Fig. 16-25).

PASSIVE CONGESTION AND CENTRILOBULAR NECROSIS

These hepatic manifestations of systemic circulatory compromise are considered together because they repre-

Figure 16-25   ■

Subcapsular hematoma dissecting under the Glisson capsule in a fatal case of eclampsia. (Courtesy of Brian D. Blackbourne, MD, Medical Examiner, San Diego, CA.)

sent a morphologic continuum. Both changes are commonly seen at autopsy, because there is an element of preterminal circulatory failure with virtually every death. Right-sided cardiac decompensation leads to passive congestion of the liver. The liver is slightly enlarged, tense, and cyanotic, with rounded edges. Microscopically, there is congestion of centrilobular sinusoids. With time, centrilobular hepatocytes become atrophic, resulting in markedly attenuated liver cell cords.

Left-sided cardiac failure or shock may lead to hepatic hypoperfusion and hypoxia. In this instance, hepatocytes in the central region of the lobule undergo ischemic necrosis. Centrilobular necrosis is visible macroscopically as slight depression of necrotic lobular centers. By microscopy there is a sharp demarcation of viable hepatocytes in the periportal region versus necrotic hepatocytes in the centrilobular region of the parenchyma. The combination of left-sided hypoperfusion and right-sided retrograde congestion acts synergistically to generate a distinctive lesion, centrilobular hemorrhagic necrosis (Fig. 16-26). The liver takes on a variegated mottled appearance, reflecting hemorrhage and necrosis in the centrilobular regions, known traditionally as the "nutmeg" liver (Fig. 16-27). An uncommon complication of sustained chronic severe congestive heart failure is so-called cardiac sclerosis. The pattern of liver fibrosis is distinctive, inasmuch as it is mostly centrilobular. The damage rarely fulfills the accepted criteria for the diagnosis of cirrhosis, but the historically sanctified term *cardiac cirrhosis* cannot easily be dislodged.

In most instances, the only clinical evidence of centrilobular necrosis is mild to moderate transient elevation

Figure 16-26 ■

Centrilobular hemorrhagic necrosis. The centrilobular region is suffused with red blood cells, and hepatocytes are not readily visible. Portal tracts and the periportal parenchyma are intact.

of serum aminotransferase levels. The parenchymal damage may be sufficient to induce mild to moderate jaundice.

PELIOSIS HEPATIS

Sinusoidal dilation occurs in any condition in which efflux of hepatic blood is impeded. Peliosis hepatis is a rare condition in which the dilation is primary. It is most commonly associated with exposure to anabolic steroids and, rarely, oral contraceptives and danazol. The pathogenesis is not known. Although clinical signs are generally absent even in advanced peliosis, potentially fatal intra-abdominal hemorrhage or hepatic failure may occur.

Figure 16-27 ■

Centrilobular hemorrhagic necrosis (nutmeg liver). The cut liver section, in which major blood vessels are visible, is notable for a variegated mottled red appearance, representing hemorrhage in the centrilobular regions of the parenchyma.

Peliotic lesions usually disappear after cessation of drug treatment.

Hepatic Vein Outflow Obstruction

HEPATIC VEIN THROMBOSIS (BUDD-CHIARI SYNDROME)

The Budd-Chiari syndrome was originally used to describe acute and usually fatal thrombotic occlusion of the hepatic veins. The definition has now been expanded to include subacute and chronic occlusive syndromes, characterized by hepatomegaly, weight gain, ascites, and abdominal pain. Hepatic vein thrombosis is associated with (in order of frequency) polycythemia vera or other myeloproliferative disorders, pregnancy, the postpartum state, the use of oral contraceptives, paroxysmal nocturnal hemoglobinuria, and intra-abdominal cancers, particularly hepatocellular carcinoma. All these conditions produce thrombotic tendencies or, in the case of liver cancers, sluggish blood flow. Some cases are caused by mechanical obstruction to blood outflow, as by a massive intrahepatic abscess or parasitic cyst, or by obstruction by thrombus or tumor of the inferior vena cava itself at the level of the hepatic veins. About 30% of cases are idiopathic.

MORPHOLOGY

With acutely developing thrombosis of the major hepatic veins or inferior vena cava, the liver is swollen, is red-purple, and has a tense capsule (Fig. 16-28). Microscopically, the affected hepatic parenchyma reveals severe centrilobular congestion and necrosis. Centrilobular fibrosis develops in instances in which the thrombosis is more slowly developing. The major veins may contain totally occlusive fresh thrombi, subtotal occlusion, or, in chronic cases, organized adherent thrombi.

Figure 16-28 ■

Budd-Chiari syndrome. Thrombosis of the major hepatic veins has caused extreme blood retention in the liver.

The mortality from untreated acute Budd-Chiari syndrome is high. Prompt surgical creation of a portosystemic venous shunt permits reverse flow through the portal vein and improves the prognosis considerably; direct dilation of caval obstruction may be possible during angiography. The chronic form of the syndrome is far less grave, and about half the patients are alive after 5 years.

VENO-OCCLUSIVE DISEASE

Originally described in Jamaican drinkers of pyrrolizidine alkaloid–containing bush tea, veno-occlusive disease now occurs primarily in the immediate weeks after bone marrow transplantation. The incidence may approach 25% in recipients of allogeneic marrow transplants, with mortality rates of over 30%. Small hepatic vein radicles are obliterated by varying amounts of subendothelial swelling and fine reticulated collagen. The presumed cause is toxic endothelial injury, as from chemotherapy and radiation therapy given before marrow transplantation. In acute disease, there is striking centrilobular congestion with hepatocellular necrosis. As the disease progresses, connective tissue is laid down in the lumen of the venule and centrilobular congestion is less evident.

TUMORS AND TUMOR-LIKE CONDITIONS

The liver and lungs share the dubious distinction of being the visceral organs most often involved in the metastatic spread of cancers. Indeed, *the most common hepatic neoplasms are metastatic carcinomas,* with colon, lung, and breast heading the list as sites of the primary tumor. The worldwide incidence of primary hepatic malignancies varies with the local prevalence of risk factors, particularly HBV infection.

Hepatic masses come to attention for a variety of reasons. They may generate epigastric fullness and discomfort or be detected by routine physical examination. Radiographic studies for other indications may pick up incidental liver masses. Important in the differential diagnosis of hepatic masses are (1) whether there is underlying liver disease, especially cirrhosis, in which there is a greater risk for primary hepatocellular carcinoma, and (2) whether the mass is solitary or multiple. Nonmalignant conditions are more likely to occur as single lesions in livers without preexistent disease, although some lesions (e.g., cysts) may be multiple.

Benign Tumors

The most common benign lesions are cavernous hemangiomas, identical to those occurring in other parts of the body (Chapter 10). These well-circumscribed lesions consist of endothelial cell–lined vascular channels and intervening stroma. They appear as discrete red-blue, soft nodules, usually less than 2 cm in diameter, often directly beneath the capsule. Their chief clinical significance is not to mistake them for metastatic tumors; blind percutaneous needle biopsy may incur severe intra-abdominal bleeding.

Solitary or multiple benign hepatocellular nodules may develop in the liver in the absence of cirrhosis. *Focal nodular hyperplasia* appears as a well-demarcated but poorly encapsulated nodule with a central fibrous scar, ranging up to many centimeters in diameter. It is believed to represent nodular regeneration in response to local vascular injury and is not a neoplasm per se. Focal nodular hyperplasia occurs most frequently in young to middle-aged adults and does not appear to pose a risk for malignancy.

LIVER CELL ADENOMA

This benign neoplasm of hepatocytes tends to occur in women of childbearing age who have used oral contraceptives, and it regresses on discontinuance of hormone use. These tumors may be pale, yellow-tan or bile-stained, well-demarcated nodules found anywhere in the hepatic substance but often beneath the capsule. They may reach 30 cm in diameter. Histologically, liver cell adenomas are composed of sheets and cords of cells that may resemble normal hepatocytes or have some variation in cell and nuclear size. Portal tracts are absent; instead, prominent arterial vessels and draining veins are distributed through the substance of the tumor. Liver cell adenomas are significant for two reasons: (1) when they present as an intrahepatic mass, they may be mistaken for the more ominous hepatocellular carcinoma; and (2) subcapsular adenomas are at risk for rupture, particularly during pregnancy (under estrogenic stimulation), causing life-threatening intra-abdominal hemorrhage. They harbor hepatocellular carcinoma only rarely.

Primary Carcinoma of the Liver

Primary carcinomas of the liver are relatively uncommon in North America and Western Europe (0.5% to 2% of all cancers) but represent 20% to 40% of cancers in many other countries. Most arise from hepatocytes and are termed *hepatocellular carcinoma (HCC).* Much less common are carcinomas of bile duct origin (cholangiocarcinomas) or tumors that are a mixture of the two cell types. Two rare forms are mentioned only: the hepatoblastoma, an aggressive hepatocellular tumor of childhood, and highly malignant angiosarcoma, which resembles those occurring elsewhere (Chapter 10). Primary liver angiosarcoma is of interest because of its association with exposure to vinyl chloride, arsenic, or Thorotrast, with latency periods of up to several decades.

Epidemiology. There are striking differences in the frequency of HCC in different nations of the world, linked strongly to the prevalence of HBV infection. Annual incidence rates of 3 to 7 cases per 100,000 population in North and South America, north and central Europe, and Australia compare with intermediate rates of up to 20 cases per 100,000 in countries bordering the Mediterranean. The highest frequencies are found in Taiwan, Mozambique, and southeast China, where annual incidence rates among males approach 150 per 100,000. A common feature of high-incidence areas is onset of the HBV carrier state in infancy, after vertical transmission from infected mothers. This chronic carrier state may confer a 200-fold increased risk for HCC by adulthood. In these regions, cirrhosis may be absent in up to half of HCC patients. In the Western world, where HBV carriers are not common, cirrhosis is present in 85% to 90% of cases of HCC, frequently arising from other chronic liver diseases.

There is a pronounced male preponderance of HCC throughout the world, on the order of 3:1 in low-incidence areas and up to 8:1 in high-incidence areas, related to the greater prevalence of HBV infection, alcoholism, and chronic liver disease among males. Within each area, blacks have attack rates approximately fourfold higher than whites. In high-incidence areas, HCC generally arises early in adult life (third to fifth decades), whereas in low-incidence areas it is most often encountered in the sixth and seventh decades.

Pathogenesis. Several factors relevant to the pathogenesis of HCC were discussed in Chapter 6. Only a few points deserve emphasis at this time.

Three major etiologic associations have been established: infection with HBV, chronic liver disease (especially including HCV and alcohol), and specific instances of hepatocarcinogens in food (primarily aflatoxins).

■ Many factors, including age, sex, chemicals, viruses, hormones, alcohol, and nutrition, interact in the development of HCC. For example, the disease most likely to give rise to HCC is, in fact, the extremely rare hereditary tyrosinemia, in which almost 40% of patients develop this tumor despite adequate dietary control.

■ The exact pathogenesis of HCC may vary between high-incidence, HBV-prevalent populations versus low-incidence Western populations, in which other chronic liver diseases such as alcoholism, HCV, and hereditary hemochromatosis are more common.

■ The development of cirrhosis appears to be an important, but not requisite, contributor to the emergence of HCC.

Extensive epidemiologic evidence links chronic HBV infection with liver cancer, and there is strong evidence implicating HCV infection. Molecular studies of HBV carcinogenesis reveal that the HBV genome does not contain any oncogenic sequences. Moreover, there is no selective site of integration of viral DNA into the host genome, precluding mutation or activation of a particular protooncogene. Rather, the following factors have been implicated:

■ Repeated cycles of cell death and regeneration, as occurs in chronic hepatitis from any cause, are important in the pathogenesis of liver cell cancers.

■ The accumulation of mutations during continuous cycles of cell division may eventually transform some hepatocytes. Genomic instability is more likely in the presence of integrated HBV DNA, giving rise to chromosomal aberrations such as deletions, translocations, and duplications.

■ Molecular analysis of tumor cells in HBV-infected individuals reveals that each case is clonal with respect to HBV DNA integration pattern, suggesting that viral integration precedes or accompanies a transforming event.

■ The HBV genome encodes a regulatory element, the HBV X-protein, that is a transacting transcriptional activator of many genes and is present in most tumors with integrated HBV DNA. It appears that in liver cells infected with HBV, the HBV X-protein disrupts normal growth control by activation of host cell protooncogenes and disruption of cell cycle control. It also exerts antiapoptotic effects.

■ As with human papillomaviruses, some (but not all) studies suggest that certain HBV proteins bind to and inactivate the tumor suppressor gene *TP53* (Chapter 6).

The association between hepatitis C infection and liver cancer is strong. Indeed, in many parts of the world, including Japan and Central Europe, chronic HCV infection is the greatest risk factor in the development of liver cancer. HCC in patients with hepatitis C occurs almost exclusively in the setting of cirrhosis.

In certain regions of the world, such as China and South Africa, where HBV is endemic, there is also high exposure to dietary aflatoxins derived from the fungus *Aspergillus flavus*. These highly carcinogenic toxins are found in "moldy" grains and peanuts. Animal studies reveal that aflatoxin can bind covalently with cellular DNA and cause mutations in protooncogenes or tumor suppressor genes, particularly *TP53*. However, carcinogenesis does not occur unless the liver is mitotically active, as is the case in chronic viral hepatitis with recurrent bouts of injury and regeneration.

None of the influences related to HCC has any bearing on the development of cholangiocarcinoma. The only recognized causal influences on this uncommon tumor are primary sclerosing cholangitis, chronic infection of the biliary tract by the liver fluke *Opisthorchis sinensis* and its close relatives, and previous exposure to Thorotrast (formerly used in radiography of the biliary tract). Most cholangiocarcinomas, however, arise without evidence of antecedent risk conditions.

MORPHOLOGY

Primary liver carcinomas, of which almost all are HCC, may appear grossly as (1) a **unifocal**, usually massive tumor (Fig. 16–29); (2) a **multifocal** malignancy, made of widely distributed nodules of variable size; or (3) a **diffusely infiltrative** cancer, permeating widely and sometimes involving the entire liver, blending imperceptibly into the cirrhotic liver background. Particularly in the latter two patterns, it may be difficult to distinguish regenerative nodules of cirrhotic liver from similar sized nodules of neoplasm. Discrete tumor masses are usually

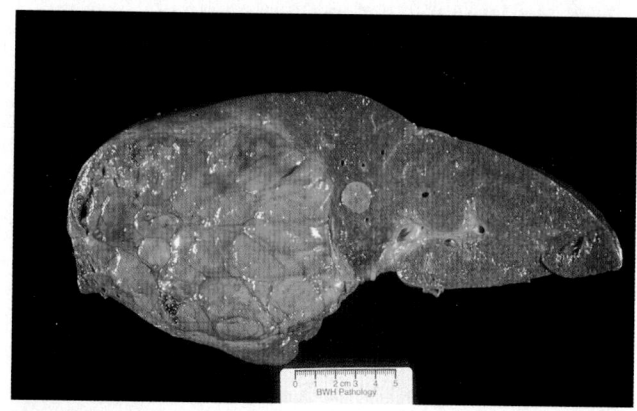

Figure 16-29   ■

Hepatocellular carcinoma, unifocal, massive type. A large neoplasm with extensive areas of necrosis has replaced most of the right hepatic lobe in this noncirrhotic liver. A satellite tumor nodule is directly adjacent.

yellow-white, punctuated sometimes by bile staining and areas of hemorrhage or necrosis. **All patterns of HCC have a strong propensity for invasion of vascular channels.** Extensive intrahepatic metastases ensue, and occasionally snakelike masses of tumor invade the portal vein (with occlusion of the portal circulation) or inferior vena cava, extending even into the right side of the heart.

Histologically, HCCs range from well-differentiated lesions that reproduce hepatocytes arranged in cords or small nests (Fig. 16-30) to poorly differentiated lesions, often made up of large multinucleate anaplastic tumor giant cells. **In the better-differentiated variants, globules of bile may be found within the cytoplasm of cells and in pseudocanaliculi between cells.** Acidophilic hyaline inclusions within the cytoplasm may be present, resembling Mallory bodies. There is surprisingly scant stroma in most HCCs, explaining the soft consistency of these tumors.

A distinctive clinicopathologic variant of HCC is the **fibrolamellar carcinoma,** which occurs in young male and female adults (20 to 40 years of age) with equal incidence, has no association with cirrhosis or other risk factors, and has a distinctly better prognosis. It usually consists of a single large, hard "scirrhous" tumor with fibrous bands coursing through it, vaguely resembling focal nodular hyperplasia. Histologically, it is composed of well-differentiated polygonal cells growing in nests or cords and separated by parallel lamellae of dense collagen bundles.

Cholangiocarcinomas appear as more or less well-differentiated adenocarcinomas, typically with an abundant fibrous stroma (desmoplasia) explaining their firm, gritty consistency. Most exhibit clearly defined glandular and tubular structures lined by somewhat anaplastic cuboidal-to-low columnar epithelial cells. **Bile pigment and hyaline inclusions are not found within the cells.**

HCC tends to remain confined to the liver until late in the course, at which time spread may occur to such extrahepatic sites as regional lymph nodes, lungs, bones, adrenal glands, and other sites. Cholangiocarcinoma has a greater propensity for extrahepatic spread to the same sites.

Clinical Features. Although primary carcinomas in the liver may present as silent hepatomegaly, they are often encountered in patients with cirrhosis of the liver who already have symptoms of the underlying disorder. In these patients, *rapid increase in liver size, sudden worsening of ascites, or the appearance of bloody ascites, fever, and pain call attention to the development of a tumor.* Laboratory studies are helpful but not diagnostic. Approximately 90% of patients have elevated serum levels of α-fetoprotein. Unfortunately, this tumor "marker" lacks specificity, because modestly elevated levels are also encountered in other conditions, such as cirrhosis, massive liver necrosis, chronic hepatitis, normal pregnancy, fetal distress or death, fetal neural tube defects such as anencephaly and spina bifida (Chapter 23), and gonadal germ cell tumors (Chapter 18). *Very high levels (above 1000 ng/mL), however, are rarely encountered except in HCC.*

The natural history of primary liver cancer (HCC and cholangiocarcinoma) is grim. The median survival is 7 months, with death from (1) profound cachexia, (2) gastrointestinal or esophageal variceal bleeding, (3) liver failure with hepatic coma, or (4) rarely, rupture of the tumor with fatal hemorrhage. The only hope for cure is surgical resection of smaller tumors, but even so there is a tumor recurrence rate of greater than 60% at 5 years. In the fortunate patient, incidental HCC is resected at the time of liver transplantation for end-stage liver disease, before it has spread beyond the organ. The best hope for controlling this dismal disease lies in comprehensive programs for immunizing high-risk world populations against HBV.

Figure 16-30   ■

Hepatocellular carcinoma. In this well-differentiated lesion, tumor cells are arranged in nests, sometimes with a central lumen, one of which contains bile *(arrow).* Other tumor cells contain intracellular bile pigment.

The Biliary Tract

Although disorders of the biliary tract do not garner the levels of attention given to other conditions, they are extremely common. Over 95% of biliary tract disease is directly attributable to cholelithiasis (gallstones) or the closely related cholecystitis (gallbladder inflammation). In the United States, the annual cost of managing cholelithiasis and its complications is $6 billion, representing 1% of the US health care budget and second only to gastroesophageal reflux disease in costs to US health care from gastrointestinal diseases.

DISORDERS OF THE GALLBLADDER

Cholelithiasis (Gallstones)

Gallstones afflict 10% of adult populations in northern hemisphere Western countries. Adult prevalence rates are higher in Latin American countries (20% to 40%) and are low in Asian countries (3% to 4%). Gallstones pose a significant health burden, as these US statistics indicate:

■ Over 20 million patients are estimated to have gallstones, totaling several tons.
■ About 1 million new patients annually are found to have gallstones, of whom two thirds undergo surgery.
■ Overall surgical mortality for biliary tract surgery is very low, but approximately 1000 patients die per year from gallstone disease or complications of surgery.

There are two main types of gallstones. In the West, about 80% are cholesterol stones, containing crystalline cholesterol monohydrate. The remainder are composed predominantly of bilirubin calcium salts and are designated pigment stones.

Pathogenesis and Risk Factors. Bile is the only significant pathway for elimination of excess cholesterol from the body, either as free cholesterol or as bile salts. Cholesterol is water insoluble and is rendered water soluble by aggregation with bile salts and lecithins cosecreted into bile. When cholesterol concentrations exceed the solubilizing capacity of bile (supersaturation), cholesterol can no longer remain dispersed and nucleates into solid cholesterol monohydrate crystals. Three conditions must therefore be met to permit the formation of cholesterol gallstones: (1) bile must be supersaturated with cholesterol, (2) nucleation must be kinetically favorable, and (3) cholesterol crystals must remain in the gallbladder long enough to aggregate into stones. Nucleation is promoted by microprecipitates of inorganic or organic calcium salts, serving as nucleation sites for cholesterol stones; a role for proteins in bile also has been proposed. Gallbladder stasis plays a key role in permitting stone formation and growth. As bile becomes more concentrated during storage in the gallbladder, cholesterol saturation of bile also may further increase.

Given the just-mentioned considerations, it is pertinent to examine the major risk factors for gallstones (Table 16–10). However, 80% of patients with gallstones have no identifying risk factors other than age and gender.

■ *Age and gender.* The prevalence of gallstones increases throughout life. In the United States, less than 5% to 6% of the population younger than age 40 has stones, in contrast to 25% to 30% of those older than 80. The prevalence in white women is about twice as high as in men.
■ *Ethnic and geographic.* Cholesterol gallstone prevalence approaches 75% in Native American populations—the Pima, Hopi, and Navajos—whereas pigment stones are rare; the prevalence appears related to biliary cholesterol hypersecretion. Gallstones are more prevalent in Western industrialized societies and uncommon in underdeveloped or developing societies.

■

Table 16–10. RISK FACTORS FOR GALLSTONES

Cholesterol Stones

Demography: Northern Europe, North and South America, Native Americans, Mexican Americans
Advancing age
Female sex hormones
   Female gender
   Oral contraceptives
   Pregnancy
Obesity
Rapid weight reduction
Gallbladder stasis
Inborn disorders of bile acid metabolism
Hyperlipidemia syndromes

Pigment Stones

Demography: Asian more than Western, rural more than urban
Chronic hemolytic syndromes
Biliary infection
Gastrointestinal disorders: ileal disease (e.g., Crohn disease), ileal resection or bypass, cystic fibrosis with pancreatic insufficiency

Figure 16–31 ■

Cholesterol gallstones. Mechanical manipulation during laparoscopic cholecystectomy has caused fragmentation of several cholesterol gallstones, revealing interiors that are pigmented because of entrapped bile pigments. The gallbladder mucosa is reddened and irregular as a result of coexistent acute and chronic cholecystitis.

- ■ *Environment.* Estrogenic influences, including oral contraceptives and pregnancy, increase hepatic cholesterol uptake and synthesis, leading to excess biliary secretion of cholesterol. Obesity, rapid weight loss, and treatment with the hypocholesterolemic agent clofibrate are also strongly associated with increased biliary cholesterol secretion.
- ■ *Acquired disorders.* Any condition in which gallbladder motility is reduced predisposes to gallstones, such as pregnancy, rapid weight loss, and spinal cord injury. In most cases, however, gallbladder hypomotility is present without obvious cause.
- ■ *Heredity.* In addition to ethnicity, family history alone imparts increased risk, as do a variety of inborn errors of metabolism such as those associated with impaired bile salt synthesis and secretion.

Although the interplay of risk factors for pigment stones is complex, it is clear that the presence of unconjugated bilirubin in the biliary tree increases the likelihood of pigment stone formation, as would occur in hemolytic anemias. Precipitation occurs primarily as insoluble calcium bilirubinate salts.

MORPHOLOGY

Cholesterol stones arise exclusively in the gallbladder and consist of 50% to 100% cholesterol. **Pure cholesterol stones** are pale yellow; increasing proportions of calcium carbonate, phosphates, and bilirubin impart gray-white to black discoloration (Fig. 16–31). They are ovoid and firm; they may be single but most often are multiple and have faceted surfaces, owing to apposition to one another. **Most cholesterol stones are radiolucent, although up to 20% may have sufficient calcium carbonate to render them radiopaque.**

Pigment stones may arise anywhere in the biliary tree and are trivially classified as black and as

brown. In general, black pigment stones are found in sterile gallbladder bile and brown stones are found in infected intrahepatic or extrahepatic ducts. The stones contain calcium salts of unconjugated bilirubin and lesser amounts of other calcium salts, mucin glycoproteins, and cholesterol. Black stones are usually small and present in great number (Fig. 16–32) and crumble easily. Brown stones tend to be single or few in number and are soft with a greasy, soaplike consistency, owing to the presence of retained fatty acid salts released by the action of bacterial phospholipases on biliary lecithins. Because of calcium carbonates and phosphates, **50% to 75% of black stones are radiopaque.** Brown stones, which contain calcium soaps, are radiolucent.

Clinical Features. Gallstones may be silent passengers for decades before symptoms develop. Indeed, 70% to 80% of patients remain asymptomatic throughout life, the remainder becoming symptomatic at the rate of 1% to 3% per year. The symptoms are striking: biliary pain tends to be excruciating, either constant or "colicky" (spasmodic) from an obstructed gallbladder or when small gallstones move downstream and lodge in the biliary tree. Inflammation of the gallbladder, in association with stones, also generates pain. More severe complications include empyema, perforation, fistulae, inflammation of the biliary tree, and obstructive cholestasis or pancreatitis. The larger the calculi, the less likely they are to enter the cystic or common ducts to produce obstruction—it is the very small stones, or "gravel," that are the more dangerous. Occasionally, a large stone may erode directly into an adjacent loop of small bowel, generating intestinal obstruction ("gallstone ileus").

Cholecystitis

Inflammation of the gallbladder may be acute, chronic, or acute superimposed on chronic and almost always occurs

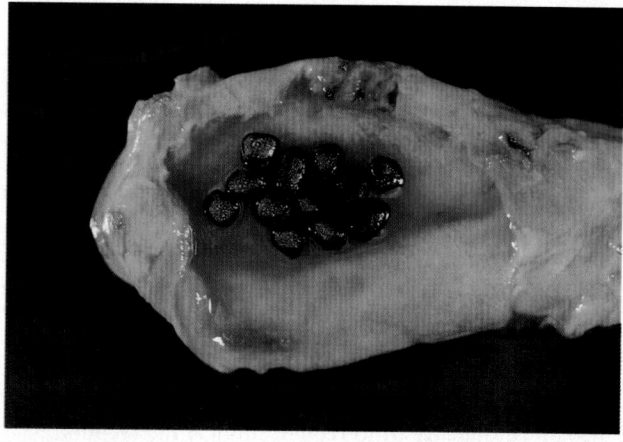

Figure 16–32 ■

Pigmented gallstones. Several faceted black gallstones are present in this otherwise unremarkable gallbladder from a patient with a mechanical mitral valve prosthesis, leading to chronic intravascular hemolysis.

in association with gallstones. In the United States, cholecystitis is one of the most common indications for abdominal surgery. Its epidemiologic distribution closely parallels that of gallstones.

MORPHOLOGY

In **acute cholecystitis,** the gallbladder is usually enlarged (twofold to threefold) and tense and assumes a bright red or blotchy, violaceous to green-black discoloration, imparted by subserosal hemorrhages. The serosal covering is frequently layered by fibrin and, in severe cases, by a suppurative exudate. In 90% of cases, stones are present, often obstructing the neck of the gallbladder or the cystic duct. The gallbladder lumen is filled with a cloudy or turbid bile that may contain fibrin, hemorrhage, and frank pus. When the contained exudate is virtually pure pus, the condition is referred to as **empyema of the gallbladder.** In mild cases, the gallbladder wall is thickened and edematous and hyperemic. In more severe cases the gallbladder is transformed into a green-black necrotic organ, termed **gangrenous cholecystitis.** Histologically, the inflammatory reactions are not distinctive and consist of the usual patterns of acute inflammation (i.e., edema, leukocytic infiltration, vascular congestion, frank abscess formation, or gangrenous necrosis).

The morphologic changes in **chronic cholecystitis** are extremely variable and sometimes minimal. The mere presence of stones within the gallbladder, even in the absence of acute inflammation, is often taken as sufficient justification for the diagnosis. The gallbladder may be contracted, of normal size, or enlarged. Mucosal ulcerations are infrequent; the submucosa and subserosa are often thickened from fibrosis. In the absence of superimposed acute cholecystitis, mural lymphocytes are the only sentinels of inflammation.

Clinical Features. Cholecystitis has many faces. Acute calculous cholecystitis may barely achieve notice or may announce itself loudly, with severe, steady upper abdominal pain often radiating to the right shoulder. Sometimes, when stones are present in the gallbladder neck or in ducts, the pain is colicky. Fever, nausea, leukocytosis, and prostration are classic; the presence of conjugated hyperbilirubinemia suggests obstruction of the common bile duct. The right subcostal region is markedly tender and rigid, owing to spasm of the abdominal muscles; occasionally a tender, distended gallbladder can be palpated. Mild attacks usually subside spontaneously over 1 to 10 days; however, recurrence is common. Approximately 25% of symptomatic patients are sufficiently ill to require surgical intervention.

In contrast, symptoms arising from acute acalculous cholecystitis (discussed next) are usually obscured by the generally severe clinical condition of the patient. Diagnosis therefore rests on keeping this possibility in mind.

Chronic cholecystitis does not have the striking manifestations of the acute forms and is usually characterized by recurrent attacks of either steady or colicky epigastric or right upper quadrant pain. Nausea, vomiting, and intolerance for fatty foods are frequent accompaniments.

The diagnosis of both acute and chronic cholecystitis usually rests on the detection of gallstones or dilatation of the bile ducts by ultrasonography, typically accompanied by evidence of a thickened gallbladder wall. Attention to this disorder is important, because of the following complications:

■ Bacterial superinfection with cholangitis or sepsis
■ Gallbladder perforation and local abscess formation
■ Gallbladder rupture with diffuse peritonitis
■ Biliary enteric (cholecystenteric) fistula, with drainage of bile into adjacent organs, entry of air and bacteria into the biliary tree, and potentially gallstone-induced intestinal obstruction (ileus)
■ Aggravation of preexisting medical illness, with cardiac, pulmonary, renal, or liver decompensation

ACUTE CALCULOUS CHOLECYSTITIS

Acute inflammation of a gallbladder that contains stones is termed *acute calculous cholecystitis* and is precipitated by obstruction of the gallbladder neck or cystic duct. It is the most common major complication of gallstones and the most common reason for emergency cholecystectomy. Symptoms may appear with remarkable suddenness and constitute an acute surgical emergency. On the other hand, symptoms may be mild and resolve without medical intervention.

Acute calculous cholecystitis is initially the result of chemical irritation and inflammation of the gallbladder wall in the setting of obstruction to bile outflow. The action of phospholipases derived from the mucosa hydrolyzes biliary lecithin to lysolecithin, which is toxic to the mucosa. The normally protective glycoprotein mucous layer is disrupted, exposing the mucosal epithelium to the direct detergent action of bile salts. Prostaglandins released within the wall of the distended gallbladder contribute to mucosal and mural inflammation. Distention and increased intraluminal pressure may also compromise blood flow to the mucosa. These events occur in the absence of bacterial infection; only later in the course may bacterial contamination develop.

ACUTE ACALCULOUS CHOLECYSTITIS

Between 5% and 12% of gallbladders removed for acute cholecystitis contain no gallstones. Most of these cases occur in seriously ill patients: (1) the postoperative state after major, nonbiliary surgery; (2) severe trauma (e.g., motor vehicle accidents); (3) severe burns; and (4) sepsis. Multiple events are thought to contribute to acalculous cholecystitis, including dehydration, gallbladder stasis and sludging, vascular compromise, and ultimately bacterial contamination.

CHRONIC CHOLECYSTITIS

Chronic cholecystitis may be the sequel to repeated bouts of acute cholecystitis, but in most instances it develops without any history of acute attacks. Like acute cholecystitis it is almost always associated with gallstones. However, gallstones do not seem to play a direct role in the initiation of inflammation or the development of pain, particularly because chronic acalculous cholecystitis exhibits symptomatology and histology similar to the calculus form. Rather, supersaturation of bile predisposes to both chronic inflammation and, in most instances, stone formation. Microorganisms, usually *Escherichia coli* and enterococci, can be cultured from the bile in only about one third of cases. Unlike acute calculous cholecystitis, stone obstruction of gallbladder outflow in chronic cholecystitis is not a requisite. Nevertheless, the symptoms of chronic cholecystitis are similar to those of the acute form and range from biliary colic to indolent right upper quadrant pain and epigastric distress. Because most gallbladders removed at elective surgery for gallstones exhibit features of chronic cholecystitis, one must conclude that biliary symptoms emerge after long-term coexistence of gallstones and low-grade inflammation.

DISORDERS OF EXTRAHEPATIC BILE DUCTS

Choledocholithiasis and Ascending Cholangitis

These conditions are considered together because they so frequently go hand in hand. *Choledocholithiasis* is the presence of stones within the biliary tree. In Western nations, almost all stones are derived from the gallbladder; in Asia, there is a much higher incidence of primary ductal and intrahepatic, usually pigmented, stone formation. Choledocholithiasis may not immediately obstruct major bile ducts; asymptomatic stones are found in about 10% of patients at the time of surgical cholecystectomy. Symptoms may develop owing to (1) biliary obstruction, (2) pancreatitis, (3) cholangitis, (4) hepatic abscess, (5) chronic liver disease with secondary biliary cirrhosis, or (6) acute calculous cholecystitis.

Cholangitis is the term used for acute inflammation of the wall of bile ducts, almost always caused by bacterial infection of the normally sterile lumen. It can result from any lesion obstructing bile flow, most commonly choledocholithiasis, and is a known complication of Roux-en-Y reconstruction of the biliary tree. Uncommon causes include tumors, indwelling stents or catheters, acute pancreatitis, and benign strictures. Bacteria most likely enter the biliary tract through the sphincter of Oddi, rather than by the hematogenous route. Ascending cholangitis refers to the fact that once bacteria are within the biliary tree they have a propensity to infect intrahepatic biliary radicals. The bacteria are usually enteric gram-negative aerobes such as *E. coli*, *Klebsiella*, *Clostridium*, *Bacteroides*, or *Enterobacter*; group D streptococci are also common, and two or more organisms are found in half of the cases. In some world populations, parasitic cholangitis is a significant problem: *Fasciola hepatica* or schistosomiasis in Latin America and the Near East, *Clonorchis sinensis* or *Opisthorchis viverrini* in the Far East, and cryptosporidiosis in patients with acquired immunodeficiency syndrome.

Bacterial cholangitis usually produces fever, chills, abdominal pain, and jaundice. The most severe form of cholangitis is suppurative cholangitis, in which purulent bile fills and distends bile ducts, with an attendant risk of liver abscess formation. Because sepsis rather than cholestasis is the dominant risk in cholangitic patients, prompt diagnosis and intervention are imperative.

Biliary Atresia

The infant presenting with neonatal cholestasis was discussed previously in the context of neonatal hepatitis. A major contributor to neonatal cholestasis is biliary atresia, accounting for one third of infants with neonatal cholestasis and occurring in approximately 1 in 10,000 live births. Biliary atresia *is defined as a complete obstruction of bile flow caused by destruction or absence of all or part of the extrahepatic bile ducts.* It is not a true atresia but rather is an acquired inflammatory disorder of unknown cause. It is the single most frequent cause of death from liver disease in early childhood and accounts for over half of the children referred for liver transplantation.

The salient features of biliary atresia include (1) inflammation and fibrosing stricture of the hepatic or common bile ducts; (2) inflammation of major intrahepatic bile ducts, with progressive destruction of the intrahepatic biliary tree; (3) florid features of biliary obstruction on liver biopsy (i.e., marked bile ductular proliferation, portal tract edema and fibrosis, and parenchymal cholestasis); and (4) periportal fibrosis and cirrhosis within 3 to 6 months of birth.

Clinical Course. Infants with biliary atresia present with neonatal cholestasis, as discussed earlier. They have normal birth weights and postnatal weight gain, a slight female preponderance, and the progression of initially normal stools to acholic stools as the disease evolves. Laboratory findings do not distinguish between biliary atresia and intrahepatic cholestasis, but a liver biopsy provides evidence of bile duct obstruction in 90% of cases of biliary atresia. Liver transplantation remains the definitive treatment. Without surgical intervention, death usually occurs within 2 years of birth.

TUMORS

Carcinoma of the Gallbladder

Among cancers of the extrahepatic biliary tract, carcinoma of the gallbladder is much more prevalent than cancer arising in the ducts (2 to 4:1). It is the fifth most common cancer of the digestive tract, is slightly more common in women, and occurs most frequently in the seventh decade of life. Only rarely is it discovered at a resectable stage, and the mean 5-year survival has remained a dismal 1% for many years. Gallstones are present in 60% to 90% of cases. However, in Asia, where pyogenic and parasitic diseases of the biliary tree are more common, gallstones are less important. Presumably, gallbladders containing stones or infectious agents develop cancer as a result of recurrent trauma and chronic inflammation. The role of carcinogenic derivatives of bile acids is unclear.

Figure 16–34 ■

Gallbladder adenocarcinoma. Malignant glandular structures are present within the gallbladder wall, which is fibrotic.

Clinical Features. Preoperative diagnosis of carcinoma of the gallbladder is the exception, occurring in less than 20% of patients. Presenting symptoms are insidious and typically indistinguishable from those associated with cholelithiasis: abdominal pain, jaundice, anorexia, and nausea and vomiting. The fortunate patient develops early obstruction and acute cholecystitis before extension of the tumor into adjacent structures or undergoes cholecystectomy for coexistent symptomatic gallstones. Preoperative diagnosis rests largely on detection of gallstones along with abnormalities in the gallbladder wall documented by imaging studies.

Carcinoma of the Extrahepatic Bile Ducts, Including Ampulla of Vater

Carcinomas of the intrahepatic bile ducts (cholangiocarcinomas) present very much like hepatocellular carcinoma and were discussed previously. In contrast, cancers arising in the extrahepatic ducts, while still called cholangiocarcinomas, are extremely insidious and generally produce painless, progressively deepening jaundice. They also occur in older individuals and, unlike cancers of the gallbladder, occur slightly more frequently in men. Attempts to relate gallstones to the genesis of these tumors have been unconvincing; gallstones are present in only about a third of cases. As with intrahepatic cholangiocarcinomas, populations at risk are those with fluke infections or preexisting primary sclerosing cholangitis or inflammatory bowel disease.

Clinical Features. Symptoms arising from these neoplasms (jaundice, decolorization of the stools, nausea and vomiting, and weight loss) are generally the result of obstruction. Hepatomegaly is present in about 50% and a palpable, distended gallbladder in about 25%. Associated changes are elevated levels of serum alkaline phosphatase and aminotransferases, bile-stained urine, and prolonged prothrombin time.

Figure 16–33 ■

Gallbladder adenocarcinoma. The opened gallbladder contains a large, exophytic tumor that virtually fills the lumen.

Differentiation of obstructive jaundice caused by benign conditions such as stone disease from neoplasia is a major clinical problem, particularly because the presence of stones does not preclude the existence of concomitant malignancy. Despite their small size, most ductal cancers are not surgically resectable at the time of diagnosis. Mean survival times range from 6 to 18 months, regardless of whether aggressive resections or palliative surgery are performed.

Two subgroups of biliary tree carcinomas merit separate mention. First, carcinomas arising at the bifurcation of the right and left hepatic ducts are called Klatskin tumors. Despite their strategic location, over half of these tumors are still inoperable at the time of diagnosis. Second, common bile duct carcinomas arising immediately upstream to the ampulla of Vater are difficult to distinguish clinically from carcinoma in the head of the pancreas (Chapter 17). Both are treated by surgical resection via the Whipple procedure.

BIBLIOGRAPHY

Albrecht J: Hepatic encephalopathy: molecular mechanisms underlying the clinical syndrome. J Neurol Sci 170:138, 1999. (A brief review.)

Apstein MD, Carey MC: Cholesterol gallstones: a parsimonious hypothesis. Eur J Clin Invest 26:343, 1996. (A definitive discussion of cholesterol gallstone pathogenesis.)

Bloor JH, et al: Alcoholic liver disease: new concepts of pathogenesis and treatment. Adv Intern Med 39:49, 1994. (An excellent review of alcoholic liver disease.)

Dufour DR, et al: Diagnosis and monitoring of hepatic injury: II. Recommendations for use of laboratory tests in screening, diagnosis, and monitoring. Clin Chem 46:12, 2000. (A discussion of liver function tests.)

Feder JN, et al: A novel MHC class I–like gene is mutated in patients with hereditary hemochromatosis. Nat Genet 13:399, 1996. (The discovery of the gene that is mutated in genetic hemochromatosis.)

Feitelson MA: Hepatitis B virus in hepatocarcinogenesis. J Cell Physiol 181:188, 1999. (A thorough discussion of the molecular pathobiology of hepatitis B–infected hepatocytes.)

Ferrell L: Liver pathology: cirrhosis, hepatitis, and primary liver tumors: update and diagnostic problems. Mod Pathol 13:679, 2000. (An excellent guide to pathologic evaluation of liver disease.)

Friedman SL: Molecular regulation of hepatic fibrosis, an integrated cellular response to tissue injury. J Biol Chem 275:2247, 2000. (A concise discussion of liver fibrogenesis.)

Gershwin ME, et al: Primary biliary cirrhosis: an orchestrated immune response against epithelial cells. Immunol Rev 174:210–225, 2000. (A thorough discussion of potential mechanisms for autoimmune destruction of the biliary tree.)

Ishak KG: Pathologic features of chronic hepatitis: a review and update. Am J Clin Pathol 113:40, 2000. (A statement of current concepts and terminology for chronic hepatitis, in what has been a changing field.)

Jones RS: Carcinoma of the gallbladder. Surg Clin North Am 70:1419, 1990. (A brief overview of pathogenesis, histology, diagnosis, treatment, and prognosis.)

Kaplan MM: Primary biliary cirrhosis. N Engl J Med 335:1570, 1996. (An excellent review that covers etiology, morphology, clinical features, and treatment.)

Kleinman S: Hepatitis G virus biology, epidemiology, and clinical manifestations: Implications for blood safety. Transfus Med Rev 15:201, 2001. (An important review of this intriguing virus.)

Lauer GM, Walker BD: Hepatitis C virus infection. N Engl J Med 345:41, 2001. (A current review of hepatitis C.)

Luyckx FH, Lefebvre PJ, Scheen AJ: Non-alcoholic steatohepatitis: association with obesity and insulin resistance, and influence of weight loss. Diabetes Metab 26:98, 2000. (Discussion of relationship of NASH to clinical management.)

Mousseau DD, Butterworth RF: Current theories on the pathogenesis of hepatic encephalopathy. Proc Soc Exp Biol Med 206:329, 1994. (A critical discussion of the causal roles of ammonia and altered neurotransmitters.)

Rapaport AM: The structural and functional units of the human liver (liver acinus). Microvasc Res 6:212, 1973. (Describes the functional anatomy of the microcirculatory unit of the liver: the lobule.)

Saxena R, et al: Microanatomy of the human liver: exploring the hidden interfaces. Hepatology 30:1339, 1999. (A discussion of the connections of the intrahepatic biliary tree to the hepatocellular parenchyma.)

Stal P: Iron as a hepatotoxin. Dig Dis 13:205, 1995. (A review that is particularly relevant to hereditary hemochromatosis.)

Taylor MB, et al: The occurrence of hepatitis A and astroviruses in selected river and dam waters in South Africa. Water Res 35:2653, 2001. (A sobering look at water purification issues.)

Tilg H, Diehl AM: Cytokines in alcoholic and nonalcoholic steatohepatitis. N Engl J Med 343:1467, 2000. (An excellent discussion of the role of TNF-α in alcoholic liver disease.)

17

The Pancreas

MICHAEL J. CLARE-SALZLER, MD
JAMES M. CRAWFORD, MD, PhD
VINAY KUMAR, MD

The pancreas is in reality two organs in one. Approximately 85% to 90% of the pancreas is an exocrine gland that secretes enzymes necessary for the digestion of food. The remaining 10% to 15% of the pancreatic substance is endocrine, consisting of the islets of Langerhans, which secrete insulin, glucagon, and a variety of other hormones. The most significant disorders of the exocrine pancreas are cystic fibrosis (Chapter 7), acute and chronic pancreatitis, and carcinoma. From the standpoints of both morbidity and mortality, diabetes mellitus (a disorder of the endocrine pancreas) overshadows all other pancreatic disorders.

EXOCRINE PANCREAS

The disorders of the exocrine pancreas are relatively uncommon in clinical practice but can be life-threatening, and therefore their recognition requires a high degree of suspicion. Only the three most common conditions are discussed. *Acute pancreatitis* may be subclinical or may produce a calamitous acute abdomen leading to death within a few days. *Chronic pancreatitis* is a cause of less severe abdominal pain, which, along with the attendant malabsorption, can be

Figure 17-1 ■

Acute pancreatitis. The microscopic field shows an advancing region of fat necrosis *(upper left)*, impinging upon preserved adipose tissue *(lower left)* and with accompanying local hemorrhage *(right)*.

disabling. *Carcinoma of the pancreas* is a silent disease that comes to attention usually only after it is advanced and beyond ready cure.

Pancreatitis

ACUTE PANCREATITIS

Inflammation of the pancreas, almost always associated with acinar cell injury, is termed pancreatitis. Clinically and histologically, pancreatitis occurs along a spectrum, both in duration and in severity. Acute pancreatitis is characterized by the acute onset of abdominal pain resulting from enzymatic necrosis and inflammation of the pancreas. Typically, there is an elevation of pancreatic enzymes in blood and urine. The release of pancreatic lipases causes fat necrosis in and about the pancreas; in the most severe form, there is damage to the vasculature with resulting hemorrhage into the parenchyma of this organ *(acute hemorrhagic pancreatitis)*. Although by no means common, severe acute pancreatitis can be a life-threatening illness that demands quick diagnosis and prompt treatment.

MORPHOLOGY

The morphology of acute pancreatitis stems directly from the actions of activated pancreatic enzymes that are released into the pancreatic substance. The four basic alterations are **(1) proteolytic destruction of pancreatic substance, (2) necrosis of blood vessels with subsequent interstitial hemorrhage, (3) necrosis of fat by lipolytic enzymes, and (4) an associated acute inflammatory reaction.** The extent and predominance of each of these alterations depend on the duration and severity of the process.

The most characteristic histologic lesions of acute pancreatitis are the focal areas of fat necrosis (Chapter 1) that occur in the stromal and peripancreatic fat and in fat deposits throughout the abdominal cavity (Fig. 17-1). These lesions result from enzymatic destruction of fat cells; the vacuolated fat cells are transformed to shadowy outlines of cell membranes filled with pink, granular, opaque precipitate. This granular material is derived from the hydrolysis of fat. The liberated glycerol is reabsorbed, and the released fatty acids combine with calcium to form insoluble salts that precipitate in situ. These deposits are evident as flocculent calcifications in abdominal radiographs, and they stain basophilic in routinely stained histologic sections.

The gross appearance of the most severe form of acute pancreatitis, **acute hemorrhagic pancreatitis,** is characterized by areas of blue-black hemorrhage interspersed with areas of gray-white necrotic softening, sprinkled with foci of yellow-white, chalky fat necrosis (Fig. 17-2). Foci of fat necrosis may also be found in intra-abdominal fat depots, such as the omentum and the mesentery of the bowel, and even outside the abdominal cavity, such as in the subcutis. In addition, in most cases the peritoneal cavity contains a serous, slightly turbid, brown-tinged fluid in which globules of fat (derived from the action of enzymes on adipose tissue) can be identified. With time, this fluid may become secondarily infected to produce suppurative peritonitis.

A common sequela of acute pancreatitis is a **pancreatic pseudocyst**. Liquefied areas of necrotic pancreatic tissue are walled off by fibrous tissue to form a cystic space, which does not contain an epithelial lining. Drainage of pancreatic secretions into this space (from damaged pancreatic ducts) may lead to massive enlargement of the cyst over months to years.

Figure 17-2 ■

Acute pancreatitis. The pancreas has been sectioned across to reveal dark areas of hemorrhage in the pancreatic substance and a focal area of pale fat necrosis in the peripancreatic fat *(upper left)*.

Table 17-1. ETIOLOGIC FACTORS IN ACUTE PANCREATITIS

Metabolic

Alcohol
Hyperlipoproteinemia
Hypercalcemia
Drugs (e.g., thiazide diuretics)
Genetic

Mechanical

Gallstones
Traumatic injury
Perioperative injury

Vascular

Shock
Atheroembolism
Polyarteritis nodosa

Infectious

Mumps
Coxsackievirus
Mycoplasma pneumoniae

Etiology and Pathogenesis. A variety of predisposing conditions for acute pancreatitis have been identified and can be grouped into four major categories (Table 17-1). Most common are gallstones and alcoholism, which together are responsible for approximately 80% of the cases. The remaining specific causes are unusual, and 10% to 20% of cases of acute pancreatitis are without apparent predisposing influences.

The anatomic changes of acute pancreatitis reflect two fundamental events: autodigestion of the pancreatic substance by inappropriately activated pancreatic enzymes, and a cellular injury response mediated by proinflammatory cytokines. The pancreas is normally protected from autodigestion by synthesis of pancreatic enzymes in the acinar cell in the proenzyme form, and by confinement of these proenzymes to membrane-bound compartments (zymogen granules) within the acinar cell before secretion. Upon stimulation of secretion, the zymogen granules release their proenzyme contents into the apical lumen for delivery via the pancreatic duct to the duodenal lumen. The proenzymes are then activated to enzymes for fulfillment of their enzymatic potential. Among many possible activators, *a major role is attributed to trypsin, which itself is synthesized in acinar cells as the proenzyme trypsinogen.* Once trypsin is formed, it activates other proenzymes such as prophospholipase and proelastase.

In acute pancreatitis, *proenzymes are activated and escape from the zymogen granule within the acinar cell.* The activated enzymes cause disintegration of acinar cells and fatty tissue in and around the pancreas, damaging the elastic fibers of blood vessels and leading to vascular leakage. Activated trypsin also converts prekallikrein to its activated form, thus bringing into play the kinin system and, by activation of Hageman factor, the clotting and complement systems as well. In this way, the small-vessel thrombosis (which may lead to congestion and rupture of already-weakened vessels) is amplified. *The other result of premature enzyme activation is the acinar cell injury response.* Damaged acinar cells release potent cytokines that attract neutrophils and macrophages. These inflammatory cells then release more cytokines such as tumor necrosis factor, interleukin 1, nitric oxide, and platelet-activating factor into the pancreatic tissue and circulation, thereby amplifying the local and systemic inflammatory response.

The key initiating step appears to be premature enzyme (especially trypsinogen) activation and retention within the acinar cell. The mechanisms by which trypsinogen is inappropriately activated are not entirely clear. Two possibilities are being explored: autoactivation within the zymogen granules, and activation by cathepsin B in the lysosomes. Autoactivation is favored by low pH and an increase in intracellular calcium, but how these changes in the intracellular milieu occur is not yet known. Activation by cathepsin B assumes that zymogen granules containing trypsinogen are inappropriately targeted to lysosomes (known to contain cathepsin B) within the acinar cells. Such mishandled traffic of trypsinogen would cause it to be activated inside the cells rather than in the lumen of the duodenum (see earlier). It is not known which of these two pathways of intra-acinar activation of trypsinogen is the predominant one. However, the central role of trypsinogen activation in acute pancreatitis is supported by recent studies into the molecular basis of a rare form of hereditary pancreatitis. In this autosomal dominant disorder, mutations in the trypsinogen gene prevent the inactivation of trypsin, thus allowing this enzyme to initiate the cascade that causes autodigestion of pancreas.

Acute pancreatitis occurs in two primary settings: pancreatic duct obstruction (e.g., by gallstones or by the intrapancreatic stones that develop in alcoholism) and direct injury to acinar cells (Fig. 17-3). *Pancreatic duct obstruction,* especially, is considered important in the pathogenesis of acute pancreatitis associated with gallstones. The common bile duct is joined by the main pancreatic duct in 70% of normal persons. Obstruction of the common outflow channel, usually by a stone impacted in the ampulla of Vater, raises the intrapancreatic ductal pressure. In 75% to 80% of patients with cholelithiasis and pancreatitis, gallstones can be found in the ampulla or in the stools. The degree of pancreatic injury appears to be proportional to the duration of ampullary obstruction by an impacted gallstone. However, reflux of bile into the pancreas does not appear to occur, nor do duodenal juices appear to enter the pancreas through a dilated ampulla after passage of a stone. Rather, mechanical obstruction of the distal biliary tree alone appears to be sufficient to produce injury. First, obstruction causes interstitial edema, which is exacerbated by the stimulation of pancreatic secretions that occurs when the bile duct is obstructed. It is proposed that edema in turn causes impaired blood flow within the pancreatic substance, leading to ischemic injury of acinar cells. The specific mechanism by which these events prematurely activate acinar proenzymes is not clear. *Primary acinar cell injury* is most clearly involved in the pathogenesis of acute pancreatitis caused by certain viruses (e.g., mumps) and drugs and after trauma.

As mentioned previously, *alcoholism* is a strong predisposing factor for acute pancreatitis; however, the manner by which alcohol precipitates pancreatitis is not known. In

Figure 17-3 ■

Proposed pathogenesis of acute pancreatitis.

some experimental models, alcohol sensitizes acinar cells to injury by other agents. Transient increases in pancreatic exocrine secretion, contraction of the sphincter of Oddi, and direct toxic effects on acinar cells have all been postulated as well. Many authorities now think that most cases of alcoholic pancreatitis are sudden exacerbations of chronic disease presenting as de novo acute pancreatitis. According to this view, chronic alcohol ingestion causes secretion of protein-rich pancreatic fluid, leading to deposition of inspissated protein plugs and obstruction of small pancreatic ducts, followed by the train of events described previously.

Clinical Features. *Abdominal pain* is the cardinal manifestation of acute pancreatitis. Its severity varies with the extent of pancreatic injury. It may be mild and tolerable, or severe and incapacitating. *Localization in the epigastrium with radiation to the back is characteristic.* Patients with extensive pancreatic necrosis and hemorrhage present with a medical emergency that must be differentiated from other causes of acute abdomen such as perforated peptic ulcer, acute cholecystitis, and infarction of the bowel. *Shock*, a common feature of acute pancreatitis, is caused not only by pancreatic hemorrhage but also by release of vasodilatory agents such as bradykinin and prostaglandins. An elevated serum level of amylase is a very important diagnostic finding. The amylase level rises within the first 12 hours and then often falls to normal within 48 to 72 hours. Although elevations of this enzyme may be produced by a variety of other diseases, including perforated peptic ulcer, carcinoma of the pancreas, intestinal obstruction, peritonitis, and indeed any disease that secondarily impinges on the pancreas, most of these conditions are associated with elevations of lesser degree than those seen with acute pancreatitis. Serum lipase levels are also increased and remain elevated after serum amylase levels have returned to normal (7 to 10 days). *Used together, the serum amylase and lipase levels are highly sensitive and specific for acute pancreatitis.* Direct visualization of the enlarged, inflamed pancreas by high-resolution computed tomography (CT) is useful in the diagnosis of pancreatitis and its complications (e.g., pseudocysts). Hypocalcemia often develops, presumably because calcium is depleted as it binds with fatty acids released from hydrolyzed fat in the abdomen. Jaundice, hyperglycemia, and glycosuria appear in fewer than half the patients.

The mortality rate with severe acute pancreatitis is high, about 20% to 40%. Death is usually caused by shock, secondary abdominal sepsis, or the acute respiratory distress syndrome. Patients who recover must be evaluated for gallstones; if these are present, cholecystectomy is indicated to prevent future acute attacks.

CHRONIC PANCREATITIS

Chronic pancreatitis is characterized by repeated bouts of mild to moderate pancreatic inflammation, with continued loss of pancreatic parenchyma and replacement by fibrous tissue. The chief distinction between acute and chronic pancreatitis is whether the pancreas is normal before a symptomatic attack or is already chronically damaged; this distinction may be impossible to apply in clinical settings. The disease is protean in its manifestations and most frequently affects middle-aged men, particularly those who are alcoholic. Biliary tract disease plays a less important role in chronic pancreatitis than in the acute form of the disease, but hypercalcemia and hyperlipoproteinemia predispose to chronic pancreatitis. Almost half of the patients have no apparent predisposing influences and are therefore said to have idiopathic pancreatitis.

The pathogenesis of chronic pancreatitis is obscure, and the distinction between the pathogenesis of acute and chronic pancreatitis remains blurred. Hypersecretion of protein from acinar cells in the absence of increased fluid secretion permits the precipitation of proteins that, when admixed with cellular debris, form ductal plugs. Such plugs are observed in all forms of chronic pancreatitis, but in alcoholic patients, these plugs may enlarge to form laminar aggregates (stones) containing calcium carbonate precipitates. One proposal suggests that in alcoholic persons there is decreased secretion of an acinar protein that normally inhibits precipitation of calcium. With reduced concentrations of this so-called lithostatin, calcification is favored, thus exacerbating small duct obstruction and atrophy of the draining pancreatic lobules. Acute pancreatitis itself initiates a sequence of perilobular fibrosis, duct distortion, and altered pancreatic secretion and ductal flow, predisposing to a chronic "necrosis-fibrosis" disorder. Lastly, protein-calorie malnutrition appears to play a role in the tropical pancreatitis of Southeast Asia and parts of Africa, where alcohol consumption is extremely low.

Recent studies have revealed that approximately one third of patients with idiopathic chronic pancreatitis have mutations in the cystic fibrosis transmembrane conductance regulator *(CFTR)* gene. As is well known, mutations in the *CFTR* gene give rise to cystic fibrosis, typically associated with pancreatic atrophy. The *CFTR* gene mediates the secretion of bicarbonate-rich alkaline pancreatic juice. With impairment of *CFTR* function, there are reduced intraluminal fluid and bicarbonate levels and lower-than-normal pH. These conditions reduce the solubility of secreted proteins and thus give rise to thickened and viscous secretions that tend to obstruct the ducts. It is interesting to note that *in patients with idiopathic chronic pancreatitis associated with CFTR mutations, other clinical features of cystic fibrosis are typically absent and the sweat chloride level is normal.* The mutations of the *CFTR* gene in such patients are distinct from those associated with cystic fibrosis. In cystic fibrosis, the secretory defects in the pancreatic ducts are much more severe, giving rise to pancreatic atrophy early in the course of the disease, rather than to chronic pancreatitis. The association between *CFTR* mutations and chronic pancreatitis highlights the heterogeneity of the clinical manifestations resulting from *CFTR* dysfunctions. Increasingly, single-organ diseases such as pancreatitis or obstructive azoospermia are being recognized in patients with specific *CFTR* mutations.

MORPHOLOGY

In chronic pancreatitis, the pancreas is transformed into a densely fibrotic organ with extensive atrophy of the exocrine glands (Fig. 17-4), sometimes with remarkable sparing of the islets. A chronic inflammatory infiltrate around lobules and ducts is usually present, and there is variable obstruction of pancreatic ducts of all sizes by protein plugs. Grossly, the gland is hard, sometimes with extremely dilated ducts and visible calcified concretions. Pseudocysts similar to those described in acute pancreatitis may be present, either internal or external to the pancreatic substance.

Clinical Features. Chronic pancreatitis has many faces. It may present as repeated attacks of moderately severe abdominal pain, as recurrent attacks of mild pain, or as persistent abdominal and back pain. Yet again, the local disease may be entirely silent until pancreatic insufficiency and diabetes develop, the latter from associated destruction of islets. In still other instances, recurrent attacks of jaundice or vague attacks of indigestion may hint at pancreatic disease.

The diagnosis of chronic pancreatitis requires a high degree of suspicion. During an attack of abdominal pain, there may be mild elevations of serum amylase and serum lipase levels; after the disease has been present for a long time, the destruction of acinar cells may preclude such diagnostic clues. A very helpful finding is visualization of calcifications within the pancreas by x-rays, CT, and ultrasonography and by identification of pseudocyst formation. Other, more sophisticated techniques attempt to

Figure 17-4 ■

Chronic pancreatitis. The exocrine pancreas has been replaced by fibrous tissue; ectatic intermediate-sized ducts and a small residuum of acinar tissue *(arrowhead)* remain.

demonstrate inadequate pancreatic enzyme responses to such stimulants as secretin and cholecystokinin. *CFTR* mutations may be detected in idiopathic cases. The condition is more disabling than life-threatening. Severe pancreatic exocrine insufficiency and chronic malabsorption can develop, as can diabetes mellitus. Severe chronic pain may become the dominant problem.

Carcinoma of the Pancreas

The term *carcinoma of the pancreas* is meant to imply carcinoma arising in the exocrine portion of the gland. (The much less common islet tumors are discussed later.) Carcinoma of the pancreas is now the fifth most frequent cause of death from cancer in the United States, preceded only by lung, colon, breast, and prostate cancers. Its incidence has remained unchanged over 50 years. Currently, 28,000 new patients are identified every year, of whom less than 5% are expected to survive 5 years. These figures are even more distressing when one considers that there are few clues as to the cause of pancreatic cancer. One consistent association has been noted: the incidence rates are several times higher in smokers than in nonsmokers. There is no convincing evidence that alcohol consumption or coffee drinking is associated with pancreatic cancer. The peak incidence occurs in persons between 60 and 80 years of age. The rare hereditary pancreatitis itself carries a risk for pancreatic carcinoma 40-fold greater than that of the general population.

As with other cancers, carcinomas of the pancreas show multiple mutations in cancer-associated genes. Most common are mutations in the *K-RAS* (formerly K-*ras*) gene and in the tumor suppressor gene *CDKN2A* (formerly *p16*), both noted in 90% of cases. Indeed, the combination of *CDKN2A* and *K-RAS* mutations is not common among other tumors and is believed to be the "molecular fingerprint" of pancreatic cancers. As usual, the *TP53* (formerly *p53*) gene is also mutated in more than half of cases. Another tumor suppressor gene, called *deleted in pancreatic cancer 4 (DPC4)*, is lost in 50% of cases. *DPC4* encodes transcription factors that regulate transforming growth factor β–mediated growth control events. The *ERBB2 (HER2/NEU)* gene, well known for its amplification in breast cancers, is also amplified in more than half of pancreatic cancers. Mutations in genes affecting DNA repair, such as *BRCA2* and *MLH1*, are noted in a smaller number of cases.

Figure 17–5 ■

Carcinoma of the pancreas. A cross-section through the head of the pancreas and adjacent common bile duct shows both an ill-defined tumorous mass in the pancreatic substance *(arrowheads)* and the green discoloration of the duct resulting from total obstruction of bile flow.

fore appear as gritty, gray-white, hard masses. In its early stages, the tumor infiltrates locally and eventually extends into adjacent structures.

With carcinoma of the head of the pancreas, the ampullary region is invaded, obstructing the outflow of bile (Fig. 17–5). Ulceration of the tumor into the duodenal mucosa may also occur. As a consequence of common bile duct obstruction, there is marked distention of the biliary tree in about half of the patients with carcinoma of the head of the pancreas. In marked contrast, **carcinomas of the body and tail of the pancreas do not impinge on the biliary tract and hence remain silent for some time. They may be quite large and widely disseminated by the time they are discovered.** They extend through the retroperitoneal spaces, infiltrate adjacent nerves, and occasionally invade the spleen, adrenals, vertebral column, transverse colon, and stomach. Peripancreatic, gastric, mesenteric, omental, and portohepatic nodes are frequently involved, and the liver is often enlarged owing to metastatic deposits. Distant metastases occur, principally to the lungs and bones.

Microscopically, there is no difference between carcinomas of the head of the pancreas and those of the body and tail of the pancreas. Most grow in more or less glandular patterns (Fig. 17–6); they may be either mucinous or non-mucin secreting. In many cases, the glands are atypical, irregular, and small, and they are lined by anaplastic cuboidal to columnar epithelial cells. Other variants grow in a totally undifferentiated pattern. Perineural or intraneural invasion almost always is present in tumors that have extended into adjacent pancreatic tissues.

MORPHOLOGY

Approximately 60% to 70% of the cancers of this organ arise in the head of the pancreas, 5% to 10% in the body, and 10% to 15% in the tail; in 20%, the tumor diffusely involves the entire gland. Virtually all of these lesions are adenocarcinomas arising from the ductal epithelium. Some may secrete mucin, and many have an abundant fibrous stroma. These desmoplastic lesions there-

Figure 17-6   ■

Carcinoma of the pancreas. Poorly formed glands are present in densely fibrotic stroma within the pancreatic substance; some inflammatory cells are present.

Clinical Features. From the preceding discussion, it should be evident that carcinomas in the pancreas usually remain silent until their extension impinges on some other structure. It is when they erode into posterior soft tissues and affect nerve fibers that pain appears. There has long been a prevalent misconception that carcinoma of the pancreas is a painless disease. Many large series have clearly documented that *pain is usually the first symptom,* although by the time pain appears these cancers are usually beyond cure. *Obstructive jaundice* is associated with most cases of carcinoma of the head of the pancreas but rarely draws attention to the invasive cancer soon enough. Spontaneously appearing phlebothrombosis (Trousseau sign), also called *migratory thrombophlebitis,* is sometimes seen with carcinoma of the pancreas, particularly that of the body and tail. However, this syndrome is not pathognomonic for cancer in this organ (Chapter 6).

Because of the insidious nature of pancreatic cancer, there has long been a search for biochemical tests to indicate its presence. Serum levels of many enzymes and antigens (e.g., carcinoembryonic antigen, CA19-9 antigen) have been found to be elevated, but no single surrogate marker has proved to be specific for pancreatic cancer. Several imaging techniques, such as ultrasonography and CT with percutaneous biopsy, have great value in diagnosis in patients who have already presented with symptoms. Instead, current hopes lie with delineation of the molecular basis of this disease. This may allow earlier diagnosis through detection of early events in the molecular carcinogenesis of the pancreatic duct epithelium, and it may also provide for more effective treatment algorithms tailored to the molecular profile of malignant lesions.

ENDOCRINE PANCREAS

The endocrine pancreas consists of about 1 million microscopic clusters of endocrine cells, the islets of Langerhans. Each islet contains about 1000 cells, differentiated by their staining properties, by the ultrastructural morphology of their granules, and by their hormone content. Of these, the four most common cell types are the beta, alpha, delta, and PP (pancreatic polypeptide) cells. The *beta cells synthesize insulin and constitute 70% of the islet cell population. Alpha cells elaborate glucagon* and account for 5% to 20% of the islet. *Delta cells contain somatostatin,* which suppresses the release of glucagon and insulin. Delta cells make up 5% to 10% of the islet cell population. *PP cells* are found not only in the islets but also scattered within the exocrine part of the pancreas. Within the islets, they constitute 1% to 2% of all cells; their polypeptide exerts a number of gastrointestinal effects, such as stimulation of secretion of gastric and intestinal enzymes and inhibition of intestinal motility.

With this background, we can turn to the two main disorders of the islet cells, diabetes mellitus and islet cell tumors.

Diabetes Mellitus

Diabetes mellitus is a chronic disorder of carbohydrate, fat, and protein metabolism. A relative or absolute deficiency in insulin secretory response, which translates into impaired carbohydrate (glucose) use, is a characteristic feature of diabetes mellitus, as is the resulting hyperglycemia.

CLASSIFICATION AND INCIDENCE

Diabetes mellitus represents a heterogeneous group of disorders that have hyperglycemia as a common feature. Traditionally, diabetes has been classified into two major categories: primary, the most common form, arising from a defect in insulin production and/or action; and secondary, arising from any disease causing extensive destruction of pancreatic islets, such as pancreatitis, tumors, certain drugs, iron overload (hemochromatosis), surgical removal of pancreatic substance, or acquired or genetic endocrinopathies in which insulin action is antagonized. In 1997, the American Diabetes Association recommended a new classification based on etiology (to the extent that it is understood). In this classification, there is no distinction between primary and secondary causes of diabetes. Descriptions based on age of onset or type of treatment have been eliminated. This classification is presented in Table 17–2. The two major variants of diabetes (types 1 and 2) differ in their patterns of inheritance, insulin responses, and origins (Table 17–3).

■ *Type 1 diabetes,* previously called insulin-dependent diabetes mellitus or juvenile-onset diabetes, accounts for 5% to 10% of all cases of diabetes. Recent studies indicate that there are two subgroups of type 1 diabetes. By far the most common form is type 1A, caused by autoimmune destruction of beta cells; type 1B is also associated with severe insulin deficiency, but there is no evidence of autoimmunity.
■ Approximately 80% of patients have the so-called *type 2 diabetes,* previously called non–insulin-dependent diabetes mellitus or adult-onset diabetes.
■ The approximately 10% of cases remaining are due to specific causes listed in Table 17–2.

Table 17-2. CLASSIFICATION OF DIABETES MELLITUS

I. Type 1 diabetes
   A. Immune mediated (type 1A)
   B. Idiopathic
II. Type 2 diabetes
III. Other specific types of diabetes
   A. Genetic defects of beta-cell function* characterized by mutations in
      1. Hepatocyte nuclear transcription factor (HNF) 4α
      2. Glucokinase
      3. Hepatocyte nuclear transcription factor 1α
      4. Insulin promoter factor
   B. Genetic defects in insulin action (e.g., type A insulin resistance)
   C. Diseases of exocrine pancreas: pancreatitis, pancreatectomy, neoplasia, cystic fibrosis, hemochromatosis
   D. Endocrinopathies: Cushing syndrome, acromegaly, pheochromocytoma, hyperthyroidism, glucagonoma
   E. Drugs or chemicals: glucocorticoids, thiazides, others
   F. Infections: congenital rubella, cytomegalovirus, coxsackievirus, others
   G. Uncommon forms of immune-mediated diabetes: "Stiff man" syndrome, anti–insulin receptor antibodies
   H. Other genetic syndromes associated with diabetes: Down syndrome, Klinefelter syndrome, others
IV. Gestational diabetes mellitus

*These were previously classified as maturity-onset diabetes of the young (MODY).

It should be stressed that although the two major types of diabetes have different pathogenetic mechanisms and metabolic characteristics, *the long-term complications in blood vessels, kidneys, eyes, and nerves occur in both types and are the major causes of morbidity and death from diabetes.*

Diabetes affects an estimated 13 million people in the United States. With an annual mortality rate of about 35,000, diabetes is the seventh leading cause of death in the United States. The lifetime risk of developing type 2 diabetes for the American adult population is estimated at 5% to 7%; for type 1, the lifetime risk is about 0.5%. The prevalence of diabetes mellitus varies widely around the world and among racial and ethnic groups, probably as a reflection of genetic and environmental factors that have yet to be totally elucidated.

PATHOGENESIS

The two types are discussed separately, but first normal insulin metabolism is briefly reviewed, because many aspects of insulin release and action are important in the consideration of pathogenesis.

Normal Insulin Physiology

The insulin gene is expressed in the beta cells of the pancreatic islets, where insulin is synthesized and stored in granules before secretion. Release from beta cells occurs as a biphasic process involving two pools of insulin. A rise in the blood glucose level calls forth an immediate release of insulin, presumably that stored in the beta-cell granules. If the secretory stimulus persists, a delayed and protracted response follows, which involves active synthesis of insulin. *The most important stimulus that triggers insulin release is glucose, which also initiates insulin synthesis.* Glucose-induced alterations in intracellular metabolism,

coupled with normal cholinergic input from the autonomic nervous system, promote beta-cell secretion of insulin. Other agents, including intestinal hormones and certain amino acids (leucine and arginine), as well as the sulfonylureas, stimulate insulin release but not insulin synthesis.

Insulin is a major anabolic hormone. It is necessary for (1) transmembrane transport of glucose and amino acids, (2) glycogen formation in the liver and skeletal muscles, (3) conversion of glucose to triglycerides, (4) nucleic acid synthesis, and (5) protein synthesis. Its principal metabolic function is to increase the rate of glucose transport into certain cells in the body. These are the striated muscle cells, including myocardial cells; fibroblasts; and fat cells, representing collectively about two thirds of the entire body weight.

Insulin interacts with its target cells by first binding to the insulin receptor; the number and function of these receptors are important in regulating the action of insulin. The insulin receptor is a tyrosine kinase that triggers a number of intracellular responses that affect metabolic pathways. *One of the important early responses to insulin involves translocation of glucose transport units (GLUTs, of which there are many tissue-specific types) from the Golgi apparatus to the plasma membrane, which facilitates cellular uptake of glucose.* Hence, removal of glucose from the circulation is a primary outcome of insulin action.

A singular feature of diabetes mellitus is impaired glucose tolerance. This is unmasked by an oral glucose tolerance test, in which blood glucose levels are sampled after overnight fasting, and then minutes to hours after an oral dose of glucose. In normal persons, blood glucose levels rise only modestly, and a brisk pancreatic insulin response ensures a return to normoglycemic levels within an hour. *In diabetic individuals and in those in a preclinical stage,*

Table 17-3. TYPE 1 VERSUS TYPE 2 DIABETES MELLITUS

	Type 1*	Type 2
Clinical	Children > adults	Adults > children
	Normal weight	Obese
	Decreased blood insulin	Normal or increased blood insulin
	Anti–islet cell antibodies	No anti–islet cell antibodies
	Ketoacidosis common	Ketoacidosis rare
Genetics	40% concordance in twins	60% to 80% concordance in twins
	HLA-D linked	No HLA association
Pathogenesis	Autoimmunity, immunopathologic mechanisms	Insulin resistance
	Severe insulin deficiency	Relative insulin deficiency
Islet Cells	Insulitis early	No insulitis
	Marked atrophy and fibrosis	Focal atrophy and amyloid deposits
	Severe beta-cell depletion	Mild beta-cell depletion

*The vast majority of type 1 diabetes is type 1A.
HLA, human leukocyte antigen.

blood glucose rises to abnormally high levels for a sustained period. This may result from an absolute lack of pancreatic insulin release or from impaired target tissue response to insulin, or both.

Currently, the following criteria are used for the laboratory diagnosis of diabetes mellitus:

1. Fasting (overnight) venous plasma glucose concentrations of 126 mg/dL or greater on more than one occasion
2. Clinical symptoms of diabetes and a random glucose level of 200 mg/dL or greater
3. After ingestion of 75 g of glucose, a 2-hour venous plasma glucose concentration of 200 mg/dL or greater

Pathogenesis of Type 1A Diabetes Mellitus

This form of diabetes results from an autoimmune destruction of beta cells. A severe, insulin-requiring form of type 1A diabetes usually develops in children and adolescents, but this autoimmune disease may manifest in adults in a milder, initially non–insulin-requiring form, so-called latent autoimmune diabetes in adults (LADA). Young type 1A patients depend on insulin for survival; hence the older term *insulin-dependent diabetes mellitus.* Without insulin, they develop serious metabolic complications such as acute ketoacidosis and coma.

Three interlocking mechanisms are responsible for the islet cell destruction: genetic susceptibility, autoimmunity, and an environmental insult. A postulated sequence of events involving these three mechanisms is shown in Figure 17–7: (1) genetic susceptibility is linked to specific alleles of the class II major histocompatibility complex (MHC) and other genetic loci that predispose certain persons to the development of autoimmunity against beta cells of the islets; (2) the autoimmune reaction either develops spontaneously or is triggered by (3) an environmental event that alters beta cells, rendering them immunogenic. Overt diabetes appears after most of the beta cells have been destroyed (Fig. 17–8). With this overview, we can discuss each of the pathogenetic influences separately.

Genetic Susceptibility. Type 1A diabetes mellitus occurs most frequently in persons of Northern European descent. The disease is much less common among other racial groups, including blacks, Hispanics, Native Americans, and Asians. Diabetes can aggregate in families. About 6% of offspring of people with type 1A diabetes develop the disease. However, over 80% of new cases occur without a family history of this disease, and among identical twins the concordance rate (i.e., both twins affected) is only 40%. Thus, both genetic and environmental factors must play an important role.

Genome-wide scans have revealed many—by some counts up to 20—chromosomal regions that regulate susceptibility to type 1A diabetes. Of these loci, the best characterized is the association with chromosome 6p21, where the MHC class II genes *(HLA-DP, -DQ, -DR)* map. This locus, termed *IDDM1,* accounts for about 45% of genetic susceptibility to this disease. It is important to note that *genes within this region provide both susceptibility and resistance to type 1A diabetes.* Within the MHC class II region, the strongest disease linkage is to specific alleles of

GENETIC PREDISPOSITION

HLA-linked genes and
other genetic loci

ENVIRONMENTAL INSULT

Immune response against
normal beta cells

AND/OR

Immune response against
altered beta cells

Viral infection:
Molecular mimicry

AND/OR

Damage to beta cells

AUTOIMMUNE ATTACK

Beta-cell destruction

TYPE 1 DIABETES

Figure 17–7   ■

Possible pathways of beta-cell destruction leading to type 1 (insulin-dependent) diabetes mellitus. An environmental insult, possibly viral infection, is thought to provoke autoimmune attack on beta cells in genetically susceptible individuals. Environmental insults may involve molecular mimicry, in which a viral antigen evokes autoimmune attack against a cross-reactive beta-cell antigen, or may cause direct damage to beta cells and thus evoke an immune response against altered beta-cell antigens.

the *HLA-DQA1* and *HLA-DQB1* genes. The analysis of the high-risk alleles of *HLA-DQA1* and *HLA-DQB1* indicates a common molecular profile: they all encode for an amino acid other than aspartate at position 57 on the β chain of the HLA molecule. Crystal structure analysis of MHC class II molecules indicates that aspartic acid at this position is important for the "shape" of the peptide-binding groove of HLA-DQ molecules and hence may influence which antigenic peptide binds to these molecules. In addition to the *HLA-DQ* genes, additional MHC-linked susceptibility is conferred by certain *HLA-DRB1* alleles. As mentioned previously, certain MHC class II molecules confer protection from diabetes. Of note, protection is dominant over susceptibility. An example of protective class II genes are certain *HLA-DR2* specificities. By contrast with susceptibility alleles, all the protective alleles have an aspartate at position 57 in the β chain. The mechanisms by which *HLA-DR* or *-DQ* genes influence susceptibility to type 1A diabetes are not clear. It is well known that the T-cell receptor of CD4+ T lymphocytes recognizes an antigen only after the peptide fragment of the antigen binds to the MHC class II molecule on the surface of the antigen-presenting cell (Chapter 5). It is possible that genetic variations in the MHC class II molecule that affect the antigen-binding cleft may allow the presentation of self-antigen to autoreactive CD4+ T cells. Thus, *class II MHC genes may affect the degree of immune*

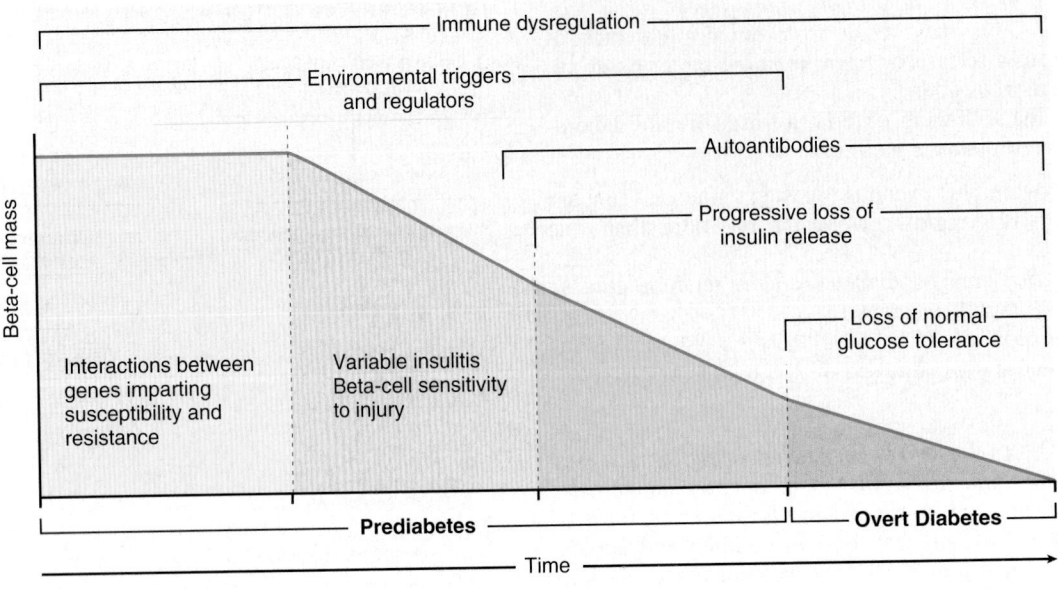

Figure 17-8

Stages in the development of type 1A diabetes mellitus. The stages of diabetes are listed from left to right; hypothetical beta-cell mass is plotted against age. (From Atkinson MA, Eisenbarth GE: Type I diabetes: new perspectives on disease pathogenesis and treatment. Lancet 358:221, 2001.)

responsiveness to a pancreatic beta-cell autoantigen, or a beta-cell autoantigen may be presented in a manner that promotes an abnormal immunologic reaction.

There are several non–MHC-linked genes that also confer susceptibility to type 1A diabetes. However, the effects of these genes are much smaller, and they are evident only in the presence of the MHC class II susceptibility genotype.

Autoimmunity. Although the clinical onset of type 1A diabetes mellitus is abrupt, this disease in fact results from a chronic autoimmune attack against beta cells that usually exists for years before disease onset (see Fig. 17–8). The classic manifestations of the disease (hyperglycemia and ketosis) occur late, after more than 90% of the beta cells have been destroyed. Several observations merit comment.

■ A lymphocyte-rich inflammatory infiltrate, often intense *(insulitis)*, is frequently observed in the islets of patients early in the course of clinically manifest disease. The infiltrate consists mostly of CD8+ T lymphocytes, with variable numbers of CD4+ T lymphocytes and macrophages. Furthermore, T lymphocytes from diseased animals can transfer diabetes to normal animals, thus establishing the primacy of T cell–mediated autoimmunity in type 1 diabetes.

■ Islet beta cells are selectively destroyed, with preservation of other cell types. Cytotoxic CD8+ lymphocytes appear to kill islets either through release of cytotoxic granules or by inducing Fas-mediated apoptosis.

■ Autoantibodies to islet cell antigens indicate a risk for type 1A diabetes. They appear as early as 9 months of age and are present in 80% of patients with new-onset disease. Among the intracellular antigens against which autoantibodies react are glutamic acid decarboxylase (GAD), insulin, and several other cytoplasmic proteins. In addition, peripheral blood T-cell responses to these same

target antigens are often detected. There is no evidence that the autoantibodies cause beta injury. They arise perhaps as a consequence of T-cell–mediated damage.

■ Asymptomatic relatives of patients with type 1A diabetes (who are at increased risk) develop islet cell autoantibodies months to years before they manifest overt diabetes.

■ Approximately 10% to 20% of persons who have type 1A diabetes also have other organ-specific autoimmune disorders such as Hashimoto thyroiditis, celiac disease, Graves disease, Addison disease, or pernicious anemia. In fact, the incidence of thyroid autoimmunity is so common that patients with type 1A diabetes are routinely tested for thyroid function.

To summarize, *overwhelming evidence implicates autoimmunity and immune-mediated injury as causes of beta-cell loss in type 1A diabetes.* Indeed, immunomodulatory and immunosuppressive therapies have been shown to ameliorate type 1A diabetes in experimental animals and in children with the disease. Large clinical trials involving at-risk relatives (i.e., those who have islet cell antibodies) are under way to test the efficacy of immune modulation in preventing the disease.

Environmental Factors. Assuming that a genetic susceptibility predisposes to autoimmune destruction of islet cells, what triggers the autoimmune reaction? *An environmental insult could trigger autoimmunity by damaging the beta cell.* Epidemiologic observations suggest that viruses may be such a trigger. Seasonal trends in the diagnosis of new cases often correspond to the prevalence of common viral infections. Several viruses are associated with type 1A diabetes, including coxsackievirus B, mumps, measles, rubella, and infectious mononucleosis. Although many viruses are beta-cell tropic, direct virus-induced injury is rarely severe enough to cause diabetes mellitus. How viral infections contribute to the pathogenesis is not clear and, indeed, is controversial. According to one view, viruses trigger the disease by "molecular mimicry." In this scenario, *an immune response is initiated against a viral protein that shares an amino acid sequence with a beta-cell protein.* In particular, T cells, reactive to GAD peptide that shares sequences with a coxsackievirus protein, can be found in patients with type 1A diabetes. According to the competing view, viruses do not trigger autoimmunity but in some way augment a preexisting autoreactive pool of T cells. In this scenario, viral infections of the pancreatic islet cells induce a local inflammatory response that generates cytokines. These then activate or expand autoreactive T cells. This is called the "bystander effect." Important in this hypothesis is the notion that viruses or other environmental agents do not trigger the disease but, rather, modulate it over the months and years that precede overt diabetes (see Fig. 17–8).

To summarize, while there is little doubt that environmental factors are essential for the development of autoimmune diabetes, their mode of action is not clear. In some undefined manner, they contribute to the immunologically mediated erosion of beta cells in individuals whose genetic background, particularly involving MHC class II antigens, is conducive to the development of autoimmunity.

Pathogenesis of Type 2 Diabetes Mellitus

Much less is known about the pathogenesis of type 2 diabetes, despite its being by far the more common type. *There is no evidence that autoimmune mechanisms are involved.* Life style clearly plays a role, as will become evident when obesity is considered. Although this was once considered a disease of adults, there is now concern over an epidemic increase in the incidence of this form of diabetes in obese children, particularly among blacks, Hispanics, Native Americans, and Asians.

Genetic factors are even more important than in type 1A diabetes. Among identical twins, the concordance rate is 60% to 80%. In first-degree relatives with type 2 diabetes (and in nonidentical twins), the risk of developing disease is five to 10 times higher than in age- and weight-matched subjects without a family history. Unlike type 1A diabetes, the disease is not linked to any HLA genes. Rather, epidemiologic studies indicate that *type 2 diabetes appears to result from a collection of multiple genetic defects,* each contributing its own predisposing risk and each modified by environmental factors. Recent and ongoing genome-wide scans of affected individuals and their family members have confirmed that no single gene of overwhelming importance regulates susceptibility to type 2 diabetes. Several genomic regions where candidate genes lie are now being vigorously pursued.

The two metabolic defects that characterize type 2 diabetes are a derangement in beta-cell secretion of insulin and an inability of peripheral tissues to respond to insulin (insulin resistance) (Fig. 17–9). The primacy of the secretory defect, in comparison with insulin resistance, is a matter of continuing debate and may in fact vary in different patients and at different stages of the disease.

Deranged Beta-Cell Secretion of Insulin. The defects in insulin secretion are subtle and quantitatively less severe than in type 1 diabetes. In fact, early in the course of the disease,

insulin levels may actually be elevated to compensate for insulin resistance. However, it is highly unlikely that insulin resistance alone gives rise to type 2 diabetes. In rare cases, mutations in the insulin receptor give rise to severe insulin resistance, which is much more severe than in patients with type 2 diabetes. However, many of these patients maintain normal blood glucose levels because normal beta cells can greatly increase insulin production.

Early in the course of type 2 diabetes, insulin secretion appears to be normal and plasma insulin levels are not reduced. However, the normal pulsatile, oscillating pattern of insulin secretion is lost, and the rapid first phase of insulin secretion triggered by glucose is obtunded. Collectively, these and other observations implicate such derangements in insulin secretion seen early in type 2 diabetes, rather than deficiencies in insulin synthesis per se.

However, later in the course of the disease, a mild to moderate absolute deficiency of insulin is present, which is less severe than that of type 1 diabetes. The cause of the insulin deficiency in type 2 diabetes is not entirely clear. On the basis of data from experimental animals with type 2 diabetes, it is thought that initially insulin resistance causes a compensatory increase in the beta cell mass and production of insulin. In those with genetic susceptibility to type 2 diabetes, this compensation fails. Later in the course of this disease, there is a 20% to 50% loss of beta cells, but this is not sufficient to account for a failure in glucose-stimulated insulin secretion. Instead, there appears to be a defect in glucose recognition by the beta cells. The molecular basis of such impairment in glu-

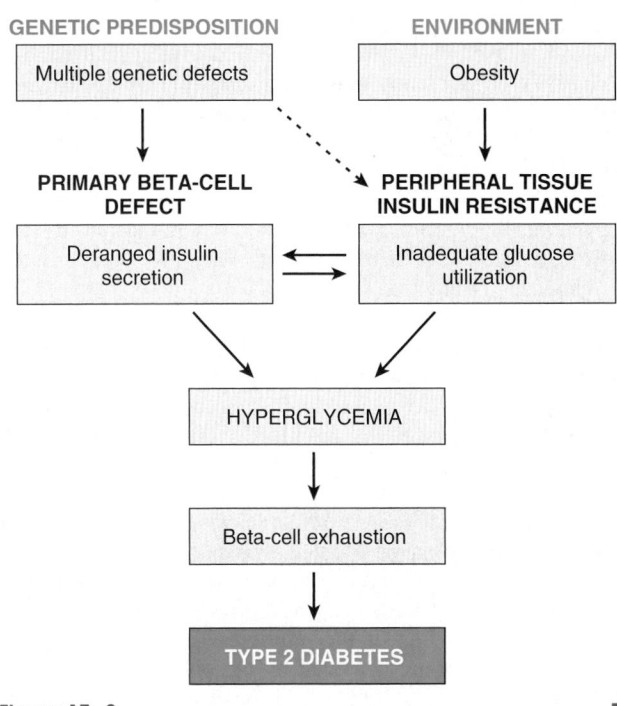

Figure 17-9   ■

Pathogenesis of type 2 diabetes mellitus. Genetic predisposition and environmental influences converge to cause hyperglycemia and overt diabetes. The primacy of deranged beta-cell insulin secretion and peripheral insulin resistance is not established; in patients with clinical disease, both defects can be demonstrated.

cose-mediated insulin secretion is not entirely clear. Recent studies implicate a mitochondrial protein that uncouples biochemical respiration from oxidative phosphorylation (thus producing heat rather than ATP). This protein, called uncoupling protein 2 (UCP2), is expressed in beta cells. High intracellular levels of UCP2 obtund the insulin response, whereas low levels accentuate it. It is hypothesized, therefore, that increased UCP2 levels in the beta cells of people with type 2 diabetes may offer an explanation for the characteristic loss of the glucose signal. Much interest is focused on this issue, since therapeutic manipulation (lowering) of UCP2 levels could be used to treat type 2 diabetes.

Another mechanism of beta-cell failure in type 2 diabetes is related to the deposition of amyloid in the islets. Some degree of amyloid deposition can be seen in 90% of type 2 diabetic patients at autopsy. Amylin, the major component of the amyloid deposited in this setting, is normally produced by pancreatic beta cells and is cosecreted with insulin in response to a glucose load. The hyperinsulinemia caused by insulin resistance in the early phases of type 2 diabetes causes a concomitant increase in the production of amylin, which then deposits as amyloid in the islets. Amylin surrounding the beta cells may render them somewhat refractory to receiving the glucose signal. More importantly, amyloid is toxic to beta cells and may thus contribute to the beta-cell loss seen in advanced cases of type 2 diabetes.

Insulin Resistance and Obesity. As discussed previously, insulin deficiency is present late in the course of type 2 diabetes; however, this is not of sufficient magnitude to explain the metabolic disturbances. Rather, the evidence suggests that *insulin resistance is a major factor in the development of type 2 diabetes.*

At the outset, it should be noted that insulin resistance is a complex phenomenon that is not restricted to the diabetes syndrome. In both obesity and pregnancy, insulin sensitivity of target tissues decreases (even in the absence of diabetes), and serum levels of insulin may be elevated to compensate for insulin resistance. Thus, either obesity or pregnancy may unmask subclinical type 2 diabetes by increasing the insulin resistance to a degree that cannot be compensated by increased production of insulin.

The cellular and molecular basis of insulin resistance are not fully understood. There are three major targets of insulin action: adipose tissue and muscle, where insulin promotes glucose uptake, and liver, where it suppresses the production of glucose. As discussed earlier, insulin acts on these targets by first binding to the insulin receptor. The resultant activation of the insulin receptor triggers a series of intracellular responses that affect metabolic pathways and lead to translocation of glucose transport units to the cell membrane, thus facilitating glucose uptake. In principle, insulin resistance could occur at the level of the insulin receptors or in any one of the multiple signaling (postreceptor) pathways that are activated by the binding of insulin to its receptors. Only in rare cases is there a qualitative or quantitative defect in insulin receptors in type 2 diabetes. Hence, *insulin resistance is believed to involve primarily postreceptor signaling.*

To understand the basis of insulin resistance, it is important to emphasize the relationship between obesity and type 2 diabetes. As stated earlier, obesity is associated with insulin resistance even in the absence of diabetes. Not surprisingly, therefore, *obesity is an important environmental risk factor in the pathogenesis of type 2 diabetes*, and it is strongly implicated in the rising incidence of this form of diabetes in children. Fortunately for many obese persons with diabetes, weight loss and physical exercise can reverse insulin resistance and impaired glucose tolerance, especially early in the course of the disease when insulin production is not much impaired.

How is obesity related to insulin resistance? Recent studies indicate that adipose tissue is not merely a storage site for triglycerides but is a versatile "endocrine" tissue that can carry out a dialogue with muscle and liver, both important targets of insulin. These long-distance effects of adipocytes occur through molecular messengers elaborated by fat cells. Such molecules include tumor necrosis factor (TNF), fatty acids, leptin, and a newly discovered factor called *resistin*. TNF, better known for its effects in inflammation and immunity, is synthesized in adipocytes and is overexpressed in fat cells from obese people. It causes insulin resistance by affecting postreceptor signaling pathways. In obesity, the free fatty acid levels are higher than normal, and they increase insulin resistance by mechanisms not entirely clear. *Leptin* is an adipocyte hormone whose genetic absence in rodents causes profound obesity and insulin resistance (Chapter 8). Returning leptin to these animals reduces obesity and, independently, insulin resistance; thus, unlike TNF, leptin ameliorates insulin resistance. The latest member to be discovered in the armamentarium of adipose tissues is *resistin*, so called because it increases insulin resistance. Resistin is produced by fat cells, and its levels are increased in a variety of rodent models for obesity. Reducing resistin levels improves insulin action, and, conversely, administration of recombinant resistin increases insulin resistance in normal animals. Quite interestingly, the therapeutic effects of certain oral antidiabetic agents used in treatment of type 2 diabetes in humans may also be linked to their ability to modulate resistin production. The thiazolidinedione class of antidiabetic agents binds to a receptor called peroxisome proliferator–activated receptor γ (PPAR-γ), expressed in the nuclei of fat cells. By binding to their receptors in adipocytes, the thiazolidinediones control the transcription of resistin or other adipose cell genes that affect insulin resistance. It is thought that PPAR-γ agonist drugs may reduce the production of resistin, thus improving insulin sensitivity. The important role of the PPAR-γ signaling in regulating insulin resistance is supported by study of rare patients who have loss-of-function mutations in the *PPAR-γ* gene. These patients have insulin resistance and diabetes. Thus, activation of the PPAR-γ receptors by drugs reduces insulin resistance, and mutations that impair PPAR-γ signaling increase insulin resistance. It is thought that a better understanding of such pathways in fat cells may provide new therapeutic targets for treatment of type 2 diabetes; as an example, drugs that neutralize resistin action may be useful in treatment of type 2 diabetes.

To summarize, type 2 diabetes is a complex, multifactorial disorder involving both impaired insulin release and

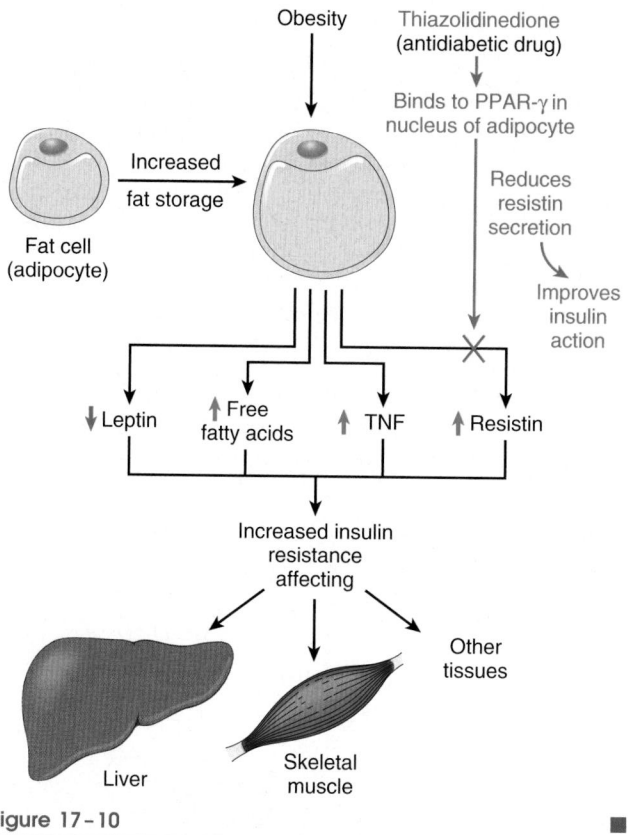

Figure 17–10 ■

The central role of fat cells in regulating insulin resistance. Adipocytes produce factors that increase or decrease insulin resistance. Certain antidiabetic drugs modify insulin resistance by affecting the synthesis of adipocyte-derived factors via the peroxisome proliferator–activated receptor γ (PPAR-γ) nuclear receptor. TNF, tumor necrosis factor.

end organ insensitivity. Insulin resistance, intimately linked with obesity (Fig. 17–10), produces excessive stress on beta cells, which eventually fail in the face of sustained need for a state of hyperinsulinism. Genetic factors are definitely involved, but how they fit into this puzzle remains unclear.

Pathogenesis of the Complications of Diabetes

The morbidity associated with long-standing diabetes of either type results from complications such as *microangiopathy, retinopathy, nephropathy, neuropathy,* and *accelerated atherosclerosis.* The basis of these chronic long-term complications is the subject of a great deal of research. *The available experimental and clinical evidence suggests that most complications of diabetes result from metabolic derangements, mainly hyperglycemia.* In addition, coexistent hypertension, common in diabetics, contributes to atherosclerosis. The most telling evidence linking metabolic abnormalities to diabetic complications comes from the finding that when transplanted from nondiabetic donors into diabetic patients, kidneys develop the lesions of diabetic nephropathy within 3 to 5 years after transplantation. Conversely, kidneys with lesions of diabetic nephropathy demonstrate a reversal of the lesion when transplanted into normal recipients. Finally, multicenter studies clearly show delayed progression of diabetic complications by strict control of the hyperglycemia.

Many mechanisms linking hyperglycemia to the complications of long-standing diabetes have been explored. Currently, two such mechanisms are considered important.

1. *Nonenzymatic glycosylation* is the process by which glucose chemically attaches to free amino groups of proteins without the aid of enzymes. The degree of nonenzymatic glycosylation is directly related to the level of blood glucose. Indeed, the measurement of glycosylated hemoglobin (HbA_{1c}) levels in blood is a useful adjunct in the management of diabetes mellitus, because it provides an index of the average blood glucose levels over the 120-day life span of erythrocytes. The early glycosylation products of collagen and other long-lived proteins in interstitial tissues and blood vessel walls undergo a slow series of chemical rearrangements to form *irreversible advanced glycosylation end products (AGEs),* which accumulate over the lifetime of the vessel wall. AGEs have a number of chemical and biologic properties that are potentially pathogenic.

   ■ *AGE formation on proteins such as collagen causes cross-links between polypeptides; this in turn may trap nonglycosylated plasma and interstitial proteins.* Trapping of circulating low-density lipoprotein (LDL), for example, retards its efflux from the vessel wall and promotes the deposition of cholesterol in the intima, thus accelerating atherogenesis (Chapter 10). AGEs may also affect the structure and function of capillaries, including those of the renal glomeruli, which develop thickened basement membranes and become leaky.

   ■ *AGEs bind to receptors on many cell types*—endothelium, monocytes, macrophages, lymphocytes, and mesangial cells. Binding induces a variety of biologic activities, including monocyte emigration, release of cytokines and growth factors from macrophages, increased endothelial permeability, and enhanced proliferation of fibroblasts and smooth muscle cells and synthesis of extracellular matrix. All these effects can potentially contribute to diabetic complications.

2. *Intracellular hyperglycemia with disturbances in polyol pathways* is the second major mechanism proposed for complications related to hyperglycemia. In some tissues that do not require insulin for glucose transport (e.g., nerves, lens, kidney, blood vessels), hyperglycemia leads to an increase in intracellular glucose, which is then metabolized by aldose reductase to *sorbitol,* a polyol, and eventually to fructose. These changes have several untoward effects. *The accumulated sorbitol and fructose lead to increased intracellular osmolarity and influx of water, and, eventually, to osmotic cell injury.* In the lens, osmotically imbibed water causes swelling and opacity. *Sorbitol accumulation also impairs ion pumps and is believed to promote injury of Schwann cells and pericytes of retinal capillaries, with resultant peripheral neuropathy and retinal microaneurysms.* In keeping with this hypothesis, experimental inhibition of aldose reductase is capable of ameliorating the development of cataracts and neuropathy.

The pathogenesis of accelerated atherosclerosis is in all likelihood multifactorial. About one third to one half of patients have elevated blood lipid levels, known to predispose to atherosclerosis, but the remainder also have an increased predisposition to atherosclerosis. Qualitative changes in the lipoproteins, brought about by excessive nonenzymatic glycosylation, may affect their turnover and tissue deposition. Low levels of high-density lipoproteins (HDLs) have been demonstrated in patients with type 2 diabetes. Because HDL is a "protective molecule" against atherosclerosis (Chapter 10), this could contribute to increased susceptibility to atherosclerosis. In addition, from 40% to 70% of patients with diabetes also have hypertension, which is a well-known risk factor for atherosclerosis (Chapter 10).

MORPHOLOGY OF DIABETES MELLITUS AND ITS LATE COMPLICATIONS

Pathologic findings in the pancreas are variable and not necessarily dramatic. Rather, the impor-

tant morphologic changes in diabetes are related to its many late systemic complications, because they are the major causes of morbidity and mortality. There is extreme variability among patients in the time of onset of these complications, their severity, and the particular organ or organs involved. In those with tight control of diabetes, the onset may be delayed. In most patients, however, after 10 to 15 years, morphologic changes are likely to be found in arteries (atherosclerosis), the basement membranes of small vessels (microangiopathy), kidneys (diabetic nephropathy), retina (retinopathy), nerves (neuropathy), and other tissues. These changes are seen in both types of diabetes. A schematic overview is provided in Figure 17–11.

PANCREAS. Lesions in the pancreas are inconstant and rarely of diagnostic value. Distinctive changes are more commonly associated with type 1 than

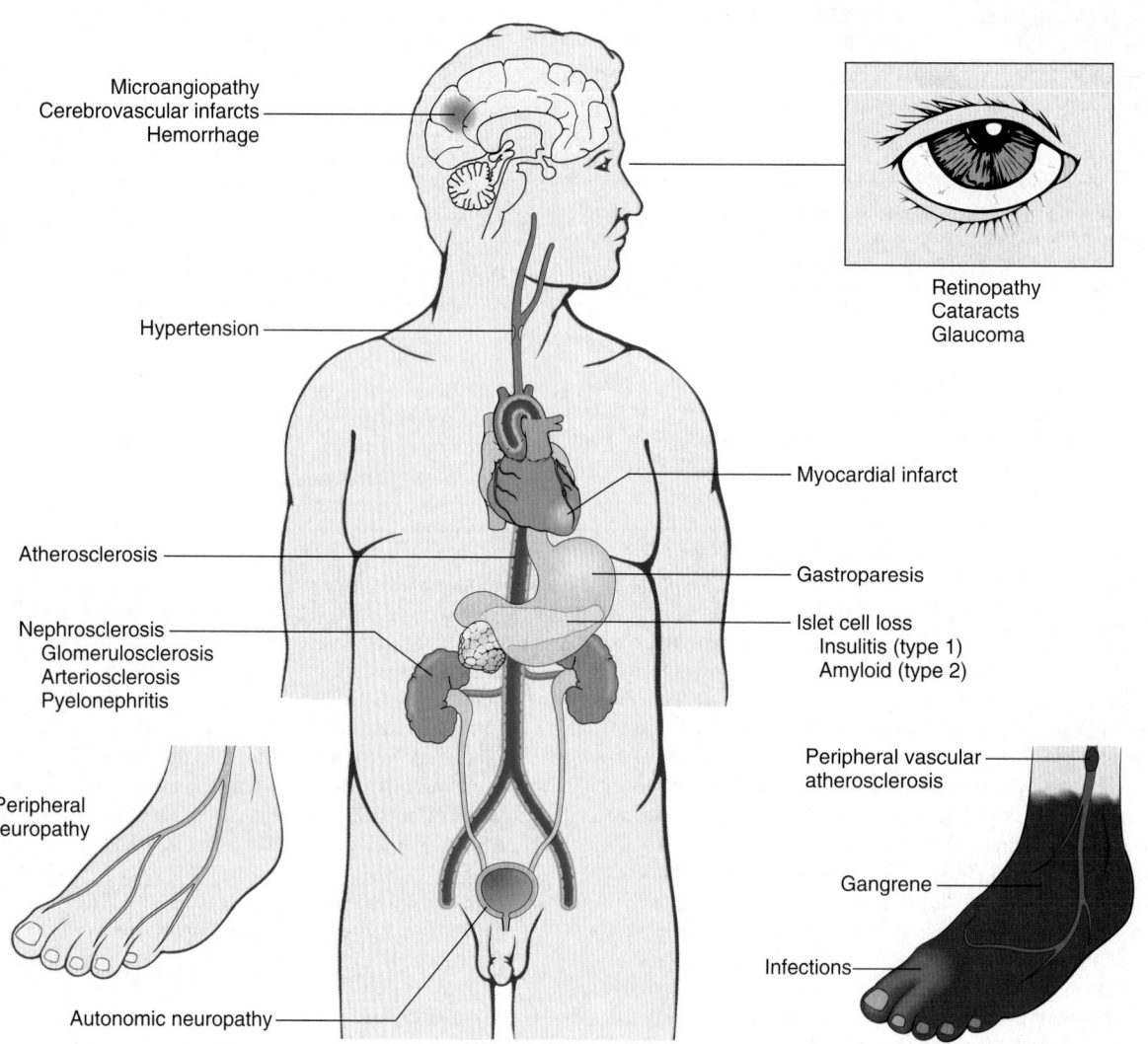

Figure 17–11

The long-term complications of diabetes.

Figure 17-12   ■

Amyloidosis of a pancreatic islet in a 65-year-old man with type 2 diabetes of 25 years' duration. (H & E.)

with type 2 diabetes. One or more of the following alterations may be present.

- **Reduction in the number and size of islets** is most often seen in type 1 diabetes, particularly with rapidly advancing disease. Most of the islets are small, inconspicuous, and not easily detected. In type 2 diabetes, loss of beta cells occurs late in the disease and is typically not more than 20% to 50%.

- **Leukocytic infiltration of the islets** (insulitis), principally by T lymphocytes, is observed in type 1A diabetes. This may be seen at the time of clinical presentation and presumably has been present for some time before the onset of overt disease. The distribution of insulitis may be strikingly uneven. Eosinophilic infiltrates may also be found, particularly in diabetic infants who fail to survive the immediate postnatal period.

- By electron microscopy, **beta-cell degranulation** may be observed, reflecting depletion of stored insulin in already-damaged beta cells. This is more commonly seen in patients with newly diagnosed type 1A diabetes, when some beta cells are still present.

- **Amyloid replacement of islets in type 2 diabetes** appears as deposits of pink, amorphous material beginning in and around capillaries and between cells. At advanced stages, the islets may be virtually obliterated (Fig. 17-12), and fibrosis may also be observed. This change is often seen in long-standing cases of type 2 diabetes. As mentioned earlier, the amyloid in this instance is partly composed of amylin fibrils derived from the beta cells. Similar lesions may be found in elderly nondiabetic persons, apparently as part of normal aging.

- **An increase in the number and size of islets is especially characteristic of nondiabetic new-** borns with diabetic mothers. Presumably, fetal islets undergo hyperplasia in response to the maternal hyperglycemia.

VASCULAR SYSTEM. Diabetes exacts a heavy toll on the vascular system. Vessels of all sizes are affected, from the aorta down to the smallest arterioles and capillaries. **The aorta and large- and medium-sized arteries suffer from accelerated severe atherosclerosis.** Except for its greater severity and earlier age of onset, atherosclerosis in diabetic patients is indistinguishable from that in nondiabetic patients (Chapter 10). **Myocardial infarction, caused by atherosclerosis of the coronary arteries, is the most common cause of death in diabetic patients. Significantly, it is almost as common in diabetic women as in diabetic men.** In contrast, myocardial infarction is uncommon in nondiabetic women of reproductive age. **Gangrene of the lower extremities,** as a result of advanced vascular disease, is about 100 times more common in diabetic persons than in the general population. The larger renal arteries are also subject to severe atherosclerosis, but the most damaging effect of diabetes on the kidneys is exerted at the level of the glomeruli and the microcirculation (see later discussion).

Hyaline arteriolosclerosis, the vascular lesion associated with hypertension (Chapter 10), is both more prevalent and more severe in diabetic than in nondiabetic persons, but it is not specific for diabetes and may be seen in elderly nondiabetic patients without hypertension. It takes the form of an amorphous, hyaline thickening of the wall of the arterioles, which causes narrowing of the lumen (Fig. 17-13). In the diabetic patient, it is related not only to the duration of disease but also

Figure 17-13   ■

Hyaline arteriolosclerosis. Note a markedly thickened, tortuous afferent arteriole in the kidney. The amorphous nature of the thickened vascular wall is evident. (Periodic acid–Schiff.) (Courtesy of Dr. M. A. Venkatachalam, Department of Pathology, University of Texas Health Science Center at San Antonio, San Antonio, TX.)

to the level of blood pressure. The cause and nature of this vascular change are still uncertain. Although at one time it was attributed to hypertension, so common among diabetic patients, it can also be seen in diabetic patients who do not have hypertension. The hyaline material consists of plasma proteins and basement membrane material. As noted earlier, it is presumed that the plasma proteins penetrate into the abnormally permeable walls of the arterioles and are trapped.

DIABETIC MICROANGIOPATHY. One of the most consistent morphologic features of diabetes is **diffuse thickening of basement membranes.** The thickening is most evident in the capillaries of the skin, skeletal muscles, retinas, renal glomeruli, and renal medullae. However, it may also be seen in such nonvascular structures as renal tubules, Bowman's capsule, peripheral nerves, and placenta. By light microscopy, the normal basal lamina consists of a relatively uniform layer of extracellular material that separates parenchymal or endothelial cells from the surrounding connective tissue stroma. In diabetic patients, this single layer is widened and sometimes replaced by concentric layers of hyaline material composed predominantly of type IV collagen. **Despite the increase in the thickness of basement membranes, diabetic capillaries are more leaky to plasma proteins than normal. The microangiopathy underlies the development of diabetic nephropathy and some forms of neuropathy.** An indistinguishable microangiopathy can be found in aged nondiabetic patients, but rarely to the extent seen in patients with long-standing diabetes.

DIABETIC NEPHROPATHY. The kidneys are prime targets of diabetes, and renal failure is second only to myocardial infarction as a cause of death from this disease. **Three important lesions are encountered: (1) glomerular lesions; (2) renal vascular lesions, principally arteriolosclerosis; and (3) pyelonephritis, including necrotizing papillitis.**

The most important glomerular lesions are capillary basement membrane thickening, diffuse glomerulosclerosis, and nodular glomerulosclerosis (Kimmelstiel-Wilson lesion). **The glomerular capillary basement membranes are thickened throughout their entire length.** This change can be detected by electron microscopy within a few years of the onset of diabetes, sometimes without any associated change in renal function.

Diffuse glomerulosclerosis consists of a diffuse increase in mesangial matrix along with mesangial cell proliferation and is always associated with basement membrane thickening. It is found in most patients with disease of more than 10 years' duration. After glomerulosclerosis becomes marked, patients manifest the nephrotic syndrome (Chapter 14), characterized by proteinuria, hypoalbuminemia, and edema.

Figure 17–14 ■

Nodular glomerulosclerosis in a patient with long-standing diabetes. (Courtesy of Dr. Lisa Yerian, Department of Pathology, University of Chicago.)

Nodular glomerulosclerosis describes a glomerular lesion made distinctive by ball-like deposits of a laminated matrix within the mesangial core of the lobule (Fig. 17–14). These nodules tend to develop in the periphery of the glomerulus, and because they arise within the mesangium, they push the glomerular capillary loops even more to the periphery. Often these capillary loops create halos about the nodule. This distinctive change has been called the **Kimmelstiel-Wilson lesion,** after the pioneers who described it. Nodular glomerulosclerosis occurs irregularly throughout the kidney and affects random glomeruli as well as random lobules within a glomerulus. In advanced disease, many nodules are present within a single glomerulus, and most glomeruli become involved. The deposits are positive on periodic acid–Schiff staining and contain mucopolysaccharides, lipids, and fibrils as well as collagen fibers, as do the matrix deposits of diffuse glomerulosclerosis.

Because tubules are perfused by vessels arising from glomerular efferent arterioles, advanced glomerulosclerosis is associated with tubular ischemia and interstitial fibrosis. In addition, patients with uncontrolled glycosuria may reabsorb glucose and store it as glycogen in the tubular epithelium. This change does not affect tubular function.

Renal atherosclerosis and arteriolosclerosis constitute only one part of the systemic involvement of blood vessels in diabetic patients. The kidney is one of the most frequently and most severely affected organs; however, the changes in the arteries and arterioles are similar to those found throughout the body. **Hyaline arteriolosclerosis affects not only the afferent but also the efferent arteriole.** Such efferent arteriolosclerosis is rarely if ever encountered in persons who do not have diabetes.

Pyelonephritis is an acute or chronic inflammation of the kidneys that usually begins in the interstitial tissue and then spreads to affect the tubules and, in extreme cases, the glomeruli. Both the acute and the chronic forms of this disease occur in nondiabetic as well as diabetic patients; they are described more fully in Chapter 14. However, these inflammatory disorders are more common in diabetic patients than in the general population, and once affected, diabetic patients tend to have more severe involvement. One special pattern of acute pyelonephritis, **necrotizing papillitis,** is much more prevalent in diabetic than in nondiabetic patients. As the term implies, necrotizing papillitis is an acute necrosis of the renal papillae, described in Chapter 14. Although this lesion is not limited to diabetic patients, they are particularly prone to develop it, owing to the combination of ischemia resulting from microangiopathy and increased susceptibility to bacterial infection.

The sclerotic lesions of the glomeruli destroy renal function and constitute potentially fatal forms of diabetic nephropathy. Nodular glomerulosclerosis is encountered in perhaps 10% to 35% of diabetic patients and is a major cause of morbidity and mortality. As with diffuse glomerulosclerosis, the appearance is related to the duration of the disease but conditioned by the genetic background. Unlike the diffuse form, which may also be seen in association with old age and hypertension, the nodular form of glomerulosclerosis, for all practical purposes, implicates diabetes. Both the diffuse and the nodular forms of glomerulosclerosis induce sufficient ischemia to cause overall fine scarring of the kidneys, marked by a finely granular cortical surface (Fig. 17–15).

DIABETIC OCULAR COMPLICATIONS. Visual impairment, sometimes even total blindness, is one of the more feared consequences of long-standing diabetes. This disease is the fourth leading cause of acquired blindness in the United States. **The ocular involvement may take the form of retinopathy, cataract formation, or glaucoma.** Retinopathy, the most common pattern, consists of a constellation of changes that together are considered by many ophthalmologists to be virtually diagnostic of the disease. **The lesion in the retina takes two forms: nonproliferative (background) retinopathy and proliferative retinopathy.**

Nonproliferative retinopathy includes intraretinal or preretinal hemorrhages, retinal exudates, microaneurysms, venous dilations, edema, and, most importantly, thickening of the retinal capillaries (microangiopathy). The retinal exudates can be either "soft" (microinfarcts) or "hard" (deposits of plasma proteins and lipids) (Fig. 17–16). The microaneurysms are discrete saccular dilations of retinal choroidal capillaries that appear through the

Figure 17–15   ■

Nephrosclerosis in a patient with long-standing diabetes. The kidney has been bisected to demonstrate both diffuse granular transformation of the surface *(left)* and marked thinning of the cortical tissue *(right)*. Additional features include some irregular depressions, the result of pyelonephritis, and an incidental cortical cyst *(far right).*

ophthalmoscope as small red dots. Dilations tend to occur at focal points of weakening, resulting from loss of pericytes. Retinal edema presumably results from excessive capillary permeability. Underlying all these changes is the microangiopathy, which is thought to lead to loss of capillary pericytes and hence to focal weakening of capillary structure.

The so-called proliferative retinopathy is a process of neovascularization and fibrosis. This lesion can lead to serious consequences, including blindness, especially if it involves the macula. Vitreous hemorrhages can result from rupture of the newly formed capillaries; the resultant organization of the hemorrhage can pull the retina off its substratum (retinal detachment).

DIABETIC NEUROPATHY. The central and peripheral nervous systems are not spared by diabetes. The most frequent pattern of involvement is a peripheral, symmetric neuropathy of the lower extremities that affects both motor and sensory function but particularly the latter. Other forms include autonomic neuropathy, which produces disturbances in bowel and bladder function and sometimes sexual impotence, and diabetic mononeuropathy, which may manifest as sudden footdrop, wristdrop, or isolated cranial nerve palsies. The neurologic changes may be caused by microangiopathy and increased permeability of the capillaries that supply the nerves as well as by direct axonal damage

Figure 17-16 ■

Diabetic retinopathy. A view of the fundus shows large areas of preretinal hemorrhage below the optic disc; pale dots represent exudates in the left side. Neovascularization is present on the right side of the optic disc. (Courtesy of Dr. Rajiv Anand, Texas Retina Associates, Dallas.)

due to alterations in sorbitol metabolism (discussed earlier).

The brain, along with the rest of the body, develops widespread microangiopathy. Such microcirculatory lesions may lead to generalized neuronal degeneration. There is in addition a predisposition to cerebrovascular infarcts and brain hemorrhages, perhaps related to the hypertension and atherosclerosis often seen in diabetic patients. Degenerative changes have also been observed in the spinal cord. None of the neurologic disorders, including the peripheral neuropathy, are specific for this disease.

Clinical Features. It is difficult to sketch with brevity the diverse clinical presentations of diabetes mellitus. Only a few characteristic patterns are presented.

Type 1A diabetes, which begins by age 35 in most patients, is dominated by polyuria, polydipsia, polyphagia, weight loss, and ketoacidosis—all resulting from metabolic derangements. Because insulin is a major anabolic hormone in the body, *a deficiency of insulin affects not only glucose metabolism but also fat and protein metabolism.* With insulin deficiency, the assimilation of glucose into muscle and adipose tissue is sharply diminished or abolished. Not only does storage of glycogen in liver and muscle cease, but also reserves are depleted by glycogenolysis. Severe fasting hyperglycemia and glycosuria ensue. The glycosuria induces an osmotic diuresis and thus *polyuria,* causing a profound loss of water and electrolytes (Na^+, K^+, Mg^{++}, PO_4^-) (Fig. 17–17). The obliga-

tory renal water loss, combined with the hyperosmolarity resulting from the increased levels of glucose in the blood, tends to deplete intracellular water, triggering the osmoreceptors of the thirst centers of the brain. In this manner, intense thirst *(polydipsia)* appears. With a deficiency of insulin, the scales swing from insulin-promoted anabolism to catabolism of proteins and fats. Proteolysis follows, and the gluconeogenetic amino acids are removed by the liver and used as building blocks for glucose. The catabolism of proteins and fats tends to induce a negative energy balance *and weight loss,* which in turn leads to increasing appetite *(polyphagia),* thus completing the classic clinical symptoms of diabetes. The combination of polyphagia and weight loss is paradoxical and should always raise the suspicion of diabetes (or possibly thyrotoxicosis, Chapter 20).

In patients with type 1A diabetes, regulation of glucose levels often requires multiple daily injections of different types of insulins. Glucose control can be difficult to obtain (brittle diabetes), in that the blood glucose level is quite sensitive to administered insulin, deviations from normal dietary intake, unusual physical activity, infection, or other forms of stress. Inadequate fluid intake or vomiting can rapidly lead to significant disturbances in fluid and electrolyte balance. Therefore, these patients are vulnerable, on the one hand, to *hypoglycemic episodes* and, on the other, to *ketoacidosis. This latter complication occurs almost exclusively in type 1A diabetes and is the result of severe insulin deficiency coupled with absolute or relative increases of glucagon* (see Fig. 17–17). The insulin deficiency causes excessive breakdown of adipose stores, resulting in increased levels of free fatty acids. Oxidation of free fatty acids within the liver through acetyl coenzyme A produces ketone bodies (acetoacetic acid and β-hydroxybutyric acid). *Glucagon* accelerates such fatty acid oxidation. The rate at which ketone bodies are formed may exceed the rate at which acetoacetic acid and β-hydroxybutyric acid can be utilized by muscles and other tissues, thus leading to ketonemia and ketonuria. If the urinary excretion of ketones is compromised by dehydration, the plasma hydrogen ion concentration increases and systemic metabolic ketoacidosis results. Release of ketogenic amino acids by protein catabolism aggravates the ketotic state. As discussed later, diabetic patients have increased susceptibility to certain types of infections. Because the stress of infection increases insulin requirements, infections often precipitate diabetic ketoacidosis.

Patients with type 2 diabetes may also present with polyuria and polydipsia but are often asymptomatic. These patients are frequently older (>40 years). However, this disease may present at any age in obese subjects, including young children. In some cases, medical attention is sought because of unexplained weakness or weight loss. Frequently, however, the diagnosis is made by routine blood or urine testing in asymptomatic persons. Although patients with type 2 diabetes also have metabolic derangements, these are easier to control and less severe. In the decompensated state, these patients develop *hyperosmolar nonketotic coma,* a syndrome engendered by the severe dehydration resulting from sustained hyperglycemic diuresis in patients who do not drink enough water to compensate for urinary losses. Typically, the patient is elderly, is disabled by a stroke or an infection that increases hyperglycemia, and has limited mobility and

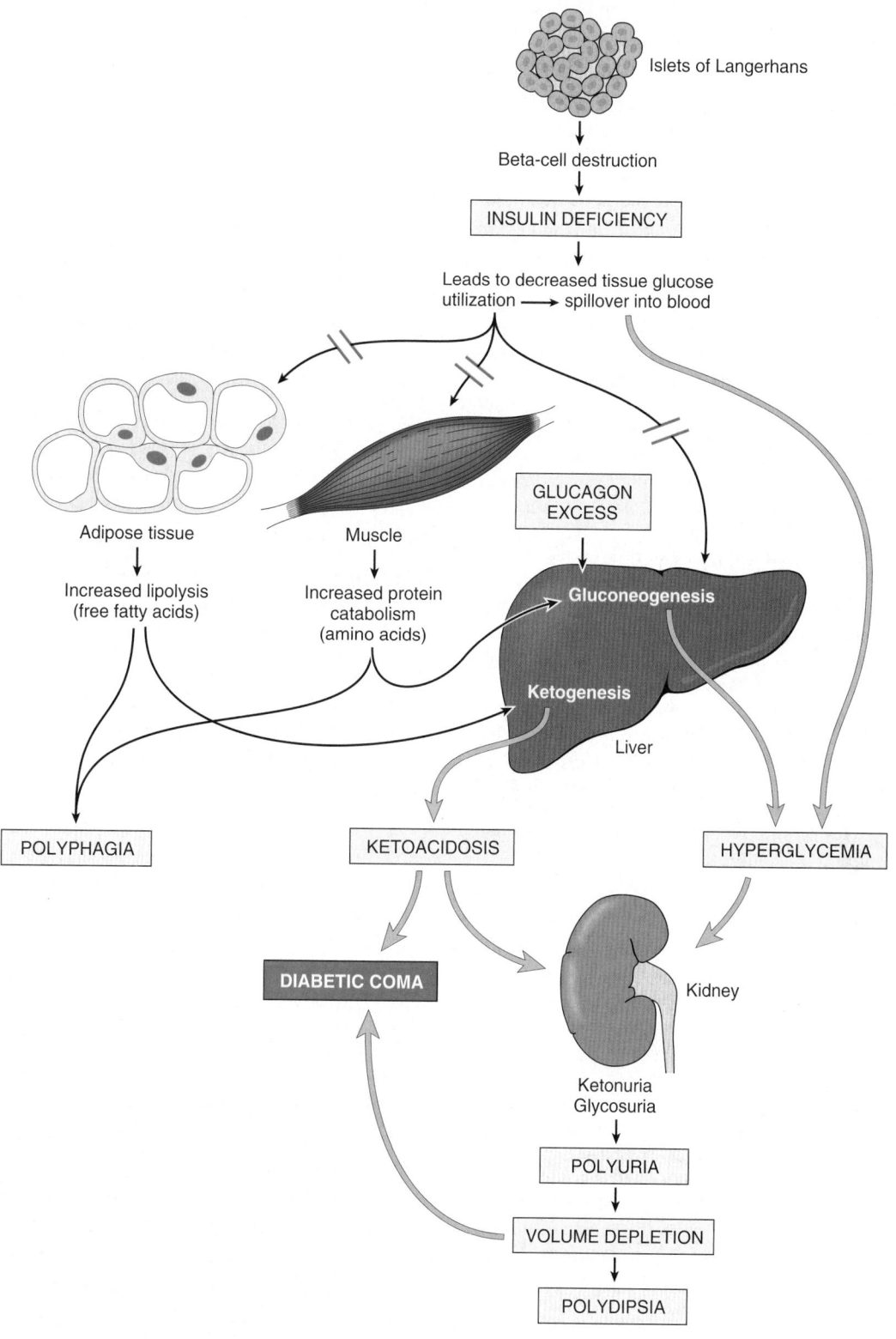

Figure 17–17

Sequence of metabolic derangements in type 1 diabetes mellitus. An absolute insulin deficiency leads to a catabolic state, eventuating in ketoacidosis and severe volume depletion. These cause sufficient central nervous system compromise to cause coma, and eventual death, if left untreated.

therefore inadequate water intake. The absence of ketoacidosis and its symptoms (nausea, vomiting) often delays the seeking of medical attention in these patients until severe dehydration occurs.

In both forms of long-standing diabetes, atherosclerotic events such as myocardial infarction, cerebrovascular accidents, gangrene of the leg, and renal insufficiency are the most threatening and most frequent complications. Diabetic patients are also plagued by enhanced susceptibility to infections with certain microbes. Contrary to popular belief, there is no generalized increase in susceptibility to all infections. Common infections include those affecting skin, lung, and urinary tract. Infections with certain microbes, such as those causing mucormycosis, occur principally in people with diabetes. Such infections cause the deaths of about 5% of diabetic patients. The basis for this susceptibility is probably multifactorial; impaired leukocyte function and poor blood supply secondary to vascular disease are involved. Phagocytosis and the bactericidal activity of neutrophils are impaired. A trivial infection in a toe may be the first event in a long succession of complications (gangrene, bacteremia, and pneumonia) that ultimately lead to death.

Patients with type 1 diabetes are more likely to die from their disease than are those with type 2 diabetes. The causes of death are myocardial infarction, renal failure, cerebrovascular disease, atherosclerotic heart disease, and infections, followed by a large number of other complications more common in the diabetic than in the nondiabetic patient (e.g., gangrene of an extremity). Hypoglycemia and ketoacidosis are uncommon causes of death today.

As mentioned at the outset, this disease continues to be one of the top 10 causes of death in the United States. It is hoped that newer forms of therapy will lead to a cure for diabetes mellitus or enable diagnosis and intervention before onset of clinical hyperglycemia. Until then, strict control of hyperglycemia and blood pressure offers the best hope for preventing the deadly complications of diabetes.

Islet Cell Tumors

Tumors of pancreatic islet cells are rare in comparison with tumors of the exocrine pancreas. Islet cell tumors may be embedded in the substance of the pancreas, or they may arise in the immediate peripancreatic tissues. They resemble in appearance their counterparts, carcinoid tumors, found elsewhere in the alimentary tract (Chapter 15). Although both share a common neuroendocrine origin, islet cell tumors have a propensity to elaborate pancreatic hormones. However, some islet cell tumors are totally nonfunctional. Among the many distinctive clinical syndromes associated with tumors of the islet cells, only three are sufficiently common to merit description: (1) hyperinsulinism, (2) hypergastrinemia and the Zollinger-Ellison syndrome, and (3) multiple endocrine neoplasia. The last of these is characterized by the occurrence of tumors in several endocrine glands and is described in Chapter 20.

HYPERINSULINISM (INSULINOMAS)

Certain islet cell tumors secrete insulin and therefore cause hypoglycemia. Patients with these tumors present

with neuropsychiatric symptoms such as nervousness, confusion, and sometimes stupor. The hypoglycemic attacks are precipitated by fasting or exercise and are promptly relieved by glucose administration or by eating. The critical laboratory findings are hypoglycemia and high circulating levels of insulin. The islet cell tumors giving rise to such symptoms are called *insulinomas*.

MORPHOLOGY

Insulinomas are most often found within the pancreas and usually are benign. Most are solitary lesions, although multiple tumors or tumors ectopic to the pancreas may be encountered. Bona fide carcinomas, comprising only about 10% of cases, are diagnosed on the basis of local invasion and distant metastases. Solitary tumors are usually small (often < 2 cm in diameter) and are encapsulated, pale to red-brown nodules located anywhere in the pancreas (Fig. 17-18). Histologically, these benign tumors look remarkably like giant islets, with preservation of the regular cords of normally oriented cells. Not even the malignant lesions present much evidence of anaplasia, and they may be deceptively encapsulated. By immunocytochemical study, insulin can be localized in the tumor cells. Under the electron microscope, neoplastic beta cells, like their normal counterparts, display distinctive, round granules that contain polygonal or rectangular dense crystals separated from the enclosing membrane by a distinct halo. It should be cautioned that granules may be present in the absence of clinically significant hormone activity.

Diffuse hyperplasia of the islets may be encountered in newborn infants of diabetic mothers. Prolonged exposure to maternal hyperglycemia seems to underlie the development of this lesion.

Figure 17-18 ■

Pancreatic islet cell tumor less than 1 cm in diameter in a focal area of pancreatic fibrosis. Despite the small size of the tumor, clinical hypoglycemia was present.

There are many other causes of hypoglycemia besides islet cell tumors. The differential diagnosis of this uncommon metabolic abnormality includes such conditions as insulin sensitivity, diffuse liver disease, inherited glycogenoses, and secretion of insulin-like growth factor 2 (IGF-2) by certain retroperitoneal fibromas and fibrosarcomas. Factitious hypoglycemia resulting from self-injection of insulin must also be kept in mind.

ZOLLINGER-ELLISON SYNDROME (GASTRINOMAS)

Marked hypersecretion of gastrin usually has its origin in gastrin-producing tumors *(gastrinomas),* which are just as likely to arise in the duodenum and peripancreatic tissues as in the pancreas. Zollinger and Ellison first called attention to the association of pancreatic islet cell lesions with hypersecretion of gastric acid and severe peptic ulceration. Ulcers are present in 90% to 95% of patients; the ratio of duodenal to gastric ulcers is 6:1 (Chapter 15).

MORPHOLOGY

Gastrinomas may arise in the pancreas, the peripancreatic region, or the wall of the duodenum. More than half of gastrin-producing tumors are locally invasive or already have metastasized at the time of diagnosis. In some instances, multiple gastrin-producing tumors are encountered in patients who have other endocrine tumors, thus conforming to multiple endocrine neoplasia I (Chapter 20). Like insulin-secreting tumors of the pancreas, gastrin-producing tumors are histologically bland and rarely exhibit marked anaplasia.

In the classic case of the Zollinger-Ellison syndrome, hypergastrinemia stimulates extreme gastric acid secretion, which in turn causes peptic ulceration. The duodenal and gastric ulcers, sometimes multiple, are identical to those found in the general population; they differ only in their intractability to usual therapies. In addition, ulcers may also occur in unusual locations such as the jejunum; whenever intractable jejunal ulcers are found, the Zollinger-Ellison syndrome should be considered. More than 50% of the patients have diarrhea, and in 30% it is the presenting symptom.

Treatment of the Zollinger-Ellison syndrome involves control of gastric acid secretion by use of proton pump inhibitors and excision of the neoplasm. Total resection of the neoplasm eliminates the syndrome. Patients with hepatic metastases have a significantly shortened life expectancy, with progressive tumor growth leading to liver failure usually within 10 years.

BIBLIOGRAPHY

Exocrine Pancreas

Bhatia M, et al: Inflammatory mediators in acute pancreatitis. J Pathol 190:117, 2000. (A discussion of the interplay between inflammatory mediators, inflammatory cells, and the pancreatic acinar cells.)
Durie PR: Pancreatitis mutations of the cystic fibrosis gene. N Engl J Med 339:687, 1998. (A concise editorial on the association between CFTR mutations and pancreatitis.)

Karne S, Gorelick FS: Etiopathogenesis of acute pancreatitis. Surg Clin North Am 79:699, 1999. (Presents the concepts of intracellular activation of acinar proenzymes.)
Steer ML: Recent insights into the etiology and pathogenesis of acute biliary pancreatitis. Am J Radiol 164:811, 1995. (A brief review of the role of gallstones in causing pancreatitis.)
Steer ML, et al: Chronic pancreatitis. N Engl J Med 332:1482, 1995. (A balanced overview of clinical and pathogenic aspects of chronic pancreatitis.)
Ulrich CD: Growth factors, receptors and molecular alterations in pancreatic cancer: putting it all together. Med Clin North Am 84:697, 2000. (A brief discussion of the current molecular studies of pancreatic carcinoma.)
Whitcomb DC: Genetic predispositions to acute and chronic pancreatitis. Med Clin North Am 84:531, 2000. (A thorough report on the mutations in trypsinogen causing hereditary pancreatitis.)

Endocrine Pancreas

Atkinson MA, Eisenbarth GS: Type I diabetes: new perspectives on disease pathogenesis and treatment. Lancet 358:221, 2001. (An excellent review of the genetic, environmental, and immunologic factors in the causation of type 1A diabetes.)
Benoist B, Mathis D: Autoimmunity provoked by infection. How good is the case for T cell epitope mimicry? Nat Immunol 2:797, 2001. (A detailed discussion of molecular mimicry versus bystander activation in the role of infections in causing autoimmune disease.)
Capella C, et al: Revised classification of neuroendocrine tumours of the lung, pancreas and gut. Virchows Arch 425:547, 1995. (A brief but sensible overview of current concepts regarding the pathobiology of the neuroendocrine system.)
Flier JS: The missing link with obesity? Nature 409:292, 2001. (A succinct description of molecular pathways that link obesity to insulin resistance.)
Goldfine AB: Type 2 diabetes: new drugs new perspectives. Hosp Pract Sep 15, 2001. (An excellent discussion of the pathogenesis of diabetes revealed by therapeutic drugs.)
Josh N, et al: Primary Care: infection in patients with diabetes mellitus. N Engl J Med 341:1906, 1999. (A very nice clinical review of infectious complications in diabetes.)
Ostenson C-G: The pathophysiology of type 2 diabetes mellitus: an overview. Acta Physiol Scand 171:241, 2001. (A good review of insulin deficiency and insulin resistance in type 2 diabetes.)
Polonsky S, et al: Non-insulin-dependent diabetes mellitus: a genetically programmed failure of the beta cell to compensate for insulin resistance. N Engl J Med 334:777, 1996. (An examination of the interplay between pathophysiology and genetics in type 2 diabetes mellitus.)
Polonsky KS, Semenkovich CF: The pancreatic β cell heats up: UCP2 and insulin secretion in diabetes. Cell 105:705, 2001. (A molecular explanation for reduced insulin synthesis in type 2 diabetes.)
Porte D Jr, Kahn SE: β cell dysfunction and failure in type 2 diabetes: potential mechanisms. Diabetes 50(Suppl 1) S160, 2001. (A discussion of β-cell dysfunction and the role of amylin in type 2 diabetes.)
Rocchini AP: Childhood obesity and a diabetes epidemic. N Engl J Med 346:854, 2002. (An editorial that discusses the diabetes epidemic in obese children.)
Schuit FC, et al: Glucose sensing in pancreatic beta-cells. A model for the study of other glucose-regulated cells in gut, pancreas, and hypothalamus. Diabetes 50:1, 2001. (Summarizes the physiology of insulin and glucose receptor function in the pancreatic beta cell.)
Saltiel AR: New perspectives into the molecular pathogenesis of type 2 diabetes. Cell 104:517, 2001. (A scholarly review of the modern understanding of molecular pathways affected in type 2 diabetes.)
Schwartz MW, Kahn SE: Insulin resistance and obesity. Nature 402:860, 1999. (A discussion of the PPAR-γ receptor, insulin resistance, and obesity.)
Shuldiner AR, Yang R, Gong D: Resistin, obesity, and insulin resistance— the emerging role of the adipocyte as an endocrine organ. N Engl J Med 345:1345, 2001. (A concise review of the role of resistin and leptin in type 2 diabetes and obesity.)
Trudeau JD, et al: Neonatal beta-cell apoptosis: A trigger for autoimmune diabetes? Diabetes 49:1, 2000. (A review of beta cell injury as it pertains to autoimmunity.)
Undlien DE, Benedicte AL, Thorsby E: HLA complex genes in type 1 diabetes and other autoimmune diseases. Which genes are involved? Trends Genet 17:93, 2001. (A detailed review of MHC-linked genes and susceptibility to type 1A diabetes.)

18

The Male Genital System

DENNIS K. BURNS, MD

Disorders of the male genital system include a variety of malformations, inflammatory conditions, and neoplasms involving the penis and scrotum, prostate, and testes. In this chapter, the major anatomic subdivisions of the male genital system are considered individually, because many of the diseases discussed tend to involve the various organs in a fairly selective fashion. The major exception to this anatomic grouping is the discussion of sexually transmitted diseases (STDs), which are described separately because of their frequent multisystem involvement. Because of many similarities in their presentations in both sexes, the manifestations of selected STDs in females are also considered in this chapter.

PENIS

The penis may be affected by many congenital and acquired disorders. Only the most common malformations, inflammatory conditions, and neoplasms are considered here. Of the inflammatory disorders affecting the penis, a significant number represent STDs, which are discussed later in the chapter.

Malformations

The most common malformations of the penis include abnormalities in the location of the distal urethral orifice, termed *hypospadias* and *epispadias*. *Hypospadias*, the more common of the two lesions, designates an abnormal opening of the urethra along the ventral aspect of the penis. The urethral orifice, which may lie anywhere along the shaft of the penis, is sometimes constricted, resulting in urinary tract obstruction and an increased risk of urinary tract infections. The abnormality occurs in approximately 1 in 300 live male births and may be associated with other genital anomalies, including inguinal hernias and undescended testes. The term *epispadias* indicates the presence of the urethral orifice on the dorsal aspect of the penis. Like hypospadias, epispadias may produce lower urinary tract obstruction; in other cases, the condition may result in urinary incontinence.

Inflammatory Lesions

A significant number of inflammatory conditions of the penis are caused by STDs. Local inflammatory processes unrelated to STDs may also involve the penis. In addition, a number of other systemic inflammatory diseases may, on occasion, produce penile lesions.

The terms *balanitis* and *balanoposthitis* refer to local inflammation of the glans penis, or of the glans penis and the overlying prepuce, respectively. Most cases occur as a consequence of poor local hygiene in uncircumcised males, with accumulations of desquamated epithelial cells, sweat, and debris, termed *smegma*, acting as a local irritant. In such cases, the distal penis is typically red, swollen, and tender; a purulent discharge may be present. *Phimosis* represents a condition in which the prepuce cannot be retracted easily over the glans penis. Although phimosis may occur as a congenital anomaly, most cases are acquired from scarring of the prepuce secondary to previous episodes of balanoposthitis. Regardless of its origin, most cases of phimosis are accompanied by evidence of ongoing distal penile inflammation. When a stenotic prepuce is forcibly retracted over the glans penis, the circulation to the glans may be compromised, with resultant congestion, swelling, and pain of the distal penis, a condition known as *paraphimosis*. Urinary retention may develop in severe cases.

Fungi may infect the skin of the penis and scrotum, because growth of fungi is favored by warm, moist conditions at this site and poor local hygiene. *Genital candidiasis* may occur in otherwise normal individuals, but it is particularly common in patients with diabetes mellitus. Candidiasis typically presents as an erosive, painful, intensely pruritic lesion involving the glans penis, scrotum, and adjacent intertriginous areas. Scrapings or biopsy specimens of the lesions yield characteristic budding yeast forms and pseudohyphae within the superficial epidermis.

Neoplasms

Most neoplasms of the penis originate from squamous epithelium. Squamous cell carcinomas of the penis are relatively uncommon, accounting for about 0.25% of all cancers in males in the United States. Most cases occur in uncircumcised patients older than 40 years of age. A number of factors have been implicated in the pathogenesis of squamous cell carcinoma of the penis, including poor hygiene, with resultant exposure to potential carcinogens in smegma, and infection with certain subtypes of human papillomavirus (HPV), particularly types 16 and 18. Exposure to environmental irritants, such as coal tar and soot, has long been recognized as an important factor in the development of squamous carcinomas of the scrotum but has not been implicated in the development of penile cancer.

As with squamous cell carcinomas at other sites, carcinomas of the penis are generally preceded by the appearance of malignant cells confined to the epidermis, termed *carcinoma in situ*. Three major variants of carcinoma in situ, all strongly associated with infection by various HPV strains, occur on the penis. *Bowen disease* is one of the more common forms of carcinoma in situ at this site, where it appears grossly as a solitary, plaquelike lesion on the shaft of the penis. Histologic examination reveals morphologically malignant cells within the epidermis with no invasion of the underlying stroma (Fig. 18–1). Bowen disease is not unique to the penis but may also occur on other mucosal surfaces, including the vulva and oral mucosa. Its major clinical importance lies in the potential for progression to invasive squamous cell carcinoma, a complication estimated to occur in 10% of cases. Bowen disease has also been associated with an increased incidence of visceral malignancies. Other variants of carcinoma in situ include *erythroplasia of Queyrat*, which occurs as an erythematous patch on the glans penis and other mucosal surfaces, and *bowenoid papulosis*, a venereally transmitted viral lesion involving the penile shaft.

Figure 18–1 ■

Bowen disease (carcinoma in situ) of the penis. Note the intact basement membrane and hyperchromatic, dysplastic epithelial cells with scattered mitoses above the basal layer. (Courtesy of Dr. Jag Bhawan, Boston University School of Medicine, Boston.)

Figure 18-2   ■

Carcinoma of the penis. The glans penis is deformed by a firm, ulcerated, infiltrative mass. (Courtesy of Dr. Kyle Molberg, Department of Pathology, University of Texas Southwestern Medical Center, Dallas.)

Squamous cell carcinoma of the penis appears as a gray, crusted, papular lesion, most commonly on the glans penis or prepuce. In many cases, the carcinoma infiltrates the underlying connective tissue to produce an indurated, ulcerated lesion with irregular margins (Fig. 18-2). In other cases, particularly the so-called *verrucous carcinomas*, the tumor may grow in a predominantly papillary pattern. The histologic appearance is usually that of an invasive squamous cell carcinoma with ragged, infiltrating margins, indistinguishable from squamous carcinomas in other sites. Verrucous carcinomas are characterized by less striking cytologic atypia and bulbous, rounded, deep margins. Most cases of squamous cell carcinoma of the penis are indolent, locally infiltrative lesions. Regional metastases are present in the inguinal lymph nodes in approximately 25% of patients at the time of diagnosis. Distant metastases are relatively uncommon. The overall 5-year survival rate averages 70%.

SCROTUM, TESTIS, AND EPIDIDYMIS

The skin of the scrotum may be affected by a number of inflammatory processes, including local fungal infections and systemic dermatoses. Neoplasms of the scrotal sac are unusual. *Squamous cell carcinoma*, the most common of these, is of historical interest in that it represents the first human malignancy associated with environmental factors, dating from Pott's observation of a high incidence of the disease in chimney sweeps. A number of disorders unrelated to the testes and epididymis may also present as scrotal enlargement. *Hydrocele*, the most common cause of scrotal enlargement, is an accumulation of serous fluid within the tunica vaginalis. It may arise in response to neighboring infections or tumors, or it may be idiopathic.

Accumulations of blood or lymphatic fluid within the tunica vaginalis, termed *hematoceles* and *chyloceles*, respectively, may also cause testicular enlargement. In extreme cases of lymphatic obstruction, caused, for example, by filariasis, the scrotum and the lower extremities may enlarge to grotesque proportions, a condition termed *elephantiasis*.

The more important disorders of the scrotum involve the testes and their adnexal structures. Testicular diseases may be congenital, inflammatory, or neoplastic. They may manifest themselves in a variety of ways, including infertility, atrophy, enlargement, and local pain. The distinctions between many of these conditions based on physical examination alone, particularly those associated with testicular enlargement, can be exceedingly difficult.

Cryptorchidism and Testicular Atrophy

Cryptorchidism represents *failure of testicular descent* into the scrotum. Normally, the testes descend from the coelomic cavity into the pelvis by the third month of gestation and then through the inguinal canals into the scrotum during the last 2 months of intrauterine life. The diagnosis of cryptorchidism is difficult to establish with certainty before 1 year of age, particularly in premature infants, because complete testicular descent into the scrotum is not invariably present at birth. A number of factors, including hormonal abnormalities, intrinsic testicular abnormalities, and mechanical problems (e.g., obstruction of the inguinal canal), may interfere with this normal descent, resulting in malpositioning of the gonad anywhere along its migration pathway. Cryptorchidism is a common feature of a number of congenital syndromes, such as the Prader-Willi syndrome (Chapter 7). In the vast majority of cases, however, the cause of the cryptorchidism is unknown. Cryptorchidism occurs in 0.7% to 0.8% of the male population.

MORPHOLOGY

Cryptorchidism involves the right testis somewhat more commonly than the left. In 25% of cases, the condition is bilateral. The cryptorchid testis may be of normal size early in life, although some degree of atrophy is usually present by the time of puberty. Microscopic evidence of tubular atrophy is evident by 5 to 6 years of age, and hyalinization is present by the time of puberty. Loss of tubules is usually accompanied by hyperplasia of interstitial (Leydig) cells. Foci of **intratubular germ cell neoplasia** (discussed later) may be present in cryptorchid testes and may be the source of subsequent tumors developing in these organs. Atrophic changes similar to those seen in cryptorchid testes may be caused by a number of other conditions, including chronic ischemia, trauma, radiation, antineoplastic chemotherapy, and conditions associated with chronic elevation in estrogen levels (e.g., cirrhosis). Intratubular germ cell neoplasia is not a feature of these latter conditions, however.

Not surprisingly, bilateral cryptorchidism causes sterility. Unilateral cryptorchidism may be associated with atrophy of the contralateral descended gonad and therefore may also lead to sterility. In addition to infertility, failure of descent is also associated with at least a four-fold increased risk of *testicular malignancy*. Patients with unilateral cryptorchidism are also at increased risk for the development of cancer in the contralateral, normally descended testis, suggesting that some intrinsic abnormality, rather than simple failure of descent, may be responsible for the increased cancer risk. Surgical placement of the undescended testis into the scrotum (orchiopexy) before puberty may decrease the likelihood of atrophy but does not guarantee fertility. The effect of orchiopexy on the risk of testicular cancer remains somewhat controversial. Most evidence suggests that patients remain at some increased risk after orchiopexy.

Inflammatory Lesions

Inflammatory lesions of the testis are more common in the epididymis than in the testis proper. Some of the more important inflammatory diseases of the testis are associated with venereal disease and are discussed later in this chapter. Other causes of testicular inflammation include nonspecific epididymitis and orchitis, mumps, and tuberculosis. *Nonspecific epididymitis* and *orchitis* usually begin as a primary urinary tract infection with secondary ascending infection of the testis through the vas deferens or lymphatics of the spermatic cord. The involved testis is typically swollen and tender and contains a predominantly neutrophilic inflammatory infiltrate. Orchitis complicates *mumps infection* in roughly 20% of adult males but rarely occurs in children. The affected testis is edematous and congested and contains a predominantly lymphoplasmacytic inflammatory infiltrate. Severe cases may be associated with considerable loss of seminiferous epithelium with resultant tubular atrophy, fibrosis, and sterility. A number of conditions, including infections and autoimmune injury, may elicit a granulomatous inflammatory reaction in the testis. Of these, *tuberculosis* is the most common. Testicular tuberculosis generally begins as an epididymitis, with secondary involvement of the testis. The histologic changes include a granulomatous inflammatory reaction and caseous necrosis, identical to that seen in active tuberculosis in other sites.

Testicular Neoplasms

Testicular neoplasms are the most important cause of firm, painless enlargement of the testis. Such neoplasms occur in roughly 2 per 100,000 males, with a peak incidence between the ages of 15 and 34 years. Tumors of the testis represent a heterogeneous group of neoplasms, 95% of which arise from germ cells. Virtually all of the latter group are malignant. Neoplasms derived from Sertoli or Leydig cells (or both) are uncommon and, in contrast to tumors of germ-cell origin, usually pursue a benign clinical course. The non–germ-cell tumors may come to attention because of their ability to synthesize and secrete steroid hormones, with resultant endocrine abnormalities.

The cause of testicular neoplasms remains unknown. As noted previously, *cryptorchidism is associated with at least a four-fold increase in the risk of cancer* in the undescended testis, as well as an increased risk of cancer in the contralateral descended testis. A history of cryptorchidism is present in approximately 10% of cases of testicular cancer. Syndromes characterized by *testicular dysgenesis*, including testicular feminization and Klinefelter syndrome, are also associated with an increased frequency of testicular cancer. Cytogenetic studies have identified a wide range of abnormalities in testicular germ cell neoplasms, the most common of which is an isochromosome of the short arm of chromosome 12. However, the role of these chromosomal aberrations in the pathogenesis of testicular neoplasms remains unclear. The risk of neoplasia is increased in siblings of patients with testicular cancers, although no consistent hereditary genetic abnormalities have been identified to account for this increased risk. The development of cancer in one testis is associated with a markedly increased risk of neoplasia in the contralateral testis. Testicular tumors are more common in whites than in blacks.

Classification and Histogenesis. A number of different classification schemes have been proposed for testicular neoplasms, based on the histologic features of the tumors and on differing theories about their histogenesis. The World Health Organization (WHO) classification is the most widely used in the United States (Table 18–1). In this schema, germ-cell tumors of the testis are divided into two broad categories, based on whether they contain a single histologic pattern (40% of cases) or multiple histologic patterns (60% of cases). This classification is based on the view that germ cell tumors of the testis arise from primitive cells that may either differentiate along gonadal lines to produce *seminomas* or transform into a totipotential cell population, giving rise to *nonseminomatous germ cell tumors*. Such totipotential cells may remain largely undifferentiated to form *embryonal carcinomas*, may differentiate along extraembryonic lines to form *yolk sac tumors* and *choriocarcinomas*, or may differentiate along somatic cell lines to produce *teratomas*. This proposed histogenesis is supported by the high frequency of mixed histologic patterns among nonseminomatous germ cell tumors. The histologic variants of testicular germ cell neoplasms are listed in Table 18–1. The morphology of the more common forms is presented below, along with a discussion of some of their more salient clinical features.

■

Table 18–1. SIMPLIFIED CLASSIFICATION OF TESTICULAR GERM-CELL TUMORS

Tumors with one histologic pattern
  Seminoma
  Embryonal carcinoma
  Yolk sac tumor
  Choriocarcinoma
  Teratomas
    Mature
    Immature
    With malignant transformation of somatic elements
Tumors with more than one histologic pattern
Miscellaneous rare variants

It is now widely believed that most testicular tumors arise from in situ lesions characterized as *intratubular germ cell neoplasms.* This lesion is present in conditions associated with a high risk of developing germ-cell tumors (e.g., cryptorchidism, dysgenetic testes). Furthermore, foci of such in situ lesions are seen in testicular tissue adjacent to a testicular tumor in 90% of cases.

MORPHOLOGY

Seminomas, sometimes referred to as "classic" seminomas to distinguish them from the less common spermatocytic seminoma discussed below, account for about 50% of testicular germ-cell neoplasms. They are histologically identical to ovarian dysgerminomas and to germinomas occurring in the central nervous system and other extragonadal sites. Seminomas are large, soft, well-demarcated, usually homogeneous, gray-white tumors that bulge from the cut surface of the affected testis (Fig. 18-3). The neoplasms are typically confined to the testis by an intact tunica albuginea. Large tumors may contain foci of coagulation necrosis, but usually there is no hemorrhage. The presence of hemorrhage should prompt careful scrutiny for an associated nonseminomatous germ-cell component to the tumor. Microscopically, seminomas are composed of **large cells with distinct cell borders, clear, glycogen-rich cytoplasm, and round nuclei with conspicuous nucleoli** (Fig. 18-4). The cells are often arrayed in small lobules with intervening fibrous septa. A lymphocytic infiltrate is usually present and may, on occasion, overshadow the neoplastic cells. A granulomatous inflammatory reaction may also be present. In 7% to 24% of cases, syncytiotrophoblast-like giant cells that stain positively for human chorionic gonadotropin (hCG) may be seen; they are presumably the source of the elevated serum hCG levels that may be encountered in some patients with pure seminoma.

Figure 18-4   ■

Seminoma of the testis. Microscopic examination reveals large cells with distinct cell borders, pale nuclei, prominent nucleoli, and a sparse lymphocytic infiltrate.

Another, less common, morphologic variant of seminoma is the so-called **spermatocytic seminoma.** These tumors, which tend to occur in older patients than do classic seminomas, contain a mixture of medium-sized cells, large uninucleate or multinucleate tumor cells, and small cells with round nuclei that are reminiscent of secondary spermatocytes. Metastases are exceedingly rare, in contrast to the situation with classic seminoma.

Embryonal carcinomas are ill-defined, invasive masses containing foci of hemorrhage and necrosis (Fig. 18-5). The primary lesions may be small, even in patients with systemic metastases. Larger lesions may invade the epididymis and spermatic cord. The constituent cells are **large and primitive looking, with basophilic cytoplasm, indistinct cell borders, and large nuclei with**

Figure 18-3   ■

Seminoma of the testis appears as a fairly well circumscribed, pale, fleshy, homogeneous mass.

Figure 18-5   ■

Embryonal carcinoma. In contrast to the seminoma illustrated in Figure 18-3, the embryonal carcinoma is a bulky, hemorrhagic mass. (Courtesy of Dr. Kyle Molberg, Department of Pathology, University of Texas Southwestern Medical Center, Dallas.)

Figure 18-6   ■

Embryonal carcinoma. Microscopic examination reveals primitive hyperchromatic cells that form sheets and occasional glands. (Courtesy of Dr. Trace Worrell, Department of Pathology, University of Texas Southwestern Medical Center, Dallas.)

prominent nucleoli. The neoplastic cells may be arrayed in undifferentiated, solid sheets or may, in other cases, contain glandular structures and irregular papillae (Fig. 18-6). In most cases other patterns of germ-cell neoplasia (e.g., yolk sac carcinoma, teratoma, choriocarcinoma) are admixed with the embryonal areas. Pure embryonal carcinomas comprise 2% to 3% of all testicular germ-cell tumors. As with other germ-cell tumors of the testes, foci of intratubular germ-cell neoplasia are frequently present in the adjacent seminiferous tubules.

Yolk sac tumors, also termed **endodermal sinus tumors,** are the most common primary testicular neoplasm in children younger than 3 years of age. In adults, yolk sac tumors are most often seen admixed with embryonal carcinoma. In the histogenetic scheme noted previously, yolk sac tumors represent **endodermal sinus** differentiation of totipotential neoplastic cells. Grossly, these tumors are typically large and may be well demarcated. Histologic examination discloses low cuboidal to columnar epithelial cells forming sheets, glands, papillae, and microcysts, often associated with eosinophilic hyaline globules (Fig. 18-7). A distinctive feature is the presence of structures resembling primitive glomeruli, the so-called **Schiller-Duvall bodies.** α-Fetoprotein can be demonstrated within the cytoplasm of the neoplastic cells by immunohistochemical techniques.

Choriocarcinomas represent differentiation of pluripotential neoplastic germ cells along **trophoblastic** lines. Grossly, the primary tumors are often small, nonpalpable lesions, even if there are extensive systemic metastases. Microscopically, choriocarcinomas are composed of sheets of small cuboidal cells irregularly intermingled with or capped by large, eosinophilic syncytial cells containing multiple dark, pleomorphic nuclei; these represent **cytotrophoblastic** and **syncytiotrophoblastic** differentiation, respectively (Fig. 18-8). Well-formed placental villi are not seen. The hormone hCG can be identified with appropriate immunohistochemical staining, particularly within the cytoplasm of the syncytiotrophoblastic elements.

Teratomas represent differentiation of neoplastic germ cells along **somatic** cell lines. Teratomas are firm masses that on cut surface often contain cysts and recognizable areas of cartilage. Histologically, three major variants of pure teratoma are recognized. **Mature teratomas** contain fully differentiated tissues from one or more germ-cell layers (e.g., neural tissue, cartilage, adipose tissue, bone, epithelium) in a haphazard array (Fig. 18-9).

Figure 18-7   ■

Yolk sac carcinoma. A, Low-power photomicrograph demonstrating areas of loosely textured, microcystic tissue and a papillary structure resembling a developing glomerulus. B, Higher-power photomicrograph demonstrating characteristic hyaline droplets within the microcystic areas of the tumor. α-Fetoprotein is present within the droplets.

Figure 18-8   ■

Choriocarcinoma. The tumor contains both cytotrophoblastic elements, with clear cytoplasm and central nuclei, and syncytiotrophoblastic cells, with multiple nuclei and abundant eosinophilic cytoplasm. Such cells elaborate human chorionic gonadotropin, which is detectable in the serum. (Courtesy of Dr. Trace Worrell, Department of Pathology, University of Texas Southwestern Medical Center, Dallas.)

Immature teratomas, in contrast, contain immature somatic elements reminiscent of those in developing fetal tissue. **Teratomas with malignant transformation** are characterized by the development of frank malignancy in preexisting teratomatous elements, usually in the form of a squamous cell carcinoma or adenocarcinoma. Most cases of malignant teratomas occur in adults; pure teratomas in prepubertal males are usually benign. As with other forms of germ-cell neoplasia, testicular teratomas in adults are often associated with the presence of other germ-cell elements. All testicular teratomas in adults therefore should be regarded as malignant neoplasms.

Mixed germ-cell tumors, as noted, account for approximately 60% of all testicular germ-cell neoplasms. Combinations of any of the described patterns may occur in mixed tumors, the most common of which is a combination of teratoma, embryonal carcinoma, and yolk sac tumors.

Figure 18-9   ■

Teratoma. Testicular teratomas contain mature cells from endodermal, mesodermal, and ectodermal lines. Pictured here are four different fields from the same tumor containing neural (ectodermal) *(A)*, glandular (endodermal) *(B)*, cartilaginous (mesodermal) *(C)*, and squamous epithelial *(D)* elements.

Table 18-2. SUMMARY OF TESTICULAR-TUMORS

Tumor	Peak Age (yr)	Morphology	Tumor Markers
Seminoma	40–50	Sheets of uniform polygonal cells with cleared cytoplasm; lymphocytes in the stroma	10% have elevated hCG
Embryonal carcinoma	20–30	Poorly differentiated, pleomorphic cells in cords, sheets, or papillary formation; most contain some yolk sac and choriocarcinoma cells	90% have elevated hCG or AFP or both
Yolk sac tumor	3	Poorly differentiated endothelium-like, cuboidal, or columnar cells	100% have elevated AFP
Choriocarcinoma (pure)	20–30	Cytotrophoblast and syncytiotrophoblast without villus formation	100% have elevated hCG
Teratoma	All ages	Tissues from all three germ-cell layers with varying degrees of differentiation	50% have elevated hCG or AFP or both
Mixed tumor	15–30	Variable, depending on mixture; commonly teratoma and embryonal carcinoma	90% have elevated hCG and AFP

AFP, α-fetoprotein; hCG, human chorionic gonadatropin.

Clinical Features. Patients with testicular germ-cell neoplasms present most frequently with *painless enlargement of the testis.* However, some tumors, especially nonseminomatous germ-cell neoplasms, may have widespread metastases at diagnosis, in the absence of a palpable testicular lesion. *Seminomas often remain confined to the testis* for prolonged intervals and may reach considerable size before diagnosis. Metastases are most commonly encountered in the iliac and para-aortic lymph nodes, particularly in the upper lumbar region. Hematogenous metastases are unusual. In contrast, *nonseminomatous germ-cell neoplasms tend to metastasize earlier,* by both lymphatic and hematogenous routes. Hematogenous metastases are most common in the liver and lungs. Metastatic lesions may be histologically identical to the primary testicular tumor, or they may contain other germ-cell elements. Testicular germ-cell neoplasms are staged by a variety of imaging techniques and studies of tumor markers as follows:

Stage I: Tumor confined to the testis

Stage II: Metastases confined to retroperitoneal nodes below the level of the diaphragm

Stage III: Metastases beyond retroperitoneal lymph nodes

Assay of *tumor markers* secreted by tumor cells is important in the clinical evaluation of germ-cell neoplasms. hCG, produced by neoplastic syncytiotrophoblastic cells, is always elevated in patients with choriocarcinoma. As noted, other germ-cell tumors, including seminoma, may also contain syncytiotrophoblastic cells without cytotrophoblastic elements and hence may elaborate hCG. Approximately 10% of seminomas elaborate hCG. α-Fetoprotein (AFP) is a glycoprotein normally synthesized by the fetal yolk sac and several other fetal tissues. Nonseminomatous germ-cell tumors containing elements of yolk sac (endodermal sinus) often produce AFP; in contrast to hCG, the presence of AFP is a reliable indicator of the presence of a nonseminomatous component to the germ-cell neoplasm, because yolk sac elements are not found in seminomas. Because mixed patterns are common, most nonseminomatous tumors have elevations of both hCG and AFP. In addition to their role in the primary diagnosis of

testicular germ-cell tumors, serial determinations of hCG and AFP are useful for monitoring patients for persistent or recurrent tumor after therapy. It should be noted, however, that AFP is also elevated in liver cancer (Chapter 16.)

The treatment of testicular germ-cell neoplasms is considered a success story of chemotherapy. Although 7000 to 8000 new cases of testicular cancer occur in the United States yearly, only 400 men are expected to die of the disease. The treatment is determined by both the histologic pattern of the tumor and the stage of disease at the time of diagnosis. Seminomas are exquisitely radiosensitive, and they also respond well to chemotherapy. The prognosis of many nonseminomatous germ-cell tumors has improved dramatically with the introduction of platinum-based chemotherapy regimens. Table 18–2 summarizes salient features of testicular tumors.

PROSTATE

The most important categories of prostatic disease are inflammatory lesions (prostatitis), nodular hyperplasia, and carcinoma.

Prostatitis

Prostatitis, or clinically apparent inflammation of the prostate, may be acute or chronic. The classification of prostatitis is based on a combination of clinical features, microscopic examination, and, in selected cases, culture of fractionated urine specimens obtained before and after prostatic massage. *Acute bacterial prostatitis* is caused by the same organisms associated with other acute urinary tract infections, particularly *Escherichia coli* and other gram-negative rods. Most patients with acute prostatitis have concomitant infection of the urethra and urinary bladder (acute urethrocystitis). In these cases, organisms may reach the prostate by direct extension from the urethra or urinary bladder or by vascular channels from more distant sites.

Chronic prostatitis may follow obvious episodes of acute prostatitis, or it may develop insidiously, without previous episodes of acute infection. In some cases of chronic prostatitis, bacteria similar to those responsible for acute bacterial prostatitis can be isolated. Such cases are designated as *chronic bacterial prostatitis.* In other instances, the presence of an increased number of leukocytes in prostatic secretions attests to prostatic inflammation, but bacteriologic findings are negative. Such cases, termed *chronic abacterial prostatitis,* or prostatodynia, account for most cases of chronic prostatitis. A number of nonbacterial agents implicated in the pathogenesis of nongonococcal urethritis, including *Chlamydia trachomatis* and *Ureaplasma urealyticum,* have also been suggested as possible causes of chronic abacterial prostatitis.

> ### *MORPHOLOGY*
>
> **Acute prostatitis** is characterized by the presence of an acute, neutrophilic inflammatory infiltrate, congestion, and stromal edema. Neutrophils are initially most conspicuous within the prostatic glands. As the infection progresses, the inflammatory infiltrate destroys glandular epithelium and extends into the surrounding stroma, resulting in the formation of microabscesses. Grossly visible abscesses are uncommon but may develop with extensive tissue destruction, as may occur in diabetic patients.
>
> The histologic features of **chronic prostatitis** are nonspecific in most cases and include a variable amount of lymphoid infiltrate, evidence of glandular injury, and, frequently, concomitant acute inflammatory changes. Evidence of tissue destruction and fibroblastic proliferation, along with the presence of other inflammatory cells, such as neutrophils, is required for a histologic diagnosis of chronic prostatitis. Isolated lymphoid aggregates occur commonly with advancing age and are not, by themselves, sufficient for a diagnosis of chronic prostatitis.
>
> A special morphologic variant of chronic prostatitis, **granulomatous prostatitis,** deserves special mention. Granulomatous prostatitis is not a single disease but is, rather, a morphologic reaction to a variety of different insults. Granulomatous inflammation may be encountered in the prostate in patients with systemic inflammatory processes associated with granulomatous inflammation (e.g., disseminated tuberculosis, sarcoidosis, fungal infections, Wegener granulomatosis). It may also occur as a nonspecific reaction to inspissated prostatic secretions and after transurethral resection of prostatic tissue. The morphologic features of granulomatous prostatitis include multinucleate giant cells and variable numbers of foamy histiocytes, sometimes accompanied by eosinophils. Caseous necrosis is a feature of tuberculous prostatitis. It is not seen in other forms of granulomatous prostatitis.

Clinical Features. The clinical manifestations of prostatitis include *dysuria, urinary frequency, lower back pain,* and poorly localized suprapubic or pelvic pain. The prostate may be enlarged and tender, particularly in acute prostatitis, in which local symptoms are often accompanied by fever and leukocytosis. Chronic prostatitis, even if asymptomatic, may serve as a reservoir for organisms capable of causing urinary tract infections. Chronic bacterial prostatitis, therefore, is one of the most important causes of recurrent urinary tract infection in men.

Nodular Hyperplasia of the Prostate

The normal prostate consists of glandular and stromal elements surrounding the urethra. The prostatic parenchyma can be divided into several biologically distinct regions, the most important of which are the peripheral, central, transitional, and periurethral zones (Fig. 18–10). The types of proliferative lesions are different in each region. For example, most *hyperplastic* lesions arise in the inner transitional and central zones of the prostate, while most *carcinomas* (70% to 80%) arise in the peripheral zones.

Nodular hyperplasia, also termed *glandular and stromal hyperplasia,* is an extremely common abnormality of the prostate. It is present in a significant number of men by the age of 40, and its frequency rises progressively with age, reaching 90% by the eighth decade. Prostatic hyperplasia is

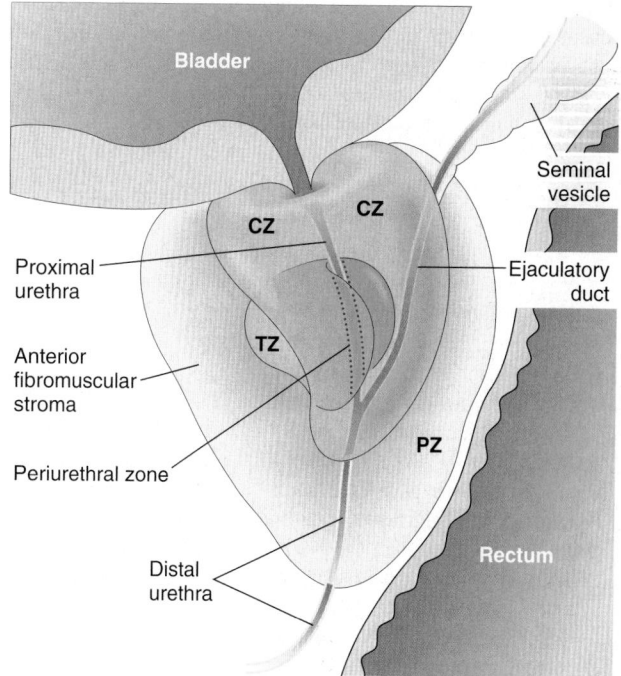

Figure 18–10   ■

Adult prostate. The normal prostate contains several distinct regions, including a central zone (CZ), a peripheral zone (PZ), a transitional zone (TZ), and a periurethral zone. Most carcinomas arise from the peripheral glands of the organ and are often palpable during digital examination of the rectum. Nodular hyperplasia, in contrast, arises from more centrally situated glands and is more likely to produce urinary obstruction early on than is carcinoma.

characterized by proliferation of both epithelial and stromal elements, with resultant enlargement of the gland and, in some cases, urinary obstruction. "Benign prostatic hypertrophy" (BPH), a time-honored synonym for nodular hyperplasia of the prostate, is both redundant and a misnomer, because all hypertrophies are benign and the fundamental lesion is a hyperplasia rather than a hypertrophy.

Although the cause of nodular hyperplasia remains incompletely understood, current evidence indicates that *androgens and estrogens play a synergistic role in its development*. It is clear that an intact testis is necessary for the development of nodular hyperplasia. Nodular hyperplasia does not occur in males castrated before the onset of puberty, in keeping with a central role for androgens in its pathogenesis. Dihydrotestosterone (DHT), an androgen derived from testosterone through the action of 5α-reductase, and its metabolite, 3α-androstanediol, appear to be the major hormonal stimuli for glandular and stromal proliferation in patients with nodular hyperplasia. DHT binds to nuclear receptors and, in turn, stimulates synthesis of DNA, RNA, growth factors, and other cytoplasmic proteins, leading to hyperplasia. This forms the basis for the current use of 5α-reductase inhibitors in the treatment of symptomatic nodular hyperplasia. Paradoxically, however, nodular hyperplasia of the prostate becomes clinically manifest in older men, at a time when testosterone levels are either stable or have begun to decline. Moreover, the administration of testosterone does not exacerbate preexisting nodular hyperplasia. These observations suggest that factors other than androgenic activity must also be considered in the pathogenesis of this condition. Experimental work suggests that age-related increases in estrogen levels may contribute to the development of nodular hyperplasia, by increasing the expression of DHT receptors on prostatic parenchymal cells and thereby enhancing the effects of DHT.

glandular elements and fibromuscular stroma. The hyperplastic glands are lined by tall, columnar epithelial cells and a peripheral layer of flattened basal cells; crowding of the proliferating epithelium results in the formation of papillary projections in some glands (Fig. 18-12). The glandular lumina often contain inspissated, proteinaceous secretory material, termed **corpora amylacea.** The glands are surrounded by proliferating stromal elements; although it is scanty in some cases, stroma is always present between the hyperplastic glands, in contrast to carcinomas (discussed later). Other nodules are composed predominantly of spindle-shaped stromal cells and connective tissue. Areas of infarction are fairly common in advanced cases of nodular hyperplasia and are frequently accompanied by foci of squamous metaplasia in adjacent glands.

Clinical Features. Clinical manifestations of prostatic hyperplasia occur in only about 10% of men with the disease. Because nodular hyperplasia preferentially involves the inner portions of the prostate, its most common manifestations are those of *lower urinary tract obstruction*. These include difficulty in starting the stream of urine (hesitancy) and intermittent interruption of the urinary stream while voiding. In some patients complete urinary obstruction may occur, with resultant painful distention of the bladder and, on occasion, hydronephrosis (Chapter 14). Symptoms of obstruction are frequently accompanied by urinary urgency, frequency, and nocturia, all indicative of bladder irritation. The combination of residual urine in the bladder and chronic obstruction increases the risk of urinary tract infections.

MORPHOLOGY

As noted, nodular hyperplasia arises most commonly in the inner, periurethral glands of the prostate, particularly from those that lie above the verumontanum. The affected prostate is enlarged, with weights in excess of 300 g reported in severe cases. The cut surface contains multiple, fairly well circumscribed nodules, which bulge from the cut surface (Fig. 18-11). This nodularity may be present throughout the prostate, but it is **usually most pronounced in the inner (central and transitional) region.** The nodules may have a solid appearance, or they may contain cystic spaces, the latter corresponding to dilated glandular elements seen in histologic sections. The urethra is usually compressed by the hyperplastic nodules, often to a slitlike orifice. In some cases, hyperplastic glandular and stromal elements lying just under the epithelium of the proximal prostatic urethra may project into the bladder lumen as a pedunculated mass, resulting in a ball-valve type of urethral obstruction.

Microscopically, the hyperplastic nodules are composed of varying proportions of proliferating

Figure 18-11 ■

Nodular hyperplasia of the prostate. Well-defined nodules bulge from the cut surface. The proximity of the nodules to the urethra accounts for the urinary obstruction associated with this lesion.

Figure 18-12   ■

Nodular hyperplasia. *A,* Low-power photomicrograph demonstrates a well-demarcated nodule at the top of the field, populated by hyperplastic glands. *B,* Higher-power photomicrograph demonstrates the morphology of the hyperplastic glands, with a characteristic inner columnar and outer cuboidal cell layer. In other cases of nodular hyperplasia, the nodularity is caused predominantly by stromal, rather than glandular, proliferation.

Carcinoma of the Prostate

Carcinoma of the prostate is the most common visceral cancer in males, ranking as the second most common cause of cancer-related deaths in men older than 50 years of age, after carcinoma of the lung. It is predominantly a disease of older males, with a peak incidence between the ages of 65 and 75 years. Latent cancers of the prostate are even more common than those that are clinically apparent, with an overall frequency of more than 50% in men older than 80 years of age.

Although the cause of carcinoma of the prostate remains unknown, clinical and experimental observations suggest that hormonal, genetic, and environmental factors may all play a role in its pathogenesis. Cancer of the prostate does not develop in males castrated before puberty, indicating that *androgens* likely play a part in its development. A hormonal influence is further suggested by the fact that the growth of many carcinomas of the prostate can be inhibited by orchiectomy or by the administration of estrogens such as diethylstilbestrol. As in the case of nodular hyperplasia of the prostate, however, the role played by hormones in the pathogenesis of carcinoma of the prostate is not fully understood.

Genetic factors have also been implicated, based on the increased risk of disease among first-degree relatives of patients with prostate cancer. Symptomatic carcinoma of the prostate is more common and occurs at an earlier age in American blacks than in whites, Asians, or Hispanics. Whether such racial differences occur as a consequence of genetic factors, environmental factors, or some combination of the two remains unknown. However, the frequency of *incidental* prostatic cancers is comparable in all races, suggesting that race plays a more important role in the growth of established lesions than in the initial development of carcinoma. Much effort is focused on finding prostate cancer genes, but no definitive data are available. There appears to be a susceptibility locus on chromosome 1, as well as on chromosome 10 where the *PTEN* tumor suppressor gene is located. Quite interestingly, racial variations in the number of CAG repeats in the androgen receptor gene seem to be linked to the higher incidence of prostate cancer in African Americans. Mechanistically these polymorphisms may be related to the action of androgens on prostatic epithelium.

A possible role for *environmental factors* is suggested by the increased frequency of prostatic carcinoma in certain industrial settings and by significant geographic differences in the incidence of the disease. Carcinoma of the prostate is particularly common in the Scandinavian countries and relatively uncommon in Japan and certain other Asian countries. Males emigrating from low-risk to high-risk areas maintain their low risk of prostate cancer; the risk of disease is intermediate in subsequent generations, in keeping with an environmental influence on the development of this disease. Among environmental factors, a diet high in animal fat has been suggested as a risk factor.

MORPHOLOGY

Of the carcinomas of the prostate, 70% to 80% arise in the outer (peripheral) glands and hence may be palpable as irregular hard nodules by rectal digital examination. Because of the peripheral location, prostate cancer is less likely to cause urethral obstruction in its initial stages than is nodular hyperplasia. Early lesions typically appear as ill-defined masses just beneath the capsule of the prostate. On cut surface, foci of carcinoma appear as firm, gray-white to yellow lesions that infiltrate the adjacent gland with ill-defined margins (Fig. 18-13). Metastases to regional pelvic lymph nodes may occur early. Locally advanced cancers often infiltrate the seminal vesicles and periurethral zones of the prostate and may invade the adjacent soft tissues and the wall of the urinary bladder. Denonvilliers fascia, the connective tissue layer sepa-

Figure 18–13

Adenocarcinoma of the prostate. The parenchyma contains a poorly defined, pale, infiltrative tumor, in contrast to the well-demarcated nodules seen in nodular hyperplasia. Compare with Figure 18–11.

rating the lower genitourinary structures from the rectum, usually prevents growth of the tumor posteriorly. Invasion of the rectum therefore is less common than is invasion of other contiguous structures.

Microscopically, most prostatic carcinomas are **adenocarcinomas** exhibiting variable degrees of differentiation. The better differentiated lesions are composed of small glands that infiltrate the adjacent stroma in an irregular, haphazard fashion. In contrast to normal and hyperplastic prostate, the glands in carcinomas are not encircled by collagen or stromal cells but rather lie "back to back" and appear to dissect sharply though the native stroma (Fig. 18–14). The neoplastic glands are lined by a single layer of cuboidal cells with conspicuous nucleoli; the basal cell layer seen in normal or hyperplastic glands is absent. With increasing degrees of anaplasia, irregular, ragged glandular structures, papillary or cribriform epithelial structures, and, in extreme cases, sheets of poorly differentiated cells are present. Glands adjacent to areas of invasive carcinoma of the prostate often contain foci of epithelial atypia, or **prostatic intraepithelial neoplasia (PIN).** Because of its frequent coexistence with infiltrating carcinoma, PIN has been suggested as a likely precursor to carcinoma of the prostate. PIN has been subdivided into high-grade and low-grade patterns, depending on the degree of atypia. Importantly, high-grade prostatic intraepithelial neoplasia shares molecular changes with invasive carcinoma, lending support to the argument that PIN is an intermediate between normal and frankly malignant tissue.

A number of histologic grading schemes have been proposed for carcinoma of the prostate. They are based on features such as the degree of glandular differentiation, the architecture of the neoplas-

tic glands, nuclear anaplasia, and mitotic activity. A commonly used tool for grading is the Gleason system. Despite the potential difficulties associated with incomplete sampling in biopsy material and the subjectivity inherent in histologic evaluation, Gleason grade has proved to correlate reasonably well with both the anatomic stage of prostatic carcinoma (discussed later) and the prognosis.

Clinical Features. Carcinomas of the prostate are often clinically silent, particularly during their early stages. Approximately 20% of localized carcinomas are discovered unexpectedly, during histologic examination of prostate tissue removed for nodular hyperplasia. In autopsy studies, the incidence approaches 60% in men older than 80 years of age. Because most cancers begin in the peripheral regions of the prostate, they may be discovered during routine digital rectal examination. More extensive disease may produce signs and symptoms of "prostatism," including local discomfort and evidence of lower urinary tract obstruction similar to that encountered in patients with nodular hyperplasia. Physical examination in such cases typically reveals evidence of locally advanced disease, in the form of a hard, fixed prostate. More aggressive carcinomas of the prostate may first come to clinical attention because of the presence of metastases. Regrettably, this is not an uncommon mode of presentation. Bone metastases, particularly to the axial skeleton, are common in prostatic carcinoma and may cause either osteolytic (destructive) or, more commonly, osteoblastic (bone-producing) lesions. *The presence of osteoblastic metastases is strongly suggestive of advanced prostatic carcinoma.*

Assay of serum levels of *prostate-specific antigen* (PSA) has gained widespread use in the diagnosis of early carcinomas. PSA is a 33-kD proteolytic enzyme produced by both normal and neoplastic prostatic epithelium. PSA is secreted in high concentrations into prosta-

Figure 18–14

Photomicrograph of well-differentiated adenocarcinoma of the prostate demonstrating crowded, "back-to-back" glands lined by a single layer of cuboidal cells. Glandular differentiation is much less obvious in some higher-grade lesions. (Courtesy of Dr. Kyle Molberg, Department of Pathology, University of Texas Southwestern Medical Center, Dallas.)

tic acini and thence into seminal fluid, where it increases sperm motility by maintaining seminal secretions in a liquid state. Traditionally, a PSA value of 4.0 ng/L has been used as the upper limit of normal. Cancer cells produce more PSA, but any condition that disrupts the normal architecture of the prostate, including adenocarcinoma, nodular hyperplasia, and prostatitis, may also cause an elevation in serum levels of PSA. Although serum PSA levels tend to be higher in patients with carcinomas than in those with nodular hyperplasia, considerable overlap in serum levels exists between the two conditions. Moreover, in a minority of cases of cancer of the prostate, especially those confined to the prostate, serum PSA levels are not elevated. Because of these problems with both specificity and sensitivity, PSA is of limited use when used as an isolated screening test for cancer of the prostate. Its diagnostic value is enhanced considerably, however, when it is used in conjunction with other procedures, such as digital rectal examination, transrectal sonography, and needle biopsy. In contrast to its limitations as a diagnostic screening test, serum PSA levels are of great value in monitoring patients after treatment for prostate cancer, with rising levels after ablative therapy correlating with recurrence and/or the development of metastases. Several refinements in the interpretation of PSA values are being tested to further enhance its diagnostic utility. These include rate of change of PSA values with time (PSA velocity), determination of the ratio between the serum PSA value and volume of the prostate gland (PSA density), and the measurement of free versus bound forms of circulating PSA. Such refinements are likely to be most useful when PSA levels are between 4 to 10 ng/mL, the "gray zone."

Anatomic staging of the extent of disease plays an important role in the evaluation and treatment of prostatic carcinoma. Prostate cancer is staged by clinical examination, surgical exploration, radiographic imaging techniques, and, in some systems, the histologic grade of the tumor and levels of tumor markers. Anatomic features employed in the revised TNM staging system are summarized in Table 18–3. The anatomic extent of disease and the histologic grade of the lesion influence the therapy for prostate cancer and correlate well with prognosis. Depending on the grade and stage, carcinoma of the prostate is treated with various combinations of surgery, radiation therapy, and hormonal manipulations. Localized disease is usually treated with either surgery or external-beam radiation therapy. Hormonal therapy plays a central role in the treatment of advanced carcinomas. Specifically, most prostate cancers are androgen sensitive and are inhibited to some degree by androgen ablation. Surgical or pharmacologic castration, estrogens, and androgen receptor-blocking agents have all been used to control the growth of disseminated lesions. Serial evaluation of serum levels of PSA, as noted, has proved to be a valuable method by which to monitor patients for recurrent or progressive disease. The prognosis for patients with limited-stage disease is favorable: more than 90% of patients with stage T1 or T2 lesions survive 10 years or longer. The outlook for patients with disseminated disease remains poor, with 10-year survival rates in this group ranging from 10% to 40%.

Table 18–3. STAGING OF PROSTATIC ADENOCARCINOMA USING THE TNM SYSTEM

TNM Designation	Anatomic Findings
Extent of Primary Tumor (T)	
T1	**Nonpalpable lesion**
T1a	Involvement of ≤5% of TURP tissue
T1b	Involvement of >5% of TURP tissue
T1c	Carcinoma present on needle biopsy
T2	**Palpable or visible cancer confined to prostate**
T2a	Involvement of ≤50% of one lobe
T2b	Involvement of >50% of one lobe, but unilateral
T2c	Involvement of both lobes
T3	**Local extraprostatic extension**
T3a	Unilateral
T3b	Bilateral
T3c	Seminal vesical invasion
T4	**Invasion of contiguous organs and/or supporting structures**
T4a	Invasion of bladder neck, rectum, or external sphincter
T4b	Invasion of levator ani muscle or pelvic floor
Status of Regional Lymph Nodes (N)	
N0	No regional nodal metastases
N1	Single regional node ≤2 cm in diameter
N2	Single regional node 2 to 5 cm in diameter, *or* multiple nodes <5 cm in diameter
N3	Regional node >5 cm in diameter
Distant Metastases (M)	
M0	No distant metastases
M1	Distant metastases present
M1a	Metastases to distant lymph nodes
M1b	Bone metastases
M1c	Other distant sites

SEXUALLY TRANSMITTED DISEASES

Venereal diseases, or STDs, have complicated human existence for centuries. Although the origins of many of the STDs remain shrouded in antiquity, ancient literature is replete with descriptions of maladies highly suggestive of venereal disease. By the twentieth century, the clinicopathologic characteristics of the classic venereal diseases—syphilis, gonorrhea, chancroid, lymphogranuloma venereum, and granuloma inguinale—were reasonably well defined. With the discovery of antibiotics and the development of aggressive public health programs, there was a sense of optimism, if not complacency, that control of the traditional venereal diseases was a realistic goal. However, STDs have continued to evolve in an unpredictable fashion. With the changing social mores of the late twentieth century, the incidence of STDs increased, a problem compounded further by the emergence of strains of sexually transmitted pathogens that are resistant to multiple antibiotics. In addition to the problems posed by the persistence of these traditional venereal diseases, the spectrum of STDs has also broadened dramatically in recent years, with the emergence of new

■

Table 18-4. CLASSIFICATION OF IMPORTANT SEXUALLY TRANSMITTED DISEASES

Pathogens	Disease or Syndrome and Population Principally Affected		
	Males	*Both*	*Females*
Viruses			
Herpes simplex virus		Primary and recurrent herpes, neonatal herpes	
Hepatitis B virus		Hepatitis	
Human papillomavirus	Cancer of penis (some cases)	Condyloma acuminatum	Cervical dysplasia and cancer, vulvar cancer
Human immunodeficiency virus		Acquired immunodeficiency syndrome	
Chlamydiae	Urethritis, epididymitis, proctitis	Lymphogranuloma venereum	Urethral syndrome, cervicitis, bartholinitis, salpingitis, and sequelae
Chlamydia trachomatis			
Mycoplasmas	Urethritis		
Ureaplasma urealyticum			
Bacteria	Epididymitis, prostatitis, urethral stricture	Urethritis, proctitis, pharyngitis, disseminated gonococcal infection	Cervicitis, endometritis, bartholinitis, salpingitis and sequelae (infertility, ectopic pregnancy, recurrent salpingitis)
Neisseria gonorrhoeae			
Treponema pallidum		Syphilis	
Haemophilus ducreyi		Chancroid	
Calymmatobacterium granulomatis		Granuloma inguinale (donovanosis)	
Shigella	*Enterocolitis		
Campylobacter	*Enterocolitis		
Protozoa	Urethritis, balanitis		Vaginitis
Trichomonas vaginalis			
Entamoeba histolytica	*Amebiasis		
Giardia lamblia	*Giardiasis		

*Most important in homosexual populations.
Modified and updated from Krieger JN: Biology of sexually transmitted diseases. Urol Clin North Am 11:15, 1984.

entities, such as human immunodeficiency virus (HIV) infection, and the recognition of venereal spread of pathogens historically transmitted by other means, such as hepatitis B virus and *Entamoeba histolytica*. The disorders currently regarded as STDs are listed in Table 18–4. A number of these entities, such as HIV infection, hepatitis B, hepatitis C, and infection with *E. histolytica*, are discussed in other chapters. Our comments here focus on some of the more important of these entities that are not conveniently addressed in other areas of this book.

Syphilis

Syphilis, or lues, is a chronic venereal infection caused by the spirochete *Treponema pallidum*. First recognized in epidemic form in sixteenth-century Europe as the Great Pox, syphilis has remained an endemic infection in all parts of the world. Although penicillin and public health programs resulted in a gratifying reduction in cases of syphilis from the late 1940s until the late 1970s, a significant resurgence of cases of both primary and secondary syphilis has been documented over the past 2 decades. In the early 1990s, in particular, significant increases in the incidence of syphilis occurred in both urban and rural areas, particularly in the southeastern part of the United States. By 1999, however, the rising tide subsided, and currently about 2.5 cases per 100,000 population are reported. There is a strong racial disparity, with African Americans affected 30 times more than whites.

T. pallidum is a fastidious spirochete whose only natural hosts are humans. The usual source of infection is an active cutaneous or mucosal lesion in a patient in the early (primary or secondary) stages of syphilis. The organism is transmitted from such lesions during sexual intercourse across minute breaks in the skin or mucous membranes of the uninfected partner. In cases of congenital syphilis, *T. pallidum* is transmitted across the placenta from mother to fetus, particularly during the early stages of maternal infection. Once introduced into the body, the organisms are rapidly disseminated to distant sites by lymphatics and the bloodstream, even before the appearance of lesions at the primary inoculation site. Two to 6 weeks after the initial infection, a primary lesion, termed a *chancre*, appears at the point of entry. Systemic dissemination of organisms continues during this period, while the host mounts an immune response. Two types of antibodies are formed: nontreponemal antibodies and antibodies to specific treponemal antigens. As discussed in detail later, detection of these antibodies plays an important part in the diagnosis of syphilis. This acquired immunity, however, fails to eradicate spirochetes introduced during the primary inoculation.

The chancre of primary syphilis resolves spontaneously over a period of 4 to 6 weeks and is followed in approximately 25% of untreated patients by the development of *secondary syphilis*. The manifestations of secondary syphilis, discussed in more detail later, include generalized lymphadenopathy and variable mucocutaneous lesions and reflect the presence of organisms disseminated throughout the body during the primary phase of the disease. *The mucocutaneous lesions of both primary and secondary syphilis are teeming with spirochetes and are highly infectious.* Like the chancre, the lesions of secondary syphilis resolve without any specific antimicrobial therapy, at which point patients are said to be in *early latent phase syphilis.* Mucocutaneous lesions may recur during this phase of the disease. In recent years the United States Public Health Service has restricted the definition of early latent syphilis to the period 1 year after infection.

Patients with untreated syphilis then enter into an asymptomatic, *late latent* phase of the illness. In about one third of cases, subsequent symptomatic lesions may develop over the next 10 to 20 years. This late symptomatic phase, or *tertiary syphilis,* is marked by the development of lesions in the cardiovascular system, central nervous system, or, less frequently, other organs. Spirochetes are much more difficult to demonstrate during the later stages of disease, and patients with late latent or tertiary syphilis are much less likely to be infectious than are those in the primary or secondary stages of disease.

Syphilis is common in HIV-infected patients. Although disease progression is more likely, there is little evidence that the clinical manifestations are more fulminant in the setting of HIV disease.

MORPHOLOGY

The macroscopic lesions of syphilis vary with the stage of disease and are discussed later. The fundamental microscopic lesion of syphilis is a **proliferative endarteritis** and an accompanying **inflammatory infiltrate rich in plasma cells.** The treponemes cause endothelial hypertrophy and proliferation, followed by intimal fibrosis and narrowing of the vessel lumen.

Local ischemia caused by the vascular changes undoubtedly accounts for some of the local cell death and fibrosis seen in syphilis, although other factors, including delayed hypersensitivity, also appear to contribute to parenchymal injury. Spirochetes are readily demonstrable in histologic sections of early lesions with the use of standard silver stains (e.g., Warthin-Starry stains). There is no evidence that the organisms cause direct toxic injury to the host tissues. Large areas of parenchymal damage in tertiary syphilis result in the formation of a **gumma,** an irregular, firm mass of necrotic tissue surrounded by resilient connective tissue. Microscopically, the gumma contains a central zone of coagulation necrosis surrounded by a mixed inflammatory infiltrate composed of lymphocytes, plasma cells, activated macrophages (epithelioid cells), occasional giant cells, and a peripheral zone of dense fibrous tissue.

PRIMARY SYPHILIS

This stage is characterized by the presence of a chancre at the site of initial inoculation. The chancre of syphilis is characteristically indurated and has been referred to in the past as a "hard chancre" to distinguish it from the "soft chancre" of chancroid (discussed later). The primary chancre in males is usually on the penis. In females, multiple chancres may be present, usually in the vagina or on the uterine cervix. The chancre begins as a small, firm papule, which gradually enlarges to produce a painless ulcer with well-defined, indurated margins and a "clean," moist base (Fig. 18–15). Spirochetes are readily demonstrable in material scraped from the ulcer

Figure 18–15 ■

A, Syphilitic chancre of the scrotum. Such lesions are typically painless, despite the presence of ulceration, and heal spontaneously. *B,* Histology of chancre with diffuse plasmacytic infiltrate and endothelial proliferation. (Courtesy of Dr. Richard Johnson, New England Deaconess Hospital, Boston.)

Figure 18-16   ■

Treponema pallidum (darkfield microscopy) showing several spirochetes in scrapings from the base of the chancre. (Courtesy of Dr. Paul Southern, Department of Pathology, University of Texas Southwestern Medical School, Dallas.)

base using darkfield microscopy (Fig. 18–16). Regional lymph nodes are often slightly enlarged and firm, but painless. Histologic examination of the ulcer reveals a loss of the overlying epidermis, with epidermal hyperplasia at its periphery. The underlying dermis contains the usual lymphocytic and plasmacytic inflammatory infiltrate and proliferative vascular changes as described previously. Even without therapy, the primary chancre resolves over a period of several weeks to form a subtle scar. *Serologic tests for syphilis are often negative during the early stages of primary syphilis* and therefore must always be complemented by darkfield microscopy or direct fluorescent antibody testing if primary syphilis is suspected.

SECONDARY SYPHILIS

Within approximately 2 months of resolution of the chancre, the lesions of secondary syphilis occur. The manifestations of secondary syphilis are varied but typically include a combination of *generalized lymph node enlargement* and a variety of *mucocutaneous lesions*. Skin lesions are usually symmetrically distributed and may be maculopapular, scaly, or pustular. *Involvement of the palms of the hands and soles of the feet is common.* In moist skin areas, such as the anogenital region, inner thighs, and axillae, broad-based, elevated lesions termed *condylomata lata* may occur. Superficial mucosal lesions resembling condylomata lata can occur anywhere, but they are particularly common in the oral cavity, pharynx, and external genitalia. Histologic examination of mucocutaneous lesions during the secondary phase of the disease reveals the characteristic *proliferative endarteritis*, accompanied by a *lymphoplasmacytic inflammatory infiltrate*. Spirochetes are present and easily demonstrable within the mucocutaneous lesions; they are therefore contagious. Lymph node enlargement is most common in the neck and inguinal areas. Biopsy of enlarged nodes reveals nonspecific hyperplasia of germinal centers accompanied by increased numbers of plasma cells or, less commonly, granulomas or neutrophils. Less common manifestations of secondary syphilis include

hepatitis, renal disease, eye disease (iritis), and gastrointestinal abnormalities. The mucocutaneous lesions of secondary syphilis resolve over a period of several weeks, at which point the patient enters the early latent phase of the disease, which lasts approximately 1 year. Lesions may recur at any time during the early latent phase, during which the disease may still be spread. *Both nontreponemal and antitreponemal antibody tests are strongly positive in virtually all cases of secondary syphilis.*

TERTIARY SYPHILIS

Tertiary syphilis develops in approximately one third of untreated patients, usually after a latent period of 5 years or more. This phase of syphilis is divided into three major categories: cardiovascular syphilis, neurosyphilis, and so-called benign tertiary syphilis. The various forms may occur singly or in combination in a given patient. *Nontreponemal antibody tests may revert to negative during the tertiary phase, although antitreponemal antibody tests remain positive.*

Cardiovascular syphilis, in the form of *syphilitic aortitis*, accounts for more than 80% of cases of tertiary disease; it is much more common in men than in women. Briefly, the disease is fundamentally an endarteritis of the vasa vasorum of the proximal aorta. Occlusion of the vasa vasorum results in scarring of the media of the proximal aortic wall, with consequent loss of elasticity. The aortic disease is characterized by slowly progressive dilation of the aortic root and arch, with resultant aortic insufficiency and aneurysms of the proximal aorta. In some cases there is narrowing of the coronary artery ostia caused by subintimal scarring with secondary myocardial ischemia. The morphologic and clinical features of syphilitic aortitis are discussed in greater detail with diseases of the blood vessels (Chapter 10).

Neurosyphilis accounts for only about 10% of cases of tertiary syphilis. Variants of neurosyphilis include chronic meningovascular disease, tabes dorsalis, and a generalized brain parenchymal disease termed *general paresis*. They are discussed in detail in Chapter 23. An increased frequency of neurosyphilis has been noted in patients with concomitant HIV infection.

A third, relatively uncommon, form of tertiary syphilis is the so-called benign tertiary syphilis, characterized by the development of gummas in various sites. These lesions are probably related to the development of delayed hypersensitivity. *Gummas occur most commonly in bone, skin, and the mucous membranes of the upper airway and mouth,* although any organ may be affected. Skeletal involvement characteristically causes local pain, tenderness, swelling, and, sometimes, pathologic fractures. Involvement of skin and mucous membranes may produce nodular lesions, or, in exceptional cases, destructive, ulcerative lesions that mimic malignant neoplasms. *Spirochetes are rarely demonstrable within the lesions.* Once common, gummas have become exceedingly rare thanks to the development of effective antibiotics such as penicillin. They are reported now mostly in patients with AIDS.

CONGENITAL SYPHILIS

T. pallidum may be transmitted across the placenta from an infected mother to the fetus at any time during pregnancy.

The likelihood of maternal transmission is greatest during the early (primary and secondary) stages of disease, when spirochetes are most numerous. Congenital syphilis is rare if maternal syphilis has been present for more than 5 years, although cases of maternal to fetal transmission have been reported even during the latent phase of the disease. Because the manifestations of maternal disease may be subtle, routine serologic testing for syphilis is mandatory in all pregnancies. The stigmata of congenital syphilis typically do not develop until after the fourth month of pregnancy, suggesting that the morphologic changes depend to some extent on the development of an immunologic response in the fetus. In the absence of treatment, up to 40% of infected infants die in utero, typically after the fourth month.

Manifestations of *congenital syphilis* include stillbirth, infantile syphilis, and late (tardive) congenital syphilis. Among infants who are stillborn, the most common manifestations are *hepatomegaly, bone abnormalities, pancreatic fibrosis, and pneumonitis*. The enlarged liver contains foci of extramedullary hematopoiesis and a mononuclear inflammatory infiltrate in the portal areas. Pancreatitis is common and may be severe. Changes in the bones include inflammation and disruption of the osteochondral junction in long bones and, on occasion, bone resorption and fibrosis of the flat bones of the skull. The lungs may be firm and pale, owing to the presence of inflammatory cells and fibrosis in the alveolar septa (pneumonia alba). Spirochetes are readily demonstrable in tissue sections.

Infantile syphilis refers to congenital syphilis in liveborn infants that is clinically manifest at birth or within the first few months of life. Affected infants present with chronic rhinitis (snuffles) and subsequently develop a desquamating rash or other mucocutaneous lesions similar to those seen in secondary syphilis in adults. Visceral and skeletal changes resembling those seen in stillborn infants may also be present.

Late, or *tardive*, *congenital syphilis* refers to cases of untreated congenital syphilis of more than 2 years' duration. Classic manifestations include the Hutchinson triad: notched central incisors, interstitial keratitis with blindness, and deafness from eighth cranial nerve injury. Other changes include a saber shin deformity caused by chronic inflammation of the periosteum of the tibia, deformed molar teeth ("mulberry" molars), chronic meningitis, chorioretinitis, and gummas of the nasal bone and cartilage with a resultant "saddle nose" deformity.

In cases of congenital syphilis, the placenta is enlarged, pale, and edematous. Microscopy reveals proliferative endarteritis involving the fetal vessels, a mononuclear inflammatory reaction (villitis), and villous immaturity. The umbilical cord may be normal, or it may contain an acute and/or chronic inflammatory infiltrate (funisitis). Spirochetes are demonstrable with the use of the appropriate special stains, particularly in sections of umbilical cord. Organisms may be more difficult to identify in other areas and may be missed if only placental villi are examined microscopically.

SEROLOGIC TESTS FOR SYPHILIS

Although polymerase chain reaction–based testing for syphilis has been developed, serology remains the mainstay of diagnosis. Serologic tests for syphilis include both non-treponemal antibody tests and antitreponemal antibody tests. Nontreponemal tests measure antibody to cardiolipin, an antigen that is present in both host tissues and the treponemal cell wall. These antibodies are detected by the rapid plasma reagin (RPR) and Venereal Disease Research Laboratory (VDRL) tests. Nontreponemal antibody tests begin to become positive after 1 to 2 weeks of infection and are usually positive by 4 to 6 weeks. Titers of these antibodies usually fall after successful treatment. The VDRL and RPR, widely used as screening tests for syphilis, are also used to monitor the results of therapy. They may be negative, however, in the late latent or tertiary phases of the disease. Nontreponemal antibodies may persist in some patients even after successful treatment. Two additional points about nontreponemal antibody tests deserve emphasis:

- *Nontreponemal antibody tests are often negative during the early stages of disease*, even in the presence of a primary chancre. Hence, darkfield microscopy should always be performed in the evaluation of a suspected chancre, even if serologic tests for syphilis are negative.
- Up to 15% of positive VDRL tests represent *biologic false-positive results*. These false-positive tests, which may be acute (transient) or chronic (persistent), increase in frequency with age. Conditions associated with false-positive VDRL results include certain acute infections, collagen vascular diseases (e.g., SLE), drug addiction, pregnancy, hypergammaglobulinemia of any cause, and lepromatous leprosy.

Treponemal antibody tests include the fluorescent treponemal antibody absorption test (FTA-Abs) and the microhemagglutination assay for *Treponema pallidum* antibodies (MHATP). These tests also become positive within 4 to 6 weeks after an infection, but, unlike nontreponemal antibody tests, they remain positive indefinitely, even after successful treatment. They are not recommended as primary screening tests, because they are significantly more expensive than nontreponemal tests; furthermore, they remain positive after treatment, and up to 2% of the general population have false-positive test results.

Serologic response may be delayed, exaggerated (false-positive results), or even absent in some patients with syphilis and coexistent HIV infection. However, in most cases, these tests remain extremely useful in the diagnosis and management of syphilis in patients with the acquired immunodeficiency syndrome.

Gonorrhea

Gonorrhea is a sexually transmitted infection of the lower genitourinary tract caused by *Neisseria gonorrhoeae*. With the exception of chlamydial infection of the genitourinary tract, discussed later, gonorrhea is the most common reportable communicable disease in the United States. The frequency of gonorrhea rose dramatically in the United States during the 1960s and early 1970s and reached a peak in 1975, when the incidence approached 500 per 100,000 in the general population. Its incidence subsequently declined into the 1990s until 1998, when a 9% increase in the number of cases of gonorrhea was reported to the Centers for Disease

Figure 18-17 ■

Neisseria gonorrhoeae. Gram stain of urethral discharge, demonstrating characteristic gram-negative, intracellular diplococci. (Courtesy of Dr. Rita Gander, Department of Pathology, University of Texas Southwestern Medical School, Dallas.)

Control and Prevention. With more than 1 million new cases still reported annually in the United States it remains a major public health problem. The gravity of gonococcal infections has increased further by the emergence of strains of *N. gonorrhoeae* that are resistant to multiple antibiotics.

Humans are the only natural reservoir for *N. gonorrhoeae*. The organism is highly fastidious, and spread of infection requires direct contact with the mucosa of an infected person, usually during sexual intercourse. There is no evidence that gonorrhea is transmitted by contact with toilet seats or other fomites. The bacteria initially attach to mucosal epithelium, particularly of the columnar or transitional type, using a variety of membrane-associated adhesion molecules and structures termed *pili* (Chapter 9). Such attachment prevents the organism from being washed away by body fluids such as urine or endocervical mucus. The organism then penetrates through the epithelial cells and invades the deeper tissues of the host.

tubo-ovarian abscesses. The acute inflammatory process is followed by the development of granulation tissue and scarring, with resultant strictures and other permanent deformities of the involved structures.

Clinical Features. In most infected males, gonorrhea is manifested by the presence of *dysuria, urinary frequency, and a mucopurulent urethral exudate* within 2 to 7 days of the time of initial infection. Treatment with appropriate antimicrobial therapy results in eradication of the organism and prompt resolution of symptoms. Untreated infections may ascend to involve prostate, seminal vesicles, epididymis, and testis. Neglected cases may be complicated by chronic urethral stricture and, in more advanced cases, by permanent sterility. Untreated men may also become chronic carriers of *N. gonorrhoeae*.

Among female patients, initial infection may be asymptomatic or associated with *dysuria, lower pelvic pain, and vaginal discharge*. Untreated cases may be complicated by ascending infection, leading to acute inflammation of the fallopian tubes (salpingitis) and ovaries. Chronic scarring of the fallopian tubes may occur, with resultant infertility and an increased risk of ectopic pregnancy. Gonococcal infection of the upper genital tract may spread to the peritoneal cavity, where the exudate may extend up the right paracolic gutter to the dome of the liver, resulting in gonococcal perihepatitis. Resolution of inflammation in such cases may result in the formation of so-called violin-string adhesions between the dome of the liver and the adjacent diaphragm.

Other sites of primary infection, more commonly encountered in male homosexuals than in heterosexuals, include the oropharynx and the anorectal area, with resultant acute pharyngitis and proctitis, respectively.

Disseminated infection is much less common than local infection, occurring in 0.5% to 3% of cases of gonorrhea. It

MORPHOLOGY

N. gonorrhoeae provokes an intense, suppurative inflammatory reaction. In males, this is manifested most often as a **purulent urethral discharge,** associated with an edematous, congested urethral meatus. Gram-negative diplococci, many within the cytoplasm of neutrophils, are readily identified in Gram stains of the purulent exudate (Fig. 18-17). Ascending infection may result in the development of acute prostatitis, epididymitis (Fig. 18-18), and orchitis. Abscesses may complicate severe cases. Urethral and endocervical exudates tend to be less conspicuous in females, although acute inflammation of adjacent structures, such as the Bartholin glands, is fairly common. Ascending infection involving the uterus, fallopian tubes, and ovaries results in acute salpingitis, sometimes complicated by

Figure 18-18 ■

Acute epididymitis caused by gonococcal infection. The epididymis is replaced by an abscess. Normal testis is seen on the right.

is more common in females than males. Manifestations include, most commonly, tenosynovitis, arthritis, and pustular or hemorrhagic skin lesions. Endocarditis and meningitis are rare manifestations. Strains that cause disseminated infection are usually resistant to the lytic action of complement.

Gonococcal infection may be transmitted to infants during passage through the birth canal. The affected neonate may develop purulent infection of the eyes (ophthalmia neonatorum), an important cause of blindness in the past. The routine administration of antibiotic ointment to the eyes of newborns has resulted in a marked reduction in the incidence of this disorder.

Culture of gonococci from discharges has been the gold standard for diagnosis. However, this is being rapidly replaced by DNA amplification techniques such as ligase chain reactions.

Nongonococcal Urethritis and Cervicitis

Nongonococcal urethritis and cervicitis are the most common forms of STDs today. A variety of organisms have been implicated in the pathogenesis of nongonococcal urethritis and cervicitis, including *C. trachomatis*, *Trichomonas vaginalis*, *U. urealyticum*, and *Mycoplasma hominis*. Most cases appear to be caused by *C. trachomatis*, and this organism is believed to be the most common bacterial cause of sexually transmitted disease in the United States.

C. trachomatis is a small gram-negative bacterium that is an obligate intracellular parasite. It exists in two forms. The infectious form, the so-called elementary body, is capable of at least limited survival in the extracellular environment. The elementary body is taken up by host cells, primarily via a process of receptor-mediated endocytosis. Once inside the cell, the elementary body differentiates into a metabolically active form, termed the *reticulate body*. Using energy sources from the host cell, the reticulate body replicates and ultimately forms new elementary bodies capable of infecting additional cells. They preferentially infect columnar epithelial cells.

C. trachomatis infections may be associated with a spectrum of clinical features that are virtually indistinguishable from those caused by *N. gonorrhoeae*. Thus, patients may develop epididymitis, prostatitis, pelvic inflammatory disease, pharyngitis, conjunctivitis, perihepatic inflammation, and, among persons engaging in anal intercourse, proctitis. *C. trachomatis* also causes lymphogranuloma venereum, discussed in greater detail in the next section. The serotypes responsible for lymphogranuloma venereum are usually different from those causing chlamydial urethritis or cervicitis.

The morphologic and clinical features of chlamydial infection, with the exception of lymphogranuloma venereum, are virtually identical to those of gonorrhea. The primary infection is characterized by a *mucopurulent discharge containing a predominance of neutrophils*. Organisms are not visible in Gram-stained sections. In contrast to the gonococcus, *C. trachomatis* cannot be isolated with the use of conventional culture media. *C. trachomatis* infection should therefore be considered in any patient with culture-negative urethritis or cervicitis. It should also be considered in patients with gonorrhea whose symptoms persist or recur after eradication of *N. gonorrhoeae*. The diagnosis is best made by nucleic acid amplification tests on voided urine. Other manifestations of chlamydial infection include a reactive arthritis, predominantly in patients who are HLA-B27 positive. This condition, designated Reiter syndrome, typically presents as a combination of urethritis, conjunctivitis, arthritis, and generalized mucocutaneous lesions (Chapter 6).

Lymphogranuloma Venereum

Lymphogranuloma venereum (LGV) is a chronic, ulcerative disease caused by certain strains of *C. trachomatis*, which are distinct from those causing the more common nongonococcal urethritis or cervicitis discussed previously. It is a sporadic disease in the United States and western Europe but is endemic in parts of Asia, Africa, the Caribbean region, and South America. As in the case of granuloma inguinale (discussed later), sporadic cases of LGV appear to be associated most often with sexual promiscuity.

MORPHOLOGY

The patient with LGV may present with nonspecific urethritis, papular or ulcerative lesions involving the lower genitalia, regional adenopathy, or an anorectal syndrome. The lesions contain a **mixed granulomatous and neutrophilic inflammatory response,** with a variable number of chlamydial inclusions in the cytoplasm of epithelial cells or inflammatory cells. Regional lymphadenopathy is common, usually occurring within 30 days of the time of infection. Lymph node involvement is characterized by a granulomatous inflammatory reaction associated with irregularly shaped foci of necrosis and neutrophilic infiltration (stellate abscesses). With time, the inflammatory reaction is dominated by nonspecific chronic inflammatory infiltrates and extensive fibrosis. The latter, in turn, may cause local lymphatic obstruction with lymphedema and strictures. Rectal strictures are particularly common in women. In active lesions, the diagnosis of LGV may be made by demonstration of the organism in biopsy sections or smears of exudate. In more chronic cases, the diagnosis rests with the demonstration of antibodies to the appropriate chlamydial serotypes in the patient's serum.

Chancroid (Soft Chancre)

Chancroid, sometimes called the "third" venereal disease, is an acute, ulcerative infection caused by *Haemophilus ducreyi*, a small, gram-negative coccobacillus. The disease is most common in tropical and subtropical areas and is more prevalent in lower socioeconomic groups, particularly among men who have regular contact with prostitutes. *Chancroid is one of the most common causes of genital ulcers in Africa and southeast Asia,* where it probably serves as an important cofactor in the transmission of HIV-1 infection. The incidence of chancroid has been increasing in the United States since the 1980s. Recent data suggest that chancroid may be underdiagnosed in the United States, because most STD clinics do not have facilities for isolating *H. ducreyi*, and the polymerase chain reaction–based tests are not widely available.

MORPHOLOGY

Four to seven days after inoculation, the patient develops a tender, erythematous papule involving the external genitalia. In males, the primary lesion is usually on the penis; in females, most lesions occur in the vagina or periurethral area. Over the course of several days, the surface of the primary lesion erodes to produce an irregular ulcer, which is more likely to be painful in males than in females. In contrast to the primary chancre of syphilis, the ulcer of chancroid is not indurated, and multiple lesions may be present. The base of the ulcer is covered by shaggy, yellow-gray exudate. The regional lymph nodes, particularly in the inguinal region, become enlarged and tender in about 50% of cases within 1 to 2 weeks of the primary inoculation. In untreated cases, the inflamed and enlarged nodes (buboes) may erode the overlying skin to produce chronic, draining ulcers.

Microscopically, the ulcer of chancroid contains a superficial zone of neutrophilic debris and fibrin, with an underlying zone of granulation tissue containing areas of necrosis and thrombosed vessels. A dense, lymphoplasmacytic inflammatory infiltrate is present beneath the layer of granulation tissue. Coccobacillary organisms are sometimes demonstrable in Gram or silver stains, but they are often obscured by the mixed bacterial growth frequently present at the ulcer base. In the majority of cases, *H. ducreyi* can be cultured from the ulcer when appropriate media are used.

Granuloma Inguinale

Granuloma inguinale is a chronic inflammatory disease caused by *Calymmatobacterium donovani*, a minute, encapsulated coccobacillus. This disease is uncommon in the United States and western Europe but is endemic in rural areas in certain tropical and subtropical regions. When it occurs in urban settings, transmission of *C. donovani* is typically associated with sexual promiscuity. Untreated cases are characterized by the development of extensive scarring, often associated with lymphatic obstruction and lymphedema (elephantiasis) of the external genitalia.

MORPHOLOGY

Granuloma inguinale begins as a raised, papular lesion involving the moist, stratified squamous epithelium of the genitalia. The lesion eventually undergoes ulceration, accompanied by the development of abundant granulation tissue, which is manifested grossly as a protuberant, soft, painless mass. As the lesion enlarges, its borders become raised and indurated. Disfiguring scars may develop in untreated cases and are sometimes associated with urethral, vulvar, or anal strictures. Regional lymph nodes typically are spared or show only nonspecific reactive changes, in contrast to chancroid.

Microscopic examination of active lesions reveals marked epithelial hyperplasia at the borders of the ulcer, sometimes mimicking carcinoma **(pseudoepitheliomatous hyperplasia).** A mixture of neutrophils and mononuclear inflammatory cells is present at the base of the ulcer and beneath the surrounding epithelium. The organisms are demonstrable in Giemsa-stained smears of the exudate as minute coccobacilli within vacuoles in macrophages (Donovan bodies). Silver stains (e.g., the Warthin-Starry stain) may also be used to demonstrate the organism.

Trichomoniasis

Trichomonas vaginalis is a sexually transmitted protozoan that is a frequent cause of vaginitis. The trophozoite form adheres to, and causes superficial lesions of, the mucosa. In females, *T. vaginalis* infection is often associated with loss of acid-producing Döderlein bacilli. It may be asymptomatic, but frequently it causes itching and a profuse, frothy, yellow vaginal discharge. Urethral colonization may cause urinary frequency and dysuria. *T. vaginalis* infection is usually asymptomatic in males but in some cases may present as nongonococcal urethritis. The organism is usually demonstrable in smears of vaginal scrapings.

Genital Herpes Simplex

Genital herpes infection, or herpes genitalis, affects an estimated 30 million people in the United States and accounts for about 5% of all visits to STD clinics. It is estimated that in the United States 500,000 new cases of genital herpes occur annually. Most cases are caused by *herpes simplex virus (HSV) type 2*, although HSV type 1 accounts for a significant number of infections as well. Genital HSV infection may occur in any sexually active population. As with other STDs, the risk of infection is directly related to the number of sexual contacts. HSV is transmitted when the virus comes into contact with a mucosal surface or broken skin of a susceptible host. Such transmission requires direct contact with an infected person, because the virus is readily inactivated at room temperature, particularly if dried.

MORPHOLOGY

The initial lesions of genital HSV infection are painful, erythematous vesicles on the mucosa or skin of the lower genitalia and adjacent extragenital sites. The anorectal area is a particularly common site of primary infection among homosexual males. Histologic changes include the presence of intraepithelial vesicles accompanied by necrotic cellular debris, neutrophils, and cells harboring characteristic intranuclear viral inclusions. The classic **Cowdry type A inclusion** appears as a light purple, homogeneous intranuclear structure surrounded by a clear halo. Infected cells commonly fuse to form multinucleated syncytia. The inclusions readily stain with antibodies to HSV, permitting a rapid, specific diagnosis of HSV infection in histologic sections or smears.

The manifestations of HSV infection vary considerably, depending on whether the infection is primary or recurrent. Among patients experiencing their first episode, locally painful vesicular lesions are often accompanied by dysuria, urethral discharge, local lymph node enlargement and tenderness, and systemic manifestations, such as fever, muscle aches, and headache. HSV is actively shed during this period, and it continues to be shed until the mucosal lesions have completely healed. Signs and symptoms may last for several weeks during the primary phase of disease. Episodes of recurrent disease are common during the first several years after the primary infection, but they tend to be milder and of shorter duration than the primary episode. As with primary infection, HSV is shed while active lesions are present.

Among immunocompetent adults, herpes genitalis is generally not life-threatening. However, HSV does pose a major threat to immunosuppressed patients, in whom fatal, disseminated disease may develop. *Neonatal herpes infection* occurs in about half of infants delivered vaginally of mothers suffering from either primary or recurrent genital HSV infection. The viral infection is acquired during passage through the birth canal. Its incidence has risen in parallel with the rise in genital HSV infection. The manifestations of neonatal herpes, which typically develop during the second week of life, include rash, encephalitis, pneumonitis, and hepatic necrosis. Approximately 60% of affected infants die of the disease, with significant morbidity occurring in about half of the survivors. The laboratory diagnosis of genital herpes relies on viral culture, but this may be replaced by polymerase chain reaction techniques.

Human Papillomavirus (HPV) Infection

HPV is the cause of a number of squamous proliferations in the genital tract, including condylomata acuminata, some precancerous lesions, and some carcinomas. *Condylomata acuminata*, also known as venereal warts, are caused by HPV types 6 and 11. They occur on the penis as well as on the female genitalia. They should not be confused with the condylomata lata seen in secondary syphilis. Genital HPV infection may be transmitted to neonates during vaginal delivery. These infants may subsequently develop recurrent and potentially life-threatening papillomas of the upper respiratory tract.

MORPHOLOGY

In males, condylomata acuminata usually occur on the coronal sulcus or inner surface of the prepuce, where they range from small, sessile lesions to large, papillary proliferations measuring several centimeters in diameter. In females, they commonly occur on the vulva (see Fig. 19–2). The microscopic appearance is that of an exuberant proliferation of stratified squamous epithelium supported by fibrovascular papillae. The more superficial epithelial cells contain irregular, hyperchromatic nuclei surrounded by a characteristic clear perinuclear halo, a change referred to as **koilocytosis** (see Fig. 19–3).

In addition to HSV and HPV, other important viral infections that are sexually transmitted include HIV-1 and HIV-2, cytomegalovirus, and hepatitis B virus, all discussed in detail elsewhere.

BIBLIOGRAPHY

Barry MJ: Prostate-specific-antigen: Testing for early diagnosis of prostate cancer. N Engl J Med 344:1373, 2001. (An excellent summary of clinical use of PSA.)

Blanchard TJ, Maybe DC: Chlamydial infections. Br J Clin Pract 48:201, 1994. (A review of the clinical spectrum of chlamydial infections, including their role as sexually transmitted pathogens.)

Cheville JC: Classification and pathology of testicular germ cell and sex cord-stromal tumors. Urol Clin North Am 26:595, 1999. (A concise summary of histologic classification of testicular neoplasms, including discussions of the roles of immunohistochemistry and serum markers in their diagnosis.)

Clyne B, Jerrard DA: Syphilis testing. J Emerg Med 18:361, 2000. (A readable, current review of laboratory methods used in the diagnosis of syphilis.)

DeMarzo AM, et al: New concepts in the pathology of prostatic epithelial carcinogens. Urology 57(Suppl 4A):103, 2001. (A review of molecular changes in prostate cancer.)

Domingue GJ, Hellstrom WJG: Prostatitis. Clin Microbiol Rev 11:604, 1998. (A comprehensive but eminently readable review of the clinical features, diagnosis, and microbiology of acute and chronic prostatitis.)

Emmert DH, Kirchner JT: Sexually transmitted diseases in women: Gonorrhea and syphilis. Postgrad Med 107:181, 189, 193, 2000. (A useful summary of current risk factors, clinical features, and therapy.)

Farnsworth WE: Estrogen in the etiopathogenesis of BPH. Prostate 41:263, 1999. (Review of the literature on the role of estrogens and, in particular, androgen/estrogen ratios in the development of nodular hyperplasia of the prostate.)

Gene M, Ledger WJ: Syphilis in pregnancy. Sex Transm Infect 76:73, 2000. (A review of the maternal and fetal complications of syphilis during pregnancy, including discussions of diagnosis and treatment.)

Kinkade S: Testicular cancer. Am Fam Physician 59:2539, 1999. (A concise, informative review of the predisposing factors, clinical features, and treatment of testicular neoplasms.)

Lipsky BA: Prostatitis and urinary tract infection in men: What's new; what's true? Am J Med 106:327, 1999. (A recent summary of clinical features and treatment of acute and chronic prostatitis.)

Looijenga LH, Oosterhuis JW: Pathogenesis of testicular germ cell tumors. Rev Reprod 4:90, 1999. (A review of recent data addressing the chromosomal and biologic differences between infantile yolk sac tumors and teratomas, seminomas and nonseminomatous germ cell tumors in older patients, and spermatocytic seminomas.)

Luger AF, et al: Significance of laboratory findings for the diagnosis of neurosyphilis. Int J STD AIDS 11:224, 2000. (A review of the laboratory tests employed in the diagnosis of suspected syphilis and their clinical application.)

McMillan A, Young H, Moyes A: Rectal gonorrhea in homosexual men: Source of infection. Int J STD AIDS 11:284, 2000. (A study of the roles of urethral or oropharyngeal gonococcal infection in the pathogenesis of rectal gonorrhea in homosexual men.)

Nandwani R, Evans DT: Are you sure it's syphilis? A review of false positive serology. Int J STD AIDS 6:241, 1995. (A review of some of the important pitfalls in the serologic diagnosis of syphilis, including a discussion of biologic false-positive tests.)

Prow DM: Germ cell tumors: staging, prognosis, and outcome. Semin Urol Oncol 16:82, 1998. (Review of current systems employed in the staging of testicular germ cell tumors.)

Stenman UH, et al: Prostate-specific antigen. Semin Cancer Biol 9:83, 1999. (Review of the physiology, diagnostic utility, and measurement of serum PSA, including a discussion of the role of levels of free [unbound] PSA in the evaluation of prostatic disease.)

Walsh PC: Treatment of benign prostatic hyperplasia. N Engl J Med 335:586, 1996. (An excellent and important editorial that relates the treatment of prostatic hyperplasia to predominant glandular or stromal proliferation. It suggests that BPH is heterogeneous, both histologically and clinically.)

19

The Female Genital System and Breast

CHRISTOPHER P. CRUM, MD
SUSAN C. LESTER, MD
RAMZI S. COTRAN, MD*

*Deceased

Fallopian Tubes

Ovaries

FOLLICLE AND LUTEAL CYSTS
POLYCYSTIC OVARIES
TUMORS OF THE OVARY
SURFACE EPITHELIAL-STROMAL TUMORS
 Serous Tumors
 Mucinous Tumors
 Endometrioid Tumors
 Cystadenofibroma
 Brenner Tumor
OTHER OVARIAN TUMORS
 Teratomas
  Benign (Mature) Cystic Teratomas
  Immature Malignant Teratomas
  Specialized Teratomas
 Clinical Correlations for All Ovarian
  Tumors

Diseases of Pregnancy

PLACENTAL INFLAMMATIONS AND
 INFECTIONS
ECTOPIC PREGNANCY

GESTATIONAL TROPHOBLASTIC DISEASE
 Hydatidiform Mole: Complete and Partial
 Invasive Mole
 Choriocarcinoma
 Placental Site Trophoblastic Tumor
PREECLAMPSIA/ECLAMPSIA (TOXEMIA OF
 PREGNANCY)

Breast

FIBROCYSTIC CHANGES
 Nonproliferative Change
  Cysts and Fibrosis
 Proliferative Change
  Epithelial Hyperplasia
  Sclerosing Adenosis
 Relationship of Fibrocystic Changes to
  Breast Carcinoma
INFLAMMATIONS
TUMORS OF THE BREAST
 Fibroadenoma
 Phyllodes Tumor
 Intraductal Papilloma
 Carcinoma
MALE BREAST
 Gynecomastia
 Carcinoma

■
■
■ Vulva

Clinically significant diseases of the vulva do not loom large in gynecologic practice. Only the uncommon carcinomas are life-threatening. Far more frequent are the inflammatory disorders (vulvitis), which are more uncomfortable than serious. Only a few other conditions need to be mentioned here: non-neoplastic epithelial disorders (discussed later); the painful Bartholin cysts caused by obstruction of the excretory ducts of the glands; and imperforate hymen in children, impounding secretions and later menstrual flow.

VULVITIS

The moist hair-bearing skin and delicate membrane of the vulva are vulnerable to many nonspecific microbe-induced inflammations and dermatologic disorders. Intense itching (pruritus) and subsequent scratching often exacerbate the primary condition. There are also many specific forms of vulval infection related to sexually transmitted diseases. Most were discussed in Chapter 18. The five most important of these infectious agents in North America are human papillomavirus (HPV), producing condylomata acuminata and vulvar intraepithelial neoplasia (both discussed in some detail later); herpes genitalis (herpes simplex virus [HSV 1 or 2]), causing a vesicular eruption; gonococcal suppurative infection of the vulvovaginal glands; syphilis, with its primary chancre at the site of inoculation; and candidal vulvitis.

NON-NEOPLASTIC EPITHELIAL DISORDERS

The epithelium of the vulvar mucosa may undergo atrophic thinning or hyperplastic thickening. For want of a better term, these alterations were collectively referred to as "dystrophies" but are now simply referred to as nonneoplastic epithelial disorders (NNEDs) to differentiate them from the premalignant lesions discussed later. There are two forms of NNED: lichen sclerosus and lichen simplex chronicus. Both may coexist in different areas in the same patient, and both may appear macroscopically as depigmented white lesions, referred to as *leukoplakia*. Similar white patches or plaques are also seen with (1) vitiligo (loss of pigment) of the skin, (2) a variety of benign dermatoses such as psoriasis and lichen planus (Chapter 22), (3) carcinoma in situ, (4) Paget disease (described later), and (5) invasive carcinoma. Thus, leukoplakia is merely a descriptive term that gives no indication of its underlying nature. Only biopsy and microscopic examinations can differentiate among these similar-looking lesions.

Lichen Sclerosus

This lesion is characterized by thinning of the epidermis and disappearance of rete pegs, accompanied by superficial hyperkeratosis and dermal fibrosis with a scant perivascular, mononuclear inflammatory cell infiltrate (Fig. 19–1). The lesions appear clinically as smooth, white plaques or papules that in time may extend and coalesce. The surface is smoothed out and sometimes parchment-like. When the entire vulva is affected, the labia become somewhat atrophic and stiffened and the vaginal orifice is constricted. It occurs in all age groups but is most common in postmenopausal women. It may also be encountered elsewhere on the skin. The pathogenesis is uncertain, but some autoimmune reaction is suspected based on the increased frequency of other autoimmune disorders in these women and the demonstration of activated T cells in the subepithelial inflammatory infiltrate. About 1% to 4% of these women have in time developed cancerous changes.

Lichen Simplex Chronicus

Previously called "hyperplastic dystrophy," this disorder is marked by epithelial thickening with significant surface hyperkeratosis. It appears clinically as an area of

LICHEN SCLEROSUS

— Hyperkeratosis
— Thinned epidermis
— Sclerosis of dermis with atrophy of adnexa

1%–4%

CARCINOMA

LICHEN SIMPLEX CHRONICUS
(Squamous Hyperplasia)

?

— Hyperkeratosis
— Thickened epidermis
— Dermis with mild chronic inflammatory infiltrate

Figure 19–1 ■

Schematic comparison of lichen sclerosus and lichen simplex chronicus of the vulvar mucosa with approximate indications of the risk of carcinomatous transformation.

leukoplakia. The epithelium may show increased mitotic activity in both the basal and prickle cell layer. Leukocytic infiltration of the dermis is sometimes pronounced. The hyperplastic epithelial changes show no atypia (see Fig. 19–1). No increased predisposition to cancer is generally associated, but suspiciously, lichen simplex chronicus is often present at the margins of established cancer of the vulva.

TUMORS

Condylomas and Low-Grade Vulvar Intraepithelial Neoplasia (VIN I)

Condylomas are essentially anogenital warts, but in the moist environment of the vulva they tend to be large. Most fall into two distinctive biologic forms, but rarer types also exist. *Condylomata lata*, not commonly seen today, are flat, moist, minimally elevated lesions that occur in secondary syphilis (Chapter 18). The more common *condylomata acuminata* may be papillary and distinctly elevated or somewhat flat and rugose. They occur anywhere on the anogenital surface, sometimes singly but more often in multiple sites. On the vulva they range from a few millimeters to many centimeters in diameter and are red-pink to pink-brown

Figure 19-2 ■

Numerous condylomas of the vulva. (Courtesy of Dr. Alex Ferenczy, McGill University, Montreal.)

(Fig. 19–2). The histologic appearance of these lesions was described earlier (Chapter 18), but particularly significant is the characteristic cellular morphology, namely, perinuclear cytoplasmic vacuolization with nuclear angular pleomorphism—koilocytosis (Fig. 19–3). Such cells are considered to be hallmarks of HPV infection. Indeed, there is a strong association with at least two types of HPV (HPV 6 and HPV 11), closely related to the virus that causes common warts. The HPV can be transmitted venereally; identical lesions occur in men on the penis and around the anus. Vulvar condylomas are not precancerous but may coexist with foci of intraepithelial neoplasia in the vulva and cervix (VIN grade I). Indeed, according to some authorities, VIN I and condylomas, both caused by HPV and of low malignant potential, should be segregated from VIN II and VIN III, discussed later. The types of HPV isolated from the cancers differ from those most often found in condylomas.

High-Grade Vulvar Intraepithelial Neoplasia (VIN Grade II or III) and Carcinoma of the Vulva

Carcinoma of the vulva represents about 3% of all genital tract cancers in women, occurring mostly in women older than age 60 years. However, there has been an increase in the frequency of VIN in the past few decades, principally among younger women (40 to 60 years of age). In all age groups, approximately 90% of carcinomas are squamous cell carcinomas; the remainder are adenocarcinomas, melanomas, or basal cell carcinomas.

Many findings suggest that there are two biologic forms of vulvar carcinoma. The most common is seen in relatively younger patients, particularly in cigarette smokers. HPV, especially type 16 and less frequently other types, is present in 75% to 90% of cases; in many cases there is coexisting vaginal or cervical carcinoma, carcinoma in situ, or condylomata acuminata, suggesting a common causal agent, probably

HPV. Often in these patients, in situ cancerous changes confined to the epithelium, so-called VIN, precede the development of the overt cancer. The VIN may be graded VIN II or VIN III (carcinoma in situ). In many instances, the VIN has preceded by many years the development of the vulvar cancer. It may be found in multiple, apparently separate foci or may coexist with an invasive lesion. Whether VIN is always destined to become an invasive cancer remains unclear, but there is good evidence that, at least in some individuals, the VIN has been present for many years, perhaps decades. Whether genetic, immunologic, or environmental influences (e.g., cigarette smoking or superinfection with new strains of HPV) determine the course is unclear. The other subgroup of vulvar carcinoma occurs in older women. It is not associated with HPV but is often preceded by years of non-neoplastic epithelial changes, principally lichen sclerosus and, rarely, lichen simplex chronicus. In some instances, atypical epithelial changes meriting the diagnosis of VIN have preceded the appearance of the overt neoplasm. Regression is infrequent in this group.

MORPHOLOGY

VIN and early vulvar carcinomas appear as areas of leukoplakia caused by epithelial thickening involving any region of the vulva or adjacent skin. In about one fourth of cases the changes are melanin pigmented. In the course of time, these areas are transformed into overt **exophytic** or ulcerative **endophytic tumors.** HPV-positive tumors are more often multifocal and appear warty or condylomatous.

Figure 19-3 ■

Histopathology of condyloma acuminatum showing acanthosis, hyperkeratosis, and cytoplasmic vacuolation (koilocytosis, *center*).

Histologically, HPV-positive neoplasms tend to be poorly differentiated squamous cell carcinoma, whereas the HPV-negative lesions, which are usually unifocal, tend to show well-differentiated keratinizing squamous cells. Although all patterns tend to remain confined to their site of origin for a few years, ultimately, direct invasion with involvement of regional nodes and lymphohematogenous spread occurs. The risk of such spread is correlated with the size of the tumor and the depth of invasion.

Figure 19-4   ■

Paget disease of the vulva, with scattered large, clear tumor cells within the squamous epithelium.

Patients with a tumor less than 2 cm in diameter have about a 75% 5-year survival after radical excision, whereas only 10% of those with larger lesions survive 10 years.

Extramammary Paget Disease

Paget disease of the vulva, like that of the breast, is essentially a form of intraepithelial carcinoma rendered distinctive by scattered single cells and small clusters of recognizable carcinomatous cells. These are set off from the surrounding more or less normal epithelium by cleared halos of periodic acid–Schiff (PAS)-positive mucopolysaccharide secreted by the cancerous cells (Fig. 19–4). The isolated intraepithelial cancer cells are believed to arise from aberrant differentiation of epithelial progenitors, but in a few instances there is an accompanying subepithelial or submucosal small tumor arising in an adnexal structure. These microscopic changes usually appear clinically as solitary or multiple well-demarcated geographic foci of red-crusted inflammatory looking areas, usually on the labia majora and easily mistaken for a form of dermatitis. When the Paget cells are confined to the epithelium, the lesion may persist for years or even decades without evidence of invasion. However, in some instances, particularly when there is an associated appendageal tumor, the Paget cells extend into the skin appendages, invade locally, and ultimately metastasize more widely to distant sites, usually within the first 2 to 5 years.

Melanoma of the Vulva

These highly aggressive neoplasms account for less than 3% to 5% of all vulvar cancers and so can be discussed briefly. In the early stages, the melanoma cells may be dispersed within the epidermis and thus create a microscopic pattern resembling Paget disease. However, the melanoma cells are not enclosed within a halo of mucopolysaccharide. The histologic characteristics are those of melanomas elsewhere and so are not discussed here (Chapter 22). The prognosis is related to depth of invasion, as it is in extravulvar melanomas, but overall the invasive lesions are treacherous neoplasms that are often fatal.

■ ■ ■ | Vagina

The vagina in adults is seldom the site of primary disease. More often, it is secondarily involved in the spread of cancer or infections arising in close proximity (e.g., cervix, vulva, bladder, rectum). The only primary disorders discussed here are a few congenital anomalies, vaginitis, and primary tumors.

Congenital anomalies of the vagina are fortunately uncommon and include entities such as total absence of the vagina, a septate or double vagina (usually associated with a septate cervix and, sometimes, uterus), and congenital small lateral Gartner duct cysts arising from persistent embryonic remnants.

VAGINITIS

Vaginitis is a relatively common clinical problem that is usually transient and not serious. It produces a vaginal discharge (leukorrhea). A large variety of organisms have been implicated at one time or another, including bacteria, fungi, and parasites. Many represent normal commensals that become pathogenic in predisposed individuals such as diabetics; with systemic antibiotic therapy that disrupts the normal microbial flora; after abortion or pregnancy; in elderly persons with compromised immune function; and, of course, in patients with the acquired immunodeficiency syndrome. In adults, primary gonorrheal infection of the vagina is uncommon. However, it may occur in a newborn born to an infected mother. The only other two organisms worthy of specific mention, because they are frequent offenders, are *Candida albicans* and *Trichomonas vaginalis*. Candidal (monilial) vaginitis produces a curdy white discharge. This organism is present in about 5% of normal adults, and so the appearance of symptomatic infection must involve predisposing influences, or sexual transmission of a new, more aggressive strain. Biopsy specimens, which are rarely obtained, reveal only superficial, nonspecific submucosal inflammation. *T. vaginalis*, which is also a frequent offender, produces a watery, copious gray-green discharge in which parasites can be identified microscopically in fresh specimens. However, *Trichomonas* can be identified in about 10% of asymptomatic women, and so active infection usually represents a sexually transmitted new strain (Chapter 18). The inflammatory reaction is confined to the superficial squamous mucosa without invasion of the underlying tissue.

Nonspecific atrophic vaginitis may be encountered in postmenopausal women with preexisting atrophy and thinning of the squamous vaginal mucosa.

VAGINAL INTRAEPITHELIAL NEOPLASIA AND SQUAMOUS CELL CARCINOMA

Extremely uncommon, these lesions usually occur in women older than age 60 years. A preexisting or concurrent carcinoma of the cervix or vulva is sometimes present. How often HPV is implicated in the development of these neoplasms is not well known, but the concurrence of neoplasms in other sites in the female genital tract strongly suggests a common, probably viral, agent. Of particular interest is vaginal clear cell adenocarcinoma, usually encountered in girls in their late teens whose mothers took diethylstilbestrol during pregnancy. Sometimes these cancers do not appear until the third or fourth decade of life. The overall risk is 1 per 1000 or less of those exposed in utero. In about one third of instances, these cancers arise in the cervix. Much more frequently, perhaps in one third of the population at risk, small glandular or microcystic inclusions appear in the vaginal mucosa—*vaginal adenosis*. These benign lesions appear as red granular foci and are lined by mucus-secreting or ciliated columnar cells. It is from such inclusions that the rare clear cell adenocarcinoma arises.

SARCOMA BOTRYOIDES

Sarcoma botryoides (embryonal rhabdomyosarcoma), producing soft polypoid masses, is another fortunately rare form of primary vaginal cancer. It is usually encountered in infants and children younger than the age of 5 years. It may occur in other sites, such as the urinary bladder and bile ducts. These lesions are described in more detail in Chapter 21.

Cervix

The cervix must serve as a barrier to the ingress of air and the microflora of the normal vaginal tract yet must permit the escape of menstrual flow and sustain the mild buffeting of intercourse and the trauma of childbirth. No small wonder it is often the seat of disease. Fortunately, most cervical lesions are relatively banal inflammations (cervicitis), but this is also the site of one of the most common cancers in women: squamous cell carcinoma.

CERVICITIS

During development, the columnar mucus-secreting epithelium of the endocervix meets the squamous epithelial covering of the exocervix at the external os; thus, the entire "exposed" cervix is covered by squamous epithelium. The endocervical columnar epithelium is not visible to the naked eye or colposcopically. In time, in most young women, there is downgrowth of the columnar epithelium below the exocervical os—ectropion; thus, the squamocolumnar junction comes to lie below the exocervix. This "exposed" mucus-secreting columnar epithelium may appear reddened and moist and has mistakenly been called cervical "erosion," but in fact it is the result of normal changes in adult women. Remodeling occurs continuously with regeneration of both squamous and columnar epithelium. The region in which this takes place is known as the *transformation zone* (Fig. 19–5). Frequently, overgrowth of the regenerating squamous epithelium blocks the orifices of endocervical glands in the transformation zone to produce small *nabothian cysts* lined by columnar mucus-secreting epithelium. In the transformation zone, there may be a mild banal inflammatory infiltrate resulting, possibly, from changes in the vaginal pH or the ever-present microflora of the vagina.

Inflammations of the cervix are extremely common and are associated with a mucopurulent to purulent vaginal discharge. Cytologic examination of the discharge reveals white cells and inflammatory atypia of shed epithelial cells, as well as possible microorganisms. These inflammations have been variously subdivided into noninfectious and infectious cervicitis. Because microorganisms are invariably present in the vagina, with or without associated inflammatory changes on cytologic examination, it is difficult to differentiate noninfectious from infectious cervicitis. Often present are indigenous and, for the most part, incidental vaginal aerobes and anaerobes, streptococci, staphylococci, enterococci, and *Escherichia coli*. Much more important are *Chlamydia trachomatis*, *Ureaplasma urealyticum*, *Trichomonas vaginalis*, *Candida* species, *Neisseria gonorrhoeae*, herpes simplex II (genitalis), and one or more types of HPV. Many of these microorganisms are transmitted sexually, and so the cervicitis represents a sexually transmitted disease. Among these pathogens, *C. trachomatis* is by far the most common and accounts for up to 40% of cases of cervicitis encountered in sexually transmitted disease clinics, thus being far more common than gonorrhea. Herpetic infections of the cervix are noteworthy because this organism may be transmitted to the infant during passage through the birth canal, sometimes resulting in a serious, sometimes fatal, systemic herpetic infection (Chapter 7).

Figure 19–5

Schematic of the development of the cervical transformation zone.

MORPHOLOGY

Nonspecific cervicitis may be either **acute** or **chronic.** Excluding gonococcal infection, which causes a specific form of acute disease, the relatively uncommon **acute nonspecific form** is limited to postpartum women and is usually caused by staphylococci or streptococci. The chronic form is the nearly ubiquitous entity usually referred to by the unqualified term **nonspecific cervicitis.**

Specific forms include herpesvirus ulcerative lesions and changes caused by *C. trachomatis.* Chronic cervicitis is not easily defined, but it consists of the process of inflammation and epithelial regeneration common in all women of reproductive age. The cervical epithelium may show hyperplasia and reactive changes. These changes may occur in both squamous and columnar mucosa.

Cervicitis commonly comes to attention on routine examination or because of marked leukorrhea. Culture of the discharge must be interpreted cautiously because commensal organisms are virtually always present. Only the identification of known pathogens is helpful. When the lesion is severe, differentiation from carcinoma may be difficult even with colposcopy and may require a biopsy. Cervicitis per se is not a precancerous lesion, but the secondary epithelial dysplastic changes may constitute a favorable subsoil for carcinogenic influences such as HPV.

TUMORS OF THE CERVIX

Cervical carcinoma, despite dramatic improvements in early diagnosis and treatment, continues to be one of the major causes of cancer-related deaths in women, particularly in the developing world. The only other "tumor" meriting mention is the endocervical polyp.

Cervical Intraepithelial Neoplasia and Squamous Cell Carcinoma

Cervical carcinoma was once the most frequent form of cancer in women around the world. Only 50 years ago it occupied this same unenviable position in the United States, but the widespread use of Papanicolaou (cytologic) screening of women has dramatically lowered the incidence of invasive tumors to about 12,900 new cases annually and the mortality to about 4400 (2001 estimate). By contrast, the incidence of precursor cervical intraepithelial neoplasia (CIN) has increased (this being in part attributable to better case finding) to its present level of over 50,000 cases annually. This growing divergence is a testament to detection of precursor lesions by the Pap smear at an early stage, permitting discovery of these lesions when curative treatment is possible.

It is important to emphasize here that most (perhaps all) invasive cervical squamous cell carcinomas arise from precursor epithelial changes referred to as CIN. However, not all cases of CIN progress to invasive cancer, and indeed many persist without change or even regress, as will be pointed out.

CERVICAL INTRAEPITHELIAL NEOPLASIA (CIN), SQUAMOUS INTRAEPITHELIAL LESION (SIL)

Cytologic examination can detect CIN (SIL) long before any abnormality can be seen grossly. The follow-up of such women has made it clear that precancerous epithelial changes may precede the development of an overt cancer by many years, perhaps as long as 20 years. However, as noted earlier, only a fraction of cases of CIN progress to invasive carcinoma. The precancerous changes referred to as CIN may begin as lower-grade CIN and progress to higher-grade CIN, or they may begin at the outset as high-grade CIN, depending on the location of the HPV infection in the transformation zone, the type of HPV infection (high versus low risk), and other contributing host factors. On the basis of histology, precancerous changes are graded as follows:

■ CIN I: Mild dysplasia
■ CIN II: Moderate dysplasia
■ CIN III: Severe dysplasia and carcinoma in situ

However, in cytologic smears the precancerous lesions are separated into only two groups: low-grade and high-grade

SIL. The low-grade lesions correspond to CIN I or flat condylomas (described later) and the high-grade lesions to CIN II or III. Progression from a lower grade to a higher grade is not inevitable. Although studies vary, with CIN I the likelihood of regression is 50% to 60%; of persistence, 30%; and of progression to CIN III, 20%. Only 1% to 5% become invasive. With CIN III, the likelihood of regression is only 33% and of progression 6% to 74% (in various studies). It is evident that the higher the grade of CIN, the greater the likelihood of progression, but it should be noted that many instances of even the higher-grade lesions do not progress to cancer.

Epidemiology and Pathogenesis. The peak age incidence of CIN is about 30 years, whereas that of invasive carcinoma is about 45 years. It is evident that precancerous changes take many years, perhaps decades, to evolve into overt carcinomas.

Prominent risk factors for the development of CIN and invasive carcinoma are as follows:

■ Early age at first intercourse
■ Multiple sexual partners
■ A male partner with multiple previous sexual partners
■ Persistent infection by "high-risk" papillomaviruses

Many other risk factors can be related to these four, including the higher incidence in lower socioeconomic groups, the rarity among virgins, and the association with multiple pregnancies. They point strongly to the likelihood of sexual transmission of a causative agent, in this case HPV. Indeed, HPV can be detected in 85% to 90% of precancerous lesions and invasive neoplasms, and more specifically, certain high-risk types, including 16, 18, 31, 33, 35, 39, 45, 52, 56, 58, and 59. By contrast, condylomas, which are benign lesions, are associated with infection by low-risk types (i.e., 6, 11, 42, and 44) (Fig. 19–6). In these lesions the viral DNA does not integrate into the host genome, remaining in the free episomal form. By contrast, HPV types 16 and 18 possess genes that, after integration into the cellular genome, encode proteins that block or inactivate tumor suppressor genes *TP53* and *RB1* in target epithelial cells and activate cell cycle-related genes such as *cyclin E*, thus permitting uncontrolled cellular proliferation (Chapter 6). Although many women harbor these viruses, only a few develop cancer, suggesting that other factors must influence cancer risk. Among the other well-defined risk factors are cigarette smoking and exogenous or endogenous immunodeficiency. For example, the incidence of carcinoma in situ is increased approximately fivefold in women infected with human immunodeficiency virus when compared with controls.

MORPHOLOGY

The cervical epithelial changes included within the term **CIN** begin with mild dysplasia called **CIN I** or **flat condyloma**. This lesion is characterized by koilocytotic changes mostly in the superficial layers of the epithelium. **Koilocytosis**, as you will recall from the discussion of condylomata acuminata (p 682), constitutes nuclear angulation surrounded by perinuclear vacuolization produced by a viral cytopathic effect, in this case HPV. In CIN II, the dysplasia is more

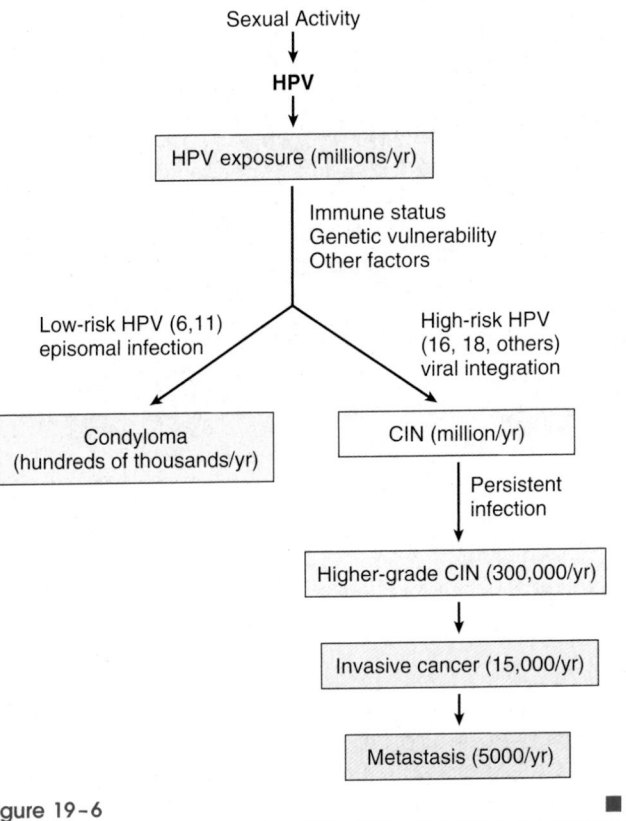

Figure 19-6 ■

An attempt to depict the sequence of events that may follow human papillomavirus (HPV) infection. CIN, cervical intraepithelial neoplasia.

perficial layer of cells is still well differentiated, but in some cases it shows the koilocytotic changes described. The next level of dysplasia, not sharply distinct from CIN II, is CIN III, marked by even greater variation in cell and nuclear size, disorderly orientation of the cells, and normal or abnormal mitoses; these changes affect virtually all layers of the epithelium and are characterized by loss of maturation. Differentiation of surface cells and koilocytotic changes have usually disappeared (Figs. 19-7 and 19-8). CIN II and III may begin as CIN I or arise de novo, depending in part on the associated HPV type. In time, dysplastic changes become more atypical and may extend into the endocervical glands, but **the alterations are confined to the epithelial layer and its glands.** It is apparent that these changes constitute **carcinoma in situ.** The next stage, if it is to appear, is invasive cancer. However, as previously emphasized, there is no inevitability to this progression nor to the development of an invasive carcinoma.

Cervical precancers produce cytologic abnormalities that often (but not always) reflect the severity of CIN. Currently, the evaluation of Pap smears is at the core of cervical cancer screening. Interestingly, the majority (over 70%) of CINs of all grades are associated with "high-risk" HPVs. Nevertheless, only a small percentage are at risk for progressing to invasive carcinoma. Moreover, up to one half of "nondiagnostic" Pap smear abnormalities (e.g., atypical squamous cells of undetermined significance) may be associated with high-risk HPVs, yet less than 25% of these changes will be followed by a biopsy-proven CIN II or CIN III. Ten to 15 percent of women with cytologically normal smears harbor high-risk HPVs. Of these, approximately 10% will eventually develop a high-grade CIN.

The previous discussion indicates that although HPV testing can identify the pool of women at risk for cervical cancer, most sexually active women will contract cervical

severe, affecting most layers of the epithelium. It is associated with some variation in cell and nuclear size and with normal-looking mitoses above the basal layer. Such changes are designated moderate dysplasia if epithelial maturation is present. The su-

Figure 19-7 ■

The spectrum of dysplastic changes in cervical intraepithelial neoplasia (CIN). *A,* There is cellular and nuclear atypicality affecting the lower half of the epithelium. *B,* The more marked atypical changes with total loss of maturation affecting the entire epithelium.

Figure 19-8

A, Cytologic smear from a CIN I, or low-grade SIL. To the left of center is a normal mature squamous cell. Grouped around it are the atypical cells with enlarged hyperchromatic nuclei and less cytoplasm; hence they are smaller. *B,* In contrast to the cells shown in *A,* the abnormal cells from CIN III or high-grade SIL are smaller, have less cytoplasm with large atypical nuclei, and have a corresponding increase in the nuclear-cytoplasmic ratio. Note the normal squamous cell at the top. (Courtesy of Dr. Edmund Cibas, Department of Pathology, Brigham and Women's Hospital, Boston.)

HPV infections at some point in their lifetime. This limits the utility of HPV testing as a screening tool for cervical cancer. Thus, cervical cytology and cervical examinations (colposcopy) remain the mainstays of cervical cancer prevention. Nevertheless, women who test HPV negative with the use of molecular probes for HPV DNA are *at extremely low risk for harboring a CIN.* Such information may be useful to strategies designed to more efficiently triage women with abnormal Pap smears.

INVASIVE CARCINOMA OF THE CERVIX

The importance of cervical cancer as a cause of morbidity and mortality around the world, in both developing and developed countries, has already been emphasized. Of these cancers, 75% to 90% are squamous cell carcinoma, which generally evolves from precursor CIN. The remainder are adenocarcinomas or variants thereof. The squamous cell lesions are appearing in increasingly younger women, now with a peak incidence at about 45 years, some 10 to 15 years after detection of their precursors. In some individuals with particularly aggressive intraepithelial changes, the time interval may be considerably shorter, whereas in other women CIN precursors may persist for life. Many factors, both constitutional and acquired, modify the course. The only reliable way to monitor the course of the disease is with careful follow-up and repeat biopsies. CIN I and even CIN II may regress, as noted earlier.

> ### MORPHOLOGY
>
> Invasive carcinomas of the cervix develop in the region of the transformation zone and range from microscopic foci of early stromal invasion to grossly conspicuous tumors encircling the os (Fig. 19-9). Thus, the tumors may be invisible or exophytic. Tumors encircling the cervix and penetrating into the underlying stroma produce a "barrel cervix," which can be identified by direct palpation. Extension into the parametrial soft tissues can fix the uterus to the pelvic structures. Spread to pelvic lymph nodes is determined by tumor depth and the presence of capillary-lymphatic space invasion, ranging from less than 1% for tumors under 3 mm in depth to over 10% once invasion exceeds 5 mm. Distant metastases, including para-aortic nodal involvement, remote organ involvement, or invasion of adjacent structures such as bladder or rectum, occur late in the course of disease.

The most common cervical carcinomas are squamous cell carcinomas (75%), followed by adenocarcinomas and adenosquamous carcinomas (20%) and small cell neuroendocrine carcinomas (less than 5%). With the exception of

Figure 19-9

Carcinoma of the cervix, well advanced.

neuroendocrine tumors, which are uniformly aggressive in their behavior, cervical carcinomas are graded from 1 to 3 based on cellular differentiation and staged from 1 to 4 depending on clinical spread.

Clinical Course. With the advent of Pap smear diagnosis, an increasing proportion of cervical carcinomas are diagnosed early in their course (stage 1). The vast majority of cervical neoplasms are diagnosed in the preinvasive phase and appear as white areas on colposcopic examination after application of dilute acetic acid. More advanced cases of cervical cancer are invariably seen in women who either have never had a Pap smear or have waited many years since the prior smear. Such tumors may be symptomatic, called to attention by unscheduled vaginal bleeding, leukorrhea, painful coitus (dyspareunia), and dysuria. Mortality is most strongly related to tumor extent and in some cases (as in neuroendocrine tumors) to cell type. Detection of precursors by cytologic examination and their eradication by laser vaporization or cone biopsy is the most effective method of cancer prevention. However, once cancer develops, the outlook hinges on stage, with 5-year survivals as follows: stage 0 (preinvasive), 100%; stage 1, 90%; stage 2, 82%; stage 3, 35%; and stage 4, 10%.

Because tumor spread is gradual, 5-year survival of patients with positive pelvic nodes approaches 50%. Recent reports indicate that chemotherapy may improve survival in advanced cases.

Endocervical Polyp

Although these lesions constitute tumors insofar as they may protrude as polypoid masses (sometimes through the exocervix), they may in reality be inflammatory in origin. They range up to a few centimeters in diameter; are soft and yielding to palpation; and are covered by a smooth, glistening surface with underlying cystically dilated spaces filled with mucinous secretion. The surface epithelium and lining of the underlying cysts are composed of the same mucus-secreting columnar cells that line the endocervical canal. The stroma is edematous and may contain scattered mononuclear cells. Superimposed chronic inflammation may lead to squamous metaplasia of the covering epithelium and ulcerations. These lesions may bleed and thus cause some concern, but they have no malignant potential.

Body of Uterus

The corpus with its endometrium is the principal seat of female reproductive tract disease. Many disorders of this organ are common, often chronic and recurrent, and sometimes disastrous. Only the more frequent and significant ones are considered here.

ENDOMETRITIS

The endometrium is relatively resistant to infections. Acute reactions are virtually limited to bacterial infections that arise after parturition or miscarriage. Retained products of conception are the usual predisposing influence. The inflammatory response is chiefly limited to the interstitium and is entirely nonspecific. Removal of the retained gestational fragments by curettage is followed by prompt remission of the infection. Chronic endometritis occurs in the following settings: (1) in association with chronic gonorrheal pelvic disease; (2) in tuberculosis, either from miliary spread or (more commonly) from drainage of tuberculous salpingitis; (3) in postpartal or postabortal endometrial cavities, usually caused by retained gestational tissue; (4) in

patients with intrauterine contraceptive devices (IUDs); and (5) spontaneously, without apparent cause, in 15% of patients. Histologically, chronic endometritis is manifested by the irregular proliferation of endometrial glands and the presence of chronic inflammatory cells: plasma cells, macrophages, and lymphocytes in the endometrial stroma.

ADENOMYOSIS

Adenomyosis refers to the growth of the basal layer of the endometrium down into the myometrium. Nests of endometrial stroma or glands, or both, are found well down in the myometrium between the muscle bundles. In the fortuitous microscopic section, continuity between these nests and the overlying endometrium can be established. The uterine wall often becomes thickened, owing to the presence of endometrial tissue and a reactive hypertrophy of the myometrium. Cyclic bleeding into the penetrating nests, producing hemosiderin pigmentation, is extremely unusual because the stratum basalis of the endometrium, from which the penetrations arise, is nonfunctional.

Marked involvement may produce menorrhagia, dysmenorrhea, and pelvic pain before the onset of menstruation.

ENDOMETRIOSIS

Endometriosis is a far more important clinical condition than adenomyosis; it often causes infertility, dysmenorrhea, pelvic pain, and other problems. The condition is marked by the appearance of foci of more or less recognizable endometrial tissue in the pelvis (ovaries, pouch of Douglas, uterine ligaments, tubes, and rectovaginal septum), less frequently in more remote sites of the peritoneal cavity and about the umbilicus. Uncommonly, the lymph nodes, lungs, and even heart or bone are involved. Three possibilities (not mutually exclusive) have been invoked to explain the origin of these dispersed lesions (Fig. 19–10). First, the *regurgitation theory* proposes menstrual backflow through the fallopian tubes and subsequent implantation. Indeed, menstrual endometrium is viable and survives when injected into the anterior abdominal wall; however, this theory cannot explain lesions in the lymph nodes or lungs, for example. Second, the *metaplastic theory* proposes endometrial differentiation of coelomic epithelium, which in the last analysis is the origin of the endometrium itself. This theory, too, cannot explain endometriotic lesions in the lungs or lymph nodes. Third, the *vascular* or *lymphatic dissemination theory* has been invoked to explain extrapelvic or intranodal implants. Conceivably, all pathways are valid in individual instances.

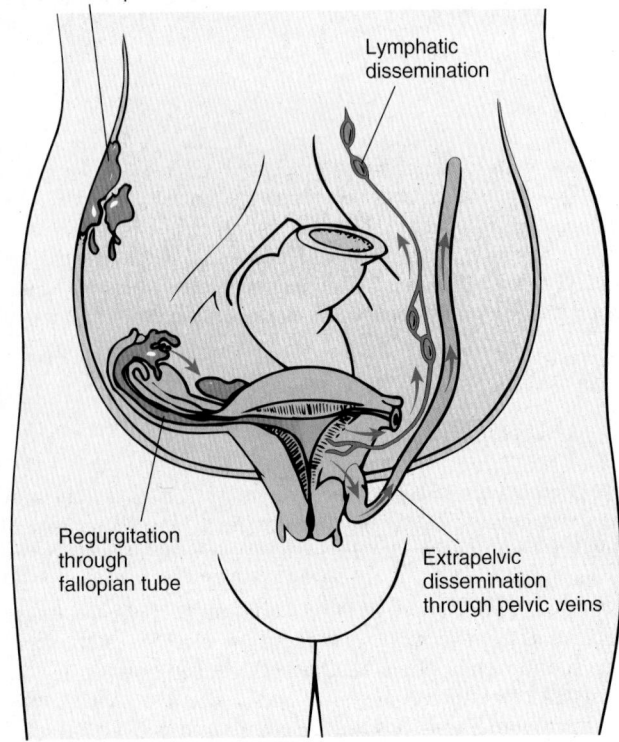

Metaplastic differentiation of coelomic epithelium

Lymphatic dissemination

Regurgitation through fallopian tube

Extrapelvic dissemination through pelvic veins

Figure 19–10

The potential origins of endometrial implants.

Figure 19–11 ■

This ovary has been sectioned to reveal a large endometriotic cyst with degenerated blood ("chocolate" cyst).

MORPHOLOGY

In contrast to adenomyosis, **endometriosis almost always contains functioning endometrium, which undergoes cyclic bleeding.** Because blood collects in these aberrant foci, they usually appear grossly as red-blue to yellow-brown nodules or implants. They vary in size from microscopic to 1 to 2 cm in diameter and lie on or just under the affected serosal surface. Often, individual lesions coalesce to form larger masses. When the ovaries are involved, the lesions may form large, blood-filled cysts that are transformed into so-called **chocolate cysts** as the blood ages (Fig. 19–11). Seepage and organization of the blood leads to widespread fibrosis, adherence of pelvic structures, sealing of the tubal fimbriated ends, and distortion of the oviducts and ovaries. The histologic diagnosis at all sites depends on finding within the lesions two of the following three features: endometrial glands, stroma, or hemosiderin pigment.

The clinical manifestations of endometriosis depend on the distribution of the lesions. Extensive scarring of the oviducts and ovaries often produces discomfort in the lower quadrant and eventually causes sterility. Pain on defecation reflects rectal wall involvement, and dyspareunia (painful intercourse) and dysuria reflect involvement of the uterine and bladder serosa, respectively. In almost all cases, there is severe dysmenorrhea and pelvic pain as a result of intrapelvic bleeding and periuterine adhesions.

DYSFUNCTIONAL UTERINE BLEEDING AND ENDOMETRIAL HYPERPLASIA

By far the most common problem for which women seek medical attention is some disturbance in menstrual function:

menorrhagia (profuse or prolonged bleeding at the time of the period), metrorrhagia (irregular bleeding between the periods), or ovulatory (intermenstrual) bleeding. Common causes include polyps, leiomyomas, endometrial carcinoma, cervical carcinoma, endometritis, endometriosis, and (of interest here) dysfunctional uterine bleeding and endometrial hyperplasia.

Dysfunctional Uterine Bleeding

Abnormal bleeding in the absence of a well-defined organic lesion in the uterus is called dysfunctional uterine bleeding. The probable cause of abnormal uterine bleeding, dysfunctional or organic (related to a well-defined lesion), depends somewhat on the age of the patient (Table 19–1).

The various causes of dysfunctional bleeding can be segregated into four functional groups:

■ *Failure of ovulation.* Anovulatory cycles are very common at both ends of reproductive life; with any dysfunction of the hypothalamic-pituitary axis, adrenal, or thyroid; with a functioning ovarian lesion producing an excess of estrogen; with malnutrition, obesity, or debilitating disease; and with severe physical or emotional stress. In many instances the basis for the failure of ovulation is mysterious, but, whatever the basis, it leads to an excess of estrogen relative to progesterone. Thus, the endometrium goes through a proliferative phase that is not followed by the normal secretory phase. The endometrial glands may develop mild cystic changes or in other places may appear disorderly with a relative scarcity of stroma, which requires progesterone for its support. The poorly supported endometrium partially collapses, with rupture of spiral arteries, accounting for the bleeding.

■ *Inadequate luteal phase.* The corpus luteum may fail to mature normally or may regress prematurely, leading to a relative lack of progesterone. The endometrium under

these circumstances reveals delay in the development of the secretory changes expected at the date of biopsy.

■ *Contraceptive-induced bleeding.* Older oral contraceptives containing synthetic estrogens and progestin induced a variety of endometrial responses, depending on the particular steroids being employed and the dosage. A common response was discordant appearance of glands and stroma—for example, a lush, decidua-like stroma and inactive, nonsecretory glands. The pills in current use have corrected these abnormalities.

■ *Endomyometrial disorders,* including chronic endometritis, endometrial polyps, and submucosal leiomyomas.

Endometrial Hyperplasia

An excess of estrogen relative to progestin, if sufficiently prolonged or marked, will induce endometrial hyperplasia ranging from simple hyperplasia to complex hyperplasia, and possibly to atypical hyperplasia (Fig. 19–12). These three categories represent a continuum based on the level and duration of the estrogen excess. Not surprisingly, in time the endometrial hyperplasia may give rise to carcinoma of the endometrium, the risk being dependent on the severity of the hyperplastic changes and associated cellular atypia.

Any basis for estrogen excess may lead to hyperplasia. Potential factors may include failure of ovulation, such as is seen around the menopause; prolonged administration of estrogenic steroids without counter-balancing progestin; estrogen-producing ovarian lesions such as polycystic ovaries (including Stein-Leventhal syndrome); cortical stromal hyperplasia; and granulosa-theca cell tumors of the ovary.

As has been indicated, endometrial hyperplasia, particularly the more severe forms, not only calls attention to some underlying basis for the abnormal endometrial changes but also causes excessive and irregular uterine bleeding. Even more important, atypical hyperplasia incurs a 20% to 25% risk of progressing to adenocarcinoma of the endometrium. It is evident that when atypical hyperplasia is discovered, it must be carefully evaluated for the possible presence of a focus of cancer and must be monitored over time by repeated endometrial biopsy to evaluate its course.

TUMORS OF THE ENDOMETRIUM AND MYOMETRIUM

The most common neoplasms are endometrial polyps, leiomyomas, and endometrial carcinomas. In addition, exotic mesodermal tumors are encountered, such as stromal sarcoma botryoides (also encountered in the vagina). All tend to produce bleeding from the uterus as the earliest manifestation.

Endometrial Polyps

These are sessile, usually hemispherical (rarely pedunculated) lesions that are 0.5 to 3 cm in diameter. Larger

Table 19–1. CAUSES OF ABNORMAL UTERINE BLEEDING BY AGE GROUP

Age Group	Cause(s)
Prepuberty	Precocious puberty (hypothalamic, pituitary, or ovarian origin)
Adolescence	Anovulatory cycle
Reproductive age	Complications of pregnancy (abortion, trophoblastic disease, ectopic pregnancy)
	Organic lesions (leiomyoma, adenomyosis, polyps, endometrial hyperplasia, carcinoma)
	Anovulatory cycle
	Ovulatory dysfunctional bleeding (e.g., inadequate luteal phase)
Perimenopause	Anovulatory cycle
	Irregular shedding
	Organic lesions (carcinoma, hyperplasia, polyps)
Postmenopause	Organic lesions (carcinoma, hyperplasia, polyps)
	Endometrial atrophy

Figure 19-12 ■

A, Nonhyperplastic anovulatory endometrium with dilatation of glands. *B,* Complex hyperplasia of a nest of closely packed glands. *C,* Atypical endometrial hyperplasia with crowding of glands, unfolding of tall columnar cells, and some loss of polarity.

polyps may project from the endometrial mucosa into the uterine cavity. On histologic examination, they are seen to be covered with columnar cells; some have an essentially normal endometrial architecture, but more often they have cystically dilated glands. It has been noted that the stromal cells in many, perhaps most, endometrial polyps are monoclonal and have a cytogenetic rearrangement at 6p21,

making it clear that the stromal cells are the neoplastic component of the polyp.

Although endometrial polyps may occur at any age, they develop more commonly at the time of menopause. Their clinical significance lies in the production of abnormal uterine bleeding and, more important, the risk (however rare) of giving rise to a cancer.

Leiomyoma and Leiomyosarcoma

Benign tumors that arise from the smooth muscle cells in the myometrium are properly termed *leiomyomas*, but perhaps because they are firm, or for some other illogical reason, they are more often referred to as *fibroids*. They are the most common benign tumor in females and are found in 30% to 50% of women during reproductive life. Genetic influences are involved, because these tumors are considerably more frequent in blacks than in whites. Estrogens and possibly oral contraceptives stimulate their growth; conversely, they shrink postmenopausally. These tumors are clearly monoclonal, and nonrandom chromosomal abnormalities have been found in about 40% of tumors, but it should be noted that 60% are karyotypically normal.

MORPHOLOGY

Macroscopically, these tumors are typically sharply circumscribed, firm gray-white masses with a characteristic whorled cut surface. They may occur singly, but most often multiple tumors are scattered within the uterus, ranging in size from small seedlings to massive neoplasms that dwarf the size of the uterus (Fig. 19-13). Some are embedded within the myometrium (intramural), whereas others may lie directly beneath the endometrium (submucosal) or directly beneath the

Figure 19-13 ■

Multiple leiomyomas of the uterus. Several large, almost pedunculated tumors protrude from the dome of the fundus. The lower uterine segment and cervix are below *(on top of the rule).* (Courtesy of Dr. Kyle Molberg, Department of Pathology, University of Texas Southwestern Medical School, Dallas.)

serosa (subserosal). The latter may develop attenuated stalks and even become attached to surrounding organs, from which they develop a blood supply and then free themselves from the uterus to become "parasitic" leiomyomas. Larger neoplasms may develop foci of ischemic necrosis with areas of hemorrhage and cystic softening, and after menopause they may become densely collagenous and even calcified. Histologically, the tumors are characterized by whorling bundles of smooth muscle cells duplicating the histology of the normal myometrium. Foci of fibrosis, calcification, ischemic necrosis, cystic degeneration, and hemorrhage may be present.

Leiomyomas of the uterus may be entirely asymptomatic and be discovered only on routine pelvic examination or post mortem. The most frequent manifestation, when present, is menorrhagia, with or without metrorrhagia. Large masses may become palpable to the patient in the pelvic region or produce a dragging sensation. There is little evidence that these benign tumors transform into sarcomas. Such transformation, if it occurs, is extremely rare.

Leiomyosarcomas arise directly from the mesenchymal cells of myometrium, not from preexisting leiomyomas. They are almost always solitary tumors, in contradistinction to the frequently multiple leiomyomas.

MORPHOLOGY

Grossly, leiomyosarcomas develop in several distinct patterns: as bulky masses infiltrating the uterine wall; as polypoid lesions projecting into the uterine cavity; or as deceptively discrete tumors that masquerade as large, benign leiomyomas. Histologically, they present a wide range of differentiation, from those that closely resemble leiomyoma to wildly anaplastic tumors. With this range in morphology, it is understandable that some well-differentiated tumors lie at the interface between benign and malignant, and sometimes these are designated **leiomyoblastomas** (a euphemism to say "we don't know whether to call it benign or malignant"). The diagnostic features of leiomyosarcoma include relatively frequent mitoses, with or without cellular atypia, or less numerous mitoses with cellular atypia.

Recurrence after removal is common with these cancers, and many metastasize widely, yielding about a 40% 5-year survival rate. Understandably, the more anaplastic tumors have a poorer outlook than the better-differentiated lesions.

Endometrial Carcinoma

In the United States and many other Western countries, endometrial carcinoma is the most frequent cancer of the female genital tract. Some years ago, it was much less common than cervical cancer. However, early detection of CIN by periodic cytologic examinations, and its appropriate treatment, have dramatically reduced the incidence of invasive cervical cancer.

Epidemiology and Pathogenesis. Endometrial cancer appears most frequently between the ages of 55 and 65 years and is distinctly uncommon under 40 years of age. A constellation of well-defined risk factors has long been noted:

- Obesity: increased synthesis of estrogens in fat depots and from adrenal and ovarian precursors
- Diabetes
- Hypertension
- Infertility: women tend to be single and nulliparous, and they often have nonovulatory cycles

Some of these risk factors point to *increased estrogen stimulation*, and indeed it is well-recognized that prolonged estrogen replacement therapy, depending on duration and dosage, increases the risk of this form of cancer, as do ovarian estrogen-secreting tumors. Many of these risk factors are the same as those for endometrial hyperplasia, and *endometrial carcinoma frequently arises on a background of endometrial hyperplasia*. These tumors are termed *endometrioid carcinomas* by virtue of their similarity to normal endometrial glands. Similarly, breast carcinoma occurs in women with endometrial cancer (and vice versa) more frequently than by chance alone. The great preponderance of endometrial carcinomas arise in the setting just described. However, a significant subset (approximately 20%) of cancers do not appear to be associated with hyperestrinism or preexisting hyperplasia. On average, these cancers arise at a later stage in life, are more poorly differentiated, and have a poorer prognosis. This less common group of tumors includes *papillary serous* and *clear cell* carcinomas, which are similar in appearance to their counterparts in the ovary. Endometrioid carcinomas are associated with microsatellite instability and mutations in the *PTEN* gene on chromosome 10. Papillary serous carcinomas frequently harbor mutations in the *TP53* tumor suppressor gene.

MORPHOLOGY

Endometrioid carcinomas closely resemble normal endometrium and may be exophytic (Fig. 19-14) or infiltrative. This group of tumors frequently exhibits a range of differentiation, including mucinous, tubal (ciliated), and squamous (occasionally adenosquamous) differentiation in the neoplastic epithelium. Tumors originate in the mucosa and may infiltrate the myometrium and enter vascular spaces, with metastases to regional lymph nodes. For this group of tumors, grading (grades 1 to 3) and staging closely parallel outcome: stage I, confined to the corpus; stage II, involvement of the cervix; stage III, beyond the uterus but within the true pelvis; stage IV, distant metastases or involvement of other viscera. One exception is synchronous endometrioid

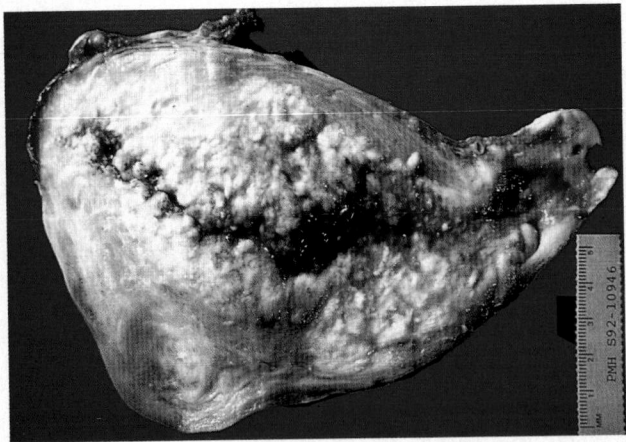

Figure 19-14 ■

Endometrial carcinoma projecting into the uterine cavity and infiltrating the myometrium. The uterine cavity is almost obliterated. (The cervix is on the right.) (Courtesy of Dr. Kyle Molberg, Department of Pathology, University of Texas Southwestern Medical School, Dallas.)

tumors arising in the uterus and ovary. This scenario often signifies two separate primary neoplasms

rather than stage III disease and has a favorable prognosis. **Papillary serous** and **clear cell carcinomas** are not graded. They behave as poorly differentiated cancers. Serous carcinomas are particularly aggressive.

Clinical Course. The first clinical indications of endometrial carcinoma are usually marked leukorrhea and irregular bleeding, raising a red flag in a postmenopausal woman. This reflects erosion and ulceration of the endometrial surface. With progression, the uterus may be palpably enlarged, and in time it becomes fixed to surrounding structures by extension of the cancer beyond the uterus. Fortunately, these are usually late-metastasizing neoplasms, but dissemination eventually occurs, with involvement of regional nodes and more distant sites. With therapy, stage I carcinoma is associated with a 90% 5-year survival rate; this rate drops to 30% to 50% in stage II and to less than 20% in stages III and IV. Prognosis for papillary serous carcinomas is strongly dependent on the extent of tumor, as determined by operative staging with peritoneal cytology. This is critical, inasmuch as very small or superficial serous tumors may nonetheless spread via the fallopian tube to the peritoneal cavity.

Fallopian Tubes

The fallopian tubes should be treasured organs to the pathology student because they are so seldom the site of primary disease. Their most common afflictions are inflammation, almost always as part of pelvic inflammatory disease. Much less often, they are affected by ectopic (tubal) pregnancy (p 701), followed in order of frequency by endometriosis (p 690) and the rare primary tumors. Only a few comments on salpingitis and tumors follow.

Inflammations of the tube are almost always bacterial in origin. With the declining incidence of gonorrhea, nongonococcal organisms, such as *Chlamydia, Mycoplasma hominis,* coliforms, and (in the postpartum setting) streptococci and staphylococci, are now the major offenders. The morphologic changes produced by gonococci conform to those already described (Chapter 18). Nongonococcal infections differ somewhat, inasmuch as they are more invasive, penetrating the wall of the tubes and thus tending more often to give rise to bloodborne infections and seeding of the

Figure 19-15 ■

Pelvic inflammatory disease, asymmetric albeit bilateral. One side has a large inflammatory mass totally obscuring the tube and ovary. The other is less involved, but the tube is widely adherent to the still recognizable ovary.

meninges, joint spaces, and sometimes the heart valves. Rarely, tuberculous salpingitis is encountered, almost always in combination with involvement of the endometrium. All forms of salpingitis may produce fever, lower abdominal or pelvic pain, and pelvic masses when the tubes become distended with either exudate or, later, burned-out inflammatory debris and secretions (Fig. 19–15). Even more serious is the potential for obstruction of the tubal lumina, which sometimes produces permanent sterility.

Primary adenocarcinomas may arise in the tubes. They are curiosities that are not usually discovered until they spread. In time they may cause death.

■ Ovaries

The ovaries are infrequently the primary site of any disease except, notably, neoplasms. Indeed, carcinomas of the ovaries account for more deaths than do cancers of the cervix and uterine corpus together. It is less the frequency of the carcinomas than their lethality (because of their silent growth) that makes them so dangerous. Non-neoplastic cysts are commonplace but generally are not serious problems. Primary inflammations of the ovary are rarities, but salpingitis of the tubes frequently causes a periovarian reaction called *salpingo-oophoritis*. As discussed earlier, the ovary is frequently secondarily affected in endometriosis. Only the non-neoplastic cysts and neoplasms are considered here.

FOLLICLE AND LUTEAL CYSTS

Follicle and luteal cysts in the ovaries are so commonplace as almost to constitute physiologic variants. These innocuous lesions originate in unruptured graafian follicles or in follicles that have ruptured and immediately sealed. Such cysts are often multiple and develop immediately subjacent to the serosal covering of the ovary. Usually they are small—1 to 1.5 cm in diameter—and are filled with clear serous fluid. Occasionally, they achieve diameters of 4 to 5 cm and may thus become palpable masses and indeed produce pelvic pain. When small, they are lined by granulosa lining cells or luteal cells, but as the fluid accumulates, pressure may cause atrophy of these cells. Sometimes, these cysts rupture, producing intraperitoneal bleeding and acute abdominal symptoms.

POLYCYSTIC OVARIES

Oligomenorrhea, hirsutism, infertility, and sometimes obesity may appear in young women (usually in girls after menarche), secondary to excessive production of estrogens and androgens (mostly the latter) by multiple cystic follicles in the ovaries. This condition is also called *polycystic ovaries*, or *Stein-Leventhal syndrome*.

The ovaries are usually twice normal in size, are gray-white with a smooth outer cortex, and are studded with subcortical cysts 0.5 to 1.5 cm in diameter. Histologically, there is a thickened fibrosed outer tunica, sometimes referred to as *cortical stromal fibrosis*, beneath which are innumerable cysts lined by granulosa cells with a hypertrophic and hyperplastic luteinized theca interna. There is a conspicuous absence of corpora lutea.

The principal biochemical abnormalities in most patients are excessive production of androgens, high levels of luteinizing hormone (LH), and low levels of follicle-stimulating hormone (FSH). The origins of these changes are poorly understood, but it is proposed that the ovaries in this condition elaborate excess androgens, which are converted in peripheral fatty depots to estrone, and these, through the hypothalamus, inhibit the secretion of FSH by the pituitary. The basis of excess ovarian androgen secretion is mysterious.

TUMORS OF THE OVARY

With more than 23,000 new cases diagnosed annually, ovarian cancer is the fifth most common cancer in US women. It is also the fifth leading cause of cancer death in women, with 13,900 deaths estimated in 2001. Tumors of the ovary are amazingly diverse pathologic entities. This diversity is attributable to the three cell types that make up the normal ovary: the multipotential surface (coelomic) covering epithelium, the totipotential germ cells, and the multipotential sex cord/stromal cells. Each of these cell types gives rise to a variety of tumors, as indicated in Figure 19–16.

It is evident that neoplasms of surface epithelial origin account for the great majority of all primary ovarian tumors, and in their malignant forms account for almost 90%

ORIGIN	SURFACE EPITHELIAL CELLS (Surface epithelial–stromal cell tumors)	GERM CELL	SEX CORD–STROMA	METASTASIS TO OVARIES
Overall frequency	65%–70%	15%–20%	5%–10%	5%
Proportion of malignant ovarian tumors	90%	3%–5%	2%–3%	5%
Age group affected	20+ years	0–25+ years	All ages	Variable
Types	• Serous tumor • Mucinous tumor • Endometrioid tumor • Clear cell tumor • Brenner tumor • Cystadenofibroma	• Teratoma • Dysgerminoma • Endodermal sinus tumor • Choriocarcinoma	• Fibroma • Granulosa-theca cell tumor • Sertoli-Leydig cell tumor	

Figure 19–16

Derivation of various ovarian neoplasms and some data on their frequency and age distribution.

of all ovarian cancers. These epithelial tumors are then the "big bananas" that require most medical attention. Germ-cell and sex cord/stromal cell tumors are much less frequent and, although they constitute 20% to 30% of all ovarian tumors, are collectively responsible for less than 10% of cancers of the ovary.

Pathogenesis. Several risk factors for ovarian cancers have been recognized. Two of the most important ones are nulliparity and family history. There is a higher incidence of carcinoma in unmarried women and married women with low parity. Interestingly, prolonged use of oral contraceptives reduces the risk somewhat. Although only 5% to 10% of ovarian cancers are familial, much is being learned about the molecular pathogenesis of these cancers by identifying the culprit genes in these cases. A majority of hereditary ovarian cancers appear to be caused by mutations in the *BRCA* genes, *BRCA1* and *BRCA2*. These, as will be discussed later, are also associated with hereditary breast cancer. Indeed, with mutations in these genes there is increased risk for both ovarian and breast cancers. The average lifetime risk for ovarian cancer approximates 30% in *BRCA1* carriers, with figures varying from 16% to 44% in different studies. The risk of *BRCA2* carriers is somewhat lower when compared with that of *BRCA1* carriers. Although mutations in *BRCA* genes are

present in the majority of the familial cases of ovarian cancer, such mutations are seen in only 8% to 10% of sporadic ovarian cancers. Thus, there must be other molecular pathways to ovarian neoplasms. For example, *ERBB2* is overexpressed in 35% of ovarian cancers, and this is associated with a poor prognosis. *K-RAS* is overexpressed in up to 30% of tumors, mostly mucinous cystadenocarcinomas. As with other cancers, *TP53* is mutated in about 50% of all ovarian cancers.

SURFACE EPITHELIAL-STROMAL TUMORS

These neoplasms are derived from the coelomic epithelium. They can be strictly epithelial (e.g., serous, mucinous tumors) or can have a distinct stromal component (cystadenofibroma, Brenner tumor). Although it is traditional to divide neoplasms into benign and malignant categories, the surface epithelial tumors also have an intermediate, borderline category currently referred to as *tumors of low malignant potential*. These appear to be low-grade cancers with limited invasive potential. Thus, they have a better prognosis than their uglier cousins do, as will be evident.

Serous Tumors

These most frequent of the ovarian tumors are usually encountered between ages 30 and 40 years. Although they may be solid, they are usually cystic, so they are commonly known as *cystadenomas* or *cystadenocarcinomas*. About 60% are benign, 15% of low malignant potential, and 25% malignant. Combined borderline and malignant lesions are the most common malignant ovarian tumors and account for about 60% of all ovarian cancers.

MORPHOLOGY

Grossly, serous tumors may be small (5 to 10 cm) in diameter, but most are large, spherical to ovoid, cystic structures, up to 30 to 40 cm in diameter. **About 25% of the benign forms are bilateral.** In the benign form, the serosal covering is smooth and glistening. In contrast, the covering of the cystadenocarcinoma shows nodular irregularities, which represent penetration of the tumor to or through the serosa. On transection, the small cystic tumor may reveal a single cavity, but larger ones are usually divided by multiple septa into a multiloculated mass (Fig. 19–17). The cystic spaces are usually filled with a clear serous fluid, although a considerable amount of mucus may also be present. Jutting into the cystic cavities are polypoid or papillary projections, which become more marked in malignant tumors (see Fig. 19–17).

Histologically, the benign tumors are characterized by a single layer of tall columnar epithelium that lines the cyst or cysts. The cells are in part ciliated and in part dome-shaped secretory cells. **Psammoma bodies** (concentrically laminated concretions) are common in the tips of papillae. When frank carcinoma develops, anaplasia of the lining cells appears, as does invasion of the stroma. Papillary formations are complex and multilayered, with invasion of the axial fibrous tissue by nests or totally undifferentiated sheets of malignant cells. Between these clearly benign and obviously malignant forms are the **tumors of low malignant potential,** with obvious epithelial anaplasia and little stromal invasion. Tumors of low malignant potential may seed the peritoneum, but typically the implants of tumor are "noninvasive." Occasionally, tumors of low malignant potential may surprise, presenting as "invasive" peritoneal implants that behave as carcinoma. Retrospective histologic studies of these tumors often reveal a greater degree of tumor complexity and cellular anaplasia. In general, malignant serous tumors spread commonly to regional lymph nodes, but distant lymphatic and hematogenous metastases are infrequent.

The prognosis of tumors of low malignant potential is determined largely by the nature of the peritoneal implants, if present. The prognosis for the patient with clearly invasive serous cystadenocarcinoma after surgery, sometimes followed by radiation and chemotherapy, is poor and depends heavily on the stage of the disease at the time of diagnosis. If the tumor appears to be confined to the ovary, the frankly carcinomatous lesions yield about a 70% 5-year survival, whereas those of low malignant potential demonstrate about 100% survival. With cancers that have penetrated the capsule, the 10-year survival rate is only 13%. In contrast, for cancers of low malignant potential with capsular penetration, the overall 10-year survival rate is about 80%, but almost 40% of such patients eventually die of their tumors.

Mucinous Tumors

Mucinous tumors are in most respects analogous to the serous tumors, differing essentially in that the epithelium consists of mucin-secreting cells similar to those of the endocervical mucosa. These tumors occur in patients in the same age range as those with serous tumors, but mucinous lesions are considerably less likely to be malignant, accounting for about 10% of all ovarian cancers. Eighty

Figure 19–17

A, Borderline serous cystadenoma opened to display a cyst cavity lined by delicate papillary tumor growths. *B,* Cystadenocarcinoma. The cyst is opened to reveal a large, bulky tumor mass. (Courtesy of Dr. Christopher Crum, Brigham and Women's Hospital, Boston.)

percent of these tumors are benign, and 10% are of low malignant potential. The remainder are malignant *(cystadenocarcinomas).*

MORPHOLOGY

Only about 5% of benign and 20% of malignant tumors are bilateral, a much lower incidence than for their serous counterparts. On gross examination, they may be indistinguishable from serous tumors except by the mucinous nature of the cystic contents. However, **they are more likely to be larger and multilocular, and papillary formations are less common. (Unlike in their serous counterparts, psammoma bodies are not found within the tips of the papillae.) Prominent papillation, serosal penetration, and solidified areas point to malignancy.**

Histologically, mucinous tumors are classified according to the character of the mucin-producing epithelial cells. Essentially three types may be identified. The first two, which are not always distinguishable, include tumors with endocervical and intestinal-type epithelia (Fig. 19–18). The latter is almost always present in mucinous tumors of low malignant potential and mucinous carcinomas. The third type is the müllerian mucinous cystadenoma, which is typically associated with an endometriotic cyst. This tumor likely represents an endometrial tumor with mucinous differentiation.

Rupture of mucinous tumors may result in mucinous deposits in the peritoneum (pseudomyxoma peritonei). However, in the vast majority of cases of pseudomyxoma the ovarian tumor is a metastasis from the gastrointestinal tract, primarily the appendix (Chapter 15). Clues to a metastatic gastrointestinal tumor include bilateral ovarian involvement and pseudomyxoma.

Figure 19–18 ■

Histologic detail of classic nonciliated, mucin-secreting, columnar lining epithelium of a mucinous cystadenoma of the ovary.

The prognosis of mucinous cystadenocarcinoma is somewhat better than that for the serous counterpart, but with modern chemotherapy, the stage rather than the histologic type is the major determinant of treatment success.

Endometrioid Tumors

These tumors may be solid or cystic, but sometimes they develop as a mass projecting from the wall of an endometriotic cyst filled with chocolate-colored fluid. Microscopically, they are distinguished by the formation of tubular glands, similar to those of the endometrium, within the linings of cystic spaces. Although benign and borderline forms exist, endometrioid tumors are usually malignant. They are bilateral in about 30% of cases, and 15% to 30% of patients with these ovarian tumors have a concomitant endometrial carcinoma.

Cystadenofibroma

The cystadenofibroma is essentially a variant of the serous cystadenoma in which there is more pronounced proliferation of the fibrous stroma that underlies the columnar lining epithelium. These benign tumors are usually small and multilocular, with simple, nonbranching papillary processes. Carcinomatous transformation is rare.

Brenner Tumor

The Brenner tumor is an uncommon, solid, usually unilateral ovarian tumor consisting of an abundant stroma containing nests of transitional-like epithelium resembling that of the urinary tract. Occasionally, the nests are cystic and are lined by columnar mucus-secreting cells. Brenner tumors are generally smoothly encapsulated and gray-white on transection and range from a few centimeters to 20 cm in diameter. These tumors may arise from the surface epithelium or from urogenital epithelium trapped within the germinal ridge. Rarely, they are formed as nodules within the wall of a mucinous cystadenoma. Although most are benign, both malignant and borderline tumors have been described.

OTHER OVARIAN TUMORS

Many other types of tumors of germ-cell or sex cord/stromal origin also arise in the ovary, but only the teratomas of germ-cell origin are sufficiently common to be described here. Table 19–2 presents some salient features of a few other neoplasms of germ-cell and sex cord origin.

Teratomas

These neoplasms of germ-cell origin constitute 15% to 20% of ovarian tumors. They display the distressing behavior

Table 19-2. SELECTED OVARIAN NEOPLASMS

	Peak Incidence	Usual Location	Morphologic Features	Behavior
Germ-Cell Origin				
Dysgerminoma	2nd—3rd decades Occur with gonadal dysgenesis	80%–90% unilateral	Counterpart of testicular seminoma. Solid large to small gray masses. Sheets or cords of large cleared cells separated by scant fibrous strands. Stroma may contain lymphocytes and occasional granuloma.	All malignant but only one third aggressive and spread; all radio-sensitive with 80% cure.
Choriocarcinoma	First three decades of life	Unilateral	Identical to placental tumor. Often small, hemorrhagic focus with two types, epithelium cytotrophoblast and syncytiotrophoblast.	Metastasizes early and widely. Primary focus may disintegrate, leaving only "mets." In contrast to placental tumors, ovarian primaries are resistant to chemotherapy.
Sex Cord Tumors				
Granulosa-theca cell	Most postmenopausal but at any age	Unilateral	May be tiny or large, gray to yellow (with cystic spaces). Composed of mixture of cuboidal granulosa cells in cords, sheets, or strands and spindled or plump lipid-laden theca cells. Granulosal elements may recapitulate ovarian follicle called Call-Exner bodies.	May elaborate large amounts of estrogen (from thecal elements) and so may promote endometrial or breast carcinoma. Granulosal element may be malignant (5%–25%).
Thecoma-fibroma	Any age	Unilateral	Solid gray fibrous cells to yellow (lipid-laden) plump thecal cells.	Most hormonally inactive. Few elaborate estrogens. About 40%, for obscure reasons, produce ascites and hydrothorax (Meigs syndrome). Rarely malignant.
Sertoli-Leydig cell	All ages	Unilateral	Usually small, gray to yellow-brown and solid. Recaps development of testis with tubules, or cords and plump pink Sertoli cells.	Many masculinizing or de-feminizing. Uncommonly malignant.
Metastases to Ovary	Older ages	Mostly bilateral	Usually solid gray-white masses up to 20 cm in diameter. Anaplastic tumor cells, cords, glands, dispersed through fibrous background. Cells may be "signet-ring" mucin-secreting.	Primaries are breast, lung, and gastrointestinal tract (Krukenberg tumors).

of arising in the first 2 decades of life, and the younger the patient, the greater is the likelihood of malignancy. However, over 90% of these germ-cell neoplasms are benign cystic mature teratomas. The immature malignant variant is rare.

BENIGN (MATURE) CYSTIC TERATOMAS

Almost all of these neoplasms are marked by ectodermal differentiation of the totipotential germ cells. Usually

Figure 19-19

Opened mature cystic teratoma (dermoid cyst) of the ovary. A ball of hair (*bottom*) and a mixture of tissues are evident. (Courtesy of Dr. Christopher Crum, Brigham and Women's Hospital, Boston.)

there is the formation of a cyst lined by recognizable epidermis replete with adnexal appendages; hence, the common designation *dermoid cysts*. Most are discovered in young women as ovarian masses or are found incidentally on abdominal radiographs or scans because they contain foci of calcification produced by contained teeth. About 90% are unilateral, more often on the right. Rarely do these cystic masses exceed 10 cm in diameter. On transection, they are often filled with sebaceous secretion and matted hair that, when removed, reveal a hair-bearing epidermal lining (Fig. 19-19). Sometimes, there is a nodular projection from which teeth protrude. Occasionally, foci of bone, cartilage, nests of bronchial or gastrointestinal epithelium, and other recognizable lines of development are also present.

For unknown reasons, these neoplasms sometimes produce infertility. More seriously, in about 1% of cases there is malignant transformation of one of the tissue elements, usually taking the form of a squamous cell carcinoma. Also, for unknown reasons, these tumors are prone to undergo torsion (10% to 15% of cases), producing an acute surgical emergency.

IMMATURE MALIGNANT TERATOMAS

These neoplasms are found early in life, the mean age being 18 years. They differ strikingly from benign mature teratomas insofar as they are often bulky, are predominantly solid or near-solid on transection, and are punctuated here and there by areas of necrosis; uncommonly, one of the cystic foci may contain sebaceous secretion, hair, and other features similar to those in the mature teratoma. Microscopically, the distinguishing feature is a variety of mature or barely recognizable areas of differentiation toward cartilage, bone, muscle, nerve, and other structures. Particularly ominous are the foci of neuroepithelial differentiation, because most such lesions are aggressive and metastasize widely. Immature teratomas are both graded and staged in an effort to predict their future. Those of grade I, stage I can often be cured with appropriate

therapy, whereas the opposite end of the spectrum carries a much graver outlook.

SPECIALIZED TERATOMAS

These curiosities are mentioned only because they tend to evoke "I don't believe it" reactions. Struma ovarii is composed entirely of mature thyroid tissue that, interestingly, may hyperfunction and produce hyperthyroidism. These tumors appear as small, solid, unilateral brown ovarian masses. Equally incongruous is the ovarian carcinoid, which in rare instances has produced the carcinoid syndrome! If you practice medicine long enough, you may come across a combined struma ovarii and carcinoid in the same ovary. More ominously, one of these elements may become malignant.

Clinical Correlations for All Ovarian Tumors

All ovarian neoplasms pose formidable clinical challenges, because they produce no symptoms or signs until they are well advanced. The clinical presentation of all ovarian tumors is remarkably similar despite their great morphologic diversity, except for the functioning neoplasms that have hormonal effects. Ovarian tumors of surface cell origin are usually asymptomatic until they become large enough to cause local pressure symptoms (e.g., pain, gastrointestinal complaints, urinary frequency). Indeed, about 30% of all ovarian neoplasms are discovered incidentally on routine gynecologic examination. Larger masses, notably the common epithelial tumors, may cause an increase in abdominal girth. Smaller masses, particularly dermoid cysts, sometimes become twisted on their pedicles (torsion), producing severe abdominal pain and an acute abdomen. Fibromas and malignant serous tumors often cause ascites, the latter resulting from metastatic seeding of the peritoneal cavity, so that tumor cells can be identified in the ascitic fluid. Mucinous cancers may literally fill the abdominal cavity with a gelatinous neoplastic mass (pseudomyxoma peritonei). Functioning ovarian tumors often come to attention because of the endocrinopathies they induce.

Unfortunately, methods of treatment remain unsatisfactory, as proved by the only modest increase of survival that has been achieved since the mid 1970s. Screening detection methods are being developed, but to this point they are of only limited value in discovering ovarian cancers while they are still curable. Among the many markers that have been explored, elevated serum levels of CA 125 have been reported in 75% to 90% of women with epithelial ovarian cancer. However, this is undetectable in up to 50% of patients with cancer limited to the ovary and, moreover, it is elevated in a variety of benign conditions, as well as nonovarian cancers. It is most valuable as a screening test in asymptomatic postmenopausal women because of the low incidence of confounding variables. However, as with carcinoembryonic antigen in colon cancer (Chapter 15), CA 125 measurements are of great value in monitoring response to therapy.

Diseases of Pregnancy

Diseases of pregnancy and pathologic conditions of the placenta are important causes of intrauterine or perinatal death, premature birth, congenital malformations, intrauterine growth retardation, maternal death, and a great deal of morbidity for both mother and child. Here we shall discuss only a limited number of disorders in which knowledge of the morphologic lesions contributes to an understanding of the clinical problem.

PLACENTAL INFLAMMATIONS AND INFECTIONS

Infections reach the placenta by two pathways: (1) ascending infection through the birth canal and (2) hematogenous (transplacental) infection.

Ascending infections are by far the most common; in most instances, they are bacterial and are associated with premature birth and premature rupture of the membranes. The chorioamnion shows leukocytic polymorphonuclear infiltration associated with edema and congestion of the vessels (acute chorioamnionitis). When the infection extends beyond the membranes, it may involve the umbilical cord and placental villi and cause acute vasculitis of the cord. Ascending infections are caused by mycoplasmas, *Candida*, and the numerous bacteria of the vaginal flora. Uncommonly, placental infections may arise by the *hematogenous spread* of bacteria and other organisms; histologically, the villi are most often affected (villitis). Syphilis, tuberculosis, listeriosis, toxoplasmosis, and various viruses (rubella, cytomegalovirus, herpes simplex) can all cause placental villitis. Transplacental infections can affect the fetus and give rise to the so-called TORCH complex (Chapter 7).

ECTOPIC PREGNANCY

Ectopic pregnancy is implantation of the fertilized ovum in any site other than the normal uterine location. The condition occurs in as many as 1% of pregnancies. In more than 90% of these cases, implantation is in the oviducts (tubal pregnancy); other sites include the ovaries, the abdominal cavity, and the intrauterine portion of the oviducts (interstitial pregnancy). Any hindrance that retards passage of the ovum along its course through the oviducts to the uterus predisposes to an ectopic pregnancy. In about half of the cases, such obstruction is based on chronic inflammatory changes in the oviduct, although intrauterine tumors and endometriosis may also hamper passage of the ovum. In approximately 50% of tubal pregnancies, no anatomic cause can be demonstrated. Ovarian pregnancies probably result from those rare instances of fertilization of the ovum within its follicle just at the time of rupture. Gestation within the abdominal cavity occurs when the fertilized egg drops out of the fimbriated end of the oviduct and implants on the peritoneum.

MORPHOLOGY

In all sites, ectopic pregnancies are characterized by fairly normal early development of the embryo, with the formation of placental tissue, the amniotic sac, and decidual changes. An abdominal pregnancy is occasionally carried to term. With tubal pregnancies, however, the invading placenta eventually burrows through the wall of the oviduct, causing **intratubal hematoma (hematosalpinx), intraperitoneal hemorrhage,** or both. The tube is usually locally distended up to 3 to 4 cm by a contained mass of freshly clotted blood in which may be seen bits of gray placental tissue and fetal parts. The histologic diagnosis depends on the visualization of placental villi or, rarely, of the embryo. Less commonly, poor attachment of the placenta to the tubal wall results in death of the embryo, with spontaneous proteolysis and absorption of the products of conception.

Until rupture occurs, an ectopic pregnancy may be indistinguishable from a normal one, with cessation of menstruation and elevation of serum and urinary placental hormones. Under the influence of these hormones, the endometrium (in about 50% of cases) undergoes the characteristic hypersecretory and decidual changes. However, the absence of elevated gonadotropin levels does not exclude this diagnosis, because poor attachment with necrosis of the placenta is common. Rupture of an ectopic pregnancy may be catastrophic, with the sudden onset of intense abdominal pain and signs of an acute abdomen, often followed by shock. Prompt surgical intervention is necessary.

GESTATIONAL TROPHOBLASTIC DISEASE

Traditionally, the gestational trophoblastic tumors have been divided into three overlapping morphologic categories: *hydatidiform mole*, *invasive mole*, and *choriocarcinoma*. They range in level of aggressiveness from the hydatidiform moles, most of which are benign, to the highly malignant choriocarcinomas. All elaborate human chorionic gonadotropin (hCG), which can be detected in the circulating blood and urine at titers considerably higher than those found during normal pregnancy, the titers progressively rising from hydatidiform mole to invasive mole to choriocarcinoma. In addition to aiding diagnosis, the fall or (alternatively) rise in the level of the hormone in the blood or urine can be used to monitor the effectiveness of treatment. Clinicians therefore prefer the term *gestational trophoblastic disease*, because the response to therapy as judged by the hormone titers is significantly more important than any arbitrary anatomic segregation of one lesion from another. Nonetheless, it is necessary to understand their individual characteristics to appreciate the spectrum of lesions.

Hydatidiform Mole: Complete and Partial

The typical hydatidiform mole is a voluminous mass of swollen, sometimes cystically dilated, chorionic villi, appearing grossly as grapelike structures. The swollen villi are covered by varying amounts of banal to highly atypical chorionic epithelium. Two distinctive subtypes of moles have been characterized: *complete* and *partial* moles. The complete hydatidiform mole does not permit embryogenesis and therefore never contains fetal parts. All of the chorionic villi are abnormal, and the chorionic epithelial cells are diploid (46,XX or, uncommonly, 46,XY). The partial hydatidiform mole is compatible with early embryo formation and therefore contains fetal parts, has some normal chorionic villi, and is almost always triploid (e.g., 69,XXY; Table 19–3). The two patterns result from abnormal fertilization; in a complete mole an empty egg is fertilized by two spermatozoa (or a diploid sperm), yielding the diploid karyotype, while in a partial mole a normal egg is fertilized by two spermatozoa (or a diploid sperm), resulting in the triploid karyotype.

The incidence of complete hydatidiform moles is about 1 to 1.5 per 2000 pregnancies in the United States and other Western countries. For unknown reasons there is a much higher incidence in Asian countries. Moles are most common before age 20 years and after age 40 years, and a history of a prior mole increases the risk for subsequent pregnancies. Although traditionally discovered at 12 to 14 weeks of pregnancy owing to a gestation that was "too large for dates," early monitoring of pregnancies by ultrasound has lowered the gestational age of detection, leading to the more frequent diagnosis of "early complete hydatidiform mole." In either instance, elevated hCG levels in the maternal blood coincide with absence of fetal parts or fetal heart sounds.

MORPHOLOGY

The uterus may be normal in size (as in early moles), but in fully developed cases the uterine cavity is filled with a delicate, friable mass of thin-walled, translucent cystic structures (Fig. 19–20). Fetal parts are rarely seen in complete moles but are common in partial moles. Microscopically, the **complete mole** shows hydropic swelling of chorionic villi and virtual absence of vascularization of villi. The central substance of the villi is a loose, myxomatous, edematous stroma. The chorionic epithelium almost always shows some degree of proliferation of both cytotrophoblast and syncytiotrophoblast (Fig. 19–21). The proliferation may be mild, but in many cases there is striking circumferential hyperplasia. Histologic grading to predict the clinical outcome of moles has been supplanted by careful following of hCG levels. In **partial moles**, the villous edema involves only some of the villi and the trophoblastic proliferation is focal and slight.

■

Figure 19–20 ■

Hydatidiform mole evacuated from the uterus. The "bunch-of-grapes" appearance of the lesion is readily apparent. (Courtesy of Dr. David R. Genest, Brigham and Women's Hospital, Boston.)

Table 19–3. FEATURES OF COMPLETE VERSUS PARTIAL HYDATIDIFORM MOLE

Feature	Complete Mole	Partial Mole
Karyotype	46,XX(46,XY)	Triploid (69,XXY)
Villous edema	All villi	Some villi
Trophoblast proliferation	Diffuse; circumferential	Focal; slight
Atypia	Often present	Absent
Serum hCG	Elevated	Less elevated
hCG in tissue	++++	+
Behavior	2% choriocarcinoma	Rare choriocarcinoma

Figure 19-21 ■

A microscopic image of a complete mole showing distended hydropic villi *(below)* and proliferation of the chorionic epithelium *(above).* (Courtesy of Dr. Kyle Molberg, Department of Pathology, University of Texas Southwestern Medical School, Dallas.)

Overall, 80% to 90% of moles remain benign after thorough curettage; 10% of complete moles become invasive, but not more than 2% to 3% give rise to choriocarcinoma. Partial moles rarely give rise to choriocarcinomas. With complete moles, monitoring the postcurettage blood and urine levels of hCG, particularly the more definitive β subunit of the hormone, permits detection of incomplete removal or a more ominous complication and leads to the institution of appropriate therapy, including in some cases chemotherapy, which is almost always curative.

Invasive Mole

Invasive moles are complete moles that are more invasive locally but do not have the aggressive metastatic potential of a choriocarcinoma.

An invasive mole retains hydropic villi, which penetrate the uterine wall deeply, possibly causing rupture and sometimes life-threatening hemorrhage. Local spread to the broad ligament and vagina may also occur. Microscopically, the epithelium of the villi is marked by hyperplastic and atypical changes, with proliferation of both cuboidal and syncytial components.

Although the marked invasiveness of this lesion makes removal technically difficult, metastases do not occur. Hydropic villi may embolize to distant organs, such as lungs or brain, but these emboli do not constitute true metastases and may actually regress spontaneously. Because of the greater depth of invasion of the myometrium, an invasive mole is usually not removed completely by curettage, and therefore hCG levels remain elevated. This alerts the clinician to the need for further treatment. Fortunately, in most cases, cure is possible by chemotherapy.

Choriocarcinoma

This very aggressive malignant tumor arises either from gestational chorionic epithelium or, less frequently, from totipotential cells within the gonads or elsewhere. Choriocarcinomas are rare in the Western hemisphere, and in the United States they occur in about 1 in 30,000 pregnancies. They are much more common in Asian and African countries, reaching a frequency of 1 in 2000 pregnancies. The risk is somewhat greater before age 20 and is significantly elevated after age 40. In about 50% of cases, choriocarcinomas follow a complete hydatidiform mole but only rarely a partial mole. About 25% arise after an abortion, and most of the remainder occur during what had been a normal pregnancy. Stated in another way, the more abnormal the conception, the greater is the risk of developing gestational choriocarcinoma. Most cases are discovered by the appearance of a bloody, brownish discharge accompanied by a rising titer of hCG, particularly the β subunit, in blood and urine, and the absence of marked uterine enlargement, such as would be anticipated with a mole. In general, the titers are much higher than those associated with a mole. In those instances that follow abortion or pregnancy, the fact that maternal age influences the frequency of this neoplasm suggests origin from an abnormal ovum rather than retained chorionic epithelium.

MORPHOLOGY

Choriocarcinomas usually appear as very hemorrhagic, necrotic masses within the uterus. Sometimes the necrosis is so complete as to make anatomic diagnosis difficult because there is deceptively little recognizable viable neoplasm. Indeed, the primary lesion may self-destruct, and only the metastases tell the story. Very early, the tumor insinuates itself into the myometrium and into vessels. **In contrast to the case with hydatidiform moles and invasive moles, chorionic villi are not formed; instead, the tumor is purely epithelial, composed of anaplastic cuboidal cytotrophoblast and syncytiotrophoblast** (Fig. 19-22).

By the time most neoplasms are discovered, there is usually widespread dissemination via the blood, most often to the lungs (50%), vagina (30% to 40%), brain, liver, and kidneys. Lymphatic invasion is uncommon.

Despite the extreme aggressiveness of these neoplasms, which made them nearly uniformly fatal in the past, present-day chemotherapy has achieved remarkable results. Nearly 100% of cases have been cured, even with neoplasms that have spread beyond the pelvis and vagina and into the lungs. Equally remarkable are reports of healthy infants born later to these survivors. By contrast, there is relatively poor response to chemotherapy in choriocarcinomas that arise in the gonads (ovary or testis). This striking difference in prognosis may be related to the presence of paternal antigens on placental choriocarcinomas, but not on gonadal lesions. Conceivably, a maternal immune response against the foreign (paternal) antigens helps by acting as an adjunct to chemotherapy.

Figure 19-22 ■

Photomicrograph of choriocarcinoma illustrating both neoplastic cytotrophoblast and syncytiotrophoblast. (Courtesy of Dr. David R. Genest, Brigham and Women's Hospital, Boston.)

Placental Site Trophoblastic Tumor

These uncommon tumors are diploid, are often XX in karyotype, and are derived from the placental site or intermediate trophoblast. They typically arise a few months following a pregnancy. Because intermediate trophoblasts do not produce hCG in large amounts, hCG levels are elevated, but only slightly. These tumors are indolent and generally have a favorable outcome if confined to the endomyometrium. However, they are not as sensitive to chemotherapy as other trophoblastic tumors, and the prognosis is poor when spread has occurred beyond the uterus.

PREECLAMPSIA/ECLAMPSIA (TOXEMIA OF PREGNANCY)

The development of hypertension, accompanied by proteinuria and edema in the third trimester of pregnancy, is referred to as *preeclampsia*. This syndrome occurs in 5% to 10% of pregnancies, particularly with first pregnancies in women older than age 35 years. In those severely affected, convulsive seizures may appear, which are then termed *eclampsia*. By long historical precedent, preeclampsia and eclampsia have been referred to as *toxemia of pregnancy*. No bloodborne toxin has ever been identified, however, and so the historically sanctified term (still in use) is clearly a misnomer. Full-blown eclampsia may lead to disseminated intravascular coagulation (DIC), with all of its attendant widespread ischemic organ injuries, and so eclampsia is potentially fatal.

However, recognition and treatment of preeclampsia has now made eclampsia and, particularly, fatal eclampsia rare.

The triggering events initiating these syndromes are unknown, but a basic feature underlying all cases is inadequate maternal blood flow to the placenta secondary to inadequate development of the spiral arteries of the uteroplacental bed. In the third trimester of normal pregnancy, the musculoelastic walls of the spiral arteries are replaced by a fibrinous material, permitting them to dilate into wide vascular sinusoids. In preeclampsia and eclampsia, the musculoelastic walls are retained and the channels remain narrow. The basis of these vascular abnormalities remains unknown, but a number of consequences ensue:

■ Placental hypoperfusion with an increased predisposition to the development of infarcts

■ Reduced elaboration by the trophoblast of vasodilators: prostacyclin, prostaglandin E_2, and nitric oxide, which in normal pregnancies oppose the effects of renin-angiotensin—hence the hypertension of preeclampsia and eclampsia

■ Production by the ischemic placenta of thromboplastic substances such as tissue factor and thromboxane, which probably account for the development of DIC

MORPHOLOGY

The morphologic changes of preeclampsia/eclampsia are variable and depend somewhat on the severity of the toxemic state.

Placental changes are most consistent. They include the following:

■ Infarcts, which are a feature of normal pregnancy, are much more numerous in about one third of patients with severe preeclampsia/eclampsia. They may, however, be absent.

■ Retroplacental hemorrhages occur in up to 15% of patients.

■ Placental villi reveal the changes of premature aging with villous edema, hypovascularity, and increased production of syncytial epithelial knots.

■ Prominent in well-advanced eclampsia is **acute atherosis** in the spiral arteries, characterized by thickening and fibrinoid necrosis of the vessel wall with focal accumulations of lipid-containing macrophages. Necrosis of these cells releases lipid, which is followed by the accumulation of lymphocytes and macrophages within and about the vessels. Such lesions accentuate the placental ischemia.

Multiorgan changes may be present, reflecting the development of DIC, which is discussed more fully in Chapter 12. Only major findings are considered here. The kidneys are variably affected, depending on the severity of the DIC. Basically, the changes consist of fibrin thrombi within the glomerular capillaries, accompanied by endothelial swelling and possibly mesangial hyperplasia. Focal glomerulitis may ensue. When numerous glomeruli are affected, blood flow to the cortex is reduced, possibly resulting in renal cortical necrosis that may be bilateral and fatal. Microvascular thrombi are also found in the brain, pituitary, heart, and elsewhere, having the potential of producing focal ischemic lesions sometimes accompanied by microhemorrhages.

Clinically, preeclampsia appears insidiously in the 24th to 25th weeks of gestation, with the development of edema, proteinuria, and rising blood pressure. Should the condition evolve into eclampsia, renal function is impaired, the blood pressure mounts, and convulsions may appear. Prompt therapy early in the course aborts the organ changes, with clearance of all abnormalities promptly after delivery or cesarean section.

■ ■ ■ Breast

Lesions of the female breast are much more common than lesions of the male breast, which is remarkably seldom affected. These lesions usually take the form of palpable, sometimes painful, nodules or masses. Fortunately, most are innocent, but as is well known, breast cancer was the foremost cause of cancer deaths in women in the United States until 1986, when it was supplanted by carcinoma of the lung. The following discussion deals largely with lesions of the female breast. The conditions to be described should be considered in terms of their possible confusion clinically with a malignancy. This problem is most acute with fibrocystic change, because it is the most common cause of breast "lumps" and because of the continuing controversy about the association of particular variants with breast carcinoma. However, a significant proportion of women have sufficient irregularity of the "normal" breast tissue to cause them to seek clinical attention (Fig. 19–23).

Before we turn to the extremely common fibrocystic change, several relatively minor lesions should be mentioned. *Supernumerary nipples or breasts* may be found along the embryonic ridge (milk line). Besides being merely curiosities, these congenital anomalies are subject to the same diseases that affect the definitive breasts. *Congenital inversion of the nipple* is of significance because similar changes may be produced by an underlying cancer. *Galactocele* is a cystic dilation of an obstructed duct that arises during lactation. Besides being painful "lumps," the cysts may rupture to incite a local inflammatory reaction, which may yield a persistent focus of induration causing some concern years later.

FIBROCYSTIC CHANGES

This designation is applied to a miscellany of changes in the female breast that range from those that are innocuous to patterns associated with an increased risk of breast carcinoma. Some of these alterations—stromal fibrosis and micro- or macrocysts—produce palpable "lumps." It is widely accepted that *this range of changes is the consequence of an exaggeration and distortion of the cyclic breast changes that occur normally in the menstrual cycle*. Estrogenic therapy and oral contraceptives (OCs) do not appear to increase the incidence of these alterations; indeed, OCs may *decrease* the risk.

Traditionally, these breast alterations have been called *fibrocystic disease;* however, physicians have expressed much dissatisfaction with this term. Most of the changes encompassed within the diagnosis of fibrocystic disease have little clinical significance except that they cause nodularity; only a small minority represent forms of epithelial hyperplasia that are clinically important. Thus, the term *fibrocystic changes* is preferred, since it does not stigmatize the subject with "a disease." Despite this semantic controversy, the

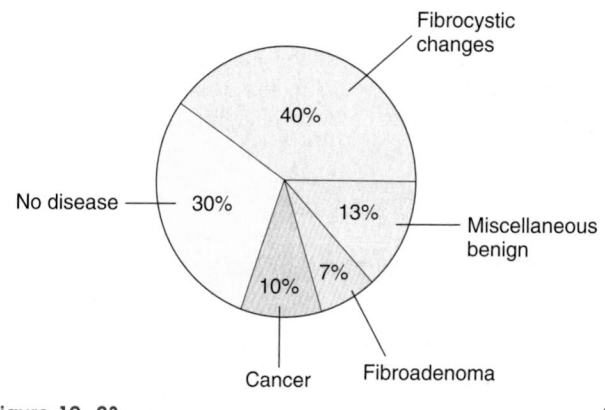

Figure 19-23   ■

Representation of the findings in a series of women seeking evaluation of apparent breast "lumps."

Figure 19–24 ■

Several biopsy specimens showing fibrocystic change of the breast. The scattered, poorly demarcated white areas represent foci of fibrosis. The biopsy specimen at the lower right reveals a transected empty cyst; those on the left have unopened blue dome cysts. (Courtesy of Dr. Kyle Molberg, Department of Pathology, University of Texas Southwestern Medical School, Dallas.)

"lumps" produced by the various patterns of fibrocystic change must be distinguished from cancer, and the distinction between the trivial variants and the not-so-trivial ones can be made by examination of fine-needle aspiration material or more definitively by biopsy and histologic evaluation. In a somewhat arbitrary manner, the alterations are here subdivided into nonproliferative and proliferative patterns. The nonproliferative lesions include cysts and/or fibrosis *without* epithelial cell hyperplasia, known as *simple fibrocystic change.* The proliferative lesions include a range of banal to atypical duct or ductular epithelial cell hyperplasias and *sclerosing adenosis.* All tend to arise during reproductive life but may persist after the menopause. The various changes, particularly the nonproliferative ones, are so common, being found at autopsy in 60% to 80% of women, that they almost constitute physiologic variants.

Nonproliferative Change

CYSTS AND FIBROSIS

Nonproliferative change is the most common type of alteration, characterized by an increase in fibrous stroma associated with dilation of ducts and formation of cysts of various sizes.

MORPHOLOGY

Grossly, a single large cyst may form within one breast, but the disorder is usually multifocal and often bilateral. The involved areas show ill-defined, diffusely increased density and discrete nodularities. The cysts vary from smaller than 1 cm to 5 cm in diameter. Unopened, they are brown to blue **(blue dome cysts)** and are filled with serous, turbid fluid (Fig. 19–24). The secretory products within the cysts may calcify to appear as microcalcifications in mammograms. Histologically, in smaller cysts, the epithelium is more cuboidal to columnar and is sometimes multilayered in focal areas. In larger cysts, it may be flattened or even totally atrophic (Fig. 19–25). Occasionally, mild epithelial proliferation leads to piled-up masses or small papillary excrescences. Frequently, cysts are lined by large polygonal cells that have an abundant granular, eosinophilic cytoplasm, with small, round, deeply chromatic nuclei, so-called **apocrine metaplasia;** this is virtually always benign.

The stroma surrounding all forms of cysts is usually compressed fibrous tissue, having lost its normal delicate, myxomatous appearance. A stromal lymphocytic infiltrate is common in this and all other variants of fibrocystic change.

Proliferative Change

EPITHELIAL HYPERPLASIA

The terms *epithelial hyperplasia* and *proliferative fibrocystic change* encompass a range of proliferative lesions within the ductules, the terminal ducts, and sometimes the lobules of the breast. Some of the epithelial hyperplasias are mild and orderly and carry little risk of carcinoma, but at the other end of the spectrum are the more florid atypical hyperplasias that carry a significantly greater risk, commensurate with the severity and atypicality of the changes. The epithelial hyperplasias are often accompanied by other histologic variants of fibrocystic change, but nonetheless they are the "cutting edge" of the histologic changes.

Figure 19–25 ■

Microscopic detail of fibrocystic change of the breast revealing dilation of ducts producing microcysts and, at right, the wall of a large cyst with visible lining epithelial cells. (Courtesy of Dr. Kyle Molberg, Department of Pathology, University of Texas Southwestern Medical School, Dallas.)

Figure 19-26   ■

A, Moderate duct epithelial hyperplasia. Note that the cells fill part of the duct lumen. *B*, More florid duct epithelial hyperplasia, with irregular lumina at the periphery, so-called *fenestrations*. (Courtesy of Dr. Stuart Schnitt, Beth Israel Deaconess Hospital, Boston.)

MORPHOLOGY

The gross appearance of epithelial hyperplasia is not distinctive and is often dominated by coexisting fibrous or cystic changes. Histologically, there is an almost infinite spectrum of proliferative alterations (Fig. 19-26). The ducts, ductules, or lobules may be filled with orderly cuboidal cells, within which small gland patterns can be discerned (so-called **fenestrations**). Sometimes the proliferating epithelium projects in multiple small papillary excrescences into the ductal lumen **(ductal papillomatosis).** The degree of hyperplasia, manifested in part by the number of layers of intraductal epithelial proliferation, can be mild, moderate, or severe.

In some instances the hyperplastic cells become monomorphic with complex architectural patterns. In short, they have changes approaching those of carcinoma in situ (described later). Such hyperplasia is called **atypical.** The line separating the epithelial hyperplasias without atypia from atypical hyperplasia is difficult to define, just as it is difficult to clearly distinguish between atypical hyperplasia and carcinoma in situ. However, these distinctions are important, as will soon become clear.

Atypical lobular hyperplasia is the term used to describe hyperplasias that cytologically resemble lobular carcinoma in situ, but the cells do not fill or distend more than 50% of the terminal duct units. Atypical lobular hyperplasia is associated with an increased risk of invasive carcinoma.

Epithelial hyperplasia per se does not often produce a clinically discrete breast mass. Occasionally, it produces microcalcifications on mammography, raising fears about cancer. Such nodularity as may be present usually relates to other concurrent variants of fibrocystic change; however, florid papillomatosis may be associated with a serous or serosanguineous nipple discharge.

SCLEROSING ADENOSIS

This variant is less common than cysts and hyperplasia, but it is significant because its clinical and morphologic features may be deceptively similar to those of carcinoma. There are in this lesion marked intralobular fibrosis and proliferation of small ductules and acini.

MORPHOLOGY

Grossly, the lesion has a hard, rubbery consistency, similar to that of breast cancer. Histologically, sclerosing adenosis is characterized by proliferation of lining epithelial cells and myoepithelial cells in small ducts and ductules, yielding masses of small gland patterns within a fibrous stroma (Fig. 19-27). Aggregated glands or proliferating ductules may be virtually

Figure 19-27   ■

Sclerosing adenosis of the breast. The epithelial hyperplasia has produced the nests of cells, which appear quite disorderly. The overgrowth of fibrous tissue enmeshes and partially obliterates many of the epithelial nests, creating a pattern very similar to the infiltrative growth of a cancer.

back to back, with single or multiple layers of cells in contact with one another **(adenosis)**. Marked stromal fibrosis, which may compress and distort the proliferating epithelium, is always associated with the adenosis; hence, the designation **sclerosing adenosis**. **This overgrowth of fibrous tissue may completely compress the lumina of the acini and ducts, so that they appear as solid cords of cells.** This pattern may then be difficult to distinguish histologically from an invasive scirrhous carcinoma. The presence of double layers of epithelium and the identification of myoepithelial elements are helpful in suggesting a benign diagnosis.

Although sclerosing adenosis is sometimes difficult to differentiate clinically and histologically from carcinoma, it is associated with only a minimally increased risk of progression to carcinoma.

Relationship of Fibrocystic Changes to Breast Carcinoma

The relationship of fibrocystic changes to breast carcinoma is a medically controversial area. Only some reasonably supportable summary statements are possible. Clinically, although certain features of fibrocystic change tend to distinguish it from cancer, the only certain way of making this distinction is by biopsy and histologic examination. With respect to the relationship of the various patterns of fibrocystic change to cancer, the following statements currently represent the best-informed opinion (Fig. 19–28):

■ *Minimal or no increased risk of breast carcinoma:* fibrosis, cystic changes (micro- or macroscopic), apocrine metaplasia, mild hyperplasia.

■ *Slightly increased risk (1.5 to 2 times):* moderate to florid hyperplasia, ductal papillomatosis, sclerosing adenosis, fibroadenomas, especially when they are associated with fibrocystic changes, proliferative breast disease, or a family history of breast cancer.
■ *Significantly increased risk (5 times):* atypical hyperplasia, ductular or lobular.
■ Proliferative lesions may be multifocal, and the risk of subsequent carcinoma extends to both breasts.
■ *A family history of breast cancer may increase the risk in all categories* (e.g., to about tenfold with atypical hyperplasia).

Only about 15% of biopsy specimens exhibit atypical epithelial hyperplasia. Thus, most women who have lumps related to fibrocystic change can be reassured that there is little or no increased predisposition to cancer. The need to differentiate among the many variants and the grounds for dissatisfaction with the unqualified terms *fibrocystic changes* or, even worse, *fibrocystic disease* are apparent. The risks inherent in the various patterns are shown in Figure 19–28.

INFLAMMATIONS

Inflammations of the breast are uncommon and during the acute stages usually cause pain and tenderness in the involved areas. Included in this category are several forms of mastitis and traumatic fat necrosis, none of which is associated with increased risk of cancer.

Acute mastitis develops when bacteria gain access to the breast tissue through the ducts; when there is inspissation of secretions; through fissures in the nipples, which usually develop during the early weeks of nursing; or from various forms of dermatitis involving the nipple.

Figure 19–28 ■

An attempt to depict by the thickness of the arrow the risk of malignant transformation of the various patterns of fibrocystic change.

MORPHOLOGY

Staphylococcal infections induce single or multiple abscesses accompanied by the typical clinical acute inflammatory changes when they are near the surface. They are usually small, but when sufficiently large they may leave in the course of healing residual foci of scarring that are palpable as localized areas of induration. Streptococcal infections generally spread throughout the entire breast, causing pain, marked swelling, and breast tenderness. Resolution of these infections rarely leaves residual areas of induration.

Mammary duct ectasia (periductal or plasma cell mastitis) is a nonbacterial inflammation of the breast associated with inspissation of breast secretions in the main excretory ducts. Ductal dilation with ductal rupture leads to reactive changes in the surrounding breast substance. It is an uncommon condition, usually encountered in women in their 40s and 50s who have borne children.

MORPHOLOGY

Usually the inflammatory changes are confined to an area drained by one or several of the major excretory ducts of the nipple. There is increased firmness of the tissue, and on cross-section dilated ropelike ducts are apparent from which thick, cheesy secretions can be extruded. Histologically, the ducts are filled by granular debris, sometimes containing leukocytes, principally lipid-laden macrophages. The lining epithelium is generally destroyed. **The most distinguishing features are the prominence of the lymphocytic and plasma cell infiltration and occasional granulomas in the periductal stroma.**

Mammary duct ectasia is of principal importance because it leads to induration of the breast substance and, more significantly, to retraction of the skin or nipple, mimicking the changes caused by some carcinomas.

Traumatic fat necrosis is an uncommon and innocuous lesion that is significant only because it produces a mass. Most, but not all, patients report some antecedent trauma to the breast.

MORPHOLOGY

During the early stage, the lesion is small, often tender, rarely more than 2 cm in diameter, and sharply localized. It consists of a central focus of necrotic fat cells surrounded by neutrophils and lipid-filled macrophages, which is later enclosed by fibrous tissue and mononuclear leukocytes. Eventually, the focus is replaced by scar tissue, or the debris becomes encysted within the scar. Calcifications may develop in either the scar or cyst wall.

TUMORS OF THE BREAST

Tumors are the most important lesions of the female breast. Although they may arise from either connective tissue or epithelial structures, it is the latter that give rise to the common breast neoplasms. Here we will describe fibroadenoma, phyllodes tumor, papilloma and papillary carcinoma, and carcinoma of the breast.

Fibroadenoma

The fibroadenoma is by far the most common benign tumor of the female breast. An absolute or relative increase in estrogen activity is thought to play a role in its development, and indeed similar lesions may appear with fibrocystic changes (fibroadenosis). Fibroadenomas usually appear in young women; the peak incidence is in the third decade of life.

MORPHOLOGY

The fibroadenoma occurs as a discrete, usually solitary, freely movable nodule, 1 to 10 cm in diameter. Rarely, multiple tumors are encountered and, equally rarely, they may exceed 10 cm in diameter **(giant fibroadenoma).** Whatever their size, they are usually easily "shelled out." Grossly, all are firm, with a uniform tan-white color on cut section, punctuated by softer yellow-pink specks representing the glandular areas (Fig. 19–29). Histologically, there is a loose fibroblastic stroma containing ductlike, epithelium-lined spaces of various forms and sizes. These ductlike or glandular spaces are lined with single or multiple layers of cells that are regular and have a well-defined, intact basement membrane. Although in some lesions the ductal spaces are open, round to oval, and fairly regular **(pericanalicular fibroadenoma),** others are compressed by extensive proliferation of the stroma, so that on cross-section they appear as slits or irregular, star-shaped structures **(intracanalicular fibroadenoma)** (Fig. 19–30).

Figure 19–29

Fibroadenoma of the breast. The tan-colored encapsulated small tumor is sharply demarcated from the whiter breast tissue.

Figure 19-30 ■

Low-power microscopic view of a fibroadenoma of the breast showing the discrete margins *(arrow)* and the intracanalicular and pericanalicular patterns.

Clinically, fibroadenomas usually present as solitary, discrete, movable masses. They may enlarge late in the menstrual cycle and during pregnancy. Postmenopausally, they may regress and calcify. Cytogenetic studies reveal that the stromal cells are monoclonal and so represent the neoplastic element of these tumors. The basis of ductal proliferation is not clear; perhaps the neoplastic stromal cells secrete growth factors that affect epithelial cells. Fibroadenomas almost never become malignant.

Phyllodes Tumor

These tumors are much less common than fibroadenomas and are thought to arise from the intralobular stroma and only rarely from preexisting fibroadenomas. They may be small (3 to 4 cm in diameter), but most grow to large, possibly massive size, distending the breast. Some become lobulated and cystic; because on gross section they exhibit leaflike clefts and slits, they have been designated phyllodes (Greek for "leaflike") tumors. In the past they had the tongue-tangling name *cystosarcoma phyllodes*, an unfortunate term because these tumors are usually benign, although some become malignant. The most ominous change is the appearance of increased stromal cellularity with anaplasia and high mitotic activity, accompanied by rapid increase in size, usually with invasion of adjacent breast tissue by malignant stroma. Most of these tumors remain localized and are cured by excision; malignant lesions may recur, but they also tend to remain localized. Only the most malignant, about 15% of cases, metastasize to distant sites.

Intraductal Papilloma

This is a neoplastic papillary growth within a duct. Most lesions are solitary, found within the principal lactiferous ducts or sinuses. They present clinically as a result of (1) the appearance of serous or bloody nipple discharge, (2) the presence of a small subareolar tumor a few millimeters in diameter, or (3) rarely, nipple retraction.

MORPHOLOGY

The tumors are usually solitary and less than 1 cm in diameter, consisting of delicate, branching growths within a dilated duct or cyst. Histologically, they are composed of multiple papillae, each having a connective tissue axis covered by cuboidal or cylindrical epithelial cells that are frequently double layered, the outer epithelial layer overlying a myoepithelial layer.

In some cases there are multiple papillomas in several ducts or intraductal papillomatosis. These lesions sometimes become malignant, whereas the solitary papilloma almost always remains benign. Similarly, papillary carcinoma must be excluded; it lacks a myoepithelial component and shows severe cytologic atypia and abnormal mitotic figures.

Carcinoma

No cancer is more feared by women than carcinoma of the breast, and for good reason. In the United States it is estimated by the American Cancer Society that in 2001, 192,200 new invasive breast cancers will be discovered in women, and there will be 40,860 deaths, making this scourge second only to lung cancer as a cause of cancer death. The data make clear that despite advances in diagnosis and treatment, almost one fourth of women who develop these neoplasms will die of the disease. However, it is also important to emphasize that although the lifetime risk is one in eight for women in the United States, 75% of women with breast cancer are older than age 50. Only 5% are younger than the age of 40. For unknown reasons (possibly related in some part to better case finding), there has been an increase in the incidence of breast cancer throughout the world. In the United States the increase was holding steady at about 1% a year, when it started to climb in 1980 to 3% to 4% a year. Fortunately, the rate has now plateaued at about 111 cases per 100,000 women. Understandably, then, there has been intense study of the possible origins of this form of cancer and of means to diagnose it early enough to permit cure.

Epidemiology and Risk Factors. A large number of risk factors have been identified that modify a woman's likelihood of developing this form of cancer. They are briefly listed in Table 19-4, which divides them into well-established and less well-established groups and indicates where possible the relative risk imposed by each. Comments about some of the more important risk factors follow.

Geographic Variations. There are surprising differences among countries in the incidence rates and mortality rates from breast cancer. The risk for this form of neoplasia is significantly higher in North America and northern Europe than in Asia and Africa. For example, the incidence and mortality rates are five times higher in the United States than in Japan. These differences appear to be environmental rather than genetic in origin, because migrants from low-incidence locales to high-incidence areas tend to acquire the rates of their adoptive countries, and vice versa. Diet, reproductive patterns, and nursing habits are thought to be involved.

Table 19-4.   BREAST CANCER RISK FACTORS

Factor	Relative Risk
Well-Established Influences	
Geographic factors	Varies in different areas
Age	Increases after age 30 yr
Family History	
First-degree relative with breast cancer	1.2–3.0
Premenopausal	3.1
Premenopausal and bilateral	8.5–9.0
Postmenopausal	1.5
Postmenopausal and bilateral	4.0–5.4
Menstrual History	
Age at menarche <12 yr	1.3
Age at menopause >55 yr	1.5–2.0
Pregnancy	
First live birth from ages 25–29 yr	1.5
First live birth after age 30 yr	1.9
First live birth after age 35 yr	2.0–3.0
Nulliparous	3.0
Benign Breast Disease	
Proliferative disease	1.9
Proliferative disease with atypical hyperplasia	4.4
Lobular carcinoma in situ	6.9–12.0
Less Well-Established Influences	
Exogenous estrogens	
Oral contraceptives	
Obesity	
High-fat diet	
Alcohol consumption	
Cigarette smoking	

Extensively modified from Bilimoria MM, Morrow M: The women at increased risk for breast cancer: evaluation and management strategies. CA Cancer J Clin 46: 263, 1995.

Age. Breast cancer is uncommon in women younger than age 30. Thereafter, the risk steadily increases throughout life, but after the menopause the upward slope of the curve almost plateaus.

Genetics and Family History. About 5% to 10% of breast cancers are related to specific inherited mutations. Women are more likely to carry a breast cancer susceptibility gene if they develop breast cancer before menopause, have bilateral cancer, have other associated cancers (e.g., ovarian cancer), have a significant family history (i.e., multiple relatives affected before menopause), or belong to certain ethnic groups. About half of women with hereditary breast cancer have mutations in gene *BRCA1* (on chromosome 17q21.3) and an additional one third have mutations in *BRCA2* (on chromosome 13q12-13). These are large, complex genes that do not exhibit close homology to each other, nor to other known genes. Although their exact role in carcinogenesis and their relative specificity for breast cancer are still being elucidated, both of these genes are thought to play a critical role in DNA repair (Chapter 6). They act as tumor suppressor genes, since cancer arises when both alleles are inactive or defective—one caused by a germ-line mutation and the second by a subsequent somatic mutation. Genetic testing is available, but it is complicated by the hundreds of different mutations detected,

only some of which confer cancer susceptibility. The degree of penetrance, the age at cancer onset, and the association with susceptibility to other types of cancers can vary with the type of mutation. However, most carriers will develop breast cancer by the age of 70, compared with only 7% of women who do not carry a mutation. The role of these genes in nonhereditary sporadic breast cancer is less clear, because mutations are infrequent in these tumors. It is possible that other mechanisms, such as methylation of regulatory regions, act to inactivate the genes in sporadic cancer. Less common genetic diseases associated with breast cancer are the Li-Fraumeni syndrome (caused by germ-line mutations in *TP53*; Chapter 6), Cowden disease (caused by germ-line mutations in *PTEN*; Chapter 15), and carriers of the ataxia-telangiectasia gene (Chapter 6).

Other Risk Factors

■ *Prolonged exposure to exogenous estrogens* postmenopausally, known as estrogen replacement therapy (ERT), is acknowledged to prevent or at least delay the onset of osteoporosis and protect against heart disease and stroke. However, it is also associated with a moderate increase in the incidence of breast cancer. The incidence is slightly *higher* in women using combined estrogens and progestagens. However, cancers in such women more commonly present at a clinically less advanced stage and are associated with a lower mortality than cancers in women who have never used hormone replacement therapy. When all the pros and cons are considered, the benefits far outweigh the possible adverse effects of ERT in terms of overall longevity for most women.

■ *Oral contraceptives* have also been suspected of increasing the risk of breast cancer. Although once again the evidence is contradictory, the newer formulations of balanced low doses of combined estrogens and progestins impose only a very slightly increased risk, which disappears 10 years after discontinuing their use.

■ *Ionizing radiation* to the chest increases the risk of breast cancer. The magnitude of the risk depends on the radiation dose, the time since exposure, and age. Only women irradiated before age 30, during breast development, appear to be affected. For example, 20% to 30% of women irradiated for Hodgkin disease in their teens and 20s will develop breast cancer, but the risk for women treated later in life is not elevated. The low doses of radiation associated with mammographic screening have little, if any, effect on the incidence of breast cancer. Any possible effect is compensated for by the demonstrated benefits of earlier detection of breast cancer.

■ *Many other less well-established risk factors*, such as obesity, alcohol consumption, and a diet high in fat, have been implicated in the development of breast cancer on the basis of population studies, but the evidence is at best inferential.

Pathogenesis. As is the case with all cancers, the cause of breast cancer remains unknown. However, three sets of influences appear to be important: (1) genetic changes, (2) hormonal influences, and (3) environmental factors.

Genetic Changes. In addition to those producing the well-established familial syndromes mentioned earlier, genetic changes have also been implicated in the genesis of sporadic breast cancer. As with most other cancers, mutations affecting protooncogenes and tumor suppressor genes in breast epithelium contribute to the oncogenic transformation process. Among the best characterized is overexpression of the *ERBB2 (HER2/NEU)* protooncogene, which has been found to be amplified in up to 30% of breast cancers. This gene is a member of the epidermal growth factor receptor family, and its overexpression is associated with a poor prognosis. Analogously, amplification of *RAS* and *MYC* genes has also been reported in some human breast cancers. Mutations of the well-known suppressor genes *RB1* and *TP53* may also be present. Most likely, multiple acquired mutations are involved in the sequential transformation of a normal epithelial cell into a cancerous cell.

Hormonal Influences. Endogenous estrogen excess, or more accurately, hormonal imbalance, clearly plays a significant role. Many of the risk factors mentioned—long duration of reproductive life, nulliparity, and late age at birth of first child—imply increased exposure to estrogen peaks during the menstrual cycle (see Table 19–4). Functioning ovarian tumors that elaborate estrogens are associated with breast cancer in postmenopausal women. Estrogens stimulate the production of growth factors by normal breast epithelial cells and by cancer cells. It is hypothesized that the estrogen and progesterone receptors normally present in breast epithelium, and often present in breast cancer cells, may interact with growth promoters, such as transforming growth factor α (related to epithelial growth factor), platelet-derived growth factor, and fibroblast growth factor elaborated by human breast cancer cells, to create an autocrine mechanism of tumor development.

Environmental Factors. Environmental influences are suggested by the variable incidence of breast cancer in genetically homogeneous groups and the geographic differences in prevalence, as discussed earlier. Other important environmental factors include irradiation and exogenous estrogens, described earlier.

MORPHOLOGY

Cancer of the breast affects the left breast slightly more often than the right. In about 4% of patients there are bilateral primary tumors or sequential lesions in the same breast. The locations of the tumors within the breast are as follows:

Upper outer quadrant	50%
Central portion	20%
Lower outer quadrant	10%
Upper inner quadrant	10%
Lower inner quadrant	10%

Breast cancers are divided into those that have not penetrated the limiting basement membrane (noninvasive) and those that have (invasive). The chief forms of carcinoma of the breast can be classified as follows:

A. Noninvasive
   1. Ductal carcinoma in situ (DCIS; intraductal carcinoma)
   2. Lobular carcinoma in situ (LCIS)
B. Invasive (infiltrating)
   1. Invasive ductal carcinoma ("not otherwise specified"; NOS)
   2. Invasive lobular carcinoma
   3. Medullary carcinoma
   4. Colloid carcinoma (mucinous carcinoma)
   5. Tubular carcinoma
   6. Other types

Of these, invasive ductal carcinoma is by far the most common. Because it usually has an abundant fibrous stroma, it is also referred to as **scirrhous carcinoma.** Comments on the more common types follow.

NONINVASIVE (IN SITU) CARCINOMA (INCLUDING PAGET DISEASE). There are two types of noninvasive breast carcinoma: ductal carcinoma in situ (DCIS) and lobular carcinoma in situ (LCIS). Morphologic studies have shown that both usually arise from the terminal duct lobular unit. DCIS tends to fill, distort, and unfold involved lobules and, thus, appears to involve ductlike spaces. In contrast, LCIS usually expands but does not alter the underlying lobular architecture. Both are confined by a basement membrane and do not invade into stroma or lymphovascular channels.

DCIS has a wide variety of histologic appearances. Architectural patterns include solid, cribriform, papillary, micropapillary, and clinging types. Necrosis may be present in any of these types. Nuclear appearance ranges from low grade and monomorphic to high grade and heterogeneous. The **comedo** subtype is characterized by cells with high-grade nuclei distending spaces with extensive central necrosis. The name derives from the toothpaste-like necrotic tissue that can be extruded from transected ducts with gentle pressure. Calcifications are frequently associated with DCIS, owing to either calcified necrotic debris or secretory material. The incidence of DCIS markedly increases from less than 5% of breast cancers in unscreened populations up to 40% of those screened by mammography, primarily owing to the detection of calcifications. These days, DCIS only rarely presents as a palpable or radiologic mass. If detection is delayed, a palpable mass or nipple discharge may be present. The cells in the better differentiated tumors express estrogen and, less often, progestagen receptors. The prognosis for DCIS is excellent, with over 97% long-term survival. Some patients develop distant metastases without local recurrence; such cases usually have extensive high-grade DCIS and probably had undetected small areas of invasion. At least one third of women with small areas of untreated low-grade DCIS will eventually develop invasive carcinoma. When invasive cancer does develop, it is usually in the same breast and quadrant as the prior DCIS. Current treatment

Figure 19-31   ■

Paget disease of the breast. Paget cells with abundant clear cytoplasm and pleomorphic nuclei dot the epithelium.

Figure 19-32   ■

A cut section of an invasive ductal carcinoma of the breast. The lesion is retracted, infiltrating the surrounding breast substance, and would be stony hard on palpation.

strategies attempt to eradicate the DCIS by surgery and radiation. Treatment with the anti-estrogenic tamoxifen may also decrease the risk of recurrence.

Paget disease of the nipple is caused by the extension of DCIS up to the lactiferous ducts and into the contiguous skin of the nipple (Fig. 19-31). The malignant cells disrupt the normal epidermal barrier, which allows extracellular fluid to be extruded onto the surface. The clinical appearance is usually of a unilateral crusting exudate over the nipple and areolar skin. In about half of cases, an underlying invasive carcinoma will also be present. Prognosis is based on the underlying carcinoma and is not worsened by the presence of Paget disease.

LCIS, unlike DCIS, has a uniform appearance. The cells are monomorphic with bland, round nuclei and occur in discohesive clusters in ducts and lobules. Intracellular mucin vacuoles (signet ring cells) are common. LCIS is virtually always an incidental finding, and, unlike DCIS, it does not form masses and is only rarely associated with calcifications. Therefore, the incidence of LCIS is almost unchanged in mammographically screened populations. Approximately one third of women with LCIS will eventually develop invasive carcinoma. Unlike DCIS, **the invasive carcinomas arise in either breast at equal frequency.** About one third of these cancers will be of lobular type (compared with about 10% of cancers in women who develop de novo lobular carcinoma), but most are of no special type. Thus, **LCIS is both a marker of increased risk of developing breast cancer in either breast and a direct precursor of some cancers.** Current treatment requires either close clinical and radiologic follow-up of both breasts or bilateral prophylactic mastectomy.

INVASIVE (INFILTRATING) CARCINOMA. The morphology of the subtypes of invasive carcinoma is presented first, followed by the clinical features of all.

Invasive ductal carcinoma is a term used for all carcinomas that cannot be subclassified into one of the specialized types described below and does not indicate that this tumor specifically arises from the ductal system. **Carcinomas of "no special type" or "not otherwise specified" are synonyms for ductal carcinomas.** The majority (70% to 80%) of cancers fall into this group. This type of cancer is usually associated with DCIS, but rarely LCIS is present. Most ductal carcinomas produce a desmoplastic response, which replaces normal breast fat (resulting in a mammographic density) and forms a hard, palpable mass (Figs. 19-32 and 19-33). The microscopic

Figure 19-33   ■

Microscopic view of so-called scirrhous carcinoma of the breast reveals the dense collagenous background in which are scattered cords and nests of tumor cells.

Figure 19-34 ■

The margin of a cancer of the breast revealing tumorous infiltration of the adjacent fatty tissue *(at right)*.

appearance is quite heterogeneous, ranging from tumors with well-developed tubule formation and low-grade nuclei to tumors consisting of sheets of anaplastic cells. The tumor margins are usually irregular (Fig. 19-34) but are occasionally pushing and circumscribed. Invasion of lymphovascular spaces or along nerves may be seen. Advanced cancers may cause dimpling of the skin, retraction of the nipple, or fixation to the chest wall. About two thirds express estrogen or progestagen receptors, and about one third overexpress *ERBB2*.

Inflammatory carcinoma is defined by the clinical presentation of an enlarged, swollen, erythematous breast, usually without a palpable mass. The underlying carcinoma is generally of no special type and diffusely invades the breast parenchyma. The blockage of numerous dermal lymphatic spaces by carcinoma results in the clinical appearance. True inflammation is minimal or absent. Most of these tumors have distant metastases, and the prognosis is extremely poor.

Invasive lobular carcinoma consists of cells morphologically identical to the cells of LCIS. Two thirds of the cases are associated with adjacent LCIS. The cells invade individually into stroma and are often aligned in strands or chains (Fig. 19-35). Occasionally, they surround cancerous or normal-appearing acini or ducts, creating a so-called bull's eye pattern. Although most present as palpable masses or mammographic densities, a significant subgroup may have a diffusely invasive pattern without a desmoplastic response and may be clinically occult. Lobular carcinomas, more frequently than ductal carcinomas, metastasize to cerebrospinal fluid, serosal surfaces, ovary and uterus, and bone marrow. Lobular carcinomas are also more frequently multicentric and bilateral (10% to 20%). Almost all of these carcinomas express hormone receptors, but *ERBB2* expression is very rare or absent. These tumors comprise less than 20% of all breast carcinomas.

Medullary carcinoma is a rare subtype of carcinoma comprising about 2% of cases. These cancers consist of sheets of large anaplastic cells with pushing, well-circumscribed borders. Clinically, they can be mistaken for fibroadenomas. There is invariably a pronounced lymphoplasmacytic infiltrate. DCIS is usually absent or minimal. Medullary carcinomas, or medullary-like carcinomas, occur with increased frequency in women with *BRCA1* mutations, although most women with medullary carcinoma are not carriers. These carcinomas uniformly lack hormone receptors and do not overexpress *ERBB2*.

Figure 19-35 ■

Lobular carcinoma. *Left,* The terminal ducts and ductules of the breast are distended with tumor cells (lobular carcinoma in situ). *Right,* Strands of tumor cells are infiltrating the fibrous pink stroma. (Courtesy of Dr. Kyle Molberg, Department of Pathology, University of Texas Southwestern Medical School, Dallas.)

Colloid (mucinous) carcinoma is also a rare subtype. The tumor cells produce abundant quantities of extracellular mucin that dissects into the surrounding stroma. Like medullary carcinomas, they often present as well-circumscribed masses and can be mistaken for fibroadenomas. Grossly, the tumors are usually soft and gelatinous. Most express hormone receptors, and rare examples may overexpress *ERBB2*.

Tubular carcinomas rarely present as palpable masses but account for 10% of invasive carcinomas less than 1 cm in size found with mammographic screening. They usually present as irregular mammographic densities. Microscopically, the carcinomas consist of well-formed tubules with low-grade nuclei. Lymph node metastases are rare, and prognosis is excellent. Virtually all tubular carcinomas express hormone receptors, and overexpression of *ERBB2* is highly unusual.

FEATURES COMMON TO ALL INVASIVE CANCERS. In all the forms of breast cancer discussed previously, progression of the disease leads to certain local morphologic features. These include a tendency to become adherent to the pectoral muscles or deep fascia of the chest wall, with consequent **fixation** of the lesion, as well as adherence to the overlying skin, with **retraction** or **dimpling** of the skin or nipple. The latter is an important sign, because it may be the first indication of a lesion, observed by the patient herself during self-examination. Involvement of the lymphatic pathways may cause localized **lymphedema**. In these cases, the skin becomes thickened around exaggerated hair follicles, a change known as **peau d'orange** (orange peel).

Spread of Breast Cancer. Spread eventually occurs through lymphatic and hematogenous channels. Nodal metastases are present in about 40% of cancers presenting as palpable masses but less than 15% of cases found by mammography. Outer quadrant and centrally located lesions typically spread first to the axillary nodes. Those in the inner quadrants often involve the lymph node along the internal mammary arteries. The supraclavicular nodes are sometimes the primary site of spread, but they may become involved only after the axillary and internal mammary nodes are affected. More distant dissemination eventually ensues, with metastatic involvement of almost any organ or tissue in the body. Favored locations are the lungs, skeleton, liver, and adrenals and (less commonly) the brain, spleen, and pituitary. However, no site is exempt. *Metastases may appear many years after apparent therapeutic control of the primary lesion, sometimes 15 years later.* Nevertheless, with each passing year the scene brightens.

Staging of Breast Cancer. The most important prognostic factors for breast cancer are the size of the primary tumor, lymph node metastases, and the presence of distant disease. Local poor prognostic factors also include invasion of the chest wall, ulceration of the skin, and the clinical appearance of inflammatory carcinoma. These features are used to classify women into prognostic groups for treatment decisions, counseling, and for clinical trials. The most commonly used staging system has been devised by the American Joint Committee on Cancer Staging and the International Union Against Cancer, as seen below. The 5-year survival for women ranges from 92% for stage 0 disease to 13% for stage IV disease.

American Joint Committee on Cancer Staging of Breast Carcinoma

Stage 0	DCIS (including Paget disease of the nipple) and LCIS
Stage I	Invasive carcinomas 2 cm or less in size and negative lymph nodes
Stage IIA	Invasive carcinomas 2 cm or less in size with metastatic disease to lymph node(s) or invasive carcinomas greater than 2 cm in size but less than 5 cm in size with negative lymph nodes
Stage IIB	Invasive carcinomas greater than 2 cm in size but less than 5 cm in size with positive lymph node(s) or invasive carcinomas greater than 5 cm in size with negative lymph nodes
Stage IIIA	Invasive carcinomas of any size with fixed lymph nodes (i.e., extranodal invasion extending between lymph nodes or invading into other structures) or carcinomas over 5 cm in size with nonfixed lymph node metastases
Stage IIIB	Inflammatory carcinoma, carcinomas invading into the chest wall, carcinomas invading into the skin, carcinomas with satellite skin nodules, or any carcinoma with metastasis to ipsilateral internal mammary lymph node(s)
Stage IV	Distant metastatic disease

Clinical Course. Breast cancer is often discovered by the patient or her physician as a deceptively discrete, solitary, painless, and movable mass. At this time, the carcinoma is typically 2 to 3 cm in size, and involvement of the regional lymph nodes (most often axillary) is already present in about half of patients. With mammographic screening, carcinomas are frequently detected before they become palpable. The average invasive carcinoma found by screening is around 1 cm in size, and only 15% of these have nodal metastases. In addition, in many women DCIS is detected before the development of invasive carcinoma. As women age, fibrous breast tissue is replaced by fat, and screening becomes more sensitive, owing to the increased radiolucency of the breast and the increased incidence of malignancy. The current controversy over the best time to begin mammographic screening must take into account the benefit to some women balanced against the morbidity of the majority of women who will be proved to have benign changes.

Prognosis is influenced by the following variables:

1. *The size of the primary carcinoma.* Invasive carcinomas smaller than 1 cm have an excellent survival in the absence of lymph node metastases and may not require systemic therapy.

2. *Lymph node involvement and the number of lymph nodes involved by metastases.* With no axillary node involvement, the 5-year survival rate is close to 90%. The survival rate decreases with each involved lymph node and is less than 50% with 16 or more involved nodes. Sentinel node biopsy has been introduced as an alternative less morbid procedure to replace a full axillary dissection. The first one or two draining lymph nodes are identified by using a dye, a radioactive tracer, or both. A negative sentinel lymph node is highly predictive of the absence of metastatic carcinoma in the remaining lymph nodes. The sentinel lymph node can be examined by more extensive procedures, such as serial sectioning or immunohistochemical studies for cytokeratin-positive cells. However, the clinical significance of the finding of micrometastases (defined as metastatic deposits measuring less than 0.2 cm in size) is still unknown.

3. *The grade of the carcinoma.* The most common grading system for breast cancer evaluates tubule formation, nuclear grade, and mitotic rate to divide carcinomas into three groups. Well-differentiated carcinomas have a significantly better prognosis as compared with poorly differentiated carcinomas. Moderately differentiated carcinomas initially have a better prognosis, but survival at 20 years approaches that of poorly differentiated carcinomas.

4. *The histologic type of carcinoma.* All specialized types of breast carcinoma (tubular, medullary, lobular, papillary, and mucinous) have a somewhat better prognosis than carcinomas of no special type ("ductal carcinomas").

5. *Lymphovascular invasion.* The presence of tumor within vascular spaces around the primary tumor is a poor prognostic factor, especially in the absence of lymph node metastases. Dermal lymphovascular invasion correlates with the clinical appearance of inflammatory carcinoma and carries a very poor prognosis.

6. *The presence or absence of estrogen or progesterone receptors.* The presence of hormone receptors confers a slightly better prognosis. However, the reason for determining their presence is to predict the response to therapy. The highest rate of response (~80%) to antiestrogen therapy (oophorectomy or tamoxifen) is seen in patients whose tumors have both estrogen and progesterone receptors. Lower rates of response (25% to 45%) are seen if only one of the receptors is present. If both are absent, very few patients (less than 10%) are expected to respond.

7. *The proliferative rate of the cancer.* Proliferation can be measured by mitotic counts, flow cytometry, or by immunohistochemical markers for cell cycle proteins. Mitotic counts are included as part of the grading system. The optimal method for evaluating proliferation has not been determined. High proliferative rates are associated with a poorer prognosis.

8. *Aneuploidy.* Carcinomas with an abnormal DNA content (aneuploidy) have a slightly worse prognosis as compared with carcinomas with a DNA content similar to normal cells.

9. *Overexpression of ERBB2.* Overexpression of this membrane-bound protein is almost always caused by amplification of the gene. Therefore, overexpression can be determined by immunohistochemistry (which detects the protein in tissue sections) or by fluorescence in situ hybridization (which detects the number of gene copies). Overexpression is associated with a poorer prognosis. However, the importance of evaluating ERBB2 is to predict response to a monoclonal antibody to the gene ("Herceptin"). This is one of the first examples whereby an antitumor antibody therapy has been developed on the basis of a specific gene abnormality present in the tumor.

Despite all prognostic indicators, it is impossible in the individual case to foresee the outcome. Sadly, only time tells the story. The overall 5-year survival rate for stage I cancer is 87%; for stage II, 75%; for stage III, 46%; and for stage IV, 13%. It should be noted that recurrence may appear late, even after 10 years, but with each passing year free of disease the outlook becomes more cheerful.

Why some cancers respond whereas others fail has always been a mystery. Clearly, similar-looking tumors may have subtle genetic differences that cannot at present be detected. However, this is about to change, because DNA chip technology (microarray analysis) allows comparison of expression of thousands of genes within individual tumors (Chapter 6). Already such DNA microarray analysis has revealed differences in breast tumors. This may allow the development of therapy that is specifically targeted to the genetic abnormalities in a given tumor.

MALE BREAST

The rudimentary male breast is relatively free of pathologic involvement. Only two disorders occur with sufficient frequency to be considered here: *gynecomastia* and *carcinoma.*

Gynecomastia

As in females, male breasts are subject to hormonal influences, but they are considerably less sensitive than are female breasts. Nonetheless, enlargement of the male breast, or gynecomastia, may occur in response to absolute or relative estrogen excesses. Gynecomastia, then, is the male analogue of fibrocystic change in the female. The most important cause of such hyperestrinism in the male is cirrhosis of the liver, with consequent inability of the liver to metabolize estrogens. Other causes include Klinefelter syndrome, estrogen-secreting tumors, estrogen therapy, and, occasionally, digitalis therapy. Physiologic gynecomastia often occurs in puberty and in extreme old age.

The morphologic features of gynecomastia are similar to those of intraductal hyperplasia. Grossly, a button-like, subareolar swelling develops, usually in both breasts but occasionally in only one.

Carcinoma

This is a rare occurrence, with a frequency ratio to breast cancer in the female of 1:125. It occurs in advanced age. Because of the scant amount of breast substance in the male, the tumor rapidly infiltrates the overlying skin and underlying thoracic wall. Both morphologically and biologically, these tumors resemble invasive carcinomas in the female. Unfortunately, almost half have spread to regional nodes and more distant sites by the time they are discovered.

BIBLIOGRAPHY

Arver B, et al: Hereditary breast cancer: a review. Semin Cancer Biol 10:271, 2000. (An excellent review of the role of *BRCA1* and *BRCA2* genes in familial breast cancer.)

Clemons M, Goss P: Estrogen and the risk of breast cancer. N Engl J Med 344:276, 2001. (An update on the relationship between estrogens and the causation of breast cancer.)

Haber D: Roads leading to breast cancer. N Engl J Med 343:1566, 2000. (A short discussion of the role of DNA damage response and breast cancer.)

Holschneider CH, Berek JS: Ovarian cancer: epidemiology, biology, and prognostic factors. Semin Surg Oncol 19:3, 2000. (An excellent review of the pathogenesis of ovarian cancers.)

Rosenfeld RL: Ovarian and adrenal function in polycystic ovary syndrome. Endocrinol Metabol Clin North Am 28:265, 1999. (A good review of this complex syndrome.)

Schnitt SJ: Breast cancer in the 21st century: *neu* opportunities and *neu* challenges. Mod Pathol 14:213, 2001. (An excellent review of the expression of *HER2/neu* and the therapeutic potential of targeting this gene.)

Sherman ME: Theories of endometrial carcinogenesis: a multidisciplinary approach. Mod Pathol 13:295, 2000. (A review of the molecular basis of endometrial cancers.)

20

The Endocrine System

ANIRBAN MAITRA, MD
VINAY KUMAR, MD

Thanks are due to Dr. Dennis K. Burns for the use of material from this chapter in the sixth edition of *Basic Pathology*.

Adrenal Medulla

PHEOCHROMOCYTOMA

NEUROBLASTOMA AND OTHER NEURONAL NEOPLASMS

Multiple Endocrine Neoplasia Syndromes

MULTIPLE ENDOCRINE NEOPLASIA TYPE 1

MULTIPLE ENDOCRINE NEOPLASIA TYPE 2
   MEN 2A (Sipple Syndrome)
   MEN 2B (William Syndrome)

The endocrine system consists of a highly integrated and widely distributed group of organs whose purpose is to maintain a state of metabolic equilibrium, or homeostasis, among the various organs of the body. To accomplish this, the endocrine glands secrete a variety of chemical messengers, or hormones, that regulate the activity of target organs. Increased activity of the target tissue, in turn, typically down-regulates the activity of the gland secreting the stimulating hormone, a process known as *feedback inhibition* (Fig. 20–1). Hormones transported to their target organs via the bloodstream are referred to as "endocrine" hormones. They include a number of steroid hormones, peptides, and amines that modify the activity of cells and tissues throughout the body.

A number of processes may disturb the normal activity of the endocrine system, including impaired synthesis or release of hormones, abnormal interactions between hormones and their target tissues, and abnormal responses of target organs to their hormones. Endocrine diseases can be broadly classified as (1) diseases of *underproduction* or *overproduction of hormones* and their resultant biochemical and clinical consequences and (2) diseases associated with the development of *mass lesions*. Such lesions may be nonfunctional, or they may be associated with overproduction or underproduction of hormones. As will become apparent, a proper understanding of endocrine diseases requires a careful integration of morphologic findings with biochemical measurements of the levels of hormones, their regulators, and other metabolites.

Figure 20-1

Diagram of the relationships among the hypothalamus, the anterior pituitary, and a peripheral endocrine gland, exemplified here by the thyroid gland. Secretion of thyroid hormones (T_3 and T_4) is controlled by trophic factors secreted by both the hypothalamus and the anterior pituitary. Decreased levels of T_3 and T_4 stimulate the release of thyrotropin-releasing hormone (TRH) from the hypothalamus and thyroid-stimulating hormone (TSH) or thyrotropin from the anterior pituitary, causing T_3 and T_4 levels to rise. Elevated T_3 and T_4 levels in turn suppress the secretion of both TRH and TSH. These interactions constitute a negative-feedback loop. (Modified from an original sketch by Dr. Ronald A. DeLellis, New England Medical Center, Boston.)

■ Pituitary

The pituitary gland is a small, bean-shaped structure that lies at the base of the brain within the confines of the sella turcica. It is intimately related to the hypothalamus, with which it is connected by both a "stalk," composed of axons extending from the hypothalamus, and a rich venous plexus constituting a portal circulation. Along with the hypothalamus, the pituitary plays a central role in the regulation of most of the other endocrine glands. The pituitary is composed of two morphologically and functionally distinct components: the anterior lobe (adenohypophysis) and the posterior lobe (neurohypophysis). Diseases of the pituitary, accordingly, can be divided into those that primarily affect the anterior lobe and those that primarily affect the posterior lobe.

The *anterior pituitary*, or *adenohypophysis*, is composed of epithelial cells derived embryologically from the developing oral cavity. In routine histologic sections, a colorful array of cells containing basophilic cytoplasm, eosinophilic cytoplasm, or poorly staining ("chromophobic") cytoplasm is present (Fig. 20–2). Detailed studies using electron microscopy and immunocytochemistry have demonstrated that the staining properties of these cells are related to the presence of various trophic hormones within their cytoplasm. The release of trophic hormones is in turn under the control of factors released by the hypothalamus; while most hypothalamic factors are stimulatory and promote pituitary hormone release, others (e.g., somatostatin and dopamine) are inhibitory in their effects (Fig. 20–3). Rarely, symptoms of pituitary disease may be caused by an excess or lack of the hypothalamic factors rather than a primary pituitary abnormality.

Symptoms of pituitary disease can be divided into the following:

■ *Hyperpituitarism:* This disorder arises from excess secretion of trophic hormones. *Its most common cause is a functional adenoma within the anterior lobe.* Other, less common causes are hyperplasias and carcinomas of the anterior pituitary, secretion of hormones by nonpituitary tumors, and certain hypothalamic disorders. The symptoms of hyperpituitarism are discussed in the context of individual tumors later in this chapter.

■ *Hypopituitarism:* This is caused by deficiency of trophic hormones and results from a variety of destructive processes, including *ischemic injury*, *surgery or radiation*, and *inflammatory reactions*. In addition, *nonfunctional pituitary adenomas* may encroach upon and destroy adjacent native anterior pituitary parenchyma and cause hypopituitarism.

■ *Local mass effects:* Among the earliest changes referable to mass effect are *radiographic abnormalities of the sella turcica*, including sellar expansion, bony erosion, and disruption of the diaphragma sellae. Because of the close proximity of the optic nerves and chiasm to the sella, expanding pituitary lesions often compress decussating fibers in the optic chiasm. This gives rise to *visual field abnormalities*, classically in the form of defects in the lateral (temporal) visual fields—a so-called *bitemporal hemianopsia*. In addition, a variety of other visual field abnormalities may be caused by asymmetric growth of many tumors. As in the case of any expanding intracranial mass, pituitary adenomas may produce signs and symptoms of *elevated intracranial pressure*, including headache, nausea, and vomiting. Pituitary adenomas that extend beyond the sella turcica into the base of the brain (invasive pituitary adenoma) produce *seizures* or *obstructive hydrocephalus*; involvement of cranial nerves can result in *cranial nerve palsy*. On occasion, acute hemorrhage into an adenoma is associated with clinical evidence of rapid enlargement of the lesion and depression of consciousness, a situation appropriately termed *pituitary apoplexy*. Acute pituitary apoplexy is a neurosurgical emergency because it may cause sudden death.

Figure 20–2   ■

Photomicrograph of normal anterior pituitary. The gland is populated by several distinct cell populations containing a variety of stimulating (trophic) hormones. Each of the hormones has different staining characteristics, resulting in a mixture of cell types in routine histologic preparations.

Figure 20–3

The adenohypophysis (anterior pituitary) releases six hormones that are, in turn, under the control of various stimulatory and inhibitory hypothalamic releasing factors: TSH, thyroid-stimulating hormone (thyrotropin); PRL, prolactin; ACTH, adrenocorticotropic hormone (corticotropin); GH, growth hormone (somatotropin); FSH, follicle-stimulating hormone; and LH, luteinizing hormone. The stimulatory releasing factors are TRH (thyrotropin-releasing hormone), CRH (corticotropin-releasing hormone), GHRH (growth hormone–releasing hormone), and GnRH (gonadotropin-releasing hormone). The inhibitory hypothalamic factors are PIF (prolactin inhibitory factor or dopamine) and growth hormone inhibitory hormone (GIH or somatostatin).

HYPERPITUITARISM AND PITUITARY ADENOMAS

In most cases, excess production of anterior pituitary hormones is caused by the presence of an adenoma arising in the anterior lobe. Functional pituitary adenomas are usually composed of a single cell type and produce a single predominant hormone. There are, however, exceptions. Some pituitary adenomas are composed of a single cell type but secrete more than one hormone (e.g., growth hormone [GH] and prolactin), and occasionally adenomas contain more than one cell population. The original classification of pituitary tumors was based on the morphologic character of the predominant cell type (i.e., acidophil, basophil, or chromophobe adenomas), but this has little functional or clinical significance. Therefore, adenomas are classified on the basis of hormone(s) produced by the neoplastic cells detected by immunohistochemical stains performed on tissue sections. The various types of anterior pituitary adenomas and their relative frequencies are listed in Table 20–1.

Pituitary adenomas account for roughly 10% of intracranial neoplasms that come to clinical attention and are discovered incidentally in up to 25% of routine autopsies. They are usually found in adults, with a peak incidence from the fourth to sixth decades. Most pituitary adenomas occur as isolated lesions. In about 3% of cases, however, adenomas are associated with the syndrome of *multiple endocrine neoplasia type 1* (MEN 1) (discussed later). Pituitary adenomas are designated, somewhat arbitrarily, *macroadenomas* if they exceed 1 cm in diameter and *microadenomas* if less than 1 cm. Nonfunctional adenomas are likely to present at a later stage than those associated with obvious endocrine abnormalities and are therefore more likely to be macroadenomas.

MORPHOLOGY

The usual pituitary adenoma is a well-circumscribed, soft lesion that may, in the case of smaller tumors, be confined by the sella turcica. Larger lesions typically extend superiorly through the sellar diaphragm into the suprasellar region, where they often compress the optic chiasm and adjacent structures (Fig. 20–4). As these adenomas expand, they frequently erode the sella turcica and anterior clinoid processes. They may also extend locally into the cavernous and sphenoidal sinuses. In up to 30% of cases the adenomas are grossly nonencapsulated and infiltrate adjacent bone, dura, and (uncommonly) brain. Such lesions are designated *invasive* adenomas. Foci of hemorrhage and/or necrosis are common in larger adenomas.

Table 20–1. PITUITARY ADENOMAS

Type	Frequency (%)
Prolactin cell adenoma	20–30
Growth hormone cell adenomas	5
Mixed growth hormone/prolactin adenomas	5
Adrenocorticotropic hormone cell adenomas	10–15
Gonadotroph cell adenomas	10–15
Null cell adenomas	20
Thyroid-stimulating hormone cell adenomas	1
Other pleurihormonal adenomas	15

Modified from Burger PC, et al: Pituitary neoplasia. In Burger PC (ed): Surgical Pathology of the Nervous System and Its Coverings, 3rd ed. New York, Churchill Livingstone, 1991.

Figure 20-4 ■

Gross view of a pituitary adenoma. This massive, nonfunctional adenoma has grown far beyond the confines of the sella turcica and has distorted the overlying brain. Nonfunctional adenomas tend to be larger at the time of diagnosis than those that secrete a hormone.

Microscopically, pituitary adenomas are composed of relatively uniform, polygonal cells arrayed in sheets, cords, or papillae. Supporting connective tissue, or reticulin, is sparse, accounting for the soft, gelatinous consistency of many lesions. The nuclei of the neoplastic cells may be uniform or pleomorphic. Mitotic activity is usually scanty. The cytoplasm of the constituent cells may be acidophilic, basophilic, or chromophobic, depending on the type and amount of secretory product within the cell, but it is fairly uniform throughout the neoplasm. **This cellular monomorphism and the absence of a significant reticulin network distinguish pituitary adenomas from non-neoplastic anterior pituitary parenchyma** (Fig. 20–5). The functional status of the adenoma cannot be reliably predicted from its histologic appearance.

Prolactinomas

Prolactinomas are the most common type of hyperfunctioning pituitary adenoma. They range from small microadenomas to large, expansile tumors associated with considerable mass effect. Prolactin is demonstrable within the cytoplasm of the neoplastic cells by immunohistochemical techniques.

Hyperprolactinemia causes amenorrhea, galactorrhea, loss of libido, and infertility. Because many of the manifestations of hyperprolactinemia (e.g., amenorrhea) are more obvious in premenopausal females than in males or postmenopausal females, prolactinomas are usually diagnosed at an earlier stage in females of reproductive age than in other patients. In contrast, hormonal manifestations may be quite subtle in men and older women, in whom the tumors may reach considerable size before coming to clinical attention. Hyperprolactinemia may be caused by conditions other than prolactin-secreting pituitary adenomas, including pregnancy, high-dose estrogen therapy, renal failure, hypothyroidism, hypothalamic lesions, and dopamine-inhibiting drugs (e.g., re-

serpine). In addition, any mass in the suprasellar compartment may disturb the normal inhibitory influence of hypothalamic dopamine on prolactin secretion, resulting in hyperprolactinemia, the so-called *stalk effect*. It should be kept in mind, therefore, that *mild* elevations of serum prolactin (<200 μg/L) in a patient with a pituitary adenoma do not necessarily indicate a prolactin-secreting neoplasm. Prolactinomas are treated with bromocriptine, a dopamine receptor agonist, which causes shrinkage of the neoplasm in most cases.

Growth Hormone (Somatotroph Cell) Adenomas

GH-producing neoplasms, including those that produce a mixture of GH and other hormones (e.g., prolactin), are the second most common type of functional pituitary adenoma. Because the clinical manifestations of excessive GH may be subtle, somatotroph cell adenomas may be quite large by the time they come to clinical attention. Microscopically, GH-producing adenomas are composed of densely or sparsely granulated cells, and immunohistochemical stains demonstrate GH within the cytoplasm of the neoplastic cells. Small amounts of immunoreactive prolactin are often present as well.

Approximately 40% of somatotroph cell adenomas have activating mutations in the GNAS1 gene on chromosome 20q13, which encodes the α subunit of a heterodimeric stimulatory G protein known as G_s. As is well known, G proteins play a critical role in signal transduction, and activation of G_s proteins is coupled to up-regulation of the intracellular enzyme adenyl cyclase and its product, cyclic adenosine monophosphate (cAMP). Cyclic AMP acts as a potent mitogenic stimulus for pituitary somatotrophs. Therefore, mutations of *GNAS1* that constitutively activate the $G_{s\alpha}$ subunit result in continued cyclic AMP production and cellular proliferation. Recently, it was shown that *GNAS1* is an imprinted gene (i.e., it is monoallelically expressed in the normal pituitary) and that "loss of imprinting" (biallelic expression) is common during tumorigenesis (Chapter 7).

Figure 20-5 ■

Photomicrograph of pituitary adenoma. The monomorphism of these cells contrasts markedly to the mixture of cells seen in the normal anterior pituitary in Figure 20–2. Note also the absence of reticulin network.

If a GH-secreting adenoma occurs before the epiphyses close, as is the case in prepubertal children, excessive levels of GH result in *gigantism*. This is characterized by a generalized increase in body size, with disproportionately long arms and legs. If elevated levels of GH persist, or present, after closure of the epiphyses, patients develop *acromegaly*, in which growth is most conspicuous in soft tissues, skin, and viscera and in the bones of the face, hands, and feet. Enlargement of the jaw results in its protrusion (prognathism), with broadening of the lower face and separation of the teeth. The hands and feet are enlarged, with broad, sausage-like fingers. In practice, most cases of gigantism are also accompanied by evidence of acromegaly. GH excess is also associated with a number of other disturbances, including *abnormal glucose tolerance* and *diabetes mellitus, generalized muscle weakness, hypertension, arthritis, osteoporosis,* and *congestive heart failure*. Prolactin is demonstrable in a number of GH-producing adenomas and in some cases may be released in sufficient quantities to produce signs and symptoms of hyperprolactinemia.

Corticotroph Cell Adenomas

Most corticotroph adenomas are small (microadenomas) at the time of diagnosis, although some tumors may be quite large. These adenomas stain positively with periodic acid–Schiff (PAS) stains, owing to the glycosylation of the adrenocorticotropic hormone (ACTH) precursor molecule. As in the case of other pituitary hormones, the secretory granules can be detected by immunohistochemical methods. By electron microscopy they appear as membrane-bound, electron-dense granules averaging 300 nm in diameter.

Corticotroph adenomas may be clinically silent or may cause *hypercortisolism* (also known as *Cushing syndrome*) because of the stimulatory effect of ACTH on the adrenal cortex. Cushing syndrome, discussed in more detail later with diseases of the adrenal gland, may be caused by a wide variety of conditions in addition to ACTH-producing pituitary neoplasms. When the hypercortisolism is caused by excessive production of ACTH by the pituitary, the process is designated *Cushing disease* because it is the pattern of hypercortisolism originally described by Dr. Harvey Cushing. Large, clinically aggressive corticotroph adenomas may develop in patients after surgical removal of the adrenal glands for treatment of Cushing syndrome. This condition, known as *Nelson syndrome*, occurs in most cases because of a loss of the inhibitory effect of adrenal corticosteroids on a preexisting corticotroph microadenoma. Because the adrenals are absent in patients with Nelson syndrome, hypercortisolism does not develop. Instead, patients present with the mass effects of the pituitary tumor. In addition, because ACTH is synthesized as part of a larger prohormone that includes melanocyte-stimulating hormone (MSH), there may also be hyperpigmentation.

Other Anterior Pituitary Neoplasms

In a significant number of pituitary adenomas, no demonstrable hormonal product can be found within the neoplastic cells by immunohistochemistry; these tumors are designated *null cell adenomas*. Such nonfunctional tumors account for approximately 20% of all pituitary adenomas. The cytoplasm of null cell adenomas often contains numerous mitochondria, whereas secretory granules are scant to absent. Null cell adenomas typically present because of mass effect. They may also compromise the residual anterior pituitary sufficiently to produce *hypopituitarism*.

Gonadotroph (luteinizing hormone [LH]- and follicle-stimulating hormone [FSH]-producing) adenomas comprise 10% to 15% of pituitary adenomas. These adenomas are diagnosed most commonly in middle-aged men and women. They may cause decreased libido in men but often produce no obvious endocrine abnormalities. They may reach large size before they are diagnosed.

Thyrotroph (thyroid-stimulating hormone [TSH]-producing) adenomas account for about 1% of all pituitary adenomas and are a rare cause of hyperthyroidism.

Pituitary adenomas may elaborate more than one hormone. As noted, somatotroph adenomas commonly contain immunoreactive prolactin. In some neoplasms, designated *mixed adenomas*, more than one cell population is present. In other cases, a single cell type is apparently capable of synthesizing more than one hormone.

Pituitary carcinomas are exceedingly rare. In addition to local extension beyond the sella turcica, these tumors virtually always have distant metastasis.

HYPOPITUITARISM

Hypofunction of the anterior pituitary may occur with loss or absence of 75% or more of the anterior pituitary parenchyma. This may be *congenital* (exceedingly rare) or may result from a wide range of *acquired* abnormalities that are intrinsic to the pituitary. Less frequently, disorders that interfere with the delivery of pituitary hormone–releasing factors from the hypothalamus, such as hypothalamic tumors, may also cause hypofunction of the anterior pituitary. *Hypopituitarism accompanied by evidence of posterior pituitary dysfunction in the form of diabetes insipidus* (see later) *is almost always of hypothalamic origin*. Most cases of anterior pituitary hypofunction are caused by the following:

■ Nonsecretory pituitary adenomas
■ Ischemic necrosis of the pituitary
■ Ablation of the pituitary by surgery or radiation

Other, less common causes of anterior pituitary hypofunction include the empty sella syndrome, inflammatory lesions such as sarcoidosis or tuberculosis, trauma, and metastatic neoplasms involving the pituitary.

Nonsecretory pituitary adenomas may compress and compromise the anterior pituitary sufficiently to result in hypopituitarism. This may occur as a consequence of gradual enlargement of the adenoma or after abrupt enlargement of the tumor as a result of acute hemorrhage (pituitary apoplexy).

Ischemic necrosis of the anterior pituitary is an important cause of pituitary insufficiency. In general, the anterior pituitary tolerates ischemic insults fairly well; loss of up to half of the anterior pituitary parenchyma is without clinical

Figure 20-6

A, View of the sella turcica in a patient dying of chronic pituitary insufficiency. A tiny nubbin of residual pituitary can be seen protruding from the posterior wall of the sella *(below). B,* Photomicrograph of the residual anterior pituitary illustrated in *A.* Most of the gland has been replaced by the dense fibrous tissue, save for a few residual cells.

consequences. However, with destruction of larger amounts of the anterior pituitary (e.g., 75% or more), signs and symptoms of hypopituitarism develop. *Sheehan syndrome,* or postpartum necrosis of the anterior pituitary, is the most common form of clinically significant ischemic necrosis of the anterior pituitary. During pregnancy, the anterior pituitary enlarges considerably, largely because of an increase in the size and number of prolactin-secreting cells. However, this physiologic enlargement of the gland is not accompanied by an increase in blood supply from the low-pressure portal venous system. The enlarged gland is thus especially vulnerable to ischemic injury in patients who develop significant hemorrhage and hypotension during the peripartum period. The posterior pituitary, because it receives its blood directly from arterial branches, is much less susceptible to ischemic injury in this setting and is therefore usually not affected. Clinically significant pituitary necrosis may also be encountered in conditions other than pregnancy, including disseminated intravascular coagulation, sickle cell anemia, elevated intracranial pressure, traumatic injury, and shock of any origin. The residual gland is shrunken and scarred (Fig. 20-6).

An "empty sella" can result from any condition that destroys part or all of the pituitary gland. The term *empty sella syndrome* is used to describe an enlarged and empty sella turcica caused by chronic herniation of the subarachnoid space into the sella turcica. In these patients, a defect in the diaphragma sellae allows the arachnoid mater and cerebrospinal fluid to herniate into the sella, with resultant expansion of the sella and compression of the pituitary. Classically, affected patients are obese women with a history of multiple pregnancies. The empty sella syndrome may be associated with visual field deficits and sometimes with endocrine abnormalities, most commonly hyperprolactinemia caused by interruption of inhibitory hypothalamic influences ("stalk effect"). It is rarely associated with generalized hypopituitarism because sufficient functioning parenchyma is preserved.

The clinical manifestations of anterior pituitary hypofunction depend on the specific hormone(s) that are lacking. Children can develop growth failure *(pituitary dwarfism)* as a result of GH deficiency. Gonadotropin or GnRH deficiency leads to amenorrhea and infertility in women and decreased libido, impotence, and loss of pubic and axillary hair in men. TSH and ACTH deficiencies result in symptoms of hypothyroidism and hypoadrenalism, respectively, and are discussed later in the chapter. Prolactin deficiency results in failure of postpartum lactation. The anterior pituitary is also a rich source of melanocyte-stimulating hormone (MSH), synthesized from the same precursor molecule that produces ACTH; therefore, one of the manifestations of hypopituitarism is pallor from loss of stimulatory effects of MSH on melanocytes.

POSTERIOR PITUITARY SYNDROMES

The posterior pituitary, or neurohypophysis, is composed of modified glial cells (termed *pituicytes*) and axonal processes extending from nerve cell bodies in the supraoptic and paraventricular nuclei of the hypothalamus. The hypothalamic neurons produce two peptides: antidiuretic hormone (ADH) and oxytocin. They are stored in axon terminals in the neurohypophysis and released into the circulation in response to appropriate stimuli. Oxytocin stimulates the contraction of smooth muscle in the pregnant uterus and those surrounding the lactiferous ducts of the mammary glands. Abnormal oxytocin synthesis and release has not been associated with significant clinical abnormalities. The clinically important posterior pituitary syndromes involve ADH. They include *diabetes insipidus* and *secretion of inappropriately high levels of ADH.*

ADH is a nonapeptide hormone synthesized predominantly in the supraoptic nucleus. In response to a number of different stimuli, including increased plasma oncotic pressure, left atrial distention, exercise, and certain emotional states, ADH is released from axon terminals in the neurohypophysis into the general circulation. The hormone acts on the collecting tubules of the kidney to promote the resorption of free water. ADH deficiency causes *diabetes insipidus*, a condition characterized by excessive urination (polyuria) caused by an inability of the kidney to properly resorb water from the urine. Diabetes insipidus can result from a number of processes, including head trauma, neoplasms, and inflammatory disorders of the hypothalamus and pituitary, and from surgical procedures involving the hypothalamus or pituitary. The condition sometimes arises spontaneously ("idiopathic") in the absence of an underlying disorder. Diabetes insipidus from ADH deficiency is designated as *central*, to differentiate it from *nephrogenic* diabetes insipidus as a result of renal tubular unresponsiveness to circulating ADH. The clinical manifestations of both diseases are similar and include the excretion of large volumes of dilute urine with an inappropriately low specific gravity. Serum sodium and osmolality are increased, owing to excessive renal loss of free water, resulting in thirst and polydipsia. Patients who can drink water can generally compensate for urinary losses; patients who are obtunded, bedridden, or otherwise limited in their ability to obtain water may develop life-threatening dehydration.

In the *syndrome of inappropriate ADH (SIADH)* secretion, ADH excess is caused by a number of extracranial and intracranial disorders. It causes resorption of excessive amounts of free water, with resultant hyponatremia. The most common causes of SIADH include the secretion of ectopic ADH by malignant neoplasms (particularly small cell carcinomas of the lung), non-neoplastic diseases of the lung, and local injury to the hypothalamus and/or neurohypophysis. The clinical manifestations of SIADH are dominated by hyponatremia, cerebral edema, and resultant neurologic dysfunction. Although total body water is increased, blood volume remains normal and peripheral edema does not develop.

■
■
■ | # Thyroid

The thyroid gland is a bilobed structure below and anterior to the larynx. The gland develops from an evagination of the pharyngeal epithelium that descends to its normal position in the anterior neck. This pattern of descent explains the occasional presence of thyroid tissue in atypical locations, such as the base of the tongue. The thyroid is composed of roughly spherical follicles, lined by low cuboidal-to-columnar epithelium, and filled with thyroglobulin-rich colloid. In response to TSH released by thyrotrophs in the anterior pituitary, the follicular epithelial cells of the thyroid pinocytize colloid and ultimately convert thyroglobulin into *thyroxine (T₄)* and lesser amounts of *triiodothyronine (T₃)*. T_4 and T_3 are released into the systemic circulation, where they are reversibly bound to circulating plasma proteins for transport to peripheral tissues. The unbound ("free") T_3 and T_4 interact with intracellular receptors to ultimately up-regulate carbohydrate and lipid catabolism and stimulate protein synthesis in a wide range of cells. The net effect of these processes is an increase in the *basal metabolic rate*. The thyroid gland also contains a population of parafollicular cells, or "C" cells, that synthesize and secrete the hormone calcitonin. This hormone promotes absorption of calcium by the skeletal system and inhibits resorption of bone by osteoclasts. Diseases of the thyroid include conditions associated with excessive release of thyroid hormones (hyperthyroidism), those associated with thyroid hormone deficiency (hypothyroidism), and mass lesions of the thyroid. First, the general features of hyperthyroidism and hypothyroidism will be considered and then specific diseases of the thyroid will be discussed.

HYPERTHYROIDISM

Thyrotoxicosis is a hypermetabolic state caused by elevated circulating levels of free T_3 and T_4. Because it is caused most commonly by hyperfunction of the thyroid gland, it is often referred to as hyperthyroidism. However, in certain conditions the oversupply is related either to excessive release of preformed thyroid hormone (e.g., in

Table 20-2. CAUSES OF THYROTOXICOSIS

Associated With Hyperthyroidism

Primary

Graves disease
Hyperfunctioning ("toxic") multinodular goiter
Hyperfunctioning ("toxic") adenoma

Secondary

Thyroid-stimulating hormone–secreting pituitary adenoma (rare)*

Not Associated With Hyperthyroidism

Subacute granulomatous thyroiditis *(painful)*
Subacute lymphocytic thyroiditis *(painless)*
Struma ovarii (ovarian teratoma with ectopic thyroid)
Factitious thyrotoxicosis (exogenous thyroxine intake)

*Associated with increased thyroid-stimulating hormone; *all other causes of thyrotoxicosis associated with decreased thyroid-stimulating hormone.*

Figure 20-7   ■

Patient with hyperthyroidism. A wide-eyed, staring gaze, caused by overactivity of the sympathetic nervous system, is one of the features of this disorder. In Graves disease, one of the most important causes of hyperthyroidism, accumulation of loose connective tissue behind the orbits also adds to the protuberant appearance of the eyes.

thyroiditis) or to an extrathyroidal source, rather than to hyperfunction of the gland (Table 20–2). *Thus, strictly speaking, hyperthyroidism is only one (albeit the most common) category of thyrotoxicosis.* With this disclaimer, we will follow the common practice of using thyrotoxicosis and hyperthyroidism interchangeably.

The clinical manifestations of thyrotoxicosis are truly protean and include changes referable to the *hypermetabolic state* induced by excess thyroid hormone as well as those related to *overactivity of the sympathetic nervous system*:

■ *Constitutional symptoms:* the skin of thyrotoxic patients tends to be soft, warm, and flushed; *heat intolerance* and excessive sweating are common. Increased sympathetic activity and hypermetabolism result in *weight loss despite increased appetite.*

■ *Gastrointestinal:* stimulation of the gut results in hypermotility, malabsorption, and diarrhea.

■ *Cardiac:* palpitations and tachycardia are common; elderly patients may develop congestive heart failure owing to aggravation of preexisting heart disease.

■ *Neuromuscular:* patients frequently experience nervousness, tremor, and irritability. Nearly 50% develop proximal muscle weakness *(thyroid myopathy).*

■ *Ocular manifestations:* a wide, staring gaze and lid lag are present owing to sympathetic overstimulation of the levator palpebrae superioris (Fig. 20–7). However, true *thyroid ophthalmopathy* associated with proptosis is a feature seen only in Graves disease.

■ *Thyroid storm* is used to designate the abrupt onset of severe hyperthyroidism. This condition occurs most commonly in patients with underlying Graves disease (discussed later), probably resulting from an acute elevation in catecholamine levels, as might be encountered during stress. Thyroid storm is a medical emergency: a significant number of untreated patients die of cardiac arrhythmias.

■ *Apathetic hyperthyroidism* refers to thyrotoxicosis occurring in the elderly, in whom old age and various comorbidities may blunt the typical features of thyroid hormone

excess seen in younger patients. The diagnosis of thyrotoxicosis in these patients is often made during laboratory work-up for unexplained weight loss or worsening cardiovascular disease.

The diagnosis of hyperthyroidism is based on clinical features and laboratory data. *The measurement of serum TSH concentration using sensitive TSH assays provides the most useful single screening test for hyperthyroidism,* because its levels are decreased even at the earliest stages, when the disease may still be subclinical. In rare cases of pituitary or hypothalamus-associated (secondary) hyperthyroidism, TSH levels are either normal or raised. A low TSH value is usually confirmed with measurement of free T_4, which is expectedly increased. In an occasional patient, hyperthyroidism results predominantly from increased circulating levels of T_3 (T_3 toxicosis). In these cases, free T_4 levels may be decreased and direct measurement of serum T_3 may be useful. Once the diagnosis of thyrotoxicosis has been confirmed by a combination of TSH assays and free thyroid hormone levels, measurement of radioactive iodine uptake by the thyroid gland is often valuable in determining the etiology. For example, there may be diffusely increased uptake in the whole gland (Graves disease), increased uptake in a solitary nodule (toxic adenoma), or decreased uptake (thyroiditis).

HYPOTHYROIDISM

Hypothyroidism is caused by any structural or functional derangement that interferes with the production of adequate levels of thyroid hormone. As in the case of hyperthyroidism, this disorder is sometimes divided into primary and secondary categories, depending on whether the hypothyroidism arises from an intrinsic abnormality in the

■

Table 20-3. CAUSES OF HYPOTHYROIDISM

Primary

Postablative (after surgery or radioiodine therapy)
Primary idiopathic hypothyroidism
Hashimoto thyroiditis*
Iodine deficiency*
Congenital biosynthetic defect (dyshormonogenetic goiter)*

Secondary

Pituitary or hypothalamic failure (uncommon)

*Associated with enlargement of thyroid ("goitrous hypothyroidism").

thyroid or results from hypothalamic or pituitary disease (Table 20-3).

The clinical manifestations of hypothyroidism include cretinism and myxedema. *Cretinism* refers to hypothyroidism developing in infancy or early childhood. In the past, this disorder was fairly common in areas of the world where dietary iodine deficiency is endemic, including the Himalayas, inland China, Africa, and other mountainous areas. It has now become much less frequent because of the widespread supplementation of foods with iodine. On rare occasions, cretinism may also result from inborn errors in metabolism (e.g., enzyme deficiencies) that interfere with the biosynthesis of normal levels of thyroid hormone (sporadic cretinism). Clinical features of cretinism include impaired development of the skeletal system and central nervous system, with severe mental retardation, short stature, coarse facial features, a protruding tongue, and umbilical hernia. The severity of the mental impairment in cretinism appears to be directly influenced by the time at which thyroid deficiency occurs in utero. Normally, maternal hormones, including T_3 and T_4, cross the placenta and are critical to fetal brain development. If there is maternal thyroid deficiency before the development of the fetal thyroid gland, mental retardation is severe. In contrast, reduction in maternal thyroid hormones later in pregnancy, after the fetal thyroid has developed, allows normal brain development.

Hypothyroidism developing in older children and adults results in a condition known as *myxedema*. Myxedema, or Gull disease, was first linked with thyroid dysfunction in 1873 by Sir William Gull in a paper addressing the development of a "cretinoid state" in adults. Manifestations of myxedema include generalized apathy and mental sluggishness that in the early stages of disease may mimic depression. Patients with myxedema are listless, cold intolerant, and often obese. Mucopolysaccharide-rich edema accumulates in skin, subcutaneous tissue, and a number of visceral sites, with resultant broadening and coarsening of facial features, enlargement of the tongue, and deepening of the voice. Bowel motility is decreased, resulting in constipation. Pericardial effusions are common; in later stages the heart is enlarged, and heart failure may supervene.

Laboratory evaluation plays a vital role in the diagnosis of suspected hypothyroidism because of the nonspecific nature of symptoms. *Measurement of the serum TSH level is the most sensitive screening test for this disorder.* The TSH level is increased in primary hypothyroidism owing to a

loss of feedback inhibition of TRH and TSH production by the hypothalamus and pituitary, respectively. The TSH level is not increased in patients with hypothyroidism caused by primary hypothalamic or pituitary disease. *T_4 levels are decreased* in patients with hypothyroidism of any origin.

GRAVES DISEASE

In 1835, Robert Graves reported on his observations of a disease characterized by "violent and long continued palpitations in females" associated with enlargement of the thyroid gland. *Graves disease is the most common cause of endogenous hyperthyroidism.* It is characterized by a triad of manifestations:

■ *Thyrotoxicosis* caused by hyperfunctional, diffuse enlargement of the thyroid is present in all cases.
■ An infiltrative *ophthalmopathy* with resultant exophthalmos is noted in up to 40% of patients.
■ A localized, infiltrative *dermopathy* (sometimes designated *pretibial myxedema*) is seen in a minority of cases.

Graves disease occurs primarily in younger adults, with a peak incidence between the ages of 20 and 40. Women are affected up to seven times more often than men. An increased incidence of Graves disease occurs among family members of affected patients, with a 50% concordance among identical twins. The occurrence of this disorder is strongly associated with the inheritance of human leukocyte antigen (HLA)-DR3.

Pathogenesis. Graves disease is an autoimmune disorder in which a variety of autoantibodies may be present in the serum. These include antibodies to the TSH receptor, thyroid peroxisomes, and thyroglobulin; of these, the *TSH receptor is the most critical autoantigen against which antibodies develop;* the effects of the generated antibody vary depending on which TSH receptor epitope it is directed against. For example, one such antibody, termed *thyroid-stimulating immunoglobulin (TSI),* binds to the TSH receptor to stimulate the adenylate cyclase/cyclic AMP pathway, with resultant increased release of thyroid hormones. Another class of antibodies, also directed against the TSH receptor, has been implicated in the proliferation of thyroid follicular epithelium (*thyroid growth-stimulating immunoglobulins,* or TGI). Still other antibodies, termed *TSH-binding inhibitor immunoglobulins (TBIIs),* prevent TSH from binding normally to its receptor on thyroid epithelial cells. In so doing, some forms of TBII mimic the action of TSH, resulting in the stimulation of thyroid epithelial cell activity, while other forms may actually *inhibit* thyroid cell function. It is not unusual to find the coexistence of stimulating *and* inhibiting immunoglobulins in the sera of the same patient, a finding that may explain why some patients with Graves disease spontaneously develop episodes of hypothyroidism.

Although the role of antibodies in the causation of Graves disease seems established, what propels B cells to make autoantibodies is not clear. There is little doubt that the antibody secretion by B cells is triggered by CD4+ helper T cells, many of which are found within the thyroid.

Intrathyroidal helper T cells are also sensitized to thyrotropin receptor, and they secrete soluble factors such as interferon-γ and tumor necrosis factor. These in turn induce expression of HLA class II molecules and T-cell costimulatory molecules on thyroid epithelial cells, thus allowing presentation of thyroidal antigen to other T cells. This may sustain the activation of TSH-receptor–specific cells within the thyroid. In keeping with the primacy of helper T-cell activation in thyroid autoimmunity, Graves disease shows an association with certain HLA-DR alleles and polymorphisms of the cytotoxic T-lymphocyte antigen 4 (CTLA-4). Activation of the latter normally dampens the T-cell response, and perhaps some alleles allow uncontrolled T-cell activation against autoantigens.

It is likely that autoantibodies to the TSH receptor also play a role in the development of the *infiltrative ophthalmopathy* characteristic of Graves disease. It is postulated that certain extrathyroidal tissues (e.g., orbital fibroblasts) aberrantly express the TSH receptor on their surface. In response to circulating anti-TSH receptor antibodies and other cytokines from the local milieu, these fibroblasts undergo differentiation into mature adipocytes and also secrete hydrophilic glycosaminoglycans into the interstitium, both of which contribute to the orbital protrusion (exophthalmos) seen in Graves ophthalmopathy. A similar mechanism has been proposed for the development of Graves *dermopathy*, with TSH receptor–bearing pretibial fibroblasts secreting glycosaminoglycans in response to stimulatory autoantibodies and cytokines.

Autoimmune disorders of the thyroid span a continuum in which Graves disease, characterized by hyperfunction of the thyroid, lies at one extreme, and Hashimoto disease, manifesting as hypothyroidism, occupies the other end. Antibodies against thyroidal antigens are common to both, but their specific epitopes are different, and hence their functional consequences differ. Not surprisingly, there is also an element of histologic overlap between the various autoimmune thyroid disorders (most characteristically, prominent intrathyroidal lymphoid cell infiltrates with germinal center formation, see later). In both disorders, the frequency of other autoimmune diseases such as systemic lupus erythematosus, pernicious anemia, type I diabetes, and Addison disease is increased.

Figure 20-8   ■

Photomicrograph of a diffusely hyperplastic gland in a case of Graves disease. The follicles are lined by tall, columnar epithelium. The crowded, enlarged epithelial cells project into the lumina of the follicles. These cells actively resorb the colloid in the centers of the follicles, resulting in the "scalloped" appearance of the edges of the colloid.

cells and mature plasma cells, are present throughout the interstitium; germinal centers are common. Preoperative therapy alters the morphology of the thyroid in Graves disease. For example, preoperative administration of iodine causes involution of the epithelium and the accumulation of colloid by blocking thyroglobulin secretion; with continued administration, fibrosis of the gland results.

Changes in extrathyroidal tissues include generalized lymphoid hyperplasia. In patients with ophthalmopathy, the tissues of the orbit are edematous, owing to the presence of hydrophilic glycosaminoglycans. In addition, there is infiltration by lymphocytes, mostly T cells. Orbital muscles are edematous initially but may undergo fibrosis late in the course of the disease. The dermopathy, if present, is characterized by thickening of the dermis, owing to deposition of glycosaminoglycans and lymphocyte infiltration.

MORPHOLOGY

In the typical case of Graves disease, the thyroid gland is diffusely enlarged because of the presence of **diffuse hypertrophy and hyperplasia** of thyroid follicular epithelial cells. The gland is usually smooth and soft, and its capsule is intact. Microscopically, the follicular epithelial cells in untreated cases are tall and columnar and are more crowded than usual. This crowding often results in the formation of small papillae, which project into the follicular lumen (Fig. 20-8). Such papillae lack fibrovascular cores, in contrast to those of papillary carcinoma. The colloid within the follicular lumen is pale, with scalloped margins. Lymphoid infiltrates, consisting predominantly of T cells, with fewer B

Clinical Features. The clinical manifestations of Graves disease include those common to all forms of thyrotoxicosis (discussed earlier), as well as those associated uniquely with Graves disease: *diffuse hyperplasia of the thyroid, ophthalmopathy, and dermopathy.* The degree of thyrotoxicosis varies from case to case and may sometimes be less conspicuous than other manifestations of the disease. Diffuse enlargement of the thyroid is present in all cases of Graves disease. The thyroid enlargement is usually smooth and symmetric, but it may be asymmetric. Increased flow of blood through the hyperactive gland often produces an audible bruit. Sympathetic overactivity produces a characteristic wide, staring gaze and lid lag. The ophthalmopathy of Graves disease, as explained previously, is caused by a combination of lymphocytic infiltration, glycosaminoglycan deposition, and adipogenesis in the orbital connective tissues, resulting in abnormal protrusion of the eyeball (exophthalmos). The proptosis may persist or progress despite successful treatment of the thyrotoxicosis, sometimes resulting in corneal injury and, if severe, in blindness. The dermopathy, sometimes designated *pretibial myxedema*, is present in a minority of cases. It is manifested most typically by localized areas of thickening and hyperpigmentation of the skin over the anterior aspect of the feet and lower legs. Laboratory findings in Graves disease include elevated free T_4 and T_3 levels and depressed TSH levels. Because of ongoing stimulation of the thyroid follicles by thyroid-stimulating immunoglobulins, radioactive iodine uptake is increased and radioiodine scans show a *diffuse uptake* of iodine.

DIFFUSE NONTOXIC GOITER AND MULTINODULAR GOITER

Goiter, or simple enlargement of the thyroid, is the most common thyroid disease. The disorder is endemic in certain areas of the world and may also occur sporadically. Whether sporadic or endemic, *the presence of goiter reflects impaired synthesis of thyroid hormone*, most often caused by dietary iodine deficiency. Impairment of thyroid hormone synthesis leads to a compensatory rise in the serum TSH level, which in turn causes hypertrophy and hyperplasia of thyroid follicular cells and, ultimately, gross enlargement of the thyroid gland.

Endemic goiter occurs in geographic areas where the soil, water, and food supply contain low levels of iodine. The term *endemic* is used when goiters are present in more than 10% of the population in a given region. Such conditions are particularly common in mountainous areas of the world, including the Himalayas and the Andes. With increasing dietary iodine supplementation, the frequency and severity of endemic goiter have declined significantly. *Sporadic goiter* occurs less commonly than endemic goiter. The condition is more common in females than in males, with a peak incidence in puberty or young adult life, when there is an increased physiologic demand for thyroxine. Sporadic goiter may be caused by a number of conditions, including the ingestion of substances that interfere with thyroid hormone synthesis at some level, such as excessive calcium and vegetables belonging to the *Brassica* and Cruciferae groups (e.g., cabbage, cauliflower, Brussels sprouts, and turnips). In other instances, goiter may result from hereditary enzymatic defects that interfere with thyroid hormone synthesis. In most cases, however, the cause of sporadic goiter is not apparent.

MORPHOLOGY

The pathogenesis of goiter involves hypertrophy and hyperplasia of thyroid follicular cells by elevated levels of TSH. In most cases, such changes result initially in diffuse, symmetric enlargement of the gland **(diffuse nontoxic goiter).** The follicles are lined by crowded columnar cells, which may pile

up and form projections similar to those seen in Graves disease. If dietary iodine subsequently increases, or if the demands for thyroid hormone decrease, the stimulated follicular epithelium involutes to form an enlarged, colloid-rich gland **(colloid goiter).** The cut surface of the thyroid in such cases is usually brown, somewhat glassy, and translucent. Microscopically, the follicular epithelium may be hyperplastic in the early stages of disease or flattened and cuboidal during periods of involution. Colloid is abundant during the latter periods. With time, recurrent episodes of stimulation and involution combine to produce a more irregular enlargement of the thyroid, termed **nodular,** or **multinodular, goiter.** The basis of nodule formation is not clear. It may be related to differential ability of normal thyroid epithelial cells to replicate in response to TSH. Conceivably, this variation in cell growth potential can cause nodule formation with cyclical and long-term exposure to increased levels of TSH.

Multinodular goiters are multilobulated, asymmetrically enlarged glands, which may reach massive size (Fig. 20–9). On the cut surface, irregular nodules containing variable amounts of brown, gelatinous colloid are present. Regressive changes are quite common, particularly in older lesions, and include areas of fibrosis, hemorrhage, calcification, and cystic change. The microscopic appearance includes colloid-rich follicles lined by flattened, inactive epithelium and areas of follicular epithelial hypertrophy and hyperplasia, accompanied by the regressive changes noted previously.

Clinical Features. The dominant clinical features of goiter are those caused by the mass effects of the enlarged gland. In addition to the obvious cosmetic effects of a large neck mass, goiters may also cause airway obstruction,

Figure 20–9 ■

Gross view of nodular goiter. The gland is coarsely nodular and contains areas of fibrosis and cystic change.

dysphagia, and compression of large vessels in the neck and upper thorax. In a significant minority of patients, a hyperfunctioning ("toxic") nodule may develop within the goiter, resulting in *hyperthyroidism*. This condition, known as *Plummer syndrome*, is not accompanied by the infiltrative ophthalmopathy and dermopathy of Graves disease. Less commonly, goiter may be associated with clinical evidence of *hypothyroidism*. Goiters are also clinically significant because of their ability to mask or to mimic neoplastic diseases arising in the thyroid.

THYROIDITIS

Inflammation of the thyroid gland, or thyroiditis, can occur in a number of different settings. Most of the common entities included under thyroiditis can be distinguished using a combination of two criteria: (1) the rapidity of onset or the duration of disease (acute, subacute, or chronic) and (2) the predominant inflammatory response (polymorphonuclear, lymphocytic, or granulomatous). For example, *acute suppurative* thyroiditis associated with microbial infections and polymorphonuclear inflammation is quite uncommon. The focus in this section will be on some of the more common types of thyroiditis, including *chronic lymphocytic* (Hashimoto) thyroiditis, *subacute granulomatous* (de Quervain) thyroiditis, and *subacute lymphocytic* thyroiditis.

Chronic Lymphocytic (Hashimoto) Thyroiditis

Hashimoto thyroiditis is the most common cause of hypothyroidism in the United States. It is an *autoimmune inflammatory disorder* of the thyroid; as in the case of Graves disease, the frequency of *other autoimmune disorders* such as systemic lupus erythematosus and rheumatoid arthritis is also increased in patients with Hashimoto disease.

Pathogenesis. Although caused primarily by a defect in T cells, Hashimoto thyroiditis involves both cellular and humoral responses (Fig. 20–10):

- Initially, activation of thyroid-specific CD4+ T cells induces formation of CD8+ cytotoxic T cells and autoantibodies. *The cytotoxic T-cell infiltration is primarily responsible for the parenchymal destruction.*
- In addition, sensitized B cells secrete *inhibitory anti-TSH receptor antibodies* that block the action of TSH, further contributing to hypothyroidism (recall that anti-TSH receptor antibodies are also formed in Graves disease, but there they mimic the action of TSH and result in *hyperthyroidism*).
- Other circulating antibodies (antithyroglobulin and antithyroid peroxidase antibodies) are probably formed as a result of tissue destruction and exposure of normally sequestered thyroid antigens to the immune system; these antibodies play a useful role in the diagnosis of Hashimoto thyroiditis but are unlikely to contribute actively to its pathogenesis.
- There is a significant *genetic component* to disease pathogenesis. Hashimoto thyroiditis occurs with increased frequency in first-degree relatives, and unaffected family members often have circulating thyroid autoantibodies. An association has also been found between disease prevalence and the HLA subtypes DR3 and DR5.

MORPHOLOGY

Grossly, the thyroid is usually diffusely and symmetrically enlarged, although more localized enlargement may be seen in some cases. The capsule is intact, and the gland is well demarcated from adjacent structures. The cut surface is pale, gray-tan, firm, and somewhat friable. Microscopic examination discloses widespread infiltration of the parenchyma by a **mononuclear inflammatory infiltrate** containing small lymphocytes, plasma cells, and well-developed **germinal centers** (Fig. 20–11). The thyroid follicles are atrophic and are lined in many areas by epithelial cells distinguished by the presence of abundant eosinophilic, granular cytoplasm, termed **Hürthle,** or **oxyphil,** cells. This is a

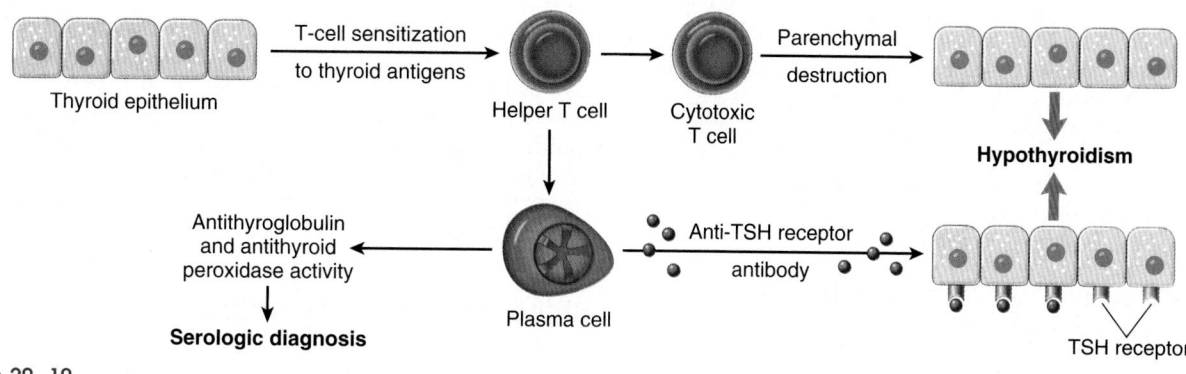

Figure 20-10

Pathogenesis of Hashimoto thyroiditis. Thyroid-specific CD4+ helper T cells induce both the cellular (CD8+ cytotoxic T cells) and the humoral (antibody-secreting mature B cells) components of the autoimmune response in Hashimoto thyroiditis. The cytotoxic T cells are primarily responsible for the parenchymal destruction, whereas B cells secrete inhibitory anti-TSH receptor and other antibodies. The antithyroglobulin and antithyroid peroxidase antibodies are unlikely to contribute to pathogenesis but serve as useful serologic markers of disease.

Figure 20–11 ■

Photomicrograph of Hashimoto thyroiditis. The thyroid parenchyma contains a dense lymphocytic infiltrate with germinal centers. Residual thyroid follicles lined by deeply eosinophilic Hürthle cells are also seen.

metaplastic response of the normally low cuboidal follicular epithelium to ongoing injury; ultrastructurally the Hürthle cells are characterized by numerous intracytoplasmic mitochondria. Interstitial connective tissue is increased and may be abundant. The fibrosis does not extend beyond the capsule of the gland. Less commonly, the thyroid is small and atrophic as a result of more extensive fibrosis.

Clinical Features. Hashimoto disease is most prevalent between 45 and 65 years of age, and it is more common in females than in males, with a female predominance of 10:1 to 20:1. It presents as painless enlargement of the thyroid, usually associated with some degree of hypothyroidism. The enlargement of the gland is generally symmetric and diffuse, but in some cases it may be sufficiently localized to raise the suspicion of a neoplasm. Hypothyroidism develops gradually, but it may be preceded by transient thyrotoxicosis ("hashitoxicosis") caused by disruption of thyroid follicles, with secondary release of thyroid hormones. During this phase, free T_4 and T_3 levels are increased, TSH is decreased, and radioactive iodine uptake is diminished. As hypothyroidism supervenes, T_4 and T_3 levels progressively decline, accompanied by a compensatory rise in TSH. Patients with Hashimoto disease are at *increased risk for the development of B-cell non-Hodgkin lymphomas within the thyroid.*

Subacute Granulomatous (de Quervain) Thyroiditis

Subacute granulomatous thyroiditis, also known as de Quervain thyroiditis, is much less common than is Hashimoto disease. de Quervain thyroiditis is most common between the ages of 30 and 50 and, like other forms of thyroiditis, occurs more frequently in women than in men. The cause is

unknown. It is often preceded by an upper respiratory tract infection, suggesting the possibility of *viral* origin.

MORPHOLOGY

The gland is firm, with an intact capsule, and may be unilaterally or bilaterally enlarged. Histologically, there is disruption of thyroid follicles, with extravasation of colloid leading to a polymorphonuclear infiltrate, which is replaced over time by lymphocytes, plasma cells, and macrophages. The extravasated colloid provokes a granulomatous reaction, with exuberant giant cells, some containing fragments of colloid. Healing occurs by resolution of inflammation and fibrosis.

Clinical Features. The onset of this form of thyroiditis is often acute, characterized by *pain* in the neck (particularly when swallowing), fever, malaise, and variable enlargement of the thyroid. Transient hyperthyroidism may occur, as in other cases of thyroiditis, owing to disruption of thyroid follicles and release of excessive thyroid hormone. Thyroid function tests are similar to those encountered in thyrotoxicosis associated with other forms of thyroiditis. The leukocyte count and erythrocyte sedimentation rates are increased. With progression of disease and gland destruction, a transient hypothyroid phase may ensue. The condition is typically self-limited, with most patients returning to a euthyroid state within 6 to 8 weeks.

Subacute Lymphocytic Thyroiditis

Subacute lymphocytic thyroiditis is also known as "silent" or "painless" thyroiditis; in a subset of patients the onset of disease follows pregnancy *(postpartum thyroiditis)*. This disease is most likely autoimmune in etiology, because circulating antithyroid antibodies are found in the majority of patients. It mostly affects middle-aged women, who present with a *painless* neck mass or features of thyroid hormone excess. There is an initial phase of thyrotoxicosis (likely to be secondary to thyroid tissue damage), followed by return to a euthyroid state within a few months. Patients with one episode of postpartum thyroiditis are at an increased risk of recurrence after subsequent pregnancies. A minority of affected individuals eventually progress to hypothyroidism. The histologic features are lymphocytic infiltration and hyperplastic germinal centers within the thyroid parenchyma; unlike Hashimoto thyroiditis, follicular atrophy and oxyphil metaplasia are not commonly seen.

Other Forms of Thyroiditis

Two uncommon variants include the following:

■ *Riedel thyroiditis*, a rare disorder of unknown etiology, is characterized by extensive fibrosis involving the thyroid and contiguous neck structures. The presence of a hard and fixed thyroid mass clinically simulates a thyroid neoplasm. It may be associated with idiopathic fibrosis in other sites in the body, such as the retroperitoneum. The presence of circulating antithyroid antibodies in most patients suggests an autoimmune etiology.

■ *Palpation thyroiditis*, caused by vigorous clinical palpation of the thyroid gland, results in multifocal follicular disruption associated with chronic inflammatory cells and occasional giant cell formation. Unlike de Quervain thyroiditis, abnormalities of thyroid function are not present, and this is usually an incidental finding in specimens resected for other reasons.

NEOPLASMS OF THE THYROID

The thyroid gland gives rise to a variety of neoplasms, ranging from circumscribed, benign adenomas to highly aggressive, anaplastic carcinomas. From a clinical standpoint, the possibility of neoplastic disease is of major concern in patients who present with thyroid nodules. Fortunately, the overwhelming majority of solitary nodules of the thyroid prove to be benign lesions, either follicular adenomas or localized, non-neoplastic conditions (e.g., nodular hyperplasia, simple cysts, or foci of thyroiditis). Carcinomas of the thyroid, in contrast, are uncommon, accounting for well under 1% of solitary thyroid nodules. Several clinical criteria provide a clue to the nature of a given thyroid nodule:

■ *Solitary nodules*, in general, are more likely to be neoplastic than are multiple nodules.
■ *Solid nodules*, in general, are more likely to be neoplastic than are cystic nodules.
■ Nodules in *younger patients* are more likely to be neoplastic than are those in older patients.
■ Nodules in *males* are more likely to be neoplastic than are those in females.
■ Nodules that do not take up radioactive iodine in imaging studies *("cold" nodules)* are more likely to be neoplastic; "hot" nodules are almost always benign.

Such statistics and general trends, however, are of little significance in the evaluation of a given patient, in whom the timely recognition of a malignancy, however uncom-

Figure 20-13 ■

Photomicrograph of follicular adenoma. Well-differentiated follicles resemble normal thyroid parenchyma.

mon, can be lifesaving. Ultimately, it is the morphologic evaluation of a given thyroid nodule, in the form of fine-needle aspiration biopsy and histologic study of surgically resected thyroid parenchyma, that provides the most definitive information about its nature. In the following sections, we will consider the major thyroid neoplasms, including adenomas and carcinoma in their various forms.

Adenomas

Adenomas of the thyroid are benign neoplasms derived from follicular epithelium. As in the case of all thyroid neoplasms, follicular adenomas are usually solitary. Clinically and morphologically, they may be difficult to distinguish, on the one hand, from hyperplastic nodules or, on the other hand, from the less common follicular carcinomas.

MORPHOLOGY

The typical thyroid adenoma is a **solitary,** spherical lesion that compresses the adjacent non-neoplastic thyroid. It is demarcated from the surrounding thyroid parenchyma by a **well-formed capsule** (Fig. 20-12), a feature that is usually lacking in hyperplastic nodules. Microscopically, the constituent cells are arranged in uniform follicles that contain colloid (Fig. 20-13). Various histologic subtypes of adenomas are recognized on the basis of the degree of follicle formation and the colloid content of the follicles (e.g., trabecular, microfollicular, macrofollicular), but these subdivisions are of no biologic significance. Papillary change is not a typical feature of adenomas and, if present, should raise the suspicion of an encapsulated papillary carcinoma (discussed later). The neoplastic cells are uniform, with well-defined cell borders. Occasionally, the neoplastic cells acquire brightly eosinophilic granular cytoplasm (oxyphil or Hürthle

Figure 20-12 ■

Follicular adenoma of the thyroid. A solitary, well-circumscribed nodule is seen.

cell change); the clinical presentation and behavior of a follicular adenoma with oxyphilia **(Hürthle cell adenoma)** is no different from a conventional adenoma. Similar to other endocrine tumors, even benign follicular adenomas may, on occasion, exhibit nuclear pleomorphism and atypia **(endocrine atypia);** on the contrary, well-differentiated follicular carcinomas can have deceptively bland cytologic features. **Careful evaluation of the integrity of the capsule is therefore critical, because the presence of capsular and/or blood vessel invasion constitutes the most reliable criteria for distinguishing follicular carcinomas from adenomas** (Fig. 20-14).

TOXIC ADENOMA. Although the vast majority of adenomas are nonfunctional, a small proportion produce thyroid hormones and cause clinically apparent thyrotoxicosis. Hormone production in functional adenomas occurs independent of TSH stimulation; hence they are called "autonomous nodules." Recent genetic analyses have shown that toxic adenomas often harbor **activating mutations of either the TSH receptor gene or GNAS1. GNAS1 encodes the α-subunit of the heterodimeric protein G_s.** Normally, the binding of TSH to its receptor activates $G_{s\alpha}$, which in turn leads to up-regulation of adenyl cyclase and its product, cyclic AMP. One of the endpoints of this tightly regulated cascade is increased transcription of thyroid hormones. In the presence of mutations that constitutively activate either the TSH receptor or the $G_{s\alpha}$ protein, there is continuous thyroid hormone production and hyperthyroidism, even in the absence of TSH stimulation.

Clinical Features. Most adenomas of the thyroid present as painless nodules, often discovered during a routine physical examination. Larger masses may produce local symptoms such as difficulty in swallowing. As previously stated, persons with toxic adenomas can present with features of thyrotoxicosis. After injection of radioactive iodine, most adenomas take up iodine less avidly than does normal thyroid parenchyma. On radionuclide scanning, therefore, adenomas appear as "cold" nodules relative to the adjacent normal thyroid gland. Toxic adenomas, however, will appear as a "warm" or "hot" nodule in the scan. Up to 10% of "cold" nodules eventually prove to be malignant. By contrast, malignancy is virtually nonexistent in "hot" nodules. Additional techniques used in the preoperative evaluation of suspected adenomas are ultrasonography and fine-needle aspiration biopsy. Although fine-needle aspiration biopsy is an excellent screening tool for initial assessment of thyroid nodules, *the definitive distinction of follicular adenomas from carcinomas can be made only after careful histologic examination of the resected specimen.* As stated previously, breach of the capsule or invasion of blood vessels indicates malignancy. Current evidence suggests that thyroid carcinomas arise de novo and that malignant transformation of adenomas does not occur.

Carcinomas

Carcinomas of the thyroid are relatively uncommon in the United States, being responsible for less than 1% of cancer-related deaths. Most cases occur in adults, although some forms, particularly papillary carcinomas, may present in childhood. A female predominance has been noted among patients developing thyroid carcinoma in the early and middle adult years, probably related to the expression of estrogen receptors on neoplastic thyroid epithelium. In

Figure 20-14 ■

Evaluating the integrity of the capsule is critical in distinguishing follicular adenomas from follicular carcinomas. In adenomas *(A),* a fibrous capsule, usually thin but occasionally more prominent, surrounds the neoplastic follicles and no capsular invasion is seen *(arrows);* compressed normal thyroid parenchyma is usually present external to the capsule *(top of the panel).* In contrast, follicular carcinomas demonstrate capsular invasion *(B, arrows)* that may be minimal, as in this case, or widespread with extension into local structures of the neck. The presence of vascular invasion is another feature of follicular carcinomas.

contrast, cases presenting in childhood and late adult life are distributed equally among males and females, largely related to exogenous influences (see later). The major subtypes of thyroid carcinoma and their relative frequencies are as follows:

■ Papillary carcinoma (75% to 85% of cases)
■ Follicular carcinoma (10% to 20% of cases)
■ Medullary carcinoma (5% of cases)
■ Anaplastic carcinomas (<5% of cases)

Most thyroid carcinomas are derived from the follicular epithelium, except for medullary carcinomas; the latter are derived from the parafollicular, or C, cells. Because of the unique clinical and biologic features associated with each variant of thyroid carcinoma, these subtypes will be described separately, after discussion of pathogenesis.

Pathogenesis. Several factors, both genetic and environmental, are implicated in the pathogenesis of thyroid cancers.

Genetic Factors. The importance of genetic factors has been underscored by the clustering of thyroid cancers in families. Familial medullary thyroid carcinomas occur in multiple endocrine neoplasia type 2 (see later) associated with germ-line *RET* protooncogene mutations; a syndrome of familial papillary thyroid carcinoma has also been recently described, although the genetic locus for this entity remains unknown. Both loss-of-function mutations of the *APC* gene in familial adenomatous polyposis and *PTEN* gene alterations in Cowden disease (multiple hamartomas syndrome) are associated with an inherited predisposition to thyroid cancers (Chapter 15). Besides familial thyroid cancers, abnormalities of the *RET* protooncogene have also been described in a small proportion of sporadic medullary and papillary thyroid carcinomas. *RET* is frequently activated in papillary thyroid carcinomas by its juxtaposition to other constitutively active genes (the fusion product arising from these somatic rearrangements of *RET* is generically known as *RET/PTC*). Recently, a chromosomal translocation, t(2;3)(q13;p25), has been identified in a proportion of follicular carcinomas of the thyroid. It causes the fusion of the gene for thyroid transcription factor *PAX8* to the *PPARγ1* gene, giving rise to a novel oncogenic protein. While this molecular master appears to be fairly specific for follicular carcinomas of the thyroid, it is expressed only in 20% of these tumors. Inactivating mutations of the *TP53* gene are uncommon in differentiated (papillary or follicular) thyroid cancers but frequent in anaplastic cancers.

Ionizing Radiation. Exposure to ionizing radiation, particularly during the first 2 decades of life, has emerged as one of the most important factors predisposing to the development of thyroid cancer. In the past, radiation therapy was liberally employed in the treatment of a number of head and neck lesions in infants and children, including reactive tonsillar enlargement, acne, and tinea capitis. Up to 9% of people receiving such treatment during childhood subsequently developed thyroid malignancies, usually several decades after exposure. The incidence of carcinoma of the thyroid is substantially higher, in addition, among atomic bomb survivors in Japan and in those exposed to ionizing radiation after the Chernobyl nuclear plant disaster. *The overwhelming majority of cancers arising in this setting are papillary thyroid cancers, and most have RET gene rearrangements.*

Preexisting Thyroid Disease. Long-standing multinodular goiter has been suggested as a predisposing factor in some cases, since areas with iodine deficiency-related endemic goiter have a higher prevalence of follicular carcinomas. As noted previously, there is little evidence that follicular adenomas progress to carcinoma. Although most, if not all, thyroid lymphomas arise from preexisting thyroiditis, there is no evidence to suggest that thyroiditis is associated with an increased risk of thyroid carcinomas.

PAPILLARY CARCINOMA

Papillary carcinomas represent the most common form of thyroid cancer (80% of all cases). They may occur at any age, and they account for the vast majority of thyroid carcinomas associated with previous exposure to ionizing radiation.

MORPHOLOGY

Papillary carcinomas may present as solitary or multifocal lesions within the thyroid. In some cases, they may be well circumscribed and even encapsulated; in other instances, they infiltrate the adjacent parenchyma with ill-defined margins. The lesions may contain areas of fibrosis and calcification and are often cystic. On the cut surface, they may appear granular and may sometimes contain grossly discernible papillary foci. The definitive diagnosis of papillary carcinoma can be made only after microscopic examination. As currently used, **the diagnosis of papillary carcinoma is based on nuclear features** even in the absence of a papillary architecture. The nuclei of papillary carcinoma cells contain very finely dispersed chromatin, which imparts an **optically clear** appearance, giving rise to the designation "ground-glass" or "Orphan Annie" nuclei (Fig. 20–15). In addition, invaginations of the cytoplasm may in cross-sections give the appearance of intranuclear inclusions (hence the term *pseudo-inclusions*). A **papillary architecture** is present in many cases, although some tumors are composed predominantly or exclusively of follicles; these **follicular variants** still behave biologically as papillary carcinomas if they have the nuclear features described (Table 20–4). When present, the papillae of papillary carcinoma differ from those seen in areas of hyperplasia. Unlike hyperplastic papillary lesions, the neoplastic papillae have dense fibrovascular cores. Concentrically calcified structures termed **psammoma bodies** are often present within the papillae. Foci of lymphatic permeation by tumor are often present, but invasion of blood vessels is relatively uncommon, particularly in smaller lesions. Metastases to adjacent cervical lymph nodes are estimated to occur in about half of cases.

Figure 20–15

Papillary carcinoma of the thyroid. *A* demonstrates the appearance of a papillary carcinoma with grossly discernible papillary structures. This particular example contained well-formed papillae *(B)*, lined by cells with characteristic empty-appearing nuclei, sometimes termed "Orphan Annie eye" nuclei *(C)*. *D* shows cells obtained by fine-needle aspiration of a papillary carcinoma. Characteristic intranuclear inclusions are visible in some of the aspirated cells. (Courtesy of Dr. S. Gokasalan, Department of Pathology, University of Texas Southwestern Medical School, Dallas.)

Clinical Features. Papillary carcinomas are nonfunctional tumors, and thus they present most often as a painless mass in the neck, either within the thyroid or as metastasis in a cervical lymph node. The presence of isolated cervical nodal metastases, interestingly, does not appear to have a significant influence on the generally good prognosis of these lesions. In a minority of patients, hematogenous metastases are present at the time of diagnosis, most commonly in the lung. Most papillary carcinomas are indolent lesions, with 10-year survival rates of up to 85%. In general, the prognosis is less favorable among elderly patients and in patients with invasion of extrathyroidal tissues or distant metastases.

FOLLICULAR CARCINOMA

Follicular carcinomas are the second most common form of thyroid cancer (15% of all cases). They usually present at an older age than do papillary carcinomas, with a peak incidence in the middle adult years. The incidence of follicular carcinoma is increased in areas of dietary iodine deficiency, suggesting that, in some cases, nodular goiter may predispose to the development of the neoplasm. There is no compelling evidence that follicular carcinomas arise from preexisting adenomas.

Table 20–4. THYROID LESIONS WITH A FOLLICULAR ARCHITECTURE

Non-neoplastic

Hyperplastic nodule in goiter

Neoplastic

Follicular adenoma*
Follicular carcinoma*
Follicular variant of papillary carcinoma†

*Differentiating follicular carcinoma from follicular adenoma requires histologic evidence of *capsular or blood vessel invasion, or documented metastasis.*

†The diagnosis of papillary carcinoma is rendered on the basis of *characteristic nuclear features,* irrespective of the presence or absence of papillae.

MORPHOLOGY

Follicular carcinomas may be grossly infiltrative or well circumscribed. Sharply demarcated lesions with minimal invasion may be impossible to distinguish from follicular adenomas on gross examination. Larger lesions may infiltrate well beyond the thyroid capsule into the soft tissues of the neck. Microscopically, most follicular carcinomas are composed of fairly uniform cells forming small follicles, reminiscent of normal thyroid. In other cases, follicular differentiation may be less apparent. Similar to follicular adenomas, Hürthle cell variants of follicular carcinomas may be seen. Extensive invasion of adjacent thyroid parenchyma makes the diagnosis of carcinoma obvious in some cases. In other cases, however, invasion may be limited to microscopic foci of capsular and/or vascular invasion (see Fig. 20–14). Such lesions may require extensive histologic sampling before they can be distinguished from follicular adenomas. The recent description of molecular abnormalities resulting in the formation of the *PAX8-PPARγ1* fusion gene may help in the diagnosis of follicular cancers. As mentioned earlier, follicular lesions in which the nuclear features are typical of papillary carcinomas should be regarded as papillary cancers (see Table 20–4).

Clinical Features. Follicular carcinomas present most frequently as solitary "cold" thyroid nodules. In rare cases, they may be hyperfunctional. These neoplasms tend to metastasize through the bloodstream to the lungs, bone, and liver. Regional nodal metastases are uncommon, in contrast to papillary carcinomas. Follicular carcinomas are treated with surgical excision. Well-differentiated metastases may take up radioactive iodine, which can be used to identify, and ablate, such lesions. Because better differentiated lesions may be stimulated by TSH, patients are usually treated with thyroid hormone after surgery to suppress endogenous TSH.

MEDULLARY CARCINOMA

Medullary carcinomas of the thyroid are neuroendocrine neoplasms derived from the parafollicular cells, or C cells, of the thyroid. Like normal C cells, medullary carcinomas secrete calcitonin, the measurement of which plays an important role in the diagnosis and postoperative follow-up of patients. In some cases, the tumor cells elaborate other polypeptide hormones such as carcinoembryonic antigen, somatostatin, serotonin, and vasoactive intestinal peptide (VIP). Medullary carcinomas arise *sporadically* in about 80% of cases. The remaining 20% are *familial* cases occurring in the setting of multiple endocrine neoplasia (MEN) syndromes 2A or 2B or familial non-MEN medullary thyroid carcinoma. Germ-line mutations in the *RET* protooncogene play an important role in the development of both MEN and non-MEN familial cancers. Somatic *RET* protooncogene mutations have also been identified in sporadic cases. Sporadic medullary carcinomas, as well as familial non-MEN cancers, occur in adults, with a peak incidence in the fifth to sixth decades. Cases associated with MEN 2A or 2B, in contrast, occur in younger patients and may even arise in children.

MORPHOLOGY

Medullary carcinomas may arise as a solitary nodule or may present as multiple lesions involving both lobes of the thyroid. **Multicentricity** is particularly common in familial cases. Larger lesions often contain areas of necrosis and hemorrhage and may extend through the capsule of the thyroid. Microscopically, medullary carcinomas are composed of polygonal to spindle-shaped cells, which may form nests, trabeculae, and even follicles. Acellular **amyloid deposits,** derived from altered calcitonin molecules, are present in the adjacent stroma in many cases (Fig. 20–16) and are a distinctive feature of these tumors. Calcitonin is readily demonstrable both within the cytoplasm of the tumor cells and in the stromal amyloid by immunohistochemical methods. Electron microscopy reveals variable numbers of intracytoplasmic membrane-bound electron-dense granules.

One of the peculiar features of familial medullary carcinomas is the presence of multicentric **C-cell hyperplasia** in the surrounding thyroid parenchyma, a feature usually absent in sporadic lesions. While the precise criteria for defining what constitutes hyperplasia are variable, the presence of multiple prominent clusters of C cells scattered throughout the parenchyma should raise the specter of a familial tumor, even if that history is not available. Foci of C-cell hyperplasia are believed to represent the precursor lesions from which medullary carcinomas arise.

Clinical Features. Sporadic cases of medullary carcinoma present most often as a mass in the neck, sometimes associated with compression effects such as dysphagia or hoarseness. In some instances the initial manifestations are caused by the secretion of a peptide hormone (e.g., diarrhea caused by the secretion of VIP). Notably, hypocalcemia is not a feature, despite the presence of raised calcitonin levels. Screening of relatives for elevated calcitonin levels or *RET* mutations permits early detection of tumors in familial cases. As discussed later, all MEN 2 kindreds carrying *RET* muta-

Figure 20–16 ■

Medullary carcinoma of the thyroid. These tumors typically contain amyloid, visible here as homogeneous extracellular material, derived from calcitonin molecules secreted by the neoplastic cells.

Table 20–5. COMPARISON OF SPORADIC AND MULTIPLE ENDOCRINE NEOPLASIA (MEN)–ASSOCIATED MEDULLARY THYROID CARCINOMAS (MTC)

	Sporadic MTC	MEN-associated MTC
Age at Onset	Elderly individuals (>5th decade)	Young adults
Centricity	Unicentric (solitary)	Multicentric, often bilateral
C-Cell Hyperplasia	Absent	Almost always present
Behavior	Less aggressive	More aggressive, particularly MEN 2B

tions are offered prophylactic thyroidectomies to preempt the development of medullary carcinomas; often, the only histologic finding in the resected thyroid of these asymptomatic carriers is the presence of C-cell hyperplasia or small (<1 cm) "micromedullary" carcinomas. In the spectrum of biologic virulence, non-MEN familial tumors are fairly indolent lesions; sporadic cases, and those associated with MEN 2A, are of intermediate aggressiveness, while MEN 2B tumors have a particularly poor outcome, with a propensity for early metastases via the bloodstream. Table 20–5 compares the features of sporadic and MEN-associated medullary carcinomas.

ANAPLASTIC CARCINOMA

Anaplastic carcinomas of the thyroid are among the most aggressive human neoplasms. They occur predominantly in elderly patients, particularly in areas of endemic goiter.

MORPHOLOGY

Anaplastic carcinomas present as bulky masses that typically grow rapidly beyond the thyroid capsule into adjacent neck structures. Microscopically, these neoplasms are composed of highly anaplastic cells, exhibiting three distinct morphologic patterns, often in combination: large, pleomorphic **giant cells; spindle cells** with a sarcomatous appearance; or cells with a vaguely **squamoid appearance.** Some tumors, previously classified as "small cell anaplastic" carcinomas in view of the resemblance of the neoplastic cells to small cell cancers in other anatomic sites, ultimately proved to be medullary carcinomas or malignant lymphomas. Foci of papillary or follicular differentiation may be present in some tumors, suggesting origin from a better differentiated carcinoma. The presence of a *TP53* mutation in anaplastic carcinomas (and its absence in differentiated thyroid cancers) is a molecular correlate of tumor progression and aggressiveness.

Clinical Features. Anaplastic carcinomas grow with wild abandon despite therapy. Metastases to distant sites are common, but in most cases death occurs in less than 1 year as a result of aggressive local growth and compromise of vital structures in the neck.

Parathyroid Glands

The parathyroid glands are derived from the developing pharyngeal pouches that also give rise to the thymus. They normally lie in close proximity to the upper and lower poles of each thyroid lobe, but they may be found anywhere along the pathway of descent of the pharyngeal pouches, including the carotid sheath and the thymus and elsewhere in the anterior mediastinum. *In contrast to several other endocrine glands, the activity of the parathyroids is controlled by the level of free (ionized) calcium in the bloodstream rather than by trophic hormones secreted by the hypothalamus and pituitary.* Normally, decreased levels of free calcium stimulate the synthesis and secretion of parathyroid hormone (PTH), which in turn

■ Activates osteoclasts, thereby mobilizing calcium from bone
■ Increases the renal tubular reabsorption of calcium
■ Increases the conversion of vitamin D to its active dihydroxy form in the kidneys
■ Increases urinary phosphate excretion
■ Augments gastrointestinal calcium absorption

The net result of these activities is an increase in the level of free calcium, which in turn inhibits further PTH secretion. Abnormalities of the parathyroids include both hyperfunction and hypofunction. *Tumors of the parathyroid glands, unlike thyroid tumors, usually come to attention because of excessive secretion of PTH rather than mass effects.*

Figure 20–17 ■

Technetium-99m-sestamibi radionuclide scan demonstrates an area of increased uptake corresponding to the left inferior parathyroid gland *(arrow)*. This patient had a parathyroid adenoma. Preoperative scintigraphy is useful in localizing and distinguishing adenomas from parathyroid hyperplasia, where more than one gland would demonstrate increased uptake.

HYPERPARATHYROIDISM

Hyperparathyroidism occurs in two major forms, *primary* and *secondary*, and (less commonly) as *tertiary* hyperparathyroidism. The first condition represents an autonomous, spontaneous overproduction of PTH, while the latter two conditions typically occur as secondary phenomena in patients with chronic renal insufficiency.

Primary Hyperparathyroidism

Primary hyperparathyroidism is one of the most common endocrine disorders and is an important cause of hypercalcemia. This condition is usually caused by a parathyroid *adenoma* or by *primary hyperplasia* of the glands. On rare occasions (less than 1% of cases), it is caused by a carcinoma of the parathyroids. Primary hyperparathyroidism is typically a disease of adults and is more common in women than in men. It may occur either sporadically or in association with one of the MEN syndromes (see later). The elevated levels of PTH produce a number of changes, including excessive bone resorption, renal disease, and, of course, hypercalcemia.

MORPHOLOGY

The morphologic changes seen in primary hyperparathyroidism include those in the parathyroid glands, as well as those in other organs affected by elevated levels of calcium. In 80% to 90% of cases, the parathyroids harbor a solitary **adenoma,** which, like the normal parathyroids, may lie in close proximity to the thyroid gland or in an ectopic site (e.g., the mediastinum). The typical parathyroid adenoma is a well-circumscribed, soft, tan nodule, invested by a delicate capsule. **By definition, parathyroid adenomas are almost invariably confined to single glands** (Fig. 20–17), and the remaining glands are normal in size or somewhat shrunken, owing to feedback inhibition by elevations in serum calcium. Most parathyroid adenomas weigh between 0.5 and 5 g. Microscopically, parathyroid adenomas are composed predominantly of fairly uniform, polygonal "chief" cells with small, centrally placed nuclei (Fig. 20–18). In most cases, at least a few nests of larger cells containing eosinophilic granular cytoplasm (oxyphil cells) are also present. A rim of compressed, non-neoplastic parathyroid tissue, generally separated by a fibrous capsule, is often visible at the edge of the adenoma (see Fig. 20–18). This constitutes a helpful internal control, since the chief cells of the adenoma are larger and show greater nuclear size variability than the normal chief cells. It is not uncommon to find bizarre and pleomorphic nuclei even within adenomas (so-called endocrine atypia), and this should not be used as a criterion for defining malignancy. Mitotic figures are rare. **In contrast to the normal parathyroid parenchyma, adipose tissue is inconspicuous within the adenoma.**

Hyperplasia is present in 10% to 20% of cases of primary hyperparathyroidism and may occur sporadically or as a component of MEN type 1 or 2A (see later). **Parathyroid hyperplasia is characteristically a multiglandular process;** in some cases, however, enlargement may be grossly apparent in only one or two glands, rendering the distinction between hyperplasia and adenoma difficult. The combined weight of all glands may exceed 1 g but is often less. Microscopically, the most common

Figure 20-18 ■

A, Solitary chief cell parathyroid adenoma *(low-power view)* revealing clear delineation from the residual gland below. *B*, High-power detail of chief cell parathyroid adenoma. There is slight variation in nuclear size and tendency to follicular formation but no anaplasia.

pattern seen is that of chief cell hyperplasia, which may involve the glands in a diffuse or multinodular pattern. Less commonly, the constituent cells contain abundant clear cytoplasm, a condition designated as water-clear cell hyperplasia. As in the case of adenomas, stromal fat is inconspicuous within foci of hyperplasia.

Parathyroid carcinomas are usually firm or hard tumors, adhering to the surrounding tissue owing to fibrosis or infiltrative growth (intraoperatively, a fibrous and adherent parathyroid is often a clue that the surgeon is dealing with a carcinoma rather than an adenoma). Parathyroid carcinomas are larger than adenomas, almost always more than 5 g and sometimes exceeding 10 g. Like their adenomatous counterparts, parathyroid carcinomas are typically single-gland disorders, and chief cells tend to predominate in most cases. The cytologic features and mitotic activity can be quite variable, showing considerable overlap with those in adenomas; therefore, neither can be reliably used to diagnose parathyroid carcinomas. The only two valid criteria for malignancy are (1) invasion of surrounding tissues and (2) metastatic dissemination.

Morphologic changes in other organs deserving special mention are found in the skeleton and kidneys. **Skeletal changes** include prominence of osteoclasts, which in turn erode bone matrix and mobilize calcium salts, particularly in the metaphyses of long tubular bones. Bone resorption is accompanied by increased osteoblastic activity and the formation of new bone trabeculae. In many cases the resultant bone contains widely spaced, delicate trabeculae reminiscent of those seen in osteoporosis. In more severe cases the cortex is grossly thinned and the marrow contains increased amounts of fibrous tissue accompanied by foci of hemorrhage and cyst formation **(osteitis fibrosa cystica).** Aggregates of os-

teoclasts, reactive giant cells, and hemorrhagic debris occasionally form masses that may be mistaken for neoplasms **(brown tumors** of hyperparathyroidism). PTH-induced hypercalcemia favors the formation of **urinary tract stones** (nephrolithiasis) as well as calcification of the renal interstitium and tubules (nephrocalcinosis). Metastatic calcification secondary to hypercalcemia may also be seen in other sites, including the stomach, lungs, myocardium, and blood vessels.

Molecular Changes in Parathyroid Tumors. Although the detailed discussion of genetic abnormalities in parathyroid tumors is beyond the scope of this book, two genes whose function is commonly affected in these tumors will be mentioned. The first of these, called *PRAD1* (for *parathyroid adenomatosis gene 1*), is located on chromosome 11q. The protein product of *PRAD1* belongs to a family of cell-cycle regulators known as cyclins (hence the protein is named cyclin D1). *Cyclin D1* promotes the transition of cells from G_1 into the S phase and thus increases cellular proliferation (Chapters 3 and 6). Overexpression of *cyclin D1* is common in parathyroid tumors (adenomas and carcinomas) as well as in hyperplasia and presumably contributes to abnormal growth. In some cases activation of *cyclin D1* gene occurs by chromosome 11 inversion that juxtaposes *cyclin D1* with the 5'-regulatory region of the parathyroid hormone gene, thus directing overexpression of cyclin D1 in the parathyroid gland. The second common abnormality involves the tumor suppressor gene *MEN1* on chromosome 11q13; loss of *MEN1* function is present in both sporadic parathyroid tumors as well as in parathyroid hyperplasia occurring in the context of familial MEN 1 syndrome (see later). Expectedly, in the latter condition, *MEN1* abnormalities are present in the germ line, as opposed to sporadic tumors, where they are somatically acquired during tumor development.

Table 20–6. CAUSES OF HYPERCALCEMIA

Elevated Parathyroid Hormone	Decreased Parathyroid Hormone
Hyperparathyroidism	Hypercalcemia of malignancy
Primary*	PTHrP mediated (lung and
Secondary†	kidney cancers)
Tertiary†	Cytokine mediated (multiple
Familial hypocalciuric hypercalcemia	myeloma)
	Vitamin D toxicity
	Immobilization
	Thiazide diuretics
	Granulomatous diseases
	(sarcoidosis)

*Primary hyperparathyroidism is the single most common cause of hypercalcemia. Hyperparathyroidism and cancer account for nearly 90% of cases of hypercalcemia.

†Secondary and tertiary hyperparathyroidism are most commonly associated with progressive renal failure.

PTHrP, parathyroid hormone–related protein.

Clinical Features. *The most common manifestation of primary hyperparathyroidism is an increase in the level of serum ionized calcium.* In fact, primary hyperparathyroidism is the most common cause of *clinically silent* hypercalcemia. It should be noted that other conditions (Table 20–6) also produce hypercalcemia. *Malignancy,* in particular, is the most common cause of *clinically apparent* hypercalcemia in adults (symptoms are usually referable to the underlying malignancy rather than the hypercalcemia) and must be excluded by appropriate clinical and laboratory investigations. In patients with hypercalcemia caused by parathyroid hyperfunction, serum PTH levels are inappropriately elevated, whereas PTH levels are low to undetectable in hypercalcemia caused by nonparathyroid diseases. In patients with hypercalcemia resulting from secretion of PTH-related protein (PTHrP) by certain nonparathyroid tumors, radioimmunoassays specific for PTH and PTHrP can distinguish between the two molecules. Other laboratory alterations referable to PTH excess include hypophosphatemia and increased urinary excretion of both calcium and phosphate. Familial hypocalciuric hypercalcemia is a rare autosomal dominant condition caused by inactivating mutations in the *calcium-sensing receptor (CASR)* gene on parathyroid cells, resulting in constitutive PTH secretion.

Primary hyperparathyroidism has been traditionally associated with a constellation of symptoms that included "painful bones, renal stones, abdominal groans, and psychic moans" (Fig. 20–19). Pain, secondary to fractures of bones weakened by osteoporosis or osteitis fibrosa cystica and resulting from renal stones, with obstructive uropathy, was at one time a prominent manifestation of primary hyperparathyroidism. Because serum calcium levels are now routinely assessed in the work-up of most patients who need blood tests for unrelated conditions, clinically silent hyperparathyroidism is detected early. Hence, many of the classic clinical manifestations, particularly those referable to bone and renal disease, are seen much less frequently. Additional signs and symptoms that may be encountered in hyperparathyroidism include the following:

- *Gastrointestinal disturbances,* including constipation, nausea, peptic ulcers, pancreatitis, and gallstones
- *Central nervous system alterations,* including depression, lethargy, and seizures
- *Neuromuscular abnormalities,* including weakness and hypotonia
- *Polyuria* and secondary polydipsia

Although some of these alterations, for example, polyuria and muscle weakness, are clearly related to hypercalcemia,

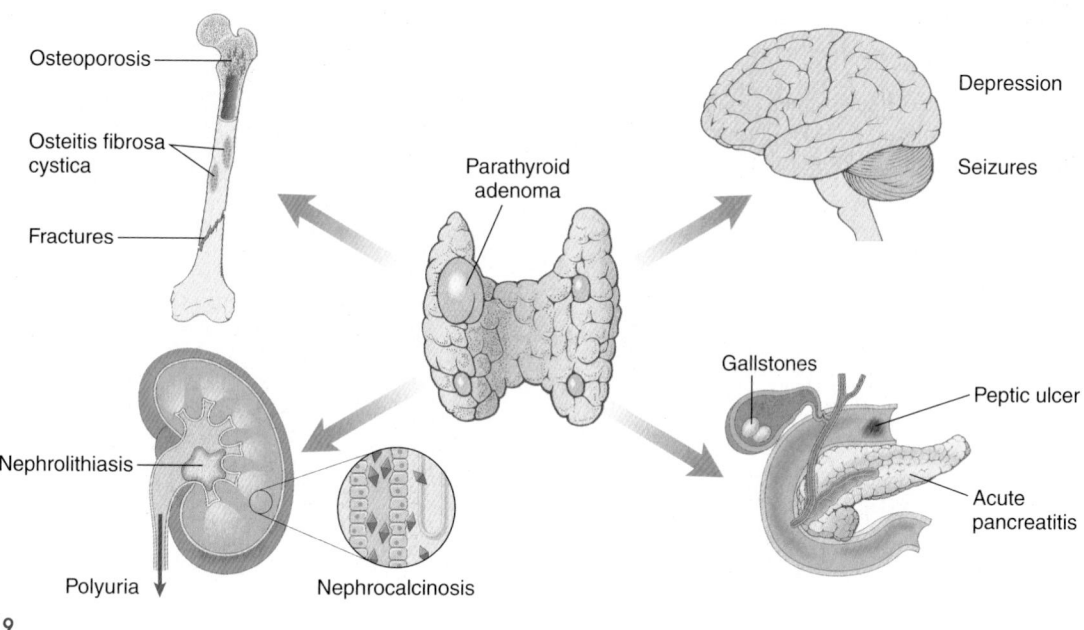

Figure 20–19

Cardinal features of hyperparathyroidism. With routine evaluation of calcium levels in most patients, primary hyperparathyroidism is often detected at a clinically silent stage. Hypercalcemia from any other cause can also give rise to the same symptoms.

the pathogenesis of many of the other manifestations of the disorder remains poorly understood.

Secondary Hyperparathyroidism

Secondary hyperparathyroidism is caused by any condition associated with a chronic depression in the serum calcium level, because low serum calcium leads to compensatory overactivity of the parathyroids. *Renal failure is by far the most common cause of secondary hyperparathyroidism.* The mechanisms by which chronic renal failure induces secondary hyperparathyroidism are complex and not fully understood. Chronic renal insufficiency is associated with decreased phosphate excretion, which in turn results in hyperphosphatemia. The elevated serum phosphate levels directly depress serum calcium levels and thereby stimulate parathyroid gland activity. In addition, loss of renal substances reduces the availability of α_1-hydroxylase necessary for the synthesis of the active form of vitamin D, which in turn reduces intestinal absorption of calcium (Chapter 8).

MORPHOLOGY

The parathyroid glands in secondary hyperparathyroidism are hyperplastic. As in the case of primary hyperplasia, the degree of glandular enlargement is not necessarily symmetric. Microscopically, the hyperplastic glands contain an increased number of chief cells, or cells with more abundant, clear cytoplasm **(water–clear cells),** in a diffuse or multinodular distribution. Fat cells are decreased in number. **Bone changes** similar to those seen in primary hyperparathyroidism may also be present. **Metastatic calcification** may be seen in many tissues, including lungs, heart, stomach, and blood vessels.

Clinical Features. The clinical manifestations of secondary hyperparathyroidism are usually dominated by those related to chronic renal failure. Bone abnormalities *(renal osteodystrophy)* and other changes associated with PTH excess are, in general, less severe than those seen in primary hyperparathyroidism. Serum calcium levels remain near normal because the compensatory increase in PTH levels sustains serum calcium. The metastatic calcification of blood vessels (secondary to hyperphosphatemia) may occasionally result in significant ischemic damage to skin and other organs, a process sometimes referred to as *calciphylaxis.* In a minority of patients, parathyroid activity may become autonomous and excessive, with resultant hypercalcemia, a process sometimes termed *tertiary hyperparathyroidism.* Parathyroidectomy may be necessary to control the hyperparathyroidism in such patients.

HYPOPARATHYROIDISM

Hypoparathyroidism is far less common than hyperparathyroidism. The major causes of hypoparathyroidism include the following:

- *Surgical ablation:* inadvertent removal of parathyroids during thyroidectomy.
- *Congenital absence:* usually occurs in conjunction with thymic aplasia and cardiac defects in DiGeorge syndrome (Chapters 5 and 6).
- *Autoimmune hypoparathyroidism:* a hereditary polyglandular deficiency syndrome arising from autoantibodies to multiple endocrine organs (parathyroid, thyroid, adrenals, and pancreas). Chronic mucocutaneous candidiasis (Chapter 13) is sometimes encountered in these patients, suggesting an underlying defect in T-cell function. This condition is discussed more extensively in the context of autoimmune adrenalitis.

The major clinical manifestations of hypoparathyroidism are referable to hypocalcemia and include *increased neuromuscular irritability (tingling, muscle spasms, facial grimacing, and sustained carpopedal spasm or tetany), cardiac arrhythmias*, and, on occasion, *increased intracranial pressures* and *seizures.* Morphologic changes are generally inconspicuous but may include cataracts, calcification of the cerebral basal ganglia, and dental abnormalities.

Adrenal Cortex

Diseases of the adrenal cortex include those associated with cortical hyperfunction or hypofunction. In addition, a variety of mass lesions may occur in the adrenal cortex that may be nonfunctional or associated with cortical hyperfunction.

ADRENOCORTICAL HYPERFUNCTION (HYPERADRENALISM)

The adrenal cortex synthesizes and secretes steroid hormones, which fall into three major categories: glucocorticoids, exemplified by cortisol; mineralocorticoids, exemplified by aldosterone; and adrenocortical androgens. Thus, hyperfunction of the adrenal cortex produces three major groups of clinical syndromes referable to excessive hormone levels. These include *Cushing syndrome*, *hyperaldosteronism*, and a number of *virilizing syndromes*. Because of the overlapping functions of some of the adrenal steroid hormones, the clinical features of these syndromes may also overlap.

Hypercortisolism (Cushing Syndrome)

This disorder is caused by any condition that produces an elevation in glucocorticoid levels. *In clinical practice, most cases of Cushing syndrome are caused by the administration of exogenous glucocorticoids.* The remaining cases are endogenous and caused by one of the following (Fig. 20–20):

■ Primary hypothalamic-pituitary diseases associated with hypersecretion of ACTH
■ Primary adrenocortical hyperplasia or neoplasia
■ The secretion of ectopic ACTH by nonendocrine neoplasms

Primary hypothalamic-pituitary disease associated with oversecretion of ACTH, also known as *Cushing disease*, accounts for more than half of the cases of spontaneous, endogenous Cushing syndrome. The disease occurs most frequently during the third to fourth decades of life and affects women about three times more frequently than men. In most of these patients the pituitary gland contains a small *ACTH-producing adenoma* (pituitary microadenoma) that does not produce mass effects in the brain; occasional tumors qualify as a macroadenoma (>10 mm). Apparently, owing to some mutations, these ACTH-producing adenomas are less sensitive to the feedback effects of the cortisol than are normal corticotrophs. In the remaining patients, the an-

terior pituitary contains areas of *corticotroph-cell hyperplasia* without a discrete adenoma. In at least some patients, the pituitary abnormality appears to result from excessive stimulation of ACTH release secondary to signals (e.g., CRH) from the hypothalamus. The adrenal glands in patients with Cushing disease are characterized by variable degrees of bilateral nodular cortical hyperplasia (discussed later), caused by elevated levels of ACTH. The cortical hyperplasia, in turn, is responsible for the hypercortisolism.

Primary adrenocortical neoplasms and hyperplasia account for between 25% and 30% of cases of endogenous Cushing syndrome. This variant of Cushing syndrome is also sometimes designated *adrenal Cushing syndrome* or, because the adrenals function autonomously, *ACTH-independent Cushing syndrome*. In most cases, adrenal Cushing syndrome is caused by a unilateral adrenocortical neoplasm, which may be either benign (adenoma) or malignant (carcinoma). Primary bilateral hyperplasia of the adrenal cortices is a rare cause of Cushing syndrome. There are two variants of this entity; the first presents as macronodules (>3 mm) and the second as micronodules (<3 mm) that are often pigmented ("primary pigmented nodular adrenocortical disease"). The micronodular variant is a familial disease, usually associated with features of overactivity in other endocrine organs such as the pituitary, thyroid, and gonads.

Secretion of ectopic ACTH by nonendocrine tumors accounts for most of the remaining cases of endogenous Cushing syndrome. Commonly, the responsible tumor is a *small cell carcinoma of the lung*, although other neoplasms, including *carcinoid tumors, medullary carcinomas of the thyroid, and islet cell tumors of the pancreas*, have also been associated with the syndrome. In addition to tumors that elaborate ectopic ACTH, an occasional neoplasm produces ectopic corticotropin-releasing hormone (CRH), which in turn causes ACTH secretion and hypercortisolism. As with Cushing syndrome associated with hypothalamic-pituitary disease, nodular cortical hyperplasia is present in the adrenals.

MORPHOLOGY

The morphology of the adrenal glands depends on the cause of the hypercortisolism. In patients in whom the syndrome results from exogenous glucocorticoids, **suppression of endogenous ACTH results in bilateral atrophy of the adrenal cortices,** owing to a

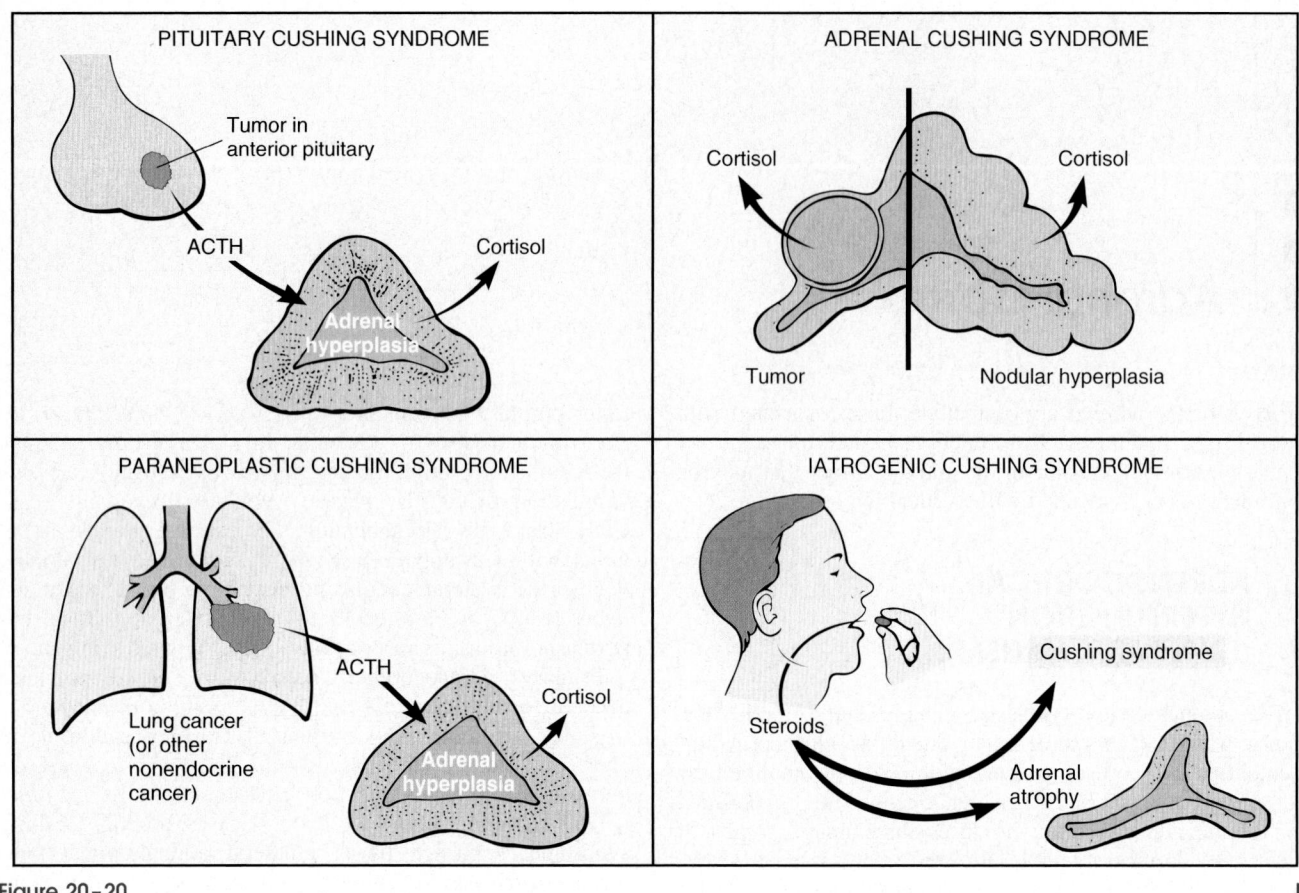

Figure 20-20 ■

Schematic representation of the various forms of Cushing syndrome, illustrating the three endogenous forms as well as the more common exogenous (iatrogenic) form. ACTH, adrenocorticotropic hormone.

lack of stimulation of the zonae fasciculata and reticularis by ACTH. The zona glomerulosa is of normal thickness in such cases, because this portion of the cortex functions independently of ACTH. In cases of endogenous hypercortisolism, in contrast, the adrenals either are hyperplastic or contain a cortical neoplasm. In Cushing syndrome caused by increased ACTH secretion by either the pituitary or an ectopic source (e.g., a small cell carcinoma of the lung), stimulation of the adrenal glands causes bilateral hyperplasia. The adrenal cortices in such cases are diffusely thickened and yellow, owing to an increase in the size and number of lipid-rich cells in the zonae fasciculata and reticularis (Fig. 20-21). The combined weight of the hyperplastic glands may be 25 to 40 g. Some degree of nodularity is common and may be pronounced (nodular hyperplasia). Primary micronodular hyperplasia is associated with brown-black pigmentation of the adrenal cortices, owing to prominent lipofuscin and neuromelanin deposits in the cells of the zona fasciculata. **Primary adrenocortical neoplasms** causing Cushing syndrome may be benign or malignant. Adrenocortical adenomas are encapsulated, expansile, yellow tumors usually weighing less than 30 g. Microscopically, they are usually

composed of lipid-rich cells similar to those encountered in the normal zona fasciculata (Fig. 20-22). Their morphology is identical to that of nonfunctional adenomas and of adenomas associated with hyperaldosteronism (discussed later). The adjacent adrenal cortex and that of the contralateral adrenal gland are atrophic, owing to suppression of endogenous ACTH by high cortisol levels. Carcinomas associated with Cushing syndrome tend to be larger than adenomas, frequently exceeding 200 to 300 g. Their morphology is identical to that of nonfunctional adrenocortical carcinomas, discussed later.

The **pituitary gland** shows changes in all forms of Cushing syndrome. The most common alteration, resulting from high levels of endogenous or exogenous glucocorticoids, is termed **Crooke hyaline change.** In this condition, the normal granular, basophilic cytoplasm of the ACTH-producing cells in the anterior pituitary is replaced by homogeneous, lightly basophilic material; this change is caused by the accumulation of intermediate cytokeratin filaments in their cytoplasm. In patients with Cushing syndrome of hypothalamic-pituitary origin **(Cushing disease),** the pituitary usually contains either an **ACTH-secreting pituitary adenoma** or foci of **ACTH-cell hyperplasia.**

Figure 20-21

Adrenocortical hyperplasia. The adrenal cortex is yellow, thickened, and multinodular owing to hypertrophy and hyperplasia of the lipid-rich zonae fasciculata and reticularis.

Clinical Features. The signs and symptoms of Cushing syndrome are an exaggeration of the known actions of glucocorticoids. Cushing syndrome usually develops gradually and, like many other endocrine abnormalities, may be quite subtle in its early stages. A major exception to this insidious onset is Cushing syndrome associated with small cell carcinomas of the lung, where the rapid course of the underlying disease precludes development of many of the characteristic features. Early manifestations of Cushing syndrome include *hypertension* and *weight gain*. With time, the more characteristic centripetal distribution of adipose tissue becomes apparent, with resultant *truncal obesity*, "moon" facies, and accumulation of fat in the posterior neck and back ("buffalo hump"). Hypercortisolism causes selective atrophy of fast-

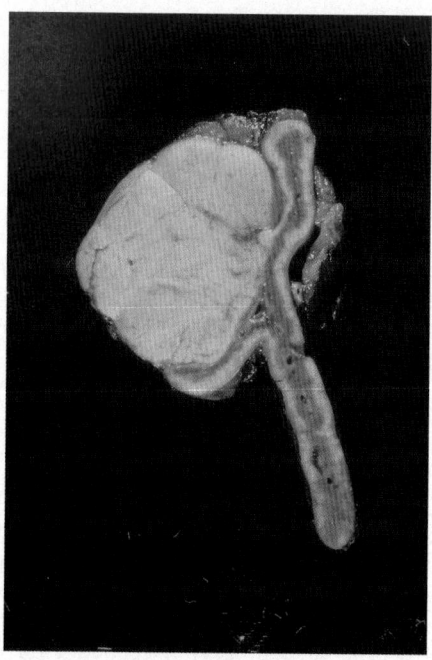

Figure 20-22

Adrenocortical adenoma. The adenoma is distinguished from nodular hyperplasia by its solitary, circumscribed nature. The functional status of an adrenocortical adenoma cannot be predicted from its gross or microscopic appearance.

Table 20-7. LABORATORY FEATURES OF CUSHING SYNDROME

Laboratory Test	Pituitary Tumor	Ectopic Tumor	Adrenal Cushing
Plasma cortisol	↑	↑	↑
Plasma adrenocorticotropic hormone	↑	↑	↓
Urinary steroids after low doses of dexamethasone	→	→	→
Urinary corticosteroids after high doses of dexamethasone	↓	→	→

↑, increased; ↓, decreased; →, no change.

twitch (type II) myofibers, with resultant *decreased muscle mass* and proximal limb weakness. Glucocorticoids induce gluconeogenesis and inhibit the uptake of glucose by cells, with resultant *hyperglycemia, glucosuria,* and *polydipsia,* simulating diabetes mellitus. The catabolic effects on proteins cause loss of collagen and resorption of bone. Thus, the skin is thin, fragile, and easily bruised; *cutaneous striae* are particularly common in the abdominal area. Bone resorption results in the development of *osteoporosis,* with consequent backache and increased susceptibility to fractures. Because glucocorticoids suppress the immune response, patients with Cushing syndrome are also at increased risk for a variety of infections. Additional manifestations include *hirsutism* and *menstrual abnormalities,* as well as a number of *mental disturbances,* including mood swings, depression, and frank psychosis. Extra-adrenal Cushing syndrome caused by pituitary or ectopic ACTH secretion is usually associated with increased skin pigmentation, because of melanocyte-stimulating activity in the ACTH precursor molecule.

The laboratory diagnosis of *Cushing syndrome* is based on (1) the 24-hour urinary free cortisol level, which is always increased; and (2) loss of the normal diurnal pattern of cortisol secretion. *Localization of the cause* of Cushing syndrome depends on (1) the level of serum ACTH and (2) measurement of urinary steroid excretion after administration of the synthetic glucocorticoid dexamethasone (Table 20–7).

■ In the most common form, pituitary Cushing syndrome, ACTH levels are elevated and cannot be suppressed by administration of a low dose of dexamethasone. Hence, there is no reduction in urinary excretion of 17-hydroxycorticosteroids. However, the cells in the corticotroph adenomas respond to a higher dose of injected dexamethasone by a reduction in ACTH secretion that is reflected by suppression of urinary steroid excretion.

■ With ectopic ACTH secretion, the ACTH level is elevated as expected, but its secretion is completely insensitive to low or high doses of exogenously administered dexamethasone.

■ When Cushing syndrome is caused by an adrenal tumor, the ACTH level is very low because of feedback inhibition of the pituitary. As with ectopic ACTH secretion, administration of both low- and high-dose dexamethasone fails to suppress cortisol production and excretion.

Hyperaldosteronism

Excessive levels of aldosterone cause *sodium retention and potassium excretion, with resultant hypertension and hypokalemia.* Hyperaldosteronism may be primary, or it may be secondary to an extra-adrenal cause. In *secondary hyperaldosteronism,* aldosterone release occurs in response to activation of the renin-angiotensin system. It is characterized by *increased levels of plasma renin* and is encountered in conditions associated with

■ Decreased renal perfusion (arteriolar nephrosclerosis, renal artery stenosis)
■ Arterial hypovolemia and edema (congestive heart failure, cirrhosis, nephrotic syndrome)
■ Pregnancy (caused by estrogen-induced increases in plasma renin substrate)

Primary hyperaldosteronism, in contrast, indicates a primary, autonomous overproduction of aldosterone, with resultant suppression of the renin-angiotensin system and *decreased plasma renin activity.* Primary hyperaldosteronism is caused either by an aldosterone-producing adrenocortical neoplasm, usually an adenoma, or by primary adrenocortical hyperplasia.

> ### MORPHOLOGY
>
> In roughly 80% of cases, primary hyperaldosteronism is caused by an **aldosterone-secreting adenoma** in one adrenal gland, a condition referred to as **Conn syndrome.** In most cases, the adenomas are solitary, small (<2 cm in diameter), encapsulated lesions, although multiple adenomas may be present in an occasional patient; carcinomas resulting in hyperaldosteronism are rare. In contrast to cortical adenomas associated with Cushing syndrome, those associated with hyperaldosteronism do not usually suppress ACTH secretion. Therefore, the adjacent adrenal cortex and that of the contralateral gland are not atrophic. Morphologically, the adenomas that cause primary hyperaldosteronism are indistinguishable from other functional or nonfunctional adrenocortical adenomas. In about 15% of cases, primary hyperaldosteronism is caused by bilateral **primary adrenocortical hyperplasia,** also termed **idiopathic hyperaldosteronism.** In most of these latter cases, the adrenal cortex is either diffusely or irregularly hyperplastic, owing to proliferation of the cells in the zona glomerulosa. The nature of the secretagogue inducing hyperplasia is not known but is postulated to be a non-ACTH pituitary glycoprotein.

Clinical Features. The clinical manifestations of primary hyperaldosteronism are those of hypertension and hypokalemia. Serum renin levels, as mentioned earlier, are low. Conn syndrome occurs most frequently in middle adult life and is more common in females than in males (2:1). Although aldosterone-producing adenomas account for less than 1% of cases of hypertension, it is important to recognize them, because they cause a surgically correctable form of hypertension. Primary adrenal hyperplasia associated with hyperaldosteronism occurs more often in children and young adults than in older adults; surgical intervention is not very beneficial in these patients, and it is best managed with medical therapy with an aldosterone antagonist such as spironolactone. The treatment of secondary hyperaldosteronism rests on correcting the underlying cause of the stimulation of the renin-angiotensin system.

Adrenogenital Syndromes

Excess of androgens may be caused by a number of diseases, including primary gonadal disorders and several primary adrenal disorders. The adrenal cortex secretes two compounds—dehydroepiandrosterone and androstenedione—which require conversion to testosterone in peripheral tissues for their androgenic effects. Unlike gonadal androgens, adrenal androgen formation is regulated by ACTH; thus, excess secretion can occur either as a "pure" syndrome or as a component of Cushing disease. The adrenal causes of androgen excess include neoplasms and an uncommon group of disorders collectively designated congenital adrenal hyperplasia. Adrenocortical neoplasms (discussed later) associated with symptoms of androgen excess *(virilization)* are more likely to be carcinomas than adenomas. They are morphologically identical to other functional or nonfunctional cortical neoplasms. *Congenital adrenal hyperplasias represent a group of autosomal recessive disorders, each characterized by a hereditary defect in an enzyme involved in cortisol biosynthesis.* In these conditions, decreased cortisol production results in a compensatory increase in ACTH secretion. The resultant adrenal hyperplasia causes increased production of androgens and cortisol precursor steroids, a number of which have virilizing activity (Fig. 20–23). *The most common enzymatic defect in congenital adrenal hyperplasia is 21-hydroxylase deficiency,* which accounts for approximately 95% of cases. Several clinical variants of 21-hydroxylase deficiency exist, each resulting from a different mutation in the 21-hydroxylase gene, located on chromosome 6.

> ### MORPHOLOGY
>
> In all cases of congenital adrenal hyperplasia, the adrenals are bilaterally hyperplastic, driven by a sustained elevation of ACTH. The adrenal cortex is thickened and nodular, populated by lipid-rich cells indistinguishable from those seen in other forms of cortical hyperplasia. Hyperplasia of corticotroph (ACTH-producing) cells is present in the anterior pituitary.

Clinical Features. The clinical manifestations of congenital adrenal hyperplasia are determined by the specific enzyme deficiency and include abnormalities related to androgen metabolism, sodium homeostasis, and (in severe cases) glucocorticoid deficiency. Depending on the nature and severity of the enzymatic defect, the onset of clinical symptoms may occur in the perinatal period, later childhood, or (less commonly) adulthood.

The biochemical consequences of 21-hydroxylase deficiency are illustrated in Figure 20–23. In this form, *exces-*

Figure 20-23

Simplified flow chart demonstrating normal adrenal steroidogenesis *(A)*. The numbers identify steps catalyzed by 21-, 17-, and 11-hydroxylases, respectively. *B,* Consequences of 21-hydroxylase deficiency. 21-Hydroxylase deficiency impairs the synthesis of both cortisol and aldosterone. The resultant decrease in feedback inhibition *(dashed line)* causes increased secretion of ACTH, resulting ultimately in adrenal hyperplasia and increased synthesis of testosterone.

sive androgenic activity causes signs of masculinization in females, ranging from clitoral hypertrophy and pseudohermaphroditism in infants to oligomenorrhea, hirsutism, and acne in postpubertal females. In males, androgen excess is associated with enlargement of the external genitalia and other evidence of precocious puberty in prepubertal patients and with oligospermia in older individuals. *Androgen deficiency* may be encountered in some rare forms of congenital adrenal hyperplasia (e.g., 17α-hydroxylase deficiency), manifested by a lack of development of secondary sexual characteristics in females and by pseudohermaphroditism in males. In some forms of congenital adrenal hyperplasia (e.g., 11β-hydroxylase deficiency), the accumulated intermediary steroids have mineralocorticoid activity, with resultant *sodium retention* and *hypertension*. In other cases, however, including about one third of patients with 21-hydroxylase deficiency, the enzymatic defect produces mineralocorticoid deficiency, with resultant *sodium wasting*. Cortisol deficiency places individuals with congenital adrenal hyperplasia at risk for *acute adrenal insufficiency* (discussed later).

Congenital adrenal hyperplasia should be suspected in any neonate with ambiguous genitalia; severe enzyme deficiency in infancy can be a life-threatening condition, with vomiting, dehydration, and salt wasting. In the milder variants, women may present with delayed menarche, oligomenorrhea, or hirsutism. In all such cases, an androgen producing ovarian neoplasm must be excluded. Patients with congenital adrenal hyperplasia are treated with exogenous glucocorticoids, which, in addition to providing adequate levels of glucocorticoids, also suppress ACTH levels and thus decrease the excessive synthesis of the steroid hormones responsible for many of the clinical abnormalities.

ADRENAL INSUFFICIENCY

Adrenal insufficiency, or adrenocortical hypofunction, may occur in a number of different clinical situations. As in the case of adrenal hyperfunction, adrenal insufficiency may reflect either primary adrenal disease (primary hypoadrenalism) or decreased stimulation of the adrenals caused by a deficiency of ACTH (secondary hypoadrenalism). *Secondary hypoadrenalism* may be encountered in any of the disorders associated with hypopituitarism discussed earlier, such as Sheehan syndrome, nonfunctional pituitary adenomas, and lesions involving the hypothalamus and suprasellar region. *Primary hypoadrenalism* may be further subdivided into chronic primary adrenal insufficiency, also known as Addison disease, and acute primary adrenal insufficiency.

Chronic Adrenocortical Insufficiency (Addison Disease)

In a paper published in 1855, Thomas Addison described a group of patients suffering from a constellation of symptoms, including "general languor and debility, remarkable feebleness of the heart's action, and a peculiar change in the color of the skin" associated with disease of the "suprarenal capsules" or, in more current terminology, the adrenal glands. Addison disease, or chronic adrenocortical insufficiency, is an uncommon disorder resulting from progressive destruction of the adrenal cortex. In general, clinical manifestations of adrenocortical in-

■

Table 20–8. CAUSES OF ADRENAL INSUFFICIENCY
Acute
Waterhouse-Friderichsen syndrome
Sudden withdrawal of long-term corticosteroid therapy
Stress in patients with underlying chronic adrenal insufficiency
Chronic
Major Contributors
Autoimmune adrenalitis
Tuberculosis
Acquired immunodeficiency syndrome
Metastatic disease
Minor Contributors
Systemic amyloidosis
Fungal infections
Hemochromatosis
Sarcoidosis

sufficiency do not appear until at least 90% of the adrenal cortex has been compromised. The causes of chronic adrenocortical insufficiency are listed in Table 20–8.

Autoimmune adrenalitis accounts for 75% to 90% of cases of Addison disease in developed countries. It may occur as a sporadic or familial disorder. In about half of the patients the autoimmune disease is apparently restricted to the adrenal glands; in the remaining patients, other autoimmune diseases, such as Hashimoto disease, pernicious anemia, type I diabetes mellitus, and idiopathic hypoparathyroidism, coexist. The terms type I or II *polyglandular syndrome* have been used to designate the various combinations of organ involvement that may be encountered. Type I polyglandular syndrome is an autosomal recessive disease, associated with mutations of the autoimmune regulator *(AIRE)* gene on chromosome 21q. In contrast, type II polyglandular syndrome and isolated autoimmune adrenalitis are multifactorial diseases, with strong linkage to certain histocompatibility antigens, particularly HLA-B8, HLA-DR3, and HLA-DQ5. Circulating antibodies to several steroidal enzymes such as 21-hydroxylase and 17α-hydroxylase have been found in patients with all varieties of autoimmune adrenalitis.

Infections, particularly tuberculosis and those produced by fungi, may also cause primary chronic adrenocortical insufficiency. Tuberculous adrenalitis, which once accounted for up to 90% of cases of Addison disease, has become less common with the advent of antituberculous therapy. However, with the resurgence of tuberculosis in many urban centers, this cause of adrenal deficiency must be borne in mind. When present, tuberculous adrenalitis is almost always associated with active infection in other sites, particularly the lungs and genitourinary tract. Among fungi, disseminated infections caused by *Histoplasma capsulatum* and *Coccidioides immitis* may also result in chronic adrenocortical insufficiency. Patients with the acquired immune deficiency syndrome (AIDS) are at risk for developing adrenal insufficiency from several infectious (cytomegalovirus, *Mycobacterium avium-intracellulare*) and noninfectious (Kaposi sarcoma) complications of their disease.

Metastatic neoplasms involving the adrenals are another potential cause of adrenal insufficiency. The adrenals are a fairly common site for metastases in patients with disseminated carcinomas. Although adrenal function is preserved in most such patients, the metastatic growths sometimes destroy sufficient adrenal cortex to produce a degree of adrenal insufficiency. Carcinomas of the lung and breast are the source of a majority of metastases in the adrenals, although many other neoplasms, including gastrointestinal carcinomas, malignant melanomas, and hematopoietic neoplasms, may also metastasize to the organ.

MORPHOLOGY

The appearance of the adrenal glands varies with the cause of the adrenocortical insufficiency. In cases of hypoadrenalism secondary to hypothalamic or pituitary disease **(secondary hypoadrenalism),** the adrenals are reduced to small, flattened structures that usually retain their yellow color, owing to a small amount of residual lipid. A uniform, thin rim of atrophic yellow cortex surrounds a central, intact medulla. Histologically, there is atrophy of cortical cells with loss of cytoplasmic lipid, particularly in the zonae fasciculata and reticularis. **Primary autoimmune adrenalitis** is characterized by irregularly shrunken glands, which may be exceedingly difficult to identify within the suprarenal adipose tissue. Histologically, the cortex contains only scattered residual cortical cells in a collapsed network of connective tissue. A variable lymphoid infiltrate is present in the cortex and may extend into the subjacent medulla. The medulla is otherwise preserved. In cases of **tuberculosis or fungal diseases,** the adrenal architecture is effaced by a granulomatous inflammatory reaction identical to that encountered in other sites of infection. Demonstration of the responsible organism may require the use of special stains. When hypoadrenalism is caused by **metastatic carcinoma,** the adrenals are enlarged and their normal architecture is obscured by the infiltrating neoplasm.

Clinical Features. The onset of chronic adrenocortical insufficiency is usually insidious. The initial manifestations often include progressive weakness and easy fatigability, which may be dismissed as nonspecific complaints. *Gastrointestinal disturbances* are common and include anorexia, nausea, vomiting, weight loss, and diarrhea. In patients with primary adrenal disease, increased levels of ACTH precursor hormone stimulate melanocytes, with resultant *hyperpigmentation* of the skin and mucosal surfaces. The face, axillae, nipples, areolae, and perineum are particularly common sites of hyperpigmentation. By contrast, hyperpigmentation is not seen in patients with adrenocortical insufficiency caused by primary pituitary or hypothalamic disease. Decreased mineralocorticoid activity in patients with primary adrenal insufficiency results in potassium retention and sodium loss, with consequent *hyperkalemia, hyponatremia, volume depletion,* and *hypotension.* The heart is often smaller than normal, presumably because of chronic hypovolemia. Hypoglycemia may occasionally occur as a result of glucocorticoid deficiency and impaired gluconeogenesis. Stresses such as infections, trauma, or surgical procedures in such patients may precipitate an acute adrenal crisis, mani-

Figure 20-24 ■

Acute adrenal insufficiency caused by severe bilateral adrenal hemorrhage in an infant with overwhelming sepsis (Waterhouse-Friderichsen syndrome). At autopsy, the adrenals were grossly hemorrhagic and shrunken; microscopically, little residual cortical architecture is discernible.

fested by intractable vomiting, abdominal pain, hypotension, coma, and vascular collapse. Death follows rapidly unless corticosteroids are replaced immediately.

Acute Adrenocortical Insufficiency

Acute adrenocortical insufficiency occurs most commonly in the clinical settings listed in Table 20-8. As noted earlier, patients with chronic adrenocortical insufficiency may develop an acute crisis after any stress that taxes their limited physiologic reserves. In patients maintained on exogenous corticosteroids, rapid withdrawal of steroids or failure to increase steroid doses in response to an acute stress may precipitate a similar adrenal crisis, owing to the inability of the atrophic adrenals to produce glucocorticoid hormones. *Massive adrenal hemorrhage* may destroy the adrenal cortex sufficiently to cause acute adrenocortical insufficiency. This condition may occur in patients maintained on anticoagulant therapy, in postoperative patients who develop disseminated intravascular coagulation, during pregnancy, and in patients suffering from overwhelming sepsis (Waterhouse-Friderichsen syndrome) (Fig. 20-24). This catastrophic syndrome is classically associated with *Neisseria meningitidis* septicemia but can also be caused by other organisms, including *Pseudomonas* species, pneumococci, and *Haemophilus influenzae.* The pathogenesis of the Waterhouse-Friderichsen syndrome remains unclear, but it likely involves endotoxin-induced vascular injury with associated disseminated intravascular coagulation (Chapter 12).

ADRENOCORTICAL NEOPLASMS

It should be evident from the discussion of adrenocortical hyperfunction that functional adrenal neoplasms may be responsible for any of the various forms of hyperadrenalism. While functional adenomas are most commonly associated with hyperaldosteronism and with Cushing syndrome, a virilizing neoplasm is more likely to be a carcinoma. However, not all adrenocortical neoplasms elaborate steroid hormones. Determination of whether a cortical neoplasm is functional or not is based on clinical evaluation and measurement of the hormone or its metabolites in the laboratory. In other words, *functional and nonfunctional adrenocortical neoplasms cannot be distinguished on the basis of morphologic features.*

MORPHOLOGY

Adrenocortical adenomas were described in the earlier discussions of Cushing syndrome and hyperaldosteronism. Most cortical adenomas do not cause hyperfunction and are usually encountered as incidental findings at the time of autopsy or during abdominal imaging for an unrelated cause. In fact, the half-facetious appellation of "adrenal incidentaloma" has crept into the medical lexicon to describe these incidentally discovered tumors. Some authorities believe that all adrenal adenomas should, by definition, demonstrate clinical or biochemical evidence of hyperfunction, and the incidentally discovered "tumors" are best classified as non-hyperfunctioning hyperplastic nodules. In either case, the typical cortical adenoma is a well-circumscribed, nodular lesion that expands the adrenal or, in some cases, lies immediately outside the adrenal capsule (Fig. 20–25). On cut surface, adenomas are usually yellow to yellow-brown, owing to the presence of lipid within the neoplastic cells. As a general rule, they are small, averaging 1 to 2 cm in diameter; in some cases, they may be difficult to distinguish from foci of nodular hyperplasia. Microscopically, adenomas are composed of cells similar

Figure 20–26 ■

Histologic features of an adrenal cortical adenoma. The neoplastic cells are vacuolated because of the presence of intracytoplasmic lipid. There is mild nuclear pleomorphism. Mitotic activity and necrosis are not seen.

to those populating the normal adrenal cortex. The nuclei tend to be small, although some degree of pleomorphism may be encountered even in benign lesions ("endocrine atypia"). The cytoplasm of the neoplastic cells ranges from eosinophilic to vacuolated, depending on their lipid content (Fig. 20–26). Mitotic activity is generally inconspicuous.

Adrenocortical carcinomas are rare neoplasms that may occur at any age, including childhood. Two rare inherited causes of adrenal cortical carcinomas include the Li-Fraumeni syndrome (Chapter 6) and the Beckwith-Wiedemann syndrome (Chapter 7). In most cases, adrenocortical carcinomas are large, invasive lesions that efface the native adrenal gland. The less common, smaller, and better-circumscribed lesions may be difficult to distinguish from an adenoma. On cut surface, adrenocortical carcinomas are typically variegated, poorly demarcated lesions containing areas of necrosis, hemorrhage, and cystic change. Invasion of contiguous structures, including the adrenal vein and inferior vena cava, is common. Microscopically, adrenocortical carcinomas may be composed of well-differentiated cells resembling those seen in cortical adenomas or bizarre, pleomorphic cells, which may be difficult to distinguish from those of an undifferentiated carcinoma metastatic to the adrenal. Adrenal carcinomas invade locally and metastasize via lymphatics and the bloodstream, with a median patient survival of about 2 years. Carcinomas of the adrenal cortex may be functional or nonfunctional. When diagnosed in childhood, these tumors are associated with virilism and are not very aggressive; by contrast, in adults the functional cancers produce a mixed Cushing-virilizing syndrome and are more aggressive.

Figure 20–25 ■

Abdominal CT scan demonstrates a well-circumscribed nodule in the left adrenal, which was biochemically and histologically confirmed as an aldosterone-secreting adrenocortical adenoma. (Courtesy of Dr. Julie Champine, Department of Radiology, Parkland Memorial Hospital, Dallas.)

Adrenal Medulla

The adrenal medulla is embryologically, functionally, and structurally distinct from the adrenal cortex. It is populated by cells derived from the neural crest, termed *chromaffin* cells, and their supporting (sustentacular) cells. The chromaffin cells, so named because of their brown-black color after exposure to potassium dichromate, synthesize and secrete catecholamines in response to signals from preganglionic nerve fibers in the sympathetic nervous system. Similar collections of cells are distributed throughout the body in the extra-adrenal paraganglion system. The most important diseases of the adrenal medulla are neoplasms, which include both neuronal neoplasms (including neuroblastomas and more mature ganglion cell tumors) and neoplasms composed of chromaffin cells (pheochromocytomas).

PHEOCHROMOCYTOMA

Pheochromocytomas are neoplasms composed of chromaffin cells, which, like their non-neoplastic counterparts, synthesize and release catecholamines and, in some cases, other peptide hormones. These tumors are of special importance because, although uncommon, they (like aldosterone-secreting adenomas) give rise to a surgically correctable form of hypertension.

Pheochromocytomas usually subscribe to a convenient "rule of 10s":

■ *10% of pheochromocytomas arise in association with one of several familial syndromes.* These include the MEN 2A and 2B syndromes (described later), type 1 neurofibromatosis (Chapters 7 and 23), von Hippel-Lindau disease (Chapters 14 and 23), and Sturge-Weber syndrome (Chapter 23).

■ *10% of pheochromocytomas are extra-adrenal,* occurring in sites such as the organ of Zuckerkandl and the carotid body, where they are usually called *paragangliomas* rather than pheochromocytomas.

■ *10% of adrenal pheochromocytomas are bilateral;* this figure may rise to 50% in cases that are associated with familial syndromes.

■ *10% of adrenal pheochromocytomas are biologically malignant,* although the associated hypertension represents a serious and potentially lethal complication of even "benign" tumors. Frank malignancy is somewhat more common in tumors arising in extra-adrenal sites.

MORPHOLOGY

Pheochromocytomas range from small, circumscribed lesions confined to the adrenal (Fig. 20-27) to large, hemorrhagic masses weighing several kilograms. On cut surface, smaller pheochromocytomas are yellow-tan, well-defined lesions that compress the adjacent adrenal. Larger lesions tend to be hemorrhagic, necrotic, and cystic and typically efface the adrenal gland. Incubation of the fresh tissue with potassium dichromate solutions turns the tumor a dark brown color, as noted previously.

Microscopically, pheochromocytomas are composed of polygonal to spindle-shaped chromaffin cells and their supporting cells, compartmentalized into small nests, or "Zellballen," by a rich vascular network (Fig. 20-28). The cytoplasm of the neoplastic cells often has a finely granular appearance, highlighted by a variety of silver stains, owing to the presence of granules containing catecholamines. Electron microscopy reveals variable numbers of membrane-bound, electron-dense granules, representing catecholamines and sometimes other peptides. The nuclei of the neoplastic cells are often quite pleomorphic. Both capsular

Figure 20-27   ■

Pheochromocytoma. A large bisected tumor affecting an adrenal gland is shown on the left. On the right, three slices of a normal adrenal gland are shown for comparison.

Figure 20-28 ■

Photomicrograph of pheochromocytoma, demonstrating characteristic nests of cells ("Zellballen") with abundant cytoplasm. Granules containing cate-cholamine are not visible in this preparation. It is not uncommon to find bizarre cells even in pheochromocytomas that are biologically benign, and this criterion by itself should not be used to diagnose malignancy.

episodes may also be associated with pain in the abdomen or chest, nausea, and vomiting. In practice, *isolated, paroxysmal episodes of hypertension occur in less than half of patients* with pheochromocytoma. In about two thirds of patients the hypertension occurs in the form of a chronic, sustained elevation in blood pressure, although an element of labile hypertension is often present as well. Whether sustained or episodic, the hypertension is associated with an increased risk of myocardial ischemia, heart failure, renal injury, and cerebrovascular accidents. Sudden cardiac death may occur, probably secondary to catecholamine-induced myocardial irritability and ventricular arrhythmias. In some cases, pheochromocytomas secrete other hormones such as ACTH and somatostatin and may therefore be associated with clinical features related to the secretion of these and other peptide hormones. The laboratory diagnosis of pheochromocytoma is based on demonstration of increased urinary excretion of free catecholamines and their metabolites, such as vanillylmandelic acid (VMA) and metanephrines. Isolated benign pheochromocytomas are treated with surgical excision, after pre- and intraoperative medication of patients with adrenergic-blocking agents. Multifocal lesions may require long-term medical treatment for hypertension.

and vascular invasion may be encountered in benign lesions. **The diagnosis of malignancy in pheochromocytomas is therefore based exclusively on the presence of metastases.** These may involve regional lymph nodes as well as more distant sites, including liver, lung, and bone.

Clinical Features. The dominant clinical manifestation of pheochromocytoma is *hypertension*. Classically, this is described as an abrupt, precipitous elevation in blood pressure, associated with tachycardia, palpitations, headache, sweating, tremor, and a sense of apprehension. Such

NEUROBLASTOMA AND OTHER NEURONAL NEOPLASMS

Neuroblastoma is the most common extracranial solid tumor of childhood. These neoplasms occur most commonly during the first 5 years of life and may arise during infancy. Neuroblastomas may occur anywhere in the sympathetic nervous system and occasionally within the brain, but they are most common in the abdomen; most cases arise in either the adrenal medulla or the retroperitoneal sympathetic ganglia. Most neuroblastomas are sporadic, although familial cases also occur. These tumors are discussed in Chapter 7, along with other pediatric neoplasms.

Multiple Endocrine Neoplasia Syndromes

The multiple endocrine neoplasia (MEN) syndromes are a group of inherited diseases resulting in proliferative lesions (hyperplasias, adenomas, and carcinomas) of multiple endocrine organs. Like other inherited cancer disorders

(Chapter 6), endocrine tumors arising in the context of MEN syndromes have certain distinct features that contrast with their sporadic counterparts:

- These tumors occur at a *younger age* than sporadic cancers.
- They arise in *multiple endocrine organs,* either *synchronously* or *metachronously.*
- Even in one organ, the tumors are often *multifocal.*
- The tumors are usually preceded by an *asymptomatic stage of endocrine hyperplasia* involving the cell of origin of the tumor (for example, patients with MEN 1 syndrome develop varying degrees of islet cell hyperplasia, some of which progress to pancreatic tumors).
- Finally, these tumors are usually *more aggressive* and *recur* in a higher proportion of cases than similar endocrine tumors that occur sporadically.

Unraveling the genetic basis of the MEN syndromes and applying the knowledge to therapeutic decision-making has been one of the success stories of translational research. The salient features of the MEN syndromes will be discussed below.

MULTIPLE ENDOCRINE NEOPLASIA TYPE 1

Multiple endocrine neoplasia type 1 is inherited in an autosomal dominant pattern. The gene (*MEN1*) is located at 11q13 and is a tumor suppressor gene; thus, loss of *MEN1* function promotes cell proliferation and tumorigenesis. Organs commonly involved include the parathyroid (95%), pancreas (>40%), and pituitary (>30%)—the "3 Ps."

- *Parathyroid:* Primary hyperparathyroidism, arising from multiglandular parathyroid hyperplasia, is the most consistent feature of MEN 1.
- *Pancreas:* Endocrine tumors of the pancreas are the leading cause of death in MEN 1. These tumors are usually aggressive and present with metastatic disease or multifocality. Pancreatic endocrine tumors are often functional (i.e., they secrete hormones). Zollinger-Ellison syndrome, associated with gastrinomas, and hypoglycemia related to insulinomas are common endocrine manifestations (Chapter 17).
- *Pituitary:* The most frequent pituitary tumor in MEN 1 patients is a prolactin-secreting macroadenoma. Some patients develop acromegaly from somatotrophin-secreting tumors.

MULTIPLE ENDOCRINE NEOPLASIA TYPE 2

Multiple endocrine neoplasia type 2 is actually two distinct groups of disorders that are unified by the common occurrence of activating mutations of the *RET* protooncogene. There is a strong *genotype-phenotype correlation* within the MEN 2 syndrome, and differences in mutation patterns possibly account for the variable features in the two subtypes. MEN 2 is inherited in an autosomal dominant pattern. The gene (the *RET* protooncogene) is located at 10q11.2.

MEN 2A (Sipple Syndrome)

Organs commonly involved include the thyroid, adrenal medulla, parathyroid:

- *Thyroid:* Medullary carcinoma of the thyroid develops in virtually all untreated cases, and the tumors usually occur in the first 2 decades of life. The tumors are commonly multifocal, and foci of C-cell hyperplasia can be found in the adjacent thyroid.
- *Adrenal medulla:* 50% of patients develop adrenal pheochromocytomas; fortunately, no more than 10% are malignant.
- *Parathyroid:* Approximately a third of patients develop parathyroid gland hyperplasia with primary hyperparathyroidism.

MEN 2B (William Syndrome)

Organs commonly involved include the thyroid and adrenal medulla. The spectrum of thyroid and adrenal medullary disease is similar to that in MEN 2A. *However, unlike MEN 2A, patients with MEN 2B*

- Do not develop primary hyperparathyroidism
- *Develop extraendocrine manifestations:* ganglioneuromas of mucosal sites (gastrointestinal tract, lips, tongue) and marfanoid habitus

Before the advent of genetic testing, family members of patients with the MEN 2 syndrome were screened with annual biochemical tests, which often lacked sensitivity. Now, routine genetic testing identifies *RET* mutation carriers earlier and more reliably in MEN 2 kindreds; *all persons carrying germ-line* RET *mutations are advised to have prophylactic thyroidectomy to prevent the inevitable development of medullary carcinomas.* Surgical intervention based on the results of a single genetic test represents a new paradigm in the practice of "molecular medicine." A similar approach is being tailored for MEN 1 families, and a consensus should emerge in the near future.

BIBLIOGRAPHY

Barbesino G, Chiovato L: The genetics of Hashimoto's disease. Endocrinol Metab Clin North Am 29:357, 2000. (A recent review on genetic susceptibilities underlying the pathogenesis of Hashimoto disease; this issue also contains excellent articles of a similar nature on Graves disease.)

Bilezikian JP, Silverberg SJ: Clinical spectrum of primary hyperparathyroidism. Rev Endocr Metab Disord 1:237, 2000. (A review on the changing face of primary hyperparathyroidism in modern times.)

Boscaro M, et al: Cushing's syndrome. Lancet 357:783, 2001. (A concise and clinically oriented review of Cushing syndrome.)

Hansford JR, Mulligan LM: Multiple endocrine neoplasia type 2 and *RET:* from neoplasia to neurogenesis. J Med Genet 37:817, 2000. (A comprehensive review of the role of *RET* proto-oncogene in normal development and tumorigenesis, including guidelines for *RET* mutation screening in MEN 2 kindreds.)

Heufelder AE: Pathogenesis of ophthalmopathy in autoimmune thyroid disease. Rev Endocr Metab Disord 1:87, 2000. (A succinct compilation of existing theories and ongoing research in this subject.)

Kroll TG, et al: *PAX8-PPARγl* fusion oncogene in human thyroid carcinoma. Science, 289:1357, 2000. (The first report of a specific molecular abnormality in follicular carcinoma of thyroid.)

Learoyd DL, et al: Molecular genetics of thyroid tumors and surgical decision-making. World J Surg 24:923, 2000. (A summary of the important genetic abnormalities in thyroid cancers classified by histologic subtype.)

Marx SJ: Hyperparathyroid and hypothyroid disorders. N Engl J Med 343:1863, 2000. (An up-to-date discussion of the etiology and manifestation of the functional derangements of parathyroid function.)

Newell-Price J, et al: The diagnosis and differential diagnosis of Cushing's syndrome and pseudo-Cushing's states. Endocr Rev 19:647, 1998. (An authoritative review on the topic, primarily from a clinician's perspective.)

Peterson P, et al: Adrenal autoimmunity: results and developments. Trends Endocrinol Metab 11:285, 2000. (A concise update on the recent developments in Addison disease, including the molecular basis of autoimmunity in this disease.)

Phay JE, et al: Multiple endocrine neoplasia. Semin Surg Oncol 18:324, 2000. (A short but complete review of all MEN subtypes, including clinical features, molecular genetics, and diagnostic considerations.)

Santoro M, et al: Gene rearrangement and Chernobyl related thyroid cancers. Br J Cancer 82:315, 2000. (A thought-provoking research paper arising out of one of the lasting human tragedies of the previous century.)

Siegel RD, Lee SL: Toxic multinodular goiter. Endocrinol Metab Clin North Am 27:151, 1998. (Review of two non-neoplastic thyroid entities—toxic adenoma and toxic multinodular goiter. This issue also contains excellent articles on clinical features of hyperthyroidism.)

Slatosky J, et al: Thyroiditis: differential diagnosis and management. Am Fam Physician 61:1047, 2000. (A lucid review on the various entities within the spectrum of thyroiditis.)

Suhardja AS, et al: Molecular pathogenesis of pituitary adenomas. Acta Neurochir (Wien) 141:729, 1999. (An update on genetic abnormalities in pituitary tumors, including an excellent discussion on the role of G proteins in tumorigenesis.)

Wajchenberg BL, et al: Adrenocortical carcinoma. Cancer 88:771, 2000. (A review of a large number of cases of this uncommon neoplasm.)

Walther MM, et al: Pheochromocytoma: evaluation, diagnosis, and treatment. World J Urol 17:35, 1999. (A discussion of the clinical aspects of pheochromocytomas that briefly covers some of the genetic aspects of this disease as well.)

Weetman AP: Graves' disease. N Engl J Med 343:1236, 2000. (An excellent review of the pathogenesis, genetics, and clinical manifestations of Graves disease.)

Wells SA, Franz C: Medullary carcinoma of the thyroid. World J Surg 24:952, 2000. (Clinical features, molecular genetics, pathology all under one roof!)

White PC, Speiser PW: Congenital adrenal hyperplasia due to 21-hydroxylase deficiency. Endocr Rev 21:245, 2000. (A scholarly work, detailing the molecular pathophysiology and clinical features of the most common cause of congenital adrenal hyperplasia.)

21

The Musculoskeletal System

DENNIS K. BURNS, MD
VINAY KUMAR, MD

Diseases of Bone

Diseases of the Joints

Diseases of Skeletal Muscle

Soft Tissue Tumors

TUMORS OF ADIPOSE TISSUE
Lipoma
Liposarcoma
TUMORS AND TUMOR-LIKE LESIONS OF FIBROUS TISSUE
Nodular Fasciitis
Fibromatoses
Fibrosarcomas

FIBROHISTIOCYTIC TUMORS
Fibrous Histiocytoma
Dermatofibrosarcoma Protuberans
Malignant Fibrous Histiocytoma
NEOPLASMS OF SKELETAL MUSCLE
Rhabdomyosarcoma
SMOOTH MUSCLE TUMORS
MISCELLANEOUS NEOPLASMS
Synovial Sarcoma

The musculoskeletal system imparts form and movement to the human body. The term *musculoskeletal disease* embraces a large number of conditions ranging from localized, benign lesions of the bone such as the osteochondroma to generalized, life-threatening disorders such as muscular dystrophy.

In this chapter we will first consider some of the more common conditions affecting the bones and joints, then discuss selected non-neoplastic diseases of skeletal muscle. We will conclude with a few brief comments about tumors arising within skeletal muscle and other soft tissues.

Diseases of Bone

The human skeleton is a complex system, well adapted to providing structural support, translating the activity of skeletal muscles into movement, and providing a protected environment for delicate internal organs. In addition, the skeleton houses the body's blood-forming (hematopoietic) elements and serves as the major reservoir of calcium and a number of other vital minerals. In this chapter we will consider those disorders of bone that do not originate within the hematopoietic tissues. Disorders of the bone marrow are discussed with other diseases of the hematopoietic and lymphoid systems in Chapter 12 and will not be considered further here.

CONGENITAL AND HEREDITARY DISEASES OF BONE

Congenital diseases of bone range from localized malformations to hereditary disorders associated with abnormalities affecting the entire skeletal system. Some of the most common congenital structural lesions include aplasia (e.g.,

congenital absence of a digit or rib), the formation of extra bones (e.g., supernumerary digits or ribs), and abnormal fusion of bones (e.g., premature closure of the cranial sutures or congenital fusion of the ribs). Such malformations may occur as isolated, sporadic lesions or as components of a more complex syndrome. Other conditions, usually hereditary, include those that interfere with bone growth and/or maintenance of a normal osteoid matrix and, as such, cause generalized skeletal abnormalities. These include achondroplasia and other forms of dwarfism, osteogenesis imperfecta, and osteopetrosis. In addition, a number of hereditary metabolic disorders not usually thought of as primary skeletal diseases, such as Hurler syndrome, may affect the bone matrix as well as other organs. These latter conditions are discussed briefly with other genetic disorders in Chapter 7.

Achondroplasia

Achondroplasia is an inherited disorder characterized by impaired maturation of cartilage in the developing growth plate. It is a major cause of *dwarfism* and is the most common of the congenital disorders of the growth plate (osteochondrodysplasias). The vast majority of cases of achondroplasia are caused by dominant mutations involving the gene coding for *fibroblast growth factor receptor 3 (FGFR3)*, located on the short arm of chromosome 4. These mutations result in a sustained activation of *FGFR3* that, in turn, inhibits the normal proliferation of cartilage at the growth plates. Although it is an autosomal dominant disorder, only 20% of patients present with a family history; the remaining 80% of cases apparently arise from a spontaneous new mutation. Achondroplasia is most commonly encountered as a nonlethal heterozygous condition. Homozygous individuals are seen only rarely, because abnormal development of the chest cavity leads to death from respiratory failure soon after birth. Achondroplasia affects all bones that are formed from cartilage. In heterozygotes, the most conspicuous changes are marked, disproportionate shortening of the proximal extremities, bowing of the legs, and a lordotic (sway-backed) posture. The cartilaginous growth plates contain hypoplastic or disorganized aggregates of chondrocytes instead of the long, orderly columns normally seen at this site.

Osteogenesis Imperfecta

Osteogenesis imperfecta (OI), or "brittle bone disease," is a group of hereditary conditions characterized by abnormal development of type I collagen. Type I collagen is present in many different tissues, including skin, joints, and eyes, and it is a major component of normal osteoid. Several different genetic defects have been shown to interfere with the normal synthesis of type I collagen. A number of the mutations appear to directly interfere with the synthesis and/or secretion of procollagen α1 and procollagen α2, the peptide precursors of the type I collagen molecule. OI is therefore not a single disease but rather is a spectrum of disorders of varying severity united by the common feature of *abnormal collagen synthesis and resultant bone fragility.* Four major forms of OI have been identified; the most common variants are inherited as autosomal dominant disorders. As explained in Chapter 7, a single mutant allele prevents normal assembly of collagen owing to a dominant negative effect. Autosomal recessive forms, exemplified by the lethal type II variant, are less common. Recognition of the various subtypes of OI is important for genetic counseling of affected families.

Whatever the subtype, OI is characterized by the presence of *multiple bone fractures.* In the more severe forms of the disease, bone fragility causes multiple fractures and fetal demise in utero or shortly after birth. In other variants, fractures may not appear until childhood and may raise concern about the possibility of child abuse. The milder forms of the disease do not appreciably shorten life. Other tissues containing type I collagen are also affected in OI, resulting in abnormal dentition; hearing loss; and a blue appearance to the sclera, caused by decreased scleral collagen.

Osteopetrosis

The term *osteopetrosis*, sometimes designated "marble bone disease," encompasses a group of uncommon heredi-

tary disorders caused by deficient osteoclastic activity. Both autosomal recessive and autosomal dominant variants have been recognized. As might be suspected from the patterns of inheritance, the molecular basis of osteopetrosis is heterogeneous. In animals, osteopetrosis can be induced by mutations in the gene for macrophage colony-stimulating factor, a cytokine required for osteoclast differentiation. Mice transgenic for *osteoprotegerin* also develop osteopetrosis. This molecule actively inhibits osteoclast formation, as is discussed later. Whether the same molecular pathways are affected in humans is unknown. Defective osteoclastic activity in these patients results in the deposition of abnormally thickened, heavily mineralized, abnormally brittle bone. In addition to an increased incidence of fractures, patients with osteopetrosis also suffer from anemia, thrombocytopenia, and an increased susceptibility to infections, caused by a dramatic decrease in the amount of marrow space available for hematopoiesis. Abnormally thickened bone may also compress nerve roots, accounting for a high frequency of cranial nerve palsies in these patients.

OSTEOPOROSIS AND ACQUIRED METABOLIC DISEASES

Many nutritional and endocrine disorders affect the skeletal system. Nutritional deficiencies causing bone disease include deficiencies of vitamin C (scurvy) and vitamin D (rickets and osteomalacia). Both of these are discussed with other nutritional diseases in Chapter 8. Hyperparathyroidism, discussed in Chapter 20, also causes significant skeletal changes, which will be briefly reviewed in this section. The major focus of our discussion here is osteoporosis, a leading form of metabolic bone disease in the Western world.

Osteoporosis

Osteoporosis is a skeletal disorder characterized by low bone mass and micro-architectural deterioration with a subsequent increase in bone fragility and susceptibility to fractures. The micro-architectural deterioration is seen as fewer and thinner bony spicules as well as the presence of horizontal "struts" that do not join to form trabeculae. It is these structural changes that render the bones fragile. The condition may be localized (as in disuse osteoporosis developing in a chronically immobilized extremity), or it may involve the entire skeletal system. Generalized osteoporosis occurs most commonly as a primary disorder, or it may be secondary to a wide range of conditions, listed in Table 21–1. When the term *osteoporosis* is used without qualification, it usually refers to the primary senile and postmenopausal forms of the disease. Primary osteoporosis is an extremely common condition that affects more than 15 million people in the United States. When the morbidity and mortality associated with osteoporosis-related fractures are included in the analysis, the cost of

■

Table 21-1. CATEGORIES OF GENERALIZED OSTEOPOROSIS

Primary

Postmenopausal
Senile
Idiopathic

Secondary

Endocrine Disorders

Hyperparathyroidism
Hyperthyroidism
Hypothyroidism
Hypogonadism
Acromegaly
Cushing syndrome
Prolactinoma
Diabetes type 1
Addison disease

Neoplasia

Multiple myeloma
Carcinomatosis
Mast cell disease

Gastrointestinal

Malnutrition
Malabsorption
Subtotal gastrectomy
Hepatic insufficiency
Vitamin C and D deficiencies

Systemic Rheumatologic Diseases

Rheumatoid arthritis
Systemic lupus erythematosus
Psoriatic arthritis

Drugs

Anticoagulants
Chemotherapy
Corticosteroids
Anticonvulsants
Lithium
Alcohol

Miscellaneous

Osteogenesis imperfecta
Immobilization
Pulmonary disease
Chronic obstructive pulmonary disease
Homocystinuria
Gaucher disease
Anemia

medical care of patients suffering from osteoporosis exceeds $13 billion annually. *Senile osteoporosis* occurs in adults of both sexes and increases in severity with age. *Postmenopausal osteoporosis*, as indicated by its designation, affects women after menopause. It is by far the more common form and is an important cause of fractures in older women.

Pathogenesis. In adults there is a dynamic equilibrium between bone formation and resorption. Osteoporosis results when this balance is tilted in the favor of bone dissolution by osteoclasts. How this imbalance occurs has remained frustratingly elusive. However, exciting recent advances in the molecular mechanisms of bone growth and remodeling have shed considerable light on this subject. Central to this understanding has been the discovery of novel members of the tumor necrosis factor (TNF) receptor family and their ligands that influence osteoclast function (Fig. 21–1). It is now known that stromal cells and osteoblasts synthesize and express on their cell membranes a TNF family member called "RANK ligand." As suggested by its name, RANK ligand binds to a receptor molecule known by the acronym RANK (receptor activator for nuclear factor κB). This name is derived from the ability of RANK to activate the NFκB transcriptional pathway. Whereas RANK ligand is produced by osteoblasts and stromal cells, its receptor (RANK) is expressed on macrophages. *The differentiation of macrophages into osteoclasts requires that RANK ligand expressed on the surface of stromal cells or osteoblasts bind to the RANK receptor on macrophages.* In addition, stromal cells also produce a cytokine called macrophage colony-stimulating factor, which attaches to a distinct receptor on macrophages. Together, RANK ligand and macrophage colony-stimulating factor collaborate to convert macrophages into bone-chewing osteoclasts. Thus, activation of the RANK receptor is a major stimulus to bone resorption. The osteoclastogenic activity of the RANK ligand–RANK pathway is regulated by a molecule called osteoprotegerin (OPG), also secreted by stromal cells/osteoblasts. OPG is a "decoy receptor" that can usurp RANK ligand and thus prevent its binding to RANK. When RANK ligand binds to OPG rather than to the RANK receptor on osteoclast precursors, formation of osteoclasts and their bone-resorbing function is curtailed. On the basis of these new findings, it is now believed that dysregulation of RANK, RANK ligand, and OPG is a major factor in the pathogenesis of osteoporosis; such dysregulation may be initiated in a variety of ways, including estrogen deficiency (discussed later). Thus, it now *appears that osteoporosis is not a single disease but rather a group of disorders with a common morphologic expression, namely, a decrease in total bone mass and density.* Some of the major factors related to the development of osteoporosis are summarized next.

Under normal conditions, bone mass increases steadily during infancy and childhood, reaching a peak in the young adult years. *The peak bone mass is an important determinant of the subsequent risk of osteoporosis.* It is determined in large part by genetic factors, although external factors, including physical activity, diet, and hormonal status, also play a role. Men achieve a higher bone density than do women, and blacks have greater peak bone mass than do whites. Hence, white females are the most vulnerable to osteoporosis and its attendant complications.

Age-related changes in bone density occur in all individuals and clearly contribute to the development of osteoporosis in both sexes. As indicated earlier, bone is a dynamic tissue, and it undergoes continuous remodeling throughout life. This remodeling is characterized by alternating periods of bone resorption and new bone formation. Maximum bone density is typically reached during the third decade of life. Thereafter, it gradually declines. The rate of bone loss averages about 0.7% per year, although the rates vary considerably from individual to individual and from one bone to another. The greatest losses generally occur in areas containing abundant

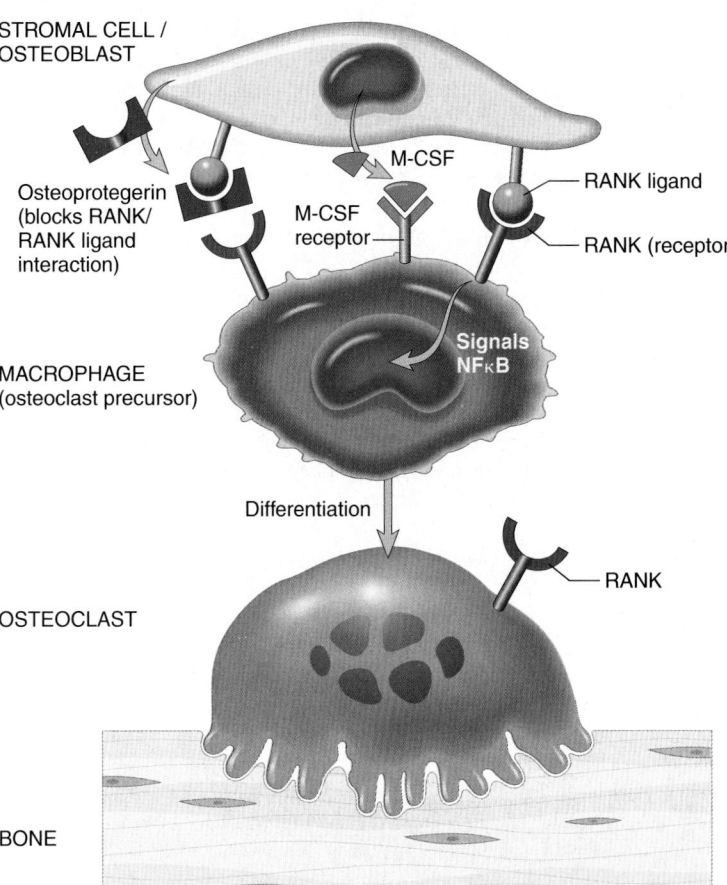

STROMAL CELL /
OSTEOBLAST

Osteoprotegerin
(blocks RANK/
RANK ligand
interaction)

M-CSF

M-CSF
receptor

RANK ligand

RANK (receptor)

Signals
NFκB

MACROPHAGE
(osteoclast precursor)

Differentiation

RANK

OSTEOCLAST

BONE

Figure 21–1   ■

Molecular mechanisms that regulate osteoclast formation and function. Osteoclasts are derived from macrophages under the influence of the RANK/RANK ligand signaling pathway. Cell membrane–associated RANK ligand binds to its receptor, RANK, on macrophages. This interaction in the presence of macrophage colony-stimulating factor (M-CSF) causes differentiation of macrophages into osteoclasts, which resorb bone. Stromal cells also secrete osteoprotegerin, which can act as a decoy receptor for RANK ligand, preventing it from binding the RANK receptor on macrophages. Thus, osteoprotegerin prevents bone resorption by inhibiting osteoclast differentiation.

cancellous (trabecular) bone, such as the spine and femoral necks. Hence, these are common sites of fractures in individuals with osteoporosis. The age-related loss of bone mass appears to be caused in large part by an *age-related decrease in osteoblastic activity as well as an increase in osteoclastic activity.* Beyond the third decade, with each bone remodeling cycle, new bone formation does not quite compensate for bone loss, resulting in a gradual attrition of bones.

Hormonal factors play a significant role in the development of osteoporosis, especially in postmenopausal women. The onset of menopause is associated with a precipitous decline in bone mass. Conversely, the administration of estrogen to postmenopausal women reduces bone loss and is associated with a decrease in the incidence of fractures. Earlier studies on the effects of estrogen on bones focused on the regulation of cytokines that affect the bone resorption and new bone formation. Decreased estrogen levels are associated with increased production of interleukin 1 (IL-1), interleukin 6 (IL-6), and tumor necrosis factor (TNF) by monocytes and other bone marrow elements. These cytokines increase bone absorption mainly by increasing the pool size of osteoclast precursors in the bone marrow. Recent studies indicate that estrogens influence the differentiation of osteoclasts via the RANK receptor pathways. Estrogen stimulates the production of OPG and thus inhibits the formation of osteoclasts; it also blunts the responsiveness of osteoclast

precursors to RANK ligand; increased levels of IL-1 and TNF (seen with estrogen deficiency) stimulate the production of RANK ligand and macrophage colony-stimulating factor, both of which promote osteoclast formation. Evidence suggests that estrogen deficiency, as well as normal aging, may also lead to decreased osteoblastic activity and, hence, decreased new bone formation. Thus, *the bone loss associated with estrogen deficiency may be caused by a combination of increased bone resorption and decreased bone formation.* Testosterone deficiency is present in about one third of men with senile osteoporosis. It also appears to contribute to increased bone turnover through local effects on cytokine production. However, this effect is not of the same magnitude as that caused by a lack of estrogen.

Genetic factors are another important piece in the osteoporosis puzzle. As noted previously, the maximum bone density that an individual reaches is determined in large part by genetic influences. Although many of the genetic factors responsible for normal bone development remain to be identified, one determinant of maximum bone density appears to be the vitamin D receptor (VDR) molecule. Certain variants of the *VDR* gene are associated with a lower maximum bone density, presumably because they impair the bone-forming effects of vitamin D. The overall role of such polymorphisms in the pathogenesis of osteoporosis remains unclear, however.

Mechanical factors, particularly weight bearing, are important stimuli for normal remodeling of bone, and reduced physical activity is associated with accelerated bone loss. This is demonstrated dramatically by bone loss in paralyzed or immobilized extremities and in the substantial decrease in bone mass noted in astronauts living in zerogravity conditions for prolonged periods. The generally sedentary life style of many older adults undoubtedly contributes to the progression of osteoporosis.

The role of diet, including calcium and vitamin D intake, in the development, prevention, and treatment of osteoporosis remains incompletely understood. A person's maximum bone density is determined in part by the total dietary calcium intake, particularly before puberty. It appears that dietary calcium intake in adolescent females is considerably less than that in males of comparable age, and this may be one factor that predisposes women to the development of osteoporosis later in life.

To summarize, osteoporosis is a multifactorial disorder. Age-related bone loss, caused in large part by reduced bone formation, is common to all forms of primary generalized osteoporosis. This loss is compounded in postmenopausal women by an increased resorption of bone, as well as by further reduction in bone synthesis brought about by declining levels of estrogen. Thus, both reduced bone formation and increased bone loss occur in osteoporosis. Although both of these factors play a role in most cases of osteoporosis, their relative contributions to bone *loss may vary depending on age, sex, nutritional status, and genetic influences.*

MORPHOLOGY

The hallmark of osteoporosis is a loss of bone, which tends to be **most conspicuous in parts of the skeleton containing abundant trabecular bone.** The bony trabeculae are thinner and more widely separated than usual, resulting in an increased susceptibility to fractures (Fig. 21-2). In postmenopausal osteoporosis, the bone loss is often particularly severe in the vertebral bodies, which may fracture and collapse. Similar bone loss is common in other weight-bearing bones, such as the femoral necks, another common site for fractures. The major microscopic changes are thinning of the trabeculae and widening of haversian canals. Osteoclastic activity is present but is not dramatically increased in microscopic sections. The mineral content of the remaining bone is normal, and thus there is no alteration in the ratio of minerals to protein matrix.

Clinical Features. In its early stages, osteoporosis is asymptomatic. Standard radiographs are an insensitive indicator of bone loss, and reliable diagnosis in early cases requires

Figure 21-2

Scanning electron micrograph of a normal bone *(A)* and a bone with osteoporosis *(B)*. Note the thinning and wide separation of the trabeculae in the osteoporotic bone. (From Dempster DW, et al: A simple method for correlative light and scanning electron microscopy of human iliac crest bone biopsies. J Bone Miner Res 1:15, 1986.)

radiographic measurements of bone density by techniques such as dual-energy x-ray absorptiometry (DEXA). In the later stages of the disease, decreased bone density becomes evident in routine radiographs, and the individual becomes prone to skeletal fractures, particularly involving the vertebral bodies, pelvis, femur, and other weight-bearing bones. Because the treatment of such fractures often requires long periods of immobilization in elderly patients, complications such as pneumonia and pulmonary thromboembolism are common and are a major cause of death.

The treatment of osteoporosis has been the subject of vigorous study. Estrogen supplementation has been shown to significantly reduce the rate of bone and calcium loss in post-menopausal women, but it does not appear to reverse the established structural changes in the bone. Adequate dietary calcium intake before the age of 30 appears to reduce the risk of osteoporosis later in life, presumably by increasing peak bone density. Calcium supplementation later in life may cause a modest reduction in the rate of bone loss. Other promising therapeutic maneuvers include the administration of a class of drugs known as bisphosphonates, which selectively decrease osteoclast-mediated bone resorption. An even newer class of drugs, the selective estrogen receptor modulators (SERMs), appears to exert a beneficial effect on bone mass similar to that of estrogens while avoiding some of the potentially dangerous side effects associated with conventional estrogen therapy. The administration of calcitonin, finally, may reduce the frequency of vertebral fractures and may be of particular benefit to those patients who are unable to tolerate estrogen therapy.

Rickets and Osteomalacia

Both rickets and osteomalacia are manifestations of vitamin D deficiency (Chapter 8). The fundamental change in these diseases is defective mineralization of bone, accompanied by an increase in nonmineralized osteoid. This is in contrast to osteoporosis, in which, although total bone mass is decreased, the mineral content of the remaining bone is normal.

In rickets, the defective mineralization involves the developing bones in children. Osteomalacia represents defective mineralization of bone that has completed its normal development. These disorders are detailed in Chapter 8.

Bone Diseases Associated With Hyperparathyroidism

As noted in the discussion of endocrine disorders in Chapter 20, parathyroid hormone (PTH) plays a central role in calcium homeostasis. The effects of PTH include the following:

- Osteoclast activation, with increased bone resorption and calcium mobilization. This effect is mediated indirectly by the increased production of RANK ligand by osteoblasts.
- Increased resorption of calcium by the renal tubules.
- Increased synthesis of active vitamin D, $1,25(OH)_2$-D, by the kidneys, which in turn enhances calcium absorption from the gut and also mobilizes calcium from the bone by inducing RANK ligand.

The net effect of these activities is to raise the level of serum calcium, which, under normal circumstances, inhibits further PTH synthesis and release. Excessive levels of PTH, whether they result from autonomous secretion (primary hyperparathyroidism) or underlying renal disease (secondary hyperparathyroidism), cause significant skeletal changes related to abnormal osteoclastic activity. While PTH appears to be directly responsible for the bone changes seen in primary hyperparathyroidism, additional factors contribute to the development of bone disease in secondary hyperparathyroidism associated with renal failure. In chronic renal insufficiency, the loss of renal tissue leads to defective synthesis of $1,25$-$(OH)_2$-D. Hyperphosphatemia also suppresses the activity of renal α_1-hydroxylase, further impairing the synthesis of active vitamin D. The resultant decrease in calcium absorption from the gut contributes further to defective mineralization of osteoid. Additional factors implicated in the development of bone disease in chronic renal failure include metabolic acidosis and aluminum deposition in bone.

MORPHOLOGY

The hallmark of PTH excess is **increased osteoclastic activity, with bone resorption.** Cortical and trabecular bone are lost and replaced by loose connective tissue. Bone resorption is especially pronounced in the subperiosteal regions and produces characteristic radiographic changes, best seen along the radial aspect of the middle phalanges of the second and third fingers. Microscopically, excessive osteoclastic activity is manifested by the presence of **increased numbers of osteoclasts and accompanying erosion of bone surfaces.** The marrow space contains increased amounts of loose fibrovascular tissue. Hemosiderin deposits are present, reflecting episodes of hemorrhage resulting from fractures of the weakened bone. In some instances, collections of osteoclasts, reactive giant cells, and hemorrhagic debris form a distinct mass, termed a **brown tumor of hyperparathyroidism.** Cystic change is common in such lesions (hence the name osteitis fibrosa cystica), which may be confused with primary bone neoplasms, particularly giant cell tumor of bone (discussed later).

OSTEOMYELITIS

The term *osteomyelitis* designates inflammation of the bone and marrow cavity. Although a number of different agents may cause bone inflammation, by convention, the use of this term is restricted to lesions caused by infectious agents. Osteomyelitis may be an acute or chronic, debilitating illness. Although any microorganism can cause osteomyelitis, the most common etiologic agents are pyogenic bacteria and *Mycobacterium tuberculosis*.

Pyogenic Osteomyelitis

Most cases of acute purulent osteomyelitis are caused by bacteria. The offending organisms reach the bone by one of three routes: (1) hematogenous dissemination, (2) direct extension from a focus of acute infection in the adjacent joint or soft tissue, or (3) traumatic implantation after compound fractures or orthopedic surgical procedures. In most patients, osteomyelitis is hematogenous in origin. In many cases the infection arises in a previously healthy individual without a known primary infection, while other cases are associated with a more obvious source of infection. *Staphylococcus aureus* is the most common causative organism. Its propensity to infect bone may be related to the fact that it expresses several receptors for bone matrix components that favor adhesion to the bone tissue. Other common pathogens include pneumococci and gram-negative rods. *Escherichia coli* and group B streptococci are important causes of acute osteomyelitis in neonates, while *Salmonella* is an especially common pathogen responsible for osteomyelitis occurring in patients with sickle cell disease. Mixed bacterial infections, including anaerobes, are responsible for many cases of osteomyelitis developing after bone trauma. In up to 50% of cases of pyogenic osteomyelitis, the causative organisms cannot be isolated because of previous antibiotic therapy, inadequate sampling for culture, or suboptimal culture methods.

MORPHOLOGY

Acute osteomyelitis is characterized by an intense, neutrophilic inflammatory infiltrate at the site of bacterial invasion. The location of infection varies with age. In children, metaphyses of long bones are typically involved, probably because blood flow is sluggish in this region, allowing bacteria to settle. In adults, hematogenous osteomyelitis primarily affects vertebral bodies that remain quite vascular. The involved bone becomes necrotic within a matter of days, owing to compression of vascular spaces by increased pressure in the marrow cavity and high concentrations of enzymes and other mediators released during the acute inflammatory reaction. In long bones, the infection spreads through the cortical bone and may reach the periosteum, sometimes creating a subperiosteal abscess. Such abscesses are particularly common in children, in whom the periosteum is more loosely anchored to the cortical bone than it is in adults. From the subperiosteal area, the infection may spread into adjacent soft tissues to create draining sinuses, or it may track along the surface of the bone for a considerable distance. Detachment of the periosteum in such cases may disrupt the blood supply to bone, resulting in even more extensive ischemic necrosis of the bone. In infants, the existence of loose periosteal attachments and connections between the vessels in the metaphysis and epiphysis allows the infection to spread to the epiphysis and joint capsule. Extension of infection to the joints is less common in adults, because the periosteum is quite firmly attached to the articular margins.

Chronic osteomyelitis develops as a sequela of acute infection. Over time, an influx of chronic inflammatory cells into the focus of osteomyelitis initiates a repair reaction that includes osteoclast activation, fibroblastic proliferation, and new bone formation. Residual necrotic bone, termed the **sequestrum,** may be resorbed by osteoclastic activity. Larger sequestra are eventually surrounded by a rim of reactive bone, termed the **involucrum** (Fig. 21–3). When a well-defined rim of sclerotic bone surrounds a residual abscess, the lesion is sometimes designated a **Brodie abscess.** Viable organisms may persist in the sequestered area for years after the original infection. Chronic osteomyelitis may be complicated by the development of draining sinuses that open on the overlying skin and by pathologic fractures. Less common complications of chronic osteomyelitis include squamous cell carcinoma developing in long-standing sinus tracts and, in exceptional cases, sarcomas and secondary amyloidosis.

Clinical Features. In its initial stages, pyogenic osteomyelitis causes systemic manifestations similar to those seen in any other acute infection, such as fever, malaise, and leukocytosis. Local signs and symptoms of bone inflammation may be subtle and easily missed, particularly in infants and young children. Conversely, local pain, swelling, and redness may occur in some adults in the absence of systemic complaints. Although radiographic studies play an important role in the diagnosis of acute osteomyelitis, bone changes may not be visible on routine radiographs for more

Figure 21–3 ■

Resected femur from a patient with chronic osteomyelitis. Necrotic bone (the sequestrum) visible in the center of a draining sinus tract is surrounded by a rim of new bone (the involucrum).

than a week after the onset of systemic manifestations. During this period significant bone destruction may occur. Radionuclide scans (e.g., gallium scans) are helpful in locating the site of infection early in the course of osteomyelitis. Infections of the bone demand vigorous and prolonged antimicrobial therapy and, in many cases, surgical debridement. Chronic osteomyelitis may supervene despite aggressive therapy in some cases, but it is particularly likely to develop when the diagnosis of osteomyelitis has been delayed or when the course of antibiotic therapy has been too brief. Complications of osteomyelitis include pathologic fractures, bacteremia, and endocarditis. Much less common complications are reactive systemic amyloidosis (Chapter 5) and squamous cell carcinomas within chronic sinus tracts.

Tuberculous Osteomyelitis

Mycobacterial infection of bone has long been a problem in developing countries of the world, and with the resurgence of tuberculosis, it is becoming an increasingly important disease in industrialized countries as well. Bone infection complicates an estimated 1% to 3% of cases of pulmonary tuberculosis. The organisms usually reach the bone through the bloodstream, although direct spread from a contiguous focus of infection (e.g., from mediastinal nodes to the vertebrae) may also occur. With hematogenous spread, *long bones and vertebrae are favored sites of localization.* The lesions are often solitary, but they may be multicentric, particularly in patients with an underlying immunodeficiency (e.g., acquired immunodeficiency syndrome [AIDS]). Because the tubercle bacillus requires fairly high concentrations of oxygen, the synovium, with its higher oxygen pressures, is a common site of initial infection. The infection spreads to the adjacent epiphysis, where it causes a typical granulomatous inflammatory reaction with caseous necrosis and extensive bone destruction. *Tuberculosis of the vertebral bodies, or Pott disease, is an important form of tuberculous osteomyelitis.* Infection at this site causes vertebral deformity and collapse, with secondary neurologic deficits. Extension of the infection to the adjacent soft tissues is fairly common in tuberculosis of the spine and often manifests as a so-called cold abscess in the psoas muscle.

PAGET DISEASE (OSTEITIS DEFORMANS)

Paget disease of bone, first described in 1882 by the British surgeon Sir James Paget, is a peculiar disorder characterized by episodes of localized, frenzied osteoclastic activity and bone resorption, followed by exuberant bone formation. The end result of these intermittent processes is skeletal deformity caused by the accumulation of excessive amounts of architecturally abnormal, unstable bone. There are three phases in the development of Paget disease: (1) an initial phase of osteoclastic activity, hypervascularity, and bone loss, followed by (2) a phase of mixed osteoclastic and osteoblastic proliferation, which gradually evolves into (3) a late, "osteosclerotic" phase, characterized by formation

of dense, mineralized bone with minimal cellular activity. Paget disease is uncommon before the age of 40, but its incidence increases steadily after that time. Males are affected slightly more often than females. Although generally occurring as a sporadic condition, the recent discovery of cases of familial Paget disease linked to the long arm of chromosome 18, as well as other familial cases not associated with chromosome 18, indicates that Paget disease may not be a single, homogeneous entity. In addition to causing bone deformities and related symptoms, Paget disease is also an important predisposing factor in the development of osteogenic sarcoma in older patients.

Pathogenesis. When first described, Paget disease was thought to be an inflammatory condition, a concept embodied in the synonym *osteitis deformans*. Although the idea that Paget disease is inflammatory in origin remained out of favor for many decades, current evidence suggests that Paget disease may in fact have an infectious etiology. Paramyxovirus-like particles and antigens have been identified within osteoclasts obtained from patients with Paget disease. More recently, nucleic acid sequences of the canine distemper virus, a paramyxovirus related to the agent responsible for measles in humans, have been identified within lesions of Paget disease. Experimental studies have shown that infection of osteoclast precursor cells with genetic material from the measles virus causes increased expression of the RANK receptor, resulting in the generation of osteoclasts with increased resorptive capacity. Paramyxoviruses are also stimulators of IL-6 production by osteoblasts, which in turn promotes osteoclast recruitment and activation. It is hypothesized, then, that Paget disease may represent a slow viral infection and that a paramyxovirus or a related agent causes abnormal recruitment and activation of osteoclasts, thereby causing pathologic bone resorption. It is important to note, however, that despite the circumstantial evidence for paramyxovirus infection in Paget disease, viruses have not yet been isolated from involved bone, even in long-term cultures. A viral etiology for Paget disease thus remains an intriguing, but still unproven, hypothesis.

MORPHOLOGY

Paget disease may present as a solitary lesion (monostotic) or may be multifocal (polyostotic). The lesions are solitary in only 10% of cases. Although any bone may be affected, the spine, skull, and pelvic bones are especially common sites of involvement. The appearance of the individual lesions varies considerably, depending on their age. As noted, three basic morphologic phases have been described (Fig. 21–4). In the **primary (osteolytic) phase** of the disease, there is focal replacement of the marrow by loose, highly vascular connective tissue. The bony trabeculae are lined by huge multinucleated osteoclasts that cause extensive resorption of bone. In the next stage, osteoblastic proliferation is superimposed, resulting in a **mixed phase,** characterized by concomitant bone resorption and new bone formation. Finally, the osteoclastic activity subsides,

Figure 21-4 ■

Diagrammatic representation of Paget disease of bone demonstrating the three phases in the evolution of the disease.

but irregular bone deposition continues in the so-called **osteosclerotic phase.** The new bone lacks the lamellar architecture of normal bone and is referred to as **woven bone.** Progressive deposition of new bone ultimately results in substantial thickening of both the cortical and trabecular bone. Because the bone formation occurs in an erratic pattern, areas of new bone are juxtaposed in a random mosaic pattern, giving the appearance of a jigsaw puzzle (Fig. 21-5). **This mosaic pattern**

of bone deposition is virtually pathognomonic of **Paget disease.** Although abnormally dense, the bone is weaker than usual and is subject to mechanical deformity and fracture.

Clinical Features. Paget disease of bone is usually asymptomatic, discovered as an incidental radiographic finding. Sometimes it comes to attention because of an unexpected elevation in serum alkaline phosphatase in routine blood tests. In some patients, the early hypervascular bone lesions cause warmth of the overlying skin and subcutaneous tissue. In patients with extensive disease, hypervascularity may cause an increase in cardiac output; in exceptional cases, high-output congestive heart failure may develop as a complication of this hypervascular state. In the proliferative phase, common symptoms include headache, enlargement of the head, visual disturbances, and deafness, all caused by deformity of the bones of the skull and impingement on cranial nerves. Back pain is common and may be associated with disabling vertebral fractures and spinal nerve root compression. The long bones of the legs are often deformed because of the inability of the pagetoid bone to adequately accommodate the mechanical stresses associated with weight bearing. Transverse fractures of the brittle long bones have been likened to breakage of chalk, giving rise to the term *chalkstick fracture*. Laboratory evaluation discloses elevated levels of serum alkaline phosphatase, reflecting increased osteoblastic activity. Serum calcium and phosphate levels are typically normal, although

Figure 21-5 ■

Photomicrograph of Paget disease demonstrating characteristic "mosaic" lines between areas of new bone formation.

urinary calcium excretion may be increased during the lytic phase of the disease. Treatment with bisphosphonates, the antiresorptive agents mentioned earlier in the discussion of osteoporosis, has been of some therapeutic benefit in Paget disease.

The development of a sarcoma in association with the osteoblastic lesions of Paget disease is a dreaded but fortunately uncommon complication, occurring in an estimated 1% of patients. The sarcomas are usually of the osteogenic type, although other histologic variants may also occur. They may develop in patients with either monostotic or polyostotic disease, and in the latter they may be multicentric. Their distribution generally parallels that of the Paget lesions, with the exception of the vertebral bodies, which rarely harbor sarcomas. Even with aggressive multimodality therapy, the prognosis of patients who develop secondary osteosarcomas is poor.

BONE TUMORS

Primary bone tumors are considerably less common than are metastatic lesions. The most common originating sites for bone metastases, in descending order of frequency, are the prostate, breast, lung, kidney, gastrointestinal tract, and thyroid. Metastases may be destructive (osteolytic) or associated with reactive new bone formation (osteoblastic). Most metastases present as osteolytic processes, although it is common for both patterns to be present in a given lesion. In some tumors, exemplified by carcinoma of the prostate, osteoblastic activity predominates. The distinction between metastatic and primary bone tumors is straightforward in most cases but may be difficult in patients who present with a solitary lesion without a history of a primary tumor in another site.

Certain conditions are associated with an increased risk of bone neoplasms. Some of these were mentioned earlier in this chapter and include Paget disease of bone, chronic osteomyelitis, and exposure to radiation. A few cases are associated with hereditary tumor syndromes, such as Gardner syndrome (osteomas) and familial retinoblastoma (osteogenic sarcomas). The cause of the vast majority of bone tumors remains unknown, however.

The relative infrequency and great diversity of primary bone tumors combine to make them a diagnostic challenge. As a group, primary bone tumors occur at all ages and may arise in any part of the body. However, certain types of tumors target particular age groups and anatomic sites, and the recognition of these patterns is very helpful in arriving at a proper diagnosis. Most osteogenic sarcomas, for example, occur in adolescents and are especially common around the knee joint, a site of rapid bone growth during normal development. Diagnosis of bone tumors requires careful integration of the clinical history and radiographic appearance with the gross and microscopic features of the tumor. The salient features of the most common primary bone tumors, excluding multiple myeloma and other hematopoietic tumors, are listed in Table 21–2. Comments about some of the more common bone tumors follow.

Bone-Forming Tumors

These neoplasms are characterized by the production of osteoid by the tumor cells. This type of intrinsic osteoid formation must be distinguished from bone formation in osteoblastic metastases, in which the osteoid is produced by reactive osteoblasts rather than by neoplastic cells. In some primary bone-forming tumors, other mesenchymal elements, such as cartilage, may also be present. Given the origin of several elements of bone from common mesenchymal stem cells, such admixtures are not entirely surprising.

OSTEOMA

Osteomas are benign lesions of bone that in many cases represent developmental aberrations or reactive growths rather than true neoplasms. They are most commonly encountered in the head and neck, including the paranasal sinuses, but may occur in other sites as well. Osteomas present as localized, usually solitary, hard, exophytic growths attached to the surface of the bone. Multiple lesions are a feature of Gardner syndrome, a hereditary condition considered further in the discussion of the fibromatoses (see "Soft Tissue Tumors"). Histologically, osteomas are composed of a bland mixture of woven and lamellar bone, which may be difficult to distinguish from normal bone. Although they may cause local mechanical problems and cosmetic deformities, they are not invasive and do not undergo malignant transformation.

OSTEOID OSTEOMA AND OSTEOBLASTOMA

Osteoid osteomas and osteoblastomas are benign neoplasms that have very similar histologic features. They are distinguished primarily by their size, site of origin, and certain radiographic features. *Osteoid osteomas* arise most often in the proximal femur and tibia during the second to third decades of life. They occur more commonly in males than in females by a ratio of 2:1. By definition, they are less than 2 cm in greatest dimension, whereas osteoblastomas are larger. Local pain is an almost universal complaint in patients with osteoid osteomas and can usually be relieved by aspirin. *Osteoblastomas* arise most often in the vertebral column, although they may occur in other sites as well. Like osteoid osteomas, they occur most often during the second to third decades and they affect males more often than females. They may also cause pain, which is often more difficult to localize than the pain associated with osteoid osteomas and is not responsive to aspirin. Local excision is the treatment of choice for most lesions; incompletely resected lesions may recur.

MORPHOLOGY

Radiographically, these neoplasms present as well-circumscribed lesions, which usually involve the cortex and rarely the medullary cavity of bone. The central area of the tumor, termed the **nidus**, is characteristically radiolucent but may become mineralized and sclerotic. A rim of sclerotic bone

Table 21-2. TUMORS OF BONE

Tumor Type	Common Locations	Age (yr)	Morphology
Bone-Forming			
Benign			
Osteoma	Facial bones, skull	40–50	Exophytic growths attached to bone surface; histologically resemble normal bone
Osteoid osteoma	Metaphysis of femur and tibia	10–20	Cortical tumors, characterized by pain; histologically interlacing trabeculae of woven bone
Osteoblastoma	Vertebral column	10–20	Arise in vertebral transverse and spinous processes; histologically similar to osteoid osteoma
Malignant			
Primary osteosarcoma	Metaphysis of distal femur, proximal tibia, and humerus	10–20	Grow outward, lifting periosteum, and inward to the medullary cavity; microscopically malignant cells form osteoid; cartilage may also be present
Secondary osteosarcoma	Femur, humerus, pelvis	>40	Complications of polyostotic Paget disease; histologically similar to primary osteosarcoma
Cartilaginous			
Benign			
Osteochondroma	Metaphysis of long tubular bones	10–30	Bony excrescences with a cartilaginous cap; may be solitary or multiple and hereditary
Chondroma	Small bones of hands and feet	30–50	Well-circumscribed single tumors resembling normal cartilage; arise within medullary cavity of bone; uncommonly multiple and hereditary
Malignant			
Chondrosarcoma	Bones of shoulder, pelvis, proximal femur, and ribs	40–60	Arise within medullary cavity and erode cortex; microscopically well-differentiated cartilage-like or anaplastic
Miscellaneous			
Giant cell tumor (usually benign)	Epiphysis of long bone	20–40	Lytic lesions that erode cortex; microscopically, contain osteoclast-like giant cells and round to spindle-shaped mononuclear cells; majority are benign
Ewing tumor (malignant)	Diaphysis and metaphysis	10–20	Arise in medullary cavity; microscopically, sheets of small round cells that contain glycogen; aggressive neoplasm

is present at the edge of both types of tumors; however, it is much more conspicuous in osteoid osteomas. Microscopically, both neoplasms are composed of interlacing trabeculae of woven bone surrounded by osteoblasts. The intervening stroma is made up of loose, vascular connective tissue instead of normal marrow elements and contains a variable number of giant cells.

OSTEOSARCOMA (OSTEOGENIC SARCOMA)

Osteosarcomas are *malignant mesenchymal neoplasms in which the neoplastic cells produce osteoid.* Excluding multiple myeloma, a tumor of B cells (Chapter 12), osteosarcoma is the most common primary malignant tumor of bone. Although once they were universally fatal, recent therapeutic advances have dramatically improved the outlook for these neoplasms. Several different variants of osteosarcoma exist; these can be distinguished from one another by clinical presentation, radiographic findings, histology, and, most importantly, prognosis. In the simplest classification scheme, osteosarcomas can be divided into *primary forms,* which arise de novo, and *secondary forms,* which arise as a complication of a known underlying process, such as Paget disease of bone or a history of radiation exposure.

A number of different forms of primary osteosarcoma have been recognized. These include the "conventional" form, which accounts for about three fourths of the cases, and several less common variants. Conventional osteosarcomas *occur most often during the second decade of life.* Although they may arise anywhere in the body, *the most common site of origin is the area around the knee, specifically the distal femur and proximal tibia.* Males are affected more often than are females. Although the cause of most primary osteosarcomas remains unknown, as with other malignant neoplasms, mutations appear to be important in their pathogenesis. Mutations in the *TP53* tumor suppressor gene, in particular, are present in many sporadic osteosarcomas. Overexpression of the *MDM2* oncogene is also noted in many cases. MDM2 protein binds to and inactivates the *TP53* gene product. Germ-line mutations in the retinoblastoma gene predispose patients to develop osteosarcomas as well as hereditary retinoblastomas. In addition, loss of heterozygosity at 3p, 13q, 17p, and 18q has also been noted. The high incidence of loss of heterozygosity at 3p suggests the existence of a tumor suppressor gene at this locus.

MORPHOLOGY

The typical osteosarcoma presents as a large, ill-defined lesion in the metaphyseal region of the involved bone (Fig. 21–6). It characteristically destroys the cortex and frequently extends inward into the marrow cavity and outward into adjacent soft tissues. The tumor often elevates the periosteum to produce the so-called **Codman triangle** on radiographs, which is formed by the angle between the elevated periosteum and the surface of the involved bone. Invasion of the epiphyseal plate is uncommon. Microscopically, **the hallmark of osteosarcoma is the formation of osteoid by malignant mesenchymal cells** (Fig. 21–7). This is seen in the form of islands of primitive bony trabeculae hugged by a rim of malignant osteoblasts. The amount of osteoid varies considerably in different tumors, but it must be present for the diagnosis of osteosarcoma to be made. Other mesenchymal elements, particularly cartilage, may also be present, sometimes in large amounts. The neoplastic mesenchymal cells in between osteoid and cartilage elements may be spindle shaped and uniform or quite pleomorphic, with bizarre, hyperchromatic nuclei and frequent mitotic figures. Giant cells, sometimes mistaken for osteoclasts, are often present.

Figure 21–7 ■

Photomicrograph of osteosarcoma. Pleomorphic, mitotically active mesenchymal cells are producing dark-staining (calcified) osteoid, an essential feature of this tumor.

Clinical Features. Osteosarcomas present as progressively enlarging, often painful masses that may come to attention because of a fracture of the involved bone. Although the combination of clinical and radiographic features may strongly suggest the diagnosis, histologic confirmation is necessary in all cases. Conventional osteosarcomas are aggressive lesions that metastasize through the bloodstream early in their course. The lungs are a common site of metastases. Approximately 20% of patients have detectable pulmonary spread at the time of diagnosis; many more have occult metastases that raise their ugly heads later in the course of the disease. However, advances in surgical techniques, combined with radiation therapy and chemotherapy for metastases, have greatly improved the prognosis of patients with these tumors.

Secondary osteosarcomas occur in an older age group than do primary conventional osteosarcomas. They most commonly develop in the setting of Paget disease or previous radiation exposure and rarely in patients with fibrous dysplasia, bone infarcts, or chronic osteomyelitis. Secondary osteosarcomas are highly aggressive neoplasms, which respond less favorably to current therapies than do conventional osteosarcomas.

Other forms of osteosarcoma include the so-called parosteal (juxtacortical), periosteal, telangiectatic, low-grade intraosseous, and small cell variants. A discussion of these less common lesions can be found in references included at the end of the chapter.

Cartilaginous Tumors

Like the bone-forming tumors of the skeleton, cartilaginous tumors span a spectrum of lesions ranging from benign, self-limited growths to highly aggressive malignancies. The more common types will be discussed here.

OSTEOCHONDROMA

Osteochondromas, sometimes called *exostoses*, are benign proliferations composed of mature bone and a cartilaginous cap. They are fairly common, accounting for about one third

Figure 21–6 ■

Osteosarcoma originating in the metaphyseal region. The tumor has grown through the cortex and elevated the periosteum.

Figure 21–8 ■

Osteochondroma. Note the glistening cartilaginous cap, characteristic of this tumor.

of all benign tumors of the bone. Like some osteomas, osteochondromas probably represent malformations rather than true neoplasms. In keeping with this, they tend to stop growing once the normal growth of the skeleton is completed. Osteochondromas occur most often as solitary, sporadic lesions, but they may be multiple in a rare familial disorder termed *multiple hereditary exostosis.* Most osteochondromas are asymptomatic, but some may cause troubling cosmetic deformities. They usually arise from the metaphysis near the growth plate of long tubular bones and present as broad-based, bony excrescences, firmly anchored to the cortex of the adjacent bone. A cap of hyaline cartilage is present (Fig. 21–8), which, in young subjects, contains a growth plate similar to that seen in the normal epiphysis. The growth plate usually disappears once epiphyseal closure has occurred in other sites. Most follow a benign course. Rare instances of sarcomatous transformation have been documented, predominantly in patients with familial disease.

CHONDROMA (ENCHONDROMA)

Chondromas are benign lesions composed of mature hyaline cartilage that occur most often in the small bones of the hands and feet. Although most common in the third to fifth decades of life, they may occur at any age and may be solitary or multiple. Several syndromes are associated with multiple chondromas: *Ollier disease* is characterized by multiple chondromas preferentially involving one side of the body, and *Maffucci syndrome* is characterized by multiple chondromas associated with benign vascular tumors (angiomas) of the soft tissues.

Chondromas are well-circumscribed lesions that usually arise within the medullary cavity of the bone (hence the term *enchondroma*). Less commonly, they may occur on the surface of the bone. Microscopically, they are composed of mature, hypocellular hyaline cartilage populated by bland chondrocytes. Cytologic atypia may be encountered in chondromas associated with Ollier disease or Maffucci syndrome, but it is not a feature of solitary lesions. Solitary chondromas are almost always innocu-

ous. In contrast, chondrosarcomas develop in about one third of patients with multiple chondroma syndromes.

CHONDROSARCOMA

Chondrosarcomas are *malignant neoplasms populated by mesenchymal cells that produce a cartilaginous matrix.* Males are affected about twice as frequently as females. Among malignant nonhematopoietic tumors of bone, they are second only to osteosarcoma in frequency. Unlike cartilage-forming osteosarcomas, the neoplastic cells in chrondrosarcomas do not form osteoid. Furthermore, as compared with osteosarcomas, chondrosarcomas occur in older patients, with a peak incidence in the sixth decade. Their distribution also differs from that of osteosarcomas. They arise in central portions of the skeleton; common sites of origin include the shoulder area, pelvis, proximal femur, and ribs, although these tumors may occur anywhere. Most chondrosarcomas arise de novo, although some occur in patients with multiple enchondromas or, more rarely, osteochondromas. As in the case of osteosarcomas, several different variants of chondrosarcoma have been described, all with particular clinical and morphologic characteristics.

MORPHOLOGY

The typical chondrosarcoma arises within the medullary cavity of the bone to form an expansile, glistening mass that frequently erodes the cortex (Fig. 21–9). Occasional lesions arise on the surface

Figure 21–9 ■

Chondrosarcoma. Cartilage formation by the neoplasm causes the glistening, gray-blue appearance visible on the cut surface. The tumor has infiltrated the medullary cavity and invaded the overlying cortex.

of the bone. Microscopically, chondrosarcomas vary greatly in appearance. The well-differentiated lesions may be quite innocuous looking, with only minimal cytologic atypia, and they are sometimes difficult to distinguish from non-neoplastic cartilage. Lesions at the other extreme may be composed of highly pleomorphic chondrocytes with frequent mitotic figures. Multinucleate cells are present, with lacunae containing two or more chondrocytes. About 10% of low-grade chondrosarcomas transform into a high-grade sarcoma and are referred to as dedifferentiated chondrosarcomas. The sarcomatous element may be an osteosarcoma or a fibrosarcoma. Other, less common, variants of chondrosarcoma include the rare mesenchymal chondrosarcoma and the clear cell chondrosarcoma.

Figure 21-10   ■

Photomicrograph of giant cell tumor of bone. Numerous osteoclast-like giant cells admixed with neoplastic mononuclear cells are visible.

Clinical Features. Chondrosarcomas present most often as progressively enlarging, sometimes painful masses involving the central portions of the skeleton. Their rate of growth and ultimate behavior are closely correlated with histologic grade, with poorly differentiated lesions behaving in a more aggressive fashion than better-differentiated tumors. Chondrosarcomas metastasize via the hematogenous route, most often to the lungs.

Other Tumors and Tumor-like Conditions of Bone

GIANT CELL TUMOR OF BONE

Giant cell tumor of bone, also known as *osteoclastoma*, is a neoplasm that contains large numbers of osteoclast-like giant cells admixed with mononuclear cells. They are fairly common tumors, accounting for about 20% of all benign tumors of the bone. Most cases arise in the epiphyses of long bones, particularly the distal femur, proximal tibia, proximal humerus, and distal radius. They occur most often between the ages of 20 and 40, with a slight female predominance. The histogenesis of giant cell tumors is incompletely understood. Current opinion suggests that the giant cell component is likely a reactive cell population derived from macrophages and that only the accompanying mononuclear cells are neoplastic.

MORPHOLOGY

Giant cell tumors present as radiolucent lesions involving the end of a long bone or, less commonly, another bone such as the sacrum. These tumors are almost always solitary. Long-standing tumors erode the cortex of the bone and may extend through the overlying periosteum. Grossly, the typical giant cell tumor has a dark-brown appearance owing to abundant vascularity. Areas of necrosis and cystic change are sometimes present. Histologically, they are composed of two

major cell populations. The most conspicuous elements are usually large **multinucleated giant cells** that closely resemble osteoclasts (Fig. 21-10). These cells appear to be derived from fusion of monocytes and are thought to be a reactive, rather than neoplastic, component of the tumor. The proliferating neoplastic component is made up of round to spindle-shaped **mononuclear cells.** This cell population contains a variable number of mitotic figures but usually has a fairly benign appearance. On rare occasions malignancy may develop, either de novo or in a previously treated giant cell tumor. In such cases it is the mononuclear cells, rather than the giant cells, that develop anaplastic features.

Clinical Features. Giant cell tumors usually present with local pain that because of the proximity of the tumors to joints may be mistaken for arthritis. Biopsy is usually necessary to establish the diagnosis. It should be noted that a wide variety of bone disorders may contain multinucleated giant cells and that their presence alone is not diagnostic of a giant cell tumor of bone. Multicentricity is exceedingly uncommon in giant cell tumors and, when present, should raise suspicion of hyperparathyroidism, in which the presence of multinucleate osteoclasts creates a more than passing resemblance to giant cell tumors. The behavior of these neoplasms is somewhat unpredictable. Although they are histologically benign, recurrences are common after simple curettage. Sarcomatous transformation is rare but, as noted, may occur de novo or in a previously benign tumor treated with radiation therapy. On occasion, a histologically benign giant cell tumor may metastasize, usually to the lung.

EWING SARCOMA FAMILY OF TUMORS

This family of tumors includes the well-known Ewing sarcoma (EWS) of the bone, extraosseous EWS, primitive neuroectodermal tumor (PNET), neuroepithelioma, and Askin tumor. Of these, EWS and PNET are the most common, and they account for 6% to 10% of all primary bone tumors, following osteosarcomas as the second most common form of bone tumor in children. The features that unite the Ewing sarcoma family of tumors are a common neural origin and the *presence of chromosomal translocations that result in the fusion of the EWS gene on 22q12 to a member of the ETS family of transcription factors*, mainly *FLI* (on 11q24) and *ERG* (on 21q22). The resulting novel chimeric proteins cause transcriptional activation of several target genes that dysregulate cell proliferation and differentiation. At a practical level, these translocations are of diagnostic importance. Thus, approximately 95% of patients with Ewing sarcoma have t(11;22)(q24;q12) or t(21;22)(q22;q12) translocations.

Ewing sarcoma occurs predominantly in children and adolescents, with a peak incidence in the second decade of life. It is a highly aggressive neoplasm that must be differentiated from other pediatric tumors composed of "small blue cells." Helpful in this regard are karyotypic studies and immunohistochemical features, described next.

MORPHOLOGY

Ewing sarcoma arises within the medullary cavity of the affected bone to produce a soft, expansile mass. **The femur, tibia, and pelvis are favored sites of origin,** although the tumor can arise in other bones and, on occasion, in the soft tissues. It occurs most often in the diaphysis, but spread to other parts is not uncommon. The tumor usually extends beyond the medullary cavity into the cortical bone and periosteum, where it may produce lamellae of reactive bone in an onion-skin pattern. Microscopically, Ewing sarcoma is composed of sheets of primitive cells with small, fairly uniform nuclei and only scant cytoplasm (Fig. 21–11A). The cytoplasm of the tumor cells contains glycogen, a feature

readily demonstrated in periodic acid–Schiff (PAS) stains or by electron microscopy. The neoplasm may be associated with reactive bone formation in the medullary cavity, but the neoplastic cells do not produce osteoid. Immunohistochemical studies are usually required to distinguish Ewing sarcoma from other small blue cell tumors such as neuroblastoma, rhabdomyosarcoma, and malignant lymphoma. Ewing sarcoma cells regularly express a neural marker, the MIC2 (CD99) antigen, which is recognized by a number of monoclonal antibodies (Fig. 21–11B). While not entirely specific for Ewing sarcoma, the identification of this antigen has proven to be of value in the diagnosis of this neoplasm, particularly when employed with a panel of other antibodies associated with other members of the small blue cell group of neoplasms.

Clinical Features. Ewing sarcoma classically presents as pain, often accompanied by local inflammation. Fever is fairly common and may initially suggest the possibility of an inflammatory lesion. The diagnosis requires biopsy, with demonstration of the characteristic morphologic and cytogenetic features of the tumor. It is important that Ewing sarcoma be distinguished from other small blue cell tumors, because each type requires a different therapy. Recent advances in treatment have significantly improved the outlook for patients with this sarcoma, with a 5-year survival rate of close to 75%.

FIBROUS DYSPLASIA

Fibrous dysplasia is an uncommon, benign, tumor-like lesion of bone in which the normal trabecular bone is replaced by proliferating fibrous tissue and disorderly islands of malformed bone. It occurs in three forms: (1) involving a single bone (monostotic fibrous dysplasia); (2) involving multiple, but not all, bones (polyostotic fibrous dysplasia); and (3)

Figure 21–11 ■

A, Photomicrograph of Ewing sarcoma, demonstrating characteristic sheets of neoplastic cells with small, primitive nuclei and scanty cytoplasm. *B,* Immunohistochemical stain with an antibody against the MIC2 glycoprotein expressed by Ewing sarcoma. The antigen is localized on the surface of the tumor cells, as indicated by a brown reaction product. (Case courtesy of Arthur G. Weinberg, MD, Department of Pathology, University of Texas Southwestern Medical School, Dallas.)

polyostotic disease with endocrine abnormalities. The pathogenesis of fibrous dysplasia is unclear. It appears to be a developmental defect in bone formation. Overexpression of the *FOS* protooncogene and somatic mutations in the gene coding for a stimulatory nucleotide binding protein have been described in the polyostotic form of the disease and may play some role in its pathogenesis.

Monostotic fibrous dysplasia is the most common form of the disease, accounting for about 70% of all cases. It usually arises during adolescence and becomes quiescent after bone growth is complete. The most common sites of involvement are the ribs, femur, tibia, bones of the jaw, and calvarium, although other bones may be affected. Although most cases are asymptomatic, in some the lesion may come to attention because of fractures or local deformity of the bone.

Polyostotic fibrous dysplasia limited to bone accounts for about 25% of cases of fibrous dysplasia. It appears at a slightly earlier age than the monostotic form of the disease and can continue to cause problems during adulthood. Craniofacial involvement is common and, when present, may cause significant facial deformity. Involvement of the pelvis, femur, and shoulder girdle is also common and may cause debilitating deformities and pathologic fractures.

Polyostotic fibrous dysplasia associated with endocrine abnormalities, the least common of the fibrous dysplasias, accounts for approximately 3% of all cases. It occurs most often in females. Affected individuals develop unilateral bone lesions, café-au-lait spots on the same side of the body, and precocious puberty. This constellation of clinical features is referred to as the *McCune-Albright syndrome*. Other endocrine abnormalities, including hyperthyroidism and Cushing syndrome, may also develop in patients with this syndrome. More recently, fibrous dysplasia has been described in association with neurofibromatosis type 1 (von Recklinghausen disease).

MORPHOLOGY

The lesions of fibrous dysplasia are circumscribed and radiolucent. They are usually surrounded by a

Figure 21–12   ■

Photomicrograph of fibrous dysplasia demonstrating slender bone trabeculae of woven bone surrounded by dense fibrous tissue (Case courtesy of Jo Ellen Krueger, MD, Department of Pathology, University of Texas Southwestern Medical School, Dallas.)

thin margin of sclerotic bone. Histologically, foci of fibrous dysplasia contain proliferating fibroblasts and abundant collagen, surrounding small, erratically distributed islands of woven bone (Fig. 21–12). Cartilaginous elements may be present but are usually only a minor component of the proliferation.

Clinical Features.   The clinical features depend on the extent of skeletal involvement. Monostotic lesions may be asymptomatic. Pathologic fractures and bone deformity may occur in any type of fibrous dysplasia, but they are a much greater problem for patients with polyostotic disease. They may require curettage and bone grafting. Sarcomas are a very rare complication of fibrous dysplasia, usually encountered in patients with the polyostotic form of the disease who have had their lesions treated with radiation therapy.

Diseases of the Joints

The joints are subject to a wide variety of disorders, including degenerative changes, infections, autoimmune diseases, metabolic derangements, and neoplasms. In this section we will confine our comments to some of the most common forms of arthritis, namely, degenerative joint disease, infectious arthritis, and gout. Rheumatoid arthritis, another important and potentially devastating disease of the joints, is discussed in detail in Chapter 5.

OSTEOARTHRITIS

Osteoarthritis, also termed *degenerative joint disease*, is the most common disorder of the joints. It is a very frequent, if not inevitable, part of aging and is an important cause of physical disability in individuals older than the age of 65. *The fundamental feature of osteoarthritis is degeneration of the articular cartilage;* the structural changes that follow in the underlying bone are secondary. In most cases it arises without obvious predisposing factors and hence is called *primary*. In contrast, *secondary osteoarthritis* refers to degenerative changes developing in a previously deformed joint, or joint degeneration that occurs in the context of certain metabolic disorders, such as hemochromatosis or diabetes mellitus. The suffix *-itis*, commonly used to refer to inflammatory disorders, is misleading, because osteoarthritis is not primarily an inflammation of joints. Inflammation occurs secondarily, however, and it may play a role in disease progression.

Pathogenesis. As mentioned earlier, articular cartilage is the major target of degenerative changes in osteoarthritis. Normal articular cartilage is strategically located at the end of bones to perform two functions: (1) bathed in synovial fluid, it ensures virtually friction-free movements within the joint; and (2) in weight-bearing joints, it spreads the load across the joint surface in a manner that allows the underlying bones to absorb shock and weight without being crushed. These functions require the cartilage to be elastic (i.e., to regain normal architecture after being compressed) and for it to have unusually high tensile strength. These attributes are provided by the two major components of the cartilage: a special type of collagen (type II) and proteoglycans, both secreted by chondrocytes. As is the case with adult bones, articular cartilage is not static; it undergoes turnover in which "worn out" matrix components are degraded and replaced. This balance is maintained by chondrocytes, which not only synthesize the matrix but also secrete matrix-degrading enzymes. Thus, the health of the chondrocytes and their ability to maintain the essential properties of the cartilage matrix determine joint integrity. In osteoarthritis, this process is disturbed by a variety of influences.

Perhaps the most important of these influences are *aging and mechanical effects*. Although osteoarthritis is not exclusively a wear-and-tear process, there is little doubt that mechanical stresses on the joint play a major role in its development. Evidence for this includes the increasing frequency of osteoarthritis with advancing age; its occurrence in weight-bearing joints; and an increase in the frequency of the disease in conditions that predispose the joints to abnormal mechanical stresses, such as obesity and previous joint deformity.

Genetic factors also appear to play a role in susceptibility to osteoarthritis, particularly in cases involving the hands and hips. The specific gene or genes responsible for this have not been identified, although linkage to chromosomes 2 and 11 has been suggested in some cases. The risk of osteoarthritis is increased in direct proportion to bone density, and high levels of estrogens have also been associated with an increased risk of the disease. The overall role played by hormones in the pathogenesis of osteoarthritis remains unclear, however.

Osteoarthritis is characterized by significant changes in both the composition and the mechanical properties of cartilage. Early in the course of the disease, the degenerating cartilage contains increased water and a decreased concentration of proteoglycans compared with healthy cartilage. In addition, there appears to be a weakening of the collagen network, presumably caused by decreased local synthesis of type II collagen, and increased breakdown of preexisting collagen. The levels of certain molecular messengers, including IL-1, TNF and nitric oxide, are increased in osteoarthritic cartilage and appear to be responsible for some of these changes in the composition of the cartilage. Apoptosis is also increased, likely responsible for a decrease in the number of functional chondrocytes. In aggregate, these changes tend to reduce the tensile strength and the resilience of the articular cartilage. In response to these regressive changes, chondrocytes in the deeper layers proliferate and attempt to "repair" the damage by producing new collagen and proteoglycans. Although these reparative changes are initially able to keep pace with the deterioration of cartilage, molecular signals causing chondrocyte loss and changes in the extracellular matrix, as noted earlier, eventually predominate. Factors responsible for this shift from a reparative to a predominantly degenerative picture remain poorly understood.

MORPHOLOGY

The earliest structural changes in osteoarthritis include enlargement and disorganization of the chondrocytes in the superficial part of the articular cartilage. This is accompanied by changes in the cartilaginous matrix, including **fibrillation** (splitting) at the articular surface (Fig. 21–13). Fissures gradually extend through the full thickness of the cartilage and into the subchondral bone. **Portions of the articular cartilage are eventually completely**

Figure 21–13 ■

Photomicrograph of osteoarthritis demonstrating characteristic fibrillation of the articular cartilage.

Figure 21-14   ■

Osteoarthritis in two femoral heads. *Left,* marked erosion of the articular cartilage; very little shiny cartilage remains. *Right,* a more advanced case, in which all cartilage is lost. Rubbing of the underlying bone has given it a polished, eburnated appearance. (Courtesy of Jim Richardson, DVM, PhD, Department of Pathology, University of Texas Southwestern Medical School, Dallas.)

eroded (Fig. 21-14), and the surface of the exposed subchondral bone becomes thickened and polished to an ivory-like consistency **(eburnation)** (see Fig. 21-14). Fragments of cartilage and bone are often dislodged to form free-floating "joint mice" in the joint cavity. Synovial fluid may leak through defects in the residual cartilage and underlying bone to form **cysts** within the bone. The underlying trabecular bone becomes sclerotic in response to the increased pressure on the surface.

Additional bone proliferation occurs at the margins of the joints to produce bony excrescences, termed **osteophytes.** As the joint begins to lose its integrity, there is trauma to the synovial membrane, which develops nonspecific inflammation. Compared with rheumatoid arthritis, the changes in the synovium are not as pronounced, nor do they occur as early.

Clinical Features. Signs and symptoms of osteoarthritis develop very gradually and usually affect only one or a few joints. The joints commonly involved include the hips, knees, lower lumbar and cervical vertebrae, proximal and distal interphalangeal joints of the fingers, first carpometacarpal joints, and first tarsometatarsal joints. Most individuals with primary osteoarthritis are asymptomatic until after the age of 50, although those with the secondary form of the disease may develop problems much earlier. Common complaints include joint stiffness and deep, aching pain, particularly in the morning. Repeated use of the joint tends to aggravate the pain. Crepitus, a crackling sound caused by exposed surfaces of bone rubbing against each other, is often present in severe cases. Some degree of joint swelling is common, and small effusions may develop. Heberden nodes, small osteophytes on the distal interphalangeal joints, are most often encountered in women with primary osteoarthritis. With time, significant joint deformity may supervene, but unlike rheumatoid arthritis, fusion of the joint does not occur. In the differential diagnosis, rheumatoid arthritis features prominently (Chapter 5). The important morphologic features of these two disorders are illustrated in Figure 21-15.

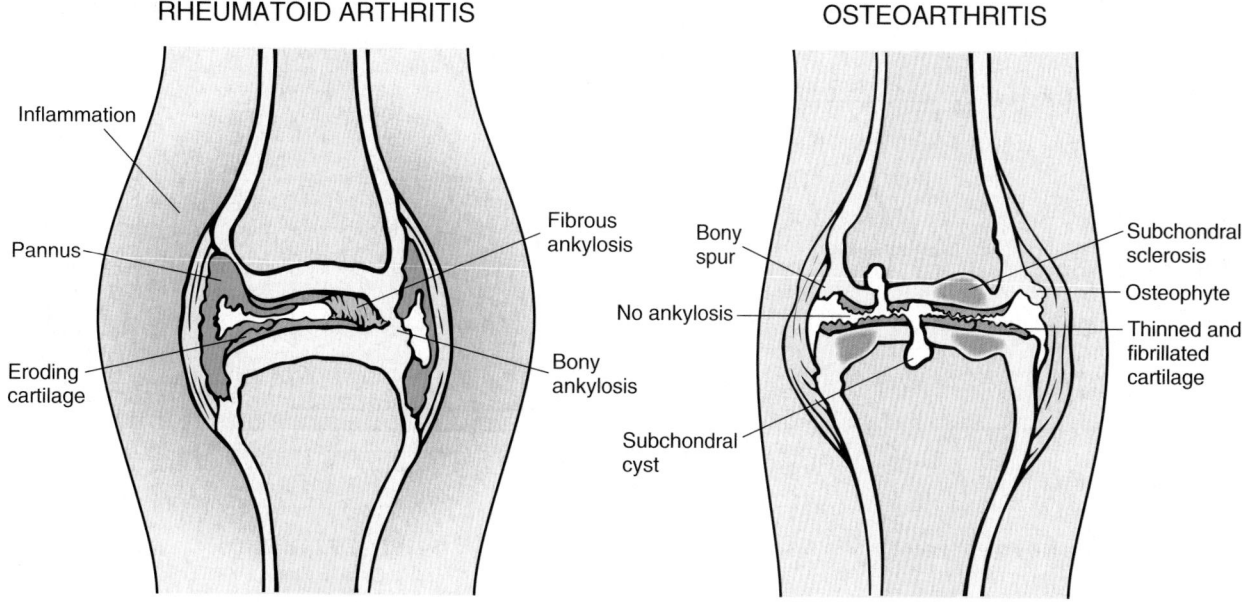

Figure 21-15   ■

Comparison of the morphologic features of rheumatoid arthritis and osteoarthritis.

■

GOUT

Gout is a disorder caused by the tissue accumulation of excessive amounts of uric acid, an end product of purine metabolism. It is marked by recurrent episodes of acute arthritis, sometimes accompanied by the formation of large crystalline aggregates termed *tophi*, and chronic joint deformity. All of these result from precipitation of monosodium urate crystals from supersaturated body fluids into the tissues. Although an elevated level of uric acid is an essential component of gout, not all individuals with hyperuricemia develop gout, indicating that factors in addition to hyperuricemia must play some role in the pathogenesis of the disorder. Gout is traditionally divided into primary and secondary forms, accounting for about 90% and 10% of cases, respectively. The term *primary gout* is used to designate cases in which the basic cause is unknown or, less commonly, when the cause is an inborn metabolic abnormality characterized primarily by hyperuricemia and gout. In the remaining cases, termed *secondary gout*, the cause of the hyperuricemia is known but gout is not the main or dominant clinical disorder. The major categories of gout are listed in Table 21–3.

Pathogenesis. Elevation of the level of serum uric acid may result from overproduction or reduced excretion of uric acid, or from both. To understand the mechanisms underlying disturbances in uric acid production or excretion, a brief review of normal uric acid synthesis and excretion is warranted. Uric acid is the end product of purine metabolism. Increased synthesis of uric acid, a common feature of primary gout, results from some abnormality in the production

Table 21–3. CLASSIFICATION OF GOUT

Clinical Category	Metabolic Defect
Primary Gout (90% of cases)	
Enzyme defects unknown (85% to 90% of primary gout)	Overproduction of uric acid Normal excretion (majority) Increased excretion (minority) Underexcretion of uric acid with normal production
Known enzyme defects (e.g., partial HGPRT deficiency [rare])	Overproduction of uric acid
Secondary Gout (10% of cases)	
Associated with increased nucleic acid turnover (e.g., leukemias)	Overproduction of uric acid with increased urinary excretion
Chronic renal disease	Reduced excretion of uric acid with normal production
Inborn errors of metabolism (e.g., complete HGPRT deficiency [Lesch-Nyhan syndrome])	Overproduction of uric acid with increased urinary excretion

HGPRT, hypoxanthine guanine phosphoribosyltransferase.

of purine nucleotides. The synthesis of purine nucleotides occurs along two pathways, referred to as the *de novo* and *salvage pathways* (Fig. 21–16):

■ The de novo pathway involves synthesis of purines and then uric acid from nonpurine precursors. The starting substrate for this pathway is ribose-5-phosphate, which is converted through a series of intermediates into purine nucleotides (inosinic acid, guanylic acid, and adenylic acid). This pathway is controlled by a complex array

Figure 21–16

Purine metabolism. The conversion of PRPP to purine nucleotides is catalyzed by amido-PRT in the de novo pathway and by APRT and HGPRT in the salvage pathway. (See text for details.) APRT, adenosine phosphoribosyltransferase; HGPRT, hypoxanthine guanine phosphoribosyltransferase; PRPP, 5-phosphoribosyl-1-pyrophosphate; PRT, phosphoribosyltransferase.

of regulatory mechanisms. Particularly important in our discussion are (1) the negative (feedback) regulation of the enzyme amidophosphoribosyltransferase (amido-PRT) and 5-phosphoribosyl-1-pyrophosphate (PRPP) synthetase by purine nucleotides and (2) the activation of amido-PRT by its substrate, PRPP.

■ The salvage pathway represents a mechanism by which free purine bases, derived from catabolism of purine nucleotides, breakdown of nucleic acids, and dietary intake, are utilized for the synthesis of purine nucleotides. This occurs in a single-step reaction whereby free purine bases (hypoxanthine, guanine, and adenine) condense with PRPP to form the purine nucleotide precursors of uric acid (inosinic acid, guanylic acid, and adenylic acid, respectively). These reactions are catalyzed by two transferases: hypoxanthine guanine phosphoribosyltransferase (HGPRT) and adenine phosphoribosyltransferase (APRT).

Circulating uric acid is freely filtered by the glomerulus and virtually completely resorbed in the proximal tubules of the kidney. A small fraction of the resorbed urate is subsequently secreted by the distal nephron and excreted in the urine.

As stated earlier, hyperuricemia may be caused by overproduction or underexcretion of uric acid or by some combination of the two processes. *Most cases of gout are characterized by a primary overproduction of uric acid, with or without excessive excretion of uric acid; in most such cases, the cause of the overproduction is unknown.* Less commonly, uric acid is produced at normal rates, and hyperuricemia occurs because of decreased excretion of urate by the kidneys. Although the cause of excessive uric acid biosynthesis is unknown in most cases, rare patients with known enzyme defects have provided valuable information on the regulation of uric acid biosynthesis. This is illustrated by patients with an inherited deficiency of the enzyme HGPRT.

Complete lack of HGPRT gives rise to the *Lesch-Nyhan syndrome.* This X-linked genetic condition, seen only in males, is characterized by excretion of excessive amounts of uric acid, severe neurologic disease with mental retardation, and self-mutilation. Because there is an almost complete lack of HGPRT, the synthesis of purine nucleotides by the salvage pathway is blocked. This has two effects: an accumulation of PRPP, a key substrate for the de novo pathway, and increased activity of the enzyme amido-PRT, a result of the dual effect of allosteric activation brought about by PRPP and reduced feedback inhibition owing to a reduction in purine nucleotides. Both of these have the effect of augmenting purine biosynthesis by the de novo pathway, resulting eventually in excess production of the end product, uric acid. It should be noted that typical gouty arthritis is neither common nor a prominent clinical feature of this disorder.

Less severe deficiencies of this enzyme (known as *partial HGPRT deficiency;* see Table 21–3) may occur, and these patients present clinically with severe gouty arthritis, beginning in adolescence, that is associated in some cases with mild neurologic disease.

In secondary gout, the hyperuricemia may be caused by increased urate production (e.g., rapid cell lysis during treatment of lymphoma or leukemia) or decreased excretion (chronic renal insufficiency), or some combination of the two. Reduced renal excretion may also be caused by drugs such as thiazide diuretics, presumably because of their effects on tubular transport of uric acid.

Whatever the cause, increased levels of uric acid in the blood and other body fluids (e.g., synovium) lead to the precipitation of monosodium urate crystals. Precipitation of the crystals in turn triggers a chain of events that culminate in joint injury (Fig. 21–17). The released crystals are chemotactic and also activate complement, with the generation of C3a and C5a leading to accumulation of neutrophils and macrophages in the joints and synovial membranes. Phagocytosis of crystals induces release of toxic free radicals and leukotrienes, particularly leukotriene B_4. Death of the neutrophils releases destructive lysosomal enzymes. Macrophages also participate in joint injury. After ingestion of urate crystals, they secrete a variety of proinflammatory mediators such as IL-1, IL-6, IL-8, and TNF. These on one hand intensify the inflammatory response and on the other hand activate synovial cells and cartilage cells to release proteases (e.g., collagenase) that cause tissue injury. Thus comes about an acute arthritis, which typically remits (days to weeks), even when untreated.

MORPHOLOGY

The major morphologic manifestations of gout are acute arthritis, chronic tophaceous arthritis and soft tissue tophi, and gouty nephropathy.

The primary morphologic change in **acute arthritis** is the deposition of **monosodium urate crystals** in the synovial tissues. These appear as pale, elongated, needle-like structures in synovial fluid aspirates and tissue sections. The crystals are accompanied by a predominantly neutrophilic inflammatory infiltrate, local congestion, and edema.

Chronic tophaceous arthritis develops after recurrent episodes of urate deposition and acute arthritis. Large, irregular deposits of chalky white sodium urate known as **tophi** are deposited on the articular cartilage and adjacent joint capsule. At these sites they provoke a chronic granulomatous inflammatory reaction. Thus, the tophus is seen in tissues as a mass of amorphous or crystalline urates surrounded by macrophages, lymphocytes, and fibroblasts. Large foreign body–type giant cells are wrapped around the urate crystals and are often very prominent (Fig. 21–18). Persistent chronic inflammation ultimately leads to fibrosis of the synovium and erosion of the articular cartilage. This may be followed by fusion of the joint (ankylosis). Tophi may also form in other sites, such as tendons, bursae, and other soft tissues, and, on occasion, in the heart and other organs. Large subcutaneous tophi may ulcerate.

Gouty nephropathy includes several different lesions. In patients with marked hyperuricemia and hyperuricaciduria, uric acid crystals may precipitate within and obstruct the renal tubules. This is a particularly important complication in patients with

Hyperuricemia

Precipitation of urate
crystals in joints

Complement
activation

Neutrophil chemotaxis

Phagocytosis of crystals
by neutrophils

Release
of crystals

Release of LTB₄,
prostaglandins,
free radicals

Phagocytosis by
monocytes

Release of IL-1,
TNF, IL-6, IL-8

Cartilage

Synovium

Lysis of neutrophils

Release of
lysosomal enzymes

Release of
proteases

Tissue injury and
inflammation

Figure 21–17   ■

Pathogenesis of acute gouty arthritis.

myeloproliferative disorders. These patients excrete large amounts of uric acid at the initiation of chemotherapy, when massive cell and nuclear lysis occurs ("tumor lysis syndrome"). In rare cases, over time, urate crystals may form within the interstitium of the medulla and may form visible tophi. Patients with gout may also develop uric acid renal stones, which may be complicated by obstructive uropathy and pyelonephritis. In advanced cases, the kidneys are shrunken and scarred, owing to a combination of tubular atrophy, obstructive uropathy, and recurrent episodes of pyelonephritis.

Clinical Features. Gout is more common in men than in women and does not usually cause symptoms before the age of 30. Four stages have been described in the evolution of gout, namely (1) asymptomatic hyperuricemia, (2) acute gouty arthritis, (3) "intercritical" gout, and (4) chronic tophaceous gout. Acute gouty arthritis is manifested by local pain, which often involves a single joint in the early stages of the disease but may subsequently become polyarticular. Although

Figure 21–18   ■

Photomicrograph of a gouty tophus. An aggregate of urate crystals is surrounded by reactive fibroblasts, mononuclear inflammatory cells, and giant cells.

any joint may be involved, the following joints, in order of frequency, are affected: great toe (90% of patients), instep, ankle, heel, and wrist. In most cases the pain is abrupt and intense. The initial acute attacks usually resolve completely and are followed by an asymptomatic interval (intercritical gout). In the absence of treatment, recurrent episodes of arthritis involve increasing numbers of joints and eventually lead to permanent joint deformity. In severe cases, chronic tophi may cause significant additional soft tissue deformity. Curiously, the tophi themselves are usually painless, despite the tendency of advanced lesions to ulcerate. Urate renal stones may cause destructive nephropathy; more chronic disease is associated with recurrent episodes of pyelonephritis and, eventually, chronic renal failure.

INFECTIOUS ARTHRITIS

Acute Suppurative Arthritis

Virtually every infectious agent has been implicated at one time or another as a cause of arthritis. The most common forms of infectious arthritis are those caused by bacteria. Infection of the joints may occur during episodes of bacteremia, through traumatic implantation, or from direct spread of an infection from the adjacent bone or soft tissues. Bacterial arthritis can occur in previously healthy individuals. However, immunodeficiency, joint trauma, or intravenous drug abuse leads to increased susceptibility. Common pathogens include gonococci, staphylococci, streptococci, *Haemophilus influenzae*, and gram-negative rods. Those individuals with a deficiency of certain complement proteins (C5, C6, C7) are particularly susceptible to dissemination of gonococci, and hence gonococcal arthritis (Chapter 18). *Salmonella* is a particularly important cause of acute bacterial arthritis in patients with sickle cell disease.

The usual reaction to infection is an acute suppurative arthritis, manifested by local pain, fever, and an intense neutrophilic inflammatory reaction within the joint and periarticular tissues. Aspiration of the joint space in such cases typically yields pus, and the responsible organisms may be visible in gram-stained smears of the exudate. Prompt diagnosis and treatment are necessary if permanent joint damage is to be avoided.

Lyme Disease

Lyme disease—named for the Connecticut town where the disease was first recognized in the mid 1970s—is caused by the spirochete *Borrelia burgdorferi*. It is transmitted from rodents to people by tiny, hard deer ticks (*Ixodes dammini*, *Ixodes ricinus*, and others); with 15,000 cases reported every year, it is the major arthropod-borne disease in the United States and is also frequent in Europe and Japan.

As in another major spirochetal disease, syphilis, clinical disease caused by Lyme spirochetes involves multiple organ systems and is usually divided into three stages. In *stage 1* (Fig. 21–19), *Borrelia* spirochetes multiply at the site of the tick bite and cause an expanding area of redness, often with an indurated or pale center. This skin lesion, called *erythema*

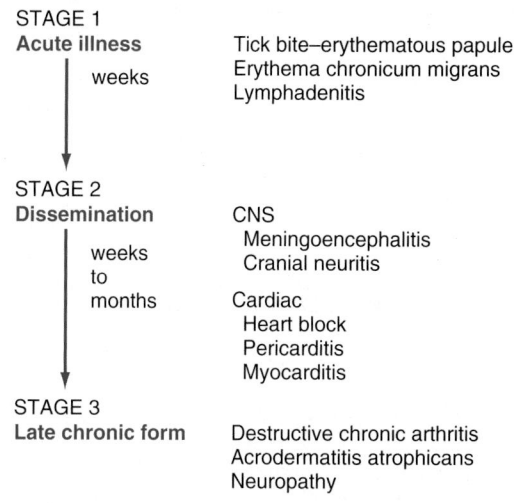

Figure 21–19   ■

The three stages and corresponding clinical features of Lyme disease.

chronicum migrans, may be accompanied by fever and lymphadenopathy but usually disappears in a few weeks' time. In *stage 2*, the *early disseminated stage*, spirochetes spread hematogenously and cause secondary annular skin lesions, lymphadenopathy, migratory joint and muscle pain, cardiac arrhythmias, and meningitis, often with cranial nerve involvement. If the disease is not treated, antibodies develop that are useful for serodiagnosis of *Borrelia* infection. Some spirochetes, however, escape host antibody and T-cell responses by sequestering themselves in the central nervous system or as intracellular forms within endothelial cells. In *stage 3*, the *late disseminated stage*, which occurs 2 or 3 years after the initial bite, Lyme *Borrelia* organisms cause a chronic arthritis, sometimes with severe damage to large joints, and an encephalitis that varies from mild to debilitating. Joint involvement is the most common manifestation of disseminated infection and eventually develops in 80% of patients. Lyme arthritis typically affects large joints such as the knee, shoulder, and elbow, but any joint may be involved. Diagnosis is based primarily on the detection of antibody response. Polymerase chain reaction testing is also available.

MORPHOLOGY

Skin lesions caused by *B. burgdorferi* are characterized by edema and a lymphocytic-plasma cell infiltrate. In early Lyme arthritis, the synovium resembles that of early rheumatoid arthritis, with villous hypertrophy, lining cell hyperplasia, and abundant lymphocytes and plasma cells in the subsynovium. A distinctive feature of Lyme arthritis is an arteritis, with onion-skin–like lesions resembling those seen in hypertension (Chapter 10). In late Lyme disease, there may be extensive erosion of the cartilage in large joints. In Lyme meningitis, the cerebrospinal fluid is hypercellular, shows a marked lymphoplasmacytic pleocytosis, and contains antispirochete immunoglobulins.

Diseases of Skeletal Muscle

The skeletal muscles are an elegant assembly of contractile proteins and their supporting membranes and organelles. Muscle development and normal activity are dependent on and closely integrated with the central and peripheral nervous systems, which together contribute to the *motor unit*. A motor unit is composed of a motor neuron in the brain stem or spinal cord; the peripheral axon emanating from the motor neuron; the neuromuscular junction; and, finally, the skeletal muscle fiber. Two major subpopulations of skeletal muscle fibers exist, namely, type I, or "slow-twitch," fibers and type II, or "fast-twitch," fibers. Whether a fiber is type I or type II is determined by the spinal motor neuron responsible for innervating the fiber. These fibers can be distinguished by special stains for specific enzymes. Diseases of the skeletal muscle may involve any portion of the motor unit. They include primary disorders of the motor neuron or its axon, abnormalities of the neuromuscular junction, and a host of primary abnormalities of the skeletal muscle itself (myopathies). For the purposes of this discussion, we will divide skeletal muscle diseases into (1) those disorders that produce predominantly myofiber atrophy, including neurogenic atrophy and type II myofiber atrophy; (2) disorders of the neuromuscular junction (exemplified by myasthenia gravis); and (3) selected primary myopathies, a highly heterogeneous group of conditions that includes inflammatory myopathies and the muscular dystrophies.

MUSCLE ATROPHY

Although virtually any skeletal muscle disease can be associated with myofiber atrophy, here we will consider those disorders in which myofiber atrophy is the predominant, and sometimes the only, abnormality. The two most common causes of simple skeletal muscle atrophy are neurogenic atrophy and type II myofiber atrophy.

Neurogenic Atrophy

As mentioned in the introductory comments, skeletal muscle development and function are dependent on intact connections with lower motor neurons in the central nervous system. If deprived of their normal innervation, skeletal muscle fibers undergo progressive atrophy. Dis-

eases involving the spinal motor neuron or the axons from that motor neuron produce similar morphologic changes in the affected skeletal muscle in older children and adults. In infants suffering from infantile spinal muscular atrophy type I (Werdnig-Hoffmann disease), a severe autosomal recessive disorder characterized by loss of spinal motor neurons, the morphologic changes in skeletal muscle differ from those seen in other neuropathic disorders.

MORPHOLOGY

Under the microscope, denervated myofibers appear sharply **angular and atrophic.** Both fast-twitch and slow-twitch fibers are involved. In many cases the atrophic fibers lie in small clusters, a pattern termed **small group atrophy** (Fig. 21–20). The activities of certain enzymes are also altered in denervated fibers. These include increased activity of certain oxidative enzymes and esterases, which are readily demonstrated by staining for the enzyme in tissue sections (see Fig. 21–20). Demonstration of these abnormalities

Figure 21–20 ■

Photomicrograph of skeletal muscle demonstrating neurogenic atrophy. The denervated cells are angular and atrophic, and they express increased esterase activity, manifested in this section as a red-orange reaction product (esterase stain). Clustering of the angular atrophic fibers, termed *small group atrophy*, is also apparent.

permits a distinction between denervation atrophy and other forms of muscle atrophy. If an injured nerve regenerates and re-establishes contact with skeletal muscle fibers, fiber size may return to normal. As a given axon regenerates, however, its sprouts tend to innervate contiguous fibers, resulting in back-to-back aggregation of muscle fibers of the same histochemical type. This loss of randomness, termed **fiber type grouping**, is readily demonstrable in enzyme histochemical preparations and may be the only clue to the presence of a previous episode of denervation. In infantile spinal muscular atrophy (Werdnig-Hoffman disease), changes in the skeletal muscle include large groups of profoundly atrophic, rounded fibers, often accompanied by the presence of scattered hypertrophic fibers (Fig. 21-21).

Clinical Features. The most consistent clinical manifestation of denervation atrophy is muscle weakness. This may vary from mild, localized weakness to severe, generalized weakness with respiratory compromise. Infantile spinal muscular atrophy is an important cause of generalized hypotonia in the neonate and is sometimes termed the *floppy infant syndrome*.

Type II Myofiber Atrophy

This pattern of muscle fiber atrophy is one of the most common abnormalities encountered in skeletal muscle. Type II atrophy is seen in patients who develop disuse atrophy when bedridden or otherwise immobilized. It is also commonly seen in patients receiving glucocorticoids and in patients with endogenous hypercortisolism of any cause.

Figure 21-21 ■

Photomicrograph of skeletal muscle from a 1-month-old infant with severe infantile spinal muscular atrophy. The denervation atrophy in this condition is characterized by large groups of profoundly atrophic, rounded fibers, associated with occasional hypertrophic fibers.

With routine histology, type II muscle fiber atrophy may be difficult to distinguish from denervation atrophy, especially in older children and adults. Like denervated fibers, the atrophic type II fibers appear angular and atrophic, although the group atrophy seen in some cases of denervation is absent. With special stains for enzymes, the detection of atrophy involving only the fast-twitch (type II) fibers reliably distinguishes this from denervation atrophy. Type II atrophy is typically associated with some degree of muscle weakness and may be suspected in patients who develop muscle atrophy under certain clinical conditions, such as Cushing syndrome or prolonged immobilization of some part of the body.

MYASTHENIA GRAVIS

Myasthenia gravis is an acquired autoimmune disorder of neuromuscular transmission characterized by muscle weakness. The disease may present at any age and affects females somewhat more frequently than males. However, males are more commonly affected in late adult life. The evidence that myasthenia gravis is immunologically mediated is substantial. Antibodies to the acetylcholine receptor (AChR) on skeletal muscle fibers are demonstrable in nearly 90% of patients with the disorder and appear to play a direct role in the pathogenesis of this disease. The antibodies either increase the internalization and down-regulation of the AChR or directly inhibit the binding of acetylcholine molecules to the receptor. With the use of appropriate stains, both immunoglobulin and various complement components are demonstrable at the neuromuscular junction. Additional observations supporting an immunologic basis for myasthenia gravis include an association between this disease and other autoimmune disorders, such as systemic lupus erythematosus, rheumatoid arthritis, and Sjögren syndrome. Thymic abnormalities are also quite common in myasthenia gravis. About two thirds of patients have hyperplasia of the thymus, and thymomas are present in 15% to 20% of patients. The relative roles played by thymic abnormalities and humoral abnormalities in the pathogenesis of myasthenia gravis are incompletely understood.

MORPHOLOGY

Myasthenia gravis is associated with minimal morphologic changes in skeletal muscle, despite the presence of profound weakness. The muscle may be normal in routine histologic sections, although a mild degree of type II myofiber atrophy may occur secondary to generalized weakness and resulting muscle disuse. Scattered **collections of lymphocytes**, sometimes designated **lymphorrhages**, may also be present in the connective tissue. Electron microscopy demonstrates simplification of the neuromuscular junction.

Clinical Features. As the name *myasthenia* suggests, the dominant clinical manifestation of myasthenia gravis is muscle weakness. The onset of this disease is typically insidious, but it may be abrupt. The muscle weakness usually becomes more pronounced with repeated contraction or stimulation and is therefore often worse during the latter part of the day than in the early morning. The most common sites of initial involvement are the *muscles of the eyelids* and the *muscles controlling eye movement*, manifested by drooping of the eyelids (ptosis) and double vision. Involvement of other facial and neck muscles commonly causes difficulty in chewing food and holding the head upright. The speech frequently assumes a nasal quality, particularly with prolonged attempts at conversation. The course of myasthenia gravis is slowly progressive, with involvement of other muscle groups. *Respiratory muscle involvement* may result in respiratory failure in untreated cases. Repetitive electrical stimulation of the skeletal muscle results in a progressive decrease in the amplitude of muscle action potentials and is a useful diagnostic test. The degree of muscle weakness varies considerably among patients, and it is not always related to the titer of anti-AChR antibodies.

Lambert-Eaton Myasthenic Syndrome

One additional disorder of the neuromuscular junction worthy of mention is the *Lambert-Eaton myasthenic syndrome*. This disorder usually develops in association with a neoplasm, particularly small cell carcinoma of the lung. Its onset may precede the diagnosis of neoplasia by a considerable amount of time. The Lambert-Eaton syndrome is distinguished from classic myasthenia gravis in electrophysiologic studies by a progressive increase in the amplitude of muscle action potentials with repetitive stimulation of the muscle. It is associated with antibodies directed against the presynaptic side of the neuromuscular junction.

INFLAMMATORY MYOPATHIES

Inflammation of the skeletal muscles can occur in a number of different settings, including infections, autoimmune disorders, and some muscular dystrophies. The idiopathic inflammatory myopathies account for most cases of significant inflammation. These disorders, which include *polymyositis* and *dermatomyositis*, are generally regarded as autoimmune diseases of skeletal muscle and are discussed with other immunologic disorders in Chapter 5. They may occur as isolated diseases or in association with other autoimmune diseases, such as systemic lupus erythematosus. *Inclusion body myositis*, also discussed in Chapter 5, is a chronic progressive myopathy associated with inflammatory infiltrates and sarcoplasmic vacuoles containing characteristic filamentous accumulations at an ultrastructural level. Despite its inflammatory appearance, however, the disease does not respond to conventional anti-inflammatory agents used in the treatment of polymyositis and dermatomyositis, suggesting that the inflammation in this condition is probably a secondary, rather than primary, abnormality.

Other important causes of skeletal muscle inflammation include infections, particularly parasitic diseases such as

toxoplasmosis, cysticercosis, and trichinosis. Of these, the most well known is trichinosis, a disease caused by the ingestion of inadequately cooked meat infected with *Trichinella spiralis* cysts. The offending meat is most often pork, although other animals may also harbor the parasite. When infected meat is ingested by humans, the cyst wall is digested, and the *Trichinella* larvae attach to the wall of the duodenum or jejunum. The larvae mature and produce additional larvae, which then migrate from the gut into the general circulation. Once in the bloodstream, the parasites may spread to a number of different sites, including the lungs, central nervous system, heart, and, ultimately, skeletal muscle. Within the skeletal muscle, the young larvae enlarge and encapsulate, provoking a variable host inflammatory reaction. The cysts may begin to calcify within a matter of months or, alternatively, may remain viable for several years. Clinical manifestations of trichinosis are referable to sites of parasite localization and include gastrointestinal disturbances, pneumonitis, altered mental status, and, in exceptional cases, myocardial failure. Skeletal muscle disease is manifested by muscle pain and weakness, often associated with facial edema.

Other pathogens may also infect skeletal muscles. A number of viruses have been implicated in the development of myositis in humans, including influenza viruses, coxsackieviruses, and human immunodeficiency virus (HIV). The manifestations of viral myositis range from nonspecific muscle aches to fulminant muscle necrosis with myoglobinuria and renal failure. Bacterial myositis is rare in the United States but is an important form of inflammatory muscle disease in tropical areas of the world

MUSCULAR DYSTROPHIES

The muscular dystrophies are a heterogeneous group of inherited diseases characterized by spontaneous, progressive degeneration of skeletal muscle fibers. In the past the diagnosis and classification of muscular dystrophies were based solely on the clinical features and patterns of inheritance of the disease. Studies in the past 2 decades have shed considerable light on the molecular basis and pathogenesis of many of the muscular dystrophies, and hence it is possible to describe many of them as specific genetic disorders. Of the various muscular dystrophies, two of the most common forms—Duchenne muscular dystrophy and the closely related Becker muscular dystrophy—are described here.

Duchenne and Becker Muscular Dystrophy

Duchenne muscular dystrophy (DMD) is an X-linked hereditary disease caused by the absence of a structural protein termed dystrophin. This disorder occurs in one of every 3500 live male births. The dystrophin gene is located on the short arm of the X chromosome (Xp21), where it spans an estimated 2400 kilobases (about 1% of the total X chromosome), making it one of the largest in the human genome. It is the enormous size of this gene that most likely renders it particularly vulnerable to deletions and other types of mutations. Dystrophin is a large protein that is expressed in a wide variety of tissues, including muscles of all types, brain, and peripheral nerves. In skeletal and cardiac muscles, dystrophin attaches portions of the sarcomere (the I and M bands) to the cell membrane, thus playing an important role in the structural and functional integrity of the myocyte. Absence or abnormalities of the dystrophin molecule are associated with impaired contractile activity and a variety of other derangements in both skeletal and cardiac muscles.

Becker muscular dystrophy (BMD) is another form of X-linked muscular dystrophy related to a mutation in the dystrophin gene. In contrast to DMD, however, dystrophin is present, but in an abnormal form. Accordingly, the resultant muscle abnormalities and clinical manifestations tend to be less severe than those of DMD.

Figure 21-22 ■

Muscular dystrophy. The muscle fibers vary considerably in size and shape. Interstitial connective tissue is increased.

MORPHOLOGY

The histologic features of DMD and BMD are similar and include **marked variation in muscle fiber size,** caused by concomitant hypertrophy and atrophy of the myofibers. Many of the residual muscle fibers exhibit a range of **degenerative changes,** including fiber splitting and necrosis, while other fibers show evidence of **regeneration,** including sarcoplasmic basophilia, nuclear enlargement, and nucleolar prominence. **Connective tissue is increased** throughout the muscle (Fig. 21-22). The definitive diagnosis is based on the demonstration of **abnormal staining for dystrophin** in immunohistochemical preparations (Fig. 21-23) or by Western blot analysis of skeletal muscle. In the late stages of the disease, extensive fiber loss and adipose tissue infiltration are present in most muscle groups. Changes that may occur in cardiac muscle in either DMD or

BMD include variable degrees of fiber hypertrophy and interstitial fibrosis.

Clinical Features. As would be expected in an X-linked disorder, most of the affected patients with either DMD or BMD are males. Affected females are rare. The cardinal manifestation of both of these disorders is muscle weakness, which initially is most pronounced in the proximal muscles. Early manifestations include a generalized clumsiness, followed by weakness in the pelvic and shoulder girdles. Some muscle enlargement may be present in the early phases of the disease, particularly in the calf muscles. This is inevitably followed by the development of muscle atrophy.

In DMD, signs and symptoms begin by about the age of 5 years and progress inexorably over the next several years to leave most patients wheelchair-bound by their teens. Most patients die in their 20s, usually as a result of progressive res-

Figure 21-23 ■

A, Photomicrograph demonstrating normal, uniform distribution of dystrophin in the skeletal muscle membrane from a patient suffering from a myopathy not related to an abnormality in dystrophin. *B,* In contrast, in a patient with Becker-type muscular dystrophy, dystrophin staining is weak and irregularly distributed. In a patient with Duchenne muscular dystrophy, staining would be completely absent.

piratory failure or pneumonia. The course may also be complicated by cardiac abnormalities, including congestive heart failure and cardiac arrhythmias.

The manifestations of BMD are variable but in general occur later and are more slowly progressive than those of DMD. Some patients may present with cardiac abnormalities even before skeletal muscle weakness is recognized. Patients with milder forms of the disease may remain ambulatory well into adult life.

Other Myopathies

As noted previously in this section, the term "myopathy" encompasses a remarkably heterogeneous group of disorders, both morphologically and clinically. Other important categories of myopathies include disorders caused by *intrinsic metabolic errors*, exemplified by glycogen and lipid storage diseases and mitochondrial abnormalities, and those arising as a consequence of an *exogenous toxic insult*. The *congenital myopathies* are an additional group of hereditary disorders characterized by a number of distinctive morphologic abnormalities in the muscles. Although a complete review of these entities is well beyond the scope of this discussion, recognition of these disorders may be of vital importance, particularly for purposes of genetic counseling. More comprehensive discussions of the congenital myopathies and other myopathic disorders can be found in specialized texts.

Soft Tissue Tumors

By convention, the term *soft tissue* is used to describe any nonepithelial tissue other than bone, cartilage, the brain and its coverings, hematopoietic cells, and lymphoid tissues. Soft tissue tumors are generally classified on the basis of the tissue type that they recapitulate, including fat, fibrous tissue, muscle, and neurovascular tissue. In some soft tissue neoplasms, however, no corresponding normal mesenchymal counterpart is known.

Soft tissue tumors may occur at any age. Most are benign lesions that are discovered incidentally or come to attention because of local mass effects. Less common are soft tissue sarcomas, characterized by aggressive local growth and widespread metastases. Occupying an intermediate position are neoplasms that may grow in a locally aggressive fashion and thus threaten a person's health but usually do not metastasize. Malignant soft tissue neoplasms are fortunately uncommon, accounting for less than 1% of all malignancies in adults. They are, however, the fourth most common type of malignancy in children, after hematopoietic neoplasms, neural tumors, and Wilms tumor.

The outlook for patients with soft tissue tumors is influenced by several factors. The distinction between benign and malignant lesions is straightforward in most cases but may be exceedingly difficult in others. The *histologic type* of the tumor, its degree of differentiation, reflected by the *histologic grade*, and the size and anatomic extent, expressed by the *stage*, all have a significant impact on the prognosis of malignant soft tissue tumors. Certain sarcomas, such as childhood rhabdomyosarcomas, respond favorably to multimodality therapy, whereas others, such as the synovial sarcomas, seem unresponsive even to aggressive therapy. In recent years, it has become increasingly clear that a significant proportion of soft tissue sarcomas have consistent chromosomal abnormalities that can be detected by standard cytogenetic or molecular techniques. Some tumors, such as Ewing sarcoma and alveolar rhabdomyosarcomas, are essentially defined by their translocations. Hence, these molecular abnormalities have an impact on diagnosis. Furthermore, in some cases the molecular changes also dictate prognosis. A classification of soft tissue tumors and tumor-like conditions is presented in Table 21–4. Only the more common forms will be described here.

TUMORS OF ADIPOSE TISSUE

Lipoma

Lipomas are the most common soft tissue tumors. They may arise anywhere in the body but are encountered most often in the subcutaneous tissues of adults. Less commonly, they may arise deep within skeletal muscle, abdominal and thoracic organs, and even the central nervous system. Most lipomas are solitary, sporadic lesions. Rare familial cases, inherited as autosomal dominant traits, are associated with the presence of multiple lipomas. Most lipomas present as slowly enlarging masses that seldom cause the patient

Table 21-4. SOFT TISSUE TUMORS

Tumors of Adipose Tissue

Lipomas
Liposarcoma

Tumors and Tumor-like Lesions of Fibrous Tissue

Nodular fasciitis
Fibromatoses
   Superficial fibromatoses
   Deep fibromatoses
Fibrosarcoma

Fibrohistiocytic Tumors

Fibrous histiocytoma
Dermatofibrosarcoma protuberans
Malignant fibrous histiocytoma

Tumors of Skeletal Muscle

Rhabdomyoma
Rhabdomyosarcoma

Tumors of Smooth Muscle

Leiomyoma
Leiomyosarcoma
Smooth muscle tumors of uncertain malignant potential

Vascular Tumors

Hemangioma
Lymphangioma
Hemangioendothelioma
Hemangiopericytoma
Angiosarcoma

Peripheral Nerve Tumors

Neurofibroma
Schwannoma
Malignant peripheral nerve sheath tumors

Tumors of Uncertain Histogenesis

Granular cell tumor
Synovial sarcoma
Alveolar soft part sarcoma
Epithelioid sarcoma

difficulty. One histologic variant, the angiolipoma, may present as local pain. Complete excision is usually curative.

MORPHOLOGY

The typical lipoma is a soft, yellow mass. Superficial lesions tend to be well circumscribed, although more deeply situated lesions (e.g., intramuscular lipomas) tend to be less well demarcated. Microscopically, most lipomas are composed of mature adipose tissue that is indistinguishable from normal fat. Several less common histologic variants also occur, including those containing fibrous tissue (fibrolipoma), large numbers of blood vessels (angiolipoma), smooth muscle (myolipoma), and bone marrow (myelolipoma). Some of the variants have characteristic chromosomal abnormalities. One additional variant is the angiomyolipoma, containing a mixture of adipose tissue, smooth muscle, and blood vessels. Angiomyolipomas occur most commonly in the kidneys of patients with tuberous sclerosis and probably represent hamartomas rather than true neoplasms. Angiomyolipomas are also notable for their tendency to undergo spontaneous hemorrhage, and they may present clinically as an acute abdominal emergency.

Liposarcoma

Liposarcomas are malignant neoplasms of adipocytes. They usually occur in adults, with a peak incidence in the fifth to sixth decades, and are one of the most common soft tissue malignancies in this age group. In contrast to lipomas, most liposarcomas arise in the deep soft tissues or in visceral sites. The lower extremities and abdomen are particularly common sites of origin. A t(12;16)(q13;p11) chromosomal translocation involving a transcriptional factor that plays a role in normal adipocyte differentiation has been identified in myxoid liposarcomas and in some cases of round cell liposarcoma, described below.

MORPHOLOGY

Liposarcomas usually present as relatively well-circumscribed lesions. A number of different histologic subtypes are recognized, including two low-grade variants, the **well-differentiated liposarcoma** and the **myxoid liposarcoma**, the latter characterized by an abundant, mucoid extracellular matrix. High-grade, aggressive variants include the **round cell liposarcoma** and the rare **pleomorphic liposarcoma.** The term **dedifferentiated liposarcoma** has been used to designate those variants that contain a mixture of better-differentiated and poorly differentiated areas. Some of the well-differentiated lesions may be difficult to distinguish histologically from lipomas, while at the other extreme, very poorly differentiated tumors may be difficult to distinguish from other high-grade malignancies.

The evolution and prognosis of liposarcomas are greatly influenced by the histologic subtype of the lesion. Well-differentiated and myxoid variants tend to grow in a fairly indolent fashion and have a more favorable prognosis than do the more aggressive round cell and pleomorphic variants. Local recurrence and hematogenous metastases, particularly to the lungs, are features of the more aggressive tumors.

TUMORS AND TUMOR-LIKE LESIONS OF FIBROUS TISSUE

Fibrous tissue proliferations are a heterogeneous and perplexing group of lesions. Some, such as nodular fasciitis, are not true tumors but are reactive, self-limited proliferations, whereas others, such as fibromatoses, are characterized by persistent local growth that may defy surgical excision. Yet others are highly malignant fibrosarcomas that not only tend to recur locally but also can metastasize. The histologic distinction between these various forms requires considerable skill and experience.

Nodular Fasciitis

Nodular fasciitis is a self-limited, reactive fibroblastic proliferation that may be mistaken for a sarcoma. The lesion is most common in young adults, in whom it presents as a rapidly enlarging, sometimes painful mass of several weeks' duration. Additional variants have also been described in children. Nodular fasciitis may arise in any part of the body but is most common in the upper extremities and trunk. In 10% to 15% of cases, there is a history of local trauma at the site of the lesion. Simple excision is curative in most cases.

MORPHOLOGY

Grossly, nodular fasciitis presents as an unencapsulated lesion in the subcutaneous tissue, muscle, or deep fascia, usually measuring less than 3 cm in diameter. Many lesions, particularly those arising in more superficial locations, are quite well circumscribed. Microscopically, nodular fasciitis is composed of plump, immature-appearing fibroblastic cells with bland, open nuclei and prominent nucleoli (Fig. 21–24). The fibroblasts are often arrayed in small fascicles in a loose, myxoid matrix. Mitotic figures are usually present and may be abundant, a feature that may result in misinterpretation of the lesion as a sarcoma. Abnormal mitotic figures are not seen.

Fibromatoses

The fibromatoses are a group of fibroblastic proliferations distinguished by their tendency to grow in an infiltrative fash-

Figure 21–24

Nodular fasciitis. The high cellularity of the lesions evident in this photomicrograph causes them to be confused with a sarcoma in some cases.

ion and, in many cases, to recur after surgical excision. While some growths are locally aggressive, unlike fibrosarcomas, they do not metastasize. The fibromatoses are divided into two major clinicopathologic groups: the superficial fibromatoses and the deep fibromatoses. The *superficial fibromatoses*, which include such entities as palmar fibromatosis (Dupuytren contracture) and penile fibromatosis (Peyronie disease), arise in the superficial fascia. The superficial lesions are generally more innocuous than their deep-seated cousins and typically they come to clinical attention because of their tendency to cause deformity of the involved structure. The *deep fibromatoses* include the so-called desmoid tumors that arise in the abdomen and muscles of the trunk and extremities. They may arise as isolated lesions, or as a component of *Gardner syndrome,* an autosomal dominant disorder characterized by adenomatous polyps of the colon, osteomas of bone, and fibromatoses. Compared with the superficial lesions, the deep fibromatoses are characterized by a greater tendency to recur and to grow in a locally aggressive manner.

MORPHOLOGY

The appearance of the fibromatoses varies considerably, depending on the site. Some lesions present as well-defined nodules. Others appear as grossly infiltrative masses without an obvious margin. Microscopically, the fibromatoses are composed of proliferating, sometimes plump fibroblasts that have a fairly uniform appearance. Some lesions may be quite cellular, particularly early in their evolution, while others, especially the superficial fibromatoses, contain abundant dense collagen.

Fibrosarcomas

Fibrosarcomas are malignant neoplasms composed of fibroblasts. Most cases occur in adults, in whom favored sites of origin include the deep tissues of the thigh, knee, and retroperitoneal area. Fibrosarcomas have no specific clinical features that allow them to be distinguished from other soft tissue tumors. As a rule, they tend to grow slowly, and they have usually been present for several years by the time they are diagnosed. As with other types of sarcomas, fibrosarcomas often recur locally after excision and may metastasize, usually by the hematogenous route to the lungs.

MORPHOLOGY

Fibrosarcomas are solitary lesions that may be grossly infiltrative or deceptively circumscribed. Histologically, the typical fibrosarcoma is composed of interlacing fascicles of fibroblasts, sometimes arrayed in a "herringbone" pattern. Nuclear atypia and mitotic activity are present but may be mild in some cases. The tumors are typically divided into four histologic grades, based on features that include the degree of cellularity, pleomorphism, and mitotic activity.

FIBROHISTIOCYTIC TUMORS

Fibrohistiocytic tumors are composed of a mixture of fibroblasts and phagocytic, lipid-laden cells with a histiocytic appearance. Like the fibroblastic tumors, the fibrohistiocytic group spans a broad range of histologic patterns and biologic behavior, from self-limited, benign lesions to high-grade sarcomas. Other lesions occupy an intermediate position, in that they recur locally but seldom metastasize.

Fibrous Histiocytoma

Fibrous histiocytomas are benign lesions that present as a well-defined, mobile nodule in the dermis or subcutaneous tissue. Most cases occur in adults. A number of histologic patterns may be encountered, including proliferations dominated by bland, interlacing spindle cells and lesions rich in foamy, lipid-rich cells with a histiocytic morphology. The borders of the lesions tend to be infiltrative, but extensive local invasion does not occur. They are cured by simple excision. These tumors have unique cytogenetic abnormalities that give rise to a fusion gene derived from the platelet derived growth factor β chain *(PDGF-β)* and collagen type 1α *(COL1A1)*. This fusion gene is believed to give rise to an autocrine loop of *PDGF-β* production.

Dermatofibrosarcoma Protuberans

This neoplasm occupies an intermediate position between the benign fibrohistiocytic tumors and the malignant fibrous histiocytomas. It presents as a slowly growing, nodular lesion, most often involving the dermis and subcutaneous tissue. Most patients are adults. The tumors are infiltrative and often recur after local excision. In exceptional cases, metastases may develop. Microscopically, dermatofibrosarcoma protuberans is composed of plump, fibroblastic cells arrayed in a "storiform" pattern. Mitotic activity is sparse in most cases, and there is little cytologic atypia.

Malignant Fibrous Histiocytoma

The term *malignant fibrous histiocytoma* (MFH) designates a heterogeneous group of clinically aggressive soft tissue sarcomas. Most occur in older adults between the ages of 50 and 70. Once considered to be the most common type of soft tissue sarcoma, current evidence suggests that many tumors previously classified as MFH represent highly pleomorphic variants of other sarcomas, such as liposarcoma and rhabdomyosarcoma. When these other types of tumors are excluded, however, there remains a small group of pleomorphic soft tissue sarcomas whose cell of origin remains obscure. MFHs tend to arise in the deep muscular tissues of the extremities or in the retroperitoneal area. Most are highly aggressive tumors that often recur locally and metastasize in about 50% of patients.

Figure 21–25　■

Photomicrograph of malignant fibrous histiocytoma containing a mixture of atypical spindle cells and bizarre neoplastic giant cells. Other sarcomas may contain similar pleomorphic cells and must be excluded by appropriate techniques before the diagnosis of malignant fibrous histiocytoma is made.

MORPHOLOGY

These tumors are usually gray-white, encapsulated masses that appear deceptively circumscribed, despite their infiltrative growth at the microscopic level. Retroperitoneal tumors may reach a very large size before coming to clinical attention. Microscopically, several different subtypes of MFH are recognized. The most common of these is the so-called storiform-pleomorphic variant, populated by cytologically atypical spindle cells arrayed in whorls, sometimes admixed with bizarre, histiocyte-like cells (Fig. 21–25). Other forms of MFH include the more vascular angiomatoid variant, inflammatory MFH, and myxoid MFH. The angiomatoid variant tends to occur in younger patients.

NEOPLASMS OF SKELETAL MUSCLE

Neoplasms of skeletal muscle include rhabdomyoma and its malignant counterpart, rhabdomyosarcoma. The rhabdomyoma is an uncommon tumor. At least one form, the cardiac rhabdomyoma associated with tuberous sclerosis, probably represents a hamartoma rather than a true neoplasm (Chapter 11).

Rhabdomyosarcoma

Rhabdomyosarcoma is a malignant mesenchymal neoplasm that exhibits skeletal muscle differentiation. In contrast to the soft tissue sarcomas discussed previously, *rhabdomyosarcoma is predominantly a neoplasm of infancy, childhood, and adolescence*, with a peak incidence in the first decade of life. It is the most common form of

Figure 21–26 ■

Rhabdomyosarcoma. *A,* The rhabdomyoblasts are round or spindle shaped, some cells having elongated cytoplasm. *B,* Immunohistochemical staining reveals desmin (brown reaction product), confirming the presence of rhabdomyoblasts. (Courtesy of Jorge Albores-Saavedra, MD, Department of Pathology, University of Texas Southwestern Medical School, Dallas.)

soft tissue sarcoma in the pediatric population. Several different but sometimes overlapping histologic variants exist, the most common of which is the *embryonal rhabdomyosarcoma.* They arise most frequently in the head and neck area, genitourinary tract, and retroperitoneum. Occasional tumors originate in the extremities. Another, less common histologic pattern is the *alveolar rhabdomyosarcoma,* a tumor encountered most often in the extremities and, less commonly, in the sinonasal tract during the adolescent years. The rare *pleomorphic rhabdomyosarcoma* arises most frequently in the deep soft tissues of adults and may be difficult to distinguish histologically from malignant fibrous histiocytoma.

Much interest has focused on the cytogenetic abnormalities in alveolar rhabdomyosarcoma: t(2;13)(q35;q14) and, less commonly, t(1;13)(p36;q14) translocations have been found in most cases. In the more common t(2;13) variant, the *PAX3* gene on chromosome 2 fuses with the *FKHR* gene on chromosome 13. Interestingly, the *PAX3* gene functions upstream of genes that control skeletal muscle differentiation. Thus, it is proposed that the pathogenesis of the tumor involves dysregulation of muscle differentiation by the chimeric PAX3-FKHR protein.

MORPHOLOGY

The gross appearance of rhabdomyosarcomas is variable. Some tumors, particularly those arising near the mucosal surfaces of the lower genitourinary tract and in the head and neck, may present as soft, gelatinous, grapelike masses, designated **sarcoma botryoides.** In other cases the pattern may be that of a poorly defined, infiltrating mass. Microscopically, the **embryonal variants,** including sarcoma botryoides, are composed of small, primitive cells, some of which contain eccentric eosinophilic "straplike" cell

processes. Such strap cells are evidence of myoblastic differentiation. The malignant cells tend to cluster immediately beneath mucosal surfaces, a configuration known as a **cambium layer.** In the absence of telltale features of myoblastic differentiation at the light microscopic level, these tumors are very difficult to distinguish from other small round cell tumors of childhood. The diagnosis of rhabdomyosarcoma is based on the demonstration of skeletal muscle differentiation, either in the form of sarcomeres under the electron microscope or by the demonstration of muscle-associated antigens such as desmin and muscle-specific actin in immunocytochemical preparations (Fig. 21–26). In the **alveolar pattern,** neoplastic rhabdomyoblasts are supported by fibrous septa to form spaces somewhat suggestive of alveolar spaces in the lung. **Pleomorphic variants,** as the name implies, are populated by highly pleomorphic malignant cells, including bizarre neoplastic giant cells. As has been noted, such cases may be difficult to distinguish from the more pleomorphic variants of MFH.

SMOOTH MUSCLE TUMORS

Benign smooth muscle tumors, or leiomyomas, are common, well-circumscribed neoplasms encountered most frequently in the uterus, although they may arise from smooth muscle cells anywhere in the body. They are discussed in detail with other tumors of the uterus in Chapter 19. Malignant smooth muscle tumors, designated *leiomyosarcomas,* occur most often in the uterus and gastrointestinal tracts, although they may arise in virtually any area of the body. Most arise de novo, rather than in a preexisting leiomyoma. They are distinguished from leiomyomas by the infiltrative growth, greater cellularity, pleomorphism, and, most importantly, greater mitotic activity.

MISCELLANEOUS NEOPLASMS

As noted in the introductory comments to this section, soft tissue tumors also include vascular neoplasms and peripheral nerve sheath tumors, which are discussed in Chapters 10 and 23, respectively. An additional group of soft tissue neoplasms includes a small number of sarcomas of uncertain histogenesis. These include the alveolar soft part sarcoma, synovial sarcoma, and epithelioid sarcoma. Only synovial sarcoma is sufficiently common to warrant a brief description here.

Synovial Sarcoma

This tumor accounts for 10% of all soft tissue sarcomas. Once thought to be a tumor of synovial origin, synovial sarcoma does not arise from synovial cells; rather, it derives from mesenchymal cells about joint cavities, and sometimes in sites totally removed from joints. A characteristic, and apparently unique, t(X;18)(p11.2;q11.2) chromosomal translocation is present in the vast majority of synovial sarcomas. The translocation has been linked to the abnormalities in several recently identified synovial sarcoma–associated genes, which appear to influence, in turn, the morphology and behavior of these tumors.

Figure 21–27 ■

Photomicrograph of synovial sarcoma showing the classic biphasic pattern composed of epithelial cells forming glands, with intervening spindle cells.

MORPHOLOGY

Synovial sarcomas range from quite small, deceptively circumscribed lesions to infiltrative sarcomatous masses. Histologically, they are characterized by a biphasic pattern that has an epithelial component forming glands, interspersed in a spindle cell pattern replicating fibroblast-like sheets (Fig. 21–27). Less commonly, the synovial sarcoma may be monophasic and composed entirely of epithelial elements that resemble a carcinoma or, alternatively, of spindle cells, which make synovial sarcoma difficult to distinguish from other sarcomas. Immunocytochemical demonstration of keratin and epithelial membrane antigen is helpful in diagnosis. The demonstration of the t(X;18) chromosomal translocation is an even more definitive diagnostic marker.

BIBLIOGRAPHY

Brown RH: Dystrophin-associated proteins and the muscular dystrophies: a glossary. Brain Pathol 6:19, 1996. (A very informative, concise summary of dystrophin and related proteins in various forms of muscular dystrophy.)

De Alava E, Pardo J: Ewing tumor: tumor biology and clinical applications. Int J Surg Pathol 9:7, 2001. (A discussion of the newly formed Ewing family of tumors.)

Dos Santos NR, et al: Molecular mechanisms underlying human synovial sarcoma development. Genes Chromosomes Cancer 30:1, 2001. (An informative review of the molecular aberrations associated with the synovial sarcoma-associated t(X;18) chromosomal translocation and their relationship to histologic patterns and clinical behavior.)

Felson DT, et al: Osteoarthritis: new insights: I. The disease and its risk factors. Ann Intern Med 133:635, 2000. (Summary of a National Institutes of Health consensus conference reviewing the epidemiology of osteoarthritis and the roles played by hormonal status, genetic factors, nutrition, and mechanical factors in its development.)

Goebel HH: Congenital myopathies. Semin Pediatr Neurol 3:152, 1996. (A review of the nosology and salient diagnostic features of the congenital myopathies.)

Hocking L, et al: Familial Paget disease of bone: patterns of inheritance and frequency of linkage to chromosome 18q. Bone 26:577, 2000. (A review article that underscores the heterogeneity of Paget disease of bone, even among familial cases.)

Kenny AM, Prestwood KM: Osteoporosis: pathogenesis, diagnosis, and treatment in older adults. Rheum Dis Clin North Am 26:569, 2000. (A concise, informative summary of current ideas regarding the pathogenesis and clinical approach to osteoporosis.)

Letson GD, Mauro-Cacho CA: Genetic and molecular abnormalities in tumors of the bone and soft tissues. Cancer Control 8:239, 2001. (A discussion of cytogenetic and molecular changes in this group of tumors.)

Lories RJV, Luyten FP: Osteoprotegerin-ligand balance: a new paradigm in bone metabolism providing new therapeutic targets. Clin Rheumatol 20:3, 2001. (A succinct review of the molecular mechanisms that regulate bone formation and resorption.)

Riggs BL: The mechanism of estrogen regulation of bone resorption. J Clin Invest 106:1203, 2000. (An excellent commentary on the effects of estrogen on the molecular pathways that regulate bone remodeling.)

Rodan GA, Martin TJ: Therapeutic approaches to bone diseases. Science 289:1508, 2000. (A review of recent developments in the treatment of osteoporosis, including a discussion of the mechanisms of action of the newer therapeutic agents.)

Ross FP: RANKing the importance of measles virus in Paget disease. J Clin Invest 5:555, 2000. (A review of the current evidence for paramyxovirus infection in the Paget disease, with additional comments about the role of RANK and the RANK ligand in its pathogenesis.)

Snaith ML: ABC of rheumatology: gout, hyperuricemia, and crystal arthritis. BMJ 310:521, 1995. (A short but lucid commentary.)

Steere AC: Lyme disease. N Engl J Med 345:115, 2001. (An update on this disease by the person who discovered it.)

Teitelbaum SL: Bone resorption by osteoclasts. Science 289:1504, 2000. (A technical but readable summary of recent developments in our understanding of the biology of osteoclast function.)

Weinberger A: Gout, uric acid metabolism, and crystal-induced inflammation. Curr Opin Rheumatol 7:359, 1995. (A good discussion of the pathways of inflammation in gouty arthritis.)

22

The Skin

GEORGE F. MURPHY, MD

Disorders affecting the skin are extremely common and range from the relatively innocuous viral warts to life-threatening malignant melanomas. It is estimated that each year approximately 30% of people in the United States develop a skin problem. Fully 10% of outpatient visits are related to a skin disorder, and more than half of these come to the attention of primary care providers such as internists, pediatricians, and family practitioners. Whereas most of the cutaneous disorders are intrinsic to the skin, many skin lesions are external manifestations of a systemic disease, such as systemic lupus erythematosus and acquired immunodeficiency syndrome (e.g., Kaposi sarcoma). Thus, skin provides an important window for the recognition of systemic disorders that are likely to be encountered by virtually every practitioner of medicine.

The structure of skin is well known to every student of medicine. However, what is not widely appreciated is that skin is not merely a passive, protective mantle. Because skin is in constant contact with the environment, it is bathed with microbial and nonmicrobial antigens. These antigens are

The author thanks Dr. John Vallone for valuable editorial assistance and advice during the preparation of this chapter.

processed by bone marrow–derived epidermal Langerhans cells that have dendritic morphology and escape casual inspection of the epidermis under the microscope. Langerhans cells possess all the attributes of antigen-presenting cells, and they communicate with the immune system by migrating to regional lymph nodes. Even the dull and uninteresting-looking squamous cells (keratinocytes) participate in maintaining the delicate homeostasis in skin by secreting a plethora of cytokines. These soluble messengers not only regulate interactions among the epidermal cells but also diffuse down and influence the dermal microenvironment. Thus, skin, simple in structure, is a complex organ in which precisely regulated cellular and molecular events govern the body's response to the external environment (Fig. 22–1). The focus in this chapter is on those diseases that are common and that are generally localized to or originate in the skin. Cutaneous manifestations of many systemic disorders are covered elsewhere in the text, along with discussions of specific diseases.

Diseases of the skin are often perplexing to students (and nonspecialists) because dermatologists and dermatopathologists use a vocabulary that is not commonly used in describing lesions in other tissues. Thus, we begin our discussion by providing a glossary of commonly used terms.

MACROSCOPIC TERMS

Macule: Circumscribed area of any size characterized by its flatness and usually distinguished from surrounding skin by its coloration

Papule: Elevated solid area 5 mm or less across

Nodule: Elevated solid area more than 5 mm across

Plaque: Elevated flat-topped area, usually more than 5 mm across

Vesicle: Fluid-filled raised area 5 mm or less across

Bulla: Fluid-filled raised area more than 5 mm across; a large vesicle

Blister: Common term used for vesicle or bulla

Pustule: Discrete, pus-filled raised area

Scale: Dry, horny, platelike excrescence; usually the result of imperfect cornification

Lichenification: Thickened and rough skin characterized by prominent skin markings; usually the result of repeated rubbing in susceptible persons

Figure 22–1

Schematic diagram of normal skin. The epidermal layer *(box)* gives rise to specialized adnexal downgrowths, including the hair follicle (h), sweat glands (g), and sebaceous lobule (s) that connects to the hair follicle. The epidermal layer (e) arises from proliferating basal cells (b) and gives rise to flattened keratinaceous scale in the superficial stratum corneum layer (sc). Other epidermal cells include melanocytes (m) and Langerhans cells (lc). The underlying dermis (d) contains lymphatic and blood vessels (v), mast cells (mc), dendritic cells (dc), and fibroblasts (f).

Excoriation: A traumatic lesion characterized by breakage of the epidermis, causing a raw linear area (i.e., a deep scratch); such lesions are often self-induced

to large edematous plaques. Sites of predilection for urticarial eruptions include any area exposed to pressure, such as the trunk, distal extremities, and ears.

MICROSCOPIC TERMS

Hyperkeratosis: Hyperplasia of the stratum corneum, often associated with a qualitative abnormality of the keratin

Parakeratosis: Mode(s) of keratinization characterized by retention of the nuclei in the stratum corneum. On mucous membranes, parakeratosis is normal

Acanthosis: Epidermal hyperplasia preferentially involving the stratum spinosum

Dyskeratosis: Abnormal keratinization occurring prematurely within individual cells or groups of cells below the stratum granulosum

Acantholysis: Loss of intercellular connections resulting in loss of cohesion between keratinocytes

Papillomatosis: Hyperplasia of the papillary dermis with elongation and/or widening of the dermal papillae

Lentiginous: Refers to a linear pattern of melanocyte proliferation within the epidermal basal cell layer; lentiginous melanocytic hyperplasia can occur as a reactive change or as part of a neoplasm of melanocytes

Spongiosis: Intercellular edema of the epidermis

ACUTE INFLAMMATORY DERMATOSES

Literally thousands of specific inflammatory dermatoses exist. In general, acute lesions last from days to weeks and are characterized by inflammation (often marked by mononuclear cells, rather than neutrophils), edema, and (in some instances) epidermal, vascular, or subcutaneous injury. Some acute lesions may persist, resulting in a transition to a chronic phase, while others characteristically never progress beyond the acute stage. The lesions discussed here are selected as examples of the more commonly encountered dermatoses within this category.

Urticaria

Urticaria (hives) is a common disorder of the skin characterized by *localized mast cell degranulation and resultant dermal microvascular hyperpermeability*, culminating in pruritic edematous plaques called wheals.

Clinically, urticaria most often occurs between the ages of 20 and 40 years, although all age groups are susceptible. Individual lesions develop and fade within hours (usually less than 24 hours), and episodes may last for days or persist for months. Lesions vary from small, pruritic papules

MORPHOLOGY

The histologic features of urticaria may be so subtle that many biopsy specimens at first resemble normal skin. Usually there is a very sparse superficial perivenular infiltrate consisting of mononuclear cells and rare neutrophils. Eosinophils may be present, often in the midreticular dermis. Collagen bundles are more widely spaced than in normal skin, a result of superficial dermal edema fluid that does not stain in routinely prepared tissue. A common and initiating feature that is not readily visible in routine stains is the degranulation of mast cells that normally reside about superficial dermal venules (see Fig. 22–1).

In most cases, urticaria results from antigen-induced release of vasoactive mediators from mast cell granules via sensitization with specific immunoglobulin E (IgE) antibodies (type I hypersensitivity; Chapter 5). This IgE-dependent degranulation can follow exposure to a number of antigens (pollens, foods, drugs, insect venom). IgE-independent urticaria may result from substances that directly incite the degranulation of mast cells, such as opiates and certain antibiotics. Hereditary angioneurotic edema is the result of an inherited deficiency of C1 esterase inhibitor that results in uncontrolled activation of the early components of the complement system (Chapter 2).

Acute Eczematous Dermatitis

Eczema is a clinical term that embraces a number of pathogenetically different conditions. All are characterized by red, *papulovesicular, oozing, and crusted lesions* at an early stage. With persistence, these lesions develop into raised, *scaling plaques*. Clinical differences permit classification of eczematous dermatitis into the following categories: (1) allergic contact dermatitis, (2) atopic dermatitis, (3) drug-related eczematous dermatitis, (4) photoeczematous dermatitis, and (5) primary irritant dermatitis (Table 22–1).

The most obvious example of acute eczematous dermatitis is an acute contact reaction to poison ivy or other contact antigens, such as laundry detergent (Fig. 22–2). Such lesions are characterized by pruritic (itchy), edematous, oozing plaques, often containing small and large blisters (vesicles and bullae) (see Fig. 22–2A). In the presence of persistent antigen stimulation, lesions may become less "wet" (fail to ooze or form vesicles) and progressively scaly (hyperkeratotic) as the epidermis thickens (acanthosis). At this juncture, the process could be more appropriately categorized as a chronic form of dermatitis.

Table 22-1. CLASSIFICATION OF ECZEMATOUS DERMATITIS

Type	Cause or Pathogenesis	Histology*	Clinical Features
Contact dermatitis	Topically applied chemicals Pathogenesis: delayed hypersensitivity	Spongiotic dermatitis	Marked itching, burning, or both; requires antecedent exposure
Atopic dermatitis	Unknown, may be heritable	Spongiotic dermatitis	Erythematous plaques in flexural areas; family history of eczema, hay fever, or asthma
Drug-related eczematous dermatitis	Systemically administered antigens or haptens (e.g., penicillin)	Spongiotic dermatitis; eosinophils often present in infiltrate; deeper infiltrate	Eruption occurs with administration of drug; remits when drug is discontinued
Photoeczematous eruption	Ultraviolet light	Spongiotic dermatitis; deeper infiltrate	Occurs on sun-exposed skin; phototesting may help in diagnosis
Primary irritant dermatitis	Repeated trauma (rubbing)	Spongiotic dermatitis in early stages; epidermal hyperplasia in late stages	Localized to site of trauma

*All types, with time, may develop chronic changes.

MORPHOLOGY

Spongiosis—the accumulation of edema fluid within the epidermis—characterizes acute eczematous dermatitis, hence the synonym "spongiotic dermatitis." Whereas in urticaria edema is localized to the perivascular spaces of the superficial dermis, in spongiotic dermatitis edema seeps into the intercellular spaces of the epidermis, splaying apart keratinocytes. Intercellular bridges become stretched and therefore more prominent, giving a "spongy" appearance to the epidermis (see Fig. 22–2B). These epidermal changes are accompanied by a superficial, perivascular, lymphocytic infiltrate associated with papillary dermal edema and mast cell degranulation. In some cases, eosinophils may also be present, a finding especially prominent in certain spongiotic eruptions provoked by drugs.

Spongiotic dermatitis caused by contact hypersensitivity (e.g., poison ivy dermatitis) is mediated by sensitized T cells (type IV hypersensitivity; Chapter 5). After initial exposure, antigens derived from poison ivy are processed by epidermal Langerhans cells, which then migrate to draining lymph nodes to present the antigen to naive T cells. This sensitization event leads to acquisition of immunologic memory, whereby on re-exposure to the antigen, the now-educated lymphocytes (memory T cells) release cytokines that recruit additional inflammatory cells and also mediate the epidermal change.

Figure 22–2

Eczematous dermatitis. *A,* Note the numerous blisters and marked redness confined to a field of contact allergy (here, the detergent used in laundering a long-sleeved shirt). *B,* The blisters are formed by fluid accumulation between epidermal cells, resulting in spongiosis and eventual separation of cell connections to form a vesicle filled with serum within the midepidermis.

Erythema Multiforme

Erythema multiforme is an uncommon, self-limited disorder that appears to be a *hypersensitivity response to certain infections and drugs*. It is associated with the following conditions: (1) infectious disorders (e.g., herpes simplex, *Mycoplasma* infections, histoplasmosis, coccidioidomycosis, typhoid, and leprosy); (2) administration of certain drugs (sulfonamides, penicillin, barbiturates, salicylates, hydantoins, and antimalarials); (3) malignancy (carcinomas and lymphomas); and (4) collagen vascular diseases (lupus erythematosus, dermatomyositis, and periarteritis nodosa).

Clinically, patients present with an array of *"multiform" lesions, including macules, papules, vesicles, and bullae, as well as the characteristic target lesion consisting of a red macule or papule with a pale vesicular or eroded center* (Fig. 22–3A). An extensive and symptomatic febrile form of the disease, more common in children, is called the Stevens-Johnson syndrome. It is marked by erosions and crusting of the mucosal surfaces of the lips, conjunctiva, oral cavity, urethra, and anogenital region. Another variant, termed *toxic epidermal necrolysis*, results in diffuse necrosis and sloughing of cutaneous and mucosal epithelial surfaces, producing a clinical situation analogous to an extensive burn.

MORPHOLOGY

Histologically, early lesions show a superficial perivascular, lymphocytic infiltrate associated with dermal edema and margination of lymphocytes along the dermoepidermal junction (Fig. 22–3B), where they are intimately associated with degenerating and necrotic keratinocytes. With time, discrete and confluent zones of epidermal necrosis occur, with concomitant blister formation.

The lesions of erythema multiforme are caused, in all likelihood, by cytotoxic T cells that may be targeting cross-reactive antigens in or near the basal cell layer of the skin and mucosae.

CHRONIC INFLAMMATORY DERMATOSES

This category focuses on those persistent inflammatory dermatoses that exhibit their most characteristic clinical and histologic features over many months to years. Unlike the normal cutaneous surface, the skin surface in some chronic inflammatory dermatoses is roughened as a result of excessive or abnormal scale formation and shedding (desquamation). Included in this category, but not described here, are cutaneous lesions of systemic lupus erythematosus (Chapter 5).

Psoriasis

Psoriasis is a common chronic inflammatory dermatosis affecting 1% to 2% of people in the United States. It is sometimes associated with arthritis, myopathy, enteropathy, spondylitic heart disease, and the acquired immunodeficiency syndrome.

Clinically, psoriasis most frequently affects the skin of the elbows, knees, scalp, lumbosacral areas, intergluteal cleft, and glans penis. *The most typical lesion is a well-demarcated, pink to salmon-colored plaque covered by loosely adherent scales that are characteristically silver-white* (Fig. 22–4). Nail changes occur in 30% of cases of psoriasis and consist of yellow-brown discoloration (often likened to an oil slick), with pitting, separation of the nail plate from the underlying bed (onycholysis), thickening, and crumbling. In the rare variant called pustular psoriasis, multiple small pustules form on erythematous plaques.

Figure 22–3

Erythema multiforme. *A,* The clinical lesions consist of a central zone of dusky pink–gray discoloration that correlates with epidermal necrosis or early blister formation, surrounded by a pink-red rim, producing the characteristic target-like appearance. *B,* Early lesions show alignment of lymphocytes along the dermoepidermal junction where basal epidermal cells have already become vacuolated as a result of the cytotoxic assault.

Figure 22-4 ■

Clinical presentations of psoriasis. Very early and active lesions, or certain rare variants *(left)*, may show multiple small pustules developing within reddened skin. More characteristic chronic plaques of psoriasis *(right)* show characteristically silvery-white scale on the surface of erythematous plaques.

MORPHOLOGY

There is increased epidermal cell turnover resulting in marked epidermal thickening (acanthosis), with regular downward elongation of the rete ridges (Fig. 22-5). **The stratum granulosum is thinned or absent, and extensive overlying parakeratotic scale is seen**. Typical of psoriatic plaques is thinning of the portion of the epidermal cell layer that overlies the tips of dermal papillae (suprapapillary plates) and dilated, tortuous blood vessels within these papillae. These blood vessels bleed readily when the scale is peeled back and the suprapapillary plates are unroofed, giving rise to multiple minute bleeding points **(Auspitz sign)**. Neutrophils form small aggregates within slightly spongiotic foci of the superficial epidermis **(spongiform pustules)** and within the parakeratotic stratum corneum **(Munro microabscesses)**.

The pathogenesis of psoriasis is not entirely clear. Like diabetes and hypertension, it seems to be multifactorial, with contributions from genetic susceptibility and environmental agents. Genome-wide scans in cases of familial psoriasis have revealed several distinct susceptibility loci. Regardless of the genetic factors, recent evidence suggests that the disease results when specifically sensitized populations of T cells enter the skin. Because certain HLA types are preferentially affected, it is likely that lesion development requires a combination of genetic and immune factors. T cells infiltrating the skin may create an abnormal microenvironment by secreting cytokines and growth factors that influence keratinocyte replication and senescence pathways, resulting in the characteristic inflammatory and proliferative lesions.

Lichen Planus

"Pruritic, purple, polygonal papules" are the presenting signs of this disorder of skin and mucous membranes. Lichen planus is self-limited and generally resolves spontaneously 1 to 2 years after onset, often leaving zones of postinflammatory hyperpigmentation. Oral lesions may persist for years.

Cutaneous lesions consist of *itchy, violaceous, flat-topped papules, which may coalesce focally to form plaques* (Fig. 22-6A). These papules are often highlighted by white dots or lines, called *Wickham striae*, and hyperpigmentation may result from melanin loss into the dermis from the damaged basal cell layer. Multiple lesions are characteristic and are symmetrically distributed, particularly on the extremities, often about the wrists and elbows, and on the glans penis. In 70% of cases, oral lesions are present as white, reticulated, or netlike areas involving the mucosa.

MORPHOLOGY

Lichen planus is characterized histologically by a dense, continuous infiltrate of lymphocytes along the dermoepidermal junction (Fig. 22-6B). The lymphocytes are intimately associated with basal keratinocytes, which show degeneration, necrosis, and a resemblance in size and contour to more mature cells of the stratum spinosum (squamatization). This pattern of inflammation causes the dermoepidermal interface to assume an angulated, zigzag contour ("sawtoothing"). Anucleate, necrotic basal cells may become incorporated into the inflamed papillary dermis, where they are referred to as colloid, or **Civatte, bodies**. Although these changes bear some similarities to those in erythema multiforme (discussed earlier), lichen planus shows changes of chronicity: epidermal hyperplasia (or

Figure 22-5 ■

Histology of psoriasis. Established plaques show marked epidermal hyperplasia with uniform downward extension of rete ridges as well as prominently increased scale that is parakeratotic and focally infiltrated by neutrophils. Blood vessels in the dermis are typically dilated and tortuous.

Figure 22-6   ■

Lichen planus. *A,* Multiple flat-topped papules have coalesced in this patient's extremity. The increased pigmentation is the result of chronic destruction of melanin-containing epidermal cells, with subsequent pigment accumulation in the underlying dermis. *B,* Histologically, there is a band of lymphocytes along a dermoepidermal junction where the rete ridges have acquired a pointed, or "sawtooth," architecture. Unlike erythema multiforme, the cytotoxic injury is chronic and the epidermis has responded with acanthosis, hypergranulosis, and hyperkeratosis.

rarely atrophy) and thickening of the granular cell layer and stratum corneum (hypergranulosis and hyperkeratosis, respectively).

The precise pathogenesis of lichen planus is not known. It is plausible that release of antigens at the levels of the basal cell layer and the dermoepidermal junction may elicit a cell-mediated cytotoxic immune response.

BLISTERING (BULLOUS) DISEASES

Although vesicles and bullae (blisters) occur as a secondary phenomenon in a number of unrelated conditions (e.g., herpesvirus infection, spongiotic dermatitis), there is a group of disorders in which blisters are the primary and most distinctive features. Blisters can occur at multiple levels within the skin, and assessment of these levels is essential to an accurate histologic diagnosis (Fig. 22-7).

Pemphigus

Pemphigus is a rare *autoimmune blistering disorder resulting from loss of the integrity of normal intercellular attachments within the epidermis and mucosal epithelium.* Most individuals who develop pemphigus are middle aged and older, and men and women are affected equally. There are four clinical and pathologic variants: (1) pemphigus vulgaris, (2) pemphigus vegetans, (3) pemphigus foliaceus, and (4) pemphigus erythematosus.

Pemphigus vulgaris, by far the most common type (accounting for over 80% of cases worldwide), involves mucosa and skin, especially on the scalp, face, axilla, groin, trunk, and points of pressure. The primary lesions are very superficial vesicles and bullae that rupture easily,

A   Subcorneal   B   Suprabasal   C   Subepidermal

Figure 22-7   ■

Schematic diagram of sites of blister formation. *A,* Subcorneal (as in impetigo and pemphigus foliaceus); *B,* suprabasal (as in pemphigus vulgaris); and *C,* subepidermal (as in bullous pemphigoid and dermatitis herpetiformis).

Figure 22–8

Pemphigus vulgaris. *A*, Eroded plaques in axilla were formed by the rapid rupture of fragile blisters with thin roofs. *B*, Suprabasal acantholysis results in an intraepidermal blister containing rounded keratinocytes that are separating from their neighbors *(inset)*.

leaving shallow erosions covered with dried serum and crust (Fig. 22–8*A*). *Pemphigus vegetans* is a rare form that usually presents not with blisters but with large, moist, verrucous (wartlike), vegetating plaques studded with pustules on the groin, axilla, and flexural surfaces. *Pemphigus foliaceus*, a more benign form of pemphigus, occurs in an epidemic form in South America, and there are isolated cases in other countries. Bullae are confined to skin, with only rare involvement of mucous membranes. They are so superficial that only zones of erythema and crusting, sites of previous blister rupture, are detected. *Pemphigus erythematosus* is considered a localized, less severe form of pemphigus foliaceus that may selectively involve the malar area of the face in a lupus erythematosus–like fashion.

MORPHOLOGY

The common histologic denominator in all forms of pemphigus is **acantholysis**. This term implies dissolution, or lysis, of the intercellular adhesion sites within a squamous epithelial surface. Detached from their moorings, acantholytic cells become rounded. In pemphigus vulgaris and pemphigus vegetans, acantholysis selectively involves the layer of cells immediately above the basal cell layer, giving rise to the **suprabasal acantholytic blister** characteristic of pemphigus vulgaris (Fig. 22–8*B*). In pemphigus foliaceus, acantholysis selectively involves the superficial epidermis at the level of the stratum granulosum. Variable superficial dermal infiltration by lymphocytes, histiocytes, and eosinophils accompanies all forms of pemphigus.

Pemphigus is caused by a type II hypersensitivity reaction (Chapter 5). Sera from patients with pemphigus contain pathogenic IgG antibodies to intercellular cement substance (desmogleins) of skin and mucous membranes.

By direct immunofluorescence, lesional sites show a characteristic netlike pattern of intercellular IgG deposits localized to sites of developed or incipient acantholysis (Fig. 22–9).

Bullous Pemphigoid

Generally affecting elderly individuals, bullous pemphigoid shows a wide range of clinical presentations, with localized to generalized cutaneous lesions and involvement of mucosal surfaces.

Clinically, *lesions are tense bullae, filled with clear fluid, on normal or erythematous skin* (Fig. 22–10*A*). The bullae do not rupture as easily as the blisters seen in pemphigus and, if uncomplicated by infection, heal without scarring.

Figure 22–9

Direct immunofluorescence of pemphigus vulgaris. There is deposition of immunoglobulin and complement *(indicated by green)* along the cell membranes of keratinocytes, producing a characteristic "fish net" appearance. Note the early suprabasal separation associated with the autoantibody deposition.

Figure 22-10

Bullous pemphigoid. *A*, Tense fluid-filled blisters result from vacuolization of basal layer, producing subepidermal blisters. *B*, Histologically, the basal cell layer is vacuolated in association with an inflammatory infiltrate containing eosinophils, lymphocytes, and occasional neutrophils.

Sites of occurrence include the inner aspects of the thighs, flexor surfaces of the forearms, axillae, groin, and lower abdomen. Oral involvement is present in up to one third of patients.

MORPHOLOGY

Bullous pemphigoid is characterized by a **subepidermal, nonacantholytic** blister. Early lesions show a perivascular infiltrate of lymphocytes and variable numbers of eosinophils, occasional neutrophils, superficial dermal edema, and associated basal cell layer vacuolization. The vacuolated basal cell layer eventually gives rise to a fluid-filled blister (Fig. 22–10*B*). Because the blister roof involves full-thickness epidermis, it is more resistant to rupture than the blister in pemphigus.

The immunopathology of bullous pemphigoid features *linear* deposition of immunoglobulin and complement in the basement membrane zone (Fig. 22–11*A*). Ultrastructural studies have shown that circulating antibody reacts with an antigen that extends into the narrow clear zone (lamina lucida) of the epidermal basement membrane that separates the underlying lamina densa from the plasma membrane of the basal cells (Fig. 22–11*B*). Reactivity also occurs in the basal cell–basement membrane attachment plaques (hemidesmosomes), where most of the bullous pemphigoid antigen, a protein involved normally in dermoepidermal bonding, is actually located. It is likely that the generation of autoantibodies to this hemidesmosome component results in the fixation of complement and subsequent tissue injury at this site by means of locally recruited neutrophils and eosinophils. Like pemphigus vulgaris, bullous pemphigoid is also caused by a type II hypersensitivity reaction, but the target antigens are different in the two conditions.

Figure 22-11

Immunopathology of bullous pemphigoid. *A*, Antibody and complement are seen by direct immunofluorescence as a linear band outlining the subepidermal basement membrane zone. *B*, The autoantibodies react with a protein in the lowermost regions of the basal cell cytoplasm, near the hemidesmosomes (HD) and the underlying lamina lucida of the basement membrane (LL). AF, Anchoring fibrils connecting the basement membrane to the underlying dermis; LD, lamina densa of basement membrane.

Dermatitis Herpetiformis

Dermatitis herpetiformis is a rare and fascinating disorder characterized by *urticaria and grouped vesicles*. Males tend to be affected more frequently than females, and the age at onset is often in the third and fourth decades. In some cases it occurs in association with intestinal celiac disease and responds to a gluten-free diet (Chapter 15).

The urticarial plaques and vesicles of dermatitis herpetiformis are extremely *pruritic*. They characteristically occur bilaterally and symmetrically, involving preferentially the extensor surfaces, elbows, knees, upper back, and buttocks. *Vesicles are frequently grouped*, as are those of true herpesvirus, hence the name "herpetiformis" (Fig. 22–12A).

MORPHOLOGY

In the early stages of the disease, fibrin and neutrophils accumulate selectively at the **tips of dermal papillae**, forming small microabscesses (Fig. 22–12B). The basal cells overlying these microabscesses show vacuolization and minute zones of dermoepidermal separation (microscopic blisters). In time, these zones coalesce to form a true **subepidermal blister**. By direct immunofluorescence, dermatitis herpetiformis shows granular deposits of **IgA** selectively localized in the tips of dermal papillae, where they are deposited on anchoring fibrils (Fig. 22–12C).

The association of dermatitis herpetiformis with celiac disease provides a critical clue to its pathogenesis. It seems that some genetically predisposed individuals develop antibodies to dietary gluten (derived from wheat). Because B cells in the gut generate many of these autoantibodies, they tend to be of the IgA class. These IgA antibodies cross-react with reticulin, a component of the anchoring fibrils that tether the epidermal basement membrane to the superficial dermis. Although it is clear that some patients with dermatitis herpetiformis and enteropathy respond to a gluten-free diet (as with celiac disease), the immunopathogenesis of the disease remains to be fully clarified.

TUMORS

Benign and Premalignant Epithelial Lesions

Benign epithelial neoplasms are common and usually biologically inconsequential. These tumors are probably derived from primitive stem cells that reside in the epidermis and hair follicles, and they tend to differentiate toward cells and structures in the epidermis and adnexa. The overwhelming majority do not undergo malignant transformation; only some, such as actinic keratosis, have malignant potential. In the ensuing discussion, some common epidermal lesions are described. Tumors differentiating toward hair follicles and other appendages (adnexal tumors) are too infrequent to merit further consideration here.

SEBORRHEIC KERATOSIS

These common epidermal tumors occur most frequently in middle-aged or older individuals. They arise spontaneously and may become particularly numerous on the trunk, although the extremities, head, and neck may also be involved.

Clinically, seborrheic keratoses appear as *round, flat, coinlike plaques that vary in diameter from millimeters to several centimeters* (Fig. 22–13A). They are uniformly tan to dark brown and usually show a velvety to granular surface. Occasionally, they become inflamed or mimic melanoma, warranting their removal.

Figure 22–12

Dermatitis herpetiformis. *A*, Clinical lesions consist of intact and eroded (usually scratched) erythematous and often grouped blisters. *B*, The blisters are associated with basal cell layer injury initially caused by accumulation of neutrophils (microabscesses) at the tips of dermal papillae. *C*, The initial event, as seen in this direct immunofluorescence image, is selective deposition of IgA autoantibody at the tips of dermal papillae.

Figure 22-13 ■

Seborrheic keratosis. *A*, Multiple coinlike brown lesions almost appear to be "stuck on" the skin. *B*, Histologically the lesions are formed by orderly proliferation of uniform, benign basaloid keratinocytes with a tendency to make keratin microcysts (horn cysts, *lower right*).

MORPHOLOGY

Histologically, these neoplasms are exophytic and are demarcated sharply from the adjacent epidermis. They are composed of sheets of small cells that most resemble basal cells of the normal epidermis (Fig. 22-13*B*). Variable melanin pigmentation is present within these basaloid cells, accounting for the brown coloration seen clinically that may mimic melanoma. Exuberant keratin production (hyperkeratosis) occurs at the surface of seborrheic keratoses, and the presence of small keratin-filled cysts (horn cysts) and downgrowths of keratin into the main tumor mass (pseudo-horn cysts) are characteristic features.

MORPHOLOGY

Histologically, keratoacanthomas are characterized by a central keratin-filled crater surrounded by proliferating epithelial cells that extend upward in a liplike fashion over the sides of the crater and downward into the dermis as irregular tongues (Fig. 22-14*A*). This epithelium is composed of enlarged cells showing evidence of reactive cytologic atypia. These cells have a characteristically "glassy" eosinophilic cytoplasm (Fig. 22-14*B*) and produce keratin abruptly, as normally occurs in the midportion of the hair follicle (without the development of the intervening granular cell layer that characterizes epidermal keratinization).

Seborrheic keratosis is an indolent and benign neoplasm that is readily treated by excision. The explosive onset of hundreds of lesions may occur as a *paraneoplastic syndrome* in rare cases. Patients with this presentation may harbor internal malignancies that produce growth factors that stimulate epidermal proliferation.

KERATOACANTHOMA

Keratoacanthoma is a rapidly developing neoplasm that clinically and histologically may mimic well-differentiated squamous cell carcinoma (see later discussion), but it heals spontaneously without treatment. Men are affected more often than women, and lesions most frequently affect sun-exposed skin of whites older than 50 years of age.

Clinically, keratoacanthomas appear as *flesh-colored, dome-shaped nodules with a central, keratin-filled plug*, imparting a crater-like topography. Lesions range in size from 1 cm to several centimeters across and have a predilection for the cheeks, nose, ears, and dorsa of the hands.

VERRUCAE (WARTS)

Verrucae are common lesions of children and adolescents, although they may be encountered at any age. They are caused by human papillomaviruses (HPVs). Transmission of disease usually involves direct contact between individuals or autoinoculation. Verrucae are generally self-limited, regressing spontaneously within 6 months to 2 years.

Warts can be classified into several types on the basis of their morphology and location. In addition, each type of wart is caused by a different HPV type. *Verruca vulgaris* is the most common type of wart. These lesions occur anywhere but are found most frequently on the hands, particularly on the dorsal surfaces and periungual areas, where they appear as gray-white to tan, flat to convex, 0.1- to 1-cm papules with a rough, pebble-like surface (Fig. 22-15*A*). *Verruca plana*, or *flat wart*, is common on the face or dorsal surfaces of the hands. These warts are slightly elevated, flat, smooth, tan papules that are generally smaller than those of verruca vulgaris. *Verruca plantaris* and *verruca palmaris* occur on the soles and palms, respectively. Rough, scaly lesions may reach 1 to 2 cm in diameter, coalesce, and be

Figure 22-14 ■

Keratoacanthoma. *A,* The tumor appears benign in profile, forming a symmetric crater-like nodule giving rise to a central plug of keratotic material. *B,* On higher magnification, apparent dermal invasion by somewhat atypical and enlarged tumor cells is observed. (*A,* From Murphy GF, Herzberg AJ: Atlas of Dermatopathology. Philadelphia, WB Saunders, 1996.)

Figure 22-15 ■

Verruca vulgaris. *A,* Multiple papules with rough, pebble-like surfaces are present at inoculation sites. *B,* Microscopically, lesions are formed by symmetric zones of papillary epidermal proliferation that often radiate symmetrically like the points of a crown. Cytoplasmic clearing (koilocytosis) and related cytopathic changes of human papillomavirus are confirmed at higher magnification *(bottom).*

confused with ordinary calluses. *Condyloma acuminatum (venereal wart)* occurs on the penis, female genitalia, urethra, perianal areas, and rectum. These lesions appear as soft, tan, cauliflower-like masses that sometimes reach many centimeters in diameter (Chapter 19).

MORPHOLOGY

Histologic features common to verrucae include epidermal hyperplasia that is often undulant in character (so-called verrucous or papillomatous epidermal hyperplasia; Fig. 22-15B, *upper panel*) and cytoplasmic vacuolization (koilocytosis) that preferentially involves the more superficial epidermal layers, producing halos of pallor surrounding infected nuclei (see Fig. 22-15B, *lower panel,* and Fig. 19-3). Infected cells may also demonstrate prominent and apparently condensed keratohyaline granules and jagged eosinophilic intracytoplasmic keratin aggregates as a result of viral cytopathic effects.

As mentioned previously, verrucae are caused by HPV, the virus associated with preneoplastic and invasive cancers of the anogenital region (Chapters 18 and 19). However, in contrast to HPV-associated carcinomas, most warts are caused by distinct HPV types that do not have the potential for causing malignant transformation in immunologically normal individuals.

ACTINIC KERATOSIS

Before the development of overt malignancy of the epidermis, a series of progressively dysplastic changes occur, a phenomenon analogous to the atypia that precedes carcinoma of the squamous mucosa of the uterine cervix (Chapter 19). Because this dysplasia in the skin is usually the result of chronic exposure to sunlight and is associated with build-up of excess keratin, these lesions are called actinic keratoses.

Figure 22-16

Actinic keratosis. *A,* Although most lesions form subtle zones of redness or sandpaper-like keratinization, this one has formed so much abnormal scale that a small "cutaneous horn" is apparent. *B,* Basal cell layer atypia (dysplasia) is associated with marked hyperkeratosis and parakeratosis. *C,* More advanced lesions show foci of full-thickness atypia, qualifying as carcinoma in situ.

Lesions of actinic keratosis are usually *less than 1 cm in diameter*; *are tan-brown, red, or skin colored*; *and have a rough, sandpaper-like consistency.* Some lesions may produce so much keratin that a "cutaneous horn" develops (Fig. 22-16A). As would be expected, skin sites commonly involved by sun exposure (face, arms, dorsum of the hands) are most frequently affected.

> ### MORPHOLOGY
>
> Cytologic atypia is seen in the lowermost layers of the epidermis and may be associated with hyperplasia of basal cells (Fig. 22-16B) or with early atrophy that results in diffuse thinning of the epidermal surface of the lesion. The dermis contains thickened, blue-gray elastic fibers (elastosis), a probable result of abnormal dermal elastic fiber synthesis by sun-damaged fibroblasts within the superficial dermis. The stratum corneum is thickened and, unlike in normal skin, nuclei in the cells in this layer are often retained (a pattern called "parakeratosis"). Some but not all lesions progress to full-thickness atypia, qualifying as squamous cell carcinoma in situ.

Whether all actinic keratoses would result in skin cancer (usually squamous cell carcinoma) if given enough time is conjectural. Indeed, it is likely that many lesions regress or remain stable during a normal life span. However, enough do become malignant to warrant local eradication of these precursor lesions.

Malignant Epidermal Tumors

SQUAMOUS CELL CARCINOMA

Squamous cell carcinoma is *the most common tumor arising on sun-exposed sites in older people.* Except for lesions on the lower legs, these tumors have a higher incidence in men than in women. Implicated as predisposing factors, in addition to sunlight, are industrial carcinogens (tars and oils), chronic ulcers and draining osteomyelitis, old burn scars, ingestion of arsenicals, ionizing radiation, and (in the oral cavity) tobacco and betel nut chewing. Indeed, the incidence of oral squamous cell carcinomas is quite high in certain regions of India, where betel nut chewing is fairly common.

Squamous cell carcinomas that have not invaded through the basement membrane of the dermoepidermal junction *(in situ carcinoma)* appear as sharply defined, red, scaling plaques. More advanced, invasive lesions are nodular, show variable keratin production appreciated clinically as hyperkeratosis, and may ulcerate (Fig. 22-17A).

> ### MORPHOLOGY
>
> Unlike actinic keratosis, squamous cell carcinoma in situ is characterized by highly atypical cells at **all levels** of the epidermis (see Fig. 22-16C). When these cells break through the basement membrane, the process has become invasive (Fig. 22-17B). Invasive squamous cell carcinomas exhibit variable differentiation, ranging from tumors formed by polygonal squamous cells arranged in orderly

Figure 22–17 ■

Invasive squamous cell carcinoma. *A,* A nodular and ulcerated lesion occurring on chronically sun-damaged skin. *B,* The carcinoma invades the dermis as irregular tongues of atypical squamous epithelium. *C,* Cytologically, the tumor cells have abundant, "squamoid" cytoplasm and contain enlarged and dark-stained nuclei with angulated contours and prominent nucleoli.

lobules that exhibit numerous large zones of keratinization (Fig. 22–17C) to neoplasms formed by highly anaplastic, rounded cells with foci of necrosis and only abortive, single-cell keratinization (dyskeratosis).

Invasive squamous cell carcinomas of the skin are usually discovered while small and resectable; less than 5% have metastases to regional nodes at diagnosis.

The most common exogenous cause of squamous cell carcinoma is exposure to ultraviolet light, with subsequent unrepaired DNA damage (Chapter 6). Individuals who are immunosuppressed as a result of chemotherapy or organ transplantation or who have *xeroderma pigmentosum* are at increased risk for developing these tumors. In addition to their effect on DNA, ultraviolet rays in sunlight also seem to exert at least a transient immunosuppressive effect on skin by impairing antigen presentation by Langerhans cells. This may contribute to tumorigenesis by impairing immunosurveillance.

BASAL CELL CARCINOMA

Basal cell carcinomas are common, *slow-growing tumors that rarely metastasize*. They have a tendency to occur at sites subject to chronic sun exposure and in lightly pigmented people. As with squamous cell carcinoma, the incidence of basal cell carcinoma rises sharply with immunosuppression and in patients with inherited defects in DNA replication or repair (xeroderma pigmentosum; Chapter 6). →

Clinically, these tumors present as *pearly papules, often containing prominent, dilated subepidermal blood vessels (telangiectasia)* (Fig. 22–18A). Some tumors contain melanin pigment and thus appear similar to nevocellular nevi or melanomas. Advanced lesions may ulcerate, and extensive local invasion of bone or facial sinuses may occur after many years of neglect, justifying the past designation "rodent ulcers."

MORPHOLOGY

Histologically, tumor cells resemble those in the normal basal cell layer of the epidermis. Because they arise from the epidermis or follicular epithelium, they are not encountered on mucosal surfaces. Two patterns are seen, either **multifocal growths** originating from the epidermis and extending over several square centimeters or more of skin surface (multifocal superficial type), or **nodular lesions** growing downward deeply into the dermis as cords and islands of variably basophilic cells with hyperchromatic nuclei, embedded in a mucinous matrix, and often surrounded by many fibroblasts and lymphocytes (Fig. 22–18B). The cells forming the periphery of the tumor cell islands tend to be arranged radially with their long axes in approximately parallel alignment (palisading). The stroma shrinks away from the epithelial tumor nests, creating clefts or separation artifacts, which assist in differentiating basal cell carcinomas from certain appendage tumors (Fig. 22–18C).

Figure 22–18   ■

Basal cell carcinoma. *A,* A prototypical lesion is a pearly, smooth-surfaced papule or nodule with associated telangiectatic vessels. *B,* The lesion is formed by multiple islands of basaloid cells infiltrating a fibrotic stroma. *C,* Cytologically, the cells have scant cytoplasm, dark-stained small nuclei, and a palisaded periphery separated from the adjacent stroma by a typical cleftlike space (separation artifact).

Tumors and Tumor-like Lesions of Melanocytes

NEVOCELLULAR NEVUS (PIGMENTED NEVUS, MOLE)

Strictly speaking, the term *nevus* denotes any congenital lesion of the skin. *Nevocellular* nevus, however, refers to any congenital or acquired neoplasm of melanocytes.

Clinically, common acquired nevocellular nevi are tan-to-brown, uniformly pigmented, small (usually 5 mm or less across), solid regions of elevated skin (papules) with well-defined, rounded borders (Fig. 22–19A). There are numerous clinical and histologic types of nevocellular nevi, and the clinical appearance may be variable. Table 22–2 provides a comparative summary of salient clinical and histologic features of the more commonly encountered forms of melanocytic nevi.

Figure 22–19   ■

Nevocellular nevus. *A,* Clinically, compound and dermal nevi are relatively small, symmetric, uniformly pigmented lesions that reach a stable size and then do not show further growth. *B,* Histologically, this compound nevus shows rounded nests formed by uniform nevus cells at the dermal-epidermal junction and within the underlying dermis.

Table 22–2. VARIANT FORMS OF NEVOCELLULAR NEVI

Nevus Variant	Diagnostic Architectural Features	Diagnostic Cytologic Features	Clinical Significance
Congenital nevus	Deep dermal and sometimes subcutaneous growth around adnexa, neurovascular bundles, and blood vessel walls	Identical to ordinary acquired nevi	Present at birth; large variants carry increased melanoma risk
Blue nevus	Non-nested dermal infiltration, often with associated fibrosis	Highly dendritic, heavily pigmented nevus cells	Black-blue nodule; often confused with melanoma clinically
Spindle and epithelioid cell nevus (Spitz nevus)	Fascicular growth	Large, plump cells with pink-blue cytoplasm; fusiform cells	Common in children; red-pink nodule; often confused with hemangioma clinically
Halo nevus	Lymphocytic infiltration surrounding nevus cells	Identical to ordinary acquired nevi	Host immune response against nevus cells and surrounding normal melanocytes
Dysplastic nevus	Large, coalescent intraepidermal nests	Cytologic atypia	Potential precursor of malignant melanoma

MORPHOLOGY

Nevocellular nevi are formed by melanocytes that have been transformed from highly dendritic single cells, normally interspersed among basal keratinocytes, to round-to-oval cells that grow in aggregates, or "nests," along the dermoepidermal junction. Nuclei of nevus cells are uniform and rounded, contain inconspicuous nucleoli, and show little or no mitotic activity. Such lesions, believed to represent an early developmental stage in nevocellular nevi, are called **junctional nevi.** Eventually, most junctional nevi grow into the underlying dermis (Fig. 22–19B) as nests or cords of cells **(compound nevi),** and in older lesions the epidermal nests may be lost entirely to leave pure **dermal nevi.** Clinically, compound and dermal nevi are often more elevated than are junctional nevi.

Progressive growth of nevus cells from the dermoepidermal junction into the underlying dermis is accompanied by a process termed *maturation.* Whereas less mature, more superficial nevus cells are larger, tend to produce melanin pigment, and grow in nests, more mature, deeper nevus cells are smaller, produce little or no pigment, and grow in cords. This sequence of maturation of individual nevus cells is of diagnostic importance in distinguishing some benign nevi from melanomas, which usually show little or no maturation.

Although nevocellular nevi are common and benign, it is important to recognize their distinctive features, lest they become confused with other skin conditions, notably malignant melanoma.

DYSPLASTIC NEVI

Dysplastic nevi may occur *sporadically or in a familial form.* The hereditary forms are inherited in an autosomal dominant fashion and are considered precursors of malignant melanoma. In the sporadic form, the risk of malignant transformation appears low.

Clinically, *dysplastic nevi are larger than most acquired nevi* (often more than 5 mm across) and may occur as hundreds of lesions on the body surface. They are flat macules to slightly raised plaques, with a "pebbly" surface. They usually show variability in pigmentation (variegation) and borders that are irregular in contour. Unlike ordinary moles, *dysplastic nevi have a tendency to occur on non–sun-exposed as well as sun-exposed body surfaces.* Dysplastic nevi have been documented in multiple members of families prone to the development of malignant melanoma (the "heritable melanoma syndrome").

MORPHOLOGY

Histologically (Fig. 22–20A), dysplastic nevi consist of compound nevi with both architectural and cytologic evidence of abnormal growth. **Nevus cell nests within the epidermis may be enlarged and exhibit abnormal fusion or coalescence with adjacent nests. As part of this process, single nevus cells begin to replace the normal basal cell layer along the dermoepidermal junction, producing so-called lentiginous hyperplasia.** Cytologic atypia consisting of irregular, often angulated, nuclear contours and hyperchromasia is frequently observed (Fig. 22–20B). Associated alterations also occur in the superficial dermis. These consist of a usually sparse lymphocytic infiltrate, loss of melanin pigment from presumably destroyed nevus cells, phagocytosis of this pigment by dermal macrophages (melanin pigment incontinence), and a peculiar linear fibrosis surrounding the epidermal rete ridges that are involved by the nevus.

The evidence that some dysplastic nevi are precursors of malignant melanoma is impressive. In individuals with a family history of malignant melanoma, the melanomas occur only in individuals who first develop dysplastic nevi. In these cases, the lifetime risk of malignant degeneration in dysplastic nevi is close to 100%.

Figure 22-20

Dysplastic nevus. *A,* The lesion has a compound nevus component *(right)* and an asymmetric "shoulder" of exclusively junctional proliferation *(left)*. The former correlates with the more pigmented and raised central zone *(inset)*, and the latter with the less pigmented flat rim at the periphery. *B,* An important feature is the presence of cytologic atypia (irregular, dark-staining nuclei) at high magnification. The dermis characteristically shows parallel bands of fibrosis.

MALIGNANT MELANOMA

Malignant melanoma is a relatively common neoplasm that not long ago was considered almost uniformly deadly. Today, as a result of increased public awareness of the earliest signs of skin melanomas, most are cured surgically. Nonetheless, the incidence of these lesions is on the rise, necessitating vigorous surveillance for their development.

Although most of these lesions arise in the skin, other sites of origin include the *oral* and *anogenital mucosal surfaces*, the *esophagus*, the *meninges*, and notably the *eye*. The following comments apply to cutaneous melanomas; intraocular melanomas are briefly discussed later.

As with other cutaneous malignancies, sunlight plays an important role in the development of malignant melanoma. The incidence is highest in sun-exposed skin and in geographic locales such as New Zealand and Australia, where sun exposure is high. Sunlight, however, does not seem to be the only predisposing factor, and the presence of a preexisting nevus (e.g., a dysplastic nevus), hereditary factors, or even exposure to certain carcinogens may play a role in lesion development and evolution. As with several other common neoplasms (e.g., of the breast or colon), melanomas occur sporadically, but a small fraction are hereditary and familial. Molecular genetic analysis of such familial as well as sporadic cases has provided important insights into the pathogenesis of melanoma. Germ-line mutations in the *CDKN2A (p16)* gene (located on 9p21), which encodes for a cyclin-dependent kinase inhibitor, are found in approximately 50% of melanoma patients with 9p linkage. In some other familial cases, the *CDNK2A* gene is silenced by methylation. Mutational loss of the *PTEN* gene on 10q23.3 is also common in certain primary melanomas. Several other tumor suppressor genes, including some located on chromosomes 1p36 and 6p, have also been implicated in some cases. Surprisingly, unlike in most malignancies, deletion of *TP53* is quite uncommon in melanomas. Perhaps this is explained by the overlapping cycle control functions of *CDNK2A* and *TP53*.

Clinically, malignant melanoma of the skin is usually asymptomatic, although itching may be an early manifestation. *The most important clinical sign of the disease is a change in the color or size in a pigmented lesion.* Unlike benign (nondysplastic) nevi, melanomas exhibit striking variations in pigmentation, appearing in shades of black, brown, red, dark blue, and gray (Fig. 22–21*A*). The borders of melanomas are irregular and often "notched." In summary, the clinical warning signs of melanoma are (1) enlargement of a preexisting mole, (2) itching or pain in a preexisting mole, (3) development of a new pigmented lesion during adult life, (4) irregularity of the borders of a pigmented lesion, and (5) variegation of color within a pigmented lesion.

Central to an understanding of the complicated histology of malignant melanoma is the concept of radial and vertical growth. Simply stated, *radial growth* indicates the initial tendency of a melanoma to grow horizontally within the epidermal and superficial dermal layers, often for a prolonged period (Fig. 22–21*B*). During this stage of growth, melanoma cells do not have the capacity to metastasize, and there is no evidence of angiogenesis. With time, the pattern of growth assumes a *vertical component*, and the melanoma now grows downward into the deeper dermal layers as an expansile mass lacking cellular maturation, without any tendency for the cells to become smaller as they descend into the reticular dermis (Fig. 22–21*C*). This event is heralded clinically by the development of a nodule in the relatively flat radial growth phase and correlates with the emergence of a clone of cells with metastatic potential; concurrently, angiogenesis is switched on. The probability of metastasis in such a lesion may be predicted by simply measuring in millimeters the depth of invasion of this vertical growth phase nodule below the granular cell layer of the overlying epidermis. *Metastases involve not only regional lymph nodes but also liver, lungs, brain, and virtually any other site that can be seeded by the hematogenous route.* Remarkably, in some cases, metastases may appear for the first time many years after surgical excision of the primary tumor, suggesting a long phase of dormancy.

Figure 22–21

Malignant melanoma. *A,* Lesions clinically tend to be larger than nevi and are irregular in contour and pigmentation. Macular areas correspond to early superficial (radial) growth, while raised areas generally indicate significant dermal invasion (vertical growth). *B,* Radial growth, showing irregular nested and single-cell spread of melanoma cells in the epidermis. *C,* Vertical growth showing nodular aggregates of malignant cells extending deeply within the dermis. *D,* Cytologically, these cells have dark-stained nuclei of nonuniform sizes and shapes with prominent nucleoli.

MORPHOLOGY

Individual melanoma cells are usually considerably larger than nevus cells. They contain large nuclei with irregular contours having chromatin characteristically clumped at the periphery of the nuclear membrane and prominent red (eosinophilic) nucleoli (Fig. 22–21D). These cells grow as poorly formed nests or as individual cells at all levels of the epidermis and, in the dermis, as expansile, balloon-like nodules, as part of the radial and vertical growth phases, respectively (see Fig. 22–21B, C).

The nature and extent of the vertical growth phase determine the biologic behavior of malignant melanomas, and thus it is important to observe and record vertical growth phase parameters. These parameters include mitotic rate and presence of tumor-infiltrating lymphocytes. By using these variables in aggregate for vertical growth phase melanomas, accurate predictive statements regarding prognosis are possible that may assist in implementation of adjunctive therapy and follow-up protocols.

Melanoma of the eye is about one twentieth as common as melanoma of the skin. Most intraocular melanomas arise in the melanocytes of the uvea (iris, ciliary body, and choroid), but they can also originate in the pigmented epithelium of the retina. Unlike the cutaneous type, ocular melanomas are composed of two distinctive cell types, spindle and epithelioid, having differing clinical implications. Lesions composed completely or predominantly of spindle cells are of low aggressiveness, do not tend to metastasize, and permit about 75% 15-year survival. In contrast, epithelioid melanomas provide only about 35% survival at 15 years despite early enucleation, owing to late metastasis.

BIBLIOGRAPHY

Costello P, FitzGerald O: Disease mechanisms in psoriasis and psoriatic arthritis. Curr Rheumatol Rep 3:419, 2001. (A summary of pathogenesis of psoriasis.)

Cotell S, Robinson ND, Chan LS: Autoimmune blistering diseases. Am J Emerg Med 18:288, 2000. (A good clinical review of pemphigus, bullous pemphigoid, and epidermolysis bullosa.)

Hertl M: Humeral and cellular autoimmunity in autoimmune bullous skin disorders. Int Arch Allergy Immunol 122:91, 2000. (A very good discussion of the immunology of blistering disease.)

Katta R: Lichen planus. Am Fam Physician 61:3319, 2000. (A review of clinical features and etiologic factors.)

Shelton RM. Skin cancer: A review and atlas for medical providers. Mt. Sinai J Med 68:243, 2001. (A clinically oriented review of common skin cancers.)

Slominski A, et al: Malignant melanoma. Arch Pathol Lab Med 125:1295, 2001. (A review that covers etiology, pathogenesis and diagnostic methods.)

23

The Nervous System

DENNIS K. BURNS, MD
VINAY KUMAR, MD

The nervous system is the major communications network in the human body. As in other vertebrates, its normal function in humans is exquisitely dependent on the maintenance of structural integrity, as well as a host of complex metabolic processes. Accordingly, processes that disrupt normal structure or metabolism, or both, are capable of producing neurologic disease.

Disorders of the nervous system are often regarded as more complex or arcane than those in other organ systems. When allowances are made for the unique structural and cellular characteristics of the nervous system, however, neuropathologic processes can be understood in the context of the principles introduced in the general pathology sections of this text.

To gain an understanding of disorders affecting the nervous system, it is appropriate to review some of the important structural features of the central nervous system (CNS) and its cellular composition. At the outset, it is important to recall that signals to and from different regions of the body are controlled by very specific areas within the nervous system. This renders the nervous system vulnerable to focal lesions that in other organ systems might produce no significant dysfunction. As an example, an isolated renal infarct would not be expected to have a significant effect on renal function. An infarct of comparable size in the posterior limb of the internal capsule of the brain, in contrast, would be expected to leave a patient with complete paralysis on the contralateral side of the body.

The nervous system has certain anatomic features that confer protection against some insults while simultaneously rendering it more vulnerable to others. An important example of this is the cranial vault, the rigid confines of which protect the brain from trauma and noxious elements in the external environment. However, this same protective shield also renders the brain vulnerable to expansile intracranial lesions, which raise intracranial pressure because of the unyielding nature of the skull and may thereby compromise the function of the organ.

The brain parenchyma is composed of neurons supported by a framework of glial cells (astrocytes, oligodendrocytes, and ependyma), blood vessels, and microglia. The processes of these cells combine to form a delicate fibrillar background termed the *neuropil*.

CELLS OF THE NERVOUS SYSTEM

Neurons

The neurons are a heterogeneous family, both morphologically and functionally, ranging from the small round cells that populate the granule cell layer of the cerebellum to the large, pyramidal Betz cells of the primary motor cortex.

A variety of morphologic alterations may be encountered in neurons, one of the most common of which is *coagulation necrosis*, a change occurring most frequently in association with hypoxic-ischemic injury (discussed later). As in the case of coagulation necrosis in other sites, neuronal necrosis is characterized by a loss of cytoplasmic ribonucleoproteins and denaturation of cytoskeletal proteins, resulting in the development of intense cytoplasmic eosinophilia ("red neurons") in hematoxylin and eosin (H & E)–stained sections. Coagulation necrosis is also accompanied by nuclear changes identical to those seen in other organs, including condensation of nuclear material (pyknosis) and loss of nuclear staining (karyolysis). A second important form of cell death discussed earlier in this book, *apoptosis*, also occurs in a number of situations in the CNS, including normal development, some forms of hypoxic-ischemic injury, and certain toxic insults. Apoptosis may also contribute to cell loss during aging and in certain neurodegenerative disorders (discussed later). Chromatolysis, a common reaction to axonal injury, is characterized by dispersion of the Nissl substance and swelling of the neuronal cell body. A wide range of neuronal alterations also occur in neurodegenerative diseases, exemplified by neurofibrillary tangles in Alzheimer disease and Lewy body formation in Parkinson disease. Finally, a number of infectious agents may produce characteristic nuclear or cytoplasmic inclusions within neurons. These inclusions and other structural changes will be considered in greater detail later in the chapter in the context of the diseases in which they occur.

Astrocytes

Astrocytes are the major supporting cells in the brain and show some of the most common reactive changes. In cases of brain parenchymal injury, astrocytes respond by producing a dense network of processes, somewhat analogous to a fibrous scar occurring elsewhere in the body. In contrast to fibroblasts, however, astrocytes do not produce collagen. The glial "scar," accordingly, is made up predominantly of cytoplasmic processes, with little or no extracellular protein. The cytoplasm of astrocytes may swell in response to injury, often in association with increased synthesis of glial fibrillary acidic protein (GFAP), the astrocyte's major cytoskeletal protein. The cytoplasm around the nucleus of such cells, termed *gemistocytic astrocytes* (Greek, *gemistos* = "full"), is eosinophilic and readily visualized in routine sections. *Rosenthal fibers* represent yet another distinctive astrocytic structure. In H & E–stained sections, they appear as brightly eosinophilic structures with an almost refractile quality. Rosenthal fibers are derived from altered GFAP filaments and are encountered in a number of slowly growing neoplasms as well as in some non-neoplastic disorders, such as chronic cystic lesions and vascular malformations. Certain metabolic disturbances, notably liver failure, produce astrocytes with enlarged, pale nuclei, termed *Alzheimer type II glia*. Finally, glycoprotein-rich materials, termed *corpora amylacea*, commonly accumulate in astrocytic processes with age. In H & E–stained sections, corpora amylacea appear as spherical, concentrically laminated basophilic bodies in regions rich in astrocytic foot processes (e.g., the subependymal, subpial, and perivascular regions), as well as within the dorsal columns of the spinal cord.

Oligodendrocytes

Oligodendroglial cytoplasmic processes wrap around the axons of neurons to form myelin in a manner analogous to the Schwann cells of the peripheral nervous system. In routine sections, oligodendroglia are recognizable by their small, rounded, lymphocyte-like nuclei, often arranged in linear arrays. Injury to oligodendroglial cells and/or their processes is a feature of acquired demyelinating disorders (e.g., multiple sclerosis) and is also seen in the leukodystrophies (discussed later). Oligodendroglial nuclei may harbor inclusions in certain conditions, such as progressive multifocal leukoencephalopathy and some neurodegenerative disorders.

Ependymal Cells

Ependymal cells line the cerebral ventricles and are closely related to the cuboidal cells that invest the choroid plexus. Disruption of ependymal cells is often associated with a local proliferation of subependymal astrocytes to produce small irregularities termed *ependymal granulations* on the ventricular surfaces. Certain infectious agents, particularly cytomegalovirus (CMV), may produce extensive ependymal injury associated with prominent intranuclear inclusions in ependymal cells.

Microglia

Despite their name, it is now generally accepted that microglia are derived from circulating monocytes rather than from the neural tube. The many functions of these ubiquitous cells are only now becoming clear. Like their counterparts outside the CNS, microglia appear to serve as antigen-presenting cells in many inflammatory conditions. Virtually any form of CNS injury is associated with the presence of activated microglial cells; these then behave as active macrophages. In the setting of tissue necrosis and demyelinating diseases, such activated macrophages may accumulate abundant intracellular lipid to form cells with foamy cytoplasm, termed *gitter cells*. In other conditions, the nuclei of microglia may elongate to form *rod cells*. Microglia may also aggregate in compact clusters in response to various insults (e.g., viral infections) to form *microglial nodules* and may engulf injured neurons in a process known as *neuronophagia*.

EDEMA, HERNIATION, AND HYDROCEPHALUS

The brain and spinal cord exist within a rigid compartment defined by the skull, vertebral bodies, and dura mater. The advantage of housing as vital and delicate a structure as the CNS in a protective environment is obvious. On the other hand, such rigid confines provide very little room for brain parenchymal expansion. A number of disorders may upset the delicate balance between brain parenchymal mass and the fixed boundaries of the intracranial vault. These include generalized brain edema, hydrocephalus, and more localized expanding mass lesions.

Cerebral Edema

Cerebral edema or, more appropriately, brain parenchymal edema indicates the presence of increased water content within the brain parenchyma. Cerebral edema may arise in the setting of several diverse diseases. Broadly speaking, it may be categorized as vasogenic edema or cytotoxic edema.

Vasogenic edema occurs when the integrity of the normal blood-brain barrier is disrupted, allowing fluid to escape from the vasculature into the interstitial space of the brain (interstitial edema). The absence of significant lymphatic drainage in the brain greatly impairs the resorption of excess extracellular fluid. The edema may be localized, as in the case of the abnormally permeable vessels encountered adjacent to abscesses and neoplasms, or it may be more generalized.

Cytotoxic edema, in contrast, implies an increase in intracellular fluid (intracellular edema) secondary to cellular injury, as might be encountered in a patient with a generalized hypoxic-ischemic insult. In these situations, energy failure at the cellular level is associated with abnormalities of ion transport, which result, in turn, in the accumulation of increased amounts of water within the cell. In practice, conditions marked by generalized edema are usually associated with elements of both vasogenic and cytotoxic edema.

Herniation

The open cranial sutures in infants and young children permit some accommodation of increases in intracranial pressure. In older children and adults, however, elevated intracranial pressure is poorly tolerated, owing to the rigid nature of the cranial vault. As noted previously, for example, the surface of the edematous brain is typically flattened, because of pressure on the brain of the inner table of the skull. In addition, as expanding brain parenchyma encounters other unyielding structures, such as dural reflections or the foramen magnum, one or more different patterns of *herniation* may develop. The three most common forms are illustrated in Figure 23-2 and are described as follows:

1. *Transtentorial (uncal gyral, mesial temporal) herniation* occurs when the medial aspect of the temporal lobe is compressed against the free margin of the tentorium cerebelli. As displacement of the temporal lobe extends, the third cranial nerve and its parasympathetic fibers are compressed, resulting in pupillary dilation and impairment of ocular movements on the side of the lesion. The posterior cerebral artery is also often compressed, resulting in ischemic injury to the territory supplied by that vessel, including the primary visual cortex.
2. *Subfalcine (cingulate gyrus) herniation* occurs when unilateral or asymmetric expansion of the cerebral

Figure 23-2 ■

Patterns of brain herniation: subfalcine (cingulate), transtentorial (uncinate, mesial temporal), and tonsillar. (Adapted from Fishman RA: Brain edema. N Engl J Med 293:706, 1975. Adapted, with permission, from The New England Journal of Medicine.)

hemisphere displaces the cingulate gyrus under the falx cerebri. This is often associated with compression of branches of the anterior cerebral artery, manifested by weakness and/or sensory abnormalities in the leg, caused by ischemic injury of portions of the primary motor and/or sensory cortex.
3. *Tonsillar herniation* refers to displacement of the cerebellar tonsils through the foramen magnum. This pattern of herniation is life-threatening because it causes brain stem compression and compromises vital respiratory centers in the medulla oblongata. Brain stem herniation is often accompanied by hemorrhagic lesions in the midbrain and pons, termed *secondary brain stem*, or *Duret*, *hemorrhages*. These linear or fountain-shaped lesions usually occur in a midline and paramedian distribution, as illustrated in Figure 23-3. Although their pathogenesis has been the source of some debate, the lesions are likely caused by kinking of penetrating branches of the basilar artery with resultant necrosis and hemorrhage in the distribution of those vessels during caudal (downward) displacement of the brain stem.

Figure 23-1 ■

Generalized brain edema. The surfaces of the gyri are flattened as a result of compression of the expanding brain by the dura mater and inner surface of the skull. Such changes are associated with a dangerous increase in intracranial pressure.

Hydrocephalus

Cerebrospinal fluid (CSF) is produced by cells of the choroid plexus, located within the lateral and fourth ventricles of the brain. The CSF normally circulates through the ventricular system, enters the cisterna magna at the base of the brain stem via the foramina of Luschka and Magendie, and then bathes the superior cerebral convexities, where it is absorbed by the arachnoid granulations. *Hydrocephalus* refers to the accumulation of excessive CSF within the ventricular system of the brain. Most such cases are caused by decreased resorption of CSF, although in rare instances (e.g., tumors of the choroid plexus), overproduction of CSF may be responsible. Whatever its origin, the increased volume of CSF within the ventricles expands them and causes an elevation in intracranial pressure. The term *noncommunicating hydrocephalus* is used when obstruction to the flow of CSF occurs within the ventricular system, as in cases of ventricular obstruction by tumor or an inflammatory process. If the obstruction occurs outside of the ventricular system (e.g., in the subarachnoid space or at the arachnoid granulations), the process is referred to as *communicating hydrocephalus*. This condition develops most frequently after episodes of meningitis or subarachnoid hemorrhage, in which organization of either inflammatory exudates or blood causes scarring of the arachnoid granulations.

If hydrocephalus develops before closure of the cranial sutures, there is enlargement of the head, manifested by an increase in head circumference. Hydrocephalus developing after fusion of the sutures, in contrast, is associated with expansion of the ventricles and increased intracranial pressure, without a change in head circumference (Fig. 23–4).

The term *hydrocephalus ex vacuo* refers to dilation of the ventricular system and a compensatory increase in CSF volume secondary to a loss of brain parenchyma. There is no increase in the rate of CSF fluid production, and the flow of CSF remains normal. Hydrocephalus ex vacuo is often associated with other evidence of parenchymal atrophy, such as thinning of cortical gyri and widening of sulci.

Figure 23–4   ■

Hydrocephalus. Obstruction of the flow of cerebrospinal fluid has caused the ventricles to expand, with a resultant increase in intracranial pressure. Obstructive hydrocephalus must be distinguished from hydrocephalus ex vacuo, in which the ventricles expand to compensate for a loss of brain parenchyma.

VASCULAR DISEASES

Under normal circumstances, the brain receives 15% of the cardiac output and uses roughly 20% of the oxygen consumed by the body. Interruption of normal blood flow to the brain and spinal cord may produce irreversible parenchymal injury within minutes. Because of this exquisite dependence on a steady supply of oxygen and other nutrients, the brain has developed mechanisms to maintain blood flow over a fairly wide range of perfusion pressures, a process termed *autoregulation*.

Although the incidence of cerebrovascular disease has declined in recent decades, vascular insults to the brain (strokes) remain the third most common cause of death in the United States, exceeded only by heart disease and cancer. Cerebrovascular diseases can be divided into three major categories:

■ Parenchymal injuries associated with a *generalized reduction in blood flow*, including global hypoxic-ischemic encephalopathy
■ *Infarcts* caused by local vascular obstruction
■ *Hemorrhages* within the brain parenchyma or the subarachnoid space

Of the three, infarcts are the most common, accounting for roughly 80% of the total.

Global Hypoxic-Ischemic Encephalopathy

As noted previously, the cerebral vasculature has a remarkable capacity to maintain normal blood flow over a wide range of perfusion pressures, constricting in response to abnormally high pressures and dilating in response to hypotension. Below a systolic pressure of approximately 50 mm Hg, however, autoregulatory mechanisms are

Figure 23–3   ■

Duret hemorrhage. Herniation of the brain stem through the foramen magnum compromises the flow of blood in small branch vessels supplying the brain stem, resulting in areas of hemorrhage and necrosis.

inadequate to compensate for the reduction in blood flow, and parenchymal injury may occur. The term *hypoxia* refers to a decrease in the oxygen available to tissues, while *ischemia* refers to a decrease in tissue perfusion. Experimental data suggest that pure hypoxia in the absence of decreased perfusion (ischemia) does not cause significant brain injury. In practice, however, the effects of pure hypoxia are difficult to separate from those of ischemia—cardiopulmonary arrest, for example, is associated with both hypoxemia and decreased perfusion pressure—and the two are usually considered together.

Within the CNS, certain regions and cell populations are more susceptible than others to hypoxic-ischemic injury. For example, neurons, as a group, are far more vulnerable to ischemic injury than are glial cells. Among the neurons, certain subpopulations, including some of the pyramidal cells in the hippocampus, the Purkinje cells of the cerebellum, and neurons within the globus pallidus of the basal ganglia, are particularly sensitive and are often sites of selective injury after generalized hypoxic-ischemic insults. The reasons for such selective vulnerability to hypoxic ischemic injury remain incompletely understood but likely include local changes in the levels and metabolism of certain neurotransmitters (e.g., glutamic acid) in the setting of ischemia. Extracellular glutamate levels, for example, increase in the setting of ischemic injury. Glutamate, in turn, is a potent excitatory neurotransmitter and may contribute to neuronal loss via overstimulation of the neurons, a phenomenon known as *excitotoxicity*.

Areas of the brain located at the junctions of arterial territories (i.e., *arterial border zones*, sometimes termed "watershed" areas) are also particularly susceptible, because these areas are the first to be deprived of blood during hypotensive episodes. Common locations for such border-zone lesions include the superior cerebral convexities at the junction of the territories of the anterior and middle cerebral arteries and the posterior aspects of the cerebellar hemispheres at the junction of the territories supplied by the superior and posterior inferior cerebellar arteries.

MORPHOLOGY

In the period immediately after a global hypoxic-ischemic insult (e.g., cardiac arrest), the brain may appear normal, both grossly and microscopically. In the case of patients who survive the acute insult, within 24 to 48 hours, the brain is softened and edematous. Irregular, mottled discoloration is often visible in gray matter; in some areas, such as arterial border zones, areas of hemorrhage may be present. The cortical mantle may contain an irregular, linear zone of softening and discoloration; this pattern, termed **laminar cortical necrosis**, reflects the vulnerability of specific (midcortical) layers of neurons to hypoxic-ischemic injury. The demarcation between gray and white matter is usually blurred, owing to the presence of edema. Fragments of soft, necrotic cerebellar parenchyma may be present in the spinal subarachnoid space. The brains of patients maintained on respiratory support after cessation of brain activity ("brain death") appear swollen, dusky, and soft, even after formalin fixation. Although the term **respirator brain** is sometimes used to designate such cases, it should be clearly understood that the use of artificial ventilatory support is not the cause of the brain injury. Microscopic changes are apparent within 12 to 24 hours and include neuronal shrinkage or swelling, followed by the development of cytoplasmic eosinophilia, nuclear pyknosis, and other cytologic features of necrosis. The parenchyma is often vacuolated, with widened perivascular and pericellular spaces, reflecting the presence of vasogenic edema, and the endothelial cells may show some swelling. In contrast to localized infarcts, there is little host inflammatory reaction, owing to the fact that effective perfusion of the brain decreases substantially in cases of irreversible global hypoxic-ischemic injury. In cases associated with prolonged survival, neurons disappear and the intervening neuropil becomes cystic and gliotic.

Clinical Features. Hypoxic-ischemic encephalopathy may occur under any circumstance that results in a global decrease in the amount of oxygenated blood available to the brain, including cardiac dysrhythmias, shock, and large increases in intracranial pressure. A number of factors may modify the degree of parenchymal injury. These include the *age* of the patient (young patients tolerate global insults better than do the elderly), the *duration* of the circulatory disturbance, and *temperature* (hypothermia increases the resistance of the brain to hypoxic-ischemic injury whereas hyperthermia worsens the effects of hypoxic-ischemic injury). The resulting deficits range from transient neurologic disturbances to "brain death," with a global cessation of electrical activity.

Infarcts

Infarcts are caused by local interruption of blood flow. Such lesions represent the most common form of cerebrovascular disease, accounting for between 70% and 80% of all cerebrovascular accidents, or "strokes." They occur most commonly in the seventh decade of life and are more common in males than in females. Cerebral atherosclerosis is the most common cause of brain infarcts, and factors that predispose individuals to atherosclerosis (e.g., hypertension, diabetes mellitus, and smoking) increase the risk of infarcts. The most severe atherosclerotic lesions are typically encountered within larger vessels, such as the internal carotid arteries, the proximal middle cerebral arteries, and the basilar artery. An important cause of vascular occlusion in patients with atherosclerosis is thrombosis of an atherosclerotic arterial segment, occurring most commonly near the carotid bifurcation or in the basilar artery. Other causes of vascular occlusion include emboli, most commonly originating from the heart or from atherosclerotic plaques in more proximal arterial segments. With the exception of the basilar arterial system, most cases of intracranial arterial occlusion are caused by emboli. Such embolic occlusions occur most commonly in branches of the middle cerebral arteries. Vasculitis and trauma are less common causes of cerebrovascular occlusion.

The location and distribution of cerebral infarcts is influenced by a number of factors, including the site of arterial occlusion, the time over which an occlusive event develops, the presence or absence of arterial anastomoses (e.g., the circle of Willis), and systemic perfusion pressure. For example, individuals with well-developed arterial anastomoses might tolerate gradual thrombotic occlusion of the internal carotid artery with minimal symptoms, whereas embolic occlusion of the middle cerebral artery might result in a massive hemispheric infarct. Collateral circulation is, in general, less well developed in more distal arterial branches, such as the small vessels that penetrate into the deeper areas of the brain; therefore, occlusion of a distal arterial branch almost always results in the development of an infarct. Patients with significant atherosclerosis may develop infarcts even in the absence of complete vascular occlusion if blood pressure drops significantly.

Figure 23-5   ■

Remote infarct. Necrotic tissue has liquefied over a period of approximately 6 months, leaving behind a permanent, fluid-filled, cystic defect in the right lateral frontal area.

MORPHOLOGY

Although cell death occurs within minutes of arterial occlusion, the gross and histologic appearance of the brain is normal for the first 4 to 12 hours. The first alterations are apparent microscopically and consist of ischemic neuronal changes (described earlier), accompanied by a neutrophilic inflammatory reaction. By 36 to 48 hours, the necrotic area becomes swollen and softer than the adjacent viable brain parenchyma. Demarcation between gray and white matter becomes blurred because of interstitial and intracellular edema. Areas of hemorrhage may be seen, particularly in infarcts involving arterial border zones or in those resulting from transient occlusion by emboli or extrinsic compression of the vessel. By the third day, macrophages begin to infiltrate the lesion and phagocytose necrotic parenchyma, resulting in progressively sharper demarcation of the infarct. By 1 month, extensive phagocytosis of necrotic parenchyma results in further softening and liquefaction of the infarct, with the development of irregular cavities. By about 6 months, most infarcts are completely liquefied (Fig. 23-5). In the case of infarcts involving the cerebral cortex, a thin rim of subpial parenchyma, supplied by small superficial leptomeningeal blood vessels, is preserved over the infarct, a feature that may be helpful in differentiating remote infarcts from old contusions (discussed later).

Clinical Features. Typically, the onset of brain infarction is fairly sudden, but it is often preceded by transient episodes of neurologic dysfunction lasting from several minutes to up to 24 hours. Such episodes, termed *transient ischemic attacks (TIAs)*, are caused by self-limited episodes of vascular obstruction by atheromatous emboli and/or platelet-fibrin aggregates. TIAs are an important predictor of subsequent infarcts, with approximately one third of patients with TIAs developing clinically significant infarcts within 5 years. Predictably, the neurologic deficits associated with brain infarction are related to the location and amount of brain damage. In addition to the deficits directly related to loss of brain parenchyma, edema of adjacent brain during the early stages also contributes to local neurologic deficits and, in the case of large infarcts, to life-threatening mass effect and brain herniation.

Infarcts occur most commonly in areas supplied by branches of the middle cerebral artery. As noted earlier, most middle cerebral artery occlusions are caused by emboli. Infarcts in this region are manifested by contralateral hemiparesis and spasticity; loss of sensation on the side of the body opposite the infarct; visual field abnormalities; and, in the case of infarcts involving the dominant cerebral hemisphere, speech abnormalities (aphasia). *Occlusion of the internal carotid artery*, usually caused by thrombosis, is less common than is occlusion of the middle cerebral artery. Internal carotid occlusion may result in massive infarction of the ipsilateral cerebral hemisphere, accompanied by monocular blindness secondary to the loss of flow to the ophthalmic artery. More often, however, arterial anastomoses, particularly at the base of the brain (circle of Willis), continue to supply blood to the internal carotid territory after occlusion of more proximal segments of that vessel. Hence, the resultant deficits are often smaller than might be expected. Branches of the *vertebrobasilar system* are also affected by atherosclerosis and are therefore potential sites of thrombosis as well as sources of atheromatous emboli. The basilar artery is especially prone to thrombotic occlusion. Occlusion of these vessels in the posterior circulation may produce lesions ranging from large, rapidly fatal infarcts involving vital brain stem areas to small, clinically silent infarcts.

Intracranial Hemorrhages

Hemorrhages may occur at any site within the CNS. In some instances parenchymal hemorrhages may develop in the setting of primary ischemic injury (infarcts), particularly when significant *reperfusion* of necrotic tissue is present, in patients on *anticoagulant therapy*, or in patients with infarcts caused by *venous occlusion*. Primary hemorrhages within the epidural or subdural space are typically related to trauma and will be discussed later with other traumatic lesions. Primary hemorrhages within the brain parenchyma and subarachnoid space, in contrast, are often a manifestation of underlying cerebrovascular disease, although trauma may also cause hemorrhage in these sites.

PRIMARY BRAIN PARENCHYMAL HEMORRHAGE

Spontaneous (nontraumatic) intraparenchymal hemorrhages occur most commonly in middle to late adult life, with a peak incidence at about age 60. Most are caused by rupture of a small intraparenchymal vessel. *Hypertension is the most common underlying cause of primary brain parenchymal hemorrhage*, accounting for more than 50% of cases of clinically significant hemorrhage. Conversely, brain hemorrhage accounts for roughly 15% of deaths among patients with chronic hypertension. Hypertension causes a number of abnormalities in vessel walls, including accelerated atherosclerosis in larger arteries; hyaline arteriolosclerosis in smaller vessels; and, in severe cases, proliferative changes and frank necrosis of arterioles. Arteriolar walls affected by hyaline change are presumably weaker than are normal vessels and are therefore more vulnerable to rupture.

In some instances chronic hypertension has been associated with the development of minute arterial aneurysms, termed *Charcot-Bouchard microaneurysms*. Charcot-Bouchard microaneurysms, not to be confused with saccular aneurysms of larger intracranial vessels, occur in vessels that are less than 300 μm in diameter, most commonly within the basal ganglia. Although their frequency is unknown, Charcot-Bouchard aneurysms have been implicated as the source of bleeding in some cases of hypertensive cerebral hemorrhage.

In addition to hypertension, *other local and systemic factors may cause or contribute to nontraumatic hemorrhage*, including systemic coagulation disorders, open heart surgery, neoplasms, amyloid deposits (cerebral amyloid angiopathy), vasculitis, saccular aneurysms, and vascular malformations. Vascular malformations and saccular aneurysms are discussed later in this section.

MORPHOLOGY

Parenchymal hemorrhages occur most commonly in the **basal ganglia,** particularly in the region of the putamen and external capsule, followed by the **thalamus, cerebral white matter, pons, and cerebellum.** Multiple hemorrhages are seen in a minority of cases. With a massive hemorrhage, the site of origin of the hematoma may be impossible to determine with certainty. Externally, the brain is asymmetrically

Figure 23-6 ■

Acute intracerebral hemorrhage. A fresh hematoma has disrupted and expanded the left cerebral hemisphere, causing the midline structures to shift to the right. Uncontrolled hypertension is an important cause of this catastrophic lesion.

distorted by the mass effect caused by the hematoma and associated edema. Various herniation patterns, described previously, are almost invariably present. On cut surface, primary intraparenchymal hemorrhages take the form of fairly well demarcated hematomas, which may dissect through adjacent parenchyma into the ventricles and/or subarachnoid space (Fig. 23-6). Some degree of softening of the adjacent neuropil is often present, although, in contrast to infarcts with secondary hemorrhage, large areas of necrosis are not seen. Large hemorrhages occurring above the tentorium cerebelli usually cause herniation of cerebellar tonsils and brain stem, with associated secondary brain stem (Duret) hemorrhages. In patients who survive the acute hemorrhage, the hematoma is resorbed over time, ultimately leaving a fluid-filled cavity lined by gliotic neuropil and hemosiderin-laden macrophages.

Clinical Features. The onset of a primary brain parenchymal hemorrhage is almost always abrupt and is accompanied by evidence of increased intracranial pressure, including severe headache, vomiting, and rapid loss of consciousness. Localizing signs may be present but are often difficult to detect in the setting of a massive elevation in intracranial pressure and coma. Progression of mass effect is associated with evidence of brain stem compression, including deep coma; irregular respirations with periods of apnea (Cheyne-Stokes respiration); dilated, nonresponsive pupils; and spasticity.

SACCULAR ANEURYSMS AND SUBARACHNOID HEMORRHAGE

The subarachnoid space may also be the site of nontraumatic intracranial hemorrhage. *The most common cause of spontaneous (nontraumatic) subarachnoid hemorrhage is rupture of a saccular aneurysm.* Saccular, or berry, aneurysms are present in approximately 1% of the general population. Their incidence is higher in patients with certain disorders, including polycystic kidney disease, fibromuscular dysplasia, coarctation of the aorta, and arteriovenous malformations of the brain. They must be distinguished from the fusiform dilations of intracranial vessels that may be seen in atherosclerosis, from infectious ("mycotic") aneurysms, and from the occasional dissecting aneurysms that may also be encountered in the intracranial compartment. Most saccular aneurysms (80%) arise at arterial bifurcations in the territory of the internal carotid artery. Common sites include branches of the middle cerebral artery, intracranial branches of the internal carotid artery, and the junction between the anterior cerebral and anterior communicating arteries (Fig. 23–7). Fifteen percent to 20% of saccular aneurysms occur within the posterior (vertebrobasilar) circulation. Although saccular aneurysms have traditionally been thought to arise as a result of congenital defects in the media of arteries at branch points, they are distinctly rare in infancy and childhood. It is more likely that they represent an acquired, degenerative lesion, perhaps related to chronic mechanical (hemodynamic) injury to the vessel wall. Saccular aneurysms enlarge with time and are at greatest risk for rupture once they reach diameters of 6 to 10 mm. Interestingly, in aneurysms greater than 25 mm in diameter, sometimes designated "giant aneurysms," the likelihood of rupture decreases and symptoms referable to their mass effects predominate.

Figure 23–8 ■

Gross view of a massive saccular aneurysm arising at the junction of the vertebral and basilar arteries. The vessels have been dissected from the brain. Multiple surgical clips, visible in the photograph, were placed on the aneurysm before death in an attempt to prevent further bleeding.

MORPHOLOGY

Asymptomatic saccular aneurysms are usually small, with diameters of less than 3 mm. They appear as rounded bulges in the arterial wall, usually at arterial bifurcations (Fig. 23–8). Multiple aneurysms are present in up to 30% of patients. The wall of the saccular aneurysm is composed of dense, collagen-rich tissue derived from the intima and adventitia of the parent vessel. The media typically ends abruptly at the neck of the aneurysm. The lumen of the aneurysm may contain a laminated thrombus. Aneurysms may compress adjacent structures and produce symptoms referable to local mass effects. Rupture of a saccular aneurysm usually occurs at the thin-walled fundus. Depending on its location, rupture may result in bleeding into the subarachnoid space and, in many cases, into adjacent brain parenchyma. **Infarcts of brain parenchyma** may also develop in the setting of subarachnoid hemorrhage, probably because of **arterial spasm,** a phenomenon demonstrable radiographically in up to 40% of cases.

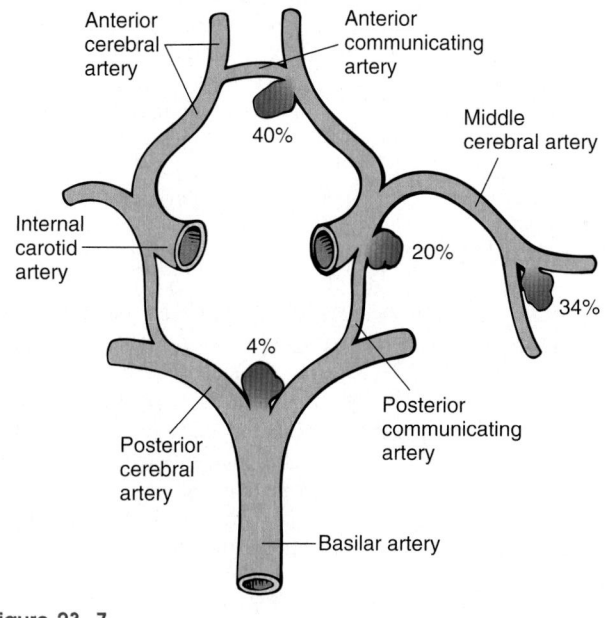

Figure 23–7 ■

Sites of saccular aneurysms and their relative frequencies. Multiple aneurysms may be present in an individual patient.

Clinical Features. Subarachnoid hemorrhage resulting from a ruptured saccular aneurysm is less common than is primary cerebral hemorrhage. Women are affected somewhat more commonly than men are, with most cases occurring before the age of 50. As in the case of primary intraparenchymal hemorrhages, the onset of subarachnoid hemorrhage is abrupt and is associated with severe headache, vomiting, and loss of consciousness. Usually, there is no history of an obvious precipitating factor. Meningeal signs, including neck rigidity, are usually present, and the CSF is grossly bloody. Roughly 50% of patients with subarachnoid hemorrhage caused by ruptured saccular aneurysm die within several days of the onset of symptoms. Other acute complications include cerebral infarcts, usually developing within 4 to 9 days after the onset of symptoms, acute hydrocephalus, and herniation. Chronic hydrocephalus may occur in patients surviving the acute insult, owing to organization of blood in the leptomeninges and/or arachnoid granulations, with resultant obstruction of CSF flow.

VASCULAR MALFORMATIONS

Vascular malformations are another important cause of intracranial hemorrhage. Most result from abnormalities in angiogenesis in the developing brain; they range from small, incidental abnormalities identified only at autopsy to large lesions associated with variable focal neurologic deficits and catastrophic intracranial hemorrhage. Four major types are usually recognized: arteriovenous malformations, capillary telangiectases, venous angiomas, and cavernous angiomas.

MORPHOLOGY

Arteriovenous malformations are the most common congenital vascular abnormalities in the brain and are the type most likely to be associated with clinically significant hemorrhage. They occur most commonly in the cerebral hemispheres and are often supplied by branches of the middle cerebral artery. Grossly, the arteriovenous malformation appears as a conglomerate of tortuous vessels, most dramatically visualized while still engorged with blood (Fig. 23-9). The microscopic appearance is that of a collection of haphazardly arranged vessels of variable caliber that include arteries, veins, and transitional forms that are neither clearly venous nor clearly arterial. The vascular channels are separated by brain parenchyma. Secondary changes, including recent and remote hemorrhages, calcification, and reactive gliosis, are almost invariably present. The most common clinical manifestation of arteriovenous malformations is spontaneous hemorrhage, which usually occurs af-

---

Figure 23-9 ■

Arteriovenous malformation. These are the most dangerous type of vascular malformation in the brain because of the associated risk of massive bleeding.

---

ter the first decade of life. Saccular aneurysms have been identified in up to 10% of people with arteriovenous malformations, usually in the vicinity of the vascular malformation.

Among the other types of vascular malformations, *cavernous angiomas* are another significant cause of spontaneous intracranial hemorrhage and seizures. They are composed of ectatic, thick-walled venous channels separated by dense fibrous stroma, with no intervening brain parenchyma. Like arteriovenous malformations, they may undergo spontaneous hemorrhage. *Capillary telangiectases* are small, punctate lesions found most commonly in the pons and cerebral white matter. These delicate capillary channels, usually encountered as incidental lesions at the time of autopsy, may leak occasionally. *Venous angiomas* occur most commonly in the meninges and spinal cord, where they appear as dilated, thin-walled veins. They are usually asymptomatic.

CENTRAL NERVOUS SYSTEM TRAUMA

Traumatic injuries remain a leading cause of death and long-term disability in Western society, with traumatic injuries to the head accounting for over one fourth of all accidental deaths. Among survivors of head injury, nearly 20% suffer from severe long-term disability, and up to 5% of cases remain in a permanent vegetative state. Most fatal or debilitating head injuries are caused by *blunt trauma* associated with motor vehicle accidents, falls, and criminal assaults (including child abuse), with *penetrating missile wounds* (bullet injuries) accounting for an additional important subset of cases. Factors that increase the risk of head trauma include alcohol abuse, previous head injury, mental retardation, and seizure disorders. Traumatic injuries to the brain caused by blunt force include three important groups: (1) epidural hematoma, (2) subdural hematoma, and (3) parenchymal injuries. Combinations of various patterns are quite common.

Epidural Hematoma

Epidural hematomas are caused most frequently by *rupture of a meningeal artery*, usually in association with a skull fracture (Fig. 23-10). The most common site of arterial disruption is a branch of the middle meningeal artery as it courses between the dura mater and squamous portion of the temporal bone. This artery is firmly attached to the periosteum of the temporal bone and hence is easily torn whenever a fracture occurs at that site. Epidural hematomas compress the subjacent dura and flatten the gyral crests of the underlying brain. If not immediately drained, they may produce uncal gyral and cerebellar tonsillar herniation; brain stem compression; and death. *A significant number of patients with epidural hematomas have a "lucid interval" immediately after injury, followed by progressive loss of*

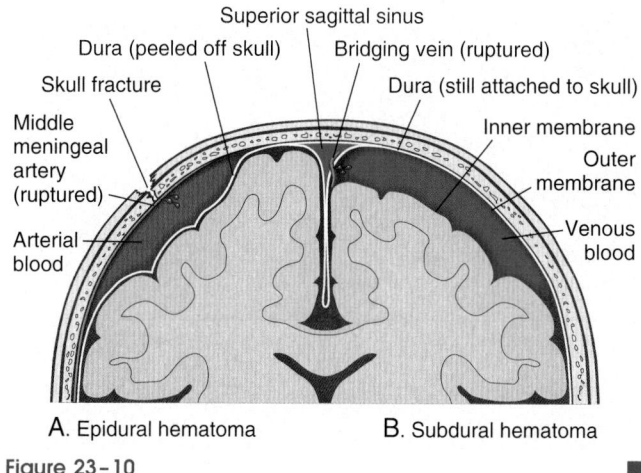

A. Epidural hematoma   **B.** Subdural hematoma

Figure 23-10 ■

Epidural and subdural hematomas. An epidural hematoma *(A)* is caused by disruption of the middle meningeal artery as it courses through the epidural space. A subdural hematoma *(B)* results from tearing of "bridging" veins between the brain and dural sinuses.

consciousness. Although at least some of this delayed deterioration is presumably related to progressive enlargement of the hematoma, concomitant swelling of the brain parenchyma underlying the hematoma may contribute to the deterioration in some cases. Because the bleeding is arterial in origin in most cases, cranial epidural hematomas expand rapidly, necessitating prompt surgical intervention.

Subdural Hematoma

Subdural hematomas are collections of blood between the internal surface of the dura mater and the arachnoid mater. In most cases, they are caused by *disruption of bridging veins* that extend from the surface of the brain to the dural sinuses (see Fig. 23–10). Any condition associated with rapid changes in head velocity (e.g., whiplash injury; blows to the head; and, in the case of infants, violent shaking of the head) may produce *tears in the delicate bridging veins* as they penetrate the overlying dura mater, with resultant hemorrhage into the subdural space. Subdural hematomas occur most often over the cerebral convexities and vary from small hemorrhages to massive lesions with substantial mass effect. They are traditionally classified as acute or chronic, depending on whether the contents of the hematoma consist predominantly of clotted blood or liquefied blood clots, respectively.

Acute subdural hematomas are usually associated with a clear history of trauma. They may be unilateral or, particularly in infants, bilateral and are frequently associated with other traumatic lesions. Acute subdural hematomas contain clotted blood, most frequently in the frontoparietal region. In contrast to the flattened convexities seen in epidural hematomas, the gyral contours are usually preserved in cases of acute subdural hematoma, owing to the fact that the pressure from the hematoma is fairly evenly distributed within the sulci and over the gyral crests. There may be considerable swelling of the cerebrum on the side of the hematoma, which contributes to the mass effect of the hematoma and to

subsequent clinical deterioration. As the hematoma enlarges, compression of the contralateral cerebral hemisphere against the inner table of the skull, as well as various forms of herniation, may occur. Because the blood in a subdural hematoma is usually of venous origin, the onset of symptoms is somewhat slower than with epidural hematomas. With time, nonfatal untreated hematomas are gradually liquefied and demarcated from the underlying brain by a reactive "neomembrane" to form chronic subdural hematomas.

Chronic subdural hematomas are less frequently associated with a well-defined history of trauma than are acute lesions. They are often associated with brain atrophy, which in turn increases the mobility of the brain within the cranial vault and renders bridging veins even more susceptible to tearing. Accordingly, traumatic episodes causing chronic subdural hematomas may be so trivial as to escape notice. They are often bilateral. Chronic subdural hematomas are composed of liquefied blood or yellow-tinged fluid separated from the inner surface of the dura mater and the underlying brain by "neomembranes" composed of granulation tissue and mature collagen, derived from the dura mater. Blood vessels within the neomembranes are abnormally permeable, owing to an incompletely developed endothelial layer, contributing to progressive accumulation of fluid and recurrent hemorrhage within the hematoma. Clinical symptoms include altered mental status, sometimes accompanied by focal neurologic deficits. Because of the slowly evolving nature of the deficits, chronic subdural hematomas may be confused clinically with dementia caused by neurodegenerative disorders such as Alzheimer disease. Appropriate imaging studies of the head (e.g., computed tomography [CT] or magnetic resonance imaging [MRI]) are invaluable in excluding the possibility of subdural hematomas in patients with slowly evolving neurologic abnormalities.

Traumatic Parenchymal Injuries

Traumatic injuries to the brain parenchyma include concussions, contusions and lacerations, diffuse axonal injury, traumatic intracerebral hemorrhage, and generalized brain swelling.

The term *concussion* refers to a transient loss of consciousness and widespread paralysis, sometimes accompanied by seizures, followed by recovery over a period of hours to days. Patients recover without sequelae, save for loss of memory about the events surrounding the injury. Concussions may be associated with minimal morphologic changes; transient injury to the reticular activating system in the brain has been proposed as the mechanism for loss of consciousness in such cases. It is likely that many cases of clinically mild concussion are associated with subtle degrees of axonal injury, however. In severe cases, more obvious diffuse axonal injury may be present.

Diffuse axonal injury is the cause of most cases of posttraumatic dementia and, in conjunction with hypoxic-ischemic injury, is responsible for most cases of persistent vegetative state. The lesions of diffuse axonal injury result from sudden deceleration and/or acceleration forces sufficient to stretch or, in extreme cases, tear nerve cell

Figure 23–11   ■

Diffuse axonal injury. *A,* Gross photograph demonstrating characteristic hemorrhagic lesions within the corpus callosum. *B,* Photomicrograph of axonal spheroids, labeled with antibody to amyloid precursor protein. The swollen axonal processes stain red in this preparation. (*A,* Courtesy of Walter Kemp, MD, Department of Pathology, University of Texas Southwestern Medical School, Dallas.)

processes within the cerebral white matter. Grossly, diffuse axonal injury may produce only minimal changes; in severe cases, there are areas of hemorrhage, most commonly in the corpus callosum and dorsal areas of the brain stem (Fig. 23–11*A*). The diagnosis rests with the *demonstration of characteristic axonal swellings* within white matter, sometimes designated *axonal spheroids* (Fig. 23–11*B*), which develop at sites where the axon has been damaged by stretch injury. Although these changes are easily missed in routine H & E–stained sections, immunohistochemical staining for a protein known as amyloid precursor protein (APP), discussed in more detail later with Alzheimer disease, has permitted identification of such axonal swellings as early as 2 hours after injury.

Contusions are hemorrhages in the superficial brain parenchyma caused by blunt trauma. They may occur at any place where the brain comes in contact with the skull or an unyielding dural reflection but are most common in the frontal poles, orbital surfaces of the frontal lobes, temporal poles, occipital poles, and posterior cerebellum. The overlying skull may contain a fracture, but it is often intact. When blunt force is applied to an immobile head, particularly with a fairly small object (e.g., a hammer), contusions are most pronounced in the area of brain immediately underneath the point of impact, a configuration referred to as a *coup contusion.* In contrast, when the head collides with a broader, hard surface, as in the case of the head striking the floor in a fall, surface contusions tend to develop in areas of the brain away from the site of impact. Falls in which the occipital area of the head strikes the floor, for example, are often associated with the development of contusions in the frontal and temporal poles. This pattern of injury is designated as a *contrecoup contusion.* It is impossible to distinguish coup from contrecoup lesions morphologically without information about the circumstances of the injury.

Cerebral contusions, particularly if accompanied by tearing of the superficial layers of the brain (lacerations), are an important cause of traumatic subarachnoid hemorrhage. In the acute phase, contusions appear as hemorrhagic lesions

involving the superficial gray matter and, on occasion, the subjacent white matter (Fig. 23–12). Microscopically, the brain parenchyma within the contusion is hemorrhagic, fragmented, and necrotic. In contrast to infarcts, which may also produce superficial hemorrhagic gray matter lesions, the subpial molecular layer is also disrupted in contusions. Healed lesions appear as depressed, firm areas on the surface of the brain. A golden brown discoloration is usually evident as a result of associated hemosiderin deposits. Remote contusions are a common cause of focal seizure activity.

Traumatic intracerebral hemorrhages are usually multiple and are most common in the frontal lobes, temporal lobes, and deep gray matter. They may occur in association with contusions, as well as deep within the brain. In many of the latter cases, they are accompanied by evidence of concomitant diffuse axonal injury. On occasion, traumatic parenchymal hemorrhages may occur without other obvious

Figure 23–12   ■

Cerebral contusions. The temporal poles are discolored by areas of hemorrhage. Such lesions represent "bruises" of the surface of the brain caused by violent contact between the delicate brain parenchyma and the hard inner surface of the skull.

evidence of trauma, in which case they may be difficult to distinguish from spontaneous intracranial hemorrhages.

Brain swelling may occur as an isolated manifestation of traumatic injury or may coexist with other traumatic lesions. It may be localized, as in the case of edema associated with an adjacent contusion or subdural hematoma, or generalized. Diffuse brain swelling occurs most commonly in children and adolescents and may follow a lucid interval immediately after trauma. Probably both cerebral congestion (i.e., engorgement of intraparenchymal vessels) and true edema play a significant role in its development.

CONGENITAL MALFORMATIONS AND PERINATAL BRAIN INJURY

Major congenital malformations occur in about 3% of newborns. Of these, malformations of the CNS account for approximately one third and are an important cause of infant mortality and long-term disability. The development of the mammalian CNS is a complex process that may be disrupted by a number of factors, including intrinsic genetic abnormalities, exogenous factors such as toxins and infections, and various combinations of the two. Some malformations have now been linked to clearly defined chromosomal and/or genetic abnormalities, and others have been associated with specific environmental factors. In the majority of cases, however, the cause of the CNS malformation is unknown.

The timing of the insult plays a critical role in its effects on the developing nervous system. Like other systems, the developing CNS is most susceptible to teratogenesis during the early stages of embryogenesis. The most common congenital malformations of the nervous system include neural tube defects, malformations associated with hydrocephalus, and primary forebrain abnormalities. Another group of conditions, the so-called neurocutaneous syndromes are also associated with a wide range of abnormalities in the nervous system. They are listed in Table 23–1 and mentioned briefly later.

In addition to primary malformations, perinatal injury is responsible for a significant proportion of CNS abnormalities in the neonatal period. Many changes, such as hemorrhages and infarcts, are clearly acquired disorders and traditionally have been distinguished from congenital malformations. As will be discussed, however, the distinction between many "acquired" abnormalities (so-called disruptions and deformations) and those regarded as "intrinsic" developmental abnormalities (true malformations) is often exceedingly difficult, particularly when the destructive event occurs before the developing brain is able to mount an effective inflammatory and repair response.

Neural Tube Defects

The brain and spinal cord are derived from ectodermal elements that differentiate and proliferate to form the neural tube. Closure of the neural tube begins on approximately the 22nd day of gestation and is complete between the 26th

Table 23–1. NEUROCUTANEOUS SYNDROMES

Syndrome (Frequency)	Site of Genetic Abnormality	Affected Gene Product (and Function If Known)	Features
Neurofibromatosis type I (1:3000)	Chromosome 17 (17q11.2)	*Neurofibromin* (tumor suppressor activity)	Neurofibromas, schwannomas, malignant peripheral nerve neoplasms, meningiomas, gliomas, hyperpigmented skin lesions (café-au-lait spots), pigmented nodules of iris (Lisch nodules)
Neurofibromatosis type II (1:40,000)	Chromosome 22 (22q12)	*Merlin* (cytoskeleton-associated protein; possible role in intracellular signaling pathways)	Schwannomas of eighth cranial nerve (often bilateral), meningiomas (often multiple), spinal neurofibromas; posterior lens opacification
Tuberous sclerosis (1:5000 to 1:10,000)	Chromosome 9 (9q34) or 16 (16p13.3)	*TSC1* on chromosome 9q34 encodes *hamartin,* and *TSC2* on chromosome 16p13.3 encodes *tuberin.* Both control the cell cycle and have tumor suppressor activity	Cerebral cortical malformations, subependymal tumors, seizures, mental retardation, cardiac rhabdomyomas, renal angiomyolipomas
von Hippel-Lindau disease (1:36,000)	Chromosome 3 (3p25-26)	*VHL* protein (may participate in regulation of transcription)	Cerebellar hemangioblastomas, retinal angiomas, renal cell carcinomas, pheochromocytomas, visceral cysts, epididymal tumors
Sturge-Weber disease (1:10,000)	Sporadic; defect unknown	Unknown	Cutaneous angiomas in distribution of seventh cranial nerve, meningeal angiomatosis, cerebral calcification, seizures, mental retardation

Figure 23–13 ■

Anencephaly, the most common and most severe of cranial neural tube defects. The orbital bones are of nearly normal size, despite absence of the brain and cranial bones, resulting in a froglike facial appearance.

and 28th day. Disorders related to abnormal closure of the neural tube are among the most common CNS malformations. Such developmental aberrations, broadly designated as *neural tube defects* or *dysraphic states*, may involve the brain or spinal cord, or both. Examples include anencephaly, cranial meningoceles and encephaloceles, and the various forms of spina bifida.

Anencephaly, with or without associated spinal abnormalities, represents the most severe form of neural tube defect and is the most common CNS malformation identified in human fetuses. Anencephaly occurs in about 1 in 500 births and is encountered worldwide, albeit with substantial regional variations in frequency. As with all neural tube defects, it is more common among lower socioeconomic groups and in infants of women older than age 40 years. Epidemiologic studies have shown a reasonably convincing association between dietary folate deficiency and an increased risk of anencephaly. For reasons that remain unclear, female fetuses are more commonly affected than are males.

MORPHOLOGY

The cranial vault in the anencephalic fetus is hypoplastic or absent, and the bones at the base of the skull are thickened. The orbits are shallow, resulting in characteristic protrusion of the eyes and "froglike" facies (Fig. 23–13). The neurohypophysis is absent, and the anterior pituitary is smaller than normal, reflecting an absence of trophic hormones from the hypothalamus. Abnormalities in the vertebral bodies or spinal cord may also be present. Other organs, including the lungs and adrenal glands, are hypoplastic.

Clinical Features. Anencephaly is incompatible with prolonged extrauterine survival, and most fetuses die within minutes to hours after birth. The diagnosis of anencephaly

can be made prenatally. Hydramnios is common in anencephalic gestations, and concentrations of α-fetoprotein and acetylcholinesterase are increased in the amniotic fluid. Ultrasonography can detect the presence of anencephaly in the later stages of the first trimester.

Encephaloceles and cranial meningoceles, representing less severe examples of cranial neural tube defects, probably develop later in gestation than does anencephaly. Encephaloceles are the more common of the two conditions and are characterized by protrusion of a variable amount of meninges and brain parenchyma through a defect in the cranial bones. This occurs most commonly in the occipital region, although any portion of the skull may be affected. Anterior encephaloceles are particularly prevalent in Southeast Asia. Cranial meningoceles are uncommon and are distinguished from encephaloceles by the presence of only meninges and CSF in the herniated tissue.

Spinal neural tube defects (spina bifida) may occur at any level but are most common in the lumbosacral region. In all cases there is absence or hypoplasia of one or more vertebral arches, with variable abnormalities in the underlying meninges and/or spinal cord. The two most common variants are meningomyelocele and spina bifida occulta.

Meningomyeloceles, or myelomeningoceles, are characterized by herniation of spinal meninges and spinal cord through a posterior vertebral defect (Fig. 23–14) to form a cystlike outpouching (spina bifida cystica). The meninges may be exposed to the external environment or covered by skin. Meningomyeloceles are frequently associated with hydrocephalus and the Arnold-Chiari malformation (see later). The cord is usually abnormal in this malformation, and the major manifestations of this defect, as might be expected, include infections, lower extremity paralysis, and disturbances in bladder and bowel control. The term *meningocele* designates a closely related but less severe form of spinal defect in which only meninges herniate through abnormally formed vertebral arches.

Figure 23–14 ■

Meningomyelocele. These defects occur because the caudal neural tube fails to close properly. In meningomyelocele, both the meninges and spinal cord parenchyma are included in the cystlike structure visible just above the buttocks. Because such lesions expose the central nervous system to the outside environment, infection is a common complication.

Spina bifida occulta is the mildest form of spinal neural tube defect. It is characterized by defective closure of the posterior vertebral arches, with intact meninges and spinal cord. The site of the defect is sometimes marked by a small skin dimple or tuft of hair. This abnormality, which occurs in about 20% of the general population, is asymptomatic.

Malformations Associated With Hydrocephalus

Many different disorders are associated with the presence of hydrocephalus. As noted earlier in this chapter, in many instances, hydrocephalus is caused by acquired lesions (e.g., tumors, hemorrhage, and inflammatory processes) that interfere with the normal flow and resorption of CSF. In other cases, primary developmental abnormalities may give rise to hydrocephalus. The more common primary malformations associated with hydrocephalus involve the cerebellum and are exemplified by the Arnold-Chiari malformation and the Dandy-Walker malformation.

The *Arnold-Chiari malformation* (sometimes designated the Chiari II malformation) is characterized by the presence of an abnormally shallow posterior cranial fossa associated with caudal extension of the medulla oblongata and portions of the cerebellar vermis through the foramen magnum. The lower brain stem appears elongated and compressed, with a thin layer of herniated, gliotic cerebellar parenchyma overlying the dorsal surface of the medulla. The cerebral aqueduct is often stenotic, and the dorsal part of the midbrain is usually malformed. Other abnormalities of the cranial vault, including focal thinning of the cranial bones, are usually present, reflecting the close embryologic relationship between the developing brain and its coverings. An associated meningomyelocele is almost invariably present in the caudal area of the cord. The malformation is usually associated with hydrocephalus. Although the pathogenesis of the hydrocephalus in the Arnold-Chiari malformation is not completely understood, it is now reasonably clear that the hydrocephalus is a secondary change and is not the cause of the Arnold-Chiari defect, as was once postulated.

The *Dandy-Walker malformation* consists of aplasia or hypoplasia of the cerebellar vermis, associated with balloon-like dilation of the fourth ventricle and an enlarged posterior fossa. The lesion is usually accompanied by hydrocephalus. Other abnormalities, including agenesis of the corpus callosum, occipital meningocele, and lesions caused by abnormal neuronal migration during embryogenesis, may also be present.

Disorders of Forebrain Development

Given the complexity of normal forebrain development, it is not surprising that a large number of malformations may be encountered in the cerebral hemispheres. Examples of such malformations include holoprosencephaly and cerebral cortical malformations.

The term *holoprosencephaly* refers to a group of malformations associated with abnormal division of the cerebral hemispheres. Such abnormalities may be seen in patients with trisomies 13 and 15 but may also occur in the absence of a specific chromosomal abnormality. In the severest form of holoprosencephaly, designated alobar holoprosencephaly, hemispheric development does not occur and a rudimentary forebrain overlies a common ventricular cavity; in less severe forms, some attempt at lobar differentiation is present (Fig. 23–15). The forebrain abnormalities are accompanied by facial abnormalities ranging in severity from cyclopia to mild facial clefts. In general, the severity of the facial malformation correlates with the severity of the underlying brain abnormality.

Cerebral cortical malformations include changes ranging from subtle, microscopic neuronal migration abnormalities, to the formation of multiple small, abnormally complex gyri *(polymicrogyria),* to a complete absence of gyri

Figure 23–15 ■

Holoprosencephaly. *A,* Gross photograph of cyclopia, the most severe of the facial abnormalities associated with holoprosencephaly. The term *cyclopia* is based on the presence of a single eye structure in the center of the face, reminiscent of the Cyclops in Greek mythology. A blind-ending structure termed a proboscis is visible just above the nonfunctional eye. *B,* Photograph of brain from patient in *A,* demonstrating lack of separation of cerebral hemispheres. A common, single ventricular cavity was present in this case. (Courtesy of Reade Quinton, MD, Department of Pathology, University of Texas Southwestern Medical School, Dallas.)

(lissencephaly). Such cerebral dysplasias account for an important subset of patients with intractable epilepsy.

Neurocutaneous Syndromes

The neurocutaneous syndromes, or phakomatoses, are a group of disorders characterized by malformations and a variety of non-neoplastic and neoplastic proliferations involving the nervous system, skin, eyes, and other organ systems. With the exception of the Sturge-Weber syndrome, most are inherited as autosomal dominant traits with variable expression. The major neurocutaneous syndromes are summarized in Table 23–1. Some, such as neurofibromatosis type 1 and von Hippel-Lindau disease, are also described elsewhere in the text (Chapters 6, 7, and 14).

Perinatal Injury

A variety of exogenous insults may injure the developing brain. Injuries that occur early in gestation may destroy brain without evoking the usual "reactive" changes in the parenchyma (e.g., gliosis or inflammation) and may be difficult to distinguish from primary malformations. Hypoxic-ischemic injury, infections, intrauterine toxin exposure, and birth trauma all contribute to the spectrum of perinatal CNS injury. Some of the more important patterns of perinatal brain injury are described here.

Germinal matrix hemorrhage is the most common cause of intraventricular hemorrhage in premature infants. The germinal matrix persists in the developing human brain until approximately 35 weeks of gestation, particularly in the subependymal region of the caudate nucleus and thalamus. The matrix is composed of primitive cells nourished by delicate, thin-walled vessels consisting of little more than an endothelial layer and basal lamina. Insults such as hypoxemia, hypercarbia, and acidosis, particularly when accompanied by fluctuations in local blood flow, may injure the endothelial cells within the germinal matrix, causing hemorrhage into the matrix. Large hemorrhages easily disrupt the ependymal layer and enter the ventricular system (Fig. 23–16). The hemorrhage may also extend into the adjacent CNS parenchyma, sometimes into an area of white matter necrosis. Many infants with matrix hemorrhage die in the neonatal period. In those surviving the acute episode, organization of the hemorrhage may cause scarring and reactive gliosis, interference with CSF drainage, and obstructive hydrocephalus.

White matter necrosis, also termed *periventricular leukomalacia*, is another important perinatal brain injury; it may be fatal or cause developmental delay and quadriplegia. In contrast to germinal matrix hemorrhages, white matter necrosis may occur in term infants as well as in premature infants, although it is more common in the latter group. Conditions associated with cardiorespiratory dysfunction, including hyaline membrane disease, shock, sepsis, and congenital heart disease, increase the risk of white matter necrosis, presumably by increasing the likelihood of local hypoxic-ischemic injury. The lesions of white matter necrosis appear as areas of chalky discoloration, sometimes associated with cavitation and hemorrhage in white matter. They are particularly common adjacent to the lateral cerebral ventricles.

Figure 23–16 ■

Germinal matrix hemorrhage. Premature infants suffering from hypoxia and related metabolic problems are susceptible to hemorrhage within the delicate germinal matrix, located just beneath the ependymal lining of the lateral ventricles. These hemorrhages commonly extend into the ventricles, as was the case in this patient, and are sometimes designated *intraventricular* hemorrhages. (Courtesy of Linda Margraf, MD, Department of Pathology, University of Texas Southwestern Medical School, Dallas.)

Gray matter injury, resulting from hypoxic-ischemic injury or, in some cases, infections, may assume the form of a typical infarct involving a well-defined vascular territory, or it may occur in areas of special vulnerability, such as the thalamus, basal ganglia, and certain brain stem nuclei. The reasons for many of the patterns of selective vulnerability remain incompletely understood but likely include combinations of local circulatory factors and regional variations in the distribution of excitatory neurotransmitters, as in the case of selective hypoxic-ischemic injury patterns in the adult brain. Gray matter injury may give rise to long-term neurologic impairment and is responsible for some cases of *cerebral palsy*, an etiologically heterogeneous group of disorders characterized by nonprogressive motor dysfunction and other neurologic deficits. Depending on the severity of the insult, the lesions of gray matter injury range from localized areas of neuronal loss and gliosis to extensive parenchymal defects accompanied by widespread gliosis, a lesion sometimes designated as *multicystic encephalopathy*. As noted earlier, destructive insults occurring early in gestation may produce large structural defects unaccompanied by gliosis or other reactive changes.

INFECTIONS OF THE NERVOUS SYSTEM

Under normal circumstances, the brain and spinal cord are shielded from the external environment by their bony coverings, connective tissue, and skin. Infectious agents may gain access to the nervous system by one of several routes. These include hematogenous spread, direct implantation in the setting of trauma or congenital CNS malformations (e.g., neural tube defects), local extension of infection in a contiguous structure (e.g., the middle ear and sinuses), and invasion via the peripheral nerves, as in the case of rabies. The development of infections within the CNS is influenced by at least two factors, acting alone or in concert: the nature of the infectious agent and the integrity of normal host defenses. For example, disruption of normal barriers, such as might be encountered in a patient with a skull fracture and meningeal tear, allows organisms of even low virulence to gain access to brain parenchyma. At the other end of the spectrum, certain organisms, because of either their highly virulent nature or their selective neurotropism (e.g., rabies virus or herpes simplex virus [HSV] type 1), are capable of producing CNS infection even in the presence of normal host defenses. Any part of the nervous system may be the site of active infection. In some instances, infections rapidly become generalized, as in the case of acute bacterial infections in the leptomeninges. In other cases, infections may be more localized, as in the case of abscesses caused by pyogenic bacteria or infections caused by agents such as poliovirus that affect neuronal subpopulations in a selective manner. Infections of the nervous system will be discussed on a regional basis, recognizing that infections affecting one compartment of the nervous system are often associated with infection of another.

Epidural and Subdural Infections

Epidural abscesses and subdural empyemas are relatively rare but have a high mortality rate. Within the skull, such lesions usually occur as a complication of primary infections in the paranasal sinuses or mastoid or as a consequence of trauma. Because the dura mater is firmly attached to the inner table of the skull, epidural infections in this region tend to remain localized, whereas those involving the subdural space may spread widely. They are caused most commonly by virulent agents such as staphylococci and streptococci. Spinal epidural infections are more common than are cranial infections, owing to the presence of intervertebral foramina connecting the epidural space with the pleura and retroperitoneum.

Leptomeningitis

Leptomeningitis, or *meningitis*, as it is more often called, refers to inflammation of the leptomeninges and subarachnoid space. Most cases result from infection, although certain chemical agents introduced into the subarachnoid space may also cause meningitis. Infectious meningitis can be divided into acute purulent meningitis, usually caused by bacteria; acute lymphocytic meningitis, usually caused by viruses; and chronic meningitis, which may be caused by a number of different infectious agents.

ACUTE (PURULENT) LEPTOMENINGITIS

Acute leptomeningitis is an important cause of morbidity and mortality at all ages. Almost all cases are caused by

bacteria, which most often reach the CNS via the bloodstream after colonizing the nasopharynx. Although identification of the specific organism responsible for the infection is critical when planning therapy, the age of the patient and other clinical features provide an important guide to empirical treatment:

■ Most cases of meningitis in the neonatal period are caused by flora in the maternal genital tract. Encapsulated group B streptococci and *Escherichia coli*, in particular, are especially important pathogens in this age group.
■ Among children older than 6 months of age, *Haemophilus influenzae* formerly accounted for most cases of acute meningitis; its frequency has declined dramatically in recent years, however, owing to the introduction of an effective vaccine. *Streptococcus pneumoniae* currently accounts for most cases of acute meningitis in young children.
■ *Neisseria meningitidis* is the most common cause of epidemics of acute leptomeningitis and the most common cause of acute meningitis in older children, adolescents, and young adults.
■ Among older adults, most cases of acute meningitis are caused by *S. pneumoniae* and various gram-negative bacilli.
■ *Listeria monocytogenes* is an important cause of acute leptomeningitis in the elderly, certain immunocompromised patients, and neonates.
■ *Staphylococcus aureus* and gram-negative rods are common pathogens in patients who develop meningitis after placement of surgical shunts to drain CSF from the cerebral ventricles into the peritoneal cavity in the treatment of hydrocephalus.

MORPHOLOGY

In the usual case of acute leptomeningitis, the meninges are intensely congested and contain a variable amount of creamy exudate in the subarachnoid space (Fig. 23–17). The distribution of

Figure 23–17   ■

Acute leptomeningitis. The leptomeninges contain abundant creamy, purulent exudate, most prominently over the superior surface of the cerebrum. The underlying brain is swollen, and the vessels are congested.

the exudate varies somewhat, depending on the cause of the meningitis. In cases of pneumococcal meningitis, for example, exudate is usually most pronounced over the cerebral convexities, while *H. influenzae* often causes a more pronounced basilar exudate. The underlying brain and spinal cord are congested and edematous. Microscopically, the leptomeninges are intensely congested and contain neutrophils and fibrin in the acute phase. Bacteria may be apparent even in tissue sections, but they are most reliably demonstrated in smears of the exudate. The inflammatory process may extend into the ventricular cavities, but infection of the underlying brain parenchyma is rare. Variable numbers of lymphocytes and other mononuclear cells may be seen in partially resolved cases.

Clinical Features. The clinical features of acute leptomeningitis include fever, headache, stiff neck, and altered mental status. The CSF, which is often turbid, contains predominantly neutrophils. CSF protein is elevated owing to increased vascular permeability, and glucose levels are markedly decreased (relative to serum levels) because of impaired transport of glucose into the CSF and, to a lesser extent, the metabolic activity of the neutrophils and microorganisms. Organisms may be visible in Gram-stained preparations of CSF in severe cases and are usually readily isolated if cultures are obtained before the initiation of antibiotic therapy. The prognosis of acute leptomeningitis is largely dependent on the rapidity with which appropriate antimicrobial therapy is initiated. Hence, rapid diagnosis is of paramount importance. Although isolation of the offending organism is always desirable, treatment of meningitis must be initiated promptly, before the results of cultures are available. Some knowledge of the clinical setting in which the meningitis occurs, as noted earlier, may provide important clues to the identity of the causative agent.

ACUTE LYMPHOCYTIC (VIRAL) MENINGITIS

Most cases of acute lymphocytic meningitis are caused by viruses. Because routine cultures are negative, viral meningitis is also referred to as *aseptic meningitis*. In contrast to acute bacterial meningitis, most cases of viral meningitis are self-limited, and patients generally have a much better prognosis. Meningitis can occur in the course of any viral infection. In some instances viral meningitis is associated with concurrent parenchymal infection (encephalitis), but often it is the only manifestation of CNS infection. Important causative agents include echovirus, coxsackievirus, mumps virus, and human immunodeficiency virus (HIV).

Clinical Features. The clinical features of viral meningitis are similar to those of acute bacterial meningitis but are usually less severe. The CSF contains predominantly lymphocytes. CSF protein concentrations are usually elevated to a modest degree, but, in contrast to acute bacterial meningitis, CSF glucose levels are usually normal.

CHRONIC MENINGITIS

Chronic leptomeningitis is most often caused by bacteria and fungi. Important etiologic agents include *Mycobacterium tuberculosis*, *Cryptococcus neoformans*, and, less commonly, *Brucella* species and *Treponema pallidum*. Cryptococcal meningitis is an especially important cause of leptomeningitis in patients with the acquired immunodeficiency syndrome (AIDS).

MORPHOLOGY

The gross and microscopic features of chronic leptomeningitis vary depending on the cause of the meningitis. In general, however, the leptomeninges, and occasionally the dura mater, are thickened and contain a dense exudate in the subarachnoid space. In some cases, notably tuberculous meningitis, the exudate is particularly abundant around the base of the brain. Dense arachnoid adhesions are often present and may cause obstructive hydrocephalus. The host inflammatory reaction depends on the cause of the meningitis. In contrast to acute leptomeningitis, however, the infiltrate is usually dominated by lymphocytes, plasma cells, and epithelioid histiocytes. In cases of tuberculous meningitis (discussed later), well-developed areas of caseous necrosis and a granulomatous inflammatory reaction may be present. In other forms of chronic meningitis, notably cryptococcal meningitis, inflammatory cells may be inconspicuous. In tuberculous leptomeningitis, as well as in some cases of fungal leptomeningitis, blood vessels in the subarachnoid space may develop exuberant proliferative changes in response to the presence of inflammatory cells. Such proliferative changes may be severe enough to compromise vessel lumens **(obliterative endarteritis),** causing **infarcts** in the underlying parenchyma.

Clinical Features. The clinical features of chronic meningitis include headache, sometimes associated with stiff neck and other signs of meningeal irritation. In many cases, however, classic "meningeal" signs may be absent. The CSF contains increased numbers of mononuclear cells, significantly increased levels of protein, and decreased levels of glucose.

Infections of the CNS in syphilis deserve special mention. *Treponema pallidum* can cause nervous system disease in both congenital and acquired syphilis. The organism frequently gains access to the nervous system during the early stages of syphilis and may cause an acute lymphocytic leptomeningitis during the secondary phase of infection. Tertiary neurosyphilis may involve the meninges, vessels, or CNS parenchyma. Combined patterns of infection are not uncommon. The morphologic features of *meningeal syphilis* are nonspecific and include meningeal thickening and a mononuclear inflammatory infiltrate, particularly at the base of the brain. On occasion, the process may preferentially involve the spinal meninges. Plasma cells are a common component of the inflammatory infiltrate and, when present, should always suggest the possibility of syphilis. Proliferative changes and/or fibrosis are often present in the meningeal vessels and may cause ischemic damage in the underlying brain parenchyma. With time, significant meningeal fibrosis may develop, followed by secondary hydrocephalus caused by CSF outflow obstruction. Meningovascular lesions involving the subarachnoid portions of the dorsal nerve roots may cause degeneration of ascending sensory fibers in the posterior columns of the spinal cord, with resultant sensory and gait abnormalities, a condition known as *tabes dorsalis*. Treponemal infection of the brain parenchyma may accompany meningeal infection, producing a condition known as *general paresis* or *general paresis of the insane*. This is characterized by cortical atrophy, neuronal loss, and proliferation of elongated microglial cells termed *rod cells*. Special stains may demonstrate the presence of spirochetes within the brain parenchyma in active cases.

Parenchymal Infections (Including Encephalitis)

Generalized infection of the brain parenchyma is termed *encephalitis*, as in some cases of neurosyphilis (discussed earlier) and in many viral infections. Parenchymal infections may be localized, as in the case of bacterial abscesses, tuberculomas, and most cases of toxoplasmosis. The discussion of parenchymal infections will be divided into brain abscesses, tuberculosis and toxoplasmosis, viral encephalitis, and the spongiform encephalopathies caused by unconventional agents known as prions.

BRAIN ABSCESSES

Brain abscesses may be caused by a variety of bacteria, including staphylococci, streptococci, and a number of anaerobic organisms. The infecting organisms may reach the brain parenchyma by *hematogenous spread* from an infection elsewhere in the body, by *contiguous spread* from adjacent foci of infection (e.g., sinusitis or chronic suppurative otitis media), or by *direct implantation* during trauma. Common sources of hematogenous spread include bacterial endocarditis, lung abscesses, and bronchiectasis. Patients with cyanotic congenital heart diseases associated with right-to-left shunts are at higher risk for the development of brain abscesses, owing to the fact that infectious material in the venous circulation may bypass the lungs and directly enter the systemic arterial circulation.

> ### *MORPHOLOGY*
>
> Brain abscesses may occur anywhere, but they are most common in the cerebral hemispheres. They are frequently solitary but may be multiple, particularly when the organisms arrive by the hematogenous route. The temporal and frontal lobes are particularly common sites of involvement when abscesses arise as complications of infections of the middle ear and paranasal sinuses, respectively. The

Figure 23–18   ■

Brain abscess that is sharply demarcated, indicating that it has been present for some time. Purulent exudate is visible in the center of the abscess. Because antibiotics penetrate very poorly into abscesses, surgical drainage is often necessary to treat such lesions.

> lesion begins as an area of softening (cerebritis), which gradually liquefies. The resultant cavity usually contains yellow-green pus, which may become quite thick (Fig. 23–18). Over the next few weeks, the abscess is delimited from the adjacent brain by proliferating fibroblasts and collagen derived from blood vessels in the adjacent brain. The surrounding brain is edematous and congested, and it contains reactive astrocytes and variable numbers of perivascular inflammatory cells.

Clinical Features. The clinical features of brain abscesses include fever, evidence of increased intracranial pressure, and variable focal neurologic deficits. The CSF contains only scanty cells, increased protein, and normal levels of glucose. Complications of cerebral abscess include brain herniation and rupture of the abscess into the ventricles or subarachnoid space.

TUBERCULOSIS AND TOXOPLASMOSIS

Tuberculosis and toxoplasmosis are important causes of brain parenchymal infections. Tuberculosis may involve the brain parenchyma as well as the meninges. CNS tuberculosis virtually always occurs after hematogenous dissemination of organisms from a primary pulmonary infection. Toxoplasmosis deserves special mention because of its occurrence in patients with AIDS. In the CNS, toxoplasmosis presents as multiple focal lesions, usually within gray matter.

> ### *MORPHOLOGY*
>
> In **tuberculosis,** organisms reach the brain and/or meninges from active pulmonary lesions via the bloodstream to establish focal lesions known as

tuberculomas. Tuberculomas may appear as small, single or multiple firm nodules or as larger, irregular lesions with a central area of caseous ("cheese-like") necrosis. Histologically, they are composed of aggregates of epithelioid histiocytes and giant cells, often associated with areas of necrosis. Stains for acid-fast bacilli are necessary to demonstrate the organisms, which may be quite scanty. Rupture of tuberculomas into the subarachnoid space results in the development of tuberculous meningitis, which may present as an acute or chronic meningitis.

Histologically, untreated lesions of **toxoplasmosis** often contain areas of necrosis associated with a variable mononuclear cell inflammatory infiltrate. *Toxoplasma gondii* organisms, in the form of pseudocysts or individual tachyzoites, are best visualized in tissue sections at the margins of necrotic areas. They may be extremely difficult to demonstrate in previously treated cases. Other important parasitic diseases responsible for focal brain lesions include cysticercosis, echinococcosis, and encephalitis caused by free-living amebae (e.g., *Naegleria* species).

VIRAL ENCEPHALITIS

Although a number of organisms are capable of producing generalized infection of the brain parenchyma (see the discussion of syphilis, earlier), viral infections are the most common cause. A large number of viruses can infect the CNS. In some instances CNS infection occurs as a minor component of systemic infection, while in other cases CNS disease represents the sole, or predominant, manifestation of infection. CNS involvement may be somewhat localized (e.g., temporal lobe encephalitis caused by HSV) or generalized. Most cases of viral encephalitis are also associated with leptomeningitis and hence are more properly designated *meningoencephalitis*. Selective infection of specific cell populations is a feature of some forms of viral encephalitis. For example, rabies virus selectively infects neurons whereas oligodendroglial cells are targets in progressive multifocal leukoencephalopathy (PML). Many forms of viral encephalitis occur in previously healthy individuals, exemplified by herpes simplex encephalitis in adults and many cases of arthropod-borne viral encephalitis. In other infections, such as PML and CMV encephalitis, viral infection occurs as a consequence of host immunosuppression.

MORPHOLOGY

The morphologic features of viral encephalitis depend to some degree on the cause of the infection. However, certain general features are shared by most forms, including perivascular inflammatory infiltrates; microglial nodules; and, in some cases, inclusion bodies. The **perivascular inflammatory infiltrates** consist of mononuclear cells, including lymphocytes, plasma cells, and macrophages. As noted, similar inflammatory infiltrates are often present in the meninges (see earlier section on acute lymphocytic meningitis). Localized aggregates of microglial cells termed **microglial nodules** are usually present and are sometimes associated with phagocytosis of neurons **(neuronophagia).** Although not seen in all cases of viral encephalitis, a number of viruses produce characteristic **inclusion bodies** within the nuclei or cytoplasm of infected cells. Examples include the intracytoplasmic Negri bodies of rabies and the prominent intranuclear inclusions of CMV.

Clinical Features. The clinical and morphologic features of some of the more common viral encephalitides are discussed in the following paragraphs.

Arbovirus (Arthropod-Borne) Encephalitides. Encephalitis caused by arthropod-borne viruses is the most common form of epidemic encephalitis in the western hemisphere. Examples include eastern and western equine, Venezuelan, St. Louis, and California encephalitis. Most cases of arbovirus encephalitis occur in late summer, when the vectors (mosquitoes) are most abundant. Histologically, nonspecific perivascular inflammation and microglial nodules, which are sometimes most pronounced in the brain stem, are seen. The prognosis varies depending on the specific virus responsible for the encephalitis and the general health of the infected individual, with very young and very old patients generally having a worse prognosis.

Herpes Simplex Encephalitis. HSV type 1 is the most common cause of sporadic viral encephalitis in the United States. The disease usually presents abruptly in previously healthy individuals. *An important feature of HSV type 1 encephalitis is its proclivity to involve the temporal lobes and orbital frontal areas,* where it produces a hemorrhagic, necrotizing encephalitis (Fig. 23–19). Microscopic features include the usual perivascular mononuclear inflammatory

Figure 23-19 ■

Herpes simplex encephalitis. The typical necrotizing, hemorrhagic lesions of herpes encephalitis are visible in the medial aspect of the left temporal lobe, and more laterally in the insular cortex. (Courtesy of Beverly Rogers, MD, and Charles L. White III, MD, Department of Pathology, University of Texas Southwestern Medical School, Dallas.)

infiltrates, microglial nodules, and smudgy inclusion bodies within the nuclei of infected glial cells and neurons. Herpesviruses can be detected in most cases by immunohistochemical stains, viral culture, or electron microscopy. Prompt treatment with effective antiviral agents has greatly reduced morbidity and mortality. *HSV type 2* is a less common cause of encephalitis in adults than is HSV type 1, but it may produce a devastating generalized encephalitis in neonates born to women with genital HSV type 2 infection.

Cytomegalovirus Encephalitis. CMV, another member of the herpesvirus group, is an important cause of encephalitis in neonates and immunocompromised patients. Its frequency has increased substantially in recent years, particularly in patients with AIDS. Although CMV may infect any portion of the brain or spinal cord, including spinal nerve roots and cranial nerves, in a significant number of cases, it affects the ependyma, causing the ependymal surfaces of the cerebral ventricles to appear frankly hemorrhagic. Microscopically, the virus evokes a typical perivascular and microglial nodule inflammatory reaction, associated with enlarged cells bearing prominent, well-defined intranuclear and occasionally cytoplasmic inclusions. The full spectrum of CMV-induced diseases is described in Chapter 13.

Human Immunodeficiency Virus Encephalitis. Neurologic disease is a frequent complication of HIV infection. As noted previously, in some instances, neurologic dysfunction occurs as a consequence of one or more opportunistic diseases. In addition to increasing susceptibility to opportunistic infections and neoplasms, HIV is also capable of directly causing disease in both the central and peripheral nervous systems, as noted in Table 23–2. Shortly after seroconversion, a minority of patients with HIV infection develop a self-limited "aseptic" meningitis, clinically indistinguishable from other forms of self-limited viral meningitis, suggesting

that infection of the nervous system occurs fairly early in the course of HIV infection. More ominously, a significant number of patients with HIV infection develop a progressive, devastating neurologic syndrome, variously designated as HIV-1 encephalitis, subacute encephalitis, or AIDS-dementia complex. Symptoms of progressive encephalopathy characteristically develop in the later stages of HIV infection, although in occasional patients, they may be the first manifestation of HIV infection. Manifestations include memory loss, cognitive impairment, and motor disturbances, the latter including impaired fine motor control, gait disturbances, and bladder and bowel incontinence. *HIV-1 encephalopathy is currently the most common cause of dementia in young adults.* Recent evidence suggests that aggressive treatment with antiretroviral agents may delay the onset, and perhaps the progression, of HIV-associated dementia.

MORPHOLOGY

The brain in HIV-1 encephalitis is often atrophic. Morphologic changes are usually most pronounced within white matter and basal ganglia and include variable degrees of myelin pallor associated with the presence of macrophages, scanty perivascular mononuclear inflammatory infiltrates, microglial nodules, and **multinucleate giant cells** (Fig. 23–20). The multinucleate giant cells, derived from fusion of HIV-infected mononuclear cells, contain viral proteins or maturing viral particles. Despite the overwhelming evidence that HIV infects the nervous system, many aspects of the pathogenesis of HIV-1 encephalitis remain unclear. Available evidence indicates that HIV-infected macrophages play a critical role in the development of the disease, both in terms of allowing the virus to gain access to the nervous system and in the development of subsequent brain dysfunction.

Table 23-2. PRIMARY HIV-ASSOCIATED NEUROLOGIC DISORDERS*

Central Nervous System

Primary HIV encephalopathies
   Multinucleate giant cell encephalitis (HIV encephalitis)
   HIV-associated white matter disease (HIV leukoencephalopathy)
   Neocortical/gray matter disease (HIV poliodystrophy)
   Mixed patterns
Vacuolar myelopathy
Lymphocytic meningitis
   Acute, monophasic meningitis
   Chronic aseptic meningitis
Cerebral vasculitis

Peripheral Nervous System

Distal symmetric polyneuropathy
Inflammatory demyelinating neuropathies
Spinal and cranial radiculitis
Vasculitic neuropathy

Skeletal Muscle

Inflammatory myopathy (polymyositis)
Mitochondrial myopathy
Nemaline myopathy

---

*Does not include opportunistic CNS infections and neoplasms also seen in HIV infection.

Figure 23-20 ■

Human immunodeficiency virus (HIV) encephalopathy. HIV infection in the brain is associated with the formation of characteristic multinucleate giant cells, created by fusion of HIV-infected macrophages. (Adapted from Burns DK, et al: The neuropathology of human immunodeficiency virus infection. Arch Pathol Lab Med 115:1112, 1991. Copyright 1991, American Medical Association.)

HIV-1 encephalopathy is often associated with **vacuolar myelopathy,** a condition characterized by vacuolation and myelin breakdown in the dorsal and lateral columns of the spinal cord. The lesions bear a striking resemblance to those of subacute combined degeneration associated with vitamin B₁₂ deficiency (see discussion of vitamin B₁₂ deficiency later in "Nutritional Diseases"). Despite its frequent association with HIV-1 encephalitis, however, the pathogenesis of vacuolar myelopathy remains obscure.

Progressive Multifocal Leukoencephalopathy. PML is a slowly evolving encephalopathy caused by a member of the papovavirus group, the JC virus (JC designates the initials of the patient from whom the virus was first isolated and bears no relationship to Creutzfeldt-Jakob disease, discussed later). PML strikes the immunocompromised and, like CMV and cerebral toxoplasmosis, has become increasingly common with the emergence of AIDS. In PML, *the virus infects oligodendroglia, resulting in areas of demyelination,* which appear grossly as irregular, gelatinous foci, most pronounced at the junction between gray and white matter. Histologic features include demyelination; enlarged, atypical astrocytes; and enlarged oligodendroglial nuclei containing smudgy, light purple inclusions.

SPONGIFORM ENCEPHALOPATHIES

The spongiform encephalopathies represent a group of uncommon, transmissible disorders that includes classic and new-variant Creutzfeldt-Jakob disease (CJD), kuru, Gerstmann-Sträussler syndrome (GSS), and fatal familial insomnia. A number of forms of spongiform encephalopathy also occur in animals, including scrapie, wasting disease of elk and mule deer, and the much-publicized bovine spongiform encephalopathy (mad cow disease). These conditions are called "spongiform" encephalopathies because of the presence of microscopic vacuolation ("spongiosis") that develops within the cell bodies of neurons and in the surrounding neuropil in most cases.

What is remarkable about this group of disorders is that they are caused by a unique family of "infectious" proteins called *prions.* For his discovery of prions, Dr. Stanley Prusiner received the 1997 Nobel Prize for Medicine or Physiology. The following four fundamental concepts have emerged from the study of prions and the diseases caused by them:

■ Prions are the only known class of infectious agents that are devoid of nucleic acids RNA or DNA.
■ Prion diseases may manifest as infectious, sporadic, or genetic disorders.
■ Prion diseases result from accumulation of an abnormally folded form of the normal prion protein.
■ Pathogenic prions can have a variety of conformations, each of which is associated with a specific disease.

Infectious prions are a modified form of a normal structural protein found in the mammalian nervous system. The normal prion protein, usually designated by the abbreviation PrP^c, is a 30-kD, membrane-associated protein encoded by a gene on chromosome 20. Although PrP^c is highly conserved and is expressed at particularly high levels in neurons, its function remains unknown.

Prion-associated diseases develop when PrP^c undergoes a conformational change to form a structurally abnormal protein known as PrP^{sc} (the "sc" designation is derived from the animal disease scrapie). Once present, PrP^{sc} is capable of inducing other normal PrP^c molecules to undergo conformational change to the PrP^{sc} form, resulting in the generation of overwhelming numbers of abnormal PrP molecules (Fig. 23–21). The polypeptide chains of PrP^c and PrP^{sc} are identical in their chemical composition but different in their three-dimensional conformations. PrP^c is rich in α helices, whereas the PrP^{sc} has much fewer α helices and many more β sheets. This structural change is the fundamental event in the pathogenesis of prion disease. In cases of *sporadic CJD,* the most common human form of spongiform encephalopathy, the initial conformational change in PrP^c to form PrP^{sc} apparently occurs slowly and spontaneously. It may have been precipitated by a somatic mutation affecting the PrP^c gene. Inoculation of PrP^{sc} from an infected animal into a normal member of the same species also initiates a similar sequence of conformational changes in the recipient, accounting for the fact that *spongiform encephalopathies are transmissible.*

Hereditary cases, as noted previously, account for an additional subset of cases of spongiform encephalopathy. Genetically transmitted forms of the disease, including fatal familial insomnia, GSS, and approximately 15% of cases of CJD are autosomal dominant disorders. They are caused by the *inheritance of a mutant PrP gene that encodes a form of PrP^c that undergoes spontaneous conformational change to the PrP^{sc} form at an abnormally high rate.* More than 20 mutations have been identified in the PrP gene. Each of these gives rise to a distinct form of the disease. However, in some cases the same mutation gives rise to a different syndrome in different families. This suggests that host factors influence the expressions of the mutant PrP gene.

Because they lack nucleic acids, prions are remarkably resistant to many agents that normally inactivate viruses, such as ultraviolet light, standard sterilizing procedures, and many of the more common disinfectants. CJD is the best known and most completely characterized of the human spongiform encephalopathies. Sporadic cases account for roughly 85% of cases of CJD, with familial forms accounting for most of the remainder. Rare instances of iatrogenic transmission have occurred in patients who have received corneal transplants and human pituitary extract or in patients who were inadvertently inoculated with PrP^{sc} through the use of improperly sterilized neurosurgical depth electrodes. A summary of the pathogenesis of prion diseases is shown in Figure 23–21.

MORPHOLOGY

In the early stages of CJD, the brain is grossly normal. Atrophy is present in cases of long duration and may be severe. The hallmark of CJD and

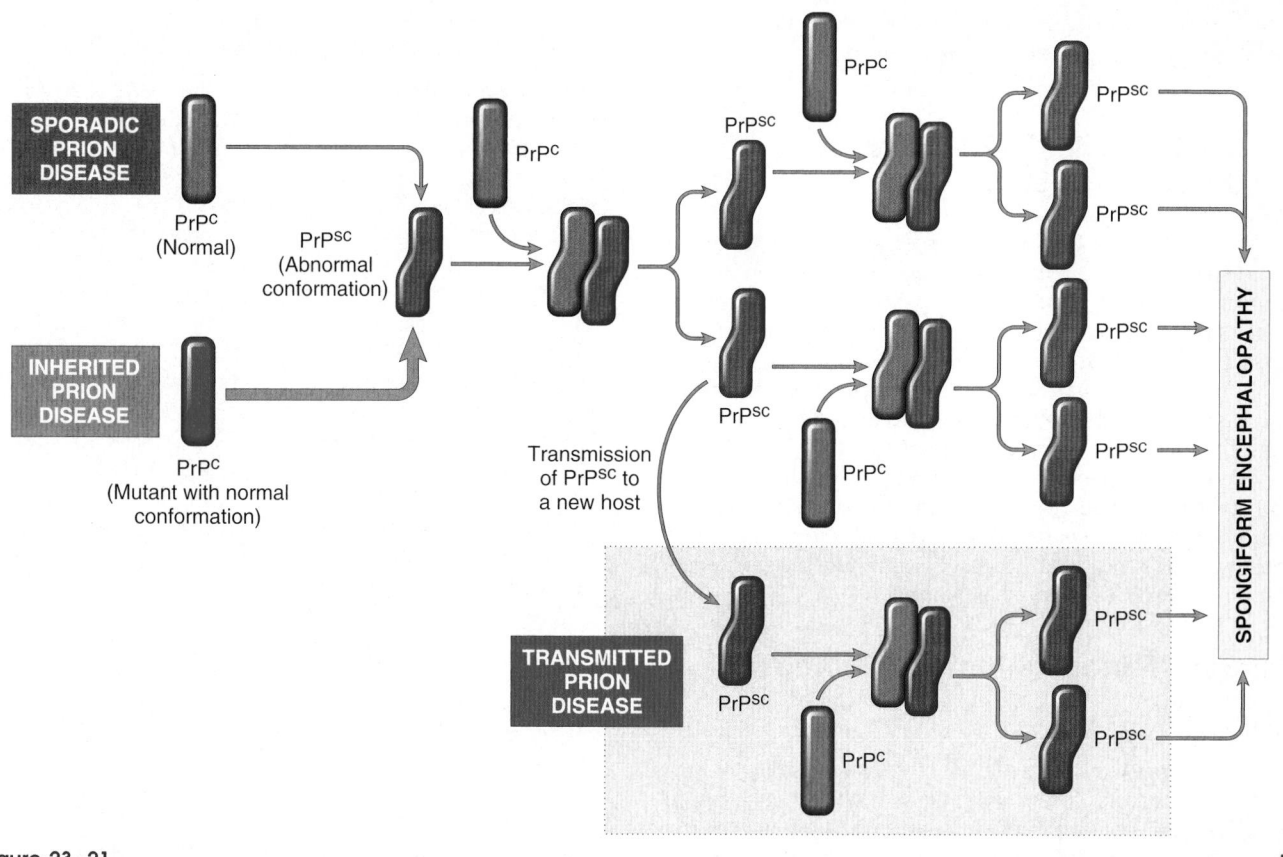

Figure 23-21   ■

Pathogenesis of the three patterns of prion disease. Sporadic prion disease occurs by slow spontaneous transformation of PrP^c to PrP^{sc}. This conversion is greatly accelerated if there is a mutation in the prion gene. Transmission of PrP^{sc} to a new host induces the disease in the recipient. Fundamental in all cases is the ability of PrP^{sc} to convert normal PrP^c protein to the abnormal, pathogenic conformation of PrP^{sc}.

other spongiform encephalopathies is the presence of vacuoles within neuropil and cell bodies in gray matter **(spongiform change)** (Fig. 23–22).

Figure 23-22   ■

Creutzfeldt-Jakob disease. This and related disorders are designated *spongiform encephalopathies* because of their tendency to produce extensive vacuolation, or "spongy" change, within the neuropil.

The vacuolation is accompanied by a variable degree of neuronal loss and reactive gliosis, the degree of which increases with the duration of the disease. Inflammatory infiltrates are usually absent. Amyloid-rich deposits known as **kuru plaques** may be encountered in some forms of spongiform encephalopathy. Although not a feature of the usual CJD case, they are prominent in the cerebral cortex of patients suffering from the so-called new-variant form of the disease (discussed below).

Clinical Features. Clinically, CJD is characterized by rapidly progressive dementia, often accompanied by gait abnormalities and abnormal jerking movements known as startle myoclonus. CJD is typically a disease of adults, with a peak incidence during the seventh decade of life. The disease is invariably fatal, with most patients succumbing within about a year after the onset of symptoms. *New-variant CJD* is a more recently recognized form of spongiform encephalopathy. This transmissible form of CJD has been linked to the ingestion of tissues from cattle with bovine spongiform encephalopathy. Cases of new-variant disease have generally occurred in younger adults than classic CJD and are dominated early in their course by behavioral and psychiatric disturbances.

NEOPLASMS OF THE CENTRAL NERVOUS SYSTEM

Neoplasms of the CNS include those originating within the brain, spinal cord, or meninges, as well as metastatic tumors originating in other sites. Primary CNS neoplasms are somewhat different from neoplasms arising in other sites, in the sense that even histologically benign lesions may result in death, owing to compression of vital structures. Furthermore, in contrast to neoplasms arising outside the CNS, even histologically malignant primary tumors of the brain rarely disseminate to other parts of the body. This discussion of primary CNS tumors will be limited to the more common neuroglial tumors (astrocytomas, oligodendrogliomas, and ependymomas), neuronal neoplasms, primitive neuroectodermal tumors (PNETs), and meningiomas.

Primary Neuroglial Tumors (Gliomas)

ASTROCYTOMAS

Astrocytomas represent the most common group of primary CNS tumors. They comprise a heterogeneous group of neoplasms, ranging from circumscribed, slow-growing lesions typified by pilocytic astrocytoma to highly malignant, infiltrating neoplasms exemplified by glioblastoma multiforme. For purposes of classification, astrocytic tumors can be subdivided into fibrillary (infiltrating) astrocytic neoplasms, pilocytic astrocytomas, and a few uncommon variants that will not be mentioned.

Fibrillary Astrocytic Neoplasms

Sometimes termed *diffuse astrocytomas*, fibrillary astrocytic neoplasms are characterized by an infiltrative growth pattern. Although most commonly encountered in adults, they may occur at any age. Tumors of this type occur most often in the cerebral hemispheres but may be found anywhere in the CNS. These neoplasms are subdivided into histologic grades based on their degree of differentiation. *As with many other neoplasms, histologic grade is an important predictor of biologic behavior.* A number of grading schemes have been proposed over the years, based on features such as nuclear pleomorphism, mitotic activity, vascular proliferation, and necrosis. One system in common use is a three-tiered scheme used in the World Health Organization grading system, which divides these tumors into three grades: well-differentiated lesions, designated *astrocytoma*; intermediate-grade tumors, termed *anaplastic astrocytoma*; and the most aggressive lesions, designated *glioblastoma multiforme*. It should be noted that fibrillary astrocytic neoplasms have a tendency to become progressively less well differentiated over time, with many well-differentiated lesions ultimately progressing to anaplastic astrocytoma or glioblastoma multiforme. In other cases, glioblastomas apparently develop as primary lesions, without a demonstrable better-differentiated precursor lesion. Mutations in the *TP53* tumor suppressor gene appear to play an important role in the development of some of these astrocytic tumors.

MORPHOLOGY

Well-differentiated astrocytomas are usually poorly defined, infiltrative lesions that expand the parenchyma and obliterate normal gray matter/white matter boundaries (Fig. 23–23). Microscopically, well-differentiated astrocytomas are characterized by the presence of increased numbers of irregularly distributed astrocytes, which tend to infiltrate around native cells such as neurons. The nuclei of the neoplastic astrocytes are mildly atypical. The cells often have discernible fibrillar processes, in keeping with their astrocytic differentiation, and may be associated with small accumulations of extracellular fluid, termed **microcysts**. The distinction between low-grade astrocytoma and reactive gliosis may be quite difficult in some cases.

Anaplastic astrocytomas are grossly indistinguishable from their better differentiated counterparts. Radiographic imaging studies, however, may provide a clue to their identity by demonstrating the presence of **contrast medium enhancement**. This results from leakage of contrast medium through abnormally permeable tumor vessels. Histologically, anaplastic astrocytomas are distinguished from well-differentiated lesions by greater cellularity, nuclear pleomorphism, and, most significantly, **mitotic activity**.

Glioblastoma multiforme presents radiographically as an irregular, contrast medium–enhancing lesion, usually associated with considerable edema in the adjacent brain parenchyma. Grossly, it is infiltrative with irregular areas of hemorrhage, necrosis, and cystic change (Fig. 23–24). **It is distinguished histologically from anaplastic astrocytoma by areas of microvascular proliferation and necrosis.** Foci of necrosis are often surrounded by a dense rim of neoplastic nuclei, a pattern designated as **palisading necrosis** (Fig. 23–25).

Figure 23–23   ■

Well-differentiated infiltrating astrocytoma. The right temporal lobe contains an infiltrative, homogeneous lesion that has expanded the lobe and obscured the normal boundaries between gray and white matter. Because of the ill-defined borders, surgical resection seldom removes all the tumor in such cases.

Figure 23-24   ■

Glioblastoma multiforme. In contrast to the well-differentiated infiltrating astrocytoma in Figure 23-23, this glioblastoma contains irregular areas of discoloration and cystic change, reflecting the presence of necrosis and hemorrhage. These lesions are widely infiltrative and associated with considerable mass effect. Note the shift of midline structures to the right.

Clinical Features. Clinically, infiltrating astrocytic neoplasms may present with evidence of increased intracranial pressure (e.g., headache) or with focal abnormalities related to their location (e.g., seizures). Their prognosis is influenced by several factors, including location, the histologic grade of the tumor, and age. Elderly patients generally fare worse than do younger patients with tumors in similar locations. Treatment is influenced by the grade of the neoplasm and currently involves surgical resection, often followed by radiation therapy and/or chemotherapy.

Pilocytic Astrocytomas

Pilocytic astrocytomas are more common in children, although they may occur at any age. Common sites include the cerebellum, third ventricle, and optic nerves, but as in the case of fibrillary astrocytomas, any part of the CNS may be involved. In general, they are distinguished from fibrillary astrocytic neoplasms by their more discrete nature and more indolent behavior.

> ### *MORPHOLOGY*
>
> Pilocytic astrocytomas are usually fairly well defined lesions. Often, they are cystic and contain a mural nodule. Pilocytic astrocytomas derive their name from the presence of astrocytes with elongated, "hairlike" cell processes (Fig. 23-26). Cystic areas, brightly eosinophilic **Rosenthal fibers,** and eosinophilic, protein-rich droplets **(hyaline granular bodies)** are often present. Although the cellular atypia and microvascular proliferation are common, they are much less aggressive than infiltrating astrocytomas. Frank malignancy is exceedingly rare.

The prognosis of patients with pilocytic astrocytomas is influenced primarily by location. Patients with surgically resectable tumors, such as those in the cerebellar hemispheres, usually have an excellent prognosis, whereas tumors in less accessible sites, such as the hypothalamus and brain stem, may cause death even in the absence of histologic evidence of malignancy.

OLIGODENDROGLIOMAS

Oligodendrogliomas are most common during adulthood and usually occur within the cerebral hemispheres. Cytogenetic abnormalities, which are common in oligodendrogliomas, include loss of heterozygosity involving the long arm of chromosome 19 and the short arm of chromosome 1.

Figure 23-25   ■

Photomicrograph of glioblastoma multiforme. Glioblastomas are characterized by hypercellularity, nuclear pleomorphism, mitotic activity, microvascular proliferation, and necrosis. The necrotic area in this example is surrounded by a dense border of tumor cells, giving rise to an appearance termed palisading necrosis.

Figure 23-26   ■

Pilocytic astrocytoma. These lesions are characterized by cells with elongated processes reminiscent, to some observers, of hair, hence the term *pilocytic.* Rosenthal fibers, brightly eosinophilic structures with an almost refractile quality, are common in pilocytic astrocytomas, as well as in a number of other indolent central nervous system neoplasms and chronic reactive processes.

Mutations involving the *TP53* gene are relatively uncommon, in contrast to infiltrating astrocytic tumors.

MORPHOLOGY

Grossly, oligodendrogliomas are usually soft and gelatinous, and they are often better circumscribed than are infiltrating astrocytomas. **Calcification is common** and, when detected radiographically, may provide an important clue to the diagnosis. Microscopically, the classic oligodendroglioma is distinguished by the presence of infiltrating cells with rounded, uniform nuclei, often surrounded by a clear perinuclear halo. The neoplastic cells tend to cluster around native neurons, a phenomenon referred to as **satellitosis.** In some cases, the tumor may extend into the subarachnoid space. Anaplastic change, characterized by increasing nuclear pleomorphism, mitotic activity, and necrosis, may be seen.

The prognosis for patients with oligodendrogliomas is less predictable than that for patients with infiltrating astrocytomas but depends, to some degree, on the histologic grade of the lesion. The age of the patient, location of the tumor, presence or absence of contrast enhancement in radiographic studies, proliferative activity, and cytogenetic characteristics all have additional influences on prognosis.

EPENDYMOMAS

Ependymomas may occur at any age. Most arise within one of the ventricular cavities or in the area of the central canal in the spinal cord. Intracranial ependymomas, in general, are most common in the first 2 decades of life, while intraspinal lesions predominate in adults. Intracranial ependymomas occur most commonly in the fourth ventricle, where they may obstruct CSF outflow and lead to hydrocephalus and increased intracranial pressure.

MORPHOLOGY

Ependymomas are generally well-demarcated lesions arising either from the ventricular walls or, in the case of intraspinal lesions, from remnants of the central canal. Intracranial lesions typically project into the ventricular cavities as solid masses, sometimes with a discernible papillary architecture (Fig. 23-27). The microscopic picture, although variable, is often dominated by elongated cells with processes radiating around blood vessels **(perivascular pseudorosettes)** or lumina **(ependymal rosettes),** the latter recapitulating the structure of normal ependyma. An additional variant, the **myxopapillary ependymoma,** is commonly encountered in the filum terminale of the spinal cord. Most ependymomas

Figure 23-27 ■

Ependymoma. These tumors may arise in both the intracranial compartment and the spine. Intracranial tumors typically originate from a ventricular surface, as in the case of this large lesion arising in the fourth ventricle.

are well differentiated, although a whole range of anaplastic changes may be encountered.

Clinical Features. The clinical manifestations of ependymoma depend on the location of the neoplasm. Intracranial tumors are often associated with hydrocephalus and evidence of increased intracranial pressure. Because of their location within the ventricular system, some tumors, particularly mitotically active anaplastic variants, may disseminate within the subarachnoid space.

Primitive Neuroepithelial Neoplasms

The primitive neuroepithelial neoplasms include a number of tumors composed of embryonal (primitive) small cells that occur predominantly, but not exclusively, in children. Such neoplasms may be undifferentiated, or they may show varying degrees of neuronal, glial, or even mesenchymal differentiation. Primitive neuroepithelial neoplasms occurring within the CNS include medulloblastomas and a number of other uncommon lesions (pineoblastoma, ependymoblastoma, and medulloepithelioma). Only medulloblastomas, the most common of these tumors, will be considered here. Neuroblastomas are described in Chapter 7. Ewing sarcoma, a primitive neuroectodermal tumor arising outside the CNS, is described in Chapter 21.

MORPHOLOGY

Medulloblastomas are lesions of the cerebellum that occur predominantly within the first 2 decades of life. The cerebellar vermis is the usual site of origin in young children, while those occurring in

Figure 23-28 ■

Photomicrograph of a medulloblastoma. These cerebellar neoplasms are composed of primitive neuroectodermal cells with inconspicuous cytoplasmic processes. These tumors may extend into the subarachnoid space and encase the entire central nervous system.

older patients often originate in the cerebellar hemispheres. The lesions obliterate normal cerebellar architecture and may project into the ventricular system, where they may mimic ependymomas. Like ependymomas, medulloblastomas may disseminate through CSF, sometimes encasing the neuraxis in sheathlike metastatic deposits. Microscopically, medulloblastomas are composed of small, primitive cells with scant cytoplasm (Fig. 23-28), reminiscent of other small blue cell tumors encountered in the pediatric population (Chapter 7). The neoplastic cells sometimes form small rosettes, termed **Homer Wright rosettes,** around a central fibrillar core. Evidence of neuronal differentiation may be present, ranging from subtle histochemical or ultrastructural evidence of neuroblastic differentiation to more mature ganglion cells.

Clinical Features. Most patients with medulloblastoma present with evidence of increased intracranial pressure and gait abnormalities, reflecting CSF obstruction and cerebellar injury, respectively. With multimodality therapy, including radiation and chemotherapy, a majority of patients survive 5 years or more.

Neuronal Neoplasms

In addition to the neuronal elements encountered in some primitive neuroepithelial tumors, neurons represent the major component of some additional interesting CNS tumors. The most common of these are the ganglion cell tumors, the dysembryoplastic neuroepithelial tumor, and the central neurocytoma.

Ganglion cell tumors, composed of mature but dysplastic ganglion cells usually admixed with variable numbers of

glial cells, are the most common form of neuronal tumor in the CNS. Most occur in children and young adults and arise within the temporal lobes, where they are an important cause of seizures. Tumors containing a mixture of mature neurons and glial cells are designated as *gangliogliomas*, with the term *gangliocytoma* reserved for tumors composed exclusively of neuronal elements. The behavior of most ganglion cell tumors is benign, although occasional examples of recurrence and aggressive growth have been reported, necessitating appropriate follow-up of all patients with these lesions.

Another important, more recently recognized, form of neuronal tumor is the so-called *dysembryoplastic neuroepithelial tumor (DNT)*. Like ganglion cell tumors, DNTs tend to occur in children and young adults, with a peak incidence during the second decade of life. They are usually associated with a long history of seizures, usually of the complex-partial type. Histologically, DNTs are composed of a mixture of mature neurons, oligodendroglioma-like areas, and astrocytes. It is important that they be distinguished from oligodendrogliomas or other forms of infiltrating glioma. Their prognosis is excellent following simple surgical excision.

The *central neurocytoma* presents as a circumscribed intraventricular mass, usually attached to the wall of the lateral ventricle, corpus callosum, or septum pellucidum. It occurs most frequently in adolescents and young adults. The tumor, which is frequently calcified, is composed of cells with round, uniform nuclei and perinuclear halos quite reminiscent of oligodendroglioma. Most cases behave in an indolent fashion; only rarely has aggressive behavior been reported.

Other Primary Intraparenchymal Neoplasms

Primary CNS lymphomas have increased in frequency in recent years, particularly in association with the emergence of AIDS; indeed, lymphoma of the brain is considered an AIDS-defining condition in HIV-positive individuals (Chapter 5). The lesions of primary CNS lymphoma may be solitary or multiple. They are often hemorrhagic and may be necrotic, even in the absence of treatment. Microscopically, their appearance is similar to that of non-Hodgkin malignant lymphomas arising in other sites, with a predominance of large cell, aggressive lesions. A characteristic feature of these tumors is their tendency to grow around and within the walls of blood vessels (angiocentric growth). Like most large cell lymphomas arising outside of the brain, CNS lymphomas are usually tumors of B lymphocytes. A significant percentage of the tumors arising in immunocompromised hosts are associated with the Epstein-Barr virus genome and *MYC* oncogene activation.

A number of *germ-cell neoplasms* may arise primarily within the intracranial compartment. Most such lesions occur in the suprasellar and pineal areas, particularly in children and young adults. The microscopic appearance of these neoplasms is identical to that of germ-cell neoplasms occurring in the gonads. Intracranial germinomas, which are morphologically identical to testicular seminomas (Chapter 18) and ovarian dysgerminomas, and teratomas are the most commonly encountered variants.

Hemangioblastomas occur in the cerebellum and, less commonly, in the meninges. In the former site, they usually present as circumscribed, cystic lesions with a mural nodule. Microscopically, they are composed of a mixture of delicate vascular channels and intervening lipid-laden, foamy stromal cells of uncertain derivation. They may occur as solitary lesions, or they may be a component of the von Hippel-Lindau syndrome (see Table 23–1). Hemangioblastomas may be extremely difficult to distinguish from metastatic renal cell carcinomas.

Meningiomas and Other Meningeal Neoplasms

Meningiomas are tumors derived from the meningothelial cells that invest the arachnoid mater. Accordingly, most lesions occur outside the brain parenchyma. Meningiomas usually occur in adults and may arise in both the cranial vault and the spinal cord. A female predominance has been noted consistently, particularly among lesions occurring in the spinal cord. This may be related to the presence of progesterone receptors on meningothelial cells and a trophic response to that hormone. Their frequency is also increased in patients with neurofibromatosis (NF) type 2, in whom they are often multiple. In patients with NF type 2, as well as in a significant number of sporadic meningiomas, there is a loss of the *NF2* gene and its product merlin. *NF2* is located on 22q11, and its loss may be due to partial or complete loss of chromosome 22.

Figure 23-29   ■

Meningioma. Most meningiomas originate from meningothelial cells in intimate association with dura mater. Like this tumor they push, rather than infiltrate, the adjacent brain parenchyma. (Adapted from Burns DK: The central nervous system. In Henson DE, Albores-Saavedra J [eds]: Pathology of Incipient Neoplasia, 2nd ed. Philadelphia, WB Saunders, 1993, p 528.)

Clinical Features. Like many other expanding intracranial masses, intracranial meningiomas present with evidence of increased intracranial pressure, sometimes accompanied by seizures and focal neurologic deficits. The overall prognosis for patients with meningiomas is influenced by the size and location of the lesion, surgical accessibility, and histologic grade.

Other primary meningeal neoplasms include hemangioblastomas (discussed earlier), the aggressive meningeal hemangiopericytoma, and rare meningeal sarcomas.

Metastatic Neoplasms

The brain is a common site for metastatic lesions. These occur predominantly in the elderly, paralleling the increase in solid visceral tumors with increasing age. However, hematopoietic neoplasms such as lymphomas and leukemias, which occur in children as well as in adults, may also spread to the CNS. Metastatic neoplasms may involve the meninges as well as brain parenchyma. Excluding leukemias and lymphomas, the most common primary sites, in descending order of frequency, are carcinomas of the lung and breast and malignant melanomas. Neurologic abnormalities may be the first clue to the presence of a visceral carcinoma, particularly in the case of carcinomas arising in the lung.

MORPHOLOGY

Meningiomas usually present as firm, lobulated lesions attached to the dura mater. A sharp interface is usually present between the tumor and the adjacent brain or spinal cord (Fig. 23–29). The overlying skull may be thickened and is sometimes invaded by tumor. A variety of microscopic patterns may be seen in meningiomas, but there is often some recapitulation of the compact cellular whorls seen in the normal arachnoid mater. Common histologic types include **syncytial** and **fibroblastic** variants; neoplasms containing a mixture of these two patterns are designated **transitional meningiomas.** Deletions of the *NF2* gene are particularly common in tumors with a fibroblastic or transitional growth pattern. Calcification, if present, usually takes the form of concentrically laminated, calcified granules termed **psammoma bodies.** A rather impressive array of other histologic variants may occur, although many are of no prognostic significance. Certain histologic features, however, are associated with more aggressive behavior, including increasing cellularity and nuclear pleomorphism, mitotic activity, necrosis, papillary architecture, and invasion of underlying brain parenchyma.

MORPHOLOGY

Carcinomas and melanomas metastatic to the brain parenchyma are well-demarcated, roughly spherical lesions that may be solitary or multiple (Fig. 23–30). A sharp interface is present between the focus of metastatic carcinoma and the adja-

Figure 23-30   ■

Metastatic melanoma. Metastatic lesions are distinguished grossly from most primary central nervous system tumors by their multicentricity and well-demarcated margins. The dark pigment in the tumor nodules in this case is characteristic of most malignant melanomas.

cent parenchyma. Considerable edema may be present around some lesions, which contributes to their mass effect. Microscopically, the morphology of metastatic carcinomas usually recapitulates the morphology of the primary lesion. Less commonly, carcinomas may metastasize to the leptomeninges. **Leptomeningeal carcinomatosis** produces a vague opacification of the leptomeninges. Malignant cells are usually demonstrable in the CSF of such patients, and concomitant metastatic lesions are sometimes present in the brain parenchyma. Carcinomas metastatic to the **dura mater** may be encountered, particularly in patients with primary lesions in the prostate, breast, or lung.

Clinical Features. Clinical features of metastatic carcinomas include evidence of increased intracranial pressure and variable focal neurologic deficits. Cranial nerve palsies are particularly common in patients with leptomeningeal carcinomatosis.

PRIMARY DISEASES OF MYELIN

In the CNS the myelin sheath is derived from the cytoplasmic processes of oligodendroglial cells, which wrap concentrically around neuronal processes in the same fashion as do Schwann cells in the peripheral nervous system. The purpose of myelin in the CNS, as in the peripheral nervous system, is to provide "insulation" for neuronal cell processes, permitting rapid conduction of electrical impulses along cell membranes. A number of disorders may interfere with the integrity of the myelin sheath, thereby disrupting the normal transmission of electrical activity within the brain and causing neurologic disease. Such processes may affect the myelin primarily, the oligodendroglial cell body,

or both. For purposes of discussion, diseases of myelin will be divided into *acquired demyelinating diseases*, typified by multiple sclerosis, in which normally formed myelin is injured, and the so-called *leukodystrophies*, in which an inborn metabolic error interferes with normal myelin development and maintenance.

Multiple Sclerosis

Multiple sclerosis (MS) is the most common demyelinating disease of the CNS. There are 250,000 to 350,000 patients with this disease in the United States. It is more frequent in temperate than in equatorial climates and in people of European extraction. MS typically presents in young adults, with a peak incidence between the ages of 18 and 40 years. Most cases are characterized by waxing and waning neurologic abnormalities involving different regions of the CNS, occurring over a number of years. The cause and pathogenesis of MS are not fully understood. However, there is a significant body of indirect evidence that it is an autoimmune disease involving T-cell–mediated injury to myelin sheaths and/or oligodendroglial cells. Both CD4+ and CD8+ cells are present within the lesions, and many are reactive against myelin basic protein. They cause injury by release of cytokines as well as direct CD8+ T-cell–mediated cytotoxicity. A disorder bearing some resemblance to human MS, termed *chronic experimental allergic encephalomyelitis*, can be induced in mice by sensitizing them to components of myelin and can be transferred into naive animals by sensitized T cells. Antibody-mediated injury also seems to play a role. Antibodies against myelin oligodendrocyte protein and myelin basic protein along with activated complement may be present in lesions undergoing demyelination. Current evidence suggests that both environmental (infectious?) and hereditary factors contribute to the development of autoimmunity in this disease. People migrating from high-risk to low-risk geographic areas, and vice versa, retain the risk of MS associated with their birthplace if migration occurs after the age of 15; if migration occurs before the age of 15, however, individuals assume the risk of MS associated with their new homes, suggesting that exposure to an environmental agent early in life contributes to the development of MS. A genetic component, in addition, is suggested by the increased risk of MS in association with HLA-DR2 genes and a higher rate of concordance in identical twins than dizygotic twins. Presumably, class II HLA genes regulate the autoimmune response (Chapter 5). The observation that the concordance rate is only 25% to 30% among identical twins, however, indicates that genetic factors alone are not responsible for the development of MS.

MORPHOLOGY

The external appearance of the brain and spinal cord is usually normal. On cut surface, MS is characterized by the presence of multiple areas of demyelination, termed **plaques**. MS plaques may occur anywhere in the brain or spinal cord,

Figure 23-31 ■

Multiple sclerosis. The typical plaque is a well-demarcated, firm, gray-pink lesion. The periventricular white matter is a common site for these lesions, although they may occur in any part of the brain or spinal cord.

immunoglobulins, known as *oligoclonal bands*, in most patients with MS. These antibodies are believed to arise in response to myelin injury and are not thought to play a primary role in the demyelination. They are also encountered in a number of conditions other than MS. *Myelin basic protein* is often present in the CSF during periods of active demyelination. Like oligoclonal bands, however, its presence is not specific for MS. Radiographic imaging, particularly magnetic resonance imaging, has proven to be an effective tool in the evaluation of suspected MS lesions, especially when interpreted in the context of the clinical signs and symptoms and ancillary CSF studies. The course of MS is somewhat unpredictable, with some patients presenting with fulminant, rapidly progressive disease and dying within weeks to months of onset (*acute MS*), and others experiencing a normal life span, with few or no chronic sequelae. In most cases, however, the disease is characterized by multiple exacerbations and remissions, with cumulative neurologic deficits developing over the course of several years to decades.

accounting for the wide range of clinical manifestations associated with the disease. Common sites include the periventricular white matter, the optic nerves, and the white matter of the spinal cord. Plaques are usually well-demarcated lesions ranging from a few millimeters to several centimeters in diameter. Acute lesions are often soft and slightly pink, while older lesions tend to be firm and pearly gray to pink (Fig. 23-31). Microscopically, plaques are characterized by areas of demyelination, initially in a **perivenous distribution,** accompanied by a variable perivascular lymphocytic inflammatory infiltrate. In active lesions, there is evidence of myelin breakdown, manifested by the presence of lipid-laden macrophages. Residual axonal processes are usually present in the areas of demyelination but are reduced in number, particularly in chronic lesions. An additional type of plaque known as the **shadow plaque** may also occur in MS. Shadow plaques contain axons invested by abnormally thin, faintly staining myelin sheaths and are believed to represent areas of remyelination. The peripheral nervous system is spared.

Clinical Features. The onset of MS may be acute or insidious. In keeping with the highly variable distribution of MS plaques, the clinical manifestations of the disease are protean. Common manifestations include visual disturbances (blurred vision, diplopia, scotomata), paresthesias, spasticity of one or more extremities, speech disturbances, and gait abnormalities. Various emotional disturbances may be seen, including depression, inappropriate euphoria, and mood lability. Cognitive impairment may be present but is usually not severe. Examination of the CSF usually reveals slightly increased protein levels and a small number of lymphocytes. The proportion of gamma globulin is increased, and CSF electrophoresis reveals discrete bands of

Other Acquired Demyelinating Diseases

Acute disseminated encephalomyelitis, sometimes designated *perivenous encephalomyelitis*, is an immune-mediated demyelinating disease that may follow certain infections (measles, chickenpox, rubella, and others) and vaccinations. This disorder is believed to represent hypersensitivity reaction, possibly triggered by exposure to selected foreign antigens; attempts to isolate virus from CNS tissues of affected patients have been unsuccessful. In contrast to the usual case of MS, acute disseminated encephalomyelitis is typically a monophasic illness of abrupt onset. Signs and symptoms include fever, seizures, coma, spinal cord dysfunction, and other focal neurologic deficits. Histologically, this reaction is characterized by areas of perivascular demyelination and mononuclear cell infiltration. The disease is fatal in 15% to 20% of cases.

Central pontine myelinolysis is a condition characterized by demyelination within the basis pontis. This condition has been associated with a number of factors, including alcoholism. Hyponatremia has been noted in a significant number of patients who subsequently develop central pontine myelinolysis, and excessively rapid correction of hyponatremia has been implicated as one possible cause of the disorder. The mechanism whereby rapid correction of hyponatremia might cause myelin injury remains unclear, however.

A number of infections may be associated with demyelination, the most well known of which is PML, discussed previously in the section "Viral Encephalitis." Herpes zoster encephalitis and CMV encephalitis may also produce areas of demyelination.

Leukodystrophies

The leukodystrophies represent a group of disorders in which an intrinsic defect interferes with the generation

Table 23–3. LEUKODYSTROPHIES

Disorder	Inheritance	Metabolic Abnormality
Metachromatic leukodystrophy	Autosomal recessive	Arylsulfatase A deficiency
Krabbe disease	Autosomal recessive	Galactocerebroside β-galactosidase deficiency
Adrenoleukodystrophy	X-linked and autosomal recessive	Peroxisomal defect; elevated levels of very-long-chain fatty acids

and/or maintenance of myelin. Most are hereditary, with both autosomal recessive and X-linked patterns of inheritance reported. In some, but not all, cases a specific lysosomal enzymatic defect has been associated with the myelin abnormality. In contrast to MS, the leukodystrophies are usually diseases of infancy and childhood, characterized by a relentlessly progressive course. They may involve peripheral nerves as well as the CNS. The most common leukodystrophies are listed in Table 23–3, along with their inheritance patterns and underlying biochemical defects.

MORPHOLOGY

Leukodystrophies are characterized by a widespread, symmetric loss of myelin throughout the brain and often the spinal cord as well. The brain is usually atrophic, and the centrum ovale and other central white matter areas appear shrunken, gray, and translucent. Some sparing of subcortical myelin ("U fibers") may be evident (Fig. 23–32). Microscopic features vary with the type of leukodystrophy

Figure 23–32   ■

Leukodystrophy. These are characterized by extensive, fairly symmetric loss of white matter, in contrast to the multifocal, demarcated areas of demyelination seen in multiple sclerosis. Sparing of the white matter immediately beneath the cerebral cortex (subcortical U fibers), as is present in this case, is seen in many leukodystrophies.

but include widespread loss of myelin, accompanied in some cases by accumulations of abnormal myelin breakdown products.

ACQUIRED METABOLIC AND TOXIC DISTURBANCES

The delicate circuitry of the nervous system may be disrupted by a number of toxic and metabolic disturbances. In some cases the changes in the nervous system are largely functional, with only subtle attendant structural abnormalities. In other instances, however, striking and sometimes highly characteristic morphologic changes are produced by the toxin or underlying metabolic abnormality. The list of acquired toxic and metabolic diseases in the nervous system is formidable; hence, only some of the more common examples will be reviewed here.

Nutritional Diseases

Thiamine and vitamin B_{12} (cobalamin) deficiencies are two of the most common nutritional disorders associated with nervous system abnormalities.

Thiamine deficiency causes the *Wernicke-Korsakoff syndrome* and is an important cause of peripheral neuropathy as well. Thiamine deficiency may occur in a number of settings, but in the United States it is most commonly encountered in chronic alcoholics. Indeed, abnormalities referable to thiamine deficiency are second only to traumatic lesions as a cause of pathologic alterations in the brains of alcoholics. *Wernicke encephalopathy* is characterized by fairly rapid onset of confusion, paralysis of extraocular muscles (particularly the lateral rectus), and ataxia. The syndrome may progress to coma and death if untreated but responds well to the administration of thiamine in the early stages. If Wernicke encephalopathy is not treated promptly, a permanent memory deficit known as *Korsakoff psychosis* may result. Korsakoff psychosis is characterized by an inability to either form new memories or retrieve old ones, often accompanied by confabulation.

MORPHOLOGY

The morphologic changes of Wernicke encephalopathy are most evident in the mamillary bodies of the hypothalamus, the dorsal medial areas of the thalamus, and the gray matter around the cerebral aqueduct, the last correlating with the eye movement abnormalities noted clinically. The earliest change is capillary endothelial proliferation associated with abnormal vascular permeability. The hemorrhages result from leakage of red cells from these abnormal capillaries (Fig. 23–33). Morphologic changes associated with Korsakoff syndrome are present in the same areas as those involved in Wernicke encephalopathy and include

Figure 23-33 ■

Wernicke encephalopathy. Thiamine deficiency in the central nervous system is associated with the development of hemorrhagic gray matter lesions, depicted here in the mamillary bodies of the hypothalamus.

gliosis and hemosiderin deposits resulting from previous hemorrhage. In contrast to changes after ischemic injury, neurons are relatively spared but are often somewhat shrunken.

Thiamine deficiency has also been implicated in the development of atrophy of the superior vermis often seen in alcoholics, termed *alcoholic cerebellar degeneration*. In the peripheral nervous system, thiamine deficiency causes a peripheral axonal neuropathy (discussed later).

Deficiency of vitamin B_{12} (cobalamin) causes pernicious anemia (Chapter 12). In the nervous system, vitamin B_{12} deficiency is associated with the development of *subacute combined degeneration of the spinal cord*, a condition characterized by myelin vacuolation in the dorsal and lateral white matter columns of the spinal cord (Fig. 23–34). In keeping with the distribution of the lesions, subacute combined degeneration is characterized by both motor and sensory abnormalities, including spasticity, weakness, and loss of proprioception. Deficiency of vitamin B_{12} may also produce a confusional state, sometimes termed *megaloblastic madness*.

Acquired Metabolic Disorders

Patients with a number of systemic derangements may develop evidence of CNS dysfunction. Probably the best characterized is that associated with hepatic failure. *Hepatic encephalopathy* is characterized by altered levels of consciousness and a characteristic "flapping" tremor termed *asterixis* (Chapter 16). Grossly, the brain may be normal or edematous. Microscopically, this condition is characterized by increased numbers of large, "naked," pale-staining astrocytic nuclei, termed *Alzheimer type II glia*, within gray matter. The astrocytic changes are likely related in some way to high levels of ammonia, the

metabolism of which occurs predominantly within astrocytes via the activity of the enzyme glutamine synthetase. Identical changes are encountered in patients with Wilson disease, an entity considered more fully in the discussion of diseases of the liver (Chapter 16).

Toxic Disorders

The list of environmental neurotoxins is so large that a complete list cannot be given here. Among the major categories of neurotoxic substances are *metals*, examples of which are arsenic, mercury, and lead; a wide variety of *industrial chemicals*, including organophosphates and methyl alcohol; and a range of *environmental pollutants* such as carbon monoxide. The most important of these were discussed in Chapter 8.

Therapeutic agents are an additional important and expanding category of neurotoxins; some of the many types of adverse effects are *peripheral neuropathies* (*Vinca* alkaloids, isoniazid) and *seizures* (metronidazole). Many neurotoxic side effects have also been associated with the administration of chemotherapeutic agents for the treatment of tumors. *Methotrexate*, an important antineoplastic agent, may cause CNS injury, particularly in patients receiving intrathecal or high-dose systemic therapy in conjunction with radiation therapy. The morphologic changes associated with methotrexate toxicity are most prominent in white matter and consist of necrosis, demyelination, gliosis, and calcification. *Ionizing radiation* can cause significant vascular injury in the CNS, as it does in other organs, leading to tissue ischemia and infarction. As in the case of methotrexate-associated lesions, the damage associated with ionizing radiation is most prominent within white matter.

Figure 23-34 ■

Subacute combined degeneration of the spinal cord. In addition to hematologic abnormalities, vitamin B_{12} deficiency may cause neurologic disease. Subacute combined degeneration of the spinal cord, the most common of these neurologic disorders, is characterized by degeneration of the lateral and dorsal columns of the spinal cord, seen here as areas of pallor surrounded by normal myelin, stained blue in this preparation.

DEGENERATIVE DISEASES

The *degenerative diseases of the CNS* encompass a heterogeneous group of disorders characterized by spontaneous, progressive degeneration of neurons in a specific region or system in the brain, spinal cord, or both. Degenerative diseases may be sporadic or familial. They show considerable clinical variability, and often there is overlapping of clinical features that clouds distinction between the various types. Our comments will focus on some of the more common degenerative diseases, including Alzheimer disease, parkinsonism, Huntington disease, and amyotrophic lateral sclerosis (motor neuron disease).

Alzheimer Disease and Related Disorders

Dementia, defined as the development of memory impairment and other cognitive deficits with preservation of a normal level of consciousness, is emerging as one of the most important public health issues in the industrialized world. Although dementia may occur at virtually any age, it is predominantly a disease of the elderly, with a prevalence of over 30% past the age of 85.

ALZHEIMER DISEASE

Alzheimer disease (AD) is the most common cause of dementia in the elderly, with cerebrovascular disease and several less common neurodegenerative disorders accounting for most of the remaining cases. Most cases of AD occur after the age of 50, with a progressive increase in incidence with increasing age. Most cases are sporadic, but in roughly 10% of patients, there is a family history of dementia. As will be discussed, these familial cases have provided important insights into the pathogenesis of AD. Morphologic changes identical to those seen in AD are also almost invariably present in patients with Down syndrome who survive beyond the age of 40. Although the cause of AD remains unknown, a number of factors have now been identified that appear to play a major role in the development of this disorder.

■ *Genetic factors* play a role in the development of some cases of AD, as evidenced by the occurrence of familial cases. Studies of familial cases have provided significant insights into the pathogenesis of familial, and possibly sporadic, AD. Mutations in at least four genetic loci have been linked conclusively to familial AD. In view of the long-recognized association between trisomy 21 and AD-like changes in the brain, it is perhaps not surprising that the first of these to be identified was a locus on chromosome 21, now known to encode a protein known as *amyloid precursor protein* (APP). As will be discussed in the next section, APP is the source of the amyloid deposits encountered in a variety of sites in the brains of patients suffering from AD. Mutations in two additional genes, termed *presenilin 1* and *presenilin 2*, located on chromosomes 14 and 1, respectively, appear to account for a much larger proportion of familial AD, particularly those of early onset. Mutations in the presenilin genes have been associated, in turn, with increased production of amyloid in the CNS (discussed later) and may also contribute to abnormal neuronal loss via apoptosis. An additional group of cases of late-onset familial AD is linked to the expression of the ε4 allele of apolipoprotein E, encoded by chromosome 19, discussed in more detail later.

■ *Deposition of a form of amyloid,* derived from breakdown of APP, is a consistent feature of AD. The breakdown product, known as β-amyloid (Aβ), is a prominent component of the senile plaques found in the brains of AD patients (discussed later), and it is usually present within the walls of cerebral blood vessels as well. Genetic or acquired defects in the processing of APP seem to be important in the causation of AD. Under normal circumstances, membrane-bound APP is cleaved by the action of a protease known as α-secretase into a large soluble version of APP and a smaller membrane-anchored fragment (Fig. 23–35A). The latter is further cleaved by γ-secretase (Fig. 23–35B). Alternatively, APP is first cleaved by β-secretase to produce a soluble fragment. However, when the remaining membrane-anchored segment is cleaved by the γ-secretase, there is the formation of less soluble Aβ peptides, which tend to aggregate into amyloid fibrils. Processing by the two pathways occurs in distinct subcellular compartments. Cleavage by β-secretase followed by γ-secretase occurs in the endosomal compartment, whereas proteolysis by the α-secretase pathway takes place in the cell membrane. Both pathways occur under normal circumstances, and there is no evidence that the β-secretase pathway dominates in sporadic cases of AD. It seems more likely that the clearance of fibrillogenic Aβ peptides is impaired in patients who develop AD. By contrast, in some familial cases of AD, mutation in APP does cause overproduction of Aβ peptides. Similarly, mutations in the presenilin genes, mentioned earlier, are also associated with increased production of Aβ. Studies indicate that presenilins may be the catalytic subunits of γ-secretase. Thus, mutations in presenilin genes that increase γ-secretase activity facilitate Aβ production. Intriguing though these observations are, however, the role played by Aβ in the pathogenesis of AD remains poorly understood. Aβ has been shown to be toxic to neurons in cell cultures, although the relationship between such in vitro activity and the lesions of AD is unclear. Whether amyloid deposition plays a primary role in the development of AD or represents a secondary phenomenon remains a topic of heated debate.

■ *Hyperphosphorylation of the protein tau* represents yet another piece of the AD puzzle. Tau is an intracellular protein that is involved in the assembly of intra-axonal microtubules. In addition to amyloid deposition, cytoskeletal abnormalities are an invariant feature of AD. Many of these structural abnormalities are associated with accumulation of hyperphosphorylated forms of tau, the presence of which may interfere with maintenance of normal microtubules. While invariably present in AD, tau-associated cytoskeletal abnormalities are not restricted

Figure 23-35 ■

Proposed scheme of the pathogenesis of Alzheimer disease. *A*, Structure of amyloid precursor protein (APP); depicted are three cleavage sites and the enzymes involved in proteolysis of APP. *B*, One proteolytic pathway involves the action of α- and γ-secretases, yielding soluble nonpathogenic fragments of APP. *C*, Another cleavage pathway of APP involves the action of β-secretase and γ-secretase; this results in the formation of Aβ peptide, which aggregates to form amyloid. Experimental studies suggest that Aβ amyloid increases the formation of tau tangles derived from abnormally hyperphosphorylated tau proteins. Together, the abnormal tau proteins and the Aβ amyloid form the senile plaques seen in Alzheimer disease.

to that disorder; they are encountered in a variety of other neurodegenerative disorders and conditions as diverse as metabolic diseases (Niemann-Pick disease), neoplasms (gangliogliomas), and hamartomas. Whether hyperphosphorylation of tau protein represents a primary event in the pathogenesis of AD, or a secondary event, remains to be established. Until very recently, there appeared to be no linkage between the formation of abnormal tau proteins and amyloid deposition. Now the proponents of the tau hypothesis ("tauists") and the β-amyloid hypothesis ("βaptists") may have found a point of convergence. It appears, at least in murine models of Alzheimer disease, that APP or its product Aβ amyloid increases the formation of neurofibrillary tangles derived from tau proteins.

■ *Expression of specific alleles of apoprotein E* (apoE) has been demonstrated in both sporadic and familial AD. Retrospective and prospective studies have demonstrated that the ε4 allele of apoE, in particular, is expressed with increased frequency in patients with late-onset AD. It has been suggested that apoE may be involved in the transport or processing of the APP molecule. ApoE con-

taining the ε4 allele is reported to bind to Aβ better than do other forms of apoE, and they may thus contribute to enhanced amyloid fibril formation. While it is clear that the presence of the ε4 allele is associated with an increased risk of AD, it should also be noted that a significant percentage of patients with documented AD do not express the apoE ε4 allele. Moreover, ε4 is expressed in some elderly individuals without AD. Together, these observations suggest that while the ε4 form of apoE may contribute to AD, its presence alone is neither sufficient nor essential for the development of AD.

As is evident from the previous discussion, the unraveling of the molecular basis of Alzheimer disease is well under way. Not only is the delineation of molecular pathways significant for understanding the pathogenesis of this debilitating disease, but it also provides targets for development of drugs that could be used to treat or halt progression of this disorder. For example, drugs that inhibit the action of γ-secretases could, by reducing Aβ amyloid production, be beneficial.

MORPHOLOGY

The brain in AD is usually atrophic, although it may be grossly normal in the earlier stages of the disease. The atrophy is most evident in the frontal, temporal, or parietal lobes but typically involves all cortical areas to some degree (Fig. 23–36). Examination of the cut surface reveals symmetric dilation of the cerebral ventricles in most cases, reflecting a generalized loss of parenchyma (hydrocephalus ex vacuo). Microscopic changes include the presence of **neurofibrillary tangles,** which appear as coarse, filamentous aggregates within the cytoplasm of neurons. They are found in the neocortex, hippocampus, basal forebrain, and some parts of the brain stem. The neurofibrillary tangles are composed of insoluble, protein-rich paired helical filaments (PHFs), the major component of which is hyperphosphorylated **tau protein.** Additional accumulations of PHFs occur within distal neuronal cell processes (neurites) to form the peripheral component of the **senile plaques,** which appear as aggregates of coarse, tortuous neurites in the neuropil of the cerebral cortex (Fig. 23–37). The senile plaques contain a central **amyloid core** composed of Aβ. In addition, β-amyloid deposits are usually present in leptomeningeal and parenchymal vessels as well, a pattern referred to as **amyloid angiopathy.** These amyloid deposits are unrelated to those encountered in other forms of systemic or localized amyloidosis (Chapter 5). The simple presence of plaques and/or tangles is not, by itself, specific for AD, because such structures are also frequently present in the brains of otherwise normal elderly individuals. It is rather the **density and widespread distribution of plaques and tangles** in neocortical areas in the setting of dementia that allows one to make a diagnosis of AD.

Figure 23–37   ■

Photomicrograph of a senile plaque from a patient with Alzheimer disease. The plaque has been labeled with immunostains against β-amyloid *(red)* and tau protein *(brown),* to demonstrate the characteristic swollen, dystrophic neurites and amyloid-rich core of the classic senile plaque. (Courtesy of Charles L. White, III, MD, Department of Pathology, University of Texas Southwestern Medical School, Dallas.)

An additional, more recently recognized morphologic change in a substantial number of cases of AD is the presence of concomitant **Lewy bodies,** structures discussed in more detail under the topic of Parkinson disease and related disorders.

Clinical Features. Persons with AD have a progressive impairment of memory and other cognitive functions. Symptoms may be subtle at first and can be easily confused with depression, another clinically important disease in the elderly. Cognitive impairment continues inexorably, usually over the course of 5 to 15 years, resulting in complete disorientation and loss of language and other higher cortical functions. In a significant minority of patients, movement abnormalities typical of parkinsonism (discussed later) may develop, usually associated with the presence of concomitant Lewy body formation. Death usually results from intercurrent bronchopneumonia or other infections.

OTHER NEURODEGENERATIVE DISORDERS ASSOCIATED WITH DEMENTIA

Although AD clearly remains the most common cause of dementia in the elderly, a number of other primary neurodegenerative diseases may also cause dementia. In some of these less common diseases, such as Pick disease and other so-called frontotemporal dementias, cognitive impairment is the dominant feature of the disorder. In yet other neurodegenerative diseases, exemplified by Parkinson disease and primary motor neuron disease (discussed later), dementia develops in association with abnormalities affecting other parts of the CNS, such as the motor system. Finally, it should be emphasized that conditions in addition to classic neurodegenerative disorders and cerebrovascular disease may present with dementia, particu-

Figure 23–36   ■

Alzheimer disease. Generalized loss of brain parenchyma has resulted in narrowing of the cerebral cortical gyri and widening of sulci. Compensatory enlargement of the ventricles (hydrocephalus ex vacuo) is usually apparent in such cases.

■

Primary Neurodegenerative Disorders

Alzheimer disease
Pick disease and other frontotemporal degenerations
Parkinson disease and diffuse Lewy body disease
Progressive supranuclear palsy
Huntington disease
Motor neuron disease

Infections

Prion-associated disorders (Creutzfeldt-Jakob disease, fatal familial
  insomnia, others)
HIV encephalopathy (AIDS dementia complex)
Progressive multifocal leukoencephalopathy
Miscellaneous forms of viral encephalitis
Neurosyphilis
Chronic meningitis

Vascular and Traumatic Diseases

Multi-infarct dementia and other chronic vascular disorders
Global hypoxic-ischemic brain injury
Chronic subdural hematomas

Metabolic and Nutritional Diseases

Thiamine deficiency (Wernicke-Korsakoff syndrome)
Vitamin B_{12} deficiency
Niacin deficiency (pellagra)
Endocrine diseases

Miscellaneous

Brain tumors
Neuronal storage diseases
Toxic injury (including mercury, lead, manganese, bromides)

larly in younger patients. Some of the more important causes of dementia are listed in Table 23–4.

Parkinsonism

Parkinsonism is a disturbance in motor functions characterized by rigidity, expressionless facies, stooped posture, gait disturbances, slowing of voluntary movements, and a characteristic "pill-rolling" tremor. Parkinsonism is not a single disease but rather is the clinical manifestation of a disturbance in the dopaminergic pathways connecting the substantia nigra to the basal ganglia. Such disturbances occur in a number of other degenerative diseases and may also be caused by trauma, certain toxic agents (notably a compound known as MPTP, a contaminant found in some batches of illicitly manufactured meperidine), vascular diseases, and encephalitis.

Perhaps the best known form of parkinsonism is that associated with Parkinson disease, also known as *idiopathic parkinsonism* or *paralysis agitans.* Parkinson disease is a degenerative disorder involving the dopamine-secreting neurons of the substantia nigra, as well as the locus ceruleus. It is a disease of adulthood, with most cases becoming manifest by the sixth decade. Although most cases arise sporadically, it is likely that genetic factors play a role in the development of the disease in some of these patients, perhaps by increasing susceptibility to an environmental toxin. Genetic abnormalities play a more obvious role in the uncommon familial cases of Parkinson disease.

Mutations in a gene coding for a protein involved in normal neuronal synapses, termed α-synuclein, account for at least some of these familial cases.

Clinical Features. The clinical onset of Parkinson disease is usually insidious. The course of the disease is one of steady progression, usually over a period of about 10 years. In addition to the motor disturbances noted previously, dementia may occur in a minority of cases. In some of these cases, the dementia is associated with the presence of Lewy bodies in cerebral cortical neurons, while in other cases, there is evidence of coexistent Alzheimer disease. Death is usually the result of intercurrent infection or trauma from frequent falls caused by postural instability.

Huntington Disease

Huntington disease (HD) is a hereditary, progressive, fatal disorder involving the "extrapyramidal" motor system,

Figure 23–38   ■

Parkinson disease, or idiopathic parkinsonism, is characterized by a loss of neurons from the substantia nigra and other pigmented nuclei. Such neuronal loss is responsible for the pallor of the substantia nigra on the left, compared with the normal midbrain on the right. (Courtesy of Eileen Bigio, MD, Department of Pathology, University of Texas Southwestern Medical School, Dallas.)

characterized by involuntary movements (chorea) and dementia. The disease is inherited as an autosomal dominant trait with complete penetrance. It usually does not become apparent until adulthood, often after affected individuals have had children, although juvenile-onset cases also occur. Early-onset cases, in particular, are more likely to be associated with inheritance of the mutation from the father than from the mother. The responsible gene (which encodes a protein called huntingtin) has been localized to the short arm of chromosome 4. The disease is caused by trinucleotide repeat mutations in the *huntingtin* gene (Chapter 7), which cause, in turn, the synthesis of a form of the huntingtin protein containing an abnormal number of glutamine residues. The normal *huntingtin* gene contains between 6 and 34 copies of the cytosine-adenine-guanine (CAG) sequence. In HD, the number of triplet repeats is increased, with most HD patients carrying between 40 and 55 CAG copies. The larger the number of trinucleotide repeats, the earlier the onset of disease; patients with juvenile-onset HD, for example, typically carry greater than 70 CAG repeats. Affected individuals can be identified before the development of symptoms by the demonstration of excessive CAG triplet repeats in the responsible gene. The identification of individuals in the presymptomatic phase of their disease obviously carries with it an immense ethical burden and should not be undertaken in the absence of appropriate counseling.

The molecular pathogenesis of HD is not fully understood. Huntingtin is expressed in all somatic tissues, and its expression is clearly essential to normal embryonic development. Nevertheless, the exact function of huntigton remains unknown. Because HD is an autosomal dominant disorder, it follows that the mutant huntingtin in some manner impairs the function of normal huntingtin produced by the normal allele. Such mutations are referred to as "gain of function" mutations. Although the exact mechanism whereby the mutant huntingtin causes brain injury remains unclear, it is likely that the presence of abnormal huntingtin causes cell loss by some combination of activation of apoptotic pathways and impairment of normal energy metabolism in susceptible neurons.

MORPHOLOGY

The brain in HD is usually small, often weighing less than 1100 g. The most distinguishing feature of the disorder is striking **atrophy of the caudate nucleus, putamen, and, in more advanced cases, the globus pallidus,** with the caudate often reduced to a thin band adjacent to the lateral ventricles (Fig. 23-39). The ventricles are symmetrically dilated, with a concave lateral wall, reflecting atrophy of the caudate nucleus. Some atrophy of other subcortical nuclei (including the substantia nigra and subthalamic nucleus) and of the cerebral cortex is usually present, although it is seldom as striking as that seen in the caudate and putamen. Microscopically, this disease is characterized by a severe loss of neurons within the caudate and putamen, accompanied by fibrillary gliosis in these areas. The smaller neurons in the corpus striatum, particularly those projecting to the lateral segment of the globus pallidus, are preferentially affected, but there is often some loss of larger neurons as well. Cortical neuronal loss is often present and correlates with the degree of dementia.

Clinical Features. The clinical onset of HD is usually in the fourth or fifth decade, although some cases present during childhood. Like other trinucleotide repeat mutations, the CAG expansions affecting the *huntingtin* gene are dynamic. During spermatogenesis, the number of CAG repeats can increase, and hence HD tends to present earlier in successive generations, a phenomenon known as *anticipation.* The initial manifestations in most patients include involuntary, writhing movements known as *choreiform movements,* a pattern sometimes designated as the *hyperkinetic* form of Huntington disease. In cases with earlier onset, seizures and rigidity may be prominent, a presentation known as the *rigid-akinetic variant* of the disease. Neuropsychiatric disturbances, including depression and

Figure 23-39 ■

Huntington disease. Coronal section of brain demonstrating characteristic atrophy of caudate nuclei in Huntington disease *(A)* compared with normal brain *(B).*

cognitive impairment, typically develop after the onset of motor abnormalities, but they may be the presenting manifestations. Symptoms progress inexorably, typically over a period of 15 to 20 years. Common causes of death include suicide and intercurrent infections. The risk of suicide, in particular, mandates the availability of proper counseling in the evaluation of presymptomatic carriers of the disease.

Diseases of Motor Neurons

The motor neurons of the brain and spinal cord are targets of injury in a fairly large number of sporadic and hereditary neurodegenerative disorders, as well as in certain infections (e.g., poliomyelitis) and some autoimmune diseases. Among the primary neurodegenerative disorders affecting motor neurons, the most common is *amyotrophic lateral sclerosis (ALS)*. This disorder, also known as Lou Gehrig disease or, in the United Kingdom, as motor neuron disease (MND), is a *degenerative disorder involving the upper and lower motor neurons of the pyramidal system, with resultant progressive muscle weakness, atrophy (amyotrophy) and spasticity*. Most cases of ALS are sporadic. Familial cases, usually inherited in an autosomal dominant fashion, account for 5% to 10% of cases. The cause and pathogenesis of most cases of ALS remain unknown, despite extensive analysis of potential environmental, toxic, infectious, and immunologic factors. A subset of familial cases has been associated with mutations in the gene coding for the enzyme *superoxide dismutase* located on the long arm of chromosome 21. As with Huntington disease, it is thought that mutations affecting superoxide dismutase cause disease by a toxic gain of function, not by the loss of the free-radical scavenging activity of this enzyme.

MORPHOLOGY

ALS is characterized by a **loss of motor neurons** in the anterior horns of the spinal cord, brain stem motor nuclei, and the primary motor cortex of the cerebrum. Grossly, the brain and cord are usually normal, although some atrophy of the primary motor cortex (precentral gyrus) may be apparent in severe cases. The anterior spinal nerve roots are usually atrophic. Microscopically, the neuronal loss in areas noted earlier is usually accompanied by some degree of fibrillary gliosis. A variety of inclusions are typically seen in residual spinal motor neurons, including **ubiquitin-positive hyaline inclusions reminiscent of Lewy bodies** and small eosinophilic cytoplasmic structures known as **Bunina bodies**. Small, ubiquitin-positive inclusions may also be seen in nonmotor areas of the cerebral cortex, particularly in cases of ALS associated with dementia. Degeneration and loss of neurons in the primary motor cortex often cause a **loss of corticospinal fibers** in the cerebral peduncles, basal pons, and medullary pyramids and especially within the lateral and anterior columns of the spinal cord. Peripheral nerves carrying motor fibers are depopulated, and affected skeletal muscles show evidence of striking denervation atrophy (Chapter 21).

Clinical Features. The onset of ALS is insidious, marked by weakness, clumsiness, and speech difficulties. The weakness, which progresses with time, is accompanied by the development of muscle atrophy and small involuntary contractions termed *fasciculations*. Extraocular muscles are not affected. Spasticity, reflecting involvement of upper motor neurons, is present in most cases. It is manifested by hyperactive deep tendon reflexes and a Babinski reflex (upgoing toes in response to a painful stimulus applied to the sole of the foot). The degree of involvement of upper and lower motor neurons varies from case to case, although most patients have evidence of both lower and upper motor neuron disease. ALS is a relentlessly progressive disease in most cases, with a median survival of about 5 years after the onset of symptoms. Death usually results from a combination of respiratory insufficiency and infections.

Other forms of progressive motor neuron diseases include the *progressive spinal muscular atrophies of infancy and childhood*. The best known of these is infantile spinal muscular atrophy type 1, or Werdnig-Hoffmann disease. This is an autosomal recessive disorder manifested by congenital hypotonia ("floppy infant" syndrome). It is characterized by a loss of motor neurons in the anterior horns of the spinal cord, resulting in atrophy of anterior spinal roots and peripheral motor nerves and denervation in multiple skeletal muscle groups (Chapter 21), including those controlling respiration. Generalized hypotonia, often present at birth, may even be evident in utero. The course of Werdnig-Hoffmann disease is relentlessly progressive, with most patients dying within the first year of life. Other forms of inherited spinal muscular atrophy (types 2 and 3) also occur, characterized by a later onset of muscle weakness and a more protracted clinical course. Deletions of a gene located on the long arm of chromosome 5, termed the survival motor neuron *(SMN)* gene, have been identified in the majority of patients with spinal muscular atrophy. In addition, abnormalities in a nearby gene known as the neuronal apoptosis inhibitory protein *(NAIP)* gene apparently also contribute to neuronal loss in a number of cases.

DISEASES OF THE PERIPHERAL NERVOUS SYSTEM

The peripheral nervous system begins a few millimeters from the pial surface of the brain and spinal cord, where Schwann cell processes replace oligodendroglial processes as the source of myelin. In the peripheral nervous system myelin shares some structural similarities with CNS myelin but also contains several proteins that are unique to the periphery. Abnormalities in some of these structural proteins have been implicated in the development of certain hereditary peripheral nerve disorders. Myelinated axons in the peripheral nerves are invested by concentric laminations of

Schwann cell cytoplasm. The myelin sheath contributed by each Schwann cell is termed a *myelin internode*, and the space between adjacent internodes is termed the *node of Ranvier*. Each myelin internode is formed by a single, dedicated Schwann cell. The normal peripheral nerve also contains many smaller-diameter unmyelinated axons, which lie in small groups within the cytoplasm of a single Schwann cell. Groups of myelinated and unmyelinated axons, in turn, are compartmentalized into discrete fascicles by concentrically arrayed *perineurial cells*. Axons are insulated from the interstitial fluids of the body by a "blood-nerve" barrier, somewhat analogous to the blood-brain barrier, formed by tight junctions between endothelial cells in small peripheral nerve vessels and tight junctions between adjacent perineurial cells. Disorders of the peripheral nervous system include peripheral neuropathies and neoplasms arising from Schwann cells and other nerve sheath elements.

Peripheral Neuropathies

A number of disorders may disrupt the normal conduction of electrical impulses in the peripheral nerves. Some of the more common causes of peripheral neuropathy are listed in Table 23–5. From a morphologic standpoint, peripheral neuropathies can be broadly subdivided into two major categories, namely, axonal degeneration and segmental demyelination. In clinical practice, mixtures of the two patterns are quite common. Each of these injury patterns will be discussed separately.

AXONAL DEGENERATION

The term *axonal degeneration* designates a pattern of nerve injury *characterized by primary injury to the axon followed by secondary disintegration of the myelin sheath*. Axonal degeneration may occur as a consequence of injury to the actual nerve cell body or to the axonal process anywhere along its length. If a proximal segment of an axon is injured, as might

Table 23–5.   CAUSES AND TYPES OF PERIPHERAL NEUROPATHIES

Nutritional and Metabolic Neuropathies

Diabetes, thiamine deficiency, pyridoxine deficiency, alcoholism, renal failure

Toxic Neuropathies

Lead, arsenic, cisplatin, vincristine, organic solvents

Inflammatory Neuropathies

Guillain-Barré syndrome, chronic inflammatory demyelinating neuropathy, vasculitic neuropathy, leprosy, sarcoidosis

Hereditary Neuropathies

Hereditary motor and sensory neuropathies (Charcot-Marie-Tooth disease, Refsum disease, Dejerine-Sottas disease), hereditary sensory neuropathies, leukodystrophies

Miscellaneous

Amyloid neuropathy, paraneoplastic neuropathies, neuropathies associated with immunoglobulin abnormalities

occur if a nerve is cut by a knife, the axon distal to the site of injury rapidly degenerates and ultimately disappears, a process termed *wallerian degeneration*. Injury to the axonal process is accompanied by complete fragmentation of its myelin sheath, resulting in the formation of characteristic lipid-rich globules termed *myelin ovoids* (Fig. 23–40*A*). After the axonal injury, axons may regenerate to some degree, a process manifested by the presence of axonal sprouts, which are invested by new myelin sheaths. Axonal regeneration may be accompanied by recovery of function in the denervated area, but this is often incomplete. In addition to traumatic injuries, vascular diseases such as vasculitis, with resultant ischemic injury to a segment of peripheral nerve, are an important cause of wallerian degeneration.

A second form of axonal degeneration, termed *distal axonal degeneration* or *distal axonopathy*, develops when there is more generalized injury of nerve cell bodies and/or

Figure 23–40   ■

Peripheral neuropathies. *A,* Electron micrograph of nerve biopsy specimen from a patient with axonal degeneration, demonstrating characteristic myelin ovoids *(arrows)* composed of degenerating fragments of axons and their myelin sheaths. Intact myelinated axons, invested by darkly staining myelin sheaths, are also present in the photograph. *B,* Electron micrograph of nerve from a patient with a primary demyelinating neuropathy. "Onion bulbs," made up of concentric lamellae of Schwann cell processes and collagen, indicate episodes of sequential demyelination and remyelination.

axonal processes, as opposed to the localized injury that leads to wallerian degeneration. In this pattern of nerve injury, axonal degeneration begins in the most distal part of the axon and extends proximally in a progressive, continuous fashion. Primary distal axonal degeneration is seen in a wide range of peripheral nerve diseases, including most nutritional neuropathies (e.g., thiamine deficiency) and many toxic insults. Myelin ovoid formation is also a feature of distal axonopathies, although it is usually less conspicuous than that seen in cases of wallerian degeneration. Like wallerian degeneration, primary distal axonal degeneration is often accompanied by some evidence of axonal regeneration.

SEGMENTAL DEMYELINATION

Segmental demyelination is characterized by primary injury to the myelin sheath, with relative preservation of axons. Morphologically, myelin injury typically affects one or more myelin internodes in a given segment of nerve. The original myelin sheath disintegrates, leaving a bare segment of axon, which conducts electrical impulses poorly. The demyelinated segment often acquires a new myelin sheath, made up of shorter, thinner myelin internodes than those that were present originally. With episodes of recurrent demyelination and remyelination, the affected axonal segment may become surrounded by concentric lamellae of Schwann cells, a process known as "onion bulb" formation (Fig. 23–40B). If the myelin injury is severe, secondary axonal degeneration often develops. The leukodystrophies, many hereditary neuropathies, and inflammatory demyelinating neuropathies (e.g., Guillain-Barré syndrome, discussed below) are characterized by primary injury to the myelin sheath.

Clinical Features of Peripheral Neuropathies. The clinical manifestations of peripheral neuropathies include some combination of motor, sensory, and occasionally autonomic deficits. The presentations vary, however, depending on the cause and type of the neuropathy. Many neuropathies, particularly primary distal axonal disorders, present with slowly evolving symmetric sensory loss, often in a "glove-and-stocking" distribution, reflecting injury of distal axonal processes. Involvement of motor fibers is manifested by the presence of muscle weakness, often accompanied by atrophy of muscle fibers (neurogenic atrophy). Deep tendon reflexes are often diminished or absent. Involvement of the autonomic nervous system may produce changes such as postural hypotension and constipation. While many peripheral neuropathies involve the body in a symmetric fashion, in other cases the presentation may be that of asymmetric neurologic deficits. This is particularly the case in neuropathies caused by vasculitis, which may affect multiple nerves in a random distribution, a pattern termed *mononeuropathy multiplex*.

GUILLAIN-BARRÉ SYNDROME

This is one of the most common life-threatening diseases of the peripheral nervous system. Its etiology is unknown, and it may develop spontaneously or after a viral prodrome, *Mycoplasma* infection, allergic reaction, or surgical procedure; an immunologic basis is considered most likely. Patients with Guillain-Barré syndrome present with rapidly progressive, ascending motor weakness that may lead to death from failure of respiratory muscles. Sensory involvement is usually much less striking than is motor dysfunction. The dominant histopathologic findings are infiltration of peripheral nerves by macrophages and reactive lymphocytes, and segmental demyelination. The CSF usually contains increased levels of protein but only a minimal cellular reaction.

Neoplasms of the Peripheral Nervous System

Neoplasms of peripheral nerve arise from Schwann cells and other elements of the peripheral nerve sheath, such as fibroblasts. The two most common primary peripheral nerve sheath neoplasms are neurofibromas and schwannomas. The frequency of both neoplasms is dramatically increased in patients with neurofibromatosis type 1 (von Recklinghausen disease), in whom such tumors may develop in childhood.

MORPHOLOGY

Schwannomas present as well-circumscribed masses attached to peripheral nerves, cranial nerves, or spinal nerve roots. The eighth cranial nerve is a particularly common site for schwannomas (also termed **acoustic neuromas**), where they present as well-demarcated masses in the angle between the cerebellum and pons. Microscopically, schwannomas classically contain areas of densely packed spindle cells, termed **Antoni A tissue,** intermixed with looser, myxoid regions termed **Antoni B tissue.** In the denser areas, cell nuclei may form orderly palisades, termed **Verocay bodies.** Degenerative changes, including vascular hyalinization and lipid-laden macrophages, are quite common. Scattered enlarged, hyperchromatic nuclei are often present and, in the absence of mitotic activity, usually represent another degenerative change. Native (non-neoplastic) peripheral nerve elements are sometimes identifiable at the periphery of the neoplasm.

Neurofibromas are peripheral nerve sheath tumors that may present as diffusely infiltrative, nodular lesions involving the skin (**cutaneous neurofibromas**) and subcutaneous tissues (**subcutaneous neurofibromas**) or as expansile intraneural lesions involving larger nerve trunks (**plexiform neurofibromas**). These tumors are discussed in more detail in Chapter 7. They may be solitary or multiple. In some sites, such as the brachial or lumbosacral plexus, neurofibromas may involve multiple nerve trunks to produce diffuse enlargement of the entire nerve plexus. In contrast to schwannomas, which are composed exclusively of Schwann cells, neurofibromas are composed of a mixture of Schwann cells, fibroblasts, and cells similar to the perineurial cells that normally surround peripheral nerve fascicles. Microscopically, neurofibromas are characterized by interlacing bundles of delicate, elongated cells with slender, frequently wavy nuclei. Native axons are usually intermingled with the neoplastic cells rather than displaced to the periphery, as in the case of schwannomas. A variety of degenerative changes similar to those seen in schwannomas may also be present in neurofibromas. Areas of increased cellularity and mitotic activity should raise concern about the possibility of malignant transformation, particularly in neurofibromas occurring in patients with **neurofibromatosis** type 1 (see Table 23-2).

Malignant peripheral nerve sheath tumors (MPN-STs) are sarcomas that arise from the peripheral nerve sheath. Approximately one half of these tumors occur in patients with neurofibromatosis type 1. They may develop in a preexisting neurofibroma, typically of the plexiform type, or they may occur in the absence of an obvious precursor lesion. Grossly, MPNSTs present as firm, incompletely demarcated lesions often marred by foci of necrosis and hemorrhage. The lesions are typically composed of fibroblast-like cells with elongated nuclei, frequent mitotic figures, and areas of necrosis. Some tumors contain evidence of glandular or mesenchymal differentiation. MPNSTs containing areas of rhabdomyosarcoma are designated as *triton tumors.*

Clinical Features. Schwannomas and neurofibromas are most common in adults, except in patients with neurofibromatosis type 1. Most sporadic lesions are solitary. The tumors may present as asymptomatic masses, or they may produce neurologic deficits, depending on their location. Schwannomas of the eighth cranial nerve are common intracranial neoplasms; they may be difficult to distinguish from meningiomas on clinical grounds. The possibility of neurofibromatosis type 1 should be entertained if MPNSTs are present. Transformation to MPNST occurs in neurofibromas but is almost never seen in schwannomas. Most cases of malignant transformation occur in patients with neurofibromatosis type 1. MPNSTs are manifested by aggressive local growth and distant metastases, particularly to lung.

BIBLIOGRAPHY

Auer RN, Benveniste H: Hypoxia and related conditions. In Graham DI, Lantos PL (eds): Greenfield's Neuropathology, 6th ed. London, Arnold, 1997, pp 263–314. (A comprehensive discussion of hypoxic-ischemic brain injury and its pathogenesis, including a discussion of excitotoxicity in the CNS.)

Esler WP, Wolfe MS: A portrait of Alzheimer secretases—new features and familiar faces. Science 293:1449, 2001. (A detailed review of the actions and secretases involved in the formation of Aβ amyloid.)

Graham DI, et al: Recent advances in neurotrauma. J Neuropathol Exp Neurol 59:641, 2000. (An informative review of the pathophysiology of cellular injury following blunt trauma.)

Ho LW, et al: The molecular biology of Huntington's disease. Psychol Med 31:3, 2001. (A concise summary of the clinical manifestations, genetics, neuropathology, and pathogenesis of Huntington disease.)

Hutton M: Molecular genetics of chromosome 17 tauopathies. Ann NY Acad Sci 920:63, 2000. (A discussion of the role played by abnormal forms of the tau protein in hereditary frontotemporal neurodegenerative disorders and in sporadic dementias.)

Kaye EM: Update on genetic disorders affecting white matter. Pediatr Neurol 25:11, 2001. (A review of the major leukodystrophies and other hereditary white matter diseases, and their radiographic features.)

King R: Atlas of Peripheral Nerve Pathology. London, Arnold, 1999. (An excellent collection of detailed photographs and accompanying text, illustrating both normal peripheral nerve morphology and the wide spectrum of axonal and myelin sheath alterations encountered in peripheral neuropathies.)

Kleihaus P, Cavanee WK: Pathology and Genetics of Tumors of the Nervous System. Lyon, IARC Press, 2000. (The most recent edition of the World Health Organization classification of central and peripheral nervous system tumors.)

Lang AE, Lozano AM: Parkinson's disease. N Engl J Med 339:1044 and 1131, 1998. (A detailed two-part review of all aspects of this disorder.)

Lee VM-Y: Tauists and βaptists United—Well almost! Science 293:1446, 2001. (A short review that synthesizes the evidence supporting a role for amyloid in the formation of tau tangles.)

Louis DN, Pomeroy SL, Cairncross JG: Focus on central nervous system neoplasia. Cancer cell 1:125, 2002. (A summary of the molecular basis of CNS neoplasms, and prospects for a molecular classification.)

Lucking CB, Brice A: Alpha-synuclein and Parkinson's disease. Cell Mol Life Sci 57:1894, 2000. (A review of the protein alpha-synuclein and its role in Parkinson disease and other neurodegenerative disorders.)

Marin-Padilla M: Developmental neuropathology and impact of perinatal brain damage: III. Gray matter lesions of the neocortex. J Neuropathol Exp Neurol 58:407, 1999. (A very comprehensive discussion of the morphology and pathogenesis of perinatal cortical brain injury.)

Mastrianni JA, Roos RP: The prion diseases. Semin Neurol 20:337, 2000. (A concise review of the basic aspects of prion biology and prion-associated disorders.)

McArthur JC, et al: Human immunodeficiency virus–associated dementia. Semin Neurol 19:129, 1999. (A comprehensive review of the pathology and pathogenesis of HIV-associated dementia and the impact of antiretroviral therapy on its frequency and evolution.)

Noseworthy JH, et al: Multiple sclerosis. N Engl J Med 343:938, 2000. (An excellent clinical and basic review of multiple sclerosis.)

Offen D, et al: Apoptosis as a general cell death pathway in neurodegenerative diseases. J Neural Transm Suppl 58:153, 2000. (An overview of the role played by pre-programmed cell death in neuronal loss in Alzheimer disease and other neurodegenerative disorders.)

Parisi JE, Scheithauer BW: Glial tumors. In Nelson JS, et al (eds): Principles and Practice of Neuropathology. St. Louis, CV Mosby, 1993, pp 123–183. (A comprehensive review of the pathology and behavior of the diverse spectrum of glial neoplasms.)

Prusiner SB: Shattuck lecture—neurodegenerative diseases and prions. N Engl J Med 344:1516, 2001. (An excellent discussion of prions and the diseases caused by them.)

Rowland LP, Shneider NA: Amyotrophic lateral sclerosis. N Engl J Med 344:1688, 2001. (A detailed discussion of the pathogenesis and clinical features of this disease.)

Sisodia S, et al: γ-secretase: never more enigmatic. Trends Neurosci 24(11 Suppl): S2. (A brief review of the role of presenilin in the pathogenesis of Alzheimer disease.)

St. George-Hyslop PH: Molecular genetics of Alzheimer's disease. Biol Psychiatry 47:183, 2000. (A concise discussion of the roles of amyloid precursor protein, the presenilins, and apolipoprotein E in the pathogenesis of Alzheimer disease.)

Steinman L: Multiple sclerosis: a coordinated immunologic attack against myelin in the central nervous system. Cell 85:299, 1996. (A brief but excellent summary of the immunopathogenesis of multiple sclerosis.)

Vonsattel JPG, DiFiglia M: Huntington disease. J Neuropathol Exp Neurol 57:369, 1998. (A comprehensive review of the clinical, genetic, and neuropathologic features of Huntington disease, including the role of huntingtin in the pathogenesis of the disorder.)

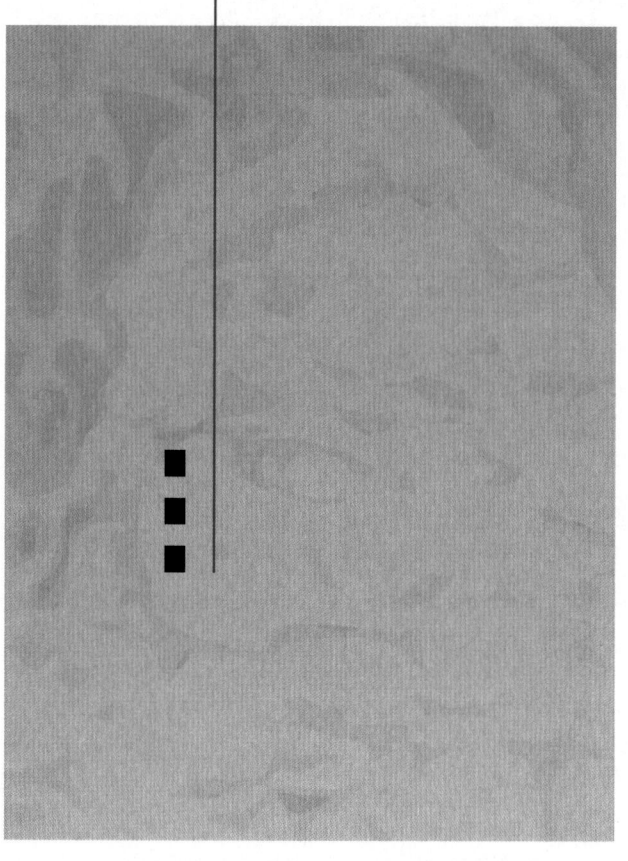

Index

Note: Page numbers in *italics* refer to illustrations; page numbers followed by t refer to tables.

Thrombosis *(Continued)*
  risk of, 91t
  venous, 93–94, 354
Thrombotic endocarditis, nonbacterial, 92, 380, *380*
Thrombotic microangiopathies, 448, 534–535
Thrombotic thrombocytopenic purpura, 448
Thromboxane A₂, 47–48, *47*, 87
Thrush, 492, *545*
Thymic hypoplasia (DiGeorge syndrome), *145*, 146
Thymoma, 451–452
Thymus, disorders of, 451–452
  in myasthenia gravis, 779
Thyroid gland, 726–738, *727*
  adenoma of, 733–734, *733*
  anaplastic carcinoma of, 735, 738
  and goiter, 730–731
  autoimmunity in, 728–730, 731–732
  follicular carcinoma of, *734*, 736–737
  Graves disease of, 728–730, *729*
  hyperfunction of, 726–727
  hypofunction of, 727–728
  in Hashimoto thyroiditis, 731–732, *732*
  inflammation of, 731–733
  medullary carcinoma of, 735, 737–738
    in MEN syndromes, 753
  nodules in, 733
  papillary carcinoma of, 735–736, *737*
  tumors of, 733–738
Thyroiditis, 731–733
  Hashimoto, 731–732, *731, 732*
  lymphocytic, 731–732, *731*
  palpation, 733
  Reidel, 732–733
  subacute (De Quervain) granulomatous, 732
Thyrotoxicosis, 726–727
Tissue inhibitor of metalloproteinases (TIMP),
    in scar remodeling, 72, *73*
  in spread of cancer, 192
Tissue-type plasminogen activator (t-PA), 89
Tobacco smoking. See *Cigarette smoking.*
Tolerance, immunologic, loss of, 128–129
  self, 126–127
Tongue, atrophic, in riboflavin deficiency, 302t
  cancer of, 546–547
Tophaceous arthritis, 775
Tophi, 774, 775
TORCH complex, 242
Total body irradiation, 287–290, *288, 290*, 290t
Toxemia, of pregnancy, 704–705
    and intrauterine growth retardation, 242
Toxic epidermal necrolysis, 793
Toxic shock syndrome, superantigens in, 111
Toxic shock syndrome toxin, 318
Toxoplasma, in TORCH complex, 242
Toxoplasmosis, nervous system in, 827–828
TP53 gene, 187–188, *187, 194*, 200, 201
  in angiogenesis, 190
  in cell cycle, 62
Trace elements, 303t
Transforming growth factor-α (TGF-α), 180
Transforming growth factor-β (TGF-β), 73, 73t
  in neoplasia, 185–186
Transfusion reactions, type II hypersensitivity
    in, 115
Transient ischemic attacks, 815
Transitional cell carcinoma, of bladder, 541
Translocation, of chromosomes. See *Chromo-some(s), translocation of.*
Transplacental infections, 242
Transplant rejection, 121–125, *123, 124*
  acute, 122–124, *124*
  antibody mediated, 122
  cardiac, 384

Transplant rejection *(Continued)*
  chronic renal, 124
  HLA complex in, 109
  hyperacute renal, 122
  of allogeneic hematopoietic cells, 125
  of lung, 474–475
  T-cell mediated, 121–122
Transposition of great arteries, 391–392
Transposons, 310
Transthyretin, 159, 160t
Transudate, 35, 80
Traumatic fat necrosis, of breast, 709
Traveler's diarrhea, 570
Trench foot, 287
Treponema pallidum infection, *321*, 670–673, *672*
  nervous system in, 826–827
Trichinosis, 312, 780
Trichomoniasis, 676, 684, 685
Trinucleotide (triplet) repeat mutations, *213*,
    234–235, *236*
  and Huntington disease, 845
  and X-linked mental retardation, 235
Trisomy 13 (Patau syndrome), *231*
Trisomy 18 (Edwards syndrome), *231*
  and hydrops fetalis, 247
Trisomy 21 (Down syndrome), 230–232, *231*
  and hydrops fetalis, 247
Trophoblastic disease, gestational, 702–704
Tropical (postinfectious) sprue, 571–572
Troponin, in myocardial infarction, 371
Trousseau sign, 354
Trousseau syndrome (migratory
    thrombophlebitis), 94, 354
Trypanosomiasis (Chagas disease), 383t, 384
Tubal pregnancy, 701
Tuberculin reaction, 119, 485
Tuberculosis, 56t, 484–490, *486, 491*
  adrenal cortex and, 748
  bone and, 763
  brain and, 827–828
  in AIDS, 156
  intestinal, 490, 568t
  laryngitis and, 506
  meningeal, 826
  miliary, 489–490
  primary, 487
  pulmonary, 487, 489, *489*
  secondary (reactivation), 488–490, *489*
  testicle and, 660
Tuberculous granuloma, 56, *57*
Tuberous sclerosis, 215t, 821t
Tubular adenoma, of colon, 580, *581*
Tubular necrosis, acute, 531–533, *532*
Tubule(s), renal, diseases of, 526–533
Tubulointerstitial nephritis, 526–531
Tumor(s), 166–210. See also *Cancer;
    Neoplasia;* and specific types, e.g.,
    Carcinoma.
  angiogenesis in, 190
  antigens, 202, *203*
  benign, nomenclature of, 166–167, 168t
    vs. malignant, *173*, 173t, 174
  clonality of, assessment of, 178, *178*
  differentiation in, 169–170, 173t
  growth of, 170–171
  heterogeneity in, 194, *195*
  initiators, 198
  malignant, nomenclature of, 167–168,
    168t
    vs. benign, 168–174, *173*, 173t
  mixed, 167, *167*
  nomenclature applied to, 166–167, 168t
  of infancy and childhood, 251–257
  progression of, 178, 194, *195*
  promoters, 196, 198

Tumor immunity, 201–205, *204*
Tumor necrosis factor (TNF), in growth
    inhibition, 73t
  in inflammation, 49–50
  in septic shock, 99–100
  in type IV hypersensitivity, 120, *121*
Tumor progression, 178, 194, *195*
Tumor suppressor genes, 183–188, *184, 185,
    187, 196.* See also specific genes.
  in familial tumors, 225
  in Wilms tumor, 256
Tumor suppressor proteins, 62
Turcot syndrome, 582
Turner syndrome (monosomy X), 233–234, *234*
  and hydrops fetalis, 247
Type I hypersensitivity (anaphylactic type),
    112–114, 112t, *113, 115*
  in asthma, 455
  in urticaria, 791
Type II (antibody-dependent) hypersensitivity,
    112t, 114–115, *116*
  in pemphigus, 796
Type II myofiber atrophy, 779
Type III (immune complex–mediated) hyper-
    sensitivity, 112t, 115–119, *117, 118*
  in glomerulonephritis, 513–516
Type IV (cell-mediated) hypersensitivity, 112t,
    119–121, *121*
  in spongiotic dermatitis, 792
  in transplant rejection, 121–122, *123*
  Mycobacterium tuberculosis infection as, 485
  sarcoidosis as, 471
Typhoid fever, 569
Typhus fever, 311

U
U1 RNP antigen, 143
UBE3A gene, 237
Ubiquitin, in cell injury, 12
Ubiquitin-proteosome pathway, 12
Ulceration, *57*, 58
Ulcerative colitis, 572, 574–577, *575*, 575t, *576*
Ultraviolet rays, as carcinogens, 199
Unconjugated hyperbilirubinemia, 594–595
Undescended testis, 659–660
Uniparental disomy, 237
Upper respiratory tract, lesions of, 506–508
Uremia, 510
Ureter, tumors of, 541–542
Urethra, tumors of, 541–542
Urethritis, nongonococcal, 675
Uric acid, and gout, 774–775
Uric acid stones, 537, 537t, 776
Urinary bladder, infection/inflammation of
    (cystitis), 528
  papilloma of, 541
Urinary collecting system, tumors of, 541–542,
    541
Urinary outflow obstruction, 536–539
Urinary tract infection, 510, 527–529, *528*
Urolithiasis, 536–537, 537t
Urothelial neoplasms, 541
Urticaria (hives), 114, 791
Uterine cervix. See *Cervix.*
Uterus, adenomyosis of, 689–690
  body of, 689–694
  carcinoma of, 693–694
  dysfunctional bleeding of, 690–691
  endometrial hyperplasia of, 690–691, *692*
  endometriosis of, 690, *690*
  endometritis of, 689
  leiomyoma of, 692–693, *692*
  leiomyosarcoma of, 692–693
  polyps of, 691–692